B. Santucci

Pathophysiology

Pathophysiology

Adaptations and Alterations in Function

SECOND EDITION

Barbara L. Bullock, R.N., M.S.N.

Cardiac Rehabilitation Program,
St. Vincent's Hospital,
Birmingham, Alabama

Pearl Philbrook Rosendahl, R.N., ED.D.

Associate Professor,
Boston University School of Nursing;
University Hospital,
Boston

Scott, Foresman/Little, Brown College Division

SCOTT, FORESMAN and COMPANY

Glenview, Illinois   Boston   London

Library of Congress Cataloging-in-Publication Data
Bullock, Barbara L.
Pathophysiology : adaptations and alterations in function.

Includes bibliographies and index.
1. Physiology, Pathological. I. Rosendahl, Pearl Philbrook. II. Title. [DNLM: 1. Pathology. 2. Physiology. QZ 4 B938p]
RB113.B85 1988 616.07 87-23355
ISBN 0-673-39710-6

2 3 4 5 6 7 8 9 10—VHJ—93 92 91 90 89 88

Printed in the United States of America

To my husband, Pete, and children,
with my love and appreciation.
—B.L.B.

Preface

Pathophysiology can be defined as the study of the physiologic and biologic manifestations of disease. This second edition of *Pathophysiology: Adaptations and Alterations in Function* provides a basis for this study by expanding the student's knowledge in the sciences and exploring how alterations in structure (anatomy) and function (physiology) disrupt the human body as a whole. Written for undergraduate and graduate students in nursing and other health-oriented disciplines, this text blends the conceptual and systems approaches: the overall mechanisms of disease are introduced and described first to set the stage for coverage of specific disease processes within each system.

Integral to the study of pathophysiology is an understanding of how the human body uses its adaptive powers to maintain the steady state. *Pathophysiology* begins its discussion of this adaptive power at the basic level, which is the cell. Because alterations cause a disruption in normal cellular processes, ultimately leading to tissue or organ alterations, the body's adaptive and compensatory mechanisms also occur at the cellular level. For this reason, the text discusses cellular processes and alterations in these processes throughout. The concept of feedback and information sharing within the body is also explored in depth. In health the body functions in a negative feedback pattern that allows return to the normal or steady state. Some pathologic processes, however, establish a positive feedback pattern that, if unchecked, will result in death.

The understanding of disease processes is continually being updated and clarified by research. Continuing studies examine the fundamental nature of life and how it is altered by pathologic conditions. In this second edition of *Pathophysiology*, every attempt has been made to provide the most current information available. Many new topics have been added and many of those carried over have been expanded. Two new chapters demonstrate how important Shock and Pain are in understanding some manifestations of disease. New chapters on Alterations in Cardiac Rhythms and Sexually Transmitted Diseases (including a major section on AIDS) reflect the growing need for knowledge about these states in the health care field. The contributors have taken great care to provide currency, detail, and concept synthesis for every topic in the book.

This new edition retains many features of the first edition, including its basic organization and presentation of topics. Physical and laboratory findings are emphasized in appropriate sections, but treatment regimens are included only to illustrate or clarify a process. The students are referred to the many current nursing and medical texts for information about treatment and nursing management.

New to this edition are several features designed to make the text easier to use. A second color, used throughout, highlights both illustrations and text. The artwork, an essential component in the first edition, is expanded and refined so that it will be more useful in helping students to visualize complex subjects. As in the first edition, students are encouraged to use the *Chapter Outlines* and *Chapter Objectives* as guides before reading each chapter and for review of content. End-of-chapter *Study Questions* have been added to provide some synthesis of the major topics. For students and faculty who wish to pursue specific topics in greater depth, each chapter is thoroughly referenced; a bibliography is provided at the end of each unit.

Pathophysiology, Second Edition, comes with a complete set of supplements to help both student and instructor. The *Instructor's Manual,* written by Anita Mikasa of Seattle University, has terms, chapter summaries, teaching strategies, and a bank of test questions. Answers to the study questions are also provided in the *Instructor's Manual.* The *Study Guide,* written by Helen Carcio of Curry College, goes beyond the usual workbook format by providing students with an outline summary of major chapter concepts and varied learning exercises encouraging students to review the text. With a *computerized test bank,* available for Apple and IBM PCs and compatibles, instructors can generate both tests from the data bank and new questions of their own. *Transparency Masters* of select illustrations in the text are also available.

Putting together a book of this magnitude requires contributions by many people. The author gratefully acknowledges the contributors to the first edition, whose material provided the beginnings of this entire project. Those contributors and their respective topics are as follows: Gloria Anderson, Erythrocyte Function; Joseph L. Andrews, Jr., Oxygen-Carbon Dioxide Exchange; Pamela Appleton, Normal Structure and Function of Skin, Traumatic Alterations to Skin; Sue H. Baldwin, Pituitary Function; Anne Roome Bavier, Motility and Motor Dysfunction of the Gastrointestinal Tract; Joan P. Buffalino, Alterations of Skin Integrity; Concepcion Y. Castro, Gastrointestinal Secretions; Jules Constant, Heart Sounds and Murmurs; Virginia Earles, Aging; Ann Estes Edgil, Genetic Disorders; Thomas Mark Fender, Skeletal System Function; Shirley Freeburn, Endocrine Mechanisms of Reproduction; Janet L. Gelein, General Systems Theory; Doris J. Heaman, Pancreatic Function and Diabetes; Reet Henze, Normal Structure and Function of the Central and Peripheral Nervous System, Adaptation and Alterations of the Special Senses, Traumatic Alterations of the Nervous System; Joan T. Hurlock, Disorders of Reproduction; Karen E. Jones, Degenerative and Other Alterations of the Nervous System; June H. Larrabee, Alterations in Movement; John A. R. Marino, Diabetes Mellitus; Gretchen S. McDaniel, Tumors and Infections of the Central Nervous System; M. S. Megahed, Alterations in Sensation, Consciousness, and Higher Cortical Function; Francis Donovan Monahan, Absorption in the Gastrointestinal System; Jennie L. Moore, Muscular System Function; Emilie Musci, Wound Healing, Neoplasia; Betty

Norris, Hypertension; Leah F. Oakley, Compromised Pumping Ability of the Heart, Alterations in Systemic Circulation; Donna Rogers Packa, Valvular Heart Disease, Pericarditis, Endocarditis; Marilyn Nelsen Pase, Infectious Agents and Leukocyte Function; Helen F. Ptak, Fluid and Electrolyte Balance, Burn Injury; Cammie M. Quinn, Normal Urinary Function, Obstruction of Genitourinary System, Renal Failure; Pearl Philbrook Rosendahl, Heart Sounds and Murmurs, Endocrine Function of the Pancreas, Alterations in Higher Cortical Function; Sharron P. Schlosser, Normal and Altered Male and Female Function; Therese B. Shipps, Nutrition and Metabolism; Eileen Ledden Sjoberg, Lung Clearance and Defense; Carol A. Stephenson, Ventilation, Diffusion, and Perfusion; Camille P. Stern, Functions of the Adrenal, Thyroid, and Parathyroid Glands; Metta Fay Street, Alterations That Result from Aging; Joan M. Vitello, Valvular Heart Disease, Pericarditis, Endocarditis; Linda Hudson Williams, Neoplasia; and Joan W. Williamson, Skeletal System Function. The contributors to the second edition refined, updated, and expanded that original material. Their efforts are also deeply appreciated.

The author also acknowledges the support and guidance provided by many talented persons at Scott, Foresman/Little, Brown College Division, specifically, Ann West, Nursing Editor, who has helped me for years to make dreams become reality. Her enthusiasm and moral support have kept me going and made me believe that I really could accomplish the task; Andrea Cava, Book Editor, for tireless attention to the details of the project. She endured my disorganization and frustrations with positive assistance; Marcia Williams, Medical Illustrator, who handled all the major revisions of select pieces of art, making many suggestions for wonderful changes. The results are truly outstanding; and Sarah Clark, Permissions Editor, who diligently followed through on my sketchy notes to properly credit publication sources.

I am also very grateful to Michele McCarren, who took on the typing and word processing of the entire manuscript and helped me to meet the deadlines. She produced virtually error-free copy and cheerfully endured my changes, revisions, and terrible handwriting. My thanks also go to the second edition reviewers, for their helpful comments and suggestions: Ruth Mauldin at the University of North Carolina at Charlotte; Ardelina Baldonado of the Marcella Nehoff School of Nursing at Loyola University in Chicago; Sarah Jane Tobiason of Arizona State University; and Rosemary H. Wittstadt of Towson State University in Towson, Maryland. Many other instructors throughout the country have provided useful feedback on their classroom experience with the first edition. I am very grateful for this input, and welcome it again for this new edition.

I could not have completed this project without the continuing support of my husband, Pete, and my children, to whom this book is dedicated.

B.L.B.

Contributing Authors

Gloria Anderson, R.N., M.S.N.
Associate Professor
University of Alabama School of Nursing, Huntsville
Huntsville, Alabama

Cheryl Bean, R.N., D.S.N., C.S.
Assistant Professor
University of Alabama School of Nursing, Birmingham
Birmingham, Alabama

Carol Bowdoin, R.N., M.S.N.
Formerly, Instructor University of Alabama School of Nursing, Huntsville
Huntsville, Alabama

Barbara L. Bullock, R.N., M.S.N.
Cardiac Rehabilitation Program
St. Vincent's Hospital
Birmingham, Alabama

Ann Estes Edgil, R.N., D.S.N.
Associate Professor
University of Alabama School of Nursing, Birmingham
Birmingham, Alabama

Thomas Mark Fender, R.N., M.S.N.
Special Units Coordinator
Crestwood Hospital
Huntsville, Alabama

Dorothy Gauthier, R.N., Ph.D.
Associate Professor
University of Alabama School of Nursing, Birmingham
Birmingham, Alabama

Doris J. Heaman, M.S.N.
Assistant Professor
University of Alabama School of Nursing, Huntsville
Huntsville, Alabama

Reet Henze, R.N., M.S.N.
Associate Professor
University of Alabama School of Nursing, Huntsville
Huntsville, Alabama

Marcia Hill, R.N., M.S.N.
Manager, Dermatologic Therapeutics
The Methodist Hospital
Houston, Texas

Bonnie Juneau, R.N., M.S.
Assistant Professor
University of Texas Health Sciences Center
School of Nursing
Houston, Texas

Marianne T. Marcus, R.N., M.Ed.
Assistant Professor
University of Texas Health Sciences Center
School of Nursing
Houston, Texas

Gretchen McDaniel, R.N., M.S.N.
Formerly, Assistant Professor
Samford University School of Nursing
Birmingham, Alabama

Richard Pflanzer, Ph.D.
Associate Professor
Indiana University/Purdue University
Indianapolis, Indiana

Sharron P. Schlosser, B.S.N., D.S.N.
Associate Professor
Samford University School of Nursing
Birmingham, Alabama

Camille Stern, Ph.D., R.N.
Assistant Professor
Samford University School of Nursing
Birmingham, Alabama

Gloria Grissett Stuart, R.N., M.S.N.
Assistant Professor
University of Alabama School of Nursing, Huntsville
Huntsville, Alabama

Joan W. Williamson, R.N., M.S.N.
Associate Professor
University of Alabama School of Nursing, Huntsville
Huntsville, Alabama

Contents

SECTION I Introduction to Pathophysiology: Adaptations and Alterations in Cellular Function *1*

UNIT 1 Cellular Dynamics *3*

Chapter 1 **Cells: Structure, Function, Organization** ***5***

Cellular Organelles *6*
Reproductive Ability of Cells *17*
Cellular Exchange *18*
Cell Movement *23*
Electrical Properties of Cells *26*
Cell Organization *28*
Study Questions *33*

Chapter 2 **Genetic Disorders** ***34***

Principles of Inheritance *35*
Classification of Genetic Disorders *36*
Single-Gene Disorders *36*
Chromosome Disorders *45*
Multifactorial Disorders *47*
Environmental Alterations in Fetal Development *47*
Study Questions *50*
References *50*

Chapter 3 **Alterations in Normal Cellular Processes Resulting in Adaptive or Lethal Change** ***51***

Stimuli That Can Cause Cellular Injury or Adaptation *52*
Intracellular and Extracellular Changes Resulting from Cellular Adaptation or Injury *53*
Cellular Changes Due to Injurious Stimuli *55*
Injury and Death of Cells Due to Lack of Oxygen *57*
Study Questions *59*
References *60*

Unit Bibliography ***60***

UNIT 2 Stress ***61***

Chapter 4 **Stress and Disease** ***63***

General Systems Theory *64*
Stress and Adaptation in the Human Body *64*
Adaptation *65*
Organ and System Function in Maintaining the Steady State *65*
Factors Related to Development of Disease *68*
Stress and Disease *69*
Study Questions *71*
References *71*

Unit Bibliography *72*

UNIT 3 Fluid, Electrolyte, and Acid-Base Balance and Shock ***73***

Chapter 5 **Normal and Altered Fluid and Electrolyte Balance** ***75***

Regulation of Fluid and Electrolyte Balance *76*
Edema *84*
Study Questions *86*
References *86*

Chapter 6 **Normal and Altered Acid-Base Balance** ***87***

Normal Acid-Base Balance *88*
Altered Acid-Base Balance *93*
Compensation *96*
Interpretation of Blood Gas Data *96*
The Anion Gap *96*
Study Questions *97*
References *97*

Chapter 7 **Shock** ***98***

Hemodynamic Homeostasis *99*
Shock—An Overview *101*
Stages of Shock *101*
Classifications of Shock *104*
Complications of Shock *111*
Study Questions *113*
References *113*

Unit Bibliography ***113***

SECTION II Bodily Defense Mechanisms: Adaptations and Alterations 115

UNIT 4 Inflammation and Repair 117

Chapter 8 Infectious Agents 119

Host-Parasite Relationships 120
Viruses 121
Rickettsia 122
Bacteria 122
Fungi 130
Protozoa 130
Helminths 132
Study Questions 132
References 134

Chapter 9 Inflammation and Resolution of Inflammation 135

Acute Inflammation 136
Chronic Inflammation 141
Local and Systemic Effects of Inflammation 141
Resolution of Inflammation 142
Study Questions 145
References 145

***Unit Bibliography* 145**

UNIT 5 Immunity 147

Chapter 10 Normal Immunologic Response 149

Organs of the Immune System 150
Immunocompetent Cells 151
Types of Immunity 157
Study Questions 159
References 159

Chapter 11 Immunodeficiency 160

Primary Immune Deficiency 161
Secondary Immune Deficiency 164
Study Questions 166
References 166

Chapter 12 Hypersensitivity and Autoimmune Reactions 167

Classification of Tissue Injury Due to Hypersensitivity 168
Classification of Immune Disorders by Source of Antigen 174
Autoimmunity 174
Study Questions 178
References 178

***Unit Bibliography* 178**

UNIT 6 Neoplasia 181

Chapter 13 Concepts of Altered Cellular Function 183

The Cell Life Cycle 184
Outer Cell Membrane Changes as an Explanation for Neoplasia 185
Inner Cell Changes in Neoplasia 187
Differentiation 188
Anaplasia 188
Study Questions 189
References 189

Chapter 14 Benign and Malignant Neoplasia 190

Definitions 192
Classification of Neoplasms 192
Benign Neoplasms 193
Malignant Neoplasms 193
Causes of Neoplasia 194
Carcinogens 194
Other Factors in Carcinogenesis 196
Growth of the Primary Tumor 197
Staging of Neoplasms 197
Metastasis 198
Host Defense Mechanisms in the Control of Neoplasia 200
Clinical Manifestations of Neoplasms 201
Study Questions 203
References 203

***Unit Bibliography* 203**

SECTION III Organ and System Mechanisms: Adaptation and Alterations 207

UNIT 7 Hematology 209

Chapter 15 Normal and Altered Erythrocyte Function 211

Hematopoiesis 214
Erythropoiesis 217
Erythrocytosis 221
Anemias 221
Laboratory and Diagnostic Tests 226
Study Questions 227
References 227

Chapter 16 **Normal and Altered Leukocyte Function** ***228***

Normal Leukocyte Function *229*
Nonmalignant White Blood Cell Disorders *234*
Malignant White Blood Cell Disorders *236*
Study Questions 240
References 240

Chapter 17 **Normal and Altered Coagulation** ***241***

Hemostasis *242*
General Mechanism of Blood Coagulation *244*
Lysis of Blood Clots *247*
Anticoagulation Factors in Normal Blood *248*
Laboratory Tests for Coagulation Problems *248*
Deficiencies in Blood Coagulation *249*
Study Questions 253
References 253

Unit Bibliography 253

UNIT 8 Circulation *255*

Chapter 18 **Normal Circulatory Dynamics** ***257***

Anatomy of the Heart *258*
Physiology of the Heart *266*
Anatomy of the Arteries, Capillaries, Veins, and Lymphatics *277*
Factors Controlling Arterial Pressure and Circulation *277*
Factors Affecting Venous Circulation *280*
Study Questions 280
References 280

Chapter 19 **Alterations in Cardiac Rhythms** ***281***

The Electrocardiogram *282*
Normal Conduction *285*
Normal Hemodynamics *287*
Cardiac Dysrhythmias *287*
Classification of Common Cardiac Dysrhythmias *290*
Study Questions 302
References 303

Chapter 20 **Compromised Pumping Ability of the Heart** ***304***

Congestive Heart Failure *305*
Cardiogenic Shock *315*
Diseases Affecting Myocardial Contractility *315*
Study Questions 317
References 317

Chapter 21 **Alterations in Specific Structures in the Heart** ***318***

Coronary Artery Disease: Ischemic Heart Disease *319*
Valvular Disease *327*
Infective Endocarditis *336*
Pericarditis *338*
Congenital Heart Disease *340*
Study Questions 345
References 346

Chapter 22 **Hypertension** ***347***

Definitions *348*
Etiology of Hypertension *348*
Pathophysiology *350*
Diagnosis of Hypertension *354*
Study Questions 354
References 354

Chapter 23 **Alterations in Systemic Circulation** ***355***

Pathologic Processes of Arteries *356*
Pathologic Processes of Veins *363*
Pathologic Processes of the Lymphatic System *365*
Diagnostic Procedures for Vascular Lesions *366*
Study Questions 367
References 367

Unit Bibliography 367

UNIT 9 Respiration *369*

Chapter 24 **Normal Respiratory Function** ***371***

Anatomy of the Pulmonary Tree *372*
Pulmonary Circulation *373*
Major Muscles of Ventilation *375*
Nervous Control of Respiration *375*
Compliance and Elastance *377*
The Mechanics of Breathing *378*
The Work of Breathing *380*
Substances Important in Alveolar Expansion *380*
Defense of the Airways and Lungs *381*
Defenses Against Infection *384*
Normal Gas Exchange *385*
Respiratory Regulation of Acid-Base Equilibrium *390*
Pulmonary Function Testing *391*
Study Questions 393
References 393

Chapter 25 **Restrictive Alterations in Pulmonary Function** ***395***

Atelectasis *396*
Infectious Diseases of the Respiratory Tract *397*
Aspiration Pneumonia *401*
Pulmonary Edema *401*
Traumatic Injuries of the Chest Wall *403*
Pleural Effusion *404*
Pneumothorax *404*

Central Nervous System Depression 405
Neuromuscular Diseases 405
Respiratory Diseases Caused by Exposure to Organic and Inorganic Dusts 406
Pulmonary Fibrosis 407
Thoracic Deformity 407
Obesity 408
Idiopathic Respiratory Distress Syndrome of the Newborn 408
Adult Respiratory Distress Syndrome 409
Study Questions 410
References 410

Chapter 26 Obstructive Alterations in Pulmonary Function 411

Acute Obstructive Airway Disease 412
Chronic Obstructive Pulmonary Disease 414
Study Questions 419
References 419

Chapter 27 Other Alterations Affecting the Pulmonary System 420

Pulmonary Embolus 421
Pulmonary Hypertension 423
Upper Respiratory Tract Alterations 423
Carcinoma of the Larynx 424
Lung Tumors 424
Respiratory Failure 426
Study Questions 427
References 427

***Unit Bibliography* 427**

UNIT 10 Urinary Excretion 429

Chapter 28 Normal Renal and Urinary Excretory Function 431

Anatomy of the Kidneys 432
Physiology of the Kidneys 435
Accessory Urinary Structures and Bladder 441
Study Questions 441
References 444

Chapter 29 Immunologic, Infectious, Toxic, and Other Alterations in Urinary Function 445

Infections of the Genitourinary Tract 446
Nephritic Glomerular Disease 447
Nephrotic Glomerular Disease 449
Tubular and Interstitial Diseases 451
Congenital Disorders Leading to Renal Dysfunction 452
Study Questions 453
References 453

Chapter 30 Obstruction of the Genitourinary Tract 454

Benign Prostatic Hyperplasia 455
Renal Calculi 456
Renal Tumors 459
Study Questions 462
References 462

Chapter 31 Renal Failure and Uremia 464

Acute Renal Failure 465
Chronic Renal Failure 470
Uremic Syndrome 473
Study Questions 475
References 476

***Unit Bibliography* 476**

UNIT 11 Endocrine Regulation 479

Chapter 32 Pituitary Regulation and Alterations in Function 481

Hormones 482
Morphology of the Pituitary Gland 483
Relationship of the Pituitary to the Hypothalamus 488
Functions of the Anterior Pituitary 490
Functions of the Neurohypophysis 492
Introduction to Pituitary Pathology 494
Pathology of the Anterior Pituitary 495
Pathology of the Posterior Pituitary 499
Tumors of the Pituitary 500
Study Questions 501
References 501

Chapter 33 Adrenal Mechanisms and Alterations 502

Anatomy of the Adrenal Glands 503
The Adrenal Cortex 504
Altered Adrenocortical Function 507
The Adrenal Medulla 511
Study Questions 513
References 513

Chapter 34 Thyroid and Parathyroid Functions and Alterations 514

Anatomy of the Thyroid Gland 515
Physiology of the Thyroid Gland 516
Calcitonin: Formation and Function 517
Functions of the Thyroid Hormones 518
Altered Thyroid Function 519
The Parathyroid Glands 525
Altered Function of the Parathyroid Glands 526
Study Questions 528
References 528

Chapter 35 Normal and Altered Functions of the Pancreas 530

Anatomy and Physiology 531
Diabetes Mellitus 537
Pancreatic Islet-Cell Disease 550

Pancreatitis 551
Carcinoma of the Pancreas 554
Cystic Fibrosis (Mucoviscidosis, Fibrocystic Disease of the Pancreas) 555
Study Questions 558
References 558

Unit Bibliography **559**

UNIT 12 **Digestion, Absorption, and Use of Food** ***561***

Chapter 36 **Normal Function of the Gastrointestinal System** ***563***

Appetite, Hunger, and Satiety 564
Anatomy of the Gastrointestinal Tract 564
Physiology of the Digestive System 570
Study Questions 576
References 576

Chapter 37 **Alterations in Gastrointestinal Function** ***577***

Diseases of the Oral Cavity 578
Esophageal Alterations 578
Alterations in the Stomach and Duodenum 581
Alterations in the Small Intestine 585
Alterations in the Large Intestine 588
Study Questions 592
References 592

Chapter 38 **Normal Hepatobiliary and Pancreatic Exocrine Function** ***593***

Anatomy of the Liver 594
Physiology of the Liver 594
Major Liver Function Tests 599
The Gallbladder 601
Exocrine Pancreatic Function 602
Study Questions 604
References 604

Chapter 39 **Alterations in Hepatobiliary Function** ***605***

General Considerations in Liver Dysfunction 606
Cirrhosis of the Liver 611
Cancer of the Liver 613
Viral Hepatitis 614
Gallbladder Disease 615
Obesity: A Major Disturbance in Nutritional Balance 616
Study Questions 617
References 617

Unit Bibliography **618**

UNIT 13 **Musculoskeletal Function** ***619***

Chapter 40 **Normal and Altered Functions of the Muscular System** ***621***

Anatomy of Striated Muscle 622
Physiology of Striated Muscle 624
Anatomy of Smooth Muscle 627
Physiology of Smooth Muscle 628
Anatomy of Cardiac Muscle 629
Alterations in Muscles of the Body 630
Pathologic Processes Affecting the Skeletal Muscles 631
Study Questions 632
References 632

Chapter 41 **Normal and Altered Structure and Function of the Skeletal System** ***633***

Normal Structure and Function of Bone 634
Normal Structure and Function of Joints 640
Fractures and Associated Soft Tissue Injuries 643
Alterations in Bone Development 650
Infectious Diseases of Bone 654
Alterations in Skeletal Structure 655
Alterations in Joints and Tendons 656
Bone Tumors 659
Study Questions 664
References 664

Unit Bibliography **664**

UNIT 14 **Protective Coverings of the Body** ***667***

Chapter 42 **Normal Structure and Function of the Skin** ***669***

Anatomy and Physiology 670
Study Questions 680
References 680

Chapter 43 **Alterations in Skin Integrity** ***681***

Inflammation 682
Common Inflammatory Diseases of the Skin 683
Viral Infections of the Skin 686
Bacterial Infections of the Skin 688
Fungal Diseases of the Skin 688
Scaling Disorders of the Skin 689
Skin Tumors 689
Traumatic Alterations in the Skin 691
Study Questions 700
References 700

Unit Bibliography **701**

UNIT 15 **Neural Control** *703*

Chapter 44* Normal Structure and Function of the Central and Peripheral Nervous Systems *705

The Neuron *706*
Excitation and Conduction in Neurons *710*
Receptors *714*
The Synapse *715*
The Central Nervous System *718*
The Peripheral Nervous System *730*
The Autonomic Nervous System *735*
The Ventricular and Cerebrospinal Fluid Systems *741*
Brain Blood Supply and Regulation *746*
Study Questions 746
References 746

Chapter 45* Adaptations and Alterations in the Special Senses *747

Vision *748*
Hearing *756*
Taste *764*
Smell *766*
Study Questions 767
References 767

Chapter 46* Common Adaptations and Alterations in Higher Neurological Function *768

Cerebrovascular Disease: Pathology and Related Clinical Signs *769*
Aphasia *773*
Apraxia *775*
Agnosia *776*
Body Image *776*
Epilepsy *776*
Study Questions 781
References 781

Chapter 47* Pain *782

Definitions of Pain *783*
Mechanisms of Pain *783*
Theories of Pain *794*
Acute Versus Chronic Pain *799*
Variations in Pain Response and Reaction *801*
Study Questions 803
References 803

Chapter 48* Traumatic Alterations in the Nervous System *805

Consciousness *806*
Alterations in Consciousness *807*
Traumatic Head Injury *812*
Assessment of Traumatic Disruption to Cranial Nerves *817*
Increased Intracranial Pressure *820*
Spinal Cord Injury *822*
Diagnostic Studies of Nervous System Alterations *827*
Study Questions 830
References 830

Chapter 49* Tumors and Infections of the Central Nervous System *831

Tumors *832*
Infections *841*
Study Questions 850
References 850

Chapter 50* Degenerative and Chronic Alterations in the Nervous System *851

Progressive Neurologic Disabilities *852*
Paralyzing Developmental or Congenital Disorders *852*
Disorders Characterized by Progressive Weakness or Paralysis *856*
Disorders Characterized by Abnormal Movements *859*
Disorders Characterized by Memory and Judgment Deficits *862*
Study Questions 863
References 864

Unit Bibliography 864

UNIT 16 **Reproduction** *867*

Chapter 51* Normal Male Function *869

Anatomy *870*
Male Reproductive Functions *872*
Physical, Laboratory, and Diagnostic Tests *877*
Study Questions 878
References 878

Chapter 52* Alterations in Male Function *879

Prostate *880*
Penis *881*
Scrotum, Testes, and Epididymis *881*
Study Questions 883
References 883

Chapter 53* Normal Female Function *884

Anatomy *885*
Female Reproductive Functions *890*
Laboratory and Diagnostic Aids *897*
Study Questions 901
References 902

Chapter 54* Alterations in Female Function *903

Menstrual Problems *904*
Reproductive Tract Infections *907*

Benign Conditions of the Female Reproductive Tract *908*
Premalignant and Malignant Conditions *910*
Study Questions *913*
References *913*

Chapter 55 Sexually Transmitted Diseases 915

Primary Sexually Transmitted Diseases *916*
Sexually Transmitted Infections *918*
Acquired Immune Deficiency Syndrome *920*
Study Questions *920*
References *920*

Unit Bibliography 921

UNIT 17 Aging 923

Chapter 56 Aging 925

Biologic Theories of Aging *926*
Biologic Effects of Aging on Body Systems *928*
Drugs and the Elderly *939*
Aging and Cancer *940*
Study Questions *940*
References *940*

Index 942

SECTION I

Introduction to Pathophysiology

Adaptations and Alterations in Cellular Function

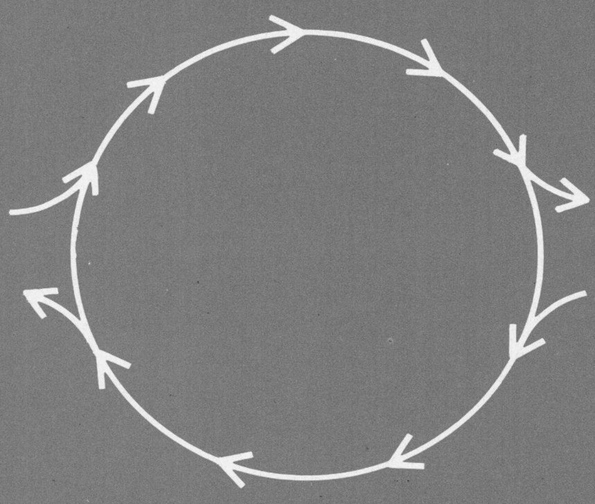

UNIT 1

Cellular Dynamics

Richard P. Pflanzer / ***Cells: Structure, Function, Organization***

Dorothy Gauthier and Ann Estes Edgil / ***Genetic Disorders***

Barbara L. Bullock / ***Alterations in Cellular Processes***

Because the cell is the basis of life, it is appropriate to begin the study of pathophysiology with a review of normal cellular processes. Understanding of these processes is necessary for the understanding of concepts in every other unit of the text. The material can be found in many anatomy and physiology textbooks, but is presented here as a convenient, accessible reference. Sources for the more detailed aspects of cellular function are listed in the bibliography at the end of Unit 1.

Chapter 1 describes normal cellular function, with special emphasis on the cellular organelles and on movement of materials across the cell membrane. Chapter 2 explains the principles of inheritance and relates them to the more common genetic disorders. Chapter 3 details the alterations in cells when they are exposed to a changing, hostile environment. Cellular adaptation, injury, and death are explored in terms of their effect on body function. Mechanisms by which the steady state can be maintained, even at the expense of altered intracellular metabolism, are explored. Altered cellular function ending in lethal change is described.

The reader is encouraged to use the learning objectives at the beginning of each chaper as a study guide outline for essential concepts. Study questions at the end of each chapter provide an assessment of learning achieved. The bibliography at the end of the unit provides general and specific resources for further study.

CHAPTER 1

Cells: Structure, Function, Organization

CHAPTER OUTLINE

Cellular Organelles

- The Plasma Membrane
- Mitochondria
  - *Formation of ATP with Oxygen*
  - *Formation of ATP Without Oxygen*
- Endoplasmic Reticulum
- Polyribosomes
- Golgi Complex
- Lysosomes
- Microtubules
- Cilia and Flagella
- Centrioles
- Nucleus
  - *Genes*
  - *Protein Synthesis*

Reproductive Ability of Cells

- Regeneration of Cells
- Reproduction of Cells
  - *The Cell Cycle*
  - *Replication*
  - *Mitosis*

Cellular Exchange

- Passive Movement Across the Cell Membrane
  - *Diffusion*
  - *Osmosis*
  - *Facilitated Diffusion*
- Active Movement Across the Cell Membrane
  - *Active Transport*
  - *Endocytosis and Exocytosis*

Cell Movement

- Ameboid Locomotion
- Muscular Contraction

Electrical Properties of Cells

Cell Organization

- Epithelial Tissue
- Muscular Tissue
- Nervous Tissue
- Connective Tissue

LEARNING OBJECTIVES

1. Differentiate between intracellular and extracellular electrolyte composition.
2. Describe in detail the structure and function of the following organelles: cell membrane, mitochondria, ribosomes, endoplasmic reticulum, Golgi apparatus, lysosomes, microtubules, centrioles, nucleus, and nucleolus.
3. Explain the major ways by which adenosine triphosphate (ATP) is formed.
4. Describe the process of protein synthesis from DNA-RNA transcription to protein manufacture.
5. Compare the function of the smooth endoplasmic reticulum with the rough endoplasmic reticulum.
6. Explain briefly the negative feedback pattern seen with the reproduction of cells of the body.
7. Classify cells by their ability to regenerate.
8. Describe briefly the process of mitosis.
9. Explain the mechanisms of transport across the cell membrane.
10. Identify facilitated passive transport, including the mechanism and what facilitates it.
11. Explain the purpose of the sodium potassium pump.
12. Compare pinocytosis and phagocytosis.
13. Describe the purpose of exocytosis.
14. Draw a cell exhibiting ameboid motion.
15. Describe the process of muscle contraction.
16. Compare smooth, cardiac, and skeletal muscle contraction.
17. Explain briefly the electrical properties of cells, including depolarization and repolarization.
18. Define the *refractory periods*.
19. Describe the differences in structure among the four major types of cells in the human body.
20. Define the purposes of the three types of epithelial cells.
21. Differentiate among skeletal, cardiac, and smooth muscle on the basis of histologic appearance.
22. Describe briefly the components of the neuron.
23. List the major types of connective tissue cells.
24. Identify the structure and function of each type of connective tissue.

The cell is the basic structural and functional unit of the body; therefore, an understanding of the basic biology of the human cell is essential to the study of pathophysiology. All pathophysiologic processes reflect changes in normal cell function, so it is appropriate to begin by reviewing fundamental concepts of cell structure, function, and organization.

Cells are the units of tissues, organs, and finally, systems of the human body (Fig. 1-1). The human body contains over 75 trillion cells, each of which performs specific functions. These functions are determined by genetic differentiation and are controlled by a highly specific information system that directs the activity of cellular organelles and inclusions.

Some cells have the major function of carrying out the activities of the organ and, as such, are called *parenchymal cells*. This means that the parenchyma of an organ actually does its function. Some examples of parenchymal cells are hepatocytes, neurons, gastric parietal cells, osteocytes, and myocardial cells. Other cells make it possible for the parenchymal cells to perform their function by providing the supporting structure or architectural framework to hold the organ in place. Examples include neuroglia, gastric capillary endothelial cells, and cardiac connective tissue cells.

Although cells have different functions, they are alike in many ways. The similarities include how nutrients are used, what type of nutrients are needed, how oxygen is used, the disposition of excretory products, and the internal organization of protoplasm.

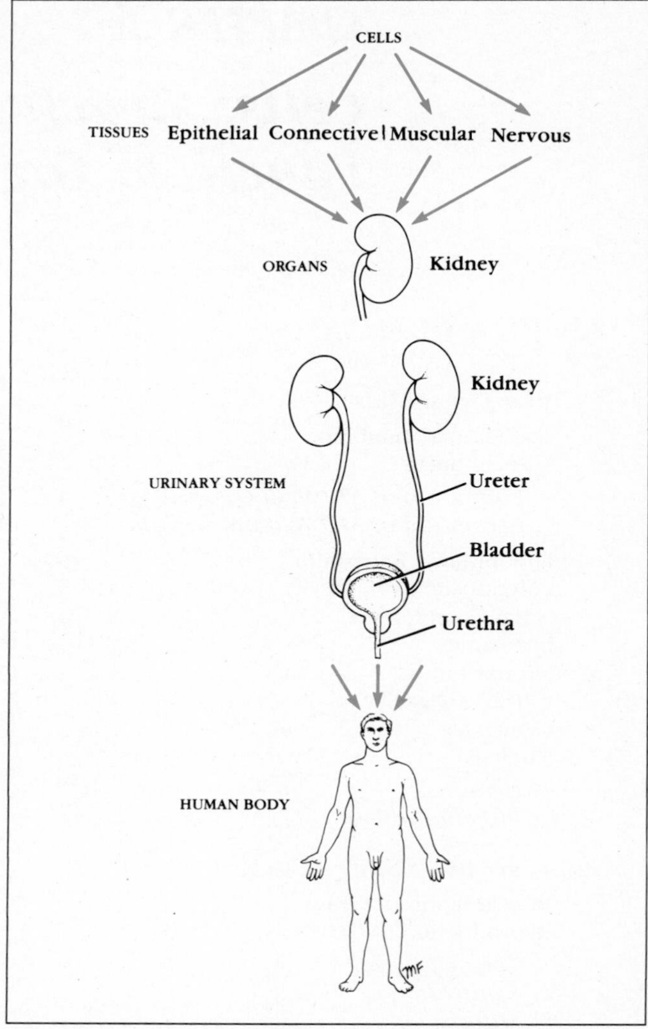

FIGURE 1-1 Structural subunits of the body: cells, tissues, organs, and systems. (From R.S. Snell, *Clinical Histology for Medical Students*. Boston: Little, Brown, 1984.)

Cellular Organelles

The cell is composed of many different structures that carry out its complex functions. Within the cell are highly organized physical structures called *organelles.* These structures are suspended in the fluid medium called *protoplasm*. This substance includes the *cytoplasm*, which is outside the nucleus of a cell, and the *nucleoplasm*, which is within the nucleus. The general structures of the cell are schematically diagrammed in Figure 1-2.

Protoplasm is composed mostly of water, but it contains specific amounts of electrolytes, proteins, lipids, and carbohydrates. The intracellular electrolyte balance is closely regulated and differs from that of extracellular fluid (Table 1-1). Proteins compose about 10 to 20 percent of the content of protoplasm and function to help the cellular inclusions maintain structural strength and form. Proteins also form the enzymes necessary for many intracellular reactions. Lipids make up a very small portion of the general cell and mainly join with proteins to keep the cell membranes insoluble in water. Lipids may be deposited in the cytoplasm of some cells when they are not needed for conversion to energy. Carbohydrates constitute a very small amount of the cytoplasm and are used mainly in forming adenosine triphosphate (ATP) for energy.

TABLE 1-1 Approximate Chemical Composition of Extracellular and Intracellular Fluid

	Extracellular	Intracellular
Na^+	142 mEq/L	10 mEq/L
K^+	3.5–5.0 mEq/L	141 mEq/L
Ca^{2+}	5 mEq/L	1 mEq/L
Mg^{2+}	3 mEq/L	58 mEq/L
Cl^-	103 mEq/L	4 mEq/L
HCO_3^-	28 mEq/L	10 mEq/L
Phosphates	4 mEq/L	75 mEq/L
Glucose	90 dl	0–20 dl
pH	7.4	7.0

Source: A.C. Guyton, *Textbook of Medical Physiology* (6th ed.). Philadelphia: W. B. Saunders Company, 1981, p. 41. Reprinted by permission.

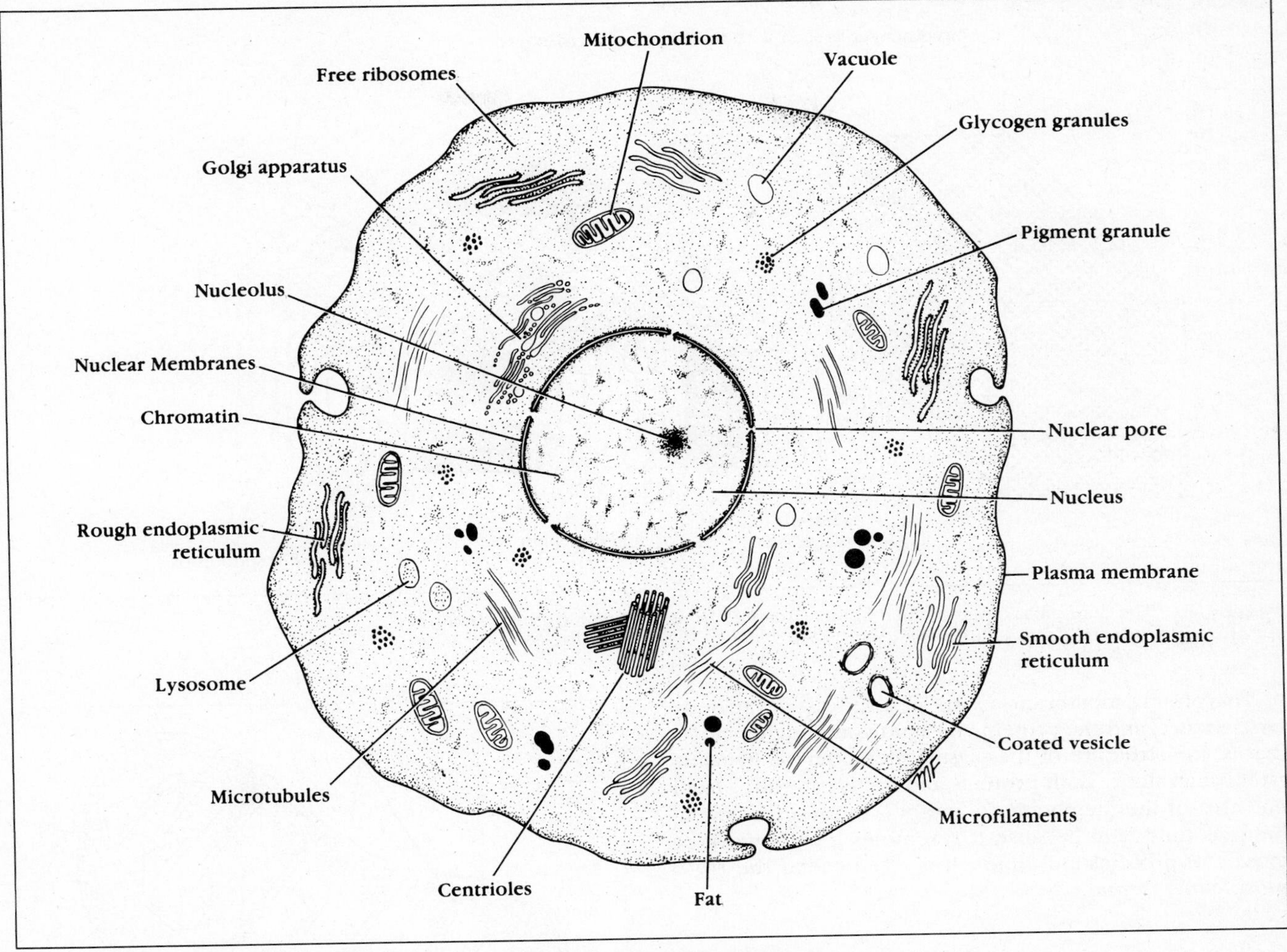

FIGURE 1-2 The general structure of a cell and its organelles. (From R.S. Snell, *Clinical Histology for Medical Students*. Boston: Little, Brown, 1984.)

The Plasma Membrane

All cells are surrounded by a limiting membrane, called the plasma membrane, that separates intracellular from extracellular fluids. Within the cell, some of the other organelles are bounded by a membrane that is similar in structure to the plasma membrane but named after the organelle (e.g., mitochondrial membrane, lysosomal membrane, etc.).

The plasma membrane consists of a double layer of lipid molecules (the lipid bilayer), with proteins bound to each layer as well as within the layers (Fig. 1-3). Lipids account for about half of the mass of the plasma membrane and consist of phospholipids (the most abundant), glycolipids, and others such as cholesterol.

The phospholipid molecules are elongated and have a polar end and a nonpolar end. Phospholipids in the bilayer are arranged so that their polar (hydrophilic) region points toward the interior or exterior of the cell and their nonpolar (hydrophobic) regions are buried in the interior of the membrane. This arrangement allows the membrane to behave as a barrier, restricting the loss of intracellular material and governing material entry.

Proteins are anchored in or on the lipid bilayer. Those bound to the inner or outer membrane surface are called *ectoproteins*. Those partially or completely embedded in the lipid bilayer are called *endoproteins*. Membrane proteins may have other types of molecules attached to them. Proteins on the outer membrane surface, for example, may have carbohydrates attached. These are called *glycoproteins*. Carbohydrates may also be attached to the polar region of the phospholipid molecules, forming *glycolipids*.

Membrane proteins not only form part of the molecular structure of the plasma membrane, but have many functional roles, such as transporting and exchanging materials between the cell and its environment. Other proteins are enzymes that help govern cell function, or receptors that communicate chemically with the cell.

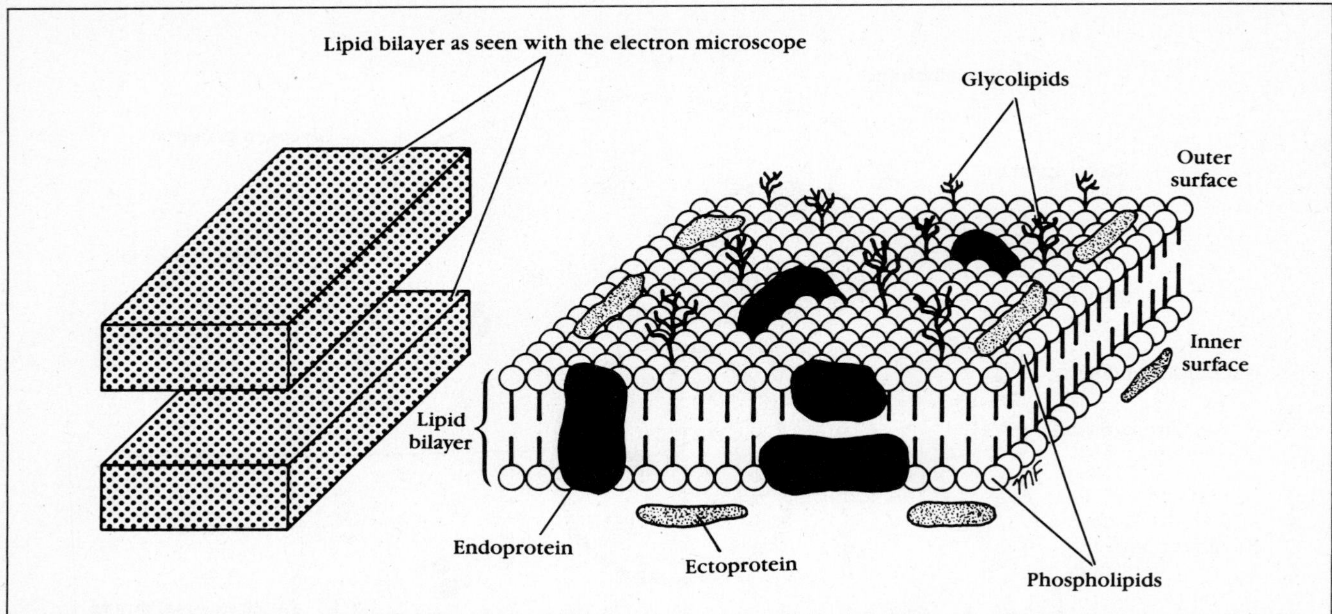

FIGURE 1-3 The fluid-mosaic plasma membrane. (Adapted from R.S. Snell, *Clinical Histology for Medical Students*. Boston: Little, Brown, 1984.)

The plasma membrane exists in a fluid state at body temperature, and the protein and lipid components move; that is, the structure of the plasma membrane is dynamic rather than static. Both proteins and lipids can move from one area of the membrane to another. Because the membrane is fluid, and because it resembles a patchwork or mosaic of proteins and lipids, it is often called the *fluid mosaic membrane*.

Mitochondria

Mitochondria (Fig. 1-4) are membranous, cigar-shaped organelles that synthesize ATP, a high-energy phosphate compound required by cells when they perform work (e.g., contraction, secretion, conduction, transport, etc.). In a sense, mitochondria are like batteries in a cell, providing energy in a form that allows the cell to function normally.

Mitochondria are bounded by a double membrane, the inner one of which is thrown into a series of shelflike folds, called *cristae*, that project into the interior of the organelle. The folded inner membrane presents a large internal surface area on which chemical reactions that generate ATP take place.

Cells that are very active and have a high energy requirement, such as skeletal muscle cells, have many mitochondria, whereas less active cells such as bone or cartilage cells have fewer mitochondria. Usually, within a given cell, mitochondria tend to be most numerous in areas that are highly energy dependent, such as around the contractile elements of the muscle cell or at the terminus of a nerve cell where transmission occurs.

Mitochondria are able to regenerate themselves under conditions of increased energy need. They contain a special type of deoxyribonucleic acid (DNA) that resembles bacterial DNA rather than cellular DNA.

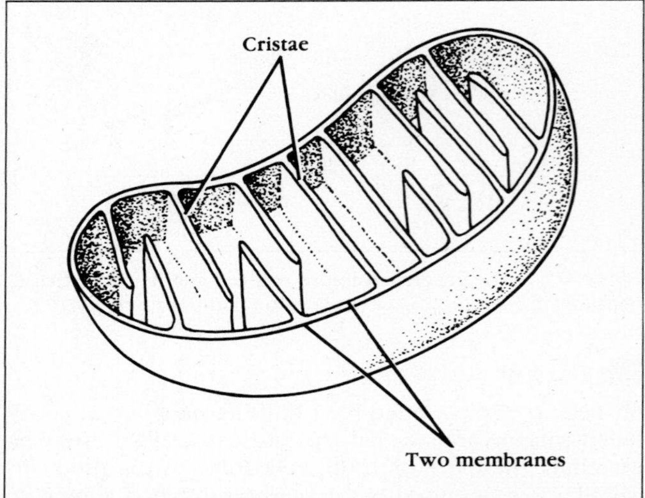

FIGURE 1-4 Schematic representation of a mitochondrion. (From R.S. Snell, *Clinical Histology for Medical Students*. Boston: Little, Brown, 1984.)

Formation of ATP with Oxygen. The process used by mitochondria to form ATP is called *oxidative phosphorylation*. It requires simple forms of carbohydrates, proteins, and fats. These substances enter the mitochondria and, using oxidative enzymes, form ATP through the citric acid or Krebs cycle (Fig. 1-5). High-energy phosphate radicals are formed that later release their energy when ATP is catabolized or reduced to adenosine diphos-

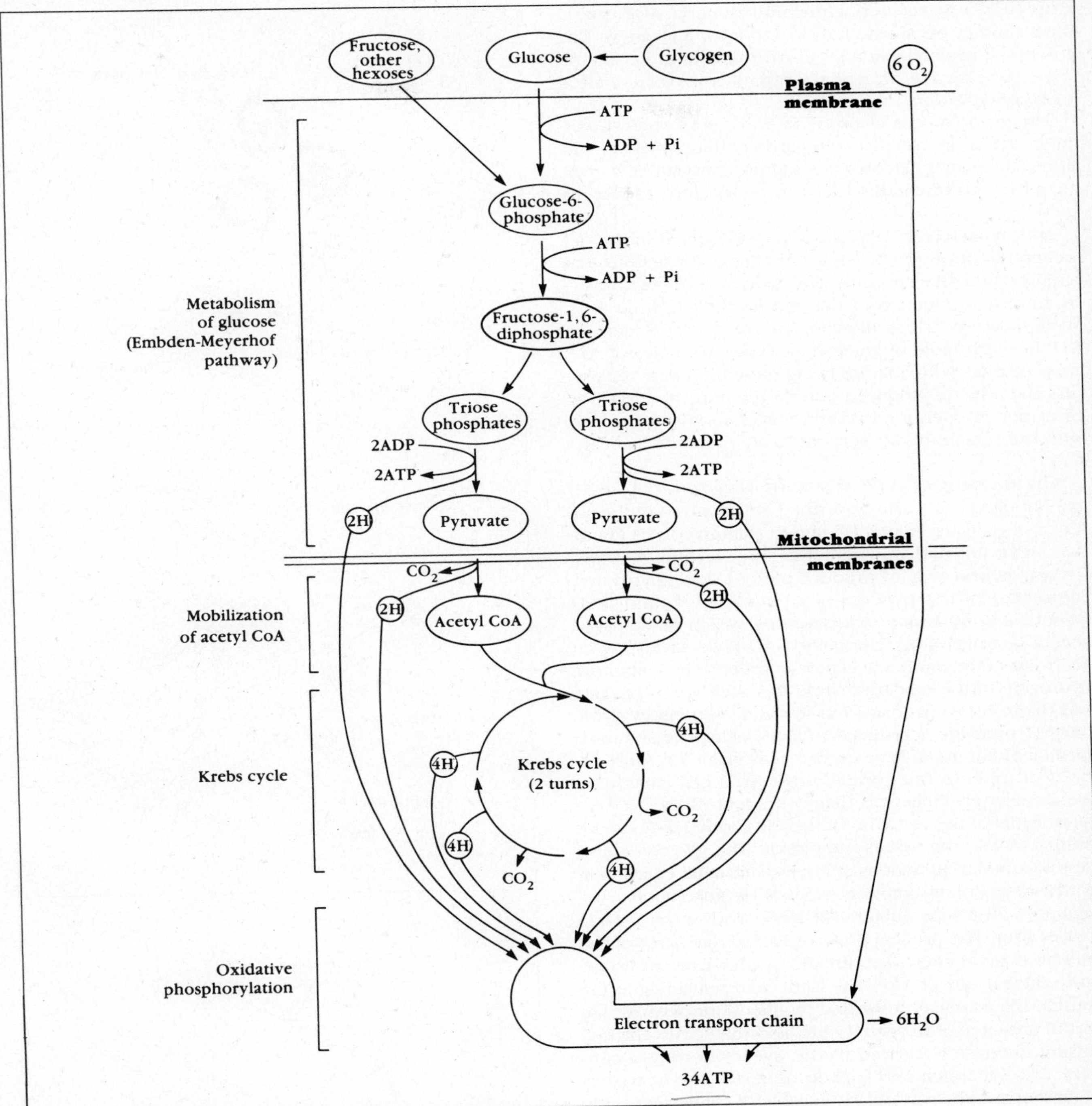

FIGURE 1-5 Metabolism of glucose in the formation of ATP. (From C.P. Hickman, Jr., L.S. Roberts, and F.M. Hickman, *Integrated Principles of Zoology* [7th ed.]. St. Louis: Mosby/Times Mirror, 1984.)

phate (ADP). By reentering the mitochondria, ADP can receive another phosphate radical and form ATP anew. The process of catabolizing ATP to ADP results in energy release. Adding the phosphate radical to ADP is called *rephosphorylation*.

The major source of *acetyl coenzyme A* (acetyl CoA), the common intermediary in carbohydrate, protein, and fat metabolism, is glucose. Fats and proteins can be metabolized to intermediates that can be fed into the Krebs cycle.

Approximately 95 percent of ATP is formed in the mitochondria through a sequence of chemical reactions that requires oxidative enzymes. The process involves glycolysis and then oxidation of the end product to form ATP. Many successive steps allow for the release of 38 moles of ATP for each mole of glucose. Actually, 40 moles of ATP are produced, with 2 moles being spent to initiate the process and 4 being produced outside the mitochondria. The efficiency in energy transformation is about 40 percent, with the remaining 60 percent being given off as heat.

Formation of ATP Without Oxygen. A small amount of ATP can also be formed by glycolysis in the absence of oxygen. Figure 1-5 shows that glycolysis (Embden-Meyerhof pathway) itself is an anaerobic process. Glycolysis proceeds to produce pyruvic acid (pyruvate). Important in the process is a coenzyme called NAD (nicotinamide-adenine dinucleotide), which functions to accept hydrogen ions. Normally, NAD picks up hydrogen and passes it to another acceptor in order to pick up more hydrogen. In the oxidative cycle this acceptor is oxygen, and the result is the formation of water. Without available oxygen, pyruvate is reduced to lactic acid. The system is inefficient but it can keep certain cells viable for short periods of time. In the normal, unstressed cell, anaerobic metabolism provides less than 5 percent of the ATP requirements of the cell. The lactic acid formed diffuses out of the cell into the tissues and plasma. This glycolytic process occurs during periods of intense muscular exertion in which oxygen consumption exceeds oxygen supply; subsequently, the accumulation of lactic acid in the muscle causes pain. The process produces an *oxygen debt* of the muscle that requires deep breathing after exercise to restore the balance of ATP. The lactic acid remaining in the muscle cell can be reconverted to glucose or pyruvic acid in the presence of oxygen. Lactic acid that leaves the cell during exercise is carried to the liver, where it is converted to glycogen and carbon dioxide. The heart has been shown to be particularly capable of converting lactic acid to pyruvic acid until extreme hypoxia occurs, when it produces more lactic acid than it can metabolize.

Endoplasmic Reticulum

In some human cells much of the cytoplasm is filled with an intricate yet ordered set of folded membranes that form small flattened sacs or tubes (Fig. 1-6). All of the membranes are interconnected, giving rise to a netlike structure, the appearance of which is reflected by its name: endoplasmic reticulum (a net within the cytoplasm).

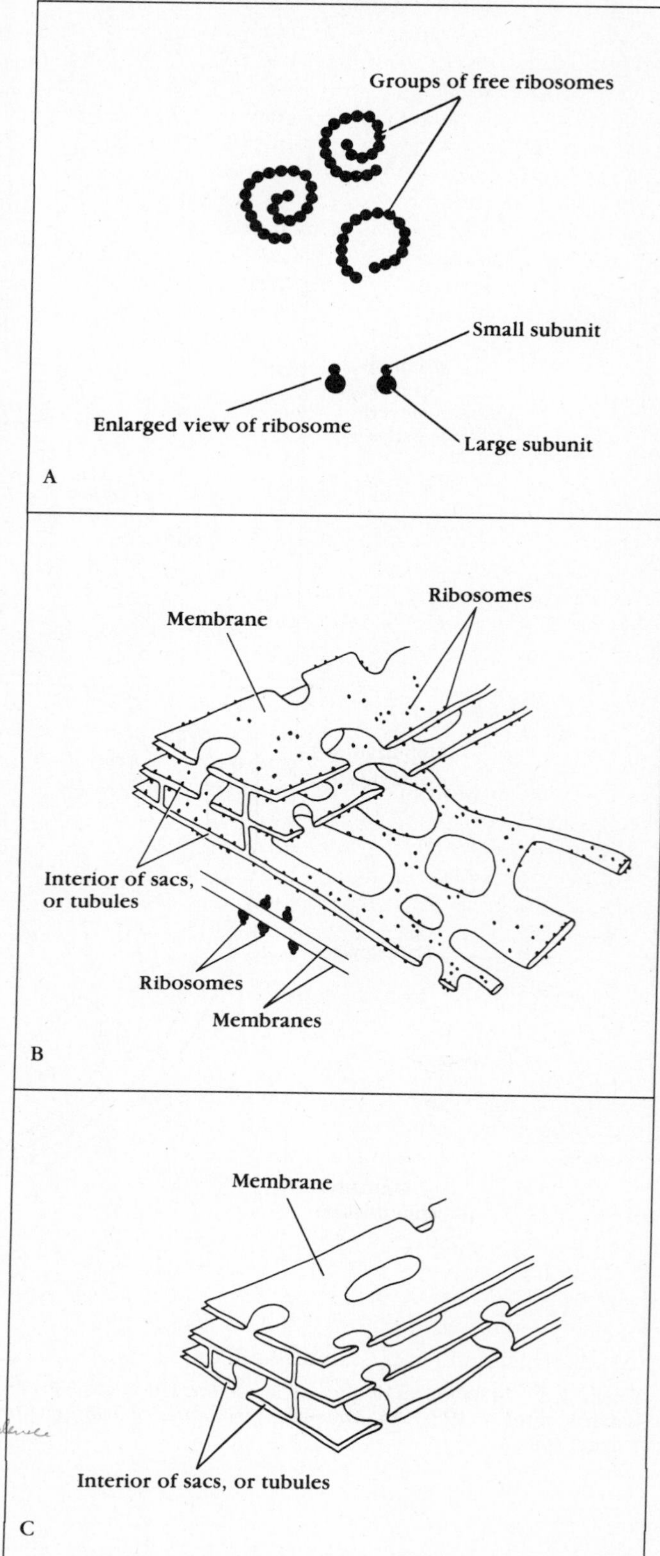

FIGURE 1-6 Electron microscopic appearance of structures of (A) Ribosomes, (B) Rough endoplasmic reticulum, (C) Smooth endoplasmic reticulum. (From R.S. Snell, *Clinical Histology for Medical Students*. Boston: Little, Brown, 1984.)

The outer membrane of the nuclear envelope is continuous with the membranes of the endoplasmic reticulum (ER), and it is believed that the nuclear envelope develops from ER membranes after cell division.

Much of the surface of the ER may be covered with small particles or granules made up of ribonucleic acid (RNA) associated with protein. The particles, called *ribosomes*, give the outer membrane of the ER a rough or granular appearance; therefore, such endoplasmic reticulum is called *granulated* or *rough ER*. Other surfaces of the endoplasmic reticulum may be free of ribosomes and hence appear relatively smooth. This type of endoplasmic reticulum is called *agranular* or *smooth ER*.

The endoplasmic reticulum, whether smooth or rough, provides a large surface within the cell on which sequences of chemical reactions can occur. Enzymes and other substances are arranged in an assembly-line sequence to provide for efficient production of various types of proteins, carbohydrates, and lipids.

The rough ER is involved primarily with the production of proteins. Proteins such as hormones, for example, which are destined to be secreted, are put together on the ribosomes of the rough ER. Also, some of the proteins that form structural parts of the cell are produced on the rough ER.

The smooth ER appears to be more involved with the formation of nonprotein substances such as the fat-soluble triglycerides, fatty acids, steroids, and phospholipids. It is also involved in biotransformation of substances and in storing calcium in some cells.

The spaces between the folded membranes of the ER forming the fluid-filled interior of the saccules and tubules are called *cisternae*. These channels or canallike spaces allow molecules to be distributed from one area of the cell to another. In a sense, the endoplasmic reticulum also functions as an intracellular circulatory system.

Polyribosomes

Some of the ribosomes within the cell are not bound to the endoplasmic reticulum; instead, a number of ribosomes involved with the production of a specific protein molecule may be linked together, much like pearls on a string, forming a chain structure called a polyribosome (literally, many ribosomes).

Polyribosomes of several different lengths may be found in the cytoplasm and all are involved with the formation or synthesis of protein molecules. Most of the proteins made on the polyribosomes are for the cell's own use in building cell components (structural proteins) or in regulating cell activities (enzymes, for example).

Golgi Complex

The Golgi complex, also called the Golgi apparatus or Golgi body, is a series of concentric, flattened saccules with membranes resembling those of the smooth endoplasmic reticulum (Fig. 1-7). In some cells the Golgi membranes appear to be connected to the smooth ER and may be a specialized part of it. Membrane-bound vesicles are

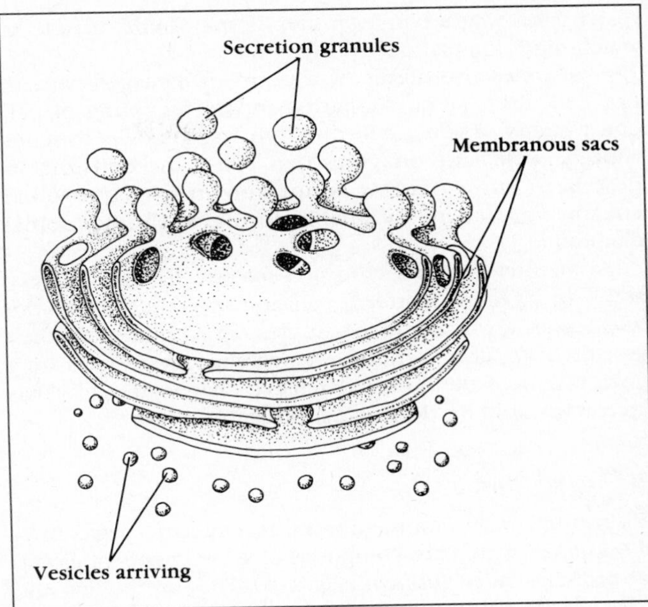

FIGURE 1-7 Probable appearance of Golgi apparatus. (From R.S. Snell, *Clinical Histology for Medical Students*. Boston: Little, Brown, 1984.)

frequently observed near the Golgi membranes and represent packaged chemicals arriving at the Golgi complex for further processing or packaged substances leaving the Golgi complex destined for secretion by way of exocytosis.

The Golgi complex is predominant in various types of secretory cells, such as pancreatic acinar cells, and plays several important roles in the process of secretion. Substances destined for secretion—a protein hormone, for example—may be produced on the rough ER and then transported through the cisternae of the ER to the Golgi apparatus. The Golgi apparatus may then prepare the hormone for release by packaging it within a membranous vacuole, which then moves toward the plasma membrane where the hormone is discharged into the extracellular environment.

Other functions of the Golgi apparatus include producing some substances such as polysaccharides, chemically modifying molecules produced by the ER (for example, activating enzymes), storing synthesized molecules, and producing digestive vacuoles called lysosomes.

Lysosomes

Lysosomes (*lyse*—destroy, *some*—body), are membrane-bound organelles that are spherical and contain digestive enzymes. They originate from the Golgi complex and endoplasmic reticulum, and participate in intracellular digestive processes.

Lysosomes contain a variety of hydrolytic enzymes that break down protein, nucleic acids, carbohydrates, and lipids. When a cell ingests material by endocytosis, lysosomes fuse their membranes with those of the endocytotic vesicle, forming a common membrane-bound vesicle in which digestion can occur (Fig. 1-8).

Lysosomes also digest "worn out" or damaged parts of the cell, thereby participating in the recycling of cell constituents. When a cell dies, the lysosomes it contains rupture, releasing enzymes that cause the cell to self-destruct (*autolysis*). It is not known why lysosomal enzymes are normally unable to digest the lysosomal membrane.

Numerous lysosomes are present in cells that are very active in ingesting matter by phagocytosis. In some of the leukocytes, for example, lysosomes are so numerous they give the cytoplasm a granular appearance. Lysosomes are a critical part of the body's defensive phagocytic cells that are responsible for destroying foreign proteins.

Microtubules

Microtubules are nonmembranous, cylindric organelles, the walls of which are composed of 13 filaments of globular proteins called *tubulin* (Fig. 1-9). They are hollow and have an internal diameter of approximately 250 angstroms (Å). An angstrom is a very small measurement equal to 10^7 mm (one ten-millionth of a millimeter).

Microtubules may function in one or more of three different ways: (1) to maintain the shape of a cell by providing structural support; (2) to act as an internal conduit for the movement of materials from one part of the cell to another; and (3) to provide for certain forms of cellular movement, such as ciliary motion.

Microtubules are commonly found in cells that possess long cellular extensions that require support; for example, embedded in the cytoplasm of the long extensions of nerve cells (axons and dendrites) where they provide a certain amount of rigidity. If microtubules are selectively destroyed by certain drugs, some cell processes lose their characteristic shape.

Because microtubules are usually oriented in the direction of material movement within the cytoplasm, they are believed to be involved with the intracellular transport of various substances. In certain nerve cells, for example, microtubules are numerous in the axon. Materials required for proper functioning of the terminals of the axon are synthesized in the cell body and transported down the

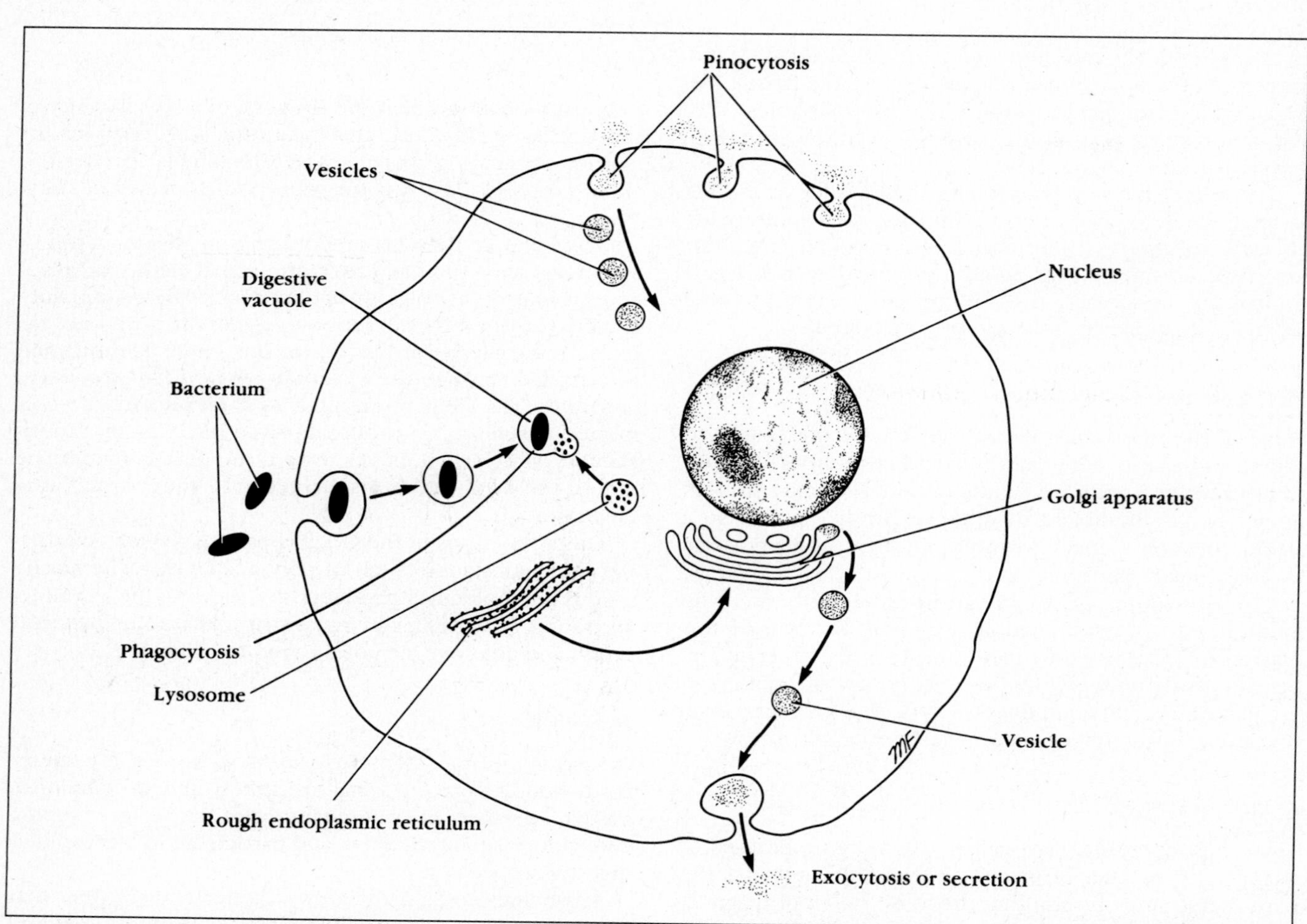

FIGURE 1-8 Schematic illustration of processes of endocytosis (pinocytosis and phagocytosis) and exocytosis. (From R.S. Snell, *Clinical Histology for Medical Students*. Boston: Little, Brown, 1984.)

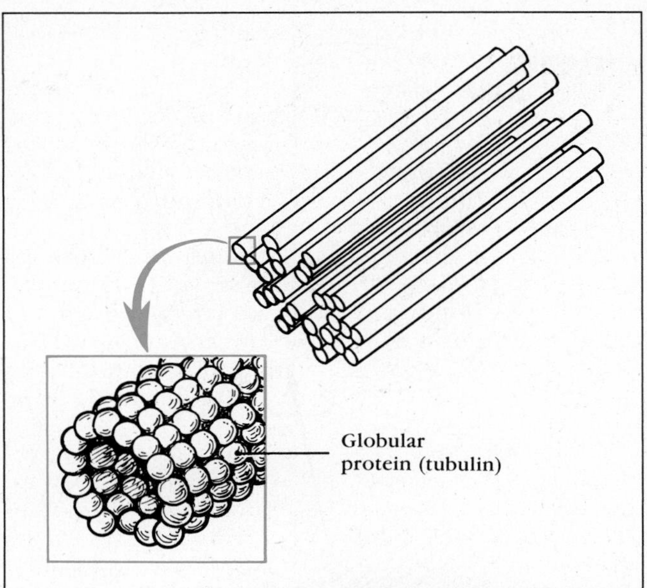

FIGURE 1-9 Microtubules. (Adapted from R.S. Snell, *Clinical Histology for Medical Students*. Boston: Little, Brown, 1984.)

axon to its terminals. If the axon is ligated (tied off), material will be observed damming up in the part of the axon nearest the cell body, and it will swell much as a river does if its flow is restricted by a dam.

Studies have shown that the globular proteins making up the wall of the microtubule move along the length of the tubule in a sequential manner as one end of the tubule is being formed while the opposite end is being broken down. Some substances that are transported by the microtubules may attach to the protein subunits at the beginning of the tubule and move in association with the protein to the other end where they may be released.

In addition to intracellular transport, microtubules form parts of cilia and flagella, cellular structures specialized for movement.

Cilia and Flagella

Cilia are short protoplasmic extensions on the free surface of some cells that line body cavities or hollow viscera. The lining of the upper respiratory tract, for example, contains ciliated cells, as does the lining of the uterine tubes.

Cilia (singular, cilium) are microtubule-containing cylinders enclosed by an extension of the plasma membrane (Fig. 1-10). Usually, a single ciliated cell projects numerous cilia on its free surface, giving that portion of the cell surface a matlike appearance. One human cell type, the spermatozoon (sperm), or male reproductive cell, has a single elongated ciliumlike extension called a flagellum (plural, flagella).

Cilia and flagella are constructed from the same basic pattern and have three major parts: the stalk, which is a sheaf of tubules enveloped by the plasma membrane; a basal granule, from which the structure originates within the cytoplasm; and rootlet fibers, which extend from the basal granule into the cytoplasm.

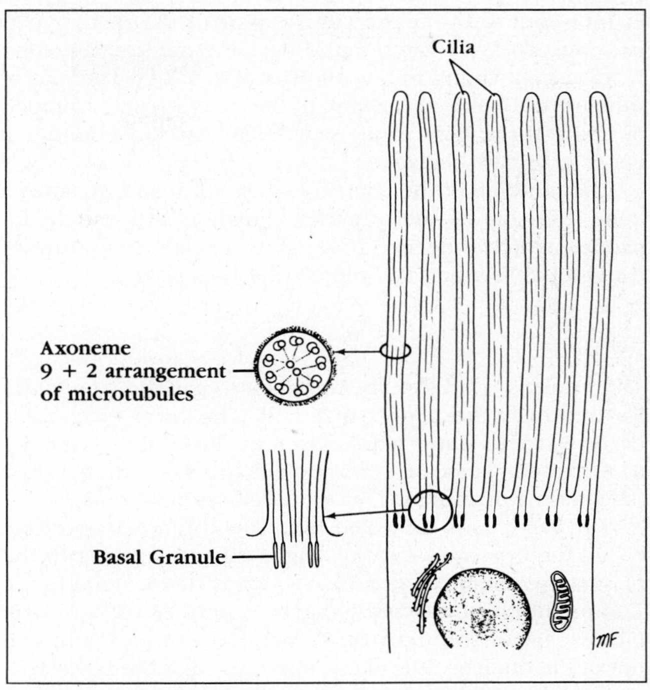

FIGURE 1-10 A ciliated cell. (From R.S. Snell, *Clinical Histology for Medical Students*. Boston: Little, Brown, 1984.)

In cross section, cilia and flagella are bounded by a sheath that encloses an array of nine double microtubules arranged in a radial fashion, with two additional microtubules in the center. This arrangement is called the 9 + 2 pattern (see Fig. 1-10), and the compound tubular structure that is formed is called an *axoneme*. Ciliary motion occurs when the microtubules, powered by ATP, slide past one another. Cilia move with a swift forward movement and a slow backward stroke (like a whip). Their movement is coordinated so that stimulation is passed from one cilium to the next. On a sheet of ciliated cells, coordinated ciliary movement resembles the effect seen when wind ripples across a field of wheat.

Ciliary movement in the upper respiratory tract is an important part of the body's defense, helping to move inhaled particulate matter trapped in mucus toward the nasal and oral cavities where it may be discharged or swallowed. In the uterine tubes, ciliary motion helps move the ovum toward the uterine cavity.

Flagellar movement is undulating (wavelike) rather than whiplike. It is responsible for propelling sperm through body fluids at a rate of 1 to 4 mm per minute in a relatively straight line.

Microtubules, cilia, and flagella are nonmembranous organelles that are structurally related to the centriole. The centriole may be the source of microtubules, cilia, and flagella.

Centrioles

Many human cells contain near the nucleus two hollow, cylindric structures called centrioles, which, like cilia, are composed of nine sets of microtubules arranged in a radial fashion, but without the central pair of tubules (9 + 0 pattern). They are often found near the nuclear envelope lying at right angles to one another (Fig. 1-11). The microtubules that make up the wall of the centriole are arranged in sets of three, lying in the same plane and embedded in a dense granular substance.

The function of the centrioles is to form and organize a complex array of microtubules known as the spindle apparatus, which is needed to separate a single cell into two daughter cells when the cell divides (see p. 18).

Nucleus

The nucleus is a large membranous organelle frequently located near the center of a cell. The term *nucleus* is derived from a Latin word meaning "little nut," referring to the resemblance of a cell nucleus to a nut within a shell (the plasma membrane), or to a seed within a pod.

The nucleus is bounded by a membranous envelope called the *nuclear envelope* (Fig. 1-12). In contrast to the plasma membrane, it consists of two distinct membranes. The membranes are fused together periodically to form circular pores through which material can pass into and out of the nucleus. It is likely, however, that the pores represent something other than simple holes in the nuclear envelope, because nuclei can be removed from cells without the loss of nuclear material.

The inner membrane of the nuclear envelope represents the actual nuclear membrane, while the outer membrane of the envelope gives rise to and is continuous with membranes of the endoplasmic reticulum.

In some cells the nucleoplasm appears homogeneous and undifferentiated. In others, distinct nuclear structures can be observed. Two commonly seen structures are the nucleolus and condensed strands of chromatin called *chromosomes*.

The *nucleolus* (little nucleus) is a collection of dense fibers and granules forming a small spherical mass that is most visible when the cell is not in the process of reproducing itself (cell division). The nucleolus (see Fig. 1-12) is composed primarily of RNA and protein, together with smaller amounts of DNA. The nucleic acids play key roles in the cellular synthesis of proteins. The granules of the nucleolus are precursors of ribosomes (particles of RNA and protein), which are the sites of protein synthesis in the cytoplasm.

Chromatin is composed of long molecules of DNA in association with protein. Chromatin fibers are too small to be seen with the light microscope. Prior to cell division, however, chromatin fibers coil and condense into compact structures that are visible when using the light microscope. These visible, x-shaped structures are called chromosomes (Fig. 1-13). There are 46 chromosomes—23 pairs—in the human cell. The pairs of chromosomes differ from one another in size and shape.

Genes. The nucleus directs and controls the activities of the entire cell through the genes. A gene is the linear sequence of nucleotides on DNA that code for the production of a single protein. The sequence is divided

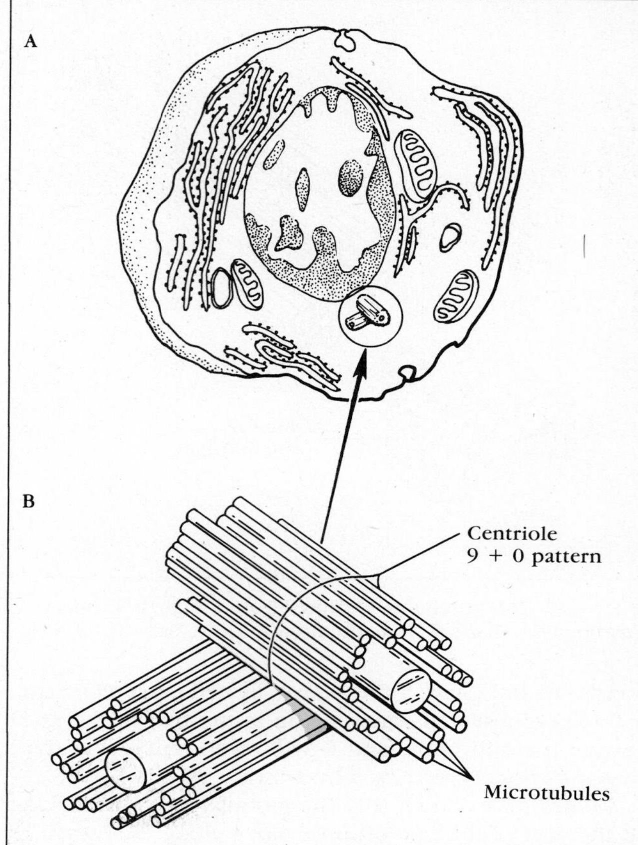

FIGURE 1-11 Centrioles. A. Placement in relationship to the nucleus. B. Appearance and composition of the centriole.

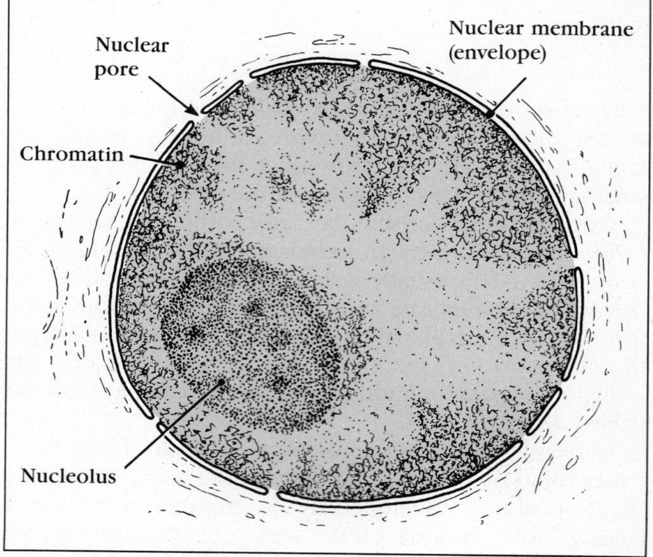

FIGURE 1-12 The nucleus.

into units of three nucleotides, each called a *triplet*. The sequence of the nucleotide bases (*guanine*, *thymine*, *cytosine*, and *adenine*) determines the unique code and ultimately codes for a single amino acid. The genes determine the specific code that is transcribed as RNA. The gene is located on one of the two DNA strands called the *master strand*, which serves as the template for *messenger RNA (mRNA)* transcription. Other parts of DNA serve as templates for *transfer RNA (tRNA)* or *ribosomal RNA (rRNA)* formation. The code, transmitted to the ribosomes, allows for the formation of several thousand types of proteins that are essential to the various functions of human cells.

Protein Synthesis. Nearly all of the chemical reactions associated with normal cell function are enzyme dependent. All known enzymes are proteins, the synthesis of which is controlled by nuclear DNA; therefore, the activity of the cytoplasmic organelles is regulated either directly or indirectly by the nucleus. In addition to enzymes, nuclear DNA contains the blueprints that specify construction of other types of proteins such as hormones or structural proteins. The synthesis of proteins occurs in two major steps known as *transcription* and *translation* (Fig. 1-14). Transcription occurs in the nucleus and involves DNA and mRNA. During transcription, the DNA molecule partially unwinds into two separate strands. One strand acts as a template upon which mRNA is synthesized; the other strand acts as a cover. The genetic message carried by DNA in the form of a series of triplets is transcribed to mRNA by complementary base-pairing; thus, the formation of mRNA results in the synthesis of a molecule having a linear sequence of bases that are complementary to DNA. The mRNA molecule separates from the DNA template as fast as it forms.

After synthesis, mRNA escapes the nucleus by way of pores in the nuclear envelope and enters the cytoplasm where it becomes associated with ribosomes, the organelle where amino acids are linked into the polypeptide chain of a protein. Within the ribosome, the genetic message carried by mRNA in the form of codons is deciphered, and correct amino acids are joined in the proper sequence to form a protein molecule. This process is translation, and it involves tRNA. One or more specific tRNA molecules exist for each type of amino acid. Transfer RNA binds itself to a specific amino acid and carries it to the site of protein synthesis in the ribosome. Transfer RNA also contains a binding site (in the form of an anticodon) for mRNA; thus, as tRNA molecules bearing specific amino acids sequentially bind to mRNA in the ribosome, the amino acids are sequenced into a protein that is then released from the ribosome.

Once the mRNA template becomes associated with the ribosome, the process of peptide synthesis occurs rapidly,

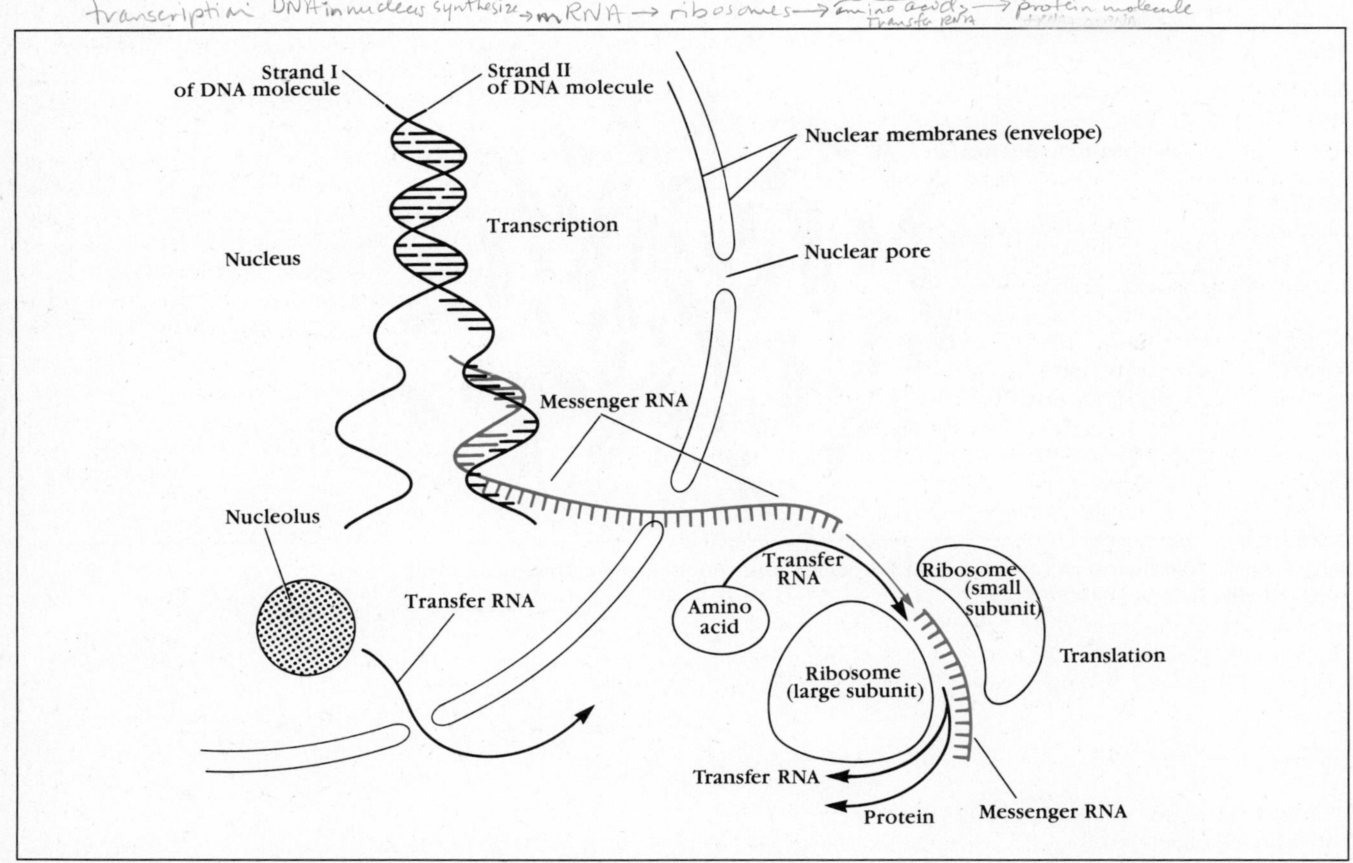

FIGURE 1-14 Highly schematic picture of protein synthesis. (From R.S. Snell, *Clinical Histology for Medical Students*. Boston: Little, Brown, 1984.)

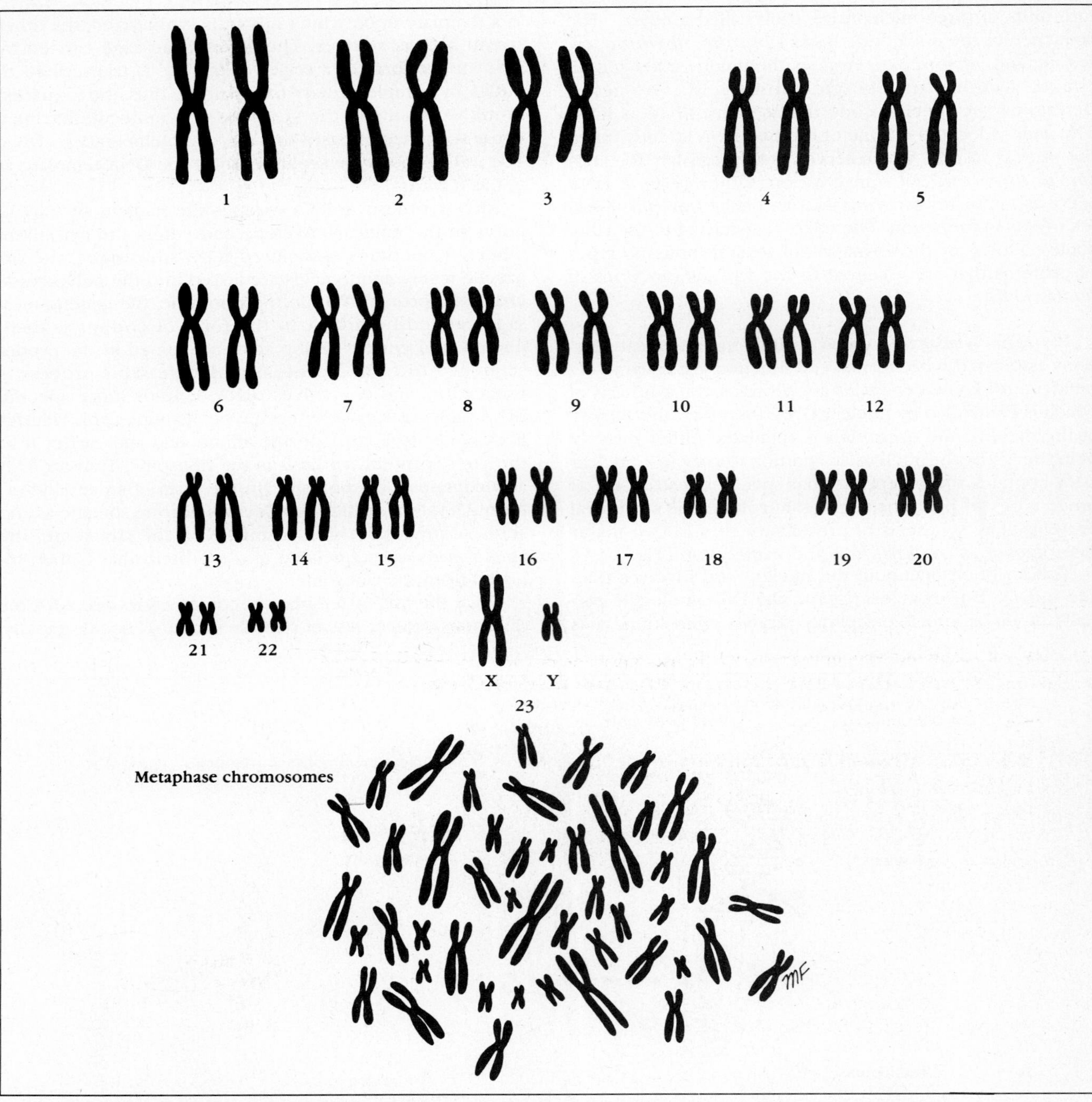

FIGURE 1-13 Chromosomes. (Adapted from R.S. Snell, *Clinical Histology for Medical Students*. Boston: Little, Brown, 1984.)

taking about one second for a new amino acid to be added to the peptide chain. Thus, the synthesis of a protein such as the hormone insulin (51 amino acids) takes about one minute. Also, several ribosomes may simultaneously translate a single strand of mRNA so that protein synthesis may occur more rapidly.

Reproductive Ability of Cells

Most cells have the ability to reproduce themselves through the complex process of *mitosis*. In the adult individual, the new cells take the place of old cells in a rigidly defined order that maintains cellular numbers but allows for the replacement of only the needed cells. The turnover rate is billions of cells per day, but rigid controls inherently limit the number of cells to be reproduced.

Specific controls on the reproductive process produce precisely the correct quantity of cells. For example, if the red blood cell (RBC) count decreases, specific stimulating factors cause the bone marrow to increase production of erythrocytes (RBCs), leading ultimately to increased numbers of circulating red blood cells (see Chap. 15). Another stage in the process of erythropoiesis (RBC production) occurs when the appropriate level of red blood cells is reached. Some factor, either diminished stimulation or an inhibitor, suppresses further production of RBC.

Regeneration of Cells

As stated earlier, almost all cells have the ability to reproduce themselves. This ability is called the regenerative capacity of cells.

Labile cells regenerate frequently and have a life span usually measured in hours or days. Some examples of labile cells are white blood cells and epithelial cells. Other cells retain the ability to regenerate or reproduce, but do so only under special circumstances. These are called *stable cells*, and their life span is measured in years or sometimes, the entire life span of an organism. Some examples of stable cells are osteocytes of bone, parenchymal cells of the liver, and cells of the glands of the body. In the normal liver cell, for example, mitotic figures are rare, but after injury, mitoses are abundant because the liver has a remarkable ability to repair itself.

The third type of cells, the *permanent cells*, live for the entire life of the organism. They include the nerve cell bodies and probably most of the muscle cells. The neuron does not divide after birth but has the ability in certain circumstances to regenerate its axon and dendrites (see Chap. 44). Myocardial muscle does not regenerate; when it dies, it is repaired by the formation of scar tissue.

Reproduction of Cells

The Cell Cycle. All human cells have a life cycle, called the cell cycle, that begins when the cell is produced by division of its parent and ends when the cell either divides to give rise to daughter cells or dies. A complete cell cycle consists of four stages labelled G_1, S, G_2, and M (Fig. 1-15).

The G_1 stage is the time interval after the formation of the cell that precedes replication of DNA. The S stage is the time during which DNA replication occurs. The G_2 stage is the time interval after DNA replication and before the beginning of the M stage (mitosis), the stage during which cell division occurs. Cells not destined for an early repeat of the division cycle are commonly arrested at the G_1 stage, or according to some systems of nomenclature, a G_0 stage (resting phase). All of the stages between mitotic divisions are collectively called *interphase*.

The process by which a cell divides to form two identical daughter cells is mitosis. Before a cell can undergo mitosis, its chromosomes must duplicate themselves, a process called *replication*.

Replication. Replication of DNA occurs during the S stage of interphase. During this time the chromosomes appear to be spread out in a tangled mass known as chromatin. In replication the two strands of the DNA molecule separate, and each serves as a template (pattern) for the formation of another strand (Fig. 1-16). Each template and its complement then form a new DNA molecule. During mitosis each daughter cell inherits a DNA molecule that consists of one new strand and one parental strand.

Each chromosome is furnished with a single centromere, an area that holds together the two daughter chromosomes produced when a chromosome replicates (see Chap. 2). After replication, the two identical, double-stranded molecules of DNA are called chromatids as long as they remain attached to each other by the centromere.

Mitosis. Mitosis is described in terms of phases through which the cell passes as it divides (Fig. 1-17). The phases are defined by the appearance of chromosomes under the light microscope and are designated (in sequence) as *prophase*, *metaphase*, *anaphase*, and *telophase*.

During prophase, the chromatin condenses into distinct chromosomes that are visible as pairs of *chromatids*

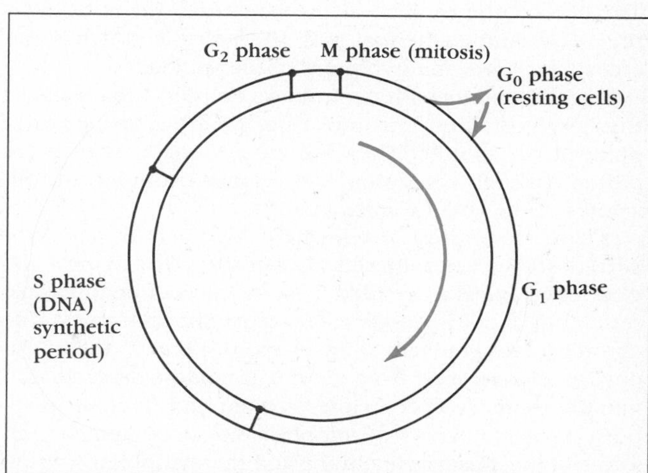

FIGURE 1-15 The cell cycle. (Adapted from J. Stein [ed.], *Internal Medicine*. Boston: Little, Brown, 1983.)

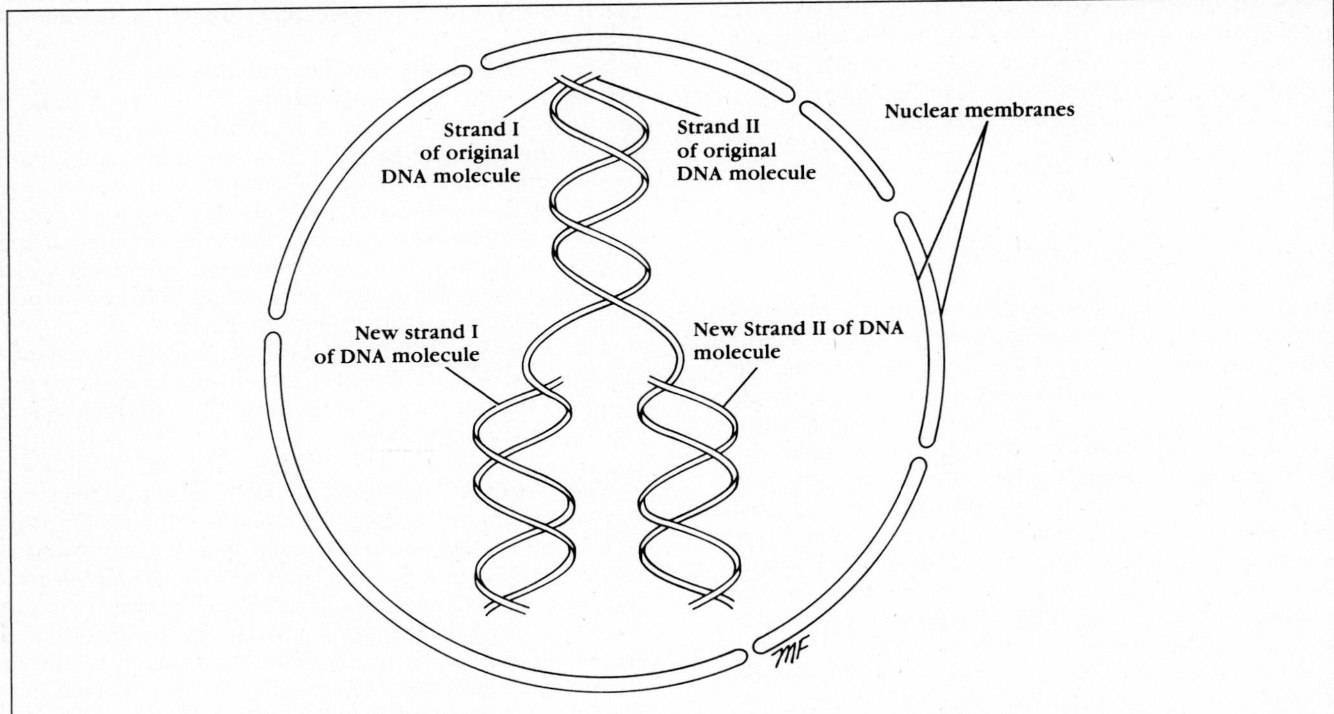

FIGURE 1-16 Replication. The two strands of a DNA molecule first separate and a new strand is synthesized alongside each one. The result is that each newly formed, double-stranded molecule is identical to the original molecule whose strands became separated. (From R.S. Snell, *Clinical Histology for Medical Students*. Boston: Little, Brown, 1984.)

joined at their centers to form an X. The point of junction of the chromatin threads is called a *centromere*. In prophase the nuclear membrane disappears, as does the nucleolus, and appears to be part of the cytoplasm. The centrioles migrate to opposite poles of the cell and a spindle of microtubules forms between the centrioles.

During metaphase, the assembly of the spindle is completed and the chromosomes align in a plane midway between the poles. This plane is called the *equatorial plane*. The chromosomes align at the equatorial plane because they experience an equal pull, through the attached microtubules, from the two poles of the spindle.

Anaphase starts with centromere division, which allows the newly divided chromosomes to move to opposite poles of the spindle. They assume a V shape as they are pulled through the cytoplasm by microtubules and filaments of the spindle apparatus.

At the beginning of telophase, two sets of daughter chromosomes are gathered at opposite poles. A new nuclear envelope is assembled from saccules of endoplasmic reticulum and surrounds each set of chromosomes. The chromosomes gradually unravel and disperse in the nucleoplasm, disappearing from view. The spindle disintegrates, but the duplicated centrioles remain and nucleoli reappear. As these events of telophase are occurring, a cleft forms in the plasma membrane and the cytoplasm is eventually divided equally between the two newly formed daughter cells by a process called *cytokinesis*.

Cellular Exchange

For the cell to produce its own protoplasm, synthesize chemicals for export, or derive energy from chemicals and convert the energy into useful work, the cell must acquire chemicals from the extracellular fluid. On the other hand, cell metabolism produces waste products that must be eliminated into the extracellular environment. In addition, hormones, enzymes, and other chemicals may be secreted into the extracellular fluid. Because the plasma membrane separates the intracellular fluid (ICF) from the extracellular fluid (ECF), all substances that either enter or leave the cell must pass through the plasma membrane.

In general, the mechanisms of cellular exchange can be divided into two categories: active and passive. *Active mechanisms* require the cell to expend energy (ATP) to effect solute movement across the plasma membrane, whereas *passive mechanisms* do not require energy expenditure by the cell.

Passive Movement Across the Cell Membrane

Diffusion. Diffusion is defined as the net movement of a substance from a region of higher concentration to a region of lower concentration. If the substance is equally distributed between two regions, no concentration gradient exists and diffusion equilibrium is present.

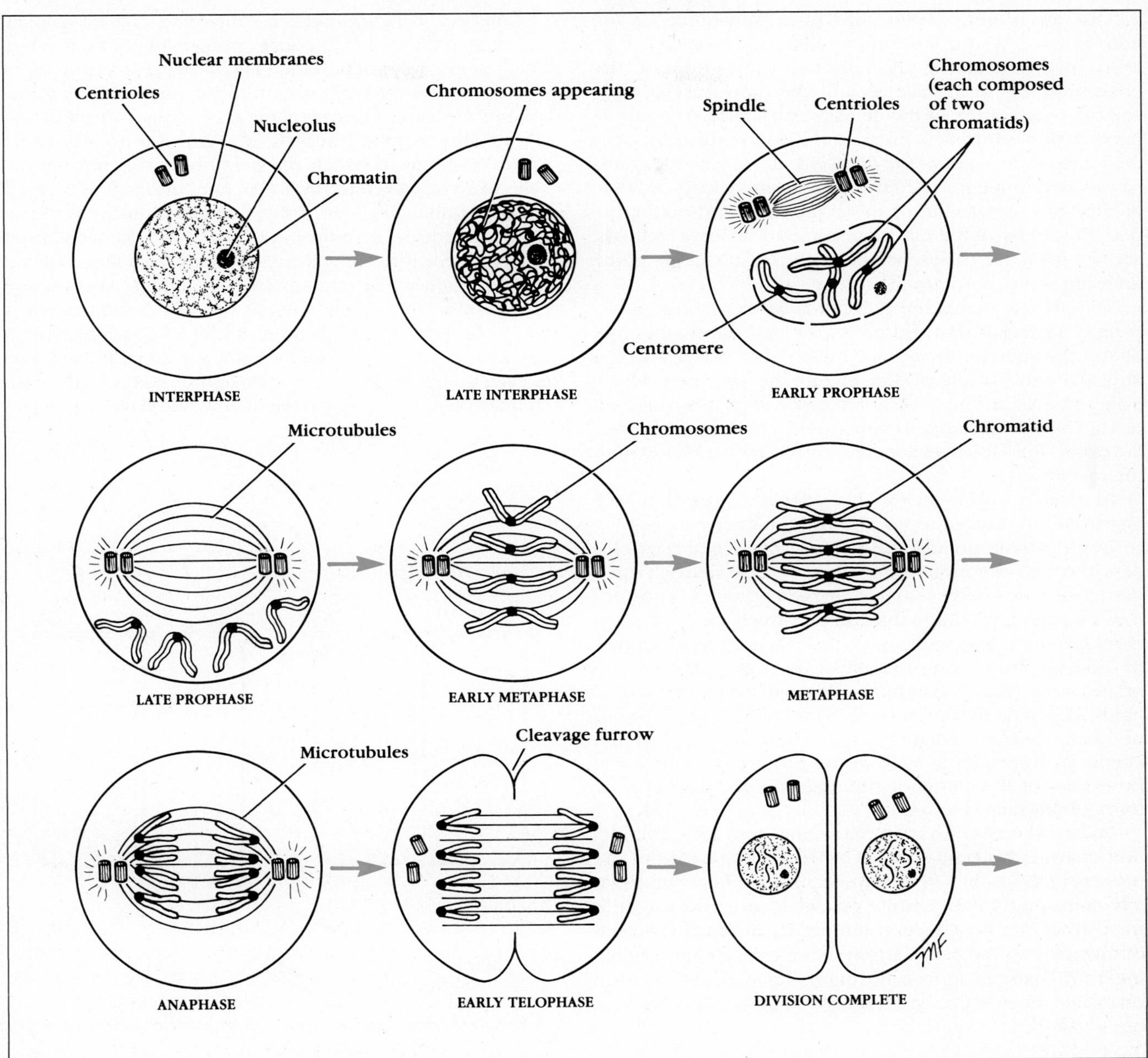

FIGURE 1-17 Mitosis. (From R.S. Snell, *Clinical Histology for Medical Students*. Boston: Little, Brown, 1984.)

The rate of net diffusion of a given substance, or the time that it takes for diffusion equilibrium to occur, is directly proportional to the concentration gradient, the cross-sectional or surface area of the diffusion pathway, and the temperature of the diffusing substance. The rate of net diffusion is inversely proportional to the square root of the molecular weight of the diffusing substance. Additional factors that influence the rates of diffusion across biologic membranes are atomic or molecular size and configuration, the ability of the diffusing solute to dissolve in lipids, and the presence or absence of an electrical charge on the diffusing solute particles.

The plasma membrane presents a barrier to the movement of materials into and out of the cell. Substances that diffuse through the membrane must either dissolve in the fluid structure of the plasma membrane and then diffuse from one side to the other, or they must pass through interruptions in the membrane called channels or *pores*. Pores are fluid-filled channels formed by proteins within the membrane.

In general, substances with a diameter greater than 8 angstroms are unable to, or else have difficulty in, passing through plasma membrane pores. Uncharged particles pass through the membrane more readily than charged particles (*ions*), and positively charged particles (*cations*) pass through less readily than do negatively charged particles (*anions*). Also, molecules that have a higher degree of lipid solubility tend to diffuse through plasma membranes more readily than molecules that are less soluble in lipids. How readily an ion or molecule diffuses into or out of a cell, therefore, depends upon both its physical and chemical properties as well as the physical and chemical properties of the plasma membrane that the molecule or ion is attempting to cross.

The movement of oxygen molecules into cells and carbon dioxide molecules out of cells is an example of the process of diffusion. Oxygen molecules are being continually consumed by metabolic processes occurring within the cell, so that the concentration gradient favors diffusion of this gas into the cell. Carbon dioxide molecules are being continually produced during cellular metabolism, so that the concentration gradient favors diffusion of this gas out of the cell.

Osmosis. Osmosis is the net diffusion of water through a selectively permeable membrane that separates two aqueous solutions with different solute concentrations. The membrane is impermeable to one or more of the solutes.

When the concentration of nondiffusible solutes (substances, dissolved in water, that cannot diffuse through the membrane) is greater on one side of the membrane than the other, net diffusion of water (osmosis) occurs through the membrane toward the area of greater solute concentration until the solute:solvent ratio is equal on both sides of the membrane, or until a force of equal magnitude opposing the force created by the movement of water is applied. Water molecules diffuse from an area of greater water concentration through a selectively permeable membrane to an area of lesser water concentration.

Consider a 500-ml beaker containing 280 ml of pure water divided into two equal compartments by a selectively permeable membrane (Fig. 1-18). For purposes of discussion, consider the system to be unaffected by atmospheric pressure. Compartment A contains 140 ml of water, as does compartment B. If 8 gm of a nondiffusible solute, a solute to which the membrane was not permeable, were dissolved in the water in compartment A and 6 gm of nondiffusible solute were dissolved in the water in compartment B, net diffusion of water would occur from compartment B to compartment A until the solute:solvent ratio of each compartment became equal. At diffusion equilibrium, the solute:solvent ratio of compartment A would be 8 gm per 160 ml and that of compartment B would be 6 gm per 120 ml, or 1 gm per 20 ml for the fluid in each compartment. A net diffusion of 20 ml water from compartment B to compartment A would have occurred.

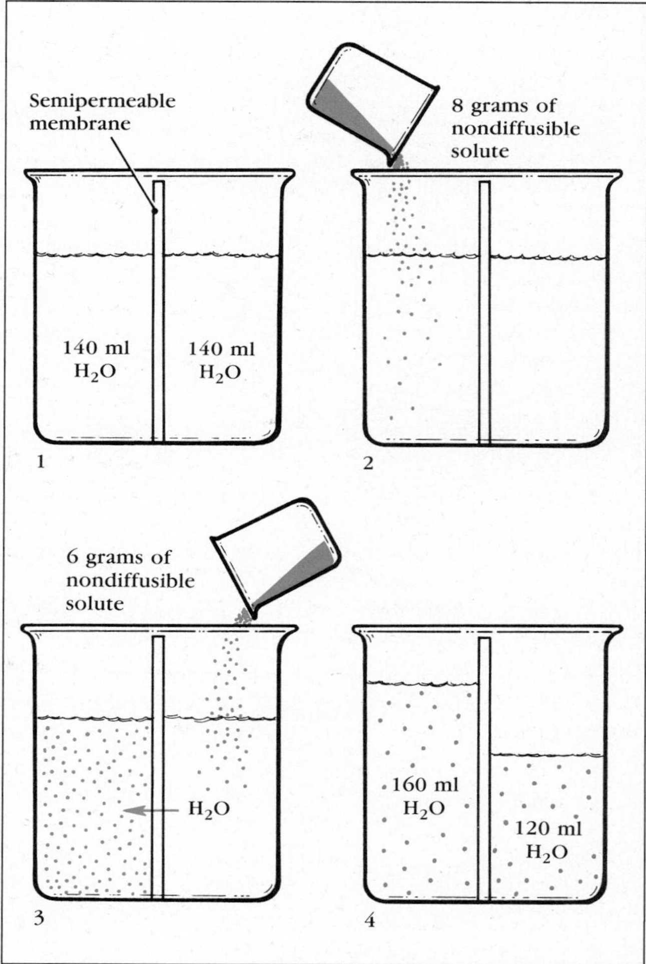

FIGURE 1-18 Osmosis. 1. A beaker of water with semipermeable membrane separating the sides. 2. Add 8 gm of a nondiffusible substance to one side. 3. Add 6 gm of a nondiffusible substance to the other side. 4. The water will move toward the more concentrated side and make the concentrations equal, with more fluid in one side than the other.

During osmosis, pressure is created on the membrane as water moves from an area of higher concentration, through the membrane, to an area of lesser concentration. This pressure is called the *osmotic pressure*. The magnitude of osmotic pressure depends upon the number of particles (solute particles) in the solution toward which water is moving. The greater the number of nondiffusible particles in that solution, the greater its osmotic pressure.

Fluids that contain osmotically active particles in the same concentration as found in the plasma of blood are *isotonic*. If a human red blood cell is placed in an isotonic solution (Fig. 1-19), it neither swells nor shrinks, because the net diffusion of water into or out of the cell is zero. An example of an isotonic solution is 0.9 percent sodium chloride in water. Fluids that contain a higher concentration of osmotically active particles than blood plasma are termed *hypertonic fluids*. Red blood cells that are placed in a hypertonic solution shrink and shrivel (*crenation*) because net diffusion of water out of the cell occurs. *Hypotonic solutions* contain a lower concentration of osmotically active particles than does plasma; therefore, red blood cells swell and hemolyze when placed in hypertonic solutions since the net diffusion of water is into the cell.

In the body, osmosis is important in maintaining plasma volume, interstitial and intracellular fluid volumes, and the volumes of other fluid compartments.

Facilitated Diffusion. This process of assisted diffusion is especially important in moving glucose from the extracellular fluid (ECF) to the intracellular fluid (ICF). Normally, there is a very small reserve of glucose for energy metabolism within the cell, so the cell is very dependent on the transport of glucose from the ECF. Glucose is not soluble in the lipid of the cell membrane and is too large to pass through the membrane pores. The mechanism of facilitated passive transport involves combining glucose with specific carrier molecules that are in the cell membrane. After combining with the carrier molecule, glucose is carried into the cell by simple diffusion (Fig. 1-20). This process requires no ATP but is assisted by the pancreatic hormone insulin, which has been shown to increase the rate of glucose transport sevenfold to tenfold. Substances move only from an area of high concentration to one of low concentration, and the process is enhanced when a greater differential exists between ECF and ICF.

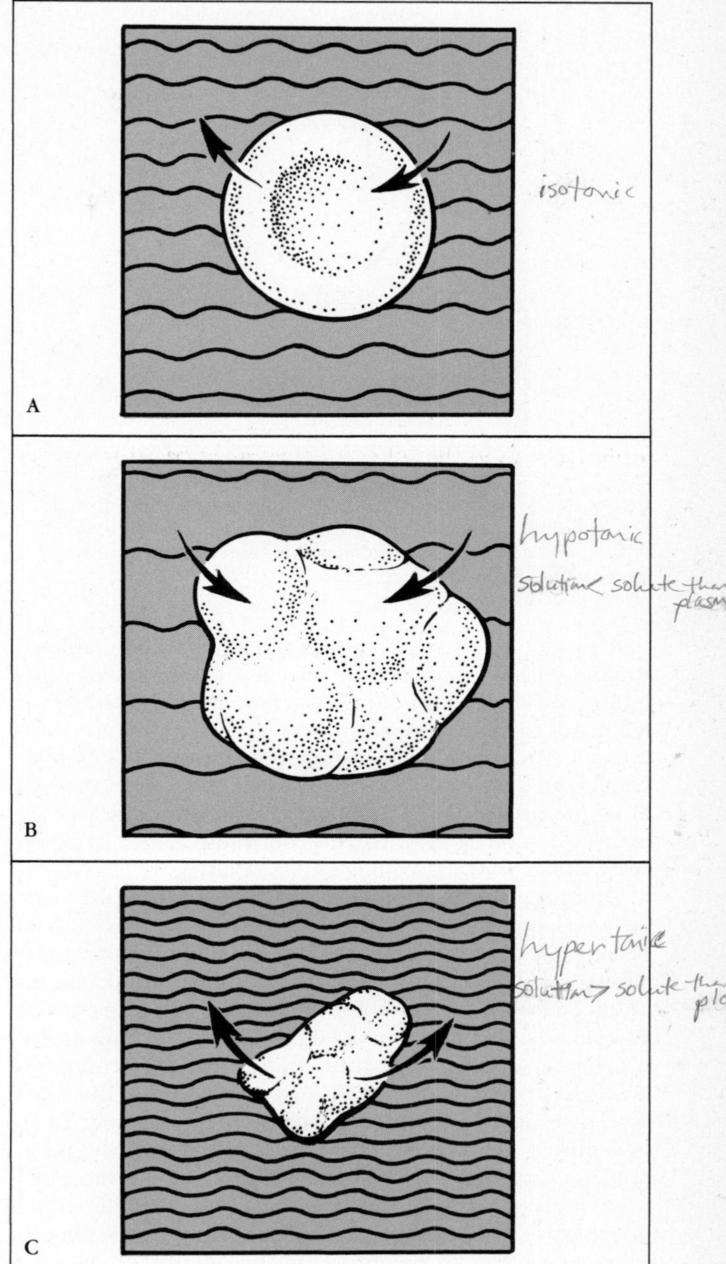

FIGURE 1-19 A. Isotonic solution (cell volume unchanged). B. Hypotonic solution (cell volume increased). C. Hypertonic solution (cell volume decreased).

Active Movement Across the Cell Membrane

Active Transport. Many carrier systems transport solutes against a chemical, electrical, or somatic gradient. These carrier-mediated transport systems always require the expenditure of energy and are often called *active transport* systems or simply *pumps*. All of the body's cells are capable of active transport in one way or another. For example, when a meal low in carbohydrate is ingested, cells that line the intestinal tract transport glucose out of the intestine and toward the blood where the concentration of glucose may be much greater.

The *sodium-potassium pump* is an important example of active transport (Fig. 1-21). This transport system pumps sodium ions out of the cell, thereby preventing their accumulation inside due to a favorable electrochemical gradient. The pump also returns potassium ions inside the cell that have diffused out due to a favorable chemical gradient. Maintenance of sodium and potassium gradients is essential for stable membrane potential.

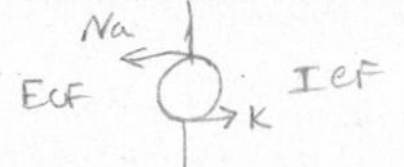

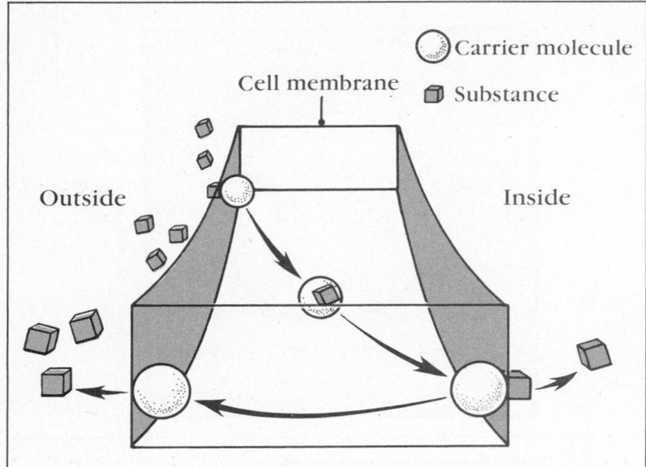

FIGURE 1-20 Example of facilitated diffusion with a substance combining with a carrier molecule and moving it to the inside of the cell and down its concentration gradient, without the expenditure of energy.

The sodium-potassium pump prevents accumulation of sodium within the cell; therefore, it also minimizes water influx and cellular swelling. Accumulation of sodium in ICF tends to cause osmosis of water toward the interior of the cell. The pumping of sodium ions out of the cell overcomes the continual tendency for water to enter the cell. Most important, when cellular metabolism ceases or decreases, adequate ATP to run the pump is not available and cellular swelling begins immediately.

Although the phenomenon of carrier-mediated transport and the characteristics of transport processes have been studied for several years, the actual molecular mechanisms involved are not clear. Many carrier molecules are believed to be membrane-bound proteins (e.g., glycoprotein) that become activated (capable of picking up and transporting) when the membrane becomes energized through the breakdown of ATP. On activation of the transport protein and its attachment to the substance to be transported, the protein changes its position in the membrane in a manner that effects the transfer of the substance from one side of the membrane to the other, as illustrated in Figure 1-21. Evidence also indicates that the binding of some substances to receptors on the membrane causes a pore or channel to form, thereby providing a less restrictive pathway for the passive movement of materials (e.g., ions) across the membrane.

Many types of solutes such as glucose, amino acids, and various inorganic ions (e.g., Na^+, $C1^-$, K^+) are transported across plasma membranes by carrier molecules. Some of these transport systems are active and others are passive. In general, carrier-mediated transport systems often display one or more of the following characteristics:

1. *Specificity*. Carrier systems are generally specific for a particular solute. For example, the system that transports glucose will not transport other organic solutes such as amino acids.

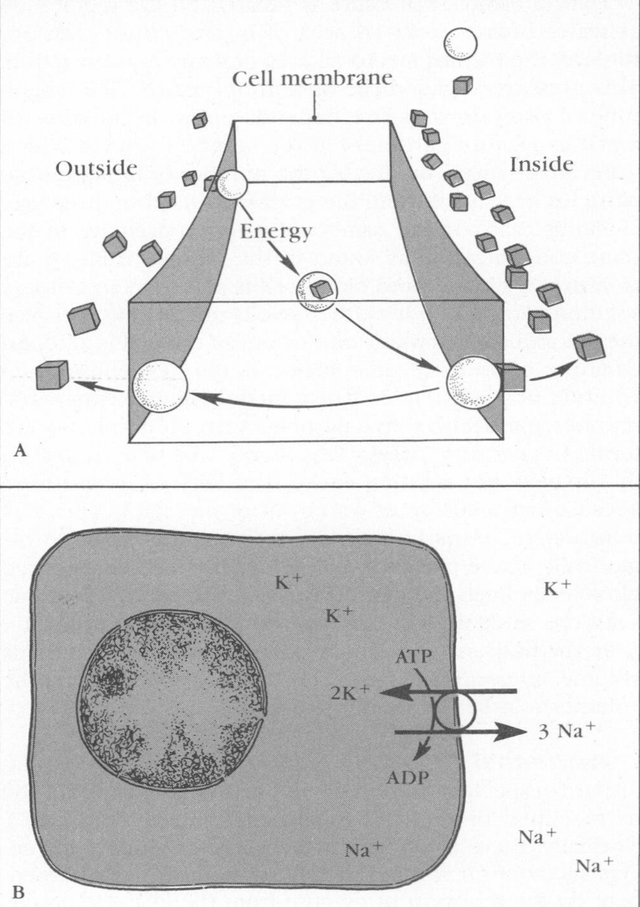

FIGURE 1-21 A. Postulated carrier system for moving substances across the cell membrane; like facilitated diffusion, except movement is against a concentration gradient and requires energy. B. Postulated mechanism for moving sodium out of the cell and potassium to the interior of the cell.

2. *Saturation*. Many systems have a maximum rate (called *transport maximum*, or *Tm*) at which a solute can be transported. If more solute is present than the system can handle, the system is said to be saturated and transporting solute at maximum rate. Below saturation level, the rate of transport varies directly with solute concentration (i.e., the higher the solute concentration, the faster the rate of transport).
3. *Competition*. If the same carrier system transports two different solutes in the same direction, the rate of transport of each will be diminished by the presence of the other. In other words, the solutes compete for transport by the carrier, and some of each solute is transported, but neither is transported at maximum rate.
4. *Energy dependency*. Many carrier systems require energy to function. Substances (metabolic inhibitors) that interfere with energy-producing reactions of the cell often stop transport processes.

Endocytosis and Exocytosis. Endocytosis and exocytosis are methods for bringing particles into the cell and releasing secretions to the exterior of the cell. These processes are schematically illustrated in Figure 1-8. Both are essential in carrying out the functional capabilities of specific cells.

Endocytosis refers to the bringing in of protein and other substances through invagination of the outer cell membrane. This process occurs in the following two ways:

1. *Pinocytosis* involves movement of complex proteins and some strong electrolyte solutions into the cell. The protein is seen to adhere to the outer cell membrane, which stimulates invagination of the membrane. The material is encased or enclosed in a vesicle and floats into the cytoplasm. Lysosomes attach to the vesicle surface, release hydrolytic enzymes into the vesicle, and the enzymes break down the complex material for use within the cells. A residual body may be left within the vesicle or excreted through the cell membrane to the ECF.
2. *Phagocytosis* involves essentially the same process, but the material brought into the cell is frequently a microorganism, especially a bacterium.

Exocytosis has been called *reverse pinocytosis* and is an active release of soluble products to the ECF. Secretion granules are formed, as described earlier, by the Golgi complex. To be secreted, the granules adhere to the inner cell membrane. This causes outpouching of the membrane and release of contents into the ECF. The secretory products are vital to maintenance of the steady state of the host and include secretions necessary for digestion, glandular secretion, neural transmission, and so on.

Both endocytosis and exocytosis require energy and are affected by cellular ability to synthesize ATP. Both processes require enzymatic activity to enhance the rate of the reactions.

Cell Movement

Many cells exhibit the ability to move. Movement may involve locomotion from one place to another or it may involve movement of microtubules and microfilaments within the cell. Ciliary and flagellar movement are examples of microtubular and microfilament movement (see p. 13). Two additional forms of cell movement are ameboid locomotion and muscular contraction.

Ameboid Locomotion

Ameboid locomotion refers to the ability of a cell to move from one location to another in a manner similar to the way a unicellar animal, called an amoeba, moves in its fluid environment. In the embryo, most of the cells exhibit ameboid motion by which they migrate to their appropriate location. This property of ameboid movement is retained by certain defensive cells of the body, especially the leukocytes, and allows them to move from the bloodstream to the tissue spaces to contact and destroy a foreign protein (see Chap. 9).

Using energy (ATP) and calcium ions, the process is accomplished by the forward projection of a portion of the cell, called the *pseudopodium* (Fig. 1-22). It probably depends on contraction of microfilaments in the outer portion of the cytoplasm to push out or project the pseudopodium. The remainder of the cell follows the projected area with a streaming motion. This process allows for the rapid movement of cells into an area.

Muscular Contraction

Approximately 50 percent of the body mass is skeletal, smooth, and cardiac muscle. Contraction of these muscles make possible both involuntary and voluntary movements. The details of muscular contraction are further described in Chapters 18, 36, and 40.

Both electrical and mechanical processes exist in muscle, with the initiation of most contractions through electrical stimulation from the nerve terminals. The electrical events are followed immediately by the mechanical events in a sequential way. Electrical activation causes depolarization, which initiates the mechanical movement of contractile proteins between each other and causes a shortening of the muscle fiber. The muscle fiber is illustrated in Figure 1-23, which shows the subunits of the fiber and the form of two contractile proteins called *actin* and *myosin*.

Skeletal muscle has a striated appearance because of its regularly ordered proteins. These proteins make up the contractile portions of the muscle fiber. The process of skeletal muscle contraction basically follows this course: A nerve stimulation causes the release of acetylcholine at the neuromuscular junction. Acetylcholine, a chemical neurotransmitter, causes a change in muscle cell ion permeability, generating an action potential that is spread throughout the muscle cell membrane and to the T tubules that carry the stimulus to the interior of the cell (Fig. 1-24). The transfer of stimulus by T tubules to the sarcoplasmic reticulum (SR) causes release of calcium

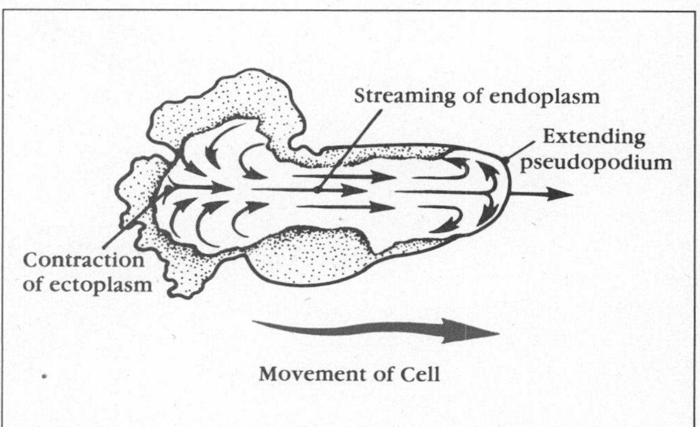

FIGURE 1-22 Method of ameboid motion of a cell, showing contraction of ectoplasm, extended pseudopodium, and streaming of endoplasm toward the projected pseudopodium.

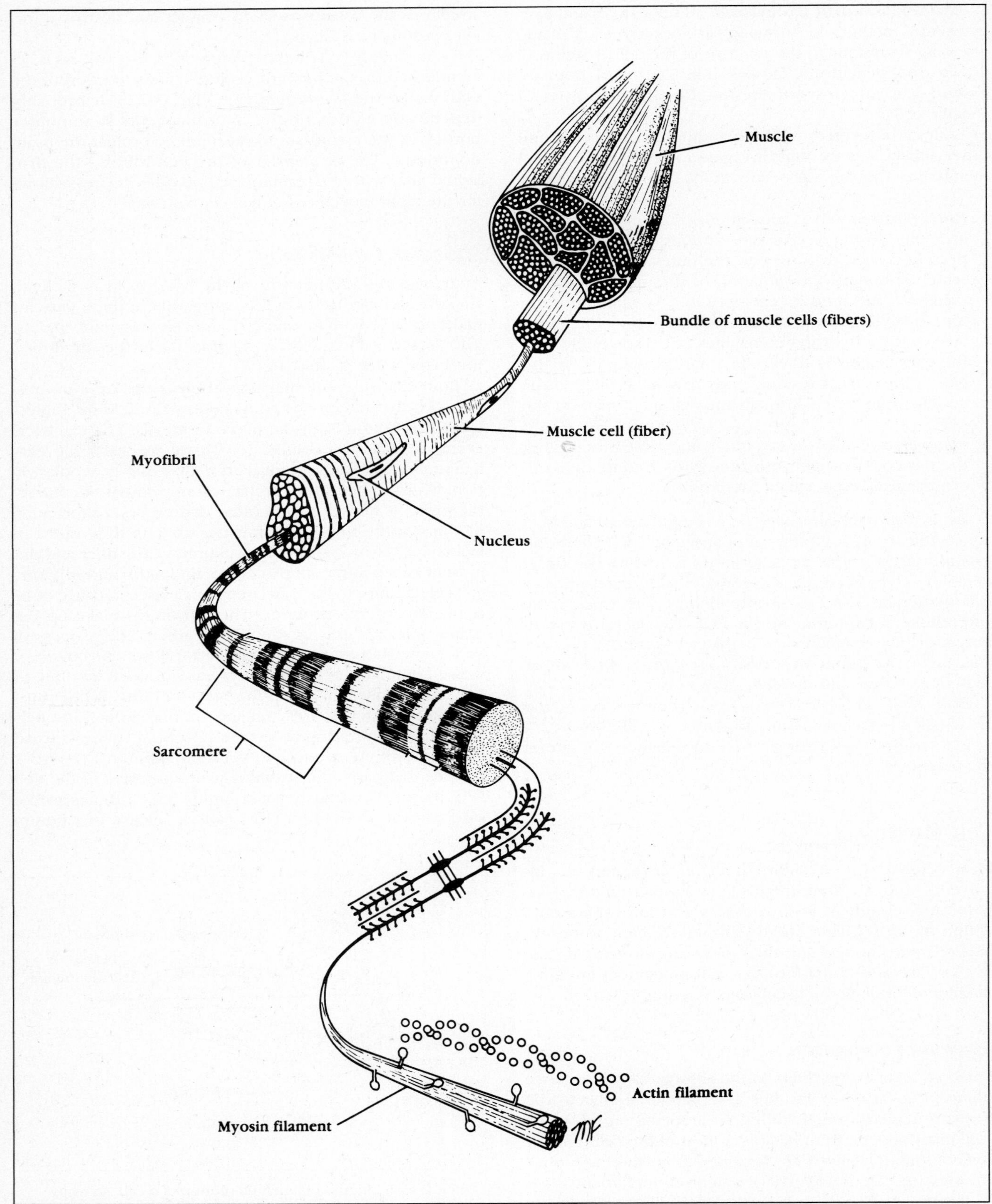

FIGURE 1-23 Gross to microscopic components of a skeletal muscle fiber. (From R.S. Snell, *Clinical Histology for Medical Students*. Boston: Little, Brown, 1984.)

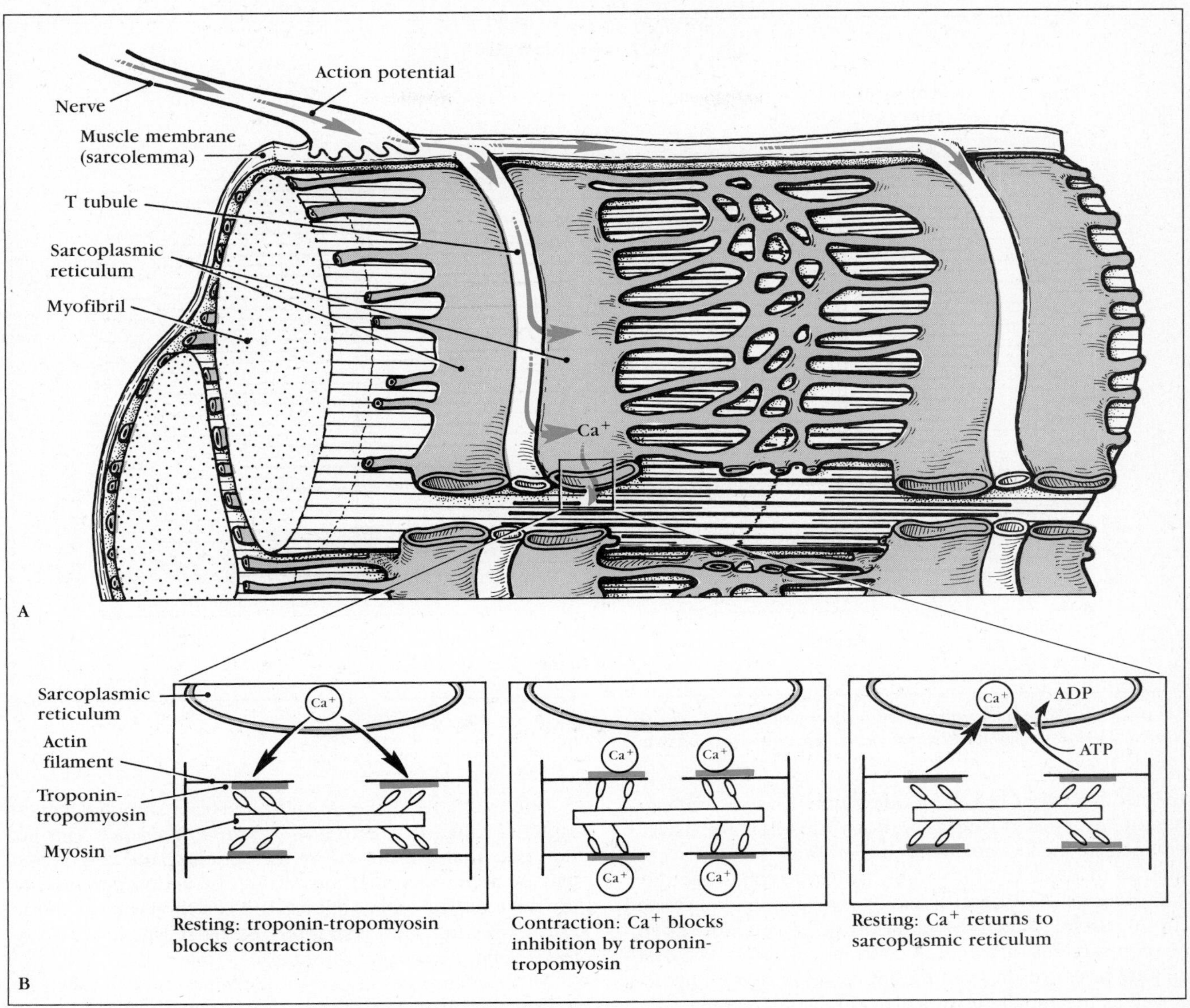

FIGURE 1-24 A. Schematic representation of depolarizing stimulus through a T tubule. B. Actin and myosin filament in the relaxed and contracted state.

from the SR. Calcium binds with the inhibitory protein *troponin*, causing troponin to interact with another protein, *tropomyosin*, resulting in the uncovering of the active sites on actin, which allows for free interaction with myosin. The actin filament is then pulled along the myosin filament, causing shortening of the entire sarcomere unit (see Fig. 1-24). Calcium is immediately taken back up into the SR, and troponin and tropomyosin regain their normal inhibitory function. Large quantities of ATP are necessary to provide energy to pump the calcium back into the sarcoplasmic reticulum. During this process sodium also leaks into the cell, and the sodium pump must be activated to prevent accumulation of water in the muscle cell.

Cardiac muscle is also striated and follows the same general pattern for contraction, but exhibits basic differences. Cardiac muscle is rapidly depolarized and contracts immediately after stimulation, but repolarizes much more slowly than skeletal muscle. This slow repolarization apparently prevents cardiac muscle from tetany, a phenomenon that may occur in skeletal muscle. Also, impulses depolarize the entire muscle mass, either atrial or ventricular, rather than individual fibers, as seen with skeletal muscle. This characteristic occurs because the individual cells within cardiac muscle are connected to one another by low-resistance electrical bridges (intercalated disks) that allow the electrical impulse to spread from cell to cell (Fig. 1-25).

Smooth muscle cells are smaller than skeletal muscle cells. They form two major types of muscle units, *multiunit* and *visceral smooth muscle*. Multiunit smooth muscle is independently innervated by nerve signals and includes the piloerector muscles of hairs ("gooseflesh"),

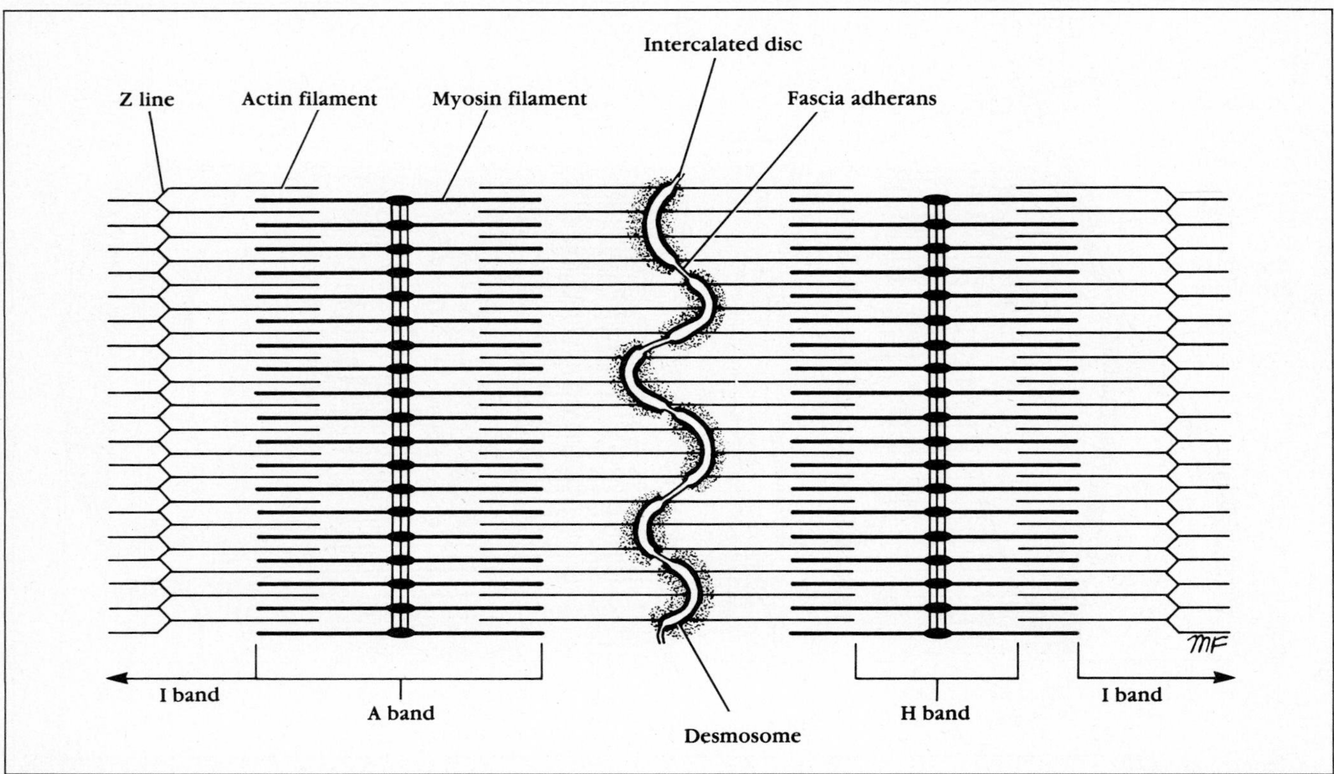

FIGURE 1-25 Schematic microscopic representation of myocardial muscle cell. (From R.S. Snell, *Clinical Histology for Medical Students*. Boston: Little, Brown, 1984.)

smooth muscle of larger blood vessels, and several muscles of the eyes. Visceral smooth muscles are usually arranged in sheets, and the cell membranes contact each other so that ions can flow freely from one cell to the next. Contractions of visceral muscles are relatively slow and can be sustained for periods of up to 30 seconds. Rhythmic contractions or waves of contractions (such as intestinal peristalsis) result from the influence of nerve impulses as well as from many chemical agents.

Electrical Properties of Cells

Differences in electrical potential across the plasma membrane are characteristic of all living cells. The membrane potential exists because of unequal distribution of ions between the inner and outer surfaces of the membrane, the membrane's different permeability to various ions, and active transport systems that maintain ionic imbalance across the membrane.

Some cells have the ability to respond to various types of stimuli, especially electrochemical stimuli. This response is called the cell's *excitability* and refers to the changing or altering of the electrical potential across the cell membrane. Two major types of cells, nerve and muscle, are considered to be excitable cells because they can change membrane potential, effect an action or response, and return to the resting state.

The excitable tissue or cell receives a stimulus, which rapidly changes its *resting membrane potential*. This action potential is followed by the action of the cell, which may be a contraction, transmitting the action potential to the next cell, or other actions. The cell then returns to the normal resting state characterized by reestablishment of the resting membrane potential.

Many changes occur in the cell membranes when an *action potential* is elicited. The following discussion of the action potential is with reference to a neuron, but applies with minor variation to other excitable cells such as skeletal muscle.

When an adequate positive stimulus is applied to the neuron, a rapid and marked change occurs in the *membrane potential* at the point on the membrane of stimulus application. The positive stimulus increases the sodium permeability of the membrane, allowing sodium to begin entering the cell at a faster rate than it can be pumped out. As more sodium passes through the membrane, the membrane potential becomes less negative (Fig. 1-26). When the membrane potential has been reduced to a critical value called the *threshold*, additional sodium channels open, increasing the membrane's sodium permeability even more, resulting in a rapid influx of sodium. The membrane potential approaches zero and then actually becomes reversed, so that the inside of the membrane is positive with respect to the outside. These changes characterize *depolarization* of the membrane.

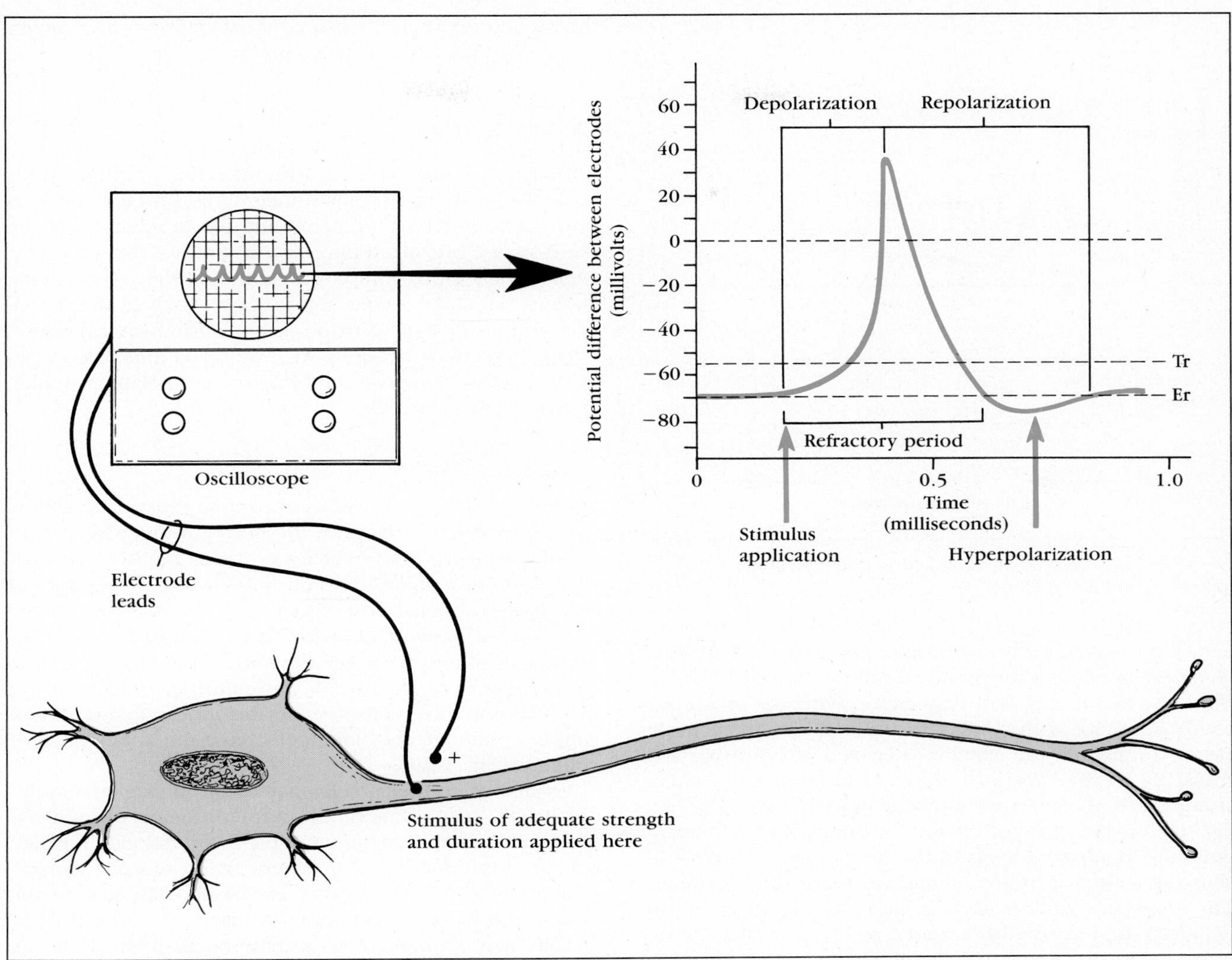

FIGURE 1-26 Recording of an action potential. (See text for explanation.)

Almost immediately after sodium influx begins to depolarize the membrane, an increase in potassium diffusion out of the cell begins and accelerates as the movement of sodium causes the inside of the membrane to become positive. Potassium leaves the cell for the same reasons that sodium entered—favorable electrical and chemical gradients coupled with an increase in membrane permeability. As potassium efflux accelerates, further diffusion of sodium into the cell is inhibited by a decrease in sodium permeability, and the net loss of positive charges (K^+) from the inside causes the membrane potential to return to zero and then become negative once again, reestablishing the resting potential. More potassium leaves the cell than is actually required to restore the resting potential, and for a short time the inside of the membrane is more negative than it normally is at rest. This increased internal negativity is termed ***hyperpolarization***. The return of the membrane potential to resting level is completed by the Na^+-K^+ pump, which exchanges internal sodium for external potassium, thereby restoring the normal internal:external ratios of these ions. The preceding activities that restore the resting membrane potential after depolarization of the membrane collectively characterize the phenomenon of ***repolarization***.

The graphic representation (voltage versus time) of membrane depolarization and repolarization is called the action potential (see Fig. 1-26). The duration of the action potential for a neuron is less than 0.5 msec. It must be remembered that the action potential represents the change in membrane potential only in the region of the membrane where an adequate positive stimulus has been applied. The entire plasma membrane does not simultaneously depolarize and then repolarize in response to an adequate stimulus. Once an action potential is generated, however, it spreads from one area of the membrane to another, resulting in the propagation of a nerve impulse.

A nerve impulse is a wave of depolarization followed by a wave of repolarization that travels along a nerve fiber away from the point of stimulation (Fig. 1-27). When an adequate positive stimulus, one of sufficient strength or

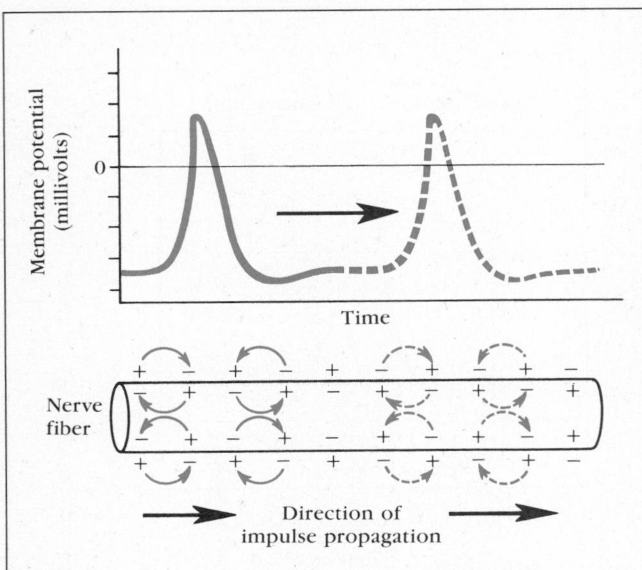

FIGURE 1-27 Propagation of an action potential along nonmyelinated nerve fiber.

duration to reduce the membrane potential to *threshold* (sometimes called a threshold stimulus), is applied to the fiber, the membrane will depolarize, with the inside becoming positive with respect to the outside. Adjacent areas of the membrane remain polarized, inside negative, resulting in the flow of electrical current as positive charges are attracted to adjacent negative charges (see Fig. 1-27). The flow of current reduces the membrane potential in adjacent areas of the membrane to threshold, allowing sodium to move in and depolarization to occur. The sequence of one area of depolarization inducing depolarization in an adjacent area results in a wave of depolarization that is propagated along the nerve fiber in a manner similar to the burning of a gunpowder fuse. As soon as the wave of depolarization passes a segment of the fiber, that segment is repolarized and its ability to respond to another stimulus is soon restored.

If an adequate (threshold) stimulus is applied to a nerve fiber, an action potential is generated at the site of stimulus and propagated away from the site. Once generated, each impulse is conducted in an identical manner without change in magnitude or velocity. Stimuli that fail individually or collectively to reduce the membrane potential to threshold fail to generate an action potential and therefore a nerve impulse. The response of a nerve fiber to a stimulus is either maximal or zero. This property is the *all-or-none law*. In other words, weak stimuli do not generate weak impulses and strong stimuli strong impulses.

After an action potential has been generated, a minimum amount of time is required before that area of the membrane becomes capable of responding in an identical manner to a second stimulus. This minimum period of time is called the *refractory period*. The length of the refractory period determines the maximum number of impulses that the fiber can conduct each second. Fibers with short refractory periods can conduct impulses at a higher frequency than fibers with long refractory periods.

Cell Organization

Although cells are the basic structural and functional units of the body, those that share a common function, such as lining a body cavity or providing for movement of the skeleton, are organized into *tissues*. In turn, tissues are organized into more complex structures known as *organs*. Organs that share a common purpose, such as the formation and excretion of urine, are grouped into *systems*, which collectively make up the body. The four basic types of tissues that compose the body are epithelial, muscular, nervous, and connective.

Epithelial Tissue

Epithelial tissue occurs as a covering of most of the internal and external surfaces of the body. In this way, it may function as a protective barrier or it may be involved with absorption of materials, excretion of waste products, and secretion of specialized products into the cavities.

Epithelial tissue is classified according to its thickness in number of layers. Simple squamous epithelium exists as single layers of flattened, pancakelike cells. Simple cuboidal epithelial cells assume the appearance of cubes. Simple columnar epithelial cells have the appearance of columns (Fig. 1-28).

Squamous epithelial cells may occur in single or multiple layers. Single layers allow for diffusion of material across the cell wall, while multiple layers provide for continuous replenishment or regeneration of cells. Simple squamous cells line the heart and blood vessels, form the alveoli, and exist in many other areas.

Cuboidal epithelial cells usually occur in single layers and frequently function in forming secretions. These cells line the ducts and are the parenchymal cells of many glands.

Columnar epithelial cells, in various forms, line the walls of the gastrointestinal and respiratory systems and are involved with the secretion of mucus. They may exist as goblet cells or have projections, called microvilli or cilia, present on their surfaces (Fig. 1-29).

Stratified squamous epithelium exists in multiple layers that replenish superficial layers as they are sloughed off. The skin is an excellent example of stratified squamous epithelium, but this tissue also lines the mouth, esophagus, vagina, and pharynx.

Transitional epithelial cells are usually considered to be cuboidal, except that their appearance varies depending on the stretch of the organ. Thus at different times they appear to be flattened or spheric. They are best exemplified by the epithelial cells in the bladder.

Muscular Tissue

The microstructure and functions of the muscle cells that make up muscle tissues are discussed in depth in Chapter

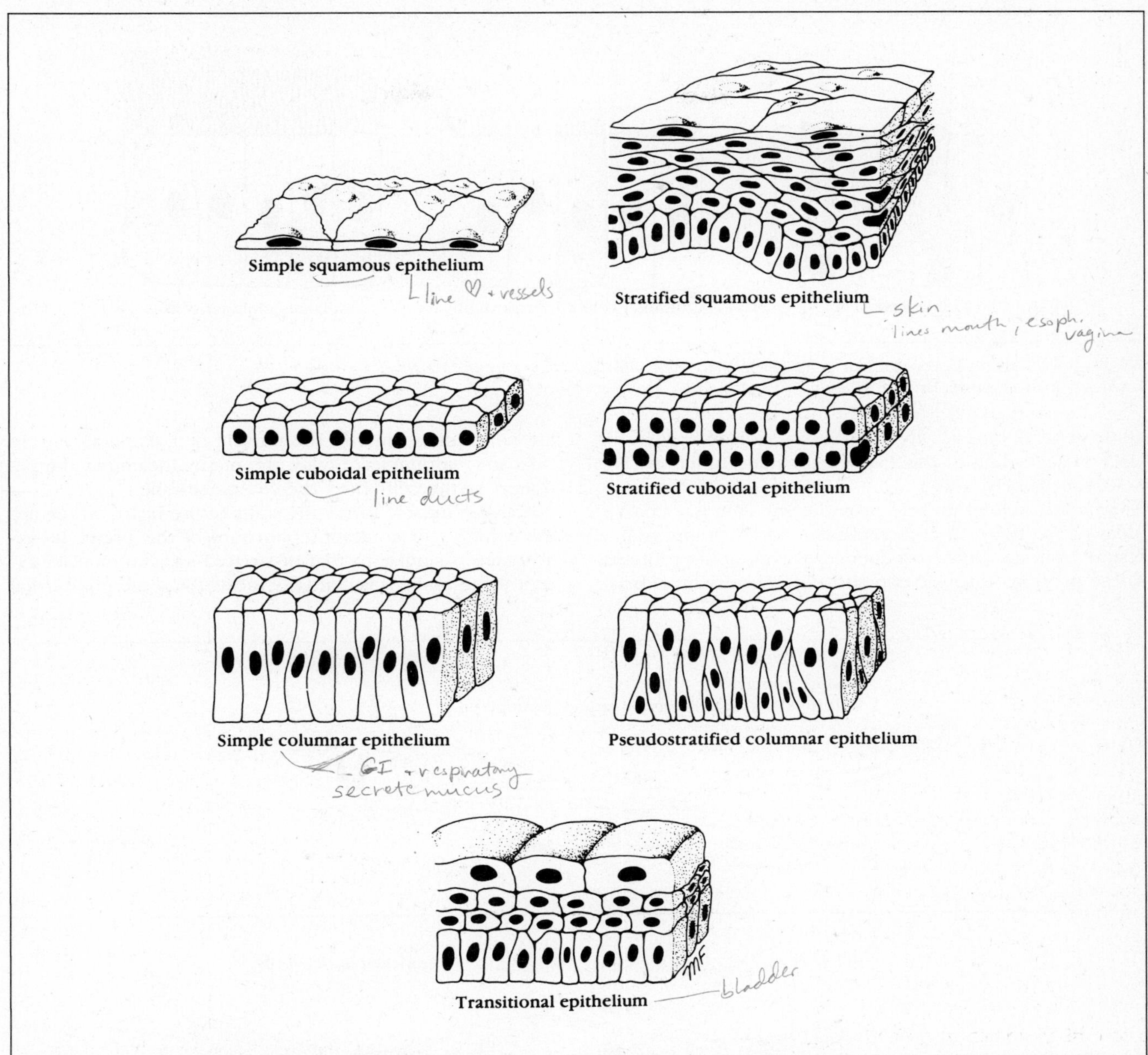

FIGURE 1-28 Different types of epithelium. (From R.S. Snell, *Clinical Histology for Medical Students*. Boston: Little, Brown, 1984.)

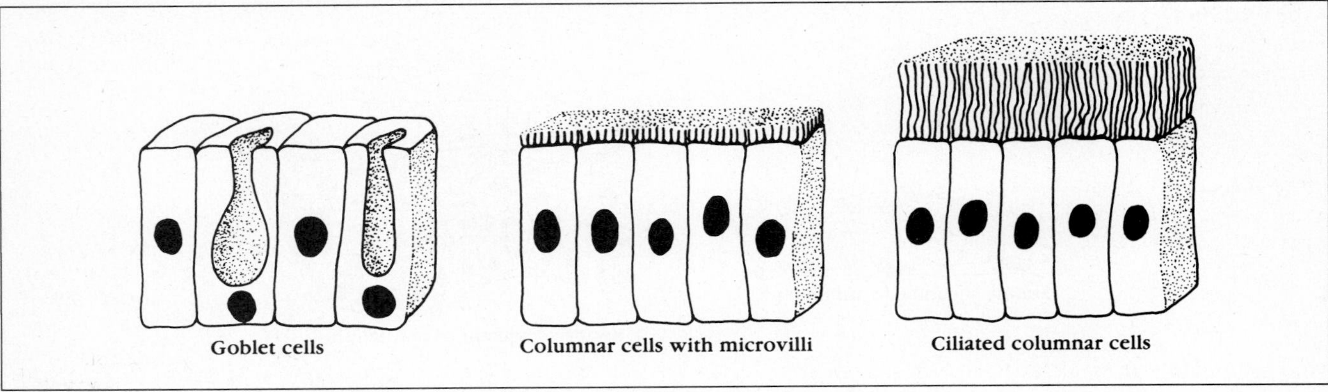

FIGURE 1-29 Specialized columnar cells. (From R.S. Snell, *Clinical Histology for Medical Students*. Boston: Little, Brown, 1984.)

40. In general, muscles are classified as skeletal, cardiac, or visceral according to their appearance and function (Fig. 1-30; see also Fig. 1-23).

Striated skeletal muscle provides for voluntary movement of the body. The characteristic striated appearance results from an ordered sequence of contractile proteins. These proteins form or constitute numerous myofibrils, the contractile units of the muscle cell. Skeletal muscle cells are multinucleate, with the nuclei located at the periphery of the cell under the cell membrane.

Cardiac muscle forms the walls of the heart, which are the working, or contractile, portions of this organ. Its appearance is similar to that of striated skeletal muscle, except that a nucleus is centrally located and the myocardial

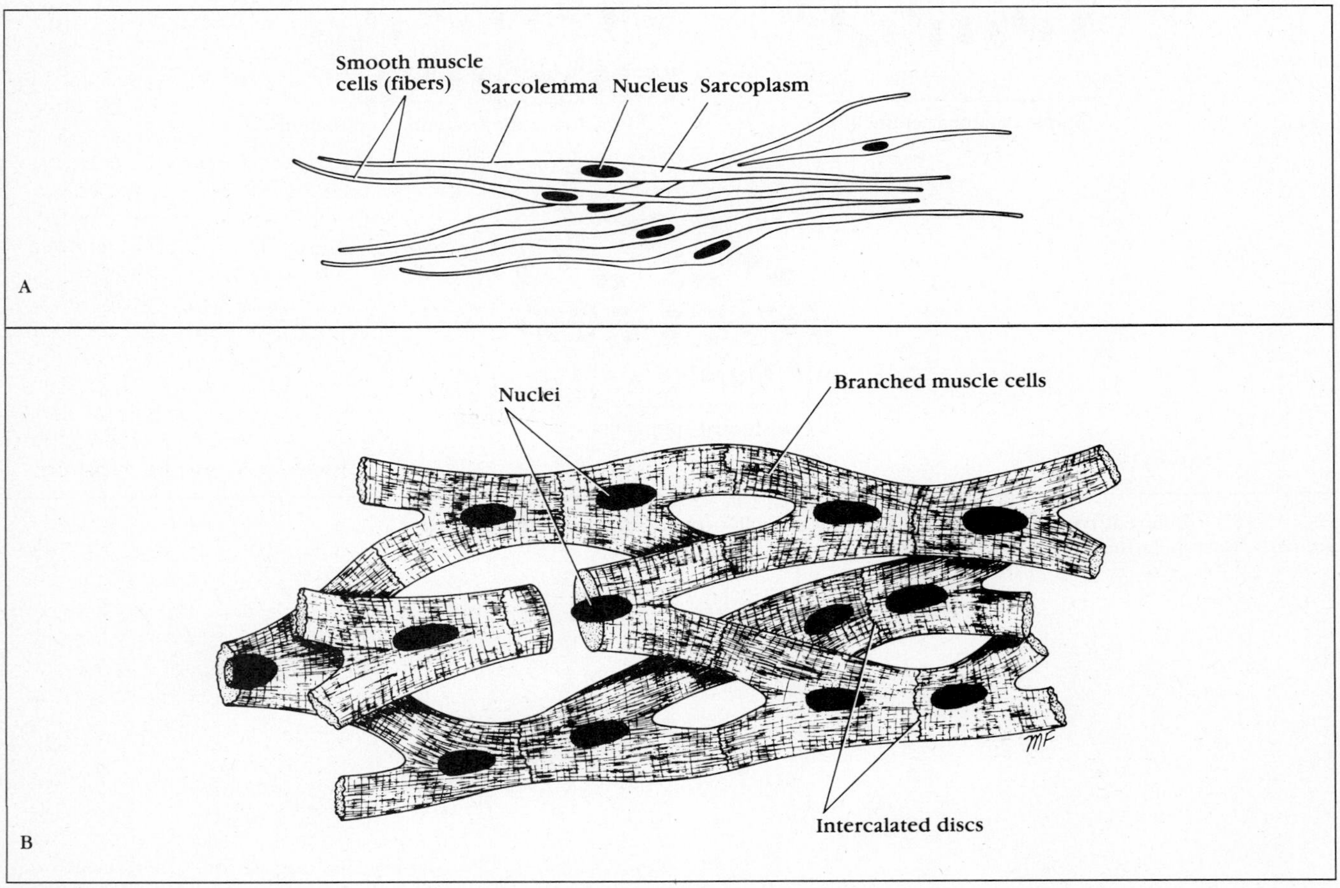

FIGURE 1-30 A. Group of smooth muscle cells (fibers) B. Group of branched cardiac muscle cells (fibers). (From R.S. Snell, *Clinical Histology for Medical Students*. Boston: Little, Brown, 1984.)

cells lie very closely approximated one to another. The importance of myocardial construction in relation to cardiac contraction is detailed in Unit 8.

Visceral, or smooth, muscle does not exhibit the characteristic striations of skeletal or cardiac muscle, but smooth muscle cells have many fibrils that extend the length of the cell. A single nucleus lies near the center of each cell. Smooth muscle cells are located in the viscera, blood vessels, uterus, and many other areas.

Nervous Tissue

Nervous tissue is made up of neurons (Fig. 1-31), the cells that conduct nerve impulses, and glial cells that provide structural and functional support for the neurons. The typical nerve cell has a large central nucleus, multiple dendrites, and a single axon. Detailed function of the neuron is described in Chapter 44.

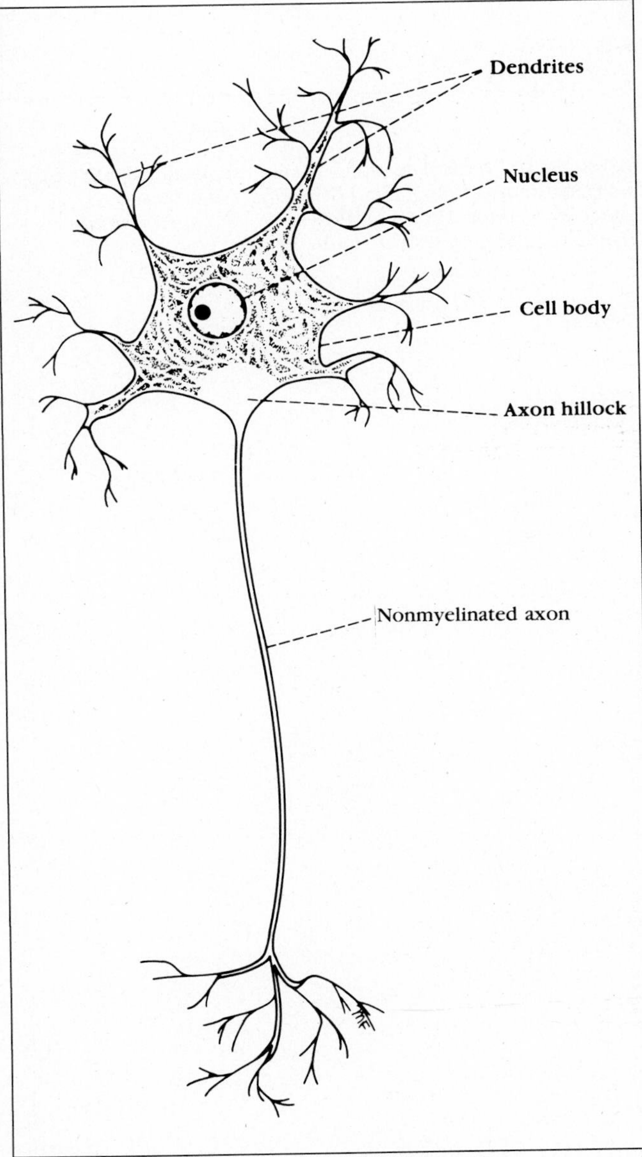

FIGURE 1-31 A neuron. (From R.S. Snell, *Clinical Neuroanatomy for Medical Students*. Boston: Little, Brown, 1984.)

Connective Tissue

Connective tissue generally forms the framework for other cells and helps to bind together various tissues and organs. Many types of cells are included in the classification of tissue (Fig. 1-32). Blood cells, described in detail in Unit 7, are specialized connective tissue cells.

Loose connective tissue (areolar tissue) contains numerous cells, especially fibroblasts and macrophages. It also attaches the skin to the body and helps to hold the organs and blood vessels in place. Spaces between cells allow for fluid storage and discharge of cellular products that are then returned to the bloodstream.

Dense irregular connective tissue is compact and forms the reticular layer of the dermis of the skin. Sheets of this tissue form sheaths of many types and can withstand stretching in the direction in which their fibers run. The layers of the dermis are composed of cells that constantly undergo synthesis and degradation. Collagen fibers interlace with each other to provide strength to the dermis. Elastic fibers lie randomly dispersed throughout this layer, which allows for flexibility.

Dense regular connective tissue is composed of white, fibrous material. The cells are mainly fibrocytes, located in a regular or ordered plane. Rows of fibrocytes with large amounts of intracellular substance, especially collagen, form the tendons that attach muscle to bone. Ligaments that attach bone to bone and fascia that provide the coverings for muscles are included in this category of connective tissue. The aponeuroses, which are similar to tendons with a wider base, attach muscles to other structures.

Adipose tissue cells are those in which the cytoplasm is filled with lipid or fatty material. This storage area for lipids serves as a protective and insulating layer in the body. Layers of adipose tissue are normally present around the kidneys and intestine. In many areas of the body, substances not metabolized within the cell are converted to fat. This process is greatly influenced by insulin, a pancreatic hormone (see Chap. 35).

Elastic connective tissue allows for the properties of elasticity and extensibility, especially in the arteries and vocal cords. This is further discussed in Units 8 and 9.

Types of cartilage, a connective tissue that is made up of cells called chondrocytes, differ depending on the number of associated collagenous fibers. It provides structural strength with some degree of flexibility. It is present in the costal cartilage, trachea, intervertebral disks, external ear, and other areas. In children, the long bones have two ends, a diaphysis and an epiphysis, separated by epiphyseal cartilage, which allows bone length to increase. Growth in length occurs as cartilage cells grow away from the shaft and are replaced by bone, resulting in increased length of the shaft. When maturity is reached, this cartilage is entirely replaced by bone, a process called closure of the epiphysis.

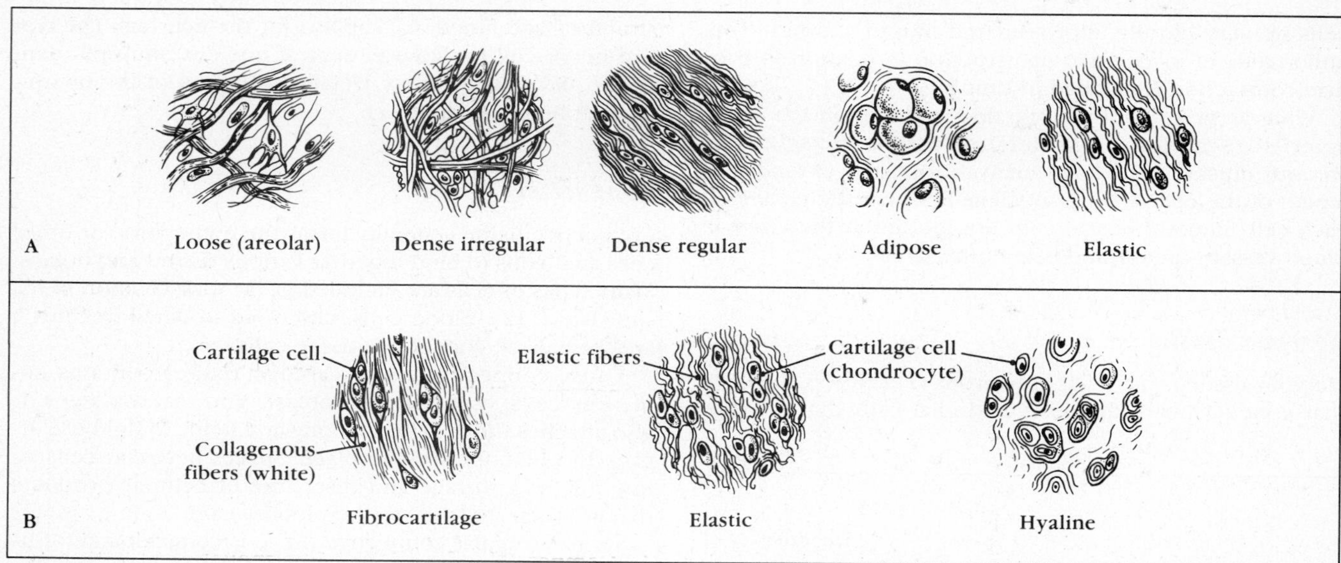

FIGURE 1-32 A. Types of connective tissues. B. Types of cartilage.

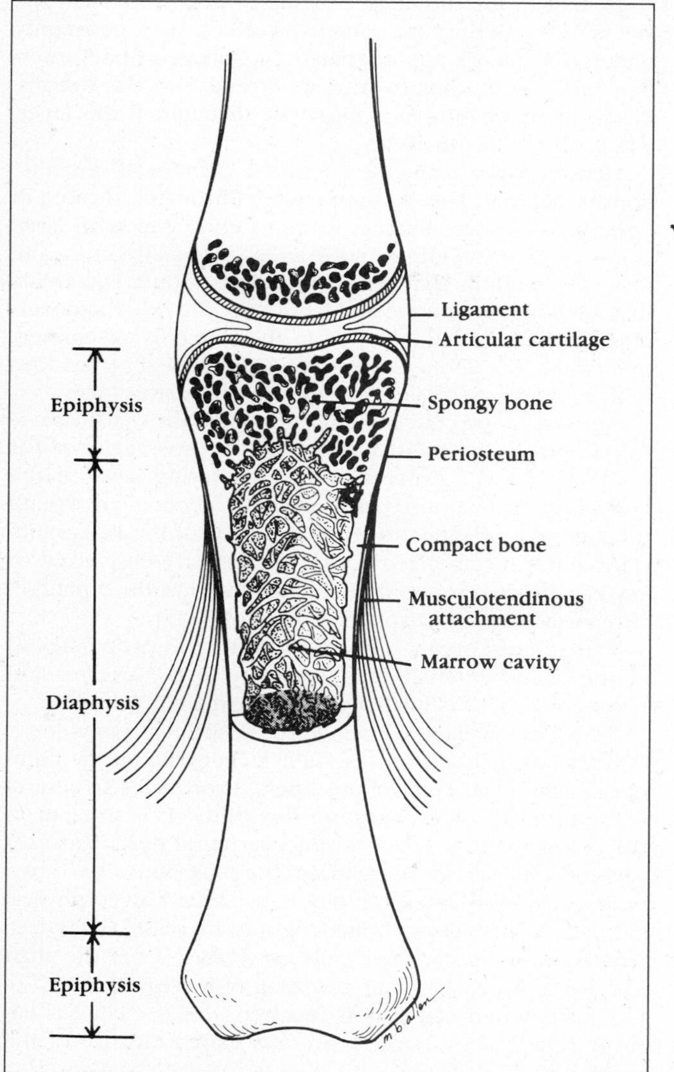

FIGURE 1-33 Vertical section through the proximal part of the femur shows the arrangement of compact and spongy (cancellous) bone. (From M. Borysenko, et al., *Functional Histology* [2nd ed.]. Boston: Little, Brown, 1984.)

Bone, the hardest of the connective tissues, provides the structural framework of the body as well as a plentiful reservoir for the minerals calcium and phosphorus. It is composed of cells, fibers, and extracellular components, which are calcified and hard. This material encloses the hematopoietic marrow, which supplies most of the blood cells of the body. Periosteum covers most bones and is lacking only in special areas. Bone tissue is organized in two ways, as compact or as cancellous (spongy) (Fig. 1-33). *Compact bone* forms a solid mass and has few spaces in its continuity. *Cancellous bone* forms a network of intercommunicating projections called trabeculae. Compact bone generally is located on the outer shell, while spongy bone is usually in the internal framework. The principal cells of adult bone are osteocytes, which with the other bone cells—osteoblasts, osteoclasts, and osteoprogenitor cells—form and repair bone tissue.

All of these distinct cells may be different functional states of the same cell type. Bone cells adjust their number in proportion to the amount of physical stress placed on them. For example, increased deposition of collagen fibers and inorganic salts occurs in response to prolonged increase in workload. Conversely, salts are pulled from bone when stress or weight bearing is decreased (see Chap. 41).

Study Questions

1. Describe the mechanism by which the cell maintains its electrolyte composition.
2. How do the individual organelles work together to achieve cellular function?
3. Differentiate between active and passive mechanisms used by the cell.
4. How does the body control cellular reproduction?
5. How do the phases of electrical potential differ between neurons and muscle cells?
6. Compare the functions of epithelial, connective and muscle cells.

CHAPTER 2

Genetic Disorders

CHAPTER OUTLINE

Principles of Inheritance
Classification of Genetic Disorders
Single-Gene Disorders

- Terminology
- Principles of Transmission
- Autosomal Dominant Inheritance
- Autosomal Recessive Inheritance
- X-Linked Inheritance
  - *X-Linked Dominant Inheritance*
  - *X-Linked Recessive Inheritance*
- Pathophysiology of Single-Gene Disorders
  - *Altered Activity of an Enzyme in a Metabolic Pathway*
  - *Loss or Alteration of Circulating Proteins*
  - *Altered Cell Membrane Components*
  - *Collagen Disorders*
  - *Single-Gene Disorders in Which the Basic Defect Is Unknown*

Chromosome Disorders

- Numeric Aberrations
- Structural Aberrations
- Mosaics
- Sex Chromosome Aberrations

Multifactorial Disorders
Environmental Alterations in Fetal Development

LEARNING OBJECTIVES

1. List the three broad types of genetic disorders.
2. Discuss briefly the chromosome set (karyotype) of human species.
3. Differentiate between the terms *homozygous* and *heterozygous*.
4. Define *allele*, *genotype*, and *phenotype*.
5. Draw a Punnett square to compute the progeny of specific genotypes.
6. Describe briefly autosomal dominant inheritance patterns.
7. Describe briefly autosomal recessive inheritance patterns.
8. Describe briefly X-linked dominant inheritance patterns.
9. Describe briefly X-linked recessive inheritance patterns.
10. Explain the three types of chromosomal aberrations.
11. Compare the inheritance pattern of multifactorial disorders with the inheritance pattern of single-gene disorders and chromosomal disorders.
12. Identify at least one disease or disorder that is determined by each type of inheritance pattern.
13. Identify the biochemical defect or structural alteration associated with phenylketonuria, albinism, sickle cell disease, and Marfan syndrome.
14. Differentiate between hemoglobinopathies and thalassemias.
15. Define teratogen and give examples of physical and chemical teratogenic agents.

Genes control the functions of a cell by determining what proteins are synthesized within the cell. Genes are also responsible for the transmission of characteristics from one generation to the next. This chapter describes the principles of inheritance, the classification of genetic disorders, and the mechanisms by which alterations in genetic material can produce structural or functional defects. Table 2-1 defines some essential terminology in the study of genetics. A large and diverse assortment of conditions has now been recognized as genetic diseases, and it is likely that the expression of any disease is influenced by the genotype of the affected person [17].

Principles of Inheritance

Gregor Mendel, an Austrian monk, is credited with discovering the basic principles of heredity. In 1865 Mendel presented the results of his experiments with garden peas, in which he crossed varieties with distinct characteristics and followed the *progeny* (offspring) of the crosses for at least two generations. Mendel proposed the idea of hereditary factors that are passed from one generation to the next, but his ideas were not accepted because the existence of chromosomes had not yet been recognized. In 1900, when chromosomes had been observed and their movements during cell division had been noted, Mendel's findings were rediscovered and accepted.

Mendel proposed two principles to describe the inheritance of characteristics in his garden peas. He concluded that the pea plant contains two inherited factors (now called *alleles*) for the determination of each characteristic. The *principle of segregation* describes the separation of these two factors during *gametogenesis*, such that one half of the gametes receive one factor and the other half the other. The *principle of independent assortment* deals with the relationship between the alleles that determine different inherited characteristics. It states that pairs of alleles segregate independently of each other. Therefore, a gamete may contain either member of one allelic pair and either member of another pair. It is known that this principle is true, provided that the alleles are located on different chromosomes. Mendel also recognized that some alleles are *dominant* and are expressed whenever one copy is present, whereas other alleles are *recessive* and require two copies for expression.

The Mendelian principles are explained by the process of *meiosis*. Chapter 1 includes a description of cell division and mitosis, in which the hereditary material of a cell is duplicated and evenly distributed between two daughter cells. During gametogenesis, however, the hereditary material is duplicated once, but the nucleus divides twice, allowing the separation of each chromosome in a pair, with distribution of each to a different gamete. This process, meiosis, is outlined for one chromosome pair (the XY pair in a male) in Figure 2-1.

Studies in biochemical genetics revealed that the unit of heredity is the *gene*, which consists of a particular sequence of nucleotides in the deoxyribonucleic acid (DNA) of the chromosome. The sequence of nucleotides in a gene either determines the structure of a polypeptide chain or has a regulatory function in protein synthesis. Thus the genes dictate which proteins are found in a cell, and these proteins determine the form and function of the cell. Each chromosome is composed of thousands of genes arranged in linear order.

The *karyotype* (characteristic chromosome makeup) of each species defines the species chromosome number and morphology. In humans, the cell most commonly used for the study of chromosomes is the lymphocyte. To study the karyotype of an individual, cytogeneticists obtain lymphocytes from a blood sample and grow them in a nutrient medium. Colchicine is added to stop cell division in metaphase, allowing a large number of cells in the same stage of cell division to accumulate. Application of a hypotonic solution causes the cells to swell, separating the chromosomes from each other. They are then placed on a glass slide, stained, and photographed. The photographs are cut out, arranged into groups, and identified by number according to the length of the chromosome and position of its centromere (the constricted portion). A normal male karyotype is shown in Figure 2-2. Normal human somatic cells contain 23 pairs of chromosomes for a total of 46. Gametes contain only one member of each chromosome pair for a total of 23.

TABLE 2-1 Genetic Terminology

Term	Definition
Progeny	Offspring
Chromosomes	Structures in the nucleus that contain DNA, which transmit genetic information
Gene	DNA, the basic unit of heredity, which is located in a particular place on the chromosome
Gamete	A mature male or female reproductive cell
Gametogenesis	Development of gametes
Alleles	One of two or more different genes that contain specific inheritable characteristics that occupy corresponding positions or loci on paired chromosomes
Homozygous	A trait of an organism produced by identical or nearly identical alleles
Heterozygous	Possessing different alleles at a given locus
Homologous	Referring to chromosomes with matching genes
Karyotype	A display of human chromosomes based on their length and the location of the centromere
Genotype	The basic combination of genes of an organism
Phenotype	The expression of the gene in an individual; e.g., physical appearance, blood type.
Pedigree chart	A schematic method for classifying genetic data
Dominant trait	Traits for which one of a pair of alleles is necessary for expression; e.g., brown hair
Recessive traits	Traits for which two alleles of a pair are necessary for expression; e.g., blue eyes

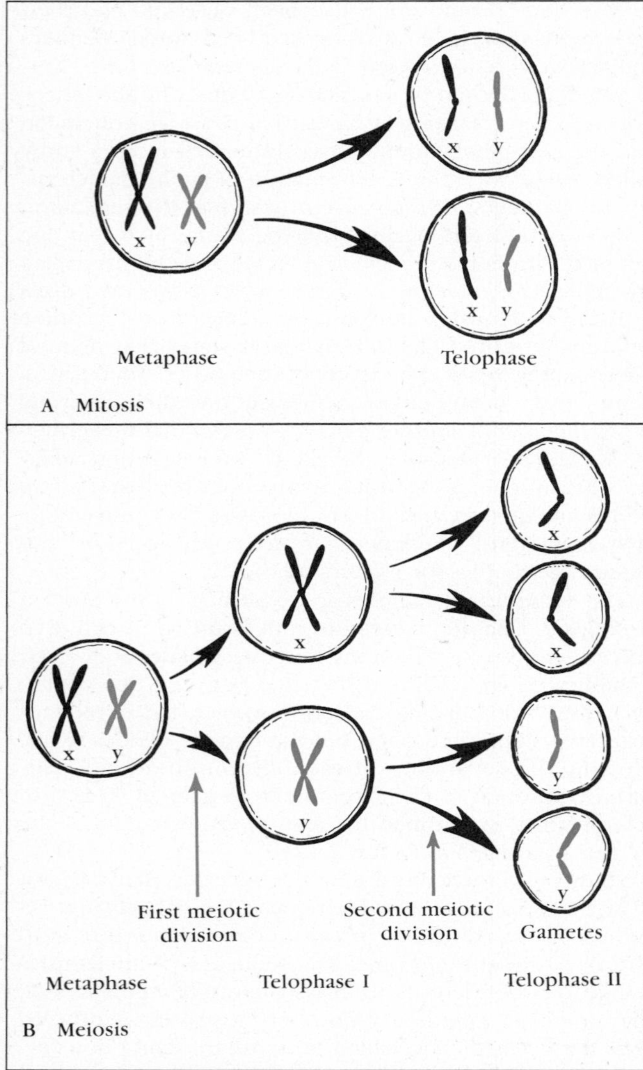

FIGURE 2-1 Selected stages in the processes of mitosis and meiosis. These are illustrated for the XY pair of chromosomes, the sex chromosomes in the male.

Classification of Genetic Disorders

Generally, genetic disorders are classified into three broad groups: (1) single-gene, (2) chromosome, and (3) multifactorial. In these three groups, altered genetic material is passed from parent to offspring. Analysis of the genetics and pathophysiology of any genetic disorder first requires its categorization into one of these types. Table 2-2 shows examples of conditions that can be caused by genetic abnormalities.

Single-gene disorders are known to be caused by mutation in a single gene. The mutated gene may be present on one or both chromosomes of a pair. In the former case, the matching gene on the partner chromosome is normal. Single-gene disorders are easily recognized as hereditary because they usually exhibit an obvious *pedigree*, the characteristic pattern of distribution of a specific trait in a family. Table 2-3 shows examples of some of the more common single-gene disorders and their frequency.

TABLE 2-2 Common Examples of Genetic Disorders

Disorder	Classification	Genetics
Huntington disease	Single-gene disorder	Autosomal dominant
Cystic fibrosis	Single-gene disorder	Autosomal recessive
Hypophosphatemia (vitamin D-resistant rickets)	Single-gene disorder	X-linked dominant
Hemophilia	Single-gene disorder	X-linked recessive
Down syndrome	Chromosome disorder	Trisomy 21
Turner syndrome	Chromosome disorder	45, X
Cleft lip/palate	Multifactorial	?

In *chromosome disorders*, the defect is due to an abnormality in chromosome number or structure. In contrast to single-gene disorders, which involve mutated genes, the structure of the genes in chromosome disorders may be normal, but the genes may be present in multiple copies or be situated on a different chromosome than is normally the case. For example, Down syndrome results from the presence of an extra chromosome 21 (trisomy 21). Chromosome disorders affect about 7 infants per 1000 births and account for about one-half of all spontaneous first-trimester abortions [8].

Multifactorial disorders result from a combination of small variations in genes that, when combined with environmental factors, produce serious defects. Although they do not show the distinct pedigree patterns of single-gene disorders, multifactorial disorders tend to cluster in families. It has been estimated that as many as 10 percent of the population is affected by these conditions [19].

Another group of disorders are *alterations in fetal development caused by the environment*. In this case, the conditions are not hereditary, but often involve a change in the expression of the cell's genetic material, which causes a defect in the structure and/or function of the cell. Environmental factors such as toxic chemicals, infectious agents, and irradiation are responsible for certain congenital abnormalities. Fetal development may also be affected by an unfavorable intrauterine environment due to maternal disease.

Single-Gene Disorders

Terminology

Transmission patterns in hereditary disorders are described in specific terms that must be defined for precise understanding. The members of a pair of matching chromosomes (those carrying genes that influence the same traits) are labeled *homologous* chromosomes. Each gene has a

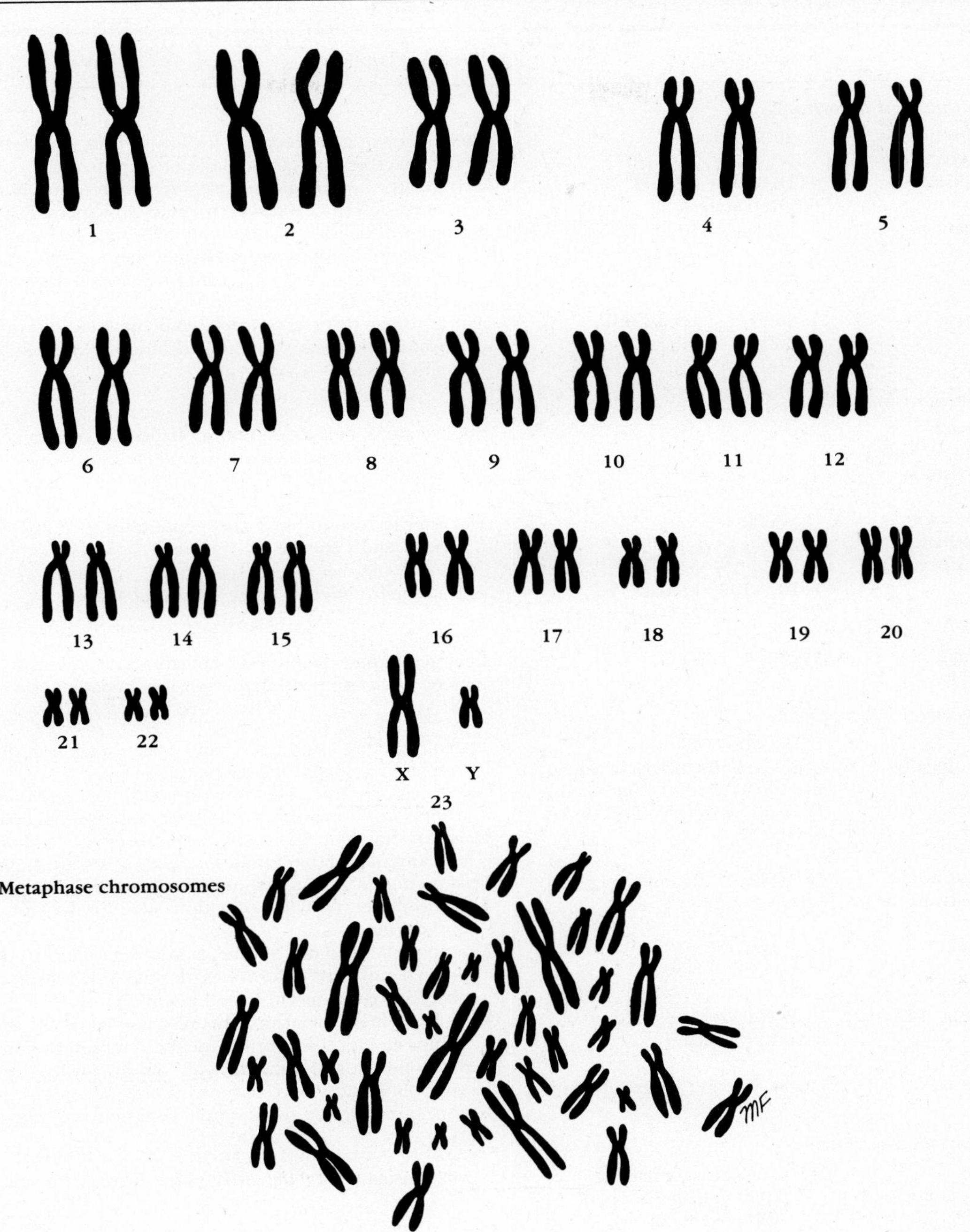

FIGURE 2-2 Structure of chromosomes in a human male karyotype. Note the identification of chromosome pairs by group and number. Each of these metaphase stage chromosomes has already been duplicated. Therefore it contains two identical strands (chromatids) attached to each other at the still undivided centromere. (From R.S. Snell, *Clinical Histology for Medical Students*. Boston: Little, Brown, 1984.)

Table 2-3 Selected Examples of Single-Gene Disorders

Disorder	Occurrence	Brief Description
Autosomal dominant inheritance		
Familial hypercholesterolemia (type II)	1:200–1:500	Deficiency in cell receptors for low density lipoproteins, hypercholesterolemia, xanthomas, coronary heart disease
Huntington disease	1:18,000–1:25,000 (United States)	Progressive neurologic disease, involuntary muscle movements, mental deterioration with memory loss, personality changes
Neurofibromatosis	1:3000–1:3300	Disorder of neural crest-derived cells with skin and central and peripheral nervous system manifestations; café au lait spots, neurofibromas, and malignant progression are common; variable expression of manifestations
Tay-Sachs disease	1:3600 (Ashkenazi Jews) 1:360,000 (others)	Lipid storage disease; progressive mental and motor retardation with onset at about age 6 months, deafness, blindness, convulsions, death by age 3–4 years
X-linked dominant inheritance		
Pseudohypoparathyroidism (Albright hereditary osteodystrophy	Rare	Short stature, delayed dentition, hypocalcemia, hyperphosphatemia, mineralization of skeleton, round facies
Vitamin D-resistant rickets (familial hypophosphatemia)	1:25,000	Disorder of renal tubular phosphate transport; low serum phosphate, rickets, short stature
Polydactyly	1:100–1:300 (blacks) 1:630–1:3300 (Caucasian)	Extra (supernumerary) digit on hands or feet
Polycystic renal disease (adult)	1:250–1:1250	Enlarged kidneys with cysts, hematuria, proteinuria, abdominal mass; may be associated with hypertension, hepatic cysts
Autosomal recessive inheritance		
Albinism (tyrosinase negative)	1:15,000–1:40,000 1:85–1:650 (American Indians)	Melanin lacking in skin, hair, and eyes; nystagmus; photophobia; increased susceptibility to neoplasia
Cystic fibrosis	1:2000–1:2500 (Caucasians) 1:16,000 (American blacks)	Abnormal exocrine gland function with pancreatic insufficiency and malabsorption, chronic pulmonary disease, excessive salt in sweat
Cystinuria	1:10,000	Defect in transport of cystine, lysine, arginine, and ornithine in intestines and renal tubules, tendency toward renal calculi
Familial dysautonomia (Riley-Day syndrome)	1:10,000–1:20,000 (Ashkenazi Jews)	Dysfunction of autonomic nervous system, sensory abnormalities, small stature, poor coordination, scoliosis, lack of tears leading to corneal ulcers
Hurler syndrome	1–2:100,000	Mucopolysaccharide disorder; mental retardation, coarse facies, skeletal and joint deformities, deafness, dwarfism, corneal clouding, onset age 6–12 months, fatal in childhood
Phenylketonuria (PKU)	1:15,000 (United States) 1:5000 (Scotland)	Deficiency in phenylalanine hydroxylase causing excess phenylalanine in blood and urine, mental retardation if untreated, normal development and life span with low phenylalanine diet
Sickle cell disease	1:400–1:600 (American blacks)	Hemoglobinopathy with chronic hemolytic anemia, growth retardation, susceptibility to infection, painful crises, leg ulcers, dactylitis
X-linked recessive inheritance		
Color blindness (red green deutan)	8:100 (Caucasian males) 4–5:100 (Caucasian females) 2–4:100 (black males)	Normal visual acuity, defective color vision with red-green confusion
Duchenne muscular dystrophy	1:3000–1:5000 males	Progressive muscle weakness, atrophy contractures, eventual respiratory insufficiency and death
G6PD (glucose-6-phosphate dehydrogenase) deficiency	1:10 black American males 1:50 black American females	Enzyme abnormality with subtypes; manifestations involve RBC since it cannot replace unstable enzyme; usually asymptomatic unless person is under stress or exposed to certain drugs or infection, which increase need for chemical-reducing power generated by action of G6PD; decreased reducing power eventually results in denaturation of hemoglobin and hemolysis
Hemophilia A	1:2500–1:4000 male births	Coagulation disorder due to deficiency of factor VIII
Hemophilia B	1:4000–1:7000 male births	Coagulation disorder due to deficiency of factor IX
X-linked ichthyosis	1:5000–1:6000 males	May be born with sheets of scales (collodion babies), dry scaling skin, corneal opacities, steriod sulfatase deficiency

Source: Adapted from F. Cohen, *Clinical Genetics in Nursing Practice.* Philadelphia: Lippincott, 1984. Pp. 78, 81, 84, 87, 91. Additional material from J. M. Connor and M. A. Ferguson-Smith, *Essential Medical Genetics.* Oxford: Blackwell Scientific, 1984. Pp. 185, 186, 198.

specific site, or *locus*, on a specific chromosome. Genes at the same locus on a pair of homologous chromosomes are called *alleles*. An individual in whom both members of a pair of alleles are the same is *homozygous* (a homozygote) with respect to that gene locus; when the members of a pair of alleles are different, the individual is *heterozygous* (a heterozygote) for that gene locus (Fig. 2-3).

Genotype is the word used to describe the genetic constitution of an individual. The trait or expression of a gene in an individual is the *phenotype*.

An allele that is expressed when it is present on one (or both) chromosomes of a pair is *dominant*. An allele that is expressed only when it is present on both chromosomes of a pair (with the exception of the XY pair) is *recessive*. The terms *dominant gene* and *recessive gene* are commonly used, and the trait (phenotype) that these genes determine can also be referred to as dominant or recessive. In genetic disorders, a *dominant disorder* is one in which the person who carries the gene (in either a heterozygous or homozygous state) is clinically affected. To be clinically affected by a *recessive disorder*, the individual must be homozygous for the gene (with the exception of genes found on the X chromosome in a male). As gene loci found on the X chromosome in the male are not matched by corresponding loci on his Y chromosome, a recessive gene on the male's X chromosome will be expressed. A disorder carried on the X chromosome is an X-linked disorder. There are no known Y-linked genetic disorders.

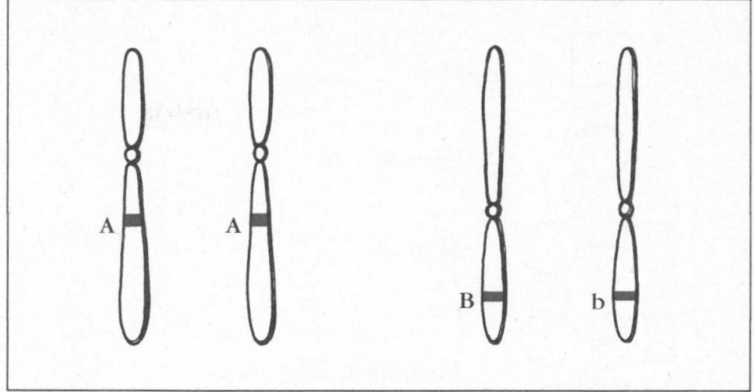

FIGURE 2-3 Two pairs of homologous chromosomes. One pair has similar allelles at locus A. The other pair has dissimilar allelles at locus B. A person with these chromosomes would be homozygous for allele A and heterozygous for allele B.

Principles of Transmission

Phenotypes determined by single genes occur in fixed proportion in the progeny of a mating. The pedigree patterns of such traits are dependent on whether the gene is located on an autosomal chromosome (any chromosome other than a sex chromosome) or on the X chromosome, and whether the gene is dominant or recessive. These factors allow four basic patterns of inheritance for single-gene traits: (1) autosomal dominant, (2) autosomal recessive, (3) X-linked dominant, and (4) X-linked recessive.

Patterns of single-gene inheritance can be exhibited in a *pedigree chart*, which is a schematic method for classifying data. Some symbols used in constructing a pedigree chart are shown in Figure 2-4. Gene symbols are always expressed in italics. Usually a capital letter is used to signify a dominant allele and the lower case of the same letter is used to signify the corresponding recessive allele. By this method, a genotype may be shown as *TT*, *Tt*, or *tt*, as in Figure 2-5.

An example of a phenotype determined by a single pair of autosomal alleles is the ability to taste phenylthiocarbamide (PTC). The bitter taste of the drug is detected by persons with the dominant gene but not by persons homozygous for the recessive allele. Therefore, those with the genotype *TT* (homozygous dominant) or *Tt* (heterozygous) would be able to taste the drug and be classified as phenotype, taster. Persons with the genotype *tt* (homozygous recessive) would not be able to taste the drug and would be classified as phenotype, nontaster.

Figure 2-5 illustrates the use of a *Punnett square* to predict the genotypes and phenotypes of the progeny of a heterozygous (*Tt*) male and female. Mendel's law of segregation and the concept of dominance are used for this prediction. As shown in the genotypes of the offspring, there is a 25 percent risk of being a dominant homozygote (*TT*) and a 50 percent risk of being a heterozygote (*Tt*). Both of these genotypes produce the phenotype, taster. There is a 25 percent risk of being a recessive homozygote (*tt*) and having the phenotype, nontaster.

Figure 2-6 illustrates all possible genotypes of offspring from matings involving a single pair of autosomal alleles. Using the same trait of PTC taster as an example, there are three possible genotypes for each male and female (*TT*, *Tt*, and *tt*) and six different combinations of genotypes that could be found in the offspring of each mating. The mating pair *Tt* × *tt* is the usual pattern of inheritance for an autosomal dominant trait, and the mating pair *Tt* × *Tt* is the usual pattern of inheritance for an autosomal recessive trait.

Autosomal Dominant Inheritance

In autosomal dominant inheritance of a genetic defect, the abnormal allele is dominant and the normal allele is recessive. The phenotype is the same whether the allele is present in either a homozygous or a heterozygous state. As previously stated, the pattern of inheritance usually seen for an autosomal dominant trait is *Tt* × *tt*. The stereotype pedigree of this pattern is shown in Figure 2-7. When either parent is heterozygous for the autosomal dominant allele (in this case the father) and the other parent is homozygous for the normal allele, each child has a 50 percent risk of receiving the dominant allele and thus being affected. Each child receives a normal allele from the normal parent. Although one-half of the children will theoretically receive the dominant allele, the chances are independent in each zygote formation, and in a small sample such as a family, the ratio of normal to affected children may be different than 1 : 1. Because the allele is autosomal and not X-linked, either sex may be affected. All affected

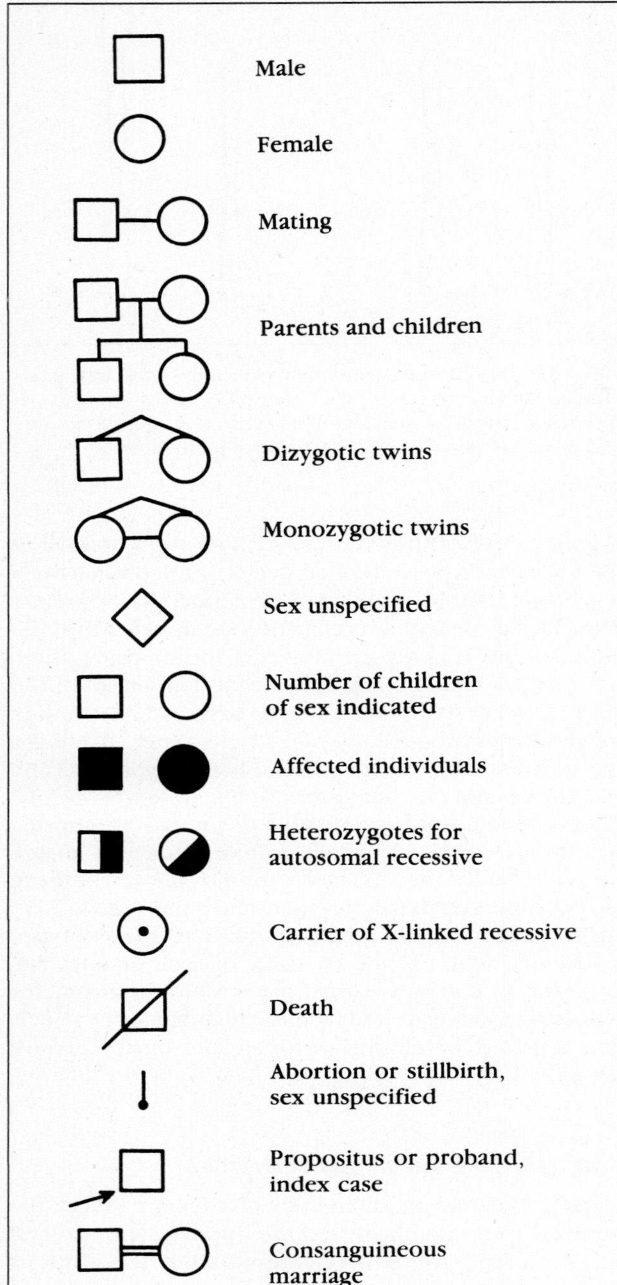

FIGURE 2-4 Symbols used in pedigree charts.

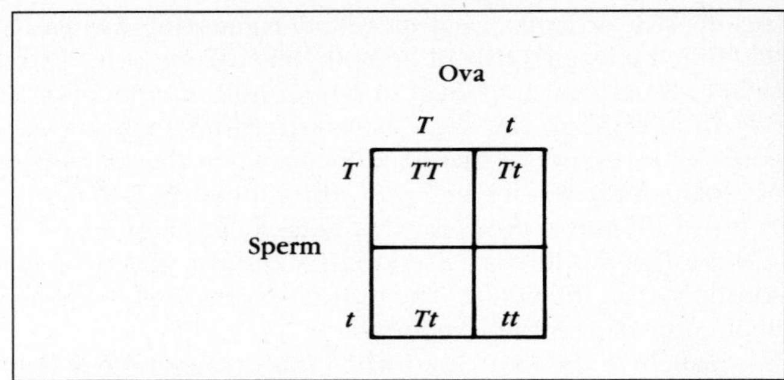

FIGURE 2-5 Progeny of *Tt* and *Tt* mating.

		Maternal genotype		
		TT	*Tt*	*tt*
Paternal genotype	*TT*	*TT*	*TT, Tt*	*Tt*
	Tt	*TT, Tt*	*TT, Tt, tt*	*Tt, tt*
	tt	*Tt*	*Tt, tt*	*tt*

FIGURE 2-6 Parental genotypes for autosomal allelles *T* and *t* and the genotypes that could be found in progeny of the various mating pairs.

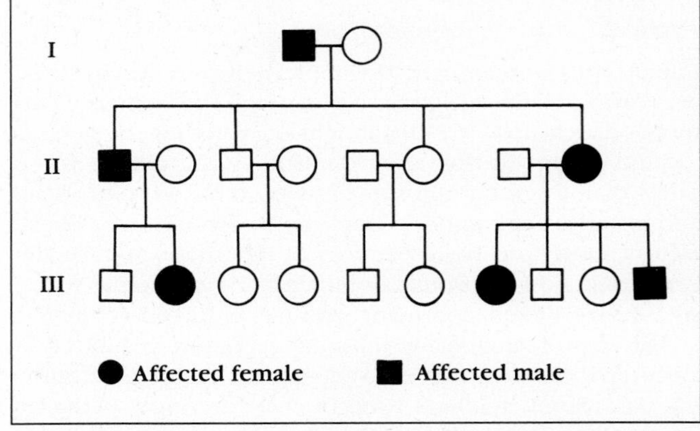

FIGURE 2-7 Stereotype pedigree of autosomal dominant inheritance.

children have an affected parent unless the disorder results from a fresh mutation.

Characteristics of autosomal dominant inheritance are summarized as follows: (1) affected persons have an affected parent; (2) affected persons mating with normal persons have affected and unaffected offspring in equal proportion; (3) unaffected children born to affected parents will have unaffected children; and (4) males and females are equally affected.

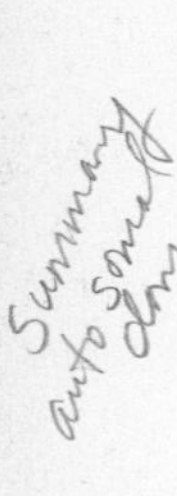

Autosomal Recessive Inheritance

In autosomal recessive disorders the abnormal allele is recessive. For the trait to be expressed, a person must be homozygous for the abnormal allele. Because the dominant or normal allele masks the trait, most persons who are heterozygous for an autosomal recessive allele go undetected. When two heterozygous individuals mate (the most common pattern in autosomal recessive inheritance) and an offspring receives the recessive allele from each parent, the trait is expressed. *Consanguineous* marriage (marriage of persons who are blood relatives) may increase this probability.

When a heterozygous person mates with a homozygous normal person, each offspring receives a normal allele from the normal parent and cannot express the trait. Figure 2-8 illustrates a stereotype pedigree of autosomal recessive inheritance. Note in line I that when a homozygous normal male mates with a heterozygous female, each offspring receives a normal gene from the father. Fifty percent of the offspring receive the recessive allele from the heterozygous mother and are therefore carriers of the trait. Line II shows a heterozygous male mating with a heterozygous female. The progeny of this mating have a 1:4 risk of receiving a recessive allele from each parent and thus being affected with the trait.

Characteristics of autosomal recessive inheritance are summarized as follows: (1) the trait usually appears in siblings only, not in the parents; (2) males and females are equally likely to be affected; (3) for parents of one affected child, the recurrence risk is one in four for every subsequent birth; (4) both parents of an affected child carry the recessive allele; and (5) the parents of the affected child may be consanguineous.

X-Linked Inheritance

Of the 23 pairs of chromosomes that determine the karyotype of the human, 22 are autosomes and 1 is the sex chromosomes. Unlike the 44 autosomes that can be arranged in 22 homologous pairs, the two sex chromosomes are of unequal size and have different placement of their centromeres (see Fig. 2-2). The two sex chromosomes in the female are XX and in the male are XY. Because the ovum must contain an X chromosome, if it is fertilized by a sperm containing an X chromosome, the product will be a female (XX). If the sperm contributes a Y chromosome, the product will be male (XY).

Transmission of genes on the sex chromosomes follows the same principles of inheritance as does transmission on the autosomes. The difference in the patterns of inheritance results from differences of morphology and gene complement in the two sex chromosomes. The X chromosome carries genes that are not matched on the Y chromosome. Because to date there are no known medically significant genes located on the Y chromosome, it seems that its major importance is sex determination. Therefore, for practical purposes, the genes located on the X chromosome are those involved in sex-linked inheritance.

Females inherit two X chromosomes, whereas males (XY) have only one. As the genes located on the male's one X chromosome have no counterparts on his Y chromosome (he is *hemizygous* for these genes), traits determined by either dominant or recessive X-linked genes are expressed in the male. The genes on the X chromosome cannot be transmitted from father to son, since fathers contribute a Y chromosome to sons, but are transmitted from father to all daughters through the one X chromosome. Recessive mutant genes on the X chromosome of a female may not be expressed because they are matched by normal genes inherited with the other X chromosome. A gene that is X-linked may be indicated as X*A* to represent a dominant gene and X*a* to represent its recessive allele.

X-Linked Dominant Inheritance. Genetic disorders caused by X-linked dominant genes are rare. The main characteristic of this inheritance pattern is that an affected male transmits the gene to all his daughters and to none of his sons. The affected female may transmit the gene to offspring of either sex (Fig. 2-9).

Characteristics of X-linked dominant inheritance are summarized as follows: (1) affected males have normal sons and affected daughters; (2) affected females (heterozygous) have a 50 percent risk of transmitting the abnormal gene to each daughter or son; and (3) the disorder tends to be more severe in males (hemizygous) than in females (heterozygous).

X-Linked Recessive Inheritance. Several genetic disorders associated with a recessive gene on the X chromosome have been identified. Again, the inheritance pat-

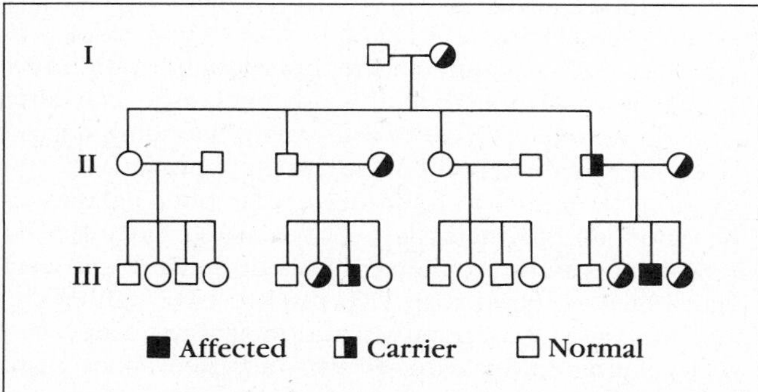

FIGURE 2-8 Stereotype pedigree of autosomal recessive inheritance.

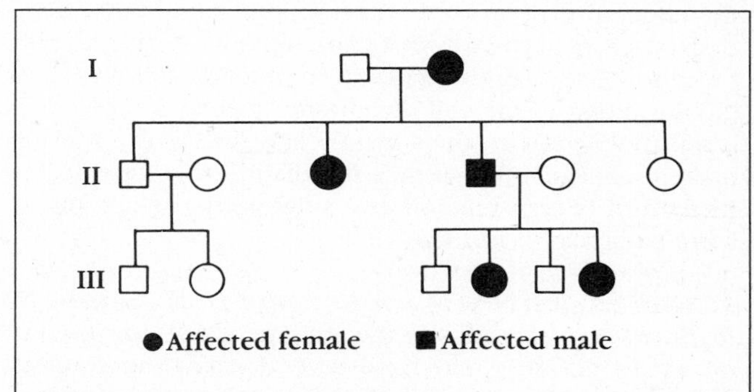

FIGURE 2-9 Stereotype pedigree of X-linked dominant inheritance.

tern of these disorders results from the morphologic difference in the X and Y chromosome. The recessive gene located on the one X chromosome of the male is not balanced by a dominant allele on the Y chromosome, and is thus expressed. The recessive gene should be expressed in the female only if she is homozygous (X*a* X*a*). Therefore, X-linked recessive disorders are rare in females. Only matings between an affected male and a carrier or affected female should result in an affected female.

Occasionally, a carrier (heterozygous) female manifests some of the signs of a recessive disorder. This is due to the fact that during early embryogenesis, one or the other of the X chromosomes in each of the somatic cells (cells other than the gametes) of all females degenerate, leaving only one functioning X chromosome in each cell [10]. Thus, approximately one-half of the cells in a normal female express the genes on one of her X chromosomes, and the other half express the genes on her other X chromosome. If this "X-chromosome inactivation" is unequal, one of the X chromosomes may have a greater effect on the female's physiology than the other, resulting in the ability of a recessive gene on that chromosome to be expressed [2].

Males affected with an X-linked recessive disorder cannot transmit the gene to sons, but transmit it to all daughters. An unaffected female who is heterozygous for the recessive gene transmits it to 50 percent of her sons and daughters. Figure 2-10 gives a stereotype pedigree of X-linked recessive inheritance.

Characteristics of X-linked recessive inheritance are summarized as follows: (1) males are predominantly affected; (2) affected males cannot transmit the gene to sons but transmit the gene to all daughters; (3) sons of female carriers have a 50 percent risk of being affected; and (4) daughters of female carriers have a 50 percent risk of being carriers.

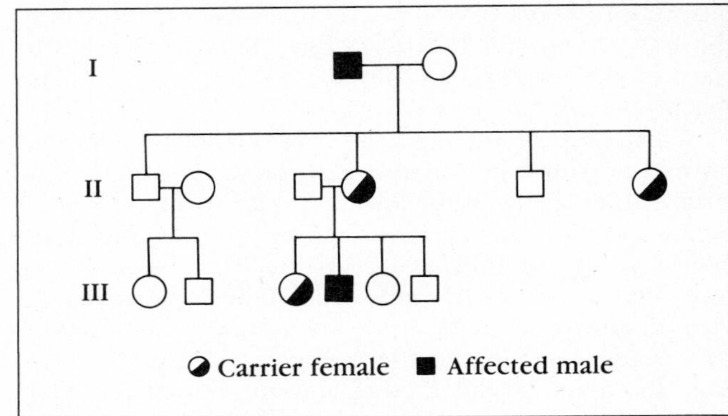

FIGURE 2-10 Stereotype pedigree of X-linked recessive inheritance.

Pathophysiology of Single-Gene Disorders

Since the genes of a cell are primarily responsible for directing the synthesis of the cell's proteins, it is not surprising that the manifestations of single-gene disorders result from alterations in protein synthesis. In many cases the affected protein is an enzyme, part of a synthetic or degradation pathway. In other instances, the altered protein is one that circulates in the blood, such as hemoglobin; is part of the cell membrane, such as a receptor of a transport protein; or is mainly supportive in function, namely collagen. Sometimes the disorder is classified by its pattern of transmission as a single-gene defect, but its basic pathology is not known.

Altered Activity of an Enzyme in a Metabolic Pathway. Alterations in the activity of one enzyme in a metabolic pathway may have several results, including a deficiency in the end product of the pathway, or the accumulation of a toxic intermediate or a toxic byproduct. These possibilities are illustrated in Figure 2-11, which shows selected pathways for the metabolism of phenylalanine and tyrosine and metabolic blocks that are responsible for three genetic disorders—albinism, alkaptonuria, and phenylketonuria.

Alterations in Amino Acid Metabolism. As indicated in Figure 2-11, both phenylalanine and tyrosine are normally available from the digestion of dietary protein. Phenylalanine is also converted to tyrosine, which has many uses in the cell, one of which is to produce melanin, the pigment in skin, hair, and eyes. In *classic albinism*, a deficiency in the enzyme tyrosinase results in decreased or absent melanin production. Manifestations of this condition are listed in Table 2-3. Another single-gene disorder, *alkaptonuria*, is due to the absence of homogentisic acid oxidase, which results in the accumulation of the pathway intermediate homogentisic acid (alkapton). Homogentisic acid is excreted in the urine and turns black in the presence of oxygen, which produces darkening of the urine. In later life, deposits of dark pigment may be noted in connective tissue and may lead to arthritis.

The most serious genetic disorder involving phenylalanine metabolism is *phenylketonuria* (PKU). In classic PKU, absence of phenylalanine hydroxylase from liver cells prevents the conversion of phenylalanine to tyrosine. Consequently, phenylalanine accumulates in the blood, and some is converted to phenylpyruvic acid, phenyllactic acid, or phenylacetic acid. These compounds are excreted in the urine, giving it a characteristic musty odor. The excess of phenylalanine and its byproducts in the blood results in various metabolic disturbances, especially alterations in nervous system development, including delayed psychomotor development, seizures, hyperactivity, and mental retardation. In addition, excess phenylalanine in the blood inhibits the activity of tyrosinase. Since this enzyme is necessary for the synthesis of melanin and catecholamines, children with PKU tend to have lighter eyes and skin than their relatives and may show a decrease in circulating epinephrine. In the untreated infant, manifestations of PKU appear at approximately 3 to 6 months of age.

Fortunately, tests are available to detect phenylalanine or its metabolites in blood or urine, and PKU screening is mandatory for newborns in most states [15]. The most

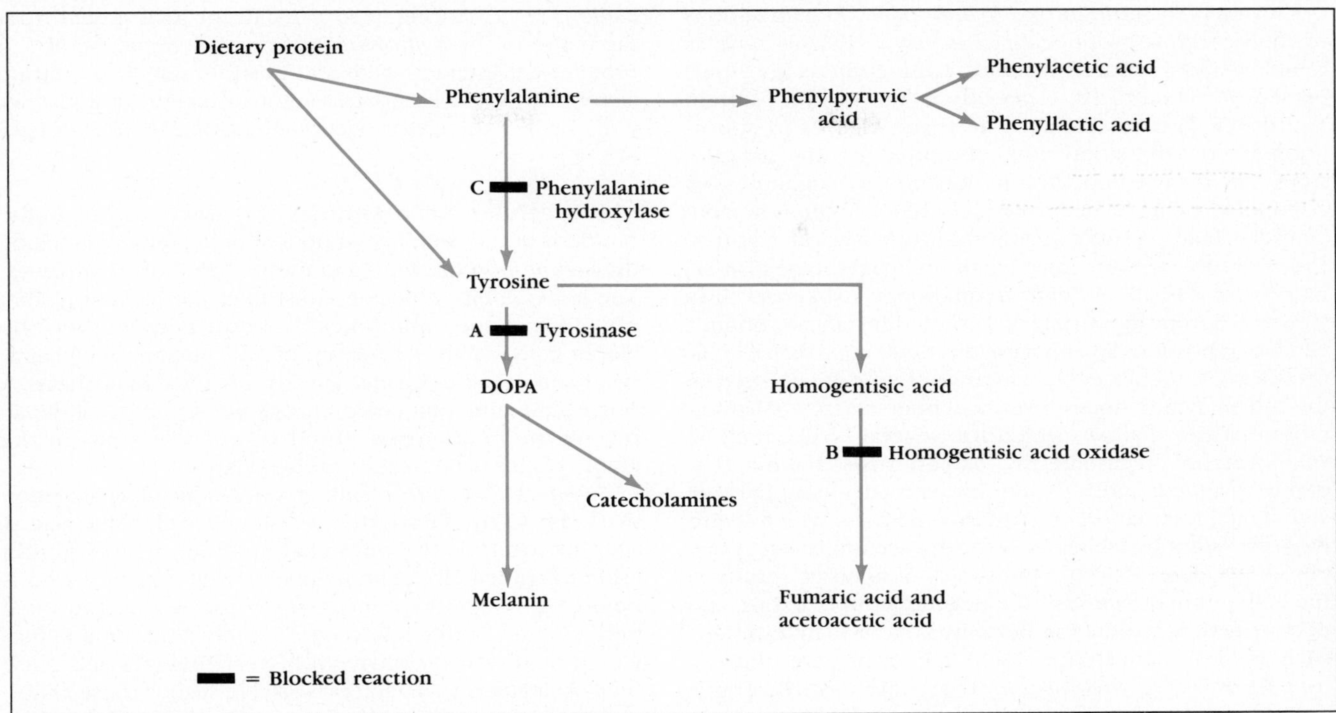

FIGURE 2-11 Metabolism of phenylalanine and tyrosine. Arrows may represent one or more chemical reactions. The indicated enzyme defects result in (A) classic albinism, (B) alkaptonuria, and (C) classic PKU.

commonly used test, the Guthrie bacterial-inhibition assay, which indicates phenylalanine level in the blood, is not positive until the infant has consumed enough protein to allow phenylalanine buildup. Therefore, if the test is performed during the first three days of life, as might occur with the current trend for early hospital discharge of mother and baby, it may have to be repeated, ideally before the infant is 3 weeks old [1]. In PKU-positive infants, neurologic damage can be prevented by restricting phenylalanine in the diet. The restrictive diet should be started as early as possible and followed until neurologic development is complete. Estimates regarding the age at which a normal diet may be allowed vary widely, from 3 years to never [2]. When a person with PKU becomes pregnant, it is also necessary for her to resume her low-phenylalanine diet to protect the fetus [2].

With the advent of widespread neonatal PKU screening, other causes of hyperphenylalaninemia have been identified, involving closely related aspects of phenylalanine metabolism. Classic PKU accounts for approximately 90 percent of all cases of hyperphenylalaninemia [2]. Other causes are deficiencies of related enzymes in the liver other than phenylalanine hydroxylase [17]. Classic PKU exhibits autosomal recessive transmission, and tests are available to detect heterozygous carriers [15].

Alterations in Carbohydrate Metabolism. Loss of activity of enzymes in the varied pathways for carbohydrate metabolism account for many single-gene disorders. These include alterations in the metabolism of glucose, galactose, or fructose, glycogen storage diseases, and disorders involving mucopolysaccharides. In *galactosemia*, deficiency of an enzyme needed for the conversion of galactose 1-phosphate to glucose 1-phosphate leads to the accumulation of galactose and galactose 1-phosphate in tissues. This interferes with normal liver and kidney function and produces other metabolic disturbances that may result in osmotic changes in the lens of the eye and cataract development.

Glucose-6-phosphate dehydrogenase deficiency, a relatively common disorder in American blacks, is described in Table 2-3. In *glycogen storage diseases*, various enzymes needed for the synthesis or breakdown of glycogen may be altered. The accumulation of glycogen in tissues, especially the liver, interferes with their functions. The most common glycogen storage disease is *von Gierke disease*, in which developing liver pathology produces hepatomegaly, acidosis, increased glucose and lipids in the blood, and retarded growth [15]. *Mucopolysaccharides* are large complex carbohydrates that form part of the extracellular matrix of connective tissue. They are constantly being turned over in the tissues and are degraded by enzymes contained in the lysosomes of a cell. A deficiency in any of the necessary lysosomal enzymes leads to the accumulation of partially degraded mucopolysaccharides within the lysosome (one type of *lysosomal storage disease*). This interferes with various activities of the cell. Manifestations of one type of mucopolysaccharidosis, *Hurler syndrome*, are listed in Table 2-3.

Disorders in Sphingolipid Metabolism. Accumulations of sphingolipids produce *lipid storage diseases* such as Gaucher and Tay-Sachs diseases. Sphingolipids are lipids present in membranes, especially in the myelin of brain and other nervous tissue. The three classes of sphingolipids are sphingomyelins, cerebrosides, and gangliosides. Like many compounds in the body, sphingolipids are continually being turned over, and a block in their metabolism can lead to their accumulation in various tissues. *Gaucher disease* is the most common lipid storage disease, exhibiting a relatively high frequency in Ashkenazi Jews (Jews of European, as opposed to Mediterranean, origin). Glucocerebrosides accumulate in reticuloendothelial cells, producing Gaucher cells, which are found most often in the spleen, lymph nodes, liver, and bone marrow. Manifestations of this disease, which has several forms, include splenomegaly, hepatomegaly, osteoporosis, anemia, tendency to bleed, and, in some forms, neurologic damage and mental retardation. In *Tay-Sachs disease*, which is also most prevalent in Ashkenazi Jews, the accumulation of one type of ganglioside in the lysosomes of neurons results in the ballooning of neurons, the degeneration of axons, and demyelination, producing nervous system manifestations such as those indicated in Table 2-3. At present, there is no treatment for this disease. Fortunately, screening is available to detect heterozygous carriers of this autosomal recessive disorder.

Other Metabolic Pathway Defects. Other biochemical pathways that are known to be altered by single-gene mutations include ones that involve the metabolism of purines, pyrimidines, or heme, and those that are used for the biotransformation of certain drugs. The synthesis of heme occurs by way of several precursors called porphyrins. The *porphyrias* are disorders in which an enzyme defect leads to the accumulation and excretion of porphyrins or porphyrin precursors. Some porphyrias are hereditary, whereas some are caused by the toxic effect of chemicals. Of the hereditary porphyrias, four types display autosomal dominant transmission and one is autosomal recessive.

General characteristics of porphyrias include the excretion of reddish urine, photosensitization of the skin and skin eruptions, excessive hair on the face and limbs, and neurologic and psychologic manifestations. This constellation of signs and symptoms may have led to afflicted persons being called the werewolves of European folklore [9]. *Drug sensitivities* that are attributed to hereditary enzyme deficiencies include sensitivity to succinylcholine and isoniazid [10].

Loss or Alteration of Circulating Proteins. Other types of single-gene disorders can involve proteins that circulate in the bloodstream. Serum albumin is deficient in *analbuminemia*, producing oncotic pressure problems. Serum globulins that may be affected by single-gene mutations include complement components, alpha$_1$-antitrypsin, alpha$_2$-macroglobulin, transferrin, or various immunoglobulins (the immunoglobulins in *X-linked agammaglobulinemia* or *severe combined immunodeficiency*) [15]. Clotting factor VIII, IX, or XI is absent from the blood in the *hemophilias*. Von Willebrand factor is a protein that interacts with and possibly stabilizes clotting factor VIII. It is also necessary for formation of a platelet plug. Lack of the factor occurs in *von Willebrand disease* [13,18].

Hemoglobin Abnormalities. Disorders involving the synthesis of the protein component of hemoglobin include the *hemoglobinopathies* and the *thalassemia syndromes*. The hemoglobin molecule consists of the protein globin, plus four heme complexes. In adult hemoglobin, the globin component is made up of four polypeptide chains: two identical alpha chains and two identical beta chains. A single-gene mutation could change the structure of the alpha or the beta chains. Hundreds of variations in the globin chains have been identified [10].

Sickle cell anemia results from a single-gene mutation that leads to the substitution of valine for glutamic acid at one location on the beta chains of adult hemoglobin (HbA), forming HbS. The hemoglobin of a person who is homozygous for the abnormal gene contains abnormal beta chains. Under low oxygen conditions, this hemoglobin tends to precipitate within erythrocytes and cause them to assume a characteristic sickle shape. These abnormal red blood cells tend to compromise blood flow to the tissues and also to lyse, resulting in anemia. A person who is homozygous for the gene is said to have *sickle cell disease*. A person who is heterozygous for the abnormal gene produces both HbS and HbA, and exhibits sickling of erythrocytes only under conditions of extremely low oxygen tension. This person may never exhibit signs of sickle cell anemia and is said to have the *sickle cell trait*, rather than the disease. Manifestations of sickle cell anemia are discussed in more detail in Chapter 15.

Whereas hemoglobinopathies such as sickle cell disease involve an alteration in the structure of the globin component of hemoglobin, the thalassemias result from reduced synthesis of normal hemoglobin molecules. They are classed as alpha- and beta-thalassemias, depending upon which polypeptide chain is synthesized in reduced amounts (see Chap. 15).

Lipoproteins. Hereditary alterations in the level and function of certain lipoproteins that are normally found in the blood occur in conditions such as *familial hypercholesterolemia*, *abetalipoproteinemia*, and *familial combined hyperlipidemia*. Although these are thought to be single-gene disorders, they are influenced somewhat by the environment, and are therefore usually classed as multifactorial conditions [15].

Altered Cell Membrane Components. Familial hypercholesterolemia involves the lack of low-density lipoprotein receptors on liver cells and is thus an example of a *cell membrane defect* produced by a single-gene mutation. Other cell membrane defects may involve proteins that participate in the active transport of substances through the membrane. Conditions that are thought to result from defective membrane-transport proteins include *cystinuria* and *vitamin D-resistant rickets*, both of which are described in Table 2-3.

Collagen Disorders. Several hereditary disorders are believed to result from abnormalities in the synthesis of collagen. This protein, which is the most abundant protein in the body, has a complex structure with several levels of organization. Eight different types of collagen are present in the various connective tissues in the body [3]. One example of a collagen disorder is *osteogenesis imperfecta*, which is discussed in Chapter 41.

Another is *Marfan syndrome*, which results from an autosomal dominant gene defect or, in 15 percent of the cases, a new mutation [3]. In this disorder, a defect in the structure of collagen or another connective tissue protein, elastin, is thought to be the basis for changes in skeletal, ocular, and cardiovascular tissues. Among the manifestations of Marfan syndrome are tall, thin stature with arachnodactyly (excessively long fingers), lax ligaments allowing hyperextension of the limbs, dislocation of the optic lenses, and a tendency toward formation of dissecting aneurysms of the aorta. The stature of Abraham Lincoln and the violin virtuosity of Paganini have been attributed to Marfan syndrome.

Single-Gene Disorders in Which the Basic Defect Is Unknown. Among the disorders that appear to be transmitted as single-gene defects are several for which the basic physiologic deficiencies are not known. These include cystic fibrosis, the muscular dystrophies, and Huntington disease, all of which are mentioned briefly in Table 2-3 and discussed in greater detail in specifically related chapters.

Preliminary studies indicate that some manifestations of cystic fibrosis may be due to faulty control of channels for the diffusion of chloride through cell membranes [6,12]. Other possible basic defects in cystic fibrosis include hypersecretion of calcium by mucous glands, increased intracellular calcium, and the production of serum glycoproteins, which inhibit the activity of cilia [17].

Huntington disease is an autosomal dominant disorder in which symptoms do not usually appear until 35 years of age or later. By the time of diagnosis, the affected person may have already reproduced, with a 50 percent chance of passing this lethal trait to each of his offspring. There is no treatment for the disease, and progressive neurologic deterioration is inevitable. Until recently, there has been no way to identify persons carrying the gene for Huntington disease before symptoms appear. Using modern techniques for analyzing DNA, researchers have noted a characteristic pattern of fragments produced when the DNA of chromosome 4 from cells of persons with the disease is cleaved by a particular enzyme, one of several called *restriction enzymes* [7]. Similar treatment of DNA from persons who do not carry the gene yields different fragments. Thus, a test is available for predicting which young persons will eventually develop the symptoms of Huntington disease [3]. Use of the predictive test must be accompanied by consideration of the impact of a positive result on the person and the family.

Chromosome Disorders

Chromosomal aberrations (deviations from normal) may be either numeric or structural and may affect either autosomes or sex chromosomes. Rarely are both simultaneously affected. Chromosome aberrations resulting in two or more cell lines with different chromosome numbers produce *mosaics*. In these situations, one or more of the cell lines are abnormal.

Numeric Aberrations

Deviations or abnormalities in chromosome number are classified in terms of loss or gain of chromosome sets. As discussed earlier, the normal chromosome number in humans is 46 (23 pairs). To compare abnormalities with the normal karyotype, several terms must be defined.

Normal somatic cells, with two sets of 23 chromosomes, are said to be *diploid* (double) or 2N; gametes, with a single set of 23, are *haploid* (single) or N. A cell with an exact multiple of the haploid number is *euploid*. Euploid numbers may be 2N, 3N (*triploid*), or 4N (*tetraploid*). Chromosome numbers that are exact multiples of N but greater than 2N are called *polyploid*. *Aneuploid* refers to a chromosome complement that is abnormal in number but is not an exact multiple of N. An aneuploid cell may be *trisomic* (2N + 1 chromosomes) or *monosomic* (2N − 1 chromosomes). Any cell with a chromosome number that deviates from the characteristic N and 2N is *heteroploid*.

Disjunction is the normal separation and migration of chromosomes during cell division. Failure of the process, or *nondisjunction*, in a meiotic division results in one daughter cell receiving both homologous chromosomes and the other receiving neither. It is the primary cause of aneuploidy. If this deviation in normal process occurs during the first meiotic division, one-half of the gametes will contain 22 chromosomes and one-half will contain 24. If joined with a normal gamete, a gamete produced in this manner will produce either a monosomic (2N − 1) or trisomic (2N + 1) zygote. Normal disjunction and nondisjunction at the first and second meiotic divisions of the ovum are illustrated in Figure 2-12. The figure also shows the union of normal sperm with gametes of varying chromosome complement. A common example of a disorder that results from an abnormality of chromosome number is *trisomy 21*, or *Down syndrome*. This disorder can result when nondisjunction of chromosome 21 occurs at meiosis, producing one gamete with an extra chromosome 21 (N + 1 = 24) and one gamete with no chromosome 21 (N − 1 = 22). Union of the 24 chromosome gamete with a normal sperm produces a 47-chromosome zygote, trisomy 21.

The overall incidence of Down syndrome is 1 per 700 live births. The incidence increases with increasing maternal age. As it has been determined that in 20 to 30 percent of cases the extra chromosome is of paternal origin, the role of increased paternal age is being investigated. Presently, it is suggested that in couples in which the father is 55 years old or older, the mother's age-specific risk

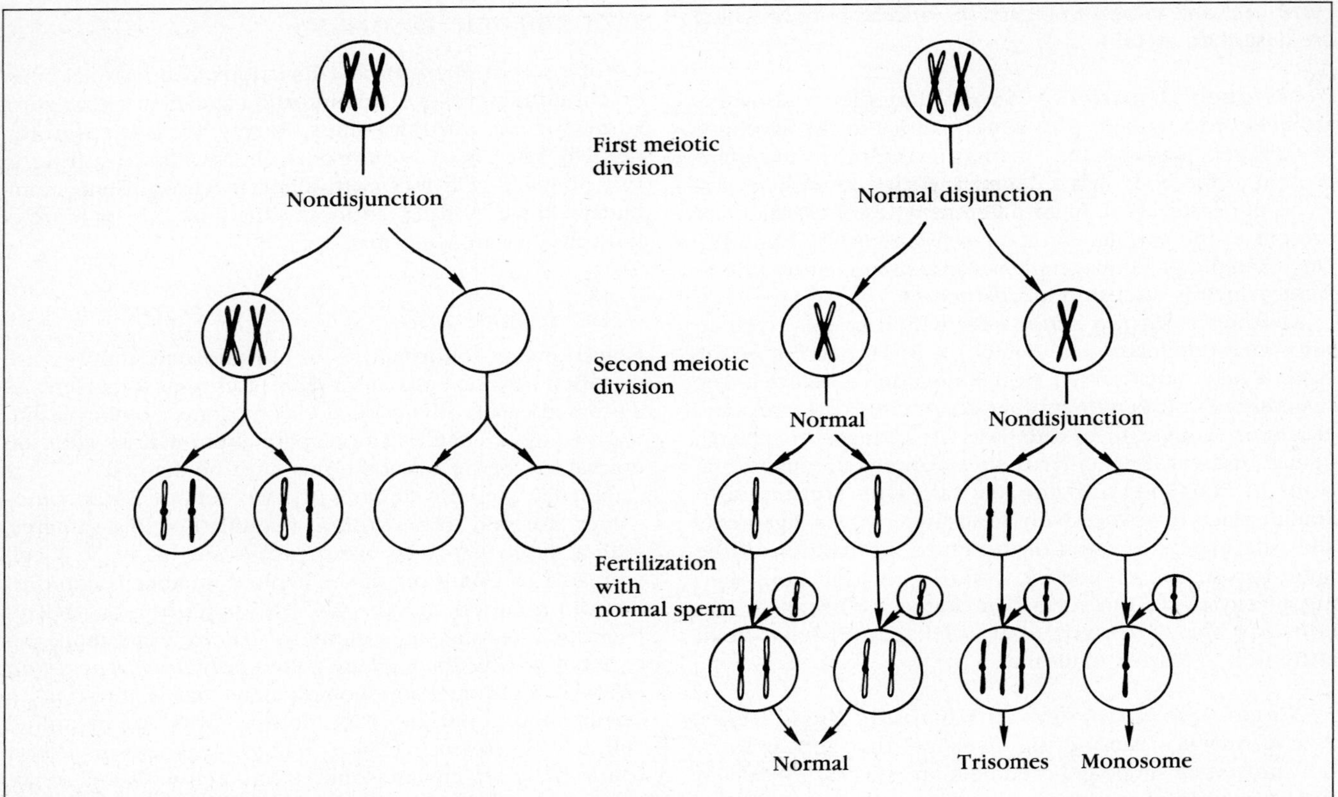

FIGURE 2-12 Process of nondisjunction at the first and second meiotic divisions of the ovum and fertilization with normal sperm.

should be doubled to estimate the couple's risk of having an infant with trisomy 21 [2].

Clinical diagnosis of trisomy 21 is often based on facial appearance. The palpebral fissures are upslanting with speckling of the edge of the iris, the nose is small, and the facial profile flat. Figure 2-13 illustrates other manifestations of trisomy 21. The simian crease (a single midpalmar fold) is found in approximately 50 percent of persons with Down syndrome and in approximately 5 to 10 percent of nonafflicted persons [2]. The presence of mental retardation is consistent in children with Down syndrome, but the degree may vary. The average IQ is approximately 50; infrequently, values may range up to 70 or 80.

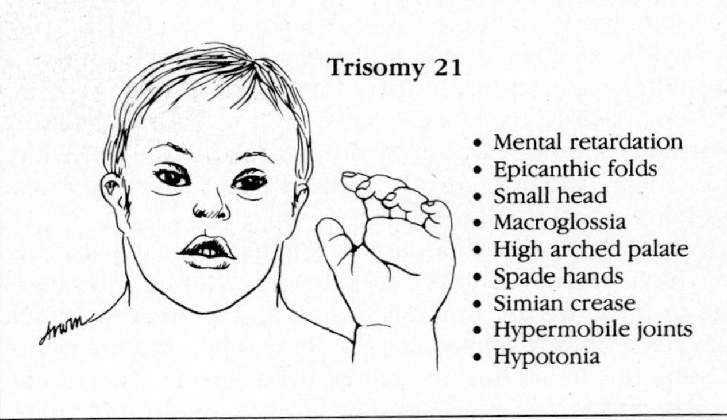

FIGURE 2-13 Down syndrome phenotype. (From R.D. Judge, G.D. Zuidema, and F.T. Fitzgerald, *Clinical Diagnosis, A Physiologic Approach* [4th ed.]. Boston: Little, Brown, 1982.)

Structural Aberrations

Deviations in the normal structure of chromosomes result from the chromosome material breaking and reassembling in an abnormal arrangement. These changes in structure may be either stable (persisting through future cell divisions) or unstable (incompatible with cell division). Stable types of structural abnormalities include the following:

1. *Deletion*, loss of a portion of a chromosome. The missing segment may be a terminal portion of the chromosome, resulting from a single break, or an internal section, resulting from two breaks.
2. *Duplication*, presence of a repeated gene or gene sequence. A deleted segment of one chromosome becomes incorporated into its homologous chromosome.
3. *Inversion*, reversal of gene order. The linear arrangement of genes on a chromosome is broken and the order of a portion of the gene complement is reversed in the process of reattachment.
4. *Translocation*, transfer of part of one chromosome to a nonhomologous chromosome. This occurs when two

chromosomes break and the segments are rejoined in an abnormal arrangement.

Mosaics

Nondisjunction occurring in cell division other than gametogenesis results in two or more cell lines with different chromosome numbers. Persons with at least two cell lines with different karyotypes are called mosaics. Although several different mosaics have been described, most of the cases of different cell lines involve sex chromosome constitution.

Sex Chromosome Aberrations

In comparison to other hereditary disorders, sex chromosome aberrations are fairly common. Of the types found in males, the incidence is about 1 in 400 births; of the types found in females, about 1 in 650 births [20].

Most sex chromosome abnormalities are due to numeric aberration resulting from nondisjunction during meiosis. The disorders are described by the total number of chromosomes present. A normal male is 46,XY and a normal female is 46,XX. Any variation from these values constitutes a disorder. The most common genotype with female phenotype is 45,X (Turner syndrome) and with male phenotype, 47,XXY (Klinefelter syndrome).

The overall incidence of *Turner syndrome* is 1 per 2500 female births. The frequency at conception is higher, but 99 percent spontaneously abort. The diagnosis may be suggested in the newborn by the presence of redundant neck skin and peripheral lymphedema. Diagnosis can also be made later during the investigation of short stature or primary amenorrhea.

The incidence of 47,XXY (*Klinefelter syndrome*) is 1 per 1000 males. The risk increases with increased maternal age [2]. Diagnosis is usually made during adult life as a result of the investigation of infertility. This syndrome is the most common cause of hypogonadism and infertility in men. Other manifestations include long lower extremities, sparse body hair with a female distribution, and, in approximately 50 percent, breast development.

Multifactorial Disorders

Multifactorial inheritance includes the disorders in which a genetic susceptibility combined with the appropriate environmental agents interact to produce a phenotype that is classified as disease.

Although the word *polygenetic* is sometimes used to describe multifactorial disorders, the former term more accurately describes disorders determined by a large number of genes, each with a small effect, acting additively [5]. To date, there is no method of establishing the exact effects of environmental factors or the additive effects of genes in determining the expression of a trait [20]. For this reason, multifactorial inheritance is more difficult to analyze than other types of inheritance. Multifactorial traits tend to cluster in families, but their genetic patterns are not clearly predictable, as they are with single-gene traits and chromosome disorders.

A characteristic of multifactorial inheritance is the unimodal distribution of a trait in the population (note the presence of only one peak in the curve in Fig. 2-14). Some normal characteristics are distributed unimodally and have family patterns that are characteristic of multifactorial inheritance [20]; for example, stature and intelligence. The correlation among relatives with such traits is proportional to their genes in common (inherited from a common ancestral source). The more distant the relationship, the fewer genes they have in common [16]. Abnormalities that are thought to be multifactorial include congenital heart disease, congenital dislocation of the hip, neural tube defects, cleft lip, cleft palate, and atherosclerotic heart disease.

The *threshold model* of multifactorial inheritance (see Fig. 2-14) can be used to explain some of the features of the family distribution of multifactorial disorders. It is based on collecting information on the frequency of the disorders in the general population and in different categories of relatives (e.g., first-degree relatives such as parents, siblings, and offspring, or second-degree relatives such as aunts, uncles, nieces, and nephews). Through this method of analysis, the empiric risk (recurrence risk based on experience) can be estimated. Knowledge of genetic and environmental factors in the pathogenesis of the disorders is not considered.

Environmental Alterations in Fetal Development

The effect of environmental influences on fetal development has been a subject of increasing concern. Reasons

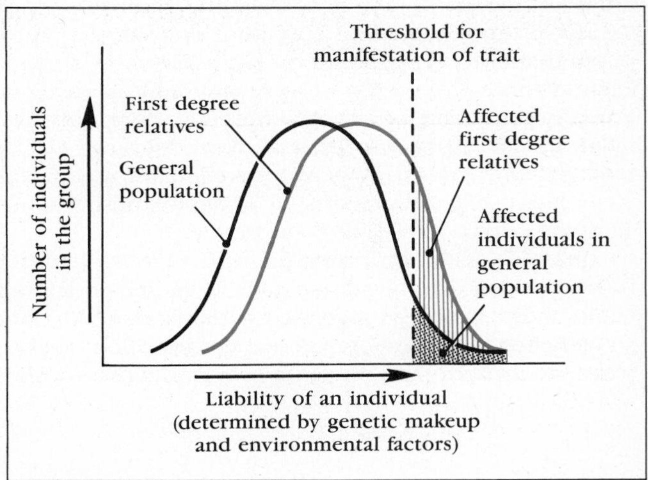

FIGURE 2-14 Threshold model for multifactorial inheritance. First-degree relatives of the affected individual have more genetic and/or environmental factors, which increase their risk of manifesting the disorder.

for this include the facts that more women have entered the workplace, the level of environmental chemical exposure is increasing for all people, and birth defects due to environmental exposure are preventable. Publicity generated by the thalidomide damage in the 1960s brought the problem to the attention of the general public.

A *teratogen* is an agent that acts on the embryo or fetus, causing abnormalities in form or function. Teratogenic agents can also be referred to as fetotoxic or developmentally toxic. Exposure to these agents results in a wide spectrum of consequences, from no apparent effect to altered fetal growth, abnormal development in one or more systems, congenital anomalies, carcinogenesis, or fetal death. Whether or not the agent causes damage is the result of both maternal and fetal factors, including dose of the agent (and virulence if it is a microorganism), timing of the exposure, and host susceptibility (that of both mother and fetus).

Exposure of the mother during the first two weeks after fertilization may not affect the fetus, since implantation has not yet occurred. Exposure of the fetus during this time may result in failure to implant or other lethal event. During the first trimester, teratogenic agents are likely to produce gross structural abnormalities as organogenesis is occurring at this time. Particularly sensitive periods for different organs are illustrated in Figure 2-15. After the first trimester, only the nervous system continues to differentiate. Fetotoxic effects in the last two-thirds of gestation mainly involve interference with the size and number of cells, producing more minor structural or functional defects.

Teratogenic effects may be produced by chemical agents, microorganisms, irradiation, and abnormalities in the maternal environment.

Although the harmful effects of alcohol consumption during pregnancy have been recognized since biblical times, it was not until 1973 that the name *fetal alcohol syndrome* (FAS) was used to describe a specific constellation of abnormalities seen in the children of chronic alcoholic mothers [11]. The Fetal Alcohol Syndrome Study Group of the Research Society on Alcoholism has proposed that FAS be diagnosed by the presence of signs in each of three categories: (1) prenatal and/or postnatal growth retardation; (2) central nervous system involvement; and (3) characteristic facial dysmorphism [14]. The term *fetal alcohol effects* (FAE) is sometimes used to describe the manifestations of fetal alcohol exposure when all of the criteria for FAS are not present.

Abundant evidence links *maternal cigarette smoking* to fetal damage. Problems include "an increased spontaneous abortion rate, an increased perinatal mortality rate, an increased incidence of maternal complications such as placenta abruptio and placenta previa, decreased birth weight and size in later childhood, an increased incidence of preterm delivery, and lower Apgar scores at 1 min and 5 min after birth" [2, p. 229]. The mechanism by which cigarette smoking produces damage is not known, but may be related to a lack of available oxygen or to toxicity of certain products of the smoke.

Microorganisms that infect a pregnant woman may damage the fetus by direct infection or by altering the maternal environment. Consequences of maternal infection include increased reproductive loss, prematurity, congenital malformations, and growth retardation. Fetotoxic effects can be produced by certain viruses, bacteria, fungi, and protozoa, with the majority attributable to viruses. Among these are cytomegaloviruses, rubella, varicella zoster, herpes simplex 1 and 2, and Venezuelan equine encephalitis virus. In the United States, most fetal damage is produced by members of the STORCH group of infections, which are composed of syphilis (a bacterial infection), toxoplasmosis (a protozoan infection), rubella, cytomegalovirus, and herpes simplex.

Exposure to *radiation* at any time during gestation can produce detrimental effects, and the question of what dose level may be considered safe is controversial. Diagnostic exposure of less than 5 rad to the fetus during the first trimester is generally considered safe with respect to teratogenic effects [4]. Exposure to 1 to 2 rad has been reported to increase the possibility of leukemia 1.5-fold to 3-fold [2]. Fifty rad can produce microcephaly, mental retardation, cataracts, abnormalities in the genital and skeletal systems, and other defects. Mechanisms of radiation damage that have been noted include the killing of brain cells (which cannot be replaced), chromosome breakage, production of aneuploidy resulting in Down or Turner syndrome, and destruction of specific tissues (e.g., the fetal thyroid by radioactive iodine).

Advances in the treatment of chronic diseases such as diabetes mellitus have resulted in an increase in the number of women with metabolic or genetic disorders who survive and become pregnant. These pregnancies are often at high risk due to the *altered maternal environment* in which the fetus must develop. Probably the hyperglycemia and ketoacidosis that accompany poorly controlled diabetes are the cause of the threefold to fourfold increase in congenital anomalies and the other problems encountered with offspring of diabetic women.

The possibility of damage to offspring of mothers with PKU was previously mentioned. Other conditions in which the maternal physiology has been known to affect the fetus include hyperthermia (from fever, sauna, or hot tub), Marfan syndrome (due to stress on the maternal cardiovascular system), homocystinuria, histidinemia, myotonic dystrophy, and acute intermittent porphyria.)

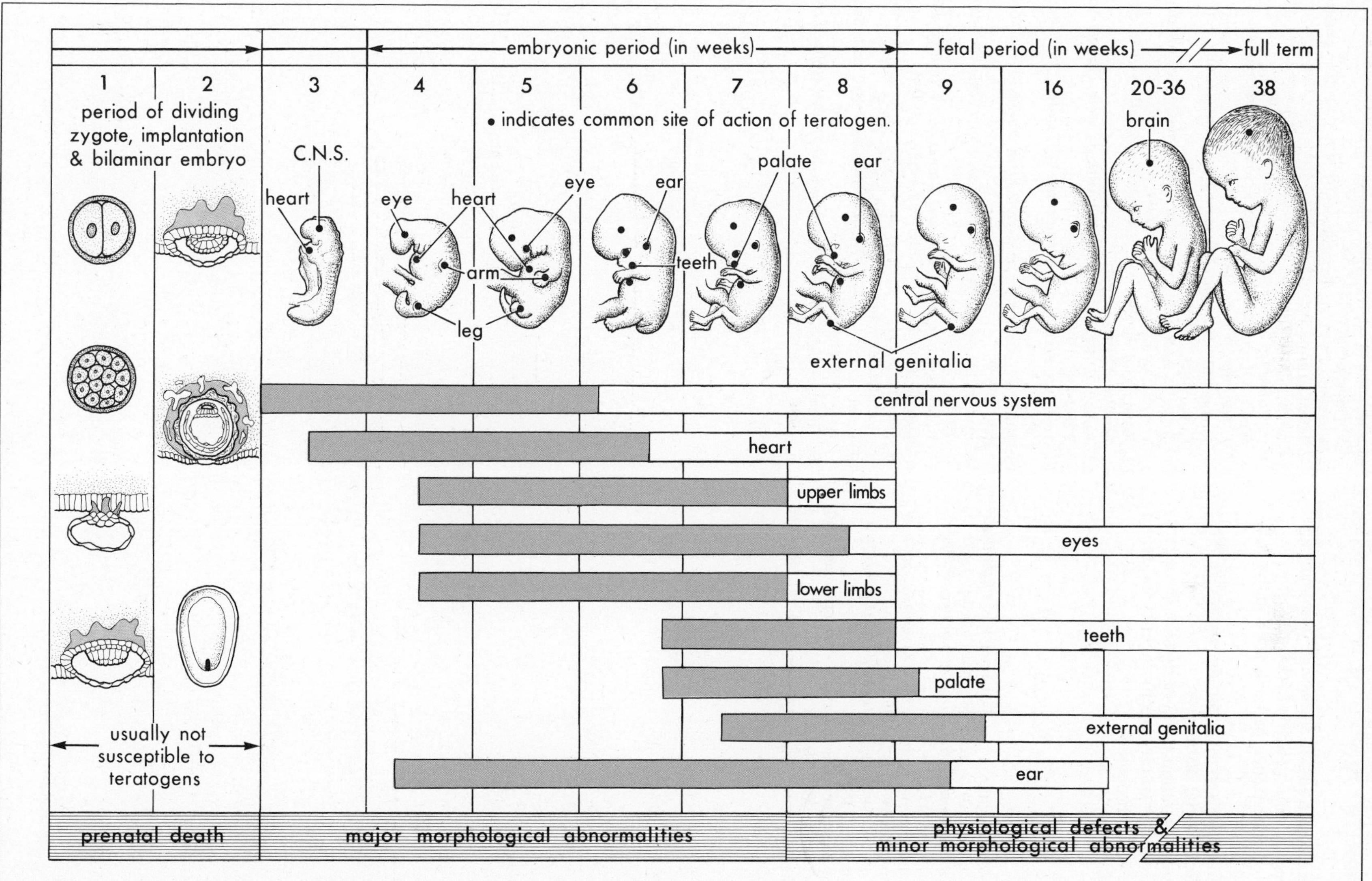

FIGURE 2-15 Schematic illustration of the sensitive or critical periods in human development. Dark bar denotes highly sensitive periods; light bar indicates stages that are less sensitive to teratogens. (From K.L. Moore, *Before We Are Born* [2nd ed.]. Philadelphia, W.B. Saunders Company, 1983, p. 111. Reprinted by permission.)

Study Questions

1. How do the manifestations of autosomal dominant and autosomal recessive inheritance patterns differ?
2. Why are X-linked inheritance patterns seen more commonly than Y-linked?
3. What are the limitations in ascertaining specific genetic patterns in multifactorial disorders?
4. Describe the most common types of genetic disorders.
5. How does knowledge of teratogenic agents influence the prevention of birth defects?

References

1. Cawson, R.A., McCracken, A.W., and Marcus, P.B. *Pathologic Mechanisms and Human Disease*. St. Louis: Mosby, 1982.
2. Cohen, F.L. *Clinical Genetics in Nursing Practice*. Philadelphia: Lippincott, 1984.
3. Connor, J.M., and Ferguson-Smith, M.A. *Essential Medical Genetics*. Oxford: Blackwell Scientific, 1984.
4. Creasy, R.K., and Resnik, R. *Maternal-Fetal Medicine*. Philadelphia: Saunders, 1984.
5. Fraser, F.C. The multifactorial/threshold concept: Uses and misuses. *Teratology* 14:276, 1976.
6. Frizzell, R.A., Rechkemmer, G., and Shoemaker, R.L. Altered regulation of airway epithelial cell chloride channels in cystic fibrosis. *Science* 233:558, 1986.
7. Gusella, J.F., et al. A polymorphic DNA marker genetically linked to Huntington's disease. *Nature* 306:234, 1983.
8. Hook, E.B., and Porter, I.H. *Population Cytogenetics: Studies in Humans*. New York: Academic Press, 1977.
9. Illis, L. On porphyria and the aetiology of werewolves. *Proc. R. Soc. Med.* 57:23, 1964.
10. Jenkins, J.B. *Human Genetics*. Menlo Park, Calif.: Benjamin/Cummings, 1983.
11. Jones, K.L., et al. Pattern of malformation in offspring of chronic alcoholic mothers. *Lancet* 1:1267, 1973.
12. Kolata, G. Research news: A new approach to cystic fibrosis. *Science* 228:167, 1985.
13. Kolata, G. Research news: Clotting protein cloned. *Science* 228:1415, 1985.
14. Lele, A.S. Fetal alcohol syndrome. *NY State J. Med.* 82:1225, 1982.
15. Muir, B.L. *Essentials of Genetics for Nurses*. New York: Wiley, 1983.
16. Porter, I.H. *Heredity and Disease*. New York: McGraw-Hill, 1968.
17. Robbins, S.L., Cotran, R.S., and Kumar, V. *Pathologic Basis of Disease* (3rd ed.). Philadelphia: Saunders, 1984.
18. Stel, H.V., et al. Von Willebrand factor in the vessel wall mediates platelet adherence. *Blood* 65:85, 1985.
19. Stern, C. *Principles of Human Genetics* (3rd ed.). San Francisco: Freeman, 1973.
20. Thompson, J.S. *Genetics in Medicine*. Philadelphia: Saunders, 1980.

CHAPTER 3

Alterations in Normal Cellular Processes Resulting in Adaptive or Lethal Change

CHAPTER OUTLINE

Stimuli That Can Cause Cellular Injury or Adaptation

Intracellular and Extracellular Changes Resulting from Cellular Adaptation or Injury

- Cellular Swelling
- Lipid Accumulation
- Glycogen Depositions
- Pigmentation
- Calcification
- Hyaline Infiltration

Cellular Changes Due to Injurious Stimuli

- Atrophy
- Dysplasia
- Hypertrophy
- Hyperplasia
- Metaplasia

Injury and Death of Cells Due to Lack of Oxygen

- Ischemia
- Thrombosis
- Embolism
- Infarction
- Necrosis
- Somatic Death

LEARNING OBJECTIVES

1. Define *adaptation*.
2. Describe alterations in cells that can occur because of stimuli.
3. List the six categories of stimuli that can cause cellular alterations.
4. Differentiate between endogenous and exogenous substances.
5. Describe the abnormal intracellular accumulations that result from noxious stimulation.
6. Discuss briefly extracellular changes resulting from cellular adaptation or injury.
7. Define the common pigments that may accumulate in the cytoplasm.
8. Discriminate among the following pathologic cellular adaptations: atrophy, dysplasia, hypertrophy, hyperplasia, and metaplasia.
9. Define *autophagic vacuoles* and *residual bodies*.
10. Differentiate between ischemia and infarction.
11. Define and describe the factors that can produce thrombosis and embolism.
12. Describe the pathologic characteristic of infarcts.
13. Specify areas in which bacterial supergrowth may occur.
14. List and describe the five major types of necrosis.
15. Explain the major changes that occur after somatic death.

The life cycle of a cell exists on a continuum that includes normal activities and adaptation, injury, or lethal changes. The pathologic changes exhibited may be obvious or very difficult to detect. The cell constantly makes adjustments to a changing, hostile environment in order to keep the organism functioning in a normal steady state. These adjustments are termed *adaptation* and are necessary to ensure the survival of the organism. *Adaptive changes* may be temporary or permanent. The point at which an adapted cell becomes an injured cell is the point at which the cell cannot functionally keep up with the stressful environment affecting it. Injured cells exhibit alterations that may affect body function and be manifested as disease.

Chapter 4 more explicitly explains the concepts of stress and stressors to illustrate how the stress response can cause the manifestations of disease. Prevention of disease is dependent upon the capacity of the affected cells to undergo self-repair and regeneration. This process of repair prevents cellular injury and death, and may prevent the death of the host.

Specifically, adaptation is a return of the internal environment of the body to the steady state or normal balance after exposure to some alteration. The rigid electrolyte and water balance between the intracellular and extracellular fluid must be maintained (see Chap. 5). The steady state may be attained at the expense of altered intracellular metabolism and may continue for a certain period of time, after which the cell, no longer able to adapt, may undergo injurious or lethal changes.

When cells are confronted with a stimulus that alters normal cellular metabolism, they may do any one or more of the following: (1) increase concentrations of normal cellular constituents; (2) accumulate abnormal substances; (3) change the cellular size or number; or (4) undergo a lethal change. These concepts are considered briefly in this chapter and delineated further in specific content areas. Categories of stimuli that can provoke changes and the types of changes that may occur are discussed in this chapter.

Stimuli That Can Cause Cellular Injury or Adaptation

Because the cell is constantly making adjustments to a changing, hostile environment, many agents potentially can cause cellular injury or adaptation. Cellular injury may lead to further injury and death of the cell, or the cell may respond to the noxious stimulation by undergoing a change that enables it to tolerate the invasion.

Stimuli that can alter the steady state are categorized as follows: (1) physical agents, (2) chemical agents, (3) microorganisms, (4) hypoxia, (5) genetic defects, (6) nutritional imbalances, and (7) immunologic reactions (Table 3-1).

Table 3-1 Stimuli That Can Cause Cellular Injury

Stimuli	Injury
Physical agents	Trauma, thermal or electrical changes, irradiation
Chemical agents	Drugs, poisons, foods, toxic and irritating substances
Microorganisms	Viruses, bacteria, fungi, protozoa
Hypoxia	Shock, localized areas of inadequate blood supply, hypoxemia
Genetic defects	Inborn errors of metabolism, gross malformations
Nutritional imbalances	Protein-calorie malnutrition, excessive intake of fats, carbohydrates, and proteins
Immunologic reactions	Hypersensitivity reactions to foreign proteins

Physical agents are such factors as mechanical trauma, temperature gradients, electrical stimulation, atmospheric pressure gradients, and irradiation. Physical stimuli directly damage cells, cause rupture or damage of the cell walls, and disrupt cellular reproduction.

Chemical agents that can cause cellular injury may include simple compounds such as glucose or complex agents such as poisons. Therapeutic drugs often chemically disrupt the normal cellular balance.

Microorganisms cause cellular injury in a variety of ways depending on the type of organism and the innate defense of the human body. Some bacteria secrete exotoxins, which are injurious to the host. Others liberate endotoxins when they are destroyed. Viruses interfere with the metabolism of the host cells and cause cellular injury by releasing viral proteins toxic to the cell (see Chap. 8).

Hypoxia is the most common cause of cellular injury and may be produced by inadequate oxygen in the blood or by decreased perfusion of blood to the tissues. The end results are disturbance of cellular metabolism and local or generalized release of lactic acid (see Chaps. 6 and 7).

Genetic defects can affect cellular metabolism through inborn errors of metabolism or gross malformations. The mechanisms for cellular disruption vary widely with the genetic defect but may result in intracellular accumulation of abnormal material (see Chap. 2)

Nutritional imbalances produce sickness and death in over one-half of the world's population. The imbalances include serious deficiencies of proteins and vitamins especially. Malnutrition may be primary or secondary, depending upon whether it is a socioeconomic problem in the underprivileged areas of the world or is self- or disease-induced. No matter the cause, nutritional deficiency is a significant cause of cellular dysfunction and death. On the other hand, excessive food intake leads to nutritional imbalances and cell injury through the production of excessive lipids in the body. Excessive intake has been shown to be associated with cardiovascular diseases, and respiratory and gastrointestinal disorders [5,6].

Immunologic agents may cause cellular injury, especially when hypersensitivity reactions occur, causing the release of excess histamine and other substances. This response is discussed in more detail in Chapter 12.

Intracellular and Extracellular Changes Resulting from Cellular Adaptation or Injury

Abnormal intracellular accumulations often result from an environmental change or inability of the cell to process materials. Normal or abnormal substances that cannot be metabolized may accumulate in the cytoplasm. These substances may be *endogenous* (produced within the body) or *exogenous* (produced in the environment) and stored by an originally normal cell. Examples of abnormal exogenous substances include carbon particles, silica, and metals that are deposited and accumulate because the cell cannot degrade them or transport them to other sites [1].

Common changes in and around cells include swelling, lipid accumulation in organs, glycogen depositions, pigmentation, calcification, and hyaline infiltration.

Cellular Swelling

Cellular swelling is the initial response to disruption of cellular metabolism. It occurs most frequently with cellular hypoxia and impairs the cell's ability to synthesize adenosine triphosphate (ATP). It results in a shift of extracellular fluid to the intracellular compartment, causing cloudy intracellular swelling with enlargement of the cell [2,4]. Ultimately, organs are affected. Cellular swelling is frequently reversible when sufficient oxygen is delivered to the cell and normal ATP synthesis resumes. Continued accumulation of water in the cells often has the appearance of small or large vacuoles of water, which may represent portions of endoplasmic reticulum (ER) that have been sequestered [3,4].

Lipid Accumulation

Lipid accumulation refers to a *fatty change process* that occurs in the cytoplasm of parenchymal cells of certain organs. Fat droplets accumulate as a result of improper metabolism and commonly are present in degenerative liver conditions. The heart and kidneys also can undergo fatty change when placed under abnormal stimulation, such as exposure to hepatotoxins or hypoxia.

Large, fatty intracellular accumulations have been shown to stimulate progressive necrosis, fibrosis, and scarring of organs. This leads to functional impairment of the involved organ (Fig. 3-1).

Fatty change of the liver is very common. Pathologically, the liver is enlarged, yellow, and greasy-looking, and infiltration may involve all or only a portion of the organ [4]. Microscopically, the cytoplasm may be filled with lipid, which pushes the nucleus and other cytoplasmic structures to one side. The predominant lipid involved in fatty change of the liver is triglyceride; its presence may be a result of increased synthesis or decreased secretion of

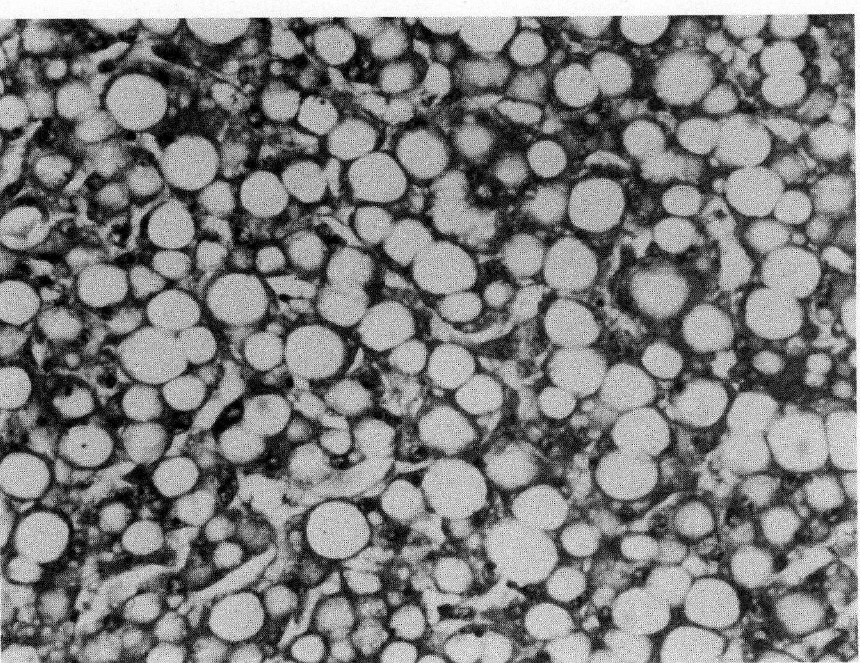

FIGURE 3-1 Fatty change of the liver. (Magnification before reduction: ×400) (From F. Miller, *Peery and Miller's Pathology* [3rd ed.]. Boston: Little, Brown, 1978.)

alcohol

this lipid from the cell. This fatty change is the initial change seen in the alcoholic liver because alcohol increases free fatty acid mobilization, decreases triglyceride use, blocks lipoprotein excretion, and directly damages ER through the liberation of free radicals. The mechanism of the process is continually being studied [6]. Protein-calorie malnutrition (PCM) causes a decrease in synthesis of cellular proteins necessary for attaching to and transporting the lipids from the cell, so that fatty change also occurs in PCM [5,6]. Other hepatotoxins such as carbon tetrachloride (CCl_4) may also cause this change [4]. The fibrous scarring of cirrhosis, discussed in Chapter 39, appears to result from a reaction to the lipid infiltration in the cytoplasm of hepatocytes.

The cells of the heart and kidneys also undergo fatty change under abnormal stimulation. It most commonly occurs in the heart after chronic hypoxia and may be patchy or diffuse. If diffuse, severe infections or toxic states are usually the causative factors. The kidneys show increased fatty change around the proximal convoluted tubules of the nephrons, often induced by exposure to certain nephrotoxins or poisons.

Associated with intracellular lipid accumulation is *interstitial fatty infiltration*, a condition that occurs with obesity. Fat cells accumulate between the parenchymal cells of an organ, probably as a result of the transformation of interstitial connective tissue cells to fat cells [4]. This condition rarely seems to affect the function of the organ and localizes most frequently in the heart and pancreas of the extremely obese individual. Other effects of obesity involve fat cells laid down during gestation, during the first year of life, and immediately after puberty. The obese child develops an increased number of fat cells that remain for life but decrease in size after weight loss [5]. Adult-onset obesity, for the most part, occurs when caloric intake exceeds energy requirements and the excess is converted to fat. Areas of subcutaneous fat distribution are related to hereditary characteristics.

Glycogen Depositions

Excess deposition of glycogen in organs and tissues occurs with different types of genetic disorders. One group, called *glycogen storage diseases*, results from specific enzyme deficiencies. Different forms of glycogen accumulate in skeletal and cardiac muscle as well as in the liver and kidneys. Glycogen disturbances also occur in diabetes mellitus with a greater than normal storage of glycogen in the proximal convoluted tubules and in the liver [4]. This disturbance is related to a deficiency in the pancreatic hormone, insulin.

Pigmentation

Pigments are substances that have color and accumulate within the cells. Many types have been described, some of which are normal components of cells and some abnormal ones that collect in cells under abnormal stimulation [6]. Pigments are often described as to source or origin: exogenous (outside the body) or endogenous (produced within the body) [4,7].

Lipofuscin pigmentation of the skin is common in the aging person. The pigment responsible is *lipofuscin* or *lipochrome*, which is the "wear-and-tear" pigment and is predominant in cells that have atrophied or are chronically injured [6]. It also may be present in the brain, liver, heart, and ovaries of an elderly individual. The pigments gradually accumulate with age and apparently do not cause cellular dysfunction.

Melanin is a pigment that is formed by the melanocytes of the skin. It is one of the pigments that impart color to the skin. It also absorbs light and protects the skin from direct sun rays. Excessive deposition of melanin in the skin is common with Addison's disease (see Chap. 33), many skin conditions, and melanomas that arise from these cells. In the aged person, melanocyte activity is decreased and the skin becomes paler, with areas of hyperpigmentation called liver spots or lentigines [4].

Hemosiderin, a derivative of hemoglobin, is a pigment that is formed from excess accumulation of stored iron. It is often a hemoglobin-derived substance, but may be formed due to excess intake of dietary iron or impaired use of iron. Hemosiderin deposits are present in many pathologic states. One example of localized hemosiderosis is the common *bruise*, which is an accumulation of hemosiderin after the erythrocytes in the injured area are broken down by macrophages. The excess hemoglobin thus released becomes hemosiderin. The colors occur as the hemoglobin is transformed first to biliverdin (green bile), then bilirubin (red bile), and the golden-yellow hemosiderin [6]. Deposits of hemosiderin in organs and tissues is called *hemosiderosis*, which may occur with excess of absorbed dietary iron, impaired use of iron, or the hemolytic anemias [4]. For the most part, accumulation of hemosiderin does not interfere with organ function unless it is extreme. In extreme hemosiderosis of the liver, fibrosis may result.

Calcification

Pathologic calcification may occur in the skin, the soft tissues, blood vessels, heart, and kidneys. Normally, calcium is deposited only in the bones and teeth under the influence of various hormones. It may precipitate in areas of chronic inflammation or areas of dead or degenerating tissue. Calcium that precipitates into areas of unresolved healing is called *dystrophic calcification* (Fig. 3-2). *Metastatic calcification* results from calcium-phosphorus imbalance associated with excess circulating calcium. Calcium precipitates into many areas, including kidneys, blood vessels, and connective tissue.

Hyaline Infiltration

Hyaline is a word that indicates a characteristic alteration within cells or in the extracellular space that appears as a homogeneous, glassy, pink inclusion on stained histologic section [4,6]. Because it does not represent a specific pattern of accumulation, different mechanisms are responsible for its formation. Intracellular hyaline changes may include excessive amounts of protein, aggregates of immunoglobulin, viral nucleoproteins, closely packed fibrils,

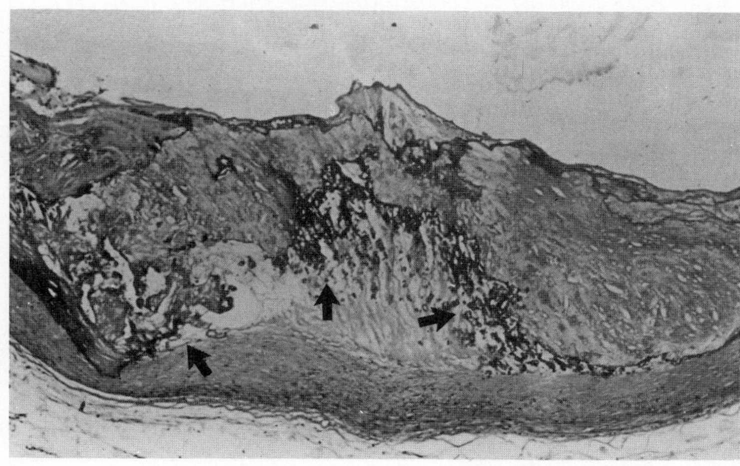

A

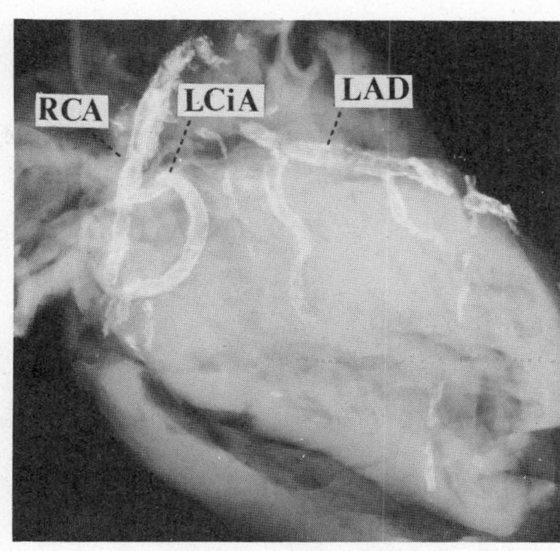

B

FIGURE 3-2 Calcification. A. Photomicrograph of section of left anterior descending coronary artery. There is marked atheromatous thickening of the intima. Calcification of the wall (*arrows*) is prominent and is found microscopically at autopsy in the coronary arteries of a majority of patients over age 60 years. B. Radiograph of postmortem heart. Dense calcification is visible in virtually all branches of the coronary arteries, including the left anterior descending, left circumflex, and right coronary arteries. Note that the lumen in the presence of calcification may be quite adequate, but that in this patient, severe atherosclerosis has occluded the distal left anterior descending coronary artery and narrowed several branches. (From H.L. Abrams [ed.], *Coronary Arteriography*. Boston: Little, Brown, 1983.)

or other substances [1,4]. Extracellular hyaline refers to the appearance of precipitated plasma proteins and other proteins across a membrane wall. This change is particularly well seen in and around the arterioles and the renal glomeruli. A variety of mechanisms causes the hyaline change, and the implications of this deposition differ depending on the underlying process.

Cellular Changes Due to Injurious Stimuli

In some cases the cell undergoes an actual change so as to adapt to an injurious agent. The changes often manifested are atrophy, dysplasia, hypertrophy, hyperplasia, and metaplasia. These adaptations are methods by which the cell stays alive and adjusts workload to demand.

Atrophy

Atrophy refers to a decrease in cell size resulting from decreased workload, loss of nerve supply, decreased blood supply, inadequate nutrition, or loss of hormonal stimulation [4]. The word implies previous normal development of the cell and that the cell has lost structural components and substance (Fig. 3-3).

Physiologic atrophy occurs with aging in many areas and allows for survival of cells with decreased function. The cells tend to reproduce less readily. Physiologic atrophy begins in the thymus gland in early adulthood and in the uterus after menopause. Many cells in other glands and muscles also undergo atrophy with aging. These cells may develop an increase in the number of autophagic vacuoles in the cytoplasm that isolate and destroy injured organelles. The triggering mechanism for autophagia is unknown, but it may result in incompletely digested material called *residual* bodies [6]. An example of this is the lipofuscin or brownish pigment seen in the aging cell. Atrophy may progress to cellular injury and death, and the cells may be replaced with connective and/or adipose tissue.

Disuse atrophy is common after an extremity has been immobilized in a cast. The decreased workload placed on the affected muscles results in decreased size of the entire muscle. When the workload is again restored, the muscle often enlarges to its preinjury size.

Loss of nerve supply may also cause muscular atrophy. An example of this is the spinal cord injury that interrupts nervous stimulation to the muscles below the level of injury. The muscles gradually atrophy, and eventually musculature is replaced by fibrous tissue (see Chap. 40). Atrophy of muscles may also be seen with chronic ischemic disease of the lower extremities. The decreased blood supply impairs the metabolism within the cell, and atrophy occurs as a protective mechanism to keep the tissue viable.

Dysplasia

Dysplasia refers to the appearance of cells that have undergone some atypical changes in response to chronic irritation. It is not a true adaptive process in that it serves no specific function. Dysplasia is presumably controlled reproduction of cells, but it is closely related to malignancy in that it may transform into uncontrolled, rapid reproduction. Epithelial cells are the most common types to exhibit

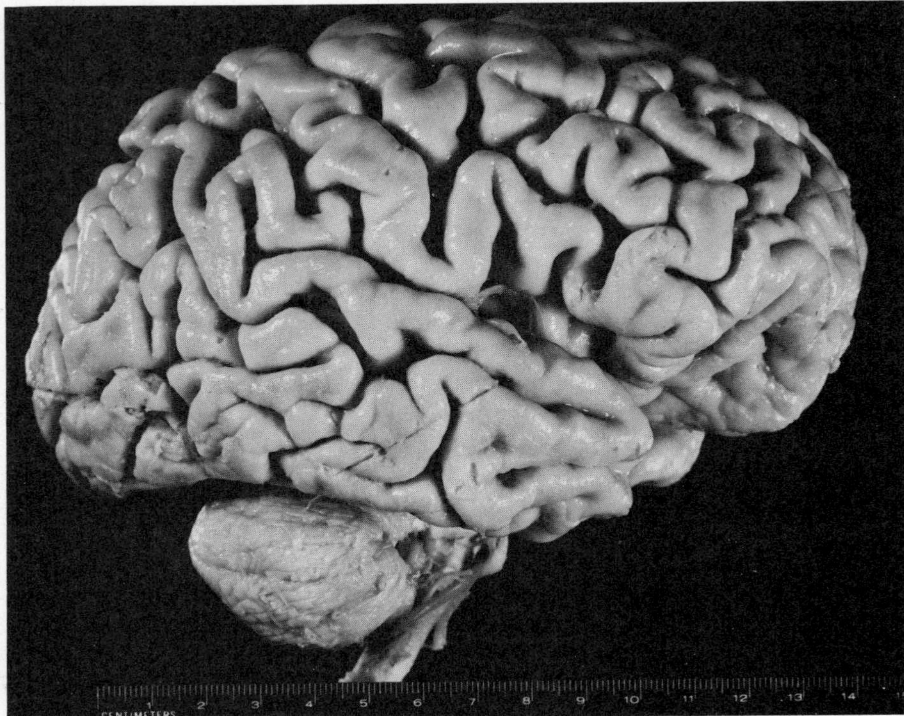

FIGURE 3-3 Atrophy of the cerebral cortex. There has been pronounced shrinking of the rounded folds that normally constitute the brain's outer surface. Severe, generalized shrinkage of this sort is uncommon, and the cause is unknown. So-called senile changes in the brain of most elderly persons are much less severe than the degree of shrinkage shown here. (From F.K. Widmann, *Pathobiology: How Disease Happens*. Boston: Little, Brown, 1978.)

dysplasia; changes include alterations in the size and shape of cells, causing loss of normal architectural orientation of one cell with the next. Dysplastic changes frequently occur in the bronchi of chronic smokers and in the cervical epithelium [6].

Hypertrophy

Hypertrophy is an increase in the size of individual cells, resulting in increased tissue mass without an increase in the number of cells. It usually represents the response of a specific organ to an increased demand for work. Hypertrophied cells increase their number of intracellular organelles, especially mitochondria. A good example of physiologic hypertrophy is the enlargement of muscles of athletes or weight lifters. The individual muscle cells enlarge but do not proliferate, and this provides increased strength. Limiting factors to hypertrophy exist, and these may have to do with limitation to the vascular supply or the capability of cells to produce energy. Hypertrophy may also be pathologic and frequently affects the myocardium (Fig. 3-4).

Hyperplasia

Hyperplasia is a common condition seen in cells that are under an increased physiologic workload or stimulation. It is defined as increase of tissue mass due to an increase in the number of cells. Cells that undergo hyperplasia are those that are capable of dividing and thus of increasing their number. Whether hyperplasia, rather than hypertrophy, occurs depends on the regenerative capacity of the specific cell.

Physiologic hyperplasia is a normal outcome of puberty and pregnancy. *Compensatory hyperplasia* occurs in organs that are capable of regenerating lost substance. An example is regeneration of the liver when part of its substance is destroyed. *Pathologic hyperplasia* is seen in conditions of abnormal stimulation of organs with cells that are capable of regeneration. Examples are enlargement of the thyroid gland secondary to stimulation by thyroid-stimulating hormone from the pituitary, and parathyroid hyperplasia due to renal failure.

Hyperplasia is induced by a known stimulus and almost always stops when the stimulus has been removed. This controlled reproduction is an important differentiating feature of hyperplasia from neoplasia. There is a close relationship between certain types of pathologic hyperplasia and malignancy (see Chap. 13).

Metaplasia

Metaplasia is a reversible change in which one type of adult cell is replaced by another type. It is probably an

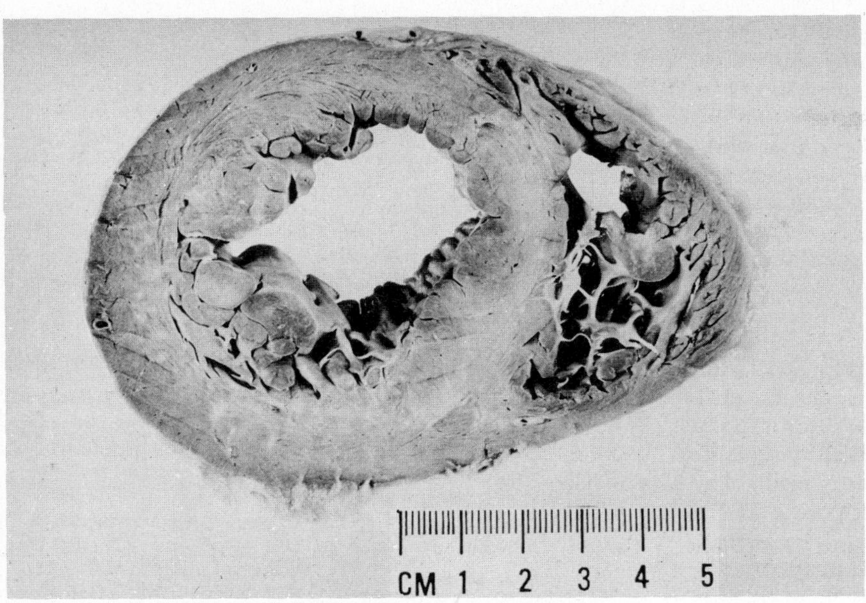

FIGURE 3-4 Hypertrophy of the myocardium. (From F. Miller, *Peery and Miller's Pathology* [3rd ed.]. Boston: Little, Brown, 1978.)

adaptive substitution of one cell type, more suited to the hostile environment, for another [2,7]. Metaplasia is commonly seen in chronic bronchitis; the normal columnar, ciliated goblet cells are replaced by stratified squamous epithelial cells. The latter cells are better suited for survival in the face of chronic, irritating smoke inhalation or environmental pollution. Metaplasia increases the chances of cellular survival but decreases the protective aspect of mucus secretion. Certain types of metaplasia are closely related to malignancy, which probably indicates that chronic irritation causes the initial change.

Injury and Death of Cells Due to Lack of Oxygen

Lack of oxygen is the most common cause of cellular injury and death. The following conditions can produce this problem: ischemia, thrombosis, embolism, infarction, necrosis, and somatic death. In some instances the injury is reversible, or it may progress to a permanent, lethal change.

Ischemia

Ischemia refers to a critical lack of blood supply to a localized area. It is reversible in that tissues are restored to normal function when oxygen is again supplied to them. Ischemia may precede infarction or death of the tissue, or it may occur sporadically when the oxygen need outstrips the oxygen supply. It is important to differentiate between ischemia, a clinical change, and infarction, a pathologic change.

Ischemia usually occurs in the presence of atherosclerosis in the major arteries. Atherosclerosis, more fully described in Unit 8, is a lipid-depositing process with fibrofatty accumulations, or plaques, on the intimal layer of the artery. The medial layer of the artery may also become involved, predisposing it to atherosclerotic aneurysm formation. Atherosclerosis often gives rise to the formation of clots or thrombi on the plaque. These changes compromise blood flow through the artery, which then impairs oxygen supply to the tissues during increased need. In later stages the blood supply is impaired even at rest.

The classic conditions resulting from ischemia are angina pectoris and intermittent claudication. The former refers to pain from ischemia affecting the heart, and the latter refers to pain from ischemia of the lower extremities. Ischemia is often relieved by rest, and the tissues return to normal function. It may be progressive and cause *ischemic infarction*, which involves cell death due to lack of blood supply or oxygen. Lack of oxygen supply to the brain, heart, and kidneys can be tolerated for only a few minutes before damage is irreversible. The fibroblasts of connective tissue, however, have been shown to survive for much longer periods.

Ischemia also occasionally occurs after vasospasm of coronary arteries or other vessels that are unaffected by atherosclerosis. Vasospasm may be induced by many factors including nicotine, exposure to cold, and in some cases, stress.

Thrombosis

The word *thrombosis* refers to the formation of a clot on the intimal lining of the blood vessels or the heart. It may decrease blood flow or totally occlude the vessel.

The most common factor in thrombosis is disruption of the endothelial lining of the blood vessels and heart. This endothelial layer is continuous from the heart throughout the vascular circuit, including the capillaries and veins. When trauma, atherosclerosis, or other factors disrupt this layer, platelets may accumulate, and the intrinsic clotting mechanism is initiated (Fig. 3-5). The body spontaneously initiates its fibrinolytic system to dissolve the clot and reopen the vessel. This may or may not be successful in reestablishing the flow of blood. Stasis of blood and increased blood viscosity also enhance coagulability of blood.

Thrombosis most frequently occurs in the deep veins of the legs, but *mural thrombosis* may occur on the endocardial lining of the heart. If this thrombosis occurs in the left ventricle, the risk for arterial embolization is quite high (Fig. 3-6). Thrombosis in an artery can disrupt blood flow to the area supplied by the vessel and cause ischemia or infarction. Thrombosis arising in the deep veins may detach, embolize, and lodge in the pulmonary arterial circuit.

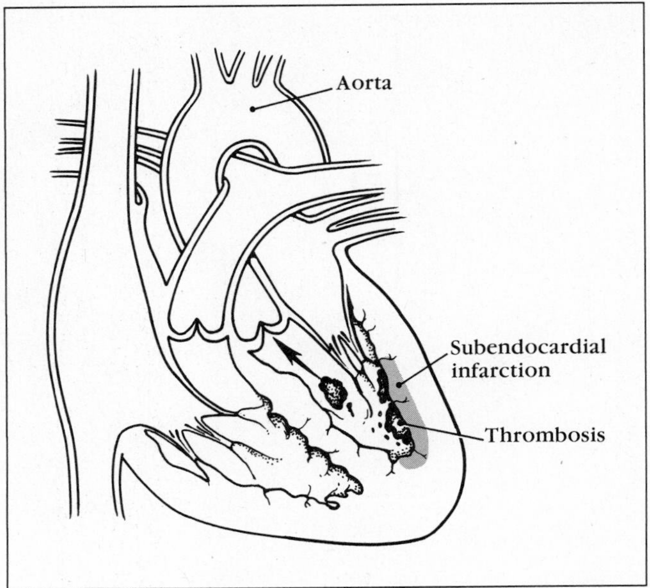

FIGURE 3-6 Disruption of the endocardial surface, such as that after a subendocardial infarction, may lead to a mural thrombosis that may become an arterial embolus.

Embolism

A thrombus may break off and become a traveling mass in the blood. This process is called *thrombotic embolization*. The most common types of emboli are derived from thrombi, but other substances such as fat, vegetations from valves, or foreign particles may embolize. The obstruction caused by an embolus is called an *embolism*.

If the embolus arises in the venous circuit, it is carried to and trapped in the vasculature of the pulmonary capillary bed. Depending on the size of the embolus, the clinical picture may vary (see Chap. 27).

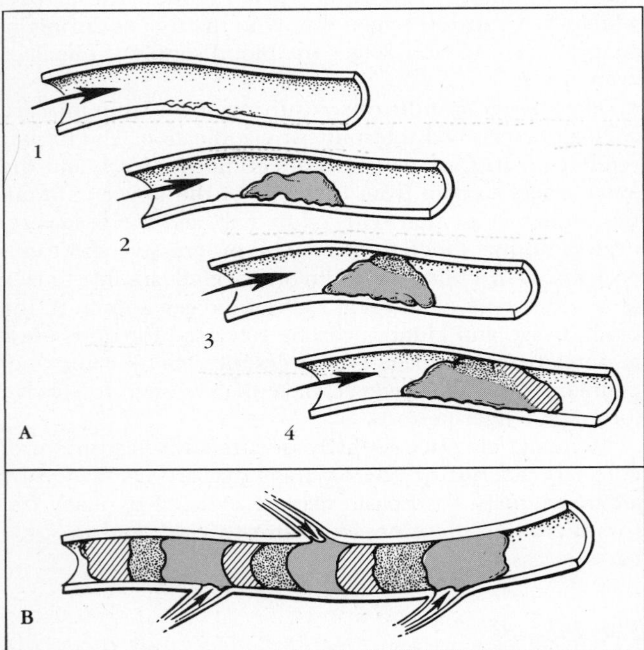

FIGURE 3-5 A. Stages in the development of phlebothrombosis: (1) intimal damage, sluggish circulation; (2) platelet aggregation; (3) occlusion of the lumen of the vein; (4) blood clot propagates. B. Clot propagates clot at each point of entry of the small veins.

If the embolus arises in the left side of the heart, it may travel to any of the arteries branching off the aorta. Arterial embolism may also occur from a larger artery, such as one affected by atherosclerosis, to a smaller artery. When it occludes the arterial tributary, it compromises blood flow to the area.

Infarction

Occlusion of the blood supply of an artery causes *infarction*, which is a localized area of tissue death due to lack of blood supply. It is also called *ischemic necrosis* and may occur in any organ or tissue.

Infarcts may have different pathologic characteristics. They are frequently classified as *pale infarcts*, *hemorrhagic infarcts*, and *infarcts with bacterial supergrowth*. Pale infarcts are seen in solid tissue deprived of its arterial circulation as a result of ischemia. Red or hemorrhagic infarcts are more frequent with venous occlusion or with congested tissues. The infarcted tissue has a red appearance, due to hemorrhage into the area, that may be poorly defined, causing difficulty in differentiating viable and nonviable tissue [2,6]. Bacterial supergrowth is common and may be present in the area or may be brought to the area.

The classification of *septic infarction* is added when there is evidence of bacterial infection in the area [6]. The lesion is converted to an abscess when it is septic and the inflammatory response is initiated. *Gangrene* is an example of infarction in which ischemic cell death is followed by bacterial overgrowth, leading to liquefaction of the tissues (Fig. 3-7). This term is frequently used to describe conditions of the extremities and the bowel [3].

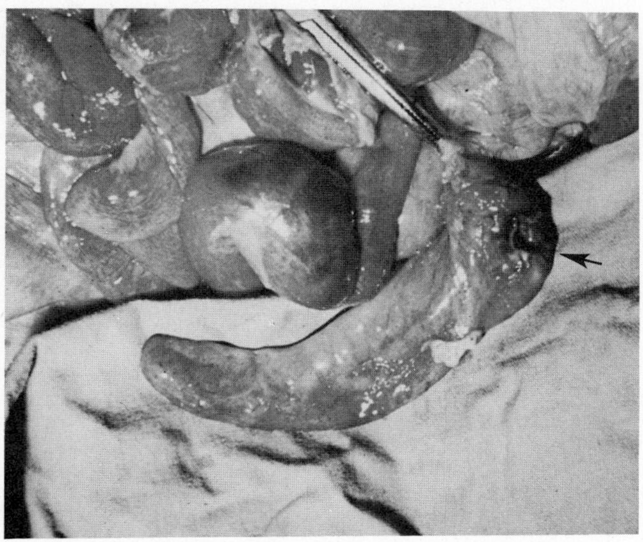

FIGURE 3-7 Acute, gangrenous appendicitis with perforation. (From F. Miller, *Peery and Miller's Pathology* [3rd ed.]. Boston: Little, Brown, 1978.)

Necrosis

The word *necrosis* refers to cell or tissue death causing characteristic cellular changes. As cells die, the mitochondria swell, functions become disrupted, membranes rupture, and the lysosomal enzymes may be released into the tissues [6]. The nucleus undergoes specific changes that may include shrinking, fragmenting, or gradual fading [3]. Necrosis is commonly described in terms of the following patterns: coagulative, caseous, and liquefactive.

Coagulative necrosis usually results from lack of blood supply to an area. It is the most common pattern of necrosis and frequently occurs in organs such as the heart and kidneys, but it may result from chemical injury. The architectural outline of the dead cell is preserved but the nucleus is lost. Eventually, the necrotic cell is removed by phagocytosis.

Caseous necrosis has long been described in relation to tuberculosis, but it may be present in a few other conditions. The central area of necrosis is soft and friable, and is surrounded by an area with a cheesy, crumbly appearance. The cellular architecture is destroyed. The area is walled off from the rest of the body and may become rimmed with calcium. Areas of caseous necrosis may localize in areas of tuberculous infestation [4].

Liquefactive necrosis most frequently occurs in brain tissue and results from fatal injury of the neuron. The breakdown of the neuron causes release of lysosomes and other constituents into the surrounding area. Lysosomes cause liquefaction of the cell and surrounding cells, leaving pockets of liquid, debris, and cystlike structures. Liquefactive necrosis is often described in brain infarction, but may be seen with bacterial lesions because of the release of bacterial and leukocytic enzymes [3,4].

Fat necrosis is a specific form of cellular death that occurs when lipases escape into fat storage areas. It occurs particularly in acute pancreatic necrosis and causes patchy necrosis of the pancreas and surrounding areas (see Chap. 35) [4,6]. *Gangrenous necrosis* is a combination of coagulative and liquefactive necroses. The cause of tissue death is ischemia, but bacteria and surrounding leukocytes cause liquefaction of the tissues. When the coagulative pattern is dominant, it is called *dry gangrene*. When the liquefactive process is more pronounced, it is called *wet gangrene* [4].

Gas gangrene is a specific type of necrosis that can occur due to *clostridia* infections. Clostridia are gram-positive anaerobes that cause such conditions as tetanus, botulism, and food poisoning [7]. Gas gangrene usually occurs in large traumatic wounds in which the organisms cause destruction of the connective tissue framework. Gas bubbles are caused by a fermentative reaction causing a blue-black semifluid appearance of involved tissues [7]. If this material reaches the bloodstream, shock and disseminated intravascular coagulation (DIC) may be produced (see Chap. 17).

Somatic Death

The body dies with the cessation of respiratory and cardiac function. The individual cells remain alive for different lengths of time, but irreversible changes occur and some of these make it difficult to determine exact premortem pathology. Postmortem changes include rigor mortis, livor mortis, algor mortis, intravascular clotting, autolysis, and putrefaction.

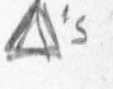

Rigor mortis develops because of depletion of ATP in the muscles, beginning in the involuntary muscles and in two to four hours affecting the voluntary muscles. The result is stiffening of the muscles, and the onset and disappearance varies among individuals. *Livor mortis* is the reddish blue discoloration of the body that results from gravitational pooling of blood. *Algor mortis* is the term used for the cooling of the body that occurs after death. The rate of cooling depends on the premortem temperature and the postmortem environmental temperature. *Intravascular clotting* results in clots that are not adherent to the lining of the blood vessels and heart. They may be layered in appearance, with streaks or layers of yellowish, fatty material. *Autolysis* refers to the digestion of tissues from released substances such as enzymes and lysosomes. Organs may be swollen and spongy in appearance. *Putrefaction* is caused by saprophytic organisms entering the dead body, usually from the intestines. This results in a greenish discoloration of the tissues and organs, and the organisms may produce gases, leading to foamy or spongy organs [2].

Study Questions

1. Describe how the body attempts to compensate for injurious stimuli. Is this compensation always of benefit to the individual?
2. Indicate how ischemia and infarction differ according to the tissue affected.
3. Which pathologic cellular adaptations are related to the development of cancer?

4. Differentiate between the effects of thrombosis and embolism.
5. How does necrosis manifest in different tissues of the body and how does this alter function?

References

1. Anderson, J.R. *Muir's Textbook of Pathology*. London: Edward Arnold, 1985.
2. Golden, A. *Pathology: Understanding Human Diseases* (2nd ed.). Baltimore: Williams & Wilkins, 1985.
3. King, D.W., Fenoglio, C.M., and Lefkowitch, J.H. *General Pathology: Principles and Dynamics*. Philadelphia: Lea & Febiger, 1983.
4. Kissane, J.M. *Anderson's Pathology* (8th ed.). St. Louis: Mosby, 1985.
5. Lewis, C.M. *Nutrition and Nutritional Therapy in Nursing*. Norwalk, Conn.: Appleton-Century-Crofts, 1986.
6. Robbins, S., and Cotran, R. *Pathologic Basis of Disease* (3rd ed.). Philadelphia: Saunders, 1984.
7. Sodeman, W.A., and Sodeman, T.M. *Sodeman's Pathologic Physiology: Mechanisms of Disease* (7th ed.). Philadelphia: Saunders, 1985.

Unit Bibliography

Anderson, J.R. *Muir's Textbook of Pathology*. London: Edward Arnold, 1985.

Ayala, F.J. and Kiger, J.A. *Modern Genetics* (12th ed.). Menlo Park, Calif.: Benjamin-Cummings, 1984.

Clarren, S.K., and Smith, D.W. The fetal alcohol syndrome. *N. Engl. J. Med.* 298:1063, 1978.

Dixon, K.C. *Cellular Defects in Disease*. Boston: Blackwell Scientific, 1982.

Elkeles, R.S., and Tavill, A.S. *Biochemical Aspects of Human Disease*. Oxford: Blackwell Scientific, 1983.

Emery, A.E.H. *Elements of Medical Genetics* (5th ed.). Edinburgh: Churchill Livingstone, 1979.

Ferguson, G.C. *Pathophysiology, Mechanisms and Expressions*. Philadelphia, Saunders, 1984.

Fisher, J.H., and Klinger, K.W. Closing in on the cystic fibrosis gene(s). *Am. Rev. Respir. Dis.* 132:1149, 1985.

Golden, A. *Pathology, Understanding Human Disease* (2nd ed.). Baltimore: Williams & Wilkins, 1985.

Guyton, A.C. *Textbook of Medical Physiology* (7th ed.). Philadelphia: Saunders, 1986.

Jensen, D. *The Principles of Physiology* (2nd ed.). New York: Appleton-Century-Crofts, 1980.

King, D.W., Fenoglio, C.M., and Lefkowitch, J.H. *General Pathology, Principles and Dynamics*. Philadelphia: Lea & Febiger, 1983.

Kolata, G. Closing in on the muscular dystrophy gene. *Science* 230:307, 1985.

MacLeod, A., and Sikora, K. *Molecular Biology and Human Disease*. Boston: Blackwell Scientific, 1984.

Moore, K.L. *Before We Are Born*. Philadelphia: Saunders, 1977.

Mottet, N.K. *Environmental Pathology*. New York: Oxford University Press, 1985.

Perez-Tamayo, R. *Mechanisms of Disease: An Introduction to Pathology* (2nd ed.). Chicago: Year Book, 1985.

Robbins, S., and Cotran, R. *Pathologic Basis of Disease* (3rd ed.). Philadelphia: Saunders, 1984.

Selkurt, E. *Basic Physiology for the Health Sciences* (2nd ed.). Boston: Little, Brown, 1982.

Sheldon, H. *Boyd's Introduction to the Study of Disease*. Philadelphia: Lea & Febiger, 1984.

Snell, R.S. *Clinical Anatomy for Medical Students* (2nd ed.). Boston: Little, Brown, 1981.

Snell, R.S. *Clinical Histology for Medical Students*. Boston: Little, Brown, 1984.

Sodeman, W.A., and Sodeman, T.M. *Sodeman's Pathologic Physiology: Mechanisms of Disease* (7th ed.). Philadelphia: Saunders, 1985.

Stanbury, J.B., et al. (eds.). *The Metabolic Basis of Inherited Disease* (5th ed.). New York: McGraw-Hill, 1983.

Taussig, M.J. *Processes in Pathology and Microbiology* (2nd ed.). Boston: Blackwell Scientific, 1984.

Thompson, J.S., and Thompson, M.W. *Genetics in Medicine* (4th ed.). Philadelphia: Saunders, 1986.

Tortora, G., Evans, R., and Anagnostakos, N. *Principles of Human Physiology*. Philadelphia: Harper & Row, 1982.

Walter, J.B. *An Introduction to the Principles of Disease* (2nd ed.). Philadelphia: Saunders, 1982.

UNIT 2

Stress

Barbara L. Bullock

This unit describes the body's physiologic response to stress and how the response can cause disease. The general systems theory is used as the framework for understanding the physiologic effects of stress. The unit also describes adaptation that allows the body to withstand tension-producing stimuli. This response occurs until a critical point is reached and exhaustion begins. The susceptibility of the individual to stress effects is related to the critical point at which these effects can cause actual disease development. The latter part of the chapter deals with some of the disease processes that are directly or indirectly related to stress effects. It is an introduction to the effects of stress in the production of disease; further information can be found in the unit bibliography. The reader is encouraged to be guided by the learning objectives at the beginning of the chapter and to review the information using the study questions at the end of the chapter.

CHAPTER 4

Stress and Disease

CHAPTER OUTLINE

General Systems Theory
Stress and Adaptation in the Human Body
Adaptation
Organ and System Function in Maintaining the Steady State

Neurologic Mechanisms
Endocrine Mechanisms

Adrenocorticotropic Hormone (ACTH)
Thyroid Stimulating Hormone (TSH)
Antidiuretic Hormone (ADH)
Aldosterone

Immunologic Mechanisms

Factors Related to Development of Disease

Genetic Predisposition
Organ Susceptibility (Weak-Organ Theory)
Unhealthful Behaviors
Personality and Attitude Toward Life

Stress and Disease

Cardiovascular Disease
Stress-Induced Immune Deficiency
Digestive Diseases
Cancer
Other Conditions

LEARNING OBJECTIVES

1. Describe the general systems theory.
2. Compare and contrast open and closed systems.
3. Illustrate examples of negative and positive feedback.
4. Define clearly the words *stress* and *stressors*.
5. Describe the general adaptation syndrome according to Hans Selye's studies.
6. Explain the chemical and hormonal mediators important in the stress response.
7. Differentiate between the general and local adaptation syndromes.
8. Define the words *adaptation* and *compensation*.
9. Describe the three physiologic mechanisms that respond to stress stimulation.
10. Identify factors that increase the risk of disease.
11. Define *genetic susceptibility*.
12. Explain briefly the weak-organ theory.
13. Identify examples of unhealthful behaviors.
14. Describe and give examples of how personalities and attitudes can contribute to the development of disease.
15. Relate diet and stressful living conditions to coronary artery disease.
16. Explain briefly the effects of catecholamines on lipids.
17. State Pelletier's theory on the relationship of stress and blood pressure.
18. Define the *type A personality*.
19. Describe the effect of stress on the immune system.
20. Relate stress to activation and progression of malignancy.
21. Relate stress to the development of stress, duodenal, and gastric ulcers.
22. Identify some effects of stress on skin, musculoskeletal, and respiratory systems.

In considering factors that cause alterations to health, it is important to realize that other variables besides direct biologic phenomena frequently cause disease or dysfunction. This chapter deals with some of the disease processes that are directly and indirectly related to stress. The physiologic factors concerning stress are also considered, and the general systems theory is used as a framework to facilitate understanding.

General Systems Theory

It is appropriate to review the systems theory in order to explain the physiologic reaction of the body to stress. Indeed, the open, physiologic organism uses relationships among its component parts to achieve a state of equilibrium, or steady state.

The general systems theory is a model for organizing and examining relationships among units. It describes *closed systems* as those that do not interact or exchange energy with their environments. The sciences of physics and physical chemistry are limited to the examination of closed systems. Conversely, *open systems* do exchange matter, energy, and information with their environments [16]. A dynamic equilibrium or relative state of balance called the *steady state* is achieved. It exists when the composition of the system is constant despite continuous exchange of components. The three fundamental qualities of open systems are structure, process, and function. *Structure* refers to the arrangement of all defined elements at a given time. *Process* is the transformation of matter, energy, and information between the system and the environment. *Function* relates to the unique manner that each open system uses to achieve its required end [9].

A feedback scheme is used to describe the fundamental qualities of open systems. This means that if a factor becomes excessive or inadequate in the body, alterations in function will be initiated to decrease or increase that factor to bring it into normal range. The processes used in this scheme include input, throughput, output, and feedback.

Input is the energy, matter, or information absorbed by the system. *Throughput* is the transformation of this energy into useful information, matter, or energy that is used by the system. The excess information, matter, or energy is discharged to the environment in a process called *output*.

Feedback, an essential component, is the process of self-regulation by which open systems determine and control the amount of input and output of the system. The two types of feedback are called *negative* and *positive feedback*. *Negative feedback* refers to a process of returning to the steady state, while *positive feedback* indicates movement away from the steady state [9]. Thus in the human body, negative feedback indicates a return to the balanced steady state; and positive feedback, unchecked, will lead to death. In the human organism, negative feedback can be readily illustrated by many functions. Figure 4-1 illustrates the feedback system used to maintain the balance of thyroid hormones. Loss of hormonal control, for example, causes disease states because the body's response becomes detrimental to the maintenance of the steady state.

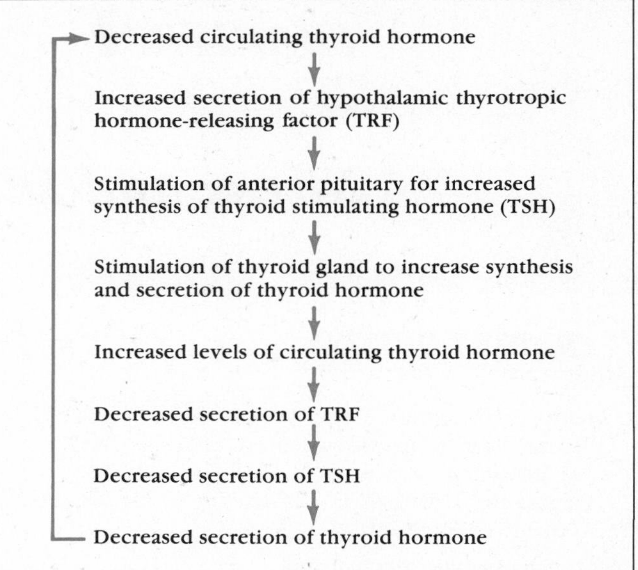

FIGURE 4-1 Feedback system illustrating functions that keep the circulating thyroid hormone in balance.

In considering the open systems theory, one must enlarge the perspective beyond the physiologic and pathophysiologic bases. The individual, as a system, has physiologic, psychosocial, environmental, and other stresses (Fig. 4-2). These factors may unite to produce a diseased or altered state, or they may have the opposite effect and reinforce adaptive behavior.

Stress and Adaptation in the Human Body

The study of the effects of stress on the human body was pioneered by Hans Selye. He studied the nonspecific response of the body to a demand and noted differences in individual abilities to withstand the same demands. He defined *stress* as a specific syndrome that is nonspecifically induced. He also defined *stressors* as tension-producing stimuli that potentially could cause disequilibrium [14]. The perception of the significance of the stressor is important and varies among individuals. It is believed that psychological stressors have as great an impact on disease states as physical stressors. Selye noted that laboratory animals reacted physiologically to different stressors by enlargement of the adrenal cortex, atrophy of the thymus gland, and development of gastric ulcers. Further study revealed a pattern including fatigue, loss of appetite, joint pains, gastric upset, and other similar nonspecific complaints.

Selye noted a similarity in sickness patterns, which at first he called "the syndrome of just being sick" and later described as the *general adaptation syndrome (GAS)* [13]. The GAS may be elicited by a variety of stimuli or stressors and may be of a physiologic, psychogenic, sociocultural, or environmental nature; or it may be from any

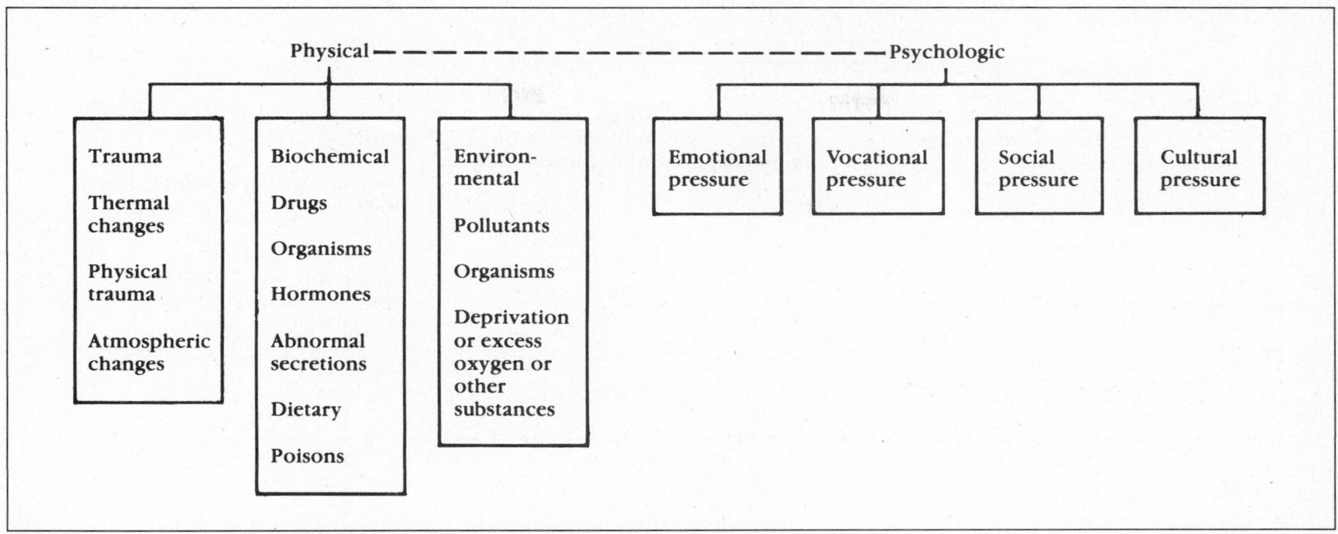

FIGURE 4-2 Stressors; types of stimuli that can provoke the stress response.

grouping of these categories. It is described in the following three stages: (1) alarm reaction, (2) stage of resistance, and (3) stage of exhaustion (Fig. 4-3).

In the *alarm stage*, the defensive abilities of the body are mobilized. The so-called *fight-or-flight* mechanism is activated mainly through the sympathetic nervous system, which releases two catecholamines, *norepinephrine* and *epinephrine*. The physiologic action of these hormones causes vasoconstriction, increased blood pressure, and increased rate and force of cardiac contraction. All of these physiologic actions prepare the body for an assault.

In the *stage of resistance,* levels of corticosteroids, thyroid hormones, and aldosterone are increased (see Fig. 4-3). The adrenal cortex enlarges and becomes hyperactive. This process increases blood sugar for available energy and stabilizes the inflammatory response. In this period, the immune system becomes depressed, causing a suppression of T cells and atrophy of the thymus gland, which leads to a depression of primary antigen-antibody response, probably due to the effect of excess corticosteroid hormone. The end result, immunologically, is suppression and atrophy of immune tissue (see Unit 5). If infection is present, it results in delayed clearing of the organisms and delayed healing.

If stage 3, *exhaustion*, occurs, it leads to depleted resistance to the stressor and ultimately to death (see Fig. 4-3). Exhaustion is frequently caused by the lack of immunologic defense, and this is considered to be an immunodeficiency secondary to stress. Selye proposed that exhaustion is a correct term for aging, a wearing down of the human body from lifelong stress [13].

Localized reaction to stressors is called the *local adaptation syndrome (LAS)*, which is well illustrated by the process of inflammation. The usual outcome of inflammation is localization and destruction of the foreign substance that triggered the process [14]. The LAS assumes the same general pattern as the GAS, with an acute phase followed by a resistance phase and exhaustion. Exhaustion of the LAS causes breakdown of the localizing mechanisms and spreading of the process, and ultimately leads to the generalized response and GAS.

Adaptation

Adaptation is defined as adjustment of an organism to a changing environment. It refers to adjustments that are made as a result of stimulation or change with the end result of modifying the original situation. An adaptive response is a type of negative feedback that maintains the organism in the steady state. Physiologic adaptation refers to the adjustments made by the organs and systems to stress or physiologic disruption. This response is often called *compensation* for abnormal stimuli. *Maladaptation* is disruptive, or tending toward positive feedback, a disordering of the physiologic response.

Organ and System Function in Maintaining the Steady State

Physiologic responses to stress stimuli (stressors) fall into three separate and interactive mechanisms: neurologic, endocrine, and immunologic. These mechanisms may promote adaptation to the stressor. Long-term application of stressors ultimately causes end-organ dysfunction through these same mechanisms [1].

Neurologic Mechanisms

Both the voluntary and autonomic divisions of the nervous system are reactive to stress. The voluntary system is mediated through the cerebral cortex, which is responsive to the stimulus. The cerebral cortex directs the muscles to move to avoid danger and effects the flight response. The combination of vasodilation in the skeletal muscle and the

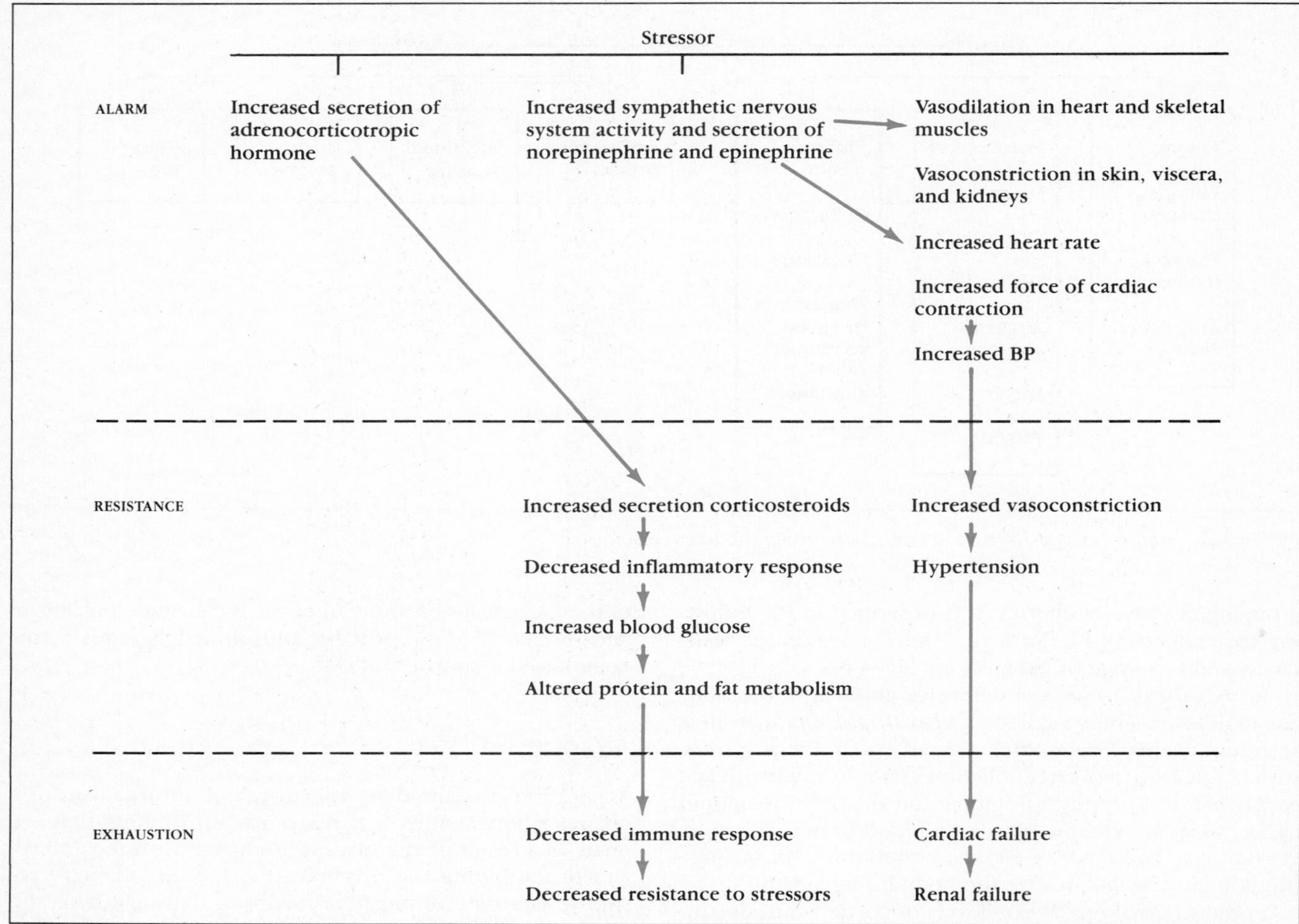

FIGURE 4-3 Stages in Selye's general adaptation syndrome.

voluntary flight response are sometimes termed the *musculoskeletal response* to a stressor.

The autonomic nervous system (ANS) is involuntary and is regulated through the hypothalamus. In the stress response, stimulation of the sympathetic nervous system (SNS) occurs, which causes an increased heart rate, constriction of many arterioles, increased respiratory rate, bronchial dilatation, dilatation of the pupils, and inhibition of the gastrointestinal tract.

Two hormones, epinephrine and norepinephrine, are necessary components of the stress response. They are classified as *catecholamines*, and their circulating levels can be measured in the urine and blood (see Chap. 33). Both are synthesized in the adrenal medulla and released when the sympathetic nervous system is activated. Norepinephrine is also synthesized and secreted at adrenergic (sympathetic) nerve terminals throughout the body and is directly released when the SNS is stimulated. Epinephrine is excreted rapidly in the urine after being biotransformed in the liver. Norepinephrine, liberated at the axon ending, is actively taken up, restored, or biotransformed here.

The primary action of epinephrine is to increase the rate and force of cardiac contraction. It is secreted as part of the stress response from the SNS stimulation of the adrenal medulla [15]. It is interesting to note that epinephrine is a potent stimulus for glycogenolysis in the liver, which leads to an increased blood glucose level [6]. In addition to accelerating the degradation of glycogen, epinephrine diverts blood from the viscera to the skeletal muscles.

Norepinephrine is secreted in small quantities in the flight-or-flight response and in acute physical or mental stress. Studies have shown a constant increase in norepinephrine levels in individuals under chronic, unremitting stress. Affected persons often feel a sense of loss of control over their lives [9]. Norepinephrine exerts its primary control over the arterioles, leading to intense vasoconstriction and increased peripheral vascular resistance (PVR), causing increased blood pressure and increased cardiac workload (Fig. 4-4) [3].

Endocrine Mechanisms

The hormones are increased in the stress response through hypothalamic stimulation of the pituitary, leading to stimulation of target organ secretion. The relationship is

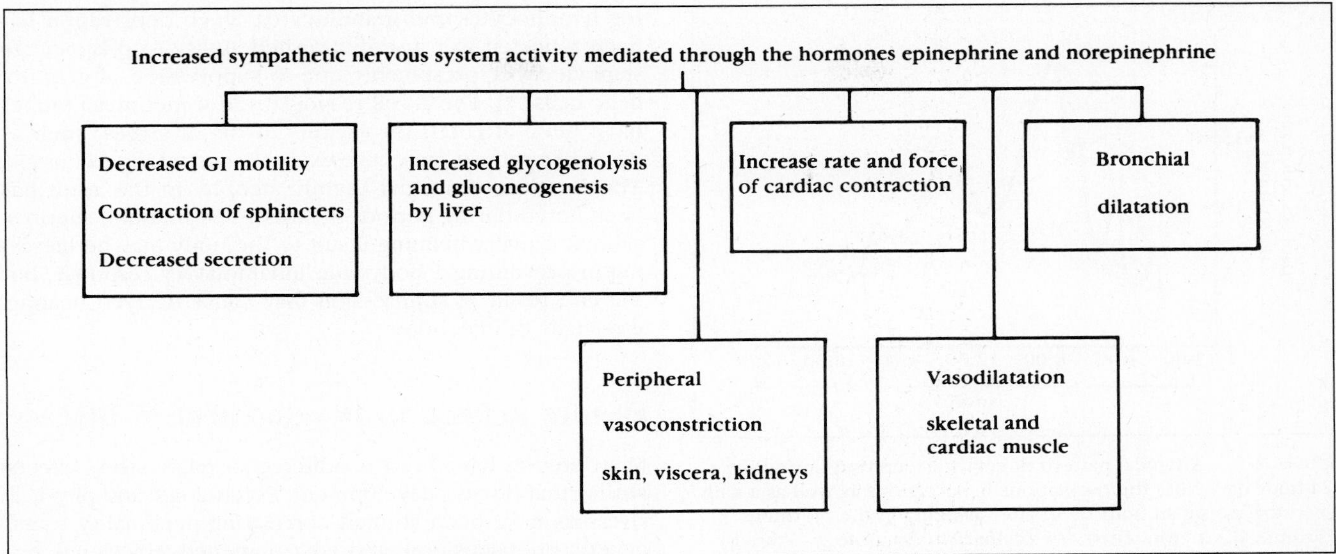

FIGURE 4-4 Sympathetic nervous system response to stress.

illustrated in Figure 4-5. Stimulation of the pituitary can increase secretion of adrenocorticotropic hormone (ACTH), antidiuretic hormone (ADH), thyroid-stimulating hormone (TSH), and others. Secretion of aldosterone is also increased from the adrenal cortex.

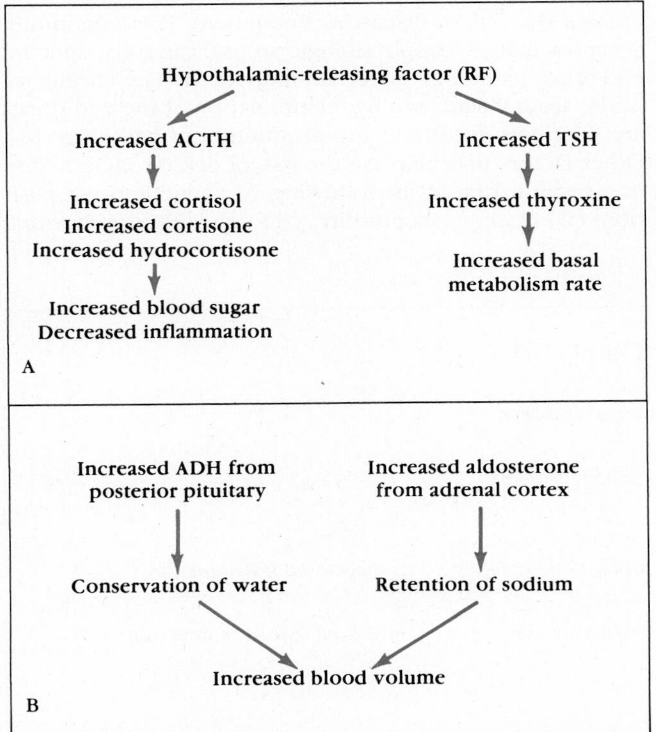

FIGURE 4-5 A. Effects of stress on hypothalamic-pituitary-target organ axis. B. Related hormonal effects of stress, possibly due to sympathetic stimulation.

Adrenocorticotropic Hormone (ACTH). The target organs of ACTH are the adrenal glands. Stimulation from this hormone causes an increased synthesis of the glucocorticoids, especially cortisol, cortisone, and small amounts of hydrocortisone. These substances increase serum glucose and alter the metabolism of carbohydrates, fat, and protein. In individuals with a day-wake–night-sleep cycle, the glucocorticoids are thought to be synchronized by light. Their concentration in blood and urine decreases during sleep and rises to its highest levels in the early morning [6]. This pattern of glucocorticoid secretion follows a particular rhythm called the *circadian rhythm* or *pattern*. The early morning high level drops about 10 A.M., increases slightly again about 2 P.M., and gradually declines until 10 P.M. (Fig. 4-6). Changes in circadian rhythm may relate to illness in that phase relationships seem to be consistent in particular maladies. For example, persons with peptic ulcer disease frequently have increased gastric acid secretion causing pain in the late night or early morning hours. Low blood levels of glucocorticoids increase the sensitivity to sounds, tastes, and smells.

Thyroid Stimulating Hormone (TSH). The stress response increases the secretion of TSH from the anterior pituitary, which leads to increased synthesis and secretion of the thyroid hormones and an increased basal metabolic rate (BMR). The effects of this increase are small and not well-coordinated with other effects of stress [3]. The thyroid hormone thyroxine apparently makes the body more responsive to the effects of epinephrine and may be the major effector of prolonged stress.

Antidiuretic Hormone (ADH). Numerous studies have shown an increase in ADH (vasopressin) secretion from the posterior pituitary in stressful situations. The general release of ADH in *any* stress reaction has not been shown consistently, but release during hypotensive

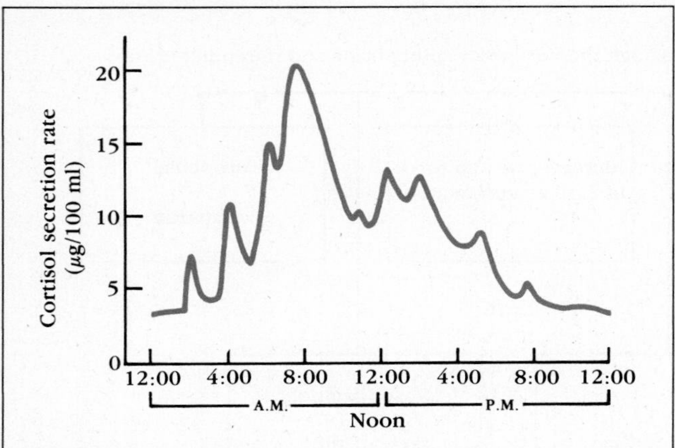

FIGURE 4-6 A typical pattern of cortisol secretion during the 24-hour day. Note the oscillations in secretions as well as a daily secretory surge an hour or so after awaking in the morning. (From A.C. Guyton, *Textbook of Medical Physiology* [7th ed.]. Philadelphia: W.B. Saunders Company, 1986. Reprinted by permission.)

episodes or in response to pain does seem to be consistent [3]. Vasopressin promotes water conservation and antidiuresis.

Aldosterone. An increased level of aldosterone is present frequently in the stress response and may, like the elevated level of ADH, be a response to hemodynamic alterations or occur when there is associated renin release. It functions in sodium and water retention (see Chap. 33).

Immunologic Mechanisms

Stress, especially chronic, unremitting stress, apparently lowers the body's defense, a response at least partly due to increased production of corticosteroids (Fig. 4-7). Corticosteroids suppress the inflammatory response by affecting lymphocytes and granulocytes. Sleep deprivation has been reported to cause diminished ability to phagocytize staphylococci, presumably due to suppression of granulocytic cells [7]. The T cell response and sometimes number have been affected by various forms of stress, such as death of a spouse, excessive exercise, and taking exams [7]. Acceleration of normal thymic atrophy in the adult has been noted during periods of stress. The immune suppression after overwhelming insult to the body may be lifesaving in preventing a bodywide inflammatory response, but the end result of suppression may cause delayed healing, especially of infections.

Factors Related to Development of Disease

Many studies have been conducted to relate stress effects with actual disease development. Psychologic and physical stressors have been studied correlating personality traits, genetic predisposition, and environmental, emotional, occupational, and social factors with specific diseases.

Some similarities in disease development have been noted around such concepts as the weak- or target-organ theory; driving or submissive personality traits; chronic, excessive, unrelenting stress factors; and/or environmental alterations. With the caution that these areas still are under study, this section describes some of the relationships between physical and/or psychological stress and specific disease phenomena. Several prominent stress-related diseases are discussed.

A maladaptive response of the body to stressors increases the risk of disease development. It is commonly accepted that psychophysiologic arousal can cause specific end-organ pathology in certain individuals. The chronicity of the arousal state and hyperstimulation of the end organ are necessary factors in the production of pathology [8]. Other factors that increase the risk of disease include one or a combination of the following: (1) genetic predisposition, (2) organ susceptibility, (3) unhealthful behaviors,

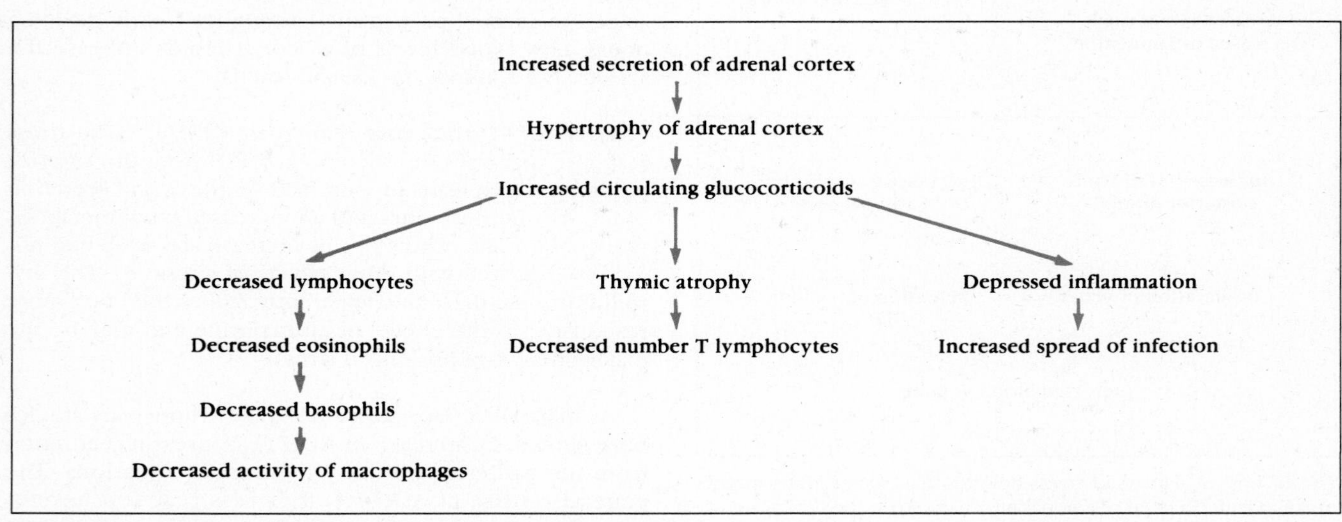

FIGURE 4-7 Effects of stress on the immune system.

and (4) personality and attitude toward life. Each can be influenced by the amount of physical and/or emotional stress placed on the individual at one time.

Genetic Predisposition

Stressors of sufficient strength or intensity can cause an alteration in normal functioning of the body. If one has a genetic or hereditary susceptibility to the stressors, the alteration may be manifested as disease.

Genetic susceptibility refers to myriad conditions that "run in the family" and seem to make the individual react in a particular way to certain stressors. A common example is an exaggerated allergic response that predisposes members of families to specific pollens. When the pollen count is seasonally high, these persons suffer different types of allergic responses. In this example, the stressor is the pollen count, but the response is heightened by a hyperactive, hereditary immune reaction (see Chap. 12).

Many other diseases seem to be familial, and development of actual disease may or may not require additional stressors to trigger the process. Coronary artery disease may develop in an individual with or without the associated risk factors of obesity, type A personality, hypertension, or others.

Organ Susceptibility (Weak-Organ Theory)

The weak-organ theory is associated with hereditary factors. In different individuals, not all organs seem to be equally resistant to stressors. Some persons under equal stress conditions develop cardiovascular disorders, while others develop peptic ulcers. Still others may suffer migraine headaches or other maladies. Why in some persons the heart is the target organ, while in others it is the stomach or other organs, is not known [18]. It is known that numerous ailments are induced, or at least aggravated, by stressful living conditions. In some cases, the major cause of the disease is not stress, although stress precipitates complications and intensity of the disease.

Unhealthful Behaviors

Some examples of unhealthful behaviors as stressors are as follows: overeating, excessive alcohol intake, smoking, drug abuse, and lack of exercise. The unhealthful behavior is a destructive force that serves as the stressor, and development of disease is correlated with the behavior. Disease does not always occur, and individuals with high stressor levels due to destructive behavior may have no residual health problems. More frequently, when a person actually develops the related disease, a pattern of behavior emerges that includes a combination of other high risk factors. An example of this is coronary artery disease with the combination of family history, obesity, high blood pressure, and smoking as major risk factors.

Personality and Attitude Toward Life

Of great interest in recent studies is the relationship between attitude and health. Social isolation, such as is often seen in aged persons, correlates with an increase in chronic disease. Children who are not loved and fondled after birth fail to thrive. The opposite effect may be seen when persons with a high number of risk factors have strong support groups and develop disease significantly less often than the general population with the same risk factors [8,10].

Faith and hope, as personality factors, have been studied in relation to cancer prognosis. Significant factors in the development of malignancy include feelings of helplessness and hopelessness, inability to express anger, self-dislike, and loss of an important emotional relationship [12]. Stress has also been implicated in the rate of progression and course of a malignancy. The same type and stage of malignancy in two individuals will behave differently as to rate of metastasis and response to therapeutic intervention [12].

Type A personality has been extensively studied in relation to the development of coronary artery disease. The type A person is described as one constantly driven to participate in a multitude of events in an ever-decreasing amount of time [17]. This so-called *hurry sickness* leads, in some cases, to increased frequency of hypertension, together with elevated serum lipoprotein levels [2]. While some studies attempted to refute a connection between personality factors and myocardial infarction, the weight of evidence seems to support the relationship. Additional support is the evidence that norepinephrine levels are increased when there is chronic, unrelenting stress, especially when the person feels a sense of loss of control over his or her life situation. Epinephrine, the other catecholamine, increases in fear and acute arousal states [8]. Other biochemical phenomena are associated with type A behavior, including elevated cholesterol, triglyceride, glucocorticoid, and insulin levels [4].

It is important to consider all of the previous information in order to understand that, while stress seems to be a significant factor in development of different diseases, and while biochemical phenomena have been described, the conclusions do not support direct relationships. Disease conditions must be considered individually with respect to the influence of stress. It must also be remembered that while some studies support the stress/disease concept, other, equally valid studies may cast some doubt on it.

Stress and Disease

Stress has been described in terms of adaptive reaction patterns and systematically related to bodily manifestations [17]. Selye referred to the production of disease as maladaptation and categorized stress-induced diseases as indicated in Table 4-1 [13]. In the subsequent material, the following are discussed in relation to their stress connection: (1) cardiovascular diseases, (2) immune deficiency diseases, (3) digestive diseases, (4) cancer, and (5) other conditions.

Cardiovascular Disease

For many years it has been recognized that stress is important in the etiology of coronary artery disease. It can be in the form of emotional, occupational, societal, cultural,

TABLE 4-1 Selye's Classification of Stress-Induced Diseases

1. Hypertension
2. Heart and blood vessel disease
3. Kidney disease
4. Eclampsia
5. Arthritis
6. Skin and eye inflammation
7. Infections
8. Allergic and hypersensitivity diseases
9. Nervous and mental diseases
10. Sexual derangements
11. Digestive diseases
12. Metabolic diseases
13. Cancer
14. Diseases of resistance

hereditary, and physical stressors. The importance of occupation has received great attention in recent years.

Several theories of the pathogenesis of coronary artery disease resulted from studies of the relationship among high-fat, stressful living situations, and development of disease. Individuals who develop hypercholesterolemia have a greater risk of developing atherosclerotic heart disease than those with normal cholesterol levels. The mechanism for the production of hypercholesterolemia is unclear. In contrast, however, studies supported the protective nature of certain serum lipoproteins called *high-density lipoproteins (HDLs)*, which may delay or prevent the development of atherosclerosis. The HDLs occur in greater serum concentrations in women than in men, which is consistent with studies showing that estrogen increases HDL levels while androgens tend to decrease them. During stressful periods, the serum cholesterol has been shown to rise, leading to the conclusion that lipid-regulating mechanisms are responsive to stress. According to some researchers, catecholamine release leads to an increased rate of lipolysis, increased serum free fatty acids, and a subsequent rise in serum cholesterol [6,11]. Correlate studies also link serum lipid levels and personality patterns. Stress-induced lipemia is considered to be the principal mechanism for stress-induced atherosclerosis. Stress can also potentiate the sequence of blood coagulation. These two factors can lead to myocardial infarction [4]. Stress may also induce coronary artery vasospasm, myocardial hypoxia, and direct myocardial injury. This may alter postinfarction adaptation [8]. Emotional stress can precipitate anginal pain and aggravate heart failure [1]. Life stressors such as bereavement and loss of employment are significant risk factors for myocardial infarction [4]. Depression significantly increases the risk of death after infarction [4].

Pelletier theorized that a relationship exists between chronic stress and blood pressure. Stress leads to increased blood pressure, which in turn leads to a weakening and tearing of the linings of the blood vessels, thus providing a focal point for the deposition of cholesterol plaques on the vessel lining. The end result is narrowing of the lumina of vessels, leading to increased peripheral vascular resistance and a further increase in blood pressure levels. To compensate for the elevated blood pressure, the left ventricle undergoes hypertrophy and requires a greater supply of blood and oxygen. A relationship between high blood pressure and coronary artery disease has not been found consistently, but the correlation is significant enough to consider hypertension as a major risk factor [1].

The increase in frequency of coronary artery disease has prompted investigations into many facets of current lifestyles in the United States. One area of study is the commonly observed personality pattern in which the individual feels a loss of control over his or her occupational or social environment. Friedman and Rosenman also identified a behavior pattern consistent with hypertension and heart attack. It includes competitiveness in work, fast work pace, time pressure, and inability to relax at work or play. Other risk factors also were studied, but the personality pattern apparently offered the greatest risk [17].

Stress-Induced Immune Deficiency

The decreased immune response after stressful situations appears to be due to increased secretion of glucocorticoids from the adrenal cortex. The major effect is suppression of T lymphocytes, which in turn decreases the cell-mediated immune response. Both T and B lymphocytes are affected by glucocorticoid release, but the lymphopenia (decreased numbers of lymphocytes) is due to redistribution rather than actual loss of T cells. Physiologically or psychologically stressful events precipitate a decrease in lymphocytes and other leukocytes [1].

The administration of glucocorticoids in conditions of hypersensitivity or exaggerated response has long been shown to be beneficial. This is especially true in such conditions as rheumatoid arthritis, acute asthmatic attacks, and specific types of malignancy, especially leukemia.

Conversely, the stress-induced response of decreased immunity can be very detrimental in conditions such as cancer. It is often seen that an individual who was declared "cured" of cancer may undergo relapse after an acute stressful situation, such as the death of a loved one. The stress-induced depression of the immune system may allow for an increased rate of malignant growth (see Unit 6).

Digestive Diseases

The relationship of stress and peptic ulcers has been studied for many years. Three types of stress-induced ulcer disease are described in this section and in further detail in Chapter 37.

Overwhelming stress frequently leads to the development of *stress ulcers*. These may be related to gastric mucosal ischemia and gastric acid secretion. The mechanism for the related gastric acid secretion is not entirely understood, but may be due to cerebral stimulation of the dorsal motor nucleus of the vagus nerve [7]. Hypersecretion has only been demonstrated clearly in the development of Cushing's ulcers, which are associated with brain lesions. Stress ulcers are very frequent in individuals who experience overwhelming conditions such as trauma, surgery, burns, or infections [1].

An increased rate of gastric secretion between meals has been demonstrated in persons having *duodenal ulcers*, while those with *gastric ulcers* often have normal or decreased secretion of hydrochloric acid. It would appear that duodenal ulcers result from a chronic increase in gastric acid secretion and affect the duodenum before the alkalinizing secretions can buffer the acid. Gastric ulcers seem to be related to gastritis and to decreased resistance of the gastric mucosa [5].

Stress has been indicated in many other digestive conditions, including such diverse ones as constipation, diarrhea, ulcerative colitis, and Crohn's disease. Personality and stress factors with ulcerative colitis and regional enteritis have been studied extensively, leading to much additional knowledge of the very complex pathogenesis of these disorders. Anger and anxiety may precipitate or exacerbate ulcerative colitis [1].

Cancer

Specific agents (stressors) are linked with cancer causation. These carcinogens are discussed in Unit 6. Numerous studies have linked psychosocial attitudes with development and progression of cancer. The findings vary, but depression, isolation, introverted personality, and feelings of hopelessness tend to support development of the disease. Individuals who suffer a major loss or chronic stressors also have increased risk of cancer development [1].

The relationship may be that depression of the immunologic responses by the stress allows cancer to be initiated [7]. Local exposure to carcinogen stressors may result in tumorigenesis. Stress can be viewed as having a twofold influence on malignancy: (1) it increases the production of abnormal cells and (2) it decreases the capability of the body to destroy these cells [14].

What is known is that all individuals are exposed daily to a host of potential carcinogens, and resistance is multifactorial, including physiologic and behavioral responses and attitudes [12].

Other Conditions

The *skin* is a target organ for stress reactivity, and when stress occurs, the vessels constrict and peripheral blood flow decreases. Some of the vasospastic conditions such as Raynaud's phenomena are partly stress induced. Other stress-related disorders include eczema, urticaria, psoriasis, and acne [1].

The *musculoskeletal* system exhibits stress effects by chronically tensed muscle, producing the common syndromes of backache, headache, and colon spasms [1]. Arthritis, especially rheumatoid arthritis, is aggravated by high degrees of stress, and symptoms may be exacerbated at these times.

The *respiratory* system participates in the acute stress reaction by hyperventilation. Stress may be exhibited also by heightened allergic sinusitis and episodes of bronchial asthma. Onset of acute asthmatic attacks may occur with sleeplessness, worry, and grief [1].

Study Questions

1. How does the clinical picture differ in the alarm, resistance, or exhaustion stages of Selye's general adaptation syndrome?
2. Describe the stereotyped response to any stressor.
3. Explain how factors that increase the risk of disease can be additive if they exist concurrently.
4. Choose one disease process and describe the physiologic changes that can produce the disease.
5. How does the current lifestyle in the United States contribute to the production of stress-induced diseases?

References

1. Asterita, M.F. *The Physiology of Stress*. New York: Human Sciences Press, 1985.
2. Carruthers, M., and Taggart, P. Behavior patterns and emotional stress in the etiology of coronary heart disease: Cardiological and biochemical correlates. In D. Wheatley, *Stress and the Heart*. New York: Raven Press, 1977.
3. Dunn, A.J., and Kramarcy, N.R. Neurochemical responses in stress: Relationships between the hypothalamic-pituitary-adrenal and catecholamine systems. In L.L. Iverson and S.D. Iverson, *Drugs, Neurotransmitters and Behavior*. New York: Plenum Press, 1984.
4. Elliott, G.R., and Eisdorfer, C. *Stress and Human Health: Analysis and Implications of Research. A Study by the Institute of Medicine National Academy of Sciences*. New York: Springer, 1982.
5. Greenberger, N.J., and Winship, D.H. *Gastrointestinal Disorders: A Pathophysiologic Approach* (3rd ed.). Chicago: Year Book, 1986.
6. Guyton, A. *Textbook of Medical Physiology* (7th ed.). Philadelphia: Saunders, 1986.
7. Irwin, J., and Anisman, H. Stress and pathology: Immunological and central nervous system interactions. In C.L. Cooper, *Psychosocial Stress and Cancer*. New York: Wiley, 1984.
8. Meerson, F.Z. *Adaptation, Stress and Prophylaxis*. New York: Springer-Verlag, 1984.
9. Miller, J. Living systems: Basic concepts. In W. Gray, et al., *General Systems Theory and Psychiatry*. Boston: Little, Brown, 1969.
10. Pelletier, K. *Mind as Healer, Mind as Slayer*. New York: Dell, 1977.
11. Robbins, S.L., Cotran, R.S., and Kumar, V. *Pathologic Basis of Disease* (3rd ed.). Philadelphia: Saunders, 1984.
12. Rosch, P.J. Stress and cancer. In C.L. Cooper, *Psychosocial Stress and Cancer*. New York: Wiley, 1984.
13. Selye, H. *The Stress of Life*. New York: McGraw-Hill, 1956.
14. Selye, H. Stress, cancer, and the mind. In S.B. Day, *Cancer, Stress and Death*. New York: Plenum Press, 1968.
15. Usdin, E., Kvetnansky, R., and Kopin, I. *Catecholamines and Stress: Recent Advances*. New York: Elsevier North-Holland, 1980.
16. von Bertalanffy, I. *General Systems Theory: Foundations, Development and Applications*. New York: Brazillier, 1986.
17. Wheatley, D. *Stress and the Heart*. New York: Raven Press, 1977.
18. Wolff, H.G. *Stress and Disease* (2nd ed.). Springfield, Ill.: Charles C. Thomas, 1968.

Unit Bibliography

Ashton, K. The many faces of stress. *Nurs. Times* 75:1297, 1979.

Bahlmann, J., and Liebau, H. *Stress and Hypertension.* New York: Karger, 1982.

Bloom, B.L. *Stressful Life Event Theory and Research*. Rockville, Md.: U.S. Dept. of Health Service, 1985.

Bogolin, L., and Harris, J. Meeting the immunological challenge: Rush-Presbyterian, St. Luke's Medical Center Symposium. *Heart Lung* 9:643, 1980.

Brockway, B.J. Situational stress and temporal changes in self-respondents and vocal measurements. *Nurs. Res.* 28:20, 1979.

Bruhn, J.G., and Wolf, S. *The Roseto Story: An Anatomy of Health*. Norman, Okla.: University of Oklahoma Press, 1979.

Burchfield, S.R. *Stress, Psychological and Physiological Interactions*. Washington, D.C.: Hemisphere, 1985.

Cox, T. *Stress*. Baltimore: University Park Press, 1980.

Cromwell, R.L., et al. *Acute Myocardial Infarction*. St. Louis: Mosby, 1977.

Cumings, S. Stress, cigarettes and ulcers. *Gastroenterology* 85(5):1232, 1985.

DePue, R. *The Psychobiology of the Depressive Disorders.* New York: Academic Press, 1979.

Dotevall, G. *Stress and Common Gastrointestinal Disorders*. New York: Praeger, 1985.

Ebersole, P., and Hess, P. *Toward Healthy Aging* (2nd ed.). St. Louis: Mosby, 1986.

Fauci, A.S., Dale, D.C., and Balow, J.E. Glucocorticosteroid therapy: Mechanisms of action and clinical considerations. *Ann. Intern. Med.* 8:304, 1976.

Folinsbee, L.J. *Environmental Stress: Individual Human Adaptations*. New York: Academic Press, 1978.

Fromm, D. Stress ulcer. *Hosp. Med.* 14:5, 1978.

Garfield, C. *Stress and Survival: The Emotional Realities of Life-Threatening Illness*. St. Louis: Mosby, 1979.

Getty, C., and Humphreys, W. *Understanding the Family*. New York: Appleton-Century-Crofts, 1981.

Glass, D. *Behavior Patterns, Stress and Coronary Disease*. Hillsdale, N.Y.: Lawrence Erlbaum, 1977.

Gunderson, E., and Rahe, R. *Life Stress and Illness*. Springfield, Ill.: Thomas, 1974.

Hemenway, J.A. Sleep and the cardiac patient. *Heart Lung* 9:453, 1980.

Henry, J.P., and Stephens, P.H. *Stress, Health and the Social Environment*. New York: Springer-Verlag, 1977.

Jalowiec, A. Stress and coping in hypertensive and emergency room patients. *Nurs. Res.* 30:10, 1981.

Jasmin, S., Hill, L., and Smith, N. The art of managing stress. *Nurs. 81* 11:52, 1981.

Marcinek, M. Stress in the surgical patient. *Am. J. Nurs.* 77:1809, 1977.

McKerns, K.W., and Pantic, V. *Neuroendocrine Correlates of Stress*. New York: Plenum Press, 1984.

Meissner, J. Measuring patient stress with the hospital stress rating scale. *Nurs. 80* 10:70, 1980.

Milsum, J.H. *Health, Stress and Illness: A Systems Approach.* New York: Praeger, 1984.

Neurnberger, P. Freedom from stress: A holistic approach. *Nurs. Life* 1:61, 1981.

Northouse, L.L. Living with cancer. *Am. J. Nurs.* 81:960, 1981.

Pohorecky, L.A., and Brick, J. *International Symposium on Stress and Alcohol Use*. New York: Elsevier, 1982.

Roundtable. When stress tips the clinical balance. *Patient Care* 15:7, 1981.

Schlesinger, Z., and Barzilay, J. Prolonged rehabilitation of patients after acute myocardial infarction and its effects on a complex of physiological variables. *Heart Lung* 9:1038, 1980.

Schmale, A.H., and Iker, H. Hopelessness as a predictor of cervical cancer. *Soc. Sci. Med.* 5:95, 1971.

Selye, H. *The Physiology and Pathology of Exposure to Stress*. Montreal: Acta, 1950.

Selye, H. *Stress Without Distress*. Philadelphia: Lippincott, 1974.

Selye, H. *Selye's Guide to Stress Research*. New York: Van Nostrand Reinhold, 1983.

Shiffman, S., and Wills, T.A. *Coping and Substance Use*. Orlando, Fla.: Academic Press, 1985.

Siegrist, J., and Halhuber, M.J. *Myocardial Infarctions and Psychosocial Risks*. New York: Springer-Verlag, 1981.

Steptoe, A., Ruddel, H., and Neus, H. *Clinical and Methodological Issues in Cardiovascular Psychophysiology*. New York: Springer-Verlag, 1985.

Stout, C., et al. Unusually low incidence of death from myocardial infarction. *J.A.M.A.* 188:845, 1964.

Stress and skin disease. *Clin. Dermatol.* 2(4):1-282, 1984.

Tierney, M.J., and Strom, S. Type A behavior in the nurse. *Am. J. Nurs.* 80:915, 1980.

Vander, A. *Nutrition, Stress and Toxic Health Controversies*. Ann Arbor: University of Michigan Press, 1981.

Vansom, S.R. Stress effects on patients in critical care units from procedures performed on others. *Heart Lung* 9:494, 1980.

Woolfolk, R.L., and Lehrer, P.M. *Principles and Practice of Stress*. New York: Guilford Press, 1984.

UNIT 3

Fluid, Electrolyte, and Acid-Base Balance and Shock

Marianne Marcus / *Normal and Altered Fluid and Electrolyte Balance*

Richard P. Pflanzer and Barbara L. Bullock / *Normal and Altered Acid-Base Balance*

Bonnie Juneau / *Shock*

The steady state of fluid, electrolyte, and acid-base balance is maintained through the complex cooperation of various systems of the body. Continual movement and exchange of water result in a regulated balance between plasma and interstitial and intracellular fluid. Because the subject encompasses many other systems, this unit provides the basis for further exploration in the specific systems of the body.

Chapter 5 summarizes water and electrolyte balance and explores the major alterations that can occur with disease states. Edema is discussed in this chapter because it represents a shift of fluid volume between compartments. Specific reference is made to electrolyte and water regulation in many other areas of the text. Chapter 6 deals with the basic concepts of the regulation of acid-base balance and how alterations in the balance can result. Respiratory alterations are described in greater detail in Unit 9 and metabolic alterations are specifically explored in Unit 10. Other systems that function in the regulation of hydrogen ion concentration are noted in Units 7, 11, 12, and 15. Chapter 7, newly incorporated into the book, covers the principles of shock by exploring the various underlying mechanisms of this disorder.

The reader is encouraged to use the learning objectives as a study guide outline and the study questions as a review; the bibliography at the end of the unit can aid in further investigation of the topic.

CHAPTER 5

Normal and Altered Fluid and Electrolyte Balance

CHAPTER OUTLINE

Regulation of Fluid and Electrolyte Balance

- Water
- Regulation of Water Balance
  - *Thirst*
  - *Renal Regulation*
  - *Antidiuretic Hormone (ADH)*
  - *Aldosterone*
  - *Prostaglandins*
  - *Glucocorticoids*
- Fluid Balance in Body Compartments
- Movement of Fluids at the Capillary Line
- Water-Sodium Deficits and Excesses
  - *Hypovolemia*
  - *Hypervolemia*
  - *Sodium*
  - *Hyponatremia*
  - *Hypernatremia*
- Potassium
  - *Hypokalemia*
  - *Hyperkalemia*
- Calcium
  - *Relationship of Calcium to Phosphate*
  - *Hypocalcemia*
  - *Hypercalcemia*
- Phosphate
  - *Hypophosphatemia*
  - *Hyperphosphatemia*
- Chloride
- Magnesium
  - *Hypomagnesemia*
  - *Hypermagnesemia*

Edema

- Decreased Colloid Osmotic Pressure
- Increased Capillary Hydrostatic Pressure
- Increased Capillary Permeability
- Obstruction of the Lymphatics
- Sodium and Body Water Excess
- Types of Edema
- Distribution of Edema

LEARNING OBJECTIVES

1. Describe the mechanisms by which water balance is normally regulated.
2. List the normal serum concentrations of the major electrolytes and plasma proteins.
3. Show the relationship of fluid and electrolyte composition between the intracellular and extracellular compartments.
4. Describe in detail the normal fluid dynamics at the capillary line.
5. Define the terms *hydrostatic pressure*, *oncotic pressure*, *colloid osmotic pressure*, and *outward and inward forces* as they relate to capillary fluid dynamics.
6. Describe briefly the role of the lymphatic system in controlling extravascular fluid volume.
7. Describe the role of sodium in controlling osmotic pressure in the extracellular fluid.
8. Differentiate between volume imbalances and osmolar imbalances.
9. Differentiate the clinical effects of hypernatremia and hyponatremia.
10. Define *dilutional hyponatremia*.
11. Discuss how SIADH can cause hyponatremia.
12. Describe the function of potassium in the body.
13. Differentiate the pathophysiologic changes resulting from hypokalemia and hyperkalemia.
14. Discuss the numerous functions of calcium in the body.
15. List several causes of hypocalcemia.
16. Describe the physiologic effects of hypocalcemia and hypercalcemia.
17. List the functions of phosphate in the body.
18. Explain the relationship between calcium and phosphates in body functions.
19. Explain how hypochloremia is related to metabolic alkalosis.
20. Describe the effects of magnesium on the body.
21. Discuss the five pathologic mechanisms that can produce edema and their relationship to each other.
22. Diagram the positive feedback mechanism associated with decreased colloid osmotic pressure.
23. Differentiate between pitting and nonpitting edema.

The volume and composition of body fluids must remain constant to support life. Continual movement and exchange of water and electrolytes occur and are regulated by the body to compensate for wide variations in intake and output that may result from environmental changes or disease states. The protein composition of plasma is also important in regulating fluid movement at the capillary line. This chapter presents a brief review of water and electrolyte balance and alterations that can occur with stress and disease.

Regulation of Fluid and Electrolyte Balance

Water

Water balance refers to an equilibrium maintained between intake and output. Water, a necessary solvent, is used in the many metabolic processes of the body and carries waste products for excretion through the urine, skin, lungs, and feces. Water cushions, protects, lubricates, insulates, and provides structure for and resilience to the skin.

Water accounts for approximately 60 percent of body weight in the adult. This amount normally decreases with age and is affected by other components of body composition. The lean individual has a greater percentage of body water than the obese person because fat cells contain less water than muscle cells. The amount of water necessary to maintain life in the adult is about 1500 ml per day. Water intake, although intermittent, is usually higher than necessary, with an average total of 2000 ml per day. Water is ingested in liquids and in foods, and is also produced by oxidation of foodstuffs. It is directly conserved by the antidiuretic hormone and indirectly conserved by aldosterone.

The composition of the body fluids is regulated by the kidneys, gastrointestinal tract, nervous system, and lungs, with input from the heart and glands. Hormones, especially aldosterone and antidiuretic hormone (ADH), regulate the composition of plasma and other fluid compartments.

The intake of water must be balanced by output. The kidneys rid the body of excess water. Obligatory urinary output to eliminate waste and maintain minimal renal function is 300 to 500 ml per 24 hours. The volume of urinary excretion can be increased tremendously, and usually totals 1500 ml per 24 hours. Water is also lost through the lungs (300 ml/24 hrs), skin (500 ml/24 hrs), and feces (200 ml/24 hrs). This loss is termed *insensible loss*. In the adult, body water gains and losses are balanced at 2500 ml per 24 hours.

Water imbalance can occur as a result of excess or depletion of body fluids. It may be closely associated with changes in sodium concentration. Body water loss is aggravated by elevated body temperature, diarrhea, vomiting, and other excessive depletion such as occurs through kidneys, skin, lungs, and gastrointestinal tract. Water excess is often associated with sodium retention, but it may occur with excess ADH secretion or excessive ingestion of water.

Regulation of Water Balance

Thirst. Thirst, defined as the conscious desire for water, is the principal regulator of water intake [3]. Osmoreceptors located in the thirst center in the hypothalamus are sensitive to changes in the osmolality of extracellular fluids. When osmolality increases, the cells shrink and the thirst sensation occurs. Thirst may also result from depleted circulatory volume due to hemorrhage or from decreased cardiac output secondary to pump failure. Thirst may be induced by dryness of the mouth in true hyperosmolar states or may occur to relieve the unpleasant dry sensation that results from reduced salivation. The sensation may be diminished or unrecognized in elderly and confused individuals, resulting in inadequate fluid consumption. Excessive water intake unrelated to thirst can occur in psychotic states.

Renal Regulation. The kidneys regulate the volume and electrolyte concentration of body fluids. Extracellular fluid is filtered through the renal glomeruli. Selective reabsorption and excretion of water and solutes occur in the renal tubules. Glomerular filtration rate and renal perfusion, reflective of cardiac output, determine the rate of this process. Hypovolemic states result in reduced urinary output.

Antidiuretic Hormone (ADH). This hormone is formed in the hypothalamus and stored in the neurohypophysis of the posterior pituitary. The area of ADH storage and release may overlap with the thirst center, which accounts for the integration of thirst and ADH release [3]. The major stimuli for ADH secretion are increased osmolality and decreased volume of extracellular fluid. Secretion may also occur with the stress of trauma, surgery, pain, and some anesthetics and drugs. The hormone increases reabsorption of water at the collecting ducts, thereby conserving water to correct osmolality and restore the volume of extracellular fluid.

Also called *vasopressin*, ADH has a minor vasoconstrictive effect on the arterioles that can increase blood pressure. A significant decrease in ADH secretion secondary to lesions or trauma of the hypophyseal tract results in diabetes insipidus, which is characterized by a massive increase in urinary output. Blood volume depletion does not result in diabetes insipidus as long as the thirst mechanism remains intact. Increased secretion of ADH, stimulated by pituitary hypersecretion or by extrapituitary tumors, results in a marked decrease in serum osmolality, an increase in blood volume, and a decrease in urinary output. This is known as the syndrome of inappropriate ADH secretion (SIADH).

Aldosterone. This hormone, secreted by the adrenal gland, acts on the renal tubules to increase the sodium uptake. The increased sodium retention causes an increase in water retention. Aldosterone release is stimulated by changes in potassium concentration, by serum sodium concentrations, and by the renin-angiotensin system (see Chap. 28). Normally, the rate or amount of aldosterone secretion is closely regulated by the potassium concentration and is very effective in controlling hyperkalemia.

Prostaglandins. The prostaglandins are naturally occurring fatty acids that are present in many of the tissues of the body and function in the inflammatory response, blood pressure control, uterine contractions, and gastrointestinal motility. In the kidneys, renal prostaglandins cause vasodilation and, in most cases, promote sodium excretion by inhibiting the response of the renal distal tubules to ADH. Prostaglandin-mediated renal vasodilation protects the kidneys from ischemia when levels of vasoconstrictors such as angiotensin II and norepinephrine increase [1].

Glucocorticoids. The glucocorticoids secreted by the adrenal cortex exert weak mineralocorticoid activity, thus promoting the resorption of sodium and water. This increases blood volume and sodium retention. Therefore, alterations in glucocorticoid levels cause alterations in the blood volume balance.

Fluid Balance in Body Compartments

Fluids are maintained in strict volume and concentration in each of the three compartments: (1) extracellular, intravascular (plasma); (2) extracellular, extravascular (interstitial fluid); and (3) intracellular. Figure 5-1 shows the relationship of fluid balance and composition of these three compartments. In normal distribution, about 70 percent of body fluid is intracellular and the rest is extracellular in the form of interstitial, plasma, and secretion or excretion fluids. The relationship of cations, anions, and volumes must be maintained rigidly to preserve life. Interstitial fluid and plasma basically contain the same electrolyte composition, but plasma contains a large amount of protein. The composition of intracellular electrolytes is quite different from that of extracellular electrolytes, but the numbers of charges (cations and anions) are basically equal in the compartments. To maintain life, fluid containing oxygen and nutrients from the blood is filtered into the interstitial spaces and carried to the intracellular fluid, while excess carbon dioxide and other cellular waste products are returned to the bloodstream to be circulated and excreted by the lungs and kidneys. The process requires the constant movement and exchange of fluids and gases (see Chap. 1).

Movement of Fluids at the Capillary Line

The capillaries are formed of endothelium, which is permeable to all of the solutes and water of the plasma. It is impermeable to the large molecules and cells in the plasma. Substances move through the gaps or spaces in the endothelial cells and some substances, such as carbon dioxide, oxygen, and small solutes, move through the endothelial membrane as well. The process occurs by diffusion, so that near equilibrium exists at the capillary line. The amount of fluid leaving the capillary nearly equals the amount resorbed. This equilibrium occurs mostly through a balance achieved between the hydrostatic pressure of the blood and the colloid osmotic pressure in the capillaries.

Blood entering the capillary comes in at a *hydrostatic pressure* that is generated by the heart. This hydrostatic pressure varies in the different systemic arterioles but is always higher at the arteriolar end of the capillary than at the venular end (Fig. 5-2). As fluid filters out of the capillary into the tissue spaces, the hydrostatic pressure decreases. The high pressure exerted at the arteriolar end of the capillary has been called a simple *outward force*, which moves fluid from the vessel to the interstitial spaces [3]. The average hydrostatic pressure at the arteriolar end is 32 mm Hg and drops to 15 mm Hg at the venous end [3]. This hydrostatic pressure provides the main outward force, but it is enhanced by a negative interstitial pressure and the interstitial fluid colloid osmotic pressure (ISCOP) as shown in Figure 5-2.

The ISCOP results from plasma proteins that are leaked into the interstitial spaces and exert a colloid, or water-pulling, effect. The pressure exerted by the plasma proteins, the *colloid osmotic (COP)* or *oncotic pressure*, is an osmotic pulling or *inward force* that draws water toward it. Because the plasma proteins cannot move into the interstitial area, they exert their colloidal effect by drawing water back into the vessel. The average COP is 25 mm Hg, a pressure that remains constant across the capillary.

Referring to Figure 5-2, note that at the arteriolar end of a schematic capillary the hydrostatic pressure exceeds the colloid osmotic pressure by about 7 mm Hg, causing fluid movement to the interstitial area. At the venous end, the hydrostatic pressure has dropped to 15 mm Hg, and is now lower than the colloid osmotic pressure, which causes the movement of fluid into the capillary. The COP in the capillaries is mainly generated by albumin because it is the most abundant of the plasma proteins. Table 5-1 lists the relative concentrations of plasma proteins.

It has been noted that while the amount of fluid filtered out of the vessel nearly equals that resorbed, a larger amount is filtered into the tissue spaces than is resorbed. Also, small amounts of protein escape into the tissue spaces during the process of fluid movement and cannot be resorbed by the blood vessels. These excesses of fluid

Table 5-1 Concentration of Major Plasma Proteins

Proteins	Concentration
Total serum proteins	6.0–8.0 gm/dl
Albumin	3.5–5.5 gm/dl
Globulin	1.5–3.0 gm/dl
Fibrinogen	200–400 mg/dl
Electrophoresis	
Albumin	45–55% of total
Globulin	
$Alpha_1$	5–8% of total
$Alpha_2$	8–13% of total
Beta	11–17% of total
Gamma	15–25% of total

Source: J. Wallach, *Interpretation of Diagnostic Tests* (3rd ed.). Boston: Little, Brown, 1978.

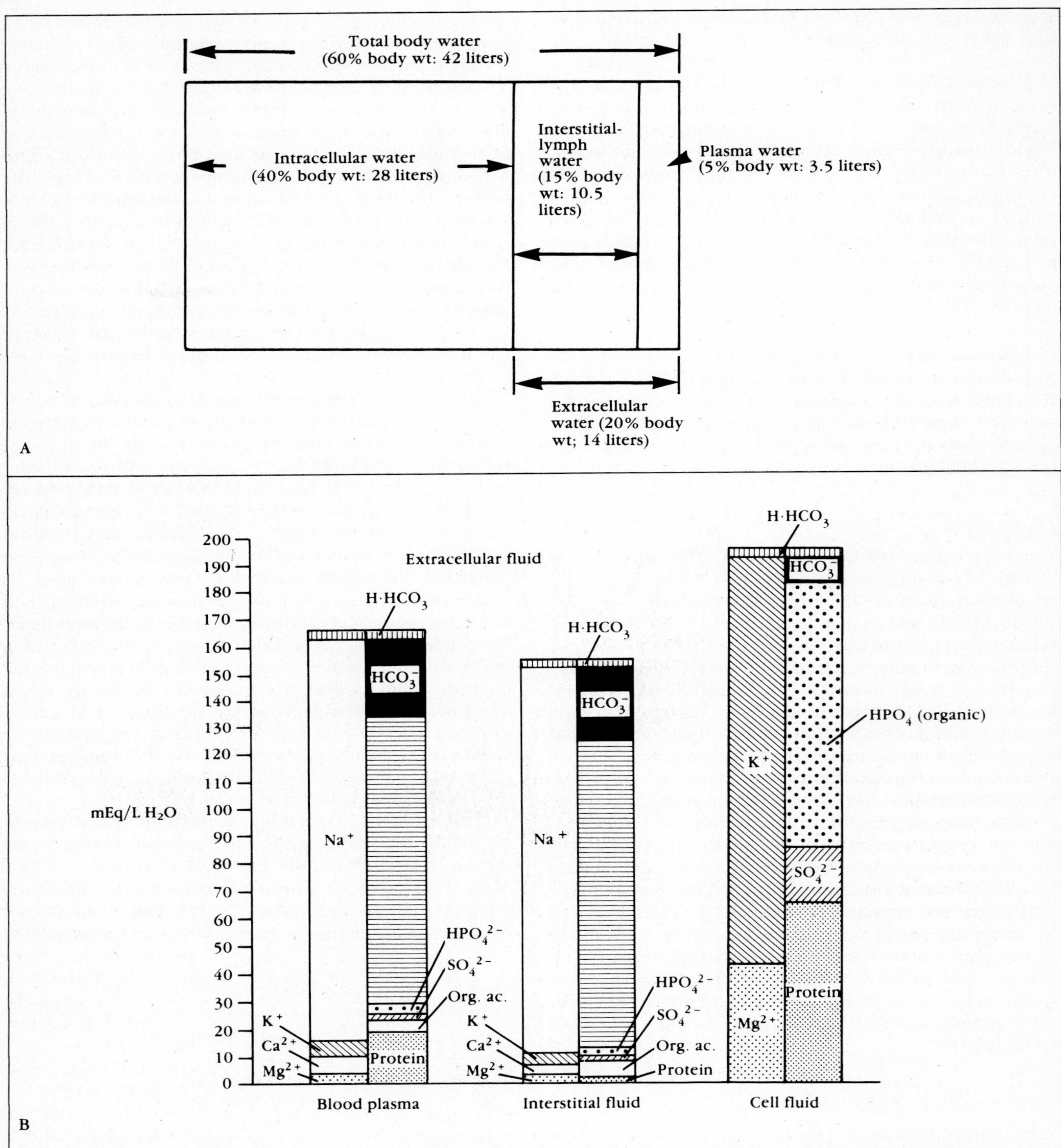

FIGURE 5-1 Fluid balance and composition. A. Distribution of water in the body. Percentages and volumes are for an idealized 70-kg young adult male. (From E. Selkurt, *Basic Physiology for the Health Sciences* [2nd ed.]. Boston: Little, Brown, 1982.) B. Electrolyte composition of the body fluid compartments.

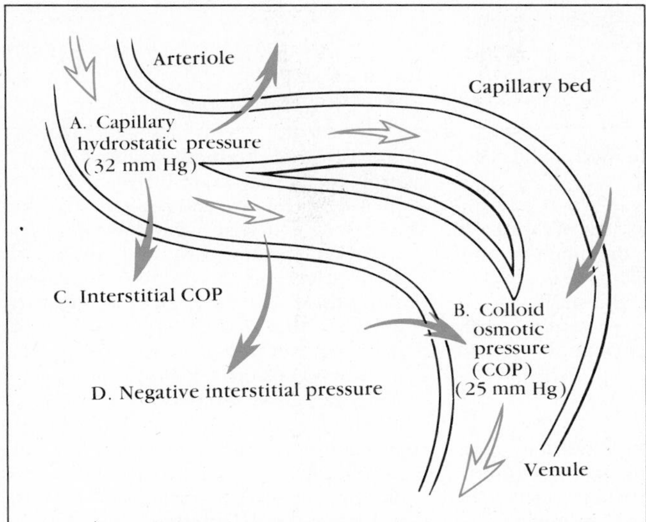

FIGURE 5-2 Fluid dynamics at the capillary line. A. Capillary hydrostatic pressure is higher at the arteriolar end and tends to push fluid out. B. Colloid osmotic pressure generated by the plasma proteins maintains a constant inward pull or force. C. Interstitial COP is an outward force. D. Negative interstitial pressure is an outward force.

and protein are absorbed by the *lymphatic system* and returned through lymphatic channels to the blood. The lymphatic system provides the only means to return plasma proteins in the tissues to the bloodstream [3].

Edema does not normally occur until there is a 17-mm Hg increase in the gradient favoring filtration, or the outward force [3]. This is because the lymph channels can increase the amount of fluid carried and thus can compensate for increased fluid escaping into the tissue spaces. Edema does result when there is significant alteration in either the inward (COP) or outward (hydrostatic) forces.

Water-Sodium Deficits and Excesses

Water and sodium imbalances are categorized as *volume* and *osmolar*. Volume, or isotonic, imbalances occur when sodium and water increase or decrease together in the same ratio that is normally found in the extracellular fluids. Osmolar imbalances result when there is an alteration in the normal relationship of water to solutes in the extracellular fluids. The serum sodium level is the best indicator of osmolality of blood because it is the most abundant solute in the vascular space [5].

Hypovolemia. Hypovolemia, or extracellular volume depletion, is an isotonic imbalance in which water and electrolytes are lost together in the same proportion as exists normally. The serum sodium level remains normal. Hypovolemia occurs when there is an abrupt decrease in intake of fluids or when fluids are removed from extracellular volume due to hemorrhage, diarrhea, vomiting, renal disease, fistulous drainage, burns, fever, intestinal obstruction, decreased aldosterone secretion, excessive diaphoresis, abscesses, draining wounds, ascites, or severe uncontrolled diabetes mellitus. Hypovolemia results in a decrease in the size of the extracellular space and circulatory collapse that eventually depletes cellular fluid. Signs and symptoms of hypovolemia are many and are related to the cause of the imbalance (Table 5-2).

Hypervolemia. Hypervolemia, or extracellular volume excess, is an isotonic imbalance in which water and electrolytes are gained together in the same proportion as exists normally in the extracellular fluid. The serum sodium level remains normal. Hypervolemia may result from excessive administration of isotonic solutions or of adrenal glucocorticoid hormones. This imbalance also may occur in disease states such as chronic renal failure, liver disease, congestive heart failure, malnutrition, and hyperaldosteronism when homeostatic mechanisms for fluid and electrolyte balance are impaired. Hypervolemia results in expansion of the extracellular space and circulatory overload. Signs and symptoms reflect the overload (see Table 5-2).

Sodium. Sodium is the major cation of extracellular fluid (ECF) (see Table 5-2). It regulates the osmotic pressure of the ECF and markedly affects the osmotic pressure of intracellular fluid (ICF). Sodium intake comes from the diet; requirements for body needs vary according to age and size. Adolescents need between 900 and 2700 mg of sodium daily. Adults can maintain sodium balance with less than 500 mg per day. One teaspoon of salt contains approximately 2 gm of sodium [4]. The average daily intake in the United States is 2.3 to 6.9 gm [4].

Sodium is also an essential component in neuromuscular excitability and is responsible for depolarization of the cell membranes of excitable cells. It participates in acid-base balance by combining with the bicarbonate radical. Sodium exists in combination with various anions, especially chloride and bicarbonate. Sodium concentration is directly regulated by aldosterone as previously described.

Hyponatremia. Deficits of serum sodium result from actual loss from body fluids or from excessive gains in extracellular water that dilutes the sodium. This imbalance may be caused by inadequate sodium intake, diuretic therapy, adrenal insufficiency, and administration of hypotonic solutions to replace fluid lost through diaphoresis, vomiting, or suctioning. Conditions that may result in water gain include psychogenic polydipsia, inadequate excretion of water secondary to renal disease or brain lesions, administration of hypotonic fluids to persons with increased ADH levels after surgery or trauma, and excessive use of tap water enemas. The cells become swollen as water moves from ECF to ICF to compensate for solute deficit. The neuromuscular system is particularly sensitive to this imbalance (see Table 5-2).

Hypernatremia. Serum sodium excess results from decreased intake or increased output of water. Overingestion of sodium may also cause this imbalance. Conditions that may lead to hypernatremia include impaired thirst sensation, dysphagia, profuse diaphoresis, watery diarrhea,

TABLE 5-2 Normal Fluid and Electrolyte Concentrations and Imbalances

Fluid and Electrolyte	Values[a]	Source and Cause of Imbalances	Functions and Clinical Manifestation
Water	Average intake 2000 ml/day	Intake of fluids, water in foods, oxidation of foodstuffs	Removes waste products; cushions, protects, lubricates, insulates, and provides structure and resilience to skin
Hypovolemia	ECF volume depletion; normal serum sodium	Decrease in fluid, intake; loss of fluids through hemorrhage, draining wounds, diarrhea, vomiting, diaphoresis, renal disease, burns, fever, fluid shifts, decreased aldosterone secretion, uncontrolled diabetes mellitus	Decrease in ECF space; thirst, weakness, abdominal pain; nausea; diminished stools, anorexia; weight loss; decreased skin turgor; decreased sweating, tearing, and salivation, decreased venous pressure; elevated pulse and respiratory rate; hypotension; oliguira, anuria, decreased body temperature (in the absence of infection)
Hypervolemia	ECF volume expansion; normal serum sodium	Excessive administration of isotonic solution; disease states that affect fluid and electrolyte homeostasis, renal, liver, congestive heart failure, malnutrition, and hyperaldosteronism; excessive administration of adrenal glucocortical hormones	Increase in ECF space; weight gain; dyspnea; cough, rales; distended abdomen; neck vein distention; bounding pulse; hypertension; hoarseness; normal skin turgor, sweating
Sodium	136–145 mEq/L	Supplied by diet; excreted by kidney; balance normally regulated by aldosterone; dominant ECF cation	Regulates fluid volume by maintaining osmotic pressure between compartments; functions in acid-base balance; functions in neuromuscular and muscular excitability
Hypernatremia	>150 mEq/L	Excess loss of water over sodium through GI system, lungs, or skin; excess administration of sodium through diet or renal insufficiency; essential hypernatremia may be due to hypothalamic lesions	Causes cellular shrinking due to hypertonic ECF, leads to CNS irritability, tachycardia, dry, flushed skin, hypotension; thirst excessive, elevated temperature, rapid pulse, weight loss, oliguria, anuria
Hyponatremia	<130 mEq/L	Dilutional hyponatremia from congestive heart failure, cirrhosis, nephrosis; sodium depletion, loss of body fluids, without replacement or replacement with hypotonic fluids; diuretic therapy	Causes cellular swelling, may lead to cerebral edema, headache, stupor progressing to coma; peripheral edema, polyuria, absence of thirst, decreased body temperature, rapid pulse, hypotension, nausea, vomiting
Potassium	3.5–5.0 mEq/L	Balance maintained by dietary intake, excess excreted by kidneys; increased potassium in plasma excreted under influence of aldosterone by kidneys; dominant cation in ICF	Regulates osmolarity of ICF, functions in neuromuscular and muscular excitability; competition with H^+ and Na^+ in renal tubule helps maintain acid-base balance
Hyperkalemia	>5 mEq/L	Renal failure or renal insufficiency—acute or chronic; hemolysis of RBC; acute increase in potassium intake	Main effect is depression of conductivity in heart, peaked T waves, widened QRS on ECG; muscle cramping, paresthesias, nausea, diarrhea, associated with metabolic acidosis
Hypokalemia	<3.5 mEq/L	Lack of dietary intake; vomiting, gastric suction, potassium-depleting diuretics, aldosteronism, salt-wasting kidney diseases; major GI surgery without replacement	Cardiac effect-increased irritability, onset of U wave on ECG, dysrhythmias, vomiting, paralytic ileus; thirst; associated with metabolic alkalosis; affect renal tubular function causing inability to concentrate urine
Calcium	4–5 mEq/L 8.5–10.5 mg/dl	Regulated by PTH and calcitonin; supplied by diet, absorbed under influence of activated vitamin D; 99% stored in bones and teeth; excreted by kidney and GI tract	Blocks sodium at cell membrane, decreases membrane excitability; enhances coagulation process; essential in complement cascade; makes up much of crystalline matrix of bone; reciprocal relationship with phosphate

TABLE 5-2 Continued

Fluid and Electrolyte	Values[a]	Source and Cause of Imbalances	Functions and Clinical Manifestations
Hypercalcemia	> 5.5 mEq/L >10.5 mg/dl	Excessive vitamin D, immobility, renal insufficiency; hyperparathyroidism, malignancies of bone or blood	Decreased neuromuscular excitability, muscle weakness, CNS depression, stupor to coma; ECG may show shortened Q–T interval; if due to increased absorption from bones, increased risk of fracture; vomiting, constipation, kidney stones
Hypocalcemia	<4.0 mEq/L <8.5 mg/dl	Hypoparathyroidism, surgical or idiopathic; malabsorption of calcium; insufficient or inactivated vitamin D; dietary lack of calcium or vitamin D; hypoalbuminemia	Increased neuromuscular excitability; Trousseau's and Chvostek's signs positive; skeletal muscle cramps, tetany, laryngospasm, asphyxiation, death
Phosphate	3.0–4.5 mg/100 ml	Supplied in diet; inverse relationship to calcium	Stored in bone; promotes acid-base balance; essential to metabolism at cellular level
Hypophosphatemia	<3.0 mg/100 ml	Increased excretion through GI tract; antacid ingestion; vitamin D deficit; diabetic ketosis, hyperparathyroidism, malnutrition, alcoholism	Anorexia; weakness, bone pain; osteomalacia; muscle weakness; tremors; hyporeflexia; confusion seizures; coma; hemolytic anemia, bleeding disorders, leukocyte malfunction
Hyperphosphatemia	>4.5 mg/100 ml	Renal failure; decreased PTH	See hypocalcemia.
Chloride	100–106 mEq/L	Major anion of ECF; supplied by diet, excreted by kidney, GI tract	Functions in acid-base balance; essential in gastric acid; follows sodium in loss and gain
Hypochloremia	<95 mEq/L	Diuretic therapy, hyponatremia, metabolic alkalosis due to chloride loss, bicarbonate gain	Signs of hyponatremia and metabolic alkalosis
Magnesium	1.5–2.5 mEq/L 1.8–3.0 mg/dl	Major cation in ICF and bones; supplied in diet, excreted by kidneys; competes at renal tubule for reabsorption; PTH increases excretion	Promotes many intracellular enzyme reactions; depresses neuromuscular excitability, peripheral vasodilation
Hypomagnesemia	<1.5 mEq/L	Malabsorption related to GI disease; excess loss of GI fluids; acute alcoholism and cirrhosis of the liver; diuretic drug therapy; pancreatitis; sometimes hyper- or hypoparathyroidism	May cause hypocalcemia, and hypokalemia; neuromuscular irritability increased, positive Chvostek's and Trousseau's signs, tetany, convulsions; tachycardia, hypertension

[a]*Source for values:* J. Wallach, *Interpretation of Diagnostic Tests* (4th ed.). Boston: Little, Brown, 1976.

polyuria due to diabetes insipidus and diabetes mellitus, excessive water loss from the lungs, and excessive administration of hypertonic solutions. Cells shrink and dehydration occurs as water moves from the ICF to the ECF to compensate for the solute excess. Brain cells are particularly sensitive to this process (see Table 5-2).

Potassium

Potassium is concentrated in the intracellular fluid. It directly affects the excitability of nerves and muscles, and contributes to intracellular osmotic pressure (see Table 5-2). Secretions and excretions contain large amounts of potassium. The source of potassium is the diet, which normally provides much more than is needed by the human body. Urine potassium concentrations vary, providing an efficient mechanism for the excretion of excess potassium in order to maintain a narrow range of normal serum concentrations.

Potassium moves into the cell during the formation of new tissues, the anabolic phase. During tissue breakdown, the catabolic phase, potassium leaves the cell. Potassium will not move into cells if there is a lack of oxygen, glucose, or insulin.

The human body very effectively excretes potassium but has little mechanism for renal conservation. Potassium deficit occurs in two to three days if there is no intake. This deficit is enhanced by conditions such as surgery that increase anabolic needs. Anything that increases the excretion of potassium, such as diuretics, may also cause depletion.

The major route for the loss of potassium is the kidneys, but some loss can occur through gastrointestinal secretions or the skin. In the kidneys the final excretion of potassium is under the control of aldosterone at the distal tubules. At this point, hydrogen, potassium, and sodium tend to compete with each other for excretion. Sodium is usually preferred for absorption in the presence of aldosterone. If the plasma hydrogen ion concentration is elevated above normal, the tubules preferentially tend to excrete hydrogen and conserve potassium, which leads to the hyperkalemia often seen in association with acidosis. The reverse is true in alkalosis: when the hydrogen concentration is low, potassium is preferentially excreted and hydrogen is conserved, thus causing hypokalemia associated with alkalosis.

Hypokalemia. A serum deficit of potassium may be caused by any of the following: (1) lack of intake; (2) diuretics (potassium-depleting); (3) major gastrointestinal surgical procedures, especially with nasogastric suctioning and incomplete replacement; (4) excessive gastrointestinal secretions; (5) hyperaldosteronism; (6) malnutrition; and (7) trauma or burns.

Hypokalemia affects every system. In the gastrointestinal system, anorexia, nausea, vomiting, and paralytic ileus may occur. In the muscles, flaccidity and weakness may be exhibited, and finally may lead to respiratory muscle weakness and arrest. Cardiac dysrhythmias are common and the electrocardiogram (ECG) may show the presence of a U wave when it was not previously present (Fig. 5-3). Ventricular tachycardia and cardiac arrest may occur when the levels are very low. Central nervous system depression and decreased deep tendon reflexes also may be noted. Hypokalemia causes decreased ability of renal tubules to concentrate waste, leading to increased water loss.

Hypokalemia causes an increased sensitivity to digitalis and may precipitate the effects of digitalis toxicity in persons taking a preparation of the drug. It enhances automaticity and may precipitate ventricular fibrillation (see Chap. 19).

Hyperkalemia. Excess potassium is usually secondary to temporary or permanent kidney dysfunction. It frequently occurs in association with renal failure. It also may be present transiently (with normal renal function) after major tissue trauma or after the rapid transfusion of stored bank blood. As blood is stored, the red blood cells begin to break down and release their potassium into the surrounding fluid. One unit of blood 1 day old has approximately 7 mEq per liter of potassium, while a unit that is 21 days old has 23 mEq per liter.

Hyperkalemia mainly affects the cardiovascular system. A decreased membrane potential causes a decrease in the intensity of the action potential, resulting in a dilated, flaccid heart. Various kinds of conduction defects may be noted together with ectopic dysrhythmias. The electrocardiogram shows tall peaked T waves, a short Q–T interval, and widening of the QRS complex (Fig. 5-3C). In the gastrointestinal system, nausea, vomiting, and diarrhea are common. Initial irritability of the skeletal muscles gives way to weakness and flaccid paralysis. Digital numbness and tingling may be described.

Calcium

Calcium is present in the body in the form of calcium salts and as ionized and protein-bound calcium (see Table 5-2). Ninety-nine percent is in the bones and teeth in the crystalline form, which gives hardness to these structures. Of the 1 percent that is circulating, approximately 40 percent

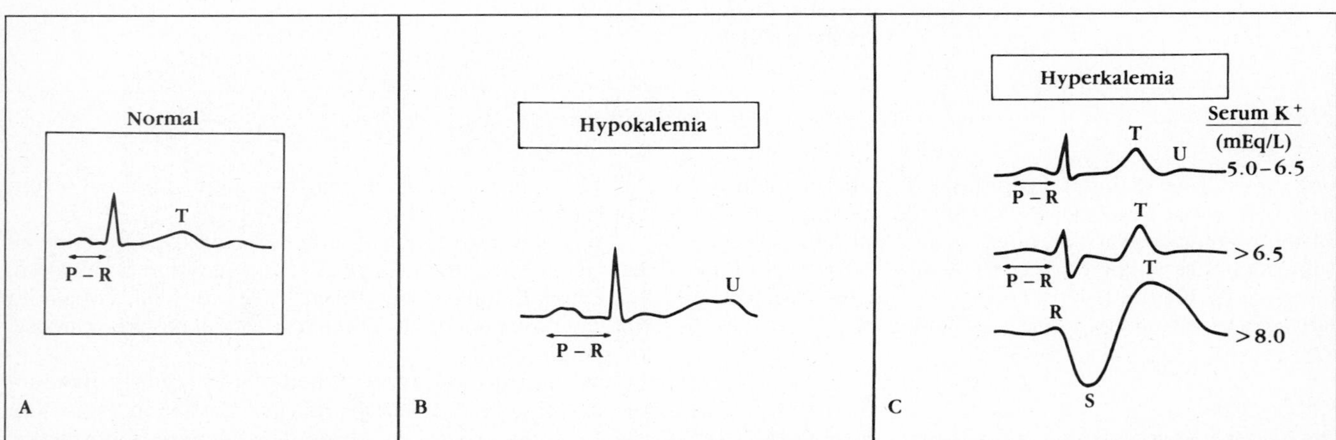

FIGURE 5-3 Altered cardiac conduction in hypokalemia and hyperkalemia. A. Normal electrocardiogram in the adult. B. In hypokalemia the T wave is flattened and the U wave is prominent. C. In hyperkalemia, the ECG changes do not always correspond to the serum potassium values given, but the progression from minor to severe changes correlates to some degree with the potassium level. With potassium concentration less than 6.5 mEq/L, the early ECG abnormality is peaking or tenting of the T waves. The next change, shown with a level of potassium concentration greater than 6.5, includes flattening of the P wave, prolongation of the P–R interval, and widening of the QRS complex, with development of a deep S wave. With severe hyperkalemia (8.0 mEq/L), ventricular fibrillation or cardiac arrest is imminent. (From R. Schrier, *Manual of Nephrology*. Boston: Little, Brown, 1981.)

is bound to plasma proteins, especially albumin. The ionized form of calcium is the active portion and functions in membrane integrity, coagulation, muscle contraction, and in the electrophysiology of the excitable cells.

Calcium can be released from its bound form, especially in the presence of a decreased serum pH. The reaction simply stated is a reversible equation:

$$Ca^{++} \text{ (protein bound)} + H^{+}$$
$$\rightleftarrows Ca^{++} \text{ (ionized)} + H^{+} \text{ (protein complex)}.$$

The reaction is driven toward the right in acidosis, causing an increase in ionized serum calcium. In alkalosis the reaction is driven more toward the left, which can cause hypocalcemia. This is the method used by the body plasma proteins to buffer hydrogen ion [7] (see Chap. 6).

Calcium concentration in the blood is under the influence of *parathyroid hormone* (PTH) and *calcitonin*. The former is released by the parathyroid glands from bone crystals and increases serum calcium levels (see Chap. 34). Calcitonin enhances the deposition (uptake) of calcium into bone when increased calcium levels are present, and it inhibits bone resorption. Calcitonin is produced by the thyroid gland and reduces serum calcium and phosphate levels.

Calcium stabilizes the cell membrane and blocks sodium transport into the cell. Because of this, decreased calcium levels increase the excitability of cells, while increased levels decrease excitability.

Vitamin D affects calcium absorption and bone deposition and resorption. Vitamin D is produced in the skin through the action of ultraviolet light and is present also in most American diets. It is changed by the liver to 25-hydroxycholecalciferol by hydroxylation and is further metabolized by the kidneys with the aid of PTH to form the most active type 1,25-dihydroxycholecalciferol. This substance is important in enhancing calcium uptake from the gastrointestinal tract and functioning with PTH in bone resorption [3,7].

Relationship of Calcium to Phosphate. Phosphate is an anion that is also regulated by PTH and activated vitamin D. Normally, the total concentration of calcium and phosphate is constant. If the calcium level increases, the phosphate level decreases. Calcium joins with phosphate to form calcium phosphate ($CaHPO_4$). When an excessive amount of $CaHPO_4$ is formed, it is not ionizable, and hypocalcemia results.

Hypocalcemia. When calcium levels decrease, the blocking effect of calcium on sodium also decreases. As a result, depolarization of excitable cells occurs more readily as sodium moves in. Therefore, when the calcium levels are low, increased central nervous system excitability and muscle spasms occur. Convulsions and tetany may be the result.

Hypocalcemia may be noted with decreased activation of vitamin D, which is often associated with renal or liver disease. Pancreatitis may cause decreased serum calcium due to the release of pancreatic lipase, which combines with fatty acids and calcium. Blood transfusions may cause hypocalcemia, as calcium binds with the citrate used in blood preparation, thus removing ionizable calcium from the blood. Hyperphosphatemia, hypoalbuminemia, parathyroid disease, administration of agents such as ACTH or glucagon, surgical removal of the parathyroid glands, gastrointestinal tract disease, and neoplastic conditions may all be associated with hypocalcemia.

The results of hypocalcemia are spasms and tetany, increased gastrointestinal motility, cardiovascular problems, and osteoporosis. Muscle tetany is both common and dangerous, especially when it involves laryngeal spasm. Trousseau's sign of hypocalcemia is elicited when a blood pressure cuff is inflated on an extremity for one to three minutes and a contraction of the fingers occurs. Chvostek's sign is elicited when the facial nerve at the temple is tapped resulting in a twitch on that side of the face (Fig. 5-4). Cardiac problems include delayed depolarization and repolarization. Sometimes decreased cardiac contractility and symptoms of heart failure result. A prolonged Q–T interval is sometimes seen in the presence of this electrolyte imbalance (Fig. 5-5).

Hypercalcemia. Excessive levels of calcium increase the blocking effect on sodium in the skeletal muscles. This leads to decreased excitability of both muscles and nerves, eventually contributing to flaccidity. Hypercalcemia is associated with decreased phosphate levels. The major cause is hyperparathyroidism, which results in increased PTH, which increases calcium uptake from the bones into the circulating blood. Some malignant tumors secrete PTH-like substances that function similarly to true PTH. Excessive ingestion of vitamin D may cause the condition, and occasionally, it occurs with prolonged immobilization.

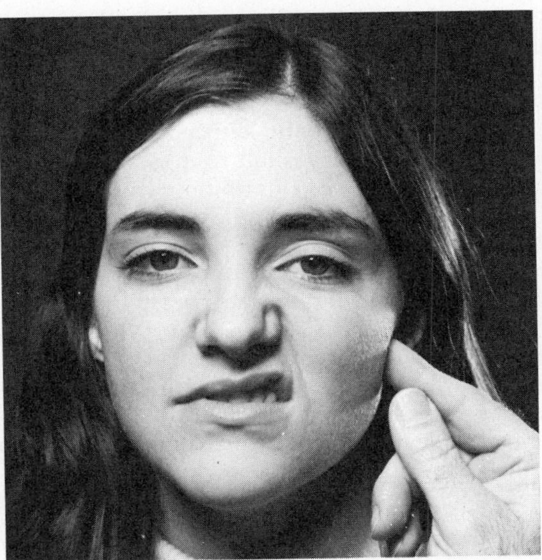

FIGURE 5-4 Facial muscle contraction in Chvostek's sign. (From M. Beyers and S. Dudas [eds.], *The Clinical Practice of Medical-Surgical Nursing* [2nd ed.]. Boston: Little, Brown, 1984.)

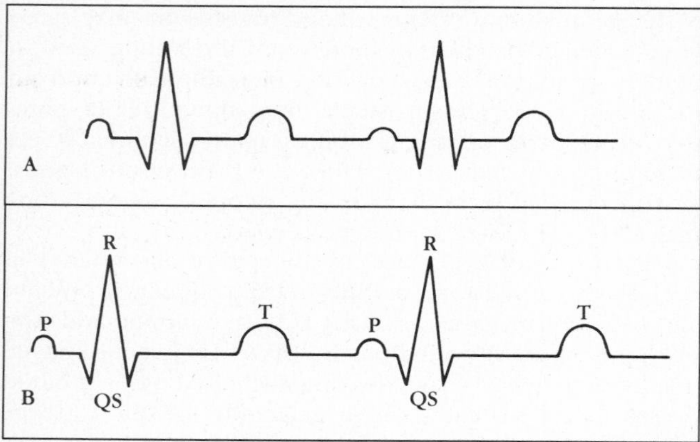

FIGURE 5-5 A. Normal electrocardiogram. B. Cardiographic changes seen with hypocalcemia; prolongation of the Q–T interval is sometimes seen.

Hypercalcemia causes skeletal muscle weakness, anorexia, nausea and vomiting, constipation, weight loss, and increased excretion of calcium in the urine. The increased circulating calcium may be deposited anywhere, but the kidneys are most vulnerable, and calcium deposition may result in kidney stones. Increased amounts may also be deposited in the arteries and cardiac valves.

Phosphate

Phosphate functions with calcium to support bone formation. Phosphate is the primary intracellular anion. It assists with energy transfers within the cells [6]. Approximately 85 percent of body phosphate is in the bones, while the remaining 15 percent is intracellular [7]. It promotes acid-base balance of the body by acting as a buffer in the extracellular fluid. It also participates in the metabolism of glucose, fat, and protein.

Hypophosphatemia. Hypophosphatemia occurs in alcoholism, malnutrition, diabetic ketoacidsis, and hyperthyroidism. A deficit may also result from antacid use because aluminum hydroxide, aluminum carbonate, and calcium carbonate combine with phosphate to promote loss of phosphate through the feces. This imbalance is characterized by hematologic malfunctions, encephalopathies, and musculoskeletal disorders (see Table 5-2).

Hyperphosphatemia. Hyperphosphatemia can occur in renal failure or when parathyroid hormone levels are decreased. Because calcium is inversely related to phosphate, the clinical manifestations of hyperphosphatemia resemble those of hypocalcemia.

Chloride

The chloride ion is the major anion of ECF (see Table 5-2). The amount of chloride in the fluid closely parallels the sodium content. Chloride is a component of hydrochloric acid in the stomach. It also serves an essential role in the transport of carbon dioxide by red blood cells (see Chap. 15). Chloride moves into the cells by passive transport.

Chloride depletion (hypochloremia) especially results from loss of gastrointestinal secretions, such as that occurring from vomiting, excessive diarrhea, and nasogastric suctioning. Diuretic therapy commonly causes hypochloremia together with hyponatremia, but urinary loss of chloride may be greater than loss of sodium. Metabolic alkalosis results as bicarbonate is conserved to maintain cation-anion balance. The clinical manifestations of hypochloremia are usually related to the associated metabolic alkalosis (see Chap. 6).

Magnesium

Magnesium is found mostly within the cells and in the bones (see Table 5-2). This cation activates a number of intracellular enzyme systems and is required for protein and nucleic acid synthesis. Magnesium is particularly essential in promoting neuromuscular integrity [6].

Hypomagnesemia. The most common cause of decreased serum magnesium is excessive ingestion of alcohol. Other causes include malnutrition, diabetes mellitus, liver failure, and poor intestinal absorption. The clinical manifestations include increased neuromuscular irritability, paresthesias, tetany, and convulsions.

Hypermagnesemia. This condition is rare but may occur in individuals with renal failure, especially if they ingest magnesium-containing antacids [6]. Clinical manifestations include lethargy, coma, cardiac dysrhythmias, respiratory failure, and death. Because dialysis in persons with chronic renal failure does not remove magnesium well, these individuals should be restricted from ingesting magnesium-containing medications.

Edema

The word *edema* refers to the expansion or accumulation of interstitial fluid volume. It may be localized or generalized, pitting or nonpitting, depending on its etiology. Edema is usually thought of as accumulation of excess fluid in the skin; however, the mechanism causing skin edema also can cause fluid shifts in other vulnerable areas of the body. These fluid shifts are sometimes termed *third-space* shifts, and include ascites, pleural or pericardial effusions, and pulmonary edema [6]. Table 5-3 summarizes the etiologic mechanisms that may lead to the formation of edema and fluid shifts. Five interrelated mechanisms are commonly described [3]:

1. Decreased colloid osmotic pressure
2. Increased capillary hydrostatic pressure
3. Increased capillary permeability
4. Lymphatic obstruction
5. Sodium and body water excess

Some forms of edema result from more than one mechanism.

TABLE 5-3 Examples of Etiologic Mechanisms for the Formation of Edema

Etiologic Mechanisms	Types of Edema
Increased capillary pressure	Congestive heart failure Phlebothrombosis Cirrhosis of the liver with portal hypertension
Vasodilatation	Inflammation Allergic reactions Burns (direct vascular injury)
Decreased colloid osmotic pressure	Liver failure Protein malnutrition Nephrosis Burns
Lymphatic obstruction	Surgical removal of lymph structures Inflammation or malignant involvement of lymph nodes and vessels Filariasis
Sodium/body water excess	Congestive heart failure Renal failure Aldosteronism Excess sodium intake

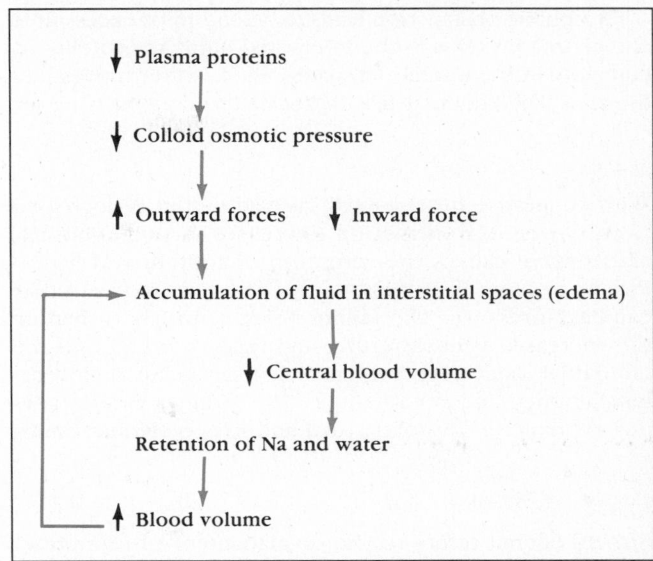

FIGURE 5-6 Positive feedback of compensatory mechanisms for decreased colloid osmotic pressure.

Decreased Colloid Osmotic Pressure

When the plasma proteins are depleted in the blood, the inward forces are decreased, allowing the filtration effect to favor movement into the tissues (see p. 77). This leads to accumulation of fluid in the tissues with a decreased central volume of plasma. The kidneys respond to the decreased circulating volume by activating the renin-angiotensin-aldosterone system, resulting in additional resorption of sodium and water.

Hypoproteinemia causes decreased colloid osmotic pressure and may result from malnutrition, neoplastic wasting, liver failure, or protein loss from burns, kidneys, or the gastrointestinal tract. Albumin is the primary protein affected because it is the most abundant and also because its molecules are rather small and can pass through damaged capillary endothelium or glomeruli. Loss of protein into the tissues causes decreased resorption of tissue fluids and edema. This is a positive feedback response because as the central blood volume becomes depleted, the kidneys conserve more sodium and water, and additional edema is formed (Fig. 5-6). This response can be terminated by restoring intravascular protein levels, which increases the intravascular colloid osmotic pressure and subsequently its volume.

The accumulation of ascitic fluid in cirrhosis of the liver is partly related to hypoproteinemia from decreased hepatic production of albumin and partly to increased hydrostatic pressure created by portal hypertension (see Chap. 39).

Increased Capillary Hydrostatic Pressure

The most common cause of increased capillary pressure is congestive heart failure in which increased systemic venous pressure is combined with increased blood volume. These manifestations are characteristic of failure of the right ventricle or right heart failure. Left heart failure may also lead to an increase in pulmonary capillary pressure (PCP). When the pressure exceeds 30 mm Hg, pulmonary edema can occur (see Chap. 20).

Other causes of increased hydrostatic pressure include renal failure with increased total blood volume, increased gravitational forces from standing for long periods of time, impaired venous circulation, and hepatic obstruction. Venous obstruction produces localized rather than generalized edema because only one vein or group of veins is usually affected.

Increased Capillary Permeability

Direct damage to blood vessels, such as with trauma and burns, may cause increased permeability of the endothelial junctions. Localized edema may occur in response to an allergen, such as a bee sting, and in certain individuals this allergen may precipitate an anaphylactic response with widespread edema initiated by the histamine or type of reaction (see Chap. 12).

Inflammation causes hyperemia and vasodilation, which lead to accumulation of fluids, proteins, and cells in an affected area. This results in edematous swelling (exudation) of the affected localized area (see Chap. 9).

Obstruction of the Lymphatics

The most common cause of lymphatic obstruction is the surgical removal of a group of lymph nodes and vessels to prevent the spread of malignancy. Radiation therapy, trauma, malignant metastasis, and inflammation may also lead to localized lymphatic obstruction. *Filariasis*, a rare parasitic infection of the lymph vessels, can cause widespread obstruction of the vessels.

Lymphatic obstruction leads to retention of excess fluid and plasma proteins in the interstitial fluid. As proteins accumulate in the interstitial spaces, more water moves into the area. The edema is usually localized.

Sodium and Body Water Excess

With congestive heart failure, cardiac output is decreased as the force of contraction decreases. To compensate, aldosterone causes the retention of sodium and water. Plasma volume increases, as does venous intravascular capillary pressure. The failing heart is unable to handle this increased venous return, and fluid is forced into the interstitial space. Hypervolemia also can occur with renal insufficiency and renal failure. The kidneys cannot adequately excrete the solute load and hypervolemia results.

Types of Edema

Pitting edema refers to the displacement of interstitial water by finger pressure on the skin, which leaves a pitted depression. This is graded 1 to 4 according to the depth of pitting noted (Fig. 5-7). After the pressure is removed, it often takes several minutes for the depression to be resolved. Pitting edema often appears in dependent sites, such as the sacrum of a bedridden individual. Similarly, gravitational hydrostatic pressure increases the accumulation of fluid in the legs and feet of an upright individual.

Nonpitting edema may be seen in areas of loose skin folds such as the periorbital spaces of the face. Nonpitting edema may occur after venous thrombosis, especially of the superficial veins. Persistent edema leads to trophic changes in the skin. These changes may progress to stasis dermatitis and ulcers that heal very slowly (see Chap. 23). Nonpitting, brawny edema is also associated with thick, hardened skin and color changes. It occurs when serum proteins become trapped and coagulated in the tissue spaces.

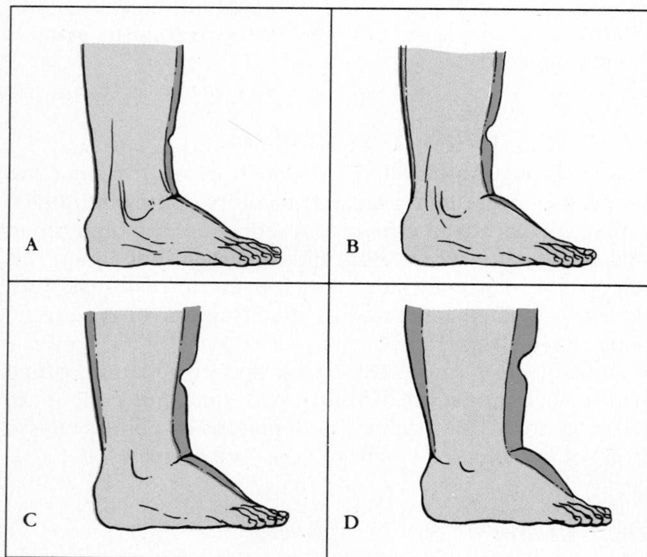

FIGURE 5-7 Grading of edema. A. 1+ slight pit, normal contours. B. 2+ deeper pit, fairly normal contours. C. 3+ deep pit, puffy appearance. D. 4+ deep pit, frankly swollen. (From R. Judge, G. Zuidema, and F. Fitzgerald, *Clinical Diagnosis* [4th ed.]. Boston: Little, Brown, 1982.)

Distribution of Edema

The distribution of edema can give clues as to its cause. If it is localized in one extremity, it is probably due to venous or lymphatic obstruction. Edema resulting from hypoproteinemia is generalized but is especially pronounced in the eyelids and face in the morning, due to the recumbent position assumed at night and the aid of gravitational forces. Edema of heart failure is usually greatest in the legs of an ambulatory individual, and it tends to accumulate throughout the day [2].

Study Questions

1. Explain the control of fluid dynamics at the capillary line.
2. How do volume imbalances differ with respect to sodium and water balance and adequate renal function?
3. What mechanisms must function adequately to maintain calcium balance in the body?
4. Relate calcium imbalance to phosphate balance.
5. Describe how the body functions in the regulation of potassium, sodium, and hydrogen ions.
6. What are the pathophysiologic effects of an imbalance in potassium in the body?
7. What is the relationship of chloride ions with other electrolytes?
8. Describe the factors necessary to determine the causative agents for edema.

References

1. Andreoli, T.E. Disorders of fluid volume, electrolyte, and acid-base balance. In J.B. Wyngaarden and L.H. Smith (eds.), *Cecil's Textbook of Medicine* (17th ed.). New York: Saunders, 1985.
2. Fishman, A.P. Heart failure. In J.B. Wyngaarden and L.H. Smith (eds.), *Cecil's Textbook of Medicine* (17th ed.). New York: Saunders, 1985.
3. Guyton, A.C. *Textbook of Medical Physiology* (7th ed.). Philadelphia: Saunders, 1986.
4. Lewis, C.M. *Nutrition and Nutritional Therapy in Nursing*. Norwalk, Conn.: Appleton-Century-Crofts, 1986.
5. Marcus, M.T. Fluid and electrolyte balance. In E.A. Mahoney and J.P. Flynn (eds.), *Handbook of Medical-Surgical Nursing*. New York: Wiley, 1983.
6. Metheny, N.M., and Snively, W.D. *Nurse's Handbook of Fluid Balance* (4th ed.). Philadelphia: Lippincott, 1983.
7. Schrier, R.W. *Renal and Electrolyte Disorders* (3rd ed.). Boston: Little, Brown, 1986.

CHAPTER 6

Normal and Altered Acid-Base Balance

CHAPTER OUTLINE

Normal Acid-Base Balance
- Fundamental Concepts
  - *Electrolytes*
- pH and Hydrogen Ion
- Metabolism: Volatile and Nonvolatile Acids
  - *Volatile Acids*
  - *Nonvolatile Acids*
- Regulation of Body Fluid pH
  - *Chemical Buffers*
  - *Respiratory Regulation of Plasma PCO_2*
  - *Renal Regulation of Plasma HCO_3^-*
- Integration of Defense Mechanisms

Altered Acid-Base Balance
- Definitions and Normal Blood Gas Values
- Acidosis and Alkalosis
- Etiology of Acidosis and Alkalosis
  - *Respiratory Acidosis*
  - *Respiratory Alkalosis*
  - *Metabolic Acidosis*
  - *Metabolic Alkalosis*
- Effects of pH Changes on Potassium, Calcium, and Magnesium Balance

Compensation

Interpretation of Blood Gas Data

The Anion Gap

LEARNING OBJECTIVES

1. Define pH.
2. List the normal values of the blood gases and pH of the different body fluids.
3. Differentiate between volatile and nonvolatile acids.
4. Diagram the dissociation of carbonic acid.
5. Describe the major buffer systems.
6. Describe specifically how the carbonic acid-bicarbonate system is affected by the respiratory and renal systems.
7. Explain how the kidneys maintain a constant hydrogen ion concentration in the plasma.
8. Describe the activity of hemoglobin as a protein buffer.
9. Differentiate between acidosis and alkalosis on the basis of physiologic disruption.
10. Describe the pathophysiology that underlies respiratory acidosis.
11. Compare respiratory acidosis and metabolic acidosis with respect to pathophysiology and compensatory mechanisms.
12. Define the term *anion gap* and relate it to an acid-base abnormality.
13. Differentiate the etiology of respiratory and metabolic alkalosis.
14. Describe the clinical manifestations of respiratory and metabolic alkalosis.

Normal Acid-Base Balance

All living cells of the human body are surrounded by a fluid environment called extracellular fluid (ECF). The chemical composition of the extracellular fluid is regulated within narrow limits that provide an optimal environment for maintaining normal cell function. The extracellular concentration of potassium ions, for example, is normally maintained within a range of 3.5 to 5.0 mEq per liter. Deviation from normal serum potassium concentration can affect transmission of nerve impulses, electrical conduction in the heart, and the contraction of skeletal, cardiac, and smooth muscles.

The most precisely regulated ion concentration in extracellular fluid is that of the *hydrogen ion*, normally ranging from 37 to 43 nEq per liter. A nanoequivalent is 10^{-9} equivalent, a very small measurement; the abbreviation saves writing a lot of zeros [2]. Deviation from normal hydrogen ion concentration can upset normal reactions of cellular metabolism by altering the effectiveness of enzymes, hormones, and other chemical regulators of cell function. It can also affect the normal distribution of other ions (such as sodium and potassium) between the intracellular and extracellular fluids, thereby disturbing a variety of cell and tissue ion-dependent functions, such as conduction, contraction, and secretion. Therefore, normal extracellular fluid hydrogen ion concentration is essential for normal body functions. The concentration is determined by the types and amounts of acids and bases present; therefore its regulation is commonly called acid-base balance.

When hydrogen ions are formed, they rapidly react with water molecules to form the *hydronium ion* ($H^+ + H_2O \rightleftarrows H_3O^+$). It is the hydronium ion that gives a solution or body fluid its acidity. In usual practice, it is referred to as if it were a single hydrogen ion [2].

Fundamental Concepts

Electrolytes. An electrolyte is a substance that *dissociates* and forms ions when mixed with water; the process is called *ionization*. It results in the formation of *cations* (positively charged electrolytes, such as sodium), and *anions* (negatively charged electrolytes, such as chloride). Ionic solutions readily conduct electric current, hence the term *electrolyte*.

An *acid* is any electrolyte that ionizes in water and forms hydrogen ions and anions. The anion formed is called the *conjugate base* of the acid. An acid is a *hydrogen ion donor* and thus elevates the hydrogen ion concentration of the solution to which it is added. The strength of an acid is determined by its degree of ionization in water. Strong acids completely ionize in water and readily liberate hydrogen ions. Hydrochloric acid (HCl) is a strong acid because 99.9 percent of its molecules ionize in pure water. Weak acids partly ionize in water and therefore do not liberate hydrogen ions as readily as strong acids. The acidity of the solution depends on how much the acid dissociates [2].

A *base* is any substance that can bind hydrogen ions. An *alkali* is a substance that contains a base. A strong base binds hydrogen ions readily. Hydroxides such as sodium hydroxide (NaOH) contain the hydroxyl (OH) ion, a strong base. A weak base binds hydrogen ions less readily. Sodium bicarbonate is a weak alkali containing the bicarbonate ion, a weak base. When *sodium bicarbonate* ($NaHCO_3$) is added to water, it completely dissociates. A small percentage of the resulting bicarbonate ions binds hydrogen ions and forms carbonic acid ($HCO_3^- + H^+ \rightleftarrows H_2CO_3$).

Since a base is a hydrogen ion acceptor, the addition of a base to a solution containing hydrogen ions lowers the hydrogen ion concentration; the opposite occurs when an acid is added.

pH and Hydrogen Ion

The pH is simply a negative logarithm of hydrogen ions (H^+) in a solution. One liter of water contains 0.0000001 gm of hydrogen ions. This figure is equal to $1/10^7$ as shown by the following equation:

$$\begin{aligned} 0.0000001 &= 1/10{,}000{,}000 \\ &= 1/(10 \times 10 \times 10 \times 10 \times 10 \times 10 \times 10) \\ &= 1/10^7 = 10^{-7} \end{aligned}$$

This simplified formula denotes the negative notation of a pH of 7 for neutral water [4]. For any given solution the numeric value of pH decreases as the hydrogen ion concentration increases. Therefore, since water is neutral at a pH of 7, when hydrogen ions are added to it, the solution becomes more acidic. The greater the hydrogen ion concentration, the more acidic the solution and the more the pH number falls. Acidic solutions range in pH between 0 and 7. Alkalotic or basic solutions, on the other hand, have less hydrogen ion concentration and range in pH between 7 and 14. The smaller the hydrogen ion concentration, the more alkaline the solution. Table 6-1 shows the Sorensen pH scale as it relates to the approximate pH compositions of body fluids. Note that the relationship between the pH and the hydrogen ion figures is logarithmic rather than linear. This means that an increase or decrease of one pH unit represents a tenfold change in hydrogen ion concentration.

In the fluids of the human body, the acceptable pH range is 7.35 to 7.45. Normal blood gas values are indicated in Table 6-2. Levels below 7.35 indicate a state of acidosis, while levels above 7.45 indicate alkalosis. When the hydrogen ion concentration is in the normal range of 40 nEq per liter, the pH is 7.40.

The broadest range of hydrogen ion concentration in extracellular fluids compatible with mammalian life is 16 to 125 nEq per liter, corresponding to a pH range of approximately 6.8 to 7.8. Cells of the human body usually function normally when the pH of extracellular fluid (interstitial fluids and plasma) remains constant at about 7.40.

TABLE 6-1 pH Scale Showing the Concentration of Hydrogen Ions from pH 1 to pH 14

H^+ Concentration (gm/liter)	Scientific Notation	pH Units	Examples
0.1	10^{-1}	$-\log 10^{-1} = 1$	Gastric juice
0.01	10^{-2}	$-\log 10^{-2} = 2$	Gastric juice
0.001	10^{-3}	$-\log 10^{-3} = 3$	Gastric juice
0.0001	10^{-4}	$-\log 10^{-4} = 4$	
0.00001	10^{-5}	$-\log 10^{-5} = 5$	Urine
0.000001	10^{-6}	$-\log 10^{-6} = 6$	Urine
0.0000001	10^{-7}	$-\log 10^{-7} = 7$	Arterial blood
0.00000001	10^{-8}	$-\log 10^{-8} = 8$	Pancreatic juice
0.000000001	10^{-9}	$-\log 10^{-9} = 9$	
0.0000000001	10^{-10}	$-\log 10^{-10} = 10$	
0.00000000001	10^{-11}	$-\log 10^{-11} = 11$	
0.000000000001	10^{-12}	$-\log 10^{-12} = 12$	
0.0000000000001	10^{-13}	$-\log 10^{-13} = 13$	
0.00000000000001	10^{-14}	$-\log 10^{-14} = 14$	

Note: The approximate pH of some of the body fluids is indicated.
Source: Adapted from M.W. Groër, *Physiology and Pathophysiology of the Body Fluids.* St. Louis: The C.V. Mosby Co., 1984, 1981.

TABLE 6-2 Normal Values for Arterial Blood Gases

Element Measured	Normal Value
pH	7.35–7.45
PCO_2	35–45 mm Hg
Total CO_2 content	21–32 mEq/L
PO_2	90–95 mm Hg
Hemoglobin saturation	95–100%

Alterations in plasma H^+ concentration alter the functioning of many enzyme and hormone systems; that is, acidosis depresses the function of epinephrine. H^+ concentration also affects neurologic functioning and the distribution of other ions.

In the processes of cellular metabolism, acid is continually being formed. Excess hydrogen is produced daily and must be eliminated from the body to maintain a steady state. The acids formed are of two types: (1) *volatile* acids that are excretable by the lungs; and (2) *nonvolatile* acids that are excreted by the kidney.

Metabolism: Volatile and Nonvolatile Acids

Volatile Acids. A volatile acid is defined as an acid that can be excreted from the body as a gas. Either the acid itself or a chemical product of the acid can be converted to a gas and excreted. Carbonic acid, produced by the hydration of carbon dioxide in body fluids, is a volatile acid. The formation can be expressed in the equation:

$$CO_2 + H_2O \underset{\text{(carbonic anhydrase)}}{\rightleftharpoons} H_2CO_3$$

Note that the enzyme carbonic anhydrase is necessary to accelerate the reaction. A normal adult produces about 300 liters of carbon dioxide per day from metabolic reactions. This results in the production of about 13,000 mEq of carbonic acid hydrogen ions, the equivalent of a liter of concentrated hydrochloric acid. Normally, the lungs excrete carbon dioxide as rapidly as cell metabolism produces it; therefore, carbonic acid is not allowed to accumulate in the body and alter extracellular fluid pH.

Nonvolatile Acids. A nonvolatile acid, also called a fixed acid, cannot be eliminated by the lungs and must be excreted by the kidneys. All metabolic acids present in body fluids except carbonic acid are classified as nonvolatile, and include sulfuric acid, phosphoric acid, lactic acid, ketoacids (acetoacetic acid, beta-hydroxybutyric acid), and smaller amounts of other inorganic and organic acids.

To some extent, fixed acids are neutralized by fixed bases in our diet. Fruits and vegetables contain such alkaline substances as potassium citrate. In a typical American diet, however, metabolic breakdown of foodstuffs leads to an excess of fixed acids (about 50–100 mEq/day), and these acids (or their conjugate bases) must be eliminated by the kidneys in order to maintain normal extracellular fluid pH.

Regulation of Body Fluid pH

As previously stated, extracellular fluid pH is normally maintained between 7.35 and 7.45. This occurs by three well-integrated mechanisms: (1) chemical buffers, (2) regulation of carbon dioxide concentration by the respiratory system, and (3) regulation of plasma bicarbonate concentration by the kidneys.

Chemical Buffers. Chemical buffers constitute the first line of defense against changes in body fluid pH. They act within a fraction of a second for immediate defense against either major increases or decreases in hydrogen ion concentration.

A chemical buffer is a mixture of two or more chemicals that minimize changes in the pH of a solution when either acids or bases are added. Buffers minimize changes in pH by taking up hydrogen ions when acids are added to body fluids, or by releasing hydrogen ions when the pH of body fluids becomes too high. The function of buffers is to convert strong acids, which would strongly decrease overall pH, into weak acids, which have a minimal effect on pH. Buffers also convert strong bases, which strongly increase overall pH, into weak bases, which have a minimal effect on pH.

The most important chemical buffers in the body fluids consist of weak acids plus the salts of their conjugate bases, together referred to as acid-base buffer pairs. In extracellular fluids, the salts are primarily sodium salts, and in the intracellular fluids, they are primarily potassium salts. Important chemical buffer pairs of the body fluids include the *bicarbonate*, *phosphate*, and *proteinate buffer systems*. The carbonic acid-bicarbonate system buffers volatile and nonvolatile acids in the interstitial fluid and in plasma. The phosphate buffer system is a major buffer of metabolic acids in the intracellular fluid (ICF). Proteinate buffers are found in plasma proteins, hemoglobin, and in ICF proteins. These buffers can react with both volatile and nonvolatile acids [2]. Figure 6-1 indicates how hemoglobin functions in the pulmonary capillary to remove CO_2 from the body and picks up CO_2 from the systemic tissue cell. Other important chemical buffers are intracellular organic phosphate complexes such as adenosine triphosphate, adenosine diphosphate, and creatine phosphate, and the hydroxyapatite crystal complex of bone.

Buffering of metabolically produced acids occurs, both intracellularly and extracellularly, in interstitial fluids as well as in blood. The majority of chemical buffering reactions takes place inside of the body's cells.

When acid or base is added to extracellular fluids, approximately half of the added ions eventually diffuse into cells where they are buffered. These ions or others that affect acid-base balance are exchanged across the cell membrane for intracellular ions or are accompanied into cells by ions of opposite charge. For example, if an acid is added to extracellular fluid, some of the hydrogen ion is buffered chemically within the extracellular fluid. Some is also diffused across cell membranes into cells. Because the hydrogen ion is positively charged, it must either be exchanged across the cell membrane for another cation, such as Na^+ or K^+, or be accompanied into the cell by an anion, such as Cl^-. Although both processes occur, the movement of cations out of the cell is quantitatively more important. In metabolic acidosis, for example, extracellular potassium levels, as measured in blood plasma, are frequently elevated, as intracellular stores are depleted to allow intracellular buffering of hydrogen ions. Often, in

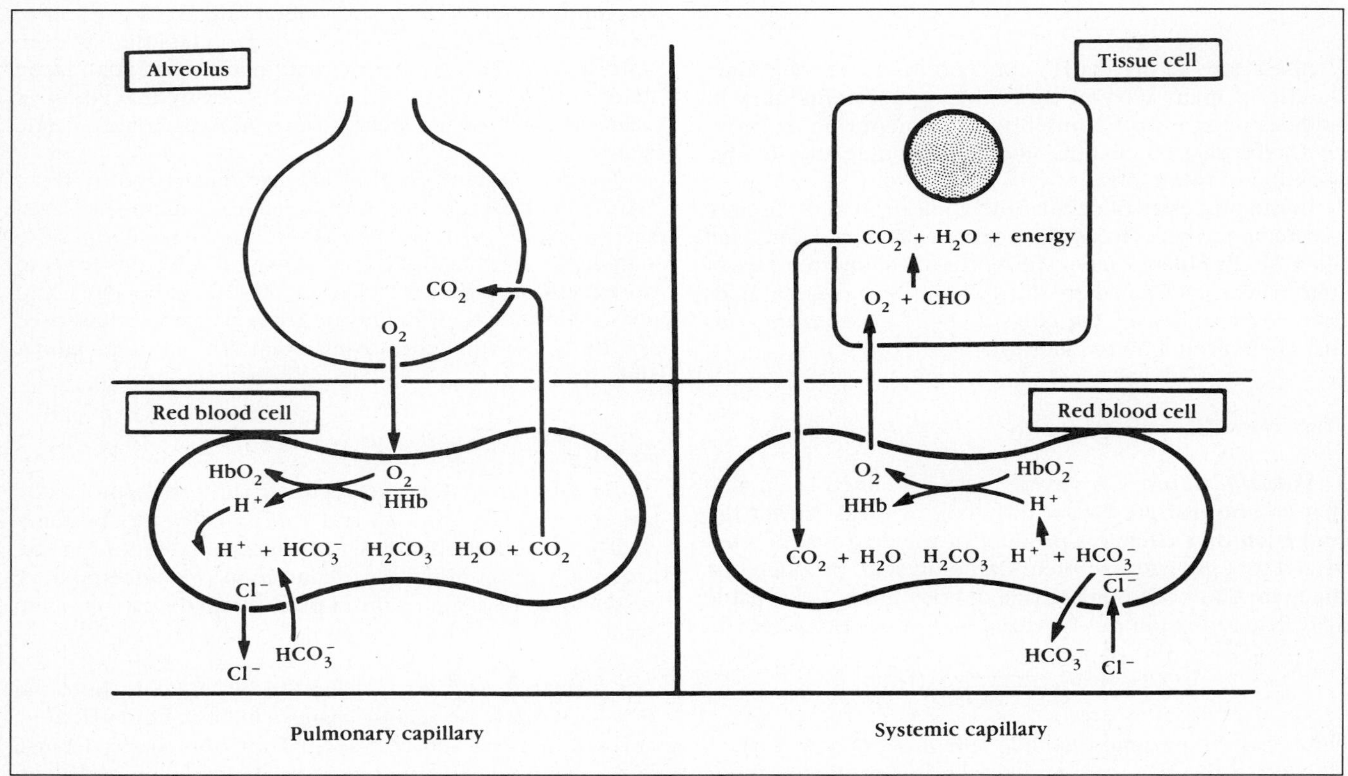

FIGURE 6-1 Hemoglobin as an important blood buffer. (From E. Selkurt [ed.], *Basic Physiology for the Health Sciences* [2nd ed.]. Boston: Little, Brown, 1982.)

metabolic acidosis, plasma chloride is also reduced. Figure 6-2 illustrates ion movement associated with intracellular buffering of extracellular hydrogen ions.

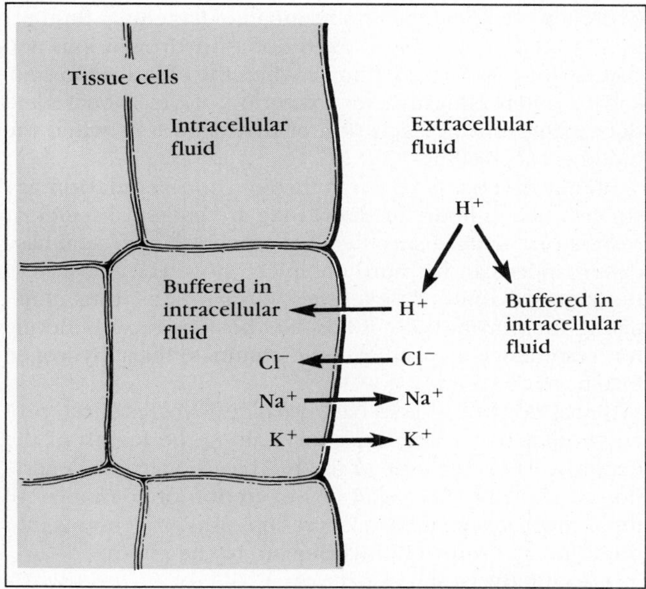

FIGURE 6-2 Ion movements associated with intracellular buffering of H^+.

The carbonic acid-bicarbonate system is the most important extracellular buffer because it can be regulated by both the lungs and the kidneys. Normally the carbonic acid (H_2CO_3)-bicarbonate (HCO_3^-) ratio is maintained at approximately 1:20 (Fig. 6-3). This ratio keeps the pH at approximately 7.40. The actual content required to maintain this balance is 1.2 mmol per liter of H_2CO_3 to 24 mEq per liter of HCO_3^-. As long as the ratio of 1:20 is maintained, the pH will also be stabilized. If, for example, a retention of carbon dioxide and a reciprocal compensatory retention of bicarbonate occurs, the amounts might be 2.0 mmol per liter of H_2CO_3 and 40 mEq per liter of HCO_3^-, which would still maintain the ratio (2:40 instead of 1:20) and the pH would remain 7.40. The respiratory system works very rapidly in the excretion or retention of CO_2, while the renal system functions much more slowly to retain or excrete HCO_3^-.

Respiratory Regulation of Plasma PCO_2. The respiratory system plays an important role in acid-base balance by controlling the partial pressure of carbon dioxide (PCO_2) in arterial blood. As excess carbon dioxide is formed during cellular processes, most of it is picked up by the red blood cells and carried to the lungs. Carbon dioxide reacts with body water to form carbonic acid, which then dissociates into hydrogen ion and bicarbonate ion, as the following reaction sequence indicates:

$$CO_2 + H_2O \underset{\text{dehydration}}{\overset{\text{hydration}}{\rightleftharpoons}} H_2CO_3 \underset{\text{association}}{\overset{\text{dissociation}}{\rightleftharpoons}} H^+ + HCO_3^- .$$

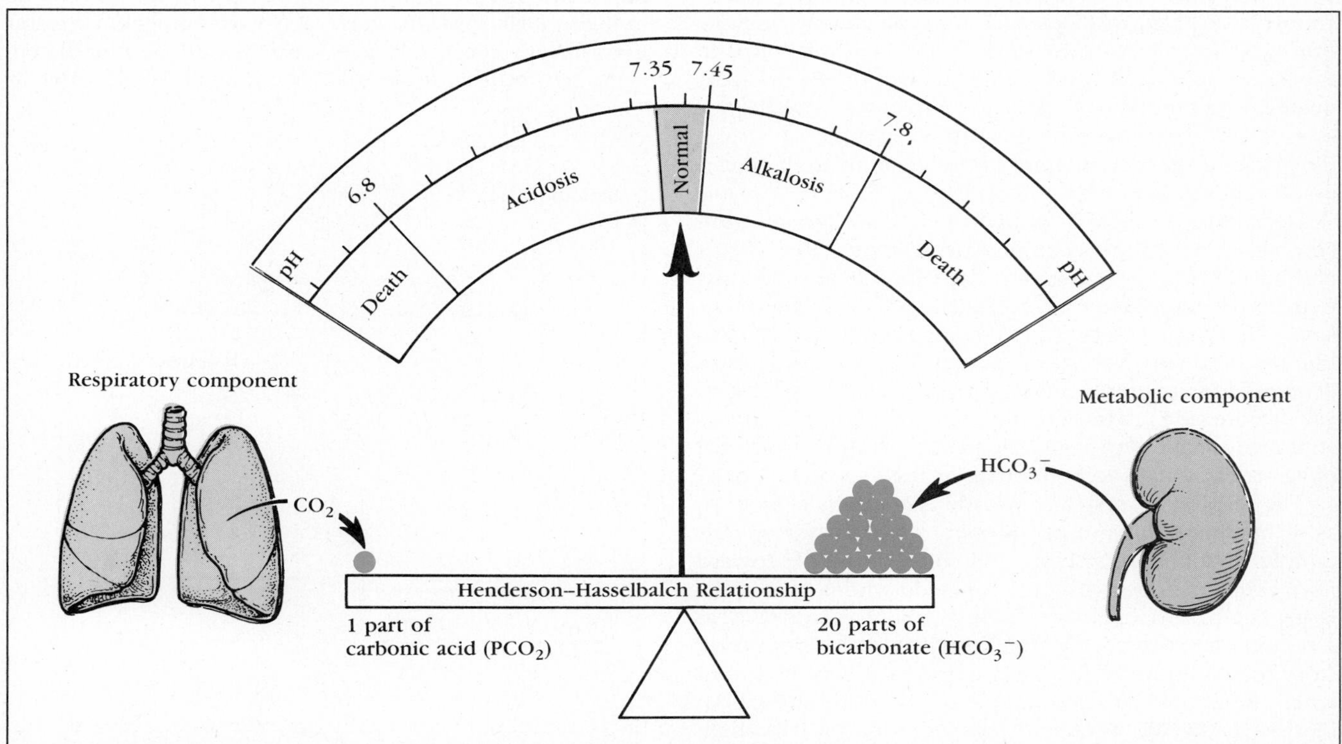

FIGURE 6-3 Mechanisms for defense against changes in body fluid pH.

These reactions are readily reversible. The hydration of dissolved carbon dioxide to form carbonic acid and the dehydration of carbonic acid to form carbon dioxide and water are slow reactions if uncatalyzed. The enzyme carbonic anhydrase, present in red blood cells, renal tubular cells, and other cells, speeds up these reactions. The dissociation of carbonic acid to hydrogen ion and bicarbonate ion, or the reaction in the opposite direction, occurs virtually instantaneously. As long as the rate at which carbon dioxide is eliminated from the body by the lungs equals the rate at which carbon dioxide is produced, no net change in the hydrogen ion concentration of the reaction sequence will occur.

An increase in carbon dioxide tension results in the liberation of hydrogen ions; thus, the pH decreases. If alveolar ventilation is decreased, metabolically produced carbon dioxide accumulates in the blood, carbonic acid concentration rises, and blood pH falls.

A decrease in carbon dioxide tension results in a fall in free hydrogen ions and consequently, a more alkaline pH. If ventilation is stimulated so that elimination of carbon dioxide temporarily exceeds its production, the blood PCO_2 moves to a lower level and alkaline blood pH results. Thus, changes in alveolar ventilation profoundly influence blood pH.

Alveolar ventilation is normally adjusted so that pH changes in the arterial blood are kept to a minimum. Increases of hydrogen ion concentration in body fluid (decreased pH), specifically in arterial blood and cerebrospinal fluid, result in a reflex increase in respiratory rate and depth. This respiratory response acts to blow off more carbon dioxide. The result is that the hydrogen ion concentration is decreased toward normal. Addition of a fixed (nonvolatile) acid to blood may increase alveolar ventilation to 5 times its normal value. Excess carbonic acid in the blood (due to failure to eliminate carbon dioxide adequately) is a powerful stimulus to ventilation. The increase in ventilation serves to diminish the retention of carbon dioxide and thereby minimizes the accumulation of carbonic acid in the blood.

Decreases of body fluid hydrogen ion concentration (increased pH) depress respiratory activity. This allows carbon dioxide to build up in the blood. Consequently, more hydrogen ions are made available, minimizing the alkaline shift in pH. A decrease in respiration due to an alkaline pH is usually not very marked. This occurs because decreased ventilation produces *hypercapnia* (high serum carbon dioxide), which stimulates ventilation. Hypoxia stimulates respiration when the partial pressure of arterial oxygen (PaO_2) falls to 60 mm Hg or less (see Chap. 24).

The respiratory system normally changes its activity so as to minimize shifts in pH. Respiratory activity responds rapidly to acid-base stresses and shifts blood pH toward normal in a matter of minutes. A person who is hypoventilating begins to accumulate carbon dioxide rapidly and, as a reflex, increases the rate and depth of breathing to restore the blood pH. Conversely, respiratory rate is slowed when the pH elevates and the pH goes toward normal. An increase in alveolar ventilation of two times normal can increase the pH of blood 0.23 pH units. Conversely, depressing ventilation to one-fourth of normal decreases the pH by 0.4 pH units [1].

Renal Regulation of Plasma HCO_3^-. The major role of the kidneys in maintaining acid-base balance is to conserve circulating stores of bicarbonate and excrete hydrogen ions. The kidneys maintain extracellular fluid pH by (1) increasing urinary excretion of hydrogen ions and conserving plasma bicarbonate when the blood is too acid, and (2) increasing urinary excretion of bicarbonate and decreasing urinary excretion of hydrogen ions when the blood is too alkaline.

Renal mechanisms for hydrogen ion regulation are slower (taking hours or days) than are chemical buffer or respiratory mechanisms. Renal compensation for acid-base disturbances can be more complete, however, because of the kidneys' ability to excrete hydrogen ions, thus eliminating them from body fluids. Neither chemical buffering nor respiratory mechanisms can eliminate these hydrogen ions from the body.

Renal control of acid-base balance involves three processes that occur simultaneously along the length of the nephron: (1) resorption of filtered bicarbonate, (2) excretion of titratable acid, and (3) excretion of ammonia. All three mechanisms involve secretion of hydrogen ions into the urine and return of bicarbonate to the plasma.

Quantitatively, the *resorption of filtered bicarbonate* is the most important process in renal acid-base regulation. Approximately 4500 mEq of sodium bicarbonate is filtered each day. Normally, all but 1 or 2 mEq of sodium bicarbonate are resorbed into the plasma.

Figure 6-4 illustrates the cellular mechanisms involved in the resorption of filtered bicarbonate. Carbon dioxide in the tubular epithelial cell reacts with intracellular water to form carbonic acid. The reaction is catalyzed by the enzyme *carbonic anhydrase*. Carbonic acid dissociates to

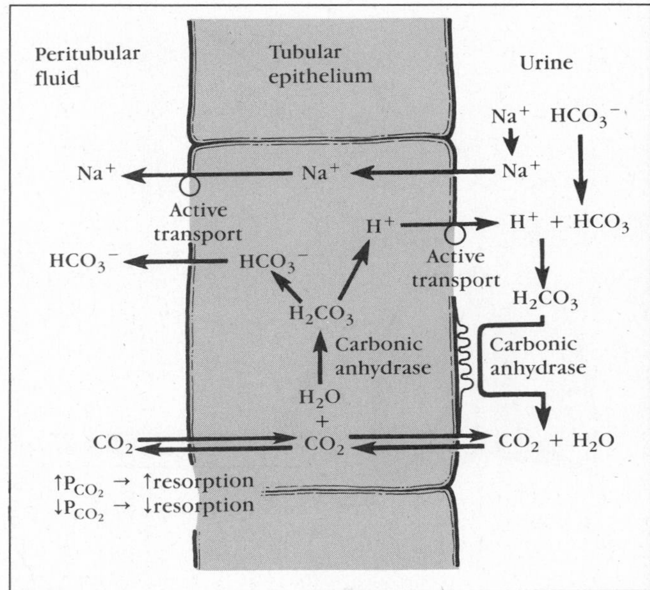

FIGURE 6-4 Resorption of filtered bicarbonate.

form hydrogen ions and bicarbonate ions. The hydrogen ions are actively secreted by the luminal cell membrane into the urine in exchange for sodium ions. The bicarbonate ion moves passively across the peritubular membrane into the blood, accompanying the actively resorbed sodium ion. In urine, hydrogen ions react with bicarbonate ions to form carbonic acid, which then dissociates into carbon dioxide and water. Water is either resorbed osmotically or eliminated in the urine, depending upon the body's water balance. Both blood and urine carbon dioxide are in equilibrium with carbon dioxide in tubular cells, and provide the main impetus for cellular generation of bicarbonate.

The kidneys also excrete hydrogen ions in the form of *titratable acids*, which consist mostly of dihydrogen phosphate ($H_2PO_4^-$) formed when hydrogen in the tubular fluid combines with monohydrogen phosphate (HPO_4^-). For each hydrogen ion excreted in the form of titratable acid, an equivalent quantity of sodium bicarbonate is added to the blood (Fig. 6-5). Approximately 10 to 20 mEq of titratable acid per day is excreted in the urine of an individual eating an average American diet.

Approximately 40 mEq of hydrogen ions is excreted per day, combined with *ammonia*. If a chronic acid load is imposed upon the body, the production and excretion of ammonia may increase more than tenfold over a period of several days.

The cellular mechanisms of ammonia excretion are illustrated in Figure 6-6. Ammonia is produced in the tubular cells from amino acid metabolism. Ammonia, readily soluble in the luminal membrane, diffuses out of the tubular cell into the urine, where it combines with hydrogen ions to form ammonium (NH_4) ions. Ammonium ions penetrate cell membranes poorly, so they are effectively trapped in urine and excreted in combination with chloride. For each hydrogen ion excreted with ammonia, an equivalent quantity of sodium bicarbonate is added to the blood. Normally, the kidneys produce up to 40 mEq of HCO_3^- per day from NH_4 formation [2].

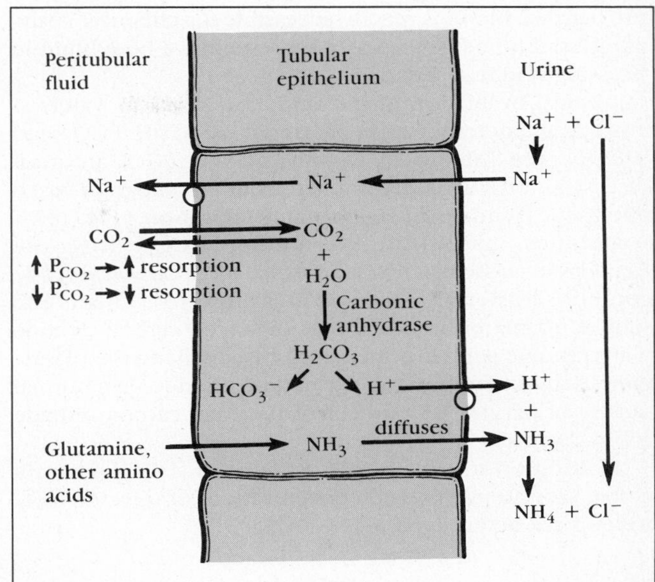

FIGURE 6-6 Excretion of ammonia.

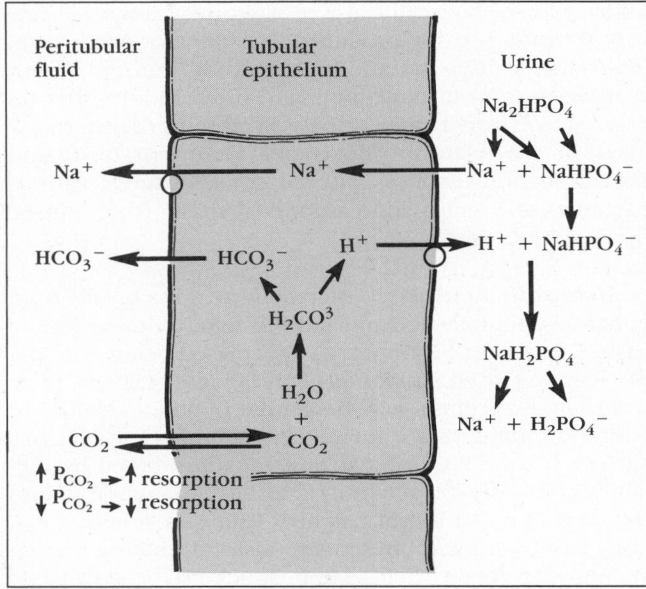

FIGURE 6-5 Production of titratable acid.

Integration of Defense Mechanisms

As previously noted, the body mechanisms for defense against changes in fluid pH consist of chemical buffers and respiratory and renal mechanisms. All of the mechanisms function simultaneously to maintain pH within normal limits, but they do not function independently of one another.

The pH of arterial blood is within normal limits (7.35–7.45) when the bicarbonate:carbonic acid ratio is 20:1 (see Fig. 6-3).

The carbonic acid concentration in plasma is very small and cannot be measured directly. It is proportional to the concentration of dissolved carbon dioxide, so PCO_2 is often used to calculate H_2CO_3 levels. Note that it is the ratio of bicarbonate to PCO_2 that determines pH, rather than the absolute amounts of bicarbonate and carbon dioxide. Plasma bicarbonate is controlled by the kidneys, while arterial PCO_2 is controlled by the lungs. Thus the effectiveness with which chemical buffers operate depends upon efficient respiratory and renal mechanisms to maintain proper buffer ratios. In this regard, the lungs and kidneys are sometimes referred to as physiological buffers. Integration of mechanisms for defense against changes in body fluid pH were described earlier (see Fig. 6-3).

Altered Acid-Base Balance

Definitions and Normal Blood Gas Values

Since the hydrogen ion concentration of blood ultimately affects the hydrogen ion concentration of all body fluids, and because blood is readily accessible for chemical analysis, arterial blood is used as a representative body fluid in assessing acid-base balance.

Clinical evaluation of the acid-base status of a person involves the determination of arterial blood pH, PCO_2, and $[HCO_3^-]$ (see Table 6-2). Usually, pH and PCO_2 are measured and $[HCO_3^-]$ is determined from a nomogram based upon the Henderson-Hasselbalch equation (Fig. 6-7). Sometimes, instead of determining $[HCO_3^-]$ from the Henderson-Hasselbalch relationship, total carbon dioxide content of arterial plasma is measured [5]. This is the sum of plasma bicarbonate plus dissolved carbon dioxide plus carbonic acid. It is measured by acidifying the plasma sample so as to remove all the carbon dioxide. In a normal sample of plasma, 95 percent of the total carbon dioxide is bicarbonate.

In addition to arterial pH, PCO_2, and $[HCO_3^-]$, hemoglobin saturation, PO_2 and concentrations of selected electrolytes are determined.

Acidosis and Alkalosis

Acidosis in the body fluids refers to an elevation of the H^+ concentration above normal or a decrease in the HCO_3^- below normal, resulting in a decrease in the pH of the body fluids to below 7.35. The source of the excess hydrogen ion or altered $H_2CO_3:HCO_3^-$ ratio can be respiratory (volatile) or metabolic (nonrespiratory or nonvolatile). *Acidemia* is defined as an acidic condition of the blood signified by an arterial pH value less than 7.35. The physiologic processes causing the acidemia define the term *acidosis* (literally, "a condition of becoming acidic").

Alkalosis refers to a decrease in the H^+ concentration of the body fluids or an excess of the HCO_3^-, thus increasing pH of the body fluids to above 7.45. The source of the depletion of hydrogen ion is either elimination of carbon dioxide (hyperventilation), or a metabolic excess of primary base bicarbonate. *Alkalemia* is defined as an alkaline condition of the blood signified by arterial pH greater than 7.45. The physiologic processes causing the alkalemia define the term *alkalosis* (literally, "a condition of becoming alkalotic").

Table 6-3 summarizes some factors that tend to cause acidosis and alkalosis. The effect of altering the ratio of bicarbonate and carbonic acid on the blood pH was described earlier (see Fig. 6-3). Other acids can similarly affect the blood pH.

Most laboratories measure pH and PCO_2 directly and calculate $HCO_3{}^-$ using the Henderson-Hasselbach equation:

$$\text{Arterial pH} = 6.1 + \log \frac{(HCO_3{}^-)}{0.03 \times PCO_2}$$

where 6.1 is the dissociation constant for CO_2 in aqueous solution and 0.03 is a constant for the solubility of CO_2 in plasma at 37°C.

FIGURE 6-7 Henderson-Hasselbalch equation. (From J. Wallach, *Interpretation of Diagnostic Tests* [4th ed.]. Boston: Little, Brown, 1986.)

Disturbances of acid-base balance may arise from respiratory or metabolic causes. Metabolic causes are sometimes termed nonrespiratory because they are not necessarily related to abnormal metabolism. The four primary types of acid-base disturbances are (1) respiratory acidosis, (2) respiratory alkalosis, (3) metabolic acidosis, and (4) metabolic alkalosis.

Etiology of Acidosis and Alkalosis

Respiratory Acidosis. Respiratory acidosis is caused by failure of the respiratory system to remove carbon dioxide from body fluids as fast as it is produced in the tissues. This leads to an increase in arterial PCO_2 above 45 mm Hg. Any condition resulting in alveolar hypoventilation leads to carbon dioxide retention and respiratory acidosis.

Causes include obstructive lung disease, interference with movements of the thoracic cage (e.g., poliomyelitis), and decreased activity of the respiratory center (due to narcotics, anesthetics, neural disease, etc.). Individuals having severe respiratory acidosis usually show signs and symptoms of respiratory insufficiency such as cyanosis; rapid, shallow breathing; and disorientation. Acute respiratory acidosis can produce carbon dioxide narcosis with symptoms of headache, blurred vision, fatigue, and weakness. Prolonged acidosis may produce severe central nervous system symptoms, including increased intracranial pressure and permanent damage [3]. When the pH falls below 7.10, dysrhythmias and peripheral vasodilatation may cause severe hypotension [3].

Respiratory Alkalosis. Respiratory alkalosis is caused by the loss of carbon dioxide from the lungs at a faster rate than it is produced in the tissues. This leads to a decrease in arterial PCO_2 below 35 mm Hg. Any condition resulting in excessive loss of carbon dioxide due to alveolar hyperventilation will cause respiratory alkalosis. Respiratory alkalosis is easily produced by voluntary overbreathing. Other causes include high altitude, anxiety, fever, meningitis, aspirin poisoning, and other factors that increase respiratory center activity. Symptoms of respiratory alkalosis are related to nervous system irritability and include lightheadedness, altered consciousness, various paresthesias, cramps and carpopedal spasm from clinical hypocalcemia (see p. 95) [3].

Metabolic Acidosis. Metabolic acidosis results from either an abnormal accumulation of fixed acids or loss of base. The plasma bicarbonate is decreased below 22 mEq per liter and arterial blood pH falls below 7.35.

Metabolic acidosis may be caused by kidney failure in which the kidneys are unable to replenish bicarbonate stores used for buffering strong acids produced by metabolism. In diabetes mellitus, ketoacid production due to incomplete oxidation of fats may lead to a severe metabolic acidosis. Anaerobic metabolism of glucose during strenuous exercise or circulatory shock may lead to lactic acidosis. Excessive administration of chloride can cause an excessive loss of HCO_3^- and metabolic acidosis. Loss of

TABLE 6-3 Disturbances of Acid-Base Balance

Arterial Blood pH	Primary Abnormality	Indicator of Primary Abnormality	Examples of Causative Factors	Compensatory Mechanisms
Alkalemia pH > 7.45	Respiratory alkalosis	↓ $PCO_2 < 35$ mm Hg	Hypoxia, anxiety, pulmonary embolus, pregnancy, other causes of hyperventilation	Kidneys retain hydrogen ions and excrete bicarbonate.
	Metabolic alkalosis	↑ $(HCO_3^-) > 26$ mEq/L	Treatment with diuretics and hormones that augment renal excretion of H^+, K^+, and Cl^-; fluid loss from stomach by vomiting or nasogastric suction; Cushing's disease, aldosteronism, excessive ingestion of alkali	Alveolar ventilation decreases, more CO_2 is retained. Kidneys increase H^+ retention and excrete bicarbonate.
Acidemia pH < 7.35	Respiratory acidosis	↑ $PCO_2 > 45$ mm Hg	Obstructive lung disease, depression of respiratory center by drugs or disease, other causes of hypoventilation	Kidneys increase H^+ excretion and bicarbonate retention.
	Metabolic acidosis	↓ $(HCO_3^-) < 22$ mEq/L	Diarrhea (loss of HCO_3^-) diabetic acidosis, lactic acidosis, renal failure, aspirin poisoning, treatment with ammonium chloride	Alveolar ventilation increases, more CO_2 is eliminated. Kidneys increase H^+ excretion and bicarbonate retention.

pancreatic bicarbonate from the intestine during chronic diarrhea or bilious vomiting produces metabolic acidosis, often with serious consequences in children. Acid-producing overdoses include acetylsalicylic acid, ethylene glycol, methyl alcohol, and paraldehyde.

Symptoms of severe metabolic acidosis include deep, rapid respiration (Kussmaul's breathing), disorientation, and coma. Clinical manifestations of metabolic acidosis depend on the pH level. Arterial pH of less than 7.10 can produce severe ventricular dysrhythmias, reduction of cardiac contractility. Production of lactic acidosis may occur with associated hypotension. Lethargy and coma can develop, but neurologic symptoms are less prominent in metabolic acidosis than in respiratory acidosis because the central nervous system is more sensitive to carbon dioxide changes than to pH shifts [3]. The chronic acidosis of renal failure retards bone growth and causes a variety of bone disturbances, probably due to buffering of acidosis by bone calcium [3].

Metabolic Alkalosis. Metabolic alkalosis results from either a loss of hydrogen ions or addition of base to body fluids. The plasma bicarbonate is elevated above 26 mEq per liter and arterial blood pH increases above 7.45.

One cause of this type of alkalosis is ingestion of excessive amounts of base (e.g., sodium bicarbonate, or baking soda) to treat stomach ulcers and indigestion. Administration of sodium bicarbonate in a cardiac arrest situation can produce a "post code" metabolic alkalosis. Another cause is vomiting of gastric contents in which hydrochloric acid is lost from the body. Endocrine disorders (e.g., Cushing disease) and treatment with certain types of drugs (e.g., thiazide) may augment renal excretion of H^+, K^+, and Cl^- and lead to metabolic alkalosis. Symptoms include apathy, mental confusion, shallow breathing, tetany, and spastic muscles. Clinical manifestations of metabolic alkalosis include weakness, muscle cramps, and dizziness which may be due to hypokalemia. Neurologic symptoms include paresthesias and lightheadedness [3].

Effects of pH Changes on Potassium, Calcium, and Magnesium Balance

Integrated into the direct effects of acidosis and alkalosis on the physiologic process are the compounding effects on potassium and calcium balance. Other electrolytes, such as magnesium and phosphate, are also affected, but the systemic effects of potassium and calcium imbalances can be life-threatening.

Hydrogen is preferentially excreted or retained over other cations by the renal system to maintain the blood pH. When the arterial pH falls, the excessive H^+ is excreted through the kidneys. It cannot be excreted unless a cation is retained. Potassium is the cation usually retained, so hyperkalemia develops in acidosis. Potassium may also shift out of intracellular fluid because more than 50 percent of the excess H^+ is buffered intracellularly. The K^+ and small amounts of Na^+ leave the cell to maintain electroneutrality [3]. The reverse is true with alkalosis. The kidney retains H^+ to normalize the blood pH and K^+ is wasted. The intracellular hydrogen is donated to the extracellular fluid and K^+ is retained intracellularly. Thus, hyperkalemia is associated with acidosis, and hypokalemia is associated with alkalosis (see pp. 81–82). Severe symptoms such as cardiac dysrhythmias and coma can result.

Changes in the arterial pH affect the ionized calcium levels in blood. The calcium in an alkalotic serum binds with serum proteins, producing the clinical effect of hypocalcemia [6]. The result can be hypocalcemia, tetany, spasm, and dysrhythmias (see pp. 83–84). In an acidic environment, more calcium may be released from the plasma proteins, and ionized calcium levels may rise transiently. The effect is not so pronounced as with alkalemia.

Serum magnesium levels also may change in response to the pH levels. Hypomagnesemia is often seen in acidosis. The symptoms include weakness, mental depression, and tetany similar to that of hypocalcemia.

Compensation

There are two ways in which an abnormal pH of arterial plasma may be returned toward normal: (1) compensation and (2) correction. In correction, the primary cause of the acid-base disturbance is repaired. For example, if respiratory acidosis is caused by partial blockage of the respiratory tree, removing or reducing the obstruction improves ventilation and allows blood pH to return toward normal. Correction of an acid-base disturbance is the primary aim of persons concerned with the delivery of health care to affected individuals.

In compensation, the system or systems not responsible for causing the acid-base disturbance make physiologic adjustments so as to return blood pH toward normal. For example, in respiratory acidosis (high PCO_2), the kidneys compensate by increasing the return of bicarbonate to the blood so as to return the $HCO_3^-:PCO_2$ ratio to normal. All processes of compensation are directed at returning the bicarbonate:PCO_2 ratio to 20:1, the normal pH of arterial plasma.

The kidneys compensate for respiratory acidosis (high PCO_2) by elevating the plasma bicarbonate above 26 mEq per liter. The kidneys compensate for respiratory alkalosis (low PCO_2) by lowering the plasma bicarbonate below 22 mEq per liter. Similar compensations are made by the kidneys in nonrenal causes of metabolic acidosis and alkalosis.

The respiratory system attempts to compensate for metabolic acidosis (low HCO_3^-) by lowering the arterial PCO_2 below 35 mm Hg through hyperventilation. It attempts to compensate for metabolic alkalosis by elevating the arterial PCO_2 above 45 mm Hg through hypoventilation.

Interpretation of Blood Gas Data

Major disturbances of acid-base balance are rarely completely compensated. Arterial pH is returned toward normal during compensation, but rarely to normal. Therefore, the arterial pH indicates whether a process of acidosis or alkalosis is present. The arterial blood PCO_2 and the plasma bicarbonate concentration indicate which process, respiratory or metabolic, is responsible for the abnormal pH and which process is compensatory.

For example, the following blood gas data indicate an acid-base abnormality: pH = 7.22; PCO_2 = 30 mm Hg; HCO_3^- = 12 mEq per liter. To interpret the data one must look at the pH to see if there is acidemia or alkalemia. In this case, the arterial pH is below normal range (7.35–7.45) and indicates acidemia. The body does not overcompensate, so the pH is reflective of the cause. The plasma PCO_2 and bicarbonate are then examined for indications of acidosis and alkalosis. Here, the bicarbonate concentration is below normal range (22–26 mEq per liter) and indicates metabolic acidosis. The arterial PCO_2 is below normal range (35–45 mm Hg) and indicates respiratory alkalosis. Since there is acidemia, the primary disturbance is one of metabolic acidosis while the compensatory process is respiratory. Therefore, the data suggest partially compensated metabolic acidosis.

Sometimes two primary disturbances of acid-base balance may be present simultaneously in the same individual. For example, a person with severely impaired pulmonary function may have a combined respiratory acidosis due to retention of carbon dioxide, and metabolic acidosis due to lactic acid production caused by inadequate oxygenation of the blood. In this example, a severe acidemia will be seen. Examples of acid-base disturbances and blood values are shown in Table 6-3.

The Anion Gap

Preliminary assessment of arterial PCO_2, $[HCO_3^-]$, and pH is helpful in determining which, if any, of the four major types of acid-base disturbances is present. Other measurements, computations, and tests are performed to confirm the preliminary diagnosis and establish the exact cause of the disturbance. The anion gap is commonly used in the differential diagnosis of metabolic acidosis.

The number of milliequivalents per liter of cations in plasma is normally balanced by an equal number of milliequivalents per liter of anions: $[Na^+] + [K^+] + [Mg^{++}] + [Ca^{++}] + [\text{other cations}] = [Cl^-] + [HCO_3^-] + [HPO_4^=] + [SO_4^=] + [\text{proteinate}^-] + [\text{other anions}]$. Only the concentrations of Na^+, K^+, Cl^-, and HCO_3^- are measured routinely; Mg^{++}, Ca^{++}, and other cations are considered unmeasured cations (UC); and $HPO_4^=$, $SO_4^=$, proteinate$^-$, and other anions are considered unmeasured anions (UA).

According to the principle of electroneutrality, plasma ionic balance can be expressed in the form of an equation between cations and anions:

$$[Na^+] + [K^+] + [UC] = [Cl^-] + [HCO_3^-] + [UA].$$

If the equation is rearranged so that measured ions are on one side and unmeasured ions are on the other side, the result is

$$[Na^+] + [K^+] - [Cl^-] - [HCO_3^-] = 16 \pm 4 \text{ mEq/L}.$$

TABLE 6-4 Differential Diagnosis of Metabolic Acidosis (After Kaehny)

Low or Normal Anion Gap (Hyperchloremic)	Increased Anion Gap
Gastrointestinal loss of HCO_3	Increased acid production
Diarrhea	Diabetic ketoacidosis
Small bowel or pancreatic drainage or fistula	Lactic acidosis
	Alcoholic ketoacidosis
Ureterosigmoidostomy, ileal loop conduit	Inborn errors of metabolism
Anion-exchange resins	
Renal loss of HCO_3^-	Ingestion of toxic substances
Renal tubular acidosis (RTA)	Salicylate overdose
Diamox	Paraldehyde poisoning
	Methal alcohol
	Ethylene glycol
Miscellaneous	Failure of acid excretion
Dilutional acidosis	Acute renal failure
Addition of HCl or its congeners	Chronic renal failure
Hyperalimentation acidosis	

Source: Schrier, R. W. *Renal and Electrolyte Disorders* (3rd ed.). Boston: Little, Brown, 1986.

Notice that $[K^+]$ is included in determining the anion gap. Since plasma $[K^+]$ is small compared to $[Na^+]$, $[Cl^-]$, and $[HCO_3^-]$, it is sometimes excluded from anion gap computations, in which case the normal value for the anion gap becomes 12 ± 4 mEq per liter. In metabolic acidosis, the anion gap may be normal, increased, or decreased, depending on the etiology (Table 6-4).

A normal anion gap in metabolic acidosis occurs in such conditions as diarrhea, ammonium chloride ingestion, and renal dysfunction. A high anion gap may be present with accumulation of organic acids such as ketoacids and lactic acids, as well as certain drugs and poisons. A normal gap is maintained by increasing chloride ions so that the sum of the HCO_3^- and Cl^- remains constant. This situation is often called ***hyperchloremic acidosis***. A high anion gap occurs when the sum of HCO_3^- and Cl^- decrease due to the accumulation of other acids.

Study Questions

1. Discuss the mechanisms that interact to maintain an equilibrium of hydrogen ion in the body.
2. Specifically explain the buffer systems.
3. What signs and symptoms relate to a clinical picture of acidosis and alkalosis?
4. How do the compensatory mechanisms of the body aid and/or hinder the resolution of acidosis?
5. Give examples of uncompensated, compensated, and mixed acid-base abnormalities.
6. Explain the anion gap and indicate its importance in understanding a specific acid-base problem.

References

1. Guyton, A. *Textbook of Medical Physiology* (7th ed.). Philadelphia: Saunders, 1986.
2. Keyes, J.L. *Fluid, Electrolyte and Acid-Base Regulation*. Monterey, Calif.: Wadsworth Health Sciences Division, 1985.
3. Rose, B.D. *Clinical Physiology of Acid-Base and Electrolyte Disorders* (2nd ed.). New York: McGraw-Hill, 1984.
4. Toporek, M. *Basic Chemistry of Life*. St. Louis: Mosby, 1981.
5. Wallach, J. *Interpretation of Diagnostic Tests* (4th ed.). Boston: Little, Brown, 1986.
6. Zaloga, G.P., and Chernow, B. Hypocalcemia in critical illness. *JAMA* 256:1924, 1986.

CHAPTER 7

Shock

CHAPTER OUTLINE

Hemodynamic Homeostasis
- Cardiac Output
- Total Peripheral Resistance
- Autonomic Response
- Intravascular Fluid Volume
- Hormones

Shock—An Overview

Stages of Shock
- Nonprogressive Shock
- Progressive Shock
- Irreversible Shock

Classifications of Shock
- Hypovolemic Shock
  - *Hemorrhage*
  - *Dehydration*
  - *Burns*
  - *Trauma*
- Cardiogenic Shock
  - *Pump Failure*
  - *Decreased Venous Return*
- Vasogenic Shock
  - *Neurogenic Shock*
  - *Septic Shock*
  - *Anaphylactic Shock*

Complications of Shock
- Lactic Acidosis
- Adult Respiratory Distress Syndrome
- Disseminated Intravascular Coagulation
- Organ Ischemia and Necrosis

LEARNING OBJECTIVES

1. Discuss the physiologic mechanisms responsible for maintaining hemodynamic homeostasis, the steady state.
2. Identify the stages of shock.
3. Discuss compensatory responses to the shock state.
4. Define irreversible shock.
5. List causes, indicators, and consequences of irreversible shock.
6. List the classifications of shock.
7. Identify the types of shock relative to their designated classification.
8. Describe the pathologic processes associated with each classification of shock.
9. List and explain the basis for symptoms associated with each classification of shock.
10. List the complications of the shock state.
11. Explain the basis for the development of each complication of shock.

The occurrence of the shock state is a most dreaded and yet predictable development in innumerable pathologic conditions ranging from hemorrhage to spinal cord injury. It is therefore absolutely imperative that the health care practitioner be thoroughly versed in all aspects relating to etiology, symptomatology, compensatory mechanisms, and consequences of this condition. This chapter provides a comprehensive account of the physiologic mechanisms that regulate hemodynamic homeostasis as well as the derangements that compromise that homeostatic state. The term *homeostasis* refers to the maintenance of constant conditions in the internal environment, the so-called steady state [7].

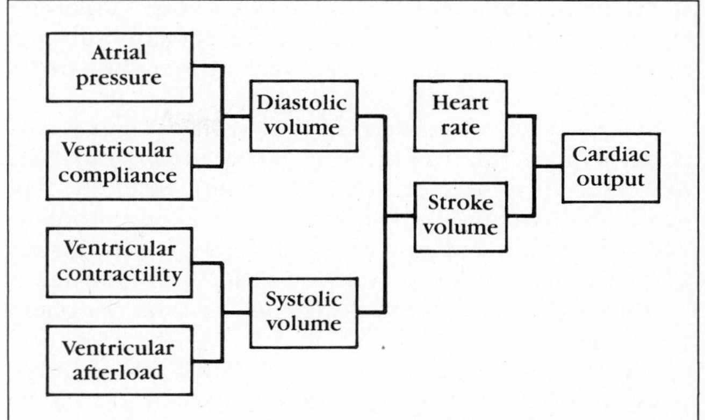

FIGURE 7-1 Physiologic determinants of cardiac output. (Reprinted with permission from R.L. Vick, *Contemporary Medical Physiology*. Menlo Park, Calif.: Addison-Wesley, 1984, p. 237.)

Hemodynamic Homeostasis

Any discussion or account relative to the state of shock must be preceded by an overview of the physiologic mechanisms that maintain and regulate normal blood pressure. Basically, blood pressure is the product of cardiac output times total peripheral resistance and can be expressed by the equation BP = CO × TPR. Any condition or derangement that increases or decreases either cardiac output or total peripheral resistance may potentially raise or lower blood pressure accordingly. Alterations in blood pressure due to an increase or decrease in either cardiac output or in total peripheral resistance are transient and momentary in healthy individuals who have intact and functional autonomic nervous systems (see Chap. 18). Because of the inverse relationship between cardiac output and total peripheral resistance in regard to blood pressure control, an increase or decrease in one component prompts an opposite response in the other so that blood pressure remains constant. For example, if cardiac output decreases, total peripheral resistance automatically increases and blood pressure returns to normal. The physiologic mechanisms responsible for activating this inverse relationship and maintaining blood pressure are generated by autonomic nervous system response.

Cardiac Output

Cardiac output is defined as the volume or load of blood ejected by the left ventricle each minute. In the average-sized adult, this volume equals 5 liters. It is usually slightly less in females due primarily to lower body weight and/or size. Cardiac output volume, although relatively consistent in most individuals, is not an absolute or constant value because it may be influenced directly or indirectly by many factors. Cardiac output is the product of stroke volume times heart rate (the equation: CO = SV × HR). Stroke volume is that quantity of blood ejected by each ventricle with each cardiac contraction. It is determined or influenced by factors such as the atrial volume (preload) and the compliance, contractility, and afterload of the ventricles [19] (see Chap. 18). The relationship between these functional factors and stroke volume as they pertain to cardiac output is represented in Figure 7-1.

In addition to the functional determinants of stroke volume, circulating blood volume with an adequate venous return plays a very significant role in determining stroke volume. Conditions that alter atrial pressure, ventricular function, or venous return affect stroke volume and consequently, cardiac output. If stroke volume increases or decreases, an automatic opposite response in heart rate serves to maintain constant cardiac output. For example, a decrease in venous return results in a decreased stroke volume. Cardiac output remains constant, however, because the decreased stroke volume indirectly prompts an increase in heart rate (see Chap. 18).

The second determinant of cardiac output is heart rate. Heart rate is mediated by autonomic nervous system (parasympathetic and sympathetic) influence on the sinoatrial (pacemaker) node. Parasympathetic innervation decreases heart rate through vagal stimulation, whereas sympathetic innervation increases heart rate.

Total Peripheral Resistance

Total peripheral resistance is determined primarily by the diameter of the arteries and, to a lesser extent, that of the veins. Resistance is high in vessels with small diameter (vasoconstriction) and low in vessels with larger diameter (vasodilation). Therefore, systemic blood pressure is increased when vessels are constricted and decreased when vessels are dilated. Like heart rate, blood vessel diameter, and hence resistance, is under the influence of the autonomic nervous system. Sympathetic stimulation results in vasoconstriction, whereas parasympathetic stimulation results in vasodilation.

Autonomic Response

The influence of the autonomic nervous system on peripheral resistance and heart rate is critical in regulating blood pressure. The effects of autonomic nervous system innervation focus on two areas in the medulla of the brainstem, the *cardiac center* and the *vasomotor center*. Both centers respond promptly to autonomic innervation through stimulation by the sympathetic branch or inhibition by the parasympathetic branch.

Sympathetic stimulation of the cardiac center results in acceleration of heart rate, while *parasympathetic stimulation* results in deceleration of heart rate. Similarly, sympathetic stimulation of the vasomotor center produces vasoconstriction and an increase in total peripheral resistance. Parasympathetic stimulation of the vasomotor center produces vasodilation and a decrease in total peripheral resistance.

The structures responsible for instigating autonomic activity are the *baroreceptors* located in the aortic arch and carotid sinuses. The baroreceptors are sensitive to changes in the degree of stretch or tension in the walls of these major arteries. Decreased stretch or tension is indicative of low cardiac output and/or decreased peripheral vascular resistance consistent with low blood pressure. Conversely, increased stretch or tension indicates elevated cardiac output and/or increased peripheral vascular resistance consistent with high blood pressure. Marked decrease in stretch in the arterial wall prompts a reflex at the baroreceptors resulting in sympathetic stimulation of the cardiac center, which then causes acceleration of heart rate, increased cardiac output, and a simultaneous stimulation of the vasomotor center, which in turn increases peripheral resistance. The net effect is an elevation in blood pressure [4,7].

In the case of increased stretch in the arterial wall, the baroreceptors respond by stimulating parasympathetic activity. Increased parasympathetic activity elicits a decelerating effect from the cardiac center, resulting in a decreased heart rate and hence cardiac output, and a concomitant decrease in total peripheral resistance through inhibition of vasomotor center activity. The overall effect is a reduction in blood pressure.

Autonomic nervous system innervation stabilizes blood pressure by modifying heart rate and thus cardiac output, and/or by changing total peripheral resistance. It performs a critically significant physiologic function in blood pressure regulation. Absence of autonomic nervous system influence in blood pressure control can lead to irreversible shock and death.

Intravascular Fluid Volume

Fluid volume ranks equally in significance with autonomic nervous system influence in blood pressure regulation. Without sufficient quantities of circulating intravascular volume, autonomic nervous system innervation would be ineffective and virtually useless in executing normal, as well as compensatory/adaptive, physiologic functions related to blood pressure control.

Normally, fluid volume contributes to blood pressure control in a maintenance-type fashion. Physiologically, adequate circulating fluid volume ensures adequate venous return, which, consequently, with other factors such as ventricular function and heart rate being normal, ensures adequate cardiac output. This provides a major contribution to blood pressure maintenance. Increases or decreases in circulating fluid volume can either raise or lower blood pressure accordingly.

An additional component in the fluid volume influence over blood pressure is the process of *autoregulation*. Autoregulation is the mechanism whereby blood vessels either constrict or dilate in response to respective increases or decreases in the amount of intravascular fluid volume circulating to the tissues [7]. In the case of increased volume, autoregulation results in vasoconstriction in order to normalize or equilibrate acceptable blood flow to tissues and organs. Vasoconstriction in peripheral vessels increases total peripheral resistance and systemic blood pressure (Fig. 7-2).

Low or inadequate fluid volume induces autoregulative vasodilation to increase the amount of blood flow to tissues and organs. Vasodilation reduces total peripheral resistance, thereby lowering blood pressure.

Intravascular fluid volume is determined in large measure by the body's sodium content by the following mechanisms. Increased sodium content activates the thirst mechanism by hypothalamic stimulation [14]. Thirst induces voluntary water intake, thereby diluting sodium levels and offsetting sodium excess. A second and probably concurrent mechanism instigated because of excessive extracellular sodium is the increased release of antidiuretic hormone (ADH or vasopressin) from the posterior pituitary. Antidiuretic hormone is released in response to either increased serum osmolarity, as would be the case in sodium excess, or to conditions of water deficit. Activity of ADH, like increased oral intake, increases water volume and raises blood pressure by increasing venous return and

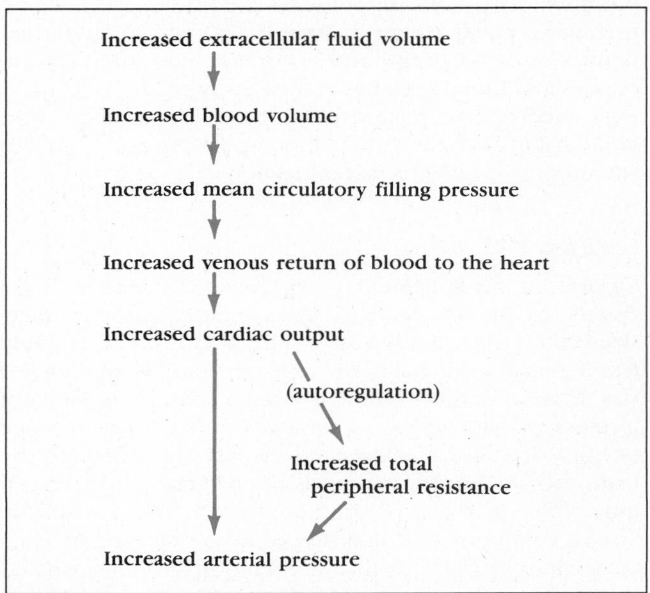

FIGURE 7-2 Effects of increased volume on blood pressure. (From A.C. Guyton, *Textbook of Medical Physiology* [7th ed.]. Philadelphia: W.B. Saunders Company, 1986, p. 261. Reprinted by permission.)

cardiac output. Increased intravascular volume also raises blood pressure.

Hormones

Hormones that are responsible for blood pressure regulation are the catecholamines (epinephrine and norepinephrine), renin-angiotensin-aldosterone, and vasopressin. Each regulates blood pressure through different but equally effective mechanisms.

The catecholamines, released by the adrenal medulla as well as by various adrenergic terminals located throughout the body, are categorized basically as short-term, immediate determinants of blood pressure and operate in the following ways. Epinephrine increases both the rate of cardiac contractions and total peripheral resistance. Both effects raise blood pressure. In instances of hypotension, epinephrine is quite effective in instituting compensatory measures to elevate blood pressure by increasing both cardiac output and total peripheral resistance. The role of norepinephrine in restoring and maintaining blood pressure is related to improving and strengthening myocardial contractility, thereby increasing stroke volume and consequently, cardiac output. Both epinephrine and norepinephrine are released into the circulation through stimulation of autonomic adrenergic sympathetic nervous system influence on the adrenal medulla and various other sympathetic terminals located throughout the body.

The role of the renin-angiotensin-aldosterone (RAA) system in blood pressure restoration is shown in Figure 7-3. This system is prompted into action by the effects of hypotensive episodes on renal perfusion. Low or decreased renal perfusion stimulates the juxtaglomerular apparatus to release renin. Renin has little or no direct effect on blood pressure, but it acts on angiotensin, a plasma protein, to produce angiotensin I, which then is converted in the lungs to angiotensin II. Angiotensin II has two profound effects on blood pressure restoration. First, it is a very potent vasoconstrictor and as such, produces a generalized increase in total peripheral resistance, thereby elevating blood pressure. Second, angiotensin II stimulates the hypothalamus to induce thirst and prompts the release of aldosterone from the adrenal cortex. Aldosterone increases the resorption of sodium from the distal tubules and collecting ducts. Increased sodium resorption obliges a concomitant resorption of water. These mechanisms increase blood pressure by elevating intravascular fluid volume.

Vasopressin is secreted by the posterior pituitary in response to hyperosmolarity, water deficit, or low blood volume. The mechanisms by which these states prompt antidiuretic hormone secretion vary, but result in quite effective compensation for each state.

Hyperosmolarity (especially due to hypernatremia) and water deficit conditions are detected by osmoreceptors located in the supraoptic nuclei of the hypothalamus. These structures in turn stimulate pituitary release of ADH. The action of the hormone in this regard is that of water conservation. It is accomplished by a poorly understood mechanism that results in increased resorption of water, mainly in the collecting ducts of nephrons. Increased resorption of water dilutes or offsets the hyperosmolar condition and corrects the water deficit. In addition, increased resorption of water raises intravascular volume, augments venous return, improves cardiac output, and thereby raises blood pressure. Increased vascular volume also raises blood pressure through autoregulation.

The second pathologic condition that stimulates secretion of ADH is low blood volume. This results in decreased stretch on the pressure sensors in the atria and in the baroreceptors in the carotid sinus and aortic arch, which in turn stimulate the secretion of ADH. In addition to its water conservation action, ADH produces a vasoconstrictive effect on arterioles, ultimately raising blood pressure [7].

In summary, hemodynamic homeostasis is maintained by a variety of physiologic mechanisms. Each serves to restore normal blood pressure by increasing total peripheral resistance, cardiac output, or circulating fluid volume. In the shock state these processes are crucial in reinstituting hemodynamic homeostasis, and their activity is evidenced by numerous physiologic signs and symptoms.

Shock — An Overview

Shock is defined as a condition in which there is an overall or generalized reduction of adequate blood flow throughout the vasculature of the body [7]. It is typically manifested by hypotension; tachycardia; oliguria; cool, moist skin; restlessness; and altered levels of consciousness. It usually is induced by such conditions as hemorrhage, heart failure, sepsis, and neurologic damage.

Regardless of its etiology or pathologic basis, every form or classification of shock is characterized by compromised or inadequate tissue and organ perfusion. In effect, a discrepancy exists between tissue need for oxygen and various nutrients, and actual supply of those elements. The ultimate result of this discrepancy is multisystem deterioration and related loss of function.

Compromised tissue and organ perfusion characteristic of shock is caused by *low cardiac output* and/or *reduced tissue perfusion pressure*. Every type of shock can easily be grouped with or related to one or sometimes both of these categories. The various forms of shock are presented separately in this chapter.

Stages of Shock

There are essentially three stages of the shock state. Various authors refer to them by different names: initial, progressive, and final [1]; nonprogressive, progressive, and irreversible [7]; early, tissue hypoperfusion, and cell and organ injury [14]; initial, compensatory, progressive, and refractory [12]. Despite the variation in nomenclature, the basic fact remains that individuals experiencing shock progress through fairly distinguishable phases ranging from compensation to various states or degrees of decompensation. The terms *nonprogressive*, *progressive*, and

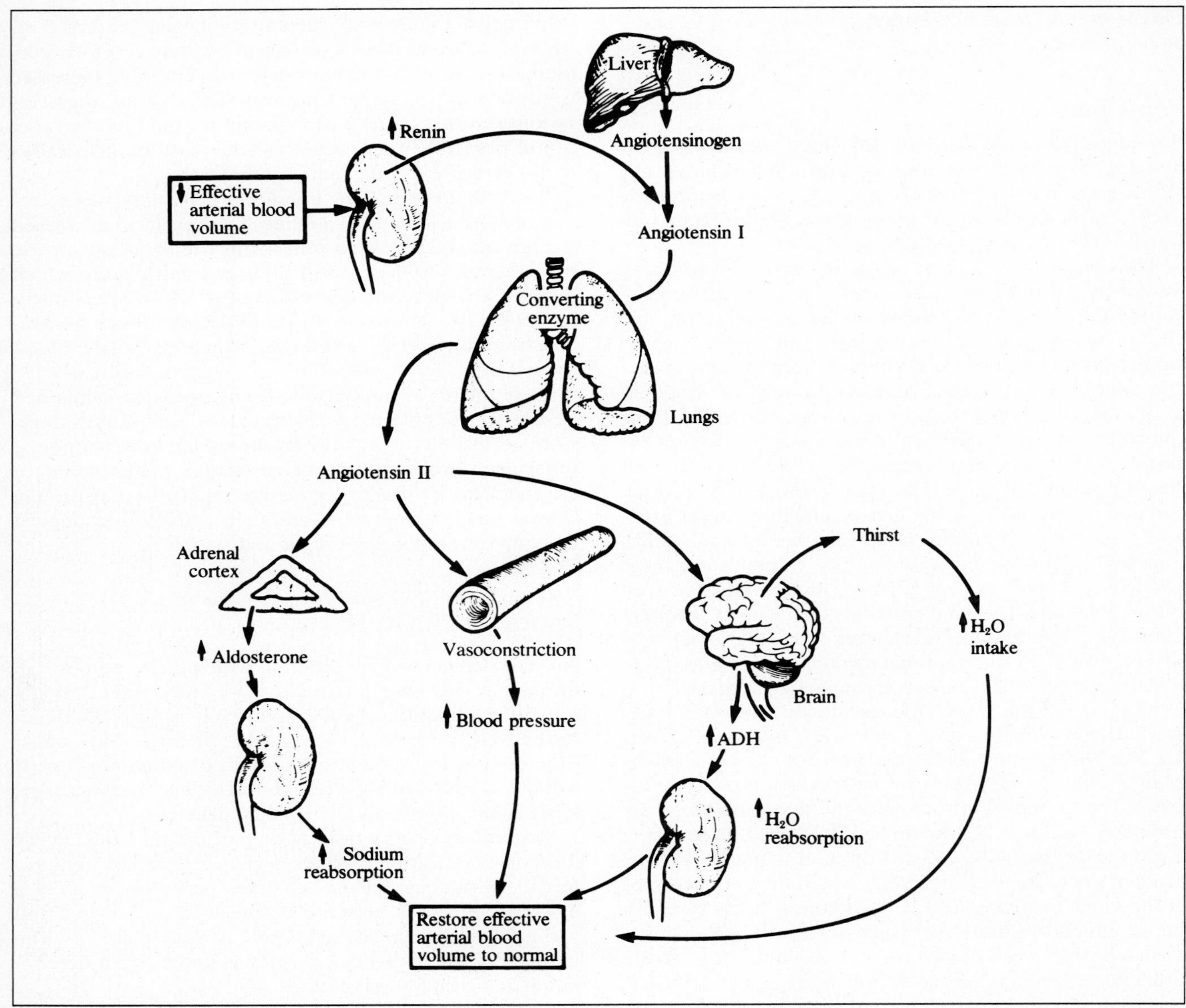

FIGURE 7-3 Influence of the renin-angiotensin-aldosterone system on blood pressure. (From E. Selkurt, *Basic Physiology for the Health Sciences* [2nd ed.]. Boston: Little, Brown, 1982.)

irreversible shock are used in this discussion. Table 7-1 indicates differences in the clinical picture according to the degree of shock.

Nonprogressive Shock

Nonprogressive shock represents the initial or early phase during which, in response to the initial insult, several physiologic compensatory mechanisms are activated. Frequently, when these mechanisms are fully operational they may compensate for the shock state, depending on the extent of the insult.

During this early phase, cardiac output and/or total peripheral resistance are decreased as a consequence of the initial insult regardless of its origin or nature. These decreases result in decreased stretch or tension in the walls of major arteries. Baroreceptors situated in these arterial walls, specifically in the aortic arch and carotid sinuses, detect the reduced stretch and activate the autonomic nervous system response.

The sympathetic branch of the autonomic nervous system (SNS) responds to baroreceptor innervation by instigating two processes. First, sympathetic activity stimulates the cardiac center to increase heart rate by inhibiting vagal tone, thereby increasing cardiac output. Second, and simultaneously, sympathetic activity stimulates the vasomotor center to increase total peripheral resistance through vasoconstriction. Both of these responses represent an effort

TABLE 7-1 Clinical Picture Exhibited According to Degree of Shock

	Nonprogressive	Progressive	Irreversible
Sensorium	Oriented to time, place, person	Remains oriented; words slurred	Disoriented
Pulse	Rate increased Quality, full to decreased	Rate, very high Quality, decreased and variable	Rate, over 150 Quality, weak, thready, difficult to feel.
Blood pressure	Normal to low (10–20% decrease but may be slightly increased as compensatory mechanism)	Decreased 40–50 mm Hg below normal (20–40% decrease)	Systolic less than 80 Diastolic may not be heard
Urinary output	35–50 ml/hr	20–35 ml/hr	Less than 20 ml/hr
Color	Pale	Pale	Mottled
Capillary refill	Circulation return slightly slowed	Circulation return slowed	Circulation return very slow; skin pale both before and after Large differences between rectal and big toe temperature
Blood gases	pH normal	pH below 7.35	pH very low, 7.0–7.2

to raise blood pressure compensatorily and thus improve or restore adequate tissue and organ perfusion. They are usually operational within several seconds to minutes.

Another compensatory mechanism set into motion in this early stage of shock is activation of the renin-angiotensin-aldosterone system (RAA system). Renin, released in response to low renal perfusion, triggers the eventual production of angiotensin II. Angiotensin II exerts its effects on blood pressure by vasoconstriction and by both stimulation of the thirst mechanism and release of aldosterone from the adrenal cortex. The vasoconstrictive effect raises blood pressure by increasing total peripheral resistance, and the other effects do so by increasing circulating intravascular fluid volume. The RAA system is fully activated about 20 minutes after the initial stimulus, so that its action follows that of the SNS.

Still another compensatory activity is increased secretion of ADH. Vasopressin (ADH) is released in response to low pressure in the atria, aortic arch, and carotid sinuses. Its action is directed primarily toward water conservation and arteriolar vasoconstriction. Both of these actions tend to elevate blood pressure.

Symptoms that predominate in this initial stage are directly related to compensatory activity. The individual is usually awake and alert but somewhat anxious. Heart rate is elevated but blood pressure is normal, indicating the presence of sympathetic activity. Without the influence of the SNS, the blood pressure would be decreased. The skin is usually pale, moist, and cool owing to sympathetic activity. Pupillary dilatation may be evident. Over time, the hematocrit becomes depressed when the condition is due to hemorrhage, because interstitial fluid is absorbed into the blood vessel, and dilutes the blood (see pp. 225–226). Respirations may be shallow, and the rate is increased in response to inadequate tissue oxygen delivery. Urinary output is slightly reduced because of impaired renal perfusion and ADH and aldosterone activity. The individual usually complains of thirst. Bowel sounds may be hypoactive, related to compensatory vasoconstriction and reduced blood delivery to nonessential organs such as the intestines. Muscle weakness and hyporeactive reflexes may be present for the same reason.

The shock state usually resolves within a matter of several hours, as long as the initiating event is not overwhelming and compensatory mechanisms are intact and functional. Otherwise, shock progresses to a more advanced stage in which compensatory mechanisms become virtually incapable of restoring blood pressure.

Progressive Shock

Progressive shock, commonly referred to as uncompensated shock, represents a condition in which compensatory responses fail to restore blood pressure and tissue perfusion. In addition, the deleterious effects of prolonged tissue and organ hypoperfusion with resultant ischemic deterioration begin to compound the worsening clinical picture. It is, in fact, during this stage that the potentially devastating complications of shock usually begin to develop (see pp. 111–112).

In the progressive stage the effects of ischemia to, as well as exhaustion of, organs generating compensatory responses become evident. The medullary vasomotor center reacts to decreased perfusion and oxygen deprivation by completely ceasing its activity. Similarly, the myocardium, subjected to inadequate coronary artery perfusion and increased work in efforts to sustain cardiac output, begins to deteriorate and is unable to generate adequate cardiac output. Additional factors responsible for myocardial ineffectiveness are related to the influence of lactic acid and the myocardial depressant factor. Lactic acid is produced both in the myocardium itself and in tissues throughout the body as a byproduct of anaerobic glycogenesis consistent with stages of oxygen deprivation. It has a very potent ability to suppress myocardial contractility. The myocardial suppressant factor also exerts a very potent negative inotropic effect. It is released by the pancreas, which suffers from comprised splanchnic organ circulation consistent with shock states [8]. Eventually, myocardial contractility is so impaired that heart failure with pulmonary edema ensues.

Renal integrity is compromised relatively early in this stage of shock. The kidneys are quite sensitive to low perfusion pressure and respond rather quickly to reduced glomerular filtration by activating the RAA system. The kidneys, like the gastrointestinal system, skin, and splanchnic organs, are targeted as nonessential organs and are further compromised by selective vasoconstriction induced by sympathetic activity. The more essential organs, the heart and brain, are not affected by sympathetic vasoconstriction. Renal effects of the shock state and preferential vasoconstriction are seen in the form of acute tubular necrosis secondary to ischemia, and rather prompt acute renal failure (see Chap. 31).

The kidneys are not the only organs affected by hypoperfusion, ischemia, and selective vasoconstriction. Lung tissue also undergoes ischemic deterioration, resulting in adult respiratory distress syndrome, or shock lung. The ischemic gastrointestinal tract undergoes necrotic changes and releases endotoxins, vasodilating substances that further compound shock. Liver function deteriorates and this organ becomes incapable of performing metabolic or biotransformation functions [7].

Symptoms associated with the progressive stage of shock are related to organ failure and the development of complications. Levels of consciousness and orientation decrease. Bradycardia and hypotension progress, urine output ceases, pulmonary and peripheral edema develop, and tachypnea with dyspnea becomes prominent. Abdominal distention and paralytic ileus are common. Central venous pressure and pulmonary artery pressure are increased. The person appears critically ill, with cold, diaphoretic, and ashen skin. The arterial pH becomes acidotic due to lactic acid accumulation. Recovery at this point depends on the underlying condition and therapeutic management.

Irreversible Shock

Irreversible shock denotes the final progression and is basically the point at which the individual becomes refractory or unresponsive to all forms of therapeutic management. Survival is virtually impossible. Figure 7-4 summarizes the different types of feedback that can lead to the progression of shock.

Classifications of Shock

It is convenient to classify shock according to either etiology or associated physiologic impairment. For example, hypovolemic shock is caused by loss of intravascular volume, cardiogenic shock is the result of cardiac decompensation, and vasogenic shock denotes widespread vasodilation. In addition, various shock states, or at least shock-promoting status, can be categorized under one of three broad classifications or headings: hypovolemic, cardiogenic, or vasogenic. Subsumed under the heading of hypovolemic shock are conditions such as hemorrhage, burns, dehydration, and trauma. Cardiogenic shock includes pump failure and decreased venous return. Vasogenic or vasodilation shock is the broad heading under which nervous system failure, septicemia, and anaphylaxis are grouped.

Hypovolemic Shock

Hypovolemic shock, or that shock state resulting from loss of circulating fluid volume, may be caused by or result from any condition that significantly depletes normal volumes of whole blood, plasma, or water. The underlying pathology, regardless of the exact type of fluid loss, is related to actual circulatory fluid pressure/volume deficits. Decreased circulating fluid volume decreases venous return, which reduces cardiac output and therefore lowers blood pressure. As a consequence, lowered blood pressure impedes tissue and organ perfusion and oxygen delivery. These consequences of lowered blood pressure are potential first steps leading eventually to ischemia, necrosis, organ malfunction, and shock. Compensatory mechanisms are activated to adjust for the reduced tissue and organ perfusion. These mechanisms, discussed on pages 102–103, include SNS stimulation to increase cardiac rate and total peripheral resistance, activation of the RAA system, and increased secretion of ADH.

These mechanisms, in toto, effectuate an increase in blood pressure. If treatment to correct or remove the underlying cause of fluid volume loss is initiated, the shock crisis is averted or resolved. If the fluid volume loss is overwhelming or therapeutic measures are not effective, this initial stage of shock may progress to the irreversible stage.

Hemorrhage. Hemorrhagic shock occurs as a result of massive loss of whole blood. Some conditions that produce drastic loss of blood include gastrointestinal bleeding, postoperative hemorrhage, hemophilia, uterine lesions, childbirth, and trauma. For the shock state to ensue, blood loss must be extensive. Minimal loss of blood, up to 10 percent of the total volume, does not produce noticeable changes in blood pressure or cardiac output. Blood losses of up to 45 percent of the total blood volume reduce both cardiac output and blood pressure to zero [7]. Symptoms depend upon the actual volume of blood lost and whether the loss was sudden and abrupt or gradual.

In addition to the compensatory mechanisms, certain humoral substances are released in hemorrhage in an attempt to restore the steady state. In shock due to abrupt hemorrhage, release of adrenocorticotropic hormone (ACTH) is increased, which in turn increases glucocorticoid levels. The *glucocorticoids* maintain capillary integrity and combat the effects of the mediators of the inflammatory response. Erythropoietin levels increase and stimulate bone marrow to produce red blood cells. Circulating volume of *2-3,diphosphoglycerate*, a substance that interacts with hemoglobin to promote the release of oxy-

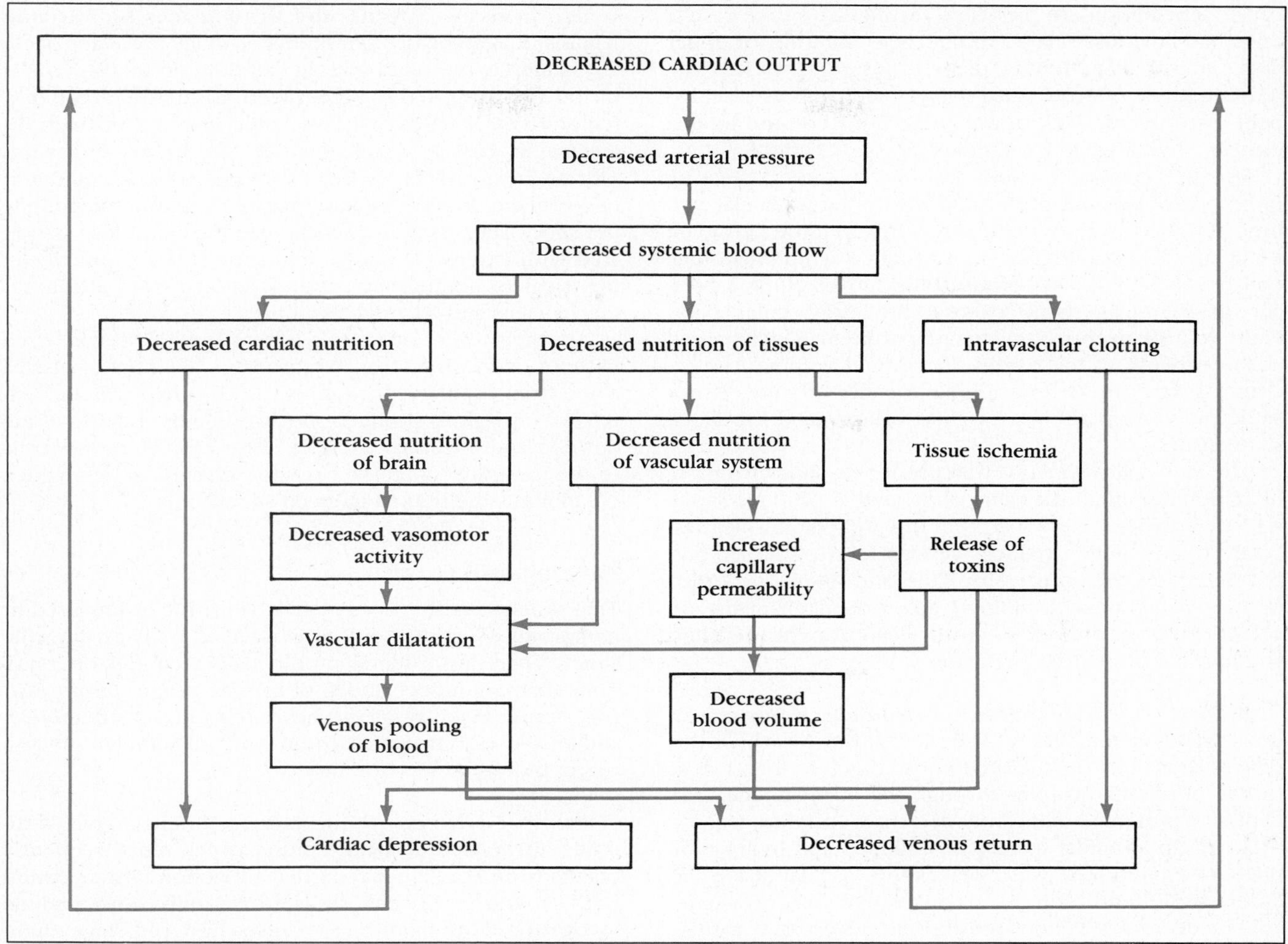

FIGURE 7-4 Different types of feedback that can lead to progression of shock. (From A.C. Guyton, *Textbook of Medical Physiology* [7th ed.]. Philadelphia: W.B. Saunders Company, 1986. Reprinted by permission.)

gen, increases. This increases the liberation of oxygen, thereby reducing the effects of the tissue and organ hypoxia characteristic of shock [16]. The *prostaglandins*—PGE_2, PG_{12}, PGF_2-alpha, and PGA_2—play a mixed role in hemorrhagic shock, exerting beneficial and detrimental effects. Both PGE_2 and PG_{12} dilate liver and renal vessels, thereby improving to some extent perfusion to these organs; PGF_2-alpha and PGA_2 constrict blood vessels. While PG_{12} retards aggregation of platelets, PGA_2 exerts the opposite effect and actually promotes platelet aggregation. This latter action has been implicated in the development of disseminated intravascular coagulation in hemorrhagic shock. Activation of the *complement system* is beneficial in hemorrhagic shock because of its role in cell lysis, but detrimental because it promotes leukocyte dysfunction, which potentiates the development of adult respiratory distress syndrome [15].

In addition to these humoral agents released in hemorrhagic shock, other substances released in response to cellular deterioration actually have the potential for perpetuating the shock state. For example, lysosomal enzymes extend cellular damage, depress myocardial contractility, and constrict coronary vessels. The kinins depress myocardial contractility, promote vasodilation, and together with histamine, make capillaries more permeable, contributing to fluid volume loss. Serotonin causes potent arteriolar constriction and thus impedes microcirculation. Lactic acid, generated by anaerobic glycogenesis, depresses myocardial contractility. Endotoxins are released in response to gastrointestinal ischemia and result in vasodilation and myocardial depression [15]. All of these substances—lysosomal enzymes, kinins, histamine, serotonin, lactic acid, and endotoxins—are released in response to cellular damage and as such, are normal byproducts of injured cells. Their overall effect in hemorrhagic shock, however, is to perpetuate the vicious cycle of decreased perfusion and hypoxia.

Dehydration. Dehydration results from extensive and profound loss of body fluid. Conditions that classically cause dehydration are profuse sweating; extensive gastrointestinal fluid loss related to diarrhea, vomiting, or upper gastrointestinal suctioning; diabetes insipidus; ascites; the diuretic phase of acute renal failure; Addison's disease; hypoaldosteronism; lack of adequate fluid volume intake; osmotic diuresis; and injudicious use of diuretics.

For dehydration to produce a shock state, it must be quite severe because of the reservoir of intravascular volume supplied by intracellular volume. Simple and even moderate dehydration does not produce symptomatology consistent with shock because fluid moves along a pressure gradient from tissue spaces to the intravascular space. Fluid volume in the vascular compartment is maintained at the expense of the tissues. Once fluid volume loss becomes severe, however, cellular transfer of water is not sufficient to maintain intravascular volume, and the shock state ensues.

The mechanisms involved in producing shock from dehydration are much the same as those that produce shock with hemorrhage. Fluid lost from the body diminishes vascular volume, which reduces venous return. Cardiac output decreases, blood pressure falls, and tissue and organ perfusion declines. Physiologic adaptive mechanisms are activated in an attempt to restore blood pressure, fluid volume, and ultimately, perfusion.

Burns. Burns, especially third-degree burns, can cause hypovolemic shock. The mechanism by which this type of shock occurs is related not so much to fluid loss as to loss of plasma proteins through the burn surface. Loss of plasma proteins significantly decreases colloidal osmotic pressure. In an effort to restore colloidal and hydrostatic pressure equilibrium, water leaves the vascular space and enters the interstitium. As a consequence, intravascular volume decreases, venous return is also decreased, cardiac output is inadequate, and blood pressure falls.

Two additional causes of shock secondary to burns are hemorrhage and sepsis. Burn surfaces promote platelet aggregation and activation of factor XII, which leads to localized intravascular clot formation. These localized clots can impair microcirculation, resulting in tissue ischemia and necrosis, and can consume factors of coagulation. Consumption of clotting factors may result in disseminated intravascular coagulation (DIC) and systemic hemorrhage [19].

Sepsis can result from extensive burns because of loss or destruction of the body's natural barrier—that is, the skin—to bacterial invasion. In addition, however, burned surfaces apparently release toxins into systemic circulation that injure intestinal capillaries, thereby permitting the release of intestinal bacteria and endotoxins into systemic circulation. The mechanisms of septic shock are discussed on pages 109–110.

Trauma. Trauma, in the forms of crushing injuries to muscles and bones, gunshot wounds, and penetration of blood vessels, the viscera, or other vital organs by knives or sharp instruments, produces the shock state primarily through extensive and sudden blood loss. An astounding amount of blood lost internally due to trauma can be concealed in tissue, organs, and third spaces for variable lengths of time before symptoms of shock are manifested. For example, the thigh muscle can hold up to 1000 ml of blood resulting from a fractured femur or a tear in a femoral vessel without a noticeable increase in thigh diameter [4]. Loss of 1 liter of whole blood represents a significant hemorrhage, especially if it goes undetected and uncorrected. It consequently perpetuates and compounds the shock state. Because of the massive blood loss associated with extensive trauma, traumatic shock is practically identical to hemorrhagic shock in terms of pathologic mechanisms and adaptive responses.

Another aspect of trauma is that loss of plasma, even without overt blood loss, often occurs [7]. Loss of plasma alone from capillary damage can lead to hypovolemia extensive enough to produce shock. Similarly, release of endotoxin and intestinal bacteria due to injury or ischemia to the gastrointestinal tract results in septic shock, which compounds the trauma-induced shock.

Cardiogenic Shock

That shock state that is directly attributable to impaired or compromised cardiac output is referred to as cardiogenic shock. There are essentially only two categories of conditions that can induce shock of cardiac origin: *pump failure*, actual inability of the heart to contract effectively, and *decreased venous return*, inability of sufficient quantities of blood to enter the heart.

Pump Failure. Pump failure shock is always directly attributable to heart failure, which most frequently results from massive myocardial infarction. Other conditions causing cardiogenic shock from pump failure include myocardiopathy from many causes and end-stage rheumatic and congenital heart diseases.

The mechanism by which myocardial infarction results in pump failure is related to extensive myocardial damage that results in greatly diminished cardiac output. The predominant and prevailing defect accounting for low cardiac output is impaired myocardial contractility with loss of functional myocardium (see Chap. 20). Pump failure results when nearly half of myocardial tissue is nonfunctional.

Decreased Venous Return. Decreased venous return is a category of cardiogenic shock that is caused not by inadequate circulating volume, but by actual impedance of blood flow into the heart. It is the consequence of conditions such as cardiac tamponade, acute pericardial effusion, and mediastinal shifts that essentially squeeze or compress the heart to such an extent that venous inflow is impaired [14]. Decreased venous return, regardless of the causes, always results in decreased cardiac output and hence lowered blood pressure with impaired tissue and organ perfusion.

In response to low cardiac output, regardless of the cause, compensatory mechanisms are activated for the purpose of improving or restoring tissue perfusion by increasing blood pressure through acceleration of heart rate and elevation of total peripheral resistance. The decreases in stroke volume, cardiac output, and perfusion brought about by impaired myocardial contractility are compounded and worsened by the autonomic sympathetic responses intended to improve them. The autonomic response increases heart rate, thus increasing oxygen demand and decreasing diastolic filling time, both of which further compromise an ischemic myocardium. In addition, autonomically mediated vasoconstriction increases afterload, forcing the failing myocardium to work even harder in its attempt to sustain adequate cardiac output. Selective vasoconstriction shunts blood away from organs such as the kidneys, skin, and splanchnic organs and toward the heart and brain, resulting in additional reduction of tissue and organ perfusion. Eventually, these selectively deprived organs experience and demonstrate the effects of inadequate perfusion. A schema depicting the sequential and intricate pattern of cardiogenic shock development is shown in Figure 7-5.

Left ventricular filling pressure and cardiac index obtained through use of a Swan-Ganz catheter are universal values for determining not only the extent of cardiac decompensation but the prognosis for survival in cardiogenic shock. Generally, those with high left ventricular end-diastolic pressure or pulmonary artery end-diastolic pressure (greater than 12–15 mm Hg) and/or low cardiac index (less than 2 L/min/m^2) have statistically higher rates of mortality (see Chap. 20). The higher the left ventricular or pulmonary artery end-diastolic pressure and the lower the cardiac index, the greater is the likelihood of death from cardiogenic shock [11].

In addition to these Swan-Ganz catheter values, other signs indicative of cardiogenic shock are varying degrees of pulmonary edema, hypotension, decompensation such as oliguria/anuria, ascites, cold and diaphoretic skin with pallor, decreased or altered sensorium, and abdominal distension with hypoactive or absent bowel sounds. Bradycardia and hypotension denote more advanced stages of shock and usually are indications that sympathetic compensatory activity has failed and that survival is not likely.

Early recognition and prompt treatment of conditions that result in cardiogenic shock may actually preclude its development. This is true especially in cardiogenic shock secondary to venous inflow impedance. If the shock state

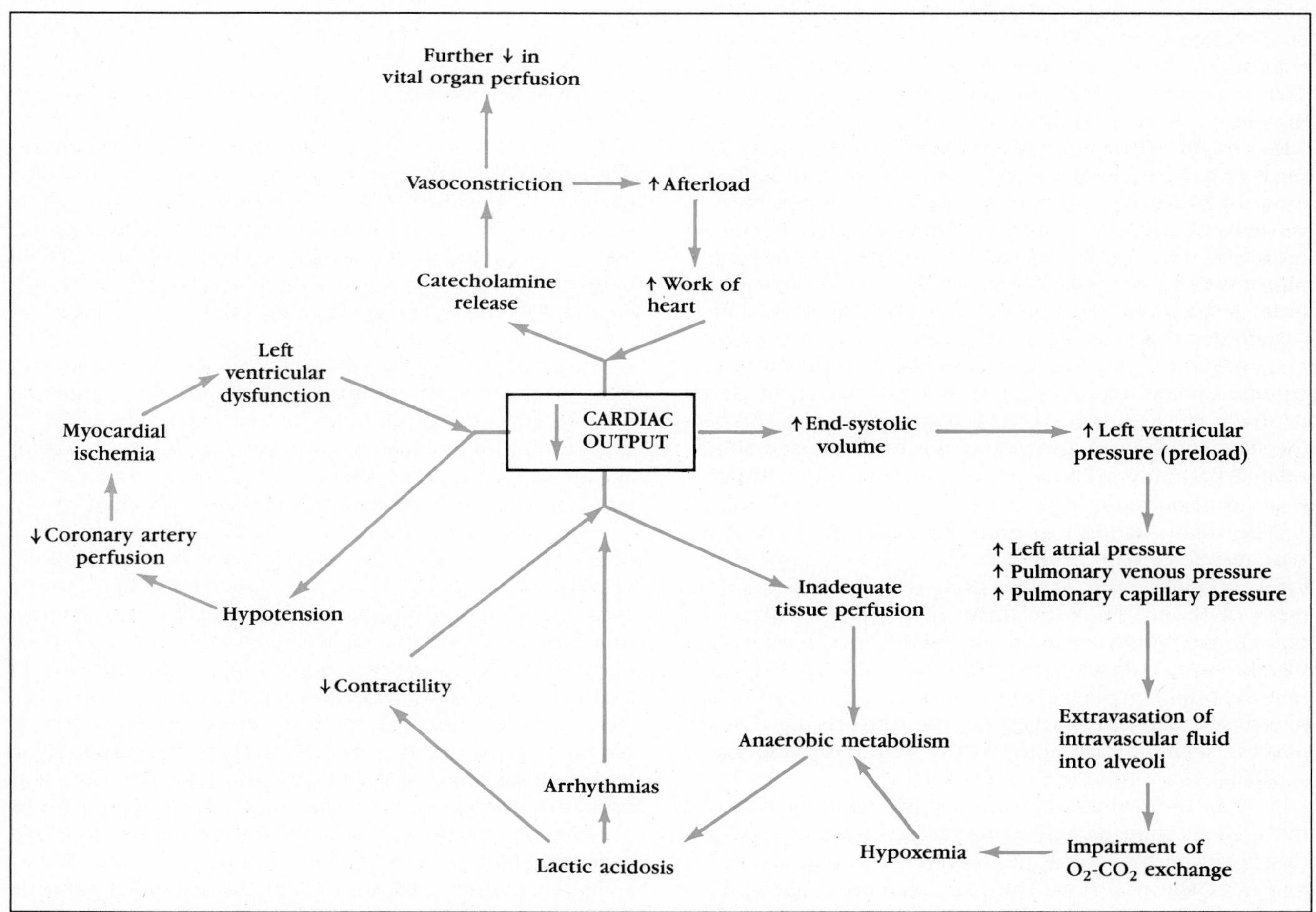

FIGURE 7-5 Pathologic development of cardiogenic shock. (From B. Hammond, Cardiogenic shock: A review. *J. Emerg. Nurs.* 9:4, St. Louis: The C.V. Mosby Co., p. 202.)

is related to acute myocardial infarction, however, prompt treatment may or may not alter the eventual outcome depending on the extensiveness of the infarct.

Vasogenic Shock

The shock state that develops as a consequence of profound and massive vasodilatation as opposed to hypovolemia or cardiac dysfunction is referred to as low-resistance [4] or distributive, that is, vasogenic, shock [13]. The primary defect is a marked increase in vascular capacity or vasodilatation relative to the amount of circulating blood volume. Blood volume per se is not reduced, but rather the circulatory capacity to accommodate that volume is increased. Categories of conditions that result in extensive vasodilatation or increased vascular capacity include vasomotor center depression, sepsis, and anaphylaxis.

Regardless of the initiating event or insult, the sequence of pathologic events that culminates in vasogenic shock is uniform and consistent. Profound arteriolar dilatation and vasodilatation related to vasomotor center depression, sepsis, or anaphylaxis lead to a relaxation or reduction of total peripheral resistance. Reduced total peripheral resistance results in a decrease in blood volume returning to the heart. This is related to blood vessel size or diameter and velocity or force of blood flow. The smaller the vessel, the more brisk is the blood flow through it. Similarly, the larger the vessel diameter, the less forceful, more sluggish, and slower is the blood flow through it. Dilated vessels are unable to generate sufficient force or pressure to propel blood adequately. Hence, in vasodilatation, blood flow toward the heart, that is, venous return, is reduced. The consequence of diminished venous return is decreased filling pressures in the chambers of the heart, with subsequent diminution of heart muscle fiber stretch or tension, such as decreased preload, which lowers stroke volume. The consequence of reduced stroke volume is impaired perfusion of tissues and organs, which deprives them of needed oxygen and nutrients. This sets the stage for the vicious cycle of positive-feedback, shock-related pathology. The sequence of events in vasogenic shock is displayed in Figure 7-6.

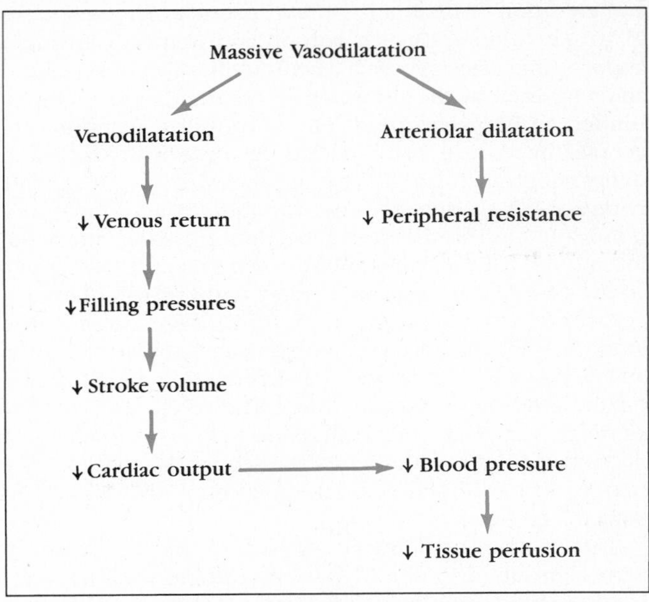

FIGURE 7-6 Sequence of events leading to vasogenic shock. (From V. Rice, Shock: A clinical syndrome. *Crit. Care Nurse* March-April:46, 1981.)

The vasodilatation that promotes or leads to the shock state interferes with or impairs tissue and organ perfusion for a variable period of time prior to the actual development of shock. Thus the onset of shock actually compounds and worsens the already existing perfusion deficit. In addition, compensatory mechanisms instituted to restore blood pressure and hence tissue perfusion are hampered and even offset by the underlying disease process, namely, vasomotor failure or potent vasodilator substances.

One of the many compensatory mechanisms activated in the shock state, namely, sympathetic vasomotor stimulation, may be futile and ineffective in vasogenic shock owing to the nature of the primary defect. As long as the initiating vasodilatatory event prevails, vasomotor response is unable to contribute to the restoration of blood pressure and tissue perfusion. Activation of the RAA system and secretion of ADH are altered in this form of shock.

Pure symptoms of vasogenic shock are very difficult to distinguish from those of the primary condition due to the predominant feature of vasodilatation. Therefore, some overlap or dual causation of symptoms is unavoidable. Symptoms include hypotension; tachycardia; cool, moist to diaphoretic skin; fever; oliguria; hypoactive bowel sounds; increased hematocrit; anxiety; and tachypnea.

Neurogenic Shock. Neurogenic shock, also known as spinal shock, is the result of loss of vasomotor tone that induces generalized arteriolar and venous dilatation [1,7]. This leads to hypotension, with pooling of blood in storage or capacitance vessels and splanchnic organ capillaries. Vasomotor tone is controlled and mediated by the vasomotor center in the medulla and the sympathetic fibers extending down the spinal cord to peripheral blood vessels, respectively. Thus, any conditions that depress medullary function or spinal cord integrity and innervation can potentially precipitate neurogenic shock. One example of such a condition is head injury that directly or indirectly adversely affects the medullary area of the brainstem. Indirect injury results from cerebral edema, with increased intracranial pressure that accompanies head trauma or ischemia of the brain. Other instances that may promote neurogenic shock from medullary brainstem depression are deep general anesthesia and drug overdose, especially barbiturates, opiates, and tranquilizers [7, 19]. Spinal cord injury and high spinal anesthesia may also induce neurogenic shock or profound vasomotor failure because of interference with or interruption of sympathetic pathways to blood vessels, which blocks vasoconstrictive responses and promotes vasodilatation. Syncopal episodes, or fainting, are considered to be a mild form of neurogenic shock that is relatively transient and inconsequential.

Septic Shock. Septic shock is defined as a severe and profound condition of generalized vascular collapse secondary to a systemic infection commonly caused by a gram-negative organism. The development of the shock state due to infection is believed to be related to the release of endotoxin from the bacterial cell wall. For this reason, septic shock is commonly referred to as *endotoxin shock* or simply *toxic shock*. Toxic shock is usually caused by gram-negative organisms but may be caused by viruses, fungi, or gram-positive bacilli. Gram-positive bacteria produce toxins on the surface of their cell walls, called exotoxins. Shock produced by these organisms is called *exotoxic shock*. Table 7-2 summarizes the most frequently occurring gram-negative bacteremias and their sites of origin.

Endotoxin, a lipopolysaccharide made up of the layers of the bacterial cell wall, is capable of interacting with and influencing the activity of other cells and plasma proteins throughout the body. The net symptomatic effects of endotoxin activity include fever, abnormal clotting, hypotension, and elevated complement levels [6]. In addition to being released by bacteria in systemic circulation, endotoxin is released from necrotic bowel [7].

The release of endotoxin by the bacterial cell wall initiates the process by which septic shock develops. Endotoxin is liberated from gram-negative bacteria through phagocytic activity of the macrophage system. If the bacterial infection is relatively minor, endotoxin is eventually neutralized and rendered harmless by the cells of the mononuclear phagocyte system. In more extreme infections, the release of greater quantities of endotoxin virtually overwhelms the defensive system, thereby allowing endotoxin activity to prevail and the shock state to develop. Endotoxin liberated into systemic circulation triggers and promotes the activation of several noxious substances, such as histamine, lysosomal enzymes, bradykinin, and serotonin, that significantly compromise capillary wall integrity. As a result of capillary damage, leakage of plasma occurs that produces marked fluid volume loss. The inevitable consequence of this plasma loss is a circulating fluid volume deficit with resultant hypotension. This capillary insult is also the basis for the development of adult respiratory distress syndrome in septic shock [17].

Recent research has identified another role of the macrophage system in producing septic shock. The macrophage system apparently activates substances known to mediate shock. These substances include acid hydrolases, complement, coagulation factors, prostaglandins, and the monokines. Monokines are initially beneficial in shock as they mobilize body nutrient stores for energy. If the shock state is protracted, however, these substances actually lead to metabolic deterioration in the form of muscle tissue catabolism, depletion of carbohydrate stores, hypoglycemia, ineffective use of fat, and retarded to absent production of ketone bodies [3].

The overall systemic effects of septic shock are shown in Figure 7-7. The process is initiated by some form of infectious agent that enters the body and overwhelms normal defenses to foreign invasion. As a consequence of host defense activity, mediators of shock such as histamine, bradykinin, complement, prostaglandins, and serotonin are liberated. The collective effects of these and other mediators are vasodilatation, capillary endothelial cell damage, platelet aggregation with microemboli formation, myocardial depression, and impaired myocardial contractility. The alterations in peripheral venules and arterioles as well as those of myocardial function impair tissue and organ perfusion, leading to hypoxia-induced lactic acid glycogenesis. Lactic acidemia further depresses myocardial contractility, total peripheral resistance, and the vital organ functions. Death ensues predictably unless this chain of events is interrupted [9].

Essentially three identifiable patterns of response or states are associated with septic shock. The initial one, referred to as the *hyperdynamic state*, presents the familiar picture of acute infection with chills, fever, and warm, dry, flushed skin (hence the synonymous term "pink shock"). Tachycardia, tachypnea with respiratory alkalosis, and little alteration of blood pressure occur in the early stage. Blood pressure is relatively normal because cardiac output remains quite high, despite early widespread vasodilatation and the beginning stage of increased capillary permeability induced by endotoxin-stimulated release of vasoactive substances. In fact, the predominant physiologic feature of the hyperdynamic state is high cardiac output, which is attributable to an intact and functional compensatory sympathetic response to decreased peripheral resistance [2].

The second or intermediate state in septic shock is called *normodynamic* and basically represents a transitional period between the first and third states. It is that

TABLE 7-2 Gram-Negative Organisms and Their Sites of Origin

Organism	Sites of Hospital-acquired Bacteremia
Escherichia coli	Urinary tract, abdominal abscesses, peritonitis
Klebsiella sp.	Lungs, abdominal wound, intravenous lines, urinary tract
Serratia sp.	Peritoneal catheter, intravenous lines, urinary tract, lungs, intravascular pressure-monitoring equipment
Pseudomonas aeruginosa	Lungs, urinary tract, cutaneous wounds, intravenous lines
Bacteroides sp.	Subphrenic abscesses, abdominal wounds, decubiti
Erwinia sp.	Intravenous infusion sets
Acinetobacter sp.	Intravenous lines
Citrobacter sp.	Urinary tract

Source: R. Gleckman and A. Esposito, Gram-negative bacteremic shock: Pathophysiology, clinical features, and treatment. Reprinted by permission from *South. Med. J.* 74(3):336, 1981.

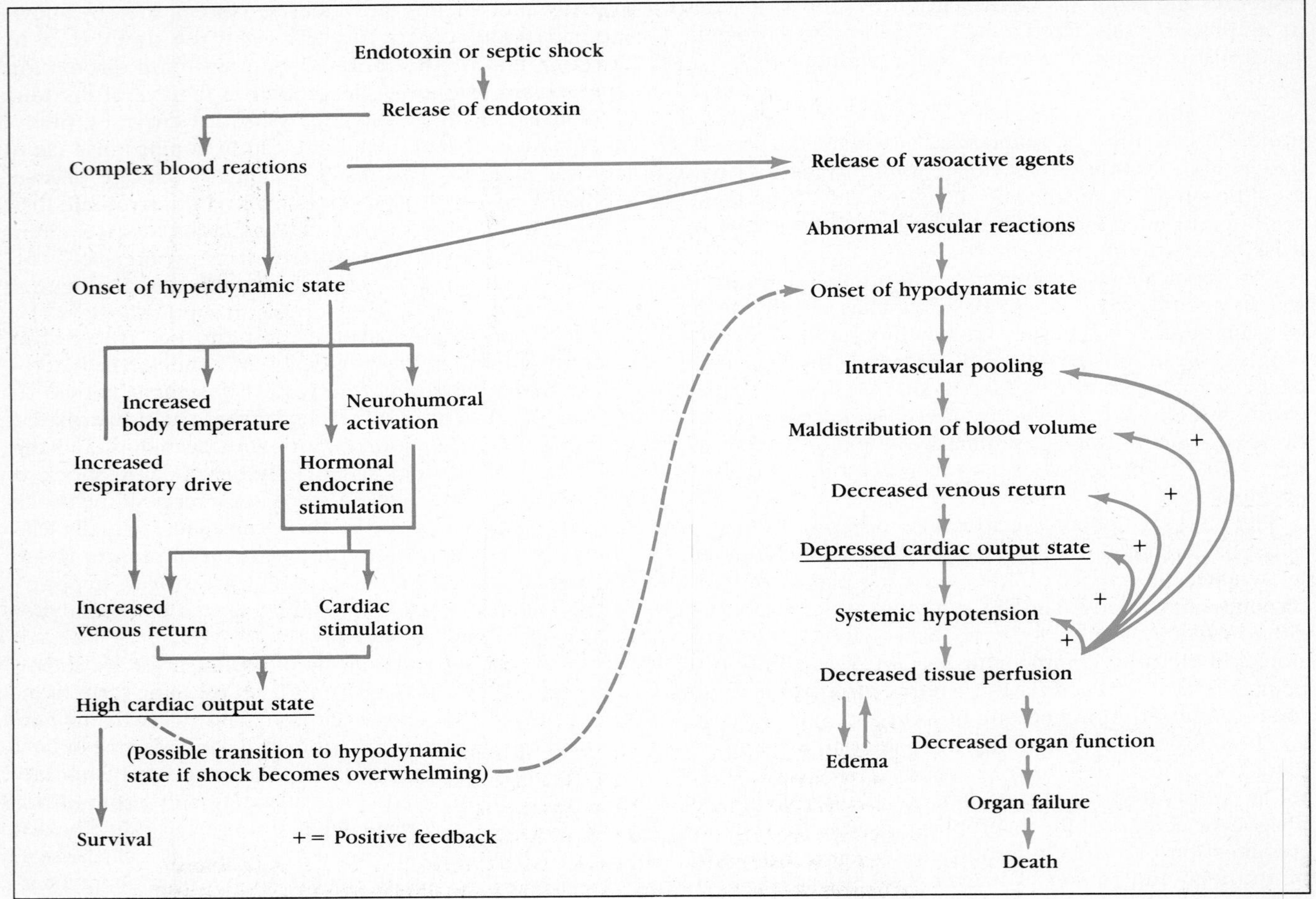

FIGURE 7-7 Septic shock may develop after either of two major pathways through a hyperdynamic (high cardiac output) or a hypodynamic (low cardiac output) state. (From L. Hinshaw, Overview of endotoxin shock. In R.A. Cowley and B.F. Trump [eds.], *Pathophysiology of Shock, Anoxia, and Ischemia*. Baltimore: Williams & Wilkins, 1982, p. 223. Copyright © 1982, The Williams & Wilkins Co., Baltimore. Reproduced with permission from the author and publisher.)

pattern or state during which the effects of endotoxin liberation begin to become manifested by signs and symptoms such as hypotension, oliguria, cool skin, and thirst. Tachycardia persists in an attempt to restore blood pressure and tissue perfusion.

The final state is called *hypodynamic* and can be equated with the irreversible stage of hemorrhagic shock. The affected person is obviously acutely ill and moribund, with cold, clammy, diaphoretic skin, anuria, severe hypotension, tachycardia, and tachypnea. Metabolic acidosis from increased tissue catabolism and lactic glycogenolysis is usual. Effects of myocardial depression are evidenced by pulmonary edema and low cardiac output. Once septic shock has progressed to this state, survival is doubtful and therapeutic measures are usually futile.

Anaphylactic Shock. Anaphylactic shock, or anaphylaxis, is the most drastic, acutely developing, and rapidly progressing of all forms of shock. Onset often occurs within a matter of seconds, and profound peripheral vascular collapse may become well established in only a few minutes. Without immediate treatment, irreversible shock develops quite promptly and death occurs in an hour or so [18]. This form of the shock state is induced by an antigen-antibody reaction that occurs when an antigen to which the individual had previously been sensitized enters the body by any one of a variety of routes. Anaphylaxis rarely occurs on initial exposure to an antigen. Antigens that are commonly known to precipitate anaphylaxis are therapeutic drugs (i.e., antibiotics, anesthetics, and contrast media, particularly those containing iodine) and foreign protein such as that found in blood products and snake and insect venom [13].

Anaphylaxis, or type I hypersensitivity reaction, is brought about or initiated by the action of immunoglobulin E (IgE). An antibody present in serum, IgE binds to mast cells and basophils when stimulated by exposure to a specific antigen. Upon a second or repeat exposure, the antigen adheres to the mast cell or the basophil, resulting in the release of substances that mediate shock [14]. These substances, which essentially include histamine, bradykinin, leukotrienes, and prostaglandins, mediate shock by different mechanisms and produce most of the overt symptomatology associated with anaphylactic shock. Histamine dilates blood vessels, constricts respiratory smooth muscle, and increases vascular permeability. Bradykinin also causes vasodilatation and makes capillaries more permeable, but apparently has little or no effect on respiratory smooth muscle. The leukotrienes C_4, D_4, and E_4 (formerly called SRS-A, or slow-reacting substances of anaphylaxis) constrict bronchial smooth muscle and increase venule permeability [5]. The prostaglandins exert a variety of effects depending on their type. They increase, decrease, or do not influence vascular permeability, blood vessel size, or respiratory smooth muscle [9].

The mechanism by which antigen-antibody reactions induce shock is directly related to the effects of the substances liberated at the outset of the reaction. Specifically, the shock state develops as a consequence of hypotension from profound vasodilatation and low cardiac output secondary to central fluid volume deficits due to increased capillary permeability and peripheral pooling of blood [10]. Compensatory mechanisms are not capable of reversing or retarding the progression of this form of shock because the initial shock-producing insult develops rapidly and acutely.

In addition to overwhelming hypotension and tissue and organ ischemia, anaphylactic shock is often characterized by severe laryngeal spasm, edema, and bronchoconstriction. These pathologic developments compound the shock state by adding further hypoxemia to the overall pattern of response. Hypoxemia perpetuates the cycle of anerobic metabolism and lactic acid production.

Signs and symptoms of anaphylaxis include profound hypotension, tachycardia, urticaria, pruritus, fever, dyspnea with hoarseness or stridor with wheezing, oliguria, cool and moist skin with pallor, cyanosis, and anxiety. The individual has a recent history of contact with a known allergen or an antigen capable of inducing the anaphylactic reaction. Respiratory complications such as stridor and inspiratory wheezing may precede respiratory arrest.

Complications of Shock

Complications that are directly caused by the shock state are devastating and often fatal. These complications stem from and are actually produced by the pathologic processes inherent in shock. The three most common processes that induce severe complications are *vasodilatation with inadequate tissue and organ perfusion*, *damage to the capillary endothelial lining*, and *activation of clotting factors*. Complications of these processes include lactic acidosis, adult respiratory distress syndrome, disseminated intravascular coagulation, and organ necrosis.

Lactic Acidosis

The basis for lactic acidosis in shock is the relentless production of lactic acid related to continual hypoxia of tissues from impaired perfusion. Impaired perfusion is secondary to vasodilatation and, to some extent, compensatory selective vasoconstriction. Hypoperfusion to tissues deprives them of oxygen. Cells are not able to metabolize nutrients appropriately without oxygen. In the absence of sufficient oxygen, cells are forced to metabolize nutrients anaerobically, which invariably results in the production of lactic acid.

Lactic acid exerts two major effects on the body. First, and probably of primary importance, it depresses myocardial contractility. Depressed contractility interferes with cardiac output, which further reduces the already compromised perfusion and oxygenation of tissue. A vicious cycle of positive feedback is thereby established. The second untoward effect of lactic acid production is that it contributes acid to the body, leading to metabolic acidosis and further impairment of cellular metabolic function (see Chap. 6).

Adult Respiratory Distress Syndrome

Adult respiratory distress syndrome (ARDS) develops secondary to shock because of at least two processes associated with the shock state. Apparently, pulmonary ischemia from hypoperfusion and aggregation of platelets in pulmonary capillaries significantly damage the endothelial lining of the pulmonary capillaries, causing them to lose selective permeability. As a consequence, water, electrolytes, red blood cells, and plasma proteins are extravasated into the interstitium of the lungs. This greatly impedes pulmonary compliance. Later, these fluids and blood components penetrate the alveoli, leading to frank pulmonary edema, further reduction in compliance, bronchospasm, atelectasis, and ultimately, significant hypoxemia [14]. A schema of the pathologic events leading to ARDS is depicted in Figure 7-8.

Disseminated Intravascular Coagulation

Disseminated intravascular coagulation (DIC) is a complex coagulopathy that occurs rather frequently among individuals who are acutely ill, especially those who have experienced some form of shock. The bases for the development of DIC are abnormal platelet aggregation and activation of factors of clotting, both of which are prominent features of shock. In response to the platelets and clotting factors, generalized coagulation occurs in the microcirculation and impedes capillary flow. In addition, the clotting process consumes fibrin, platelets, and other factors of clotting, and initiates fibrinolysis. Active fibrinolysis produces and releases fibrin degradation products, which are the end products of fibrin, fibrinogen, and plasmin lysis. The presence of these fibrin degradation products plus the consumption of platelets and other clotting factors precludes subsequent coagulation leading to widespread bleeding [14].

Symptoms of microcirculation (capillary) coagulation are present, including cool skin with mottling and cyanotic nail beds, and concomitant signs of profuse bleeding, especially from puncture sites, incisions, and the gas-

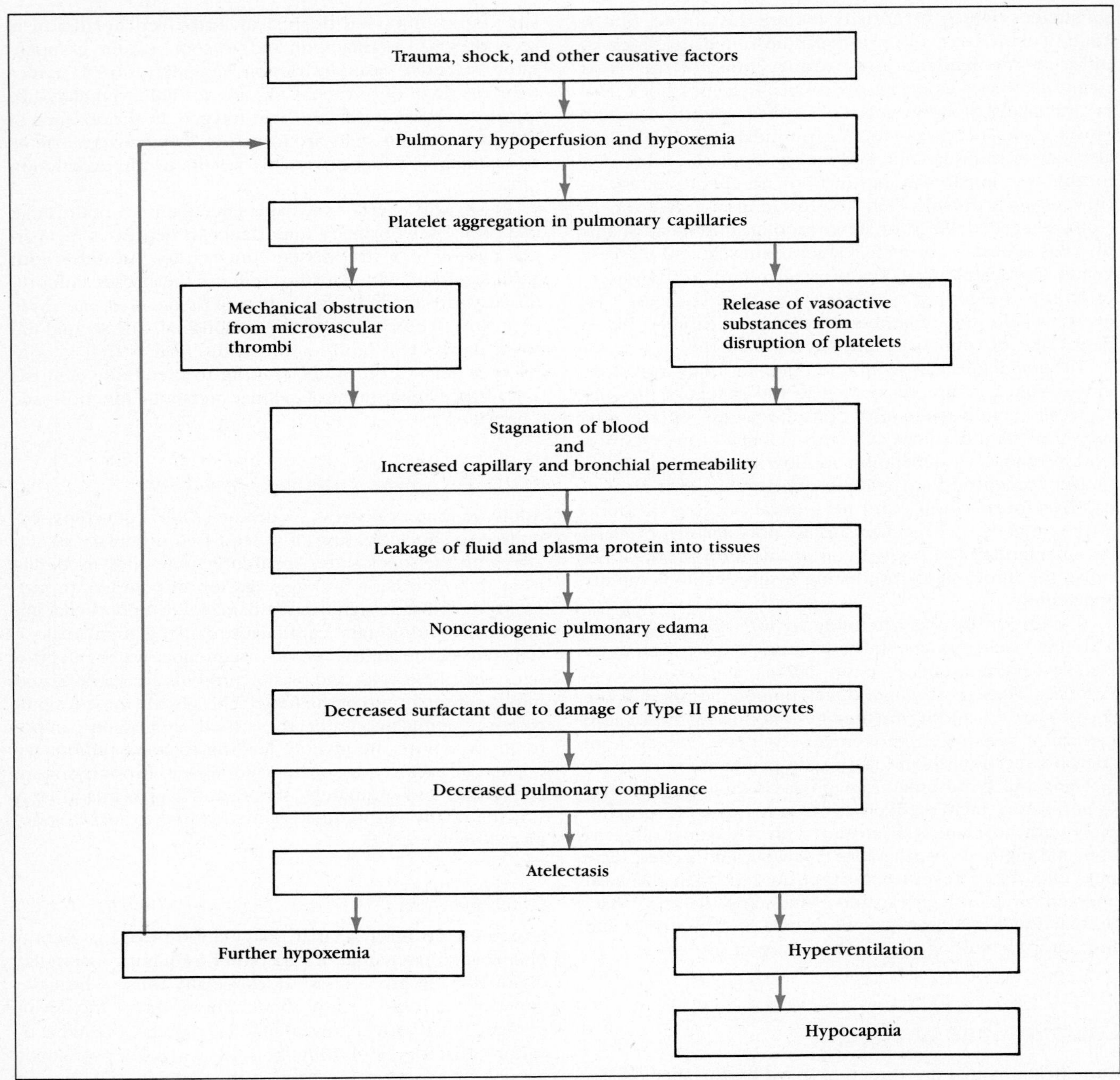

FIGURE 7-8 Sequential development of adult respiratory distress syndrome. (Reprinted with permission from the February issue of *Nursing 82*. Copyright © 1982 Springhouse Corporation, 111 Bethlehem Pike, Springhouse, PA 19477. All rights reserved.)

trointestinal tract. The overall picture of DIC is one of a vicious cycle of coagulation and anticoagulation (see Chap. 17).

Organ Ischemia and Necrosis

Organ ischemia with resultant necrosis and loss of function are the inevitable consequences of shock, particularly if the condition is protracted or progresses to the irreversible stage. Organ ischemia occurs secondary to shock as a consequence of hypotension, selective vasoconstriction of sympathetic activity, platelet aggregation with microcirculation clotting, and capillary endothelial damage. Organ systems that undergo the most pronounced damage are the heart, brain, kidneys, liver, and lungs. Necrotic lesions secondary to the shock state have been identified in liver, myocardial, renal, and lung tissue with resultant dysfunction or complete loss of function [7].

Study Questions

1. Discriminate among the mechanisms that can produce shock and indicate the differences in clinical pictures that may be seen.
2. What features help in identifying the stages of shock?
3. When do the complications of the shock begin and how can they be prevented?
4. Describe the normal mechanisms for maintaining the steady state and explain how their breakdown produces shock.
5. Draw a schematic indicating the progression of shock for each of the major mechanisms of causation.

References

1. Abel, F. Heart and circulation. In E.E. Selkurt, *Basic Physiology for the Health Sciences* (2nd ed.). Boston: Little, Brown, 1982. 273-322.
2. Baumgartner, J.D., Vaney, C., and Perret, C. An extreme form of the hyperdynamic syndrome in septic shock. *Intensive Care Med.* 10:245, 1984.
3. Filkins, J.P. Monokines and the metabolic pathophysiology of septic shock. *Fed. Proc.* 44:300, 1985.
4. Ganong, W.F. *Review of Medical Physiology* (12th ed.). Los Altos, Calif.: Lange, 1985.
5. Gaunder, B.N., Winkle, D. Anaphylaxis: Managing and preventing a true emergency. *Nurse Practitioner* May:17, 1984.
6. Gleckman, R., Esposito, A. Gram-negative bacteremic shock: Pathophysiology, clinical features, and treatment. *South. Med. J.* 74:335, 1981.
7. Guyton, A.C. *Textbook of Medical Physiology*. Philadelphia: Saunders, 1986.
8. Lefer, A.M. The pathophysiologic role of myocardial depressant factor as a mediator of circulatory shock. *Klin. Wochenshr.* 60:13, 1982.
9. Parker, M.M., Parrillo, J.E. Septic shock hemodynamics and pathogenesis. *JAMA* 250:3324, 1983.
10. Perkins, R.M., Anas, N.G. Mechanisms and management of anaphylactic shock not responding to traditional therapy. *Ann. Allergy* 54:202, 1985.
11. Rackley, C.E., Russell, R.O. Jr., Mantle, J.A., and Rogers, W.J. *Cardiovasc. Clin.* 11:15, 1981.
12. Rice, V. Shock, a clinical syndrome. I. Definition, etiology and pathophysiology. *Crit. Care Nurse* March/April:44, 1981.
13. Rice, V. Shock, a clinical syndrome. II. The stages of shock. *Crit. Care Nurse* May/June:4, 1981.
14. Robbins, S.L., Cotran, R., Kumar, V. *Pathologic Basis of Disease* (3rd ed.). Philadelphia: Saunders, 1984.
15. Runciman, W.B., Skowronski, G.A. Pathophysiology of hemorrhagic shock. *Anesthesia and Intensive Care* 12:193, 1984.
16. Schrier, R.W. *Renal and Electrolyte Disorders* (3rd ed.). Boston: Little, Brown, 1986.
17. Schumer, W. Pathophysiology and treatment of septic shock. *Am. J. Emergency Med.* 2:74, 1984.
18. Silverman, H.J., VanHook, C., Haponik, E. Hemodynamic changes in human anaphylaxis. *Am. J. Med.* 77:341, 1984.
19. Vick, R.L. *Contemporary Medical Physiology*. Menlo Park, Calif.: Addison-Wesley, 1984.

Unit Bibliography

Cawley, R.A., and Dunhan, C.M. *Shock Trauma/Critical Care Manual: Initial Assessment and Management*. Baltimore: University Park Press, 1982.

Cerra, F.B., Mazuski, J.E., Chute, E., Nuwer, N., Teasley, K., Lysne, J., Shronts, E.R., Konstantinides, F.N. Branched chain metabolic support. *Ann. Surg.* 3:286, 1984.

Corbett, J.V. *Laboratory Tests in Nursing Practice*. Norwalk, Conn.: Appleton-Century-Crofts, 1982.

Falkner, B., and Gazdick, M.A. Fluids and Electrolytes. In S.S. Zimmerman and J.H. Gildea, *Critical Care Pediatrics*. Philadelphia: Saunders, 1985.

Gann, D.S., and Amaral, J.R. Pathophysiology of trauma and shock. In G. Zuidema, R. Rutherford, and W. Ballinger, *The Management of Trauma* (4th ed.). Philadelphia: Saunders, 1985.

Gonick, H.C., and Buckalew, V.M. *Renal Tubular Disorders: Pathophysiology, Diagnosis and Management*. New York: Dekker, 1985.

Gröer, M.W. *Physiology and Pathophysiology of the Body Fluid*. St. Louis: Mosby, 1981.

Guyton, A. *Textbook of Medical Physiology* (7th ed.). Philadelphia: Saunders, 1986.

Hassett, I., and Border, J.R. The metabolic response to trauma and sepsis. *World J. Surg.* 7:125-131, 1983.

Hazinski, M.F. *Nursing Care of the Critically Ill Child*. St. Louis: Mosby, 1984.

Kee, J.L. *Laboratory and Diagnostic Tests with Nursing Implications*. Norwalk, Conn.: Appleton-Century-Crofts, 1983.

Kenner, C.V., Guzzetta, C.E., and Possey, B.M. *Critical Care Nursing: Body, Mind, Spirit* (2nd ed.). Boston: Little, Brown, 1985.

Kenney, P.R., Allen-Rowlands, C.F., and Gann, D.S. Glucose and osmolality as predictors of injury severity. *J. of Trauma* 23:712, 1983.

Keyes, J.L. *Fluid, Electrolyte and Acid-Base Regulation*. Monterey, Calif.: Wadsworth, 1985.

Lewis, C.M. *Nutrition and Nutritional Therapy in Nursing*. Norwalk, Conn.: Appleton-Century-Crofts, 1986.

Linton, A.L. Electrolyte disturbances. In W.J. Sibbald, *Synopsis of Critical Care* (2nd ed.). Baltimore: Williams & Wilkins, 1984.

Lowry, S.F. Nutritional support of the traumatized patient. In G.T. Shires, *Principles of Trauma Care* (3rd ed.). New York: McGraw-Hill, 1985.

Mann, J.K., and Oates, A.P. *Critical Care Nursing of the Multi-injured Patient*. Philadelphia: Saunders, 1980.

Moore, G.L. Metabolic and nutritional problems in trauma. Unpublished presentation at First Annual Symposium on Trauma. Vanderbilt University, Nashville, 1985.

Moylan, J.A. Fluid and nutritional support for the injured child. In J.G. Randolph, M.M. Ravitch, C.D. Benson, and E. Aberdeen, *The Injured Child: Surgical Management*. Chicago: Yearbook Medical, 1975.

Munster, A.M. Immunologic manipulation of the injured patient. In J.R. Ninneman, *Traumatic Injury*. Baltimore: University Park, 1983.

Pelos, G., et al. Anticatabolic properties of branched chain amino acids in trauma. *Resuscitation* 10:153, 1983.

Robbins, S.L., Cotran, R.S., and Kumar, V. *Pathologic Basis of Disease* (3rd ed.). Philadelphia: Saunders, 1984.

Robinson, C.H., and Weigley, E.S. *Basic Nutrition and Diet Therapy* (5th ed.). New York: Macmillan, 1984.

Rose, B.D. *Clinical Physiology of Acid-Base Electrolyte Disorders* (2nd ed.). New York: McGraw-Hill, 1984.

Schoengrund, L., and Balzer, F. *Renal Problems in Critical Care*. New York: Wiley, 1985.

Schrier, R.W. *Renal and Electrolyte Disorders* (3rd ed.). Boston: Little, Brown, 1986.

Seldin, D.W., and Giebisch, G. *The Kidney—Physiology and Pathophysiology*. New York: Raven Press, 1985.

Shires, G.T. *Principles of Trauma Care* (3rd ed.). New York: McGraw-Hill, 1985.

Shires, G.T. *Shock and Related Problems*. Edinburgh: Churchill Livingstone, 1984.

Sodeman, W.A., and Sodeman, T.M. *Sodeman's Pathologic Physiology: Mechanisms of Disease* (7th ed.). Philadelphia: Saunders, 1985.

Vander, A.J. *Renal Physiology* (3rd ed.). New York: McGraw-Hill, 1985.

Watson, R.R. *Handbook of Nutrition in the Aged*. Boca Raton, Fla.: CRC Press, 1985.

Weil, M.H. et al., Difference in acid-base state between venous and arterial blood during cardiopulmonary resuscitation. *NEJM* 315:153, 1986.

Woolfolk, R.L., and Lehrer, P.M. *Principles and Practice of Stress*. New York: Guilford, 1984.

Zuidema, G., Rutherford, R., and Ballinger, W. *The Management of Trauma* (4th ed.). Philadelphia: Saunders, 1985.

SECTION II

Bodily Defense Mechanisms

Adaptations and Alterations

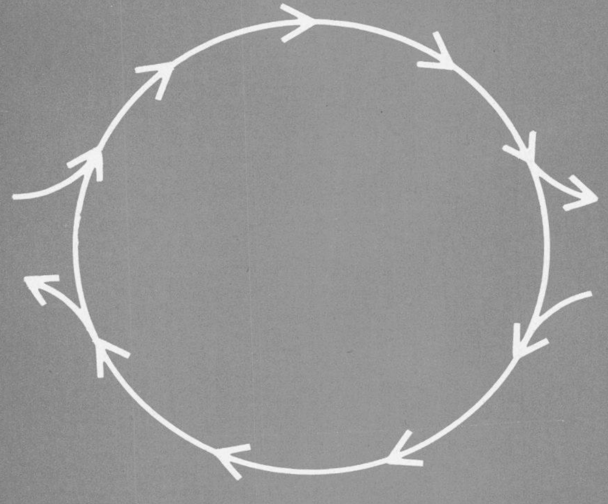

UNIT 4

Inflammation and Repair

Barbara L. Bullock

The inflammatory response is the body's reaction to tissue injury. It is usually initiated by an injurious substance and results in removal of the foreign material. It is a beneficial response that must be present for the maintenance of life. The most common causes of inflammation are infectious agents. Chapter 8 presents a condensed review of the classifications of organisms that can cause inflammation. It also describes the normal mechanisms used by the body to prevent or inhibit an organism's entrance. The student may wish to expand the study of microbiology as it relates to pathophysiology; a reference list is included. Chapter 9 details acute and chronic inflammation, and their resolution. Normal and aberrant resolutions are presented. Effects of the inflammatory process as they alter specific organs and systems are studied in other sections of this textbook.

The reader is encouraged to study Units 4 and 5 together to maximize understanding of inflammation and immunity. Use of the learning objectives will facilitate understanding by providing an organized approach to the topic. Study questions at the end of each chapter provide an opportunity for synthesis of learning. The bibliographies at the end of the units provide additional sources for investigation.

CHAPTER 8

Infectious Agents

CHAPTER OUTLINE

Host-Parasite Relationships
Viruses
Structure, Reproduction, and Pathogenesis

Rickettsia
Bacteria
Pathogenesis

Fungi
Protozoa
Helminths

LEARNING OBJECTIVES

1. Describe the major defense mechanisms of the host.
2. Define *organotropism*, *opportunistic infections*, and *pathogenic and nonpathogenic organisms*.
3. List the major characteristics of each type of infectious agent.
4. Explain how infectious agents are classified.
5. Describe the mode of viral infection and how viruses multiply.
6. List the events that occur as a cell is infected by a virus.
7. Describe at least six viral infections, differentiating DNA and RNA viruses, incubation periods, mode of transmission, and clinical effects.
8. Describe the pathologic effects of the rickettsial organism in spotted and typhus fevers.
9. Discuss the role of toxins produced by bacterial organisms.
10. Describe at least six gram-positive and gram-negative bacterial infections in terms of pathogenesis and clinical effects.
11. List three major classifications of fungi that are infectious to humans and describe the relationships among them.
12. List the protozoa that may be pathologic to humans.
13. Explain how protozoa move and reproduce.
14. Describe briefly three infections that may result from protozoa.
15. Categorize the types of helminths and describe how each can cause pathology in humans.

Infectious diseases are produced by living organisms: viruses, rickettsia, bacteria, fungi, protozoa, and nematodes. These diseases have been present in enormous numbers and have caused epidemics by their contagiousness. Although developments in nutrition, insect control, immunization, sanitation, and drug therapy have decreased the mortality and morbidity of infectious diseases, these microbial infections have not been eliminated [8]. Microbes have developed mutant strains that are resistant to once-effective antimicrobial therapy. Infectious diseases still occur in great numbers and often are fatal to very young or debilitated victims. Persons in less developed countries have a much greater risk of developing and dying from infectious organisms than do those in industrialized countries [8].

Host-Parasite Relationships

The occurrence of infectious diseases depends on many factors, including virulence of the organism, number of invading organisms, defense mechanisms of the body, and pathogenesis of the infection. *Virulence* is the ability of the infecting organism to cause disease, requiring a receptive host in which it can settle and multiply. The mechanisms by which an organism can cause disease are epithelial attachment, penetration into tissues, production of toxins, and ability to cause alterations in the genome of the new host [1]. The number of invading organisms must be sufficient to overwhelm the host's defenses. *Organotropism* is the term used for the high selectivity of infectious organisms for specific tissues [1]. Some organisms are *opportunistic*, that is, normally *nonpathogenic* but *pathogenic* when the immune defense of the host is compromised [1].

The defense mechanisms of the human body reside on the external and internal surfaces and include physical, chemical, and immune barriers. Whether or not the organism can cause disease depends largely on the success or failure of these mechanisms and barriers to provide adequate defense. The main physical, external barrier to infection is the skin, an intact epidermis being almost impervious to infection. The mucous membranes lining various organs also remove organisms by secreting mucus that provides a washing effect and prevents organisms from adhering to membranes. Chemical secretions, such as hydrochloric acid in the stomach and the usually acid-pH urine, contribute to the sterile environment in the organs. The immune system targets pathogens for destruction. When organisms gain access to the body, lymphocytes recognize and destroy them, often without producing disease manifestations. The competence of the immune system also plays a major role in the outcome of infectious disease (see Chap. 10).

The defense mechanisms can be grouped into physical or chemical characteristics, immune factors, and nature of the host (Table 8-1). Clinically apparent infections occur when the defense mechanisms have not been sufficient to hold the growth of the organism in check.

TABLE 8-1 Defense Mechanisms of the Body

Mechanism	Characteristics of Defense
Physical	Intact epidermis
	Mucus-secreting membranes
	Mucus blanket movement in respiratory tract
	Connective tissue
Chemical	Hydrochloric acid in stomach
	Acid pH of urine
	Lysozyme enzyme present in many secretions
	Resident flora in mouth, on skin, in large intestine
Immune	Specific autigen-antibody reactions
	Immunoglobin A
	Inflammatory response
Host factors	Age
	Sex
	Genetic susceptibilities
	Nutritional balance
	Stress—physiologic or emotional
	Presence of other diseases

Pathogenesis of infection depends on the capability of the specific organism and its ability to bypass or inactivate the defense mechanisms of the body. Manifestations of infections can be ascribed to injury, dysfunction, destruction of host cells, and alterations in the steady state [6]. Once actual infection is established, it often causes nonspecific signs and symptoms that characteristically include fever, chills, muscle pain, lymph node enlargement, and variable elevation in the white cell count (see Chap. 9). Each microorganism is distinct and has its own means of invasion and reproduction. The major classifications of living organisms are described in this chapter. The effects of the resultant diseases are also described in the chapters relating to specific organs and systems.

Infections may produce illness, as described above, or they may be inapparent or *subclinical*, in which state they are so mild that signs and symptoms are not seen. A particular form of subclinical infection is the *carrier state* in which the individual remains a reservoir of infection and retains the ability to infect others [1]. Another important form of infection is *latent infection* in which bouts of disease occur, interrupted by periods of no disease manifestation or infectivity. Herpes viral infections are common latent infections that can be reactivated by stress, other infection, or other factors [1].

All infectious organisms are *communicable* (transmissible) from one member of the same species to another. The modes of transmission vary and depend on the source, quantity of organisms, transit survival, and a susceptible new host [1].

The human organism has the ability to contact and combat a multitude of potential pathogens in the environment. This is evidenced by the state of relative disease freedom in most individuals. This active defense is maintained through the complex immune system, which demonstrates a high degree of selectivity for organisms. The defensive ability of this system is affected by age, genetic factors, psychologic factors, and environmental and nutritional factors [1] (see Chap. 10).

Viruses

Viruses are the smallest infectious agents known. They are not complete cells in themselves and exist essentially as parasites on living cells. These organisms use the biochemical products of other living cells to replicate.

Structure, Reproduction, and Pathogenesis

Viruses vary in size, appearance, and behavior (Fig. 8-1). They are classified as either DNA or RNA viruses according to their genetic material. Many contain nucleic acid, which is protected by a closed protein shell called the *capsid*. Some have a surrounding lipid envelope.

Mature virus particles are called *virions* [4]. The virion can be thought of as a block of genetic material, either DNA or RNA, surrounded by a protective coat [7]. Viruses appear to be species and organ specific and apparently can replicate only in permissive or receptive cells. Some viruses enter a receptive cell by pinocytosis, after which the process of multiplication can begin.

The structure of the virus has been studied with the electron microscope and is described according to its appearance. The complete infective particle is called a *virion*. The *capsid* is the protein coat, which is made up of protein subunits called *capsomeres*. Complex virions may contain additional layers, or envelopes.

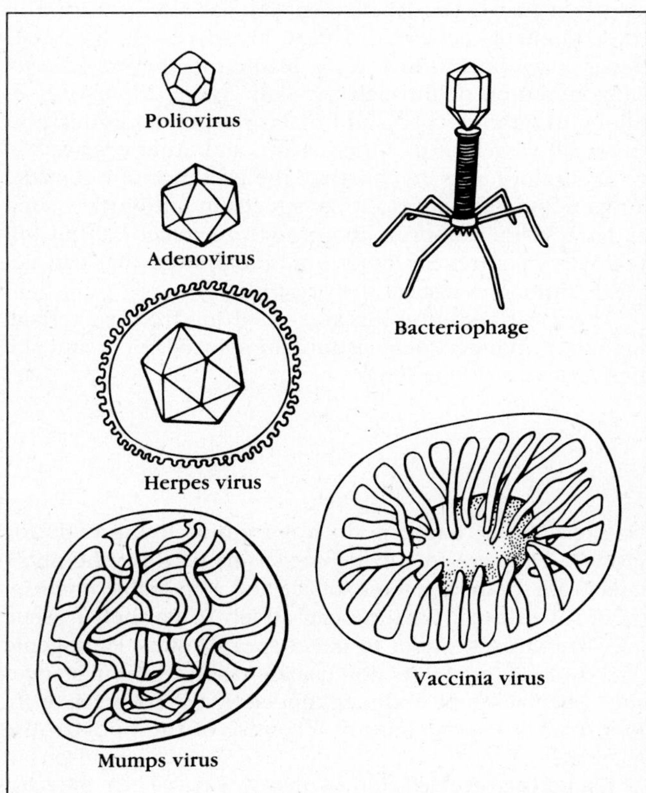

FIGURE 8-1 Various forms of viruses.

The protein covering of the virus is type specific. The surface structure is responsible for attachment to particular cell receptors. Infection depends on the compatibility of the viral surface with the host cell receptors and the ability of viral nucleic acid to use the host cell to manufacture viral products. All viruses are similar in their method of attachment to the specific receptors on the host cell membrane, the so-called lock-and-key attachment. Some have amino acids that are similar to the actively transported substances in the cell membrane of the host. Viruses can fool the cell, attach themselves to receptor sites on the host cell, and block the movement of normally transported materials.

Viruses affect and infect specific cells. Some B lymphocytes, for example, carry receptors for the Epstein-Barr virus, while cells in the tracheal lining have receptors for the influenza virus. Viruses produce specific diseases involving specific tissues, but their modes of transmission and diseases produced are numerous. Cells respond to viral infection in different ways. There may be no apparent cellular change because viral DNA may adopt a symbiotic relationship with the host cell. Cellular pathologic effects, such as death or virus-induced hyperplasia, may occur. Cytopathic effects are common, and include aggregation of host cells into clusters with shrinkage, lysis, and fusion of the cells. The effects differ and are influenced by the effects of the virus on cellular synthesis of macromolecules, alteration in cellular organelles such as lysosomes, and changes in the host cell membrane.

While no one virus is typical, the replication and transmission of this organism have been assessed extensively by studying the bacteriophage (virus that attacks bacteria). The genetic material of the bacteriophage is enclosed in an angular head or protein-containing capsid. This hollow head contains the viral genetic material and connects with a hollow cylinder of protein surrounded by protein contractile fibers. The contractile fibers coil around the cylinder like a spring. At the end of the tail, the fibers and an enzyme are important in attaching the virion to the host cell (Fig. 8-2).

Viral multiplication usually occurs in several steps. The first step is recognition and attachment of the virus to the host cell. The mechanism varies with the type of virus. The accumulation of viral particles in the cell ultimately results in lysis of the cell and viremia [8]. The tail of the virus may adsorb to specific receptor sites on the host cell and then digest a part of the host cell wall through lysosomelike enzymes. The hole produced by the virus allows viral genome to be injected into the recipient cell. The viral shell (capsid and tail) remains attached to the host cell (as a "ghost" on the outside of the cell wall) after the genetic material has been injected. Within the host cell, the viral particles may alter protein synthesis, cause chromosomal changes, or alter the genes of the host [7]. Synthesis of new viral DNA, proteins, and shells occurs, and new

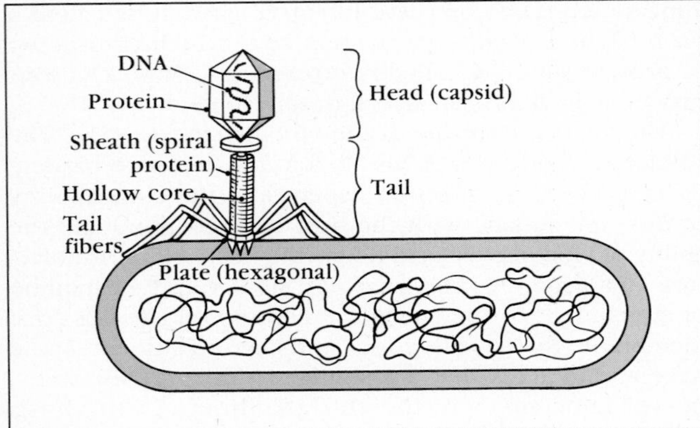

FIGURE 8-2 A bacteriophage.

DNA is assembled into the hollow protein shells, a process that continues until the host cell ruptures and releases swarms of new infective viruses (Fig. 8-3). For example, in a few hours the poliovirus can produce 100,000 poliovirus particles [3]. The formed particles can survive outside the host cell for variable periods of time, often until a new susceptible host cell can be found.

Viral infections stimulate the immune system's antibody production. Neutralizing antibodies are formed during viremia, but the main host defense is through cell-mediated immunity [8] (see pp. 158–159). The initial response to viral infestation is usually by the mononuclear cells such as monocytes and lymphocytes. At the site of entry of viruses into the body, the immunocompetent (antigen-specific) cells accumulate and initiate the process of inflammation. Macrophages often attach to the virus and enhance T and B cell interaction (see Chap. 10). Exposure to viral agents initially causes the synthesis of specific IgM antibodies, which is followed after about 10 days by IgG antibodies. When the virion is sufficiently coated with antibody, it is rendered noninfectious. The specific T lymphocytes provide for long-term immunity. Viruses and other substances stimulate the production of *interferon*, an antiviral protein that inhibits viral spread from cell to cell [5].

After attachment, an *eclipse* stage may be entered, during which viral DNA becomes part of the host chromosome and remains *latent*. The greater the capability to initiate a rapid reproductive cycle, the more virulent the virus.

Activation or induction causes the latent viruses to become active and reprograms the cell for viral reproduction. It has been suggested that activation may be initiated by cold temperatures, carcinogens, or materials in food, air, or water. Each virus responds to a specific induction mechanism. Sometimes a few cells with viruses within them escape induction so that not all affected cells are lysed. In this way, the host cell carries viral DNA as part of its own DNA, and the virus can remain latent in the host tissues throughout the life of the cell.

Viral infections produce many diseases, including hepatitis, meningoencephalitis, pneumonia, rhinitis, skin diseases, and numerous other disorders affecting almost every system of the body. Research is being conducted in many other disease conditions, such as multiple sclerosis, diabetes mellitus, and cancer, in the hopes of finding a viral connection [8]. Although there are multitudes of types of viruses, most of them can be classified into DNA or RNA structural viruses. Table 8-2 presents this classification, listing the common disease-producing groups, their modes of transmission, and the resulting symptomology.

Rickettsia

Rickettsia, once thought to be related to viruses because of their small size, are obligate, parasitic organisms. They possess all of the features of bacteria except that they can multiply only within certain cells of susceptible hosts [8]. Their normal reservoir is most often the arthropods, especially ticks, mites, lice, and fleas, in which they multiply without causing disease. Most rickettsial diseases are transmitted to humans through the bite or feces of the infected arthropod. An exception to this is Q fever, which is probably spread person to person by respiratory droplet. The classification of rickettsia is based on the clinical features and epidemiologic aspects of the diseases they cause. The organisms are often organized into the (1) spotted fever group, (2) typhus group, and (3) others, including Q fever.

All rickettsial diseases cause fever, and most cause a skin rash that is the result of rickettsial multiplication in the endothelial cells of the small blood vessels. The cells become swollen and necrotic, leading to the vascular lesions noted on or through the skin. Aggregations of lymphocytes, granulocytes, and macrophages accumulate in the small vessels of the brain, heart, and other organs.

Laboratory tests demonstrate the presence of rickettsial antigen and antibodies. Broad-spectrum antibiotics, such as tetracycline, suppress the growth of rickettsia, but full recovery requires an intact immune system that can develop antibodies against the organism.

The most common diseases resulting from rickettsial infection include Rocky Mountain spotted fever and the typhus fevers (Table 8-3).

Bacteria

Unlike viruses, bacteria do not require living cells for growth. They are free-living organisms that use the nutrients of the body as a food source and a favorable environment for growth. Bacteria can attach to epithelial tissue and, like viruses, prefer to infect specific sites. Pathogenic effects of bacterial infection usually result from substances such as enzymes or toxins produced by the bacteria, or injury from the inflammatory response of the body to the bacteria.

Bacteria are classified in many ways. They may be gram-positive or gram-negative depending on the chemical composition of their cell walls and absorption of staining dye. *Gram-positive bacteria* stain purple because their

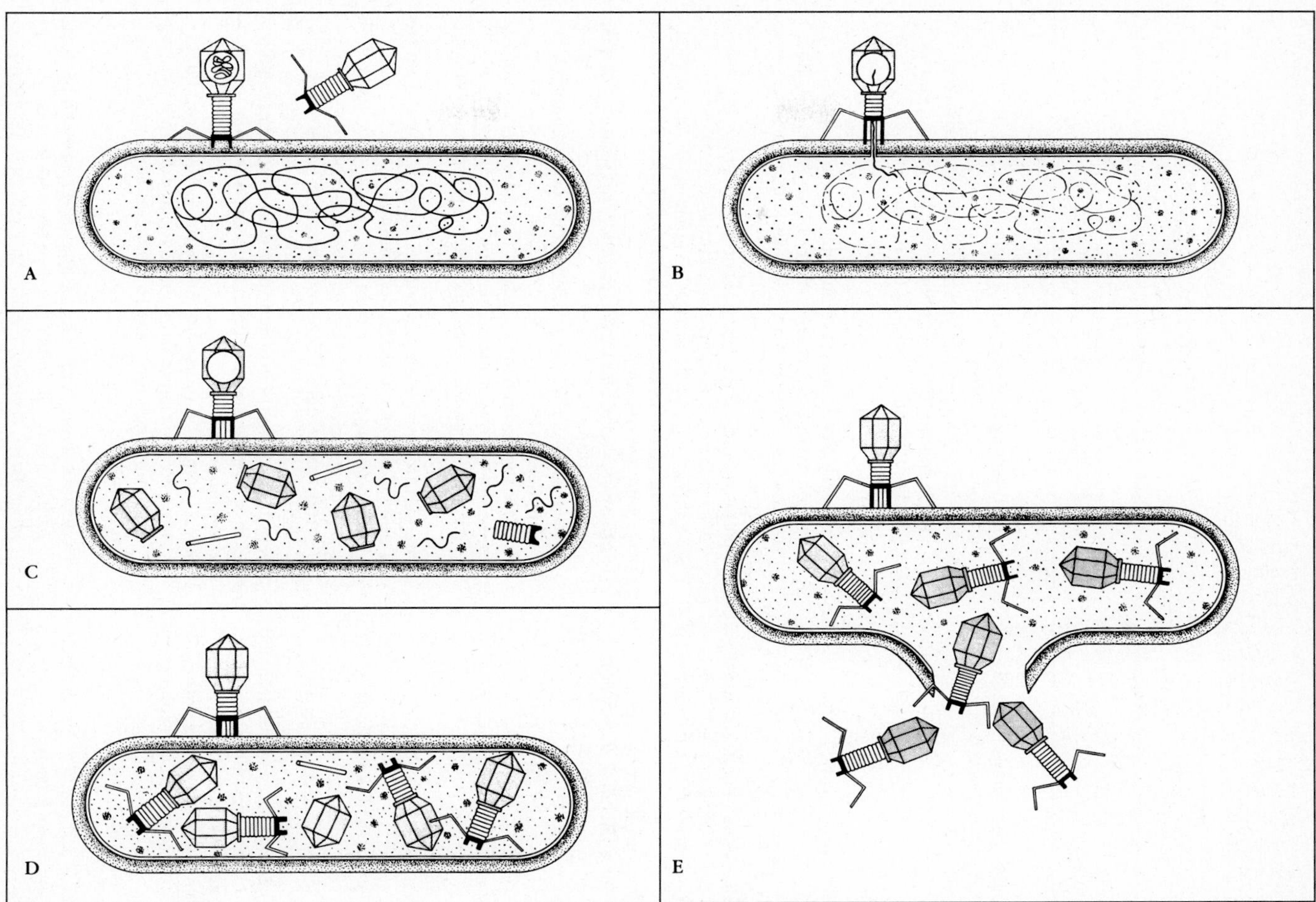

FIGURE 8-3 Development of a virulent phage in a susceptible bacterium. A. The polyhedral head of the phage is attached to the outer surface of the bacterium by its tail and tail fibers. B. Within a few seconds or minutes the bacterial cell wall and membrane have been perforated by the lytic enzymes in the tail, and the DNA of the phage has entered the bacillus through the phage tail. Note the retraction of the tail sheath. The opening through the cell wall is resealed. The inert protein coat of the phage remains on the outside of the cell. Disintegration of cell DNA begins at once. The phage, as such, is no longer demonstrable. C. During the next 12 minutes phage protein heads, tails, and phage DNA replicons are being synthesized. D. About 12 minutes later, after a brief period of maturation during which some of the heads, tails, and DNA molecules have been assembled, infective phage virions are first demonstrable by artificial rupture of the cell. E. About 12 minutes later the assembly of parts into phage virions is complete, and the now eviscerated cell, an inert sac, ruptures by enzymic lysis of the cell wall, liberating many new phage particles. Their number is characteristic of the burst size of the phage involved; in this case, six. The whole process, A-E, occupies about 30 to 40 minutes in this particular virus-cell system. In this diagram the phage virions have been drawn about 3 times larger proportionately in order to show more clearly certain structural details. (From M. Frobisher et al., *Fundamentals of Microbiology* [9th ed.]. Copyright © 1974 by W.B. Saunders Company. Reprinted by permission of Holt, Rinehart and Winston, CBS College Publishing.)

TABLE 8-2 Common Viruses That Cause Pathologic Effects in Humans

Type	Nucleic Acid Present	Incubation Period	Epidemiology	Clinical Manifestations
Herpesviruses				
Varicella (chicken pox)	DNA	10–21 days	Highly contagious through respiratory droplets.	Fever, disseminated vesicular eruption profuse on trunk and on oral mucosa.
Zoster (shingles)	DNA	Variable		Follows chickenpox, may occur years after a primary attack; spreads down peripheral nerves of skin, active ganglionitis causes burning or dull pain, vesicles follow nerve fibers.
Herpes simplex				
Type 1	DNA	2–12 days	Skin contact (oral).	Fever, vesicular eruption of mucous membranes, conjunctivitis, oral lesions (fever blisters); encephalitis occasionally results when virus ascends to central nervous system.
Type 2	DNA	2–5 days	Skin contact (genital); attack rate with sexual contact 1:3.	Genital vesicles, fever, burning, urinary urgency in males, dysuria, vulvar burning, dyspareunia in females.
Epstein-Barr	DNA	30–50 days	Respiratory droplet, transfusion.	Sore throat, lymphadenopathy, splenomegaly, supraorbital edema; virus has been isolated from Burkitt's lymphoma.
Cytomegalovirus (CMV)	DNA	?20–50 days	Saliva, urine, feces, semen transplacental, transfusion.	Vary with age of onset: *Congenital:* failure to thrive, jaundice, respiratory distress, may be fatal. *Postnatal:* infection may cause anemia, hepatomegaly, lymphocytosis. *Adult form:* fever, lymphocytosis, Guillain–Barré syndrome. *Immunosuppressed individuals:* interstitial pneumonia, increased frequency of rejection of transplanted organs.
Pox viruses				
Variola (smallpox)	DNA	7–17 days	Respiratory droplets.	High fever, vesicles on mucous membranes, papules on face and trunk, bone marrow depression.
Vaccinia	DNA	Approximately 2 weeks after vaccination	Inoculation for smallpox.	Vaccinia virus probably a hybrid of variola or cowpox virus; may cause widespread eczematous reaction or encephalomyelitis that causes death in 30–40% of individuals.
Adenovirus (many strains identified)	DNA	5–10 days	High frequency in children and military recruits; respiratory aerosol or droplet.	Febrile pharyngitis; headache, regional lymphadenopathy, nasal obstruction and discharge, conjunctivitis, *pneumonia.*
Papovavirus (warts)	DNA	1–20 months	Skin contact, contact with contaminated secretions.	Solid, rounded tumors with horny projections 1–2 cm in size; often asymptomatic unless located on area of irritation; often found on hands, neck, shins, and forearms.
Picornavirus				
Coxsackieviruses A & B (many strains)	RNA	2–5 days	Fecal-oral contact, insects may be passive vectors.	Depend on type; acute myocarditis, fever, muscle, pleuritic pain, vesicular lesions on soft palate and tonsils, pharyngitis, associated with many systemic problems.

Rhinovirus (many strains)	RNA	1–2 days	Respiratory droplet.	Common respiratory illness; fever, cough, croup, and pneumonia may develop in children; sore throat, nasal congestion, and nasal discharge without fever common in adults.
Poliovirus	RNA	2–5 days	Fecal-oral contact.	Undifferentiated febrile illness may spread to involve anterior horn cells of spinal cord and motor nuclei of cranial nerves; causes various muscle paralyses, hemiplegia, paraplegia; bladder and respiratory muscle dysfunction; poliovaccines can prevent disease.
Myxovirus				
Influenza A, B, and C	RNA	18–36 hours, up to 7 days	Epidemic, new strains evolve frequently; transmitted by infected respiratory secretions.	Respiratory symptoms, cough, headache, muscle pain, fever, chills, sneezing, nasal discharge, prostration common; symptoms among strains similar.
Mumps	RNA	15–21 days	Very communicable in crowded conditions; transmitted by upper respiratory secretions.	Painful enlargement of salivary glands; orchitis occurs in 20–35% postpubertal males; small percentage develop meningitis or may affect other glands.
Arenavirus				
Rubella	RNA	14–21 days	Very communicable; disease confers immunity; nasopharyngeal transmission.	Rash begins on face, spreads to trunk and extremities; lasts 1–5 days; enlarged lymph nodes common; joint pains and encephalomyelitis rare complications.
Rhabdovirus				
Rabies	RNA	Variable average 2–6 weeks in humans	Animal bite of nonimmunized domestic dogs or cats, or of wild animals such as skunks, foxes, raccoons, wolves, bats.	Virus introduced through mucous membranes or epidermis; replicates in striated muscle then spreads up peripheral nerve bundles to central nervous system; passes to all organs but major effects on CNS; acute encephalitis, brainstem dysfunction and death; rapidly fatal if not treated; hydrophobia (excessive salivation) characteristic.
Arbovirus				
Four groups cause CNS disease	RNA	4–14 days	Mosquito bite transmits to humans; can multiply in horses, birds, bats, snakes, insects.	Age-related; younger individuals often have high fever and convulsions; headache, fever, drowsiness, confusion, disorientation; some manifest mainly by lethargy, "sleeping sickness"; muscle weakness; residual effects range from none to convulsions; speech difficulties.
Unclassified				
Hepatitis A	RNA similar to picornaviruses	15–45 days	Fecal-oral enhanced by poor hygiene, overcrowding, contaminated food, water; sexual; percutaneous.	Onset acute, most frequent in young individuals; causes anorexia, malaise, and other symptoms followed by jaundice; dark urine, clay-colored stools; recovery usually complete.
Hepatitis, non A, non B	RNA	15–160 days	Not known, possible fecal-oral or percutaneous.	Clinical course variable; debilitation and liver dysfunction not infrequent.
Hepatitis B	DNA-type	45–160 days	Percutaneous, sexual, fecal-oral.	Chronic active hepatitis may occur; jaundice, liver dysfunction may progress to liver failure; recovery slow.
Human immunodeficiency virus (HIV)	RNA retrovirus	Not known	Homo- or heterosexual contact; blood contamination; percutaneous African monkey bites.	May be dormant; may cause AIDS related complex (ARC) or clinical AIDS; immunodeficiency affects resistance to cytomegalovirus and Epstein-Barr virus with high percentage affected; pneumonia due to *Pneumocystic carinii*; series of opportunistic infections; Kaposi's sarcoma; with ARC, swollen lymph glands, fatigue, weight loss occur; clinical AIDS usually results in death.

TABLE 8-3 Common Rickettsia That Cause Pathologic Effects in Humans

Rickettsia	Morphology	Epidemiology	Clinical Effects
Spotted fevers *R. rickettsii* (Rocky Mountain spotted fever)	Small organism, stains purple; usually gram-negative cell wall antigen; elaborates endotoxinlike substance.	Multiply in nucleus and cytoplasm of infected cells of ticks and mammals; commonly occurs in Western Hemisphere; transmitted by bite of infected tick or through skin abrasions contacting tick feces or tissue juices; incubation 3–12 days.	Swelling and degeneration of endothelial cells, vascular damage, myocarditis pneumonitis; peripheral vascular collapse may cause death; impairment of hepatic function and consumption coagulopathy may occur; severe headache, muscle pain, fever for 15–20 days; characteristic rash begins as small discrete, nonfixed, pink lesions on wrists, ankles, forearms, etc., becomes petechial; mortality approximately 7–10%.
Typhus fevers *R. prowazekii* (epidemic typhus)	Small, gram-negative organism, always multiplies within cytoplasm of cells.	Inhalation of dried louse feces; louse feces often rubbed into broken skin as with scratching of bite; incubation approximately 1 week.	Intense headache, continuous pyrexia for 2 weeks, macular rash in axilla spreads to extremities, becomes petechial; peripheral vascular collapse as with Rocky Mountain spotted fever.
R. mooseri (endemic typhus)	Similar to *R. prowazekii.*	Transmitted by fleas, widespread in U.S., especially Southeastern and Gulf Coast States.	Headache, fever, chills; fever up to 12 days; rash generalized, dull red macular, over thorax and abdomen; prognosis good with or without treatment.
Q. fever *Coxiella burnetti*	Appearance similar to other rickettsiae.	Inhalation of infected dust, of ticks on body and lice feces; sheep, goats, cows often affected; incubation 2–4 weeks; present throughout the world.	Fever, headache, weakness, interstitial pneumonitis; dry cough, chest pain; hepatitis and endocarditis may follow; rash not characteristic.

cell walls resist decolorization by acetone-alcohol. *Gram-negative bacteria* are decolorized and then stained with a red dye to make them stand out.

Bacteria are also classified by their morphology. Spherical bacteria are *cocci*, rod-shaped are *bacilli*, and spiral are *spirochetes*. They can be pyogenic (pus producing), granulomatous, aerobic, or anaerobic. Organisms such as *Mycobacterium tuberculosis* elicit a granulomatous inflammatory response that involves a chronic inflammatory process with a nodule of granulation tissue and actively growing fibroblasts and capillary buds (see Chap. 25).

Pathogenesis

All bacteria are capable of localizing in specific organs and often produce acute inflammatory reactions. The degree of tissue damage depends on the number of bacteria present, the virulence of the organisms, the site of infestation, and the resistance of the host to the organism. The bacteria must resist engulfment by the defensive neutrophil cell. Some elaborate toxins that kill or depress the phagocytic cell; others develop resistant strains to escape recognition. Some of these organisms are *facultative intracellular bacteria* that counteract the defensive phagocyte after being interiorized. In this way, latent foci can be reactivated years after the initial infection [8]. The most common example of this is tuberculosis. Table 8-4 presents a classification of some of the more common bacteria that affect humans. The list is necessarily incomplete because there are thousands of bacterial organisms.

The virulence of bacteria is enhanced by the elaboration of endotoxins and exotoxins. *Endotoxins* are produced by many gram-negative organisms and when released, are pyrogenic and confer antigenic specificity to the toxin [8]. These enhance chemotaxis and some activate complement by the alternative pathway (see Chap. 9). *Exotoxins* are usually produced by gram-positive bacteria. These toxins have specific effects on target organs; for example, elaboration of diphtherial toxin causes the forma-

TABLE 8-4 Bacteria That Cause Pathologic Effects in Humans

Bacteria	Gram's Stain	Morphology	Epidemiology	Clinical Effects
Pseudomonas aeruginosa	Gram-negative	Motile rod; greenish yellow pigment formed; saprophytic but can establish infection and invade when host resistance is decreased.	Commonly present on skin and mucous membranes; often attacks debilitated, immunosuppressed, burned, premature, or elderly individuals; transmitted by contact, especially to urinary tract, lungs, or damaged skin.	Purulent drainage from wounds; characteristic greenish mucus from site of infection; bacteremia carries a 75% mortality; high fever, confusion, chills followed by circulatory collapse and sometimes leukopenia.
Proteus	Gram-negative	Actively motile rod; hydrolyzes urea; actively decomposes protein.	Commonly present in decaying matter, soil, water, and human intestine; affects skin, urinary tract, ears, and other areas secondarily in susceptible individuals.	Localized purulent infections may spread and cause bacteremia, symptoms of bacteremia; usually sensitive to penicillin therapy.
Enterobacter, Klebsiella	Gram-negative	Short, plump, nonmotile rods; type-specific capsular antigens.	Urinary tract and respiratory infections, especially pneumonia; often found in immunosuppressed, alcoholics, or individuals with diabetes mellitus.	Symptoms of pneumonitis: productive cough, weakness, anemia; may resemble TB; responds well to aminoglycoside therapy.
Shigella	Gram-negative	Nonmotile rods; aerobic or nearly anaerobic.	GI tract resident; transmitted through fecal-oral route, or through contaminated food, water, swimming pools; common in countries where sanitation is poor; incubation usually less than 48 hours.	Fever, colicky abdominal pain, diarrhea; liquid, greenish stools may contain various amounts of blood; dehydration may result.
Escherichia coli	Gram-negative	Non-spore-forming rods; different strains characterized by their antigens.	Normal inhabitant of colon; may spread to urinary tract directly or through bloodstream; opportunistic organism in debilitated individuals.	Accounts for more than 75% of urinary tract infections (UTI); abscesses may form on any area; bacteremia characterized by fever, chills, dyspnea; may develop endotoxic shock.
Salmonella S. typhi (typhoid fever)	Gram-negative	Motile; type identified by specific antigens.	Ingestion of contaminated foods, water, or milk; transmitted through fecal contamination of foodstuffs; totally transmitted by human carriers; incubation period about 10 days.	Rare in U.S.; onset of fever, chills, abdominal pain, and distention; rash of small macules on upper abdomen and thorax; without treatment often causes intestinal bleeding and perforation.
Other *Salmonella* organisms	Gram-negative		Food contamination; disease onset within hours of food ingestion.	Enteritis, massive vomiting, diarrhea, dehydration, fever; antibiotic treatment normally not helpful.
Hemophilus *H. influenzae*	Gram-negative	Small, pleomorphic nonmotile, aerobic non-spore-forming.	Respiratory transmission especially to very young and aged individuals.	Nasopharyngitis may be epidemic especially in impoverished and rural populations; often outbreaks during winter months may develop into pneumonia, ear infections, rarely meningitis.
H. pertussis *(Bordetella pertussis)*	Gram-negative	Small, aerobic, slow-growing.	Respiratory droplets; very contagious; incubation approximately 1 week.	"Whooping cough"; characterized by catarrhal stage followed by paroxysmal cough and laryngeal stridor; without immunization, epidemics occur; immunization or disease does not provide lifelong immunity.

(continued)

TABLE 8-4 Continued

Bacteria	Gram's Stain	Morphology	Epidemiology	Clinical Effects
Staphylococcus	Gram-positive	Spherical, grapelike clusters of organisms on solid media.		
S. aureus	Gram-positive	Coagulase positive; remains viable on surfaces of furniture or clothing.	Commonly resides on skin and mucosal surfaces, invades skin through hair follicles, thence to bloodstream; occasionally through urinary or respiratory tract.	Most common cause of ***skin infections***, furuncles, boils, and carbuncles; may have localized lymphadenopathy; impetigo results from exfoliative toxin from a form of *S. aureus*. ***Pneumonia*** more common in hospitalized individuals; causes fever, tachycardia with localized areas of pneumonia; also may cause empyema; ***bacteremia*** may produce fever, tachycardia with abscess throughout the body; often fatal, nearly 50% mortality; ***acute osteomyelitis*** commonly caused by this organism; may result from skin or bloodborne infection or from open or closed trauma of affected bone; high fever and bone pain; may cause much osseous destruction; usually responds well to antimicrobials; UTI most frequently result from contamination of indwelling catheter, ascend to kidneys from bladder.
Streptococci	Gram-positive	Spherical, anaerobe nonmotile, non-spore-forming.		
Group A, *S. pyogenes* (at least 60 subtypes), B hemolytic	Gram-positive		Respiratory, droplet.	Streptococcal ***pharyngitis*** very common in crowded living situations, greatest frequency ages 5–15 years; fever, extremely painful and inflamed pharynx, tonsils, uvula; ***scarlet fever*** may result when a specific strain of ***Streptococcus*** A produces a toxin causing rash, diffuse erythema, with petechiae on soft palate, scarlet "strawberry" tongue in early stages; later, tongue becomes beefy in appearance, called "raspberry" tongue; desquamation of skin occurs up to 3–4 weeks after the disease; may occur prior to rheumatic fever; ***rheumatic fever*** may follow acute streptococcal infection and apparently is immune reaction to organism; ***acute glomerulonephritis*** also may follow streptococcal infection; ***erysipelas***, an acute infection of the skin and SQ tissue from *S. pyogenes*, causes malaise, itching, erythema that spreads rapidly with edema and encrustation; localized skin lesions, cellulitis, and pneumonia may also result.
Group B, *S. agalactiae*	Gram-positive		Frequently colonize in the female genital tract, throat, and rectum; may be transmitted to susceptible individual directly or by respiratory contact.	May occur in puerperium to cause septicemia, pulmonary involvement, and meningitis in newborns.
S. pneumoniae Pneumococcus	Gram-positive	Diplococcal form, lancet-shaped.	Transmitted by respiratory tract droplet; rapidly progressive once established.	Preceded by "cold" or "sinus" complaints; fever, chills, pleuritic pain, cough productive of rusty sputum; hypoxia occurs with infiltration of lung tissue; progresses to atelectasis in one or more lobes; responds well to antibiotic therapy.
Neisseria				
N. meningitides	Gram-negative	Single cocci, grows well in media with small amount of oxygen.	Resides in nasopharynx of carriers, spreads through respiratory droplets; transmitted by bloodstream to meninges.	***Meningococcemia*** begins with cough, headache, sore throat followed by high fever and sometimes manifestations of endotoxic shock; ***meningitis*** evidenced by presence of meningococcus in cerebrospinal fluid and neurologic symptoms.

N. gonorrhoeae (gonorrhea)	Gram-negative	Diplococcus.	Humans only natural hosts; transmitted almost solely through sexual intercourse; incubation period usually less than 1 week.	Men develop dysuria, urethral discharge; because of penicillin treatment complications are rare; women have dysuria, vaginal discharge, abnormal menstrual bleeding, Bartholin's gland may be involved; pelvic inflammatory disease may result.
***Corynebacterium diphtheriae* (diptheria)**	Gram-positive	Nonmotile red, club-shaped; elaborates exotoxin.	Most frequently transmitted through respiratory tract but may be transmitted by skin, genitalia; incubation 1 day–1 week.	Respiratory effect on pharynx, larynx, and trachea, formation of thick, leathery membrane on these structures causing respiratory obstruction; exotoxin effects: heart, causing myocarditis; nervous system, causing peripheral neuritis, motor denervation; peripheral vascular collapse occurs in late stages; without antitoxin protection, mortality about 35% with 90% of those having laryngeal involvement.
***Clostridium tetani* (tetanus)**	Gram-positive	Anaerobic, motile rod, spore-bearing; exotoxin production.	Found in soil and intestinal tract of humans and some animals; puncture or laceration of skin usual mode of entry; incubation variable, usually about 14 days.	Exotoxin attacks CNS causing muscle rigidity and spasms; pain and stiffness of jaw early symptoms; *lockjaw* refers to inability to open jaw; laryngospasm may lead to hypoxia; overall mortality 40–60%.
Mycobacterium				
M. tuberculosis (tuberculosis)		Aerobic, acid-fast; resists decolorization with acid or acid alcohol; curved, spindle-shaped.	Respiratory droplet; reinfection or activation of dormant infection; incubation 4–8 weeks if not walled off.	*Primary TB:* usually lung involvement, macrophages wall viable organisms off; these may be seen on radiograph as rims of calcification; *clinical TB:* fever, pleurisy, night sweats, cough, weight loss; can spread to bone or cause liquefaction and cavitation of lung.
M. leprae		Hansen's bacillus; acid-fast rod.	Prolonged exposure, especially familial; skin or nasal mucosa may be portal of entrance; incubation approximately 3–5 years; little immunity has been demonstrated; endemic regions: tropical countries and few states in U.S.	Destructive lesions of skin, peripheral nerves, upper respiratory passages, testes, hands and feet; treatment may be curative.
***Treponema pallidum* (syphilis)**		Spiraled organism, with fibrils, 3 at each end, contractile elements for motility.	Almost always transmitted by sexual contact; incubation averages 3 weeks.	Organism can penetrate any mucous membrane, enters blood and lymphatics; primary lesion at site of infection, heals; secondary effects are lymphadenopathy, skin rash, arterial inflammation; tertiary syphilis involves CNS changes, dementia, inflammatory changes of aorta, etc.

tion of a thick membrane on the respiratory structures and toxic effects on the heart and nervous system.

Coagulase, an enzyme produced by many staphylococcal organisms, can initiate the coagulation sequence and produce coagulation in various areas. Coagulase may also cause the deposition of fibrin on the surface of staphylococci that may inhibit the ability of defensive phagocytes to destroy the bacteria. Laboratory tests often note whether or not a bacterium is coagulase positive.

Fungi

Fungal or mycotic diseases are caused by yeasts and molds. They are often divided into three groups according to the part(s) of the body they infect. *Systemic* or *deep mycoses* affect the internal organs or viscera. The pathogens involved can attack major systems and organs and may cause death. *Subcutaneous mycoses* infect the skin, subcutaneous tissue, fascia, and bone. Infection usually occurs from direct contamination with fungal spores or mycelia (mycelia are filamentous parts of fungi) fragments into wounds or broken areas of the skin. *Superficial mycoses* involve only the epidermis, hair, and nails. The principal habitat of the organisms is mammalian skin [4].

Unlike bacteria, most pathogenic fungi produce no extracellular toxic substances. They usually stimulate hypersensitivity to their antigenic components or metabolites that is thought to cause their pathogenicity. Of the many thousands of species of fungi, only about 50 cause pathology in humans. The structure of pathogenic fungi is similar to that of other fungi. Long, branching filaments called *hyphae* are produced, which may divide into a chain of cells by forming walls or septa. As hyphae grow and branch, they form a mesh of growth called a *mycelium*. Fungi reproduce sexually by spores when there is fusion, or asexually by nuclei when there is no fusion [7].

Saprophytic fungi that grow in the soil usually cause a systemic mycosis. The infection is transmitted from the soil or the droppings of fowl to humans through the inhalation of spores. Most deep mycoses are caused by free-living organisms and are limited to certain geographic locations. The severity of the disease depends on the degree of hypersensitivity of the host. The usual pathologic lesion is a chronic inflammatory granuloma that can produce abscess and necrosis.

Saprophytic fungi in the soil or on vegetation can also cause subcutaneous mycotic infection. This infection is opportunistic in that it occurs by direct implantation through a crack or sore on the skin. As with the systemic mycoses, necrotic, granulomatous lesions of any area may occur.

The superficial mycoses may represent allergic reactions to fungi. These organisms do not invade deeper tissues or become disseminated.

Table 8-5 summarizes some of the common human fungal infections. The reaction to these organisms often depends on host resistance and nutritional balance. Fungal infections are more commonly seen in individuals in poor health.

Protozoa

Protozoa are complex, unicellular organisms that may be spherical, spindle-shaped, spiral, or cup-shaped [7]. Many absorb fluids through the cell membrane and all possess the ability to move from place to place. Pathogenesis caused by protozoa often occurs in the gastrointestinal tract, genitourinary tract, and circulatory system. Table 8-6 summarizes several common protozoal diseases in humans.

The protozoa may be divided into four groups or *subphyla*. The *flagellates* (Mastigophora) have flagella, or undulating membranes. They are considered to be some of the more primitive protozoa. This group includes members of *Giardia*, *Trichomonas*, and *Enteromonas* genera, which infect the intestinal or genitourinary tracts [2]. Other flagellates such as *Leishmania* tend to be localized to skin, tissue, or mucous membranes. *Trypanosoma* organisms cause a systemic disease that is frequently fatal [8]. *Trichomonas vaginalis*, a common protozoal infection in women, is discussed in Chapter 55.

Typical ameboid characteristics are seen in the subphylum Sarcodina. Species of the genera *Entamoeba*, *Endolimax*, and *Iodamoeba* are representative of this group.

Organisms in the Sporozoa subphylum have a definite life cycle that usually involves two different hosts, one of which is often the arthropod and the other a vertebrate. *Plasmodium*, genus of the malaria parasites, is representative of this group.

Together with the Sporozoa, organisms in the subphylum Ciliata are the most complex of the protozoa. These organisms have cilia distributed in rows or patches and two kinds of nuclei in each individual. *Balantidium coli* is the only representative that is pathogenic to humans. It is a rare cause of infection, with only a few cases being recorded [4].

The motility of the protozoa is accomplished by pseudopod or by the action of flagella or cilia. In *pseudopod* movement, characteristic of many ameboid cells, the projection is actively pressed forward and rapidly followed by the rest of the organism. The movement is usually directional, toward a specific focus. *Flagella* are whiplike projections that cause very rapid movement of the organism from place to place. *Cilia* are shorter and more delicate, and cover the entire outer surface of the organism. The synchronous action of these structures allows the organism to move rapidly.

Reproduction may be sexual or asexual depending on the species. The sexual cycle, when it occurs, occurs in the *definitive* host, while the asexual cycle occurs in the intermediate host [7]. Protozoa capable of sexual reproduction are called *gametes* and those of asexual reproduction are called *zygotes*. Protozoa also have the ability to form cysts, which means that they can surround them-

TABLE 8-5 Common Fungi That Cause Pathologic Effects in Humans

Fungus	Morphology	Epidemiology	Clinical Effects
Superficial Dermatophytoses: tinea pedis (athlete's foot), tinea capitis (scalp ringworm), tinea corporis (body ringworm)	Branching hyphae on microscopic examination; found on keratinized portion of skin, nail plate, and hair.	Contact with fungus through skin; maceration or poor hygiene favor acquisition.	Fissuring of toe webs, itching, irritation, areas of alopecia, and scaling; circumscribed lesion with round borders of inflammation leads to designation of *ringworm;* treatment curative.
Systemic Candidiasis *(C. albicans)*	Small, yeastlike cells; blastospores with budding; forms clusters of round growths on cornmeal agar.	Contact with normal flora of mouth, stool, vagina; may be superficial or systemic in susceptible immunosuppressed individuals.	*Oral* lesions: white plaques on mouth and tongue, may cause fissures and open sores; *urinary tract infection* after broad-spectrum antibiotic therapy or individual with diabetes mellitus; *vaginal* discharge may be profuse and irritating; *Candida* in serum may cause disseminated abscesses.
Coccidioidomycoses *(C. immitis)*	Yeastlike cells, no budding is formed, divide into multiple small cells.	Soil saprophyte in southern U. S., Mexico, South America; infection occurs with inhalation of arthrospores; symptoms begin 10–14 days after inhalation.	*Primary form:* respiratory infection causes flulike symptoms, sometimes pneumonia; pleural effusion may occur; *progressive form:* dissemination to regional lymph nodes, skin, meninges, etc. may occur especially with immunosuppressed, other than Caucasian; fever, cough, chest pain, pulmonary coin lesion.
Histoplasmosis *(H. capsulatum)*	Dimorphic fungus, forms cottony white growth on glucose agar.	Grows as mold, prefers moist soil; airborne exposure by cleaning chicken coops, working with soil.	Cough, fever, weight loss, hilar adenopathy; progressive fibrosis of mediastinal structures; difficult to diagnose; treatment with amphotericin B may or may not be helpful.

TABLE 8-6 Common Protozoa That Cause Pathologic Effects in Humans

Protozoa	Morphology	Epidemiology	Clinical Effects
Amebiasis *Entamoeba histolytica*	Motile trophozoite usually seen in active disease; cysts form usual means of disease transmission; anaerobic.	Cysts transmitted from human feces; contaminated food, poor personal hygiene.	Chronic, mild diarrhea to fulminant dysentery; stools may contain mucus and blood, may persist for months or years; numerous trophozoites found in stools; fever, abdominal cramps, and hepatomegaly common.
Malaria *Plasmodium vivax* *Plasmodium ovale* *Plasmodium malariae* *Plasmodium falciparum*	Asexual phase passed in human body; multiply in liver, called *exoerythrocytic* cycle; then enter RBC and multiply, *trophozoite* stage; as RBCs hemolyze, segments called *merozoites* released into blood.	Transmitted by bite of infected female *Anopheles* mosquito; incubation period varies with type of organism from 10 days–7 weeks.	Anemia due to loss of RBCs; hemolyzing process with release of parasites causes chills and fever; immunologic mechanisms cause normal as well as infected RBC hemolysis; debilitation progressive; hepatic complications may cause permanent damage.
Toxoplasmosis *Toxoplasma gondii*	Intracellular protozoa exist in trophozoites; cysts and oocysts form; trophozoites invade all cells; cysts often take the form of transmission; *oocysts* transmitted through cycle by cat; form not seen in humans.	Transplacental transfusion or fecal-oral cysts; may be in lamb or pork.	Focal areas of necrosis, especially of eyes but may cause CNS or disseminated effects; lymphadenopathy common in immunosuppressed individuals, CNS involvement leads to high mortality; may infect fetus of affected mother.

selves with a resistant membrane. This prevents destruction and allows them to live for a long time.

Helminths

The word *helminth* means worm and usually refers to pathogenic worms, which are often parasitic. The common intestinal helminths are often divided into three general groups: *nematodes* or roundworms, *trematodes* or flukes, and *cestodes* or tapeworms. Helminths are very complex organisms in both their structure and life cycle. Many spend part of their developmental life in several locations and in various hosts such as fish, hogs, rats, snails, and humans. Often their eggs or larvae are eliminated in the feces or urine of humans and may be found in the feces on microscopic examination. The mode of infection for intestinal helminths is often through fecal-oral transmission or through broken skin.

Table 8-7 summarizes some common disease caused by helminths. These conditions, although not often fatal, are an important source of disability worldwide.

Study Questions

1. In what major ways can a person maintain freedom from infectious agents?
2. Discuss the differences among mechanisms of infection by bacteria, viruses, rickettsia, fungi, protozoa, and helminths.
3. How does the mechanism of host interaction differ for DNA and RNA viruses?
4. What are the differences between gram-positive and gram-negative bacterial infections?
5. How does host resistance affect susceptibility to infectious diseases?
6. Differentiate the clinical manifestations of viral and bacterial infections.

TABLE 8-7 Common Helminths That Cause Pathologic Effects in Humans

Helminths	Morphology	Epidemiology	Clinical Effects
Trematodes (flukes) Schistosomiasis	Blood flukes grow and mature in portal venous system, may attain 1–2 cm in length; life span 4–30 years.	Eggs of worm pair excreted in feces or urine of humans, hatch miracidia that penetrate a specific snail host and transform into infective larvae; these penetrate human skin and are carried to rest finally in portal venous circulation; worldwide distribution.	Usually asymptomatic; may cause dermatitis at focus of entry; cause mild fever and malaise; acute fever begins 1–2 months after exposure often associated with lymph-adenopathy; eosinophill levels elevate markedly; mucosa of bowel may become ulcerative and ova may be recovered from stool specimens.
Cestodes (tapeworms) *Taenia saginata* (beef) *Taenia solium* (pork) *Hymenolepis nana* (dwarf) *Dipylidium caninum* (dog)	Segmented ribbon-shaped hermaphroditic worms; absorb food through their surface; attach to host intestinal mucosa by sucking cups; length varies with species from 1 cm–10 m.	Transmitted when raw or poorly cooked beef or pork eaten; other types may be transmitted by fecal-oral route, man to man or dog to man; usually matures in adult intestines.	Weight loss, hunger, epigastric discomfort. In *T. solium,* encysted larvae may deposit in muscles, eyes, and brain; leads to eosinophilia, weakness, muscular pain; anemia may result from tapeworm competition for nutrition.
Nematodes	Elongated, cylindric, unsegmented organisms from a few millimeters to a meter in length; life span 1–2 months to 10 years.		
Trichinosis *(T. spiralis)*		Encysted larvae of *T. spiralis* ingested in poorly cooked pork or bear meat; larvae released in intestinal mucosa, multiply, and new larvae migrate into vascular channels throughout body; lodge in skeletal muscle, become encysted and grow for 5–10 years.	Severe inflammation of muscles in major infestation of muscle; may begin with diarrhea and fever; muscle pain, conjunctivitis, and rash may develop; eosinophilia common.
Enterobiasis (pinworm, threadworm)	Female 10 mm, male 3 mm; live attached to mucosa of bowel; female deposits eggs on perianal skin at night, then dies.	Fecal-oral transmission, transfer of eggs from anus to mouth; contamination of bed linens, remains viable 2–3 weeks; common infection in humans.	Pruritus of anal and genital region common, especially at night; bladder infection or other foci relatively rare; simultaneous treatment of entire families and groups essential.
Hookworm *(Ancylostoma duodenale, Necator americanus)*	Four prominent hooklike teeth attach worm to upper part of small intestine; adults about 1 cm in length.	Affects about 700 million persons worldwide, greatest incidence in Africa, Asia, tropical Americas; transmitted by invasion of exposed skin by larvae, migrates through lungs and resides in GI tract; excretion of larvae in fecal material perpetuates cycle.	Iron-deficiency anemia and hypoalbuminemia result from chronic intestinal blood loss; most infections asymptomatic but may have GI distress or ulcerlike pain; eosinophilia common.

References

1. Bellanti, J.A. Host-parasite relationships. In J.A. Bellanti, *Immunology III*. Philadelphia: Saunders, 1985.
2. Benenson, A.S. *Control of Communicable Diseases in Man* (14th ed.). Washington, D.C.: American Public Health Association, 1985.
3. Braunstein, H. (ed.). *Outlines of Pathology*. St. Louis: Mosby, 1982.
4. Fuerst, R. *Frobisher and Fuerst's Microbiology in Health and Disease* (14th ed.). Philadelphia: Saunders, 1978.
5. Jawetz, E., and Grossman, M. Introduction to infectious diseases. In M.A. Krupp, M.J. Chatton, and L.M. Tierney, *Current Medical Diagnosis and Treatment 1986*. Los Altos, Calif.: Lange, 1986.
6. Root, R.K. Infectious diseases: Pathogenic mechanisms and host responses. In L.H. Smith and S.O. Thier, *Pathophysiology: The Biological Principles of Disease* (2nd ed.). Philadelphia: Saunders, 1985.
7. Smith, A.L. *Principles of Microbiology* (10th ed.). St. Louis: Mosby, 1985.
8. von Lichtenberg, F. Infectious Diseases. In S.L. Robbins, R.S. Cotran, and V. Kumar, *Pathologic Basis of Disease* (3rd ed.). Philadelphia: Saunders, 1984.

CHAPTER 9

Inflammation and Resolution of Inflammation

CHAPTER OUTLINE

Acute Inflammation

- Vascular Phase
- Cellular Phase
  - *Margination and Pavementing*
  - *Emigration*
  - *Recognition and Phagocytosis*
- Complement and Other Mediators of the Inflammatory System
  - *Complement*
  - *Autocoids (Arachidonic Acid Metabolites)*
  - *Kinins*
  - *Coagulation System*
  - *Histamine and Serotonin*
  - *Lymphokines*
  - *Neutrophils*
- Exudates
- Summary of the Acute Inflammatory Response

Chronic Inflammation

Local and Systemic Effects of Inflammation

- Lymphadenopathy
- Fever
- Erythrocytic Sedimentation Rate
- Leukocytosis

Resolution of Inflammation

- Simple Resolution
- Regeneration
- Repair by Scar
  - *Healing by First Intention*
  - *Healing by Second Intention*
- Aberrant Healing
  - *Exuberant Granulations and Keloids*
  - *Contracture*
  - *Debiscence and Evisceration*
  - *Stenosis and Constriction*
  - *Adbesions*

LEARNING OBJECTIVES

1. Define and describe different types of mechanical and physical wounds.
2. List factors that can cause inflammation.
3. Describe the vascular and cellular phases of acute inflammation.
4. Define *chemotaxis* and *chemotactic gradient*.
5. Explain leukocyte response in inflammation.
6. Describe directional emigration.
7. Draw or describe the process of phagocytosis.
8. Explain briefly how organisms are actually killed.
9. Describe the functions of the major mediators of the inflammatory system.
10. Draw the classic and alternate pathways for complement activation.
11. Define the types of exudates and show familiarity with how they are named.
12. Differentiate chronic inflammation from acute inflammation.
13. Describe the reasons for the effects of inflammation, including fever, leukocytosis, lymphadenopathy, lymphangitis, lymphadenitis, and neutropenia.
14. Explain briefly the process of simple resolution in inflammation.
15. Explain why regeneration occurs in some tissues and not in others.
16. Describe the process of repair by scar tissue.
17. Define *cicatrization*.
18. Differentiate between healing by first intention and healing by second intention.
19. Define *epithelialization* in wound healing.
20. Describe exuberant granuloma and keloid scar formation.
21. Define *contracture* as a normal and abnormal part of wound healing.
22. Define *stenosis*, *constriction*, *adhesion*, *dehiscence*, and *evisceration*.

In the process of living, injury to the body tissues and organs inevitably occurs. Healing and repair of these tissues and organs must proceed for life to be maintained. Wound healing and inflammation are part of many disease processes, and are modified or altered by many environmental and individual factors. Healing is normally preceded by inflammation, which provides a cellular environment conducive to healing.

A *wound* is a break or interruption of the continuity of a tissue caused by *mechanical* or *physical* means (Table 9-1). A mechanical wound is caused by some kind of trauma that damages the tissues. Physical wounds may result from organisms, chemical or thermal agents, or death of tissues or organs. Each type of wound results in inflammation, which is the reaction of the body to tissue injury. Many diseases result in chemical changes that alter the process of healing and/or decrease resistance to infection. Examples of a few such diseases are atherosclerosis, diabetes mellitus, cirrhosis of the liver, and renal failure.

Inflammation is usually a beneficial response to invasion by microbial agents and/or to tissue injury. It normally proceeds on a continuum from the inflammatory phase to the healing phase. Inflammation can be defined as a tissue reaction to injury that characteristically involves vascular and cellular responses working together in a coordinated manner to destroy substances recognized as being foreign to the body. The tissue is then restored to its previous state or repaired in such a way that the tissue or organ can retain viability. The process of inflammation is closely related to the process of immunity (see Chap. 10).

Healing ideally involves the return of tissue exactly to its previous state. Tissue regeneration also participates in the healing process. If the amount damaged is excessive, scar tissue may result.

Inflammatory states may be classified as *acute* or *chronic*. The most common causes of inflammation include (1) infection from microorganisms in the tissues; (2) physical trauma, often causing free blood in the tissues; (3) chemical, irradiation, mechanical, or thermal injury, causing direct irritation to the tissues; and (4) immune reactions causing hypersensitivity responses in the tissues.

TABLE 9-1 Types of Mechanical and Physical Wounds

Wound	Definition
Mechanical	
Incision	Caused by cutting instrument; wound edges are in close proximity, aligned.
Contusion	Caused by blunt instrument, usually disrupting skin or organ surface; causes hemorrhage or ecchymosis of affected tissue.
Abrasion	Caused by rubbing or scraping of epidermal layers of skin or mucous membranes.
Laceration	Caused by tissue tearing, with blunt or irregular instrument; tissue nonaligned with loose flaps of tissue.
Puncture	Caused by piercing of tissue or organ with a pointed instrument, accidentally, such as with a nail, or intentionally, such as a venipuncture.
Projectile or penetrating	Caused by foreign body entering tissues at high velocity; fragments of foreign missile may scatter to various tissues and organs.
Avulsion	Caused by tearing of a structure from its normal anatomic position; damage to vessels, nerves, and other structures may be associated.
Physical	
Microbial agents	Living organisms may affect skin, mucous membranes, organs, and bloodstream; secrete exotoxins; or release endotoxins or affect other cells.
Chemical agents	Agents toxic to specific cells include pharamaceutic agents, substances released from cellular necrosis, acids, alcohols, metals, and others.
Thermal agents	High or low temperatures can produce wounds of various thicknesses; these in turn may lead to cellular necrosis.
Irradiation	Ultraviolet light or radiation exposure affects epithelial and/or mucous membranes; large doses of whole-body radiation cause changes in CNS, blood-forming system, and GI system.

Acute Inflammation

Vascular Phase

When injury occurs, large amounts of strong chemical substances are released in the tissue. These substances create a "chemical wall" called a *chemotactic gradient*, which provides a source toward which fluids and cells begin to move. The initial reaction to injury is a neural reflex causing vasoconstriction, which decreases the blood flow initially. It is rapidly followed by arteriolar and venular dilatation, which allows more fluids to cross from the capillaries into the tissue spaces. The increased permeability allows protein-rich fluid high in fibrinogen to move into the area of high concentration. This fluid may dilute the injurious chemicals and bring complement, antibodies, and other chemotactic substances to the area. The plasma proteins leaked into the tissues provide an osmotic gradient, or pull, that brings more water in from the plasma (Fig. 9-1A).

Cellular Phase

The components of the fluid exudate cause a characteristic response by the leukocytes commonly described as margination and pavementing, directional emigration, aggregation, recognition, and phagocytosis. The properties of the leukocytes allow for the destruction of the foreign material and the removal of cellular debris (see Chap. 16).

Margination and Pavementing. Margination refers to the movement of granulocytes and monocytes toward the endothelial lining of the vessel. Because of the increased capillary permeability resulting from the initial

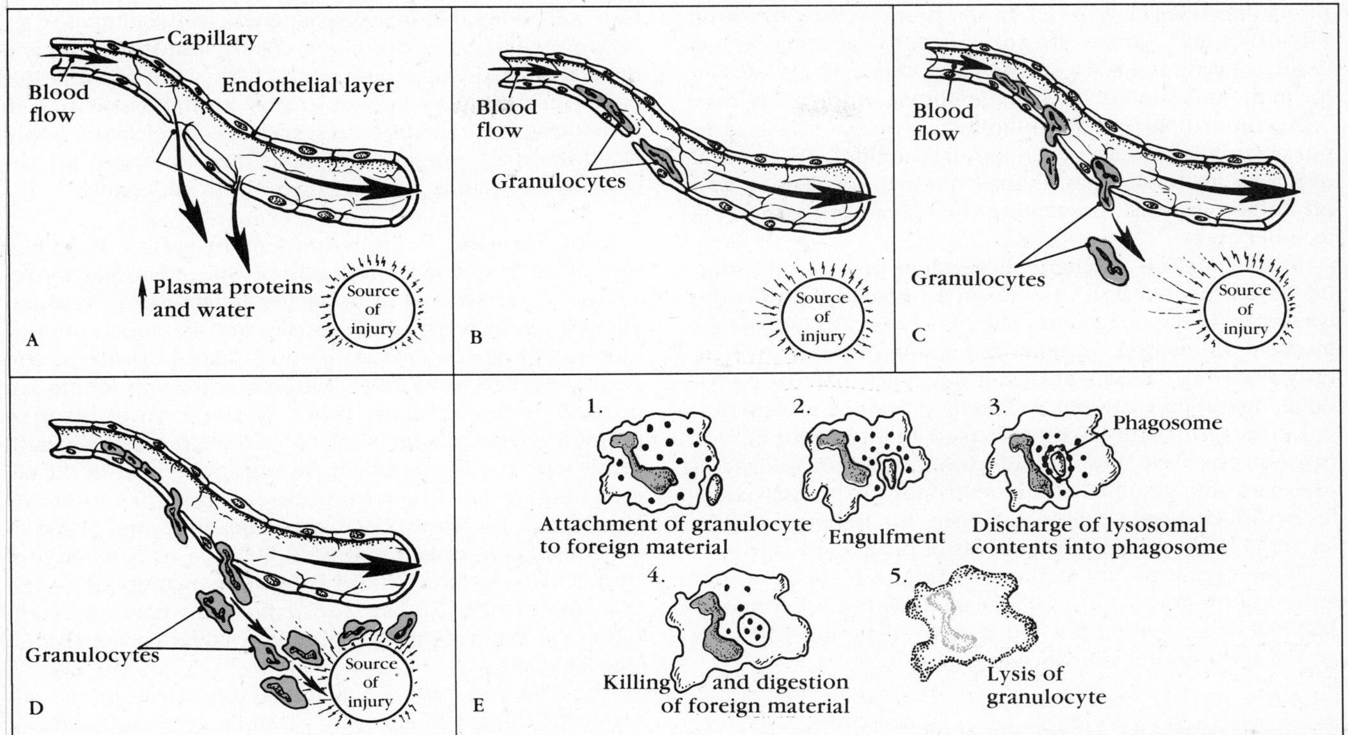

Figure 9-1 Acute inflammation. A. Vascular phase. Increased permeability of endothelial junctions allows the movement of plasma proteins into interstitial spaces, pulling water into the area and leading to edema. This increased permeability is induced by chemical mediators given off by the foreign agent or by cells' reaction. It occurs immediately after the injury and primarily affects the venulae. B. Cellular phase. Granulocytes marginate to the wall of the blood vessel. This is also probably a response to the chemical messengers. As groups stick to the endothelium, a pavementing pattern is seen. The leukocyte then begins to move by ameboid action toward the endothelial junctions. C. Emigration. Granulocytes move by ameboid action through the endothelial gaps toward the chemotactic source. D. Chemotaxis. Large numbers of granulocytes accumulate in the area of injury. E. Phagocytosis engulfs and destroys foreign material. Many granulocytes are also destroyed, and may release their lytic enzymes into surrounding tissues.

injury, the movement of blood is slowed. The polymorphonuclear leukocytes (PMNs) drop to the side of the venulae to form a layer closely approximated to the endothelial lining. This layer assumes a particular appearance called *pavementing* (Fig. 9-1B). The platelets and a few red blood cells may also join the PMNs on the endothelial lining. Normally, the endothelial cells are charged so that blood cells are repelled, but the changes occurring during inflammation appear to inhibit this property.

Emigration. White blood cells move to the area of injury by the process of emigration. Neutrophils move by ameboid motion toward the chemotactic signal by projecting a pseudopodium into the gap between two endothelial cells. This active process is followed by the cytoplasm streaming toward the projected extension (Fig. 9-1C) [10]. The entire leukocyte then arrives in the tissue spaces; the first ones on the scene are neutrophils. Monocytes (macrophages) and lymphocytes arrive later. Red blood cells may also leak into the tissues passively after the PMNs or after hydrostatic pressure changes.

Directional orientation for the movement of the PMNs is through chemotaxis. *Chemotaxis* is the directional movement of ameboid cells along a concentration gradient composed of substances such as bacterial toxins, products of tissue breakdown, activated complement factors, and other factors. The gradient provides a directional force that draws phagocytic cells to the area (Fig. 9-1D).

Recognition and Phagocytosis. Phagocytosis is a highly specific process that requires recognition of the foreign particle by the phagocyte before actual attack and engulfment can take place. The major phagocytes are neutrophils and macrophages. Neutrophils generally require the foreign material to be coated with a substance called *opsonin*. Opsonins include immunoglobulins, especially IgG and the opsonic fragment of C3 [10] (see pp. 152–154). Once the foreign particles are recognized, their receptors are attached by the leukocyte and phagocytosis occurs. Macrophages may respond to opsonized or other foreign material.

Phagocytosis involves the engulfment of foreign material. The cytoplasm of the phagocyte flows around the foreign particle and ingests it. Cytoplasmic lysosomes attach to the ingested particle and release hydrolytic enzymes into it, which often kills the microorganisms or dissolves foreign proteins (Fig. 9-1E). In the process, the phagocyte often dies and releases its enzymes into the surrounding tissue, causing injury to surrounding cells and also resulting in the digestion of the cell membrane of the phagocyte.

Accumulations of large numbers of phagocytes lead to pus accumulations and eventual destruction and removal of foreign material. Phagocytosis tends to localize or wall off foreign material, preventing the spread of the process to other areas.

Phagocytosis is an energy-dependent process and stimulates the production of hydrogen peroxide within the lysosomes of the phagocyte. The pH of the lysosome drops to about 4.0, which enhances the action of the hydrolytic enzymes [10]. The quantities of hydrogen peroxide produced are apparently not sufficient to induce a bactericidal effect, but they are increased in the presence of myeloperoxidase and a halide ion. Myeloperoxidase is present in the granules of the neutrophils [8]. Superoxide, formed during oxidative metabolism, has been studied in bacterial killing during the process of phagocytosis [6].

Some organisms are virulent and quite resistant to destruction by phagocytes. Others, such as the tuberculosis bacillus, are engulfed but not destroyed by macrophages and live within the cells for years [10].

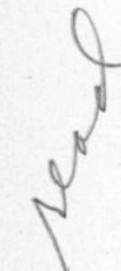

Complement and Other Mediators of the Inflammatory System

Many mediators of the inflammatory system enhance and depress the response to prevent excessive tissue damage. General factors that promote a beneficial inflammatory reaction include adequate blood supply, nutrition, age, and general health. This section deals with some of the major chemical mediators known to play an important role in promoting inflammation. Research has disclosed complicated interplay among the various mediators, and the cooperative system is just beginning to be understood.

Complement. The complement system has been identified as a major mediator of the inflammatory response. It is essential in the acute inflammatory reaction elicited by bacteria, some viruses, and immune complex disease [9]. It contains at least 18 distinct proteins and their cleavage products. Complement components are normally present in the blood in the form of inactive proteins called zymogens [9]. These are sequentially activated, with each component activating the next in the series (Fig. 9-2). The complement system enhances chemotaxis, increases vascular permeability, and in the final conversion, causes cell lysis. Fixation or activation of complement at the C1 level is by antigen-antibody (ATG-ATB) interaction [5]. This *classic pathway* continues a reaction pattern until the C8 and C9 enzymes are activated (see Chap. 10).

The *alternate pathway* is initiated by cleavage or activation of the C3 portion by plasmin, trypsin, bacterial proteases, and other enzymes in the tissues [5]. The C5 fragment also can be activated by many of these same substances. These may be important pathways for mediating the inflammatory process to clear agents that have little

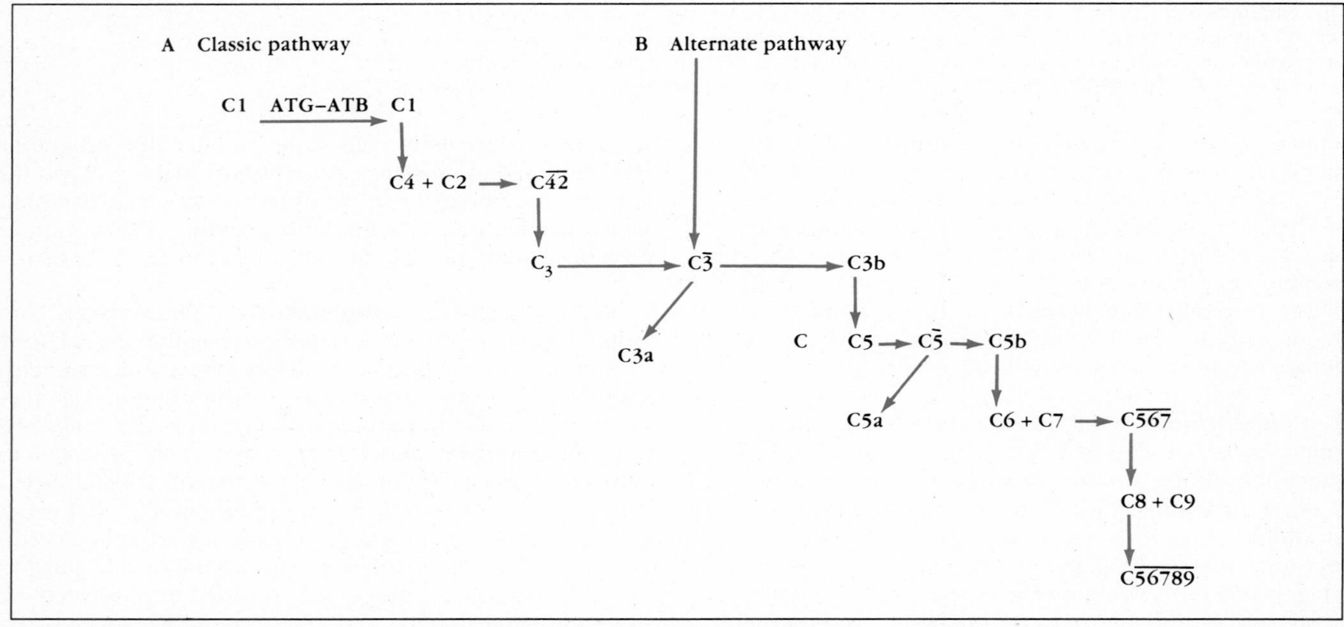

FIGURE 9-2 Complement activation. A. Classic pathway activated by ATG-ATB reaction.
B. Alternate pathway at C3 activated by endotoxins, trypsin, plasmin, and tissue proteases.
C. Alternate pathway at C5 activated by trypsin, bacterial proteases, and macrophages.
C3a increases vascular permeability; anaphylotoxin causes liberation of histamine from mast cells and platelets; C3b is an opsonic factor; C5a increases chemotaxis and vascular permeability; C$\overline{567}$ complex is chemotactic; C$\overline{89}$ causes breakdown of cell membrane (cell lysis).

immunologic specificity, such as some bacterial products and proteases present in normal tissue [9].

The inflammatory process is greatly diminished in the absence of complement enzymes. Deficiency of C3 especially causes a depression of the response and poor clearing of infection [4].

Autocoids (Arachidonic Acid Metabolites). Prostaglandins and related substances belong to a group of so-called autocoids or local, short-range hormones that exert their effects locally and are rapidly broken down [10]. These substances can be synthesized by most connective tissue, blood, and parenchymal cells. Through a complex conversion process, another group of active substances, called *leukotrienes*, is formed. Some of these substances (previously called slow-reacting substances of anaphylaxis, or SRS-A) are potent mediators of smooth muscle contraction and increased chemotaxis (Fig. 9-3) [3]. During cell injury, phospholipids become available for conversion to prostaglandins. Other mediators of inflammation such as bradykinin also have been shown to stimulate prostaglandin synthesis. Some of the prostaglandins function as vasodilators by enhancing vascular permeability. This leads to edema, with increased concentrations of these substances in the fluids and exudates of inflammatory reactions. The mechanism by which prostaglandins increase fever is not known, but local production is thought to affect the hypothalamus, which then transmits the information to the vasomotor system, resulting in stimulation of the sympathetic nervous system.

Kinins. Substances called kinins can cause vasodilation. *Bradykinin*, a small polypeptide, is activated by the enzyme *kallikrein*. Kallikrein, present in the body fluids in an inactive form, can be activated by a decrease in pH of body fluids, changes in temperature, contact with abnormal surfaces, and activation of the Hageman factor (XII) of the clotting system. The Hageman factor may be activated by endotoxins, cartilage contact, and contact with basement membrane tissue. Bradykinin is a powerful vasodilator; kallikrein, which can be converted to bradykinin, has been shown to have chemotactic properties.

Coagulation System. Factor XII, the Hageman factor, activated by surface-active agents, causes the activation of the coagulation proteins as well as conversion of

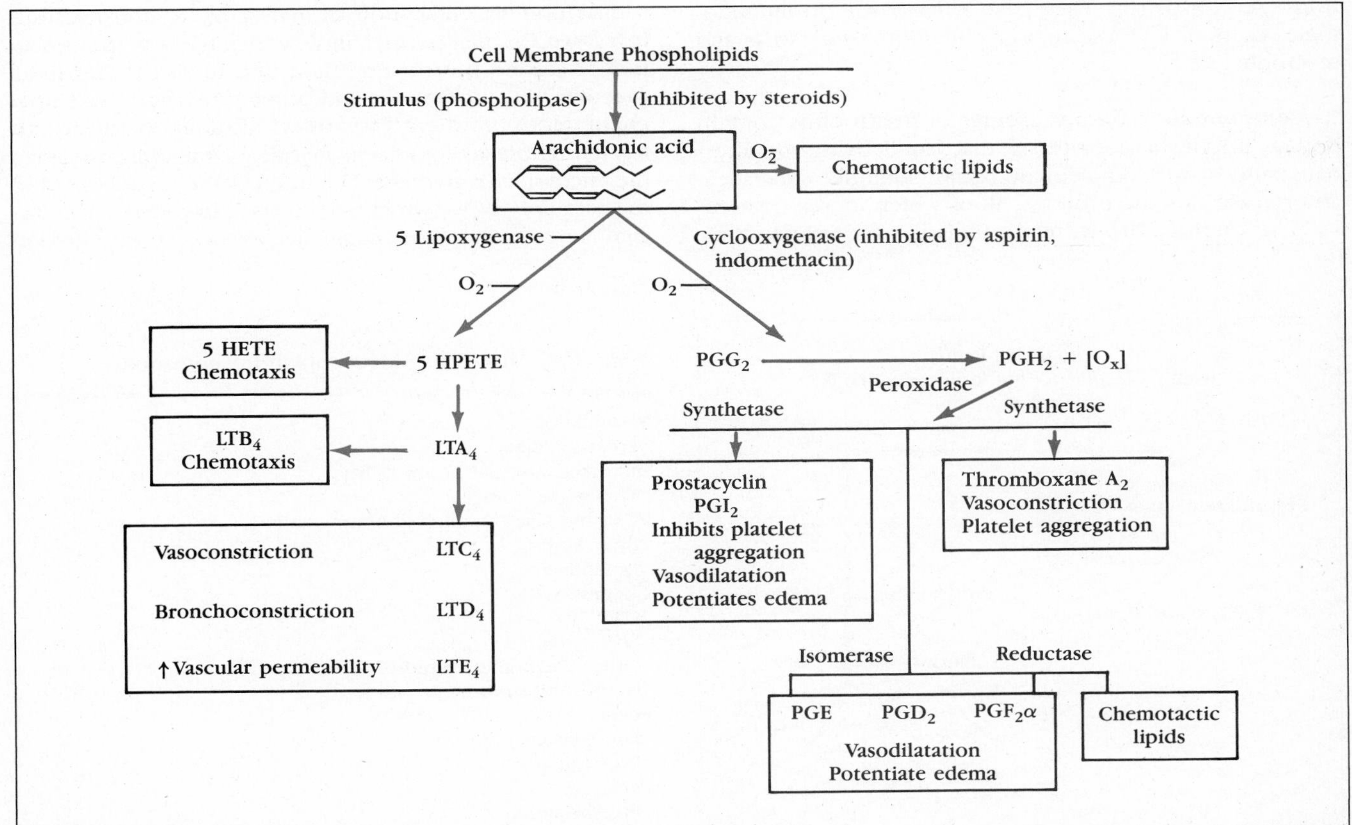

FIGURE 9-3 Arachidonic acid metabolites in inflammation. The principal mediators are the leukotrienes (LTA4, LTB4, LTC4, LTD4, and LTE4), the prostaglandins (PGG_2, PGH_2, PGI_2, PGE, PGD_{2a}, PGF_2), and thromboxane A_2. Arachidonic acid may be converted to HPETE, which is a hydroperoxy derivative (hydroperoxy eicosatetranoic acid). It then may undergo peroxidation to HETE, which is a chemotactic stimulus for neutrophils. (From S.L. Robbins, R.S. Cotran, and V. Kumar, *Pathologic Basis of Disease* [3rd ed.]. Philadelphia: W.B. Saunders Company, 1984, p. 55. Reprinted by permission.)

prekallikrein to kallikrein. Kallikrein then causes further activation of the Hageman factor [10] (Fig. 9-4.) Complement also works in the coagulation system through activation of the Hageman factor. The process is not fully understood but may be an underlying factor in disseminated intravascular coagulation (DIC) (see p. 250) [9]. Plasminogen may be activated to plasmin in the process that lyses fibrin clots and also activates the alternate pathway of complement. Several factors in this system lead to increased vascular permeability.

Histamine and Serotonin. In the immediate post-injury phase, histamine and serotonins are the major mediators of increased vascular permeability. Histamine is present mostly in mast cells, basophils, and platelets. Its release from tissue may result from such varied things as mast cell/IgE reaction, C3 and C5a fragments, trauma, heat, and lysosomes of neutrophils.

Some serotonin is present in the platelets, but the major source of this amine is the mucosal layer of the gastrointestinal tract. It is not present in mast cells of humans.

Lymphokines. This group of vasoactive substances is released from T lymphocytes during immunologic reactions (see Chap. 10). They have a major role in immunologic reactions and also induce chemotaxis for PMNs and macrophages.

Neutrophils. The lysosomes of neutrophils contain potent proteins and proteases that can activate the alternate pathway for complement, release kininlike substance, and release cationic proteins, all of which increase vascular permeability [10]. As neutrophils die and release their products into the surrounding tissue, chemotaxis and vasodilation are enhanced. Table 9-2 summarizes the most common chemical mediators of inflammation.

Exudates

In the process of inflammation, different types of exudates are formed, the analysis of which may offer clues as to the nature of the process. An exudate is fluid and/or matter collecting in a cavity or tissue space. The simplest exudate, the *serous* exudate, is the protein-rich fluid that escapes into the tissues in the early stages of inflammation. Because of its high protein content, it draws water and thus is responsible for the edema at the site of an inflammatory reaction. Depending on the source of the inflammation, other types of exudates may be seen. These are described in Table 9-3, which shows that the nomenclature depends on the constituents of the exudates.

Summary of the Acute Inflammatory Response

Acute inflammation begins with the invasion of the body by an agent recognized as being foreign. The initial response is often vasoconstriction followed closely by vasodilatation. Vasodilatation, or hyperemic response, causes increased vascular permeability, which leads to the exudation of serous, protein-rich fluid into the area. This fluid, together with histamines and other substances, sets up a chemotactic gradient toward which leukocytes are attracted. These ameboid cells marginate and emigrate along the chemotactic gradient. The first cells to be delivered to the area are PMNs, which attack and phagocytize the foreign material once it is recognized as foreign. Recognition

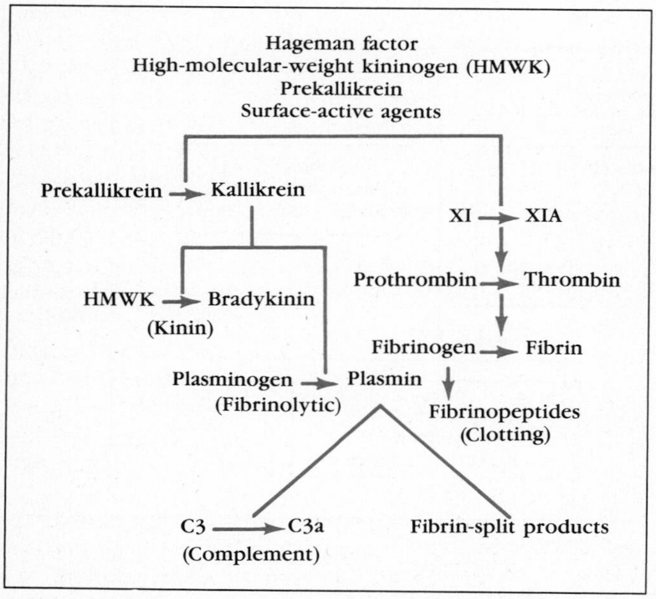

Hageman factor
High-molecular-weight kininogen (HMWK)
Prekallikrein
Surface-active agents

Prekallikrein → Kallikrein
XI → XIA
Prothrombin → Thrombin
HMWK → Bradykinin
(Kinin)
Fibrinogen → Fibrin
Plasminogen → Plasmin
(Fibrinolytic)
Fibrinopeptides
(Clotting)
C3 → C3a
(Complement)
Fibrin-split products

FIGURE 9-4 Interactions of kinin, clotting, fibrinolytic, and complement systems. (From S.L. Robbins, R.S. Cotran, and V. Kumar, *Pathologic Basis of Disease* [3rd ed.]. Philadelphia: W.B. Saunders Company, 1984, p. 54. Reprinted by permission.)

TABLE 9-2 Most Likely Mediators in Inflammation

Vasodilation
Prostaglandins
Increased vascular permeability
Vasoactive amines
C3a and C5a (through liberating amines)
Bradykinin
Leukotrienes C, D, E
Chemotaxis
C5a
Leukotriene B_4
Other chemotactic lipids
Neutrophil cationic proteins
Fever
Endogenous pyrogen
Prostaglandins
Pain
Prostaglandins
Bradykinin
Tissue Damage
Neutrophil and macrophage lysosomal enzymes
Oxygen metabolites

Source: Robbins, S., Cotran, R., and Kumar, V. *Pathologic Basis of Disease* [3rd ed.]. Philadelphia: W.B. Saunders Company, 1984, Reprinted by permission.

TABLE 9-3 Types of Exudates

Type	Description
Serous	Exudate fluid high in proteins; without cells.
Fibrinous	Exudate has high content of fibrin; may lead to development of adhesions.
Hemorrhagic	Usually suppurative exudation also containing red blood cells.
Purulent	Exudate that contains pus.
Suppurative	Exudate with pus and tissue damage from breakdown of neutrophils and macrophages; PMNs major cells in early suppurations; macrophages in old exudates.
Abscess	Area of pus, usually located in an organ.
Furuncle	Abscess of the skin.
Carbuncle	Extensive abscess of skin that tends to spread.
Cellulitis	Suppurative exudation with diffuse spread along tissue planes.
Serofibrinous	Serous exudate with high fibrin content.
Fibrinopurulent	Purulent exudate with high fibrin content.

occurs through opsonization, which is the coating of the foreign material by antibody or through fragments of the complement factors. Complement enhances hyperemia, chemotaxis, and opsonization, and causes cell lysis. When the foreign agent is destroyed, the cellular debris is removed by macrophages and neutrophils and the inflammation resolves (see pp. 142–144).

Chronic Inflammation

When an inflammatory process persists in the tissues and is not cleared by the body, certain patterns of response occur. The chronically inflamed area is usually infiltrated by mononuclear leukocytes, mostly macrophages and lymphocytes, while the acute process mostly contains PMNs. Certain types of chronic inflammations, such as osteomyelitis, contain neutrophils for months, while some types of acute inflammations have increased numbers of lymphocytes in the early phase. When macrophages are the predominant cells, they divide and multiply, and release chemotactic substances that attract more macrophages. The inflammatory process may begin as a low-grade, poorly cleared inflammation or it may begin as an acute inflammation that is not totally resolved by the body.

Chronic inflammation results in infiltration of the site with fibroblasts, increased amounts of collagen deposits, and varying amounts of scar tissue formation. The scar tissue and smoldering inflammation often cause organ dysfunction.

A distinctive pattern of chronic inflammation is the *granulomatous* inflammation, which is characterized by the accumulation of large *macrophages* or *histiocytes*. The offending foreign material is walled off from the rest of the body but not removed. In tuberculosis, the resulting granuloma is called a *tubercle*, which is characterized by caseous necrosis and calcium infiltration at the rim of the granuloma [10]. Calcium infiltration is usual in a chronic inflammatory process.

Local and Systemic Effects of Inflammation

All types of inflammation have in common five cardinal signs, which were described many centuries ago: calor (heat), dolor (pain), rubor (redness), tumor (swelling), and loss of normal function. These result from vasodilatation, exudation, and irritation of nerve endings. The vasodilatation is associated with the release of chemical mediators, as described earlier. Exudation results from fluid and white blood cell movement into the affected area.

Lymphadenopathy

Lymphadenopathy is a sign of a severe, localized infection. It results when the local lymph nodes and vessels drain the infected material, which becomes enmeshed in the follicular tissue of the nodes.

Increased lymphatic flow is characteristic of localized inflammation. If an inflammation of the lymphatic vessel occurs, it is termed *lymphangitis*. If it affects the lymph nodes, it is termed *lymphadenitis*. The lymph system helps to keep infections localized and away from the bloodstream.

Fever

Fever is an almost universal phenomenon of illness, particularly of inflammation. It is thought to be caused by the release of *endogenous pyrogens* from macrophages and possibly from eosinophils, which are activated by phagocytosis, endotoxins, immune complexes, and other products [1]. These pyrogens (fever producing substances) act on the temperature-regulating centers in the hypothalamus to elevate the thermostat set point. In response to the pyrogens, the body generates arachidonic acid and the prostaglandin PGE_1, which actively mediate the central responses and may further increase the hypothalamic set point (see Table 9-2 and Fig. 9-3) [11]. The body then initiates heat conservation measures, including vasoconstriction, piloerection (gooseflesh), and shivering, to drive the body temperature up to a new level. These mechanisms, along with conscious heat conservation measures, such as covering the person up with blankets, aid the body in attaining the new set point. Therefore, the new set point may be 38–40°C. Above 40°C the temperature control regulation can become seriously impaired, causing central nervous system damage.

When the set point is reached or the stimulus is removed, the body initiates cooling measures, including vasodilation (flush) and sweating, in order to maintain the set point. If the set point returns to normal, the fever rapidly dissipates. This rapid resolution has often been termed "breaking of the fever" and may signify that the causative agent has been destroyed. Effective antibiotic therapy can rapidly destroy a pyrogen that produces bacteria, and cause a rapid recovery of the temperature control mechanism. Also, antipyretic agents such as aspirin and acetominophen can interfere with prostaglandin synthesis and reduce fever.

The purpose of fever is unknown, but in the presence of elevated body temperature, the phagocytes act more quickly to accomplish their purpose. The metabolism of the body is increased, which may promote phagocytosis by increased blood flow. Fever in viral infections may stimulate interferon production and thus may limit the course of the viral infection [12].

Erythrocyte Sedimentation Rate

The erythrocyte sedimentation rate (ESR) is the rate that red blood cells settle in a test tube. The rate is elevated probably because of alterations in plasma components that occur during the inflammatory process.

Leukocytosis

Leukocytosis refers to an elevation in the white blood cell count. The rise in number of cells is selective according to the causative agent. For example, pyogenic bacteria often cause an increase in the neutrophil count, while helminthic infections may cause eosinophilia (see Chap. 16).

In advanced or overwhelming infections, neutropenia may occur. This depletion of neutrophils indicates that the system is unable to mount an adequate defense.

Resolution of Inflammation

For the body to maintain a steady state, foreign material must be removed or isolated to prevent deleterious effects on the body. This is accomplished through (1) simple resolution, (2) regeneration, and/or (3) replacement by a connective tissue scar.

Simple Resolution

Simple resolution involves no destruction of normal tissue and probably goes on continuously in the human body. The offending agent is neutralized and destroyed. The vessels return to their normal permeability and excess fluid exudation is resorbed. Any defensive cells in the area are either resorbed or cleared by tissue macrophages.

Regeneration

The term *regeneration* refers to the replacement of lost or necrotic tissue by tissue of the same type. It is a part of the reparative process to heal and reconstitute damaged tissue [10]. Intact, healthy, neighbor cells surrounding the dead cells undergo mitosis and proliferate to replace the cells lost in the tissue. This process generally occurs to the greatest degree in epithelial tissue. Certain glands and organs can regenerate functional parenchymal cells if the architectural structure remains intact.

In the healthy human body, how cell growth and reproduction occur is still essentially unknown. Certain cells such as hematopoietic and epithelial cells reproduce continuously. Many others, such as bone and fibrous tissue, do not reproduce for years unless stimulated to do so. Cells such as neurons do not reproduce at all during the entire lifetime of an individual. If a person develops a deficiency of some cell types, these reproduce rapidly until a precisely adequate number is available. Other cells do not reproduce even when their numbers are depressed.

Very little is known about mechanisms and controls that keep adequate numbers of cells in the human body. Control substances are probably secreted by cells that act as a feedback mechanism to stop or slow growth when an adequate number of cells is produced [4]. Cells removed from the body can be grown in a laboratory culture if the medium is suitable. These cells stop growing when small amounts of their own secretions are allowed to collect in the culture medium. Thus the secretions are probably the control substances that limit cell growth and reproduction.

Cells are often classified according to reproductive capability. Differences in reproductive ability cause these cells to react differently during wound healing. All of the *labile* cells undergo complete regeneration by the proliferation of reserve cells. *Stable* cells regenerate if they are stimulated to do so. For example, bone injury causes fibroblasts to differentiate into osteoblasts and osteocytes. Studies of muscle regeneration have shown that smooth muscle shows little regenerative ability, while voluntary muscle may partially regenerate if conditions are optimal [7]. Synovial cells in the tendons may be reformed under optimal healing conditions. *Permanent* cells do not regenerate, so their death requires replacement by scar tissue.

If tissue cells are to regenerate, they must preserve (1) a part of the original structure, and (2) the architectural framework of the injured tissue.

Repair by Scar

Repair by scar occurs when dead tissue cells are replaced by viable cells that are different from the original cells. The new cells form granulation tissue, which later matures to fibrous scar tissue.

Wound healing begins with inflammation; there is no distinct line between the processes. Healing follows several typical steps or stages. The first stage requires a cleanup of cellular debris, organisms, or clot, which is carried out mostly by macrophages and a few neutrophils. Replacement of necrotic material, clot, or exudate by granulation tissue is called *organization*. *Granulation tissue* is proliferative connective tissue that is highly vascularized. The gradual laying down of *collagen* by these connective tissue cells eventually causes a dense fibrous scar to form [7]. Collagen is a group of proteins composed mostly of fibrous tissue, basement membrane, bone, cartilage, and other specialized tissues. It is the main component that provides strength to healing wounds [4,10]. The scar begins as collagen, bridges the defect, and provides the initial strength to a wound. Epithelialization also occurs from the wound margins across the surface of the wound (Fig. 9-5).

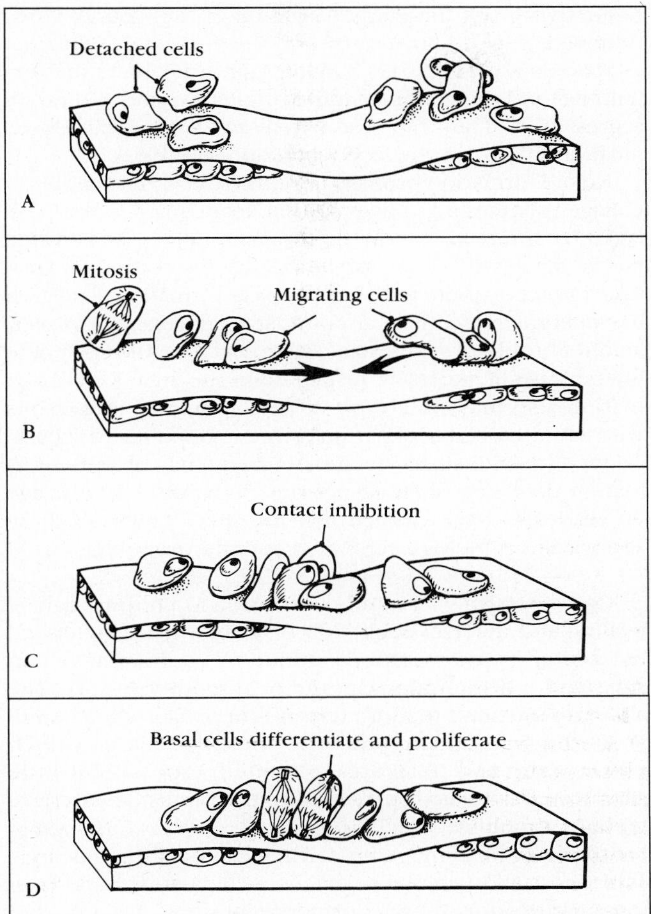

FIGURE 9-5 Epithelialization of a wound. A. With injury, epidermal cells detach from basement membrane and enlarge. B. Undifferentiated basal cells migrate toward center of wound defect. C. Contact inhibition occurs when migrating cells meet in the center and touch. D. Basal cells proliferate to restore epidermis.

As granulation tissue forms, it is very vascular and bleeds readily. As the scar forms, it tends to mold to the shape of the surrounding tissue and increases in tensile strength by compressing the collagen. In the early weeks the scar is red due to the many blood vessels infiltrating it. The new vessels originate by a budding or sprouting process called *angiogenesis* or *neovascularization*. The new vessels are leaky and allow fluid and protein to pass into the extravascular spaces. This leakiness accounts for long-term edema after the acute inflammation has subsided. The red color fades as vessels become smaller, until the scar assumes a white, fibrous appearance. Wound remodeling occurs throughout healing. Contraction or shortening is effective in pulling the wound edges closer together in the early stages of scar formation.

Cicatrization denotes formation of mature scar tissue. It has been described as the erratic contracting of dense collagenous scar tissue. Extensive scarring may produce a large cicatrix, which causes deformity or immobilization in an area.

Healing by First Intention. First-intention healing refers to scar tissue that is laid down across a clean wound whose edges are in close apposition. The edges are sealed together by a blood clot, which dries to protect and seal the wound. The best example is a clean surgical wound closed by sutures (Fig. 9-6).

An acute inflammatory reaction occurs within the first 24 hours, with neutrophilic infiltration of the area. By the third day, macrophages have moved in to clear up cellular debris, and fibroblasts begin to synthesize collagen on the margins of the incision. By the fifth day the collagen fibrils begin to bridge the defect. Maximum vascularization occurs at this time. Collagen continues to accumulate to form a firm, tough scar, progressively increasing in strength by the end of the first month. Epithelialization across the superficial layers restores a smooth contour. The scar is vascular initially and fades to a thin, white line as vascularity decreases.

Healing by Second Intention. This type of healing parallels first-intention healing except that it occurs in larger wounds in which large sections of tissue have been lost or in wounds complicated by infection. Much more time is necessary to remove the necrotic debris and infection from this type of wound. The inflammatory reaction is greater and occurs over a longer period of time.

Large amounts of granulation tissue must be formed. The wound must granulate from the margins and base, with collagen gradually filling the defect. Epithelialization across the granulation tissue occurs to provide a smooth surface. Wound contraction results, due mostly to fibroblast contraction that tends to pull the wound edges into closer proximity (Fig. 9-7).

Healing by second intention is similar to healing by first intention except that more cellular debris must be cleared, much more granulation tissue is formed, and a

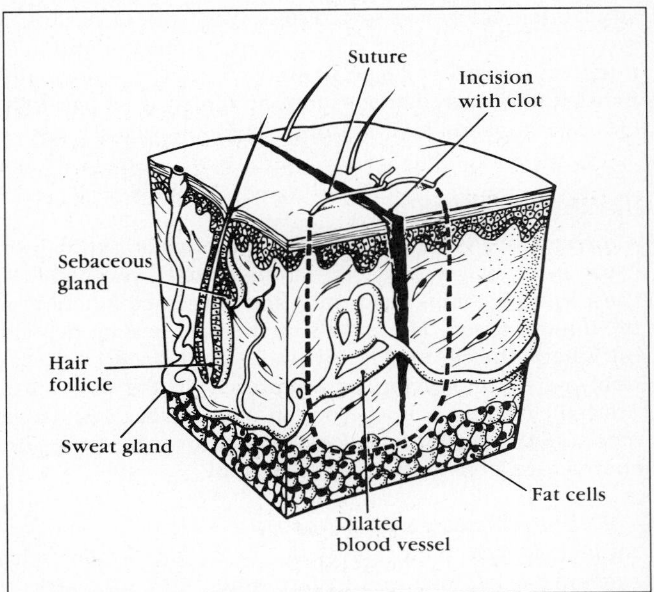

FIGURE 9-6 Initial stage of healing by first intention.

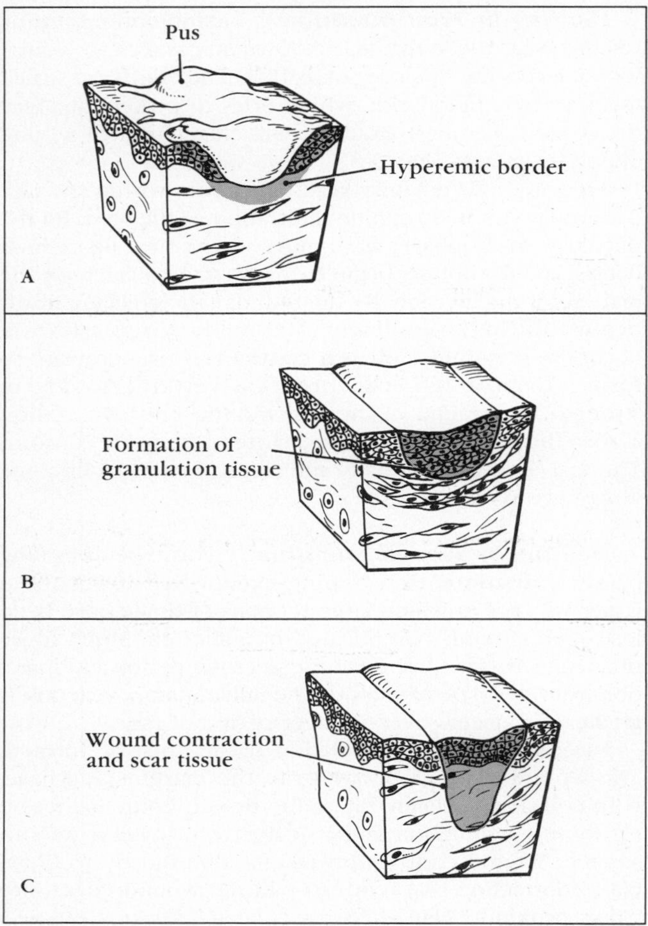

FIGURE 9-7 Healing by second intention. A. Hyperemic border around infected area. B. Formation of granulation tissue. C. Wound contraction and scar tissue.

large, often deforming scar results. This type of healing is required in third-degree burns, deep skin ulcerations, and infected and other large wounds. Structures normally found in the scarred area cannot be replaced, so hair follicles, sweat glands, and melanin-producing cells are lost.

Aberrant Healing

Aberrant means deviating from the normal, typical, or usual. In healing wounds, deviations from the normal may cause complications, deformity, and decreased function of the injured tissue. The results of aberrant healing depend on where the wound is located, the degree of deviation, and the modifying factors present in the individual. Aberrant healing results from an abnormality in healing mechanisms that leads to formation of excess scar tissue, contracture, constrictions, or adhesions.

Exuberant Granulations and Keloids. Exuberant granulations, or "proud flesh," occur when there is an excessive accumulation of scar tissue. They may vary in size from small to very large protrusions of granulation tissue that block the epithelialization of the wound. Once removed, they do not return.

Keloids are excessive, bulging, tumorous scars that extend beyond the confines of the original wound and rarely regress [10]. They can result with any wound but occur most often around the face, neck, and shoulders.

Keloid formation probably results from abnormalities in collagen synthesis and degradation. Inadequate lysis of collagen by *collagenase* may be the main defect, or elevated levels of propylhydroxylase, necessary for collagen formation, may contribute to the excess scar formation. Research has demonstrated that, in contrast to normal fibroblasts, keloid fibroblasts synthesize collagen at a rapid rate, possibly because of excessive histamine in the area. Keloid formation also may be a type of autoimmunity in persons with elevated levels of serum immunoglobulins [2]. Dark-skinned individuals have a greater frequency of keloid formation than light-skinned persons. Individuals below age 30 years also have a propensity for development of these abnormalities. Keloids tend to recur after removal.

Contracture. Wound contraction is a normal part of healing and involves migration of wound margins toward the center. Some wounds continue to contract after closure, and a disfiguring scar and/or disability results. The ability of a wound to close depends in part on the flexibility of the surrounding skin. The ability of skin to stretch on the scalp and tibial area is limited, especially if little subcutaneous tissue is present. Contractures may interfere with joint mobility or with other body movements such as breathing or head movement. They can occur in any area, skin, and subcutaneous tissue, as well as after bone fractures and tendon, muscle, or nerve injuries.

Dehiscence and Evisceration. Dehiscence is the surface disruption that results in the bursting open of a previously closed wound. This can occur as a result of interruption of primary or secondary healing. Dehiscence occurs when the strength of the collagen framework is not adequate to hold against the forces imposed on the wound. Poor collagen synthesis is often related to poor circulation.

Evisceration refers to the internal organs moving through a dehiscence. This most frequently occurs with the abdominal organs, but others may also eviscerate.

Stenosis and Constriction. If scar tissue forms in and around tubular areas, such as the ureter or esophagus, a stricture may develop, leading to narrowing or obstruction of an opening. Scarring may occur around an incision line or as a consequence of inflammation.

Adhesions. When serous or mucous membrane surfaces are inflamed, the exudate may cause scar tissue to bind or adhere to adjacent surfaces. Adhesions commonly occur in the peritoneal cavity between loops of bowel or abdominal viscera, especially after abdominal surgical procedures. Partial or complete intestinal obstruction can result from the fibrinous bands extending from organ to organ or from organ to peritoneal wall. Adhesions often develop after pleuritis, causing dense fibrous pleural adhesions that obliterate the pleural space and restrict respiratory excursion.

Study Questions

1. List and describe the interactions among the various chemical mediators of infection.
2. How do neutrophils contact, recognize, and destroy foreign material?
3. Diagram how complement factors participate in the inflammatory response.
4. How do the mediators of inflammation cause fever?
5. Compare simple and reparative resolution of inflammation.
6. Describe some aberrations of healing and indicate how they might be prevented.

References

1. Bodel, P. Studies on the mechanism of endogenous pyrogen production. *J. Exp. Med.* 140:73, 1974.
2. Cohen, I.K., and Diegelmann, R.F. The biology of keloid and hypertrophic scar and influence of corticosteroids. *Clin. Plast. Surg.* 4:2, 1977.
3. Goetzl, E.J., and Stobo, J.D. Immunology. In L.H. Smith and S.O. Thier, *Pathophysiology: The Biological Principles of Disease*. Philadelphia: Saunders, 1985.
4. Guyton, A. *Textbook of Medical Physiology* (7th ed.). Philadelphia: Saunders, 1986.
5. Haeney, M. *Introduction to Clinical Immunology*. London: Butterworths, 1985.
6. Johnston, R.B., and Lehmeyer, J.S. *Superoxide and Superoxide Dismutase*. New York: Academic Press, 1978.
7. Kissane, J.M. *Anderson's Pathology* (8th ed.). St. Louis: Mosby, 1985.
8. Klebanoff, S.J. Antimicrobial mechanisms in neutrophilic polymorphonuclear leukocytes. *Semin. Hematol.* 12:117, 1975.
9. Laurell, A.B. The complement system. In L.A. Hanson and H. Wigzell, *Immunology*. London: Butterworths, 1985.
10. Robbins, S.L., Cotran, R.S., and Kumar, V. *Pathologic Basis of Disease* (3rd ed.). Philadelphia: Saunders, 1984.
11. Root, R.K. Infectious diseases: Pathogenetic mechanisms and host responses. In L.H. Smith and S.O. Thier, *Pathophysiology: The Biological Principles of Disease*. Philadelphia: Saunders, 1985.
12. Walter, J.B. An Introduction to the Principles of Disease (2nd ed.). Philadelphia: Saunders, 1982.

Unit Bibliography

Bettoli, E.J. Herpes: Facts and fallacies. *Am. J. Nurs.* 82:924, 1982.

Bodel, P. Studies on the mechanisms of endogenous pyrogen production. *J. Exp. Med.* 140:73, 1974.

Braunstein, H. *Outlines of Pathology*. St. Louis: Mosby, 1982.

Cawson, R.A., McCracken, A.W., and Marcus, P.B. *Pathologic Mechanisms and Human Disease*. St. Louis: Mosby, 1982.

Cohen, I.K., and Diegelmann, R.F. The biology of keloid and hypertrophic scar and influence of corticosteroids. *Clin. Plast. Surg.* 4:2, 1977.

Cohen, I.K., et al. Immunoglobulin, complement, and histocompatibility antigen studies of keloid patients. *Plast. Reconstr. Surg.* 63:689, 1979.

Dineen, P., and Hildick-Smith, G. *The Surgical Wound*. Philadelphia: Lea & Febiger, 1981.

Flynn, M.E. Influencing repair and recovery. *Am. J. Nurs.* 82:1550, 1982.

Flynn, M.E., and Rovee, D.T. Promoting wound healing. *Am. J. Nurs.* 82:1543, 1982.

Fox, R.A. *Immunology and Infection in the Elderly*. Edinburgh: Churchill Livingstone, 1984.

Fuerst, R. *Frobisher and Fuerst's Microbiology in Health and Disease* (14th ed.). Philadelphia: Saunders, 1978.

Guyton, A. *Textbook of Medical Physiology* (7th ed.). Philadelphia: Saunders, 1986.

Ham, A.W., and Cormack, D.H. *Histology* (8th ed.). Philadelphia: Lippincott, 1979.

Hickman, C.P., et al. *Integrated Principles of Zoology*. St. Louis: Mosby, 1979.

Johnston, W.B., and Lehmeyer, J.S. *Superoxide and Superoxide Dismutase*. New York: Academic Press, 1978.

Kissane, J.M. *Anderson's Pathology* (8th ed.). St. Louis: Mosby, 1985.

Klebanoff, S.J. Antimicrobial mechanisms in neutrophilic polymorphonuclear leukocytes. *Semin. Hematol.* 12:1117, 1975.

Lynch, J.M. Helping patients through the recurring nightmare of herpes. *Nurs. 82* 12:52, 1982.

McAdams, C.W. Interferon: The penicillin of the future. *Am. J. Nurs.* 80:714, 1980.

Morello, J.A., Mizer, H.E., and Wilson, M.E. *Microbiology in Patient Care*. New York: Macmillan, 1984.

Phaff, H.J. Industrial microorganisms. *Sci. Am.* 245:76, 1981.

Robbins, S.L., Cotran, R.S., and Kumar, V. *Pathologic Basis of Disease* (3rd ed.). Philadelphia: Saunders, 1984.

Simons, K., Garoff, H., and Helenius, A. How an animal virus gets into and out of its host cell. *Sci. Am.* 246:58, 1982.

Smith, A.M. *Principles of Microbiology* (10th ed.). St. Louis: Mosby, 1985.

Taylor, D.L. Wound healing: Physiology, signs, and symptoms. *Nurs. 83* 13:44, 1983.

Weissmann, G. *The Cell Biology of Inflammation*, Amsterdam: Elsevier North-Holland, 1980.

Weissman, G. (ed.). *Mediators of Inflammation*. New York: Plenum Press, 1974.

Wilson, G., Miles, A., and Parker, M.T. *Topley and Wilson's Principles of Bacteriology Virology and Immunity*. Baltimore: Williams & Wilkins, 1983–4.

UNIT 5

Immunity

Barbara L. Bullock

An intact, functioning immune system is essential to protect the human body from invasion by microorganisms and damage by foreign substances. The cells of the immune system are called immunocompetent cells and are developed during fetal life, during which time they develop self-tolerance, thus distinguishing self from nonself. Chapter 10 covers the basic immunologic response, including components of the immune system and the development of immunity. Chapter 11 describes the alterations in defense that can occur with primary or secondary immunologic deficiency. Chapter 12 discusses the hypersensitivity or exaggerated immune responses. Autoimmune disease is considered to be a hypersensitive response and is discussed in this chapter.

The topic of immunity is vast and knowledge of the system's functioning is constantly expanding. It requires readers to be familiar with a new terminology. In studying immunity, the reader is encouraged also to review or study the inflammatory process. The learning objectives are helpful as a study guide outline for learning. Study questions at the end of each chapter provide an opportunity for synthesis of learning. The bibliography at the end of the unit gives some direction for further research.

CHAPTER 10

Normal Immunologic Response

CHAPTER OUTLINE

Organs of the Immune System

Lymphoid Organs and Tissues

Lymph Nodes
Thymus
Spleen
Tonsils

Immunocompetent Cells

B Lymphocytes

IgM
IgG
IgA
IgD
IgE

Formation of Specific Antibodies
T Lymphocytes

Major Histocompatibility Complex (MHC)
Killer Cells
Helper T Cells
Suppressor T Cells

Macrophages
Null Cells
Antigen, Immunogen, or Hapten Recognition

Types of Immunity

Humoral Immunity

Primary Response
Secondary Response
Complement Activation in Humoral Immunity

Cell-Mediated Immunity

LEARNING OBJECTIVES

1. Identify the functions of the organs and cells of the immune system.
2. Differentiate between T and B lymphocytes on the basis of function.
3. Trace the development of immunocompetent T and B cells.
4. Compare antibody-mediated immunity with cell-mediated immunity.
5. Define *self* and *nonself* as they are used in immunology.
6. Differentiate between primary and secondary immune responses.
7. Compare the functions of the different classes of immunoglobulins.
8. Describe briefly the role of macrophages and polymorphonuclear leukocytes in the immune response.
9. Explain one theory of specificity in the immune reaction.
10. Define the process of *immunosurveillance*.

The immune system consists of cells and organs that defend the body against invasion by microorganisms and damage by foreign substances. The inherent capacity to distinguish what is foreign from what belongs to the body is effected by particular cells called *immunocompetent* cells. These cells distinguish *self* from *nonself*. The development of *self-tolerance* involves the recognition of self proteins and is gained during fetal development. All other proteins to which the body is exposed are treated as foreign agents and are targeted for destruction.

This chapter describes the processes for the development of immunity and for the recognition of foreignness. Table 10-1 lists some of the essential terminology used in describing this system. Knowledge in the area of immunology is expanding rapidly through both research and many applications to clinical situations. Chapters 11 and 12 detail the major abnormalities of the immune system.

Organs of the Immune System

Lymphoid Organs and Tissues

The lymphoid organs include the lymph nodes, thymus, spleen, and tonsils. The lymphoid tissues are composed of lymphocytes and plasma cells, which are present throughout the body, especially in the gastrointestinal tract and bone marrow. Lymphocytes travel throughout the lymphoid tissues and organs, entering and leaving the tissue spaces with ease. Two major classes of lymphocytes exist, the T and B lymphocytes. Their function is discussed on pages 151–156. A network of lymphatic vessels conducts the lymph fluid to the vascular circulation and drains areas throughout the entire body.

TABLE 10-1 Terms Frequently Used to Explain Immune Responses

Term	Definition
Antibody	A protein produced as the result of introduction of an antigen; also called immunoglobulins; secreted from plasma cells.
Antigenic determinants	Specific areas or combining sites on the surface of the cell membrane of an antigen; determine specificity.
Antigens	Foreign substances, usually proteins, that are capable of stimulating an immune response.
Autoimmunity	Immunity to self-antigens; loss of self-tolerance.
Complement	A series of enzymes, normally inactive, circulating in the bloodstream that, when activated by an antigen-antibody reaction, participate in the inflammatory response.
Immunocompetent cells	Those cells that can recognize and react with antigen; T and B lymphocytes.
Memory	Ability to respond to an antigenic challenge due to previous exposure to the antigen and development of a bank of specific immunocompetent cells to that antigen.
Specificity	The property of reacting with one antigen only; both the antigen and the T or B lymphocyte have surface receptors that allow them to recognize each other specifically.
Tolerance	A state of unresponsiveness developed to a specific, known antigen.

Lymph Nodes. These encapsulated organs are distributed throughout the body and receive the lymph circulation. A lymph node consists of an outer portion, called the *cortex*, and an inner portion, called the *medulla*. Lymphocytes are formed and/or seeded from the thymus, especially in the cortical areas. In the middle and deep cortex is an area called the *thymus-dependent zone*, which is believed to contain chiefly T lymphocytes. The *germinal centers* contain mostly B lymphocytes but may contain a few T lymphocytes and macrophages.

The node consists of a stroma in which different types of free cells are held in place by reticular and collagen fibers. The lymph sinusoid is a thin-walled vessel through which lymph flows. The lymph sinus in the subcapsular space is like a hollow space that conducts the lymphatic flow [7]. Basically, lymph nodes serve as a series of in-line filters so that all lymph in the lymph vessels is filtered by at least one node. Lymph nodes receive lymph from an afferent lymphatic vessel, and the lymph then passes through the cortical, paracortical, and medullary regions (Fig. 10-1). Many lymphocytes and macrophages reside in

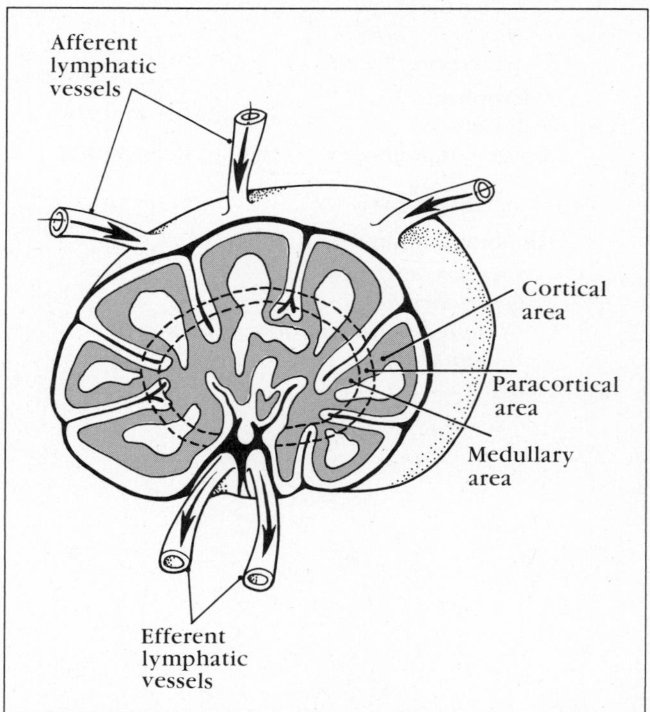

FIGURE 10-1 Regions and lymphatic vessels of a representative lymph node.

these areas. The T lymphocytes are found in the paracortical region, with many plasma cells in the medullary sinuses.

Thymus. The thymus gland, located in the mediastinal area, processes lymphocytes, and rapid production of lymphocytes occurs in this region from the early years of life until puberty. In the medullary area, lymphocytes appear to become more differentiated, after which they enter the circulation (Fig. 10-2). Many of the cells that are produced by the thymus die in the gland. The thymus and other lymphatic tissues undergo marked changes in size in relation to age (Fig. 10-3). The thymus grows rapidly in children, reaching maximum size at puberty, after which it gradually begins the process of involution, beginning in the cortical zone and progressing to the medullary area [1]. The gland never completely disappears, but in elderly people it is a collection of reticular fibers, some lymphocytes, and connective tissue. During stress reactions, the cortical cells rapidly involute in size due to the effect of corticosteroids (see Chap. 4) [1].

Lymphocyte maturation is regulated by transformation of lymphocyte precursor cells into antigen-specific lymphocytes (see p. 154). This process occurs in the cortical and medullary areas under the influence of the *thymic hormones*. A group of hormones that affect cell activities has been identified, but not all of their effects are known [1]. *Thymopoietin* secreted by the thymus and circulating in body fluids has been shown to enhance T cell immunity [6].

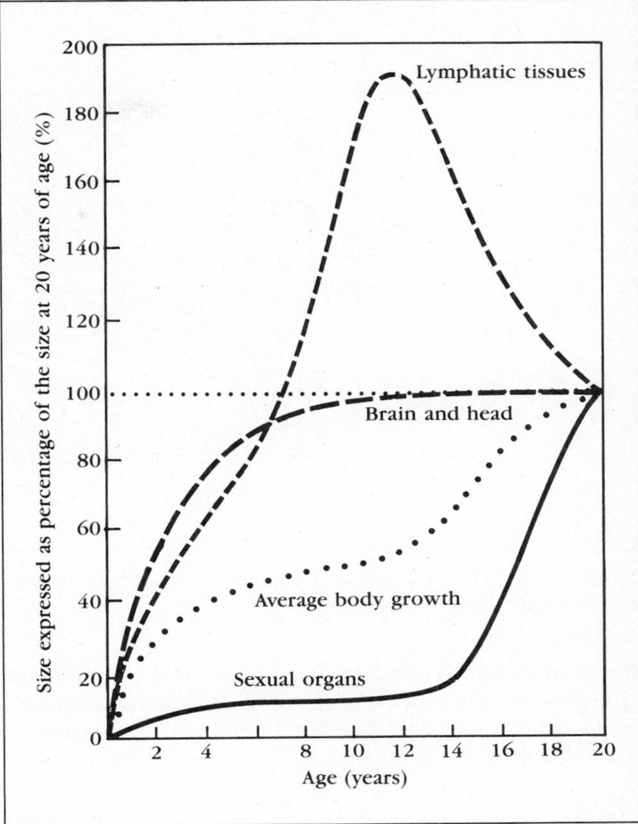

FIGURE 10-3 A comparison of the growth curves for various tissues. Note that the lymphatic tissues achieve maximum growth and function in the early adolescent years. (From L.A. Hanson and H. Wigzell, *Immunology*. Almqvist and Wiksell Publishers, 1985. Figure 1.9, p. 14. Reprinted with permission.)

Spleen. This organ, the largest lymphatic organ, can function as a reservoir for blood in two areas, the venous sinuses and the pulp (Fig. 10-4). As the spleen enlarges, the quantity of red blood cells within its *red pulp* (so called because of its dark red tissue that is rich in blood) also can increase. One of the main functions of the spleen is to process the red blood cells that squeeze through its pores. Those red cells nearing the end of their life span often break down here (see Chap. 15). The macrophages in the splenic tissue clear the cellular debris and process hemoglobin.

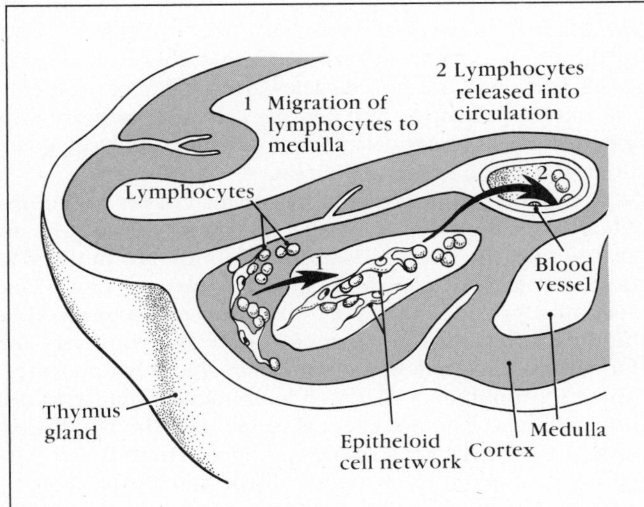

FIGURE 10-2 A thymus lobule. Note that the medulla extends into each lobule. The lymphocytes in the cortex rapidly divide and are immature. Those in the medulla are immunologically mature and are released from this area into the circulation.

Many phagocyte cells, especially macrophages, line the pulp and sinuses of the spleen. Groups of lymphocytes and plasma cells that can be seen with the naked eye throughout the parenchyma of the spleen are called the *white pulp*. These cells function in the process of immunity.

Tonsils. Tonsils are aggregations of lymphoid tissue and are named according to their location (Fig. 10-5). Those of the mouth and pharynx are called *palatine*, *lingual*, and *pharyngeal*. They are composed of lymphoid tissue and many lymphocytes.

In the intestinal area, *Peyer's patches* are accumulations of lymphoid tissue, as is the vermiform appendix.

Immunocompetent Cells

Mononuclear and the polymorphonuclear leukocytes are involved in the immune response. Mononuclear T and B

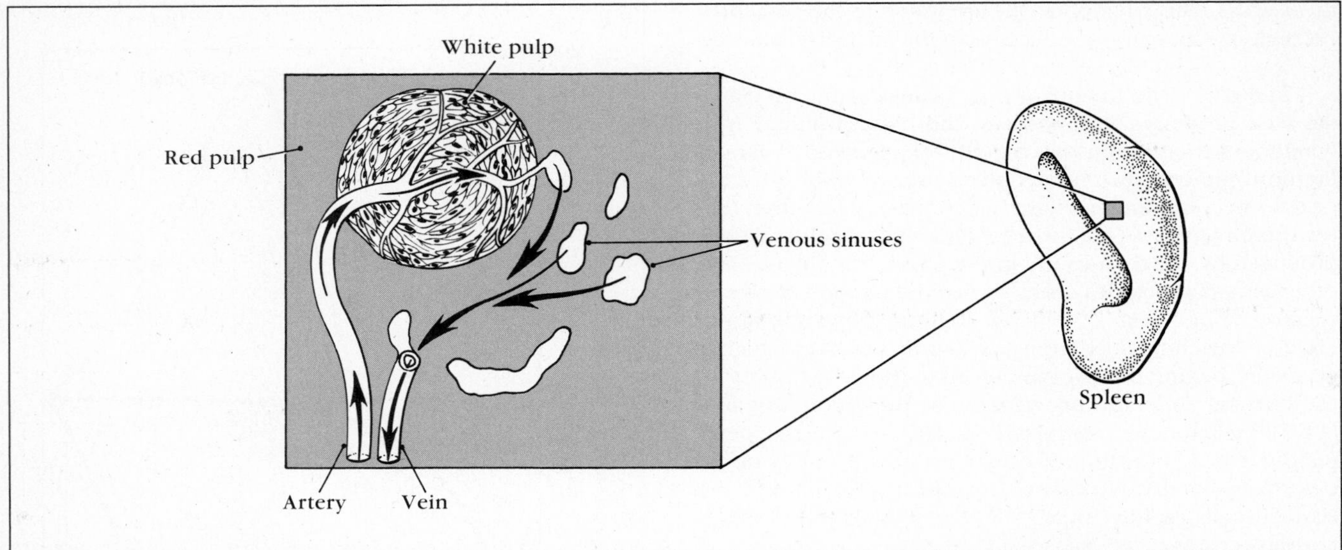

FIGURE 10-4 The structure of the spleen allows for the processing of red blood cells and can serve as a storage area for blood.

lymphocytes are considered to be the only immunocompetent cells. They provide for specificity, or recognition, of specific antigens by specific lymphocytes. An *antigen* is a substance recognized by the immunocompetent cells as being foreign, against which an immune reaction is initiated.

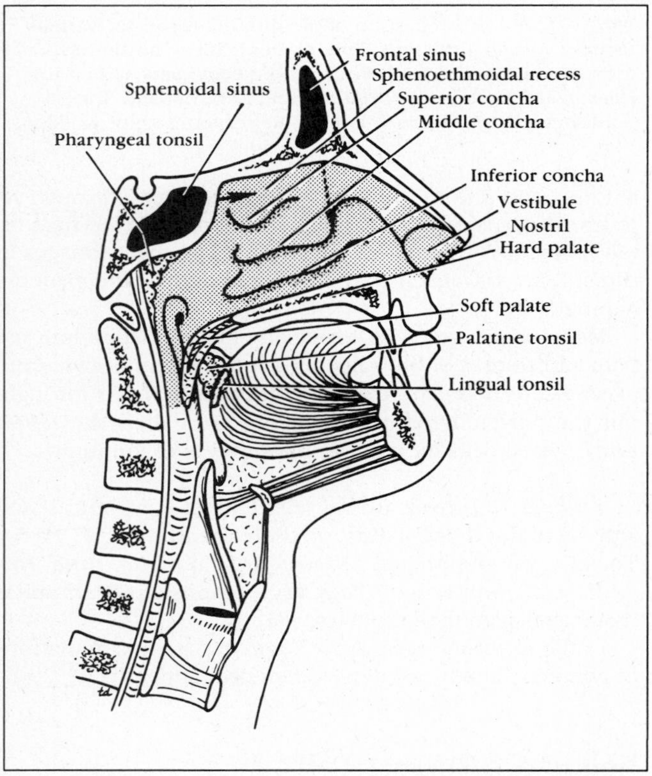

The polymorphonuclear leukocytes (PMLs) are *nonspecific* and interact with the lymphocytes to produce an inflammatory reaction (see Chap. 9). Phagocytic macrophages also play an important role in the immune response in that macrophages can be used to process antigen. This role is further described in later sections of this chapter.

The interaction among B cells, T cells, and macrophages with antigen provides the basis for the development of immunity.

B Lymphocytes

The B lymphocytes are responsible for *humoral-* or *immunoglobulin-*mediated immunity. These cells originate in the bone marrow and mature either there or in some other portion of the system. They are capable of proliferating and differentiating into *plasma cells* and *memory cells* when exposed to antigen. Plasma cells secrete large quantities of specific immunoglobulin.

Immunoglobulin secreted by plasma cells is called *antibody*. Antibody has exquisite specificity for antigen, so that within the many classes of antibody are molecules that recognize only their specific antigen [14]. The specificity resides in a portion of the molecule having binding affinity for antigen [3]. Some lymphoblasts are formed by activation of a clone of specific B lymphocytes. These form numbers of new B lymphocytes similar to the original clone. The net effect is to increase the population of specific B cells for a specific antigen. These B cells circulate throughout the lymphoid tissue and are available to combat antigen whenever it is encountered. An expanded clone causes a rapid response when new contact occurs [6]. These are the methods for fighting infection through the primary and secondary immune response described on pages 157–158.

FIGURE 10-5 The tonsils of the mouth and pharynx. (From R. Snell, *Clinical Anatomy for Medical Students* [2nd ed.]. Boston: Little, Brown, 1981.)

The basic unit of every immunoglobulin molecule is a symmetric arrangement of four polypeptide chains. Two of the polypeptide chains, called *heavy chains (H)*, are identical and have a greater molecular weight than the two *light chains (L)*. These heavy (H) and light (L) chains are kept together as a symmetric four-chain molecule (H_2L_2) [3]. The chains are held together by disulfide bonds. Figure 10-6 shows a representative model of an immunoglobulin. The Fab (fragment, antigen-binding) portion is the *variable* portion, while the Fc (fragment, crystalizable) portion is the *constant* portion of the immunoglobulin class. The constant portion, or heavy chain, almost certainly directs the biologic activity of the antibody and perhaps the distribution or location of the immunoglobulin in the body [14]. The variable portion, or light chain, provides individual specificity for binding antigen and varies among immunoglobulin molecules.

Five major classes of immunoglobulins have been identified: IgG, IgM, IgA, IgE, and IgD. The classification depends on the structure of the heavy chain portion of the molecule [14]. Table 10-2 lists the main properties of each major classification. The ability of the antibody to combine with a specific antigen resides in the Fab portion of the molecule, whereas the biologic properties that determine how the antigen is destroyed or rendered harmless are found in the Fc portion of the molecule [14].

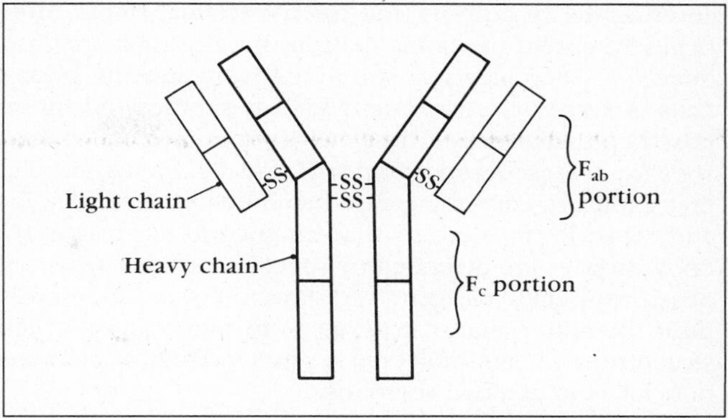

FIGURE 10-6 Schematic of an immunoglobulin showing two light and two heavy polypeptide chains. The constant portion, or Fc, accounts for the biologic activity, while the variable portion, or Fab, provides for the binding of specific antigen. SS = disulfide bonds.

IgM. Often called the macroglobulin, IgM is the first immunoglobulin produced during an immune response. It is made up of five units held together by a short peptide chain called the J chain. Immunoglobulin M is efficient in agglutinating antigen as well as lysing cell walls. It is present in high concentrations in the bloodstream and also early in the course of an infection. It can react in an efficient manner with bacteria and viruses. The level of IgM normally decreases in about a week as the IgG response increases [3,14]. Immunoglobulin M activates (fixes) complement and has five binding sites for antigen.

IgG. Immunoglobulin G makes up about 80 percent of the antibodies in plasma. During the secondary response, it is the major immunoglobulin to be synthesized. This antibody freely diffuses into the extravascular spaces to interact with antigen. The amount of IgG synthesized is closely related to the amount of *antigenic* stimulation presented to the host. In prenatal life it diffuses across the placental barrier to provide the fetus with passive immune protection until the infant can produce an adequate immune defense. Various subtypes of IgG exist, each with slightly different biologic characteristics [3,14]. It has been shown to carry the major burden in neutralizing bacterial toxins partly through its ability to fix complement. This property functions in accelerating phagocytosis.

IgA. Most IgA (80–90%) is in the form of *secretory* IgA in the external body secretions, such as saliva, sweat, tears, mucus, bile, and colostrum. It provides a defense against pathogens on exposed surfaces, especially those

TABLE 10-2 Immunoglobulin Classification

	IgG	IgA	IgM	IgD	IgE
Serum concentration (mg/dl)	700–1500	150–400	60–170	3.0	0.03
Binds to mast cells	–	–	–	–	+
Fixes complement	++	–	+++	–	–
Total (%)	80	13	6	1	0.002
Crosses placenta	+	–	–	–	–
Function	Major antibody formed in secondary response; most common antibody in response to infection	External secretions and surfaces, saliva, tears, mucus, bile, colostrum	Antibody formed in primary response	Not known; found with IgM	Reaginic antibody binds to mast cells; causes allergic symptoms

Key: – = negative; + = positive; ++ = active; +++ = highly active.
Source: From L. Roitt, *Essential Immunology* (3rd ed.). Oxford: Blackwell Scientific Publications, Ltd., 1977. Reprinted by permission.

entering the respiratory and gastrointestinal tracts. More than 85 percent of plasma cells in the intestinal area produce IgA. Secretory IgA is derived from specific plasma cells. A *secretory component (SC)* is synthesized by exposed epithelial cells. These two factors interact to form specific defense against bacterial and viral antigens. The first exposure causes increased amounts of secretory IgA and SC to be formed, so that on second exposure, the body surfaces are defended by specific antibody when exposed to specific antigen [4,5]. Antibodies to IgA may inhibit the adherence of pathogens to mucosal cells. The structure of the IgA molecule appears to facilitate its transport into the external secretions.

IgD. Immunoglobulin D is present in plasma and is readily broken down (half-life in plasma 2–8 days). Its function is not exactly known, but the fact that it has been found on the lymphocyte surfaces together with IgM suggests that it may be the receptor that binds antigens to the cell surface. Its levels are elevated in chronic infections, but it has no apparent affinity for particular antigens [3].

IgE. Immunoglobulin E is called the reaginic antibody because it is involved in immediate hypersensitivity reactions. Concentrations are normally low in the serum, and the antibody apparently remains firmly fixed on the tissue surfaces, probably bound to mast cells. Contact with an antigen triggers the release of the mast cell granules. The released vasoactive amines cause the signs and symptoms of allergy and anaphylaxis (see Chap. 12). High serum levels of IgE occur in allergy-prone individuals and in those infected with certain parasites, especially helminths.

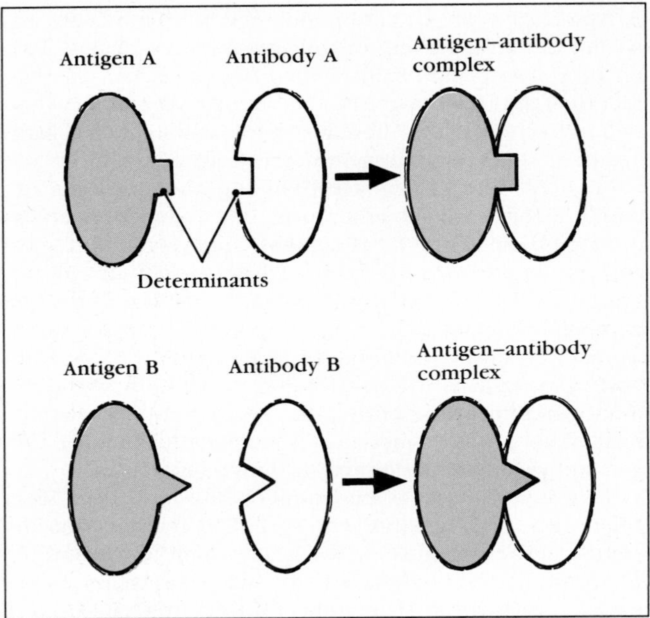

FIGURE 10-7 Highly schematic appearance of specificity of antibody for antigen, the so-called lock-and-key response. The determinants on the surface of the antigen and antibody provide for recognition of antigen by antibody (ATG-ATB interaction).

Formation of Specific Antibodies

To be specific, an antigen and antibody must fit together precisely, the way the right key fits into a lock (Fig. 10-7). The antigen-binding, or variable, region of the antibody bind others of similar structure. A person is confronted every day with many different antigens, both environmental and synthetic, against which the body must provide defense.

Each immunoglobulin molecule has a *constant region (C)* and a *variable region (V)*. The constant region is similar in molecules of each class of immunoglobulin. The variable region must be able to bind many different antigens and provides for specificity. Several theories have been proposed to try to explain immunoglobulin specificity.

One of these, the *selective theory*, proposes that each lymphocyte contains all the genetic information necessary to produce all possible antibodies. Thus, the gene for specific antibody is activated by contact with the antigen, and large amounts of the antibody are formed [14]. "The binding of antigen stimulates the selected B cells to divide, producing daughter cells of the same specificity" [14, p. 8]. Expanding this theory, the *clonal-selection model* assumes that large amounts of antigenic stimulation trigger the immunocompetent lymphocyte to divide and make large amounts of specific antibody [13].

When the B cell first encounters its specific antigen, it may become a *memory cell* or a *plasma cell*. Memory cells are a method of stockpiling a specific clone of B cells, so that immediate production of large quantities of the specific immunoglobulins results with exposure to a particular antigen.

T Lymphocytes

The long-lived T lymphocytes account for approximately 70 to 80 percent of the blood lymphocytes. They live from a few months to the lifetime of an individual and account for long-term immunity. The T lymphocytes are thought to originate from stem cells in the bone marrow but are matured under the influence of the thymus gland. They are sometimes called *thymocytes* because they mature in the thymus gland. The process proceeds from stem cell to prothymocyte to immature thymocyte to the mature, immunocompetent T lymphocyte [14]. These cells develop distinctive receptors on their cell surfaces, which makes their functions different from those of B cells. The T lymphocytes proliferate rapidly in the thymus and produce large numbers of antigen-specific cells.

The T lymphocytes leave the thymus to enter special regions called thymus-dependent zones, mainly in the paracortical region of the lymph nodes and part of the white pulp of the spleen. They may remain in the lymphoid tissue, enter the blood circulation, or enter the extravascular spaces to encounter antigens that correspond to the membrane receptors on their surfaces. If a T cell encounters its specific antigen, it divides and proliferates to form a clone of T cells that can destroy the antigen. The

T lymphocytes can be functionally divided into three subgroups: killer, helper, and suppressor cells.

Major Histocompatibility Complex (MHC). The maturation of T cells requires the influence of thymic hormones. The mature T lymphocyte has the ability to recognize products of genes in the *major histocompatibility complex (MHC)* [5]. A low reaction to *self*-MHC proteins is acquired, while a high reaction to *nonself* or foreign proteins is developed. The T cell becomes a major defender against infected host cells or nonself cells such as transplanted tissue [10].

All nucleated cells contain histocompatibility antigens that are genetically determined and expressed on their membranes. The MHC genes are critical in initiating and regulating immunity. The MHC is found in the HLA (human leukocyte antigen) on chromosome 6. These HLA antigens are so named because they were first seen on the leukocyte population. The products of the MHC are expressed on the cell surface of nucleated cells, which are a part of the genetic makeup of the individual [5,10,14].

Killer Cells. Killer T lymphocytes (cytotoxic T cells) bind to the surface of the invading cell, disrupt its membrane, and kill it by altering its intracellular environment. Killer T cells secrete *lymphokines*, which include such substances as chemotactic factor (CF), migratory-inhibition factor (MIF), macrophage activation factor (MAF), blastogenic factor (BF), transfer factor (TF), lymphotoxin, and interferon [14]. These substances may be *chemotactic*, establishing a chemical gradient that helps to bring leukocytes and other substances into the area.

Cytolytic T lymphocytes (CTL) directly kill cells and are essential in killing virally infected cells. This is accomplished by binding to virally infected host cells and secreting cytotoxic substances into the host cytoplasm. This kills the cells and stops the spread of viral particles [2]. The recognition mechanism of the T cells must be tightly controlled to discriminate between self and nonself because they recognize the membrane proteins of the host cell rather than free antigen. Therefore, CTLs are the chief mechanisms to react to and reject foreign tissue [10]. The lymphokines secreted draw macrophages to the area and stimulate the production of interferon. Interferon has been shown to suppress the spread of viruses from cell to cell (Fig. 10-8).

Helper T Cells. Helper T cells stimulate B lymphocytes to differentiate into antibody producers. A message from antigen-sensitized T lymphocytes induces also sensitized B cells to divide and mature into plasma cells, which begin to synthesize and secrete immunoglobulins. It has been noted that the synthesis of IgM seems to be the least dependent on T cell activity, while the IgA response is the most dependent.

Suppressor T Cells. These cells also reduce the humoral response. The production of immunoglobulins

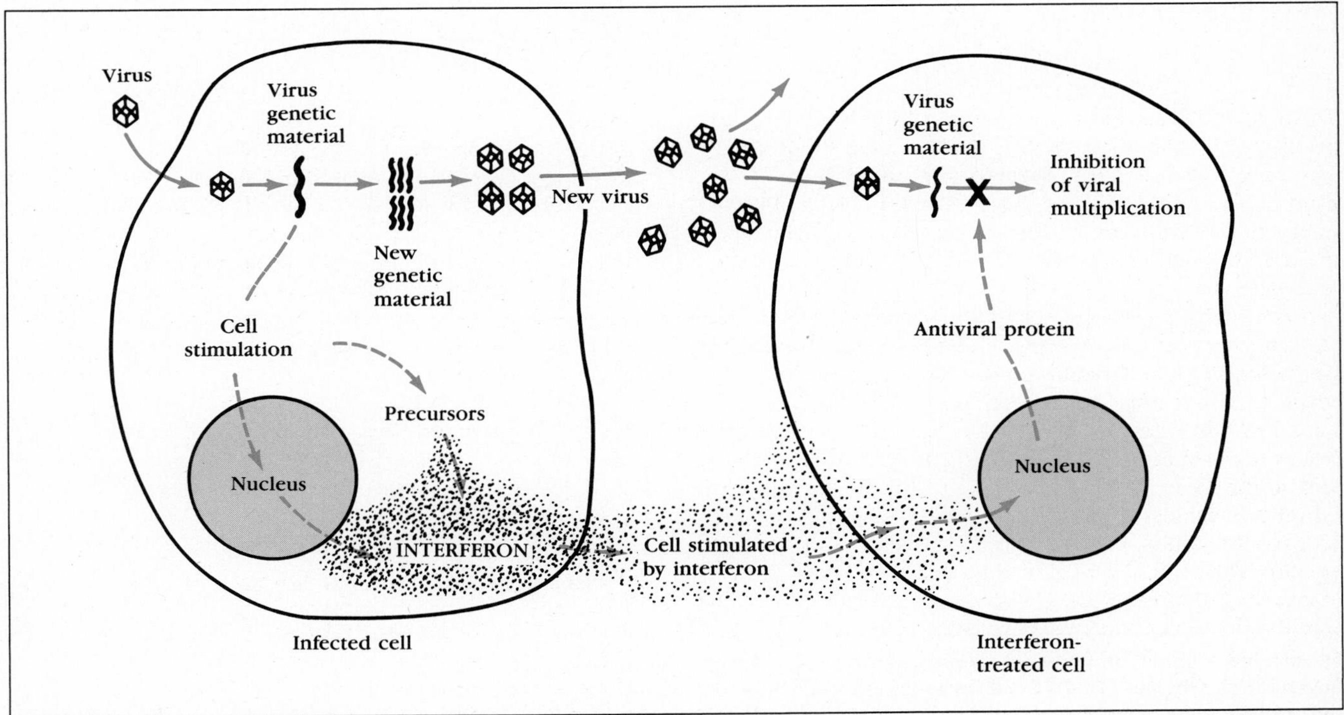

FIGURE 10-8 Schematic representation of interferon activity. (From J.A. Bellanti, *Immunology III*. Philadelphia: W.B. Saunders Company, 1985. Figure 16-5, p. 292. Reprinted by permission.)

against a particular antigen can be reduced or totally abolished in the presence of suppressor T cells. The mechanism of action may be to control the production of immunoglobulins either by regulating the proliferation of B cells or by inhibiting the activity of helper T cells.

Figure 10-9 shows the comparative formation and differentiation of T and B lymphocytes.

Macrophages

Macrophages are mature forms of blood monocytes. They migrate into the different tissues of the body and function as phagocytes. Tissue macrophages make up a network of phagocytic cells throughout the body. These have special names in different areas: Kupffer cells in the liver, alveolar macrophages in the lungs, peritoneal macrophages in the peritoneal cavity, histiocytes in the connective tissue, and others. In the central nervous system the special cells of the neuroglia classification called *microglia* have the ability to undergo changes and develop the property of phagocytosis during pathologic states [8].

Macrophages serve an essential function in removing foreign and devitalized material from the body. They are active at a site of injury during the process of wound healing, and in removing microorganisms, cellular debris, and necrotic material.

Macrophages also have an important cooperative role in the immune response, but how they function is not entirely understood. These cells trap and process antigens to present them to lymphocytes. They may play a secondary or accessory role in promoting lymphocyte activity, and may function as an intermediary between specific T cells and specific B cells [14].

The macrophage moves by ameboid motion toward a chemical concentration of soluble substances released into its environment by antigens or by lymphocytes. This is called movement toward a *chemotactic gradient*, or signal, that is elicited by soluble substances such as lymphokines (see Chap. 9). The macrophage migration-inhibition factor and macrophage-activating factor, which respectively tend to retain the macrophage in an area and increase its phagocytic activity, are especially important lymphokines [14].

Null Cells

Some cells cannot be classified as T or B cells or macrophages because they lack the surface markers characteristic of these cells and are not phagocytic. Called null cells, they resemble small or medium-sized lymphocytes. Often classified within this group are *K cells*, which are noted to lyse antibody-coated target cells. Also included are *NK cells*, which, like killer cells, lyse tumor cells, virus-infected cells, and sensitized normal cells. These types of cells are large, granular lymphocytes [12]. Some lyse opsonized antigen and function in graft rejection, lyse certain

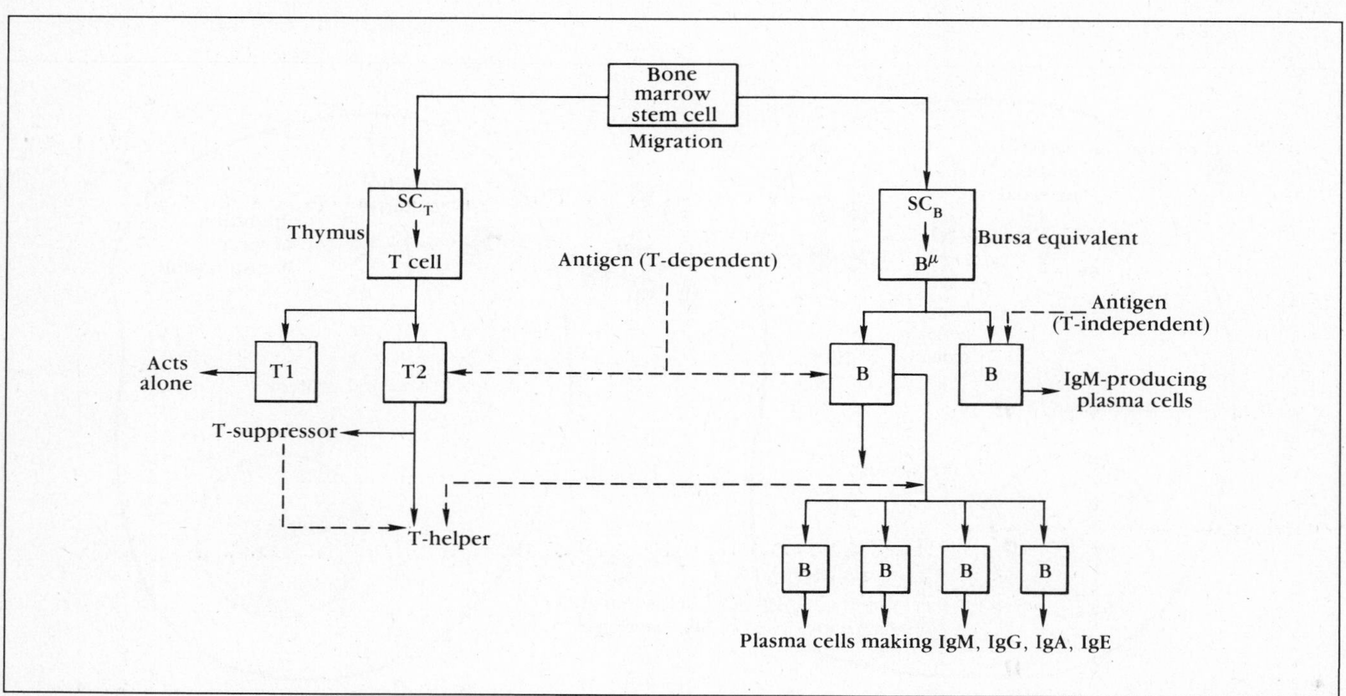

FIGURE 10-9 Both T and B lymphocytes arise from the bone marrow stem cell (SC) and migrate to the thymus gland (T cell) or to an unknown bursa equivalent area (B cell) where they mature to immunocompetent cells. The T cells may act in cooperation with B cells or alone. Some antigens can stimulate B cells without T cell interaction, a process that imparts little or no memory. Some T cells can suppress the activity of other T cells, while some T cells enhance the activity of B cells.

tumors, or destroy specific viruses. They appear to be marrow dependent and are called NK cells, K cells, or M cells according to their function.

Antigen, Immunogen, or Hapten Recognition

An *antigen* is defined as a molecule capable of inducing a detectable immune response when introduced into the body. When an antigen stimulates an immune response, it is said to have *immunogenicity* [14]. It then stimulates the immune response, denoting an active production of antibodies or sensitized cells. Most antigens and immunogens are proteins, but other large molecules such as polysaccharides and nucleoproteins may also function in this way.

Several characteristics appear to determine whether a molecule can stimulate an immune response, and these include such aspects as size, foreignness, shape, and solubility. Some molecules become antigenic only when they are combined with a carrier. Called *haptens*, these substances fail to elicit an immune response because they are small. These molecules cannot serve as complete antigens until they are combined with protein carriers (Fig. 10-10). An example is the contact allergens, which probably attach to proteins of the skin and stimulate the proliferation of a T cell population sensitized to the substance. Later exposure to the allergen leads to a more rapid reaction [11]. Other examples include drugs, dust particles, dandruff, industrial chemicals, and poisons [6].

Types of Immunity

Humoral Immunity

Humoral immunity refers to immunity effected by antibody synthesis or the production of specific immunoglobulin that coats the antigen and targets it for destruction by polymorphonuclear neutrophils. The interaction of antigen with antibody causes the activation of the classic pathway of the complement system (see Chap. 9).

Most antigens are recognized by T helper cells, which promote the activation of specific B cells. These B cells are "turned on" either by direct T cell interaction or by T cell secretions. In some cases a macrophage serves as an intermediary between the T and B cells. The B cell then divides and differentiates into a plasma cell that secretes specific immunoglobulin to target the antigen for destruction. Antigen recognition by T or B cell is often enhanced by macrophage interaction, which processes the antigen and presents it to the appropriate cell (Fig. 10-11).

Certain antigens, designated as ***thymus-independent antigens***, elicit strong B cell responses without T cell interaction. Examples include *Escherichia coli*, pneumococcal polysaccharide, dextrans, and other large polymers [14].

Humoral immunity is often described in terms of the *primary* and *secondary* immune responses. This terminology refers to the time lapse between the introduction of antigen and the humoral or immunoglobulin response.

Primary Response. The first time a particular antigen enters the body, a characteristic pattern of antibody production is induced. As the antigen binds to specific B

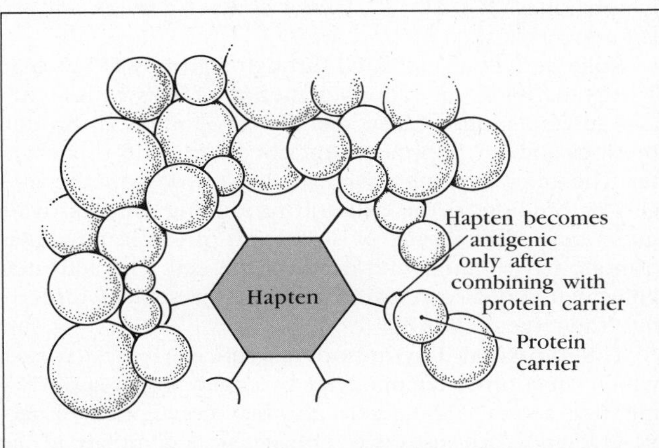

FIGURE 10-10 Some molecules become antigenic only after they have combined with a carrier, usually a protein. These molecules, called haptens, when combined with a carrier are fully antigenic.

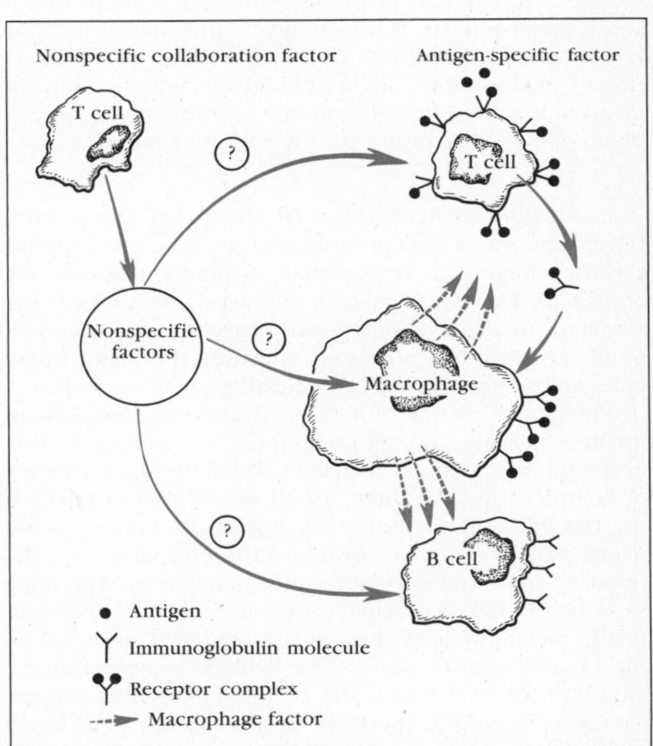

FIGURE 10-11 The macrophage often enhances antigen recognition and probably serves as an intermediary between T and B cells.

cells, activation occurs and causes the cells to proliferate and differentiate into specialized antibody-producing plasma cells. After about six days, antibodies specific to the antigen can be measured in the blood. The first antibodies or immunoglobulins to be produced in measurable quantities are usually IgM. These are produced in large quantities with levels, increasing up to 14 days and then gradually declining in production to very little IgM production after a few weeks [5].

After the initial IgM elevation, IgG immunoglobulins appear at about day 10, peak at several weeks, and maintain high levels much longer. During the course of the primary immune response, the immunoglobulins improve in their ability to bind the inducing antigen. The mechanisms responsible for this change are not known, but probably more firm binding occurs because of greater precision in matching surface receptors. Immunoglobulin G is considered to be the highest-affinity antibody that binds antigenic groupings firmly [6,12].

Secondary Response. The secondary response differs from the primary response in that the production of specific antibodies for the antigen begins almost immediately. More antibody is produced, and specific immunoglobulin is produced early and in large amounts.

The secondary response is called the memory response because the immune system responds much faster to a second exposure to a particular antigen. Both T and B memory cells are involved because in the primary response, lymphocytes proliferate and differentiate into T and B memory cells. If the antigen is introduced into the host a second time, these cells begin immediate production of antibodies of a higher binding capacity than in the primary response. Small amounts of antigen stimulate a highly specific response with the specific antibody [13].

Complement Activation in Humoral Immunity. Complement is a system of at least 18 different proteins and their fragments that circulate as functionally inactive molecules. They are capable of interacting with each other in a sequential activation cascade. They are designated by numbers, with nine numbers indicating the major molecules and symbols or names indicating the components.

The classic pathway for the activation of complement involves binding the first component, C1, with a portion of the immunoglobulin molecule. This begins the cascade of complement activation, which is essential in promoting the inflammatory process. Figure 10-12 shows the major pathway of activation and the end results of the process. The system promotes inflammation by increasing vascular permeability, chemotaxis, and phagocytosis, and finally causing lysis of the foreign cell [9]. The results of the cascade tend to cause some damage to normal tissue around the foreign tissue and, in some cases, this process can be damaging to the host. In most cases, an antigen-antibody reaction is required for the activation of complement. The complement factors then can participate in the process of inflammation with the result of destroying foreign material.

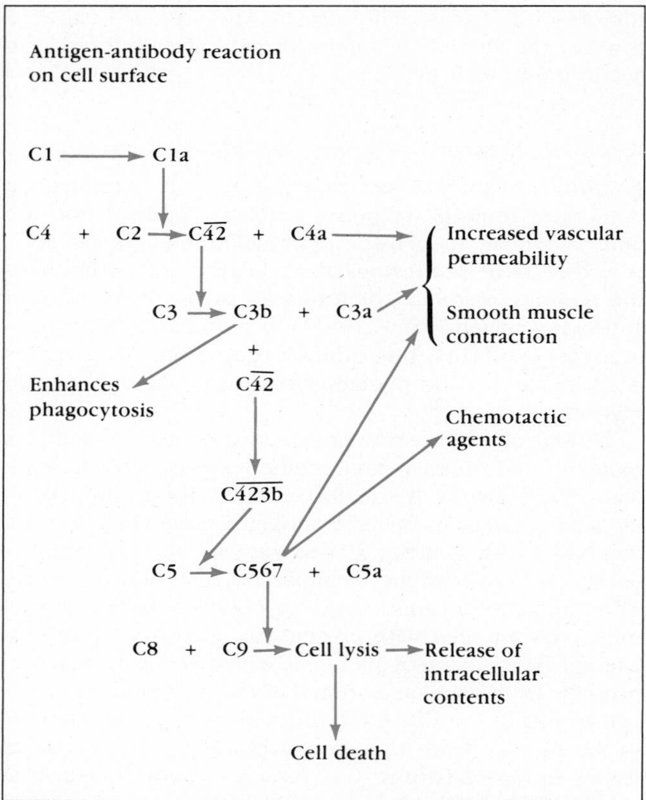

FIGURE 10-12 Classic pathway of complement activation.

Cell-Mediated Immunity

Cell-mediated immunity (CMI), due to T lymphocyte activity, is mediated through contact between T cells and antigen, with subsequent destruction of the antigen. The T lymphocyte recognizes antigen by receptors on the surface of the T cell [5]. Destruction may occur through the release of soluble chemical compounds directly into the target cell membrane or through the secretion of lymphokines (Fig. 10-13). Direct contact with an antigen is frequently called ***killer activity***.

Killer activity is mediated through a group of cytotoxic T cells that function in the destruction of cells with identified surface antigens. The specific recognition is through the lock-and-key approach described earlier in this chapter. The killer T lymphocyte may directly destroy the antigen by binding to the cell and producing a break in its membrane. This results in disruption of the intracellular osmotic environment and death of the cell. The activated killer cell may also release cytotoxic substances directly into the target cell [10].

The activated T lymphocytes release lymphokines, which affect other lymphocytes by enhancing or suppressing their activity. These cells also may create a chemotactic gradient that causes macrophages to accumulate in the area. The chemotactic gradient also attracts eosinophils, basophils, and neutrophils to the area.

Cell-mediated immunity, often termed *delayed hypersensitivity*, involves the direct intervention of T cells in a

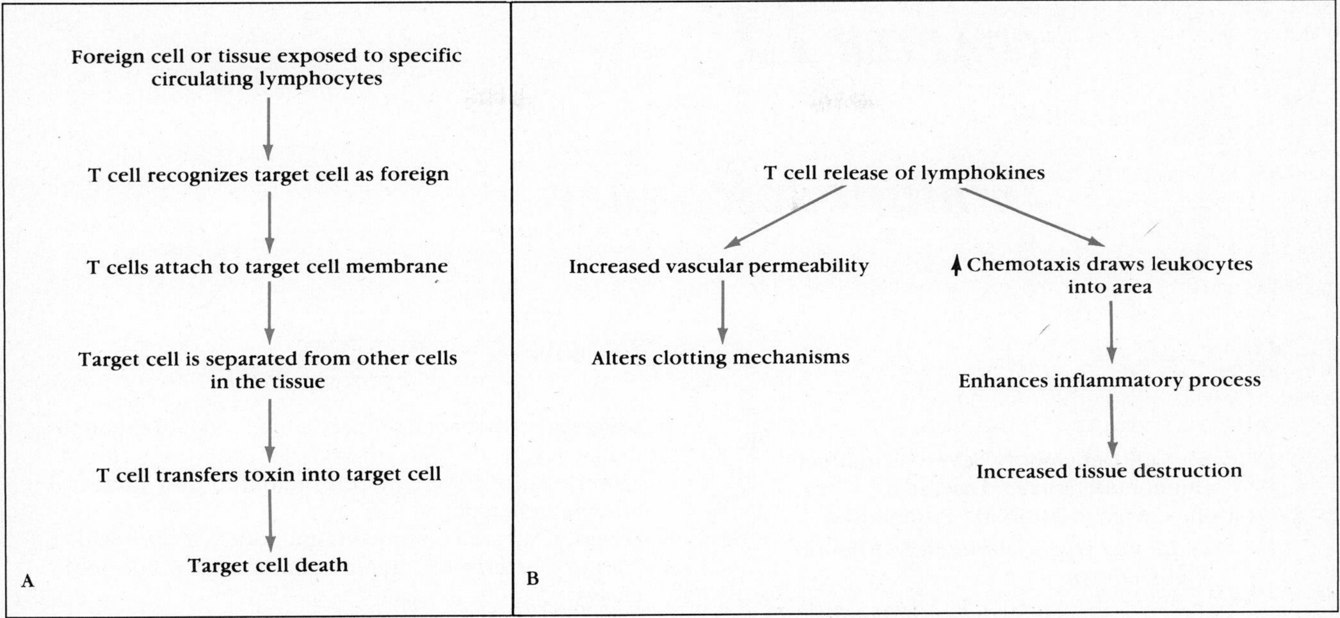

FIGURE 10-13 Cell-mediated response. A. Direct killing of foreign cells by T cells. B. Killing of foreign cells through lymphokine release.

response without a corresponding humoral immunity. It results in the accumulation of macrophages around the small blood vessels, resulting in destruction of vessels. This may lead to minor vascular lesions, for example, the wheal-and-flare response, or it may result in major destruction and massive necrosis. The antigen may initially react with a few specific T cells in the area, and produce the chemotactic response and also macrophage-inhibiting factor, which tends to keep macrophages in the area. The response seems to be dose related in that the greater the amount of antigen present, the greater the development of sensitized T lymphocytes. The end result is cytolysis of the antigenic cell. This mechanism, which involves the T cells and associated macrophages, is responsible for rejecting transplanted organs and, in this process, is called *cell-mediated lymphocytolysis* [10].

The T cells function in *immunosurveillance* to detect cells in the host that have foreign antigens on their surface. They can be thought of as defensive cells that patrol the blood and tissue spaces. This self-protective function prevents the transplantation of tissue from one person to another unless the antigens on the surface of the cells in the tissue are similar enough for the host tissue to accept the transplanted tissue as self.

Study Questions

1. Describe how the human body develops resistance against organisms in the environment.
2. Draw the interaction between T and B lymphocytes with and without macrophages.
3. How do the various classes of immunoglobulins protect the individual from various pathogens?
4. Using the information from Chapter 9, trace the development of immunity to the organism, starting with the entrance of the pathogen.
5. What are the similarities and differences between cell-mediated and humoral immune responses?

References

1. Alm, G., and Wigzell, H. Anatomy of the immune system. In L.A. Hanson and H. Wigzell, *Immunology*. London: Butterworths, 1985.
2. Bellanti, J.A. *Immunology III*. Philadelphia: Saunders, 1985.
3. Bennich, H. Immunoglobulins. In L.A. Hanson and H. Wigzell, *Immunology*. London: Butterworths, 1985.
4. Ganong, W.F. *Review of Medical Physiology* (14th ed.). Los Altos, Calif.: Lange, 1985.
5. Goetzl, E.J., and Stobo, J.D. Immunology. In L.H. Smith and S.O. Thier, *Pathophysiology: The Biological Principles of Disease* (2nd ed.). Philadelphia: Saunders, 1985.
6. Guyton, A.C. *Textbook of Medical Physiology* (7th ed.). Philadelphia: Saunders, 1986.
7. Ham, A.W., and Cormack, V.H. *Histology* (8th ed.). Philadelphia: Lippincott, 1979.
8. Jensen, D. *The Principles of Physiology* (2nd ed.). New York: Appleton-Century-Crofts, 1980.
9. Laurell, A.B. The complement system. In L.A. Hanson and H. Wigzell, *Immunology*. London: Butterworths, 1985.
10. Marrack, P., and Kapplar, J. The T cell and its receptor. *Sci. Am.* 254:2, 1986.
11. Perlmann, P., and Hammarstrom, S. Antigen-antibody reactions. In L.A. Hanson and H. Wigzell, *Immunology*. London: Butterworths, 1985.
12. Robbins, S.L., Cotran, R.S., and Kumar, V. *Pathologic Basis of Disease* (3rd ed.). Philadelphia: Saunders, 1984.
13. Roitt, I. *Essential Immunology* (5th ed.). Oxford: Blackwell, 1985.
14. Unanue, E.R., and Benacerraf, B. *Textbook of Immunology* (2nd ed.). Baltimore: Williams & Wilkins, 1984.

CHAPTER 11

Immunodeficiency

CHAPTER OUTLINE

Primary Immune Deficiency

- Stem Cell Deficiency (Severe Combined Immunodeficiency Disease)
- Deficiencies of Antibody Production
  - *X-Linked Hypogammaglobulinemia*
  - *IgA Deficiency*
- Deficiency of Cell-Mediated Immunity (DiGeorge Syndrome)
- Complement Abnormalities

Secondary Immune Deficiency

- Multifactorial Secondary Immune Deficiency
- Acquired Immune Deficiency Syndrome

LEARNING OBJECTIVES

1. Differentiate between primary and secondary immunodeficiency.
2. Differentiate between cell-mediated and humoral immunodeficiency.
3. Describe severe combined immunodeficiency (SCID).
4. Identify briefly the genetic basis for immunodeficiency.
5. Characterize the age of onset of signs and symptoms in the major described primary immunodeficiencies.
6. Explain the different symptoms that can occur according to the types of cells affected.
7. Describe briefly complement abnormalities and how these affect the immune response.
8. List at least six disorders that can cause secondary immunodeficiency.
9. Describe why secondary immunodeficiency increases the risk for the host.
10. Describe specifically how stress alters the immune response.
11. Explain the effect of aging on T and B cell response.
12. List several immunosuppressive agents, giving benefits and drawbacks of their use.
13. Describe how cancer can disrupt the immune mechanism.
14. List three causes of malnutrition and/or protein depletion and explain how these can disrupt the immune response.
15. Describe the acquired immune deficiency syndrome (AIDS).

The development of an immunocompetent system is essential to protect the human organism from foreign invasion. Therefore, any deficiency in any of the components of the immune system can alter the activity of the body's entire defense system. The effects of phagocytic dysfunction are described in Chapter 16. The major classifications of immunodeficiency are *primary* and *secondary*. Primary immunologic deficiency is a developmental abnormality that results in failure of humoral immunity, the cell-mediated response, or both. Complement abnormalities are briefly described as one category of immune deficiency. Secondary immunologic deficiencies are acquired conditions that may be associated with disease states or result from medical treatment.

Primary Immune Deficiency

A primary defect in the immunologic system results from the failure of an essential part of the immune system to develop. The defect can occur at any point during the development of the immune system and may involve organ or cellular defects. Many different types of primary immunodeficiency states have been described according to the cell type affected and the developmental stage of the cellular system (Table 11-1). The more common disorders are described in the text.

Stem Cell Deficiency (Severe Combined Immunodeficiency Disease)

Severe combined immunodeficiency disease (SCID) is thought to arise from a deficiency of the stem cell population that forms the lymphocytes. It is manifested by T and B cell deficiency associated with a hypoplastic thymus. A tremendous decrease in the number and maturity of lymphocytes provides for little, if any, immune response to antigen. The loss of T cells is usually greater than that of B cells, and T cell immaturity may be manifested by failure to differentiate to a mature form upon antigen stimulation [5]. There are evidently two mechanisms for the development of SCID: (1) a defect in stem cell population and (2) abnormal differentiation of T cells due to abnormalities in the thymus gland [7]. The result is deficiency of both humoral and cell-mediated responses.

This disease severely depresses the individual's ability to mount any type of immune response. The thymus is small and embryonic, resembling that of a 6- to 8-week-old fetus [7]. The few lymphocytes present are not activated by antigen. Few plasma cells are present, so all classes of immunoglobulins are depressed, resulting in lack of production of specific antibodies.

An infant with this condition is affected from birth and is unable to cope with an environment laden with germs. The child is vulnerable to all forms of infections and often dies within the first year of life. The initial problem in early infancy is failure to thrive, which is followed in the first few weeks of life by serious infections such as pneumonia and infectious diarrhea. Any type of infection may develop and none responds well to treatment. If SCID is suspected within hours of birth, the child may be placed in a germ-free environment with a later attempt to perform bone marrow transplantation.

In some cases, full immunologic ability can be attained if graft-versus-host disease (GVHD) does not limit the success. This disorder occurs when immunocompetent cells are transplanted to recipients lacking the usual immune defense. The normal cells react against those of the recipient. Involvement of the skin, liver, and intestinal mucosa is most common (Fig. 11-1). Graft-versus-host disease can be ameliorated by close matching of bone marrow for transplantation and, in some cases, pretreating bone marrow cells (Fig. 11-2) [2].

Table 11-1 Classification of Immunodeficiency Disorders

Antibody (B cell) immunodeficiency diseases
- X-linked (congenital) hypogammaglobulinemia
- Transient hypogammaglobulinemia of infancy
- Common, variable, unclassifiable immunodeficiency (acquired hypogammaglobulinemia)
- Immunodeficiency with hyper-IgM
- Selective IgA deficiency
- Selective IgM deficiency
- Selective deficiency of IgG subclasses

Cellular (T cell) immunodeficiency diseases
- Congenital thymic aplasia (DiGeorge's syndrome)
- Chronic mucocutaneous candidiasis (with or without endocrinopathy)

Combined antibody-mediated (B cell) and cell-mediated (T cell) immunodeficiency diseases
- Severe combined immunodeficiency disease (autosomal recessive, X-linked, sporadic)
- Cellular immunodeficiency with abnormal immunoglobulin synthesis (Nezelof's syndrome)
- Immunodeficiency with ataxia-telangiectasia
- Immunodeficiency with eczema and thrombocytopenia (Wiskott-Aldrich syndrome)
- Immunodeficiency with thymoma
- Immunodeficiency with short-limbed dwarfism
- Immunodeficiency with enzyme deficiency
- Episodic lymphopenia with lymphotoxin
- GVH disease

Phagocytic dysfunction
- Chronic granulomatous disease
- Glucose 6-phosphate dehydrogenase deficiency
- Myeloperoxidase deficiency
- Chédiak-Higashi syndrome
- Job's syndrome
- Tuftsin deficiency
- "Lazy leukocyte syndrome"
- Elevated IgE, defective chemotaxis, eczema, and recurrent infections

Complement abnormalities and immunodeficiency diseases
- C1q, C1r, and C1s deficiency
- C2 deficiency
- C3 deficiency (type I, type II)
- C4 deficiency
- C5 dysfunction, C5 deficiency
- C6 deficiency
- C7 deficiency
- C8 deficiency

Source: D. P. Stites, et al., *Basic and Clinical Immunology* (5th ed.). Los Altos, Calif.: Lange Medical Publishers, 1984. Reprinted by permission.

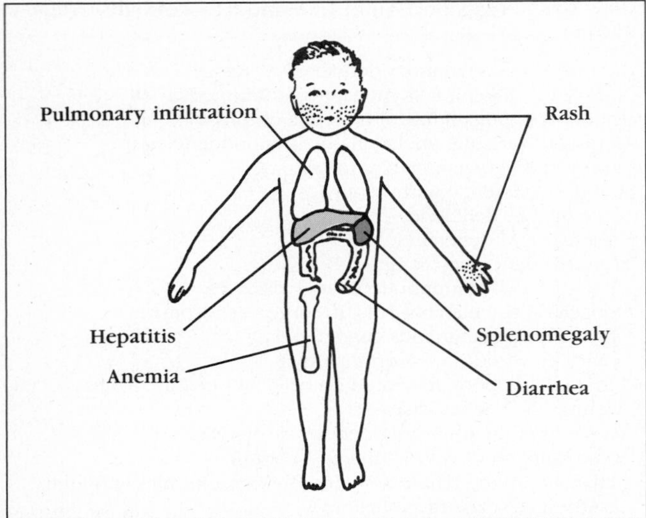

FIGURE 11-1 Major clinical features of GVHD in humans. (From M. Haeney, *Introduction to Clinical Immunology*. Update-Siebert Publications Limited, 1985. Figure 7.11. Reprinted with permission.)

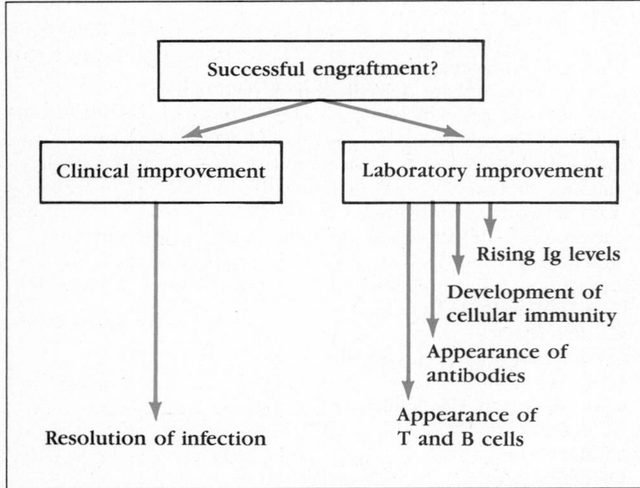

FIGURE 11-2 Indirect evidence that bone marrow grafting is successful. (From M. Haeney, *Introduction to Clinical Immunology*. Update-Siebert Publications Limited, 1985. Figure 7.12. Reprinted with permission.)

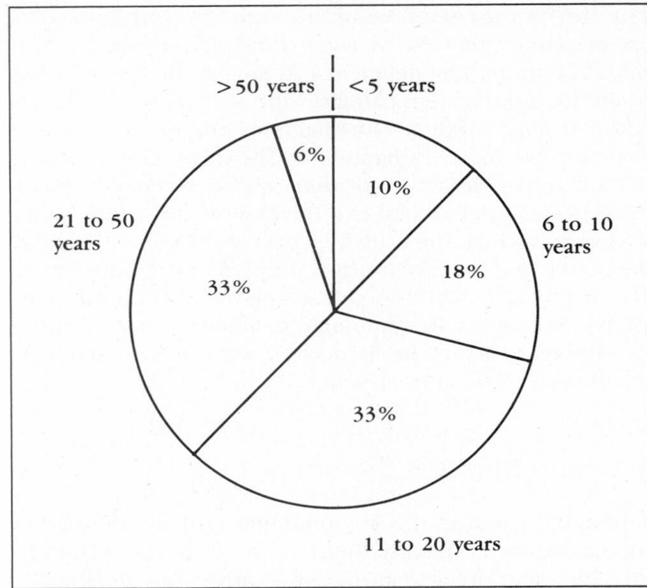

FIGURE 11-3 Age at diagnosis of individuals with primary defects of antibody synthesis. (From M. Haeney, *Introduction to Clinical Immunology*. Update-Siebert Publications Limited, 1985. Figure 6.8. Reprinted with permission.)

Deficiencies of Antibody Production

Several pathophysiologic defects in the immune system result in abnormal immunoglobulin synthesis or a deficiency of immunoglobulins. These can affect production of all of the immunoglobulins or of only specific classes.

Antibody deficiency is suspected in individuals with persistent, recurrent, severe, or unusual infections. Different types of deficiencies can arise at any age (Fig. 11-3). Examples include transient hypogammaglobulinemia of infancy, sex-linked hypogammaglobulinemia, IgA deficiency, selective IgM or subclass IgG deficiency. Both X-linked hypogammaglobulinemia and IgA deficiency are discussed in more detail below.

X-Linked Hypogammaglobulinemia. A defect in the maturation of stem cells into B cells occurs in X-linked hypogammaglobulinemia (*Bruton-type agammaglobulinemia*). This is a congenital disease that first appears in male infants at about age 5 to 6 months when the maternally transmitted level of antibodies has decreased. The B cells are virtually absent from the blood and the basic defect seems to be failure of B cells to mature [7].

Levels of immunoglobulins IgM, IgG, and IgA are low. Antigens, both T cell-dependent and T cell-independent, are not cleared well from the body, causing infants with this condition to be extremely susceptible to bacterial infections, especially those caused by *Staphylococcus aureus*, *Streptococcus pyogenes*, *Hemophilus influenzae*, and the *pneumococcus organisms*. The result is a very high frequency of respiratory, sinus, and throat infections [7].

The cellular immune system remains competent. Allograft rejection and the ability to resist viral, fungal, and parasitic infections are apparently normal. Autoimmune disease occurs frequently, especially rheumatoid arthritis and systemic lupus erythematosus [2].

IgA Deficiency. Selective IgA deficiency, which occurs in apparently healthy persons who may have normal serum levels of the other immunoglobulins, is the most common immunodeficiency disorder (1 of every 600 individuals). These persons lack IgA in serum and external secretions. The disease has a hereditary basis [7].

The presence of normal numbers of B cells with IgA expressed on their surface suggests failure in the synthesis and release of IgA rather than absence of IgA B lymphocytes. The defect appears to be in differentiation of IgA B lymphocytes; perhaps due to hyperactivity of IgA suppressor cells that prevents the differentiation. A defect in the helper cells specific for IgA synthesis may also be present. Acquired IgA deficiency may occur in individuals treated with the drugs phenytoin and penicillamine.

The most common symptoms relate to those surfaces that are normally covered with mucosal secretions. Infections of the sinuses and respiratory tract are common. Related gastrointestinal problems include ulcerative colitis, pernicious anemia, and malsorption states. About 50 percent of persons with IgA deficiency also have some atopic disease [8]. The prevalence of autoimmune disease, such as systemic lupus erythematosus and rheumatoid arthritis, increases; many persons with these diseases have anti-IgA antibodies. A high frequency of malignancies in the respiratory and gastrointestinal tracts and lymphoid system has been reported.

The reason for this increased suceptibility to atopic disease, autoimmune disease, and malignancy is not known, but one theory is that IgA normally interacts with many antigens on the mucosal surfaces and prevents their entry into the body. A deficiency of IgA would allow the body to be exposed to more antigens than it can successfully combat. Because of increased antigenic stimulation, more antigen can react with IgE and produce allergic manifestations. Increased risk of production of antibody that will cross-react with a self antigen increases the risk of autoimmune disease. Chronic irritation and inflammation due to the large amount of antigen could predispose the exposed tissue to malignant transformation [7].

Deficiency of Cell-Mediated Immunity (DiGeorge Syndrome)

Selective immunodeficiency affecting T cells but not B cells is rare. The complete DiGeorge syndrome consists of (1) low-set ears and slanted eyes, (2) hypoparathyroidism, (3) congenital heart defects, such as septal defects and truncus arteriosus, and (4) cellular immunodeficiency [2]. The complete DiGeorge syndrome is associated with failure of the embryonic third and fourth pharyngeal pouches to develop, which results in hypoplasia or aplasia of the thymus gland. No familial history is found, so it is thought that the defect is due to an environmental agent or drug exposure before the eighth week of gestation. If the defect is not complete, T cell function may become adequate by age 5 years [2].

There are other causes of deficiency of cell-mediated immunity. The most common is an enzyme defect (purine nucleoside phosphorylase, or PNP) that results in accumulation of byproducts within T lymphocytes causing a blockage of DNA synthesis. The congenital thymic hypoplasia causes a decrease or absence of T cells, and the neonate is extremely susceptible to fungal and viral infections. This defect has been successfully treated by transplantation of the thymus gland. If the disease is untreated, death due to overwhelming infection occurs in infancy.

The immune defect is due to the developmental failure of the thymus and parathyroid glands. Lack of the thymus gland and thus lack of the thymic hormone result in failure of T cells to mature.

Individuals with this condition are unable to reject allografts or to react to skin test antigens. They have little or no resistance to intracellular infections by viruses, fungi, and some gram-negative bacteria. A decrease of T cell helper function may depress the humoral response. The corresponding failure of parathyroid development may lead to tetany due to hypocalcemia.

Complement Abnormalities

Complement factors are necessary to promote the inflammatory process. Complement deficiency has been shown in an increased number of individuals with autoimmune disease (Table 11-2). Various symptoms occur depending on the complement factor that is deficient.

Deficiency of complement inhibitors also can result in allergic reactions; the most frequent is *hereditary angioedema* caused by a genetic deficiency of C1 esterase inhibitor. This produces uncontrolled activation of the complement system, causing angioedema in the skin, larynx, and gastrointestinal and genitourinary tracts [7].

Deficiencies of complement 2 and 3 (C2 and C3) are fairly common. Deficiency of C2 is transmitted as an autosomal dominant trait, and individuals with this condition have a high frequency of systemic lupus erythematosus and other connective tissue disorders [2,11].

Deficiency of C3 results in impairment of the inflammatory response and difficulty in clearing pyogenic and gram-negative infection. The deficiency can be inherited

TABLE 11-2 Clinical Problems Associated with Complement Deficiencies

Complement Protein	Clinical Problems
C1q	High frequency of immune complex disease
C1r	High frequency of immune complex disease
C2	High frequency of immune complex disease
C3	Recurrent pyogenic infection
C4	High frequency of immune complex disease
C5	Recurrent neisserial infection, high frequency of systemic lupus erythematosus
C6	Recurrent neisserial infection
C7	Recurrent neisserial infection
C8	Recurrent neisserial infection
C9	Asymptomatic
C1INH	Angioneurotic edema
Factor (C3bINA)	Recurrent pyogenic infection
Factor H	Recurrent pyogenic infection
Properdin (P)	Recurrent neisserial infection

Source: E. R. Unanue and B. Benacerraf, *Textbook of Immunology* (2nd ed.). Table 15.1, p. 306. Baltimore: Williams & Wilkins, 1984.

or acquired. The substance is used faster than it can be made in major systemic infections or in a nutritionally depleted host [7].

Secondary Immune Deficiency

Multifactorial Secondary Immune Deficiency

Secondary immune deficiency states result from the loss of a previously effective immune system. They include any disorder that exhibits loss of immunocompetence as a result of another condition. A broad classification includes immune deficiency secondary to any of the following: stress, malnutrition, systemic infection, cancer, renal diseases, radiation therapy, immunosuppressive drugs, and aging (Table 11-3). These conditions may lead to a loss of immunoglobulins, inadequate synthesis of immunoglobulins, loss of specific lymphocytes responsible for cell-mediated immunity, loss of phagocytic inflammatory cells, or a combination of these.

Even though decreased effectiveness of the immune system is frequently not life threatening, it often results in decreased ability of the organisms to mount an inflammatory or immune response. Therefore, susceptibility to infection by bacteria, viruses, fungi, or all three is increased. In some cases the loss of immunocompetence causes enough alteration in host resistance to increase morbidity and mortality.

Stress response has been the target of a great deal of research with respect to how it disrupts the physiologic functioning of the body (see Chap. 4). Stress appears to alter the immune response by neural interruption from the hypothalamus, which ultimately decreases the functioning of the thymus through secretion of glucocorticoids. These hormones mainly diminish the inflammatory response by suppressing macrophages, decreasing the number of white blood cells, and causing regression of lymphatic tissue. This can enhance the spread of infection [7].

The inevitable result of aging is immunologic deterioration. This relates to an increased rate of malignancy and increased frequency of autoimmune disease, and causes antibody deficiency, impaired hypersensitivity response, and decreased lymphocyte regeneration [4]. Thymic involution occurs in senescence together with a decreased T cell- and B cell-mediated immune response, resulting in increased susceptibility to infection [4].

Immunosuppression usually refers to pharmacologic suppression of the immune system. Drugs have been used extensively to decrease the rejection phenomenon in transplanted tissue, the rate of growth of malignant tumors, and the inflammation involved with autoimmune disorders. Agents used to achieve these effects are cytotoxic drugs such as methotrexate and corticosteroids such as hydrocortisone. The cytotoxic drugs are toxic to cells that divide rapidly, including T and B lymphocytes as well as polymorphonuclear leukocytes. Corticosteroids suppress the inflammatory response. The result of immunosuppression is increased sensitivity to the environmental antigens. Superimposed infections may develop and spread readily. Many pharmacologic agents cause depression of the bone marrow formation of leukocytes and thus affect all types of white blood cells [11].

Systemic infection can deplete the host defense to the point at which further antigen stimulation may result in decreased resistance. Thus, host resistance is decreased and opportunistic organisms may cause serious problems.

Cancer usually causes malnutrition due to protein wasting. Decreased synthesis of lymphocytes results. Immune deficiency due to B lymphoproliferative disorders such as chronic lymphocytic leukemia (CLL) and multiple myeloma results in impairment of the antibody responses, causing secondary infections with pyogenic bacteria.

Radiation therapy, usually instituted against malignancy, affects rapidly proliferating cells and results in a decrease in all of the cells of the inflammatory response, including the T and B lymphocytes. Opportunistic infections, especially those due to gram-negative bacteria, viruses, and fungi, occur with increased frequency [8].

Renal disease probably causes most of its immunosuppressive effects from proteinuria leading to hypoproteinemia or acid-base disruptions that can affect the formation of lymphocytes, especially T cells. Many pathologic processes of the kidneys are treated with corticosteroids, and immunosuppression may be a result of drug therapy.

TABLE 11-3 Conditions Causing Secondary Immunosuppression

Immunosuppressive therapy
Antimetabolites
Corticosteroids
Antibiotics
Radiation therapy
Cancer
Malnutrition
B cell lymphoproliferative disorders
T cell deficiency
Stress
Aging
Systemic infections
Renal disease
Malnutrition
Cirrhosis
Tumor cachexia
Dietary deficiency
Burns
Trauma
Surgery

Acquired Immune Deficiency Syndrome

The life-threatening disease acquired immunodeficiency syndrome (AIDS) was first described in 1981, and the reported incidence has been increasing every month since that time. At the current rate of infection it is estimated that by 1991, 268,000 persons in the United States will be diagnosed as having AIDS [3]. The Centers for Disease Control issue weekly surveillance reports on the epidemic status of AIDS, with a reported 37,019 men, women, and children being diagnosed as of June 15, 1987. The total number of deaths reported as of that date is 21,460 [1].

The causative agent has been identified as a retrovirus (RNA type) called *human immunodeficiency virus* (HIV) [3]. The mode of transmission is almost exclusively through sexual or blood contact.

While a virus has been implicated, exposure to it may not be enough to cause clinical AIDS. The at-risk population includes homosexual or bisexual males, intravenous-drug abusers of either sex, promiscuous heterosexual males or females, and persons receiving transfusions of blood or blood components such as those with hemophilia or coagulation disorders (Table 11-4). Children with the disease are thought to have been infected transplacentally or during birth, or they may have received blood transfusions for complications of hemophilia or trauma.

In 1985 a screening test, the enzyme-linked immunosorbent assay (ELISA), was distributed nationwide in this country. It was first used to screen blood and blood products for the antibody, and later was available to local health departments to screen individual blood samples. A positive result can be interpreted to mean that the person has been exposed to the virus, but it does not necessarily indicate active infection. A second test, called the Western blot, can be used to confirm antibody reactivity.

Three forms of AIDS have been described and the prognosis for an individual depends upon the form. The first is the antibody-positive form, called HIV antibody-positive, asymptomatic. The second is *AIDS-related complex (ARC)*, in which the individual exhibits fever, lymphadenopathy, idiopathic thrombocytopenic purpura, chronic diarrhea, fatigue, and even senile dementia. These individuals may be antibody positive or negative, and the condition may or may not proceed to clinical AIDS. Of the estimated 60,000 to 120,000 persons with ARC in the United States, approximately 6 to 20 percent may develop clinical AIDS within two years [9]. The third form is clinical AIDS, which causes severe immune deficiency and inability to combat environmental antigen. The individual usually has fever, weight loss, and lymphadenopathy. The concurrent demonstration of opportunistic infection and severe suppression of T cell function leads to the diagnosis of clinical AIDS [10]. The mortality with this disease is alarming, with most deaths resulting from opportunistic infections, especially the rare *Pneumocystis carinii* pneumonia (Table 11-5). A rare malignancy called Kaposi's sarcoma is also a common cause of death in these individuals.

Immune defense totally collapses due to decreases in the number and function of T4 lymphocytes. The T cells make up subsets on the basis of function, and the designated T4 subset has helper and inducer roles. The T4 cells function with macrophages, which prepare the antigen for recognition. Normally, activated T cells produce lymphokines, some of which stimulate proliferation of T cells into larger clones of mature cells specific to that antigen. Memory T cells accelerate reactions with subsequent encounters with antigen. The T4 cells secrete *interleukin 2*, an important lymphokine that stimulates macrophages to engulf viruses. The AIDS virus, however, avoids destruction by steadily undergoing genetic changes, and the anti-

TABLE 11-4 Percentages of Adult AIDS by Risk Group and Sex

Risk Group	Males	Females
Homosexual or bisexual men	79	—
Intravenous-drug users	15	53
Hemophilia/coagulation disorders	<1	<1
Heterosexual contact with persons in a high-risk category	<1	17
Transfusions with blood or blood products	1	9
None of the above/other	5	20
Totals	100	100

Because the percentages have been rounded off to whole numbers, they do not total 100.
Source: J. Turner and K. Williamson, AIDS: A challenge for contemporary nursing. *Focus on Critical Care* 13:3, June 1986, pp. 53–61. Reprinted by permission.

TABLE 11-5 Opportunistic Infections That Accompany AIDS

Type of Infection	Examples
Viral	Cytomegalovirus
	Disseminated
	Pneumonia
	Retinitis
	Encephalitis
	Herpes simplex
	Progressive
	Herpes zoster
	Limited cutaneous
	Progressive multifocal leukoencephalopathy
Fungal	*Candida albicans*
	Oral thrush
	Esophagitis
	Disseminated
	Cryptococcus neoformans
	Meningitis
	Disseminated
	Histoplasma capsulatum
	Disseminated
	Petriellidium boydii
	Pneumonia
	Aspergillus
	Pulmonary
Protozoal	*Pneumocystis carinii*
	Pneumonia
	Retinal infection
	Toxoplasma gondii
	Encephalitis
	Cryptosporidium
	Enteritis
	Isospora belli
	Enteritis
Mycobacterial	*Mycobacterium avium intracellularis*
	Disseminated
	Mycobacterium tuberculosis
	Disseminated
Others	*Nocardia*
	Legionella

Source: Reproduced with permission from M.S. Gottlieb et al., The acquired immunodeficiency syndrome. *Ann. Intern. Med.*, 99:208, 1983.

gen-specific immune response misses its mark [6]. The AIDS virus destroys the immune system by infecting T4 cells and killing them. Normally, T4s make up 60 to 80 percent of T cell population, but in clinical AIDS they are often not even present in the blood. Without the T4 cells, B cells are unable to produce specific antibody, but large amounts of nonspecific immunoglobulin are secreted. The AIDS virus also may be harbored by macrophages, platelets, and B cells. A small fraction of carriers do not produce enough antibody to cause a positive ELISA result, so that transfusions with their donated blood may be still somewhat of a risk.

It is estimated that 1 to 2 million persons in the United States alone are infected with the AIDS virus. Vaccination has not been successful because of the genetic variability of the virus. Almost every person with the combination of opportunistic infections and AIDS dies within four years of onset of illness. The drug azidothymidine (AZT) has been shown to slow the progress of the disease but does not produce a cure. By the end of 1986, researchers discovered a subgroup of white blood cells (suppressor T cells) that can control the AIDS virus in cell cultures [3]. Research is continuing to clarify this puzzling epidemic.

Study Questions

1. Why doesn't the individual with SCID reject transplanted bone marrow?
2. Explain graft-versus-host disease.
3. How do primary immunodeficiencies differ from secondary immunodeficiencies?
4. What are the most common secondary immunodeficiencies and how could they be prevented?
5. Identify the causative agent in AIDS and describe the variable clinical syndromes presented.

References

1. Centers for Disease Control. *Acquired Immunodeficiency Syndrome (AIDS) Weekly Surveillance Report.* Atlanta, Ga.: CDC, 1987.
2. Haeney, M. *Introduction to Clinical Immunology*. Boston: Butterworths, 1985.
3. Hermanson, R. Moving through the AIDS maze. *The Mission* 14:2, 1987.
4. Kenney, R.A. *Physiology of Aging*. Chicago: Yearbook, 1982.
5. Kissane, J.M. and Scotti, J. *Anderson's Synopsis of Pathology* (11th ed.). St. Louis: Mosby, 1985.
6. Laurence, J. The immune system in AIDS. *Sci. Am.* 253:12, 1985.
7. Robbins, S.L., Cotran, R.S., and Kumar, V. *Pathologic Basis of Disease* (3rd ed.). Philadelphia: Saunders, 1984.
8. Stites, D.P., et al. *Basic and Clinical Immunology* (5th ed.). Los Altos, Calif.: Lange, 1984.
9. Turner, J., and Williamson, K.M. AIDS: A challenge for contemporary nursing, Part I. *Focus on Critical Care* 13:53, 1986.
10. Turner, J., and Williamson, K.M. AIDS: A challenge for contemporary nursing, Part II. *Focus on Critical Care* 13:41, 1986.
11. Unanue, E.R., and Benacerraf, B. *Textbook of Immunology* (2nd ed.). Baltimore: William & Wilkins, 1984.

CHAPTER 12

Hypersensitivity and Autoimmune Reactions

CHAPTER OUTLINE

Classification of Tissue Injury Due to Hypersensitivity

- Type I: Anaphylaxis or Atopy
  - *Anaphylaxis and Anaphylactic Shock*
  - *Bronchial Asthma*
  - *Atopic Eczema*
- Type II: Cytotoxic Hypersensitivity
  - *Hemolytic Reactions*
  - *Specific Target Cell Destruction*
- Type III: Immune Complex Disease
  - *Serum Sickness*
  - *Arthus Reaction*
  - *Other Type III Conditions*
- Type IV: Cell-Mediated Hypersensitivity
  - *Delayed Hypersensitivity*
  - *Cytotoxic Cell-Mediated Responses*
  - *Contact Dermatitis*
- Transplant or Graft Rejection

Classification of Immune Disorders by Source of Antigen

Autoimmunity

- Systemic Lupus Erythematosus
- Rheumatoid Arthritis

LEARNING OBJECTIVES

1. Define *hypersensitivity reactions*.
2. Discuss the types of agents that can elicit hypersensitivity reactions.
3. Describe the types of hypersensitivity reactions according to underlying pathophysiologic mechanisms and how they are manifested as disease.
4. Differentiate between anaphylaxis and atopy.
5. Identify the mechanisms of red cell destruction seen with cytotoxic hypersensitivity reactions.
6. Describe the results of hemolysis with respect to transfusion reactions, erythroblastosis fetalis, and warm and cold antibody diseases.
7. Describe the development of Goodpasture's syndrome as a result of cytotoxic hypersensitivity.
8. Explain the underlying pathophysiology of immune complex disease.
9. Describe the mechanisms occurring in serum sickness.
10. Identify the pathophysiologic mechanism of Arthus reaction.
11. Describe the relationship of hypersensitivity reactions and autoimmune disorders.
12. Describe the pathophysiologic mechanisms by which delayed hypersensitivity can result.
13. Identify the histology of contact dermatitis.
14. Describe transplant graft rejection using the transplanted kidney as an example.
15. Describe the classification of immune disruptions according to homologous, exogenous, and autologous sources of antigen.
16. List at least six conditions that are probably the result of autoimmunity.
17. Name the main clinical finding that supports diagnosis of the autoimmune phenomena.
18. Describe systemic lupus erythematosus (SLE) in terms of pathology and resultant clinical effects.
19. List 10 of the 14 criteria issued by the American Rheumatism Association for the diagnosis of SLE.
20. Describe the basis for classifying rheumatoid arthritis as an autoimmune disease.
21. Explain the pathophysiologic results of rheumatoid arthritis on the joints and other systems of the body.
22. Describe the syndrome of rheumatoid arthritis.

Immune disorders have been classified in various ways to clarify their pathophysiologic basis. Four mechanisms of immunologically mediated disorders have been described according to the manner in which tissue injury occurs [6,12]. These conditions also may be classified according to the source of the offending antigen. Both classifications are discussed in this chapter.

The classic term for immunologic, tissue-damaging reactions is *hypersensitivity reactions*, which refers to an exaggerated response of the immune system to an antigen. The antigen eliciting the response is frequently called an *allergen*. Allergens produce different responses depending on an individual's genetic predisposition for an exaggerated response. In some cases the antigen producing the response is unknown.

Classification of Tissue Injury Due to Hypersensitivity

The types of hypersensitivity reactions are described in this section according to the underlying pathophysiologic mechanisms and how they manifest themselves in different diseases (Table 12-1).

Type I: Anaphylaxis or Atopy

Anaphylaxis refers to an acute reaction usually associated with a wheal-and-flare type of skin reaction and vasodilation that may precipitate circulatory shock. Atopy, which results from the same mechanism, chronically recurs in responses that depend on the antigen, frequency of contact, route of contact, and sensitivity of the organ system to the antigen.

Atopy, or anaphylactic disease, is the most common of the immediate hypersensitivity reactions. These diseases, commonly called *allergies*, occur in organs exposed to environmental antigens [2]. The skin, respiratory tract, and gastrointestinal system are especially affected. Many different types of antigens or allergens can initiate the hypersensitivity state in susceptible individuals. The most common of these are the environmental allergens such as pollens, dander, foods, insect bites, and certain household cleaning agents. Drug sensitivity reactions can effect the same response. Other disease states that are classified in this group include hay fever, urticaria (hives), asthma, and atopic eczema. Susceptibility to allergy is inherited and may result from excessive IgE production [14].

Pathophysiologically, the immune response is activated when antigen binds to IgE antibodies attached to the surface of mast cells. Mast cells are present in profusion in connective tissue, skin, and mucous membranes. The reaction proceeds when the IgE molecule specific for a particular antigen becomes cross-linked on the surface of the mast cell and triggers the release of intracellular granules. These granules contain large quantities of histamine and other chemotactic substances. Histamine causes peripheral vasodilation and an increase in vascular permeability, resulting in local vascular congestion and edema. It also causes constriction of smooth muscle in the bronchioles, which accounts for the bronchiolar constriction often associated with the allergic reaction (Fig. 12-1).

Testing for a reaction to a particular allergen is done with a needle prick to the skin. Sensitivity to the allergen on the needle is exhibited by a rapid wheal-and-flare reaction. A provocation test also may be performed in which the allergen is dropped on the mucous membrane of the eyes or nose [8].

Anaphylaxis and Anaphylactic Shock. Anaphylaxis is defined as an allergic hypersensitivity reaction of the body to a foreign protein or a drug. Anaphylactic shock

TABLE 12-1 Classification of Hypersensitivity States

Type	Cause	Responsible Cell or Antibody	Immune Mechanism	Examples of Disease States
I Anaphylaxis Atopy	Foreign protein (antigen)	IgE	IgE attaches to surface of mast cell and specific antigen, triggers release of intracellular granules from mast cells.	Hay fever Allergies Hives Anaphylactic shock
II Cytotoxic	Foreign protein (antigen)	IgG or IgM	Antibody reacts with antigen, activates complement, causes cytolysis.	Transfusion Hemolytic drug reactions Erythroblastosis fetalis Hemolytic anemia Vascular purpura Goodpasture's syndrome
III Immune complex	Foreign protein (antigen)	IgG	Antigen-antibody complexes precipitate in tissue, activate complement, cause inflammatory reaction.	Rheumatoid arthritis Systemic lupus erythematosus Serum sickness
IV Delayed cell-mediated	Foreign protein, cell, or tissue	T lymphocytes	Sensitized T cell reacts with specific antigen to induce inflammatory process by direct cell action or by activity of lymphokines.	Contact dermatitis Transplant graft reaction

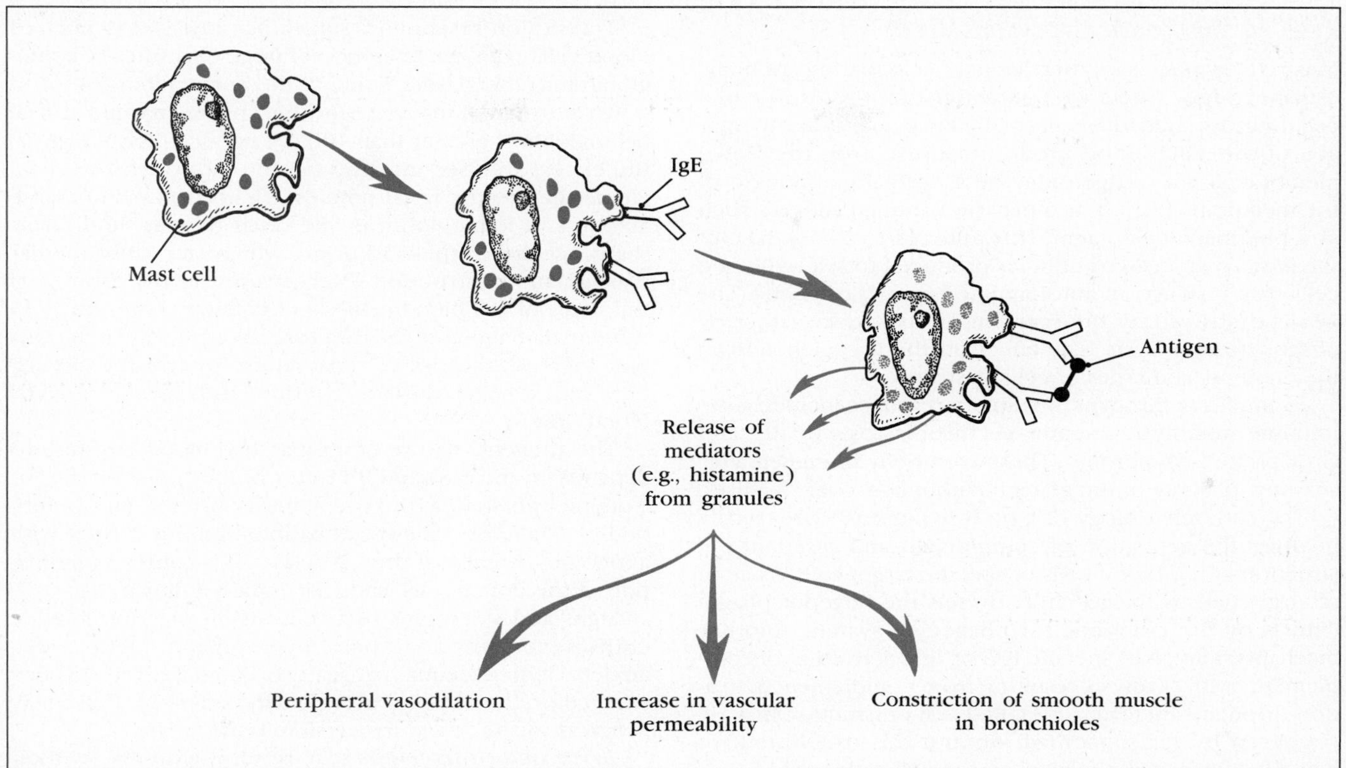

FIGURE 12-1 Type I hypersensitivity reaction. The mast cell and IgE antibody are attached by a specific antigen that causes release of the vasoactive substances histamine and SRS-A.

occurs when the reaction becomes systemic and thus a life-threatening event. In either case, the subject has been previously sensitized to the antigen. The antigen-antibody reaction occurs on the mast cells in the connective tissue and around small blood vessels. It causes the mast cells to release histamine and other mediators, which results in contraction of smooth muscle and increased vascular permeability. This causes bronchospasm and the loss of intravascular fluid into the tissue spaces in some cases. Edema follows and is particularly noticeable around the eyes. This edema, called *angioneurotic edema* or *angioedema*, may appear in the skin or mucous membranes. Laryngeal edema associated with bronchospasm often causes acute dyspnea and air hunger [16].

Hives, or urticaria, may appear on any skin surface as cutaneous localized swellings. These are sudden, generalized eruptions of papules or wheals, and intense itching is exhibited.

Fluid shift from increased vascular permeability may be significant enough to result in decreased blood pressure and shock. Signs and symptoms of anaphylactic shock include urticaria, angioedema, dyspnea, hypoxia, and hypotension [2]. Some individuals experience vascular collapse without signs of respiratory distress. Other signs that are associated with anaphylaxis include leukopenia, decreased body temperature, and bradycardia.

Bronchial Asthma. Atopic allergy may cause bronchial asthma, frequently induced by the inhalation of environmental antigens (see Chap. 26). The mechanism for bronchial asthma, like atopy, may result from interaction of antigen with specific IgE antibodies. The inflammation produces mucosal edema, increased secretion of mucus, and bronchospasm, all of which cause narrowing of the airways and increased airway resistance. The early signs and symptoms of asthma are dyspnea and wheezing. Repeated attacks result in hypertrophy of the smooth muscle, which can exaggerate bronchoconstriction and increase the severity of each subsequent attack. Bacterial or viral infections may precipitate asthmatic attacks.

Atopic Eczema. This acute or chronic, noncontagious, inflammatory condition may occur after contact with irritants to which a person has a specific sensitivity [7]. In some cases it results from a cell-mediated reaction (see p. 173) and in others it is mediated by IgE, with liberation of chemotactic mediators into dermal areas.

Atopic eczema causes urticaria and angioedema. Urticaria involves the superficial capillaries, while angioedema involves the capillaries of the deeper skin layers. The wheals of urticaria have well-defined margins, erythema, and vesicles filled with clear fluid. Pruritus is frequently severe. Angioedema causes nonpitting swelling of localized areas of the skin [10]. This skin reaction to an allergen is frequently associated with respiratory hypersensitivity, especially hay fever or other type of allergy. Drug reactions may result in the same dermatologic manifestations, probably due to the same mechanisms [16].

Type II: Cytotoxic Hypersensitivity

In type II hypersensitivity response, a circulating antibody, usually an IgG, reacts with an antigen on the surface of a cell. Because individuals normally have antibodies to antigen of the ABO blood group not present on their own membranes, the antigen may be a normal component of the membrane [12]. It also may be a foreign antigen, such as a pharmacologic agent, that adheres to the surface of the host's own cells. Antibodies produced to self red blood cells may produce an autoimmune hemolytic anemia. The cell is destroyed by the reaction on its surface either by phagocytosis or lysis. The effect on the host depends on the numbers and types of cells destroyed.

Examples of this hypersensitivity response include autoimmune hemolytic anemia, erythroblastosis fetalis, and Goodpasture's syndrome. These are briefly discussed after a review of some of the general pathophysiologic features.

The pathophysiology of type II hypersensitivity usually involves the activation of complement and resultant destruction of red blood cells or specific target cells. Coating of target cells with IgG antibody sets the stage for phagocytosis by the mononuclear phagocyte system. Another mechanism involves specific IgG or IgM activation of complement, with cytolysis resulting from complement activation through C89 (Fig. 12-2). Red cell destruction may be triggered by IgG opsonization and the attachment of lymphocytes or macrophages to the cell surface [11].

Hemolytic Reactions. Examples of reactions that destroy red blood cells are transfusion reactions, erythroblastosis fetalis, autoimmune hemolytic anemia, and drug-induced hemolysis. The reaction of host antibody with the surface antigens on the red blood cells of an incompatible donor results in hemolysis. The surface antigens that make up the ABO and Rh systems are common sources of incompatibility.

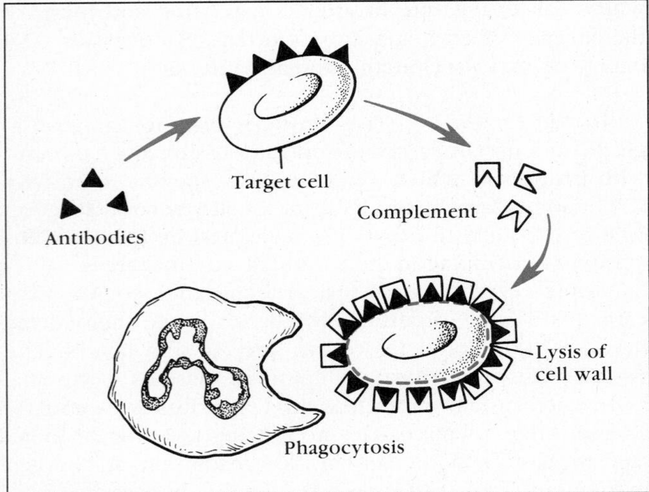

FIGURE 12-2 Type II hypersensitivity response. The target cell is covered with antibody that activates complement and sets the stage for phagocytosis.

Transfusion reactions result in hemolysis of donor red blood cells with the liberation of large quantities of hemoglobin into the plasma. Some of the hemoglobin is broken down into unconjugated bilirubin. If the amount of free hemoglobin is greater than 100 mg per deciliter of plasma, the excess diffuses into the tissue or through the renal glomeruli into the renal tubules [8]. Precipitation of large amounts of hemoglobin in the renal tubular fluid forms sharp needles in the acid urine, which can cause tubular damage and obstruction. Precipitation in the tubules of the shells of red blood cells also frequently contributes to tubular damage and renal failure. Transfusion reactions may increase the risk of renal failure by causing circulatory shock, renal vasoconstriction, and decreased renal blood flow.

The antigenic nature of mismatched blood transfusions depends on the type and Rh factor of the donor blood. For example, persons with type A blood possess anti-B antibodies. Therefore, the incompatible blood is coated with antibodies, usually of the IgM class. This causes agglutination of the donor cells, and lysis rapidly follows [1].

Signs and symptoms of a transfusion reaction include chills, fever, low back pain, hypotension, tachycardia, anxiety, hyperkalemia, nausea and vomiting, red or port-wine-colored urine, and occasionally, urticaria. These may progress to shock and irreversible renal failure.

Erythroblastosis fetalis may result if a mother without Rh antigens carries a child with Rh antigens or if mother and fetus have ABO incompatibility. A mother who *lacks Rh antigens* on her red blood cells (Rh-negative) can be sensitized to the Rh antigen carried on the cells of the fetus by mixing her red blood cells with fetal red blood cells. If the woman again becomes pregnant with a fetus having Rh antigens, her anti-Rh antibodies may cross the placenta and enter the fetal circulation. The result is destruction of fetal red blood cells through a hemolytic reaction. More commonly, *ABO blood group incompatibility* causes the free passage of antibodies from the mother through the placenta to the fetus [11]. Blood types interact in different ways, but the result is attachment and hemolysis of fetal red blood cells by maternal antibodies [1,12].

Hemolysis of fetal red blood cells results in severe *anemia*, which may lead ultimately to heart failure. Also, the release of high concentrations of bilirubin from hemoglobin may result in brain damage, called *kernicterus*, as unconjugated bilirubin passes across the still permeable blood-brain barrier, causing edematous swelling of brain parenchyma. The mechanism by which unconjugated bilirubin crosses the blood-brain barrier is not clearly understood. The barrier is apparently more permeable in neonates and premature infants [11]. *Hyperbilirubinemia* is common in an affected infant who survives for more than several days. This increased bilirubin level is usually manifested as jaundice and is termed *icterus gravis*. The red cell activity in bone marrow increases, and extramedullary hematopoiesis begins in the liver, spleen, and perhaps in other organs to compensate for lost red blood cells.

The risk of erythroblastosis fetalis in subsequent pregnancies can be reduced by administering anti-Rh antibodies to the mother within 72 hours after the birth of the first Rh-positive infant. More difficult to predict is ABO erythroblastosis, but the condition can be monitored if both parents are aware of their blood incompatibility.

Two types of hemolytic anemias with a probable autoimmune basis are *warm antibody disease* and *cold antibody disease*. Warm antibody disease is called *autoimmune hemolytic anemia* and is usually due to IgG antibody that attacks the host's own red blood cells. The disease can be life-threatening depending on the amount of hemolysis. The red blood cells develop a very limited life span, and the resulting anemia can be severe. Autoimmune hemolytic disease may develop for no known reason, or it may be associated with other autoimmune diseases, malignancy, or systemic infection [11]. Cold antibody disease results when an autoantibody, usually IgM, binds to erythrocytes at temperatures below 31° C. These temperatures may be reached in the fingers or toes during very cold weather. The red blood cells thus coated with cold antibodies reenter the general circulation, activate complement, and hemolyze the red blood cells. These hemolytic attacks occur only after exposure to cold and tend to be self-limiting [11]. The major diagnostic criterion for hemolytic anemia is the Coombs' antiglobulin test. In this test, agglutination of red blood cells occurs when immunoglobulins are attached to the red blood cell membranes [3,11].

Drug-induced hemolysis may result from drug-antibody complexes that bind passively to red blood cells and initiate the complement reaction. Other drugs may act as haptens and bind to a red blood cell carrier. Antibody is formed and induces hemolysis of the red blood cells. Some drugs produce changes in the surface antigens of the red blood cells, resulting in antibody production against the host's own erythrocytes. Most drug-induced hemolytic reactions stop once use of the drug is discontinued.

Specific Target Cell Destruction. The best illustration of specific target cell hypersensitivity reaction is *Goodpasture's syndrome*, which is a rapidly occurring condition characterized by the development of *antiglomerular basement membrane antibodies (anti-GBM)*. These antibodies are directed at the glomerular basement membrane of the kidneys as well as the basement membrane of the pulmonary alveoli. The initiator is unknown, but the condition may progress rapidly to death due to destruction of the basement membranes, which frequently leads to hemoptysis or uremia. Improvement in prognosis has been reported with use of plasma exchange to remove anti-GBM antibodies. Both pulmonary and glomerular improvement have been seen [11]. Bilateral nephrectomy has also been shown to arrest the pulmonary course of the disease [11].

Type III: Immune Complex Disease

Immune complex disease results in the formation of antigen-antibody complexes that activate a variety of serum factors, especially complement [11]. This results in precipitation of complexes in vulnerable areas, leading to inflammation as a consequence of complement activation. The end result is an intravascular, synovial, endocardial, and other membrane inflammatory process affecting the vulnerable organs. Each person apparently has some unique vulnerability in target organs.

Antigen-antibody complexes may be present in the plasma but may not cause disease manifestations. If the complexes are not removed by the mononuclear phagocyte system, they may lodge in the tissue where they initiate an inflammatory reaction that leads to tissue destruction. Frequently, the complexes are small; and their size seems to determine whether they will be cleared and whether they can lodge at a place where significant damage can occur. The antigen-antibody complexes that remain in solution cause reactions when they circulate through the body and lodge in the tissue and small vessels. Increased vascular permeability allows the complexes to be deposited in the extravascular spaces. Deposition also appears to be greater at points of high pressure, high flow, and turbulence [7]. Once precipitated, the immune complexes initiate the inflammatory process by activating complement and releasing vasoactive substances from the defense cells (Fig. 12-3). Table 12-2 summarizes the pathogenesis of inflammatory lesions in type III reactions.

Serum Sickness. Serum sickness results from injection of large doses of foreign material and can cause various types of arthritis, glomerulonephritis, and vasculitis. First reported after passive immunization with horse serum (equine tetanus antitoxin), which contains at least 30 different antigens, serum sickness can cause an acute reaction or a chronic condition. Antigen-antibody complexes form in the bloodstream and precipitate into vulnerable areas.

If the antigen concentration is greater than the antibody concentrations, the resulting antigen-antibody complexes tend to be small and remain in solution for as long

TABLE 12-2 Pathogenesis of Inflammatory Lesions in Type III Reactions

Formation of antigen-antibody complexes (generally in antigen excess)
Fixation of complement by complexes
Release of complement components chemotactic for leukocytes
Damage to platelets, causing release of vasoactive amines
Increased vascular permeability
Localization of antigen-antibody complexes in vessel walls
Further fixation of complement and release of chemotactic factors
Infiltration with polymorphonuclear leukocytes
Ingestion of immune complexes by neutrophils and release of lysosomal enzymes
Damage to adjacent cells and tissues by lysosomal enzymes
Deposition of fibrin
Regression and healing if lesion is due to a single dose of antigen, or chronic deposition and inflammation if there is continuing formation of immune complexes

Source: D.P. Stites et al., *Basic and Clinical Immunology* (5th ed.). Los Altos, Calif.: Lange Medical Publishers, 1984. Reprinted by permission.

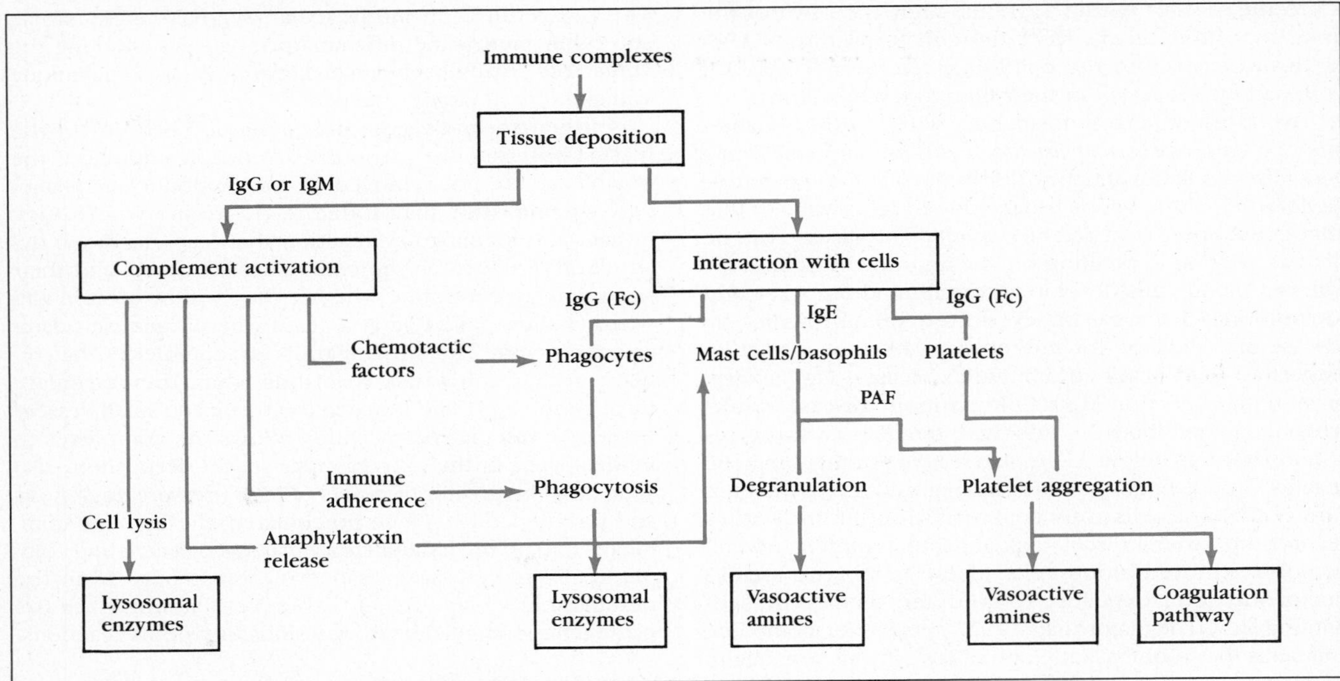

FIGURE 12-3 Simplified view of the major pathways by which immune complex deposition may produce tissue damage. PAF = platelet aggregating factor. (From M. Haeney, *Introduction to Clinical Immunology.* Update-Siebert Publications Limited, 1985. Reprinted with permission.)

as 8 to 15 days after initial injection. Immune complexes are deposited throughout the vasculature of the body; complement is activated, and neutrophils and macrophages move into the area in response to chemotactic signals. Phagocytosis of the immune complexes begins with the release of lysosomal enzymes into the area, which causes acute vasculitis with destruction of the elastic lamina of the arteries. Once phagocytosis of the immune complexes is complete, the inflammatory process decreases, leaving some scarring of the blood vessel walls [11].

Renal glomerular deposits of complexes occur even when the immune complex concentrations are not high, probably because of the efficient filtering action of the kidneys. The complexes form characteristic deposits in the glomerular walls that activate complement and lead to destruction of glomerular tissue. Increased permeability of the glomerular basement membrane often produces hematuria and proteinuria.

Arthus Reaction. Another type III disorder, the Arthus reaction, involves inflammation and cellular death at the site of injection of antigen into a previously sensitized person. Pathologically, it causes an acute, localized vasculitis that occurs from antibody precipitation and complement activation. It then involves all of the effects of inflammation, with activation of the complement fragments through $\overline{C89}$, which destroys antigen and surrounding tissue. The vasculitis causes platelets to adhere to vessels, and thrombosis at the site of vessels.

Hypersensitive pneumonitis probably is an Arthus reaction from the inhalation of organic dusts [16]. This reaction is closely involved with the anaphylactic type I response except that IgG immunoglobulin seems to be necessary for Arthus' reaction and IgE is involved with the type I reaction. It has been postulated that some relationship exists between the reactions [11].

Other Type III Conditions. Many of the common autoimmune conditions are classified as immune complex disorders. The mechanism for inflammation and damage is the precipitation of immune complexes into vulnerable areas. Immune complex disorders are dynamic, constantly changing processes that are manifested in the tissues in which they become lodged. Systemic lupus erythematosus, rheumatoid arthritis, and some types of glomerulonephritis are examples. Systemic lupus erythematosus and rheumatoid arthritis are discussed more fully on pages 175–178. Glomerulonephritis is described in detail in Chapter 29.

Type IV: Cell-Mediated Hypersensitivity

Type IV response is the result of specifically sensitized T lymphocytes. Two types have been described: delayed hypersensitivity and cytotoxic cell-mediated.

Delayed Hypersensitivity. Delayed hypersensitivity responses are due to the specific interaction of T cells with antigen. The T cells react with the antigen and release lymphokines that draw macrophages into the area. The lymphokines include the macrophage migration-inhibitory factor (MIF), the macrophage-activating factor (MAF), chemotactic factors, lymphotoxin, transfer factor, and other factors. These substances enhance the inflammatory response that destroys the foreign material (Fig. 12-4).

The tuberculin response is the best example of the delayed hypersensitivity response and is used to determine whether an individual has been sensitized to the disease. Reddening and induration of the site begin within 12 hours of injection of tuberculin and reach a peak in 24 to 72 hours. This response can only be elicited when lymphocytes are present [9,11].

Cytotoxic Cell-Mediated Responses. Cytotoxic cell-mediated responses occur as a result of T cell contact and destruction of antigen. Three stages of the lytic cycle have been described: (1) cell-to-cell interaction, (2) lesion insertion, and (3) target cell membrane destruction. The T cell binds specifically to the target cell. The T cell "sits" on the target cell and causes membrane permeability changes, a process that is dependent on the presence of calcium but not on energy production. The T cell-mediated lysis causes rupture of the target cell membrane and destruction of the cell [9] (Fig. 12-5). The surrounding nontargeted cells are not damaged. The T cell may also activate macrophages, and these cells may lyse other cells such as tumor cells.

Contact Dermatitis. This common allergic skin reaction seems to be a T cell response with a delayed reaction. It occurs on contact with certain common household chemicals, cosmetics, and plant toxins. These may alter the normal skin protein so that it becomes antigenic, or they may act as haptens that combine with proteins in the skin.

The area of contact becomes red and indurated, and vesicles begin to appear. Lymphocytes and macrophages infiltrate the area and react against the epidermal cells. Sterile, protein-rich fluid fills the blebs. If the blebs are opened, the antigen may be spread to a new area. The affected cells are destroyed, slough off, and are replaced by regenerating new cells.

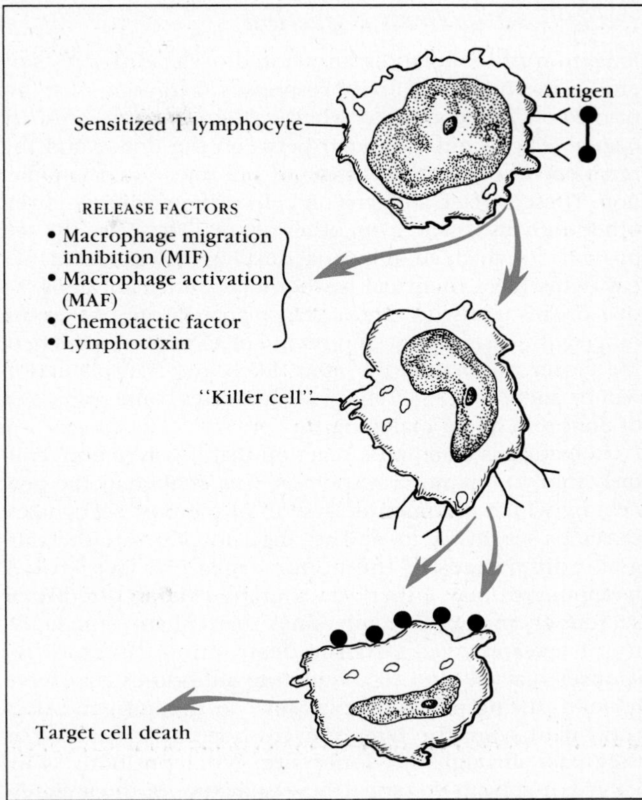

FIGURE 12-4 Type IV cell-mediated hypersensitivity. The T lymphocyte contacts the foreign material, and through direct intervention or secretion of substances toxic to the foreign material, destroys the foreign protein.

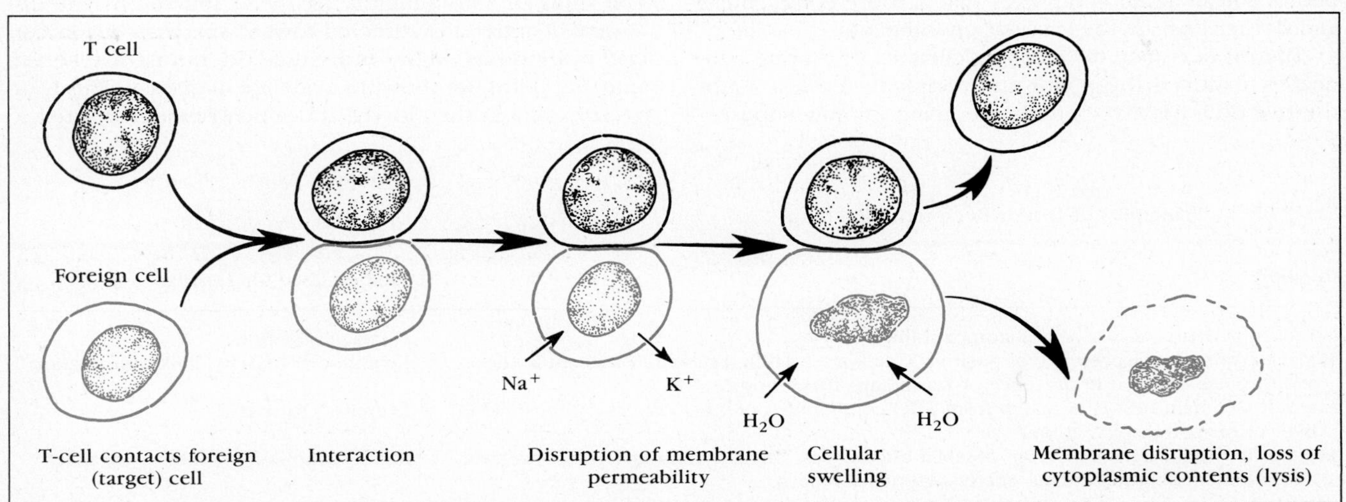

FIGURE 12-5 Method of T cell-induced lysis of foreign cells in type IV reaction.

Transplant or Graft Rejection

Rejection of tissue and transplanted organs involves several of the hypersensitivity responses. Targeting of transplanted organs depends on whether the *histocompatibility antigens* are similar enough between the donor and the recipient to prevent activation of the rejection phenomenon. These surface antigens on cells distinguish them from other individuals and from other organs. These are the self proteins to which an individual develops tolerance. Identical twins have identical histocompatibility antigens, so that organs or tissue can be transplanted from one to the other with ease. Donor and recipient tissues are matched; the closer the match, the more likely the transplantation will be successful [5]. Table 12-3 indicates some principles of donor-recipient matching.

Rejection is a complex reaction that involves both cell-mediated and humoral responses. It is defined as the process by which the immune system of the host recognizes, develops sensitivity to, and attempts to eliminate the antigenic differences of the donor organ [5]. Cytolytic T lymphocytes may either attack grafted tissue directly or secrete chemotactic lymphokines that enhance the activity of macrophages in tissue destruction. Humoral responses may be due to circulating antibodies that were formed during previous exposure to the antigen. After transplantation, the lymphocytes become sensitized as they pass through the donor site. When antibody is involved, it appears to target the vasculature of the graft, especially at the graft site [5,11].

The rejection phenomenon of a transplanted kidney has been studied extensively. It appears to involve both humoral and cell-mediated hypersensitivity. The sensitized lymphocytes interact with the graft proteins and release mediators that attract macrophages and polymorphonuclear (PMN) leukocytes to the area. The lysosomal enzymes released by these cells cause endothelial destruction, especially of the blood vessels, that leads to decreased glomerular filtration rate and renal failure.

The T lymphocytes are directly cytotoxic to the donor cells. They also may activate B lymphocytes to form antibodies and immune complexes that activate complement and further damage the vascular endothelium.

The process may be acute or chronic. The more adequately matched the donor and recipient, the less acute the reaction. Also, recipients are given immunosuppressive drugs that delay the rejection. Chronic changes usually affect the vasculature and lead to renal ischemia and eventual failure.

Graft rejection is very common, and most cadaver grafts are rejected within five years. Long-term survival of grafts has not been achieved except in twin or relative donors.

Classification of Immune Disorders by Source of Antigen

Immunologically mediated disorders may also be classified according to the underlying causes — exogenous, homologous, and autologous. Some antigens are environmental, some result from antigenic dissimilarities among individuals, and some seem to arise from loss of tolerance to self antigens.

The *exogenous* diseases are basically atopic reactions to environmental allergens such as pollens and contact irritants. These can be prevented if the person has no contact with the substances. The strength of the reaction is determined by individual sensitivity to the allergen, with one person exhibiting no response and another suffering an anaphylactic reaction. The predisposition for the type of reaction appears to be genetically programmed, but the entire mechanism is not well understood.

Homologous disorders are exemplified by transfusion reactions, erythroblastosis fetalis, and transplant rejection. The commonality in these disorders is antigenicity among individuals, which means that the material (e.g., blood, tissue) is recognized by the recipient as foreign and the reaction is elicited to destroy the donor material. Antigenicity is a protective mechanism to ensure individual survival.

The *autologous* diseases include any of the disorders in which the body loses recognition of self antigen and makes antibody against a self protein. This means that there is loss of *self-tolerance* resulting in an *autoimmune* reaction.

Autoimmunity

The study of autoimmunity has been spurred by the discovery of antibodies directed toward specific cells in certain individuals. Many individuals demonstrate serum autoantibodies but show no evidence of disease. This is especially true in the elderly, and much research related to

TABLE 12-3 Principles of Donor-Recipient Matching

Principle	Method Used for Testing
No transplantation across ABO incompatibility	Hemagglutination
No transplantation in presence of positive T cell crossmatch, i.e., anti–T cell antibodies; avoid transplantation in presence of warm anti–B cell bodies	Lymphocytotoxicity, leukagglutination
Attempt to obtain best HLA match from ABO-compatible potential donors (not critical in liver or heart transplantation)	Lymphocytotoxicity
Attempt to obtain transplant from donor inducing least mixed lymphocyte response from ABO-compatible, satisfactorily matched, potential donors	Mixed lymphocyte culture reactivity

Source: J. A. Bellanti, *Immunology III.* Philadelphia: W.B. Saunders Company, 1985. Figure 20–19. Reprinted by permission.

the loss of self-tolerance with aging is being conducted. Even persons who have suffer myocardial infarction may exhibit myocardial autoantibodies but experience no further myocardial disruption. In diabetes mellitus, autoantibodies to the islet cells of the pancreas are often demonstrated, which leads to the theory that some forms of diabetes mellitus may be a result of an autoimmune attack on these cells [13].

A wide spectrum of autoimmune responses has been divided clinically into systemic, nonorgan-specific and organ-specific diseases [15]. Many of these are described in other sections of the book. The relationships of destructive autoimmune reactions are most clearly demonstrated in myasthenia gravis, Graves' disease, rheumatoid arthritis, systemic lupus erythematosus, and others (Table 12-4). The possibility of autoimmunity as a causative factor has been speculated in conditions as diverse as multiple sclerosis, hepatitis, and malignancies. Autoantibodies have not been consistently demonstrated in malignancies. The appearance of *autoantibodies* and the symptomatology of a disease lend support for an autoimmune classification. Table 12-5 lists some of the pathologic lesions that may occur with autoantibodies [12].

Observations of autoimmune phenomena have resulted in the following generalizations:

1. Specific autoimmune phenomena occur with greater frequency in certain families, which suggests a genetic disorder related to a fundamental disorder of thymic immune control.
2. Autoimmune diseases are more common in females than in males, which indicates a relationship between the sex hormones and the immune response.
3. Elderly persons have a greater prevalence of autoantibodies, which may be the result of genetic errors due to the immune system wearing out through the aging process.
4. Viruses may play a role in the occurrence of autoimmunity because of their ability to disrupt the immune system at any one of several levels.
5. Sequestered tissue (tissue and protein not normally in contact with T and B cells) may be exposed to these cells through disease or disruption.
6. Tissue self antigen is altered by disease or injury so that the host no longer recognizes it as self [11,15].

Systemic Lupus Erythematosus

Systemic lupus erythematosus (SLE) is a multisystem, chronic, rheumatic disease that may assume several forms. It is frequently fatal in persons who develop significant involvement of the glomerular capillaries. Greatest frequency of the disease is found in women 20 to 40 years of age.

Pathologically, widespread degeneration of connective tissue occurs, especially in the heart, glomeruli, blood vessels, skin, spleen, and retroperitoneal tissue. Skin changes include atrophy, dermal edema, and fibrinoid infiltration. The renal glomeruli characteristically demonstrate fibrinoid changes, necrosis with scarring, and deposits of immunoglobulin and complement in the basement membrane [10]. Antinuclear antibody (ANA) is demonstrated in the serum of 80 to 100 percent of persons with SLE. The ANA may represent antibodies to DNA, to nucleoproteins, or to other nuclear components. The LE (lupus erythematosus) cell is present in approximately 76 percent of affected persons. It is basically a mature polymorphonuclear leukocyte that has engulfed nuclear material. These cells may be seen to be clustered around masses of nuclear material and are then called LE rosettes [11]. The LE cell is the result of targeting by antinuclear antibodies.

The American Rheumatism Association issued a list of 14 criteria indicative of SLE [17]. If the person exhibits four or more of these, the diagnosis is probable (Table 12-6).

Stiffness and pain in the hands, feet, or large joints are common complaints. The joints appear red, warm, and tender but do not exhibit the deformities of rheumatoid arthritis. The exposed skin shows signs of a patchy atrophy. An erythematous rash frequently occurs in a butterfly pattern over the nose and cheeks. The dermis becomes edematous and infiltrated by lymphocytes, plasma cells, and histiocytes.

Renal involvement, a serious complication, results from the precipitation of immune complexes in the renal glomeruli. The complexes on the endothelial side of the basement membrane cause inflammatory lesions, thickened basement membrane, tubular atrophy, and interstitial spaces filled with lymphocytes and plasma cells. The course of renal involvement is characterized by remissions and exacerbations ranging in severity from mild proteinuria to massive hematuria and proteinuria finally resulting in total renal failure [4].

Systemic problems including fever, fatigue, anorexia, and weight loss are common. Cardiopulmonary and neurologic manifestations are also seen. Besides antibody demonstration, hematologic abnormalities include anemia and leukopenia.

Rheumatoid Arthritis

Rheumatoid arthritis is a chronic, systemic, inflammatory disease that specifically affects the small joints of the hands and feet in its early stages, and involves the larger joints in later stages. It is nonsuppurative but finally results in the destruction of cartilage and joints. It may also produce lesions of the heart valves, pericardium, myocardium, and pleura [10].

The pathophysiologic manifestations of rheumatoid arthritis appear to result from the development of antibody against IgG. These antibodies, called *rheumatoid factor (RF)*, belong to the IgM, IgG, and IgA classes [11]. The RF is present in 85 to 90 percent of persons with rheumatoid arthritis and may be stimulated by a self antigen, an antigen in the synovial cavity, or an infectious antigen. The RF continues to interact with IgG even in the absence of any specific antigen [11]. Chronic antigen stimulation, such as occurs in chronic respiratory infections, causes the production and destruction of large amounts of antibody. The RF-IgG complexes are present in the rheumatoid lesions and apparently activate complement and/or prostaglandins or other substances that promote the inflammatory response (Fig. 12-6).

TABLE 12-4 Autoimmune Diseases

Condition	Autoantibody	Method of Detection
Organ-specific diseases		
Myasthenia gravis	Anti-acetylcholine	Immunoprecipitation of ^{125}I-α-bungarotoxin–conjugated acetylcholine receptors
Graves' disease (diffuse toxic goiter)	Thyroid-stimulating immunoglobulin (TSI) or anti-TSH receptor autoantibody	Bioassay; measurement of adenylate cyclase activity after incubation of thyroid tissue with immunoglobulin from patient's serum, radioreceptor assay for antibodies competing with TSH for the receptor on thyroid membranes
Hashimoto's thyroiditis	Antibodies to thyroglobulin and to microsomal antigens	Radioimmunoassay, tanned erythrocyte agglutination, complement fixation, immunofluorescence assay
Insulin-resistant diabetes associated with acanthosis nigricans	Antiinsulin receptor	Inhibition of ^{125}I-insulin binding to receptors on monocytes or adipocytes; activation of lipogenesis in adipocytes
Insulin-resistant diabetes associated with ataxia-telangiectasia	Antiinsulin receptor	
Allergic rhinitis, asthma, functional autonomic abnormalities	Antibodies to β_2-adrenergic receptors	Binding of ^{125}I-protein A to lung membranes preincubated with sera; ability of plasma to inhibit binding of ^{125}I-iodohydroxybenzylpindolol (HYP) to calf lung membranes; immunoprecipitation of soluble receptors complexed with ^{125}I-HYP in the presence of propranolol
Juvenile insulin-dependent diabetes	Antibodies to islet cells; antiinsulin antibodies	Immunofluorescence assay; competitive inhibition of insulin binding, stimulation of adipocytes
Pernicious anemia	Antibody to gastric parietal cells and to vitamin B_{12}-binding site of intrinsic factor	Immunofluorescence assay; radioimmunoassay
Addison's disease	Antibodies to adrenal cells	Immunofluorescence assay
Idiopathic hypoparathyroidism	Antibodies to antigens of parathyroid cells	Immunofluorescence assay
Spontaneous infertility	Antibodies to sperm	Agglutination and immobilization of spermatozoa
Premature ovarian failure	Antibodies to interstitial cells and corpus luteum cells	Immunofluorescence assay
Pemphigus	Antibodies to intercellular substance of skin and mucosa	Immunofluorescence assay
Bullous pemphigoid	Antibodies against basement membrane zone of skin and mucosa	Immunofluorescence assay
Primary biliary cirrhosis	Antibodies to mitochondrial antigens	Immunofluorescence assay
Autoimmune hemolytic anemia	Antired blood cell antibodies	Direct and indirect Coombs' tests
Idiopathic thrombocytopenic purpura	Antiplatelet antibodies	Immunofluorescence assay
Idiopathic neutropenia	Antineutrophil antibodies	Agglutination, immunofluorescence assay
Vitiligo	Antimelanocyte antibodies	Immunoprecipitation, immunofluorescence assay
Osteosclerosis and Meniere's disease	Anticollagen type II antibodies	Radioimmunoassay
Chronic active hepatitis	Antinuclear antibodies; antihepatocyte antibodies	Immunofluorescence assay
Systemic diseases (nonorgan-specific)		
Goodpasture's syndrome	Antibasement membrane antibodies	Immunofluorescence assay, radioimmunoassay
Rheumatoid arthritis and Sjögren's syndrome	Antigammaglobulin antibodies; antibodies to EBV-related antigens	Sensitized-SRBC agglutination, latex-immunoglobulin agglutination, radioimmunoassay, immunofluorescence assay, immunodiffusion
Systemic lupus erythematosus	Antinuclear antibodies	Immunofluorescence assay
	Anti-dsDNA and anti-ssDNA	Farr assay, solid phase enzyme and radioimmunoassay, hemagglutination, counterelectrophoresis
	Anti-Sm antibodies	Hemagglutination, immunodiffusion, radioimmunoassay
	Antiribonucleoprotein antibodies	Hemagglutination, radioimmunoassay
	Antilymphocyte antibodies	Immunofluorescence assay, cytotoxicity
	Antired blood cell antibodies	Coombs' test
	Antiplatelet antibodies	Immunofluorescence assay
	Antineuronal cell antibodies	Immunofluorescence assay
	Antigammaglobulins	Radioimmunoassay

Source: D.P. Stites, et al., *Basic and Clinical Immunology* (5th ed.). Los Altos, Calif.: Lange Medical Publishers, 1984. Reprinted by permission.

TABLE 12-5 Direct Pathogenic Effects of Humoral Antibodies

Disease	Autoantigen	Lesion
Autoimmune hemolytic anemia	Red cell	Erythrocyte destruction
Lymphopenia (some cases)	Lymphocyte	Lymphocyte destruction
Idiopathic thrombocytopenic purpura	Platelet	Platelet destruction
Male infertility (some cases)	Sperm	Agglutination of spermatozoa
Pernicious anemia	Intrinsic factor	Neutralization of ability to mediate B_{12} absorption
Hashimoto's disease	Thyroid surface antigen	Cytotoxic effect on thyroid cells in culture
Thyrotoxicosis	TSH receptors	Stimulation of thyroid cells
Goodpasture's syndrome	Glomerular basement membrane	Complement-mediated damage to basement membrane
Myasthenia gravis	Acetylcholine receptor	Blocking and destruction of receptors
Acanthosis nigricans (type B) & ataxia-telangiectasia with insulin resistance	Insulin receptor	Blocking of receptors

Source: L. Roitt, *Essential Immunology* (5th ed.). Oxford: Blackwell Scientific Publications, Ltd., 1984. Table 10–4. Reprinted by permission.

TABLE 12-6 Criteria Indicative of SLE

Facial erythema (butterfly rash)
Hemolytic anemia, leukopenia, thrombocytopenia
Photosensitivity
Chronic false positive for syphilis
Alopecia
Psychosis or neurologic deficits or convulsions
Cellular casts
Oral or nasopharyngeal ulceration
Pleuritis or pericarditis
Arthritis without deformity
Discoid lupus
Raynaud's phenomenon
Proteinuria (over 3.5 gm/day)
LE cell

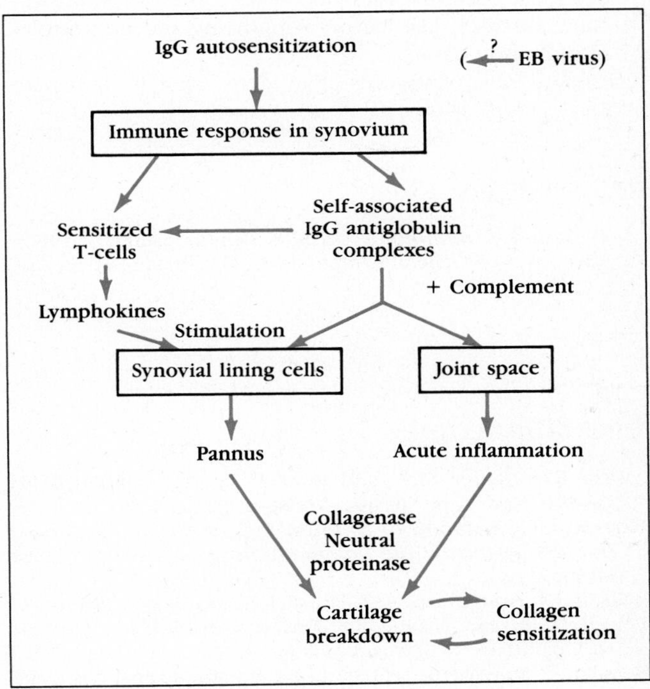

FIGURE 12-6 Hypothetical scheme showing how initial autosensitization to IgG can lead to the pathogenetic changes characteristic of rheumatoid arthritis. (From L. Roitt, *Essential Immunology* [5th ed.]. Oxford: Blackwell Scientific Publications, Ltd., 1984. Figure 9–14. Reprinted by permission.)

Acute attacks of rheumatoid arthritis occur as the RF-IgG complexes precipitate in the synovial fluid. Complement is activated and attracts polymorphonuclear leukocytes, whose main function appears to be phagocytosis of the complexes. The lysosomal enzymes released by these cells intensify the inflammatory reaction and increase destruction of the articular cartilage. Granulation tissue and inflammatory cells form a mass of tissue called *pannus* that erodes the articular cartilage. The joint space is destroyed, and the resultant scarring may completely immobilize the joint or cause bleeding and thrombosis in the area.

Rheumatoid subcutaneous nodules are often seen and are described as firm, nontender, oval masses, up to 2 cm in diameter. These are present on the forearms and sometimes the Achilles tendons, or attached to underlying periosteum or tendons.

Other systems are also affected. A necrotizing arteritis may lead to thrombosis of small arteries. Fibrinous pericarditis, cardiomyopathy, and valvular lesions may affect the heart. Pleuritis and interstitial fibrosis may affect the lungs. The rheumatoid nodules may occur on bone, and other effects are seen in the nervous system and the eyes [4].

The signs and symptoms of rheumatoid arthritis are due to both systemic and local inflammatory lesions. Fatigue, weakness, joint stiffness, and vague arthralgias are early symptoms. The individual complains of morning stiffness, which gradually improves after rising. Joints in the hands or feet may be inflamed and swollen; these symptoms tend to spread symmetrically so that the corresponding joints on the contralateral extremity become involved.

Laboratory values, besides the positive RF, include mild leukocytosis with eosinophilia and elevated erythrocyte sedimentation rate.

The course of rheumatoid arthritis is variable, with remissions and exacerbations. Some persons have a relatively benign disease, while others progress rapidly to severe deformity and total disability.

Study Questions

1. List the four types of hypersensitivity reactions and describe the pathophysiologic mechanisms that underlie each.
2. What is the underlying concept in autoimmunity?
3. Describe transplant graft rejection and indicate how it could be prevented.
4. Describe the target organs affected in SLE and its mechanism of damage.
5. Compare rheumatoid arthritis with the other autoimmune diseases. List factors supporting and negating an autoimmune basis.
6. Prepare a list of sources of antigens. Classify their reactions as type I–type IV.

References

1. Bellanti, J.A. *Immunology III*. Philadelphia: Saunders, 1985.
2. Chatton, M.J. General Symptoms. In M.A. Krupp, et al., *Current Medical Diagnosis and Treatment 1986*. Los Altos, Calif.: Lange, 1986.
3. Corbett, J.V. *Laboratory Tests in Nursing Practice*. Norwalk, Conn.: Appleton-Century-Crofts, 1982.
4. Fishman, M.C., et al. *Medicine* (2nd ed.). Philadelphia: Lippincott, 1985.
5. Gelfand, M.C. Organ Transplantation. In J.A. Bellanti, *Immunology III*. Philadelphia: Saunders, 1985.
6. Gell, P.G., Coombs, R.R., and Lachmann, R. *Clinical Aspects of Immunology* (3rd ed.). Oxford: Blackwell, 1975.
7. Haeney, M. *Introduction to Clinical Immunology*. Boston: Butterworths, 1985.
8. Hanson, L.A., and Wigzell, H. *Immunology*. London: Butterworths, 1985.
9. Henney, C.S. T Cell-Mediated Cytotoxicity. In D.P. Stites, et al., *Basic and Clinical Immunology* (5th ed.). Los Altos, Calif.: Lange, 1984.
10. Kissane, J.M. *Anderson's Pathology* (8th ed.). St. Louis: Mosby, 1985.
11. Robbins, S.L., Cotran, R.S., and Kumar, V. *The Pathologic Basis of Disease* (3rd ed.). Philadelphia: Saunders, 1984.
12. Roitt, I. *Essential Immunology* (5th ed.). Oxford: Blackwell, 1984.
13. Rose, N. Autoimmune disease. *Sci. Am.* 244:383, 1981.
14. Strober, S., Grumet, C., and Stites, D.P. Immunologic Disorders. In M.A. Krupp, et al., *Current Medical Diagnosis and Treatment 1986*. Los Altos, Calif.: Lange, 1986.
15. Theofilopoulos, A.N. Autoimmunity. In D.P. Stites, et al., *Basic and Clinical Immunology* (5th ed.). Los Altos, Calif.: Lange, 1984.
16. Wells, J.V. Immune Mechanisms in Tissue. In D.P. Stites, et al., *Basic and Clinical Immunology* (5th ed.). Los Altos, Calif.: Lange, 1984.
17. White, J. Systemic lupus erythematosus. *Nurs. 78* 8:26, 1978.

Unit Bibliography

Albert, E.D., Bauer, M.P., and Mayr, W.R. *Histocompatibility Testing*. New York: Springer-Verlag, 1984.

Barrett, J.T. *Textbook of Immunology: An Introduction to Immunochemistry and Immunobiology* (4th ed.). St. Louis: Mosby, 1983.

Bellanti, J.A. *Immunology III*. Philadelphia: Saunders, 1985.

Benacerraf, B., and Unanue, R.E. *Textbook of Immunology* (2nd ed.). Baltimore: Williams & Wilkins, 1984.

Bogolin, L., and Harris, J. Meeting the immunological challenge: Rush-Presbyterian-St. Luke's medical symposium. *Heart Lung* 9:643, 1980.

Bowry, T.R. *Immunology Simplified* (2nd ed.). Oxford: Oxford University Press, 1984.

Bullock, W.W. ABA-T determinant regulation of delayed hypersensitivity. *Immunol. Rev.* 39:3, 1978.

Cohen, S. The role of cell-mediated immunity in the induction of inflammatory responses. *Am. J. Pathol.* 88:502, 1977.

Cooper, M.D., and Lawton, A.R., III. The development of the immune system. *Sci. Am.* 231:58, 1974.

Dean, J.H., et al. *Immunotoxicology and Immunopharmacology*. New York: Raven Press, 1985.

Fahey, J.L. Antibodies and immunoglobulins: Structure and function. *JAMA* 194:41, 1965.

Ganong, W.F. *Review of Medical Physiology* (12th ed.). Los Altos, Calif.: Lange, 1985.

Gershwin, M.E., Beach, R.S., and Hurley, L.S. *Nutrition and Immunity*. Orlando, Fla.: Academic Press, 1985.

Giese, A.C. *Cell Physiology*. Philadelphia: Saunders, 1979.

Glasser, R. How the body works against itself. *Nurs. 77* 7:38, 1977.

Guyton, A.T. *Textbook of Medical Physiology* (7th ed.). Philadelphia: Saunders, 1986.

Haeney, M. *Introduction to Clinical Immunology*. Boston: Butterworths, 1985.

Hanson, L.A., and Wigzell, H. *Immunology*. London: Butterworths, 1985.

Herberman, R.B., and Callewaert, D.M. *Mechanisms of Cytotoxicity by NK Cells*. Orlando, Fla.: Academic Press, 1985.

Hitzig, W.H. Congenital immunodeficiency disease: Pathophysiology, clinical appearance and treatment. *Pathobiol. Annu.* 6:163, 1976.

Hood, L.E., et al. *Immunology* (2nd ed.). Menlo Park, Calif.: Benjamin-Cummings, 1984.

Hudgel, D., and Madsen, L. Acute and chronic asthma: A guide to intervention. *Am. J. Nurs.* 80:1791, 1980.

Jensen, D. *The Principles of Physiology* (2nd ed.). New York: Appleton-Century-Crofts, 1980.

Katz, D.H. Control of IgE antibody production by suppressor substances. *J. Allergy Clin. Immunol.* 62:44, 1978.

Kissane, J.M. *Anderson's Pathology* (8th ed.). St. Louis: Mosby, 1985.

Klaustermeyer, W.B. *Practical Allergy and Immunology*. New York: Wiley, 1983.

Koren, M.E. Cancer immunotherapy: What, why, when and how? *Nurs. 81* 11:34, 1981.

Lachmann, P.J., and Peters, D.K. *Clinical Aspects of Immunology*. Boston: Blackwell, 1982.

MacDonald, D.M. *Immunodermatology*. London: Butterworths, 1984.

McDuffie, F.C. Immune complexes in the rheumatic diseases. *J. Allergy Clin. Immunol.* 62:37, 1978.

Mitchell, M.S. *The Modulation of Immunity*. Oxford: Pergamon Press, 1985.

Niemtzow, R.C. *Transmembrane Potentials and Characteristics of Immune and Tumor Cells*. Boca Raton, Fla.: CRC Press, 1985.

Notkins, A.L., and Koprowski, H. How the immune response to a virus can cause disease. *Sci. Am.* 228:22, 1973.

Parker, C. Food allergies. *Am. J. Nurs.* 80:262, 1980.

Paul, W.E. *Fundamental Immunology.* New York: Raven Press, 1984.

Robbins, S.L., Cotran, R.S., and Kumar, V. *Pathologic Basis of Disease* (3rd ed.). Philadelphia: Saunders, 1984.

Roitt, I. *Essential Immunology* (5th ed.). Oxford: Blackwell, 1985.

Rose, N. Autoimmune diseases. *Sci. Am.* 244:80, 1981.

Ryan, G.B., and Majno, G. Acute inflammation. *Am. J. Pathol.* 86:184, 1977.

Schwartz, R.S. The immunological basis of auto-immunization. *J. Allergy Clin. Immunol.* 60:69, 1977.

Selekman, J. Immunization: What's it all about? *Am. J. Nurs.* 80:1441, 1980.

Sodeman, W.A., Jr., and Sodeman, W.A. *Sodeman's Pathological Physiology: Mechanisms of Disease* (7th ed.). Philadelphia: Saunders, 1985.

Stinnett, J.D. *Nutrition and the Immune Response*. Boca Raton, Fla.: CRC Press, 1983.

Stites, D.P., et al. *Basic and Clinical Immunology* (5th ed.). Los Altos, Calif.: Lange, 1984.

Unanue, E.R. The regulation of lymphocyte functions by the macrophage. *Immunol. Rev.* 40:225, 1978.

Waldmann, T.A., and Broder, S. Suppressor cells in the regulation of the immune response. *Prog. Clin. Immunol.* 3:155, 1977.

Wallach, J. *Interpretation of Diagnostic Tests* (4th ed.). Boston: Little, Brown, 1986.

Walter, J.B. *An Introduction to the Principles of Disease* (2nd ed.). Philadelphia: Saunders, 1982.

Watkins, J. *Trauma, Stress, and Immunity in Anesthesia and Surgery*. Boston: Butterworths, 1982.

Watson, J.D., and Marbrook, J. *Recognition and Regulation in Cell-Mediated Immunity*. New York: Dekker, 1985.

Watson, R.R. *Nutrition, Disease Resistance and Immune Function*. New York: Dekker, 1984.

White, J. Teaching patients to manage systemic lupus erythematosus. *Nurs. 78* 8:26, 1978.

UNIT 6

Neoplasia

Barbara L. Bullock

The response of cells to the daily barrage of stimuli they receive may be growth or degeneration, alteration of normal metabolism, or even death. Cellular growth and proliferation often occur on a continuum from near normal to grossly abnormal. Neoplasia refers to an alteration in cellular growth and development. This unit examines some of the factors related to neoplasia. Chapter 13 describes cell membrane changes in neoplasia and some related alterations in cellular characteristics. Chapter 14 describes the process of carcinogenesis and mechanisms for growth and spread of malignancy.

The topic of neoplasia is inclusive, and investigative studies are revealing much new, important data. The extensive bibliography at the end of this unit is an attempt to provide current and important historical documentation for this vast subject.

Chapter 13 serves as an introduction to Chapter 14 and should be reviewed first to facilitate understanding. The reader is encouraged to study the unit by using the learning objectives at the beginning of each chapter and then assess the learning achieved using the study questions at the end of the chapters. The unit bibliography provides sources for further investigation.

CHAPTER 13

Concepts of Altered Cellular Function

CHAPTER OUTLINE

The Cell Life Cycle
Outer Cell Membrane Changes as an Explanation for Neoplasia
- Appropriate Cell Recognition
- Cellular Adhesion
- Intercellular Communication

Inner Cell Changes in Neoplasia
- Changes in the Cytoplasm
- Changes in the Nucleoplasm

Differentiation
Anaplasia

LEARNING OBJECTIVES

1. Define *neoplasia*, *neoplasm*, *benign*, and *malignant*.
2. Identify the steps in the cell's life cycle.
3. Explain the physiology of each step in the cell's life cycle.
4. Relate the cell's life cycle to neoplasia.
5. Name three areas of potential change in the outer cell membrane that may alter cellular growth.
6. Explain the difference between neoplastic and normal cells in relationship to contact inhibition.
7. Identify the three types of intercellular connections.
8. Discuss the role of each intercellular connection in cellular adhesion.
9. Discuss alterations in intercellular connections of neoplastic tissues.
10. Describe factors other than intercellular connections that are involved in cellular adhesion.
11. Define *contact inhibition*.
12. Explain the role of contact inhibition in intercellular communication.
13. Discuss the role of the gap junction in intercellular communication.
14. Explain the relationship between alterations of the gap junction and intercellular communication in neoplasia.
15. Relate second messengers in the cytoplasm to growth and neoplasia.
16. Discuss the nucleus as the site of all hereditary information in relation to neoplasia.
17. Define *cellular differentiation*.
18. Relate cellular differentiation to neoplasia.
19. Define *anaplasia*.
20. Discuss the histologic features of an anaplastic cell.

The cell is constantly confronted by factors in its environment that stimulate or inhibit its activity. It responds to these factors by growth and proliferation, and/or regression and degeneration. These two responses may occur simultaneously in a given cell population, or one may follow the other [1]. When cells are confronted with a stimulus that alters their normal metabolism, they may increase concentrations of normal cellular constituents, accumulate abnormal substances, change cellular size and number, and/or undergo lethal change. The stimuli that cause these alterations are grouped as follows: (1) physical agents, (2) chemical agents, (3) microorganisms, (4) hypoxia, (5) genetic factors, and (6) immunologic factors.

Alterations in cellular growth and proliferation may be viewed as occurring on a continuum from near-normal changes to grossly abnormal alterations. Hypertrophy, hyperplasia, metaplasia, and dysplasia are usually classified as controlled adaptive cellular responses (see Chap. 3). They make the cell vulnerable to injurious agents that cause alterations in its normal controls of growth and development.

Neoplasia is defined as the development of an abnormal mass of tissue that is unresponsive to normal growth control mechanisms [7]. A *neoplasm* is a group or clump of neoplastic cells. *Benign neoplasia* refers to neoplastic cells that do not invade the surrounding tissue and do not metastasize. *Malignant neoplasia* refers to neoplastic (cancer) cells that grow by invading surrounding tissue and metastasize to receptive tissue. All malignant neoplasms are classified as cancers and then further delineated as to their origin (see Chap. 14).

The Cell Life Cycle

The cell life cycle is composed of all the steps in the process of reproduction or that period extending from one mitosis to the next [1]. In a normal cell population, inhibitory controls slow or stop reproduction, while stimulating factors cause the process to proceed more rapidly. Therefore, the actual length of a cell life cycle varies. The four phases are designated G_1, S, G_2, and M, with a fifth phase, G_0, being composed of cells leaving the normal cell cycle, which can be induced to reenter the cycle by specific stimuli (Fig. 13-1) [6]. The letter G is an abbreviation for "gap" and refers to the time between mitosis and synthesis (G_1) and synthesis and mitosis (G_2).

The symbol G_0 is used to describe the cell that performs all metabolic activities except for reproduction (mitosis). The cell remains at this level until some stimulus, such as the death of other cells of the same population, triggers the beginning of G_1. A cell may remain in the G_1 phase for long periods until some key process occurs to signal its entrance into the S phase of DNA synthesis [6].

Ribonucleic acid (RNA) and protein are synthesized in the G_1 *interval*. The length of the G_1 interval varies with each cell type, being shorter in cell populations with great activity. At a certain point in G_1 the decision is made between proliferation and resting; this is called a *restriction point* [3]. The cell, stimulated to begin the synthesis of deoxyribonucleic acid (DNA), enters the S step. Synthesis of DNA occurs in the S step with replication of the chromosomes. The length of the S step varies and is followed by a period of inactivity called G_2. Very little is known about this phase except that some RNA is synthesized in preparation for mitosis. Mitosis (M) occurs next, with cellular division creating two daughter cells that have identical genetic information (see Chap. 1). These daughter cells can mature and repeat the process or can enter a G_1 or G_0 interval until they are stimulated to reproduce.

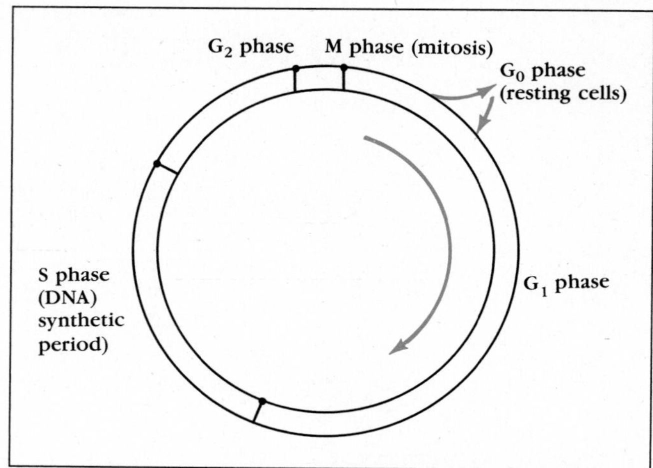

FIGURE 13-1 The cell cycle. Interphase (G_1), DNA synthesis (S), intermediate phase (G_2), and mitosis (M) interval are shown. The G_0 period may be entered from G_1, and reentry from G_0 to G_1 may occur.

The concept of the cell life cycle has helped in the basic understanding of the causes and effects of neoplasia. Neoplastic cell populations ignore normal growth limitations and enter the cell cycle repeatedly at different rates. The following terms identify this tendency in neoplastic tumors: growth fraction, cell cycle time, cell loss, and doubling time. *Growth fraction* refers to the proportion of cells in a given cell population undergoing cell cycle activity at any given time. Rapidly growing neoplasms have a larger number of cells in active reproduction at any given time than do slow-growing neoplasms. *Cell cycle time* is usually shorter in rapidly growing neoplasms than in normal cells. *Cell loss* refers to the number of cells lost because of death or some other event. These three factors, when taken together, account for the *doubling time*, which is the rate at which a neoplasm doubles its cell population.

Cell replication depends on the degree and specialization of the particular cell. In general, the greater the degree of specialization, the less the tendency of the cell to reproduce. Neurons and cardiac muscle cells have lost the ability to reproduce entirely. Cells such as the skin, gastrointestinal mucosal cells, and blood cells continually reproduce to replace lost cells throughout life.

Outer Cell Membrane Changes as an Explanation for Neoplasia

All cells are surrounded by a limiting membrane that constantly exists in a dynamic state (see Chap. 1). The parts of the membrane have the capacity to redistribute and change the cell surface properties, which may have an effect on the cell's growth, metabolism, and behavior [10].

The outer cell membrane is the point of contact between cells (Fig. 13-2). Interactions involving the outer cell membrane have been shown to function in the control of normal cellular growth [1]. Changes in the membrane are apparent in neoplastic cells and have been implicated in the failure of neoplastic cells to respond to normal growth-control mechanisms. They involve alterations in appropriate cell recognition, cellular adhesion, and intercellular communication. Escape from growth control could involve breakdown at any of these points [8].

Appropriate Cell Recognition

The mechanisms used by specific cells to recognize each other are not well defined. That recognition exists can be demonstrated by mixing cells of different types in culture media; specific cells eventually segregate themselves. Membrane enzymes and surface sugar residues are thought to contribute to recognition. One hypothesis is that sugar-binding enzymes, glycosyltransferases, in the outer cell membrane recognize sugar residues on glycoproteins in the membrane of neighboring cells [8]. In neoplastic cells, glycolipids are altered (Fig. 13-3). Glycoproteins and/or glycolipids may be missing from the membrane or have abnormal structure [1].

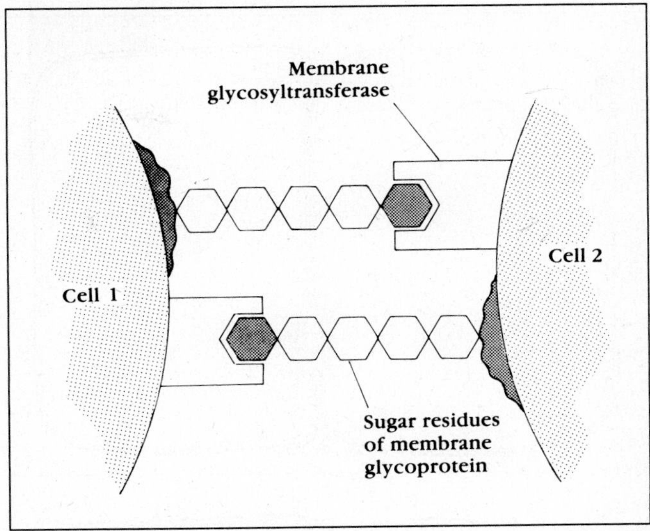

FIGURE 13-3 Cell recognition through sugar-binding enzymes and sugar residues on glycoprotein in the membrane of neighboring cells. (From M.J. Taussig, *Processes in Pathology.* Oxford: Blackwell Scientific Publications, Ltd., 1979. Figure 4–6.)

Cellular Adhesion

Cellular adhesion is a complex process that involves the development of connections between cells. Three types of connections have been described (Fig. 13-4).

1. The *desmosome* is a mechanical way of holding cells together. Because it is composed of fibrous protein, it can be destroyed by a proteolytic enzyme, such as

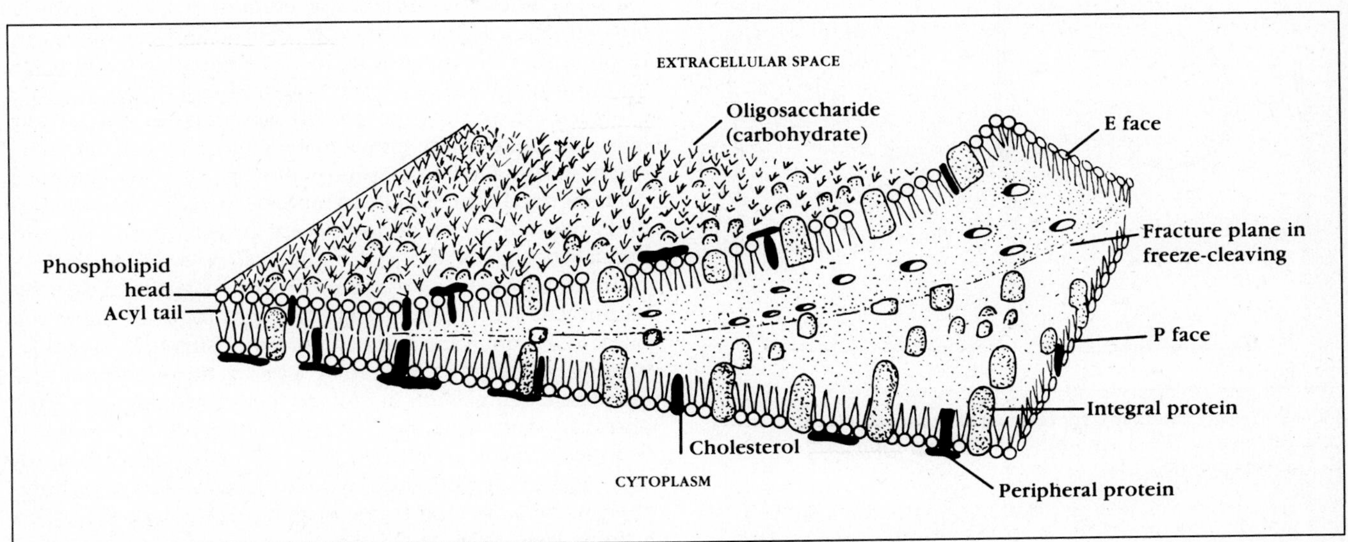

FIGURE 13-2 Outer cell membrane demonstrating integrated structures that are associated with various surface properties of the cell. (From M. Borysenko et al., *Functional Histology* [2nd ed.]. Boston: Little, Brown, 1984.)

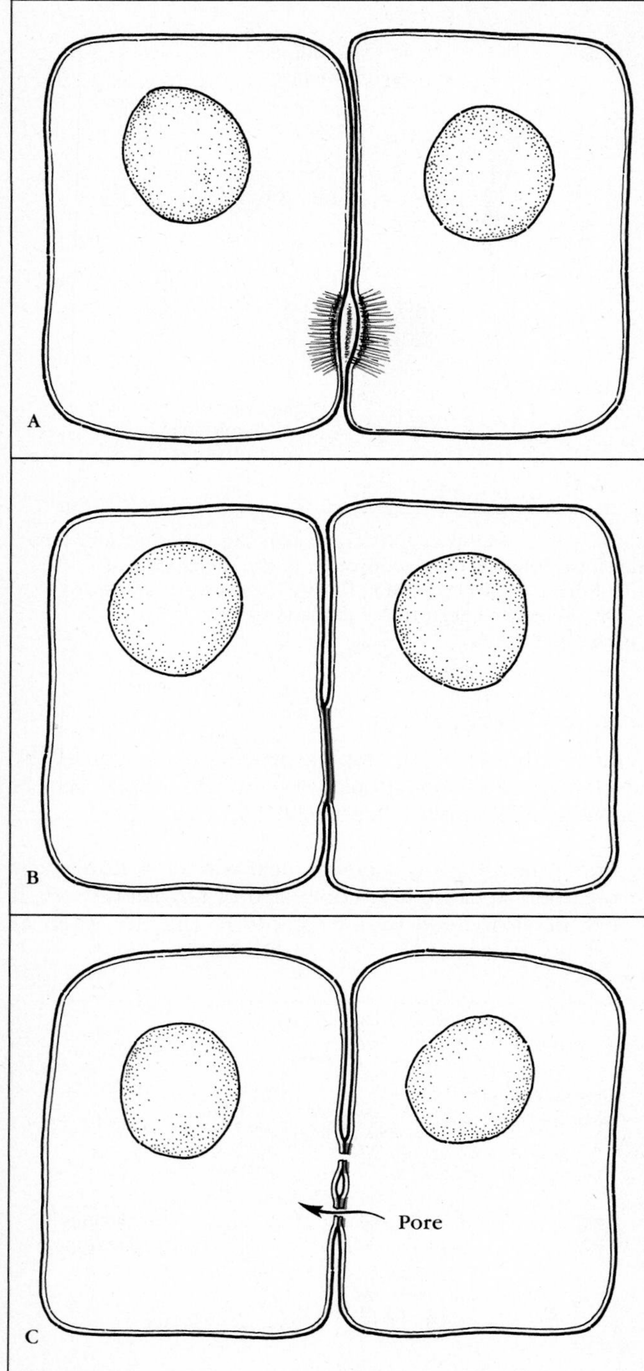

FIGURE 13-4 Schematic representation of intercellular connections. A. The desmosome. B. The tight junction. C. The gap junction.

trypsin. Once the desmosome is gone, the cells separate (see Chap. 14).

2. The *tight junction* involves the actual fusion of two cell membranes forming impermeable barriers [8]. Thus, it is present where sharp physical separation is needed, such as in the endothelial lining of the cerebral blood vessels that forms the blood-brain barrier.
3. The *gap junction*, a pore passing through the outer cell membrane, permits the movement of low-molecular-weight substances from one adjoining cell to the next.

A decrease in the number of desmosomal, tight, and gap junctions often occurs in the neoplastic cell population. This causes a decrease in cellular adhesion. The communication of cells is evidently dependent on the junctions described. When cells cannot communicate in this way, the loss of contact inhibition can lead to neoplastic change [8]. This reduction in tight cell connections disrupts the extracellular environment.

Junctional changes may not be involved in the early disruption of cellular adhesion. Research indicates that glycosyltransferase, serum factors, cell surface proteins, cytoskeletal elements, and membrane glycoproteins all play a role in early cellular membrane changes [1,8].

Cellular adhesion properties also include the electrical charge of the outer cell membrane. Under physiologic conditions, all mammalian cell surfaces have a negative charge, but this charge becomes more negative in neoplasia. The more aggressive the behavior of the neoplasm, the more negative the cell surface charge. This tends to push the cells away from each other [8].

Intercellular Communication

Contact inhibition, or density-dependent growth control, is observed when normal cells are grown in culture media. The cells move around freely in the culture media until they touch one another. On contact, they adhere to one another and form parallel lines. They then grow on a single layer until they reach the edge of the culture dish. Growth then stops. The cells of a neoplasm, however, respond by continuing to divide and migrate until they are several layers deep. Clearly, normal cells respond to a crowded environment, but neoplastic cells do not, as they have lost their ability either to receive or to send the necessary information to stop growth (Fig. 13-5) [8]. Robbins characterized cancer cells as "antisocial, fairly autonomous units that appear to be indifferent to the constraints and regulatory signals imposed on normal cells" [7, p. 230].

In addition to contact inhibition, agglutination by lectins has been used by researchers to study both the outer cell membrane and cell growth. Using lectins (sugar-binding proteins) as molecular markers during normal and neoplastic cell growth in culture media, investigators have observed that when the outer layer of protein is removed from their outer membrane, normal cells begin to reproduce and are agglutinated by lectin. Neoplastic cells, however, when subjected to a nonagglutinating lectin grow to a single layer (Fig. 13-6) [8].

Lectins have been used to study the cell cycle and growth signals. On entering mitosis, normally growing cells appear to experience a change on the outer cell membrane that leads to the next round of cell division by a messenger, or *go*, signal. Sometime after that, but before

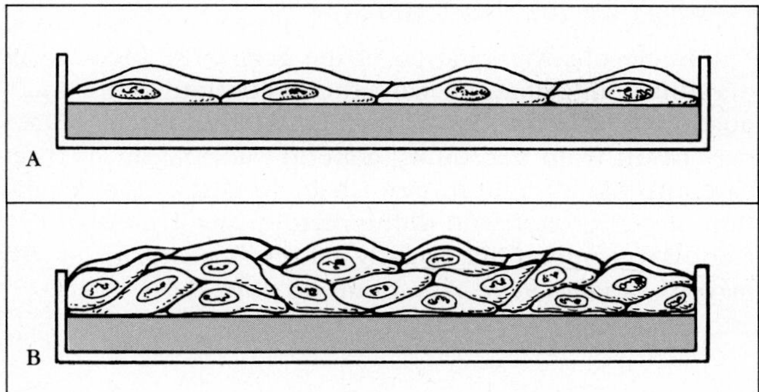

FIGURE 13-5 A. Normal cells are inhibited by a crowded environment. B. Neoplastic cells continue to grow despite cell contact.

the outer cell membrane returns to the nonagglutinable state, another messenger, or *stop* signal, is received that causes the cell to enter G_0, the resting phase. If the stop signal is not received, the cell is committed to another round of division. Therefore, normal growth apparently involves signals to stop division; these signals may be blocked in the neoplastic cell.

In a related phenomenon, cells removed from the body and placed in culture medium grow and reproduce if the medium is constantly replenished. Growth and reproduction stop when secretions of the cells are allowed to collect in the medium. This supports the theory that substances produced by the cell provide a feedback mechanism that slows or stops growth (Fig. 13-7). These substances are called *chalones* or hormonelike mitosis inhibitors. Chalones have not been isolated in pure form, but are thought to be proteins or glycoproteins. They apparently are specific with regard to different cell types [5], but have not been identified for all organs. Other substances also apparently have a part in the inhibition of mitosis [7]. If chalones are important to cell reproduction, neoplasms have developed a way to escape their control. Neoplasms either produce no chalones or are not sensitive to them [8].

Messengers carrying information on growth control move into the cell through the gap junction. With loss of gap junction, as occurs in neoplasia, the cell may become isolated from the growth-control messengers of its normal neighboring cells as well its own (Fig. 13-8).

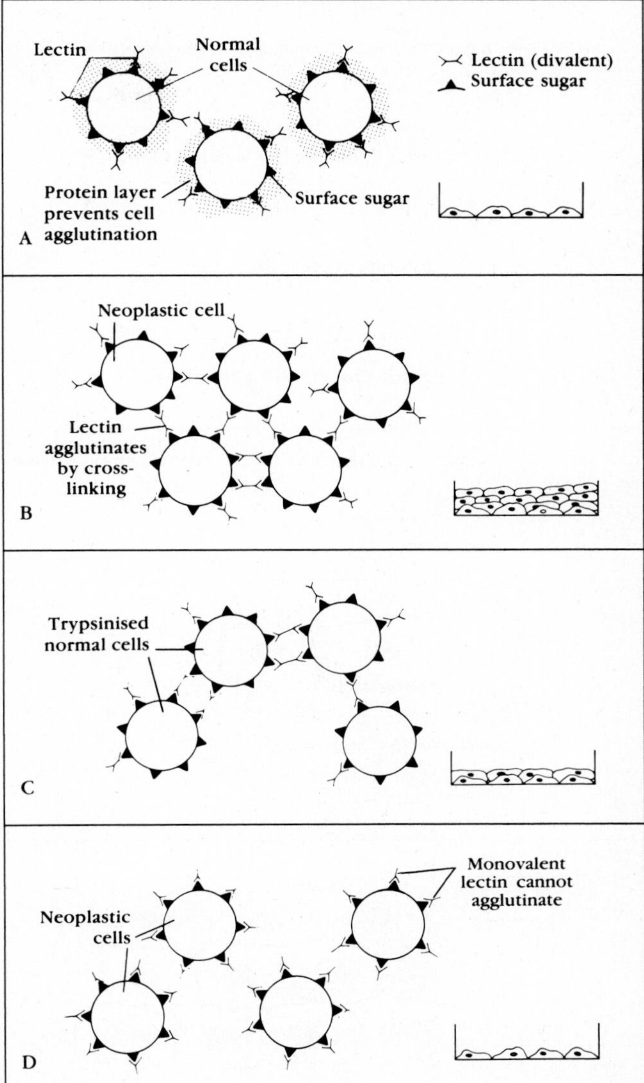

FIGURE 13-6 Effects of lectins on normal and neoplastic cells. A. Normal cells grow to a monolayer in culture and are not agglutinated by lectin. B. Neoplastic cells grow as multilayers and are agglutinated by lectin. C. Normal cells after trypsin treatment enter further replication and are lectin agglutinable. D. Neoplastic cells treated with monovalent (nonagglutinating) lectin grow to monolayer. (From M.J. Taussig, *Processes in Pathology.* Oxford: Blackwell Scientific Publications, Ltd., 1979. Figure 4–6.)

Inner Cell Changes in Neoplasia

Just as changes occur in the outer cell membrane in neoplasia, changes occur within the cell. It is difficult to ascertain whether they are a function of the neoplasia or of the increased growth rate. The changes involve both the cytoplasm and the nucleoplasm.

Changes in the Cytoplasm

The cytoplasm is a medium through which second messengers related to growth must move to reach the nucleus of the cell where they interact with DNA. The exact nature of the second messengers remains unclear. Protein growth factors, cyclic nucleotides (cyclic adenosine monophosphate, or cAMP, and cyclic guanosine monophosphate, or cGMP) and ions (Ca, Mg, Na, and K) are possible second messengers. Cyclic nucleotides mainly activate protein kinases. A mutant cell that has no protein kinase cannot be stopped in G_1. Two cAMP-dependent protein kinases that correlate with cell growth are produced during specific phases of the cell life cycle [2].

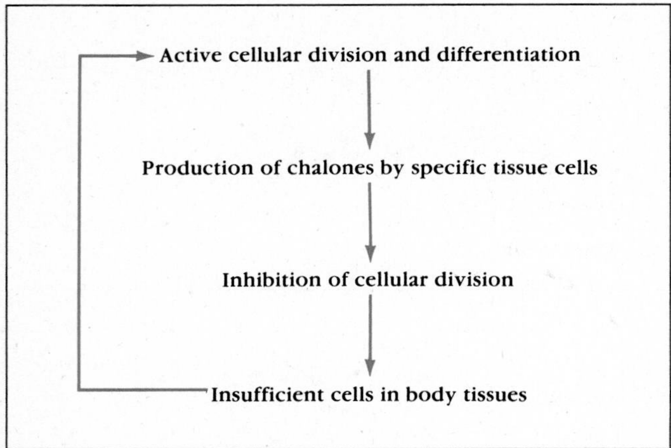

FIGURE 13-7 Negative feedback of tissue mass regulation using specific chalones.

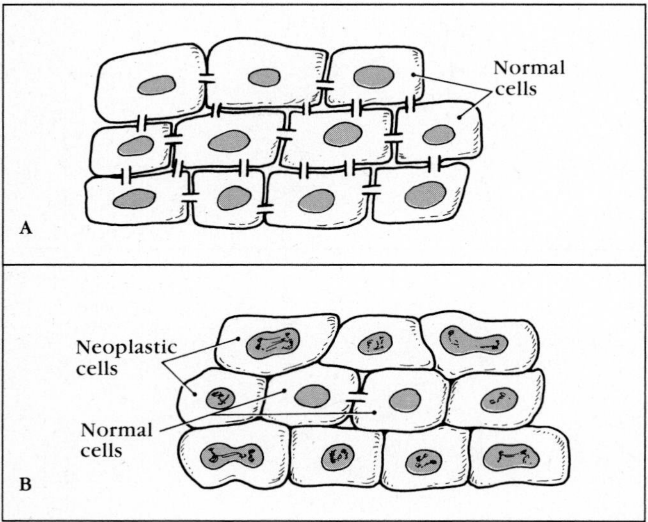

FIGURE 13-8 A. Demonstration of normal growth control information by the gap junction. B. Isolation of normal cells from neighboring cells.

The cytoplasm also contains many enzymes active in anabolism and catabolism. Both enzyme and chromosome changes are present in rapidly growing neoplastic cells. Enzyme alterations do not occur in all neoplastic cells [7].

Cytoplasmic ribosomes are responsible for the synthesis of protein. In general, neoplastic cells entrap nitrogen compounds very quickly, take up amino acids, and use these acids to make new proteins through an active anabolic process. They also have key enzymes necessary for making raw products into nucleic acids [9]. Neoplastic cells make proteins more rapidly than nonneoplastic cells.

The mitochondria provide for aerobic energy production. The rate of glucose use and lactic acid production in the presence of oxygen is increased in some neoplasms. Some neoplasms may use glucose faster than normal cells because it is moved into the cells rapidly [1].

Changes in the Nucleoplasm

The nucleus is the location of the genes, the locus of all hereditary information, with the exception of the small quantity of DNA in the organelles. Altered nuclear DNA may result from hereditary genetic information or from carcinogenic alteration (See Chap. 14). Also, the regulation of cell growth and differentiation involves DNA [3]. Neoplastic nuclei are usually larger than normal, with marked variations in shape from the normal [4].

Differentiation

During fetal development, cells undergo changes in their physical and structural properties as they form the different tissues of the body. This is cellular differentiation. Differentiated cells become specialized and differ from one another physically and functionally. Nerve cells, for example, are like other nerve cells, but they look and act quite different from other types of cells. The more specialized and differentiated a cell is, the less likely it is to divide, and, therefore it is less susceptible to neoplastic change.

The controlling factors of cell differentiation are not well understood, but probably involve selective repression of genetic information. Repressor substances in the cytoplasm are apparently responsible for differentiation, with the repressor substance in one cell acting to repress one genetic characteristic, and that of another cell acting to repress a different genetic characteristic. The full set of genetic information is always present, but parts of it are repressed [4]. Cells that look like the cell of origin (parent cells) are called *well-differentiated cells*. The cells of a neoplasm are not as well-differentiated as the cells of normal tissue. Neoplasms composed of cells resembling the mature cells of the tissue of origin are called *well-differentiated tumors* [7]. Neoplasms composed of cells that bear little or no resemblance to the tissue of origin are called *poorly differentiated* or *undifferentiated tumors*.

Anaplasia

Anaplasia is a word that describes the regression of a cell population from being well differentiated to being less differentiated. Anaplastic cells vary in morphology, and in some of the better differentiated lesions, may reproduce a structure resembling the tissue of origin [7]. Less differentiated (more anaplastic) tumor cells lose orientation to each other and bear very little resemblance to the tissue of origin. The functional efficiency of anaplastic cells correlates with the level of morphologic differentiation [7].

Robbins illustrated the point by noting that well-differentiated cancer cells may elaborate normal products of the tissue of origin, while poorly differentiated cancer cells may lose all specialized functional characteristics [7]. Very anaplastic tumors may elaborate product completely foreign to the tissue of origin. An example is the elaboration of antidiuretic hormone (ADH) from the small cell (oat cell) carcinoma of the lung (see Chap. 27).

The anaplastic cell is usually *pleomorphic*, which means that it has many shapes and sizes. Large hyperchromatic nuclei with irregular membranes are exhibited, having larger and more numerous nucleoli [1].

The cytoplasmic organelles of the anaplastic cell are less numerous than those of a normal cell and are abnormal in form. Pseudopodia, microfilaments and clumps of membranous sacs, and tubules are usually present. Less endoplasmic reticulum and fewer mitochondria are present, so that less cell work occurs. The nuclear membrane appears convoluted, irregular, and doubled onto itself [1].

Mitoses of anaplastic cells are frequently abnormal, and various chromosomal defects result. Most cells exhibit atypical and bizarre mitotic figures [7]. Few mitoses faithfully reproduce the abnormality, and new aberrations with chromosome deletions or translocations occur [1].

Study Questions

1. What is the fundamental difference between neoplastic and normal tissue?
2. How do cell types differ in their ability to become malignant?
3. How do changes in outer cell membrane promote a malignancy?
4. Discuss the interaction of chalones in cellular physiology.
5. Describe anaplasia and indicate how it relates to malignant growth.

References

1. Cheville, N.F. *Cell Pathology* (2nd ed.). Ames: Iowa State University Press, 1983.
2. Das, M. Mitogenic hormone-induced intracellular message: Assay and partial characterization of an activator DNA replication induced by epidermal growth factor. *Proc. Natl. Acad. Sci. USA* 77:112, 1980.
3. DeVita, V.T., Hellman, S., and Rosenberg, S.A. *Cancer: Principles and Practice of Oncology* (2nd ed.). Philadelphia: Lippincott, 1985.
4. Guyton, A. *Textbook of Medical Physiology* (7th ed.). Philadelphia: Saunders, 1986.
5. Ham, A.W., and Cormack, D.H. *Histology* (8th ed.). Philadelphia: Lippincott, 1979.
6. Pitot, H.C. *Fundamentals of Oncology* (3rd ed.). New York: Dekker, 1986.
7. Robbins, S.L., Cotran, R.S., and Kumar, V. *Pathologic Basis of Disease* (3rd ed.). Philadelphia: Saunders, 1984.
8. Taussig, M.J. *Processes in Pathology and Microbiology* (2nd ed.). Boston: Blackwell, 1984.
9. Weber, G. Enzymology of cancer cells. *N. Engl. J. Med.* 296:541, 1977.
10. Weiss, L. *Histology, Cell and Tissue Biology* (5th ed.). New York: Elsevier, 1983.

CHAPTER 14

Benign and Malignant Neoplasia

CHAPTER OUTLINE

Definitions
Classification of Neoplasms
Benign Neoplasms
Malignant Neoplasms
Causes of Neoplasia

- Mutational Theories
- Nonmutational Theories

Carcinogens

- Chemical Carcinogens
- Physical Carcinogens
- Oncogenic Viruses

Other Factors in Carcinogenesis

- Diet
- Sexuality
- Habits
- Hormones
- Predisposing Lesions

Growth of the Primary Tumor
Staging of Neoplasms
Metastasis

- Invasion
- Cell Detachment
- Dissemination
  - *Lymphatic Dissemination*
  - *Bloodstream Dissemination*
- Arrest, Establishment, and Proliferation
- Sites of Metastasis

Host Defense Mechanisms in the Control of Neoplasia
Clinical Manifestations of Neoplasms

- Local Manifestations
- Systemic Manifestations

LEARNING OBJECTIVES

1. Define *neoplasm*, *tumor*, *aberrant cellular growth*, *benign*, *malignant*, *cancer*, *carcinoma*, *sarcoma*, and *metastasis*.
2. Define cancer at the clinical, cellular, and molecular levels.
3. Explain the morphologic differences in the subgroups of cancer.
4. Explain staging of malignancies.
5. Compare the characteristics of benign and malignant neoplasms.
6. Describe the mutational and nonmutational causes of neoplasia.
7. Describe the role of DNA and RNA viruses in altering the genetic code.
8. Explain how reverse transcriptase may cause RNA coding of DNA.
9. Identify three viruses associated with specific human cancers.
10. Define *carcinogen*.
11. Identify the two broad groups of carcinogens.
12. Classify chemical carcinogens and identify the neoplasms with which they are associated.
13. Discuss irradiation as a cause of malignant neoplasms.
14. List sources of irradiation and the malignant neoplasms it causes.
15. Relate dietary factors, sexuality, habits, hormones, and predisposing lesions to the development of malignant neoplasms.
16. Explain important factors in primary tumor growth.
17. Describe the TMN classification for staging neoplasms.
18. List the phases of metastasis.
19. Discuss the role of vascularization and collagenase IV in the ability of the malignant cell to break through the basement cell membrane.

LEARNING OBJECTIVES continued

20. Explain how malignant cells detach from the primary neoplasm.
21. Explain dissemination of malignant cells through the lymph and blood vessels.
22. Discuss the role of the immune system in the destruction of malignant cells.
23. Define *tumor-specific antigens*.
24. Explain the mechanisms responsible for the development of local symptoms of neoplasms.
25. Identify symptoms that result from interference with blood supply, interference with function, and mobilization of compensatory mechanisms and immune responses.
26. Define *paraneoplastic syndromes*.
27. Discuss briefly paraneoplastic syndromes of the endocrine, nervous, hematologic, renal, and gastrointestinal systems.
28. Explain the anorexia-cachexia syndrome.

The capacity to undergo mitosis is inherent in all cells. Mitosis is repressed or controlled until a specific stimulation for growth occurs. Every time a normal cell passes through a cycle of division, the opportunity exists for it to become neoplastic. Cancer cells lack repression and therefore lose control of mitosis. The wonder, then, is not that we have so many neoplasms, but that we have so few. Neoplastic disease affects one person in four and causes worldwide problems of morbidity and mortality (Fig. 14-1).

Malignant neoplasms constitute more than 100 distinct disease entities. Cancer can strike at any age. It kills more children aged 3 to 14 years than any other disease [2]. The three leading death-producing cancers in adult males are cancer of the lung, colon and rectum, and prostate gland. For adult females, the most common malignancies are those of the breast, lung, and colon and rectum. Advancing age increases the risk of developing cancer. The frequency rises sharply as age increases, with the death rate from

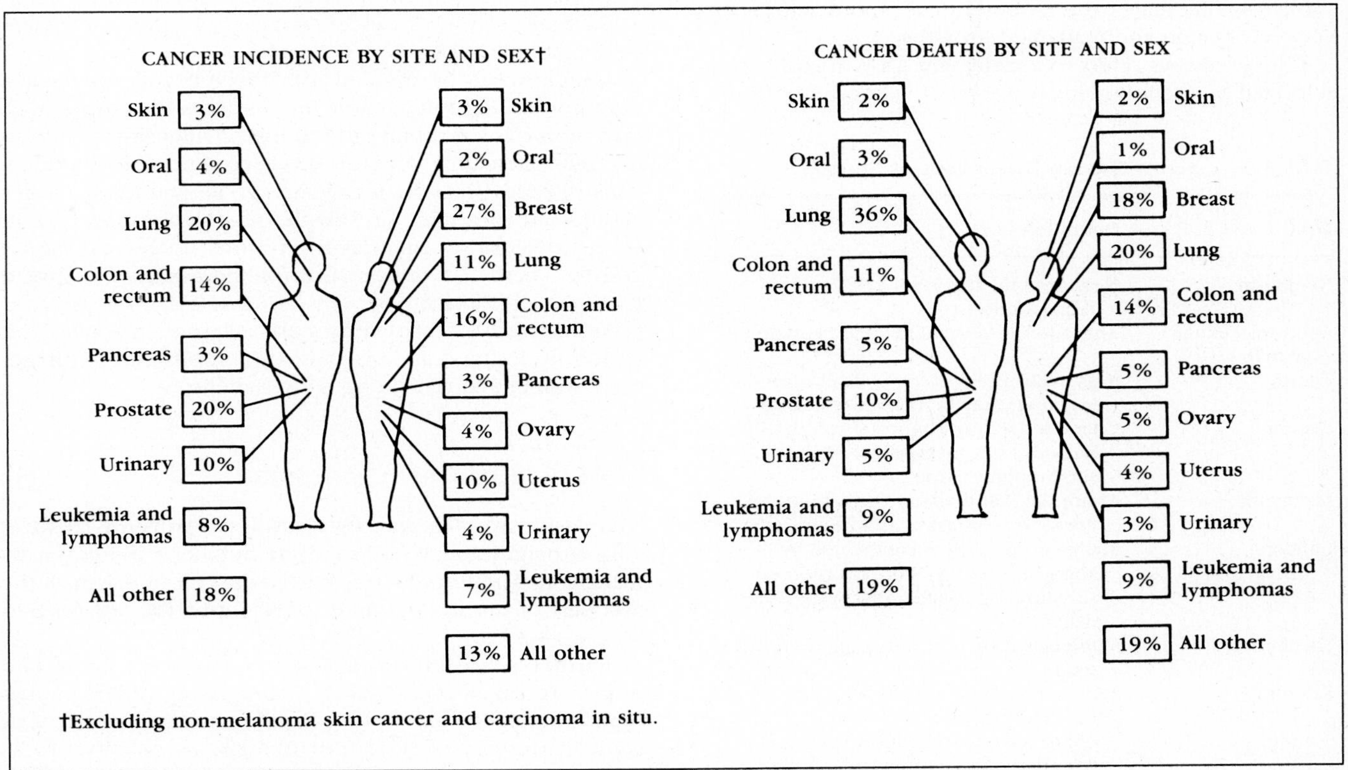

FIGURE 14-1 Cancer incidence and deaths by site and sex, 1986 estimates. The incidence chart excludes nonmelanoma skin cancer and carcinoma in situ. (From *Cancer Facts and Figures 1987*. Rochester, N.Y.: American Cancer Society, 1987.)

cancer of the large intestine, for example, increasing 1000-fold between the ages of 20 and 80 years. Cancer follows heart diseases as the second leading cause of death in the United States, with both morbidity and mortality being greater in blacks than in Caucasians [2].

This chapter compares benign and malignant neoplasms. Various causative factors are discussed and the process of metastasis is explored. The local and systemic effects of neoplasms on the individual are explained using benign and malignant tumors as examples. Neoplasms of specific organs are described in the chapters relating to each system.

Definitions

Terms commonly used in discussions of abnormal cellular growth include neoplasm, tumor, aberrant cellular growth, benign, malignant, cancer, carcinoma, sarcoma, and metastasis (Table 14-1). A *neoplasm* refers to a new growth that is abnormal, and the word is usually used synonomously with *tumor*. *Aberrant cellular growth* refers to an alteration in normal cell growth. The transformation of a normal cell into one that escapes the host's usual controls on growth and differentiation is involved in all aspects of neoplasia.

Malignant and *benign* are words that describe the ability or inability of abnormally dividing cells to invade normal tissues and spread to distant sites in the host. Table 14-2 indicates the commonly accepted differences between benign and malignant growths.

Cancer always refers to a malignant growth and is characterized by the following features: (1) abnormal cell division, (2) invasion of surrounding normal tissues, and (3) spread to distant sites in the host. In humans, cancer consists of a large group of diseases with a variety of local and systemic signs and symptoms. Untreated, widespread systemic effects can cause the death of the host.

TABLE 14-1 Terms Used in Discussions of Neoplasia

Term	Definition
Neoplasm	New growth, abnormal cellular reproduction
Aberrant cellular growth	Alteration in normal cellular growth
Tumor	A growth of neoplastic cells clustered together; may be benign or malignant
Benign	Characterized by abnormal cell division but does not metastasize or invade surrounding tissue
Malignant	Abnormal cell division with ability to invade, metastasize, and recur
Cancer	Malignant growth accompanied by abnormal cell division, invasion of surrounding tissues, and metastasis to distant sites
Carcinoma	Malignant growth originating in epithelial tissue
Sarcoma	Malignant growth originating in mesodermal tissues that form connective tissue, blood vessels, lymphatic organs
Metastasis	Ability to establish secondary tumor growth at a new location away from the primary tumor

TABLE 14-2 A Comparison of Benign and Malignant Neoplasms

Benign	Malignant
Similar to cell of origin	Dissimilar from cell of origin
Edges move outward smoothly (encapsulated)	Edges move outward irregularly
Compresses	Invades
Slow growth rate	Rapid to very rapid growth rate
Slight vascularity	Moderate to marked vascularity
Rarely recur after removal	Frequently recur after removal
Necrosis and ulceration unusual	Necrosis and ulceration common
Systemic effects unusual unless it is a secreting endocrine neoplasm	Systemic effects common

At the cellular level, cancer consists of diseases caused by abnormal cellular growth resulting from defective controls on cell reproduction. Cells lose their differentiation characteristics and become less like the normal parent cell. The loss of differentiation is called anaplasia, which is a characteristic feature of malignancy (see pp. 188–189). At the molecular level, cancer is caused by abnormal nucleic acid metabolism [3].

Cancers may be divided into three broad subgroups: carcinomas, sarcomas, and leukemias and lymphomas. *Carcinoma* is a term often used interchangeably with cancer, but it actually refers to a group of abnormally dividing cells of epithelial origin that invade surrounding tissues and spread to distant sites in the host. *Sarcomas* arise in connective tissues, such as the fibrous tissues and blood vessels. These also invade surrounding tissues and spread to distant sites in the host. The *leukemias* and *lymphomas* arise in the blood-forming cells of bone marrow and lymph nodes, and then invade the mononuclear phagocytic system and remaining body structures.

Classification of Neoplasms

Neoplasms are customarily classified according to their cell of origin and whether their behavior is benign or malignant. The terminology places the cell of origin as the first part of the name, while "oma" forms the last portion (Table 14-3).

Epithelial benign tumors of squamous and basal cell origin are called *papillomas*. Glandular epithelial benign tumors are called *adenomas*. Papillomas or adenomas that grow at the end of a stem or pedicle are referred to as *polyps*, and they may or may not be neoplastic. As stated earlier, malignant neoplasms of epithelial origin are carcinomas. Those of glandular epithelial origin are called *adenocarcinomas*, such as adenocarcinoma of the breast.

TABLE 14-3 Classification of Common Benign and Malignant Neoplasms

Cell	Benign	Malignant
Epithelial		Carcinoma
Squamous	Squamous cell papilloma	Squamous cell carcinoma
Basal cell	Basal cell papilloma	Basal cell carcinoma
Glandular	Adenoma	Adenocarcinoma
Pigmented	Benign melanoma	Malignant melanoma
Muscle		
Smooth muscle	Leiomyoma	Leiomyosarcoma
Striated muscle	Rhabdomyoma	Rhabdomysarcoma
Nerve		
Nerve sheath	Neurilemmoma	Neurofibrosarcoma
Glial cells	Glioma	Glioblastoma
Ganglion cells	Ganglioneuroma	Neuroblastoma
Meninges	Meningioma	Malignant meningioma
Connective tissue		
Fibrous	Fibroma	Fibrosarcoma
Fatty	Lipoma	Liposarcoma
Bone	Osteoma	Osteosarcoma
Cartilage	Chondroma	Chondrosarcoma
Blood vessels	Hemangioma	Angiosarcoma
Lymph vessels	Lymphangioma	Lymphangiosarcoma
Bone marrow		Multiple myeloma Leukemia Ewing's sarcoma
Lymphoid		Malignant lymphoma Lymphosarcoma Reticulum cell sarcoma Lymphatic leukemia Hodgkin's disease
Other blood cells		
Erythrocytes	Polycythemia vera	
Granulocytes		Myelogenous leukemia
Monocytes	Mononucleosis	
B lymphocytes		Plasma cell myeloma Multiple myeloma

Neoplasms of muscle cell origin are named according to muscle type; for example, *leiomyoma*, which means "smooth muscle tumor." Malignant neoplasms of muscle cell origin are *sarcomas*, an example of which is *leiomyosarcoma*. Neoplasms of nerve cells and connective tissue cells are named in a similar manner. Neoplasms of the blood-forming cells and lymph nodes are named according to the type of blood cell affected.

Pigmented and embryonic cells are also indicated in the nomenclature of neoplasms. In normal embryologic development three different layers of cells become apparent. The outer layer is the *ectoderm*, which forms the skin and other structures in the adult human. The middle layer, or *mesoderm*, forms the supporting structures of bone, muscle, fat, blood, and connective tissue. Malignant tumors of these mesodermal or mesenchymal structures are called sarcomas. The inner layer is the *endoderm*, which ultimately forms the gastrointestinal tract and other structures [15]. Sometimes *blastoma* is used to denote that the tissue has a primitive or embryonic appearance. A *teratoma* is another embryonic-appearing tumor that comes from all three germ layers but appears as a highly disorganized array of cells. The teratoma is considered to be benign while the *teratocarcinoma* is malignant. The teratocarcinoma also contains embryonal carcinoma cells that are a population of stem cells whose proliferation is responsible for the malignancy of these tumors [11]. Neoplasms of pigmented cells are named for their cell of origin, the melanocyte. Neoplasms of embryonic cell origin also may contain bits of the germinal layers, such as hair or teeth.

Benign Neoplasms

Benign neoplasms consist of cells that are similar in structure to the cells from which they are derived. The cells of benign neoplasms are more cohesive than those of malignant neoplasms. Growth occurs evenly from the center of the benign mass, usually resulting in a well-defined border. The edges move outward, smoothly pushing adjacent cells out of the way (Fig. 14-2). As this occurs, most of these tumors become encapsulated. The capsule, composed of connective tissue, separates the tumor from surrounding tissues. A benign neoplasm usually grows slowly and is limited to one area. Its blood supply is less profuse than that of a malignant neoplasm. A benign neoplasm rarely recurs after surgical removal and rarely ulcerates, undergoes necrosis, or causes systemic problems. An exception is a secreting endocrine neoplasm, which causes symptoms resulting from excess hormone secretion.

Malignant Neoplasms

Malignant neoplasms have atypical cell structure, with abnormal nuclear divisions and chromosomes. The malignant cell loses its differentiation or resemblance to the cell of origin. The tumor cells are not cohesive and consequently, the pattern of growth is irregular; no capsule is

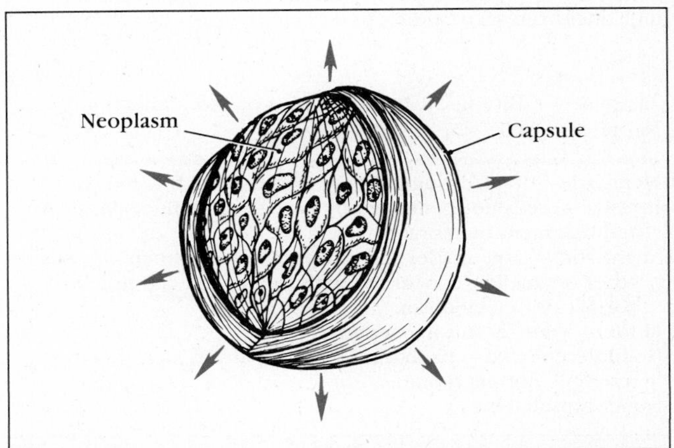

FIGURE 14-2 An encapsulated benign neoplasm. Arrows indicate equal expansion from the center.

formed, and distinct separation from surrounding tissues is difficult (Fig. 14-3). Malignant cells invade adjacent cells rather than pushing them aside. Tumors have varying growth rates and develop a greater blood supply than normal tissues or benign neoplasms (see p. 197). The hallmark of a malignant neoplasm is its ability to metastasize or spread to distant sites. Table 14-4 summarizes the biologic characteristics of the tumor. It frequently recurs after surgical removal and can cause systemic problems.

Causes of Neoplasia

Most research related to the etiology of neoplasia concerns malignant tumors. Because cancer is not 1 disease but more than 100 entities, it probably has a phenomenal number of etiologies. None of the theories that attempt to explain the peculiarities of the cancer cell has been completely successful. Cancer is revealing itself as a highly logical, coordinated process by which cells turn the usual benign life purposes to the most dangerous of ends [16]. Many areas of study have evolved to explain the nature of the different disease processes. These include mutational theories, which suggest that cancer genes (oncogenes) can cause a genetic mutation or rearrangement that makes a cell become cancerous. The nonmutational theories suggest that cancers arise from epigenetic mechanisms, or activation of genes normally repressed [3]. The neoplastic cells fail to respond to normal cellular signals of differentiation.

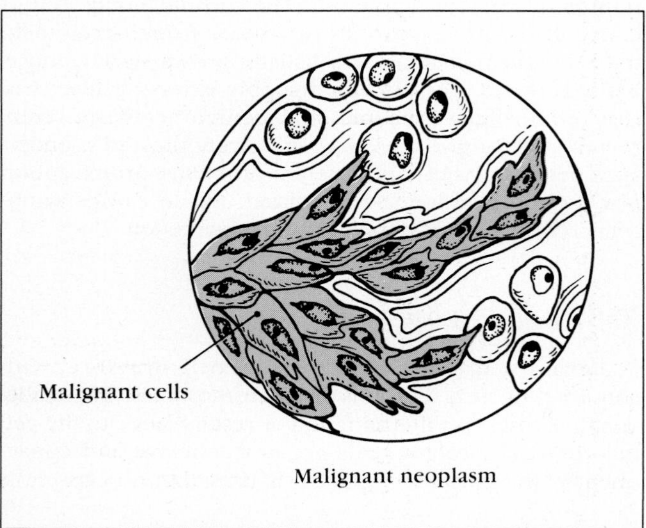

FIGURE 14-3 A malignant neoplasm with irregular borders, indistinct from surrounding tissues.

TABLE 14-4 Biologic Characteristics of the Malignant Neoplastic Cell

Metastatic — transferring to other tissues by blood and lymph.
Invasive — cells not contained by barriers of connective tissue and basement membrane.
Anaplastic — large nuclei and nucleoli; fewer mitochondria and other organelles; concerned with replication and not with normal cell metabolism.
Mitotic — greater mitotic activity.
Nondifferentiated — haphazard growth pattern, does not resemble normal tissues.
Nonencapsulated.

Source: Reprinted by permission from *Cell Pathology* (2nd ed.) by N.F. Cheville. © 1983 by Iowa State University Press, 2121 South State Avenue, Ames, Iowa, 50010.

Mutational Theories

The theory of somatic cell mutation was formulated by Bauer in 1928. It supports the concept that genetic abnormalities can be induced by mutational carcinogenic agents and hereditary susceptibility. There is strong evidence that this mutational process is progressive and involves many steps [17]. Some cancers can develop as a result of more than one carcinogenic influence.

Numerous substances have been identified as having cancer-causing abilities. These include physical and chemical agents, as well as oncogenic viruses (see p. 196). The substances must undergo molecular modification inside the cell to cause the cancer. Foreign substances are normally modified and detoxified by different enzymes, but certain individuals have enzymes that modify the carcinogens in such a way as to bind to the nuclear DNA. This modification is called *activation* and it becomes the first step in cancer-causing mutations [16]. The individuality of enzyme systems may be one factor that accounts for susceptibility to different forms of cancers. In many cases the DNA disruption can be repaired and the process does not progress. The mutation that is produced also must affect particular genes to initiate the cancerous process [16].

In the 1940s Berenblum described a two-step mutational model that involved *initiation* and *promotion*. The initial mutation, called *initiation*, increases the sensitivity of the cell to surrounding promoters and a larger population of initiated cells is formed. The processes of initiation and promotion probably must go on for several cycles with subsequent mutations of initiated cells before a tumorous mass can be formed.

Nonmutational Theories

Some tumors arise from epigenetic mechanisms that cause neoplastic transformation in the process of normal differentiation. The cells identified often have a very embryonic appearance. The frequency of malignant neoplasms often increases during periods of alteration in growth and development [17].

Carcinogens

Since 1775, when Sir Percival Pott linked the occurrence of scrotal cancer in chimney sweeps and their exposure to soot, it has been known that certain substances are capable of inducing neoplastic growth. These substances are *carcinogens* or *oncogens*. Carcinogens are known to increase the likelihood that exposed individuals will develop a neoplasm. *Cocarcinogens* increase the activity of carcinogens. Some substances in higher doses and exposure rates are carcinogenic, while at lower doses and exposure rates they may be cocarcinogenic. *Procarcinogens* are carcinogens that must be activated or modified in the cell [15]. Many procarcinogens in their original form cannot induce cellular changes, but require metabolic activation in the body. Three types of carcinogens are examined in the subsequent pages: (1) chemical, (2) physical, and (3) viral.

Chemical Carcinogens

Many agents are capable of causing neoplasms either in humans or animals [17]. Chemical carcinogens can be grouped as polycyclic aromatic hydrocarbons, aromatic amines, alkylating agents, nitrosamines and other nitrosocompounds, naturally occurring products, drugs, metals, and industrial carcinogens (Table 14-5).

Polycyclic aromatic hydrocarbons are some of the most powerful carcinogens. They are present in the condensates of tobacco smoke, automobile exhaust, and other products of combustion. Cancers of the lips, tongue, oral cavity, head, neck, larynx, lungs, and bladder are associated with exposure to polycyclic aromatic hydrocarbons.

Aromatic amines and *azodyes* are another significant group of carcinogens. These include certain foods, naphthalene (a coal tar used in moth repellents and insecticides), and 2-acetylaminofluorene, an insecticide. The aromatic amines have been linked with cancer of the bladder [17].

TABLE 14-5 A Summary of Chemical Carcinogens and Their Sites of Action

Carcinogens	Source	Sites of Action
Polycyclic aromatic amines	Soots, tars, cigarette smoke, benzpyrene	Lips, tongue, oral cavity, head, neck, larynx, lungs, bladder
Aromatic amines	Dyes, naphthalene, 2-acetylamino-fluorene	Bladder
Alkylating agents	Nitrogen mustard and mustard gas, drugs (cyclophos-phamide, melphalan)	Lungs, larynx, bladder, hemopoietic system
Nitrosamines and nitroso-compounds	4-Nitrobiphenyl	
Naturally occurring products	Aflatoxin B, betel nut	Liver, oral cavity
Drugs	Griseofulvin, hycanthone, metronidazole, diethylstilbestrol	Cancers in rats, vagina, bladder, hemopoietic system

Alkylating agents in controlled circumstances are used for therapeutic purposes but can be carcinogenic. Two common alkylating agents are nitrogen mustard (cyclophosphamide) and mustard gas. Both are implicated in the causation of leukemia and lymphoid neoplasms [17].

Nitrosamines and other nitrosocompounds develop under physiologic conditions from chemical interactions between nitrites and other secondary amines. Numerous drugs and nicotine may supply the amines for the process of converting nitrites to nitrosamines. Nitrites are present in foods as additives. These agents require activation and may be contributors to gastric carcinomas [18].

Naturally occurring products implicated in the causation of malignant neoplasm include aflatoxin and the betel nut. Aflatoxin B is a mold, *Aspergillus flavus*, found on corn, barley, peas, rice, soybeans, fruit, some nuts, milk, and cheddar cheese. It has been linked to liver cancer in humans. In animals, aflatoxin B has been shown to cause liver, stomach, colon, and kidney cancer [17]. Chewing the betel nut has been implicated in cancer of the oral cavity.

Several *drugs* besides the alkylating agents are known to have carcinogenic effects. Griseofulvin, an antifungal agent used to treat mycotic disease of the skin; hycanthone, an antischistosomal agent; and metronidazole, an antiprotozoal used to treat *Trichomonas vaginalis* and *Entamoeba histolytica* cause cancer in rats. Diethylstilbestrol (DES), used during the 1950s to prevent spontaneous abortion, increased the frequency of cancer of the vagina in the daughters of women who received this treatment. Studies also have shown increased prevalence of malignancy in male offspring of treated mothers (see Chap. 52).

Alcohol deserves special mention as a cancer-causing drug. Heavy consumption is associated with cancer of the mouth, pharynx, esophagus, larynx, and liver [11]. Alcohol apparently enhances the effects of procarcinogens and carcinogens such as nicotine by increasing their solubility, altering liver metabolism, altering the intracellular metabolism of epithelial cells, and causing nutritional deficiencies [11].

Asbestos, cadmium, chromium, and nickel are some of the *metals* involved in carcinogenesis. All are associated with cancer of the lung. Chromium and nickel may also cause nasal cavity tumors. Cadmium may be associated with cancer of the prostate gland. Asbestos may cause malignancy of the pleural cavity and gastrointestinal tract.

Industrial compounds have been implicated in carcinogenesis. One example of these is polyvinyl chloride, which is used in the manufacture of plastics and may cause angiosarcomas of the liver [10].

Physical Carcinogens

Ionizing radiation is a recognized cause of cellular mutations. Damage to DNA may be direct or indirect. Direct damage results from interaction of the electron itself with the DNA of the cell. Indirect damage occurs when a secondary electron interacts with a water molecule, giving rise to a free radical, which then damages DNA [16]. A long latent period often exists between exposure and the development of clinical disease. Firm evidence links exposure to large doses of irradiation to leukemia.

Overexposure to irradiation from atomic bomb detonation has been extensively studied in survivors of Hiroshima and Nagasaki, Japan. The high prevalence of leukemia in these persons supports the relationship between leukemia and irradiation.

Even low doses of irradiation may cause cancer in susceptible individuals. The frequency of breast cancer increases with small, widely spread doses of irradiation, and that of thyroid cancer increases with head and neck radiograms during childhood. Radiograms of the fetus in utero increase its chances of developing childhood cancer.

Ultraviolet radiation from the sun is a major cause of skin cancers. Fair-complexioned individuals are more likely to develop skin cancers than their darker-complexioned counterparts because of the lack of melanin, which protects the latter from injurious effects of the sun (see Chap. 43) [12].

Plastic films implanted at various body sites in rodents have been shown to be carcinogenic. A profuse foreign body reaction occurs before the tumor develops. Sarcomas have been observed in relation to foreign body reactions in humans, but no conclusive evidence is available regarding cancer and prosthetic insertions.

Schistosoma haematobium infestations, common in inhabitants of the Nile Valley, Mozambique, and Rhodesia, are associated with squamous cell carcinoma of the bladder. The development of this cancer is also preceded by chronic inflammation and fibrosis of the bladder wall.

Injections of mineral oil into the peritoneal cavity of mice causes a granulomatous inflammation of the peritoneum, followed by plasma cell tumors [9]. This seems to support the role of chronic inflammation or foreign body reactions in the development of neoplasms [6].

Asbestos fibers are associated with bronchogenic and gastrointestinal carcinomas in humans continuously exposed to the substances. The fibers are thought to function as promoters for other carcinogens such as cigarette smoke [17]. Chronic pulmonary tuberculosis is also associated with an increased frequency of lung carcinoma. Chronic injury of the mucosa of the lips and gums from dentures or pipe smoking leads to increased occurrence of oral cancer.

Oncogenic Viruses

Viruses are thought to cause human malignant neoplasms and have been directly associated with tumor induction in animals. Viruses implicated in human cancers are called oncogenic viruses. Current evidence favors the view that viruses alter the genome of the infected cell, which then alters the progeny (offspring) of the host cell [17].

The two types of oncogenic viruses are deoxyribonucleic acid (DNA) and ribonucleic acid (RNA). The DNA viruses are incorporated into the genes of the host and are then transmitted to subsequent generations. The genes are then expressed without the usual symptoms that accompany infections [15]. The RNA viruses, or *retroviruses*, also contribute genetic information to the host cell. The mechanism for this viral transmission appears to involve a reversal of the normal processes. Thus, the transcription and synthesis of DNA results from an RNA template using an enzyme called reverse transcriptase [17]. This explanation clarifies the process by which genes are expanded and new DNA sequences are developed without the parent structures being altered (Fig. 14-4). As part of the genome of the host cell, the virus is not attacked and destroyed by the immune system. Present evidence favors the view that *reverse transcriptase* acts to accomplish *reverse transcription*, to degrade RNA in the new DNA-RNA complex and to form the new DNA double strand [17].

Some viruses associated with human malignant neoplasms are the C-type and B-type RNA viruses, and certain DNA viruses. Although the mechanism is not clearly established, the C-type RNA viruses are implicated as causative agents in the development of certain types of leukemias; the B-type RNA viruses may be factors in causing breast cancer and herpesviruses may be associated with cervical cancer. The Epstein-Barr virus, a DNA virus of the herpes type, has been closely associated with Burkitt's lymphoma and nasopharyngeal carcinoma [17]. Table 14-6 summarizes the viruses most closely implicated in the development of malignant neoplasia.

Other Factors in Carcinogenesis

Epidemiologic studies have revealed other factors in the occurrence of neoplasms besides chemical and physical

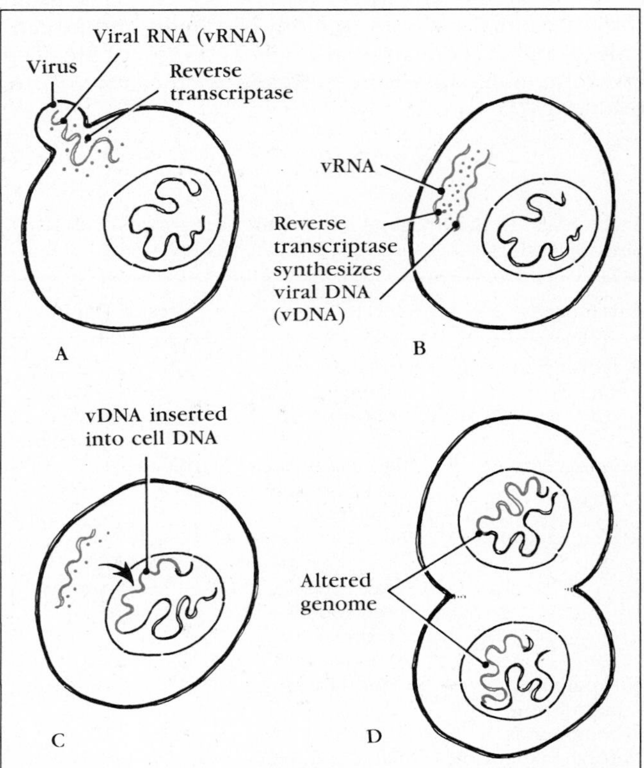

FIGURE 14-4 Schematic showing how RNA viruses change the genome of the cell and cause replication of new cells with altered genome. A. Virus infects the cell. B. Alteration of cell RNA by virus (vRNA). C. Alteration of cell DNA. D. Duplication of the cell, with altered DNA going to the progeny.

Table 14-6 Viruses Implicated in Malignant Neoplasia

Virus	Associated Malignancy
C type RNA	Leukemia
B type RNA	Breast cancer
Herpes II	Cancer of cervix
Epstein-Barr	Burkitt's lymphoma, nasopharyngeal cancers

carcinogens. These factors are primarily related to habits of daily living and religious or cultural traditions. Some predispose persons to the development of neoplasms, while others serve a protective function. For example, cancer of the stomach is more common in Japan than in the United States, while cancers of the intestine, breast, and prostate are less common. These differences are lost within a generation or two after Japanese individuals take residence in the United States.

Diet

Dietary customs have been the subject of a great deal of research. Diets high in fat and low in fiber content have been implicated in cancers of the colon and breast. The mechanisms postulated for these connections include the estrogen hormone for breast cancer and the slowing of transit time in colon cancer. Food preservation seems to play a role in carcinogenesis. The nitrates used in some food preservatives can be activated, and nitrates in water and soil can be reduced to nitrites by the body [18]. Foods preserved by salting, drying, or charring increase the consumer's risk of cancer of the stomach [20].

Sexuality

Customs and religious beliefs involving sexuality seem to have a role in carcinogenesis. Cancer of the cervix is more likely to occur in women who begin having sexual intercourse at a young age and who have many sexual partners. The frequency of cervical cancer is lowest in nuns, virgins, and Jewish women. The last is thought to be due to hygiene practices and circumcision. Cancer of the penis is also lowest among Jewish men who are circumcised shortly after birth. Cancer of the breast is more prevalent in women who have no children, who begin menses early, or who enter menopause late [2,20]. Kaposi's sarcoma, a virus-associated tumor, occurs mainly in victims of acquired immune deficiency syndrome. This is a disease mainly of homosexual males and intravenous-drug abusers (see pp. 164–166).

Habits

A person who consumes 6 oz. of 80-proof alcohol a day over a period of time increases the risk of developing cancer of the esophagus 2 to 3 times. The risk is even greater for those who also smoke cigarettes. A person who smokes cigarettes increases the risk of lung cancer fourfold by smoking 9 to 10 cigarettes a day, or 10 or more times by smoking a pack or more a day. There also seems to be a relationship between polluted air and cigarette smoking, and the development of cancer [2].

Hormones

Alterations in hormonal balance resulting in increased hormone levels over a prolonged time may cause neoplasms in the target cells. Cancer of the breast, endometrium, vagina, prostate, thyroid, and adrenal cortex are thought to be related to altered hormonal influences.

Predisposing Lesions

Many neoplastic changes in tissues are known to be precancerous. For example, chronic cystic disease of the breast predisposes the individual to cancer of the breast. Adenomatous polyps of the colon and rectum remain questionably precancerous.

Growth of the Primary Tumor

Benign tumors are considered to grow more slowly than malignant tumors. The rate of growth of a benign neoplasm is variable and depends upon such factors as hormone dependence and adequate blood supply.

The growth rate of malignant tumors does tend to correlate with their level of differentiation. Therefore, the more undifferentiated or anaplastic a tumor, the greater is its potential for aggressive growth and dissemination.

The primary tumor usually grows for years before producing a clinically overt mass [17]. It depends upon the cellular reproduction of tumor cells. Each time a cell reproduces, it doubles the tumor mass; from 1 to 2 to 4 to 8, and so on. It is estimated that a typical tumor has doubled 30 times before it becomes clinically observed. A 40-time doubling often proves to be fatal to the host. The growth fraction is the ratio of proliferating to nonproliferating cells. As the total volume of the tumor increases, the growth fraction usually decreases. Another factor is the number of cells of the primary tumor that are lost through death or shedding into a hostile environment [14].

The rate of tumor growth is affected by many influences, including blood supply, nutrition, immune responsiveness, and, in some tumors, endocrine support. Studies have shown that many tumors elaborate a *tumor angiogenesis factor (TAF)* that promotes directional blood vessel growth into the tumor mass [7]. If a tumor outgrows its blood supply, central ischemic necrosis may occur. In a nutritionally depleted host, the tumor growth may slow due to a decrease in the supply of adequate nutrients [17].

Staging of Neoplasms

Staging is an effort to describe the extent of a neoplasm in terms that are commonly understood. The purposes of staging are to: (1) determine treatment, (2) evaluate survival rates, (3) establish the relative merits of different methods of treatment, and (4) facilitate the exchange of information among treatment centers. The TMN classification varies slightly with different types of malignancy, but provides some general principles of staging (Table 14-7).

The three capital letters are used to denote the following: T—the tumor or primary lesion and its extent, N—lymph nodes of the region and their condition, and M—distant metastasis [15]. *Tumor in situ*, or localized tumor, is abbreviated TIS. The term T_x is used when the extent of tumor cannot be assessed adequately. Using the letter *T* and adding ascending numbers indicates increasing tumor size. The spread of malignancy to regional lymph nodes is indicated by N_1, referring to "few," with N_2 referring to many nodal metastases [17]. The presence or absence of distant metastasis is designated by a M_0, M_1, or M_2. When the amount or extent of metastasis cannot be assessed, M_x is used.

Metastasis

The ability of a malignant neoplasm to spread to distant sites is *metastasis*. A clump of malignant cells, no longer attached to the original neoplasm, travels to and becomes established at a new site. The original malignancy is the primary neoplasm, tumor, or site. Metastasis involves the release of many malignant cells, only some of which are able to survive the defense mechanisms and hostile environment [19]. Five phases are involved in the process of metastasis: (1) invasion, (2) cell detachment, (3) dissemination, (4) arrest and establishment, and (5) proliferation (Fig. 14-5) [14].

TABLE 14-7 TNM System of Clinical Staging of Neoplasms

Neoplasm	Description
Tumor	
T_o	No evidence of primary tumor.
TIS	Carcinoma in situ.
T_1, T_2, T_3, T_4	Progressive increase in tumor size and involvement.
T_x	Tumor cannot be assessed.
Nodes	
N_o	Regional lymph nodes not demonstrably abnormal.
N_1, N_2, N_3, etc.	Increasing degrees of demonstrable abnormality of regional lymph nodes. (For many primary sites the subscript "a," e.g., N_{1a}, may be used to indicate that metastasis to the node is not suspected; and the subscript "b," e.g., N_{1b}, may be used to indicate that metastasis to the node is suspected or proved.)
N_x	Regional lymph nodes cannot be assessed clinically.
Metastasis	
M_o	No evidence of distance metastasis.
M_1, M_2, M_3	Ascending degrees of distant metastasis, including metastasis to distant lymph nodes.

Source: Adapted from "Clinical Staging System for Carcinoma of the Lung," published by the American Joint Committee for Cancer Staging and End Results Reporting, Chicago: American Joint Committee, September, 1973. By H.C. Pitot in *Fundamentals of Oncology*, (3rd ed.), Marcel Dekker, Inc., New York, 1986. Reprinted from *Fundamentals of Oncology*, Table 7.4, by courtesy of Marcel Dekker, Inc.

Invasion

To invade normal adjacent cells, the malignant cells grow out from their original location into the neighboring location. To infiltrate a body cavity or blood vessel, the malignant cells must break through the basement cell membrane. They may escape into the bloodstream through gaps between endothelial cells as rapidly growing capillary tubes penetrate the basement membrane of the capillaries.

A major structural component of the basement cell membrane is type IV collagen. It has been suggested that an enzymatic action causes dissolution of the basement membrane so that tumor cells can penetrate it. This enzyme, *collagenase type IV*, actively attaches to and dissolves type IV collagen [7]. Greatly damaged endothelium has high levels of collagenase IV, which may be significant as malignant cells select invasion sites [7].

Cell Detachment

After invading the neighboring tissues, body cavities, and blood vessels, malignant cells separate from the primary neoplasm and penetrate lymphatic or blood vessels. As discussed on pages 185–186, the tumor cells lack the property of adhesion and are easily shed into surrounding tissues, blood, and lymph.

Dissemination

The most common route that malignant cells take to distant sites from the primary neoplasm is through the lymphatic and blood vessels. Malignant cells move from lymphatic to blood vessels and vice versa. A malignant neoplasm of just a few grams may shed several million cells into the circulation each day. A very large proportion of these cells die, and few possess the factors necessary for survival in the hostile, turbulent circulatory system [13]. To survive in the circulatory system and to effect arrest in the endothelium, malignant cells undergo a variety of cellular interactions involving immunity and adherence.

Lymphatic Dissemination. As the tumor invades surrounding tissue it penetrates the small lymphatic vessels. Tumor cell emboli are shed into the vessels and trapped in the first lymph node encountered [5]. The lymph nodes of a group may become involved with disease or some may be skipped [7]. The lymph node often enlarges, which may be due to a localized reaction to the tumor cells or growth of the tumor within the node. Stimulation of the immune defense system may contain the material or filter the tumor cells from the circulation. This may decrease the net spread of tumor [8].

There are numerous venous-lymphatic communications by which tumor cells can pass between the blood

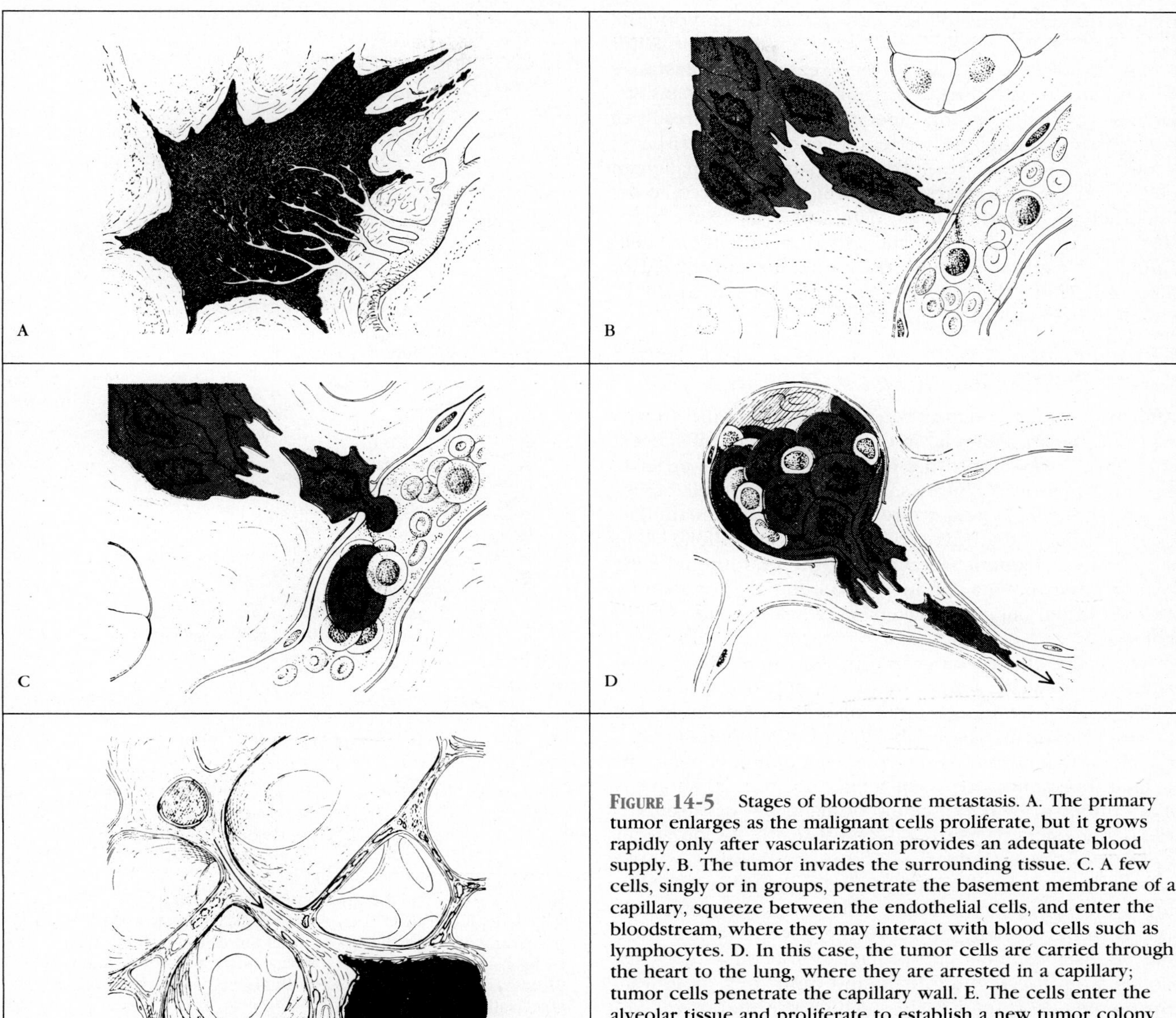

FIGURE 14-5 Stages of bloodborne metastasis. A. The primary tumor enlarges as the malignant cells proliferate, but it grows rapidly only after vascularization provides an adequate blood supply. B. The tumor invades the surrounding tissue. C. A few cells, singly or in groups, penetrate the basement membrane of a capillary, squeeze between the endothelial cells, and enter the bloodstream, where they may interact with blood cells such as lymphocytes. D. In this case, the tumor cells are carried through the heart to the lung, where they are arrested in a capillary; tumor cells penetrate the capillary wall. E. The cells enter the alveolar tissue and proliferate to establish a new tumor colony. (From G.L. Nicolson, Cancer metastasis. *Sci. Am.* 240:70, 1979. Reprinted with permission.)

vessels and lymph systems. The main communication lies at the thoracic duct where lymphatic fluid empties directly into the venous circulation. Tumor cells brought to the lungs by the thoracic duct may be trapped in the pulmonary capillary bed or break into the pulmonary veins and reach the systemic circulation [5].

Bloodstream Dissemination. Just as the tumor spreads into and sheds its cells into the lymphatic system, it also can spread into the microcirculation. The spreading is facilitated when collagenase IV is present because this enzyme dissolves the capillary basement membrane and enhances dissemination. Tumor then may grow at the site of vascular spread or it may embolize to other parts of the body. Most tumor cells do not survive the turbulence of circulating blood. The chances for survival improve if the tumor cells aggregate with one another or with host cells such as platelets or leukocytes.

Metastasis requires entrapment in the capillary bed of distant organs [8]. Fibrin deposits often form around the new tumor and may protect it from destruction by immune defensive cells. After the tumor is carried to the lungs, it may invade branches of the pulmonary veins and be released into the systemic circulation to travel to the brain or viscera [5]. If the tumor is shed into the portal venous system, it often ends in liver metastasis.

The *vertebral vein plexus* provides some answers regarding the odd distributions of metastases of certain tumors. This plexus of veins has no valves and communicates with all major vein systems [5]. It obviously carries neoplastic cells from the prostate gland to the vertebra, pelvis, and femur in the absence of evidence of other metastatic disease. Cancer of the breast may metastasize specifically to the dorsal vertebra, as do lung cancers. Even some of the cerebral metastases may be a result of cells passing through the vertebral venous plexus [5].

Adherence is also involved in the survival of malignant cells in the circulatory system, as well as their arrest in the endothelium of the capillary. Malignant cells form clumps that enter the capillary bed and adhere to endothelial cells lining the capillary, where they become entrapped or arrested. There the clump surrounds itself with fibrin, which protects it during growth.

Arrest, Establishment, and Proliferation

After becoming trapped in the small vessels of the arteries or veins, the aberrant clump of malignant cells must break through the vessel into the interstitial spaces in order to continue to grow. Cell-free spaces in the endothelial lining of the capillary appear to be induced by the malignant cells, a process that involves alterations in cellular adhesion and consequent retraction of the endothelial cells. A new environment conducive to cellular growth must be established once the malignant cells are in the interstitial spaces.

Once the clump has grown to exceed about 2 cm in diameter, it can no longer supply its nutritional needs by diffusion. Its own blood supply becomes essential for further development. The establishment of a blood supply is the factor that changes a self-contained clump of malignant cells into a rapidly growing metastatic tumor. As in primary tumor growth, the clump of malignant cells secretes tumor-angiogenesis factor, which causes the blood vessels to send out new capillaries. These new capillaries grow toward and eventually penetrate the malignant cells, creating a blood supply through which the malignant cells receive nourishment and have their waste products removed. Establishment and proliferation of these cells also depends on the immunologic and outer cell membrane properties discussed earlier. Thus, the malignant cell adjusts its environment to further its own growth. Figure 14-6 illustrates the possible outcomes of metastasis from the primary tumor.

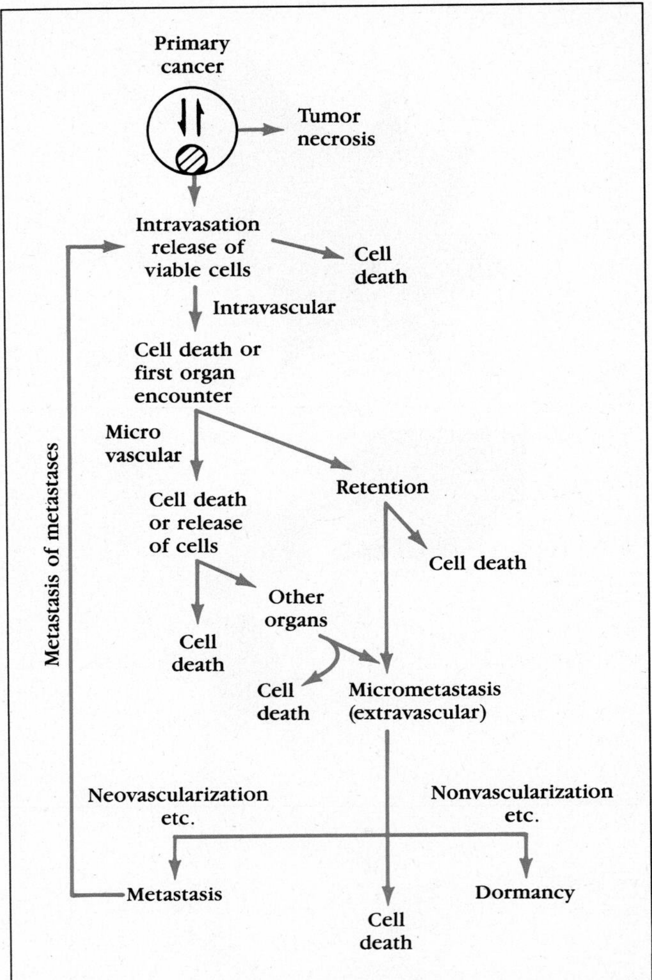

FIGURE 14-6 The metastatic process showing cell loss and gain. This illustration shows intravascular metastasis to organ involvement. Note that more cells die in the process than survive and grow. (From L. Weiss and H. A. Gilbert, *Liver Metastasis.* Copyright © 1982. Reprinted by permission of G.K. Hall.)

Sites of Metastasis

Primary tumors have a great tendency to metastasize to and grow in specific organs. Because a small tumor can release several million cells a day into the bloodstream, eventually some will arrest and survive at a receptive site [8]. Patterns of metastasis apparently are determined by individual cellular characteristics and by environmental factors [13].

Certain primary malignant neoplasms metastasize more readily to specific sites. For example, cancer of the breast metastasizes to the lungs and brain, while cancer of the prostate or adrenals metastasizes to the bone. The site of the metastatic neoplasm is not randomly chosen but may be based on mechanical considerations involving cell size, pressure, vessel size, and other physical features. Also, the site of metastasis may be similar to the site that fostered the primary growth. Vascularity of the secondary site is a well-established need. The lungs may well be a popular site simply because malignant cells entering the venous system enter their first capillary network there.

Host Defense Mechanisms in the Control of Neoplasia

Investigations have shown that some human tumors have tumor-specific antigens on their cell surfaces. Various nonmalignant tissues also elaborate a number of different antigens. Among these are the oncofetal antigens, lineage-associated antigens, differentiation antigens, and histocompatibility determinants [1]. In a malignant neoplasm the

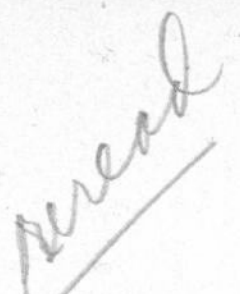

antigen-bearing cells are expanding, so that as the tumor grows, the total tumor-associated antigen (TAA) also increases. If treatment decreases the pool of TAA, measuring the amount of TAA can be very helpful in plotting the course of certain cancers. The use of TAA as a target for clinical treatment is limited because its expression varies among cells within a tumor.

Oncofetal antigens are those normally present during embryonic development and reexpressed in some neoplastic tissue. Useful markers of this classification include the carcinoembryonic antigen (CEA), alphafetoprotein (AFP), and gross cystic disease protein (GCDP).

Studies are continuing into the significance of the differentiation antigens that are present mainly in the lymphocytic and lymphoblastic leukemias [1].

Lineage-associated determinants have been noted in several solid tumors and may prove useful in the future for monitoring gastrointestinal and ovarian tumors.

Histocompatibility antigens are being studied in neoplastic tissue with the goal being to use a host-versus-tumor reaction to destroy the tumor or metastasis. If the immune system can recognize the tumor as foreign, the immunization prepared from host tumor or tumor cell membranes of a donor may cause the host to reject the tumor. In animal studies these processes have been quite successful, but in humans the response has been variable [4].

The immune system has natural defenses for tumor destruction. When the tumor cell antigen is recognized by the immune system as being foreign, it may be destroyed by T cell cytotoxic response, by natural killer (NK) cells, by macrophage intervention, or by B cells and complement activation. Apparently, T cells and NK cells contact the foreign material directly and destroy its membrane. Activated macrophages bind to and destroy neoplastic cells more readily than normal cells. In antibody reactions the antibody apparently serves as a bridge between the effector (NK cells, macrophages, polymorphonuclear leukocytes, etc.) and target cells (Fig. 14-7). When complement is involved, the final activated complement can cause the destruction of tumor cells [1].

If the immune system is capable of destroying neoplastic tissue, how do tumor cells escape destruction? Many human tumors lack tumor-specific antigens or the antigen is not expressed at the cell surface to be recognized as foreign. Some tumors can modulate the expression of antigen after exposure to the immune system. Immune suppression in individuals debilitated by systemic disease or irradiation or chemotherapy predisposes them to a higher than normal frequency of later malignancies, especially leukemia and lymphoma. Persons with malignancies may have specific and nonspecific suppressor factors particularly active against T cells [1].

Tumor immunology is very complex and is in the early stages of understanding. Deficiency in lymphocyte function has been described with certain malignancies, and further deficiency has been imposed with various forms of cancer treatment. Certain malignancies do seem to evoke an immune response, but as of now, immunotherapy has been disappointing. Monoclonal antibodies may become useful in radioimmunoassays for tumor markers or to localize tumor mass. These antibodies may be carriers of molecules lethal to tumor cells in future treatment methods [4].

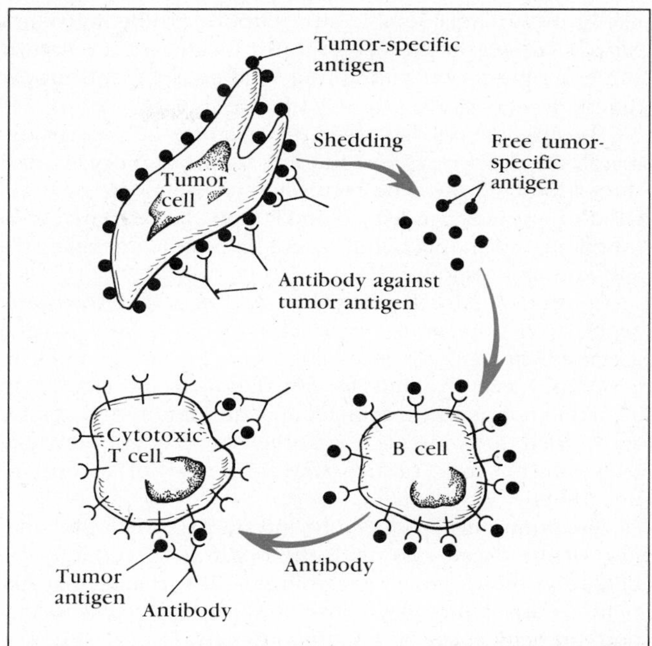

FIGURE 14-7 Postulated humoral and cellular immunity reactions in tumor destruction.

Certain malignancies can be followed by biochemical methods. The choriocarcinoma elaborates a particular form of human choriogonadotropin (HCG) and AFP. High levels of AFP have been associated with liver and embryonal carcinomas. Carcinoembryonic antigen has been used as an indicator of colon, liver, stomach, and even lung metastasis, and is useful in following affected persons for recurrence of disease. Other substances useful in biochemical studies of specific malignancies include calcitonin, parathyroid hormone, prostaglandins, adrenocorticotropic hormone (ACTH), and antidiuretic hormone (ADH) [4].

Clinical Manifestations of Neoplasms

In their earliest stages of development, benign and malignant neoplasms are asymptomatic. The mass of cells simply is not large enough to interfere with any bodily function. As it increases in size, however, local alterations in function occur. As malignant neoplasms metastasize, they interfere with function at distant sites and disrupt the biochemical balance of the body.

Local Manifestations

The nature and development of local symptomatology depends on the location of the neoplasm and on the size and distensibility of the space it occupies. A neoplasm located in the abdomen, which is large and distensible, may grow to considerable size without producing symptoms. A neoplasm the size of a pea located in the cranial vault, a rigid space containing vital sensory and motor functions, may cause major symptoms.

The mass of cells that makes up a primary or a metastatic neoplasm compresses surrounding tissues and organs, and their blood supply. The resulting symptomatology is related to interference with blood supply, interference with function, and mobilization of compensatory mechanisms and immune responses.

Compression by the neoplasm interferes with the blood supply to tissues and/or organs and decreases their oxygen and nutrient supply, resulting in ischemia and necrosis. In addition, waste products are not removed, and lactic acid accumulates. As lactic acid accumulates and blood vessels are eroded, the individual experiences pain and bleeding. Ischemic necrotic tissues may form sites of secondary infections.

The symptoms produced by interference with the function of the organ vary with the organ involved and the degree of interference. A carcinoma of the lung that obstructs a bronchus may cause atelectasis, abscess formation, bronchiectasis, or pneumonitis distal to the site. The obstruction inhibits removal of secretions and bacteria from the area distal to it. The person experiences coughing, which may or may not be productive, together with signs and symptoms of infection. Infection is common in structures obstructed by a neoplasm. Neoplasms of the colon obstruct the bowel. If the obstruction is incomplete, the individual experiences pencil-thin stools, constipation, and cramping. Activated function, rather than an altered function, may occur. For example, compression of nerves or stretching of a nerve-rich membrane by a tumor stimulates the nerve and produces pain.

Compensatory mechanisms also vary with the organ involved. The cramping associated with obstruction of the bowel is the result of increased peristalsis in an attempt to force a fecal mass past the obstruction. Mobilization of the immune system awakens the inflammatory response. As a result, the individual experiences increased pulse rate, elevated temperature, and elevated white blood cell count.

Systemic Manifestations

Neoplasms have systemic as well as local effects. Systemic symptoms may be the first indication that a person has a neoplasm, or they may accompany more advanced metastatic disease. They include anorexia, nausea, weight loss, and malaise, as well as signs and symptoms of anemia and infection. These signs and symptoms occur away from the primary tumor or metastasis and are not a direct effect of either one. The term used to describe them is *paraneoplastic syndromes* [17]. Up to 75 percent of all persons with a malignant neoplasm experience a paraneoplastic syndrome sometime during their illness. Significant paraneoplastic syndromes involve the endocrine, nervous, hemotologic, renal, and gastrointestinal systems.

Only those hormones produced by nonendocrine neoplastic tissues are considered to be paraneoplastic. Symptoms that occur as a result of endocrine paraneoplastic syndromes vary with the hormone produced. For example, all types of lung cancer and small-cell lung cancer can produce ACTH, causing the person to experience symptoms of Cushing's syndrome—moon face, salt retention, water retention, and so on. Another example is the hypercalcemia or hypocalcemia that can be caused either by the production of a parahormonelike agent or calcitonin by ectopic neoplastic tissues. This type is commonly found in multiple myeloma and breast and lung cancer [7].

Persons with malignant tumors may experience neurologic difficulties that frequently are due to direct effects of the neoplasm, its metastasis, or endocrine, fluid, and electrolyte alterations. A few neurologic symptoms are paraneoplastic, however, and may be the primary signs of a malignancy. The possible neurologic symptoms can be grouped according to the area involved: cerebral, spinal cord, or peripheral nerve. Examples of cerebral symptoms are ataxia, dysarthria, hypotonia, abnormal reflexes, and dementia. Examples of spinal cord symptoms are muscular weakness, atrophy, spasticity, hyperreflexia, extensor-plantar responses, and paralysis. The syndromes associated with the spinal cord may resemble amyotrophic lateral sclerosis. Examples of peripheral nerve symptoms are sensory loss, weakness, wasting, and areflexia.

Hematologic alterations also most frequently result from the direct effects of the malignant neoplasm, its metastasis, or therapy. Some of these alterations may be paraneoplastic, and include an increase in red blood cells (associated with an erythropoietin-secreting tumor), anemia, increase or decrease in granulocytes, increase or decrease in thrombocytes [7]. Symptoms are related to the specific alteration. For example, in the case of anemia, the person may experience fatigue, cold feet, increased respirations, and palpitations. Coagulation alterations also occur frequently, resulting in either hemorrhage or thrombosis. Disseminated intravascular coagulation (DIC) often results from tumor secretions (see Chap. 17). Nonbacterial thrombotic endocarditis, in either the presence or absence of DIC, is another cause of thrombosis or hemorrhage.

Renal paraneoplastic syndromes result from lesions of the glomeruli and obstructions that are caused by neoplastic products. The nephrotic syndrome with proteinuria may be experienced. Hodgkin's disease is the most common neoplastic cause of the nephrotic syndrome. Tumor antigens and other products of the immune response have also been identified in the glomeruli.

Gastrointestinal paraneoplastic syndromes include loss of protein into the gut, malabsorption, liver dysfunction, and anorexia-cachexia. Over 90 percent of persons with advanced disease have a low serum albumin level. Loss of albumin into the gastrointestinal tract occurs as a result of (1) inflammation and ulceration of the mucosa, (2) intestinal lymph channel abnormalities (usually neoplastic obstruction), (3) congestive heart failure, and (4) causes of unknown origin. Hypoalbuminemia causes edema. The liver may enlarge in the absence of metastatic involvement. Other abnormalities, such as elevated levels of alkaline phosphatase, hyperglobulinemia, and hypocholesterolemia, and prolonged prothrombin time may occur. Anorexia, cachexia, weight loss, and taste changes are experienced by most individuals with advanced malignant neoplasia.

The anorexia-cachexia syndrome may occur either early or late in the course of disease. This condition may be the manifestation of an undiagnosed malignancy. A wide range of other events may cause anorexia-cachexia, such as chemotherapy, radiation therapy, obstruction of the gastrointestinal tract, and toxicity. About one-third of persons with malignant neoplasms experience negative nitrogen balance. The person experiencing the anorexia-cachexia syndrome has anorexia; loss of strength; loss of body fat, protein, and other nutrients; anemia; water and electrolyte imbalance; and increased metabolic rate and energy use.

Taste plays an important role in appetite. Persons with malignant neoplasms may have altered taste perception. A dislike for meats and other protein foods correlates with a lower threshold for bitter taste, while satisfaction with sweets indicates an elevated threshold for sugars. Besides taste, hunger and satiety are controlled by other complex mechanisms, such as the satiety and feeding centers of the hypothalamus, and insulin, glucagon, and amino acid levels. The cause of the anorexia-cachexia syndrome is likely to involve alterations in these mechanisms as a result of the neoplasm.

Paraneoplastic syndromes occur in all organ systems. Other paraneoplastic phenomena may not be related to an organ system, and include lactic acidosis, hyperlipidemia, amylase elevation, and various muscle and joint pains [17]. Fever occurs frequently; paraneoplastic fever refers to an unexplained temperature elevation that subsides with destruction of the malignancy but recurs with its reappearance. It occurs with a variety of neoplasms, for example, Hodgkin's disease, myxomas, hypernephroma, and osteogenic sarcoma.

Study Questions

1. How do the stages of malignant neoplasms help to determine the clinical course of the disease?
2. Describe the effect of various carcinogens on the production of cellular alterations and malignancy.
3. How are viruses implicated in cancer causation?
4. Identify tumors that have tumor-specific antigens.
5. Describe the local effects of benign and malignant neoplasms.
6. Describe the paraneoplastic syndromes and their significance for the host.
7. How does immune deficiency facilitate the growth of malignant cells?

References

1. Bast, R.C. Principles of cancer biology: Tumor immunology. In V.T. DeVita, S. Hellman, and S.A. Rosenberg, *Cancer: Principles and Practice of Oncology* (2nd ed.). Philadelphia: Lippincott, 1985.
2. *Cancer Facts and Figures 1986*. Rochester, N.Y.: American Cancer Society, 1985.
3. Cheville, N.F. *Cell Pathology* (2nd ed.). Ames: Iowa State University Press, 1983.
4. Coombes, R.C., and Neville, A.M. Methods of tumor detection. In A.J.S. Davies and P.S. Rudland, *Medical Perspectives in Cancer Research*. Chichester, England: Ellis Horwood, 1985.
5. del Regato, J.A., Spjut, H.J., and Cox, J.D. *Ackerman and del Regato's Cancer: Diagnosis, Treatment and Prognosis* (6th ed.). St. Louis: Mosby, 1985.
6. DeVita, V.T., Hellman, S., and Rosenberg, S.A. *Cancer: Principles and Practice of Oncology* (2nd ed.). Philadelphia: Lippincott, 1985.
7. Fidler, I.J., and Hart, I.R. Principles of cancer biology: Cancer metastasis. In V.T. DeVita, S. Hellman, and S.A. Rosenberg, *Cancer: Principles and Practice of Oncology* (2nd ed.). Philadelphia: Lippincott, 1985.
8. Fidler, I.J., and Hart, I.R. Biological diversity in metastatic neoplasms: Origin and implications. *Science* 217:998, 1982.
9. Fry, R.J.M. Principles of cancer biology: Physical carcinogenesis. In V.T. DeVita, S. Hellman, and S.A. Rosenberg, *Cancer: Principles and Practice of Oncology* (2nd ed.). Philadelphia: Lippincott, 1985.
10. Jakobovits, A., Banda, M.J., and Martin, G.R. Embryonal carcinoma-derived growth factors: Specific growth-promoting and differentiation-inhibiting activities. In J. Feramisco, B. Ozanne, and C. Stiles, *Cancer Cells*. New York: Cold Spring Harbor Laboratory, 1985.
11. Lewis, C.M. *Nutrition and Nutritional Therapy in Nursing*. East Norwalk, Conn.: Appleton-Century-Crofts, 1986.
12. Miller, E.C., and Miller, J.A. Mechanisms of chemical carcinogenesis. *Cancer* 47:5, 1055, 1981.
13. Nicholson, G.L. Tumor metastasis. In A.J.S. Davies and P.S. Rudland, *Medical Perspectives in Cancer Research*. Chichester, England: Ellis Horwood, 1985.
14. Pardee, A.B. Principles of cancer biology: Biochemistry and cell biology. In V.T. DeVita, S. Hellman, and S.A. Rosenberg, *Cancer: Principles and Practice of Oncology* (2nd ed.). Philadelphia: Lippincott, 1985.
15. Pitot, H.C. *Fundamentals of Oncology* (3rd ed.). New York: Dekker, 1986.
16. Rensberger, B. Cancer: The new synthesis: Cause. *Science* 84 5(7):28, 1984.
17. Robbins, S.L., Cotran, R.S., and Kumar, V. *Pathologic Basis of Disease* (3rd ed.). Philadelphia: Saunders, 1984.
18. Tannenbaum, S.N. Ins and outs of nitrites. *Science* 20:7, 1980.
19. Weiss, L. *Principles of Metastasis.* Orlando, Fla.: Academic Press, 1985.
20. Whelan, E.M. What is your cancer risk? What factors increase your risk of cancer? How can you protect yourself? *Med. Times* 105:96, 1977.

Unit Bibliography

Allison, A.C. Immunological surveillance of tumors. *Cancer Immunol. Immunother.* 2:1, 1977.

Althouse, R., et al. An evaluation of chemicals and industrial processes associated with cancer in humans based on human and animal data: SARC monographs, volumes 1 to 20: Report of an ARC working group. *Cancer Res.* 40:1, 1980.

Baltimore, D. Tumor viruses. *Cold Spring Harbor Symp. Quant. Biol.* 39:23, 1975.

Barrett, J.C., and Ts'o, P.O. Relationship between somatic mutation and neoplastic transformation. *Proc. Natl. Acad. Sci. USA* 75:3297, 1978.

Becker, F.F. *Cancer, A Comprehensive Treatise*. New York: Plenum Press, 1978.

Blackman, M.R., et al. Ectopic hormones. *Adv. Intern. Med.* 23:85, 1978.

Bosmann, H.B. Cell surface enzymes: Effects on mitotic activity and cell adhesion. *Int. Rev. Cytol.* 50:1, 1977.

Cairns, J. The cancer problem. *Sci. Am.* 233:64, 1975.

Cancer Facts and Figures 1986. New York: American Cancer Society, 1985.

Carter, R.L. *Precancerous States*. New York: Oxford University Press, 1984.

Chevilie, N.F. *Cell Pathology* (2nd ed.). Ames: Iowa State University Press, 1983.

Chu, E.H.Y., et al. Mutational approaches to the study of carcinogenesis. *J. Toxicol. Environ. Health* 2:1317, 1977.

Clayson, D.B. Nutrition and experimental carcinogenesis: A review. *Cancer Res.* 35:3292, 1975.

Creasey, W.A. *Diet and Cancer*. Philadelphia: Lea & Febiger, 1985.

Das, M. Mitogenic hormone-induced intracellular message: Assay and partial characterization of an activation of DNA replication induced by epidermal growth factor. *Proc. Natl. Acad. Sci. USA* 77:112, 1980.

Davies, A.J.S., and Rudland, P.S. *Medical Perspectives in Cancer Research*. Chichester, England: Ellis Horwood, 1985.

del Regato, J.A. Pathways of metastatic spread of malignant tumors. *Semin. Oncol.* 4:33, 1977.

del Regato, J.A., Spjut, H.J., and Cox, J.D. *Ackerman and del Regato's Cancer: Diagnosis, Treatment and Prognosis* (6th ed.). St. Louis: Mosby, 1985.

DeVita, V.F., Hellman, S., and Rosenberg, S.A. *Cancer: Principles and Practice of Oncology* (2nd ed.). Philadelphia: Lippincott, 1985.

DeWys, W.D. Working conference on anorexia and cachexia of neoplastic disease. *Cancer Res.* 30:2816, 1970.

Diamond, L., O'Brien, T.G., and Bard, W.M. Tumor promoters and the mechanism of tumor promotion. *Adv. Cancer Res.* 32:1, 1980.

Doll, R. The epidemiology of cancer. *Cancer* 45:2475, 1980.

Fidler, I.J. Tumor heterogeneity and the biology of cancer invasion and metastasis. *Cancer Res.* 38:2651, 1978.

Fidler, I.J., Gerstein, D.M., and Hart, I.R. The biology of cancer invasion and metastasis. *Adv. Cancer Res.* 28:149, 1978.

Fidler, I.J., Gerstein, D.M., and Riggs, C.W. Relationship of host immune status to tumor cell arrest, distribution, and survival in experimental metastasis. *Cancer* 40:46, 1977.

Fogel, M., et al. Differences in cell surface antigens of tumor metastasis and those of the local tumor. *J. Natl. Cancer Instit.* 62:585, 1979.

Folkman, J. The vascularization of tumors. *Sci. Am.* 234:58, 1976.

Folkman, J., and Cotran, R. Relation of vascular proliferation to tumor growth. *Int. Rev. Exp. Pathol.* 16:207, 1976.

Fraumeni, J.F. *Genetics of Human Cancer*. New York: Raven Press, 1977.

Fraumeni, J.F. *Radiation, Carcinogenesis, Epidemiology, and Biological Significance*. New York: Raven Press, 1984.

Fraumeni, J.F. *Cancer Epidemiology and Prevention*. Philadelphia: Saunders, 1982.

Garfinkel, L., et al. Cancer in black Americans. *CA* 30:39, 1980.

Gelfant, S. A new concept of tissue and tumor cell proliferation. *Cancer Res.* 37:3845, 1977.

Gospodarowicz, D., and Ill, C.R. Do plasma and serum have different abilities to promote cell growth? *Proc. Natl. Acad. Sci. USA* 77:2726, 1980.

Gottlieb, A.A. *Fundamental Aspects of Neoplasia*. New York: Springer-Verlag, 1975.

Graham, S., et al. Diet in the epidemiology of cancer of the colon and rectum. *J. Natl. Cancer Inst.* 61:709, 1978.

Gropp, C., Havermann, K., and Scheuer, A. Ectopic hormones in lung cancer patients at diagnosis and during treatment. *Cancer* 46:347, 1980.

Haddox, M.K., Magun, B.E., and Russell, D.H. Differential expression of type I-type II cyclic AMP-dependent protein kinases during cell cycle and cyclic AMP-induced growth arrest. *Proc. Natl. Acad. Sci. USA* 77:3445, 1980.

Hall, T.C. (ed.). Paraneoplastic syndromes. *Ann. N.Y. Acad. Sci.* 230:565, 1974.

Harris, H. Some thoughts about genetics, differentiation, and malignancy. *Somatic Cell Genet.* 5:923, 1979.

Herberman, R.B., et al. Natural killer cells: Characteristics and regulation of activity. *Immunol. Rev.* 44:43, 1979.

Jakobovits, A., Banda, M.J., and Martin, G.R. Embryonal carcinoma-derived growth factors: Specific growth-promoting and differentiation-inhibiting activities. In J. Feramisco, B. Ozanne, and C. Stiles, *Cancer Cells*. New York: Cold Spring Harbor Laboratory, 1985.

Kerbel, R.S. Implications of immunological heterogeneity of tumors. *Nature* 280:358, 1979.

Labarthe, D., et al. Design and preliminary observations of National Cooperative Diethylstilbestrol Adenosis (DESAD) Project. *Obstet. Gynecol.* 51:453, 1978.

Liotta, L.A., et al. Metastatic potential correlates with enzymatic degradation of basement membrane collagen. *Nature* 284:67, 1980.

Lowenstein, W.R. Junctional intercellular communication and the control of growth. *Biochim. Biophys. Acta* 560:1, 1979.

Maclure, K.M., and MacMahon, B. An epidemiologic perspective of environmental carcinogenesis. *Epidemiol. Rev.* 2:19, 1980.

McKeehan, W.L., and McKeehan, K.A. Serum factors modify the cellular requirement for Ca^{2+}, K^{+}, Mg^{2+}, phosphate ions and 2-oxocarboxylic acids for multiplication of normal human fibroblasts. *Proc. Natl. Acad. Sci. USA* 77:3417, 1980.

Miller, D.G. On the nature of susceptibility to cancer. *Cancer* 46:1307, 1980.

Miller, E.C., and Miller, J.A. Mechanisms of chemical carcinogenesis. *Cancer* 47:1055, 1981.

Miller, R.W. The discovery of human teratogens, carcinogens and mutagens: Lessons for the future. In A. Hollaender and F.J. de Serres (eds.), *Chemical Mutagens*. New York: Plenum Press, 1978.

Moses, H.L., et al. Comparisons of RNA metabolism in G_1 arrested and stimulated nontransformed and chemically transformed mouse embryo cells in culture. *Cancer Res.* 39:4516, 1979.

Mulvihill, J.J. *Genetics of Human Cancer*. New York: Raven Press, 1977.

Nicolson, G.L. Cancer metastasis. *Sci. Am.* 240:66, 1979.

Nicolson, G.L., Brunson, K.W., and Fidler, I.J. Specificity of arrest, survival and growth of selected metastatic variant cell lines. *Cancer Res.* 38:4105, 1978.

Pilot, H.C. *Fundamentals of Oncology* (3rd ed.). New York: Dekker, 1986.

Pott, P. *Chirurgical Observations Related to the Cataract, the Polypus of the Nose, the Cancer of the Scrotum, the Different Kinds of Rupture, and the Mortification of Toes and Feet.* London: Hawes, Clarke, and Collins, 1775.

Rapp, F. Viruses as an etiologic factor in cancer. *Semin. Oncol.* 3:49, 1976.

Recklies, A.D., et al. Secretion of proteinases from malignant and nonmalignant human breast tissue. *Cancer Res.* 40:550, 1980.

Rodgers, J.E. Catching the cancer strays. *Science 83* 4:42, 1983.

Rotkin, I.D. Sexual characteristics of a cervical cancer population. *Am. J. Public Health* 57:815, 1967.

Rubin, P. *Clinical Oncology for Medical Students and Physicians* (2nd ed.). Rochester, N.Y.: American Cancer Society, 1983.

Sandberg, A.A. *The Chromosomes in Human Cancer and Leukemia.* New York: Elsevier North-Holland, 1980.

Saunders, G.F. *Symposium on Fundamental Cancer Research*. Houston: M.D. Anderson Hospital and Tumor Institute, 1982.

Siracky, J. An approach to the problem of heterogeneity of human tumour-cell populations. *Br. J. Cancer* 39:570, 1979.

Smets, L.A. Cell transformation as a model for tumor induction and neoplastic growth. *Biochim. Biophys. Acta* 605:93, 1980.

Spratt, J.S. The primary and secondary prevention of cancer. *J. Surg. Oncol.* 18:219, 1981.

Temin, H.M. On the origin of RNA tumor viruses. *Harvey Lect.* 69:173, 1975.

Viola, M.V., et al. Reverse transciptase in leukocytes of leukemic patients in remission. *N. Engl. J. Med.* 294:74, 1976.

Weber, G. Enzymology of cancer cells. *N. Engl. J. Med.* 296:541, 1977.

Yalow, R.S., et al. Plasma and tumor ACTH in carcinoma of the lung. *Cancer* 44:1789, 1979.

SECTION III

Organ and System Mechanisms

Adaptations and Alterations

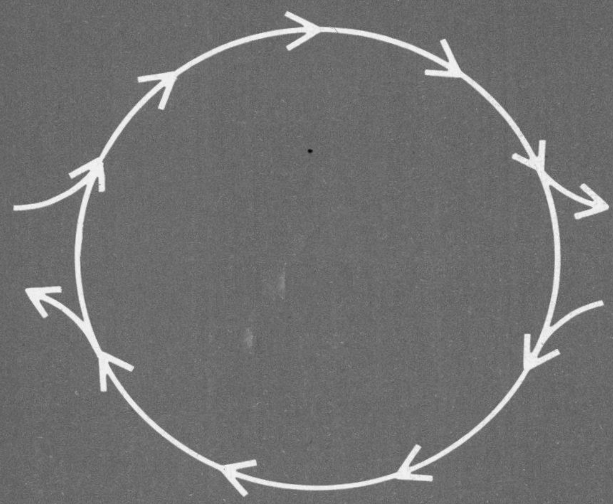

UNIT 7

Hematology

Gloria Anderson and Barbara L. Bullock / ***Erythrocyte Function***

Barbara L. Bullock / ***Leukocyte Function***
Coagulation

This unit consists of three chapters that deal with the major functions of blood cells. Activities of some of the white blood cells were previously discussed in Units 4 and 5.

Chapter 15 details erythrocyte activities with special emphasis on the pathologic processes of erythrocytosis and anemia. Chapter 16 expands on leukocyte function and emphasizes nonmalignant and malignant disorders of the white blood cells. Blood coagulation is explained in Chapter 17, providing a basis for understanding the normal clotting process and disorders of coagulation deficiency. Descriptions of crucial hematologic studies are included in all three chapters. The detailed contents of this unit provide for increased understanding of pathologic processes involving blood cell disorders.

The reader is again encouraged to use the learning objectives as study guides and the study questions as a review. The unit bibliography presents resources for additional study.

CHAPTER 15

Normal and Altered Erythrocyte Function

CHAPTER OUTLINE

Hematopoiesis
- Bone Marrow
- Stem Cell Theory
- Spleen

Erythropoiesis
- Description of Erythrocytes
- Development of Erythrocytes
- Hemoglobin
- Substances Needed for Erythropoiesis
- Energy Production in Erythrocytes
- Function of Red Blood Cells in Oxygen and Carbon Dioxide Transport
- Factors Influencing Erythropoiesis
- Antigenic Properties of Erythrocytes
- Destruction of Erythrocytes

Erythrocytosis
- Polycythemia Vera

Anemias
- Aplastic Anemia
  - *Red Blood Cell Aplasia*
- Hemolytic Anemia
  - *Abnormalities of the Red Cell Membrane*
  - *Increased Rigidity Causing Abnormal Flow*
  - *Direct Physical Trauma*
- Maturation-Failure Anemia
  - *Pernicious Anemia*
  - *Folic Acid Anemia*
- Microcytic, Hypochromic Anemia
  - *Iron-Deficiency Anemia*
- Posthemorrhagic Anemia

Laboratory and Diagnostic Tests
- Hematologic Studies
  - *Hemoglobin*
  - *Red Blood Cells*
  - *Packed Cell Volume or Hematocrit*
  - *Erythrocyte Sedimentation Rate (ESR)*
  - *Mean Corpuscular Volume (MCV)*
  - *Mean Corpuscular Hemoglobin (MCH)*
  - *Mean Cell Hemoglobin Concentration (MCHC)*
  - *Reticulocyte Count*
  - *Bone Marrow Studies*
- Diagnostic Test
  - *Schilling Test*

LEARNING OBJECTIVES

1. Describe the composition of whole blood.
2. List three physical characteristics of blood.
3. List four factors that affect blood volume.
4. Give five primary functions of blood.
5. Explain the stem cell theory.
6. Describe the development of erythrocytes.
7. Explain the structure and function of hemoglobin.
8. List five substances needed for erythropoiesis.
9. Review energy production in the erythrocyte.
10. Name two factors thought to influence erythropoiesis.
11. Explain the meaning of the terms *AB blood*, *Rh negative*.
12. Describe the process of red blood cell destruction.
13. Describe the factors that may cause erythrocytosis.
14. Differentiate between physiologic erythrocytosis and polycythemia.
15. Contrast erythrocytosis and hemoconcentration.
16. List and differentiate the morphologic characteristics of five types of anemia.
17. Explain how aplastic anemia can develop.
18. Describe the hemolytic anemias.
19. Describe the precipitating etiology of and environment that produces sickle cell anemia.
20. Explain why iron-deficiency anemia is common in children and young women.
21. Relate the lack of iron to the morphologic characteristics of iron-deficiency anemia.
22. Explain the relationship of intrinsic factor deficiency to the development of pernicious anemia.
23. Differentiate the etiologies of pernicious anemia and folic acid anemia.
24. Explain briefly why posthemorrhagic anemia may not occur immediately after an acute hemorrhage.
25. Describe briefly the laboratory findings and diagnostic tests that are helpful in diagnosing disorders of red blood cells.

All living cells require materials to survive and to perform functions that are necessary to maintain life. Blood and interstitial fluid provide the means by which essential substances are delivered to the cells and materials not needed are removed from the cells. Transportation of cellular and humoral messages by the blood helps to integrate physiologic processes, thus enabling the body to function as a unified whole.

Since ancient times there has been much interest in and curiosity about blood and its relationship to life. Blood was known to be essential to human existence; loss of large amounts became associated with loss of life. The first description of red blood cells (RBCs) came with the discovery of the microscope by Leeuwenhoek (1632–1723). He examined the blood and described the red corpuscles [12]. Sophisticated and advanced technology now makes it possible to examine and describe blood components and their functions in minute detail.

The primary roles of blood are to integrate body functions and to meet the needs of specific tissues. Two functions basic to meeting these goals are transportation and distribution of (1) respiratory gases to and from the tissues, (2) hormones to body tissues or organs, and (3) nutrients to the cells. In addition, blood is involved in regulating acid-base balance, thermoregulation, and electrolyte distribution. As detailed in Chapter 16, the leukocytes provide a defense mechanism for the body against invading microorganisms. Platelets aid in the coagulation process by affecting clot formation (see Chap. 17).

Blood consists of a clear yellow fluid called *plasma*, in which cells and many other substances are suspended. Proteins are the major solutes in plasma and consist primarily of albumins, globulins, and fibrinogen. The composition of plasma is very similar to that of interstitial fluid, except that it has a much higher protein concentration. This higher concentration of proteins in the blood maintains the intravascular volume by the exertion of colloid osmotic pressure. In addition to holding water in the intravascular spaces, plasma proteins bind substances such as lipids and metals such as iron, contribute to viscosity of blood, and participate in the coagulation of blood (see Chap. 17). They are also important in regulating acid-base balance.

Blood accounts for about 8 percent of total body weight [4]. The total blood volume is divided into two main categories, plasma and cells. Ninety-nine percent of the cells are red blood cells. Table 15-1 summarizes the substances present in blood.

The blood volume is the sum of volumes of plasma and formed elements of blood in the vascular system. It can be calculated from either plasma volume or cell volume, which in the healthy adult male average 45 ml per kg and 30 ml per kg body weight, respectively [4].

A wide variation in normal blood volumes exists because of several factors.

1. *Weight*. Because fatty tissue contains little water, the total blood volume correlates more closely with lean body mass than with total body weight.
2. *Sex*. Because females usually have a higher ratio of fat tissue to lean tissue, the blood volume per kilogram for them is generally lower than that for males.
3. *Pregnancy*. Total blood volume gradually rises as a pregnancy progresses, with the greatest increase occurring primarily in plasma volume.
4. *Posture* or *position*. Volume tends to increase when a person is in bed for a period of time and decreases

TABLE 15-1 Some Compounds Present in Human Blood

Compound[a]	Concentration and Fraction[b]	Compound[a]	Concentration and Fraction[b]
Acetoacetic acid + acetone (ketone bodies)	0.2–2.0 mg/100 ml (S)	Iodine, protein-bound	3.5–8.0 μg/dl (S)
Adenosine diphosphate	100 μm (E)	Iron	50–150 μg/dl (S)
Adenosine monophosphate	13 μm (E)	Lactic acid	0.6–1.8 mEq/L (B); 1 mm (P)
Adenosine triphosphate	1 μm (E)	Lead	3 μm (E)
Aldosterone	3–10 mg/dl (P)	Lipase	Below 2 units/ml (S)
Alpha-amino acid nitrogen	3.0–5.5 mg/dl (P)	Lipids, total	450–1000 mg/dl (S)
Amino acid, total	300 mg/dl (P), 120 mg/dl (E)	Magnesium	1.5–2.0 mEq/L; 1–2 mg/dl (S)
Ascorbic acid	0.4–1.5 mg/dl (fasting B)	Nitrogen, nonprotein	15–35 mg/dl (S)
Bicarbonate	25 mM	Phosphatase, acid, total[c]	Male: 0.13–0.63 sigma units/ml (S); female: 0.01–0.56 sigma units/ml (S)
Bilirubin	Direct: 0.1–0.3 mg/dl (S); indirect: 0.2–1.2 mg/dl (S)	Phosphatase, alkaline[c]	2.0–4.5 Bodansky units/ml (S)
Calcium	8.5–10.5 mg/dl; 4.3–5.3 mEq/L (S)	Phospholipids	145–225 mg/dl (S)
Carbon dioxide	26–28 mEq/L (S)	Phosphorus, inorganic	3.0–4.5 mg/dl (adult, S); 0.9–1.5 mm/L (adult, S)
Carotenoids	0.08–0.4 μg/ml (S)	Potassium	4 mm (P); 111 mm (E)
Ceruloplasmin	27–37 mg/dl (S)	Protein	
Chloride	100–106 mEq/L (S); 102 mm (P); 78 mm (E)	Total	6.0–8.0 gm/dl (S)
Cholesterol	150–240 mg/dl (S)	Albumin	3.5–4.5 gm/dl (S)
Cholesterol esters	≅60–75% of total cholesterol (S)	Globulin	2.0–3.0 gm/dl (S)
Cobalt	17 μm (E)	Pyruvic acid	0–0.11 mEq/L (P)
Copper, total	100–200 μg/dl (S); 17 μm (E)	Riboflavin	500 nanomol (E)
Cortisol (17-hydroxycorticoids)	5–18 μg/dl (P)	Sodium	136–145 mEq/L; 310–340 mg/dl (S); 140 mm (P); 6 mm (E)
Creatine	40 μm (P): 600 μm (E)	Sulfate	0.5–1.5 mEq/L (S)
Creatinine	0.7–1.5 mg/100 ml (S); 450 μm (P); 160 μm (E)	Transaminase (serum glutamic oxaloacetic transaminase [SGOT])[c]	10–40 units/ml (S)
2,3-Diphosphoglycerate (DPG)	4 mm (E)	Urea nitrogen (blood urea nitrogen, BUN)	8–25 mg/dl (B)
Glucose (folin)	80–120 mg/dl (fasting, B)	Uric acid	3.0–7.0 mg/dl (S)
Glucose (true)	70–100 mg/dl (B)	Vitamin A	0.15–0.6 μg/ml (S)

[a]The substances and the values listed for them in this table give an indication of the biochemical complexity of blood and are not to be construed as absolute. Blood levels of specific components can vary among normal individuals or in the same individual at different times. Furthermore, the normal values for specific blood constituents can differ greatly among different laboratories, depending on the technique used for their determination.
[b]Abbreviations used for the several blood fractions are: B = whole blood; P = plasma; S = serum; E = erythrocytes.
[c]Activities of over 50 specific enzymes have been detected in various blood fractions, only 3 of which are listed here.
Source: From D. Jensen, *The Principles of Physiology* (2nd ed.). New York: Appleton-Century-Crofts, 1980. Table 32-2.

when he or she assumes the erect position. This variation in blood volume may result from alterations in capillary pressure that lead to changes in glomerular filtration.

5. *Age*. Percentage of blood volume is higher in the newborn and decreases with increasing age.
6. *Nutrition*. Lack of nutrients may cause a decrease in RBCs or plasma formation, thus decreasing the total blood volume.
7. *Environmental temperature*. The volume of blood increases when the environmental temperature is increased.
8. *Altitude*. At high altitudes the environmental oxygen pressure is greatly decreased and greater numbers of red blood cells are produced for oxygen transport.

Although numerous factors affect blood volume, it remains relatively stable in the healthy person. Several compensatory mechanisms contribute to this stability; for example, decreased RBC volume is followed by increased plasma volume, thus returning total blood volume to its normal level. Capillary dynamics and renal mechanisms play major roles in maintaining plasma volume.

General physical characteristics of the blood are summarized in Table 15-2. Oxygenated arterial blood is bright red, changing to dark red or crimson when oxygen is lost and carbon dioxide is added. The pH is regulated within the narrow limits of 7.35 to 7.45 (see Chap. 6). The relatively high viscosity of blood is primarily due to the suspension of cells and plasma components, which causes it to flow more slowly than water.

TABLE 15-2 Physical Characteristics of Blood

Characteristic	Normal	Example of Alterations
Color	Arterial: bright red Venous: dark red or crimson	Anemia
pH	Arterial: 7.35–7.45 Venous: 7.31–7.41	Decreases in acidosis; increases in alkalosis
Specific gravity	Plasma: 1.026 RBC: 1.093	
Viscosity	3.5–4.5 times that of water	Increases in polycythemia; decreases in anemia
Volume	5000 ml (70-kg male) Approximately 3 L in plasma 2 L blood cells	Decreases in dehydration Increases in pregnancy

The circulation of blood provides for maintenance of a steady state in individual body cells. The constituency of blood rapidly and continuously changes, but the overall concentration of substances remains relatively constant. This constancy in the environment of individual body cells is essential for life.

Hematopoiesis

Bone Marrow

In the adult, the bone marrow produces all of the blood cells and platelets. At birth, *red marrow* is present in all bone marrow cavities, and blood cells are formed there as well as in the liver and spleen [3]. In the first three years of life there is enough red marrow to produce only adequate amounts of red cells. After age 3, the red marrow actively produces blood cells. After age 5 years, red marrow becomes infiltrated with fat and is called *yellow marrow* [3]. By age 20 to 25 years, red marrow is present in the cranial bones, vertebrae, sternum, ribs, clavicles, scapulae, pelvis, and proximal ends of the femora and humeri. In the aged person, it begins to leave the cranial bones and lower vertebrae [4]. The marrow then contains mostly blood, hematopoietic cells, and fat.

The blood supply to the marrow comes from large-lumina, thin-walled arteries that branch into a network of capillaries to become a bed of sinusoids. Between the sinuses lies the hematopoietic tissue in which blood cells are formed. The new cells enter the sinuses through small openings in the walls. Blood cells gain access to the sinusoids at a critical moment in their maturation phase, and maturation is completed in the circulatory system and tissues. Loss of integrity of the sinus walls or increased need may allow the release of immature cells into the circulation.

Hematopoiesis is a dynamic, constant process, with rapid turnover of blood cells and a constant need for new cells. Bone marrow can meet the body's changing needs for various types and numbers of cells. It maintains a reserve supply of cells for stressful and unexpected situations that create an increased demand. Normally, 75 percent of cells in the marrow are precursors to white blood cells, while 25 percent are maturing red blood cells [11].

Stem Cell Theory

Most of the formed elements of the blood have a limited life span. Erythrocytes live approximately 120 days. Granulocytes circulate in the blood for an average of six hours, then move into the tissues where they may live for several days [3,11]. Other cells, such as macrophages and lymphocytes, may live months or years. A continual supply of cells is needed to replace lost cells.

The origin of cells that develop into mature erythrocytes, leukocytes, and platelets has been investigated for many years. The *stem cell theory* helps to explain the various stages of cell differentiation in the bone marrow [11]. The cellular elements finally present in blood are the more differentiated and mature cells. The pluripotential stem cells transform to committed precursors and finally differentiate (mature) into recognizable precursors of mature cells (Fig. 15-1). Stem cells can be *pluripotent*, from which any type of blood cell can form, or *unipotent*, from which only one type of cell develops [11]. The appearance of these cells cannot be distinguished by ordinary microscopic techniques.

Stem cells may be described based on their morphology, kinesis, and operation (function). *Morphologically*, they are small mononuclear cells resembling lymphocytes. Occasional stem cells are normally present in the blood. The *kinetic* definition recognizes the stem cell pool (compartment) as able to maintain itself and to produce cells that can become committed to a certain line of blood cells. The *operational* definition regards stem cells as a colony-forming unit (CFU). Complex feedback loops of humoral regulation of hemopoiesis are beginning to be recognized. Colony-stimulating and -inhibiting factors are important in regulating the proliferation and differentiation of blood cells [11]. Marrow cells have been injected intravenously into irradiated mice in which the spleen and marrow were reduced to stroma, hematologically empty. Colonies developed in the spleen, and later, specific differentiation took place. These colonies contained cells for erythrocytes, neutrophils, and megakaryocytes [1]. The stem cell maintains its pool and apparently can recover if it is not lethally damaged [12]. Red blood cell formation is discussed on page 217 and is the most well understood of the hemopoietic systems. The reader is referred to Chapters 10, 16, and 17 for discussions of the other blood cells.

Spleen

The spleen is a large, highly vascular organ with elements of the lymphoid and mononuclear phagocyte systems. It is located in the left upper abdominal cavity, directly beneath the diaphragm, above the left kidney, and behind the fundus of the stomach (Fig. 15-2). The spleen is covered by peritoneum and held in position by the peritoneal folds. It has a connective tissue capsule from which trabeculae

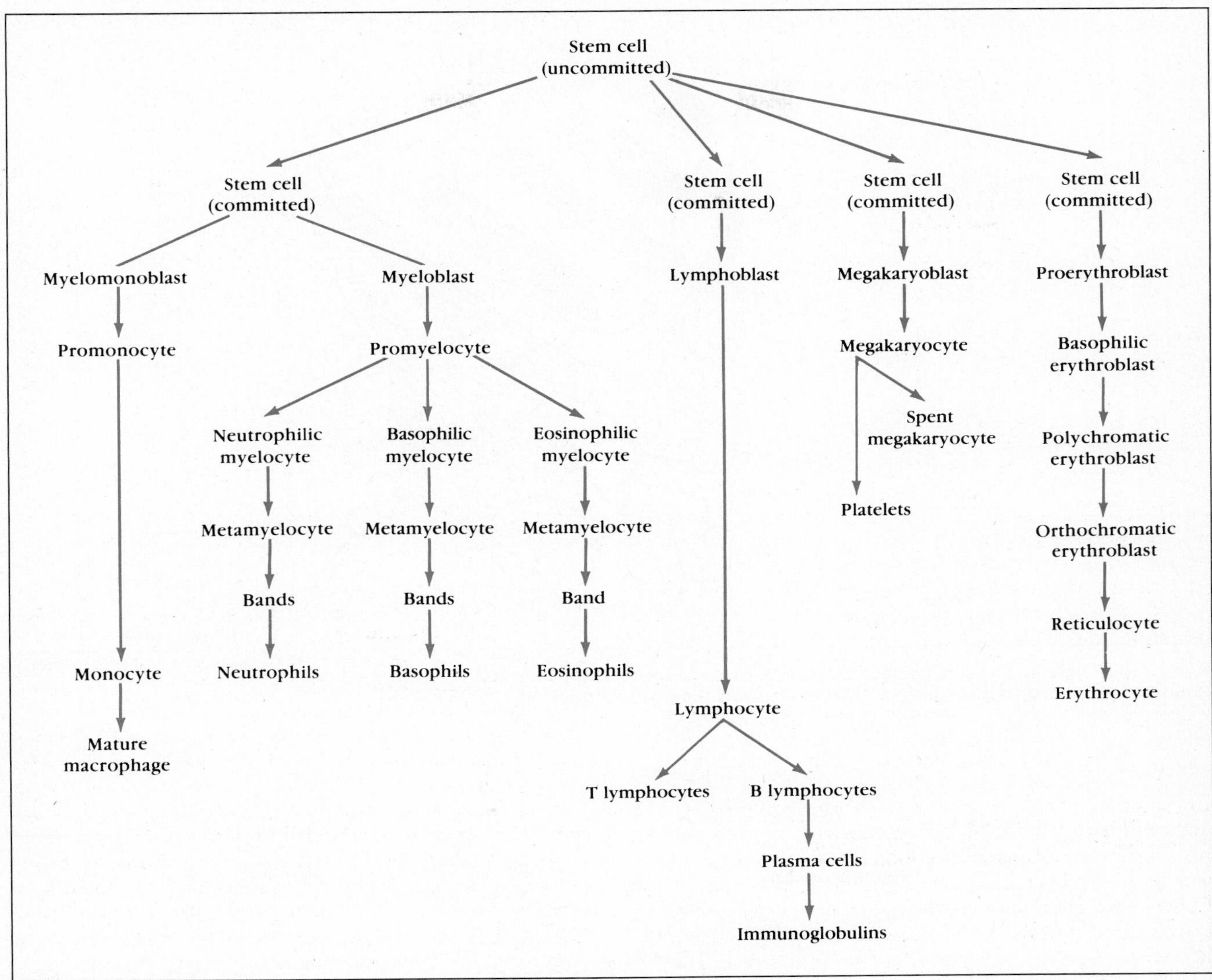

FIGURE 15-1 Differentiation of stem cells in the bone marrow. (From M. Wintrobe et al., *Clinical Hematology* [7th ed.]. Lea and Febiger, 1984.)

(supporting strands) extend inside the organ and form a framework. Splenic pulp is present in the small spaces of this framework (Fig. 15-3). The major areas of spleen are as follows:

1. *White pulp* sequesters lymphocytes, macrophages, and antigen, and permits them to interact. Mature plasma cells are present in the marginal zone.
2. *Red pulp* stores and tests the viability of red cells, granulocytes, and platelets.
3. *Marginal zone* lies between the white pulp and red pulp and receives the terminal branches of most of the arterial vessels. Large blood flow and meshwork structure make this area the major filtration site of blood in the spleen [5].

Blood is brought to the spleen by the splenic artery, which divides into several branches before entering the concave side of the spleen; a small amount of splenic blood passes directly into the sinusoids. This is called the *rapid-transit pathway* because it goes almost unobstructed to the venous collecting system. The greatest amount of splenic circulation travels the *slow-transit pathway*, which brings it into close contact with the marginal zone, red pulp, and phagocytic cells of the white pulp. Much of the plasma and many leukocytes are diverted into right-angle branches that lead to the white pulp. Therefore, the blood that reaches the marginal zone and the red pulp becomes concentrated. The arterial capillaries empty their contents into the vascular spaces of the reticular meshwork of the marginal zone and the red pulp. In the red pulp, the capillaries are quite permeable so that blood, including erythrocytes, passes from them into and through the venous sinuses. The capillaries empty into thin-walled veins that finally terminate in the splenic vein, which itself terminates in the portal vein.

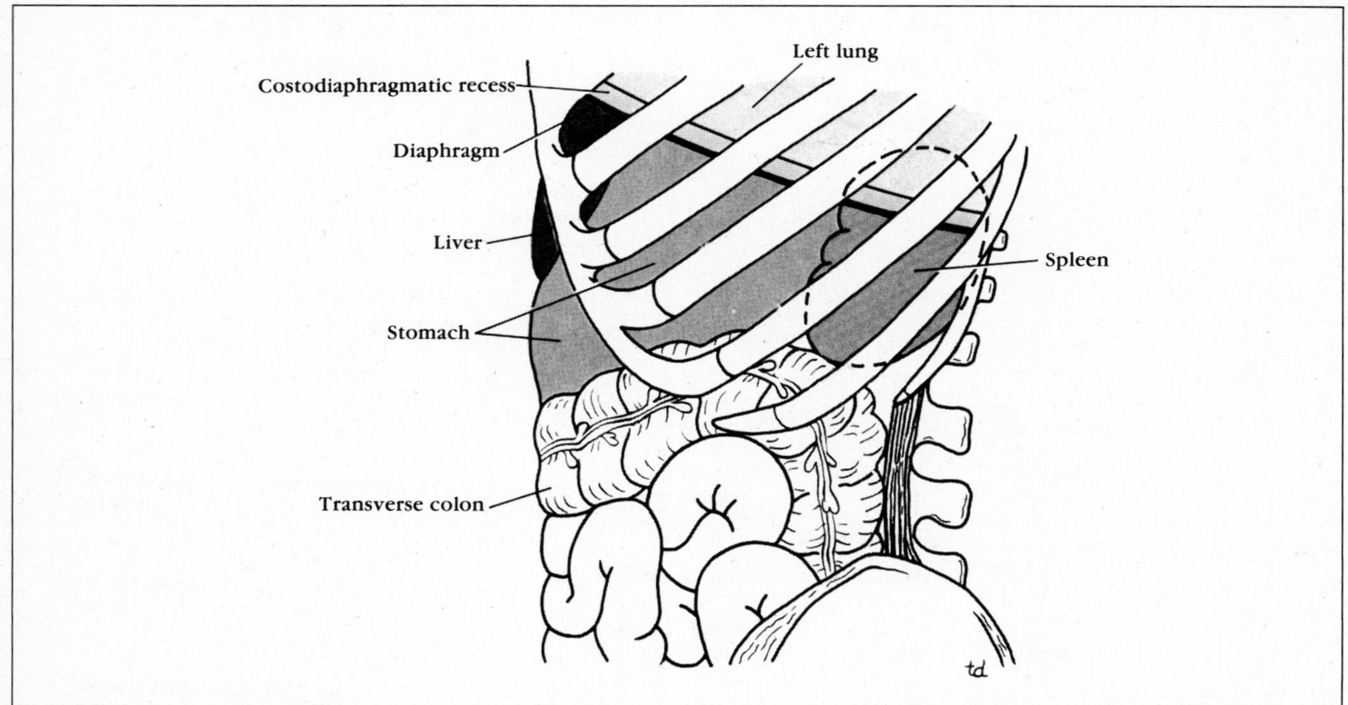

FIGURE 15-2 Spleen, showing notched anterior border and its relation to adjacent structures. (From R. Snell, *Clinical Anatomy for Medical Students* [2nd ed.]. Boston: Little, Brown, 1981.)

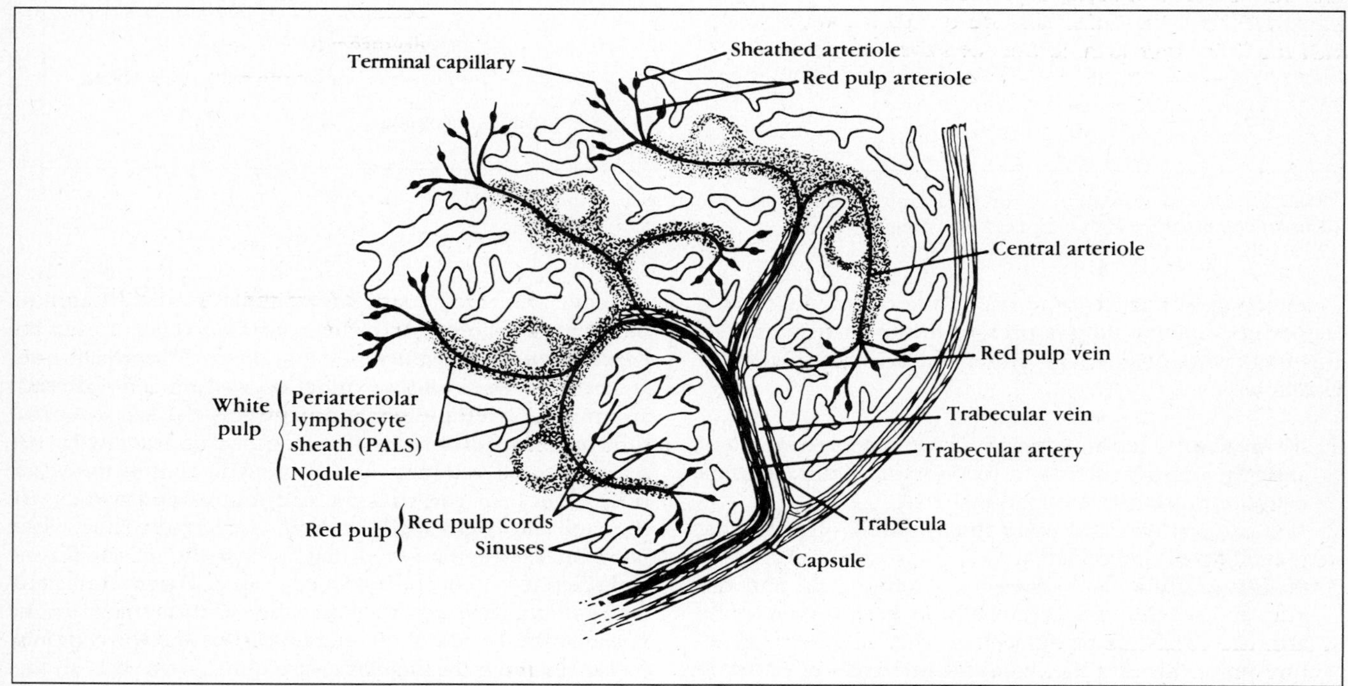

FIGURE 15-3 A schematic representation of part of the spleen showing the relationship of the vasculature to the red and white pulp. (From M. Borysenko, *Functional Histology* [2nd ed.]. Boston: Little, Brown, 1984.)

Although the spleen is not necessary for survival, it is involved in four general functions: (1) production of lymphocytes in the white pulp, (2) destruction of erythrocytes in the red pulp, (3) filtration and trapping of foreign particles in both areas, destroying bacteria and viruses, and (4) storage of blood [5]. In fetal life the spleen is active in hematopoiesis, a function that mostly ends at or before birth. The stasis of blood flow through the marginal zone and the red pulp provides an opportunity for phagocytosis by the phagocytic cells. The destruction of old and imperfect red blood cells is sometimes referred to as "culling." Reticulocytes and many platelets are stored in the spleen. The normal adult spleen holds about 150 to 200 ml of blood, but this volume can increase in pathologic states such as congestive heart failure [4].

The spleen is a nonmuscular organ and consequently does not contract in times of stress. The storage and release of blood are thought to be related to passive dilatation of the organ, and/or dilatation and constriction of vessels in it.

Erythropoiesis

Description of Erythrocytes

Erythrocytes are nonnucleated, biconcave disks. This shape provides a large surface:volume ratio that permits distortion of the cells without stretching of their membrane. Red blood cells are able to traverse very small capillaries, and normal RBCs adapt to the sinusoids of the spleen, escaping without being trapped and destroyed. The unique shape of erythrocytes is also conducive to gas exchange. The membrane is made of lipids and proteins, with the lipid layer located between the two protein layers. Erythrocytes contain hemoglobin, which binds loosely with oxygen and carbon dioxide to carry essential gases to and away from tissues (see p. 219).

Development of Erythrocytes

Erythrocytes are formed in the blood islands of the yolk sacs during the first several weeks of gestation. During the second trimester of pregnancy, fetal RBCs are produced in the liver, spleen, and lymph nodes. After birth the bone marrow becomes the principal site of RBC production. After adolescence, the red marrow of the membranous bones, especially the pelvic bone, sternum, ribs, and vertebrae, take over the major erythropoietic function. This marrow cell pool provides a constant supply of peripheral red blood cells.

The forerunner of the mature RBC is derived from a stem cell, which proceeds through several divisions and differentiations prior to reaching the final stage of maturity (Fig. 15-4). During maturation, the nucleus decreases in size, the total size of the cell shrinks, the amount of ribonucleic acid (RNA) lessens, and hemoglobin synthesis increases.

The maturational process of the RBC appears to follow an established sequence.

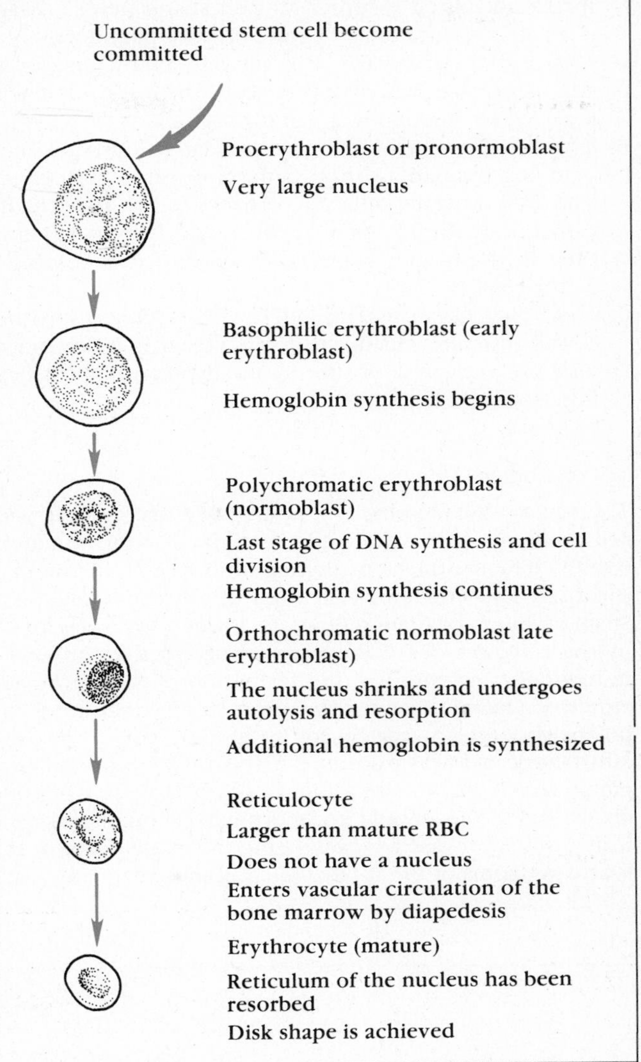

FIGURE 15-4 Development of red blood cells.

1. *Proerythroblast*. This is the most immature cell of erythropoiesis and is formed from the stem cell located in bone marrow. The nucleus, which occupies the greatest portion of this cell, is large, centrally located, and contains from one to five nucleoli that are not clearly separated from the rest of the nucleus.
2. *Basophilic erythroblast*. The nucleus becomes smaller and hemoglobin synthesis begins. The cell contains small pinocytic vesicles that are thought to be involved in the uptake of ferritin, which is necessary in the formation of hemoglobin.
3. *Polychromatic erythroblast*. The nucleus becomes even smaller and more dense. This cell contains a mixture of basophilic material and red hemoglobin, giving it the name polychromatic.
4. *Late orthochromatic normoblast*. Hemoglobin synthesis is almost complete, reaching a concentration of 34 percent of cell volume. The nucleus continues to

shrink and often assumes an odd shape before disappearing. The nucleus migrates into a pseudopodlike protrusion of cytoplasm. It is surrounded by a cytoplasmic membrane, which degenerates; the freed nucleus is ingested by surrounding macrophages.

5. *Reticulocyte*. This large, nonnucleated immature cell contains remnants of the Golgi apparatus, mitochondria, and other cytoplasmic organelles [4]. It normally remains in the marrow approximately one day and then in the bloodstream one day before becoming a mature RBC.
6. *Mature erythrocyte*. This cell develops after resorption of the reticulum in the reticulocyte. It is a biconcave disk that is capable of altering its shape without damaging its membrane.

Hemoglobin

The protein hemoglobin is a conjugated, oxygen-carrying red pigment with a molecular weight of approximately 64,500. The synthesis of hemoglobin begins in the erythroblast and continues through the normoblast stage. Small amounts of hemoglobin are formed for a day or so by the reticulocytes. Two parallel processes are involved in hemoglobin synthesis: the formation of the porphyrin structure (heme) that contains iron, and formation of the polypeptide chains that make up globin (Fig. 15-5). The adult hemoglobin molecule (HbA) is composed of a globin (made of two alpha and two beta, large polypeptide chains) with four heme (iron porphyrin) complexes. One iron atom is present for each heme molecule. Each of the four iron atoms of the molecule combines reversibly with an atom of oxygen, forming oxyhemoglobin. When oxygen concentration is high, as in the lungs, oxygen combines with hemoglobin; but when the concentration is lower, as in the tissues, oxygen is released. In the lungs about 95 percent of hemoglobin becomes saturated with oxygen. The high density of hemoglobin in each red blood cell allows a large amount of oxygen to be transported. The disk shape of the erythrocytes provides a large surface area per unit mass of hemoglobin, enhancing gas exchange in the capillary system.

Substances Needed for Erythropoiesis

Several substances are essential for the proper formation of red blood cells and hemoglobin. Among these are amino acids, iron, copper, pyridoxine, cobalt, vitamin B_{12}, and folic acid. Iron is essential for the production of heme, and approximately 65 percent of body iron is present in hemoglobin. The total amount of iron in the body equals about 4 gm, with 15 to 30 percent of this amount being stored as *ferritin*, primarily in the liver. Ferritin (storage iron) is formed from a combination of iron with a protein called *apoferritin* [4]. It is readily available for hemoglobin synthesis when needed through the aid of a beta-globulin called *transferrin*. Transferrin has specific binding capabilities that facilitate the transfer of iron across the membranes of immature erythrocytes. Transferrin also carries the iron released from worn-out erythrocytes to the bone marrow, where it is reused for hemoglobin synthesis.

Daily losses of iron are replaced by dietary intake. Iron is absorbed mostly in the duodenum by an active process that apparently continues until all of the transferrin is

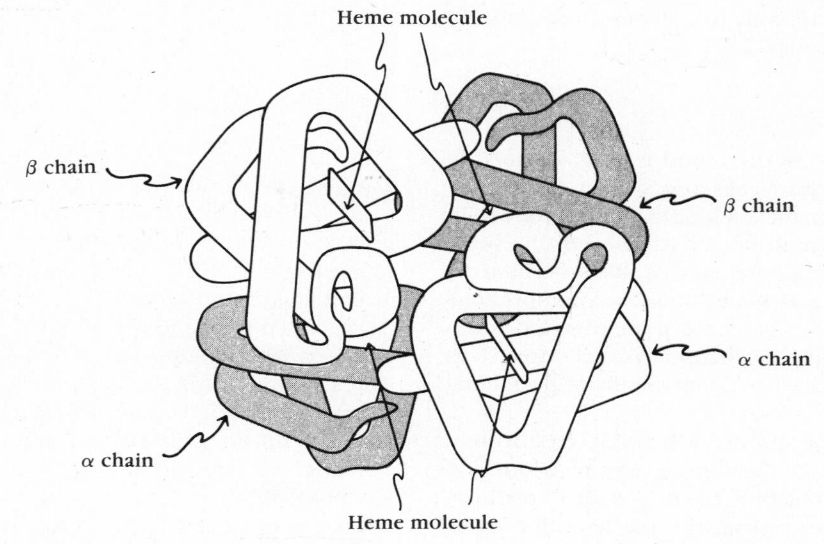

FIGURE 15-5 Structure of the hemoglobin molecule. The hemoglobin molecule is made up of four polypeptide chains. Two identical chains are called α chains, and the other two identical chains are called β chains. Each chain encloses a heme molecule. (From G. Schmid, *The Chemical Basis of Life: General, Organic, and Biological Chemistry for the Health Sciences.* Boston: Little, Brown, 1982.)

saturated. When transferrin can accept no more iron, absorption of iron almost entirely ceases in the duodenum. Conversely, if the stores are depleted, larger amounts of iron are absorbed. The result is a feedback mechanism that keeps a stable level of iron for hemoglobin synthesis [4]. Lack in the diet or poor absorption of iron leads to iron-deficiency anemia (see p. 225).

Vitamin B_{12} (cyanocobalamin) is essential for the synthesis of deoxyribonucleic acid (DNA) molecules in the forming RBCs. This large molecule does not easily penetrate the mucosa of the gastrointestinal tract but must be bound to a glycoprotein known as the *intrinsic factor (IF)* for its absorption. The IF is secreted by the parietal cells of the gastric mucosa and binds to vitamin B_{12} to protect it from the digestive enzymes. After absorption from the gastrointestinal tract, vitamin B_{12} is stored in the liver and is available for the production of new erythrocytes. Longstanding lack of B_{12} leads to maturation-failure anemia (pernicious anemia) (see p. 225).

Folic acid (pteroylglutamic acid) is also necessary for the synthesis of DNA and promotes red cell maturation. Lack of folic acid causes folic acid anemia, a type of maturation-failure anemia that readily responds to dietary replacement.

Energy Production in Erythrocytes

Immature erythropoietic cells are comparable to other tissue cells in their metabolic activity, but the mature erythrocytes cannot synthesize nucleic acids, complex carbohydrates, lipids, or proteins. Because there are no mitochondria for oxidative metabolism, the energy of mature red blood cells is generated from the metabolism of glucose by the Embden-Meyerhof (anaerobic) pathway and at least three other pathways that use oxygen in different ways. Even without a nucleus, the RBC is metabolically active and requires energy to provide for the following functions: (1) maintenance of osmotic stability through intact membrane pumps and active transport of sodium and potassium; (2) maintenance of iron in the reduced state by using the NADH coenzyme system (see p. 10); and (3) modulation of hemoglobin function by generating 2,3-diphosphoglycerate in the process of generating energy [8].

Function of Red Blood Cells in Oxygen and Carbon Dioxide Transport

Most of the oxygen that crosses the alveolocapillary membrane to the blood combines with the heme portion of hemoglobin. This combination is in a loose bond called *oxyhemoglobin*. Hemoglobin saturation with oxygen is usually 95 percent in arterial blood, and oxygen is rapidly released when it reaches the tissues, which have an oxygen pressure (PO_2) of about 40 mm Hg. In normal venous blood the PO_2 is approximately 40 mm Hg, with a hemoglobin saturation of approximately 70 percent (see Chap. 24) [4].

Transport of carbon dioxide from the tissues of red blood cells occurs in two major ways: (1) in combination with hemoglobin as carbaminohemoglobin (20–25%) and (2) in the dissolved form of bicarbonate (70%). When carbon dioxide is released from the tissue cell it diffuses into the RBC and combines with water, with carbonic anhydrase as the catalyst, to form carbonic acid. Carbonic acid (H_2CO_3) almost immediately dissociates into free hydrogen and bicarbonate ions. Free hydrogen attaches to hemoglobin because it is a powerful acid-base buffer, and bicarbonate is free to diffuse into the plasma or attach to a positive ion within the RBC. When bicarbonate diffuses into the plasma, it is usually replaced by chloride in the *chloride shift*. This is made possible by a bicarbonate-chloride carrier protein that moves these ions in opposite directions very rapidly. The end result is a greater amount of chloride in venous RBCs than in arterial cells [4].

Factors Influencing Erythropoiesis

The normal life span of adult red blood cells is 120 days. Old RBCs are continuously destroyed, and new ones are regenerated daily for replacement. There is normally little variation in the rate of destruction and production, so that the total red blood cell mass in the body remains relatively constant. Erythropoiesis is controlled by the number of circulating red blood cells; decreased numbers stimulate the activity of the bone marrow to increase production of RBCs. Erythropoiesis also is stimulated by a decrease in the PO_2 of arterial blood. Over a long period of time, hypoxemia produces an increase in the number of circulating RBCs.

Erythropoietin hormone stimulates the bone marrow to produce increased numbers of RBCs through conversion of certain stem cells to proerythroblasts. These stem cells are derived from pluripotent stem cells but are more sensitive to erythropoietin than other stem cells. These cells are referred to as erythropoietin-responsive cells (ERC), which are part of a fast cycling system for RBC production. These cells also mature faster than other precursor cells [3,11]. Erythropoietin principally comes from renal glomerular epithelial cells, but some may be released from liver epithelium. The usual stimulus for erythropoietin secretion is hypoxia, but androgens and possibly other hormones have an effect on its secretion. The androgen connection accounts for the higher RBC count in males than in females [3]. A negative feedback system is established, with hypoxemia being a stimulus for erythropoietin and resulting in increased production of red blood cells (Fig. 15-6). The hypoxic stimulus is relieved, so that both the stimulus for erythropoietin synthesis and the rate of erythropoiesis decrease. Conversely, if the volume of circulating red blood cells is increased, erythropoiesis is delayed.

Antigenic Properties of Erythrocytes

More than 30 common red blood cell antigens have been identified. The distinct RBC antigenic properties are genetically determined, with antigens and antibodies almost never being precisely the same among individuals [4]. The antigens in the blood of one person may react

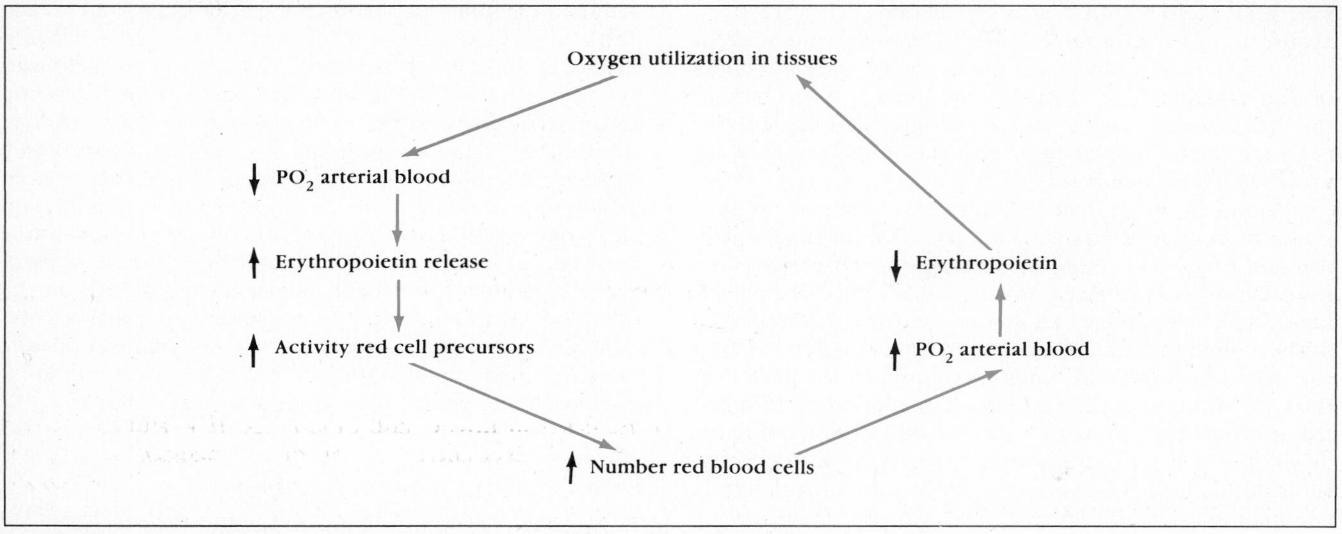

FIGURE 15-6 Feedback mechanism for maintaining the red blood cell population.

with plasma or cells of another, especially during or after a blood transfusion. The antibody to the RBC antigen attaches to the antigenic sites and may cause hemolysis or agglutination of the RBCs.

Blood is classified into different groups and types according to the antigens present on the red cell membrane. Antigens most commonly present on RBC membranes are antigens A, B, and Rh. These make up the O-A-B system of antigens and the Rh system (Table 15-3). A person may inherit neither of these antigens (type O), or may inherit one (A or B) or both (A and B). Type O blood is commonly referred to as the universal donor because it lacks A or B antigens. Type AB blood, commonly referred to as the universal recipient, contains neither anti-A nor anti-B antibodies. Either may contain other agglutinins that can account for a blood transfusion reaction.

The Rh type is determined by the presence or absence of particular antigens on the red blood cell. Type Rh negative refers to the absence of these antigens, while Rh positive refers to the presence of the antigens. There are six types of Rh factors: C, D, E, c, d, and e. The most common is D, which, when present, accounts for the Rh^+ designation. Blood that does not have the D antigen is called Rh^- (negative). The other factors are considered in blood transfusion reactions. Eighty-five percent of Caucasians and 95 percent of blacks in the United States are Rh^+ [4,8].

TABLE 15-3 Blood Types

Percentage of Population	Type
47	O: neither antigen A nor B
41	A: antigen A on RBC; no anti-A antibodies; contains anti-B antibodies
9	B: antigen B on RBC; no anti-B antibodies; contains anti-A antibodies
3	AB: both antigen A and antigen B on RBC; no anti-A; no anti-B antibodies in plasma

Types A and B surface antigens are called *agglutinogens*, and plasma antibodies that can cause agglutination are called *agglutinins* [11]. Antibodies to the agglutinogens are almost always present if the agglutinogen is not present on a person's RBCs [3,4]. For example, anti-A agglutinins are present in the plasma of someone who does not have a type A agglutinogen. Table 15-3 provides a summary of the ABO blood system.

Destruction of Erythrocytes

When red blood cells are released into the circulation from bone marrow, they have a limited life span of approximately 120 days [4]. The metabolism of glucose begins to fail in the aging erythrocytes, causing a gradual decrease in the amount of available adenosine triphosphate (ATP). Without an adequate supply of ATP, the cells are no longer able to maintain functions that are essential for life. The fragile cell membrane may rupture when passing through a tight spot in the circulation such as the spleen, or it may be phagocytized by cells in the spleen, liver, or bone marrow. After lysis of the RBC, hemoglobin is reduced, releasing iron, which is then recycled. After the iron is removed, the remainder of the components in the heme molecule are converted to bilirubin. Bilirubin is taken to the liver to be conjugated with glucuronide (see Chap. 38).

A few RBCs undergo intravascular destruction. When the RBC membrane is damaged, hemoglobin moves out of the cells and quickly becomes bound with a plasma globulin called *haptoglobin*. The resulting complex prevents renal excretion of hemoglobin. The complex is then taken up by phagocytic cells in the liver and processed. When the amount of hemoglobin presented for uptake exceeds renal absorptive capacity, free hemoglobin and methemoglobin appear in the urine [8]. The membranous remains of RBCs are called "ghosts" when they are present in blood samples.

Erythrocytosis

No general agreement has been reached regarding the use of the term *erythrocytosis* versus the term *polycythemia*. Some authorities use the words interchangeably, while others make the clear distinction that polycythemia implies an excess of *all* types of blood cells, and erythrocytosis refers to an increase in erythrocytes only [1]. The term *myeloproliferative disorders* includes a large group of syndromes whose common denominator is the ability to proliferate hemopoietic elements [6]. Table 15-4 lists the conditions grouped as myeloproliferative disorders.

The most commonly recognized causes of erythrocytosis are as follows.

1. *Hypoxemia*. A decrease in oxygen availability to the tissue cells causes an increase in blood levels of erythropoietin, stimulating the marrow to produce more red blood cells and causing release of increased numbers of reticulocytes. In the process of acclimatization to high altitudes, plasma volume reduces, red cell volume slowly rises, and total hemoglobin increases, resulting in an increase in total blood volume. Hypoxemia is frequently noted in persons with pulmonic disease, and many of these affected persons have an associated erythrocytosis. Heavy smokers often have an increased hematocrit level, which is probably due to either an increase in red cell mass or a decrease in plasma volume, or both. This probably results from the high carbon monoxide levels in cigarette smoke that displace oxygen from the hemoglobin and reduce oxygen content.
2. *Overproduction of erythropoietin*. Inappropriate production of erythropoietin has been associated with renal disease, tumors, or other conditions in which there is a disturbance of renal blood flow.

The elevated RBC count that occurs with dehydration and burns results from loss of plasma. The count returns to normal with reexpansion of the plasma volume. This is more properly called *hemoconcentration* rather than erythrocytosis. Table 15-5 shows the classifications of the polycythemias.

Table 15-4 Myeloproliferative Disorders

Polycythemia vera	Leukoerythroblastosis
Myelofibrosis	Thrombocytosis
Myelosclerosis	Leukemoid reactions
Agnogenic myeloid metaplasia	Di Guglielmo's syndrome
	Leukemia (nonlymphocytic)

Source: Reproduced by permission from J.B. Maile, *Laboratory Medicine: Hematology* (6th ed.). St. Louis: The C.V. Mosby Co., 1982. Table 16-6, p. 700.

Polycythemia Vera

Polycythemia vera is a myeloproliferative disorder in which there is increased production of all the formed elements (RBCs, granulocytes, and platelets) of blood. The etiology of this condition is unknown. It is relatively rare, occurring most frequently in males between ages 40 and 60 years.

The abnormal proliferation often initially involves both white and red elements of the marrow. Thrombocytosis and erythrocytosis may be double the normal values. Current evidence supports the belief that the disease is a neoplastic disorder that suppresses normal stem cells [2,8].

The results of the proliferating cellular elements are increases in RBC count, blood viscosity, and blood volume. The liver and spleen become congested and packed with RBCs. The thick blood causes stasis and thrombosis in many areas, which may lead to infarction in any area. Vascular thrombosis results mainly from associated elevated platelet levels [1]. The course of the disease may change, resulting in aplastic, fibrotic, or even leukemic bone marrow [6]. The leukemic change has been questioned, but the frequency of leukemia after polycythemia varies between 14 and 20 percent. Almost all of these are of the chronic granulocytic type, but the terminal episode is usually an acute leukemia (see p. 237) [6,9].

The clinical onset of polycythemia vera is insidious. Most symptoms appear to be related to the increased blood volume, increased blood viscosity, and changes in cerebral blood flow. Lightheadedness, visual disturbances, headaches, and vertigo may be described. Ruddy cyanosis of the face is usually apparent. Pruritus is a common complaint and may be the reason for seeking medical advice. Increased cardiac work may be manifested by eventual congestive heart failure. Thrombophlebitis and thrombosis of digital arteries, accompanied by gangrene, may occur. Associated laboratory values are increased hematocrit, hemoglobin, red cell mass, leukocytes, thrombocytes, leukocyte alkaline phosphatase, serum B_{12} and B_{12}-binding protein, and uric acid. The RBC count may be 7 to 9 million per μl or higher; erythrocyte sedimentation rate is decreased and the blood volume is elevated.

Anemias

Anemia ordinarily refers to a decrease in hemoglobin concentration, the number of circulating RBCs, or volume of packed cells (hematocrit) compared to normal values. Anemias are generally categorized according to etiology and/or morphology (Table 15-6). The approach to diagnosis is first to determine the underlying mechanism of the disease; for example, decreased production, abnormal maturation, or early destruction of RBCs. The reticulocyte count is of primary importance in diagnosis, as are the size, shape, color, and hemoglobin content of RBCs as determined on blood smear. Morphologic characteristics of red blood cells are usually used in the classification of anemias. The terms used include the following:

TABLE 15-5 Classification of the Polycythemias

Disease Type	Characteristics
Relative (decreased plasma volume)	Water deprivation or febrile dehydration
	Loss of water and electrolytes: gastrointestinal disease (vomiting or diarrhea), renal disease, adrenocortical insufficiency, stress (?), Gaisböck's syndrome, vigorous diuretic therapy, etc.
	Loss of plasma: burns, enteropathy, etc.
Absolute	
Secondary	
With compensatory erythropoietin elaboration	Low arterial oxygen saturation
	Low PO_2 in inspired air: high altitude
	Low PO_2 in umbilical vein in fetus
	Ventilation perfusion imbalance and alveolar hypoventilation: insensitivity of respiratory center, restrictive and/or obstructive pulmonary disease, obesity and/or recumbent posture, kyphoscoliosis, sarcoid, pulmonary fibrosis, berylliosis
	V-A shunting: intracardiac septal defects, great vessel anomalies, intrapulmonary A-V aneurysm, hemangiomata
	Normal arterial oxygen saturation
	Decreased oxygen transport by hemoglobin: methemoglobinemia, carboxyhemoglobinemia, M hemoglobins (?)
	Increased affinity for oxygen by abnormal hemoglobins: Chesapeake, Rainier, Little Rock, etc.
	Failure of tissue perfusion: low-output cardiac failure
	Decreased tissue oxygen use: $CoCl_2$ administration
With inappropriate erythropoietin elaboration	Renal diseases: hydronephrosis, cysts, hypernephroma
	Cerebellar hemangioblastoma (?)
	Hepatoma
	Adrenal virilizing adenoma
	Uterine fibroid (?)
	Thyroid or androgen administration
Primary	Polycythemia vera

Source: From W.S. Beck, *Hematology* (4th ed.). Cambridge, Mass.: MIT Press, 1985. Reprinted with permission of The MIT Press.

1. *Normocytic, normochromic*. Normal size and color of red blood cells imparted from hemoglobin concentration
2. *Microcytic, hypochromic*. Decreased size and color of red blood cells due to inadequate hemoglobin concentrations
3. *Macrocytic*. Large size of red blood cells
4. *Anisocytosis*. Variations in red blood cell size
5. *Poikilocytosis*. Variations in red blood cell shape

Alterations in RBC size or hemoglobin content are common in anemias related to deficiencies of iron, folate, or vitamin B_{12}. The shape of the cells gives valuable clues in diagnosis of inherited membrane abnormalities, hemolytic anemias, and hemoglobinopathies. In addition, the blood smear provides information regarding red cell inclusions. Increased stimulus for erythrocyte production is indicated by an increased number of reticulocytes (polychromatophilia) or normoblasts in the peripheral blood.

Aplastic Anemia

Aplastic anemia occurs as a result of reduced bone marrow function and causes a decline in levels of all blood elements. The blood-forming cells do not mature. A severe anemia results, with the formed RBCs sometimes appearing morphologically as slightly macrocytic. The cells also may be normocytic and normochromic.

The cause of aplastic anemia is poorly understood, and in over one-half of cases it is not known [10]. Genetic failure of bone marrow development or injury to stem cells may prohibit the cells' reproduction and differentiation. Physical agents such as whole-body irradiation have been implicated. Chemical agents that may cause aplastic anemia include cytotoxic drugs used for treatment of malignant disease, antimicrobial agents such as chloramphenicol, anticonvulsants, and antiinflammatory drugs. Aplastic anemia may also occur as a complication of infections; for example, viral hepatitis.

A routine blood examination and marrow aspiration and biopsy provide essential information regarding bone marrow function. The marrow is hypocellular or, in rare cases, hypercellular. Marrow biopsy reveals large areas of fat with clusters of lymphocytes, reticular cells, and plasma cells. Uptake of iron by the marrow is decreased and serum iron level is increased. Smears show normocytic, normochromic RBCs that are profoundly decreased in number [8,10].

The onset of symptoms is variable and usually is gradual. Symptoms are often associated with the progressive

TABLE 15-6 Classification of Anemias

Type	Morphologic Characteristics	Causes
Aplastic	Normocytic, normochromic RBCs, depletion of leukocytes and platelets	1. Drug toxicity 2. Genetic failure 3. Radiation 4. Chemicals 5. Infections
Hemolytic	Normocytic, normochromic, increased number of reticulocytes	1. Mechanical injury 2. RBC antigen-antibody reaction 3. Complement binding 4. Chemical reactions 5. Hereditary membrane defects
Macrocytic or megaloblastic; pernicious or folic acid	Macrocytic with variation in size (anisocytosis) shape (poikilocytosis) of RBCs	1. Inadequate diet 2. Lack of intrinsic factor for pernicious anemia 3. Impaired absorption
Microcytic; iron-deficiency; chronic blood loss	Microcytic, hypochromic	1. Inadequate diet 2. Blood loss, chronic 3. Increased need
Posthemorrhagic; acute hemorrhage	Normocytic, normochromic, ↑ number reticulocytes within 48–72 hours	1. Loss of blood leading to hemodilution from interstitial fluid within 48–72 hours 2. Internal or external hemorrhage leading to blood volume depletion

Key: ↑ = increased.

anemia and concomitant decrease in oxygen transport. Weakness, dyspnea, headaches, and syncope are common. Symptoms resulting from leukopenia include decreased immunologic defense and recurrent infections. The thrombocytopenia is variable, with bleeding tendencies ranging from formation of small petechiae to severe bleeding.

Bone marrow transplantation may be a practicable option for the younger individual if a compatible family donor is available. Blood components may be replaced by blood transfusions to allow time for bone marrow to recover in cases of transient marrow failure. Therapy with drugs and other chemical agents should be discontinued until recovery of the bone marrow begins. Splenectomy may be indicated if active hemolysis is associated.

The prognosis of aplastic anemia varies depending on the causative agent. Gradual recovery of hematopoiesis can occur once the agent is discontinued. Severe, progressive anemia is a poor prognostic sign, although infection and hemorrhage are the most frequent causes of death.

Red Blood Cell Aplasia. Pure red blood cell aplasia is much less common than aplastic anemia. It is characterized by severe normocytic, normochromic anemia. It may be immunologically mediated, drug induced, or preleukemic, or occur after a viral infection. Red blood cell aplasia is frequently secondary to end-stage renal failure [10,11].

Hemolytic Anemia

The life span of the RBC may be shortened by intrinsic or extrinsic factors that adversely affect the cell; the shortening may be compensated for by an increase in erythrocyte production. When erythrocyte survival is shortened to 20 days or less, increased erythropoiesis becomes unable to compensate for the rapid RBC destruction [7].

There are a number of ways to classify hemolytic anemias. Categories often overlap and no classification seems to be completely satisfactory. A common presentation of mechanisms of hemolysis is seen in Table 15-7.

Abnormalities of the Red Cell Membrane. These are primarily inherited and acquired disorders of the red cell membrane and include such conditions as hereditary spherocytosis, acquired immune hemolytic anemia, and glucose-6-phosphate dehydrogenase deficiency.

Hereditary spherocytosis (HS) is an inherited autosomal dominant condition that results in a red cell membrane defect. The red cells are spheric and are prematurely destroyed in the spleen. The cells rapidly hemolyze in a hypotonic solution [8]. Clinical signs depend upon the amount of hemolysis present and can include jaundice, splenomegaly, and signs of anemia. Crises in HS are related to associated problems such as infections and gallstones.

Acquired immune hemolytic anemia results from destruction of the red blood cells by the immune system. It is diagnosed by the Coombs' test. A *positive direct Coombs' test* means that a plasma protein, usually IgG or complement, has become fixed to the surface of a RBC. The type involving IgG is associated with lymphoma, systemic lupus erythematosus (SLE), and drug reactions, or it may be idiopathic. Some persons with this type of disease have an antibody against a specific antigen on their own RBCs.

The IgG-related Coombs' test agglutination of red blood cells is sometimes called *warm antibody disease* because antibody-coated cells adhere to macrophages in the spleen and precipitate RBC destruction at 37°C [11]. *Cold antibody disease* is mediated through the IgM antibodies, which at temperatures below 30°C trigger the

TABLE 15-7 Hemolytic Anemias

Cause	Examples
Abnormalities of red cell membrane	Hereditary spherocytosis Immune defects Glycolytic defects
Increased rigidity leading to abnormal flow	Sickle cell anemia Thalassemias
Direct physical trauma	Direct external trauma Turbulent flow Fibrin strands

complement sequence that destroys RBC membranes, leading to loss of hemoglobin. Most cold antibody disease is idiopathic, but it has been described with some of the myeloproliferative disorders. Hemolysis is localized to those body parts exposed to cold temperatures [8,11].

The *indirect Coombs' test* employs normal RBCs exposed first to the suspected serum, then crossed with the Coombs' serum, which induces agglutination of RBCs if antired cell antibodies are present in the suspected serum. It is often used as a screening test to detect the presence of antibodies especially in cross-matching blood for transfusions. Both direct and indirect Coombs' tests may be positive, especially in relation to drugs such as penicillin, quinidine, quinine, and methyldopa [10]. The signs and symptoms of anemia, hemolysis, and fever are often temporal and remit after the drug is withdrawn.

Glucose-6-phosphate dehydrogenase (G6PD) deficiency is a deficiency of this X-linked red cell enzyme. It occurs in 13 percent of American black males, and 25 percent of black females are carriers. Levels of the enzyme reflect the susceptibility of the carrier to hemolysis. One in four carriers is subject to hemolysis. Oxidant drugs such as sulfonamides and primaquin may precipitate the development of hemolysis. Conditions that may precipitate an acute hemolytic episode include viral or bacterial infections and diabetic ketoacidosis. Two main variants of the disease have been described, with profound hemolytic anemia occurring in affected African blacks and persons of Mediterranean descent. Once the infection is controlled or the triggering drug discontinued, recovery usually occurs [10].

Increased Rigidity Causing Abnormal Flow. Two related genetic disorders are described as *sickle syndromes*: *sickle cell trait* and *sickle cell anemia*. These syndromes occur almost exclusively in blacks and are demonstrated by the curved shape of the RBCs when they are exposed to decreased oxygen tension. About 10 percent of American blacks carry the gene HbS on the hemoglobin molecule and approximately 0.2 percent exhibit the actual disease [8]. The sickle cell trait is carried by heterozygous individuals; sickle cell anemia occurs when the individual is homozygous.

Persons with the sickle cell trait usually have no symptoms unless they suffer a hypoxic episode during which some hemolysis and anemia may be noted. Heterozygous red blood cells require very low oxygen tension to precipitate the characteristic sickling effect, so that RBC life span is usually not affected.

Sickle cell anemia causes shortened life expectancy, with symptoms beginning at approximately 6 months of age. It involves the substitution of an amino acid on the beta chain of the globin molecule. The resulting hemoglobin, called HbS, when deoxygenated, undergoes gelation or crystallization, which distorts the red blood cell into a sickle or holly-leaf shape. When there is a significant disparity between the oxygen needed by the cells and the amount available, the cells become rigid and take on abnormal shapes. Small blood vessels become blocked by aggregates of these sickle cells, and the blood supply to all parts of the body may be compromised. The damaged RBCs are trapped in the spleen, and eventually the entire organ may become infarcted.

Infections or hypertonic plasma greatly increase the chances of sickling. As the RBCs obstruct blood flow to the tissues, further deoxygenation and more sickling occurs. The characteristic shape usually returns to normal when oxygen again becomes available.

Hemolysis occurs when RBCs assume the sickle form, and average RBC survival time becomes 10 to 15 days. Bilirubin is released from the hemoglobin during hemolysis, and jaundice may become evident when increased conjugated and unconjugated bilirubin accumulates in the plasma.

The bone marrow often becomes hyperplastic, with evidence of increased erythropoiesis. Reticulocytes and even normoblasts may be released into the circulating blood.

Signs and symptoms of sickle cell anemia vary in severity from sickle crisis in acute hemolysis to impairment of growth and maturity. Because of increased susceptibility to infections, especially those caused by pneumococci, repeated episodes of painful crisis occur. These result from microinfarcts from the vasoocclusive phenomenon [8,10]. Anemia is usually severe, with most of the hemolysis occurring in the extravascular spaces. Chronic leg ulcers, attacks of abdominal pain, and neurologic complications of sudden onset are common. Joint pains may mimic osteomyelitis and joint effusions are frequent. Any organ may be permanently damaged. Splenic function is markedly impaired. Severe renal impairment characteristically contributes to the dehydration and sometimes leads to frank renal failure (see Chap. 31). The prognosis for sickle cell anemia is improving, and more individuals are surviving to adulthood with supportive care.

Thalassemias are intrinsic, congenital disorders that result from defects in the synthesis of hemoglobin and cause a hypochromic, microcytic anemia. They are classified as *major* and *minor* according to the features of the disease. Defects of both beta and alpha chains are known. Disease involving defects of beta chain synthesis occurs most frequently in inhabitants of the Mediterranean area, Central Africa, Asia, the South Pacific, and parts of India [8]. Defects in alpha chain synthesis are most frequent among southern Orientals. The effects vary markedly, depending on whether they are heterozygous or homozygous.

Thalassemia major is homozygous and exhibits ineffective erythropoiesis and peripheral hemolysis, which stimulates enlargement of the red marrow to increase RBC formation. Sometimes the liver also becomes involved in erythropoiesis, resulting in hepatomegaly. Clinical manifestations include profound anemia, wasting, jaundice, hepatomegaly, and characteristic "chipmunk" facies. Typical expansion of the bone marrow leads to thin cortical bone, causing enlargement of the bones of the face and jaws. The long bones become vulnerable to fracture. Growth retardation is common, as are marked splenomegaly and hepatomegaly. Death often occurs at about age 17 years [8].

Thalassemia minor is a heterozygous disorder that offers some resistance against malaria. Affected persons are usually asymptomatic with a mild anemia. It is diagnosed by blood smear and must be differentiated from iron-deficiency anemia [9].

Direct Physical Trauma. Direct physical trauma to red cells can induce hemolytic anemias. External trauma from blows, as may be inflicted in the martial arts, is usually self-limiting. Turbulent blood flow can also cause trauma to the RBCs. Trauma to circulating RBCs has been reported from prolonged exercise, artificial cardiac valves, extracorporeal circulation devices, and conditions in which fibrin deposited in the microvasculature causes fragmentation of RBCs. The results include mild to severe hemolysis and bilirubinemia. The degree of hemolysis is related to the severity of the symptomatology; for example, artificial cardiac valves may be replaced if significant hemolysis continues.

Maturation-Failure Anemia

Pernicious Anemia. Vitamin B_{12} deficiency may occur as a result of decreased dietary intake or of malsorption factors. Pernicious anemia, which results from this deficiency, occurs most frequently in persons over age 60 years who have fair complexions and a family history of the disease. Support for an autoimmune reaction comes from the demonstration of 75-gamma-autoantibody against the intrinsic factor in 40 percent of persons with the disease [10].

Normally, vitamin B_{12} binds chemically with the intrinsic factor that promotes its absorption. In certain conditions, such as atrophy of the gastric mucosal cells, lack of secretion of the intrinsic factor leads to malsorption of vitamin B_{12}. Normal erythrocyte maturation is dependent on adequate amounts of vitamin B_{12} for the synthesis of deoxyribonucleic acid (DNA) molecules. Without B_{12} a macrocytic or megaloblastic anemia results, with marked anisocytosis and poikilocytosis. Ineffective erythropoiesis and increased erythroblast destruction result in hyperbilirubinemia. Although the most pronounced changes arise in the RBCs, mild neutropenia and thrombocytopenia may also occur.

The onset of symptoms is usually insidious, but may be hastened by conditions such as infection. Persons with pernicious anemia do not secrete hydrochloric acid (on gastric analysis) even after parenteral stimulation with histamine. Many of the signs and symptoms of pernicious anemia are common to any of the anemic states. Anorexia, fatigue, shortness of breath, and irritability are common. Soreness of the tongue characteristically occurs early in the illness and progressively grows worse. The soreness is quickly relieved after adequate vitamin B_{12} treatment. Symmetric numbness and tingling of the toes and fingers occur in 10 percent of persons and indicate early neurologic disease. Ataxia and loss of vibration sense also may be noted. Neurologic symptoms may not entirely remit after treatment.

Folic Acid Anemia. A deficiency of folic acid produces anemia with characteristics similar to those of pernicious anemia. The two conditions cannot be distinguished morphologically. The RBCs are large (megaloblastic) with fragile membranes. A definite dietary deficiency can be demonstrated, and the anemia develops one to two months after the dietary lack. It is common in alcoholism and chronic malnutrition. Increased frequency during pregnancy relates also to poor nutrition [10]. Folic acid anemia usually responds well to oral dietary replacement unless malsorption is a problem.

Microcytic, Hypochromic Anemia

Iron-Deficiency Anemia. This disease is characterized by deficient hemoglobin synthesis due to a lack of iron. With severe deficiency, the RBCs become microcytic and hypochromic because of low concentrations of hemoglobin. This is the most common type of anemia and occurs in all geographic locations and in all age groups. The main causes of iron deficiency are increased loss, as in chronic or acute bleeding, and decreased dietary intake. The blood lost during menstruation accounts for a high frequency of iron deficiency in women. Iron deficiency is common among preschool children, presumably because of increased dietary need and poor dietary supply.

Because iron is absorbed mostly in the duodenum and its ionization and absorption are enhanced by gastric hydrochloric acid, iron-deficiency anemia may accompany pernicious anemia or gastrectomy. Also, malsorption syndromes impair absorption of iron along with other nutrients.

Laboratory values reflect decreased levels of serum iron and apoferritin (iron-binding protein produced by the liver) in the early stages. Normal serum iron levels range from 12 to 300 μg per ml but 20 percent of affected adults have normal iron indices [10]. Anemia, characterized by microcytic and variably sized hypochromic RBCs, is a relatively late manifestation [11].

Clinical manifestations are nonspecific and their onset is insidious. Fatigue, tachycardia, irritability, and pallor with epithelial abnormalities such as sore tongue or stomatitis may occur. Thinning or spooning of the nails (koilonychia) is encountered occasionally. Pica may be striking, with affected individuals craving dirt, starch, or ice [6]. Late manifestations may include cardiac murmurs, congestive heart failure, loss of hair, and pearly sclera.

Posthemorrhagic Anemia

Posthemorrhagic anemia may occur after acute or chronic blood loss, although chronic blood loss usually results in iron-deficiency anemia. Plasma and red blood cells are both lost during hemorrhage, so laboratory values may reveal a normal hemoglobin level and red blood cell count immediately after a hemorrhage.

Blood volume is restored by the movement of fluid from the interstitial spaces into the capillaries, causing dilution of the remaining red blood cells (dilutional anemia) with a maximum effect in 48 to 72 hours. This dilute blood carries too few RBCs to oxygenate the tissues efficiently. Anemia of a normocytic and normochromic type becomes apparent. The bone marrow is stimulated to produce increased numbers of red blood cells, but this process requires a period of time that varies according to the amount of blood lost. Within seven days the reticulocyte count can be elevated to 10 to 15 percent [11]. In acute massive bleeding, this compensatory effect may not occur in time to be lifesaving without transfusions of whole blood.

Laboratory and Diagnostic Tests

Hematologic Studies

Examination of the blood provides valuable information in the diagnosis and treatment of blood disorders. Normal hematologic values, summarized in Table 15-8, are based on the examination of statistically significant numbers of healthy persons. They vary with age, environment, sex, genetics, and physiologic state. The most important erythrocyte studies are discussed in this section.

Hemoglobin. The primary function of hemoglobin is to carry oxygen in the form of oxyhemoglobin; therefore, the oxygen-combining capacity of blood is directly proportional to the hemoglobin concentration. The hemoglobin level varies significantly with sex and age (Table 15-8). Levels may be decreased in anemia or circulatory overload and are increased in polycythemia.

Red Blood Cells. Erythrocytes are the mature circulating red blood cells whose primary function is to transport oxygen and carbon dioxide. Increases and decreases in red cell counts usually vary in the same direction as the hemoglobin, as previously mentioned.

Packed Cell Volume or Hematocrit. The packed cell volume is the ratio of packed cells to total volume in a sample that has been centrifuged. The packed cell volume is used to determine red blood cell indices, calculate blood volume and total red blood cell mass, and measure roughly the concentration of red blood cells [11]. Levels increase in conditions associated with hemoconcentration (burns, shock, and trauma), hypovolemia, and polycythemia. The hematocrit decreases in hypervolemic states (cardiac failure, overhydration with intravenous fluid), hemorrhage, and hemolysis.

Erythrocyte Sedimentation Rate (ESR). Blood is a suspension of formed elements in plasma; therefore, when it is mixed with an anticoagulant and stands, the heavier red blood cells sink to the bottom. The rate at which the RBCs settle is a function of fibrinogen and globulin. These proteins enhance clumping of erythrocytes, thus increasing the rate at which the cells fall. Other factors that affect the rate are alterations in the positive charge of plasma, the ratio of plasma protein fractions to each other, and changes in the erythrocyte surface.

The ESR is a nonspecific test, but because the sedimentation rate is increased in many inflammatory conditions, it can serve in the differential diagnosis in such conditions as acute myocardial infarction, angina pectoris, rheumatoid arthritis, and osteoarthritis. A moderately increased ESR is often noted in persons over age 60 years.

Mean Corpuscular Volume (MCV). The MCV measures the volume and size of each red blood cell. The MCV increases in megaloblastic anemias (large cells) and decreases in iron deficiency (small cells) [11].

Mean Corpuscular Hemoglobin (MCH). The MCH gives the amount of hemoglobin by weight in the average red blood cell. Macrocytic cells with large volume of hemoglobin show increased levels, as in macrocytic anemia. Levels of MCH are decreased in conditions related to hemoglobin deficiency, as in iron-deficiency anemia.

Mean Cell Hemoglobin Concentration (MCHC). This measurement gives the average percentage of hemo-

TABLE 15-8 Normal Hematologic Values

Red blood cells	
Infant, first day	5.1 ± 1 million/μl
Child, 1 year	4.5 ± 1 million/μl
Child, 6–10 years	4.7 ± 1 million/μl
Adult	
Female	4.8 ± 0.6 million/μl
Male	5.4 ± 0.8 million/μl
Hemoglobin	
Infant, first day	19.5 ± 5.0 gm/dl
Child, 1 year	11.2 ± 2.3 gm/dl
Child, 6–10 years	12.9 ± 2.3 gm/dl
Adult	
Female	14.0 ± 2.0 gm/dl
Male	16.0 ± 2.0 gm/dl
Volume packed RBC (hematocrit)	
Infant, first day	54 ± 10 ml/dl
Child, 1 year	35 ± 5 ml/dl
Child, 6–10 years	37.5 ± 5 ml/dl
Adult	
Female	42 ± 5 ml/dl
Male	47 ± 5 ml/dl
Erythrocyte sedimentation rate (ESR) (Westergren method)	
Female	0–20 mm/hour
Male	0–13 mm/hour
Mean corpuscular volume (MCV)	
Female and male	87 ± 5 cuμ
Mean corpuscular hemoglobin (MCH)	
Female and male	29 ± 2 μg
Mean corpuscular hemoglobin concentration (MCHC)	
Female and male	34 ± 2%
Reticulocyte count	0.5–1.5% of erythrocytes

Source: J. Wallach, *Interpretation of Diagnostic Tests* (4th ed.). Boston: Little, Brown, 1986.

globin saturation or concentration of hemoglobin in the average red cell. Decreased levels occur in hemoglobin deficiency.

Reticulocyte Count. The reticulocyte is a young, nonnucleated cell of the erythrocyte line. An elevated reticulocyte count is indicative of increased bone marrow activity, with early release of increased numbers of reticulocytes, as in hemolytic anemias.

Bone Marrow Studies. Bone marrow may be obtained for examination by aspiration or biopsy. Data obtained from bone marrow examination are very useful in the diagnosis, progression, and prognosis of blood disorders.

Diagnostic Test

Schilling Test. This test measures the absorption of vitamin B_{12}. Radioactive B_{12} is administered orally and a 24-hour urine collection is begun. The presence of radioactivity in the urine indicates gastrointestinal absorption of vitamin B_{12}. Above 8 percent excretion of the radioactive dose is normal. This test is used in the diagnosis of pernicious anemia.

Study Questions

1. Explain the differences in cellular development among leukocytes, erythrocytes, and platelets.
2. Discuss the process of erythropoiesis and explain how it maintains a sufficient population of red blood cells.
3. Review the antigenic nature of red blood cells and explain why it is important in blood transfusions.
4. Describe the morphologic differences among the five types of anemias. How do the clinical manifestations compare?
5. Explain the differences between physiologic and pathologic polycythemia.
6. Discuss the importance of the Coombs' test in isolating the types of anemias.
7. Describe the major erythrocyte studies and list several reasons for performing each.

References

1. Castle, W.B. The polycythemias. In W.S. Beck, *Hematology* (4th ed.). Cambridge, Mass.: MIT Press, 1985.
2. Dietschy, J.M., et al. (eds.). *Hematology and Oncology*. New York: Grune & Stratton, 1980.
3. Ganong, W.F. *Review of Medical Physiology* (12th ed.). Los Altos, Calif.: Lange, 1985.
4. Guyton, A.C. *Textbook of Medical Physiology* (7th ed.). Philadelphia: Saunders, 1986.
5. Junqueira, L.C., and Carneiro, J. *Basic Histology* (4th ed.). Los Altos, Calif.: Lange, 1983.
6. Maile, J.B. *Laboratory Medicine: Hematology* (6th ed.). St. Louis: Mosby, 1982.
7. Reich, P.R. *Hematology: Physiopathologic Basis for Clinical Practice* (2nd ed.). Boston: Little, Brown, 1984.
8. Robbins, S.L., Cotran, R.S., and Kumar, V. *Pathologic Basis of Disease* (3rd ed.). Philadelphia: Saunders, 1984.
9. Thompson, R.B. *Disorders of the Blood*. New York: Churchill Livingstone, 1977. P. 713.
10. Wallerstein, R.O. Blood. In M.A. Krupp, M.J. Chatton, and L.M. Tierney, *Current Medical Diagnosis and Treatment*. Los Altos, Calif.: Lange, 1986.
11. Weatherall, D.J., and Bunch, C. The blood and blood-forming organs. In L.H. Smith and S.O. Thier, *Pathophysiology: The Biological Principles of Disease* (2nd ed.). Philadelphia: Saunders, 1985.
12. Wintrobe, M.M. *Blood, Pure and Eloquent.* New York: McGraw-Hill, 1980.

CHAPTER 16

Normal and Altered Leukocyte Function

CHAPTER OUTLINE

Normal Leukocyte Function

- Characteristics of Leukocytes
- White Cell Count
- Differential White Cell Count
- Genesis of Leukocytes
- Life Span of White Blood Cells
- Properties of Leukocytes
  - *Functional Classification*
  - *Phagocytosis*
  - *Degranulation*
  - *Killing*
  - *Diapedesis*
  - *Chemotaxis*
  - *Pinocytosis*
  - *Recognition of the Particle*
- Function of Phagocytes
- Function of Basophils and Eosinophils
  - *Basophils*
  - *Eosinophils*
- Mononuclear Phagocyte System

Nonmalignant White Blood Cell Disorders

- Quantitative Alterations of Granulocytes
  - *Neutrophils*
  - *Eosinophils*
  - *Basophils*
- Qualitative Alterations of Granulocytes
- Monocyte Abnormalities
- Lymphocytic Disorders
  - *Infectious Mononucleosis*
  - *Lymphadenopathy*

Malignant White Blood Cell Disorders

- Leukemia
  - *Classification*
  - *Clinical Manifestations*
  - *Progression of the Disease*
- Malignant Lymphomas
  - *Classification*
  - *Hodgkin's Disease*
- Multiple Myeloma

LEARNING OBJECTIVES

1. List and describe the five types of leukocytes.
2. Differentiate leukocytes on the basis of morphology and function.
3. Define the normal white cell count per microliter of blood and explain its significance.
4. Describe the differential white count and list the relative proportion of each cell type.
5. Describe phagocytosis and discuss its significance with respect to the destruction of microorganisms and immunologic integrity.
6. Compare the average life span of the five types of leukocytes.
7. Explain locomotion, diapedesis, degranulation, killing, chemotaxis, and opsonization with respect to phagocytosis and immunologic integrity.
8. Explain the function of the mononuclear phagocyte system.
9. Compare quantitative and qualitative alterations of granulocytes and list several examples of conditions that influence these alterations.
10. Compare qualitative and quantitative alterations of monocytes and lymphocytes. List several examples of conditions that influence these alterations.
11. Describe the characteristics of a myeloproliferative disorder.
12. Differentiate between malignant and nonmalignant disorders in leukocytes.
13. Describe the qualitative and quantitative alterations of leukocytes in leukemia.
14. Explain the basis of classification of leukemias.
15. Differentiate between acute and chronic leukemia.
16. Differentiate generally between reactive lymphadenopathies and malignant lymphomas.
17. Differentiate Hodgkin's disease and other lymphomas on the basis of laboratory findings.
18. Describe the qualitative and quantitative alterations of leukocytes in infectious mononucleosis.
19. Discuss the causative agent of infectious mononucleosis and its significance with respect to malignancy and immunosuppression.
20. Explain the significance of Sternberg-Reed cells with respect to Hodgkin's disease.
21. Discuss the clinical features and pathologic alterations in multiple myeloma.

Leukocytes, larger and less numerous than erythrocytes, play a key role in the defense mechanisms of the body. As the name implies, leukocytes are almost white (the Greek *leukos* means "white"). Examination of a centrifuged tube of whole blood reveals a fuzzy gray-white layer between the packed red cells and the clear yellow plasma. This layer, called the *buffy coat*, contains leukocytes and platelets. The white buffy color is due to the leukocytes.

The most important function of the leukocytes is to defend the body against invasion by foreign organisms and to produce, transport, and distribute defensive elements such as antibodies or other factors that are necessary for the immune response. The various types of leukocytes work together in an integrated system. Each type performs different functions in the defense mechanisms, and all functions are necessary for a total integrated and effective defense.

Normal Leukocyte Function

Characteristics of Leukocytes

There are normally about 5000 to 10,000 leukocytes per μl of adult human blood [1]. Of these, *granulocytes* (polymorphonuclear leukocytes, or polys) make up the largest portion of the total number, approximately 65 percent. The *agranulocytes* comprise the remaining 35 percent. Granulocytes have large granules and horseshoe-shaped nuclei that differentiate and become multilobed, with two to five distinct lobes connected by thin strands. The background cytoplasm stains blue to pink with Wright's stain, which enhances their morphologic identification (Table 16-1).

Granulocytes are subdivided into three cell types: neutrophils, eosinophils, and basophils. The *neutrophils* are the most numerous, making up 50 to 70 percent of the total white cell count. They have small, fine, light pink or lilac acidophilic granules when stained, and a segmented, irregularly lobed, purple nucleus.

Eosinophils constitute approximately 1 to 5 percent of the normal white cell count. They have large, round granules that contain red-staining, basic mucopolysaccharides and multilobed, purple-blue nuclei [2,5].

Like eosinophils, *basophils* constitute a small percentage of the white cells, ranging from 0 to 1 percent of the total count. The coarse, basophilic, blue granules often conceal the segmented nucleus. The content of these granules includes histamine, heparin, and acid mucopolysaccharides [5].

Lymphocytes and monocytes are the remaining white blood cell types normally present in peripheral blood. They are often called *agranulocytes* because they were originally thought to have no granules. Their granules are very small and stain quite differently than the large granules of granulocytes. Lymphocytes and monocytes are also called mononuclear leukocytes because they do not have the multilobed nucleus as the granulocytes do.

Lymphocytes, also called immunocytes, are cells with large, round, deep-staining nuclei and very little cytoplasm. The cytoplasm is slightly basophilic and stains pale blue. They make up approximately 20 to 40 percent of the total white cell count.

The *monocyte* is a large mononuclear leukocyte with a prominent, multishaped nucleus that is sometimes kidney-shaped. The chromatin in the nucleus looks like lace, with small particles linked together by fine strands. Chromatin is less clumped than in the mature granulocyte or lymphocyte. The gray-blue cytoplasm is filled with many fine lysosomes that stain pink with Wright's stain. Monocytes constitute about 1 to 6 percent of the total white cell count. Figure 16-1 illustrates the different types of white blood cells.

Table 16-1 Staining Characteristics of Leukocytes

Leukocyte	Cytoplasm	Cytoplasmic Granules	Nucleus
Neutrophil	Blue to pink	Lilac	Purple-blue
Eosinophil	Blue to pink	Red	Purple-blue
Basophil	Blue to pink	Blue-black	Purple-blue
Lymphocyte	Pale blue		Dark blue
Monocyte	Gray-blue	Pink	Blue lighter than lymphocytes

White Cell Count

The white cell count is determined by counting cells in a diluted blood sample. The procedure can be done manually, but usually an electronic enumerator counts the leukocytes suspended in a dilute fluid that lyses the erythrocytes to prevent interference. Normal values range between 5000 and 10,000 white cells per μl. The count is important as a diagnostic tool in cases of infection, malignancy, and other disorders that cause alterations of these cells. Significant increases or decreases of the count are known as *quantitative alterations*.

Differential White Cell Count

Each of the leukocytes has a specific function in the body's defense system. An attack by a foreign agent often elicits a response by a certain type of leukocyte. For example, a pyogenic bacterial infection may elicit an increase in neutrophils, or a parasitic infection might elicit an increase in eosinophils. Therefore, an increase or decrease in the normal percentage of leukocytes may have significant diagnostic value. The relative proportion of leukocyte cell types is called the differential count.

The differential count is determined on a smear of blood one cell-layer thick. This layer is stained with a polychrome solution containing both basic and acidic dyes, usually Wright's stain. The leukocyte cellular structure absorbs the dye differentially and permits evaluation not only of the relative proportions of the white cells, but of cellular elements and platelets. Differentials may be done manually or electronically (Table 16-2).

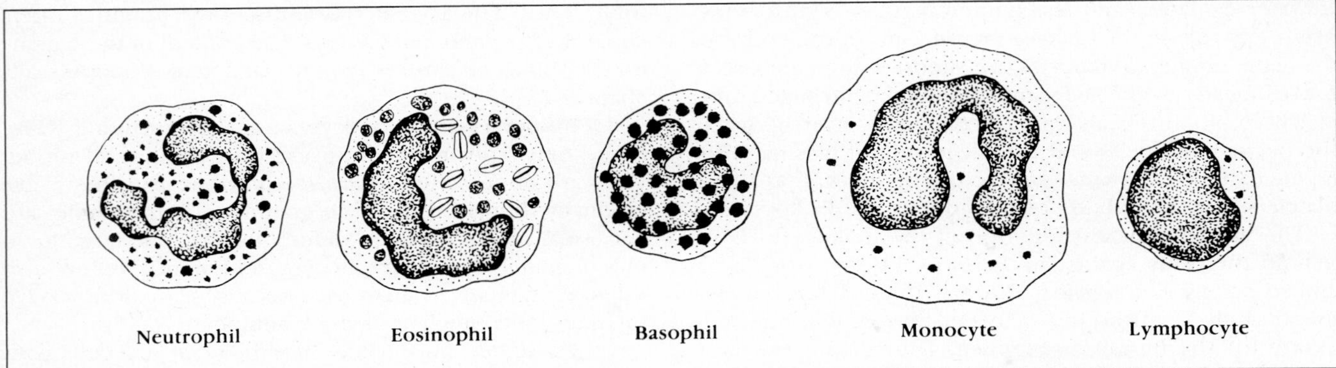

FIGURE 16-1 Characteristics of different types of leukocytes. (From M. Borysenko, *Functional Histology* [2nd ed.]. Boston: Little, Brown, 1984.)

TABLE 16-2 Normal Differential Count of Leukocytes

Leukocytes	Count (%)
Neutrophils, segmented	50–70
Neutrophils, bands or stabs	0–5
Eosinophils	1–4
Basophils	0–1
Lymphocytes	20–40
Monocytes	1–6

Normal differential white cell proportions vary with age. The neutrophils, for example, are significantly increased at birth, but fall below the normal adult level by 2 weeks of age. Lymphocytes, higher at birth and in early childhood, decrease in numbers until adult levels are reached. The relative proportion, however, is higher from age 4 weeks to 4 years (Table 16-3) [10].

Often an *absolute count* of a particular leukocyte is necessary for diagnosis. This can be obtained by using a special diluting fluid that lyses the erythrocytes and either lyses or does not stain the other white cells present. The specific leukocyte can then be counted without including the other cells.

TABLE 16-3 Normal Age-Related Leukocyte Differential Count in Peripheral Blood

Cell type	Percentage	Number
Segmental neutrophils		
Infant, first day	47 ± 15	8870
Child, 1 year	23 ± 10	2600
Child, 10 years	46 ± 15	3700
Adult, over 21	51 ± 15	3800
Band neutrophils		
Infant, first day	14.2 ± 4	2580
Child, 1 year	8.1 ± 3	990
Child, 10 years	8.0 ± 3	645
Adult, over 21	8.0 ± 3	620
Eosinophils		
Infant, first day	2.4	450
Child, 1 year	2.6	300
Child, 10 years	2.4	200
Adult, over 21	2.7	200
Basophils		
Infant, first day	0.5	100
Child, 1 year	0.4	50
Child, 10 years	0.5	40
Adult, over 21	0.5	40
Lymphocytes		
Infant, first day	31 ± 5	5800
Child, 1 year	61 ± 15	7000
Child, 10 years	38 ± 10	3100
Adult, over 21	34 ± 10	2500
Monocytes		
Infant, first day	5.8	1100
Child, 1 year	4.8	550
Child, 10 years	4.3	350
Adult, over 21	4.0	300

Source: J. Wallach, *Interpretation of Diagnostic Tests* (4th ed.). Boston: Little, Brown, 1986.

Genesis of Leukocytes

The multipotential or uncommitted stem cells in bone marrow are essentially responsible for blood cell and platelet formation. They differentiate into unipotential, or committed, stem cells that ultimately become white blood cells, platelets, and erythrocytes (Fig. 16-2).

Neutrophils, basophils, and eosinophils are formed in the bone marrow and can be stored there until needed. If the need is greater than the supply, immature forms may be released.

Granulocytes and monocytes are thought to be derived from a common committed stem cell. The promonocyte is also formed and differentiated in bone marrow and is released into the circulation as a mature monocyte. The monocyte can leave the blood for the tissues, where it enlarges and is transformed or matured into a lysosome-filled macrophage. The macrophage is much larger than the monocyte, which is important for the phagocytosis of large particles and debris [3,5]. Both granulocytes and monocytes have phagocytic properties.

Lymphocytes are thought to be formed from a separate committed stem cell in the bone marrow. In the fetus, proliferating stem cells migrate from the yolk sac to the liver, which is a major blood-forming organ during gesta-

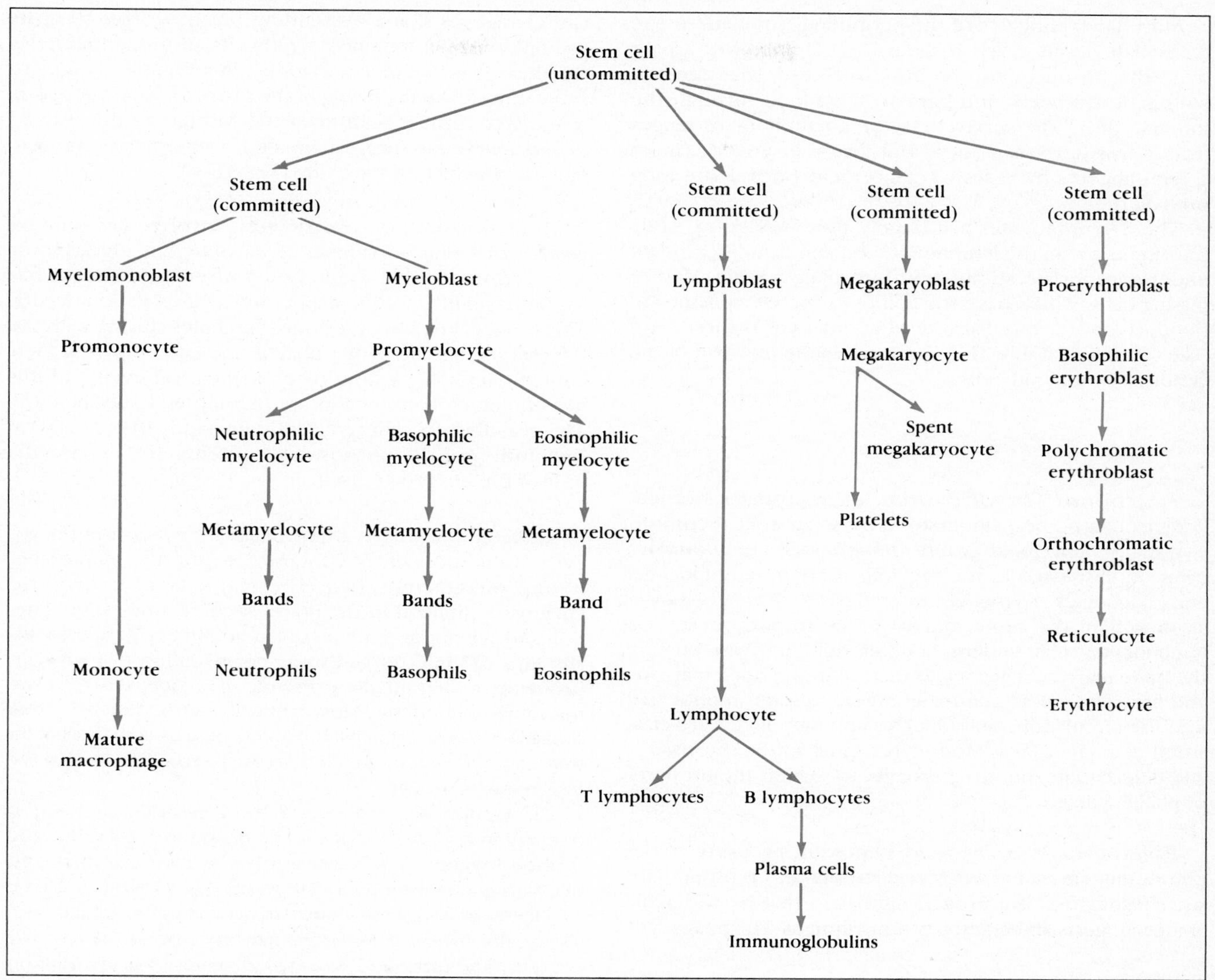

FIGURE 16-2 Differentiation of stem cells in the bone marrow. (From M. Wintrobe et al., *Clinical Hematology* [7th ed.]. Lea and Febiger, 1984.)

tion [3]. Unlike granulocytes and monocytes, most lymphocytes are differentiated not in the bone marrow but in the lymphoid tissue, thymus, or spleen. Only large and small lymphocytes and plasma cells can be identified by morphology. Identification of B and T lymphocytes involves such laboratory techniques as cell marker studies and cytochemistry. Differentiation of the B and T lymphocytes in the lymphoid tissue is an important aspect of the immunologic response (see Chap. 10).

Life Span of White Blood Cells

The life span of white blood cells in the circulating blood is generally short. The average half-life of a neutrophil is approximately six hours [8]. During a serious infection, granulocytes often live two hours or less, until they are used or destroyed. Granulocytes mature in the bone marrow. After myelocytes (precursors of granulocytes) stop dividing, maturing granulocytes accumulate as a reserve in the bone marrow. Under normal conditions, there is about a five-day supply of granulocytes in this reserve. Once the granulocytes leave the marrow, they spend an average of 12 hours in the circulation and about 2 to 3 days in the tissues before they are destroyed.

Monocytes spend less time in the bone marrow pool than granulocytes. The life span of the monocyte in the circulation is approximately 36 hours, or about 3 times as long as that of granulocytes [8]. After the monocyte has been transformed into a mobile or fixed macrophage in the tissues, its life is long, ranging from months to years.

The life span of the lymphocytes varies tremendously. A small population of extremely long-lived cells may survive for many years. These cells are necessary for maintaining immunologic memory and have the special ability to reenter cell division through specific stimulation by an antigen.

Most T lymphocytes of the peripheral lymphatic tissue recirculate about every 10 hours [3]. They follow a path from the blood to the lymphatic tissue, through the lymphatic channels, and back to the blood through the thoracic duct. The survival rate of T lymphocytes ranges from a few days to months and years. In general, most T lymphocytes have slow replacement rates and a long survival time.

The B lymphocytes are largely noncirculating. They remain mainly in the lymphoid tissue and can differentiate under appropriate stimulation into plasma cells. Mature plasma cells, which have the ability to secrete specific antibodies, have a survival rate of about two to three days (see Chap. 10). Table 16-4 summarizes the life span of the various white blood cells.

Properties of Leukocytes

Functional Classification. The properties of leukocytes can be best understood by separating them into two major functional groups: *phagocytes* and *immunocytes*. As discussed in the previous section, immunocytes and phagocytes are thought to be derived from a common stem cell in the bone marrow. The immunocytes, or lymphocytes, may undergo a differentiation phase outside the bone marrow. Phagocytes mature in the bone marrow, and are released as mature granulocytes and monocytes into the circulation. Granulocytes and monocytes are classified as phagocytes. Monocytes must enter the tissues and differentiate into macrophages to exhibit the property of phagocytosis.

Phagocytosis. The most important property of the phagocytes (granulocytes and macrophages) is phagocytosis. Phagocytosis is a process similar to that by which an amoeba ingests and digests its nourishment. The phagocyte can change its shape by sending out processes from its protoplasm. Microorganisms, old cells, or foreign particles can then be enveloped or engulfed in a vacuole, or *phagosome*, formed by the fusing of the processes of protoplasm. Associated with ingestion of the foreign or devitalized material are rapid increase in cellular energy and the generation of hydrogen peroxide (Fig. 16-3).

Degranulation. Phagocytosis involves not only ingestion of a microorganism or particle, but digestion or destruction of this foreign body. After the material has become engulfed in the phagosome, degranulation occurs. This process involves lysosomes (granules) fusing with the internal membrane of the phagosome and emptying their contents into its vacuole. The biochemical events of this morphologic phenomenon are incompletely understood. The granules contain hydrolytic enzymes that cause the dissolution of the phagosome contents and eventually, lysis of the phagocyte itself.

Killing. Killing is the process by which the phagocytized microorganism contained within the membrane-bound phagosome dies. The majority of hydrolytic enzymes contained in the granules serve a digestive function and are not directly involved in killing [5]. What actually kills the microorganism is peroxidation of hydrogen peroxide, which, in the presence of iodide, destroys the microbial membrane. Most bacteria can be killed by this process. Some organisms, however, such as acid-fast bacilli that cause tuberculosis and leprosy, are able to survive inside the phagocyte.

Dissolution is complex and involves integrated action of many hydrolytic enzymes. The phagocyte, as well as the foreign invader, is often lysed by its own enzymes and becomes part of the degradation products (see Fig. 16-3).

The degradation products that remain after phagocytosis usually intensify the inflammatory process to varying degrees. The released lysosomal enzymes of degranulation or toxins released by the bacteria may cause damage to the surrounding tissues. Degradation products include thromboplastic products that lead to vascular clotting (see Chap. 17).

Phagocytosis is promoted by other factors such as temperature and electrical charge. Elevated body temperatures or increased heat at the site of infection enhances phagocytosis. Fever during an infection may serve as a protective mechanism within limits. The electrical charge on antigen surfaces may also enhance phagocytosis, as the charge on dead or foreign particles is different from that on living tissues and is considered to be a dominant factor in specificity [3].

Increased glucose metabolism and cellular oxygen consumption are needed for phagocytosis, because increased energy is necessary for the production of large amounts of hydrogen peroxide used to kill bacteria. Energy in the form of adenosine triphosphate (ATP) is supplied by glycolysis in the white blood cell itself.

Diapedesis. Phagocytes have the ability to accumulate at the site of invasion or injury. Like the amoeba, they

TABLE 16-4 Life Span of White Blood Cells

Cell Type	In Circulating Blood	Tissue Life
Granulocytes	6–8 hours; time shortened in acute infection.	2–3 days
Monocytes	Short transit time, often less than 36 hours.	Months or years as tissue macrophages.
T lymphocytes	Remain in the blood a few hours but recirculate about every 10 hours.	Varies from a few days to years.
B lymphocytes	Few circulate.	Most remain in lymphoid tissue; when they become secreting plasma cells, they survive 2–3 days.
Platelets	Most circulate; are totally replaced every 10 days.	

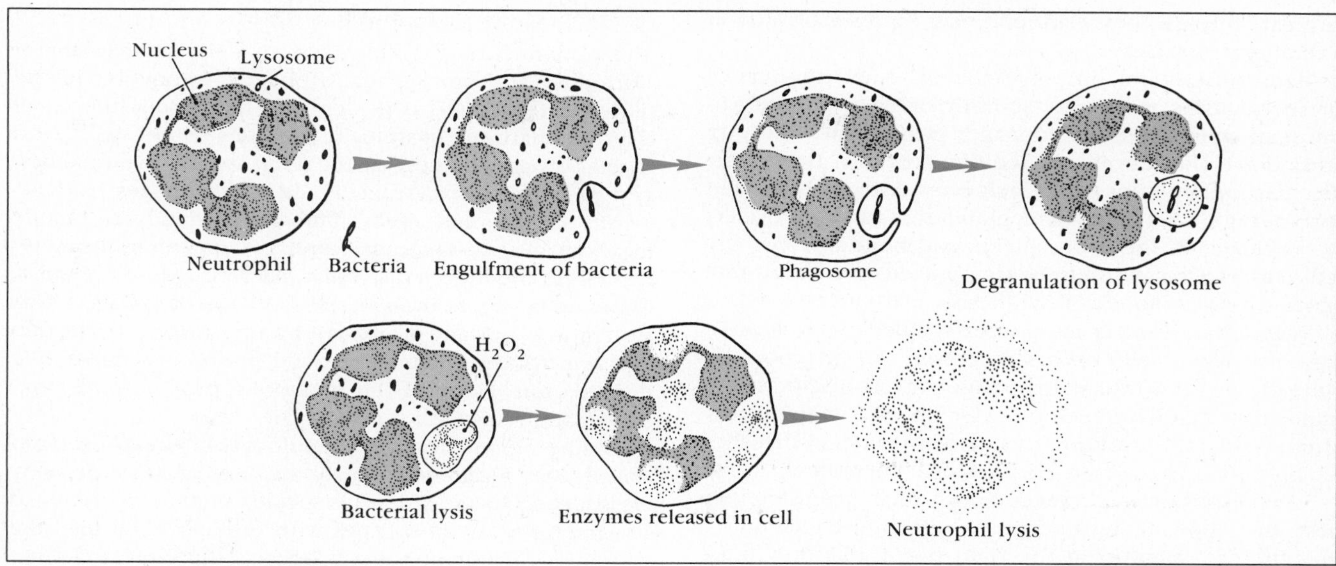

FIGURE 16-3 Phagocytosis of bacteria.

form pseudopodlike processes that allow them to move through avenues of the body. Granulocytes and monocytes can leave the circulation and enter tissue by a process called diapedesis. Diapedesis refers to the ability of the phagocyte to slip through the walls of the capillary vessel by amoeboid motion. A small portion of the phagocyte slides through at a time until the entire cell leaves the circulation. Diapedesis allows phagocytes to accumulate at the invasion site (see Chap. 9).

Chemotaxis. The phagocytes must be able to find the site of a bacterial invasion or recognize that infection has taken place. Specific phagocytes break down and digest necrotic material. Chemical substances, called chemotactic agents or mediators, are released from the infected or necrotic tissues and provide a signal for the leukocytes to move toward the source of the chemotactic agent. This process, called chemotaxis, is dependent on a concentration gradient. A greater concentration of the chemical causes more leukocytes to move toward the source. Other chemotactic agents include the complement system, plasminogen, the fibrinolytic system, kallikrein (the kinin system), and substances released from the phagocytes.

Pinocytosis. Pinocytosis is the cellular engulfment by the phagocyte of tiny particles included in a droplet of fluid. It differs from phagocytosis in that in phagocytosis the membrane sends out processes to grasp a relatively large particle using a biochemical mechanism similar to muscle action. In pinocytosis, macrophages ingest and break down macromolecules. The role of pinocytosis in many macrophage activities is not totally understood [3].

Recognition of the Particle. Before a phagocyte can ingest a bacterium or particle, it must recognize the particle. Recognition of the foreign invader is achieved through mediation in one of two ways: opsonization and surface properties [9].

Opsonization of the antigenic surface is necessary for the phagocyte to attach to the antigen. Opsonization is mediated by activation of the complement protein system or by specific antibodies. Activation of complement results in attachment of C3b to the surface of the particle, which, with specific antibody, allows it to be recognized and phagocytized by the leukocyte [9].

Some particles have special ***surface properties*** that cause them to adhere to the phagocyte and subsequently undergo phagocytosis. These physiochemical properties allow the particle to adhere to the cell membrane of the phagocyte while pseudopodia surround and engulf the particle. This type of phagocytosis is seen in the early phases of an illness and is most effective with tightly packed leukocytes. The exact mechanism of attachment of the phagocyte to the antigen before antibody formation, complement activation, or cell devitalization is not known.

Function of Phagocytes

The functions of granulocytes and monocyte-macrophages overlap, but in general, granulocytes are the first line of defense against microbial invasion; neutrophils are adept at recognizing, ingesting, and killing pyogenic bacteria; and monocyte-macrophages are important in the final removal or cellular clean-up of debris after phagocytosis and cell lysis.

Monocyte-macrophages are able to ingest bigger particles and larger amounts of debris because of their larger size. Inert materials as large as wood or steel fragments can be engulfed by macrophages and removed from the site of inflammation. If a particle is very large, multinucleated foreign-body *giant cells* may be produced. The characteristic foreign-body giant cell may represent fusion of several macrophages.

Macrophages not only provide the final removal of microorganisms, but clear the body of its own aged and damaged cells. Some macrophages possess the ability to break down and recycle old red blood cells. A type of tissue macrophage possesses heme oxidase activity that enables it to break down hemoglobin that can be recycled. Macrophages of the liver, spleen, and bone marrow can return iron to transferrin to be transported to the erythroid marrow for red blood cell synthesis.

Phagocytes contain antibacterial substances, peroxidase, and lysosomal enzymes necessary for phagocytosis and other activities. Macrophages are thought to kill tumor cells that have been processed by the lymphocytes. Monocytes and granulocytes also interact with other biologically active substances such as complement.

For the phagocytes to accomplish their defensive purpose, the following must occur: (1) they must accumulate in sufficient numbers at the right place; (2) they must attach to the foreign material or agent; (3) they must envelop or engulf the agent; and (4) they must dispose of the debris [5,9]. Alterations in any of these functions results in defective phagocytosis, which then results in a defective defensive response.

Function of Basophils and Eosinophils

The precise function of basophils and eosinophils is not well understood, but it is known that these cells participate in the inflammatory and allergic reactions.

Basophils. Basophils contain histamine, heparin, and small quantities of bradykinin and serotonin. They are present in small numbers in the blood and in larger numbers in the connective tissue and pericapillary areas. Their function seems to be largely to prevent clotting in the microcirculation and to mediate allergic reactions [5]. It has been noted that persons with allergies often have elevated levels of immunoglobulin E (IgE). Receptor sites for IgE have been found on the basophils. When these receptor sites are attacked, histamine and other substances are released that increase chemotaxis and also enhance the allergic response (see Chap. 12). The number of basophils increases in some of the myeloproliferative diseases, such as polycythemia vera.

Eosinophils. These cells weakly exhibit phagocytosis and chemotaxis [5]. They are present in large numbers in the mucosa of the intestinal tract and of the lungs. Because of this they probably help to detoxify foreign proteins. The circulating level of eosinophils is increased in persons with allergies, perhaps as a result of the cells removing and digesting the antigen-antibody complex. Eosinophilia is associated with worm infestation or parasitic infections. In trichinosis the numbers of eosinophils can increase 25 to 50 percent. The relationship of basophils and eosinophils to allergy or hypersensitivity is discussed in Chapter 12.

Mononuclear Phagocyte System

The mononuclear phagocyte system is the large system of stationary and mobile macrophages. Important in the body's defense; it is considered to be more a functional than an anatomic system. It includes all the fixed and mobile phagocytic cells in the liver, spleen, lymph nodes, and gastrointestinal tract. Fixed macrophages in these organs seem to exist in dynamic equilibrium with mobile macrophages. All tissue macrophages, including the Kupffer cells of the liver and alveolar macrophages in the lungs, originate from the mobile circulating macrophages. This system is important in preventing the spread of infection and removing cellular debris and products of metabolic degradation. Many of the metabolic products are conserved and recycled.

Unlike monocytes and granulocytes, lymphocytes do not possess phagocytic capabilities but protect the body against specific antigens. This specific immunity, discussed in Chapter 10, is integrated with other general immune responses. The lymphocytes occupy the same anatomic area, the lymphoid tissues, as the macrophages.

Nonmalignant White Blood Cell Disorders

Quantitative Alterations of Granulocytes

Quantitative alterations of granulocytes result from several conditions that cause a significant increase or decrease in the number of leukocytes. This is usually measured by calculating the number of leukocytes in blood. Each cell type is often considered and counted individually in order to identify the causative condition.

Neutrophils. A normal physiologic shift in the number of neutrophils can be influenced by several conditions. Leukocytosis (increase in number of leukocytes above 10,000 per μl), can be caused by exercise, emotional stress, menstruation, sunlight, cold, and anesthesia. During pregnancy the number of polymorphonuclear leukocytes increases consistently. This increase is even more exaggerated during labor and the first postpartum week. The newborn infant also has increased neutrophil levels.

Neutrophilic leukocytosis is defined as an absolute neutrophil count greater than 7500 per μl blood [1]. The total white count in this condition is usually greater than 10,000 per μl [11]. A *shift to the left* occurs with increases in the number of leukocytes of nonsegmented neutrophils in circulating blood. When increased numbers of neutrophils are released in an inflammatory process, some may be in immature forms called bands or stabs, which have a very short life span. An increased number of these cells in the peripheral blood is often a good indicator of an inflammatory process, especially an acute bacterial infection. If the percentage of immature forms decreases in the peripheral blood smear, there is a *shift to the right*. Generally, a leftward shift indicates progression of infection, while a rightward shift indicates a subsiding infection [9]. Neutrophilic leukocytosis occurs in such pathologic conditions as acute pyogenic infections, hemorrhage, hemolysis, tissue necrosis, and metabolic chemical toxic poisonings.

Neutrophilic leukopenia (neutropenia) occurs when the absolute neutrophil count is less than 2500 per μl of blood [1]. Irradiation, anaphylactic shock, and systemic lupus erythematosus are specific causes of this decrease. Chemical agents that affect the hematopoietic system cause a decrease in the neutrophils. Antithyroid drugs, phenothiazines, and chemotherapeutic agents are only a few of the many drugs that can cause neutropenia. Disorders that affect the hematopoietic system, such as aplastic anemia and acute leukemia, cause a neutrophilic leukopenia.

Nonpyogenic bacterial, viral, and rickettsial infections can cause a decrease in the neutrophil count. Any overwhelming bacterial infection may lead to a neutrophilic leukopenia because the vast number of cells used to fight the infections is much greater than the reserve supply. The body's reserve ability to form neutrophils is exhausted and the neutrophil count falls.

Eosinophils. *Eosinophilic leukocytosis (eosinophilia)*, is defined as an absolute eosinophil count exceeding 500 per μl of blood and is often associated with allergy [1]. It is believed that this increase with allergic conditions is due to the tissue reactions associated with allergy-released products that specifically increase the production of eosinophils in bone marrow.

Eosinophilic leukocytosis also occurs in response to parasitic infection. This is probably the most common cause of extremely large numbers of eosinophils. The mechanism by which the parasitic infections cause the increased count is not known. Eosinophilic leukocytosis can also be caused by pulmonary disorders, skin diseases, and malignancy [13].

Eosinophilic leukopenia (eosinopenia) occurs when the absolute eosinophil count is less than 50 per μl of blood [1]. The decrease may be due to severe infection, shock, or adrenocortical stimulation. Peripheral blood eosinophils are very sensitive to adrenocortical hormones and may be reduced or absent in stress, with Cushing's disease, or in individuals being treated with corticosteroids [13].

Basophils. Basophilic leukocytosis *(basophilia)*, is defined as an absolute basophil count exceeding 50 to 100 per μl of blood [1]. This is usually greater than 2 percent of the white cell differential and is associated with myeloproliferative disorders, chronic granulocytic leukemia, and occasionally, ulcerative colitis and certain skin diseases [13].

Basophilic leukopenia (basopenia), occurs when the absolute basophil count is less than 20 per μl of blood [1]. It is often associated with suppression of other granulocytes in drug-induced suppression, as well as severe infection, shock, and adrenocortical stimulation.

Qualitative Alterations of Granulocytes

When granulocytes display defective physical and chemical functions, they are said to have qualitative abnormalities. Most of these defective functions are related to phagocytosis. The defects may be in phagocyte locomotion or in the phagocyte itself, such as that in the "lazy leukocyte" syndrome. There may be deficient chemotaxis generation and complement abnormalities. The latter are associated with collagen vascular disorders and occasionally with bacterial infections.

Normal human serum contains a low concentration of heat-stable globulin that impairs both chemotaxis and phagocytosis in vitro. This inhibitor is elevated in the sera of the majority of patients with cancer.

Ethanol has been shown to cause a significant decrease in leukocyte migration and chemotaxis during acute intoxication. Chemotaxis can also be decreased by the use of some antibiotics such as gentamicin in therapeutic doses [13].

Granulomatous diseases are qualitative defects of the granulocytes, especially neutrophils, and result in defective bactericidal activity. In chronic granulomatous disease (CGD), there is an inherited absence of neutrophil oxidase. This enzyme is necessary for the actual killing of bacteria; without it, leukocytes are unable to oxidize or destroy certain bacteria. Diagnosis can be made by the nitroblue tetrazolium (NBT) reduction test. Normally, NBT is reduced to a blue-black material called blue formazan, but in CGD this reduction is not seen. The disease results in severe recurrent infections of skin, lymph nodes, lungs, liver, and bones [3].

Several qualitative abnormalities of the granulocytes are inherited. Altered nuclear structure and appearance, excessive granulation of cytoplasm, and hypersegmentation of neutrophils may all occur. These alterations may affect the process of phagocytosis or may have no clinical implications.

Monocyte Abnormalities

Monocytosis infers an absolute monocyte count greater than 750 per μl in children and 500 to 600 per μl in adults [1]. This disorder arises in nonpyogenic bacterial infections such as active tuberculosis, subacute bacterial endocarditis, syphilis, and brucellosis. It is associated with recovery from such disorders as agranulocytosis, hematologic disorders, malignancy, and collagen disease.

Monocytopenia refers to a decrease in the blood monocyte counts. It is frequently secondary to acute stress reactions and/or glucocorticoid administration. Overwhelming infections and immunosuppressive agents also decrease the monocyte count.

Lymphocytic Disorders

Lymphocytosis must be defined according to the individual's developmental stage. The absolute lymphocyte count from birth to age 3 years is 9000 per μl of blood. From 4 to 12 years it is 7000 per μl and in adults it is 4000 per μl [1]. Viral disorders that produce lymphocytosis include mumps, rubella, rubeola, hepatitis, and varicella. Lymphocytosis also occurs in pertussis and chronic lymphocytic leukemia. Numbers of atypical lymphocytes are increased in infectious mononucleosis, cytomegalic inclusion disease, and toxoplasmosis.

Lymphopenia is defined as an absolute lymphocyte count of less than 1400 per μl in the child and less than 1000 per μl in the adult [1]. This condition may be caused by such factors as stress, adrenocortical stimulation, alkylating agents, and irradiation. It is associated with Hodgkin's disease, lymphosarcoma, terminal uremia, and acute tuberculosis.

Infectious Mononucleosis. This disease that often strikes young adults is characterized by cervical lymphadenopathy, fever, sore throat, and splenomegaly. Exudative tonsillitis is common.

The designation mononucleosis is misleading because the proliferating cells present in the lymph nodes, spleen, tonsils, and other organs are lymphocytes and monocytes. Serology shows an increase in lymphocytes and monocytes, with 10 to 20 percent of these being abnormal. The disease is classified as a *leukemoid* reaction, which refers to a condition of quantitative and qualitative changes of the WBCs. A differential diagnosis to rule out leukemia is sometimes necessary [8].

Mononucleosis is caused by the Epstein-Barr virus (EBV). This is the same herpesvirus that causes the malignant Burkitt's lymphoma that occurs in some areas in Africa. It has been found that if cultured infectious mononucleosis lymphocytes are transplanted into immunosuppressed animals, a malignant lymphoproliferative disorder results. Genetically determined defects in the immune response may be the key to this malignancy [9].

The Epstein-Barr virus subclinically infects from 50 to 80 percent of the world's population [9]. Large epidemiologic studies have shown that only persons without antibodies against EBV are at risk for developing infectious mononucleosis. The active disease is associated with the brief appearance of IgM antibodies against the Epstein-Barr virus. The IgM antibody increase represents a primary response and indicates recent exposure to the virus.

Infectious mononucleosis affects particularly the adolescent and young adult age groups. It has been postulated that, in low-socioeconomic groups, exposure to the Epstein-Barr virus occurs early in life and is almost entirely asymptomatic [7]. Exposure later in adolescence or young adulthood may result in infectious mononucleosis in up to two-thirds of the exposed population.

Hematologic changes are characteristic of mononucleosis. At first there may be a mild leukopenia, but by the second week the white cell count reaches 15,000 to 30,000 per μl of blood. Atypical lymphocytes make up 15 to 60 percent of the white cells in the second through the fourth weeks. The atypical lymphocytes may take one of several forms, but the most common picture includes nuclear chromatin that is finely divided or clumped. The nucleolus is usually absent and vacuoles are often present in the cytoplasm. If atypical lymphocytes are present in large numbers, the disease may resemble acute leukemia or Hodgkin's disease hematologically [9].

The Epstein-Barr virus induces an increase in antibody formation by B lymphocytes. The presence of this antibody forms the basis for laboratory diagnostic testing. The heterophil antibody titer and MonoSpot tests are used for differential diagnosis. No correlation has been noted between the levels of EBV or antibody titer and severity of the disease [4].

Symptoms of infectious mononucleosis disappear before the abnormal hematologic findings do. Clinical characteristics include fever, malaise, sore throat, and weakness. Splenomegaly and hepatic dysfunction may be present. Gradual recovery usually occurs in two to four weeks with no residual effects.

Lymphadenopathy. Lymphadenopathies are characterized by enlarged lymph nodes. The nodes may be tender or nontender and movable or fixed. Nodes involved by lymphomas or leukemias tend to be large, firm, and movable, while those of metastatic spread of malignancy tend to be adherent to surrounding structures. In acute infections the nodes are generally asymmetric with associated redness and edema.

Localized lymphadenopathy usually indicates drainage of an inflammation that may be due to infection, neoplasm, or early lymphoma. Generalized lymphadenopathy is less frequently caused by infection in the adult and may be due to a malignant or nonmalignant process.

Lymph node enlargement may be due to reactive follicular hyperplasia of nonspecific origin. There is usually hyperplasia of follicular center cells, which may be due to stimulation of B cells in viral diseases, syphilis, or autoimmune diseases such as rheumatoid arthritis or systemic lupus erythematosus.

Lymphadenopathies show individual pathologic features depending on the causative agent. Suppurative lymphadenitis is characterized by neutrophils in the sinusoids of the lymph nodes. These nodes serve as filtration units for the regions infected by pyogenic bacteria. Many other conditions may be associated with lymph node enlargement, including autoimmune diseases, metastatic carcinomas, and systemic infections.

Malignant White Blood Cell Disorders

Leukemia

Leukemia is the name of a group of malignant diseases characterized by both qualitative and quantitative alterations in circulating leukocytes. It is associated with diffuse abnormal growth of leukocyte precursors in the bone marrow. The word *leukemia* is derived from the Greek *leukos* and *aima*, meaning "white" and "blood," referring to the abnormal increase in leukocytes. This uncontrolled increase eventually leads to anemia, infection, thrombocytopenia, and in some cases, death.

Classification. Classification of leukemia is usually based on (1) *the course and duration of the illness* and (2) *the abnormal type of cells and tissue involved*. The course of the illness has been subclassified into acute and chronic.

Acute leukemia is associated with rapid onset, massive number of immature leukocytes, rapidly progressive anemia, severe thrombocytopenia, high fever, infective lesions of the mouth and throat, bleeding into vital areas, accumulation of leukocytes in vital organs, and severe infection. Laboratory studies usually show some degree of anemia and thrombocytopenia. Most advanced laboratory methods can now identify the cell type causing acute leukemia, but a small percentage of cases cannot be classified, except that the predominant cell is an undifferentiated stem cell (Table 16-5) [8]. Demonstration of leukemic cells in the peripheral blood cannot always be relied on. Open surgical biopsy of the bone marrow generally demonstrates the abnormal cells.

Chronic leukemia is characterized by gradual onset and leukocytes that are more mature. This disease mostly strikes older persons. The clinical course progresses more slowly than, but can end with the onset of acute leukemia. Laboratory analysis usually reveals a well-differentiated leukemic cell that can be classified as lymphocytic or granulocytic (Table 16-6).

Leukemia is further classified by the type of tissue and abnormal cell involved. Three broad categories based on tissue origin are (1) *myeloid*, which includes the granulocytes (neutrophils, eosinophils, or basophils), (2) *monocytic*, and (3) *lymphocytic*. If abnormal proliferation of granular leukocytes or their precursors is found in the blood or bone marrow, the leukemia may be called granulocytic, myelocytic, or myelogenous. With abnormal proliferation of lymphocytes or monocytes, the disease is called lymphocytic or monocytic, respectively.

TABLE 16-5 French-American-British (FAB) Classification of Acute Leukemias

Acute lymphoblastic or lymphocytic (ALL)
- L_1: small cell, homogenous, some with T lymphocyte markers
- L_2: larger cell, more heterogenous, some with T lymphocyte markers
- L_3: large cell, homogenous, B lymphocyte markers

Acute myelogenous or acute myeloid (AML)
- M_1: myeloblastic without maturation, nongranular
- M_2: myeloblastic with maturation to promyelocyte stage or beyond
- M_3: hypergranular, abnormal promyelocytes
- M_4: granulocytic and monocytic differentiation
- M_5: monocytic or monoblastic
- M_6: abnormal erythroblasts, myeloblasts, promyelocytes

Source: From S.L. Robbins, R. Cotran, and V. Kumar, *Pathologic Basis of Disease* (3rd ed.). Philadelphia: W.B. Saunders Company, 1984. Reprinted by permission.

TABLE 16-6 Chronic Leukemias

Chronic granulocytic (CGL), chromosome marker (Philadelphia chromosome) in marrow and peripheral blood

Myeloproliferative, intermediate maturity, thrombocytosis, WBC count 150,000/μl; may convert to AML

Chronic lymphocytic (CLL) proliferation of mature appearing, nonfunctional lymphocytes, B lymphocyte proliferation with hypogammaglobulinemia; WBC count: usually 100,000/μl

Source: S.L. Robbins, R. Cotran, and V. Kumar, *Pathologic Basis of Disease* (3rd ed.). Philadelphia: W.B. Saunders Company, 1984. Reprinted by permission.

If the majority of cells are immature, the suffix "blastic" is used instead of "cytic." For example, lymphoblastic, myeloblastic, or monoblastic indicate immaturity of leukocytes.

Classification of the chronic leukemias has not been a diagnostic problem because sufficient abnormal mature cells are often present from which to make a diagnosis. Diagnosis and classification of acute leukemia present a greater challenge. Because of cellular immaturity, it is sometimes difficult to identify the cell type. Research and technologic advances have led to a more sophisticated identification and classification system that includes the use of cell marker studies, cell secretory activity, and cytochemistry, as well as morphology and response to therapy.

Many factors are thought to influence the development of leukemia. These can be generally divided into three groups: (1) genetic factors, (2) acquired diseases, and (3) chemical and physical agents.

Genetic factors present in an identical twin pose a great risk if the other twin has leukemia or Bloom's syndrome. Bloom's syndrome is caused by an autosomal recessive trait characterized by dwarfism, photosensitivity, and butterfly telangiectatic erythema of the face with numerous defects of the skin pigment and keratin development. Siblings of a person with leukemia and individuals with Down syndrome are also at significant risk for developing leukemia. Several chromosomal abnormalities have been associated with the onset of leukemia. The Philadelphia chromosome, now thought to be chromosome 22 rather than 21 as previously reported, is associated with chronic granulocytic leukemia. Acute leukemias often show abnormalities of chromosomes 8 and 21 [13].

Acquired diseases with high risk factors for leukemia include myelofibrosis, polycythemia vera, and sideroblastic refractory anemia. Multiple myeloma and Hodgkin's disease also represent increased risk for development of the disease.

Physical and chemical agents that pose significant risk include irradiation and long-term exposure to benzene. Some risk also is associated with the chemotherapeutic agent chloramphenicol and alkylating agents. Viral causation of leukemia in humans has been studied extensively, particularly because it has been noted in lower animals. Induction of leukemic changes in tissue cultures of human cells by RNA viruses supports the possibility of viral transmission of certain forms of leukemia [6,8].

Clinical Manifestations. Pathologic alterations due to the disease process create characteristic signs and symptoms. *Acute lymphocytic leukemia (ALL)* usually occurs abruptly, with fever, bleeding, signs of bone marrow dysfunction, and bone pain. Anemia is present in 90 percent of persons with ALL [6]. The WBC count is variable, sometimes normal to low. The bone marrow is crowded with lymphoblasts that may be morphologically indistinguishable from myeloblasts [6].

Acute nonlymphocytic leukemia (ANLL) also arises abruptly with symptoms similar to those of ALL. Laboratory studies differentiate various forms of acute myelocytic (AML), myelomonocytic, promyelocytic, and erythroleukemia (Di Guglielmo's disease). Di Guglielmo's disease is often classified in early stages with the polycythemias, but as it progresses, it reaches an erythromyelocytic phase that usually evolves into AML [6,12]. The WBC and RBC counts are similar to those of ALL.

Chronic myelocytic leukemia (CML) is the least common type and may be discovered on routine physical examination, especially with evidence of an enlarged spleen. Bleeding, anemia, and infection are late manifestations. The WBC count is very high, from 50,000 to 500,000 per μl. A great majority of affected persons have the Philadelphia chromosome [9].

Chronic lymphocytic leukemia (CLL) is a long-term disease usually of elderly individuals, especially among Western peoples [6,12]. It is characterized by generalized lymphadenopathy and often is otherwise asymptomatic. Anemia, fatigue, and night sweats may be described. The WBC count may range from 20,000 to 150,000 per μl.

Infection due to marrow failure and granulocytopenia is the most common cause of fatality in all types of leukemia. It may appear in any organ or area and may be manifested by fever, chills, inflammation, and weakness. Bleeding of the skin, gingivae, or viscera often occurs due to thrombocytopenia. Disseminated intravascular coagulation (DIC) due to reduced platelets and coagulation factors may cause significant hemorrhage (see Chap. 17). Probably DIC is triggered by proteolytic enzymes or factors released by the leukemic cells that activate the clotting process.

Reduced appetite and hypermetabolism result in weight loss, weakness, fatigue, and pallor associated with anemia. The progression varies with the specific disease process. Calcium and magnesium abnormalities can be seen in serologic laboratory tests.

Leukemic infiltration of the meninges, central nervous system, and cranial nerves results in such clinical manifestations as headache, visual disturbances, nausea, and vomiting. Bone infiltration leads to bone tenderness and pain. Hepatosplenomegaly and infiltration of other viscera are manifested by abdominal tenderness and anorexia. Lymphadenopathy and neoplastic masses are due to local infiltration.

Progression of the Disease. Chemotherapy has markedly increased the survival rates for acute leukemias. Untreated ALL is usually fatal within three months. Studies show that over 50 percent of children who receive chemotherapy are alive after five years [9]. Acute myeloblastic leukemia has a poorer record, even with treatment, with average survival of one to two years.

The chronic leukemias have a variable course that can be controlled by oral alkylating agents or irradiation. Progressive anemia and susceptibility to infection are hazards, and CML may terminate by transforming into AML.

Malignant Lymphomas

Malignant lymphomas are solid neoplasms containing cells of lymphoreticular origin. *Lymphoreticular organs* include the lymph nodes, spleen, bone marrow, thymus, liver, and submucosa of the gastrointestinal and respiratory tracts.

Pathologically, lymphadenopathy is characteristic, with eventual involvement of the liver, spleen, and viscera. Diffusely diseased nodes are gray, with capsular infiltration occurring later in the process. The enlarged nodes may become adherent to each other and to surrounding organs and tissues [9].

Classification. The classification of malignant lymphomas is usually based on the predominant cell type and its degree of differentiation. The disease may be further divided into nodular and diffuse types depending on the predominant pattern of cell arrangement. Table 16-7 shows the cellular origins of malignant lymphomas. With more specific antiserums, the lymphocyte origin of B cells, T cells, and monocytes can be delineated.

The diffuse lymphomas are more invasive than the nodular lymphomas. The more undifferentiated the cell, the more aggressive the tumor becomes. As with leukemia, most individuals with lymphomas develop immunodeficiencies that are followed by infection. A common staging classification for lymphomas is used; the later the stage, the greater the involvement, and the worse the prognosis (Table 16-8).

Hodgkin's Disease. Hodgkin's disease is a malignant lymphoma that occurs in various distinct forms. It is characterized by proliferation of malignant cells of unknown origin. Peculiar giant cells called Sternberg-Reed cells are produced. Infiltration of the nodes with eosinophils and plasma cells occurs, and this is associated with necrosis and fibrosis.

The histologic criteria in malignancy of Hodgkin's disease are similar to those in non-Hodgkin's lymphomas. The Sternberg-Reed cell, which is a multinucleated odd-looking giant cell with a prominent nucleolus, must be present to confirm the diagnosis. Hodgkin's disease appears to involve a defect in the T cells, and the total lymphocyte count is depressed. Infection often causes major complications.

Hodgkin's disease has been classified into four types: (1) lymphocyte predominant, in which there is diffuse replacement by lymphocytes; (2) mixed type, which includes several distinct cell patterns, both lymphocytic and histiocytic; (3) lymphocyte depletion, with a predominant pattern of large malignant cells; and (4) nodular sclerosing, which has extensive scarring [9].

Staging of Hodgkin's disease uses the same classification as other lymphomas (see Table 16-8). Bone marrow examination and examination of the spleen for pathology after splenectomy are often the bases for staging. As with other lymphomas, the later the stage, the poorer the prognosis [10].

TABLE 16-7 Cellular Origins of Malignant Lymphomas

Neoplasms of B Cell Origin	Neoplasms of T Cell Origin	Neoplasms of Histiocytic or Reticulum Cell Origin
Chronic lymphocytic leukemia (98%)	Chronic lymphocytic leukemia (2%)	Malignant histiocytosis (histiocytic medullary reticulosis)
Small lymphocytic (well-differentiated lymphoma)	Mycosis fungoides/Sézary syndrome	Monocytic leukemia
Lymphocytic lymphoma, intermediate and/or small cleaved cell type	Diffuse aggressive lymphomas of adults (25%) Mixed cell type Large cell, immunoblastic	Large cell lymphomas (<5%) Hodgkin's disease
Follicular lymphomas	Adult T cell leukemia or lymphoma	
Diffuse aggressive lymphomas of adults (65%) Mixed cell type Large cell type Large cell immunoblastic Small noncleaved cell	Antiocentric lymphomas (lymphomatoid granulomatosis) (polymorphic reticulosis)	
Burkitt's (small noncleaved cell) lymphoma		
Acute lymphocytic leukemia (70%)	Acute lymphocytic leukemia (25%)	
Lymphoblastic lymphomas (10%)	Lymphoblastic lymphomas (85%)	

Source: Reproduced with permission from E. Braunwald et al. *Harrison's Principles of Internal Medicine* (11th ed.). McGraw-Hill. Reprinted with permission of McGraw-Hill Publishers.

TABLE 16-8 Staging Classification for Lymphomas

Stage	Definition
I	Involvement of a single lymph node region (I) or of a single extralymphatic organ or site (I_E).
II	Involvement of two or more lymph node regions on the same side of the diaphragm (II) or localized involvement of an extralymphatic organ or site and of one or more lymph node regions on the same side of the diaphragm (II_E).
III	Involvement of lymph node regions on both sides of the diaphragm (III), which may also be accompanied by involvement of the spleen (III_S) or by localized involvement of an extralymphatic organ or site (III_E) or both (III_{SE}).
III_1	Involvement limited to the lymphatic structures in the upper abdomen, that is, spleen, or splenic, celiac, or hepatic portal nodes, or any combination of these.
III_2	Involvement of lower abdominal nodes, that is, paraaortic, iliac, or mesenteric nodes, with or without involvement of the splenic, celiac, or hepatic portal nodes.
IV	Diffuse or disseminated involvement of one or more extralymphatic organs or tissues, with or without associated lymph node involvement.

Note: E = extralymphatic site; S = splenic involvement. The presence of fever, night-sweats, and/or unexplained loss of 10 percent of body weight in the 6 months preceding admission is denoted by the suffix letter B. The letter A indicates the absence of these symptoms. Biopsy-documented involvement of stage IV sites is also denoted by letter suffixes; marrow = M+; lung = L+; liver = H+; pleura = P+; bone = O+; skin and subcutaneous tissue = D+.
Source: Reproduced with permission from E. Braunwald et al. *Harrison's Principles of Internal Medicine* (11th ed.). © 1987 McGraw-Hill. Reprinted with permission of McGraw-Hill Publishers.

Common clinical manifestations of Hodgkin's disease are enlarged, palpable lymph nodes, fever, weight loss, and loss of energy. Node enlargement may cause compression on the spinal cord or other organs. The tumor may invade the vasculature or the lung parenchyma.

Anemia and immunodeficiency with lymphocytopenia occur in the later stages. Biopsy may demonstrate Sternberg-Reed cells [9]. These cells have been demonstrated in other conditions as well. Immunodeficiency, exacerbated by chemotherapy, leads to ineffective control of microbial invasion, especially fungal and protozoal. Infection is a common complication, both of the disease and the tumor.

Treatment with chemotherapy and radiation therapy has markedly improved the prognosis for Hodgkin's disease, with 90 to 100 percent remission being reported.

Multiple Myeloma

Multiple myeloma or *plasma cell myeloma* is a malignant neoplasm of plasma cells that causes damage to the bone marrow and skeletal structure. The aberrant myeloma cells arise from a single clone of plasma cells that are B cell-derived and secrete anomalous circulating immunoglobulins, also called *paraproteins*. Most often, the immunoglobulins are of the IgG class, but may be IgA, IgM, or, rarely, IgD or IgE (see Chap. 10) [9].

Laboratory examination of the bone marrow shows proliferation of both mature and immature plasma cells, with about 20 percent or more having multinucleated forms. These cells often completely replace the bone marrow. Serum protein electrophoresis and immunoelectrophoresis are abnormal. Bence Jones proteinemia and proteinuria, which are proliferations of light chains of immunoglobulin molecules, are present in about 50 percent of affected individuals. A higher frequency of renal failure correlates with the amount of protein found in the urine [3]. About 1 percent of the affected plasma cells do not secrete antibodies.

The malignant neoplasm that arises in bone usually does not metastasize outside bone. The destructive lesions erode the bone and cause punched-out lytic lesions observable radiographically. These lesions can be visualized in any bone but are most frequent in the vertebral column, ribs, skull, pelvis, femurs, clavicles, and scapulae [9]. The bones can become so fragile that simple movements can cause fractures. Pathologic fractures usually occur due to the lesions, especially of the weight-bearing regions.

Calcium metabolism is often abnormal, causing some persons to have elevated serum calcium levels. There is often a normocytic, normochromic anemia, with variable depression of white cell and platelet counts.

Bone or back pain is the most common symptom. Pallor and weakness due to secondary anemia may occur.

In some cases, myeloma nephrosis occurs due to the infiltration and precipitation of the light chains (Bence Jones protein) in the distal tubules as the urine is concentrated. The laminated, crystalline casts in the distal tubules damage the kidney cells and obstruct the tubules. Pathologic interstitial inflammation and fibrosis further impair kidney function, leading to uremia and a poor prognosis.

Anemia, thrombocytopenia that leads to bleeding, and neutropenia resulting in infection are common results of the disorder. Vascular insufficiency may occur in the peripheral areas and is apparently related to increased blood viscosity due to high levels of circulating immunoglobulins. Survival statistics remain poor and depend largely on the person's response to the chemotherapeutic regimen, with two to five years as the norm. In about ten percent of cases, the disease progresses very slowly, taking many years to run its course.

Study Questions

1. Explain the classification of leukocytes on the bases of morphology and function.
2. How does the mononuclear phagocyte system function in defending the body from invasion?
3. Define the various terms used for increased and decreased levels of leukocytes in the blood.
4. Compare the acute and chronic leukemias in reference to cells of origin, effect on the body, and clinical manifestations.
5. Describe the usual effects of infectious mononucleosis. What are its potential effects?
6. Compare Hodgkin's and non-Hodgkin's lymphomas.
7. Discuss the morphology and resultant pathology of multiple myeloma. How does Bence Jones proteinuria develop from it?

References

1. Braunstein, H. (ed.). *Outlines of Pathology*. St. Louis: Mosby, 1982.
2. Corbett, J.V. *Laboratory Tests in Nursing Practice*. Norwalk, Conn.: Appleton-Century-Crofts, 1982.
3. Goetzl, E.J., and Stobo, J.D. Immunology. In L.H. Smith and S.O. Thier, *Pathophysiology: The Biological Principles of Disease* (2nd ed.). Philadelphia: Saunders, 1985.
4. Grossman, M., and Jawetz, E. Infectious diseases: Viral and rickettsial. In M.A. Krupp, M.J. Chatton, and L.M. Tierney, *Current Medical Diagnosis and Treatment 1986*. Los Altos, Calif.: Lange, 1986.
5. Guyton, A.C. *Textbook of Medical Physiology* (7th ed.). Philadelphia: Saunders, 1986.
6. Harmon, D.C. The leukemias. In W.S. Beck, *Hematology* (4th ed.). Cambridge, Mass.: MIT Press, 1985.
7. LoBuglio, A.F. (ed.). *The Medical Clinics of North America: Symposium on Hematologic Disorders*. Philadelphia: Saunders, 1980.
8. Maile, J.B. *Laboratory Medicine: Hematology* (6th ed.). St. Louis: Mosby, 1982.
9. Robbins, S.L., Cotran, R.S., and Kumar, V. *Pathologic Basis of Disease* (3rd ed.). Philadelphia: Saunders, 1984.
10. Rosenthal, D.S. The malignant lymphomas. In W.S. Beck, *Hematology* (4th ed.). Cambridge, Mass.: MIT Press, 1985.
11. Wallach, I. *Interpretation of Diagnostic Tests* (4th ed.). Boston: Little, Brown, 1986.
12. Wallerstein, R.O. Blood. In M.A. Krupp, M.J. Chatton, and L.M. Tierney, *Current Medical Diagnosis and Treatment 1986*. Los Altos, Calif.: Lange, 1986.
13. Weatherall, D.J., and Bunch, C. The blood and blood-forming organs. In L.H. Smith and S.O. Thier, *Pathophysiology: The Biological Principles of Disease* (2nd ed.). Philadelphia: Saunders, 1985.

CHAPTER 17

Normal and Altered Coagulation

CHAPTER OUTLINE

Hemostasis
- Vasoconstriction
- Hemostatic Platelet Plug Formation
- Characteristics and Physiology of Platelets

General Mechanism of Blood Coagulation
- Clotting Factors
- Formation of the Prothrombin Activator
- Intrinsic Pathway
- Extrinsic Pathway
- Enzymatic Complexes
- Final Common Pathway to Clot Formation
- Clot Formation
  - *Blood Clot Composition*
  - *Clot Retraction*

Lysis of Blood Clots
Anticoagulation Factors in Normal Blood
Laboratory Tests for Coagulation Problems
- Clotting or Coagulation Time
- Prothrombin Time
- Partial Thromboplastin Time
- Tests for Specific Deficiencies
- Platelet Count
- Bleeding Time
- Clot Retraction

Deficiencies in Blood Coagulation
- Single Coagulation Factor Deficiencies
  - *Hemophilia*
- Vitamin K Deficiency
- Disseminated Intravascular Coagulation
- Primary Fibrinolysis
- Antibody Anticoagulants
- Platelet Disorders
  - *Thrombocytopenia*
  - *Thrombocytosis*
  - *Qualitative Platelet Disorders*
  - *Hypercoagulation*

LEARNING OBJECTIVES

1. Define *hemostasis* and list the four major events included in this process.
2. Explain the role of vasoconstriction in hemostasis and the mechanism of stimulation.
3. State the purpose of hemostasis and coagulation.
4. Describe the function of the platelets and explain their role in the hemostatic process.
5. Describe the sequence of events in the coagulation process.
6. Describe briefly the essential clotting factors, where they are formed, and how they act.
7. Explain the common pathway of blood coagulation.
8. Differentiate between the intrinsic pathway and the extrinsic pathway in prothrombin activation.
9. Define a *zymogen* and describe its role in cascade activation.
10. Diagram the interrelationships of the major components involved in hemostasis.
11. Describe the composition of the blood clot.
12. Explain the action of the fibrinolytic system.
13. List several factors normally present in the blood that inhibit clotting.
14. Differentiate factors that enhance coagulation and those that inhibit coagulation in normal blood.
15. Explain the basis of common laboratory tests used to determine coagulation problems.
16. Explain briefly the role of liver function with respect to normal coagulation.
17. Differentiate the factor deficiencies that cause the various types of hemophilia.
18. Explain how uncontrolled bleeding occurs in disseminated intravascular coagulation (DIC).
19. Differentiate between thrombocytosis and thrombocytopenia, and list some causative conditions for each.
20. Describe some platelet disorders that are associated with hypercoagulability.

Coagulation is an essential, protective part of hemostasis that prevents blood loss when a vessel is damaged. Hemostasis refers to the arrest of bleeding. Coagulation is the ability of blood to change from a fluid to a semisolid mass. It involves the conversion of *fibrinogen*, a soluble macromolecule composed of three polypeptide chains, to *fibrin* monomers by action of the proteolytic enzyme *thrombin*. Polymerization of the monomers follows and spontaneously bonds fibrin monomers together. A fibrin-stabilizing factor acts on fibrin to cause cross-linkage bonding, which forms an insoluble, threadlike mesh on which a clot forms. This mechanism for clot initiation and formation involves a series of sequential cascadelike reactions that employ several factors in the blood and injured tissues.

Hemostasis

Hemostasis, the arrest of bleeding or circulation of the blood, is often divided into four main events: (1) vasoconstriction, (2) formation of a hemostatic platelet plug, (3) blood coagulation, and (4) clot formation. The interaction of all four events is essential for normal hemostasis. The general dynamic interaction of these events is illustrated in Figure 17-1.

Vasoconstriction

Vasoconstriction is the result of many events that occur during an injury. Immediately after the wall of a vessel is injured, contraction of the vessel decreases the flow of blood into and out of the vessel. This contraction is due mainly to two factors: (1) nervous reflexes and (2) local myogenic spasms [3]. Nervous reflexes are probably initiated by pain impulses created by the tissue or vascular trauma. Local myogenic spasm is initiated by direct damage to the vascular wall and by the release of serotonin from platelets.

The greater the portion of vessel traumatized, the greater the degree of spasm. A sharply cut vessel bleeds longer than a crushed one [3]. A clean cut by a sharp razor blade, for example, bleeds longer than a scrape or jagged cut.

Hemostatic Platelet Plug Formation

When a blood vessel is damaged, the endothelial lining is disrupted, exposing the underlying collagen. When platelets are exposed to collagen or other foreign surfaces such as antigen-antibody complexes, thrombin, proteolytic enzymes, endotoxins, or viruses, they undergo a dynamic change called ***viscous metamorphosis***. They begin to swell and form irregular shapes with processes protruding from their surfaces. They become sticky and adhere to the collagen and basement membrane of the vessel. The platelets release adenosine diphosphate (ADP), which attracts other platelets and aids in platelet adhesion and aggregation. Adenosine diphosphate also is released from disrupted red blood cells and damaged tissue. Enzymes

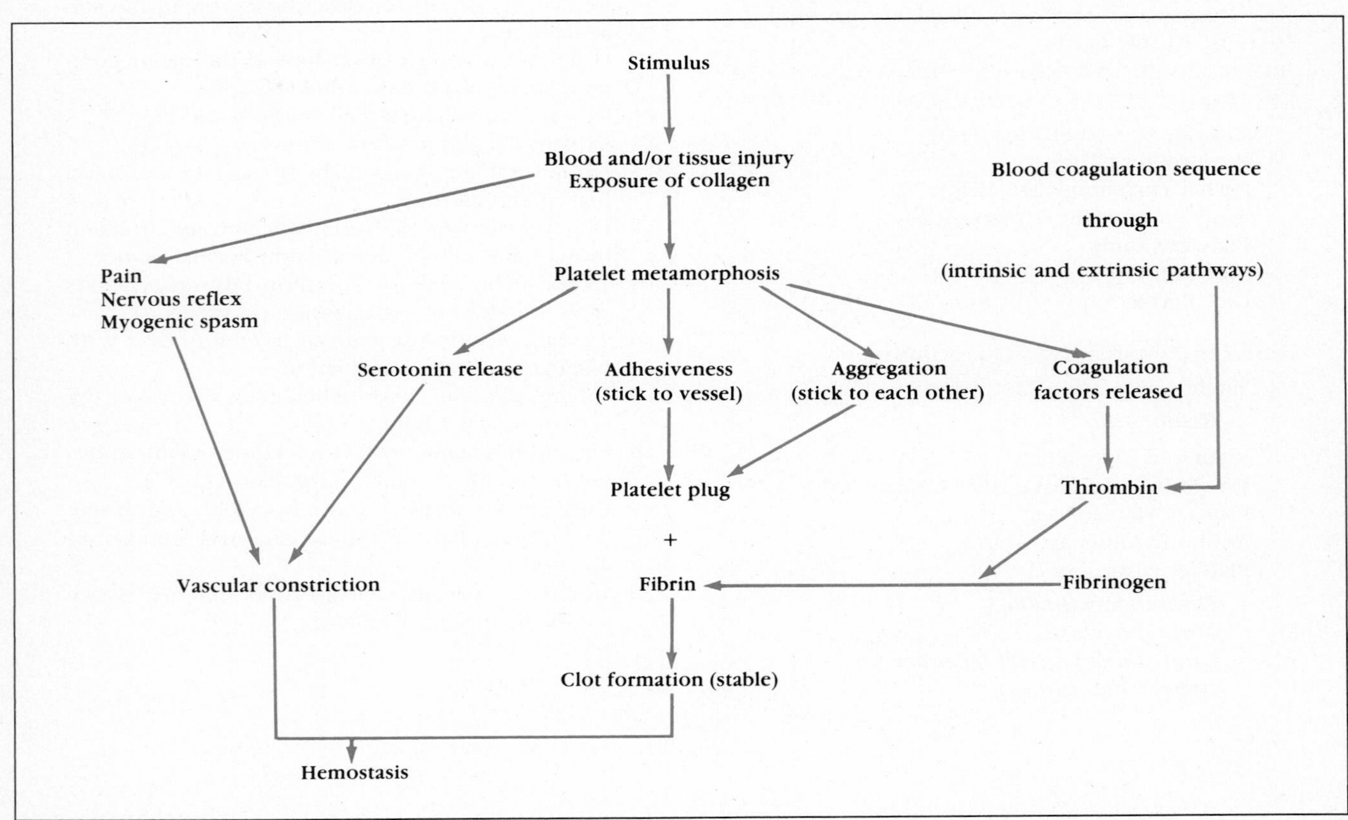

FIGURE 17-1 Hemostatic mechanism.

released from the platelets cause the formation of thromboxane A in the plasma. Both ADP and thromboxane A activate nearby platelets that stick to the original platelets, thus creating a cycle of platelet activation. The *platelet plug* results, causing the damaged endothelial vessel wall to adhere to the collagen fibers. This plug is loose and arrests circulation only if the tear in the vessel is small. Later, a tight plug is formed by fibrin threads that result from the process of coagulation.

Hundreds of minute ruptures occur in the capillaries each day. The platelet plug is important because it can stop bleeding completely if the damage is small. A significant decrease in the number of platelets can lead to small hemorrhagic areas under the skin and in the internal tissue [3]. Usually the plugging mechanism seals the tear in the vessel rather than occluding the lumen.

Characteristics and Physiology of Platelets

Platelets are fragments of megakaryocytes formed in the bone marrow and released into the circulation. The normal platelet concentration in the blood is about 140,000 to 340,000 per μl [13]. Adequate numbers must be present for normal hemostasis and clotting.

Each platelet has four major functional regions, the peripheral, sol-gel, organelle, and membrane systems zones (Fig. 17-2) [14]. The *peripheral zone* includes the cell membrane and closely associated structures in which are found the receptors for the various stimuli that trigger platelet activation, the substrate for adhesion and aggregation reactions, and a surface for coagulant protein interaction. Adhesion involves the platelet-collagen interaction that results in platelets sticking to the site of injury on the blood vessel. Aggregation is a calcium-requiring process of platelet to platelet association. The peripheral zone translates the signals of stimuli into chemical messages and initiates the physical alterations required for platelet activation [15].

The sol-gel zone is composed of the platelet cytoplasm matrix. Here are the fiber systems that support the disklike shape of the unstimulated platelets and provide the contractile systems that allow the platelets to change shape, form pseudopods, and perform contraction and secretion functions. *The organelle zone* contains the cellular organelles, which are embedded in the sol-gel matrix and serve metabolic purposes. This zone is an important storage area for enzymes, serotonin, calcium, and protein constituents. The *membrane systems region* is comprised of canalicular systems or tiny surface-connected canallike structures that have access to the interior. In this region, plasma substances are able to enter, and cellular products may be released or secreted. Products stored in secretory organelles are extruded to the outside through an energy-dependent process [14].

Contractile physiology dominates the platelet response and is critical to the development of the hemostatic plug. The contractile ability allows shape changes and internal transformation. It facilitates the process of secretion and converts loosely clumped platelets into tightly packed masses that can seal a vascular rent. Contraction of the platelets provides the force for contraction of the platelet-fibrin meshwork and allows for retraction of a clot.

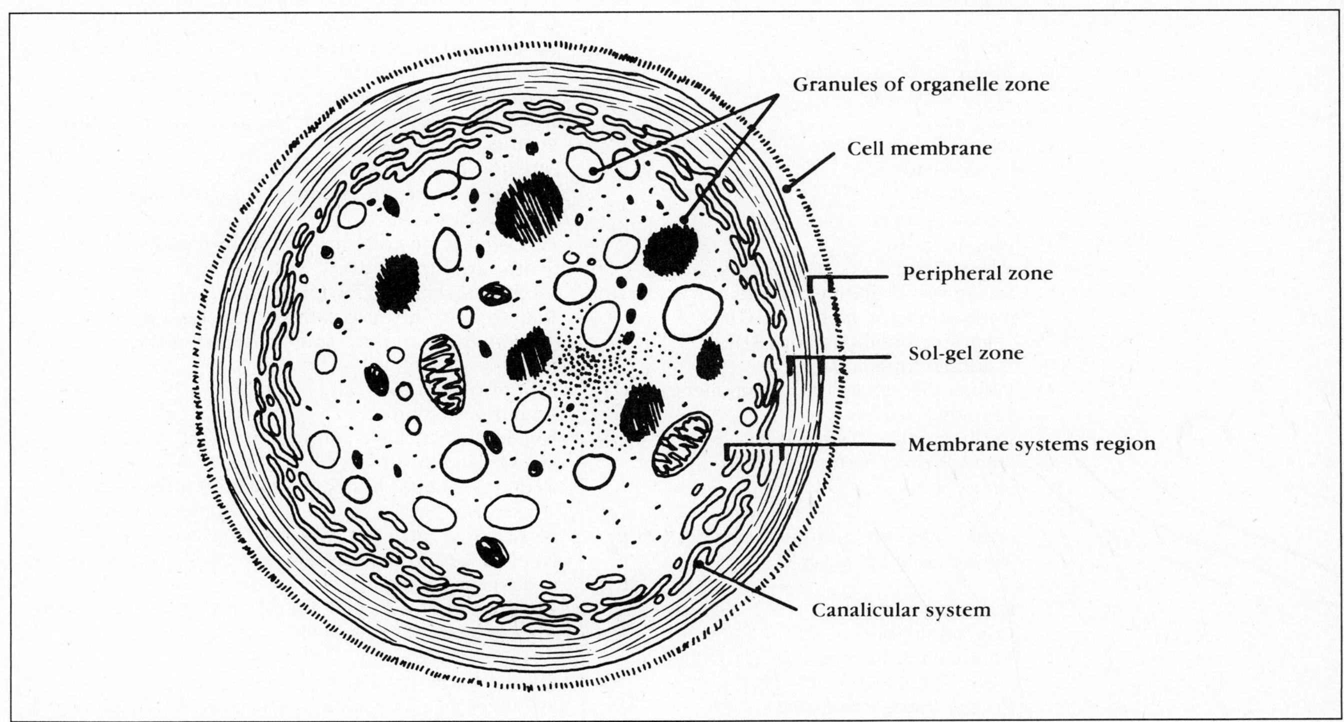

FIGURE 17-2 Major functional regions of the platelet.

General Mechanism of Blood Coagulation

Three basic reactions constitute the sequential pathway for blood coagulation: (1) a prothrombin activator is formed by the intrinsic or extrinsic pathway in response to tissue or endothelial damage; (2) prothrombin activator catalyzes the conversion of prothrombin to thrombin; and (3) thrombin catalyzes the conversion of soluble fibrinogen to solid fibrin polymer threads. These fibrin threads form the meshwork on which plasma, blood cells, and platelets aggregate to make the clot (Fig. 17-3). Before these three reactions can occur, other responses must take place. A group of reactants called clotting factors begin the process that terminates in the formation of the blood clot.

Clotting Factors

The clotting factors are a series of plasma proteins that are generally inactive forms of proteolytic enzymes. Table 17-1 summarizes these factors and indicates the international nomenclature used for each. The enzymatic proteolytic actions cause successive reactions of the clotting process in a cascadelike sequence. One activated factor is important for the activation of the next factor. The inactive precur-

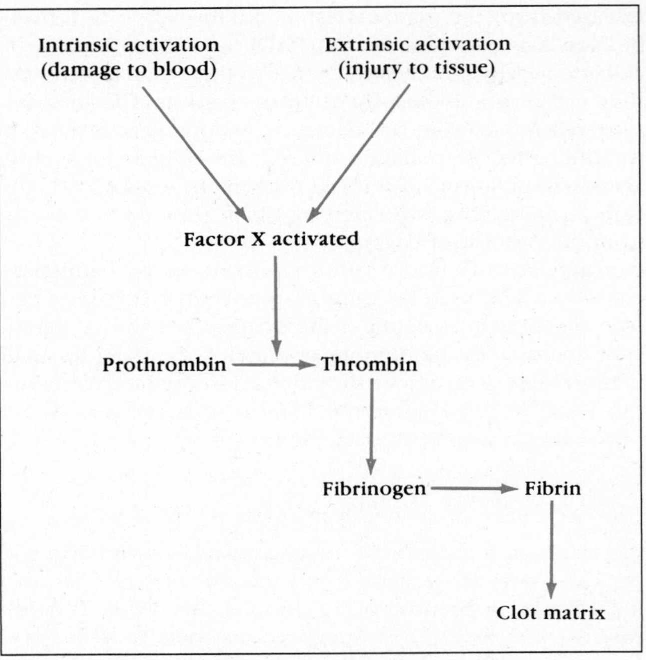

FIGURE 17-3 Common pathway of blood coagulation.

TABLE 17-1 Blood Coagulation Factors

Factor (International nomenclature)	Common Synonyms	Remarks
I	Fibronogen	Soluble macromolecule, synthesized in liver, fibrin precursor
II	Prothrombin	Synthesized in liver, vitamin K required for formation
III	Tissue thromboplastin	Phospholipid
	Thrombokinase	Involved in activation of extrinsic pathway
IV	Calcium	Involved in several complexes in coagulation process
V	Proaccelerin	Synthesized in liver
	Labile factor	Modifier protein, not enzyme
	Ac-globulin; Ac-G	Required in prothrombin activator complex
(VI)	Obsolete term	Same as factor V
VII	Proconvertin	Part of enzyme complex in extrinsic pathway
	Stable factor	Synthesized in the liver
	Serum prothrombin conversion accelerator	Vitamin K required for formation
VIII	Antihemophilic globulin (AHG); antihemophilic factor (AHF); antihemophilic factor A	Required for intrinsic pathway function; possibly synthesized in liver, spleen, RES, or kidneys
IX	Plasma thromboplastin component (PTC)	Synthesized in liver
	Christmas factor	Requires vitamin K
	Antihemophilic factor B	Needed for intrinsic pathway function
X	Stuart-Prower factor	Synthesized in the liver
	Stuart factor	Requires vitamin K, needed for both intrinsic and extrinsic pathways
XI	Plasma thromboplastin antecedent (PTA)	Substrate in intrinsic activator enzymatic complex
	Antihemophilic factor C	Needed for intrinsic system activation, area of synthesis unknown
XII	Hageman factor	Involved in first step of activation of intrinsic system
	Contact factor	Area of synthesis unknown
	Antihemophilic factor D	
XIII	Fibrin stabilizing factor (PSF)	Causes amide cross-linkage fibrin
	Plasma transglutaminase	Stabilizes clot formation, synthesized by platelets and possibly other proteins, may be activated by liver

sor enzyme is activated by peptide bond cleavage. A low level or lack of even one of these inactive proteolytic enzymes can lead to abnormal bleeding and hemorrhage [9].

Fibrinogen, prothrombin, and factors VII, IX, and X are essential procoagulation factors. *Fibrinogen* (factor I) is synthesized in the liver at a rate that usually corresponds to the rate of use or need. The levels of fibrinogen may be increased by adrenocorticotropic hormone (ACTH), growth hormone, endotoxin, pregnancy, and occlusive arterial disease. *Prothrombin* (factor II) and factors VII, IX, and X are also synthesized exclusively in the liver by a process that requires vitamin K. These factors are affected by pregnancy, oral contraceptives, and diethylstilbestrol [11].

Formation of the Prothrombin Activator

The coagulation process begins with the formation of the prothrombin activator, a substance or complex of substances [11]. The mechanism is initiated by trauma to the tissues or blood, or contact of the blood with damaged endothelial cells, collagen, or other substances outside the blood vessel endothelium. This injury or contact leads to the formation of the prothrombin activator, which then leads to the conversion of prothrombin to thrombin.

The prothrombin activator is formed in one of two ways: (1) through the extrinsic pathway, initiated by trauma to the vessel wall or tissues outside the vessel, or (2) through the intrinsic pathway, which begins with trauma to blood components, and thus alters the platelets and factor XII.

Interplay of both the intrinsic and extrinsic systems is needed for normal clotting. Deficiency of a single protein in one of these pathways may lead to a clotting disorder. The intrinsic and extrinsic pathways converge on a final common pathway, leading to the formation of a fibrin clot (see Fig. 17-3). Each precursor protein is important in the clotting process because it is necessary for the activation of the next.

The clotting process occurs by a cascade of zymogen activation. A *zymogen* is an inactive precursor that is converted to an active enzyme by the action of another enzyme [11]. The activated form of one factor sequentially catalyzes the activation of the next in cascade fashion, leading to clot formation.

Intrinsic Pathway

In 1863 Joseph Lister noted that blood stayed fluid longer in the excised veins of an ox than in a glass container [12]. The abnormal surface of the glass activated components that were already in the blood. This means of activation was called the intrinsic pathway, because clotting was triggered by substances that were normally present in the blood.

The intrinsic mechanism for initiating clotting begins inside the vessel. When the blood comes into contact with collagen or damaged endothelium, an intrinsic activator-enzyme complex is formed. An important part of this complex is the Hageman factor (activated factor XII), a proteolytic enzyme. This complex enzymatically activates factor XI. Sequential events continue in cascade fashion. Activated factor XI enzymatically activates factor IX. Factor IX forms factor X activation complex, which consists of activated factor IX, factor VIII, calcium, and phospholipids. Activated factor X then combines with factor V, calcium, and phospholipids to form the prothrombin activator. Within seconds, the prothrombin activator initiates the proteolytic cleavage of prothrombin bonds to form thrombin. The amount of thrombin formed is closely related to the amount of prothrombin activator present. Once thrombin is formed, the final clotting process is set in motion (Fig. 17-4).

If factor VIII or the platelets are not at an adequate level, activation of factor X is impaired. Decreased factor VIII is the major problem in classic hemophilia, and decreased platelets result in bleeding disorders such as thrombocytopenia (see p. 251). All of the clotting factors are essential to the normal coagulation sequence.

Extrinsic Pathway

The extrinsic pathway for coagulation is triggered by factors not normally present in the blood, such as substances released from damaged tissues or other foreign materials. When the blood comes in contact with a traumatized vascular wall or extravascular tissue, substances called tissue factor and tissue phospholipids are released. Tissue factor is a proteolytic enzyme with cleavage ability, and tissue phospholipids are mainly those of the cell membrane.

The tissue factor, factor VII, calcium, and phospholipids form a complex. This complex acts enzymatically on factor X to form activated factor X. Activated factor X then becomes part of the prothrombin activator complex, which enzymatically converts prothrombin to thrombin. Thrombin, in turn, enzymatically converts fibrinogen to fibrin (see Fig. 17-4).

Enzymatic Complexes

The cascade hypothesis used to describe the relationships among the protein constituents associated with blood coagulation has been the object of much study over the years. Most of the enzymes involved in the process and their precursors have been isolated and identified. The specificity of the proteolytic cleavages and activation processes in the coagulation transformations is quite well understood. Recently, progress has been made in isolating and understanding nonenzyme cofactor proteins, which are necessary for the blood coagulation. Four principal enzymatic complexes involving these cofactors have been isolated [7]:

1. *The "intrinsic" activator*, which includes the Hageman factor (factor XII), prekallikrein, high-molecular-weight kininogen, and the substrate for the reaction factor XI
2. *Factor VII, tissue factor, calcium, and phospholipids*
3. *Factor X activation*, which is composed of activated factor IX, cofactor, factor VIII, calcium, and phospholipids
4. *The prothrombinase complex*, which includes activated factor X, activated factor V, calcium, and phospholipids

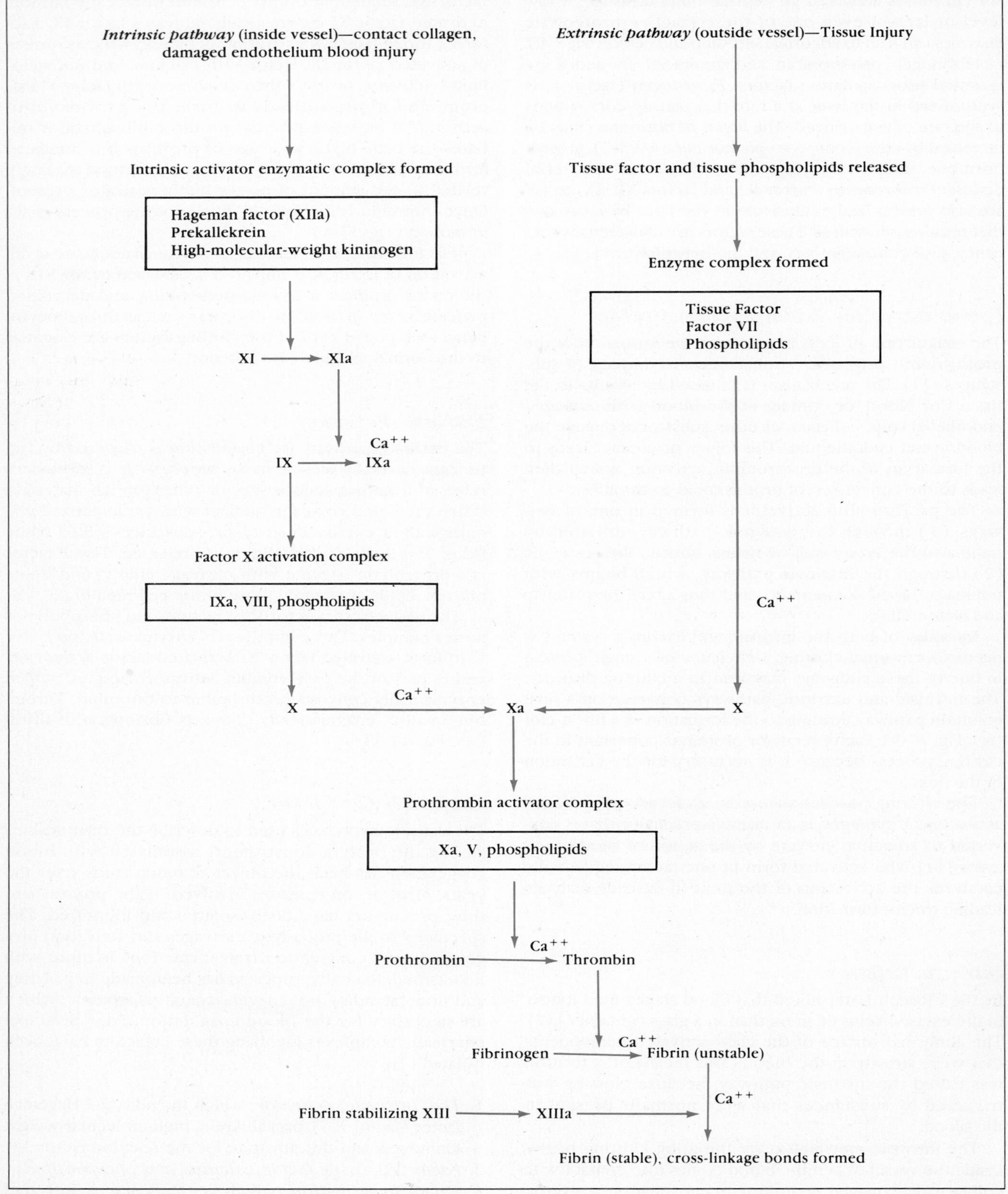

FIGURE 17-4 Blood coagulation sequence. Key: a = activated enzyme; Ca^{++} = calcium, necessary in several reactions.

The significance of the cofactors and complex formation may be illustrated by the prothrombinase complex. The cofactors in this complex at physiologic concentrations lead to amplification of the reaction rate by 300,000 times [7,11]. It is obvious that without these cofactors and the interactions of the components in the complex, conversion of prothrombin to thrombin would be slowed tremendously.

Final Common Pathway to Clot Formation

With the activation of factor X and formation of the prothrombin activator complex, the final common pathway for clot formation begins. Prothrombin activator complex causes the conversion of prothrombin to thrombin. Thrombin, in turn, enzymatically converts fibrinogen to fibrin. These reactions constitute the final coagulation pathway for both the intrinsic and extrinsic systems (see Fig. 17-3). The rate of the blood coagulation reaction is generally related to the amount of prothrombin activator formed and the degree of activation of factor X. If either is inhibited or stopped because of the absence of a clotting factor or other reasons, the coagulation process becomes altered and excess bleeding results.

Clot Formation

Blood coagulation occurs faster with severe trauma to the vascular wall than with minor trauma. The general sequence of physical events takes place in a comparatively short time. After the vessel is severed, the platelets agglutinate and fibrin appears. A fibrin clot can form in as little as 15 seconds up to 6 minutes. Clot retraction follows and may take 30 minutes to an hour. After the clot is formed, it either dissolves or organizes into a fibrous mass.

Blood Clot Composition. The blood clot is composed of a meshwork of polymerized fibrin threads that have become attached to blood cells, platelets, and plasma products. The fibrin threads adhere to the damaged vessel surface, holding the clot in place and preventing blood loss. The meshwork is produced by spontaneous aggregation of fibrin monomer to form polymer threads. Transglutaminase (factor XIII) acts on the fibrin to form covalent cross-links. This stabilizes the clot and makes it resistant to dissolution [11,14].

Clot Retraction. The contractile physiology of the platelet response is critical in clot retraction. Failure of a clot to retract often indicates a decrease in the number of platelets. The platelets entrapped in the clot continue to release fibrin-stabilizing factor. Stronger bonding of the fibrin threads occurs and causes the threads to contract. Clot retraction pulls the edges of a broken vessel closer together, which allows the vascular wall to mend. After contraction is completed, blood serum, which includes plasma and the clotting factors, is expressed from the clot.

Lysis of Blood Clots

Plasmin or *fibrinolysin*, a proteolytic enzyme that resembles trypsin, is formed from inactive circulating plasminogen by the action of thrombin, which stimulates the production of *tissue-type plasminogen activator* [11]. It digests fibrin threads and causes lysis of the clot along with destruction of blood-clotting factors. Large amounts of the inactive enzyme plasminogen are incorporated into the clot and activated by vascular endothelial factors such as thrombin, activated factor XII, and lysosomal enzymes in damaged tissue (Fig. 17-5) [3]. Urokinase, a definite activator, is synthesized by renal cells and is present in urine [14]. Bacterial organisms, especially streptococci, produce activators. In the case of the streptococcus organism, the activator is *streptokinase*, which has been used therapeutically to dissolve clots. Plasmin largely mediates the fibrinolytic system. This built-in, self-destructing system for clots breaks down and limits excessive clot formation. Plasmin is self-limiting and localizes the fibrinolytic activity to the region of the resolving clot. Inhibitors of plasmin prevent excessive proteolytic action. Specific substances such as alpha$_2$-antiplasmin and alpha$_2$-macroglobulin inhibit plasmin action. Alpha$_2$-antiplasmin binds to fibrin by factor XIII during clot formation, so that the rate of fibrinolysis depends upon a balance of amounts of plasminogen, plasminogen activators, and antiplasmins within the clot [14]. The fibrinolytic system breaks down the clot so that healing can occur. Intravascularly, it assures patency of the vascular system.

The degradation products produced from fibrinolysis are called fibrinogen degradation products (FDP). They inhibit the formation of thrombin and limit the formation of the clot. A balance between the formation of thrombin and plasmin must be present for normal coagulation and clotting to occur.

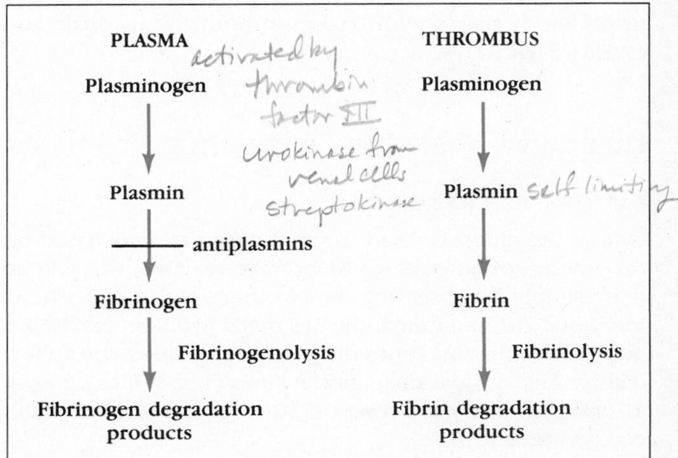

FIGURE 17-5 Plasminogen activation in plasma and in a thrombus, and digestion of fibrinogen and fibrin. (From R.G. Petersdorf et al. [eds.], *Harrison's Principles of Internal Medicine* [10th ed.]. New York: McGraw-Hill, 1983. Reprinted by permission of McGraw-Hill Publishers.)

Anticoagulation Factors in Normal Blood

Anticoagulants inhibit coagulation and are important in keeping the blood fluid. Factors that aid in the prevention of clotting include the smooth endothelial lining of the vessel, rapid blood flow through an area, negatively charged proteins on the endothelial surface, and anticoagulant substances in the blood.

A smooth endothelium and a monomolecular layer of negatively charged proteins adsorbed on the endothelium are essential for maintaining the fluidity of blood [3]. Rapid blood flow dilutes the factors that promote coagulation, thus preventing initiation of the clotting process. An intact, smooth endothelium prevents contact activation of the intrinsic pathway, and the layer of negatively charged proteins repels clotting factors and platelets that might stick to the vessel wall.

Several plasma proteins can dampen the activity of proteolytic enzymes generated in the coagulation and fibrinolytic systems. These include antiplasmin, activated protein C inhibitor, antithrombin III, and alpha$_2$-macroglobulin [10]. These plasma proteins localize coagulation action at the site of injury and prevent propagation of the coagulation effect throughout the vascular system.

The most powerful anticoagulants in the blood are those that remove the excess thrombin formed during coagulation. These are *fibrin threads* and *antithrombin III*. During clot formation, 85 to 90 percent of thrombin becomes adsorbed to fibrin threads [3]. This adsorption effectively stops the action of thrombin on fibrinogen. Excess thrombin not adsorbed combines with the plasma protein antithrombin III, which blocks the effect of thrombin on fibrinogen and inactivates the thrombin.

Heparin, a potent anticoagulant, is present in the granules of the circulating basophils and the tissue mast cells. Its concentration in blood is very slight. Heparin acts as an anticoagulant mainly by inhibiting factor IX, factor X, and thrombin. It reacts with factors in both the intrinsic and extrinsic pathways.

Laboratory Tests for Coagulation Problems

Clotting or Coagulation Time

One of the oldest tests for normal coagulation is based on the amount of time drawn blood takes to clot. This can be done simply by observing the clotting time in a test tube. Increased clotting time indicates that a problem exists, but normal clotting time does not rule out a hemostatic abnormality. The normal coagulation time (Lee-White) is 6 to 17 minutes in a glass tube or 19 to 60 minutes in a siliconized tube [13].

Causes of prolonged clotting time include deficiencies of any factor in the intrinsic clotting system or in the common pathway, fibrinogen deficiency, or excessively rapid fibrinolysis. This test has long been used for persons receiving heparin therapy but is now being replaced by the partial thromboplastin time (PTT), which is a more sensitive measurement of coagulation factors [2].

Table 17-2 lists the laboratory tests for coagulation problems.

Prothrombin Time

To perform the test for prothrombin time (PT), animal tissue extract and calcium are added to freshly drawn and separated citrated plasma. The time the mixture takes to clot is given in seconds. The tissue extract bypasses the intrinsic clotting system so that only factors VII, X, and V, prothrombin, and fibrinogen affect the test. Normal prothrombin time (11–16 seconds) is increased if any of the above factors is deficient [13]. The PT is often reported as a percentage of normal activity, which is a way of expressing the activity of factors in comparison to a normal control. Normal is always considered to be 100 percent. If the individual measures at 20 percent, only about one-fifth of normal clotting activity exists. A person having faster clotting activity than the control can have greater than 100 percent activity. An *increased* PT refers to a longer time for clotting to occur, with clotting ability being less than normal [2]. A *decreased* PT refers to the reverse. Deficiencies of factors XII, XI, IX, and VIII do not affect the prothrombin time.

The PT is often used to monitor the effects of coumarin anticoagulants. Coumarin depresses the synthesis of factors VII, IX, X, and prothrombin.

Partial Thromboplastin Time

Partial thromboplastin time (PTT) is a relatively simple test for mild to moderate deficiencies of intrinsic clotting factors. It is useful for detecting many types of bleeding disorders due to decreased amounts of factors composing the intrinsic system. It is a general test that is used to monitor heparin therapy. Chemicals are often added to achieve an activated PTT, or APTT. The resulting clotting time is accelerated.

TABLE 17-2 Normal Blood Coagulation Values

Test	Normal Values
Clotting or coagulation time	6–17 min (glass tube) 19–60 min (siliconized tube)
Prothrombin time	11–16 sec
Partial thromboplastin time (PTT)	60–90 sec
Activated partial thromboplastin time (APTT)	25–37 sec
Platelet count	140,000–340,000/μl (Rees-Ecker) 200,000–350,000/μl (Coulter Counter model B)
Bleeding time	4 min (Ivy method) 1–4 min (Duke method)
Clot retraction	Begins: 30–60 min Complete: 12–24 hours

Source: J. Wallach, *Interpretation of Diagnostic Tests* (4th ed.). Boston: Little, Brown, 1986.

The PTT increases (becomes longer) in both hereditary factor deficiencies and in acquired conditions such as disseminated intravascular coagulation (DIC) (see p. 250) [2]. Therapeutic heparin is used to keep the PTT at 1.5 to 2.5 times the normal level (see Table 17-2). Deficiencies of all the factors prolong the PTT with the exception of factor VII. A person with a factor VII deficiency has a normal PTT and a prolonged PT. Partial thromboplastin time can be used to demonstrate circulating anticoagulants in plasma. If a mixture of test plasma mixed with normal plasma has a longer PTT than normal plasma alone, it indicates that something in the test plasma has inhibited coagulation.

Tests for Specific Deficiencies

Special tests can determine the absence of specific clotting factors. Small amounts of blood are added to samples of plasma known to be deficient in a particular factor. If, for example, the added plasma corrects the partial thromboplastin time to normal for plasma known to be deficient in a particular factor, that factor is not deficient in the sample. The process is repeated until the tested plasma does not correct the PTT. This identifies the missing factor. Several special tests for coagulation factors are based on this laboratory method.

Platelet Count

One of the most common laboratory tests, the complete blood count (CBC), usually includes the platelet count. Platelets normally range from about 140,000 to 340,000 per μl (Rees-Ecker) or 200,000 to 350,000 per μl (Coulter Counter Model B) [13]. Platelets are difficult to count because of their inherent tendency to clump, adhere to the vessel, and aggregate. Electronic means of counting them offer the greatest accuracy.

Thrombocytosis (elevated platelet count) may occur in association with certain malignancies and with polycythemia vera [6]. Thrombocytopenia (decreased platelet count) may be secondary to many conditions or it may be idiopathic (see p. 251).

Bleeding Time

To measure "bleeding time" an incision is made either on the earlobe (Duke method) or on the inner surface of the forearm (Ivy method). The time needed for active bleeding from the clean, superficial wound to stop is called the bleeding time. Normal bleeding time is less than four minutes by the Ivy method and one to four minutes by the Duke method [13]. The variables involved are vascular contractility and platelet aggregation.

Secondary bleeding time can be measured by noting how long it takes for bleeding to cease after a scab is removed. Secondary bleeding time is prolonged in persons with deficiencies of factors in the intrinsic pathway or factor XIII, the fibrin-stabilizing factor.

Clot Retraction

Measuring the clot retraction time consists of observing the time in which a clot retracts and expresses serum, and the degree of retraction. Whole blood is left in a test tube at 37°C. Clot retraction normally begins in about 30 minutes, and by 4 hours a well-defined clot is surrounded by clear serum. Complete retraction requires about 12 to 24 hours if measured at room temperature. The norm is 50 to 100 percent in 2 hours [2]. If platelet function or number is decreased, clot retraction is impaired.

Deficiencies in Blood Coagulation

Deficiency of any of the clotting factors can result in a defect or impairment of blood coagulation. This impairment may result from genetic deficiencies of clotting factors, or suppression or consumption of the major clotting components. Coagulation does not occur as an isolated, independent event, but continually interacts with other mechanisms of the body such as the inflammatory process. Alterations in the process can result in injury, hemorrhage, or death.

Single Coagulation Factor Deficiencies

Single coagulation factor deficiencies are usually hereditary. The most common deficiencies are of factors VIII, IX, and XI. All cause bleeding that may involve any of the soft tissues or the joints.

Hemophilia. Hemophilia loosely defines several different hereditary deficiencies of coagulation factors of the intrinsic pathway. The most common cause of this coagulation disorder is a deficiency in factor VIII, accounting for about 83 to 85 percent of cases of hemophilia [1,9]. Usually factor VIII is produced, but it is abnormal and does not promote coagulation.

The classic factor VIII deficiency is genetically transmitted through a sex-linked recessive gene. It affects males almost exclusively. Females are usually asymptomatic carriers, but in rare cases may manifest the disease [9]. This type of hemophilia is called *classic hemophilia* or *hemophilia A*, and is characterized by spontaneous or traumatic subcutaneous and intramuscular hemorrhages. Hematuria and bleeding from the mouth, gums, lips, and tongue are common manifestations. Joint hemorrhages cause extreme pain and deformity. Transfusion of normal factor VIII or fresh plasma relieves the bleeding tendency for a short time.

Von Willebrand's disease is characterized by a quantitative and qualitative deficiency of factor VIII. Because of this deficiency, adhesion of platelets to the injury-exposed collagen is impaired. This condition produces a prolonged bleeding time. Von Willebrand factor is one of the products of factor VIII (VIII R) [14]. This condition, thought to be hereditary, has been shown to be associated with some of the autoimmune or lymphoproliferative conditions.

Factor IX deficiency, called *hemophilia B or Christmas disease*, is sex-linked, recessive, and accounts for about 10 to 15 percent of cases of hemophilia [9]. Bleeding tends to be severe, with crippling joint deformities. This condition is sometimes seen in association with severe protein-wasting glomerulopathies [9].

Factor XI deficiency, called *hemophilia C or Rosenthal's disease*, is a mild bleeding disorder manifested by bruising, epistaxis, and menorrhagia. It is transmitted as an autosomal recessive trait and accounts for about 2 percent of hemophiliacs. The mildness of this disease is thought to be due to activation of factor XI through other mechanisms [14].

Vitamin K Deficiency

Many disorders can lead to deficiencies of several coagulation factors. One example is fat-soluble vitamin K, which is required for the synthesis of factors II, VII, IX, and X. These vitamin K-dependent factors can be monitored by prothrombin time. Factor VII has a very short half-life and prolongs the PT more quickly than the other factors. Deficiencies of vitamin K may result from several conditions. A newborn infant is normally deficient in vitamin K due to an immature liver and lack of intestinal bacteria that are important for the synthesis of the vitamin. The newborn is often given injections of vitamin K to help prevent any possible bleeding disorder that might occur.

Obstructive liver disease and malsorption disorders can also cause a deficiency in vitamin K. Obstructive liver disease blocks the flow of bile necessary for the absorption of fat-soluble vitamins, and malsorption disorders do not allow enough vitamin K to be absorbed into the circulation.

Coumarin anticoagulants are competitive inhibitors of vitamin K. Vitamin K can be injected as an antidote in case of excessive bleeding or possible hemorrhage due to overdose of these drugs.

Disseminated Intravascular Coagulation

Disseminated intravascular coagulation (DIC) involves both bleeding and clotting. It occurs as a complication of several clinical conditions. The process begins with activation of the sequence causing coagulation. This *hypercoagulable state* produces thrombosis, especially in the small vessels [5]. Widespread coagulation activation leads to consumption of clotting factors such as platelets and fibrin. Also, secondary activation of the fibrinolytic system occurs. Table 17-3 indicates some of the diverse factors that can initiate the coagulation sequence.

Persons who develop DIC are often critically ill as a result of the underlying pathology. Then DIC often develops insidiously, so that widespread bleeding becomes the initial sign.

The clotting sequence is triggered either by endothelial damage that activates the intrinsic coagulation cascade or by release of thromboplastic substances. The resultant clotting causes occlusion of a large proportion of the small peripheral blood vessels. The clotting sequence activates the fibrinolytic system and thus causes diffuse fibrinolysis. The conversion of plasminogen to plasmin in the fibrinolytic system inhibits the proteolysis of fibrinogen by thrombin and may inhibit platelet aggregation. Fibrin degradation products are formed by the lysis of plasmin, fibrinogen, and fibrin. These end products form a complex with the fibrin monomer, which prevents the laying down of the fibrin thread and platelet aggregation. Therefore, despite widespread clotting, the major problem is bleeding (Fig. 17-6).

Uncontrolled bleeding occurs because of consumption of the clotting factors. Normal hemostasis is prevented, so that varying degrees of ecchymoses, petechiae, and bleeding from any opening may occur. The onset may be acute, such as that after acute obstetric emergencies, or it may gradually develop, as with disseminated cancers. Bleeding problems usually predominate, and venipuncture sites or incisions may bleed profusely. Acrocyanosis often occurs in the digits, and is seen in cold, mottled fingers and toes. Hypoxemia may cause dyspnea, cyanosis, and air hunger. Neurologic or renal symptoms may result from microthrombi that occlude the small vessels.

Laboratory tests that are helpful include the prothrombin time, partial thromboplastin time, fibrinogen level, and platelet count. Both the PT and PTT are prolonged, while fibrinogen and platelet levels are depressed. Levels of fibrin split or degradation products (FSP) are elevated.

TABLE 17-3 Etiology of Disseminated Intravascular Coagulation

Causative Agent or Condition	Probable Massive Coagulation Stimulus
Infection	
Gram-negative bacteria	Endotoxemia; endothelial damage
Gram-positive bacteria	Fulminating sepsis; endothelial damage
Rickettsia rickettsii (Rocky Mountain spotten fever)	Parasitization of endothelial cells; rupture walls of small vessels
Plasmodium falciparum (falciparum malaria)	Injury to red cells and platelets; possible antigen-antibody reaction
Complications of pregnancy	
Amniotic fluid embolism	Circulating thromboplastins absorbed
Saline abortion	
Hydatidiform mole	
Puerperal sepsis	Vascular damage
Toxemia	
Large hemangiomas	Turbulence of blood, stasis Endothelial damage
Disseminated carcinoma	Circulating tissue thromboplastins from malignant tissue
Hemolytic transfusion RX, anaphylaxis, hemolytic-uremic syndrome	Antigen-antibody reactions
Tissue damage	
Massive trauma	Thromboplastins released
Heat stroke	
Extensive burns	
Snake bites	
Extracorporeal circulation	Blood injury

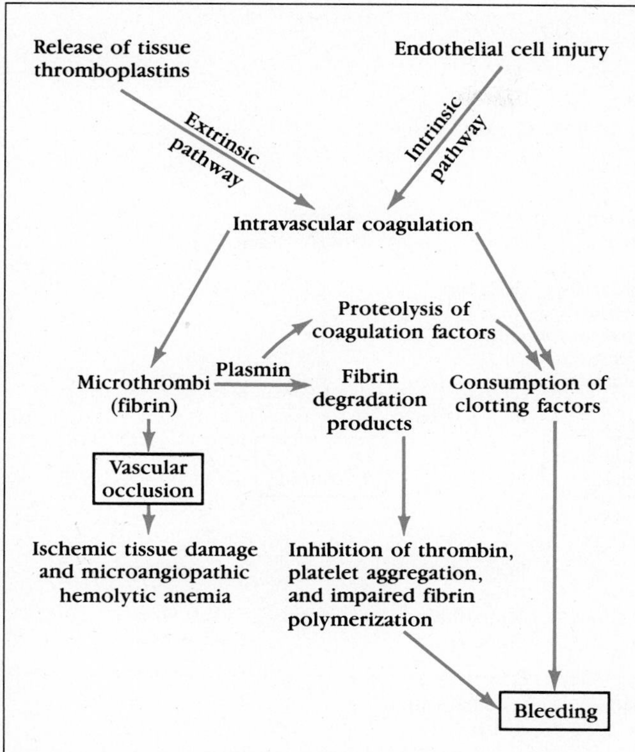

FIGURE 17-6 Pathophysiology of DIC (From S.L. Robbins, R.S. Cotran, and V. Kumar, *Pathologic Basis of Disease* [3rd ed.]. Philadelphia: W.B. Saunders Company, 1984. Reprinted by permission.)

Primary Fibrinolysis

Primary fibrinolysis results when massive amounts of plasminogen activator are released into the system. The activator, such as streptokinase, may be administered therapeutically to dissolve pulmonary emboli. Plasminogen activators can also be released by activator-rich neoplastic tissue such as prostatic carcinoma. Severe anoxia, shock, or surgical procedures may also precipitate their release.

Disseminated intravascular coagulation and primary fibrinolysis reactions are similar. Both are associated with increased fibrinolytic activity, but primary fibrinolysis results in increased amounts of plasminogen activator in the plasma, while in DIC it is a secondary response to a hypercoagulable state.

Antibody Anticoagulants

Antibodies to various coagulation factors have been observed in many disease states. About 10 percent of persons treated for hemophilia A develop an antifactor antibody to factor VIII [1]. Antibodies to paraproteins in those with multiple myelomas and antibodies to multiple coagulation factors in persons with systemic lupus erythematosus are other examples of antibodies that act as circulating anticoagulants. The development of antibodies to coagulation factors results in an increased risk of hemorrhage.

Platelet Disorders

Thrombocytopenia. This quantitative platelet disorder involves the presence of a very low number of platelets in the circulatory system. If the platelet number falls below 50,000, there is a potential for hemorrhage associated with trauma such as surgery or accidents. A platelet count of about 20,000 is associated with petechiae, ecchymoses, and sometimes bleeding from mucous membranes. With a count below 5000, a great risk exists for fatal hemorrhage through the intestinal tract or central nervous system [1].

An abnormal decrease in the number of platelets may occur in several disorders, such as defective platelet production, increased platelet destruction, sequestration of platelets, and loss of platelets from the system. The two major types of thrombocytopenia are idiopathic thrombocytopenic purpura (ITP) and secondary thrombocytopenia. Table 17-4 classifies causes of thrombocytopenia by mechanism. Figure 17-7 illustrates the evaluation of thrombocytopenia to determine the cause.

Idiopathic thrombocytopenia purpura is apparently an autoimmune condition that causes an increased rate of destruction of platelets. The result is either acute destruction of platelets, which often follows a viral infection, or

TABLE 17-4 Classification of the Thrombocytopenias

Type of Disease	Etiology
Decreased production	
Hypoproliferation	Toxic agents Radiation, infection Constitutional factors (Fanconi's anemia, etc.) Idiopathic aplastic anemia Paroxysmal nocturnal hemoglobinuria Myelophthisis (tumor, fibrosis, etc.)
Ineffective thrombopoiesis	Megaloblastic anemia Di Gugliemo's syndrome Familial thrombocytopenia
Abnormal distribution	Congestive splenomegaly Myeloid metaplasia, lymphoma Gaucher's disease
Dilutional loss	Massive blood transfusion
Abnormal destruction	
Consumption	Disseminated intravascular coagulation, vasculitis Thrombotic thrombocytopenia (TTP)
Immune mechanism	Idiopathic thrombocytopenic purpura (ITP) Drug-induced thrombocytopenia Chronic lymphocytic leukemia, lymphoma, LE Neonatal thrombocytopenia Posttransfusion purpura

Source: Reprinted with permission from W.S. Beck, *Hematology* (4th ed.). Cambridge, Mass.: MIT Press, 1985.

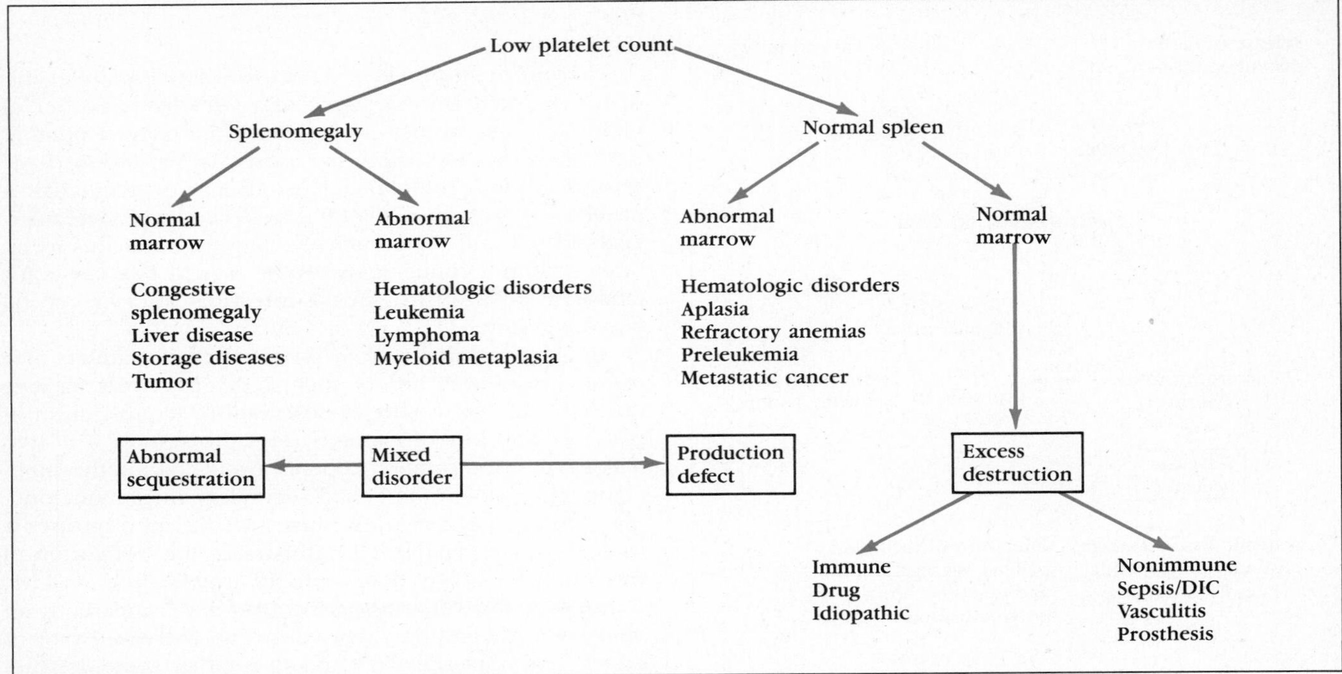

FIGURE 17-7 A schematic approach to the clinical evaluation of thrombocytopenia. (Reprinted by permission from W.S. Beck, *Hematology* [4th ed.]. Cambridge, Mass.: MIT Press, 1985.)

chronic ITP, which may be associated with another autoimmune disease such as autoimmune hemolytic anemia [4]. The pathogenesis appears to involve the production of autoantibodies directed against the platelets. Clinical manifestations include diffuse petechiae, ecchymosis, epistaxis, hemorrhages into the soft tissues, melena, or hematuria.

Secondary thrombocytopenia commonly occurs in association with drug hypersensitivity, viral infections, and some of the autoimmune conditions. The platelet count is depressed as a result of a superimposed hemorrhagic problem caused by the underlying condition. Some of the drugs that may induce secondary thrombocytopenia are chlorothiazide derivatives, gold thiomalate, diphenylhydantoin, acetaminophen, quinidine, sulfonamides, chloramphenicol, antimetabolites, and antihistamines. The drug usually acts as a hapten, and the antibody-drug complex binds to platelets, fixes complement, and causes intravascular damage [4].

Thrombocytosis. Thrombocytosis is an increased number of platelets in the peripheral blood. Counts of 400,000 to 1 million per μl are usually asymptomatic, but counts greater than 1 million per μl may result in thrombosis or bleeding, due to malfunctions of platelets [1]. Physiologic thrombocytosis occurs in response to infection, trauma, and other conditions. It almost always occurs after splenectomy, when all of the platelets are circulated in the blood because they can no longer pool in the spleen. Idiopathic thrombocythemia refers to a sustained platelet count of greater than 800,000 per μl. The condition is generally regarded as one of the myeloproliferative disorders due to its responsiveness to chemotherapy. It occurs with splenic enlargement and may be associated with other myeloproliferative disorders such as chronic myelogenous leukemia and polycythemia vera. Affected individuals often exhibit peripheral thrombosis and episodes of spontaneous bleeding.

Qualitative Platelet Disorders. Qualitative platelet disorders include alterations that have a prolonged bleeding time with a normal platelet count in most instances. The disorders are due to a variety of defects of platelet function, such as in platelet adhesion in von Willebrand's disease, or in platelet aggregation as in thrombasthenia, a congenital disorder.

Qualitative platelet disorders can also be acquired. Drugs such as aspirin may impair the aggregation of platelets. In uremia a dialyzable factor is formed that inhibits platelet aggregation.

Hypercoagulation. Hypercoagulation may involve accelerated rates of coagulation, hyperviscosity, and increased platelet activity or antithrombin III deficiency. Atherosclerosis associated with vascular clotting and myocardial infarction has been found to involve increased platelet turnover, and increased platelet release of factor IV and beta-thromboglobulin [8]. Giant hemangiomas have an increased platelet and fibrinogen turnover, which is thought to be the result of massive blood turbulence and stasis in the large bed of vascular tissue. A very extensive hemangioma may lead to a pattern of disseminated intravascular coagulation, thrombocytopenia, and low levels of circulating fibrinogen, factor V, and factor VII, with an increase in fibrin degradation products [8].

Thrombotic thrombocytopenic purpura, a rare disorder, is characterized by thrombocytopenia, anemia, neurologic deficits, and renal failure. Endothelial cell damage may be the activator in the disorder, with an immune vasculitis affecting the endothelial cells. Platelet adhesion and aggregation lead to obstruction of the vessel and ischemia of the surrounding tissues [8].

Blood stasis in the small vessels is enhanced when the blood is more viscous. Polycythemia increases viscosity and affects the rate of blood flow. An increased number of any of the formed elements may increase the viscosity of blood.

Hyperfunction of platelets in the absence of thrombocytosis has been postulated as a mechanism for various pathologies. It is theorized that strokes and transient ischemic attacks in younger persons who have no evidence of arterial abnormalities or degenerative changes could be the result of hyperfunction of the platelets. Platelet clumping in small vessels may result in alterations of blood supply [14].

Platelet activation and release of thromboxane A_2 may lead to coronary artery spasm, ischemia, and infarction. Platelet function in these cases can be examined by laboratory means for increased sensitivity to aggregating agents and increased release of thromboxane A_2 and other platelet factors.

Several cases of sudden deafness have been associated with increased platelet sensitivity. A single artery supplies the cochlea and may constrict, obstructing blood flow. The sudden deafness is often preceded by an acute viral infection. Under experimental conditions, myxoviruses have been shown to cause platelet damage and acceleration of the release of platelet factor III. The viral action may be the mechanism responsible for initiating this deafness syndrome [8].

Antithrombin III deficiency is an inherited familial disorder that results in thrombosis. The antithrombin III inactivates most of the active proteases involved in thrombin formation. A modest decrease in this inhibitor allows the proteases to remain active for a longer period, which results in the rapid formation of thrombi. Antithrombin III deficiency can also occur as an acquired disorder and is associated with liver disease or DIC. Oral contraceptives and heparin also reduce antithrombin III levels.

Study Questions

1. Compare the processes of hemostasis and coagulation.
2. Discuss the intrinsic and extrinsic pathways for coagulation. How are they alike and how are they different?
3. What are the components of the fibrinolytic system and how do they react following coagulation?
4. Why does blood not clot in the vascular system in the normal individual?
5. Compare the usefulness of the common laboratory tests for the coagulation process.
6. Why do individual factor deficiencies cause bleeding, such as that in hemophilia?
7. Explain how septicemia can initiate DIC.
8. Contrast primary and secondary thrombocytopenia.

References

1. Braunstein, H. *Outlines of Pathology*. St. Louis: Mosby, 1982.
2. Corbett, J.V. *Laboratory Tests in Nursing Practice*. Norwalk, Conn.: Appleton-Century-Crofts, 1982.
3. Guyton, A.C. *Textbook of Medical Physiology* (7th ed.). Philadelphia: Saunders, 1986.
4. Handin, R.J. Hemorrhagic disorders II: Platelets and purpura. In W.S. Beck, *Hematology* (4th ed.). Cambridge, Mass.: MIT Press, 1985.
5. Handin, R.J., and Rosenberg, R.D. Hemorrhagic disorders III: Disorders of primary and secondary hemostasis. In W.S. Beck, *Hematology* (4th ed.). Cambridge, Mass.: MIT Press, 1985.
6. Maile, J.B. *Laboratory Medicine: Hematology* (6th ed.). St. Louis: Mosby, 1982.
7. Mann, K.G. Complex formation in blood-clotting reactions. *Clin. Chem.* 27:721, 1981.
8. Penner, J.A. Hypercoagulation and thrombosis. *Med. Clin. North Am.* 64:542, 1980.
9. Robbins, S.L., Cotran, R.S., and Kumar, V. *Pathologic Basis of Disease* (3rd ed.). Philadelphia: Saunders, 1984.
10. Rosenberg, R.D. Inhibition of clotting. *Clin. Chem.* 27:879, 1981.
11. Rosenberg, R.D. Hemorrhagic disorders I: Protein interactions in the clotting mechanisms. In W.S. Beck, *Hematology* (4th ed.). Cambridge, Mass.: MIT Press, 1985.
12. Stryer, L. *Biochemistry*. San Francisco: Freeman, 1975.
13. Wallach, J. *Interpretation of Diagnostic Tests* (4th ed.). Boston: Little, Brown, 1986.
14. Weatherall, D.J., and Bunch, C. The blood and blood-forming organs. In L.H. Smith and S.O. Thier, *Pathophysiology: The Biological Principles of Disease* (2nd ed.). Philadelphia: Saunders, 1985.
15. White, J.G. Calcium prostaglandins and granules in platelet function. *Clin. Chem.* 27:618, 1981.

Unit Bibliography

Anderson, J.R. *Muir's Textbook of Pathology* (12th ed.). London: Arnold, 1985.

Beck, W.S. *Hematology* (4th ed.). Cambridge, Mass.: MIT Press, 1985.

Braunwald, E., et al. (eds.). *Harrison's Principles of Internal Medicine* (11th ed.). New York: McGraw-Hill, 1987.

Donovan, E.V. *Essentials of Pathophysiology*. New York: Macmillan, 1985.

Ferguson, G.C. *Pathophysiology, Mechanisms and Expressions*. Philadelphia: Saunders, 1984.

Fishman, M.C., et al. *Medicine* (2nd ed.). Philadelphia: Lippincott, 1985.

Ganong, W.F. *Review of Medical Physiology* (12th ed.). Los Altos, Calif.: Lange, 1985.

Golden, A., Powell, D., and Jennings, C.D. *Pathology, Understanding Human Disease* (2nd ed.). Baltimore: Williams & Wilkins, 1985.

Guyton, A.C. *Textbook of Medical Physiology* (7th ed.). Philadelphia: Saunders, 1986.

Hardisty, R.M., and Weatherall, D.J. *Blood and Its Disorders* (2nd ed.). Boston: Blackwell, 1982.

Hocking, W.G. *Practical Hematology*. New York: Wiley, 1983.

Hughes-Jones, N.C. *Lecture Notes on Haematology* (4th ed.). Oxford: Blackwell, 1984.

Kaufman, C.E., and Papper, S. *Review of Pathophysiology*. Boston: Little, Brown, 1983.

Kissane, J.M. *Anderson's Pathology* (8th ed.). St. Louis: Mosby, 1985.

Krupp, M.A., Chatton, M.J., and Tierney, L.M. *Current Medical Diagnosis and Treatment 1986.* Los Altos, Calif.: Lange, 1986.

Miale, J.B. *Laboratory Medicine: Hematology* (6th ed.). St. Louis: Mosby, 1982.

Rifkind, R.A., et al. *Fundamentals of Hematology* (3rd ed.). Chicago: Year Book, 1986.

Selkurt, E.E. *Physiology* (5th ed.). Boston, Little, Brown, 1984.

Sheldon, Huntington. *Boyd's Introduction to the Study of Disease* (9th ed.). Philadelphia: Lea & Febiger, 1984.

Smith, L.H., and Thier, S.O. *Pathophysiology: The Biological Principles of Disease* (2nd ed.). Philadelphia: Saunders, 1985.

Sodeman, W.A., and Sodeman, T.M. *Sodeman's Pathologic Physiology* (7th ed.). Philadelphia: Saunders, 1985.

Spivak, J.L. *Fundamentals of Clinical Hematology* (2nd ed.). Philadelphia: Harper & Row, 1984.

Thompson, R.B. *A Concise Textbook of Hematology* (6th ed.). Baltimore: Urban & Schwarzenberg, 1984.

Williams, W.J., et al. *Hematology* (3rd ed.). New York: McGraw-Hill, 1983.

Wintrobe, M.M., et al. *Clinical Hematology* (8th ed.). Philadelphia: Lea & Febiger, 1981.

UNIT 8

Circulation

Gloria Grissett Stuart and Barbara L. Bullock

Carol Bowdoin / *Alterations in Cardiac Rhythm*

The study of circulation requires an understanding of both normal dynamics and alterations of related structures that lead to the effects of compromised tissue perfusion.

Chapter 18 examines the anatomy of the heart and vessels. The physiology of the system is reviewed in sufficient depth to support the contents of subsequent chapters. An attempt has been made to relate the electrophysiology of the heart to electrocardiography. The major dysrhythmias that may occur are covered in Chapter 19. The material presented in these two chapters provides a physiologic basis for much of the subsequent information.

Chapter 20 details heart failure, a result of many other conditions. To simplify the concept, the author has classified the condition into left and right heart failure on the basis of clinical manifestations. Both left and right heart failure are interrelated, and that which affects one side of the heart ultimately affects the other. Chapter 21 details specific diseases of the heart and pericardium. The more common congenital heart defects are included in this chapter. Chapter 22 classifies and clarifies hypertension. Chapter 23 discusses arterial and venous peripheral vascular disease.

It is suggested that the reader use the learning objectives and study questions in each chapter and the bibliography at the end of the unit to enhance learning.

CHAPTER 18

Normal Circulatory Dynamics

CHAPTER OUTLINE

Anatomy of the Heart
- Atria
- Ventricles
- Atrioventricular Valves
- Semilunar Valves
- Veins
- Arteries
- Coronary Arteries
- Coronary Veins
- Conduction System
- Myocardial Cellular Structure

Physiology of the Heart
- Contraction of Cardiac Muscle
  - *Action Potential*
- Metabolism of Cardiac Muscle
- Automaticity
- Rhythmicity
- Excitability
- Conductivity
- Electrical Events of the Cardiac Cycle
- Mechanical Events of the Cardiac Cycle
  - *Preload*
  - *Afterload*
  - *Contractility*
  - *Heart Rate*
- Phases of the Cardiac Cycle
  - *Atrial Filling and Contraction*
  - *Ventricular Filling and Contraction*
  - *Heart Sounds*
- Autonomic Influences on Cardiac Activity
  - *Sympathetic Nervous System (SNS)*
  - *Parasympathetic Nervous System (PSNS)*
- Baroreceptors
- Chemoreceptors

Anatomy of the Arteries, Capillaries, Veins, and Lymphatics
- Arteries
- Capillary Network
- Veins
- Lymph Vessels

Factors Controlling Arterial Pressure and Circulation
- Arterial Blood Pressure
- Pulse Pressure
- Direct and Indirect Determinants of Blood Pressure
  - *Cardiac Output*
  - *Vascular Resistance*
  - *Aortic Impedance*
  - *Diastolic Arterial Volume*

Factors Affecting Venous Circulation

LEARNING OBJECTIVES

1. Locate the major structures of the heart, including the chambers, valves, and vessels.
2. List the three layers that compose the atrial and ventricular walls.
3. Show the positions of the trabeculae carneae, the papillary muscles, and the chordae tendineae.
4. Differentiate the structures of the atrioventricular valves and the semilunar valves.
5. Locate the origin and the branches of both the right and left coronary arteries.
6. Trace the conduction system of the heart.
7. Differentiate structurally a myocardial muscle cell and a skeletal muscle cell.
8. Define *intercalated disk* and *syncytium*.
9. Review the general mechanism for skeletal muscle contraction.
10. Compare skeletal and cardiac muscle contraction.
11. Define *absolute* and *relative refractory periods* in cardiac muscle.
12. Describe cardiac metabolism and cardiac work.
13. Describe clearly the properties of the heart: automaticity, rhythmicity, excitability, and conductivity.
14. Define *diastolic depolarization* in the sinoatrial node and indicate why the SA node is considered to be the pacemaker of the heart.
15. Relate the events of the cardiac cycle to the waveforms seen on an ECG tracing.
16. Describe the four interrelated factors of cardiac contraction: preload, afterload, contractility, and heart rate.
17. Define *ventricular compliance*.
18. Define *inotropic* and *chronotropic effects*.
19. Describe the events of the cardiac cycle.
20. Differentiate isovolumic contraction, ejection, and isovolumic relaxation as phases in ventricular systole.
21. Explain how a different stroke volume between the ventricles is compensated for or equalized.
22. List the normal pressure and oxygen saturations in the chambers of the heart and in the vessels.
23. Describe the factors responsible for generating heart sounds.
24. Explain sympathetic and parasympathetic influences on the heart.
25. Locate and define the function of the chemoreceptors and baroreceptors.
26. Differentiate between the elastic and nutrient arteries.
27. Define *exchange vessel* and *capacitance vessel*.
28. Describe the structure and function of the lymphatic system.
29. Describe briefly the generation of Korotkoff sounds.
30. List some factors that can affect pulse pressure.
31. Describe clearly the four direct determinants of blood pressure.

Understanding the dynamics of normal cardiac contraction provides the basis for understanding the effects of alterations to structures within the heart, myocardial muscle, and vessels. The first part of this chapter is devoted to normal cardiac anatomy and physiology; the second part deals with the dynamics of circulation.

Anatomy of the Heart

The heart is a double pump that pumps its blood to the lungs and to the systemic arteries. It provides for oxygenation and nourishment of all of the tissues of the body.

The heart is composed of four pumping chambers: the right and left atria and the right and left ventricles. The right atrium and ventricle receive blood from the systemic veins and pump it to the lungs through the pulmonary artery. The left atrium and ventricle pump blood received from the pulmonary veins to the systemic arteries through the aorta. Figure 18-1 shows the general anatomy of the heart and blood vessels.

Atria

The *right atrium* is a low-pressure, thin-walled chamber that receives blood from the superior and inferior vena cava and from the veins draining the heart. The *left atrium* is slightly smaller than the right and receives blood from the four pulmonary veins that carry oxygenated blood from the lungs back to the heart.

The atrial walls are composed of three layers: (1) *epicardium*, a thin outer layer that is continuous with the outer layer of the ventricles; (2) *myocardium*, the middle, or muscular, layer of the atria, discontinuous with that of the ventricles; and (3) *endocardium*, a thin, continuous, inner layer that covers the inner surface of the atria, the valves, ventricles, and vessels entering and leaving the heart. The muscular layer of the atria is much thinner than that in the ventricles and accounts for the lower pressures maintained in these chambers. The atria serve mostly as storage reservoirs and as conductive passageways for the movement of blood to the ventricles.

Dividing the atria is the membranous atrial septum, a separation that prevents the communication of blood between the atria. This septum houses the fossa ovalis, which originated as a fetal communication, the foramen ovale.

Ventricles

The ventricular walls are also composed of three layers: epicardium, myocardium, and endocardium (Fig. 18-2). The *right ventricle* has been described as looking like a

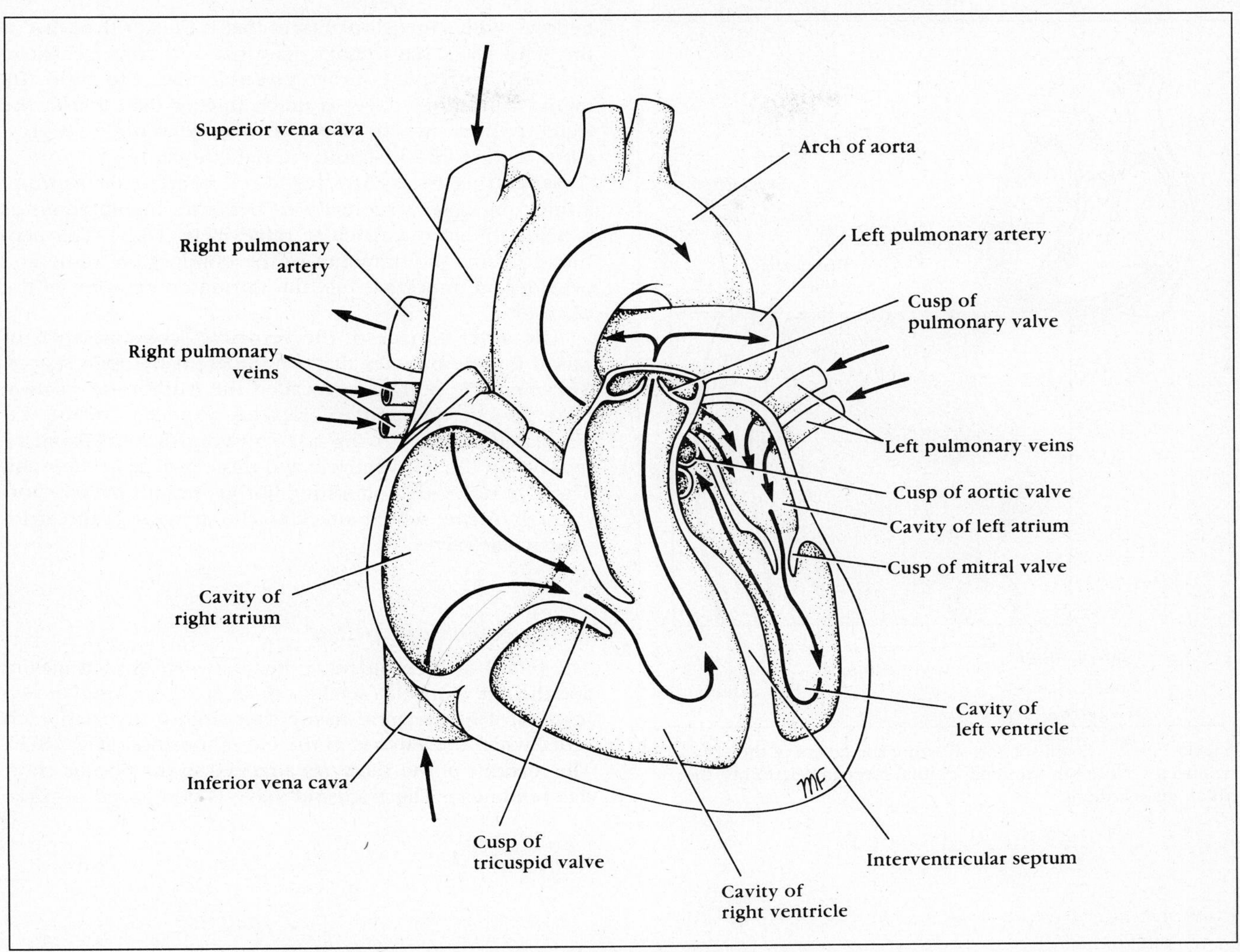

FIGURE 18-1 Anatomy of the heart and great vessels. Arrows show the flow of blood through the heart. (From R.S. Snell, *Clinical Histology for Medical Students*. Boston: Little, Brown, 1984.)

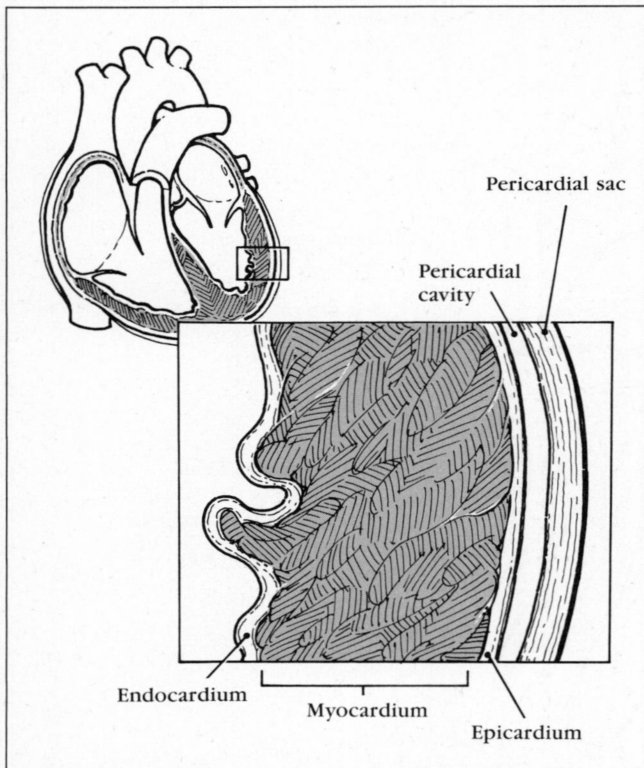

FIGURE 18-2 Cross-section showing the layers of the ventricles. Note the thin endocardial layer in relation to the thick myocardium.

bellows, with a myocardial layer that is thicker than that in the atrial walls, but thinner than that of the left ventricle. The *left ventricle* is more circular than the right. Its myocardial muscle layer is much thicker than that in the right ventricle, which allows it to achieve the high pressures required for systemic arterial circulation.

Separating the ventricles is the ventricular septum, a thick muscular structure that becomes membranous as it nears the atrioventricular valves (Fig. 18-3). This septum contains the branches of the conduction tissue and provides an important fulcrum during contraction of the ventricles.

The inner surface of the ventricles contains areas of raised muscle bundles that are undercut by open spaces. These muscle bundles are called the *trabeculae carneae* (Fig. 18-4). The papillary muscles project from the trabeculated surface, giving rise to two groups of papillary muscles in the left ventricle and three groups in the right. These muscles give off strong fibrous strands called *chordae tendineae*, which attach to the margins of the atrioventricular valves.

Atrioventricular Valves

The mitral or bicuspid valve lies between the left atrium and the left ventricle (see Fig. 18-4). It is composed of two leaflets of fibroelastic tissue that slightly overlap each other when the valve is in the closed position (Fig. 18-5). The margins of the valve are attached to the fibrous chordae tendineae. The tricuspid valve is composed of three

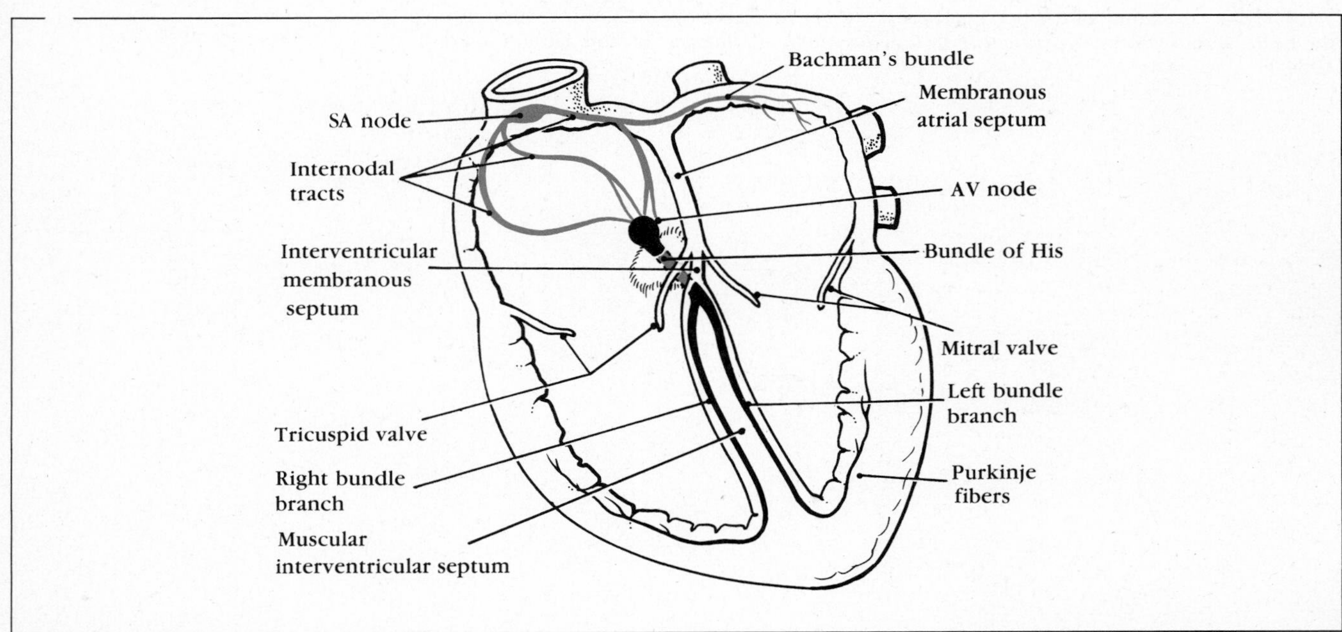

FIGURE 18-3 Interventricular septum and branches of the conduction system.

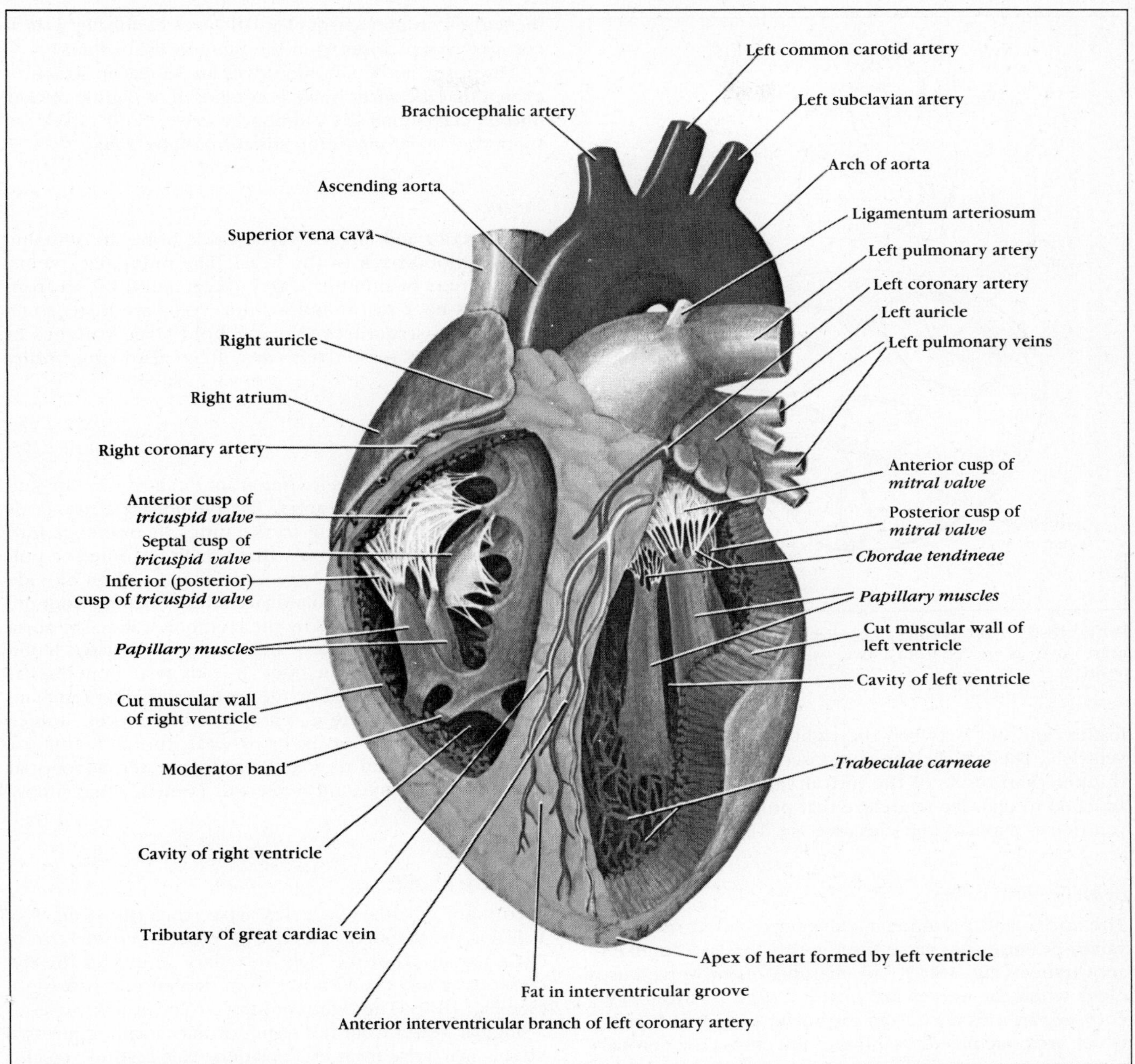

FIGURE 18-4 The heart viewed from the left side. The anterior wall of the right ventricle and posterior wall of the left ventricle have been removed. Note the trabeculae carneae, or raised muscle bundles, are more prominent in the left ventricle than the right. (From R.S. Snell, *Atlas of Clinical Anatomy*. Boston: Little, Brown, 1978.)

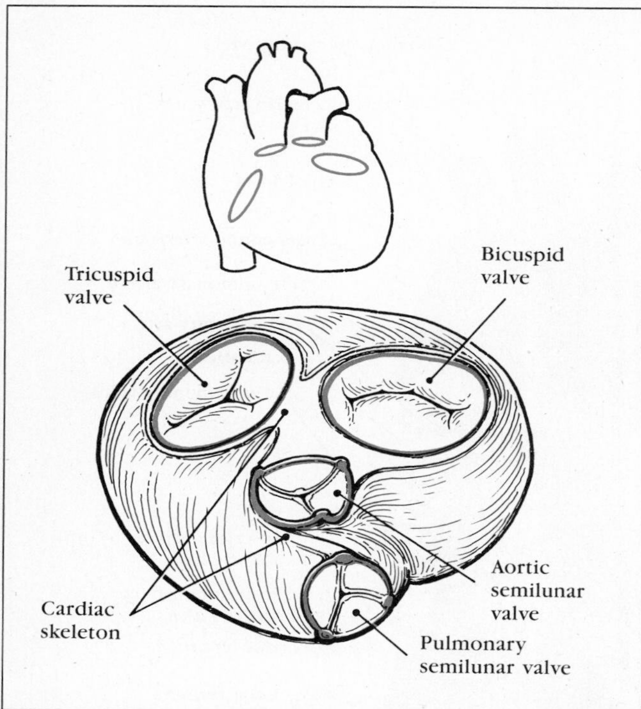

FIGURE 18-5 Fibrous rings of cardiac skeleton surround the heart valves as viewed from above. Valves are in the closed position.

leaflets and lies between the right atrium and the right ventricle. The leaflets, also composed of fibrous tissue, are thinner than those of the mitral valve. These are also attached to chordae tendineae that project from the right ventricular papillary muscles (see Fig. 18-4).

Semilunar Valves

The aortic and pulmonary valves are called semilunar valves because they have three cusps that are cuplike in appearance (Fig. 18-6). The margins of the valve cusps meet when the valves are in the closed position. Two coronary arteries arise from the aortic sinuses of Valsalva, which are pouchlike dilatations of the cusps. The coronary ostia, or openings, are located in the upper one-third of the aortic coronary cusps (Fig. 18-7). Occasionally, a third coronary artery arises from the right coronary sinus.

The aortic and pulmonic valves are similar in structure except that the aortic valve is composed of slightly thicker fibrous cusps than the pulmonary valve. Both valves are supported by strong fibrous tissue, or valve rings.

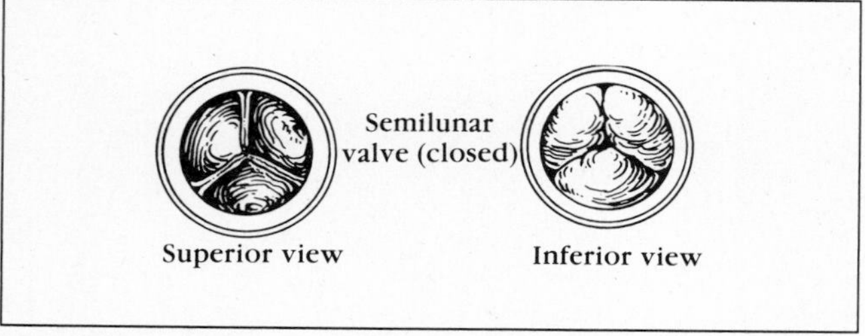

FIGURE 18-6 Appearance of the semilunar valves from superior and inferior positions. The valves are in the closed position. (Reprinted from J. Kernicki, B. Bullock, and J. Matthews, *Cardiovascular Nursing*. New York: G.P. Putnum, 1971.)

Veins

The superior and inferior venae cavae bring the systemic venous blood back to the heart. The pulmonary veins, usually four in number, carry oxygenated blood from the lungs back to the left atrium. Veins are distensible, thin-walled structures that can hold large volumes of blood. For this reason veins are often called *capacitance vessels* [13].

Arteries

The two major arteries leading from the heart are the pulmonary artery and the aorta. The pulmonary artery leads from the right ventricle to the lungs. It branches into smaller and smaller vessels that finally become the pulmonary capillary bed where oxygen and carbon dioxide exchange occurs. The pulmonary artery opening from the right ventricle is guarded by the pulmonic valve. The aorta is the main systemic artery and carries oxygenated blood to all of the tissues of the body. It leads away from the left ventricle and is guarded by the aortic valve. The aorta and pulmonary arteries are composed of three layers: tunica intima, or endothelial layer or coat; tunica media, or muscular layer; and tunica externa, or outer, adventitial coat. The aorta gives off numerous branches that supply systemic tissues.

Coronary Arteries

Two main coronary arteries arise from the sinuses of Valsalva of the aortic valve. The *right coronary artery* (RCA) arises from the right coronary sinus and the *left coronary artery* (LCA) arises from the left coronary sinus (see Fig. 18-7). The right coronary artery usually arises as a singular vessel from the right coronary ostium, but two vessels may arise from this position. This second vessel is usually called the *conus artery*. When a single coronary artery arises on the right side, the conus artery is the first branch off the right main coronary artery [9]. The RCA travels in the atrioventricular groove, or sulcus, and turns downward in the posterior surface to the posterior interventricular sulcus. Smaller arterial vessels branch off the main artery. In about 55 percent of human hearts, the RCA supplies blood to the sinoatrial (SA) node and in about 90 percent it supplies the atrioventricular (AV) node. In some hearts the right coronary artery supplies the posterior surface of the right and left ventricles and the posterior interventricular septum. It may extend to supply part of the lateral and apical surfaces of the heart. A variation in the amount of myocardial tissue supplied by the right coronary artery accounts for the difference in myocardial pathology when the RCA is diseased.

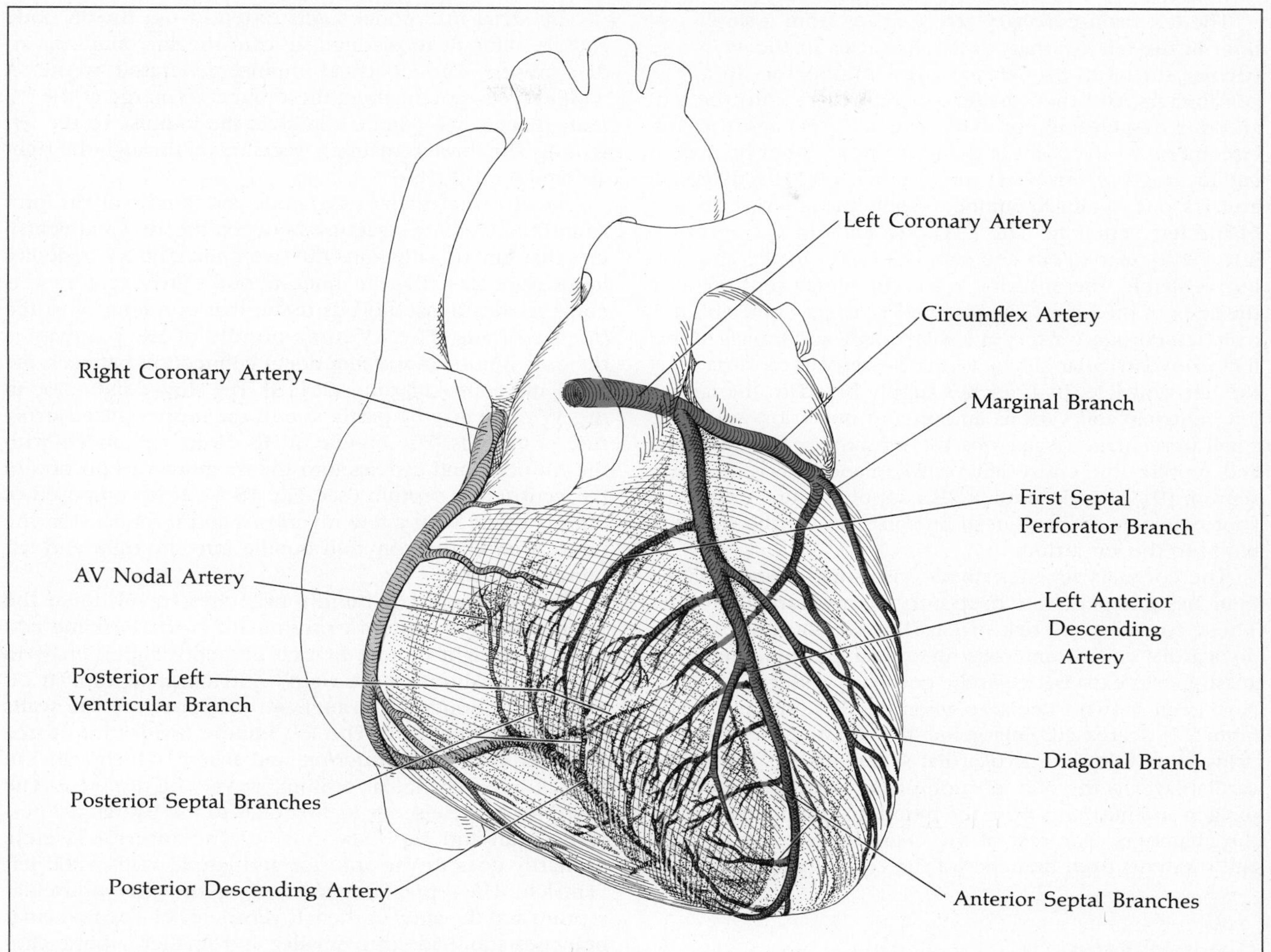

FIGURE 18-7 Coronary arteries. The right and left coronary arteries arise from the aorta immediately above the aortic valve. The right coronary artery runs in the AV groove toward the posterior surface of the heart. In its course, it gives off branches that supply the right atrium and ventricle. At the posterior border of the interventricular septum the right coronary artery gives off the AV nodal artery, which supplies the atrioventricular node and then divides into a posterior descending artery and a posterior left ventricular branch. Septal branches arising from the posterior descending artery supply blood to the posterior one-third of the interventricular septum. Soon after its emergence from the aortic sinus, the left main coronary artery divides into the left anterior descending artery, which runs downward to the cardiac apex, and the circumflex artery, which winds around the left side of the heart in the AV groove. The left anterior descending artery in turn gives rise to a first septal perforator branch, which is a major supplier of nutrient blood to the right bundle branch and the anterior fascicle of the left bundle branch; a diagonal branch, which courses laterally to nourish the anterolateral aspects of the left ventricle; and anterior septal branches, which supply the anterior two-thirds of the interventricular septum. The circumflex artery gives off a marginal branch that nourishes the lateral aspect of the left ventricle. (© 1987 Scientific American, Inc. All rights reserved. From *Scientific American Medicine*, Figure 1, Section 1, Subsection IX.)

The left main coronary artery arises from a single ostium in the left coronary sinus. It travels in the atrioventricular sulcus to the left for a few millimeters to a few centimeters, and then divides, or bifurcates, into the left anterior descending coronary artery (LAD) and the left circumflex. At the point of the bifurcation, other branches, called *diagonal arteries*, may branch off. The diagonal arteries, one to four in number, supply the anterior surface of the left ventricle. The LAD descends in the anterior interventricular sulcus and supplies blood to the anterior left ventricle, the anterior interventricular septum, and the apex of the heart. The circumflex artery comes off the main left coronary artery at a sharp angle and travels in the left atrioventricular sulcus to the posterolateral surface of the left ventricle. Its branches supply blood to the lateral left ventricle and various amounts of posterior wall. In a small percentage of persons the circumflex is dominant, and supplies the entire left ventricle and interventricular septum [9]. The circumflex also supplies the SA node in approximately 45 percent of persons and usually supplies blood to the left atrium.

The coronary arteries divide into smaller and smaller branches that penetrate deep into the myocardial muscle. These form a network of capillaries that supply the myocardial cells. Numerous functional and nonfunctional anastomoses exist between the coronary vessels, and these have been shown to enlarge when the flow in one arterial branch is decreased. Enlargement of anastomoses can improve blood flow to myocardial segments [9]. The endocardial layer is the only portion of the heart that receives oxygen and nutrients from the blood that circulates within the chambers. The rest of the heart receives its oxygen and nutrients from branches of the coronary arteries.

Coronary Veins

The coronary veins provide for drainage of the myocardium and empty into the right atrium. The majority of drainage from the left ventricle is received by the coronary sinus and its branches. The coronary sinus is basically an extension of the great coronary vein. The anterior cardiac veins drain the right ventricle and usually empty directly into the right atrium. The remaining venous blood empties into the heart through the small thebesian veins.

Conduction System

Normal contraction of the heart is initiated by specialized conductive tissues, which are actually myocardial muscle cells with fewer myofibrils than the other myocardial cells. Figure 18-8 shows the location of the conductive structures in the heart: the SA node, atrial internodal tracts, AV node, bundle of His, right and left bundle branches, and terminal or Purkinje network.

The sinus (SA) node is a small mass of cells located near the entrance of the superior vena cava into the right atrium. It normally serves as the pacemaker of the heart because of its ability to generate an impulse through automatic diastolic depolarization (see p. 267).

The atrial internodal tracts extend from the SA node and are difficult to distinguish from the surrounding cardiac muscle. The electrical impulse generated by the SA node travels rapidly along these tracts to merge at the AV node. Bachman's bundle conducts the impulse to the left atrium. The three remaining tracts travel through the right atrium (see Fig. 18-8).

The atrioventricular (AV) node and bundle of His form an interconnecting structure between the atria and ventricles that functionally joins the two units. The AV node lies in the right atrium at the juncture of the atrial septum. It is composed of dense fibrous tissue that continues into the bundle of His. The AV node/bundle of His pathway is the only muscular and functional connection between the atrial and ventricular muscles [8]. The slow conduction in the AV node may be partly due to the unspecialized structure of its cells. The bundle of His directly connects with the AV node and crosses into the membranous portion of the ventricular septum (see Fig. 18-8). It is composed of fibrous tissue with a few myofibrils and terminates in the bifurcation of the common bundle into the right and left bundle branches.

The right and left bundle branches travel down the interventricular septum to terminate in the Purkinje network. The right bundle branch descends superficially in the endocardium of the right ventricular septum. It divides into numerous branches that penetrate the walls of the right ventricle. The left bundle divides into three *fascicles*, *posterior*, *anterior*, and *septal*, which travel in the left interventricular septum for varying distances. The posterior fascicle sends its branches to the lateral and posterior wall and papillary muscle. The anterior fascicle primarily goes to the anterior and lateral wall of the left ventricle. The septal fascicle travels to the interventricular septum and the apex of the left ventricle [9]. The fascicular branches subdivide into smaller and smaller subbranches and terminate in the Purkinje network.

The Purkinje network is composed primarily of Purkinje cells that have few myofibrils and are joined end to end by intercalated disks that aid in the property of accelerated conduction of the impulse [9]. A Purkinje fiber is composed of many Purkinje cells in a series. These fibers penetrate about one-third of the way into myocardial muscle, thus facilitating excitation of the right and left ventricles.

Myocardial Cellular Structure

Cardiac muscle cells are similar to skeletal muscle cells in many ways but have some fundamental differences. Cardiac muscle cells have a single central nucleus, while skeletal cells have peripheral nuclei. The muscle cells are closely approximated so that impulses generated in one myocardial cell can be passed easily to the next.

The myofibril is the contractile unit of the myocardial muscle cell. Its action occurs through the movement of actin on myosin in the sarcomere unit. The thin actin filament also contains two inhibitory proteins, *tropomyosin* and *troponin*. The activity of these proteins in muscle contraction is described in detail in Chapter 40.

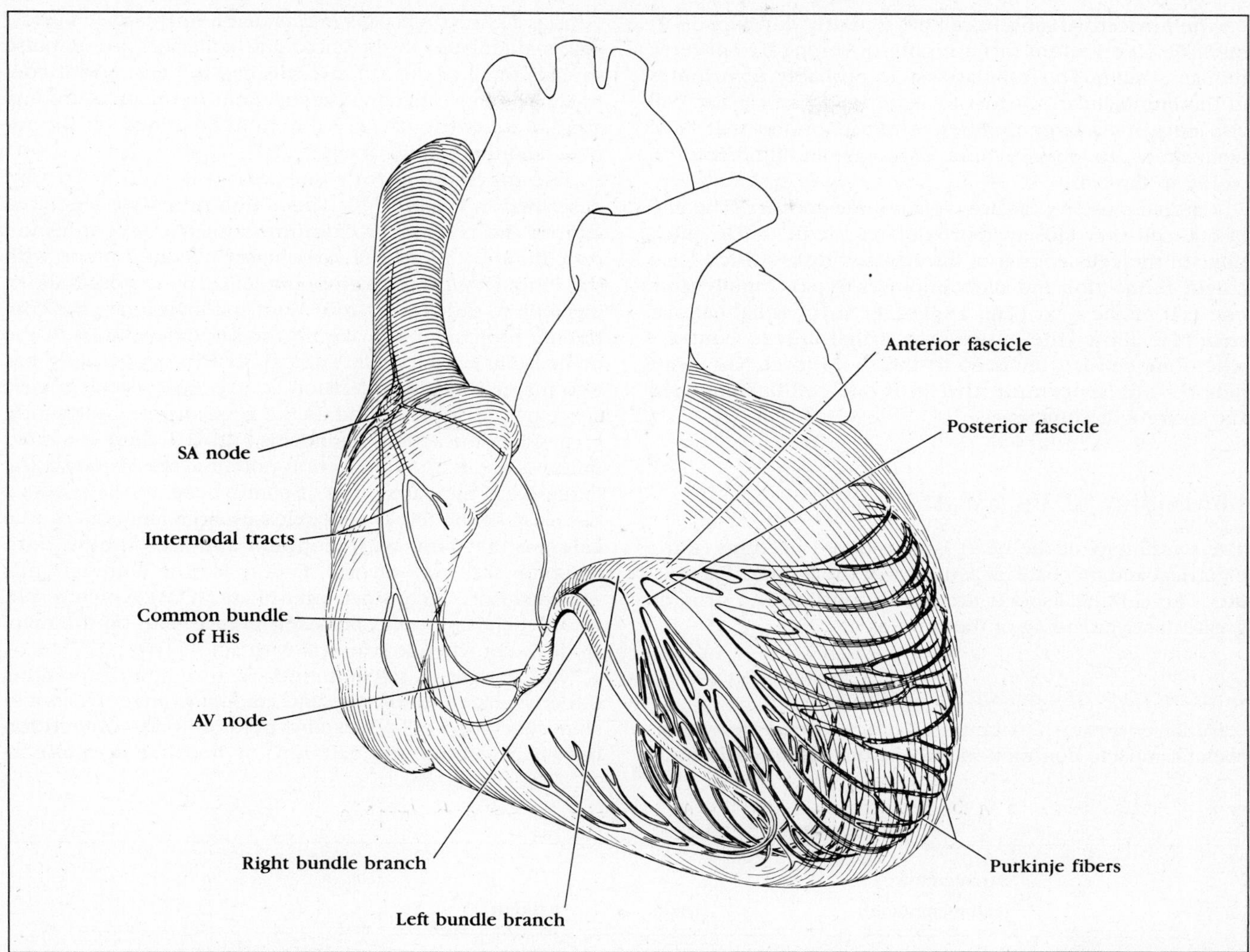

FIGURE 18-8 Cardiac conduction system. The cardiac impulse originates in the sinus node and is conducted to the ventricles by way of the internodal tracts, the AV node, the bundle of His, and the right and left bundle branches, which terminate in the network of Purkinje fibers. The left bundle branch subdivides into an anterior and a posterior fascicle. (© 1987 Scientific American, Inc. All rights reserved. From *Scientific American Medicine*, Figure 6, Section 1, Subsection VI.)

The myocardial muscle cell has a poorly developed sarcoplasmic reticulum but a highly developed transverse tubular system. This tubular system probably contributes to the intracellular release of calcium [3]. The cardiac cell also contains a large number of mitochondria that have been shown to store calcium. Glycogen and lipid are also stored in the cells.

Cardiac muscle cells are close to one another. The end of one cell very closely approximates the next. The junctions of the cells consist of intercalated disks, which form a tight connection and allow impulses to pass rapidly from one cell to the next (Fig. 18-9). The myocardial cellular structure allows the entire myocardial unit to contract when one cell is stimulated to threshold level. The heart behaves as a *syncytium*; that is, if one cell is stimulated the entire unit contracts.

Physiology of the Heart

The physiology of the heart is considered in terms of the electrical and mechanical activities of the myocardial muscle. The cellular aspects are briefly outlined to provide greater understanding of the process.

Contraction of Cardiac Muscle

Cardiac contraction occurs in much the same way as skeletal muscle contraction except that the muscle functions as a syncytium. This means that if one cardiac muscle cell is stimulated to threshold and contracts, the impulse spreads to all of the muscle cells and the entire unit contracts. The two separate syncytial units in the myocardium, atrial and ventricular, are functionally joined by the AV node and the bundle of His.

The mechanism for contraction is similar to that described in Chapter 40. The action potential generated causes the release of calcium from the sarcoplasmic reticulum (SR) into the sarcoplasm. Calcium binds with the inhibitory proteins troponin and tropomyosin, allowing actin to slide on myosin. Actin and myosin are the contractile proteins that make up the sarcomere units of the myocardial muscle cell. The calcium ion apparently has two major roles in excitation-contraction, as the trigger substance or initiator and as the regulator of contraction [10]. When the action potential is initiated, there is a rapid influx of sodium. As the action potential travels down the extensive T tubular system, it comes close to the terminal cisternae of the SR. The SR releases large amounts of free calcium that bind with troponin and thus inhibit both troponin and tropomyosin. Energy for the contraction is obtained from adenosinetriphosphate (ATP), which is split by an adenosinetriphosphatase (ATPase) site on the myosin filament when it interacts with actin [10].

The amount of calcium available to inhibit troponin is directly related to the rate and amount of myocardial tension developed [11]. It is also possible that competition between sodium and calcium for binding sites affects

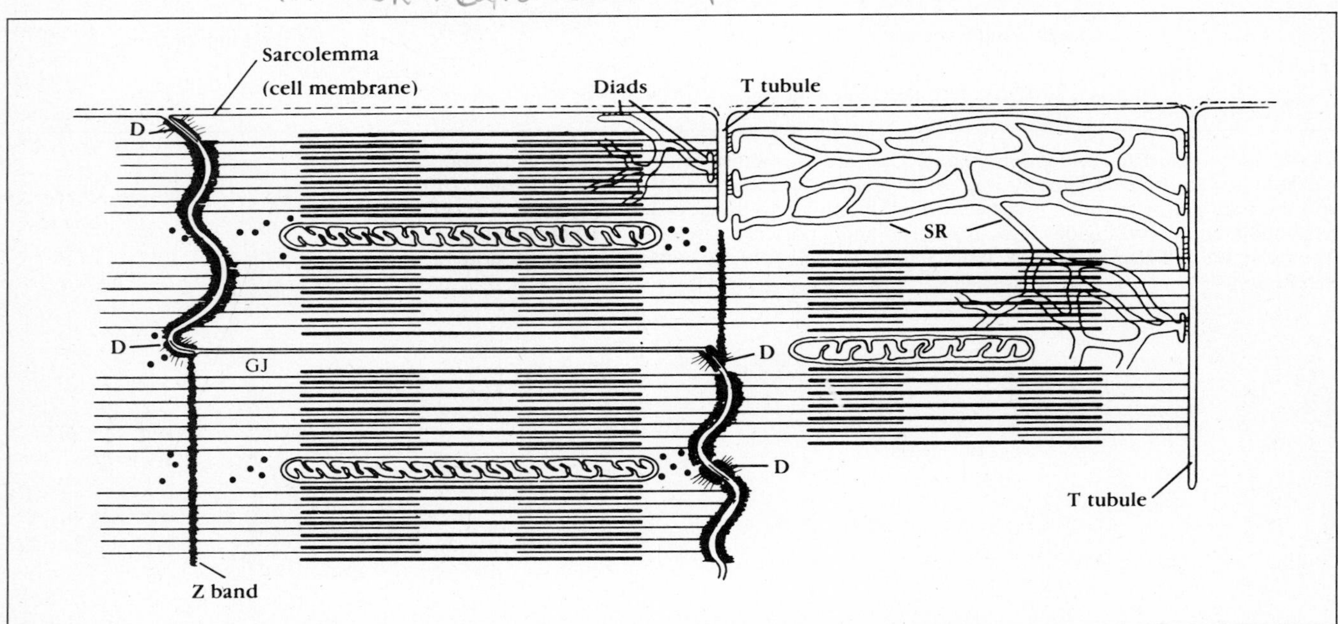

FIGURE 18-9 A thin section through cardiac muscle as it might appear on electron microscopy. Portions of two cardiac muscle fibers are depicted in the area where their plasmalemmas associate to form the intercalated disk. Desmosomes (D) provide structural integrity to the disk. The gap junctions (GJ) are located in the horizontal part of the disk. The disk occurs where a Z band would have been. The T tubules occur at the Z lines. The sarcoplasmic reticulum (SR) forms a sleeve around the myofibrils, but here it is depicted alone to show its pattern more clearly. (From M. Borysenko et al., *Functional Histology* [2nd ed.]. Boston: Little, Brown, 1984.)

myocardial contractility. Calcium must be returned to the sarcoplasmic reticulum through a continually active calcium pump that decreases the free calcium. A decreased level of calcium in the sarcoplasmic fluid restores the inhibition of actin and myosin by the troponin-tropomyosin complex [6]. The sarcomere unit then returns to the resting position.

Action Potential. When the myocardial muscle cell is at rest, the resting membrane potential is approximately −85 to −95 mV. When an action potential occurs, it changes the membrane potential from the negative to a slightly positive value. The action potential in cardiac muscle remains in plateau longer than in other excitable cells, which allows for a longer contraction in cardiac muscle. After the action potential, contraction occurs, and is followed by repolarization and a return to the resting state. As noted in Figure 18-10, these changes in potential and state of cardiac muscle can be described in terms of discrete phases: phase 0 denotes depolarization; phase 1 indicates complete depolarization and contraction; phase 2 is a plateau phase of maximum cardiac contraction; phase 3 is the period of repolarization; and phase 4 indicates the myocardium at rest [11].

Restimulation during phases 1 and 2 does not cause the muscle to contract again. This is called the refractory period, and occurs in both atrial and ventricular muscle. The *absolute refractory period* is the time during which the membrane is completely depolarized and/or contracting, when no stimulus can cause it to respond or contract again. The *relative refractory period* (phase 3) occurs when the muscle membrane is repolarizing, and a strong stimulus will cause it to contract.

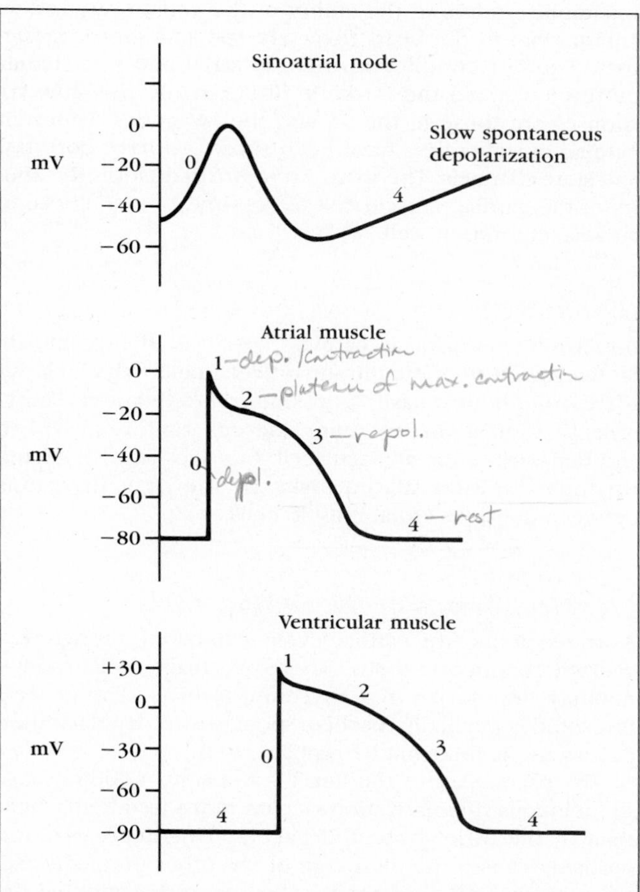

FIGURE 18-10 Differentiating feature of pacemaker cells. (From W.E. James [ed.], *Clinical Electrocardiography*. Parker, Colo.: Postgraduate Institute for Medicine, 1981.)

Metabolism of Cardiac Muscle

Cardiac muscle requires constant production of ATP. Little is stored in cardiac muscle, so oxygen and nutrients for energy production must be constantly supplied. Most ATP is produced in the numerous myocardial mitochondria using fatty acids and other nutrients, especially lactate and glucose. If one substance is not available, cardiac muscle can efficiently use the other.

The amount of ATP produced is equivalent to the work needed to pump incoming blood into the arteries with sufficient pressure to maintain vital body functions. Myocardial work is generated by the ventricular wall tension during systole and diastole. The wall tension generated during systole creates the pressure to eject blood into the arteries. Cardiac work is often expressed in terms of myocardial oxygen consumption. The amount of oxygen consumed is closely related to the amount of stress developed in the ventricular wall. The major factors that affect oxygen consumption include the amount of myocardial muscle mass, the contractile or inotropic state, heart rate, and intramyocardial tension generated [10]. The oxygen supply for this work is totally delivered from the coronary arteries. Increased oxygen is needed in stress situations because of the enhanced contractility and tachycardia induced by the catecholamines.

The myocardial muscle takes up a large amount of the oxygen delivered to it from the coronary arteries. Oxygen extraction of up to 70 percent leaves little oxygen reserve. Increased energy needs can be met only by increasing the heart rate (Fig. 18-11).

Automaticity

The spontaneous property of generating an action potential by the conduction tissue is called *automaticity*. This occurs through a slow, sliding depolarization that creeps toward threshold. When the threshold level is reached, spontaneous depolarization occurs. The action potential usually arises in the SA node where an inward leakage phenomenon allows sodium to drift into the cell. Self-initiation of the action potential, or diastolic depolarization, then occurs. All parts of the conduction system retain the property of automaticity. Figure 18-12 shows that this phenomenon normally occurs because of an unstable membrane potential, with gradual, slow depolarization at the end of the cycle (phase 4). The rate of depolarization in phase 4 is more rapid in the SA node and thus, it fires

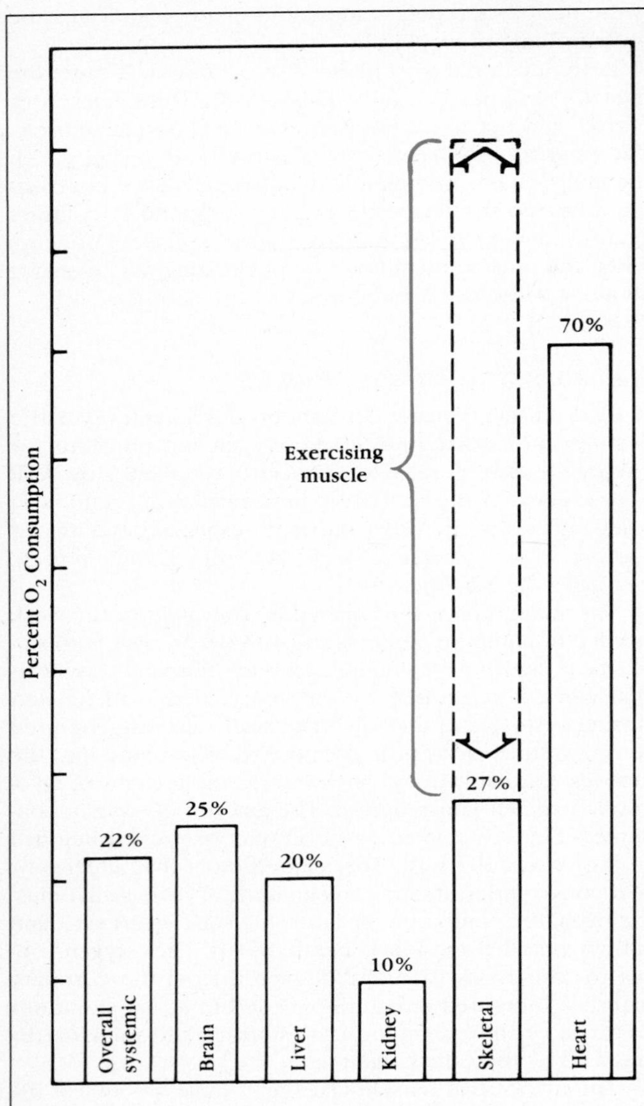

FIGURE 18-11 Oxygen extraction by the heart and other organs. (From M. Jackle and M. Halligan, *Cardiovascular Problems*. Bowie, Md.: Brady, 1980.)

more frequently. These SA node impulses dominate other automatic regions simply because they are formed with greater frequency. The importance of this phenomenon is further illustrated by Figure 18-13, which shows how the action potential can be affected by altering the threshold at which the cell can respond. The term *enhanced automaticity* usually refers to increased irritability of cells of the conduction tissue outside the SA node.

Pharmaceutic agents, hypoxemia, and injury are examples of factors that can alter the threshold for myocardial response. Some drugs, for example, raise the threshold for generation of the action potential and thus decrease the rate of diastolic depolarization. This is especially effective if ectopic impulses are causing ventricular dysrhythmias (see Chap. 19).

Parasympathetic influences through the vagus nerve slow the rate of diastolic depolarization and decrease the rate of SA node automaticity. Sympathetic influences increase the automaticity and rate of diastolic depolarization.

Rhythmicity

Rhythmicity is an important property of the conduction tissue that is characteristic of all of the potential pacemakers of the heart. It refers to the rhythmic or regular generation of an action potential. The leakage phenomenon described above remains regular, allowing for the same amount of time from one depolarization to the next. Therefore, the action potential discharges regularly. Rhythmicity also may be affected by the sympathetic nervous system and the parasympathetic system. A cyclic increase and decrease in cardiac rate due to respiratory influences on the vagus nerve result in an increased cardiac rate on inspiration and a decreased rate on expiration in certain persons. Rhythmicity may be interrupted by enhanced automaticity of influences such as nervous system stimulation, electrolyte imbalances, and pharmaceutic agents.

Excitability

Excitability refers to the ability of the cell to respond to stimulation. In the heart there are fast and slow conductors. The fast conductors include atrial and ventricular muscle cells and the Purkinje fibers, while the slow responses are those in the SA and the AV nodes. Different cardiac muscle fibers have been shown to have both fast and slow channels. The word *excitability* denotes the ability of the cardiac muscle cell to respond to an impulse in an adjacent muscle cell [11].

Conductivity

Impulse transmission in cardiac muscle is affected mostly by the structure of the intramyocardial cells, which allows the current to flow easily from one cell to the next. Therefore, threshold current from one cell rapidly passes to and depolarizes the adjacent cell. Conductivity is effected through the intercalated disks, or the tight junctions between the myocardial muscle cells.

Electrical Events of the Cardiac Cycle

As stated above, the cardiac cycle is initiated through specialized conduction tissue. These pacemaker cells spontaneously depolarize in a rhythmic fashion. The critical threshold is gradually reached; spontaneous depolarization occurs and is followed by repolarization.

The pacemaker of the heart is the sinus node because spontaneous depolarization occurs more frequently here than in the other potential pacers. This depolarization probably causes the discharge of the other potential pacers, a mechanism sometimes called *overdrive suppression* [12]. The conduction tissue has been referred to as a cascade of potential pacers that fire at different rates and can

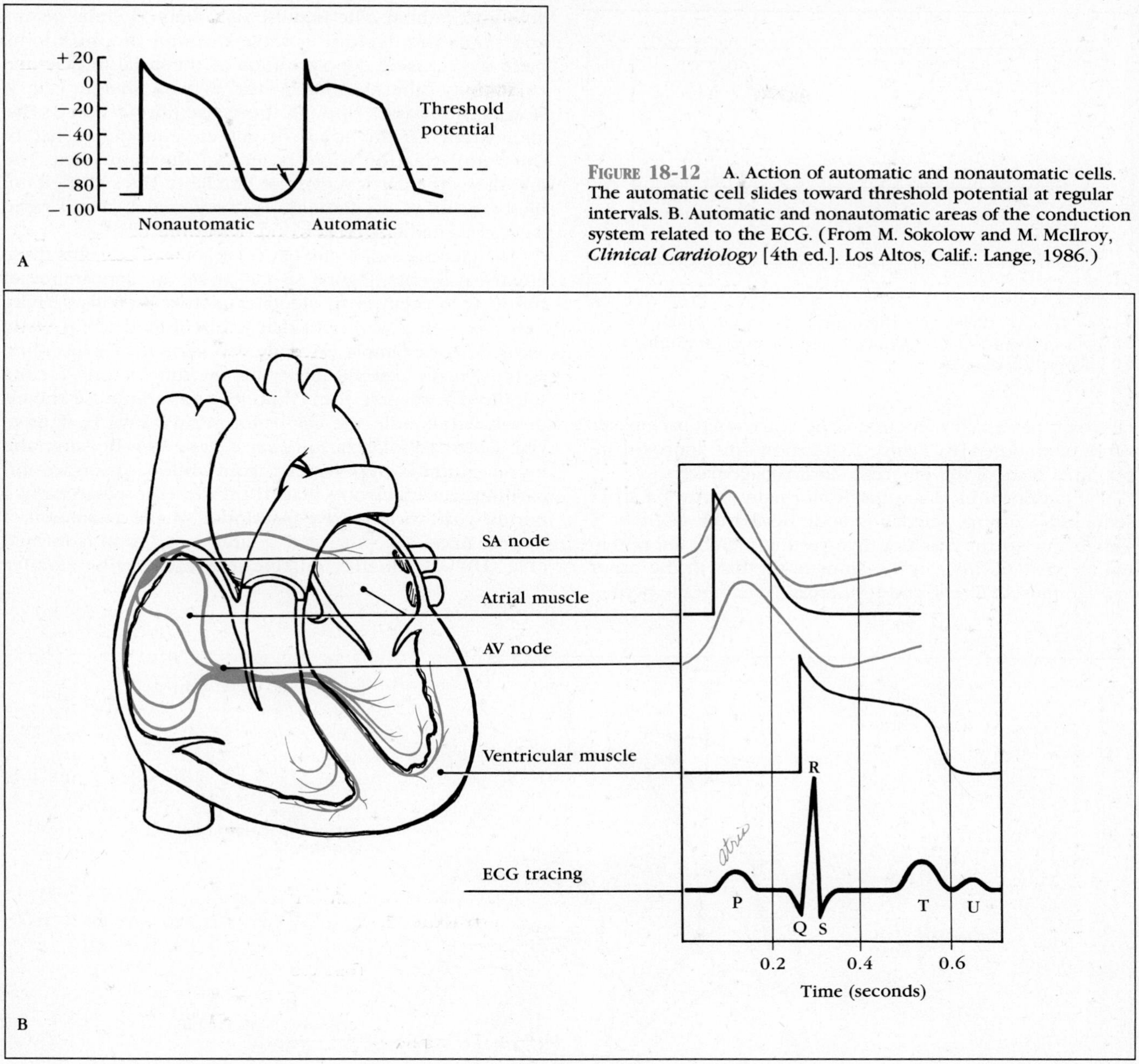

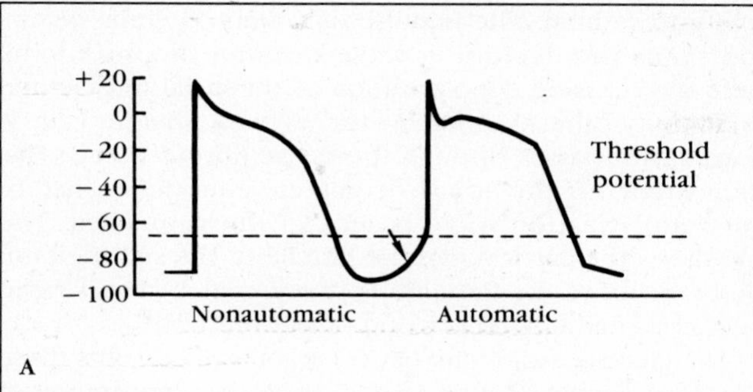

FIGURE 18-12 A. Action of automatic and nonautomatic cells. The automatic cell slides toward threshold potential at regular intervals. B. Automatic and nonautomatic areas of the conduction system related to the ECG. (From M. Sokolow and M. McIlroy, *Clinical Cardiology* [4th ed.]. Los Altos, Calif.: Lange, 1986.)

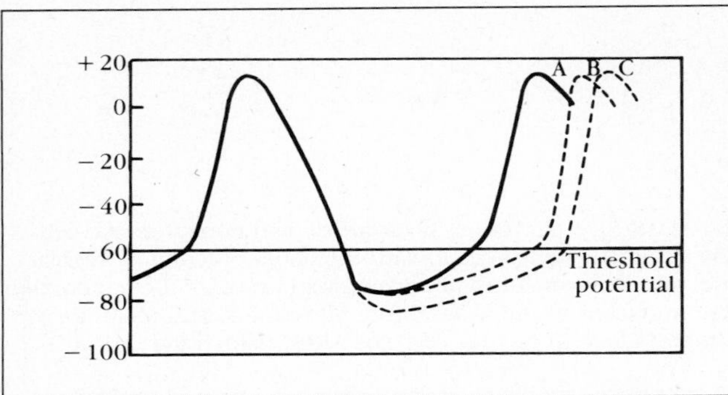

FIGURE 18-13 Changes in rhythmicity can result from (A) changes in threshold, (B) reduced diastolic depolarization, or (C) hyperpolarization.

take over pacemaker function if the more rapid pacemaker is not operational [8]. Figure 18-14 shows the approximate potential rates of the inherent cardiac pacemakers.

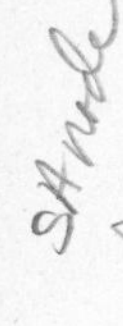

Excitation of cardiac muscle normally follows a strict sequential pattern. The sinus node begins the excitation. This is due to the less negative resting membrane potential (−55−−60 mV) in the sinus node than in the other cardiac muscle fibers, and to increased membrane permeability to sodium. The impulse or action potential occurs and sends the excitation wave through the internodal pathways, causing depolarization of the atrial muscle and excitation of the AV node. At the AV node, the impulse is slowed as it passes through the dense fibrous tissue. This allows time for the atria to complete contraction before the depolarization wave is sent to the ventricles. The impulse is then sent down the bundle of His and the bundle branches to the Purkinje network, which causes rapid depolarization and contraction of the ventricles.

The electrocardiogram (ECG) graphically depicts these electrical events. Figure 18-15 shows the appearance of the ECG in relation to electrical activities. This activity creates an electrical field that is distributed to the body surfaces. For example, SA node depolarization is inscribed as the P wave. The PR interval is the time it takes for the impulse to traverse the AV node. As the impulse travels down each bundle, the QRS is formed. Finally, the T wave represents repolarization (see Chap. 19). Because the myocardium is depolarized from endocardium to epicardium, an electrode placed on the epicardial surface normally shows a positive inscription. If a large amount of muscle mass is depolarized, a large inscription is formed (Fig. 18-16). Smaller muscle masses inscribe smaller R waves.

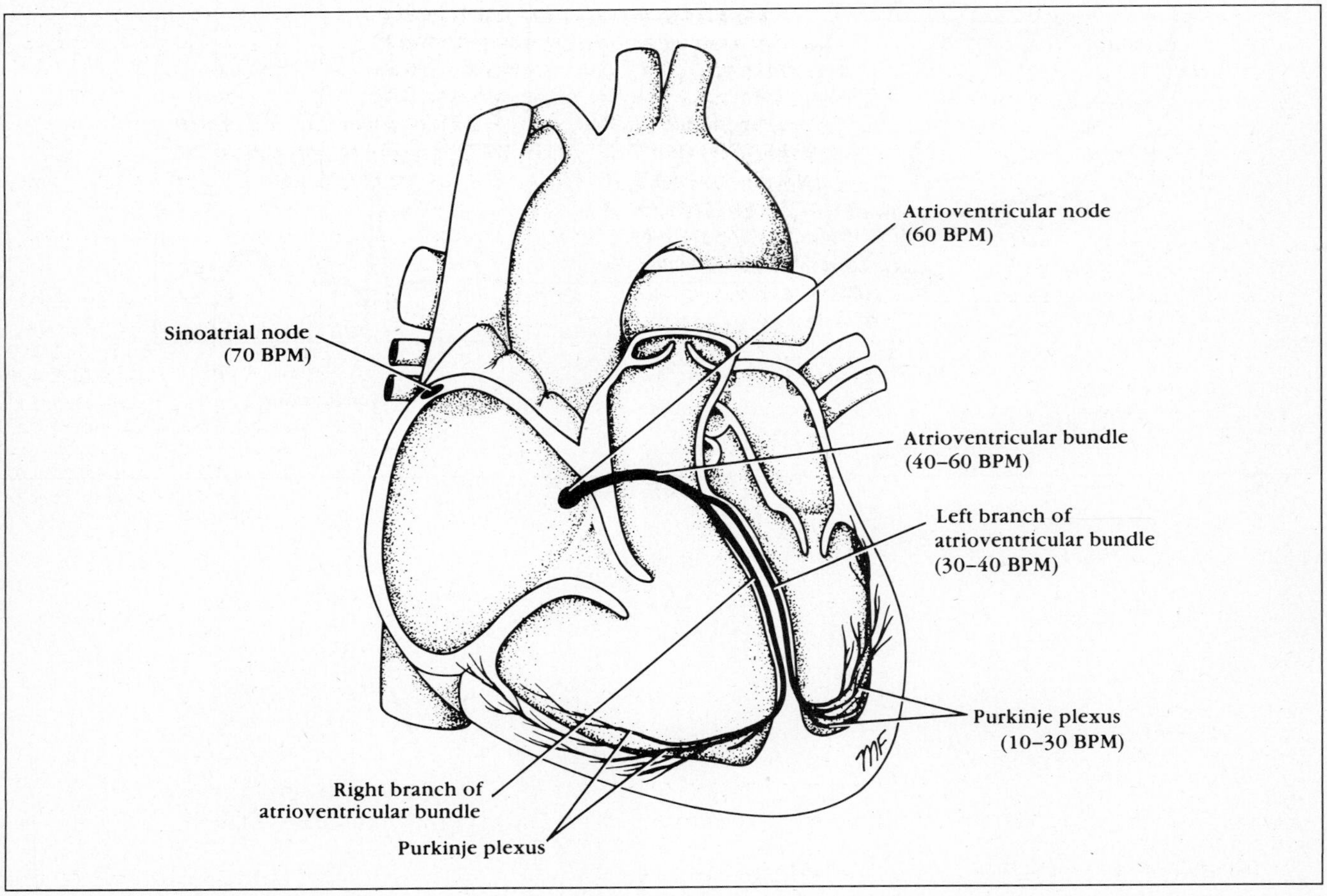

Atrioventricular node (60 BPM)
Sinoatrial node (70 BPM)
Atrioventricular bundle (40–60 BPM)
Left branch of atrioventricular bundle (30–40 BPM)
Purkinje plexus (10–30 BPM)
Right branch of atrioventricular bundle
Purkinje plexus

FIGURE 18-14 Approximate rates of inherent cardiac pacemakers.

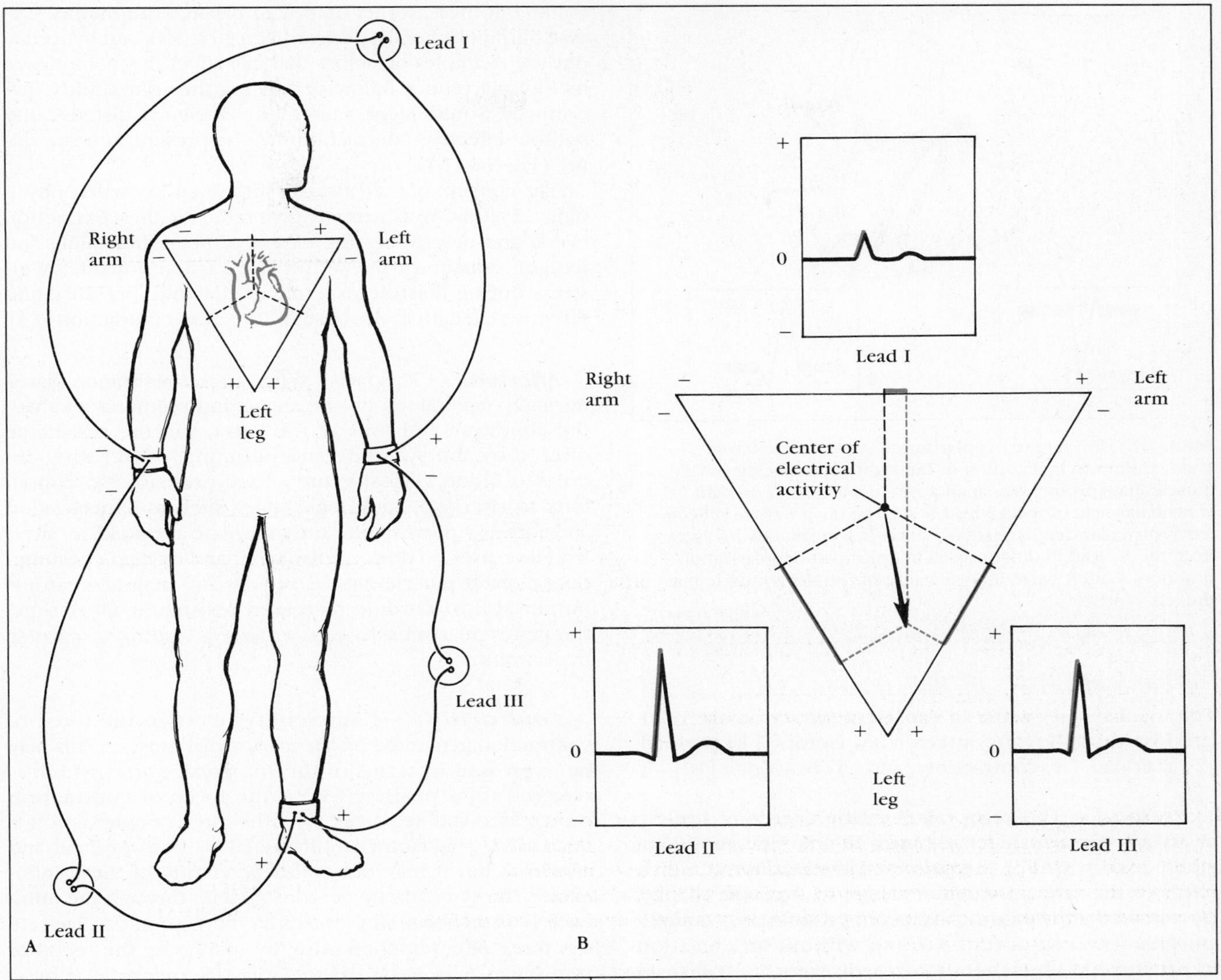

Lead I
Right arm
Left arm
Left leg
Lead III
Lead II
A

Lead I
Right arm
Left arm
Center of electrical activity
Left leg
Lead II
Lead III
B

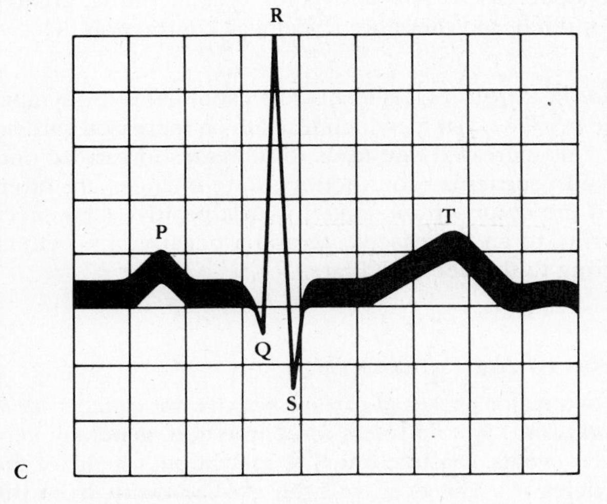

FIGURE 18-15 A. The standard electrocardiographic leads with their attachments to the body. B. Electrocardiograms recorded with leads I, II and III. C. The normal electrocardiogram from lead II. Each small square represents 0.04 seconds on the horizontal plane. Measurements are made of time required for impulses to pass through different portions of the conduction system. The P wave indicates SA node initiation of the impulse. The QRS indicates ventricular depolarization and the T wave reflects ventricular repolarization.

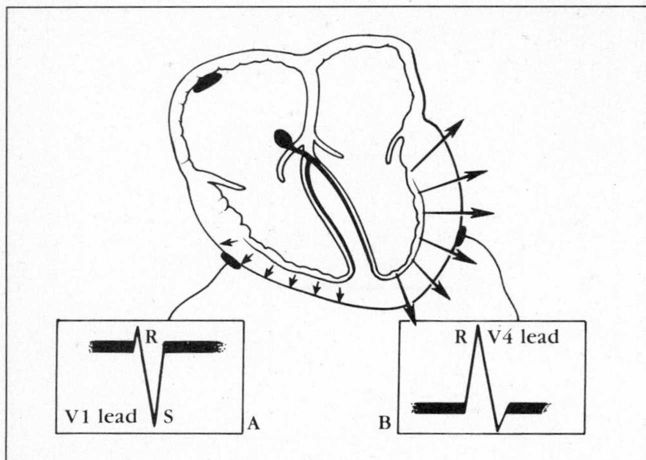

FIGURE 18-16 As the depolarization wave spreads from endocardium to epicardium in the right ventricle, the small muscle mass produces a small positive wave in V_1 or right ventricular lead of the 12-lead ECG. The deep S wave reflects left ventricular depolarization, which is seen as moving away from the V_1 lead. B. Endocardial-to-epicardial depolarization produces a tall R wave in V_4 because of the thick muscle mass of the left ventricle.

Mechanical Events of the Cardiac Cycle

The mechanical events of cardiac contraction are regulated by the following interrelated factors: (1) preload, (2) afterload, (3) contractility, and (4) heart rate [10].

Preload. This term refers to the degree of stretch, or myocardial muscle length, prior to contraction. A commonly used word for this property is *compliance*, which refers to the ratio of volume change to pressure change. Decreased compliance means increased stiffness; a compliant chamber can accept volume without an elevation in pressure [11]. Ischemia of cardiac muscle causes a decrease in compliance, while a normally functioning ventricle can increase volume without a significant increase of pressure, such as during exercise stress.

The inherent property of cardiac muscle that allows for an increased force of contraction due to increased initial fiber length is called the *Frank-Starling law of the heart*. The increased fiber length is related to increased volume of blood, which causes the initial stretch. When the fiber is stretched, it responds with an increased force of contraction. This has been related to the all-or-nothing law of the heart, which means that despite the strength of stimulus applied, cardiac muscle responds either to its fullest or not at all.

In the normal, compliant ventricle, changes of volume can be accommodated quite readily. Ventricular compliance refers to the ability of the ventricle to accept more diastolic volume. Normally, right ventricular output equals that of the left, even though the stroke volumes between the chambers may vary slightly. Respiratory excursion, for example, may cause a temporary increase in right ventricular output, but when the ventricle receives this increased volume, it increases its output to balance the minute cardiac output. Ischemia, pericardial restriction, and hypertrophy are examples of factors that can affect this compliance by limiting venous inflow or limiting the contractility that normally would occur. Increased ventricular distensibility without effective contraction may be present in heart failure (Fig. 18-17).

The concept of *wall stress* is important in cardiac physiology. Systolic wall stress is generated by the contraction event, and determines the extent of fiber shortening and oxygen consumption within the cardiac muscle. Wall stress during diastole determines diastolic pressure and sarcomere length at the onset of the next contraction [13].

Afterload. This factor refers to the resistance that is normally maintained by the aortic and pulmonary valves, the condition and tone of the aorta, and the resistance offered by the systemic and pulmonary arterioles. Increased blood viscosity and added preload also contribute to afterload. Pathologic states such as hypertension and aortic stenosis significantly increase afterload. As afterload increases, so does cardiac work and oxygen consumption. Greater muscle mass is required to maintain cardiac output against chronic increased resistance. Over time, the ventricular muscle mass enlarges, leading to cardiac hypertrophy.

Contractility. Contractility refers to the force of contraction generated by the myocardial muscle. This may be expressed in terms of the *inotropic state*, which is referred to as positive (+) if the force of contraction is increased and negative (−) if the force of contraction is decreased. This factor is influenced by both preload and afterload, but it may occur independently of these influences. The sympathetic nervous system, through the influence of catecholamines, causes an increase in cardiac rate and force of contraction. Also, by increasing the recoil of ventricular muscle on diastole, diastolic ventricular pressure is decreased. This allows for greater filling, greater fiber stretch, and therefore a stronger contraction [9].

Heart Rate. Stress in any form stimulates the sympathetic nervous system, which leads to an increased cardiac rate. This increased rate leads to increases in cardiac output and ventricular contractility. Rate changes are often called the *chronotropic effect*, with a positive (+) effect referring to an increased rate and a negative (−) effect referring to the decreased rate.

Phases of the Cardiac Cycle

The two major phases of cardiac activity are called *systole* and *diastole*. Systole refers to contraction, generally ventricular events. Diastole refers to relaxation, usually of the ventricles [6]. The events of the cardiac cycle, from the atria through the ventricles, relating systole and diastole are discussed in this section. Table 18-1 summarizes the commonly used terms in the cardiac cycle.

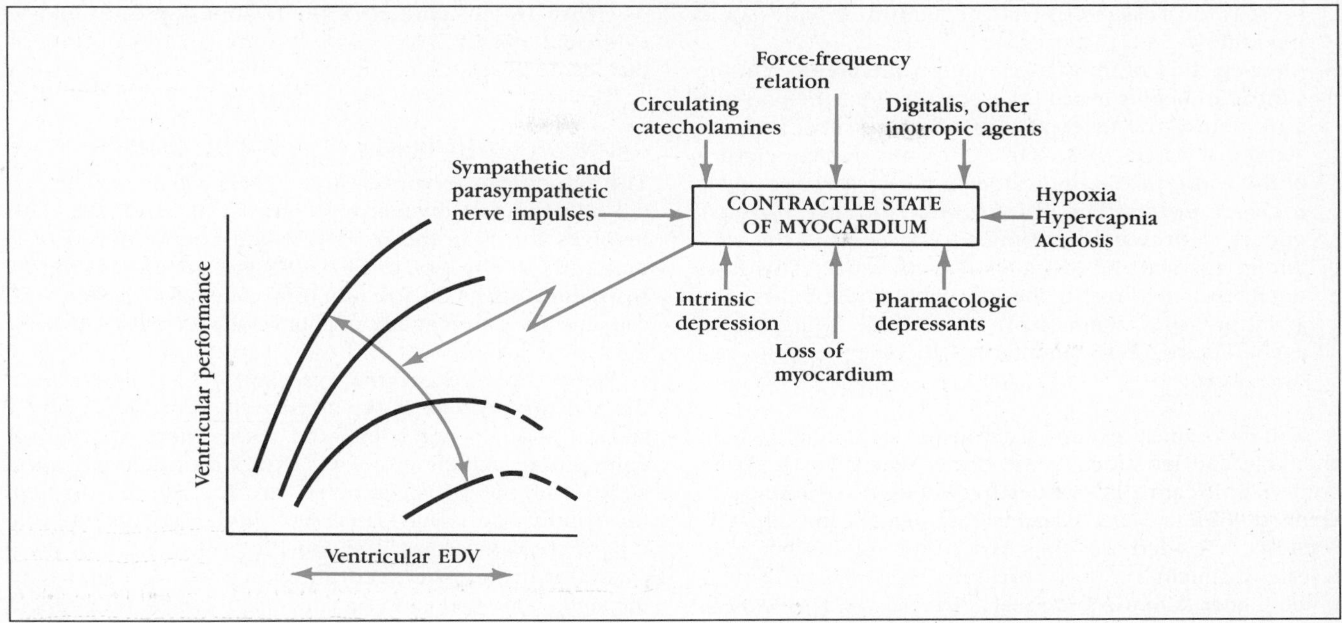

FIGURE 18-17 Effects of changes in myocardial contractility on the Frank-Starling curve. The major factors influencing contractility are summarized on the right. The dashed lines indicate portions of the ventricular function curves where maximum contractility has been exceeded; that is, they identify points on the "falling limb" of the Frank-Starling curve. EDV = end-diastolic volume. (From E. Braunwald, J. Ross, and E.H. Sonnenblick, Mechanisms of contraction of the normal and failing heart. *N. Engl. J. Med.* 1967; 277:794. Courtesy of Little, Brown.)

TABLE 18-1 Terms Used to Define the Cardiac Cycle

Term	Definition
Cardiac output	Amount of blood pumped from heart/minute; cardiac output = stroke volume × heart rate.
Stroke volume	Amount of blood ejected from each ventricle/beat. This is not all of the blood in each ventricle, but about 60–75% of the volume, and is called the *ejection fraction.*
End-diastolic volume	Amount of blood in the ventricle just before systole.
Isovolumic contraction	Period of ventricular pressure rise prior to opening of semilunar valves.
Ejection	Period of time when ventricular pressure exceeds arterial pressure, and blood is ejected from heart.
Incisura	Inscription of a pressure recording that occurs when aortic valve closes; caused by a momentary reversal of pressures between aorta and left ventricle.
Isovolumic relaxation	Rapid drop of pressure in ventricles toward diastolic pressure. Occurs prior to opening of atrioventricular valves and ventricular filling.
Systole	Contraction of the heart.
Diastole	Relaxation of the heart.

Atrial Filling and Contraction. As the atria receive blood from the incoming veins, blood accumulates in these structures until ventricular pressures fall below atrial pressures. As the atrial pressure rises, the flow of blood passively opens the atrioventricular valves and blood flows into the ventricles. Approximately 70 percent of blood flow from the atria to the ventricles occurs passively. Atrial contraction, which follows atrial depolarization from the sinoatrial pathways, provides the "atrial kick" to move the remaining blood into the ventricles.

Ventricular Filling and Contraction. Rapid ventricular filling occurs after the atrioventricular valves open. Blood moves into the ventricles passively and then actively in response to the atrial kick. Ventricular depolarization and contraction occur from the conduction pathways and Purkinje activation of the muscle. Ventricular systole occurs in discrete phases:

1. Ventricular pressure begins to rise, causing increased tension around the AV valve structures and closure of the mitral and tricuspid valves. This is called the *isovolumic contraction* period and occupies the time between onset of ventricular contraction and opening of the semilunar valves.
2. Blood is ejected from the ventricles when the pressure in the ventricles exceeds the diastolic pressures maintained in the aorta and the pulmonary artery. This

increased pressure opens the semilunar valves and blood flows into the arteries.

3. After ejection of the stroke volume, the pressure in the ventricles begins to fall. At a certain point the pressure falls below the arterial diastolic pressure, and the semilunar valves close. On a pressure tracing, closure of the aortic valve is indicated by the *incisura* or *aortic dicrotic notch*. The *isovolumic relaxation phase* occurs as pressure continues to descend in the ventricles toward the low diastolic pressure. This lasts until the pressure in the ventricles falls below the atrial pressure, when rapid ventricular filling begins again. Figure 18-18 summarizes the events of the cardiac cycle.

The mechanical events occur at the same time in both the right and left sides of the heart. Figure 18-19 shows some significant differences between the chambers in terms of pressure and oxygen saturation. It can be readily seen that left-sided pressures exceed the right. While both arteries maintain a diastolic pressure, the aortic pressure is much higher than the pulmonary. The diastolic pressure in both ventricles is normally very low, nearing zero.

Heart Sounds. Two major distinct sounds are produced in the normal heart: S1, often called the mitral sound, and S2, which occurs with the closure of the semilunar valves. The S1 occurs when the ventricles begin contraction or during cardiac systole. It has always been attributed to closure of the atrioventricular valves, but that may or may not be a component of the sound. The S1 is probably produced by the acceleration and deceleration of blood with tensing of the valve structures and cardiac vibrations [7]. Normally, this sound is best heard in the fifth intercostal space, in the midclavicular line.

The second heart sound is mainly due to closure of the semilunar valves. It has two components, the aortic and pulmonary closure sounds. During the inspiratory phase of respiration there is an increase in venous return to the right side of the heart, which increases the volume in the right ventricle, thereby increasing ejection time; the pulmonary valve closes slightly after the aortic valve, producing a physiologic splitting sound. This split is more obvious in young persons and during hyperventilation. This sound is best heard in the aortic and pulmonary areas at the second intercostal spaces (Fig. 18-20).

The third heart sound, S3 (ventricular gallop), may be normally heard in young children, but is usually pathologic in adults. When heard, it occurs after the S2. It results from tensing of the chordae and atrioventricular ring during the end of the rapid filling phase [7]. It is most frequently heard when there is a dilated ventricle or volume overload.

The fourth heart sound, S4 (atrial gallop), occurs with increased ventricular pressure during atrial contraction. It is heard immediately before S1 and may be associated with hypertension or decreased ventricular compliance. Both S3 and S4 are heard best at the apex with the bell portion of the stethoscope.

Figure 18-18 summarizes the relationship of S1 and S2 to cardiac events. Also shown are the periods of the cardiac cycle as related to the ECG.

Autonomic Influences on Cardiac Activity

The autonomic nervous system (ANS) provides an external influence on myocardial contractility and rate. This involves adjusting the heart rate and contractility to the demands of the body. The ANS has an enhancing or restraining effect on the inherent pacemaker system and can alter the automaticity of abnormal pacemaker systems.

Sympathetic Nervous System (SNS). Fibers from the SNS are present in the atrial wall, ventricles, and SA and AV nodes. When stimulated, these fibers release norepinephrine, which stimulates the rate of depolarization and the rate at which impulses are transmitted through the conduction tissue. Therefore, increased sympathetic tone increases cardiac rate and the contractility of myocardial muscle. The predominant effect is usually on the sinus node and causes a sinus tachycardia as occurs in response to exercise or fear. Stimulation of the SNS also can increase the irritability of myocardial muscle cells, causing abnormal or early depolarization, such as with premature atrial or ventricular contractions (see Chap. 19). These are usually referred to as *ectopic foci* because they are outside the SA node.

The effects of the SNS on the coronary arteries are somewhat more complex. Norepinephrine has been shown to cause coronary artery vasoconstriction and causes increased oxygen extraction by the myocardial cell. Some individuals have a hyperactive response to norepinephrine and exhibit coronary artery vasospasms during stressful situations. Ischemia results and causes the liberation of metabolites that, in turn, can cause vasodilation. Epinephrine, most of which is released from the adrenal glands, has a secondary dilating action on the coronary arteries. Prostaglandins, a group of chemically related substances, may be stimulated secondarily in the stress response. They are synthesized by the myocardial cells and arteries and usually dilate the coronary arteries [6].

Normally, autoregulation of coronary blood flow appears to counteract the effects of neural stimulation. Studies reveal that an increased release of fluid adenosine, a powerful coronary artery vasodilator, results from increased myocardial oxygen need [1]. When ANS stimulation induces coronary vasoconstriction, coronary autoregulation usually overrides the mechanism and ischemia is prevented [4]. This mechanism seems to affect the small coronary arteries but is ineffective in the larger vessels.

Parasympathetic Nervous System (PSNS). The PSNS is mediated through the chemical transmitter acetylcholine, which is released from the vagal fibers. The major effect of vagal stimulation is on the SA node, atrial muscle, and the AV node. The result of stimulation is a restraining influence on the conduction tissue, with only a slight

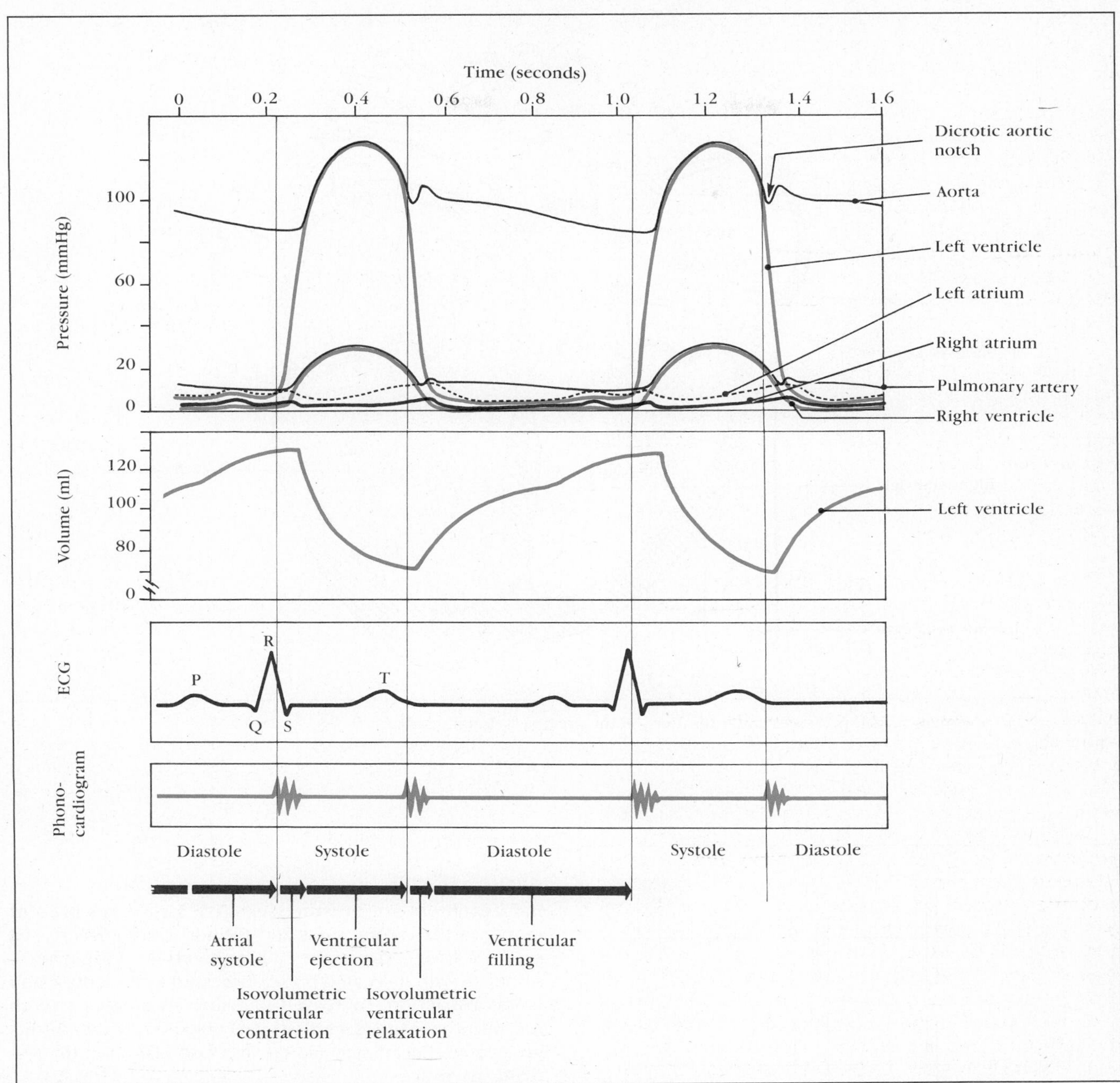

FIGURE 18-18 Events of the cardiac cycle indicating changes in volume and pressure related to the ECG and heart sounds.

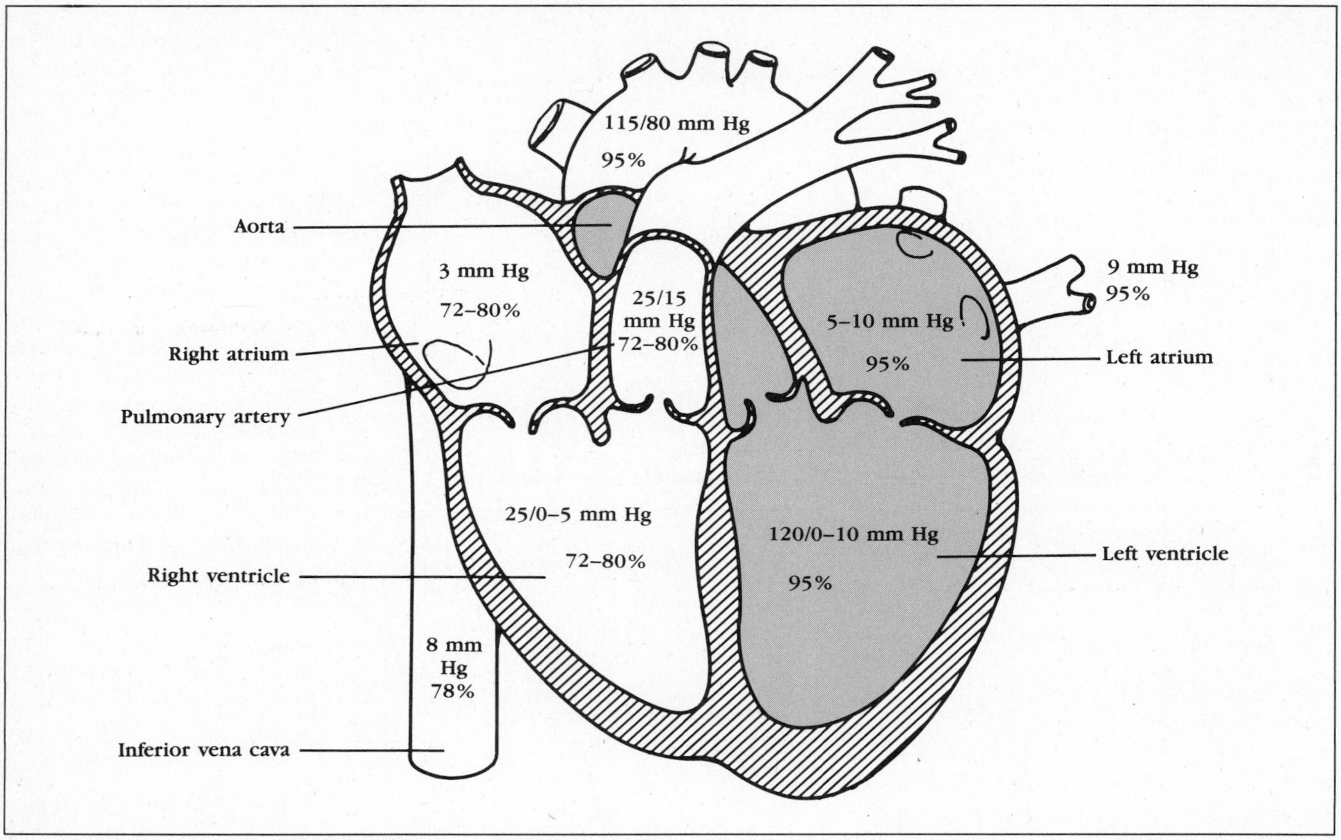

115/80 mm Hg
95%
Aorta
3 mm Hg
72–80%
25/15
mm Hg
72–80%
5–10 mm Hg
95%
9 mm Hg
95%
Right atrium
Pulmonary artery
Left atrium
25/0–5 mm Hg
72–80%
120/0–10 mm Hg
95%
Right ventricle
Left ventricle
8 mm
Hg
78%
Inferior vena cava

FIGURE 18-19 Normal oxygen pressures and saturations in the great vessels and cardiac chambers.

S1
S2
Expiration
Inspiration
AC PC

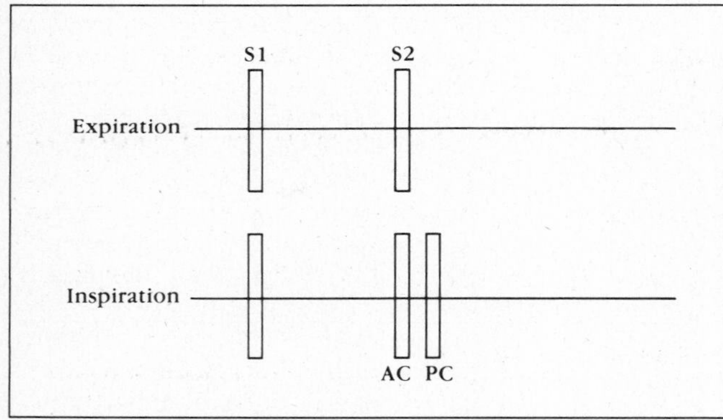

FIGURE 18-20 Illustration of splitting of the second heart sound on inspiration. Note that aortic closure (AC) occurs first; pulmonic closure (PC) follows. On inspiration two separate sounds may be heard.

decrease in ventricular contractility. Vagal stimulation slows the heart rate by restraining the rate of diastolic depolarization in the conduction tissue.

Baroreceptors

Baroreceptors are pressure-sensitive structures present mostly in the carotid sinus and the aortic arch. Decreased systolic blood pressure causes a reflex sympathetic response with increased pulse, increased contractility, and vasoconstriction. Increased pressure stimulates stretch receptors and causes a reflex vagal response, which results in decreased heart rate and passive vasodilation in the systemic arterioles.

Chemoreceptors

The major chemoreceptor of the body is the medulla oblongata, but special receptors are also located in the carotid and aortic bodies. Chemical changes in the blood, especially of pH and carbon dioxide and oxygen levels, alter cardiac activity. A decreased pH or PO_2 causes a reflex sympathetic discharge that results in tachycardia, vasoconstriction, and increased myocardial contractility. A decreased PCO_2 and increased pH serve to reduce the vasoconstrictor effect, leading to passive vasodilatation [8].

↓pH or PO_2 → sympathetic discharge → tachy, constriction

Anatomy of the Arteries, Capillaries, Veins, and Lymphatics

Arteries

The arteries are composed of three layers: tunica intima, tunica media, and tunica externa or adventitia (Fig. 18-21). The layers contain variable amounts of collagen and muscle fibers according to the type of artery, but basically the outer coat supports or gives shape to the vessel, the middle or muscular coat regulates the diameter of the vessels, and the inner coat provides a smooth passageway for blood flow. The large arteries are called *elastic vessels* because they can stretch or increase their diameter to receive the stroke volume of the heart and then contract or resume their original shape, which pushes the blood forward. The *nutrient arteries* are branches of the elastic vessels and supply oxygen and nutrients to the organs and tissues. The smallest branch of an artery is the *arteriole*, which leads into the capillary bed (Fig. 18-22). The arteriole offers varying degrees of resistance to circulating blood by constricting or dilating its diameter. This mechanism regulates the volume and pressure in the artery and the capillary bed.

Blood pressure changes as blood courses down the arteries, being highest in the aorta and lowest in the capillary system (see Fig. 18-22). Vasoconstriction causes increased diastolic pressure (increased peripheral vascular resistance) and decreased capillary pressure. Vasodilatation causes decreased diastolic pressure (decreased peripheral vascular resistance) and increased capillary pressure. The terminal portion of the arteriole contains precapillary sphincters that constrict and relax with autonomic stimulation or with local changes in temperature, pH, and oxygen levels.

Capillary Network

A network of tiny blood vessels provides the microcirculation through which materials enter or leave the circulating blood. A capillary consists of a single layer of endothelial cells. These cells are lined up in such a way as to allow for the exchange of fluids, dissolved gases, and small molecules [8]. Large molecules, such as the plasma proteins, are held back in the capillaries and provide osmotic pressure. Capillary pressures differ in different organs and systems.

Veins

The smallest veins are the venuoles, which receive their blood from the capillaries. These vessels have very thin walls through which some nutrients and oxygen may leave and waste products may enter. Capillaries and venuoles are often called *exchange vessels* [8]. Venuoles join together to form the veins. Many more veins than arteries are formed. These vessels contain approximately 75 percent of circulating blood volume at any one time. Because they have the capability to stretch and hold blood, they are called *capacitance vessels*. The larger veins have valves that are endothelial flaps or folds interspersed along the inner surface of the veins. These prevent the backflow of blood and are numerous in the lower extremities, especially in skeletal muscle areas.

Lymph Vessels

Lymph vessels begin as blind-ended capillaries. They connect the lymph nodes and provide a secondary circulatory system. Approximately 2 liters of fluid is left in the interstitial spaces every day, and this diffuses into the lymph capillaries. The lymph vessels effectively remove any excess plasma proteins that have leaked into the interstitial area.

The movement of lymph through the large lymphatic vessels occurs because of arterial pulsations and muscle movement. Backflow is prevented by the lymphatic vessel valves. Lymph flow in the thoracic duct is approximately 1.3 ml per kg of body weight per hour [5]. If the lymphatic circulation is decreased or blocked, *lymphedema* (edema of high protein content) occurs.

Factors Controlling Arterial Pressure and Circulation

Arterial Blood Pressure

Arterial blood pressure is determined by cardiac output and resistance to blood flow. The highest pressure is the *systolic pressure*, which is achieved by the contracting left ventricle in the ejection of its stroke volume. The *diastolic pressure*, maintained or stored as potential energy in the aorta during diastole, permits a continuous forward flow of blood. The difference between the systolic and diastolic pressures is the *pulse pressure*.

The sounds described in auscultating blood pressure are called *Korotkoff sounds* (Fig. 18-23). They are generated after a cuff is placed around an extremity and pressure sufficient to occlude the blood flow is applied. As the cuff pressure is released, the beating sounds begin when the pressure falls below the systolic blood pressure. As the cuff pressure is continually released, the sounds become muffled and disappear at the point of diastolic pressure. It is generally appreciated that an error of 8 to 10 mm Hg (systolic pressure underestimated by 4 to 5 mm Hg and diastolic pressure overestimated by the same amount) occurs with this indirect measurement [5]. The sounds are basically produced by turbulence of blood flow through the constricted segment. Flow of blood in an unconstricted artery is silent [5].

Pulse Pressure

The pulse pressure is the difference between the systolic and diastolic pressures and normally is about 50 mm Hg [5]. Changes are affected by changes in the systolic or diastolic level. High systolic and low diastolic pressures in-

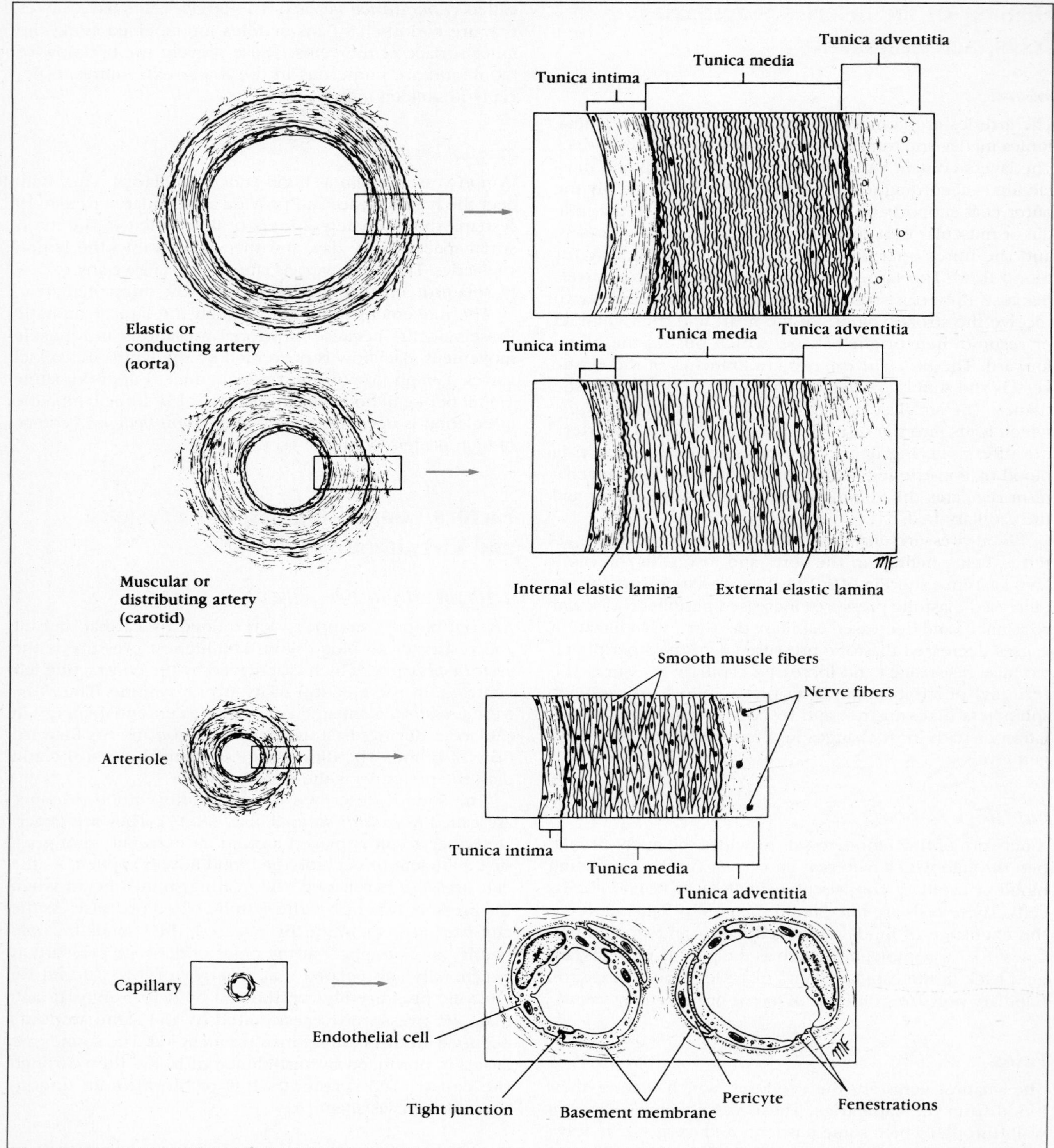

FIGURE 18-21 Layers of the aorta, artery, arterioles, and capillary.

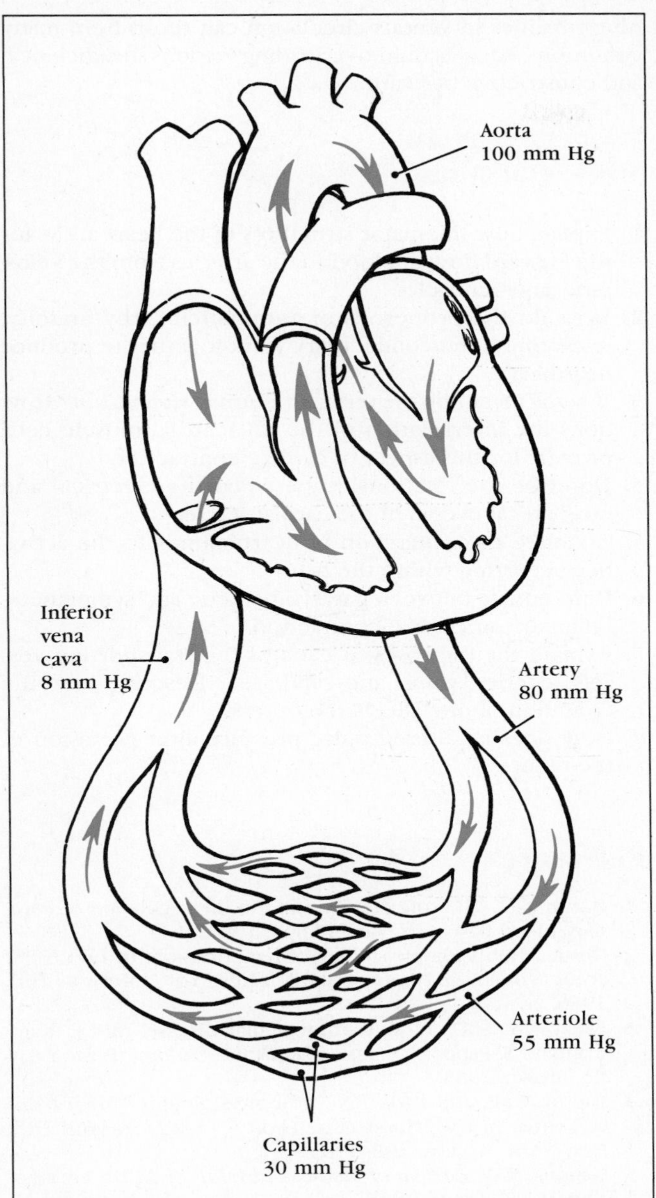

FIGURE 18-22 Changes in pressure of blood from the aorta to the capillary bed to the great veins.

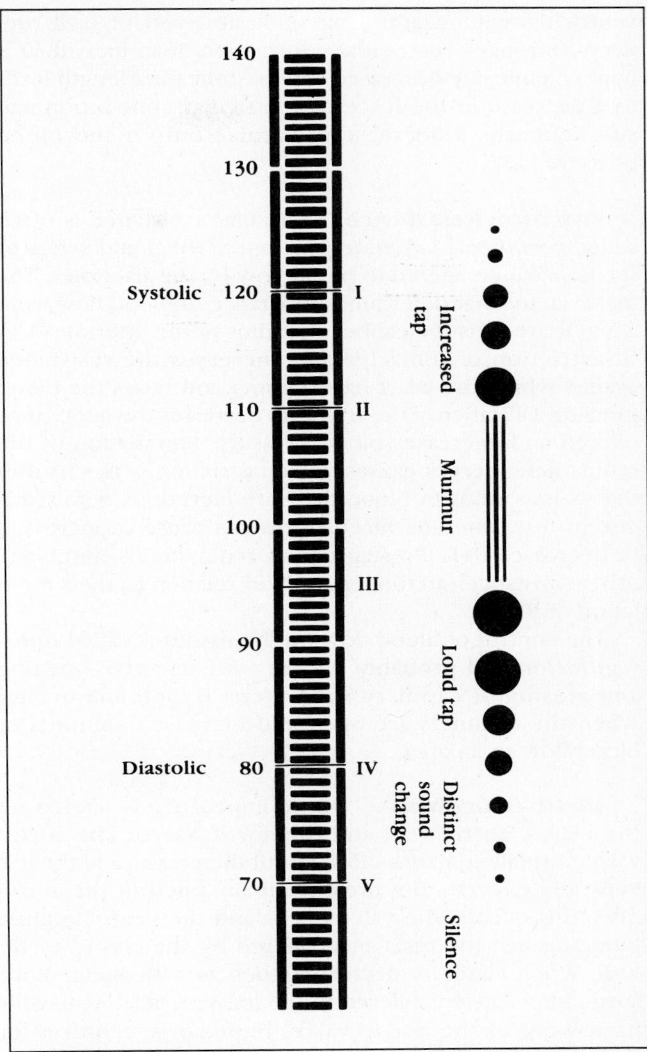

FIGURE 18-23 Korotkoff sounds. (From C. Kenner, C. Guzzetta, and B. Dossey, *Critical Care Nursing: Body, Mind, Spirit*. Boston: Little, Brown, 1981.)

crease or widen the pulse pressure. Low systolic and high diastolic pressures decrease or narrow the pulse pressure. Either component can be altered with a net effect of pulse pressure alteration.

Increased pulse pressure is usually the result of increased stroke volume, decreased peripheral volume, or decreased peripheral vascular resistance, factors that might occur during exercise, fever, with aortic insufficiency, or sometimes with atherosclerosis. A narrowed pulse pressure can occur with increased peripheral vascular resistance, decreased cardiac output, hypovolemia, or other conditions; this often indicates pathology [13].

Direct and Indirect Determinants of Blood Pressure

Contraction of the left ventricle moves its stroke volume into the aorta. The left ventricle pumps against the elastic resistance of the aortic wall, the resistance offered by the arterioles, and the residual volume in the aorta. Therefore, direct determinants of arterial blood pressure include cardiac output, vascular resistance, aortic impedance (resistance to flow), and diastolic arterial volume [2]. Indirect determinants of blood pressure include the activity of the autonomic nervous system and the renin-angiotensin-aldosterone system.

Cardiac Output. The amount of blood ejected from the heart is partly determined by the length of end-diastolic fibers or the Frank-Starling mechanism. Changes in stroke volume vary in healthy persons, and increased ventricular volume at the end of diastole will, of itself, produce a stronger ventricular contraction. If an individual is hypovolemic, the decreased end-diastolic fiber length leads to a decrease in the force of ventricular contraction and subsequently, a decrease in cardiac output and blood pressure [13].

Vascular Resistance. Vascular resistance is often called *peripheral vascular resistance (PVR)* and refers to the impedance offered to blood flow by the arterioles. The major factor that determines resistance to blood flow from a major artery is the caliber or radius of the arteriole [13]. Constriction of the arterioles increases the resistance against which the heart has to pump and raises the blood pressure. Dilatation of the arterioles decreases the impedance offered and decreases blood pressure. Stimulation of the sympathetic nerves causes vasoconstriction, a mechanism that is important in blood pressure elevations with exercise or fear. Humoral mechanisms can cause an increased or decreased PVR. Prostaglandins, renin, kinins, and many other substances are under study in relation to their regulation of PVR.

The control of blood flow by the tissues is called *autoregulation* and probably occurs with selective opening and closing of capillary sphincters. Hyperemia occurs when the channels are open and increased amounts of blood flow to an area.

Aortic Impedance. Aortic impedance is offered by the elastic aortic wall and the aortic valve. The aortic valve normally remains closed until the pressure in the left ventricle exceeds the pressure maintained in the aorta. After this occurs, the valve opens and the ventricle must pump against the resistance offered by the elastic aortic wall. When elasticity decreases, such as with aging, more aortic impedance is offered to the left ventricle. Also, with narrowing of the aortic valve, impedance requires an increased ventricular force to eject its contents.

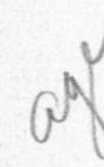

Diastolic Arterial Volume. The amount of blood remaining in the aorta on diastole is related to all of the factors mentioned in the previous paragraph. If cardiac output is increased and peripheral vascular resistance is also elevated, increased amounts of blood remain in the arterial circuit during diastole. This usually increases the diastolic pressure and the resistance against which the ventricle has to pump. If cardiac output is increased and peripheral vascular resistance is decreased, the "run-off" decreases the diastolic volume and volume resistance against which the heart is pumping.

Factors Affecting Venous Circulation

Blood in the veins does not normally pulsate as it does in arteries. Movement of blood through the systemic veins is due to pressure differences; skeletal, thoracic, and visceral muscle pressures; and valves that prevent the backflow of blood. Pulsations may be seen in the jugular veins; these reflect the activity of the right atrium and ventricle. Abnormalities in venous circulation can result from many conditions, such as fluid overloading, venous insufficiency, and constrictive pericarditis.

Study Questions

1. Explain how the major structures of the heart allow for the forward flow of blood to the arteries from the veins, atria, and ventricles.
2. How do the properties of automaticity, rhythmicity, excitability, and conductivity work together to produce heartbeat?
3. What is meant by the term *functional syncytium*? How does the interrelation of the myocardial muscle cells provide for this aspect of cardiac contractility?
4. Describe the relationship between the electrical and mechanical events of the cardiac cycle.
5. Compare the generation of heart sounds to the activities occurring within the heart.
6. Differentiate between parasympathetic and sympathetic influence on cardiac contraction.
7. Explain the purposes of each of the transporting vessels: arteries, veins, and capillaries. Describe how the condition of one affects the others.
8. How does an altered pulse pressure alter perfusion of the tissues?

References

1. Berne, R.M. The role of adenosine in the regulation of coronary blood flow. *Circ. Res.* 47:807, 1980.
2. Dustan, H.P. Pathophysiology of hypertension. In J.W. Hurst et al. (eds.), *The Heart* (6th ed.). New York: McGraw-Hill, 1986.
3. Ezekowitz, M.D., et al. Cardiovascular disease. In C.E. Kaufman and S. Papper, *Review of Pathophysiology*. Boston: Little, Brown, 1983.
4. Factor, S.M., and Kirk, E.S. Pathophysiology of myocardial ischemia. In J.W. Hurst et al. (eds.), *The Heart* (6th ed.). New York: McGraw-Hill, 1986.
5. Ganong, W.F. *Review of Medical Physiology* (12th ed.). Los Altos, Calif.: Lange, 1985.
6. Guyton, A.C. *Textbook of Medical Physiology* (7th ed.). Philadelphia: Saunders, 1986.
7. Leatham, A., et al. Auscultation of the heart. In J.W. Hurst et al. (eds.), *The Heart* (5th ed.). New York: McGraw-Hill, 1982.
8. Little, R.C. *Physiology of the Heart and Circulation* (3rd ed.). Chicago: Yearbook, 1985.
9. Schlant, R.C., and Silverman, M.E. Anatomy of the heart. In J.W. Hurst et al. (eds.), *The Heart* (6th ed.). New York: McGraw-Hill, 1986.
10. Schlant, R.C., and Sonnenblick, E.H. Pathophysiology of heart failure. In J.W. Hurst et al. (eds.), *The Heart* (6th ed.). New York: McGraw-Hill, 1986.
11. Sokolow, M., and McIlroy, M.B. *Clinical Cardiology*. Los Altos, Calif.: Lange, 1986.
12. Wallace, A.G. Electrical activity of the heart. In J.W. Hurst et al. (eds.), *The Heart* (6th ed.). New York: McGraw-Hill, 1986.
13. Wallace, A.G., and Waugh, R.A. Pathophysiology of cardiovascular disease. In L.H. Smith and S.O. Thier, *Pathophysiology: The Biological Principles of Disease* (2nd ed.). Philadelphia: Saunders, 1985.

CHAPTER 19

Alterations in Cardiac Rhythms

CHAPTER OUTLINE

The Electrocardiogram
Normal Conduction
Normal Hemodynamics
Cardiac Dysrhythmias
Classification of Common Cardiac Dysrhythmias

- Disturbances in Impulse Formation
  - *Sinoatrial Rhythms*
  - *Ectopic Rhythms*
- Disturbances in Conduction of Cardiac Impulses
  - *Sinoatrial Block*
  - *Atrioventricular Block*
  - *Intraventricular Block*
- Disturbances in Both Conduction and Impulse Formation

LEARNING OBJECTIVES

1. Identify the limb and precordial leads of the ECG.
2. Identify the leads for examining changes indicative of anterior MI and inferior MI.
3. Discuss the effects of digitalis toxicity and hyperkalemia on conduction of electrical impulses in the heart.
4. Trace the path of a normal sinus impulse from the SA node to the ventricles.
5. Define *dysrhythmia* and *escape rhythms*.
6. Discuss the factors that alter hemodynamic stability during dysrhythmias.
7. List etiologic factors commonly associated with dysrhythmia development.
8. Discuss the two major mechanisms responsible for altered cardiac rhythms.
9. Identify and state the ECG characteristics of the following dysrhythmias: sinus bradycardia, atrial fibrillation, and junctional rhythm.
10. List the three classifications of dysrhythmias and give an example of each.
11. Discuss the pathophysiology for each of the following dysrhythmias: atrial tachycardia, Wolff-Parkinson-White syndrome, and ventricular tachycardia.
12. Discuss the role of electrophysiologic mapping in detecting and treating dysrhythmias.
13. List the dysrhythmias classified as disturbances in impulse formation.
14. Discuss the R-on-T phenomenon.
15. Define *hemiblock*.
16. Discuss the relationship between dysrhythmias and coronary artery supply in the setting of acute myocardial infarction.
17. Compare and contrast the clinical significance of Mobitz type I and Mobitz type II AV block.
18. Identify the characteristic waveforms associated with atrial flutter.
19. Discuss the clinical significance of complete heart block.

continued on next page

LEARNING OBJECTIVES continued

20. Define circus movement and give one example of dysrhythmia initiated by it.
21. List the factors that alter automaticity in the cardiac pacemaker cells.
22. Identify the rhythm most commonly noted in myocardial infarction and indicate its etiology.
23. Discuss the significance of the bifascicular block: right bundle branch block with left anterior hemiblock.
24. Explain the hemodynamic effect of paroxysmal atrial tachycardia.
25. Identify the dysrhythmias described as lethal and discuss the rationale for immediate intervention.
26. Differentiate between active and passive rhythms, and give an example of each.

An alteration in the normal cardiac rhythm can be an unwelcome symptom or a life-threatening event. Cardiac rhythm abnormalities may be symptomatic of developing or chronic disease processes or occur in otherwise healthy individuals. This chapter presents the common alterations in cardiac rhythms, known as cardiac dysrhythmias, the pathophysiology of these events, and their hemodynamic consequences.

The Electrocardiogram

Any discussion of alterations in cardiac rhythms must be prefaced with an overview of the basic concepts, purpose, and use of the electrocardiogram (ECG). Electrocardiographic tracings are indispensable to differentiate between normal and abnormal cardiac rhythms. The rhythm identified can provide evidence not detected through the usual diagnostic techniques. It should be noted that ECGs are not to be depended on solely to diagnose pathologic conditions. A comprehensive evaluation of an individual's history, physical examination, and other diagnostic tests are necessary to make a differential diagnosis.

The ECG is a graphic recording of the heart's electrical activity. The waveforms produced are (1) the electrical activity (action potential) generated as electrical impulses spread through the conduction system and (2) the recovery of myocardial cells after depolarization (Fig. 19-1). These waveforms, called P, Q, R, S, and T waves, are recorded on graph paper with horizontal time and vertical voltage scales (Fig. 19-2). Positive waveforms are those occurring above the line, while negative waveforms occur below the 0 or isoelectric line. The technology used to transmit and record this data consists of electrodes, monitoring cables, amplifier, and oscilloscope (monitor).

The electrical impulses are sensed by positive and negative electrodes placed at various locations on the body surface. One positive and one negative electrode make a lead. Leads record the magnitude, direction, and surface potential of impulses generated by cardiac cells. Electrical impulses moving toward a positive electrode produce a predominantly positive deflection of the QRS complex (R wave), while impulses traveling away from a positive electrode or toward a negative electrode produce predominantly negatively deflected QRS (QS) complexes.

The two types of leads are *bipolar* and *unipolar*. Bipolar leads were first identified by Einthoven as a triangular lead system composed of a positive and a negative electrode placed an equal distance from the heart [12]. Electrodes placed on the left arm, right arm, and left leg are *limb leads* (Fig. 19-3). In lead I, the positive electrode is on the left arm and the negative on the right; lead II, the negative electrode is on the right arm and the positive on the left leg; and lead III, the positive electrode is on the left leg and the negative on the left arm. The bipolar leads view the heart from the frontal plane, gathering data from the superior, inferior, right, and left surfaces. The basic electrodes necessary for monitoring in the limb leads are the positive, negative, and ground electrodes [22]. For ECG machines and some monitoring systems, a fourth electrode is placed on the right leg to serve as an electrical ground.

The unipolar leads consist of the augmented limb leads and the precordial chest (V) leads. The augmented limb leads are so called because the electrical voltage is so small that it must be amplified in order to be seen. These leads also look at the frontal plane of the heart. A positive electrode is placed on the left arm (aV_L), right arm (aV_R), or left leg (aV_F) with a common reference point at the heart (see Fig. 19-3) [16].

Precordial leads provide six views (V_1 through V_6) of electrical activity of the heart on the horizontal plane. Due to the position of the electrodes in the precordial area, these leads are particularly useful in detecting ventricular activity and chamber hypertrophy, and also in providing a mirror image of posterior heart activity. As the positive electrode is placed on the chest, the majority of electrical impulses move away from the electrode in V_1, producing a small positive R wave and deep negative S wave. Due to the placement of V_2 through V_6 electrodes and the flow of the forces, the R wave appears to grow, becoming more positive and reaching maximum height in leads V_3 and V_4. This is known as *R wave progression* and is characteristic of normal ECGs. The R waves in V_5 and V_6 then become smaller (Fig. 19-4).

The 12-lead ECG is composed of the 6 limb and 6 precordial leads, giving a comprehensive view of the heart in two dimensions. Figure 19-5 illustrates a normal 12-lead ECG. It is useful in diagnosing acute myocardial infarction (MI), atrial and ventricular hypertrophy, and congenital

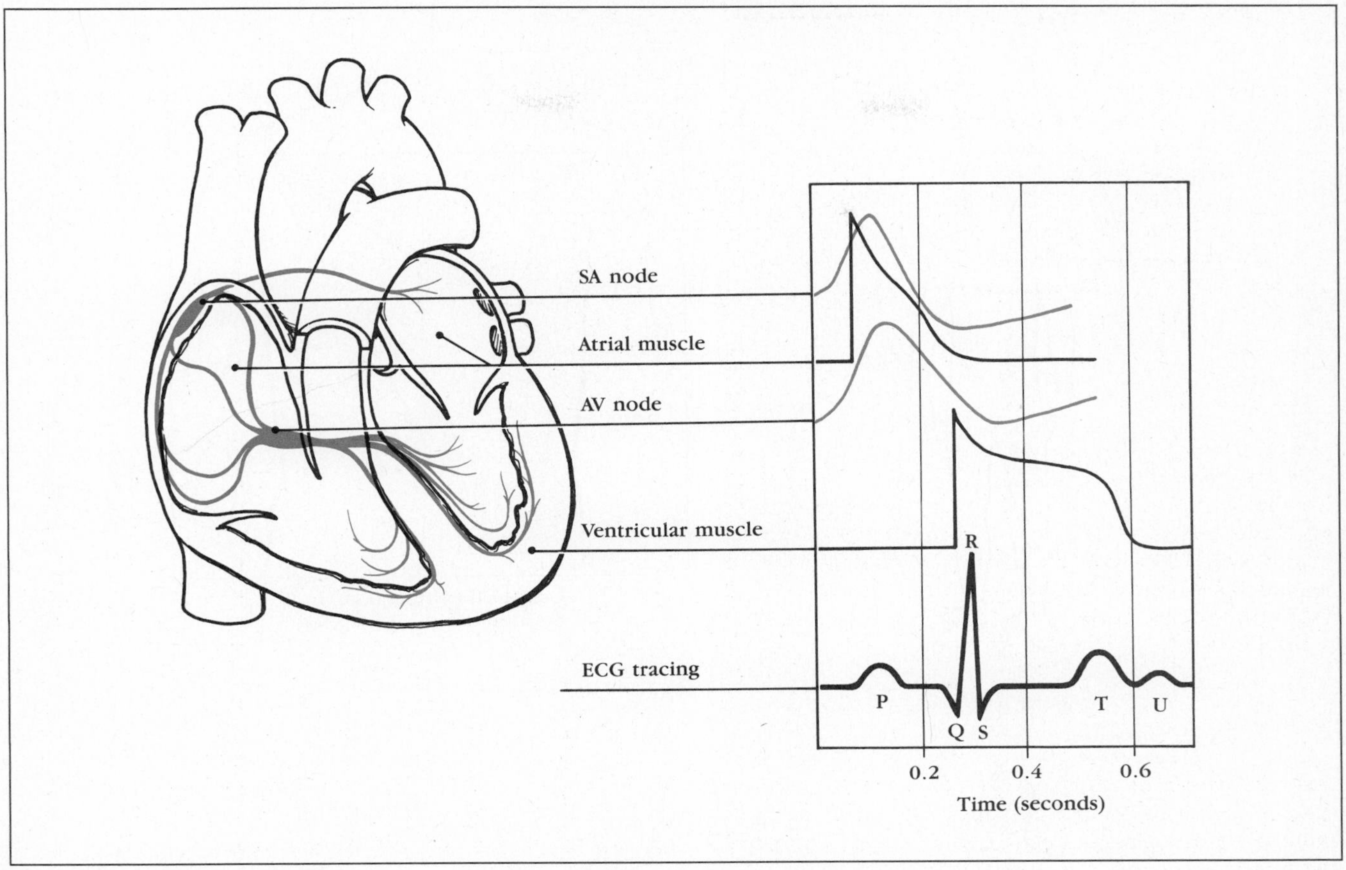

FIGURE 19-1 Action potentials.

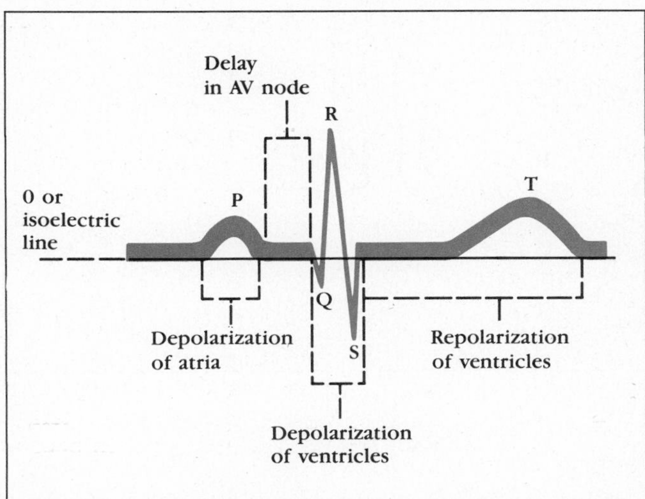

FIGURE 19-2 Correlation between the waves of the electrocardiogram and impulses that spread through the heart. (From J. Constant, *Learning Electrocardiography*. Boston: Little, Brown, 1973.)

defects, and it can detect the dysrhythmias associated with acute or chronic heart disease. Suspect cardiac rhythms must be evaluated in all 12 leads. An ectopic rhythm is not identified from a single monitoring lead unless the rhythm requires immediate intervention [21]. Figure 19-6 exemplifies the need to view a dysrhythmia in all 12 leads to identify it. In a single lead, this rhythm appears to be a bradycardia; however, on examination of all the leads, the undulating waves of atrial fibrillation can be seen (see pp. 294).

In the diagnosis of acute MI, the 12-lead ECG assesses anatomic areas or surfaces of the heart perfused by the right and left coronary arteries. Patterns reflecting ischemia, injury, and necrosis can be detected by examining these areas (Fig. 19-7). Leads II, III, and aV_F view the inferior and posterior portions of the myocardium normally perfused by the right coronary artery. Leads I and aV_L view the lateral portion of the left ventricle perfused by the left anterior descending artery. Leads V_1 through V_6 view the anterior septal, anterior, and anterolateral areas perfused by the left main and circumflex arteries. Loss of R wave progression is characteristic of infarction in these areas. In

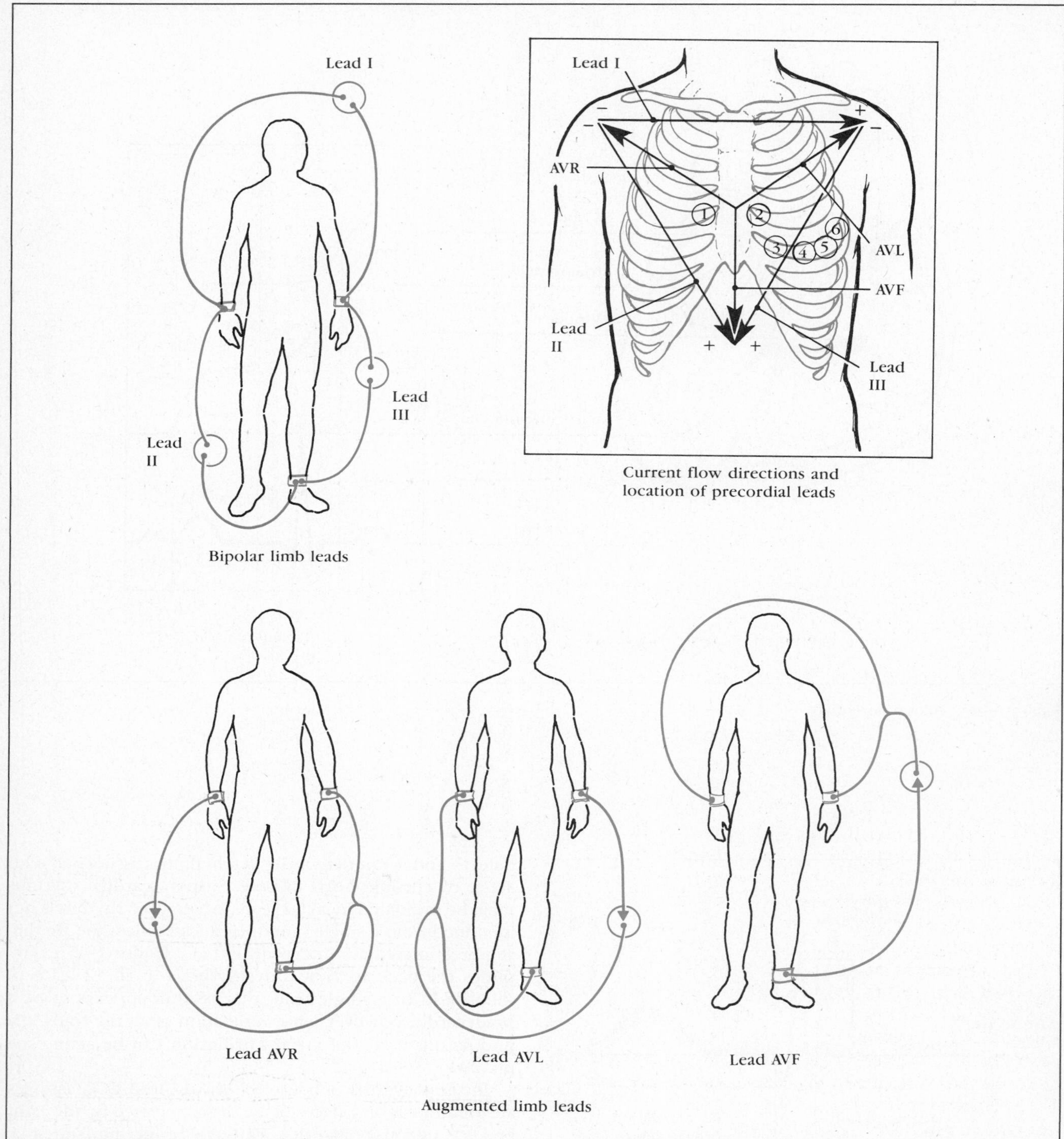

FIGURE 19-3 The ECG leads and 12-lead placement.

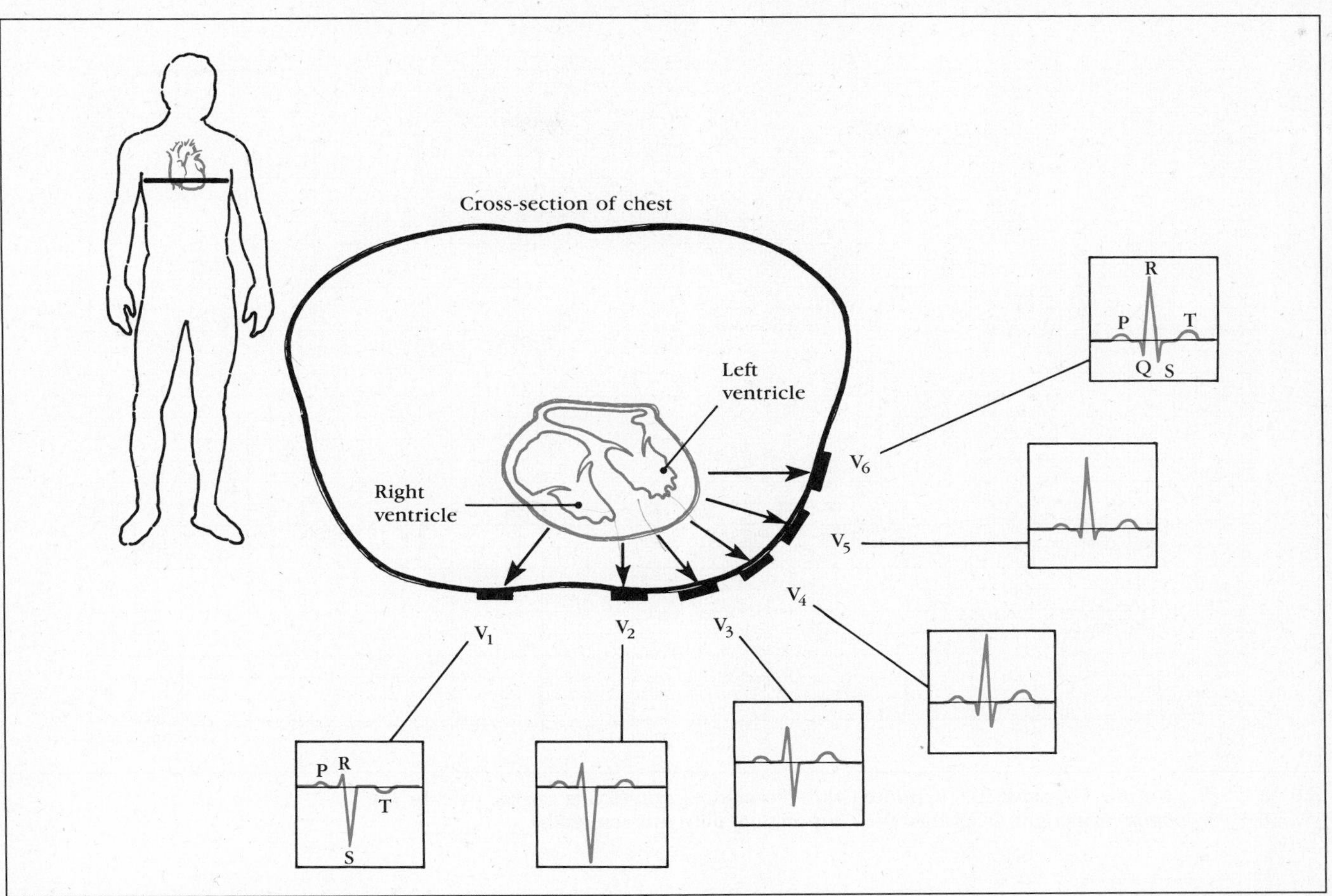

FIGURE 19-4 Appearance of QRS complexes in precordial leads of 12-lead ECG.

addition, the precordial leads may indicate posterior infarction by their ability to mirror electrical activity from the posterior surface of the left ventricle. In this mirror image, R waves are positively deflected with inverted ST segments. Figure 19-8 illustrates ECG changes indicative of inferior MI with a complicating third-degree block.

The movement of depolarization forces (a wave of impulses) through the myocardium is called a *vector*. The sum of these forces is the *electrical axis* [12]. The strength of contraction and the rate at which it occurs is determined by the density of the myocardial muscle mass. Thus, in the normal myocardium, the left ventricular forces dominate the right. Determining the electrical axis using the bipolar lead I and unipolar aV_F is important in the critical care setting to detect hemiblocks and to differentiate various types of ventricular dysrhythmias.

Normal Conduction

Chapter 18 details the normal cardiac anatomy, physiology, and electromechanical events. Normal cardiac rhythm is composed of many single cardiac events, each the result of an electrical impulse originating in the sinoatrial (SA) node. Figure 19-9 shows normal cardiac conduction and correlates these electrical events occurring in the myocardium to ECG representation.

From the SA node the impulse spreads to the atria through the intranodal pathways. Whether or not the Bachmann, Wenkebach, and Thorel tracts are conduction pathways between the sinus and atrioventricular (AV) nodes remains a source of controversy among researchers [1,4,8,25]. It is undisputed, however, that sinus impulses are conducted by specialized cells, resulting in atrial depo-

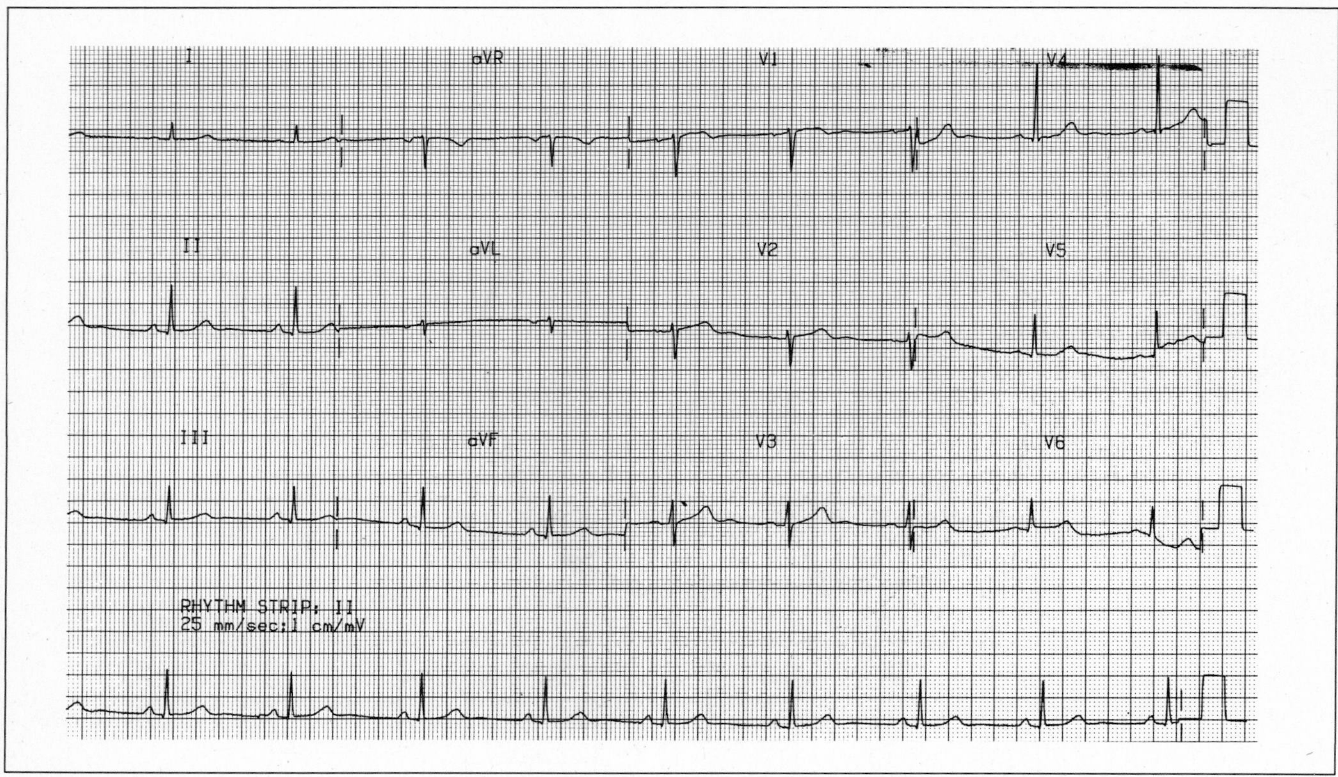

FIGURE 19-5 Normal 12-lead ECG. (Reprinted with permission from Giving cardiac care. In *The Nursing Photobook*. Copyright © Springhouse Corporation. All rights reserved.)

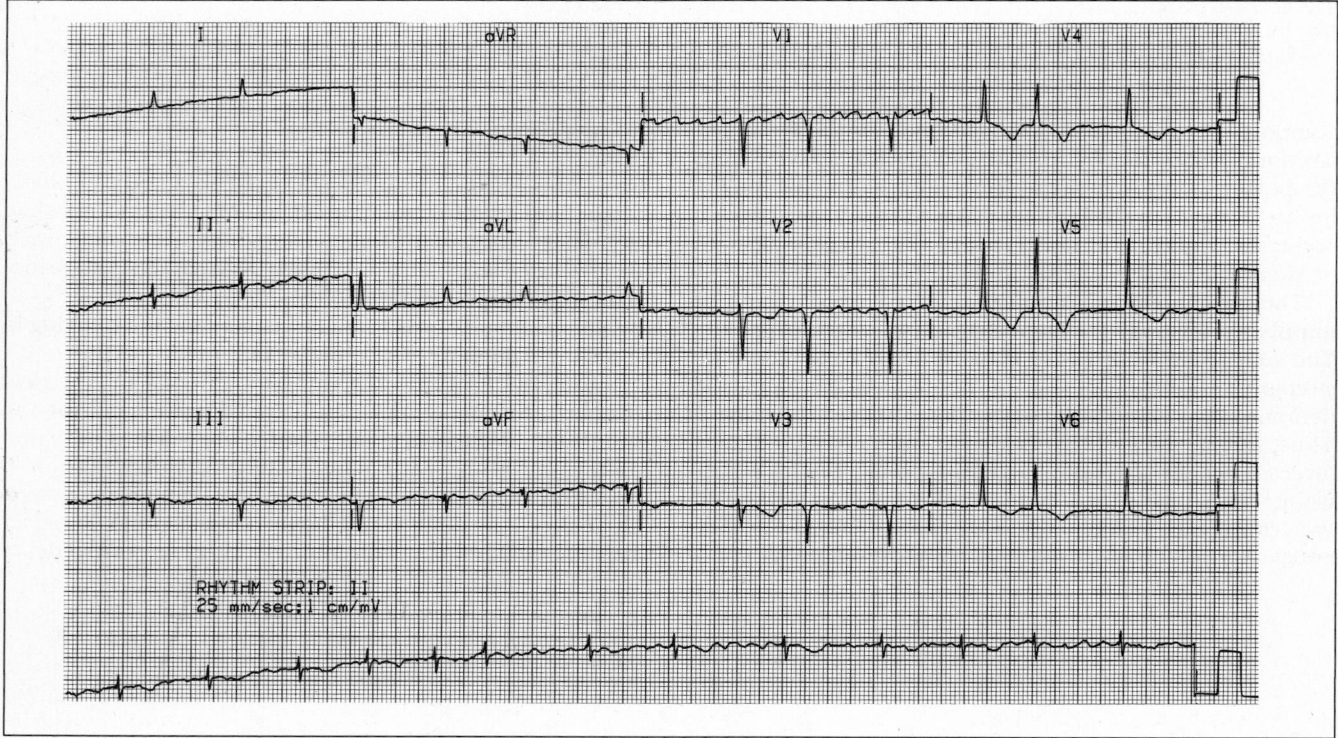

FIGURE 19-6 The 12-lead ECG used to detect dysrhythmias: atrial fibrillation.

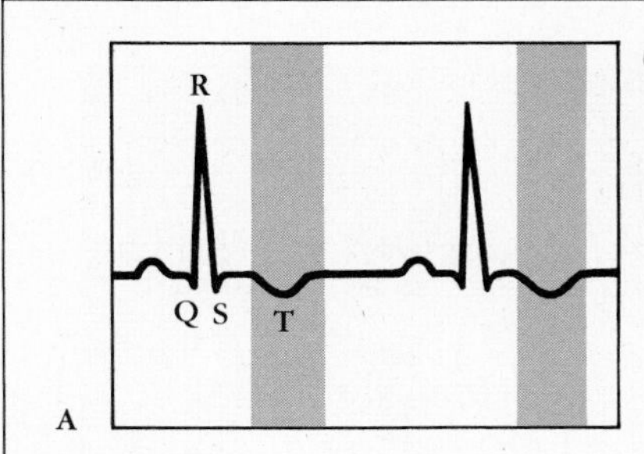

Ischemia causes inversion of T wave as a result of altered repolarization.

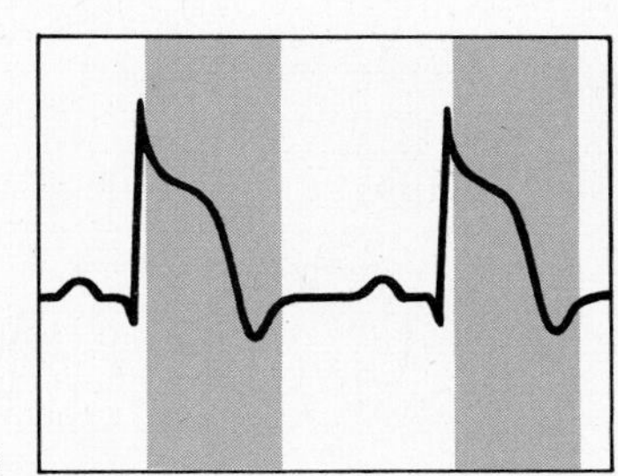

Injury to cardiac muscle causes elevation of S-T segment—"hyperacute S-T segment."

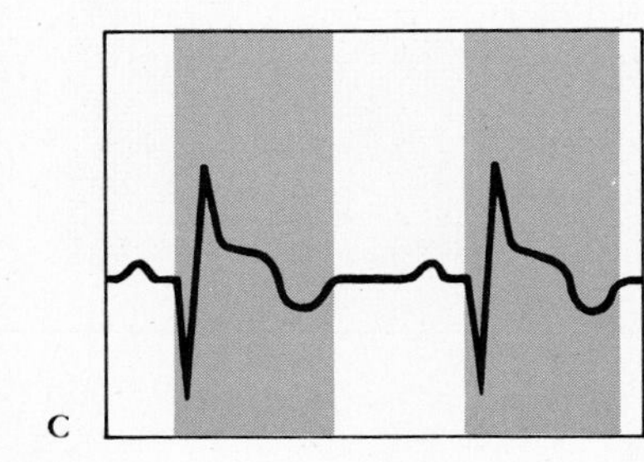

Necrosis (cardiac muscle death) causes deep Q wave as a result of scarring. Necrotic tissue does not conduct electrical impulses.

FIGURE 19-7 These ECG patterns reflect (A) ischemia, (B) injury, and (C) necrosis.

larization and contraction. The electrical event is reflected on the ECG as the P wave.

At the AV node, the impulse slows as it passes through the nodal fibers, thereby allowing the atria time to completely contract. This event constitutes the PR interval of the ECG complex. The impulse then flows through the bundle of His to the left and right bundle branches to reach the Purkinje fibers embedded in the ventricular muscle. Stimulation of the ventricles results in ventricular depolarization and contraction. The QRS complex represents this electrical event. Repolarization of the ventricles is reflected by the T wave.

These electromechanical events make up one cardiac cycle or one heartbeat. Sixty to 100 cardiac cycles per minute constitute a normal cardiac rate (Fig. 19-10). A series of normal regular cardiac electrical events is known as normal sinus rhythm.

Normal Hemodynamics

The electrical events of the heart precede the mechanical events. The mechanical events of the cardiac cycle, systole and diastole, are responsible for adequate perfusion and oxygenation of systemic organs and tissues. Normal cardiac output (4–8 L/min) is dependent upon stroke volume and heart rate (see Chap. 18). Any condition that alters these two components alters the steady state. Most of the dysrhythmias discussed in this chapter alter cardiac output and coronary perfusion either directly or potentially.

Cardiac Dysrhythmias

An alteration in the normal rhythm of the cardiac cycle is often called dysrhythmia, arrhythmia, or ectopic rhythm. The term most widely accepted is dysrhythmia. A dysrhythmia is defined as an abnormality of the formation or conduction of an electrical impulse that causes an alteration in heart rate or regularity [8,19]. A dysrhythmia occurs when pathologic mechanisms alter the normal action potential of the heart. The two primary mechanisms that initiate alterations in normal cardiac rhythm are *abnormal automaticity* and *reentry phenomena* [26].

Automaticity may be enhanced or depressed. In *enhanced automaticity*, the rate of pacemaker discharge is increased secondary to an accelerated rise of phase 4 (see p. 267). Conversely, *depressed automaticity* results from a slowing of the rise of phase 4. Factors influencing automaticity are listed in Table 19-1.

During conditions that enhance automaticity, a second action potential may be generated at the end of phase 2 or early in phase 3. If this after-potential is conducted, a premature beat ensues. The enhanced automaticity and secondary action potentials may trigger repetitive impulse conduction, producing *tachydysrhythmias*.

Reentry develops when an impulse has the ability to reexcite tissue that was previously depolarized by way of anatomic or functional circuits [12,26]. The rate of impulse conduction and the length of the refractory period influence the presence of reentry phenomena. As illustrated in Figure 19-11, when all criteria are present, single or multiple impulses may enter the circuit, generating ectopic beats or recurrent tachydysrhythmias. Continuous excitement of the myocardium by normal or anomalous paths is described as *circus movement* [27]. Sustained tachydysrhythmias are associated with the combination of reentry and circus movement. Electrophysiologic mapping techniques have provided much new insight into the mechanisms responsible for dysrhythmias seen clinically. The techniques remain imprecise, however, and the findings are controversial [8,11,14].

Alterations in cardiac rhythms can result from many etiologies (Table 19-2). The most common include disease or injury to the cardiac muscle, structures, or conduction system; systemic diseases; drug intoxication; electrolyte imbalances; and exercise [4]. Figure 19-12 exemplifies the effect of some drugs and electrolytes on the ECG.

Dysrhythmias are clinically significant as indicators of underlying heart disease or they may produce life-threatening electrical events with catastrophic hemodynamic results. Dysrhythmias may be present with or without clinical signs or symptoms and in individuals with

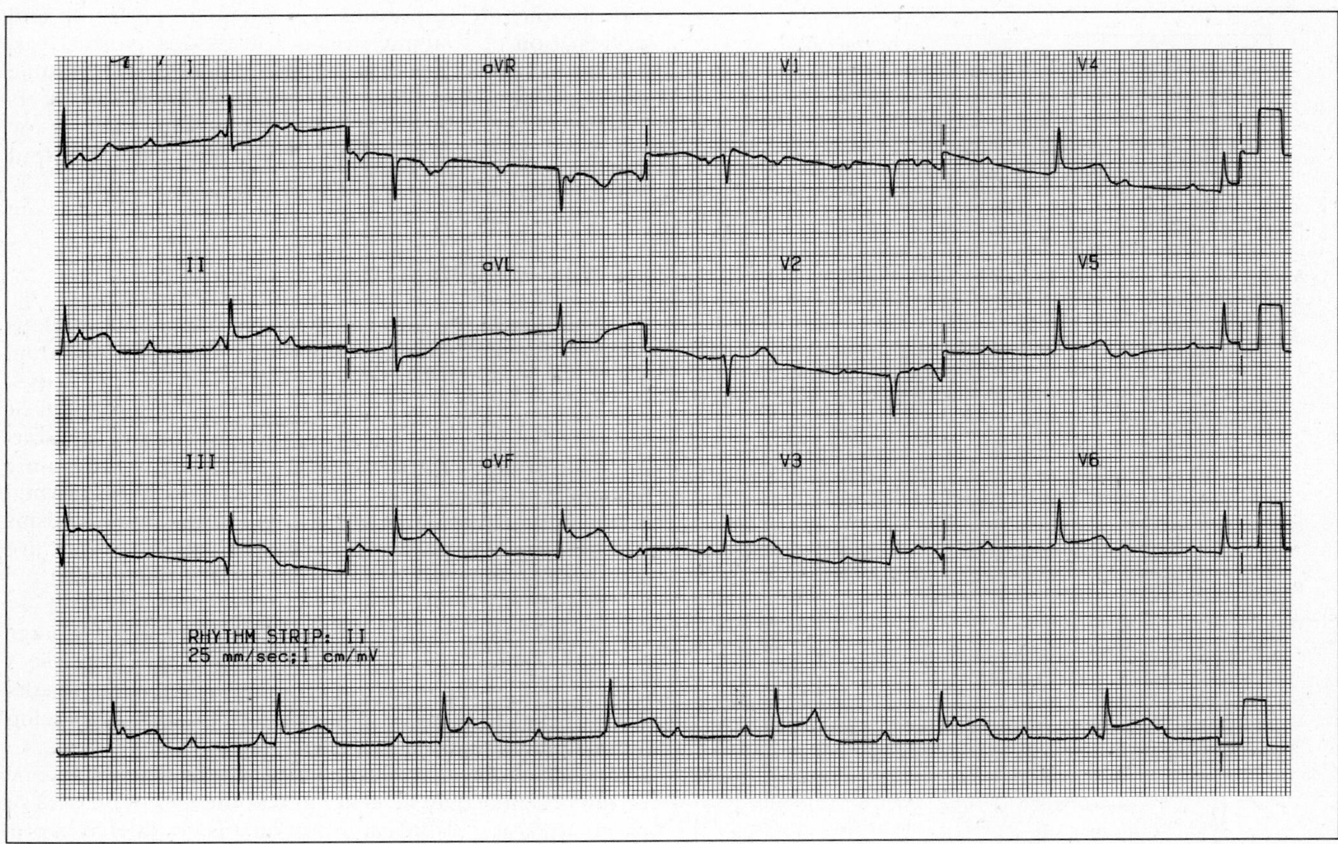

FIGURE 19-8 Inferior MI with third-degree AV block. Note elevated ST segments in Leads II, III, and aV_F. Some elevation of ST segments in V leads suggests possible septal injury.

TABLE 19-1 Factors That Enhance and Depress Automaticity

Enhancing Factors	Depressing Factors
Sympathetic nervous system stimulation	Parasympathetic nervous system stimulation
Fever	Vagotonia
Pain	Hyperkalemia
Anxiety	Drugs
High-output states	
Hyperthyroidism	
Anemia	
AV fistula	
Congestive heart failure	
Hypoxia	
High metabolic rates	
Toxic states	
Exercise	
Drugs	
Vagolytics (atropine)	
Sympathomimetics (epinephrine, norepinephrine)	
Catecholamines	
Hypokalemia	

TABLE 19-2 Etiologies of Dysrhythmias

Etiology	Examples
Underlying cardiac disease	Coronary artery disease
	Cardiomyopathies
	Valvular lesions
	Congenital defects
	Rheumatic heart disease
Acute myocardial infarction	
Systemic/metabolic diseases	Diabetes
	Hypertension
	Pulmonary disorders
	Hyperthyroidism
	Anemia
Electrolyte imbalance	
Anesthesia	
Drug intoxication	Digitalis
	Other prescription and illegal drugs
Central nervous system disorders	
Psychoneurogenic disorders	
Exercise	

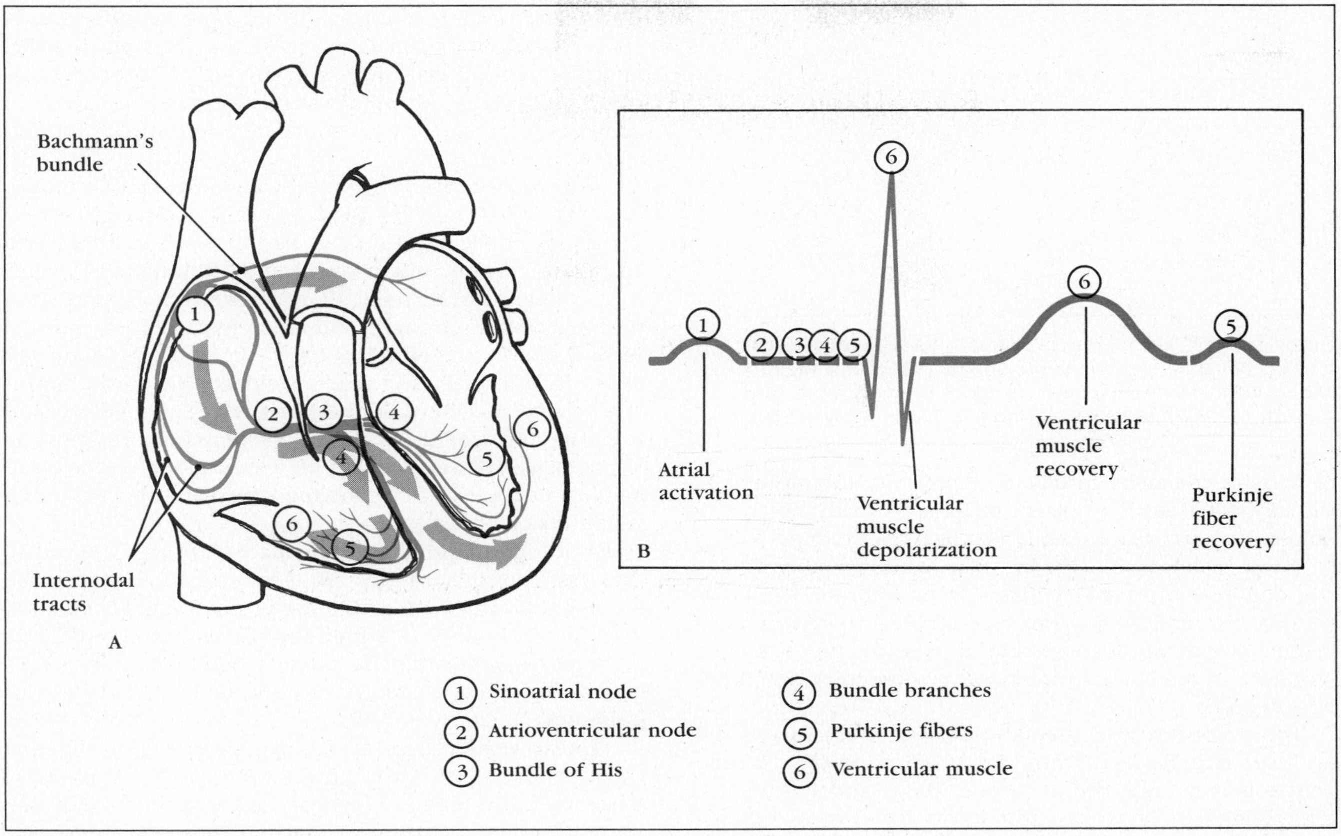

Bachmann's bundle

Internodal tracts

A

Atrial activation

Ventricular muscle depolarization

Ventricular muscle recovery

Purkinje fiber recovery

B

(1) Sinoatrial node
(2) Atrioventricular node
(3) Bundle of His
(4) Bundle branches
(5) Purkinje fibers
(6) Ventricular muscle

FIGURE 19-9 A. Normal cardiac conduction. B. Correlation of electrical events of the heart and ECG tracing.

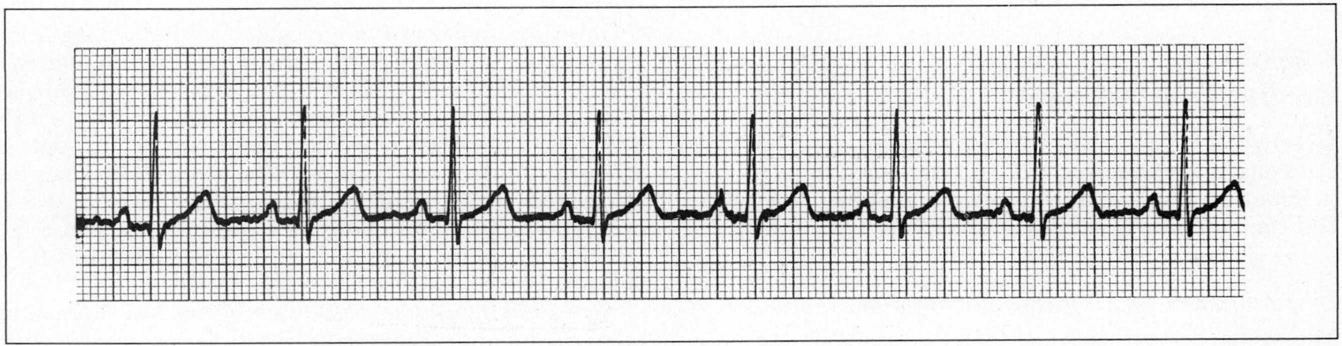

FIGURE 19-10 Normal sinus rhythm.

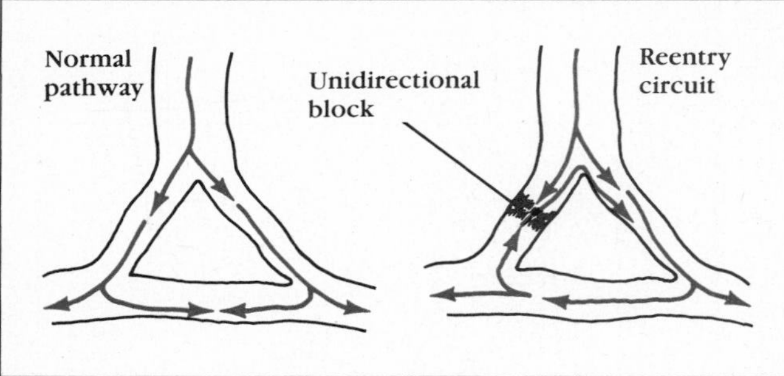

FIGURE 19-11 Mechanism of reentry. In the reentry circuit, a unidirectional block permits the impulse to reenter the tissue and set up a circus movement. (From B.H. Yee and S.L. Zorb, *Cardiac Critical Care Nursing*. Boston: Little, Brown, 1986.)

or without advanced cardiac disease. Clinical symptoms in the individual with a normal heart are usually not noted unless the heart rate exceeds 180 beats per minute (BPM) or slows to below 40 BPM [4]. Due to the inability of normal compensatory mechanisms to equilibrate, these extremely fast or slow rhythms can significantly reduce both cardiac output and systemic blood pressure, thus reducing perfusion of the brain, heart, kidneys, mesentery, and other vital centers.

The hemodynamic effects of dysrhythmias vary based on heart rate; heart rhythm; synchronization of atrial and ventricular events; the presence, stage, and etiology of underlying cardiac disease; the existence of drug toxicity; and state of vasomotor compensatory mechanisms [6,18].

Dysrhythmias in the pediatric population, while similar in appearance to adult dysrhythmias, differ in subcellular mechanisms, rates, and prognosis [9]. Discussion in this chapter is limited to adults.

Classification of Common Cardiac Dysrhythmias

Dysrhythmias are classified into three major groups according to their mechanisms and etiologies: disturbances in impulse formation, disturbances in impulse conduction, and combinations of the two [5,7,11,12].

Disturbances in Impulse Formation

The primary disturbances of impulse formation are sinoatrial, ectopic, and ventricular rhythms.

Sinoatrial Rhythms. Sinus bradycardia and sinus tachycardia are dysrhythmias associated with *abnormal rates*. The PR and QRS intervals are normal.

In sinus bradycardia the heart rate is less than 60 BPM and is a regular sinus rhythm (Fig. 19-13). Sinus bradycardia is usually not associated with pathologic findings unless it is a sequela of sick sinus syndrome. Usually it occurs as a normal compensatory mechanism to reduce cardiac output secondary to increased vagal stimulation. With automaticity in the SA node decreased, the heart rate slows. This rhythm is normal for the athletic individual at rest. If sinus bradycardia occurs after acute myocardial infarction, junctional or escape rhythms may be precipitated. Bradycardia is thought to be due to a vagal reflex, a chemoreflex triggered by chemical stimuli from the left ventricular wall [23].

Sinus tachycardia (ST) occurs when the heart rate is in the range of 100 to 150 BPM. There is no change in QRS waveform or PR interval (Fig. 19-14). With the increased rate there may be a slight variation in RR interval. This feature is helpful in distinguishing between atrial and sinus tachycardias at fast rates. Sinus tachycardia is a normal response to increased stress on the body. Such conditions as fever, exercise, and fear stimulate the normal sinus mechanism and increase the heart rate. Sinus tachycardia is commonly seen as a normal compensatory response in hypotensive states requiring increased tissue perfusion. It may also develop after drinking caffeinated beverages or using tobacco products.

Pathology in sinus tachycardia is rare and limited to that associated with sick sinus syndrome. Because the accelerated firing of the SA node is due to enhanced automaticity secondary to stimulation from the sympathetic nervous system, it may be an early occurrence with congestive heart failure (CHF), myocardial infarction (MI), or pulmonary infarct (PI) [25].

Clinical significance of ST is dependent upon whether or not there is an underlying disease process. Elevated heart rates can increase myocardial oxygen demand, thus increasing any existing myocardial ischemia. Increased heart rate in the presence of myocardial ischemia may also lead to increased ventricular irritability and trigger ventricular tachycardia.

Sinoatrial rhythms with *irregular impulse* formation include sinus dysrhythmia and sick sinus (tachy-brady) syndrome.

Sinus dysrhythmia is an irregular rhythm arising from the SA node. Commonly called the respiratory rhythm, the cycles vary with respiratory rate, increasing with inhalation and decreasing with exhalation (Fig. 19-15) [6,24]. The PQRS complexes and intervals remain normal unless altered by other mechanisms. The irregularity can be attributed to factors that enhance vagal tone, and the dysrhythmia becomes clinically significant when the RR intervals are slow enough to allow atrial, junctional, or ventricular ectopic beats to escape.

Sick sinus syndrome (SSS) is a syndrome of alternating tachycardic and bradycardic rhythms associated with cerebral hypoperfusion and syncopal episodes [24]. It is one of the most common causes of hypoperfusion and is usually treated with pacemaker insertion. Pathology may be linked to (1) dysfunction of the SA node secondary to inflammatory, collagen, or metastatic diseases; (2) influence of the autonomic nervous system, such as abnormal vagotonia; (3) effect of drugs, such as beta blockers and antihypertensives; or (4) surgical injury [5,24].

The tachycardia associated with this syndrome may be a supraventricular (SVT) escape mechanism rather than one arising from the SA node [5,13]. The escape mechanism is triggered by the bradycardic rate as a compensa-

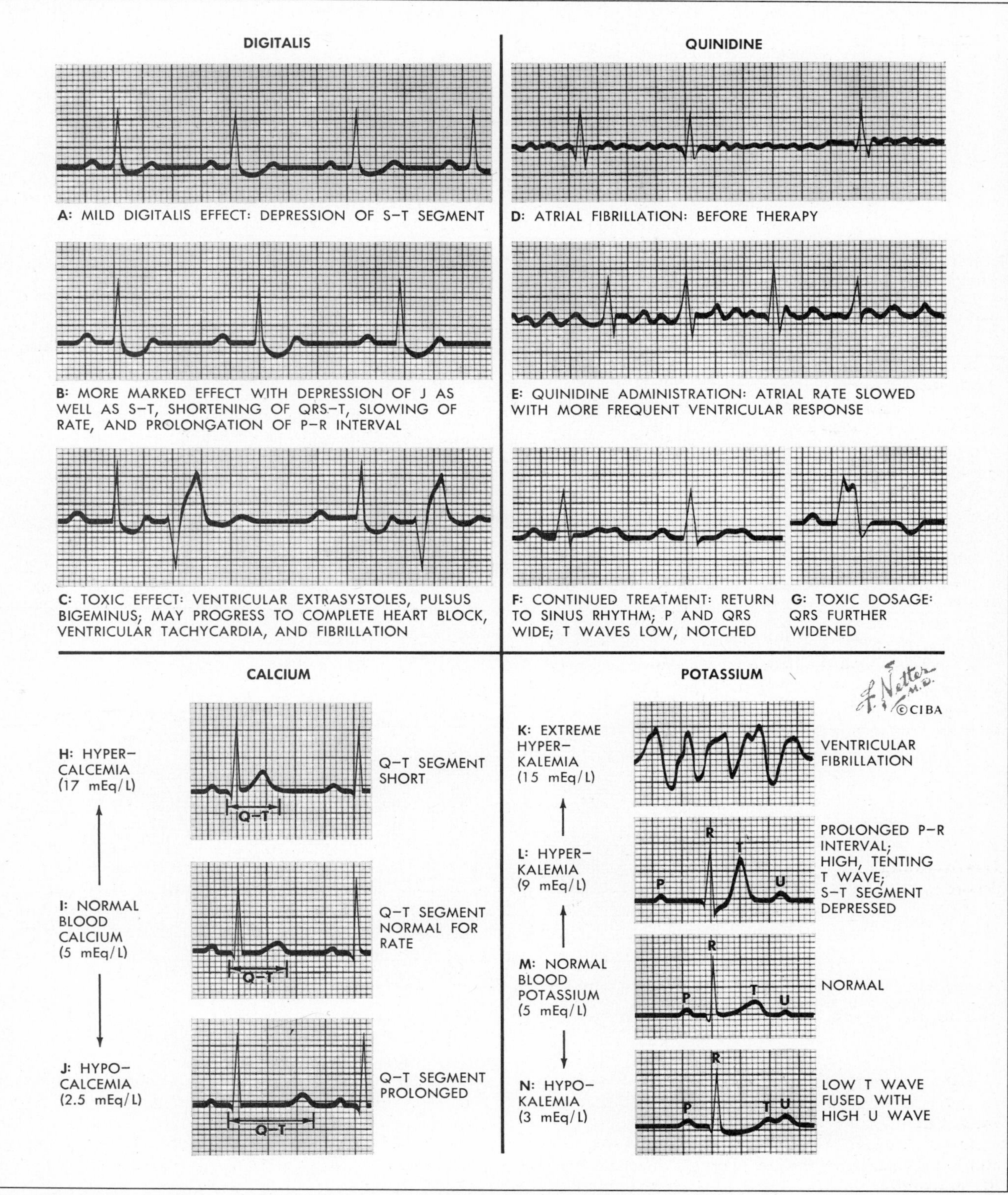

FIGURE 19-12 Effects of drugs and electrolytes on the electrocardiogram. (© Copyright 1969, CIBA Pharmaceutical Company, division of CIBA-GEIGY Corporation. Reprinted with permission from *The CIBA Collection of Medical Illustrations*, illustrated by Frank H. Netter, M.D. All rights reserved.)

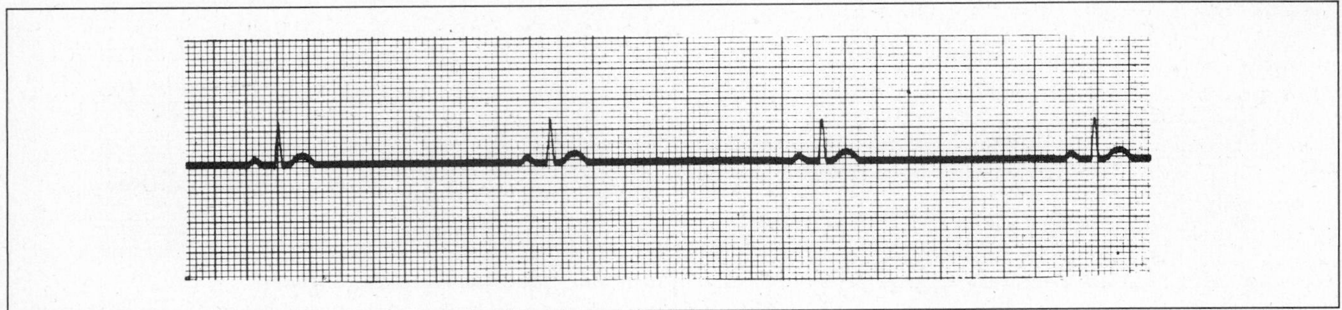

FIGURE 19-13 Sinus bradycardia. (From B.H. Yee and S.L. Zorb, *Cardiac Critical Care Nursing*. Boston: Little, Brown, 1986.)

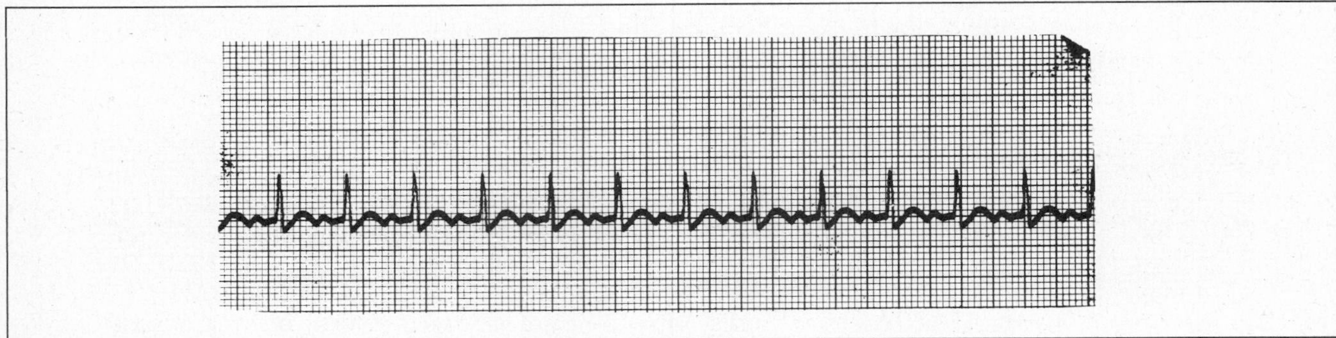

FIGURE 19-14 Sinus tachycardia. (From B.H. Yee and S.L. Zorb, *Cardiac Critical Care Nursing*. Boston: Little, Brown, 1986.)

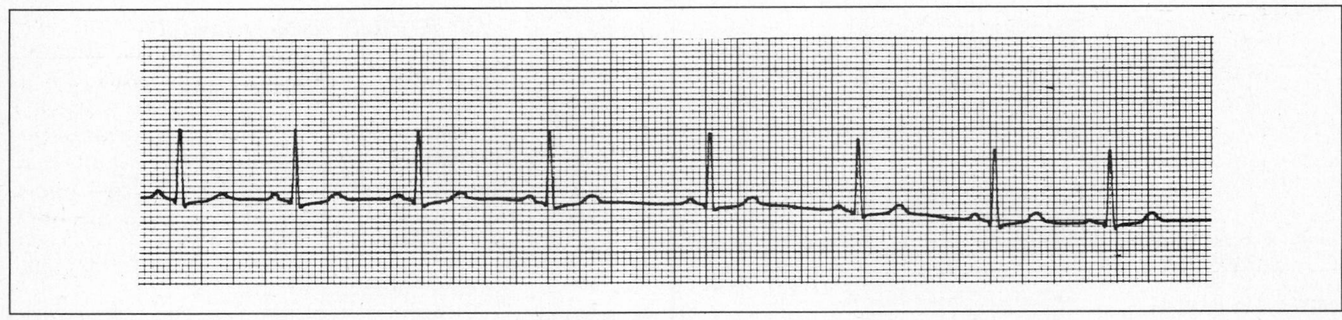

FIGURE 19-15 Sinus dysrhythmia. (From B.H. Yee and S.L. Zorb, *Cardiac Critical Care Nursing*. Boston: Little, Brown, 1986.)

tory mechanism. Without this escape mechanism, profound bradycardia and cerebral hypoperfusion occur. The fast and slow rhythms may alternate with palpitations and symptoms of extreme tachycardia, and with a slow rate and inadequate perfusion.

Sinus arrest is a rhythm produced by a marked depression of sinus node activity secondary to coronary artery disease, acute infectious processes, enhanced carotid sinus and vagal tone, and the toxic effects of digitalis, quinidine, and salicylates [24]. Sinus arrest is notable for long pauses in cardiac rhythm and absent P waves (Fig. 19-16). The rate and PQRST complexes of the underlying rhythm are normal unless altered by other mechanisms. The pauses generated by failure of the SA node to fire produces an irregularity in the underlying rhythm. This dysrhythmia is clinically insignificant unless SA node depression is prolonged and atrial standstill results. The AV node may assume the pacemaking function, or an escape rhythm may surface to maintain the ventricular rate.

Ectopic Rhythms. Ectopic rhythms are those that originate outside the SA node. Usually these arise due to the inability of the primary pacemaker (SA node) to generate an electrical impulse. Thus, automatic cells within the atria or one of the latent pacemakers (the AV node or ventricles) initiate impulses to stimulate the myocardium to sustain the ventricular rate [24]. The dysrhythmias in this category are atrial rhythms, junctional escape rhythms, and ventricular rhythms.

Atrial rhythms. The primary ectopic beats that originate from the atria are *premature atrial contractions (PACs)*. These impulses result from enhanced automaticity and arise secondary to emotional distress, use of tobacco and caffeine, electrolyte imbalance, atrial hypertrophy, hypoxia, digitalis toxicity, and chronic lung disease [4,6,12].

The PACs appear on the ECG as premature beats that interrupt the underlying cardiac rhythm (Fig. 19-17). They may appear alone or alternate with the intrinsic rhythm. The shape of the P wave of the PAC appears different from the sinus P wave and varies depending upon the origin of the ectopic focus in the atria. Occasionally, the PAC arises so soon after the sinus beat that it is nonconducted, producing a blocked PAC. The PR interval and QRS complex of the PAC is usually normal unless affected by other mechanisms that alter conduction through the AV junction and the ventricles. A pause follows the PAC due to the early depolarization of the atria and the resetting of the SA node [4,12].

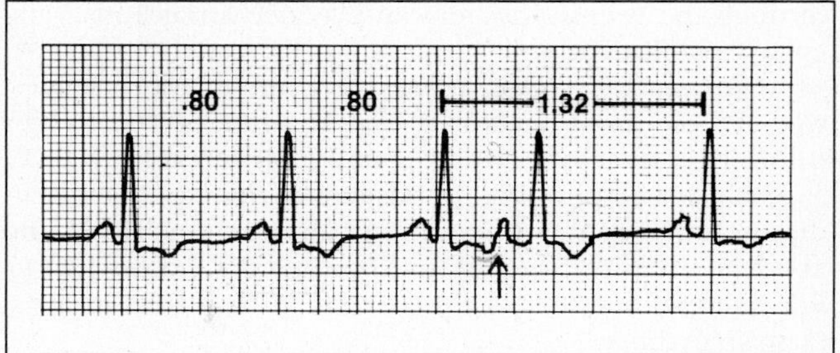

FIGURE 19-17 Premature atrial complexes. Multiple PACs are present, resulting in irregular rhythm. (Reproduced with permission from *Textbook of Advanced Cardiac Life Support*. © American Heart Association.)

An individual who has a normal heart may experience PACs. Frequent PACs may produce palpitations and discomfort, but they are otherwise clinically insignificant. In the presence of a diseased myocardium, PACs may precipitate atrial tachycardia, atrial flutter, and atrial fibrillation. Both PACs and subsequent atrial dysrhythmias are dangerous to the individual with an acute MI. A decrease in cardiac output may further decrease myocardial perfusion and increase ventricular irritability. In the acute MI period, PACs may also indicate impending CHF or electrolyte imbalance.

Premature atrial contractions can occur at a critical time, the so-called *critical coupling interval*, and can establish a reentry circuit, thus producing atrial tachycardia [23].

Reentry from the premature atrial beat through the AV node back to the atria has been projected as the most common cause of PACs. Other reentry circuits may include the SA node, the atria, or accessory bypass tracts. The wave of depolarization proceeds through the fiber with slowed conduction; then it returns to a nearby fiber, causing reexcitation [23]. Increased rapidity of firing

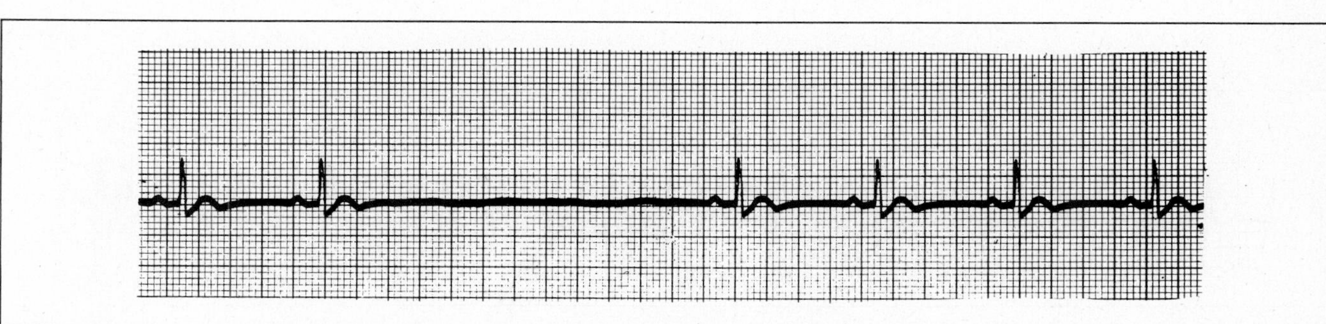

FIGURE 19-16 Sinus arrest. (From B.H. Yee and S.L. Zorb, *Cardiac Critical Care Nursing*. Boston: Little, Brown, 1986.)

through the reentry circuit can produce atrial flutter and even atrial fibrillation.

Atrial tachycardia is defined as three or more successive ectopic atrial beats in a row at a rate of 160 to 250 BPM. This dysrhythmia is usually initiated by a PAC. Mechanisms responsible for sustaining the atrial tachycardia include reentry phenomena already described and abnormal impulses generated by digitalis excess [3,11]. Repeated stimulation of this reentry path results in atrial tachyarrhythmia.

Onset of tachyarrhythmia may be abrupt, thus the term *paroxysmal atrial tachycardia (PAT)*. The condition may be transient or chronic. Termination is often spontaneous or in response to vagal stimulation (Valsalva maneuver, carotid sinus stimulation, gag reflex, etc.).

Factors contributing to development of atrial tachycardias include hypoxia, alkalosis, increased catecholamine levels, hypokalemia, recent myocardial infarction, cardiomyopathy, atrial septal defects, hypertension, atrial dilatation, and acute alcohol ingestion [6,23]. The PAT often occurs in individuals with no known cardiac disease and in those under emotional duress. Rheumatic heart disease, mitral valve disease, pericarditis, coronary artery disease, and thyrotoxicosis are less common causes. Wolff-Parkinson-White syndrome often manifests episodes of PAT (see p. 302).

Atrial tachycardia presents on the ECG as a continuous run of PACs (Fig. 19-18). The P wave configuration differs from the sinus P due to its ectopic atrial origin. The PR intervals may vary depending upon atrial rate and degree of AV block. The QRS and T waves are normal. Persistently rapid ventricular rates or the preexistence of a bundle branch block (see pp. 300–301) may cause the QRS complex to take on an aberrant configuration.

At rapid rates it is often difficult to distinguish between PAT and junctional tachycardia due to the merging of the P wave with the T wave of the previous beat. In these circumstances the rhythm is often identified as a supraventricular tachycardia (SVT, or PSVT if paroxysmal).

Atrial tachycardias have clinical significance for both diseased and healthy hearts. Symptoms associated with these dysrhythmias (weakness, palpitations, diaphoresis, shortness of breath, and hypotension) are related to the fall in cardiac output secondary to rapid ventricular rates. Therefore, the major factors to be considered are the duration of the dysrhythmia and the existence of cardiac disease. Atrial tachycardia in the presence of a diseased myocardium precipitates congestive heart failure and coronary insufficiency. It has been noted that congestive heart failure can also develop in the nondiseased myocardium undergoing long-term, rapid atrial tachycardia [12].

The focus or foci for *atrial flutter* may originate anywhere within the atria. It occurs most commonly in individuals over age 40 years who have underlying cardiac disease, especially infective endocarditis, coronary artery disease, and mitral stenosis. It also may occur after cardiac surgery and with digitalis toxicity.

The mechanisms most often attributed to atrial flutter are (1) enhanced automaticity of an ectopic focus and (2) circus movement through the atria [3,12,22]. These mechanisms activate rapid depolarization and contraction of the atria. This is noted on the ECG as a characteristic sawtooth pattern (Fig. 19-19). Atrial rates range from 250 to 350 BPM with ventricular rates 125 to 175, depending upon the efficiency of conduction through the AV node. The ratio of atrial to ventricular conduction is usually 2:1 to 4:1 [11]. The QRS complexes usually remain normal. Atrial flutter may progress to atrial fibrillation or it may respond to vagal stimulation or electric countershock.

Clinical significance of atrial flutter is dependent upon the cardiac rate and degree of underlying heart disease. Ventricular rates of 100 or less are usually asymptomatic. Higher rates may reduce coronary perfusion in individuals with ischemic heart disease.

Atrial fibrillation (AF) is commonly associated with numerous disease processes that enhance automaticity or increase atrial size, such as rheumatic heart disease, pericarditis, hyperthyroidism, coronary artery disease, hypertension, chronic obstructive pulmonary disease, and digitalis toxicity [19,23]. It is the most common atrial dysrhythmia in the elderly population.

Atrial fibrillation is an irregular rhythm that can be established or paroxysmal. In the latter case attacks may last from hours to days. Paroxysmal attacks of AF may spontaneously convert to sinus rhythm or may do so with electric cardioversion. The acute attack may continue and become established as chronic atrial fibrillation. The degree of hemodynamic disruption depends upon the underlying heart disease, the cardiac rate, and whether or not congestive heart failure ensues.

Atrial fibrillation can be identified on the ECG monitor as an irregularly irregular ventricular rhythm with chaotic

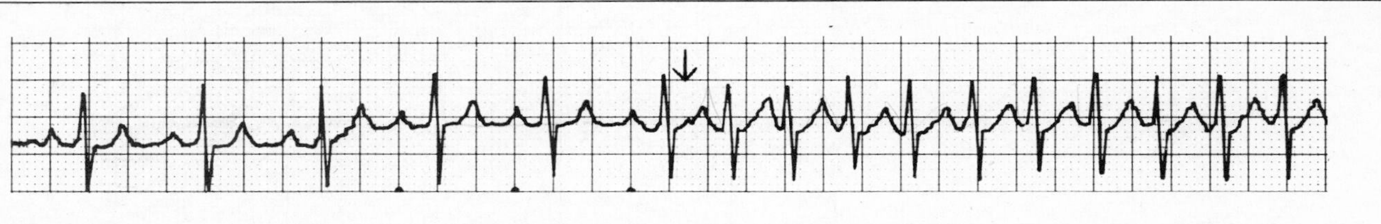

FIGURE 19-18 Atrial tachycardia beginning with normal sinus rhythm. A PAC initiates an episode of atrial tachycardia with a rate of 185 beats per minute. (Reproduced with permission from *Textbook of Advanced Cardiac Life Support*. © American Heart Association.)

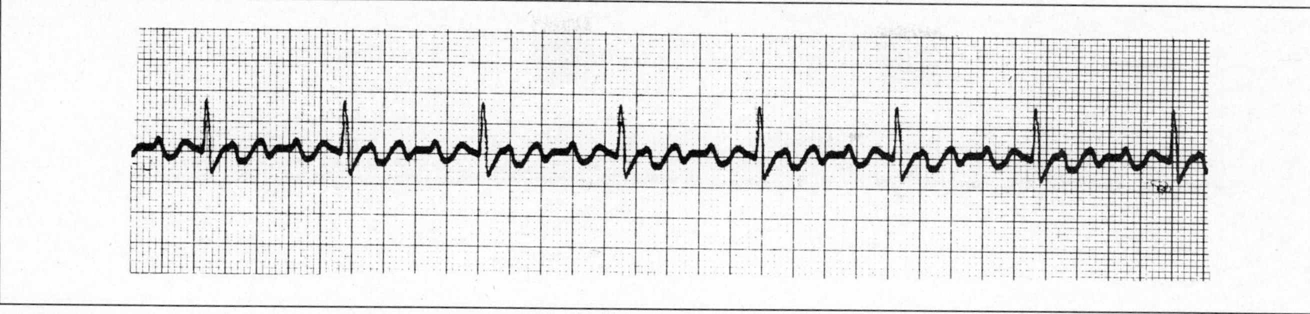

FIGURE 19-19 Atrial flutter. (From B.H. Yee and S.L. Zorb, *Cardiac Critical Care Nursing*. Boston: Little, Brown, 1986.)

atrial fibrillatory waves (Fig. 19-20). Atrial rate usually exceeds 350 BPM, with ventricular rates between 50 and 200 BPM, depending on the degree of AV conduction. Elevated ventricular rates almost invariably occur unless the rhythm is treated with a digitalis preparation. The pulse manifests as an irregular rhythm with the apical rate being faster than the radial pulse. This *pulse deficit* is produced because the more rapid beats may not lead to a stroke volume sufficient to cause a perceptible pulse [23]. With very rapid rates the apical rate may be much higher than the radial rate. Because of the irregularity of the beat, it may become difficult to distinguish S1 and S2 heart sounds, so that ascertaining the apical beat is difficult.

Pulmonary or arterial embolization occurs in 30 to 40 percent of individuals with atrial fibrillation [3]. Emboli result from thrombus formation in the atria that loosen and travel in the arterial circuit. The atrial appendages often contain thrombus formation or the entire atrial chambers may become filled with thrombi, a condition occurring especially in rheumatic mitral stenosis (see Chap. 21).

Escape Rhythms. Escape rhythms arise from the AV junction and act as secondary pacemakers when the SA node fails. They include premature junctional contractions, junctional (nodal) rhythm, junctional tachycardia, and supraventricular tachycardia.

Premature junctional contractions (PJCs) occur less commonly than their atrial and ventricular cousins. They originate as either premature or escape beats emitting from the bundle of His. The mechanisms involved include enhanced automaticity of the junctional sites and an AV nodal reentry phenomena as a result of digitalis toxicity, acute inferior MI, rheumatic fever, or profound slowing of the cardiac cycle [4,6].

As with PACs, PJCs occur earlier in the cardiac cycle than the sinus beat. The atrial impulse is conducted in a retrograde fashion, producing an inverted P wave in lead II that may precede, follow, or be buried in a normal QRS complex (Fig. 19-21). The PR interval may vary depending on the location of the focus and the rate of conduction. A PJC may be followed by a partial or full compensatory pause.

Junctional rhythm is considered to be a physiologically passive rhythm occurring when a sinus impulse fails to be generated or conducted. The impulse arises in the atrial-nodal junction or the nodal-His bundle junction [23]. The rhythm then becomes the pacemaker of the heart and controls ventricular activity.

Junctional rhythm may be attributed to the presence of SA node disease or trauma, enhanced vagotonia, digitalis toxicity, hyperkalemia, acute MI, or the presence of sinus block, sinus arrest, sinus bradycardia, and second- and third-degree heart block [6].

The ECG characteristics include a rate of 40 to 60 BPM, abnormal or absent P waves, and variable PR intervals with normal QRS complexes (Fig. 19-22). Hemodynamic effects depend on the underlying cause and duration of this rhythm, the ventricular rate, and the presence of car-

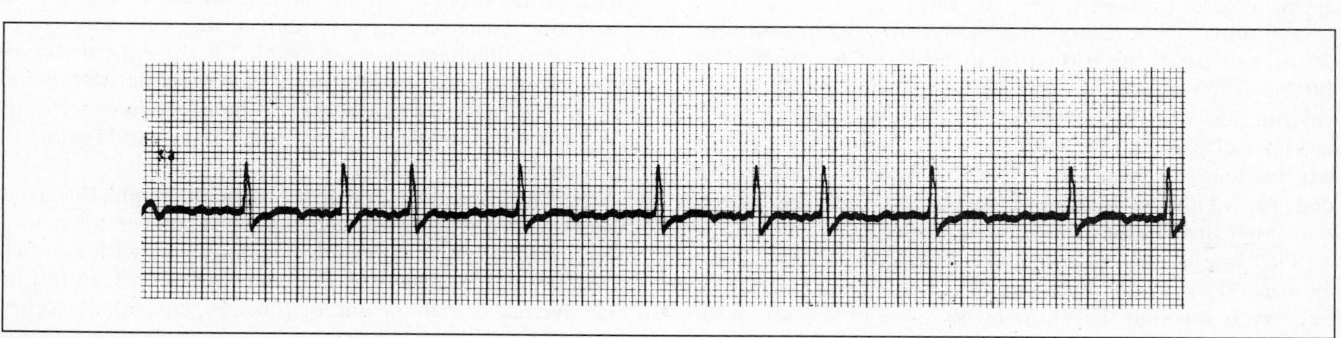

FIGURE 19-20 Atrial fibrillation. (From B.H. Yee and S.L. Zorb, *Cardiac Critical Care Nursing*. Boston: Little, Brown, 1986.)

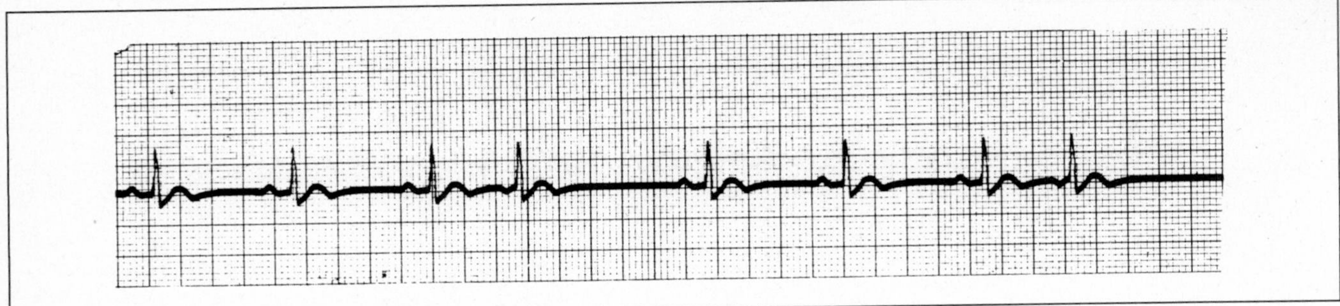

FIGURE 19-21 Premature junctional contraction. (From B.H. Yee and S.L. Zorb, *Cardiac Critical Care Nursing*. Boston: Little, Brown, 1986.)

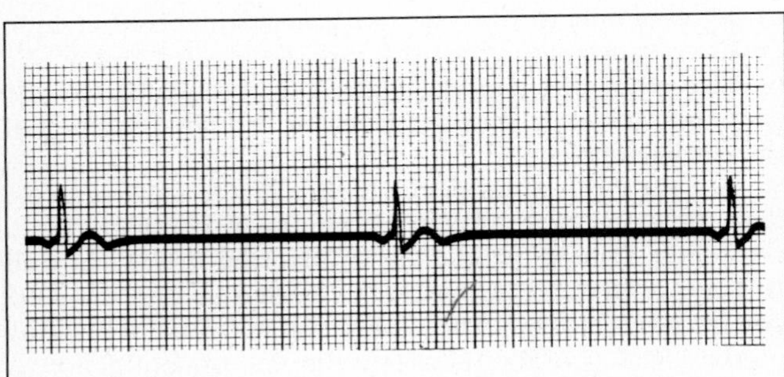

FIGURE 19-22 Junctional rhythm. (From B.H. Yee and S.L. Zorb, *Cardiac Critical Care Nursing*. Boston: Little, Brown, 1986.)

diac disease. Junctional rhythm predisposes those with a diseased myocardium to myocardial ischemia, intractable congestive heart failure, and Stokes-Adams attacks [4].

Junctional tachycardia, by definition, may begin in any site within AV junctional tissue and is stimulated by an ectopic focus. It appears on the ECG as a series of PJCs. Junctional tachycardia, may be paroxysmal or nonparoxysmal, depending on onset, rate, and clinical significance [4].

Paroxysmal junctional tachycardia usually occurs in the individual with a nondiseased myocardium. It is initiated by a premature junctional ectopic focus. The rate ranges between 160 and 250 BPM. The individual may describe palpitations, dizziness, or weakness, or may be asymptomatic even with very fast rates.

Nonparoxysmal junctional tachycardia causes rates of 60 to 150 BPM. Junctional tachycardia of less than 100 BPM is often termed *accelerated junctional* or idionodal rhythm. Most of these tachycardias result from increased automaticity of the junctional tissues, which may result from released metabolites from ischemic and hypoxic cells [23]. This dysrhythmia is therefore closely associated with myocardial disease.

Paroxysmal supraventricular tachycardia (PSVT) can be caused by an AV nodal reentry mechanism [12]. Here, reentry is through the alpha (slow) and beta (fast) pathways within the AV node. The impulse is conducted first down the alpha paths to the ventricles and returns up the beta paths to the atria. The impulse reactivates the ectopic focus and the process repeats until it is therapeutically interrupted or spontaneous cessation occurs. As discussed on page 294, it is difficult to differentiate atrial and supraventricular tachycardia due to the distortion caused by rapid rates. Usually PSVT ranges between 170 and 250 BPM, the P waves are indistinguishable, and the QRS is normal unless altered by conduction defects in the bundle branches. The PSVT can be initiated by any of the ectopic foci. In the presence of acute myocardial infarction, the resultant decrease in cardiac output and increased myocardial energy consumption exacerbates further ischemic episodes.

Ventricular Rhythms. Ventricular dysrhythmias arise from ectopic foci within the ventricles. The main dysrhythmias are premature ventricular contractions, idioventricular rhythms, ventricular tachycardia, and ventricular fibrillation.

Premature ventricular contractions (PVCs) originate from single or multiple foci below the level of the bundle of His [4]. These premature depolarizations interrupt the underlying cardiac rhythm. The hallmark of the PVC is a wide (greater than 0.12 second), irregular QRS complex with no associated P wave. The T wave is directed in opposition to the T wave of the sinus beat, with a full compensatory pause afterward (Fig. 19-23). The PVCs may occur singly, in multiples, or in regularly occurring combination with the underlying rhythm, such as ventricular bigeminy or trigeminy. All PVCs of six or more per minute, paired (coupled) or multifocal, must be treated if there is underlying cardiac disease. This dysrhythmia is frequently a precursor of the lethal dysrhythmia of ventricular tachycardia, ventricular fibrillation, and sudden death syndrome.

The two mechanisms responsible for the appearance of PVCs are *enhanced automaticity* of ventricular tissue and *reentry*. The reentry phenomenon involves microcircuits in the His-Purkinje tissue or macrocircuits in the bundle of His branch fibers [15,20].

The PVCs are detected in both healthy and diseased hearts. Premature ventricular ectopy is seldom seen in a young person but occurrence does increase with age [4]. In healthy individuals, ventricular ectopy is attributed to excessive use of caffeine and/or tobacco, emotional excitement, and exercise. The effects of catecholamines, drugs (e.g., isoproterenol, aminophyllin), digoxin toxicity, elec-

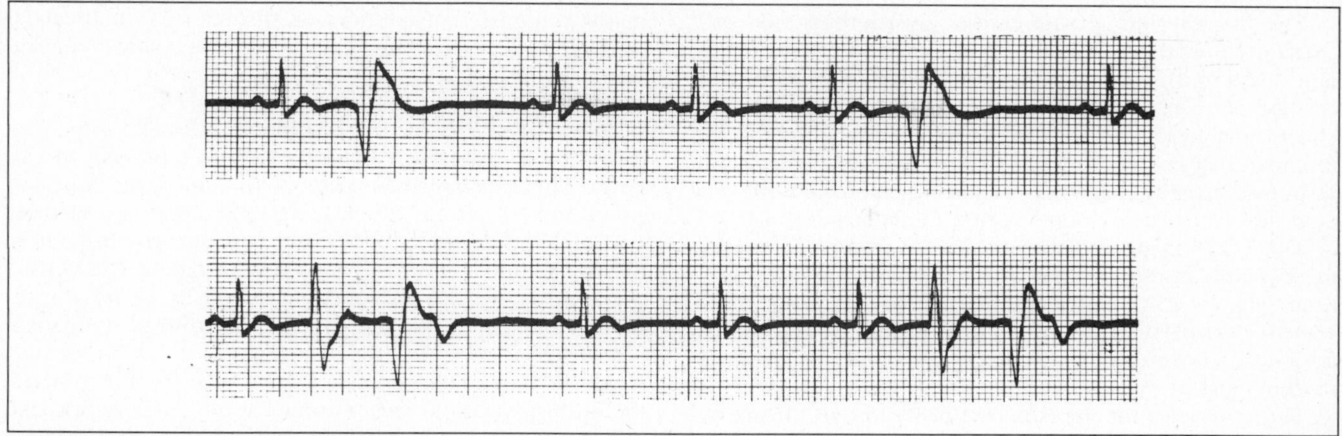

FIGURE 19-23 Premature ventricular contractions, multifocal couplet. (From B.H. Yee and S.L. Zorb, *Cardiac Critical Care Nursing*. Boston: Little, Brown, 1986.)

trolyte imbalances (hypokalemia, hypomagnesemia), hypoxia, myocardial ischemia, mitral valve prolapse, advanced anemia, and myocardial hypertrophy or aneurysm can produce PVCs in the diseased heart [22,23]. In myocardial ischemia, the ventricular myocardium is irritable due to the hypoxia and acidosis associated with decreased coronary artery perfusion. Thus, PVCs are the most common dysrhythmia associated with acute MI.

The hemodynamic effects of PVCs are usually transient and clinically insignificant. The PVCs are associated with shortened left ventricular filling time, decreased stroke volume, and decreased contractility, thereby reducing cardiac output with each abnormal beat [18]. Thus, the frequency and the presence of associated cardiac disease are the important factors in determining the significance of the dysrhythmia.

Six or more consecutive premature ventricular beats constitute the ventricular dysrhythmia called *ventricular tachycardia*. Ventricular tachycardia appears on the ECG as a series of slightly irregular, wide, undulating waves. The only identifiable waves are the wide, distorted QRS (greater than 0.12 second), ST segments, and T wave (Fig. 19-24). The ventricular rate ranges between 100 and 250 BPM [6,12]. Ventricular tachycardia may be transient or may continue until the underlying cause is treated.

Ventricular tachycardia is often triggered by a PVC falling during the vulnerable period of ventricular diastole (R-on-T phenomenon) [11]. Often this ectopic focus is a product of enhanced automaticity of the ventricular myocardium. Acidosis, hypoxia, hypotension, and hypokalemia are instigating factors. Advanced heart disease in the forms of coronary vasospasm, cardiomyopathy, mitral valve prolapse, and congestive heart failure are commonly associated with the occurrence of ventricular tachycardia. Recent studies demonstrate the appearance of ventricular tachycardia after coronary reperfusion [15]. Electrophysiologic mapping techniques have demonstrated that scarring and left ventricular aneurysm formation after acute MI cause a delay in ventricular depolarization and repolarization [20]. These delays set the stage for microcircuit reentry and repetitive firing of ectopic foci to occur [10]. Mapping techniques allow the anatomic sites of ectopic activity to be pinpointed for possible surgical or pharmacologic intervention.

Ventricular tachycardia is clinically significant and requires immediate intervention. Loss of consciousness and hypotension are indicators of the substantial reduction of cardiac output associated with this dysrhythmia. Untreated, ventricular tachycardia usually progresses to ventricular fibrillation.

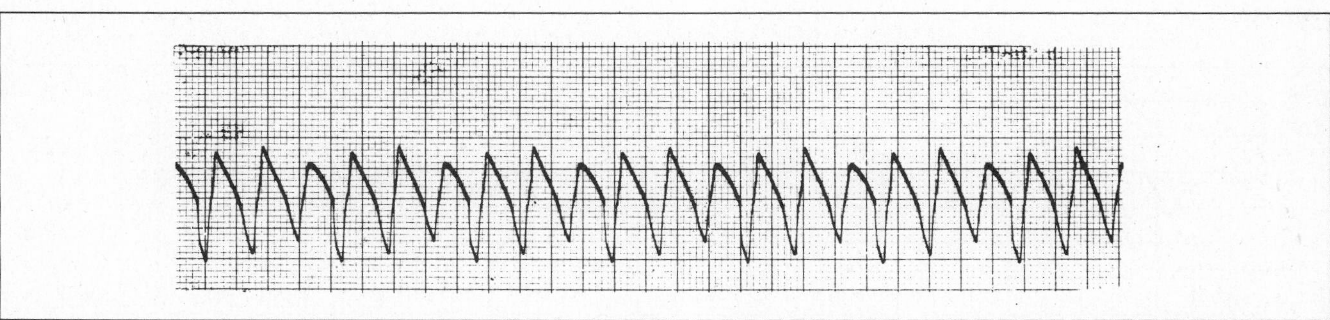

FIGURE 19-24 Ventricular tachycardia. (From B.H. Yee and S.L. Zorb, *Cardiac Critical Care Nursing*. Boston: Little, Brown, 1986.)

The most serious of the cardiac dysrhythmias is *ventricular fibrillation*. It is the most common cause of sudden death and is often the terminal rhythm in advanced cardiac disease. Single or multiple ectopic foci fire in a chaotic manner, producing an asynchronous quivering of the myocardium. It is thought that several mechanisms are responsible for this activity, including macro-reentry circuits and circus movements within the ventricles [4,10].

The ECG reveals indistinguishable waveforms undulating about the isoelectric line with varying degrees of amplitude (Fig. 19-25). Ventricular fibrillation can range from 150 to 500 BPM [4]. It often profoundly disintegrates into slow idioventricular rhythm (*agonal* or dying heart rhythm) just prior to death.

The etiologies for ventricular fibrillation are primarily the same as for PVCs and ventricular tachycardia. In addition, cardiac pacing, cardiac catheterization, electric shock, and hypothermia are known to stimulate this rhythm.

Because of its life-threatening potential this dysrhythmia must be detected and treated immediately. Due to the quivering of the ventricles, no pump action takes place and therefore no cardiac output is produced. Brain damage occurs within four to six minutes without oxygenated perfusion to its tissues.

Disturbances in Conduction of Cardiac Impulses

Disturbances in conduction of cardiac impulses are described as various types of heart block. There are three major categories of conduction disorders: (1) sinoatrial (SA) block, (2) atrioventricular (AV) block, and (3) intraventricular block.

Sinoatrial Block. The SA block is thought to be produced by the blockage of sinus impulses leaving the SA node. This mechanism occurs at the sinoatrial junction and is called an exit block [12]. Exit blocks are usually transient and produce pauses in the cardiac rhythm where the sinus impulse normally would have fallen. The PQRST waveforms are normal unless altered by other conditions. Ventricular rate and rhythm vary due to the pauses (Fig. 19-26).

An SA block can be caused by a variety of etiologies, including excessive vagal stimulation, acute myocardial infectious processes, digitalis or quinidine intoxication, hyperkalemia, thyroid disorders, metastatic cancer, and degenerative diseases of the SA node [11]. The block occurs frequently after an acute inferior MI because the right coronary artery supplies the blood supply to the SA node in 60 percent of individuals.

An SA block can occur in healthy as well as diseased hearts. The duration of the pause during which no cardiac output is produced, as well as the presence and degree of underlying cardiac disease, determines the clinical significance of this dysrhythmia. Prolonged pauses or episodes in which secondary pacemakers or escape mechanisms fail may produce symptoms associated with a fall in cardiac output. Lengthy pauses lead to ventricular standstill and death.

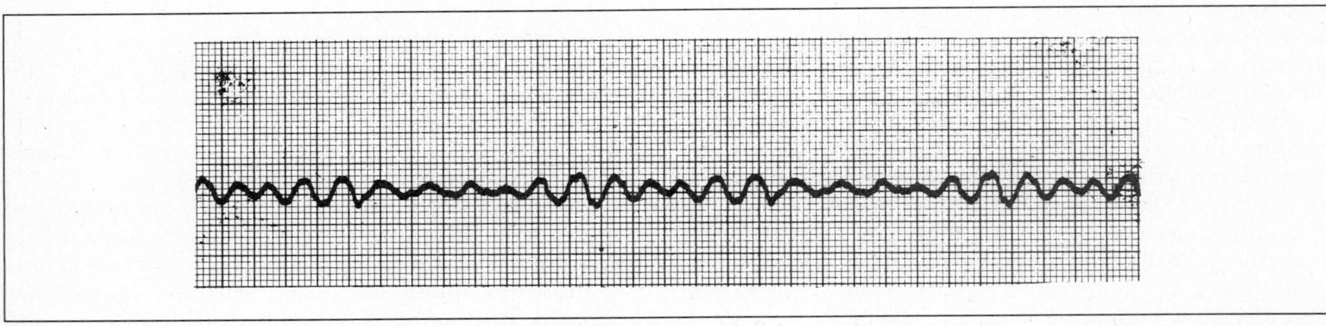

FIGURE 19-25 Ventricular fibrillation. (From B.H. Yee and S.L. Zorb, *Cardiac Critical Care Nursing*. Boston: Little, Brown, 1986.)

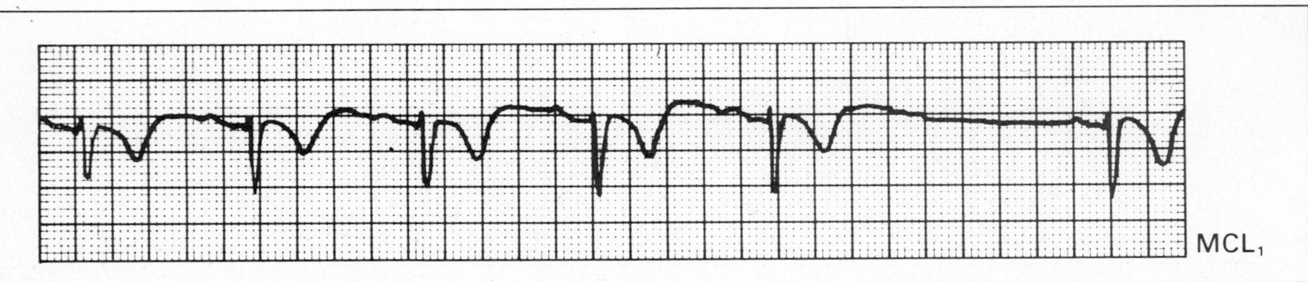

FIGURE 19-26 Sinoatrial (sinus exit) block. (From S. Underhill et al., *Cardiac Nursing*. J.B. Lippincott/Harper & Row. Copyright © 1982. Reprinted by permission.)

Atrioventricular Block. Atrioventricular block can occur as either a physiologic or pathologic mechanism. The physiologic function protects the ventricular rate of the heart by blocking impulses during states such as atrial fibrillation. The pathologic mechanism blocks impulses from reaching the ventricles in varying degrees based on the area of the AV junction involved [12]. The AV blocks caused by pathology in the AV node are transient and ischemic. Infranodal blocks involving bundle of His and bundle branches are permanent and require intensive management [4]. The AV block is classified in degrees reflecting the extent of the conduction disturbance.

First-degree AV block is a result of delayed conduction at the AV node between the SA node and the ventricles (Fig. 19-27). The ECG reveals a sinus rhythm with a prolonged PR interval (greater than 0.20 second).

First-degree AV block is often seen in healthy elderly adults secondary to degenerative changes in the AV node and is generally clinically insignificant. It becomes significant for persons taking digoxin or beta blockers as it may signal toxic drug levels. First-degree AV block in those with inferior wall MI is usually transient but may progress to the Wenkebach phenomenon. The occurrence of this dysrhythmia in persons with anterior wall MI may progress rapidly to third-degree heart block and trifascicular bundle branch block [4]. This dysrhythmia is also associated with acute myocarditis, uremia, hyperkalemia, and rheumatic fever.

In *second-degree AV block*, the degree of block increases so that not every sinus impulse reaches the ventricle. The two major types of second-degree AV blocks are Mobitz type I (Wenkebach) and Mobitz type II.

Mobitz type I block produces a progressive delay in conduction at the AV node until a sinus impulse is completely blocked. This is seen on the ECG as gradual lengthening of the PR interval until a QRS complex is dropped (Fig. 19-28). The underlying rate is normal, the rhythm irregular, and the QRS complex of sinus beats normal. Mobitz type I is usually a temporary dysrhythmia associated with ischemic heart disease, digoxin toxicity, and right coronary artery pathology [6]. In persons with acute inferior MI, it may progress to third-degree AV block.

Mobitz type II block is an infranodal conduction delay [4]. Some sinus impulses are blocked within or distal to the bundle of His and do not reach the ventricles. The degree of block occurs at variable intervals. Thus the ECG monitor shows constant PR intervals of the conducted beats with varying ratios of P waves to QRS complexes (Fig. 19-29). Due to the level of conduction defect, the QRS complex may be widened. Overall ventricular rhythm is regular with a normal or bradycardic rate.

The causes of Mobitz type II block include degenerative collagen diseases, Lev's disease (fibrocalcific changes in the conduction system), myxedema, and progressive ischemic conduction system disease [22]. By far the most clinically significant condition is left coronary artery

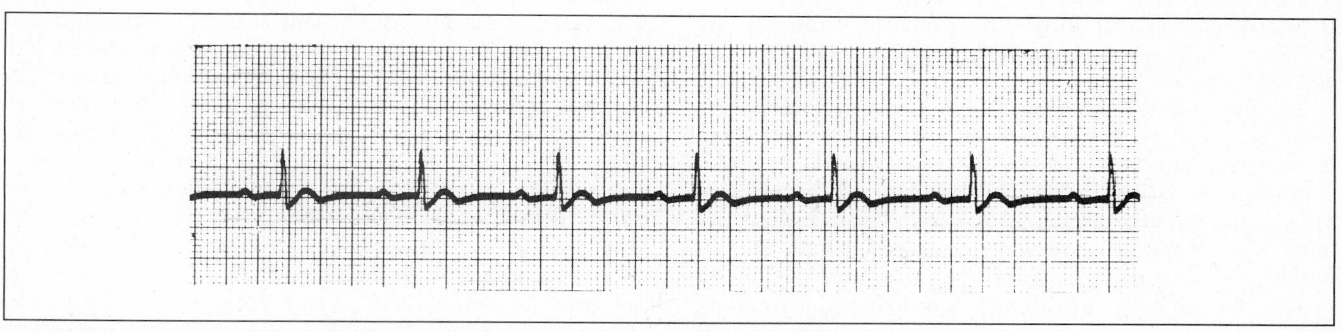

FIGURE 19-27 First degree AV block. (From B.H. Yee and S.L. Zorb, *Cardiac Critical Care Nursing*. Boston: Little, Brown, 1986.)

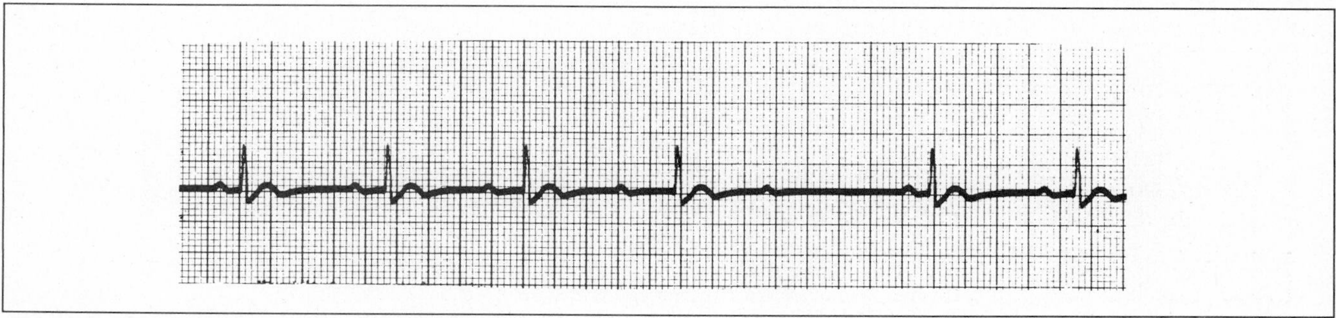

FIGURE 19-28 Second-degree AV block, Mobitz type I. (From B.H. Yee and S.L. Zorb, *Cardiac Critical Care Nursing*. Boston: Little, Brown, 1986.)

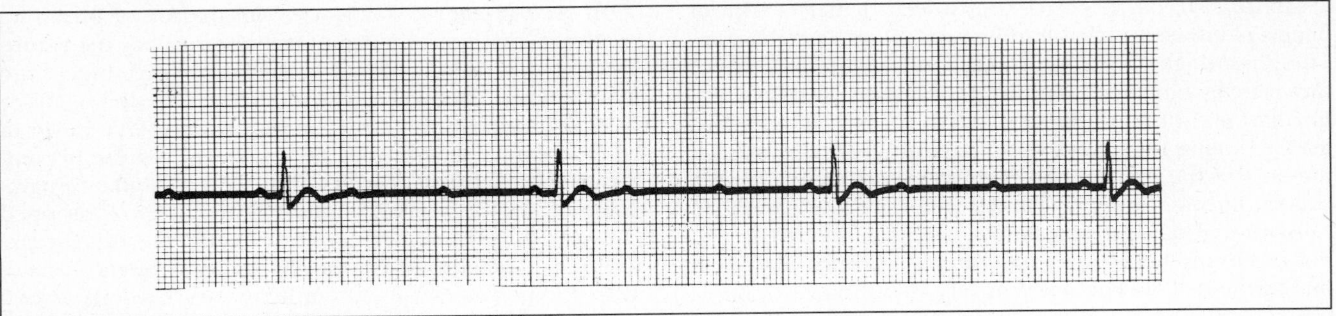

FIGURE 19-29 Second-degree AV block, Mobitz type II. (From B.H. Yee and S.L. Zorb, *Cardiac Critical Care Nursing*. Boston: Little, Brown, 1986.)

pathology associated with acute anterior MI. The degree of block is usually irreversible and progresses to complete heart block, which requires pacemaker insertion.

Third-degree or *complete AV block* occurs when no sinus impulses reach the ventricles. The most prominent characteristic is the independent activity of the atria and ventricles (Fig. 19-30). A slower idioventricular rhythm established in the bundle branches or lower system is responsible for ventricular contraction.

The most common cause of third-degree AV block is anterior MI. Extensive necrosis of the intraventricular septum and damage to the bundle branches can result from occlusion of the left coronary artery [22]. Other causes include open heart surgery, degenerative fibrosclerosis of the cardiac skeleton, fibrosis of the conduction system, coronary artery disease, cardiomyopathies, scleroderma, and Lev's disease [2].

Persons with third-degree AV block may or may not be symptomatic depending on onset, etiology, and ventricular rate. Acute onset with a slow ventricular rate and a symptomatic fall in cardiac output require immediate pacemaker insertion. Stokes-Adams syndrome occurs when the established idioventricular pacemaker fails to initiate a ventricular beat, resulting in variable periods of ventricular asystole. Cerebral symptoms resulting from this include transient giddiness, loss of consciousness, convulsions, and sudden death, depending upon the duration of the asystole [23].

Intraventricular Block. Intraventricular blocks are conduction defects occurring in the bundle branch network. These give rise to several types of blocks: left bundle branch, right bundle branch, bifascicular, and trifascicular. Intraventricular blocks may be chronic and relatively benign, or acute with serious implications in the setting of myocardial infarction.

Left bundle branch block (LBBB) occurs when a lesion blocks the common left bundle. Due to its dual blood supply from the left and right coronary arteries and its size, this block usually represents advanced cardiac disease [6]. Impulses are conducted normally from the atria until the area of block is reached. The impulse is then conducted down the right bundle normally, but the impulse is delayed at the left bundle and may be passed from muscle fiber to muscle fiber rather than through the normal channels to effect left ventricular depolarization. The block may be intermittent and develop over a period of years [23]. A characteristic wide (greater than 0.12 second), notched QRS complex is produced. This is best seen as a negative QS complex in lead V_1 and a positive RR complex in V_6. The most common cause of this defect is cardiovascular atherosclerosis, but it may be associated with Lenegre's

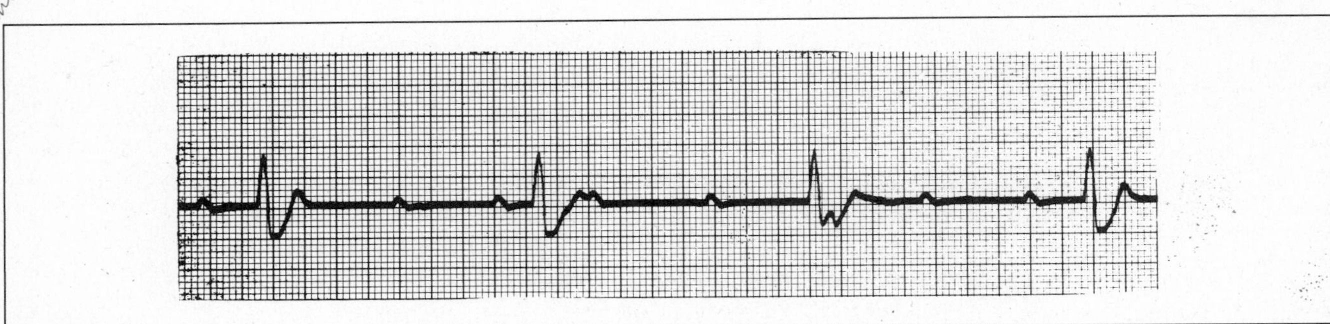

FIGURE 19-30 Third-degree AV block. (From B.H. Yee and S.L. Zorb, *Cardiac Critical Care Nursing*. Boston: Little, Brown, 1986.)

disease (idiopathic fibrosis of the His-Purkinje system), Lev's disease, coronary artery disease, syphilis, trauma, tumors, congenital lesions, aortic stenosis, and acute infections [2,6,22]. It also may be idiopathic [23].

Left bundle branch block may be chronic and clinically insignificant. Sudden onset in the presence of anterior MI, however, may indicate further progression in the intraventricular conduction system.

A *hemiblock* represents a blockage of one of the divisions of the left bundle branch. It is identified on ECG by examining the frontal leads and QRS axis.

A block in the anterosuperior division produces left anterior hemiblock. This fascicle is particularly vulnerable due to its location, size, and blood supply from the left coronary artery.

Left posterior hemiblock develops from a block in the posteroinferior branch of the left bundle. Its development is significant in that it may indicate compromise of both the right and left coronary arteries. Due to the greater density of its fascicle, location, and dual blood supply, it is relatively rare. In addition to the etiologies previously listed, pulmonary disorders are responsible for this block.

Right bundle branch block (RBBB) may occur in both healthy and diseased hearts. Because of the small size of the right fascicle, it can be affected by small insults such as altered blood flow from the left anterior descending artery. In right bundle branch block, conduction proceeds from the atria to the septum and left bundle in the normal fashion. Conduction occurs from left to right, producing an rS_R pattern in V_1 and QRS pattern in V_6 characteristic of this conduction defect.

Etiologies of right bundle branch block include acute MI and any of the conditions that can cause LBBB. It can also be produced after surgery to repair atrial-septal defects and tetralogy of Fallot [6]. In the event of anterior MI, RBBB should be observed closely for the development of bifascicular block.

Bifascicular block is a combination of right bundle branch block and either type of hemiblock. The most common combination is with left anterior hemiblock because they share a common blood supply. This combination in the presence of anterior MI may be a precursor to trifascicular block [17].

Trifascicular block results from the blocking of all fascicles of the bundle branch system, suggesting profound interruption to blood flow from the coronary arteries. If this is incomplete, a supraventricular escape rhythm with first-degree or type II second-degree block emerges. If block is complete, an escape rhythm below the block develops, with a ventricular rate incompatible with life [6].

Disturbances in Both Conduction and Impulse Formation

Dysrhythmias classified as disturbances in both conduction and impulse formation are frequently complicated, involving mechanisms not fully understood. The more common disorders are AV dissociation, preexcitation syndromes, and ventricular standstill.

Atrioventricular dissociation may result from various mechanisms. Usually two separate pacemakers, one sinus and the other junctional, coexist and produce independent rhythms. It is thought to be produced by a slowing or failure of the SA node, accelerated impulse formation in the AV junction or ventricles, and/or complete SA or AV block [4]. This condition usually occurs as a symptom of rhythm disturbance rather than as a separate entity.

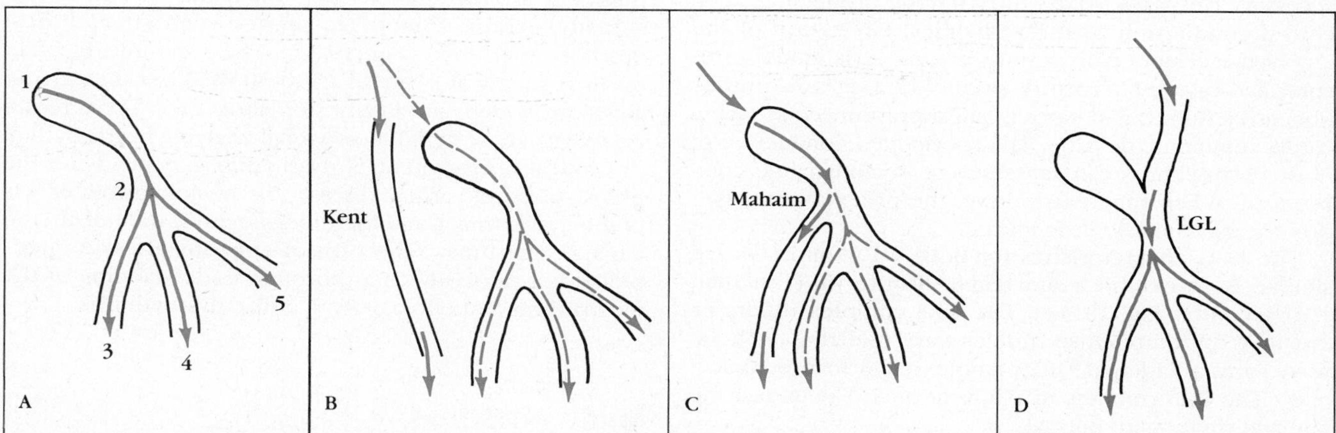

FIGURE 19-31 Diagrammatic illustrations of accessory pathways. A. Normal conduction from atrium to (1) AV node, (2) bundle of His, (3) right bundle branch, (4) left anterior fascicle, and (5) left posterior fascicle. B. Lateral accessory pathway. This bypasses the AV node and enters a site in the ventricular myocardium (typical WPW). C. Mahaim fibers connecting the distal AV node or His bundle with a portion of the ventricular myocardium. D. Accessory pathway connecting the atrium with the distal AV node or His bundle (LGL). (Reprinted with permission from M.J. Goldman, *Principles of Clinical Electrocardiography* (10th ed.). Los Altos, Calif.: Lange, 1979, Figure 16-1, p. 266.)

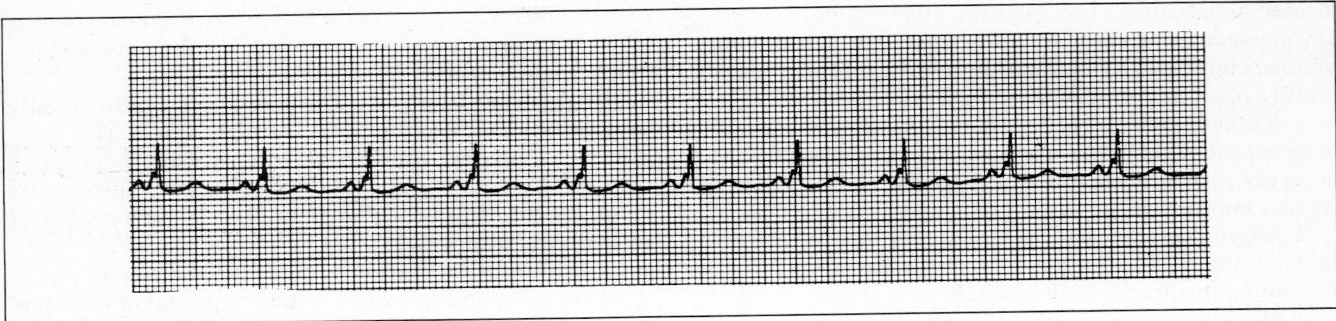

FIGURE 19-32 Preexcitation. (From B.H. Yee and S.L. Zorb, *Cardiac Critical Care Nursing*. Boston: Little, Brown, 1986.)

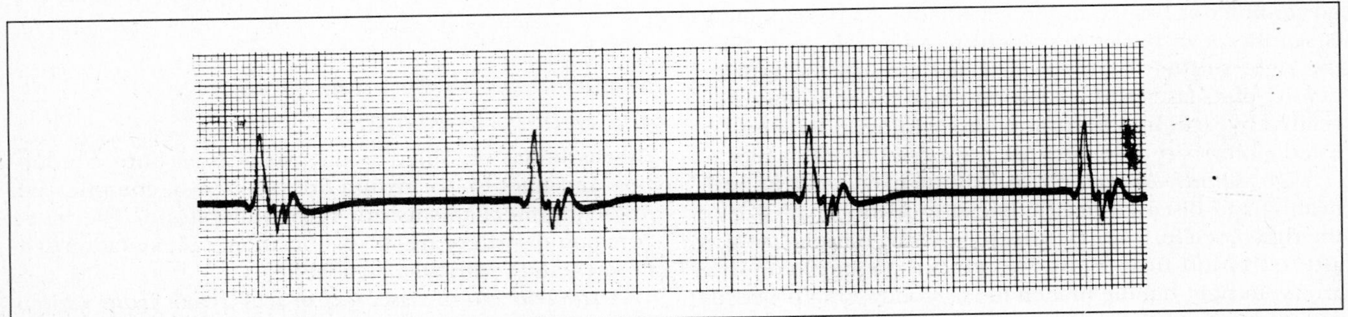

FIGURE 19-33 Idioventricular rhythm. (From B.H. Yee and S.L. Zorb, *Cardiac Critical Care Nursing*. Boston: Little, Brown, 1986.)

Preexcitation syndrome arises secondary to the existence of accessory pathways between the atria and ventricles (Fig. 19-31). *Wolff-Parkinson-White (WPW)* and *Lown-Ganong-Levine (LGL)* syndromes are the most common forms of this condition. In these syndromes, the accessory pathways bypass the AV node producing accelerated conduction to the ventricles. Excitation of the involved accessory path permits ectopic atrial impulses to enter and establish a reentry circuit [12,25]. Atrial fibrillation, atrial flutter, and paroxysmal supraventricular tachycardia commonly develop. The accelerated conduction of these dysrhythmias can cause severe hemodynamic compromise. When they exist alone, the preexcitation syndromes are clinically insignificant.

The ECG characteristics for both WPW and LGL are similar. Both exhibit a shortened PR interval (less than 0.10 second) (Fig. 19-32). The QRS complex differs in that in WPW there exists a delta wave (slurring of the R wave) and a widened QRS complex (less than 0.10 second). The QRS complex in LGL is normal. The underlying rate and rhythm are normal.

Preexcitation syndromes have been observed in persons with psychoneurotic disorders, hyperthyroidism, mitral valve prolapse, rheumatic heart disease, congenital defects, atrial-septal defects, and idiopathic subaortic stenosis [12].

Ventricular standstill occurs when lower-level pacemakers fail to produce escape rhythms and no ventricular activity ensues. This often terminal dysrhythmia of a dying heart may occur after numerous conditions, especially acute MI, digitalis toxicity, and unsuccessful conversion of ventricular fibrillation [4]. At onset the ventricles cease to contract. The P waves continue for a time before also ceasing. Intervention must be immediate as no cardiac output is produced and death will quickly ensue. Occasionally, erratic complexes surface even after clinical death is established (Fig. 19-33). These complexes often occur regularly at a rate of 15 to 30 BPM but then gradually slow, widen, and finally stop altogether. These terminal events are referred to as agonal or dying heart rhythm.

Clinical management of dysrhythmias depends on the preexistence of cardiac disease, the hemodynamic effects of the dysrhythmia, and the timely identification of altered cardiac rhythms. Selection of appropriate treatment modalities necessitates a thorough understanding of the mechanisms and etiologies of cardiac dysrhythmias.

Study Questions

1. Describe the electrophysiology of the heart. How is it transmitted to an electrocardiographic recording?
2. Trace the conduction of an impulse through the heart and locate the resultant lead configurations on a 12-lead ECG.
3. Discuss the major precipitating factors in the development of both common and life-threatening dysrhythmias.

4. Describe the reentry phenomenon and list at least two dysrhythmias probably associated with it.
5. Compare the three classifications of dysrhythmias according to precipitating cause, hemodynamic results, and prognosis.

References

1. Anderson, R.H., and Becker, A.E. Gross anatomy and microscopy of the conducting system. In W.J. Mandel (ed.), *Cardiac Arrhythmias*. Philadelphia: Lippincott, 1980.
2. Andreloi, K.G. (ed.). *Comprehensive Cardiac Care* (5th ed.). St. Louis: Mosby, 1983.
3. Benditt, D.G., et al. Atrial flutter, atrial fibrillation and other primary atrial tachycardias. *Med. Clin. North Am.* 68:895, 1984.
4. Chung, E.K. *Principles of Cardiac Arrhythmias* (3rd ed.). Baltimore: Williams & Wilkins, 1983.
5. Chung, E.K. Sick sinus syndrome: Current views. *Mod. Concepts Cardiovasc. Dis.* 49:67, 1980.
6. Conover, M.B. *Pocket Nurse Guide to Electrocardiography*. St. Louis: Mosby, 1986.
7. Friedberg, C.K. *Diseases of the Heart*. Philadelphia: Saunders, 1966.
8. Gallagher, J.J. Mechanisms of arrhythmias and conduction defects. In J.W. Hurst (ed.)., *The Heart* (6th ed.). New York: McGraw-Hill, 1986.
9. Garson, A. Arrhythmias in pediatric patients. *Med. Clin. North Am.* 68:1171, 1984.
10. German, L.D., and Ideker, R.E. Ventricular tachycardia: Mechanisms, diagnosis, and management. *Med. Clin. North Am.* 68:970, 1984.
11. Gilmour, R.F., and Zipes, D.P. Basic electrophysiologic mechanism for the development of arrhythmias. *Med. Clin. North Am.* 68:795, 1984.
12. Goldman, M.J. *Principles of Clinical Electrocardiography* (10th ed.). Los Altos, Calif.: Lange, 1979.
13. Kaplan, B.M. Tachycardia-bradycardia syndrome. *Am. J. Cardiol.* 31:497, 1973.
14. Kruthcher, K.L. Cardiac electrophysiologic mapping techniques. *Focus Crit. Care* 12:26, 1985.
15. Loeb, J.M. Cardiac electrophysiology. *Crit. Care Q.* 7:9, 1984.
16. Marriott, H.J. *Practical Electrocardiography* (7th ed.). Baltimore: Williams & Wilkins, 1983.
17. Marriott, H.J., and Myerberg, R.J. Recognition of arrhythmia and conduction abnormalities. In J.W. Hurst (ed.), *The Heart* (6th ed.). New York: McGraw-Hill, 1986.
18. McCarthy, E. Hemodynamic effects and clinical assessment of dysrhythmias. *Crit. Care Q.* 4:9, 1981.
19. Mead, R.H., and Harrison, D.C. Clinical management of common cardiac abnormalities. In D.A. Zschoche (ed.), *Mosby's Comprehensive Review of Critical Care* (3rd ed.). St. Louis: Mosby, 1986.
20. Rowe, M.A. The use of electrophysiologic mapping studies in treating sustained ventricular tachycardia. *Crit. Care Q.* 4:67, 1981.
21. Schamroth, L. *An Introduction to Electrocardiography* (6th ed.). Boston: Blackwell, 1982.
22. Sidel, J.C. *Basic Electrocardiography*. St. Louis: Mosby, 1986.
23. Sokolow, M., and McIlroy, M.B. *Clinical Cardiology* (4th ed.). Los Altos, Calif.: Lange, 1986.
24. Sweetwood, H.M. *Clinical Electrocardiography for Nurses*. Rockville, Md.: Aspen, 1983.
25. Swiryn, S., McDonough, T., and Hueter, D.C. Sinus node function and dysfunction. *Med. Clin. North Am.* 68:935, 1984.
26. Watanabe, Y., Drefifus, L., and Sodeman, W.A., Sr. Arrhythmias: Mechanisms and pathogenesis. In W.A. Sodeman and T.M. Sodeman (eds.), *Pathologic Physiology: Mechanisms of Disease* (7th ed.). Philadelphia: Saunders, 1985.
27. Winkle, R.A. Cellular basis of cardiac arrhythmias. In R.A. Winkle (ed.), *Cardiac Arrhythmias: Current Diagnosis and Practical Management*. Menlo Park, Calif.: Addison-Wesley, 1983.

CHAPTER 20

Compromised Pumping Ability of the Heart

CHAPTER OUTLINE

Congestive Heart Failure

- Pathophysiology of Heart Failure
  - *Sympathetic Response to Heart Failure*
  - *Renin Release from the Kidneys*
  - *Anaerobic Metabolism*
  - *Oxygen Extraction from the Red Blood Cells*
  - *Frank-Starling Law of the Heart*
  - *Hypertrophy of the Myocardium*
  - *Dilatation of the Heart*
  - *Summary of Compensatory Mechanisms*
- Classification of Heart Failure
- Left Heart Failure
  - *Causes*
  - *Pathophysiology*
  - *Signs and Symptoms*
- Right Heart Failure
  - *Causes*
  - *Pathophysiology*
  - *Signs and Symptoms*
- Diagnosis of Congestive Heart Failure
  - *Radiologic Changes*
  - *Hemodynamic Monitoring*
  - *Arterial Blood Gases*
  - *Other Laboratory Tests*

Cardiogenic Shock

- Causes of Cardiogenic Shock
- Pathophysiology of Cardiogenic Shock
- Diagnosis of Cardiogenic Shock

Diseases Affecting Myocardial Contractility

- Cardiomyopathy
  - *Congestive or Dilated Cardiomyopathy*
  - *Restrictive Cardiomyopathy*
  - *Hypertrophic Cardiomyopathy*
- Myocarditis

LEARNING OBJECTIVES

1. Differentiate between cardiac and circulatory failure.
2. Describe *preload* and *afterload*.
3. Discuss compensatory mechanisms of cardiac failure.
4. Describe cause and effect of dilatation of the heart chambers.
5. List the underlying factors that can precipitate heart failure.
6. Describe the pathophysiology of right and left heart failure.
7. Describe the basis for the clinical manifestations of left heart failure.
8. Describe the basis for the clinical manifestations of right heart failure.
9. Discuss radiologic changes in right and left heart failure.
10. Identify the purposes of the Swan-Ganz catheter in monitoring congestive heart failure.
11. Identify blood tests used to aid in the diagnosis of congestive heart failure.
12. List causes of cardiogenic shock.
13. Discuss the mechanism of compensated shock.
14. Identify clinical signs and symptoms of cardiogenic shock.
15. Discuss irreversible or decompensated shock.
16. Define *cardiomyopathy*.
17. Differentiate primary and secondary cardiomyopathies.
18. Describe congestive, restrictive, and hypertrophic cardiomyopathies.

Many conditions may lead to impairment of myocardial contractility. The result of such impairment is congestive heart failure. This chapter examines heart failure, its sequelae, cardiogenic shock, and cardiomyopathy.

Congestive Heart Failure

Heart failure refers to a constellation of signs and symptoms that result from the heart's inability to pump enough blood to meet the body's metabolic demands. The pump itself is impaired and unable to supply adequate blood to meet the cellular needs. Cardiac failure is one type of *circulatory failure*, a term that also includes hypoperfusion resulting from extracardiac conditions such as hypovolemia, peripheral vasodilatation, and inadequate oxygenation of hemoglobin.

The clinical result of heart failure includes *circulatory overload* or *congestive heart failure (CHF)*. This is a clinical syndrome characterized by abnormal retention of sodium and water resulting from renal compensation for the decreased cardiac output. Circulatory overload is enhanced by the resulting excess blood volume and increased venous return.

The causes of heart failure are varied and include intrinsic myocardial disease, malformation or injury, and secondary abnormalities (Table 20-1). Myocardial failure is often the cause of death in terminal illness of noncardiac etiology.

TABLE 20-1 Intrinsic and Secondary Causes of Heart Failure

Intrinsic[a]	Secondary
Cardiomyopathy	Pulmonary embolism
Myocardial infarction	Anemia
Myocarditis	Thyrotoxicosis
Ischemic heart disease	Systemic hypertension
Congenital heart defects	Arteriovenous shunts
Pericarditis/cardiac tamponade	Blood volume excess
	Metabolic/respiratory acidosis
	Drug toxicity
	Cardiac dysrhythmias

[a] *Intrinsic* refers to myocardial, endocardial, and pericardial disease, and congenital malformations that increase ventricular volume load and ischemia or infarction of the ventricular myocardium.

Pathophysiology of Heart Failure

The onset of heart failure may be acute or insidious. It is often associated with systolic or diastolic overloading and with myocardial weakness. As the physiologic stress on the heart muscle reaches a critical level, the contractility of the muscle is reduced and cardiac output declines, but venous input to the ventricles remains the same. The responses to the decreasing cardiac output are predictable, and include (1) reflex increase in sympathetic activity, (2) release of renin from the juxtaglomerular cells of the kidneys, (3) anaerobic metabolism by affected cells, and (4) increased extraction of oxygen by the peripheral cells. The responses of the heart to increased volume of blood in the ventricles are also predictable and include both short- and long-term mechanisms.

In *acute* or *short-term mechanisms*, as the end-diastolic fiber length increases, the ventricular muscle responds with dilatation and an increased force of contraction (Frank-Starling effect). In *long-term mechanisms*, ventricular hypertrophy increases the ability of the heart muscle to contract and push its volume into the circulation. The pathology of the predisposing condition determines whether heart failure is acute or insidious in onset, as compensation often occurs for long periods of time before the manifestations of heart failure develop.

An example of long-term compensation is that which results from *systemic hypertension*. Because the ventricles must pump against increased pressure (increased afterload), the ventricular myocardium hypertrophies, the heart pumps with more force, and the heart rate is often elevated. These mechanisms may maintain normal cardiac output for years prior to the onset of failure. Symptoms of CHF signal that the pump can no longer keep up with cellular demands. Gradually, the manifestations of heart failure become apparent.

An example of acute onset of heart failure is an extensive myocardial infarction, which causes direct impairment of cardiac contractility, a sudden decrease in cardiac output, and insufficient available time for the development of hypertrophy.

Sympathetic Response to Heart Failure. A decrease in cardiac output results in decreased blood pressure, which causes a reflex stimulation of the sympathetic nervous system (SNS). The SNS causes an increase in the rate and force of contraction of the ventricles both through the conduction system and through an increase in ventricular irritability. It also results in vasoconstriction of the arterioles throughout the body.

The SNS activity is mediated through epinephrine and norepinephrine. Epinephrine mostly increases the rate and force of cardiac contractions, while norepinephrine functions mainly in arteriolar vasoconstriction.

Renin Release from the Kidneys. When blood pressure decreases, the decline is perceived by the renal juxtaglomerular cells, which release renin. Renin acts on angiotensinogen, a plasma protein produced by the liver, to form angiotensin I. Angiotensin I is converted to angiotensin II by an enzyme present mostly in the lungs (Fig. 20-1). Angiotensin II is a potent vasoconstrictor that constricts renal arterioles, stimulates the thirst center in the brain, and stimulates the secretion of aldosterone by the adrenal glands [1]. These actions cause vasoconstriction, which leads to increased blood pressure and expansion of the blood volume through the aldosterone effect of sodium preservation. Angiotensin II is rapidly destroyed by *angiotensinase*, a term used for various blood tissue enzymes [1].

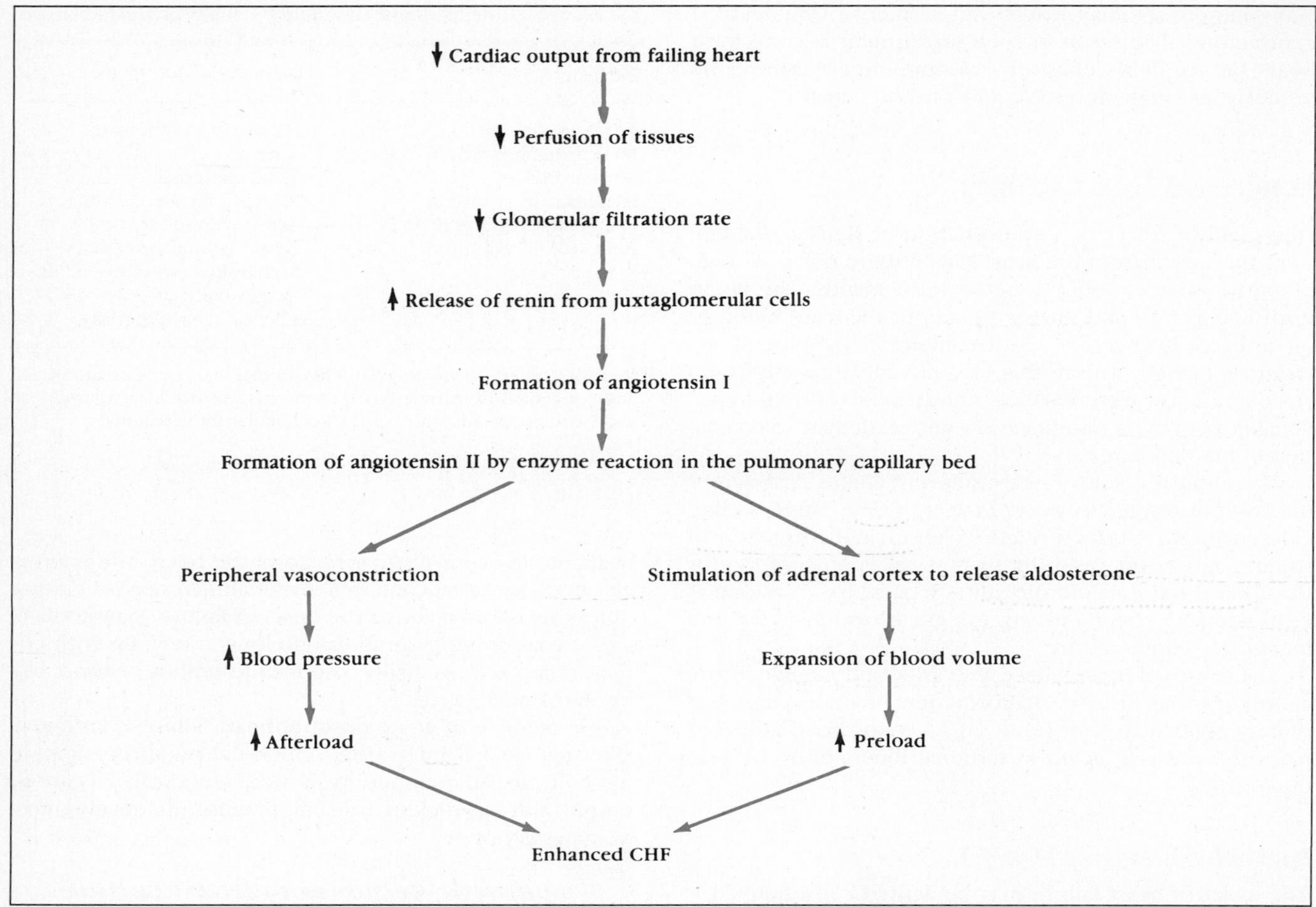

FIGURE 20-1 Renin-angiotensin-aldosterone (RAA) system in CHF. Note the positive feedback created as the body attempts to adjust to decreased cardiac output.

Anaerobic Metabolism. When cells do not receive adequate circulation or oxygen, metabolism decreases and alternative methods are used to produce energy. The major alternative method is the anaerobic production of adenosine triphosphate (ATP), which is an inefficient process but accomplishes the purpose of keeping cells alive for a limited period of time. This compensatory mechanism is activated only in severe circulatory failure and shock.

Oxygen Extraction from the Red Blood Cells. Oxygen extraction from the red blood cells (RBCs) to the tissues increases when the circulation is inadequate and perfusion is diminished. Normally, about 30 percent of oxygen is extracted from RBCs by the peripheral tissue, but greater amounts can be extracted during periods of poor perfusion. Unfortunately, this mechanism is not very useful to the myocardium because myocardial muscle normally extracts the maximum amount possible, 65 to 75 percent of the oxygen it receives [1].

Frank-Starling Law of the Heart. When the heart is not pumping all of its contents out, increased amounts of blood are left within the organ. This residual volume increases diastolic fiber length. The inherent compensatory mechanism is an increase in the force of recoil so that the heart responds with increased stroke work and volume (see Chap. 18). In the failing heart, diastolic fiber length is continually increased, causing the heart to enlarge. With activation of the renin-angiotensin-aldosterone (RAA) system, blood volume is increased, adding to this diastolic preload (see Fig. 20-1).

Hypertrophy of the Myocardium. When increased stress is placed on any chamber of the heart, hypertrophy can result. This stress response is due to chronically increased workload. The individual myocardial muscle cells increase in size but not in number. Hypertrophy probably results when the wall tension of the chamber must continuously increase on systole to eject the contents of the chamber. Ventricular hypertrophy is more common than atrial hypertrophy and provides for compensatory adaptation to a chronically increased workload.

Hypertrophy may be classified as concentric or eccentric. *Concentric hypertrophy* reveals a thickened ventricular wall without apparent enlargement of the heart. This often occurs with aortic stenosis and sometimes with systemic hypertension. *Eccentric hypertrophy* exhibits a proportionate increase in the wall size and diameter of the left ventricle [7]. This type of hypertrophy often occurs in conditions associated with increased preload. Hypertrophy maintains or increases contractility until heart failure ensues.

Dilatation of the Heart. Dilatation refers to enlargement of cardiac chambers. It often occurs because of increased volume of blood that enters the heart. The ventricles are always dilated in acute congestive heart failure. Dilatation often coincides with hypertrophy, especially if the stressful event causing the failure is chronic, such as systemic hypertension.

Radiographic enlargement of the cardiac shadow characterizes heart failure. In the normal heart, increased input to the ventricle results in increased ventricular force of contraction, but no permanent enlargement occurs. As the cardiac reserve fails, the ventricle is unable to pump out all of its contents and thus enlarges.

Dilatation imposes a mechanical disadvantage on the ventricles. As ventricular volume increases, a large portion of the mechanical energy of contraction is expended in imparting tension to the fibers and a smaller portion for fiber recoil or shortening. An example of this concept can be illustrated by comparing the contractile power of two left ventricles. If one ventricle had twice the diameter of another, it would take 4 times the contractile power to produce the same systolic pressure in the larger ventricle [8,11].

A heart that is greatly dilated also works at a metabolic disadvantage because its need for oxygen is increased. More blood to the myocardium is required, which may not be supplied by the coronary arteries.

Dilatation is characteristic of cardiomyopathy in which separation of the trabeculae carneae may occur together with fibrosis of the myocardium. Usually, the greater the dilatation the more ineffective the cardiac contraction. Ineffective left ventricular contraction is often called *hypokinesis* of the left ventricle.

In persons with valvular insufficiency, septal defects, or other abnormal communications, the diastolic inflow to one or both ventricles is permanently augmented. In such conditions, dilatation of cardiac chambers occurs to maintain normal or near normal circulation even if a defect is quite large.

Summary of Compensatory Mechanisms. The compensatory mechanisms described above may preserve the life of the individual, but they usually aggravate the underlying condition.

Sympathetic regulation tends to preserve circulation to the brain and heart, but it increases the cardiac workload by increasing the afterload, which may depress the effectiveness of cardiac contraction. Activation of the RAA system also increases afterload because of the peripheral vasoconstriction produced. The aldosterone effect increases blood volume and thus increases preload. Anaerobic metabolism causes metabolic acidosis, which depresses myocardial contractility. The Frank-Starling effect increases the energy requirements of the myocardium. Hypertrophy increases the oxygen need of each myocardial muscle cell, which is a problem if the blood flow is reduced from coronary artery disease.

The ability of the heart to increase its output under stress is called the *cardiac reserve*. This reserve is accomplished by increasing the stroke volume and increasing the heart rate. The normal heart can increase its output 4 to 5 times normal under conditions of stress [1]. As heart failure ensues, the reserve falls so that the individual may first have symptoms of heart failure when placed under significant stress; later in the course of the disease symptoms develop when only minor stress is encountered. Heart failure manifestations at rest indicate that there is no cardiac reserve for any stressful situation at all.

Classification of Heart Failure

Heart failure has been classified as left-sided and right-sided on the basis of clinical manifestations. It has further been divided into forward and backward effects in order to explain its low-output and venous congestion components. In some cases the forward or low-output syndrome dominates, while in others the congestive phenomenon is the major manifestation. In reality, both features are present in heart failure just as both left- and right-sided effects necessarily must be present. This discussion divides left and right heart failure into separate entities, but the reader must keep in mind that the heart and lungs are interconnected, so what affects one side of the heart eventually affects the other (Fig. 20-2).

Left Heart Failure

Left-heart failure (LHF) occurs when the output of the left ventricle is less than the total volume of blood received from the right side of the heart through the pulmonary circulation. As a result, the pulmonary circuit becomes congested with blood that cannot be moved forward, and the systemic blood pressure falls.

Causes. The most common cause of predominantly left ventricular failure is myocardial infarction. Other causes include systemic hypertension, aortic stenosis or insufficiency, and cardiomyopathy. Mitral stenosis and mitral insufficiency also cause the symptoms of LHF (Fig. 20-3) [8].

Pathophysiology. Because the left ventricle cannot pump out all of its blood, blood dams back to the left atrium into the four pulmonary veins and the pulmonary capillary bed (PCB). As the volume of blood in the lungs increases, the pulmonary vessels enlarge. The pressure of blood in the PCB increases, and when it reaches a certain point (approximately 25–28 mm Hg), fluid passes across the pulmonary capillary membrane into the interstitial spaces around the alveoli and finally into the alveoli (Fig. 20-4). Acute pulmonary edema (APE) results, which impairs gas exchange and can be life-threatening. Higher PCB pressures may cause rupture of the capillary mem-

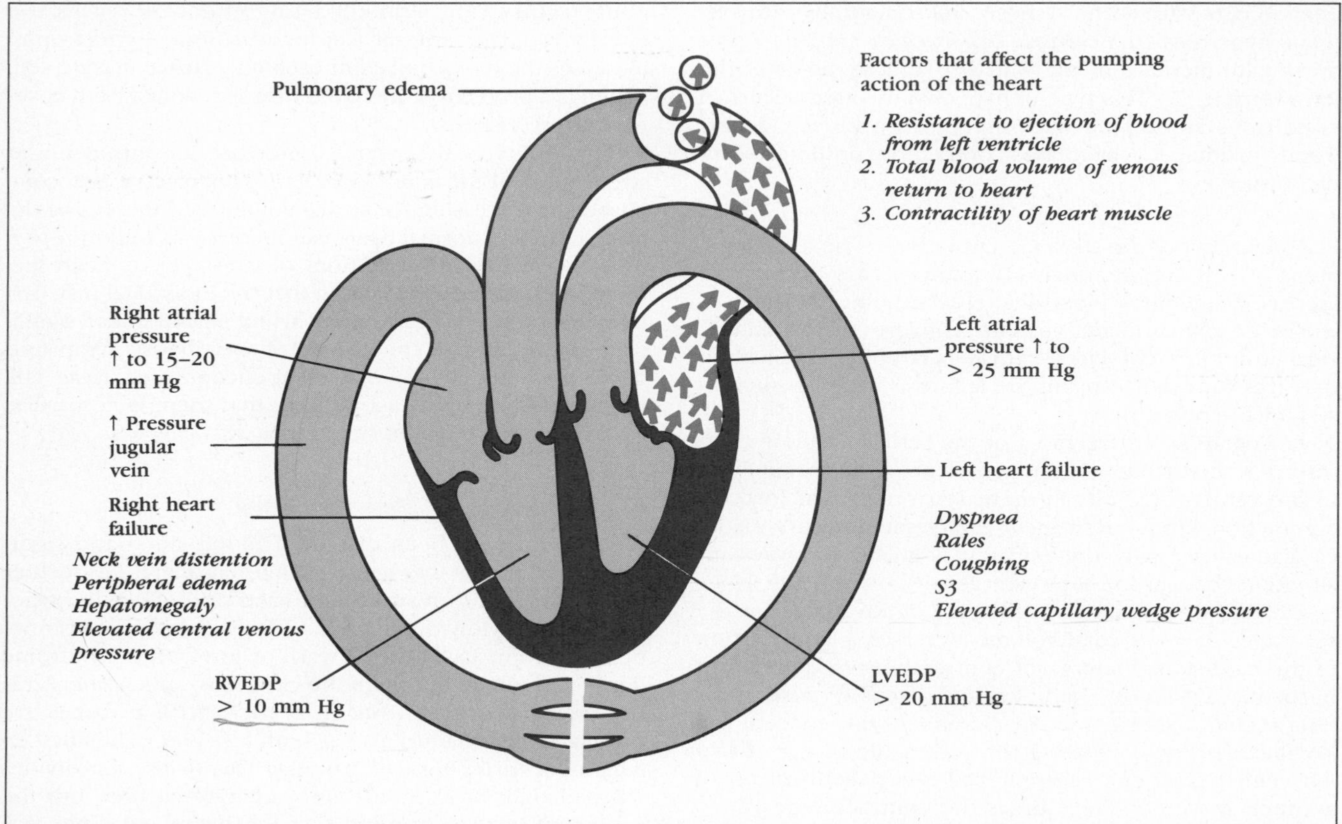

FIGURE 20-2 Biventricular failure usually results when left ventricular failure occurs, with elevated pulmonary pressures and subsequent elevation of the right-sided pressures leading to right-sided failure. (Adapted from C. Kenner, C. Guzzetta, and B. Dossey, *Critical Care Nursing: Body, Mind, Spirit* (2nd ed.). Boston: Little, Brown, 1985.)

branes leaking small or large amounts of blood into the alveolar sacs. All of these changes are called the *backward effects of LHF*.

The left ventricle also cannot pump its normal stroke volume out the aorta. Thus, the systemic blood pressure decreases. This decrease is sensed by the pressoreceptors that cause a reflex stimulation of the SNS. The result of SNS stimulation is increased heart rate and peripheral vasoconstriction. The RAA system is stimulated, leading to further vasoconstriction together with sodium and water retention (see Fig. 20-4). These are the main manifestations of the *forward effects of LHF*.

Chronic LHF often occurs in mitral valve disease, and it may progressively occur in cardiomyopathy and postmyocardial infarction. In the last two conditions pulmonary congestion may be evidenced, but APE does not occur unless additional stress increases the cardiac demand. Individuals with mitral stenosis, for example, have been shown to have a pulmonary pressure greater than 30 mm Hg without symptoms of APE. In conditions of sudden onset, however, this level would cause acute manifestations.

Signs and Symptoms. In the early stages of LHF, dyspnea is exhibited when the cardiac reserve is exceeded. As fluid begins to accumulate in the PCB, the formation of interstitial edema causes a defect in oxygenation [12]. The oxygen saturation of blood decreases, causing the chemoreceptors to stimulate the respiratory center. The respiratory rate increases, at first during exercise and later even at rest.

Because of decreased cardiac output and decreased oxygen saturation of the blood, hypoxia of the body tissues occurs, which results in easy fatigue, weakness, and dizziness. Dizziness is the result of hypoxia to the brain. As failure and hypoxia worsen, disorientation, confusion, and ultimately unconsciousness can occur. Loss of potassium induced by increased levels of aldosterone also causes muscle weakness.

Inability to breathe in a supine position is called *orthopnea*. In chronic left heart failure, interstitial and alveolar pulmonary edema may be present all of the time, and the upright position is assumed so that fluid gravitates to the bases of the lungs.

Auscultation of the heart reveals an S3 gallop and a paradoxic split of the second sound on expiration. A *pulsus alternans*, characterized by alternating weaker and stronger pulsations in the peripheral arteries, often occurs and indicates a poorly functioning ventricle.

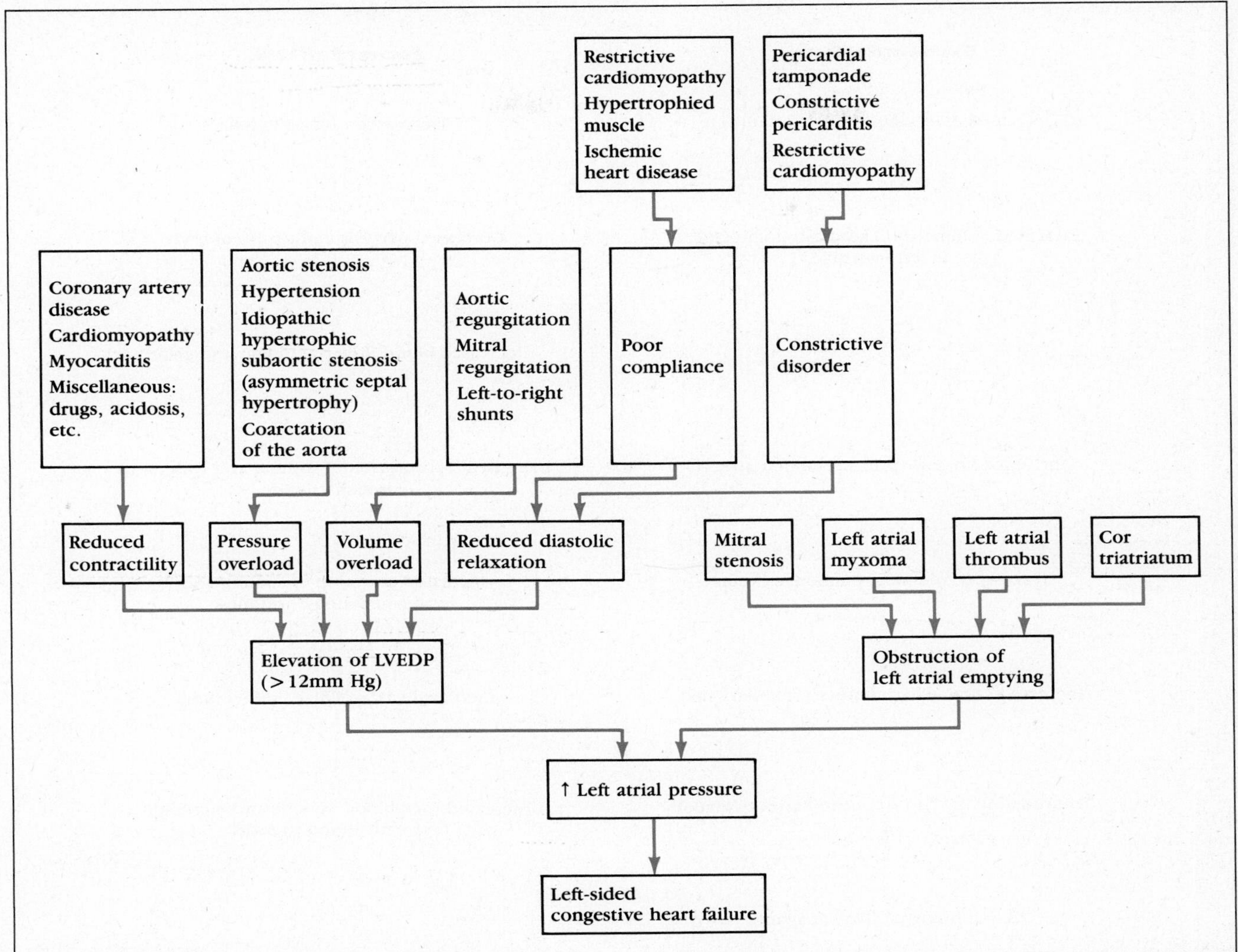

FIGURE 20-3 Various pathologic conditions may ultimately cause an elevation in left atrial pressure and thereby precipitate left-sided congestive heart failure. In general, the rise in left atrial pressure can be attributed either to mechanical obstructions that interfere with diastolic emptying of the left atrium or to those clinical syndromes that produce an elevation in left ventricular end-diastolic pressure (LVEDP). (© 1987 Scientific American, Inc. All rights reserved. From *Scientific American Medicine*, Figure 3, Section 1, Subsection II.)

Lt ♡ failure

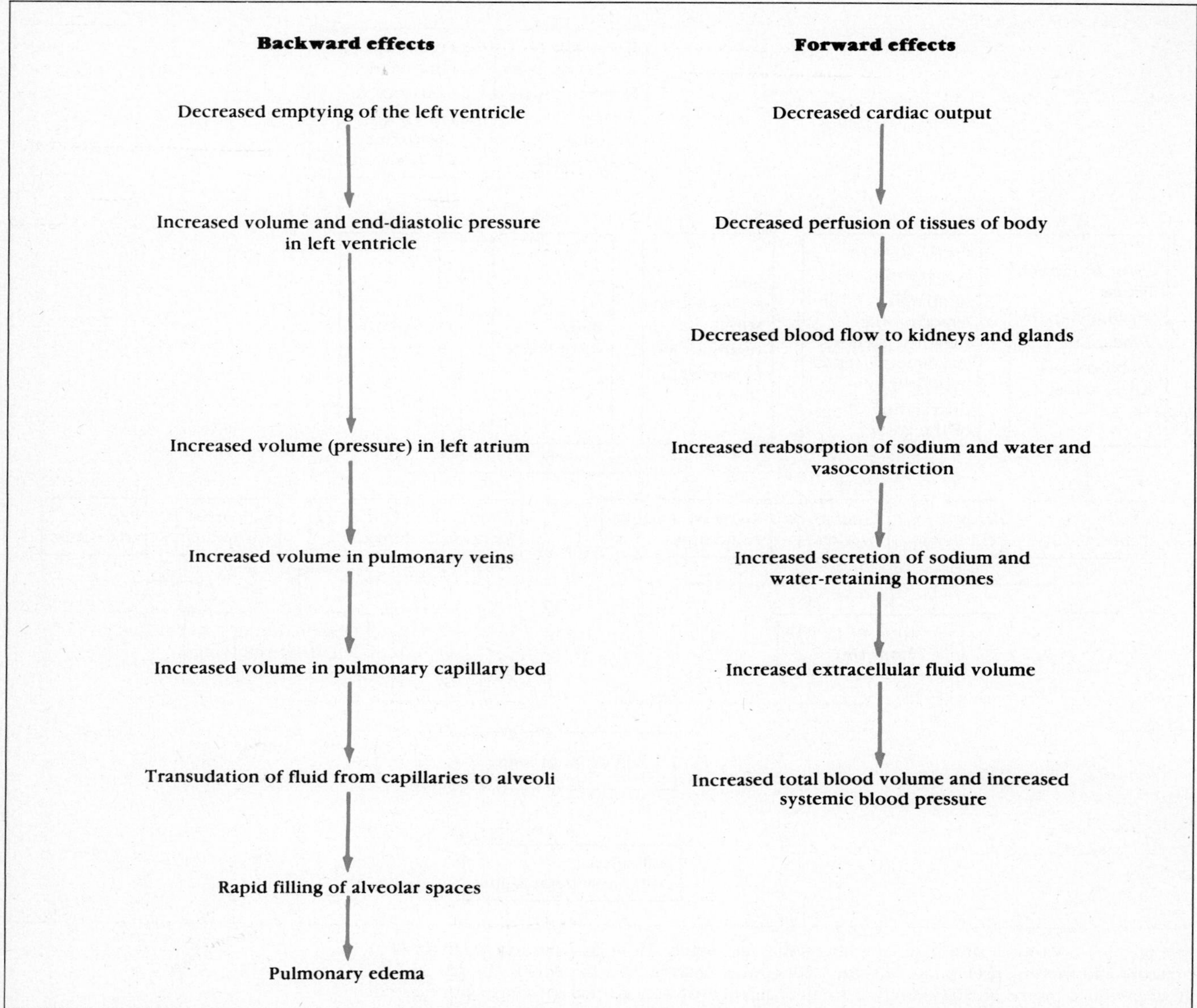

Figure 20-4 Highly schematic representation of the pathophysiology of left heart failure.

Paroxysmal nocturnal dyspnea (PND) refers to the onset of acute episodes of dyspnea at night. This condition is thought to result from improved cardiac performance at night, during recumbency. This causes increased resorption of fluid which has accumulated in the lower half of the body into the systemic circuit. The increased fluid overloads the left ventricle, causing acute pulmonary congestion until the individual assumes the orthopneic position. Acute breathlessness and a feeling of smothering are described [9].

Pulmonary edema is an acute, life-threatening condition that usually results from left heart failure and may also result from abnormal permeability of the alveolocapillary membrane. Signs and symptoms of APE include dyspnea of sudden onset, basal rales, gasping respirations, extreme anxiety, rapid weak pulse, increased venous pressure, and decreased urinary output. The skin is cool and moist to the touch, ashen-gray, or cyanotic. A cough accompanied by expectoration of frothy, pink-tinged, or bloody sputum is usually present. Most attacks gradually subside in one to three hours, but they may progress rapidly to shock and death [9].

Right Heart Failure

Right heart failure (RHF) occurs when the output of the right ventricle is less than the input from the systemic venous circuit. As a result, the systemic venous circuit is congested and output to the lungs decreases.

Causes. The major cause of RHF is LHF; the right ventricle fails because of the excessive pulmonary pressures generated by failure of the left heart. Other causes include chronic obstructive lung disease (COPD), pulmonary embolus, right ventricular infarction, and congenital heart defects, especially those that involve pulmonary overloading and pulmonary hypertension (Fig. 20-5).

Pathophysiology. In RHF the right ventricle cannot pump all of its contents forward, so blood dams back from the right ventricle to the right atrium, causing an increased pressure in the systemic venous circuit. The increased volume and pressure are transmitted to distensible organs such as the liver and spleen. Increased pressure in the peritoneal vessels leads to transudation of fluid into the peritoneal cavity. Increased pressure at the capillary line causes fluid to move into the interstitial space, and systemic edema results (Fig. 20-6). The cardinal signs of RHF are jugular venous distention, hepatomegaly, splenomegaly, and peripheral, dependent edema. These are considered the *backward*, or *congestive*, effects of RHF.

The right ventricle also cannot maintain its output to the lungs. This results in a decreased pulmonary circulation and decreased return to the left side of the heart. These *forward effects of RHF* cause all of the forward effects of LHF (see Fig. 20-6).

Signs and Symptoms. The signs and symptoms of RHF reflect both forward and backward effects. Dependent, pitting edema is characteristic and may be noted in the sternum or sacrum of a bedridden patient as well as the feet and legs of an individual in the sitting position.

Enlargement of the spleen and liver can cause pressure on surrounding organs, respiratory impingement, and organ dysfunction. Inadequate deactivation of aldosterone by the liver may lead to additional fluid retention. Jaundice and coagulation problems may result with severe, decompensated RHF. Ascites also occur when RHF is severe, and may cause respiratory embarrassment and abdominal pressure.

Jugular venous distention occurs and can be measured at the bedside. It is measured in centimeters when the head is elevated to a 30-, 45-, or a 90-degree angle (Fig. 20-7).

Diagnosis of Congestive Heart Failure

Radiologic Changes. Radiologic evidence of pulmonary congestion usually precedes the development of audible rales in LHF. Cardiac enlargement is noted by an increased size of the left ventricular shadow. The left ventricle extends past the midclavicular line, and fluid effusion may be present throughout the lung fields (Fig. 20-8). In RHF the right ventricular shadow can be seen extending out from the right sternal border. Pulmonary markings may be decreased due to decreased pulmonary circulation (Fig. 20-9) [3].

Hemodynamic Monitoring. The balloon-tipped flow-directed catheter (Swan-Ganz) is an effective monitoring system for assessing pulmonary and systemic circulations. The Swan-Ganz catheter is threaded into the pulmonary artery where it finally halts in a vessel slightly smaller than the inflated balloon tip, blocking the flow of blood from the right ventricle [10]. A pressure reading at this time reflects the diastolic pressures of the left ventricle if there is no concomitant mitral valve disease. This pulmonary artery wedge pressure (PAWP) reflects its pressures because of the continuous circuit to the left heart. Thus pressure measurements reflect the left ventricular end-diastolic pressure (LVEDP).

The end-diastolic volume (EDV), normally 70 ml per m^2 of body surface, is elevated in the failing heart. Because an increase in EDV is often associated with an increase in end-diastolic pressure (EDP), the EDP can be used as an indicator of ventricular function. The EDP of the left ventricle is usually 12 mm Hg or less and in the right ventricle 5 mm Hg or less. A high LVEDP can be the result of increased left ventricular volume or reduced left ventricular compliance, or both. In the absence of increased pulmonary vascular resistance and mitral valve disease, mean pulmonary capillary wedge pressure and pulmonary artery diastolic pressure reflect LVEDP. When the balloon tip is deflated, the catheter tip usually locates in the right or left main pulmonary artery [10]. The Swan-Ganz catheter also measures central venous pressure (right atrial pressure) and pulmonary artery pressure. Most Swan-Ganz catheters also can be used to measure cardiac output by the thermodilution method, in which a computer analyzes a temperature differential between two points on the catheter.

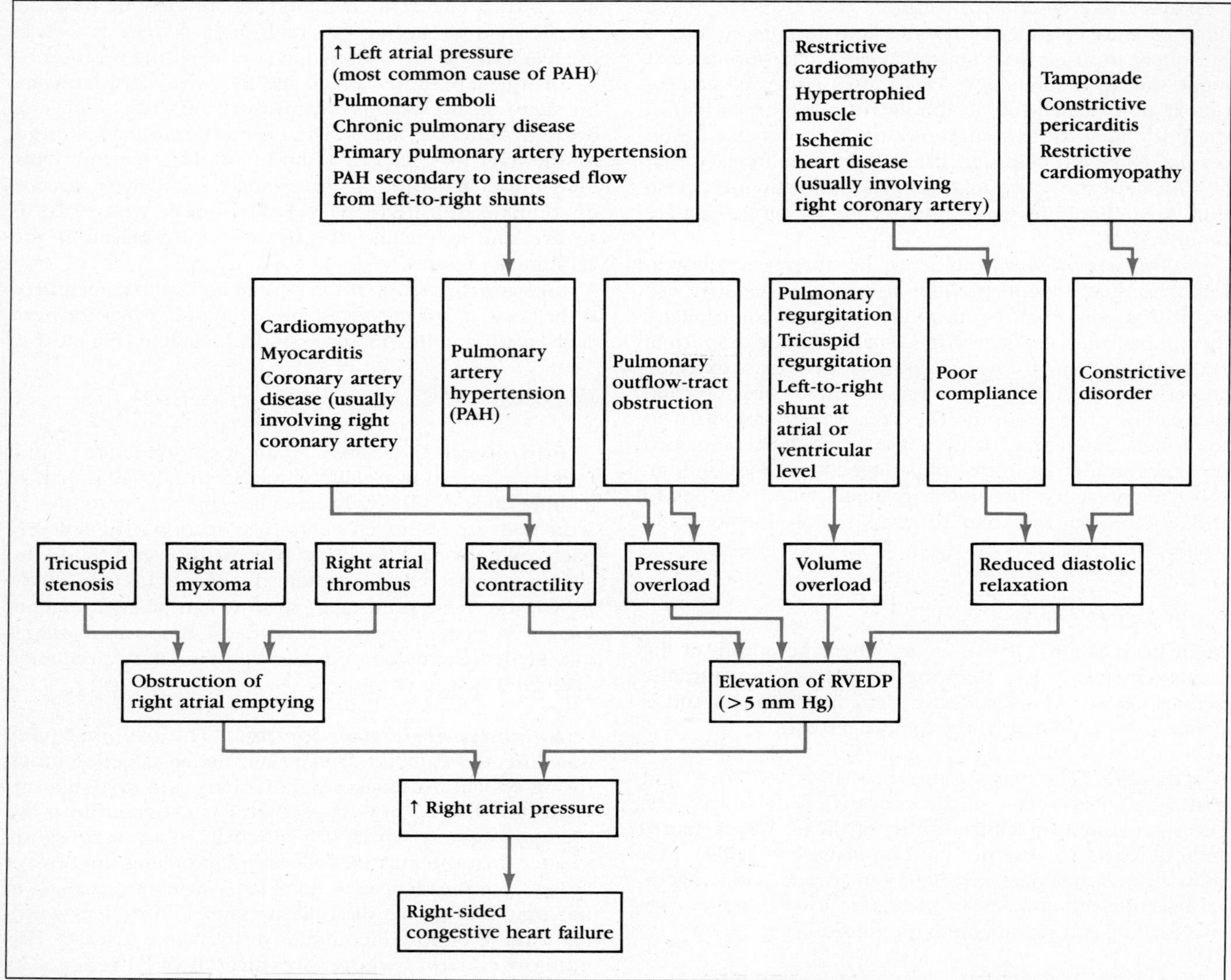

FIGURE 20-5 Various pathways may lead to an increase in right atrial pressure and consequently provoke right-sided congestive heart failure. Elevation of right atrial pressure can be induced either by mechanisms that cause an increase in the right ventricular end-diastolic pressure (RVEDP) or by lesions that obstruct blood flow from the right atrium. The most common cause of right ventricular failure is left ventricular failure, which produces a rise in left atrial pressure. This in turn leads to pulmonary artery hypertension, which imposes a pressure overload on the right ventricle and may trigger right ventricular failure. (© 1987 Scientific American, Inc. All rights reserved. From *Scientific American Medicine*, Figure 4, Section 1, Subsection II.)

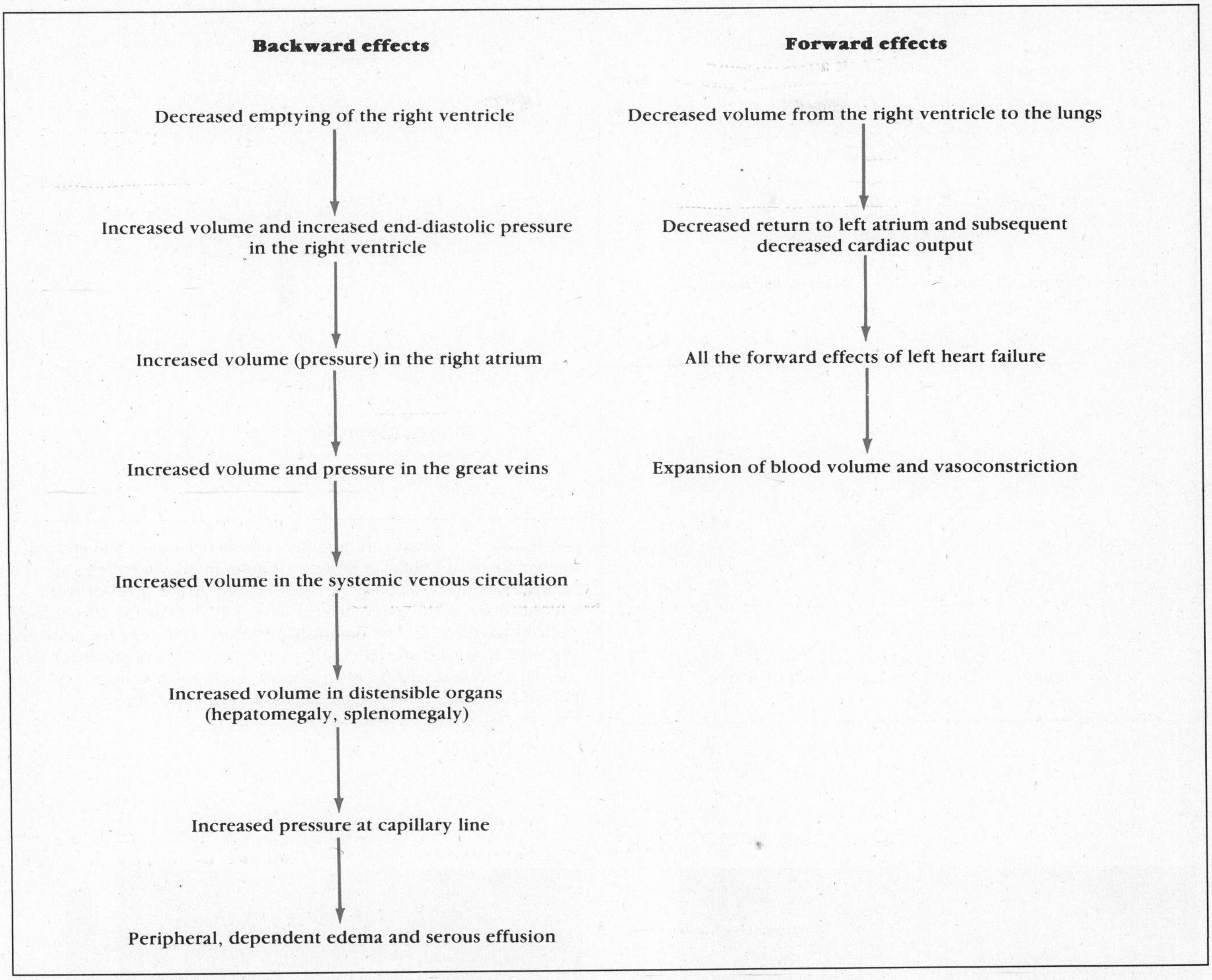

Backward effects	**Forward effects**
Decreased emptying of the right ventricle	Decreased volume from the right ventricle to the lungs
↓	↓
Increased volume and increased end-diastolic pressure in the right ventricle	Decreased return to left atrium and subsequent decreased cardiac output
↓	↓
Increased volume (pressure) in the right atrium	All the forward effects of left heart failure
↓	↓
Increased volume and pressure in the great veins	Expansion of blood volume and vasoconstriction
↓	
Increased volume in the systemic venous circulation	
↓	
Increased volume in distensible organs (hepatomegaly, splenomegaly)	
↓	
Increased pressure at capillary line	
↓	
Peripheral, dependent edema and serous effusion	

FIGURE 20-6 Highly schematic illustration of the pathophysiology of right heart failure.

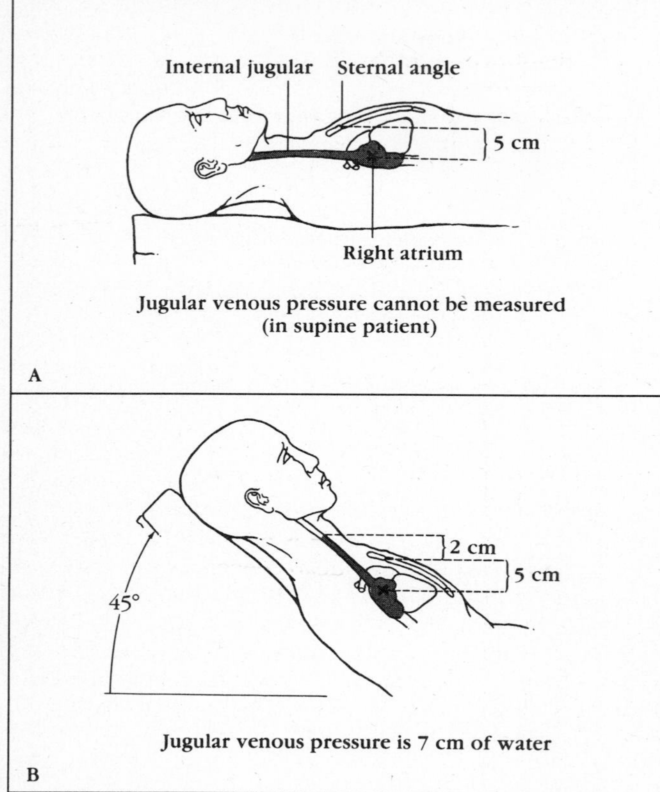

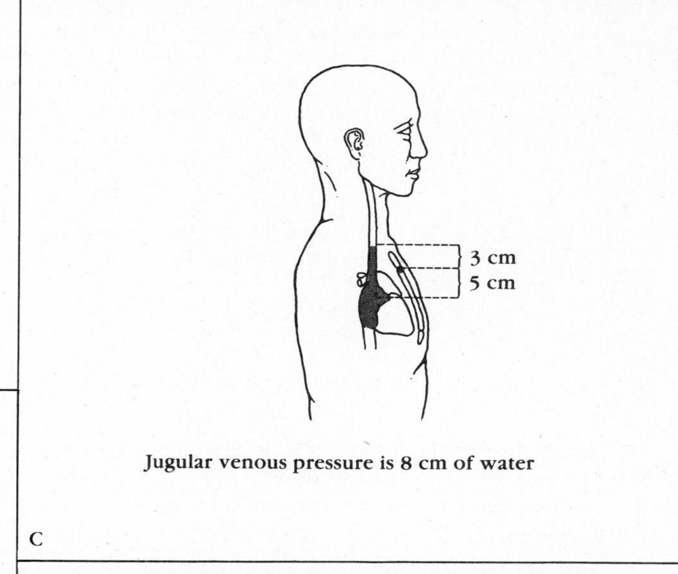

FIGURE 20-7 Measuring jugular venous pressure. The sternal angle (angle of Louis) is a bony ridge palpable between the manubrium and the body of the sternum at the level of the second intercostal space. It is always 5 cm vertically above the midright atrium. In any position therefore, one may measure the distance from the sternal angle to the meniscus of the internal jugular vein and add 5 cm to obtain the jugular venous pressure. (From R. Judge, G. Zuidema, and F. Fitzgerald, *Clinical Diagnosis*. Boston: Little, Brown, 1982.)

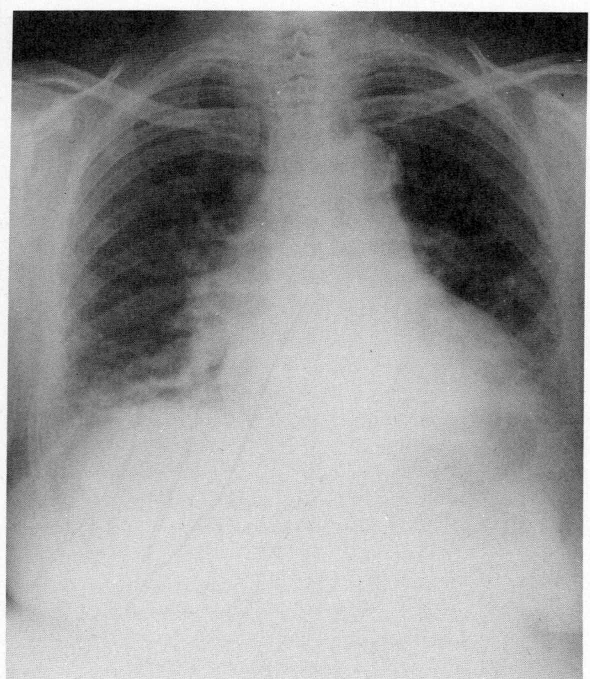

FIGURE 20-8 Radiologic changes in LHF. Note left ventricular enlargement and fluid effusion in lung fields.

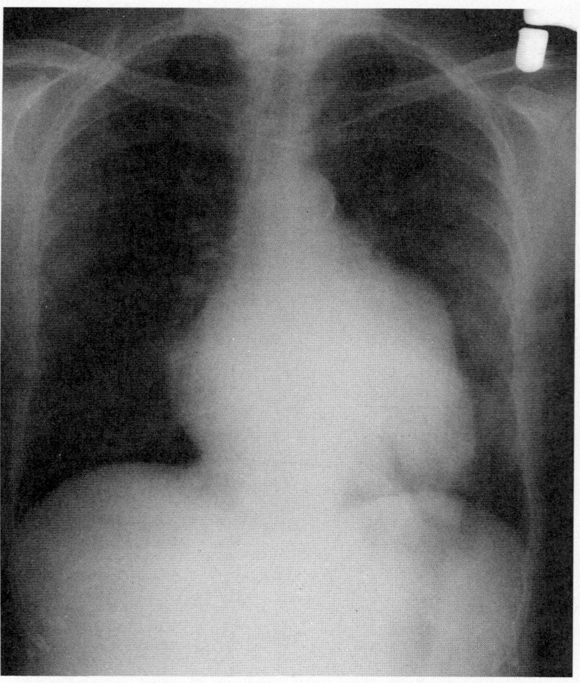

FIGURE 20-9 Radiologic changes in RHF. Note right ventricular shadow extending out from the right sternal border.

The normal cardiac output is approximately 4 to 8 liters per minute. The level of decreased cardiac output in persons with CHF helps to determine the necessary treatment. Levels of 2.2 to 3.0 liters per minute or below may indicate cardiogenic shock depending on the size and age of the individual.

Arterial Blood Gases. The normal arterial and venous blood gases are presented in Table 20-2. Hypoxemia (decreased partial pressure of oxygen, or PO_2) is often the only change that is noted with CHF. Oxygen saturation often remains normal until decompensation is severe. The partial pressure of carbon dioxide (PCO_2) may be low due to hyperventilation. In endstage CHF the PCO_2 may be elevated.

Other Laboratory Tests. *Serum sodium* levels are often low in CHF even though body sodium levels are almost always elevated. This lab picture results from the retention of sodium and water described on pp. 79–81. *Serum potassium* may be decreased due to the aldosterone effect and potassium-depleting diuretics (see Chap. 5).

Cardiogenic Shock

Causes of Cardiogenic Shock

Heart failure may lead to cardiogenic shock with a low-output component and/or the congestive phenomena. The most common cause of cardiogenic shock is myocardial infarction, but cardiomyopathy, dysrhythmias, cardiac tamponade, pulmonary embolism, or any factor that can depress myocardial function may precipitate this syndrome.

Cardiogenic shock always carries a grave prognosis. If it develops after myocardial infarction (MI), mortality is approximately 60 to 80 percent, which correlates well with the amount of ventricular mass lost. A 30 to 40 percent loss of left ventricular mass by infarctions, both new and old, is often correlated with cardiogenic shock [2].

Pathophysiology of Cardiogenic Shock

Cardiogenic shock results from decreased ability of the left or right ventricle to maintain adequate cardiac output. This results in decreased systolic blood pressure, with reduced peripheral perfusion manifested by cold, clammy skin, diaphoresis, tachycardia, mental confusion, and decreased urinary output. The cold, clammy skin and tachycardia result from sympathetic stimulation. The effects of SNS stimulation increase the taxation on an already overtaxed heart but enhance cerebral and coronary blood flow.

Anaerobic metabolism begins in peripheral cells as vital oxygen deprivation occurs. The effect of this energy production is to keep cells viable, but the production of lactic acid as a byproduct can lead to metabolic acidosis (see Chap. 6).

Cardiogenic shock is often described in stages. If the compensatory mechanisms can restore arterial pressure and urinary output, it is termed *compensated shock*. If the underlying cause of the shock is not corrected, the response of the body to poor tissue perfusion results in continuation of the shock state, which is called *progressive shock*. When arteriolar tone is finally destroyed and peripheral pooling occurs, death becomes inevitable; this condition is called *irreversible* or *decompensated shock*. Pooling is enhanced by loss of arteriolar tone prior to loss of venular tone, which encourages fluid movement into the interstitial spaces. Anaerobic energy production and lactic acidosis eventually cause cellular failure and death [6].

TABLE 20-2 Arterial and Venous Blood Gas Studies (Normal values in healthy adults)

	Arterial Blood	Mixed Venous Blood
pH	7.40[a] (7.35–7.45)	7.36[a] (7.30–7.41)
PO_2	80–100 mm Hg	35–40 mm Hg
O_2Sa	95%	70–75%
PCO_2	35–45 mm Hg	41–51 mm Hg
HCO_3	22–26 mEq/L	22–26 mEq/L
Base excess	−2–+2	−2–+2

[a] Mean.

Diagnosis of Cardiogenic Shock

Diagnosis of cardiogenic shock is often one of exclusion. Sometimes hypovolemic shock must be ruled out. Physical examination reveals gallop rhythms, sometimes venous engorgement, and effects of acute hypotension. The ECG often shows cardiac dysrhythmias and evidence of myocardial infarction. The Swan-Ganz catheter reveals elevated pulmonary wedge pressures and decreased cardiac output.

Diseases Affecting Myocardial Contractility

The word *cardiomyopathy* refers to a group of myocardial diseases that primarily affect the pumping ability of the heart (Table 20-3). *Myocarditis* is the word used for myocardial disease associated with inflammation of the myocardium.

Cardiomyopathy

Primary or idiopathic myocardial disease refers to conditions affecting the ventricular muscle that have no known origin. *Secondary* cardiomyopathy designates conditions in which the causative factors are known. The cardiomyopathies have been classified as congestive, restrictive, and hypertrophic [11].

Congestive or Dilated Cardiomyopathy. Congestive or dilated cardiomyopathy is usually of unknown etiology, but it has been described in association with beriberi, thyrotoxicosis, alcoholism, childbirth or the postpartum period, diabetes mellitus, drug toxicity (especially

TABLE 20-3 Morphologic and Hemodynamic Characteristics of the Cardiomyopathies

	Dilated (congestive)	Hypertrophic	Restrictive
Morphologic	Biventricular dilatation	Marked hypertrophy of left ventricle, occasionally also of right ventricle, and usually but not always, disproportionate hypertrophy of septum	Reduced ventricular compliance; usually caused by infiltration of myocardium (e.g., by amyloid, hemosiderin, or glycogen deposits)
Hemodynamic			
Cardiac output	↓ ↓	Normal	Normal to ↓
Stroke volume	↓ ↓	Normal or ↑	Normal or ↓
Ventricular filling pressure	↑ ↑	Normal or ↑	↑ ↑
Chamber size	↑ ↑	Normal or ↓	Normal or ↑
Ejection fraction	↓ ↓	↑ ↑	Normal to ↓
Other findings	May have associated functional mitral or tricuspid regurgitation.	Obstruction may develop between interventricular septum and septal leaflet of mitral valve. Mitral regurgitation may be present.	Characteristic ventricular pressure tracings resemble those recorded in constrictive pericarditis, with early diastolic dip-and-plateau configuration.

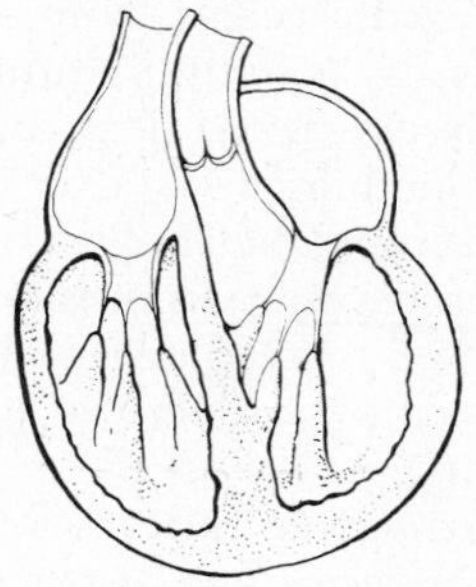

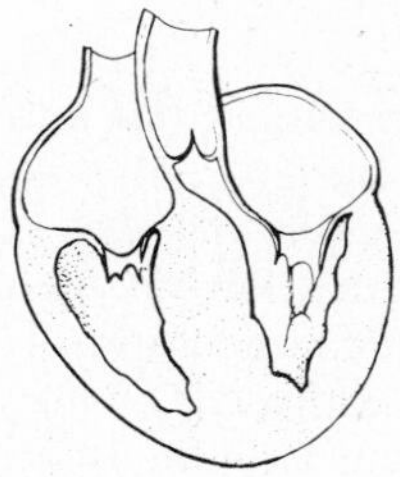

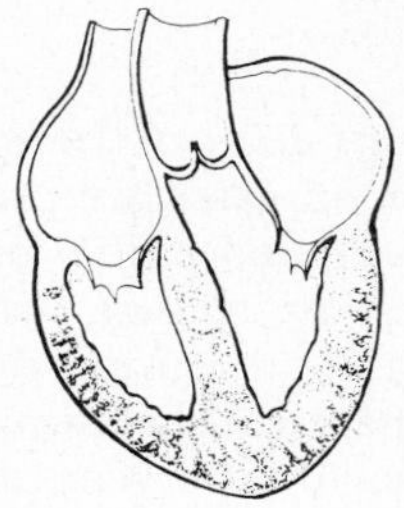

Source: From *Scientific American Medicine*, Table 1, Section 1, Subsection XIV.

from daunorubicin), cobalt therapy, and certain neuromuscular disorders. The striking effect of this type of cardiomyopathy is immense cardiomegaly. The enlargement is a combination of dilatation and hypertrophy of the heart. This dilatation leads to a hypokinetic myocardium with the usual onset of biventricular CHF. Symptoms include exertional dyspnea, fatigue, paroxysmal nocturnal dyspnea, and pulmonary edema with symptoms of RHF late in the course of the disease. Atrial and ventricular gallops may be noted on auscultation. Peripheral edema and hepatomegaly are signs of RHF.

Restrictive Cardiomyopathy. Restrictive cardiomyopathy describes the clinical picture of constrictive pericarditis, the underlying cause of which is actually myocardial. The etiology is generally unknown, but it has been described in association with such diverse conditions as amyloidosis, hemosiderosis, and glycogen storage disease. The myocardial muscle becomes infiltrated with abnormal substances that apparently cause dysfunction of the ventricle.

Congestive and restrictive cardiomyopathies are mostly differentiated on the basis of the presence or absence of cardiomegaly. Symptoms of biventricular failure are common. Ventricular filling is impeded and the end-diastolic pressure of the ventricles usually becomes exceedingly high. The prognosis for survival is poor, and death often results from CHF.

Hypertrophic Cardiomyopathy. Hypertrophic cardiomyopathy usually refers to an asymmetric increase in ventricular muscle mass. It has also been termed *idiopathic hypertrophic subaortic stenosis* (IHSS) and *hypertrophic obstructive cardiomyopathy*.

The etiology of this condition is unknown. Familial occurrence is noted, with no predominance for one sex or another. Certain studies support a prenatal disorder of myocardial development [4]. The pathologic features include greater hypertrophy of the ventricular septum than of the ventricular chambers. Small or normal ventricular chamber size and disorganization of septal muscle cells, especially of the myofibrils, may occur.

Other significant abnormalities associated with this condition include fibrous plaque on the endocardium, abnormal septal arteries, and mitral valve insufficiency [10].

Because of the septal hypertrophy, the left ventricular cavity is misshapen and, on contraction, the hypertrophied septum causes obstruction to the flow of blood from the ventricle. Any condition that enhances contractility increases the degree of obstruction. The associated left ventricular hypertrophy causes impairment of ventricular filling during diastole and reduced ventricular compliance [5].

The signs and symptoms are mainly those of LHF, including exertional dyspnea, angina, periods of syncope, and orthopnea. Right-sided effects occur later in the course of the disease.

Myocarditis

Inflammation of the myocardium may result from an infectious process or from radiation therapy or chemical agents. Viruses, especially the coxsackieviruses, have been implicated in the etiology. Myocarditis is often a self-limiting condition that is manifested by tachycardia, symptoms of heart failure, and gallop rhythm or auscultation. Many types of myocarditis resolve with bedrest, fluid restriction, and limited drug therapy. In a small percentage of affected persons, the disease is progressive and leads to all of the manifestations of dilated, congestive myocardiopathy.

Study Questions

1. Explain why the compensatory mechanisms activated in heart failure are a positive feedback system.
2. Describe the differences between the underlying causative factors in left and right heart failure. How do they interact?
3. Discuss the changes in preload and afterload encountered with conditions that can precipitate heart failure.
4. Diagram the sequence of events from compensated to irreversible heart failure.
5. Discuss the significance of cardiogenic shock.
6. Which tests are most helpful in diagnosing congestive heart failure?
7. Compare the major classifications of cardiomyopathies on the basis of underlying pathology and clinical course.

References

1. Guyton, A.C. *Textbook of Medical Physiology* (7th ed.). Philadelphia: Saunders, 1986.
2. Houston, M.C., Thompson, W.L., and Robertson, D. Shock: Diagnosis and management. *Arch. Intern. Med.* 144:1433, 1984.
3. Lorell, B., and DeSanctis, R.W. Right ventricular infarction. *Primary Cardiol.* 4:117, 1981.
4. Manasek, F.J. Histogenesis of the embryonic myocardium. *Am. J. Cardiol.* 25:149, 1970.
5. Martin, L.B., and Cohen, L.S. Cardiomyopathy. *D.M.* 28:13, 1981.
6. Messer, J.V. Cardiogenic shock: Etiological and pathophysiological considerations, monitoring and management. *Cardiol. Pract.* 86:283, 1978.
7. Robbins, S.L., Cotran, R.S., and Kumar, V. *Pathologic Basis of Disease* (3rd ed.). Philadelphia: Saunders, 1984.
8. Schlant, R.C., and Sonnerblick, E.H. Pathophysiology of heart failure. In J.W. Hurst et al. (eds.), *The Heart* (6th ed.). New York: McGraw-Hill, 1986.
9. Sokolow, M., and McIlroy, M.B. *Clinical Cardiology* (4th ed.), Los Altos, Calif.: Lange, 1986.
10. Swan, H.J. Techniques of monitoring the seriously ill patient. In J.W. Hurst et al. (eds.), *The Heart* (6th ed.). New York: McGraw-Hill, 1986.
11. Wenger, N.K., Goodwin, J.F., and Roberts, W.C. Cardiomyopathy. In J.W. Hurst et al. (eds.), *The Heart* (6th ed.). New York: McGraw-Hill, 1986.
12. Wallace, A.G., and Waugh, R.A. Pathophysiology of cardiovascular diseases. In L.H. Smith and S.O. Thier, *Pathophysiology: The Biological Principles of Disease* (2nd ed.). Philadelphia: Saunders, 1985.
13. Wasserman, K. Dyspnea on exertion: Is it the heart or lungs? *JAMA* 248:2039, 1982.

CHAPTER 21

Alterations in Specific Structures in the Heart

CHAPTER OUTLINE

Coronary Artery Disease: Ischemic Heart Disease

Pathogenesis of Coronary Artery Disease
Angina Pectoris or Myocardial Ischemia
Clinical Manifestations
Diagnostic Tests
Exercise ECG or Graded Exercise Test (GXT)
Nuclear Cardiology
Coronary Arteriography
Unstable or Preinfarctional Angina
Myocardial Infarction
Pathophysiology
Diagnostic Tests
Myocardial Infarction Imaging
Complications of Myocardial Infarction

Valvular Disease

Diagnostic Tests
Chest Radiography
Electrocardiography
Echocardiography
Cardiac Catheterization
Acute Rheumatic Fever: A Major Cause of Valvular Disease
Pathophysiology
Clinical Manifestations
Mitral Stenosis
Pathophysiology and Compensatory Mechanisms
Clinical Manifestations
Diagnostic Tests
Course and Complications
Mitral Regurgitation or Insufficiency
Pathophysiology and Compensatory Mechanisms
Clinical Manifestations
Diagnostic Tests
Course and Complications
Mixed Mitral Stenosis and Regurgitation
Diagnostic Tests
Mitral Valve Prolapse
Aortic Stenosis
Pathophysiology and Compensatory Mechanisms
Clinical Manifestations
Diagnostic Tests
Aortic Regurgitation, Insufficiency, or Incompetence
Pathophysiology and Compensatory Mechanisms
Clinical Manifestations
Mixed Aortic Stenosis and Regurgitation

Infective Endocarditis

Pericarditis

Congenital Heart Disease

Embryology
Consequences of Congenital Heart Disease
Left-to-Right Shunt
Right-to-Left Shunt
Patent Ductus Arteriosus
Atrial Septal Defects
Ventricular Septal Defects
Tetralogy of Fallot
Transposition of the Great Vessels
Coarctation of the Aorta
Other Defects

LEARNING OBJECTIVES

1. Describe the following diagnostic procedures: coronary arteriogram, thallium scan, exercise ECG, multigated blood pool scan, cardiac catheterization, and echocardiography.
2. Differentiate the pathologic and clinical manifestations of angina and myocardial infarction.
3. Describe the development of an atherosclerotic plaque in a coronary artery.
4. Identify the most common sites of coronary artery lesions.
5. List the risk factors for coronary atherogenesis.
6. Describe the process of healing after a myocardial infarction.
7. List and explain the significance of the characteristic ECG changes of angina and myocardial infarction.
8. Describe briefly why heart pain occurs and why it radiates to other areas.
9. Explain how a myocardial infarction impairs myocardial contractility.
10. Differentiate the significant changes of *each* of the cardiac enzymes.
11. Describe at least four common complications of myocardial infarction.
12. Relate the pathophysiologic consequences of acute rheumatic fever to chronic valvular disease.
13. State the major pathophysiology and compensatory mechanisms that are used in mitral stenosis, mitral insufficiency, mitral valve prolapse, aortic stenosis, and aortic regurgitation.
14. Describe the clinical manifestations of mitral stenosis, mitral insufficiency, mitral valve prolapse, aortic stenosis, and aortic regurgitation.
15. Describe how pulmonary hypertension can develop from mitral stenosis.
16. Describe briefly the major characteristics of cardiac murmurs produced by valvular defects.
17. Identify the pathophysiologic alterations in and clinical manifestations of infective endocarditis.
18. State the pathophysiologic alterations in and clinical manifestations of pericarditis.
19. Describe the embryologic events leading to cardiac structure.
20. Differentiate the consequences of left-to-right and right-to-left shunts.
21. Identify the pathophysiologic results of these common congenital defects: patent ductus arteriosus, atrial and ventricular septal defects, tetralogy of Fallot, transposition of the great vessels, and coarctation of the aorta.

Coronary Artery Disease: Ischemic Heart Disease

Atherosclerosis of the coronary arteries is the leading cause of coronary artery disease in the United States. Although the mortality from ischemic heart disease (IHD) has declined about 25 percent since the late 1960s, it is still the cause of one-third to one-half of all deaths in the United States [21]. Improved mortality figures may reflect widespread application of cardiopulmonary resuscitation, better medical control of emergencies, control of hypertension, lower-cholesterol diets, or numerous other factors [25].

There are numerous theories of the pathogenesis of atherosclerosis, most agreeing that it begins early in life and progresses over a period of decades (see Chap. 23). Many factors probably interact to accelerate the atherogenic process. These have been identified as risk factors in epidemiologic studies since they seem to reflect an increase in the probability of a person developing coronary atherosclerosis but do not predict the severity or extent of an atherosclerotic lesion [25].

The risk factors that cannot be altered include age, sex, race, and genetic heritage. Susceptibility to coronary artery disease (CAD) increases with age; especially noted is the protection of women from the disease during the childbearing years. After the menopausal years, women become as susceptible as men to atherosclerosis of the coronary arteries. The likelihood of premature atherosclerotic heart disease is increased in persons who have a positive family history and in those afflicted with diabetes mellitus.

Risk factors that can be altered by lifestyle changes include (1) elevated levels of dietary serum lipids, (2) hypertension, (3) cigarette smoking, (4) diets high in saturated fats, (5) sedentary lifestyle, (6) stressful lifestyle, and (7) obesity. Dietary intake and exercise has been extensively studied with apparent alteration of the serum lipoproteins. The risk of coronary heart disease has been shown to decrease as the cholesterol level decreases. Athletic individuals often have high blood levels of cholesterol of the high density type, called high density lipoprotein or HDL. As illustrated in Figure 21-1, increased HDL levels correspond with a decrease in the risk of coronary heart disease. Therefore, modifying all of the risk factors has the potential of retarding the atherogenic process. A considerable time lag exists between the occurrence of pathologic coronary artery narrowing and the appearance of symptomatic disease. During this latent period, modification of risk factors can have a preventive effect.

Geographic differences seem markedly to affect the predisposition to CAD. For example, in men between ages

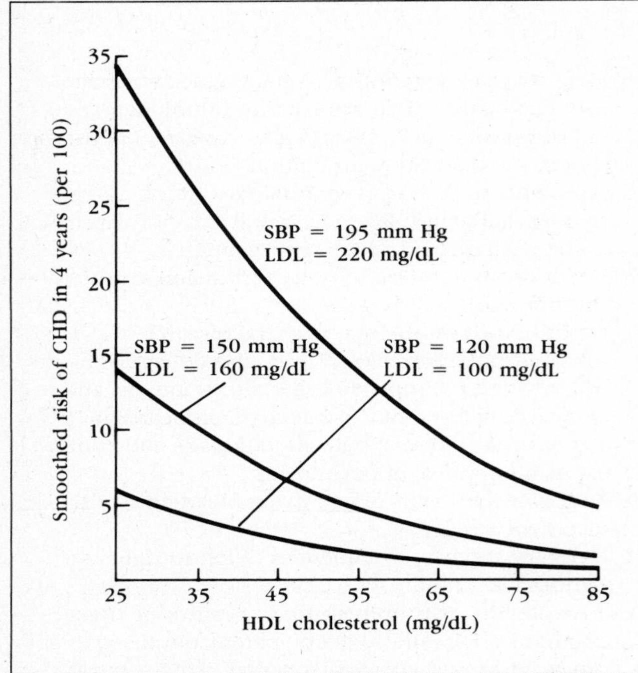

FIGURE 21-1 Risk of coronary heart disease according to levels of high-density lipoprotein cholesterol in 55-year-old men. Framingham study 24-year follow-up. CHD = coronary heart disease; SBP = systolic blood pressure; LDL = low-density lipoprotein; HDL = high-density lipoprotein. (Reproduced with permission from W.B. Kannel, W.P. Castelli, and T. Gordon, Cholesterol in the prediction of atherosclerotic disease. *Ann. Intern. Med.;* 90:85, 1979.)

35 and 64 years, the mortality for myocardial infarction is 4 to 5 times higher in the United States than in Japan [19]. The effect of the geographic differences appears to be environmental rather than genetic. Perhaps differences in diet, physical activity, and lifestyle are determinative of frequency.

Pathogenesis of Coronary Artery Disease

The lesions of coronary atherosclerosis develop progressively in much the same manner as those of atherosclerosis of the other major arteries (see Chap. 23). The initial change occurs early in life and consists of a fatty streak that may develop into a fibrous plaque or atheroma. This atheromatous plaque is white, becomes elevated, and partially occludes the lumen of the artery. The core of the plaque becomes necrotic, and hemorrhage and calcification may result. Thrombosis on or around the plaque may also occur, partially or completely occluding the lumen of the vessel (Fig. 21-2).

Lesions do not usually cause symptoms until the atherosclerotic process is well advanced, occluding 60 percent or more of the vascular supply to an area. Sometimes total occlusion of a vessel does not cause ischemia to a supplied area because of the development of collateral circulation.

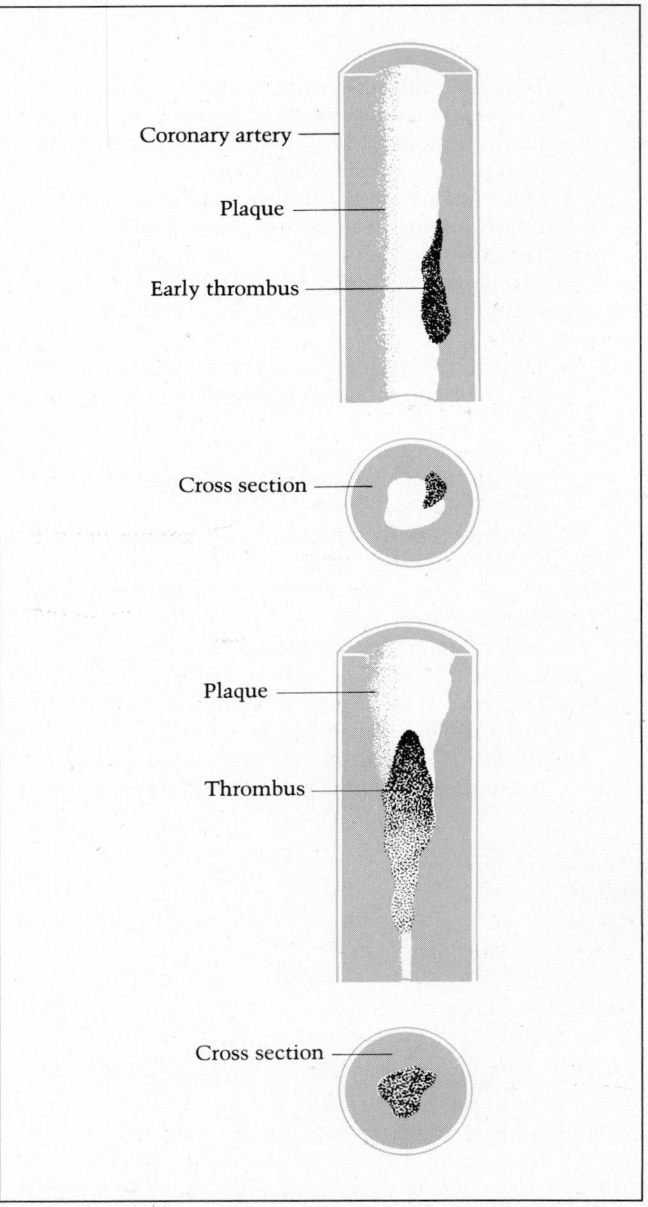

FIGURE 21-2 The arterial thrombus most frequently begins at areas of luminal narrowing caused by atherosclerotic plaques. The chief components are platelets, followed by platelets and fibrin. (From C. Kenner, C. Guzzetta, and B. Dossey, *Critical Care Nursing: Body, Mind, Spirit*. Boston: Little, Brown, 1981.)

Atherosclerotic plaques tend to appear at bifurcations, curvatures, and tapering areas of arteries. The right and left main coronary arteries branch sharply off the aorta and thus become a prime target for the development of atheromas. The vessels then bifurcate and taper rapidly so that these areas also can become affected quickly.

As the coronary artery lumen narrows with increasing plaque formation, resistance to blood flow increases and myocardial muscle blood supply is compromised. As was noted in Chapter 18, normal myocardial oxygen uptake is quite efficient, taking 60 to 75 percent of the oxygen supplied for use by myocardial muscle. As the amount of blood flow through the vessel decreases, oxygen uptake cannot increase significantly, resulting in compromise of the oxygen supply to the tissues. When this compromise causes myocardial ischemia, angina pectoris results. Further compromise or lack of blood supply may cause necrosis of the myocardial muscle.

A considerable latent period usually exists between the onset of arterial lumen narrowing and symptomatic disease. This can be two to four decades, with symptoms beginning when the lumen is obstructed over 75 percent. The final event that produces infarction may be sudden and involve hemorrhage into an atherosclerotic plaque, thrombosis on an established plaque, or coronary artery spasm.

Angina Pectoris or Myocardial Ischemia

Myocardial ischemia is manifested by angina pectoris, which is a squeezing, substernal pain described as a feeling of tightness or fullness. The pain results from an imbalance between myocardial oxygen supply and demand. In other words, insufficient oxygen is supplied to the myocardial cell for it to function effectively. This condition is almost always related to atherosclerotic narrowing of the coronary arteries. Ischemia suggests, however, that the changes are reversible and cellular function can be restored with restoration of oxygen to the affected muscle. Anaerobic metabolism is used to produce adenosine triphosphate (ATP) during oxygen insufficiency, but the resulting accumulation of lactic acid impairs left ventricular function. This results in decreased strength of cardiac contraction and impaired wall motion. The degree of impairment depends on the size of the ischemic area and the general contractility of the left ventricular myocardium. Depression of left ventricular function may lead to decreased stroke volume and changes in systemic blood pressure.

The heart is unique in that it can be manipulated or operated on without pain; however, ischemia of cardiac muscle causes intense pain. The cause of this pain is not known, but ischemic myocardial muscle releases acidic substances (lactic acid) that may then stimulate the nerve endings in the muscle, conducting pain through the sympathetic nerves to the middle cervical ganglia and through the thoracic ganglia to the spinal cord. The referred nature of the pain (to the left or right arm or neck) probably has to do with interconnections in the sympathetic nerves. These nerve fibers enter the cord all the way from C3 to T5 [11]. When ischemia is very severe, cardiac pain may be described as crushing and substernal. The source of pain also is not entirely understood, but may be from sensory nerve endings from the heart to the pericardium that reflect pain sensation to the great vessels [11].

The ischemic episodes causing the chest pain of angina pectoris usually subside in minutes if the imbalance is corrected. Ischemia is totally reversible, and a return to normal metabolic, functional, and hemodynamic balance occurs.

Clinical Manifestations. The clinical features of angina pectoris are related to the pain and the person's physiologic response to it. Anginal pain is typically described as substernal, a feeling of tightness or fullness, or oppression. It may radiate down one or both arms or into the neck and jaws. Characteristically, the person becomes immobile and also may exhibit pallor, profuse perspiration, and dyspnea. The dyspnea may be a compensatory result of temporary cardiac failure induced by left ventricular hypokinesis (see Chap. 20).

Classically, angina is precipitated by activity (physical or emotional stress) and is relieved within minutes by rest or the administration of a coronary vasodilator such as nitroglycerin. During the anginal attack, typical electrocardiographic (ECG) changes occur, including T wave inversion and ST segment depression (Fig. 21-3). It also indicates the artery involved and, to some extent, the amount of myocardium in jeopardy (Table 21-1). Approximately 50 to 70 percent of persons with angina pectoris who have had no previous myocardial infarction have a normal resting ECG. Levels of cardiac enzymes in blood drawn during or after an anginal attack are usually normal.

Diagnostic Tests. The ECG, cardiac enzymes, and other routine tests may be performed to differentiate angina pectoris from a myocardial infarction. Other tests are also used for differential diagnosis and to determine the degree of cardiac impairment. These include the exercise ECG, myocardial imaging, and cardiac catheterization with a coronary arteriogram. Establishing that the cause of chest pain is angina rather than another condition is extremely important. Major therapeutic decisions depend on the diagnosis.

Exercise ECG or Graded Exercise Test (GXT). The exercise test with a treadmill or stationary bicycle allows for the evaluation of exercise-induced symptoms and electrocardiographic changes. Exercise-induced ST segment displacement is the only reliable ECG change of diagnostic significance in myocardial ischemia [3]. Exercise is conducted according to a controlled program so that the heart rate increases progressively, or until 85 percent of the individual's maximum heart rate is achieved.

Exercise testing helps to evaluate the severity of CAD. For example, a person who becomes hypotensive with marked ST abnormalities during exercise has a poorer prognosis than one who maintains a good cardiac output with less significant ST changes. Exercise testing may be

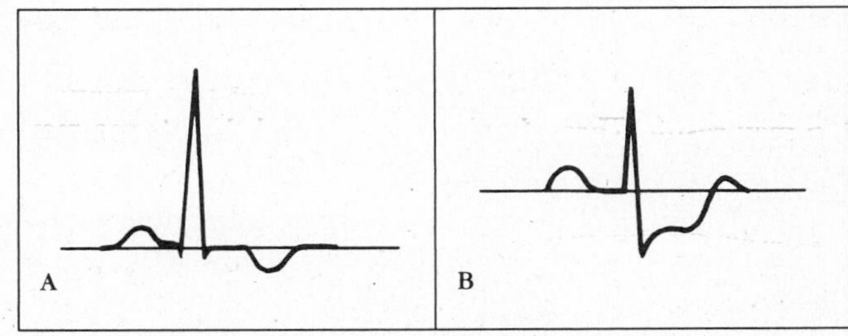

FIGURE 21-3 A. Inversion of T wave. B. Depression of ST segment.

TABLE 21-1 Correlation Between ECG Location of Ischemic Changes and Area of Myocardium and Coronary Artery Involved

ECG Leads Reflecting Ischemic Changes	Area of Myocardium Involved	Coronary Artery
II, III, aV_F	Inferior	Right coronary artery
V_1, V_2 (reciprocal changes)	Posterior	Right coronary artery
V_2–V_4	Anteroseptal	Left anterior descending branch of left coronary artery
V_3–V_5	Anterior	Left anterior descending branch of left coronary artery
I, aV_L	High lateral	Marginal branch of circumflex artery or diagonal branch of left coronary artery
V_5, V_6	Apical	Usually left anterior descending branch of left coronary artery; may be posterior descending branch of right coronary artery

Source: © 1987 Scientific American, Inc. All rights reserved. From *Scientific American Medicine,* Table 2, Section 1, Subsection IX.

used to screen apparently healthy individuals. A 10 to 15 percent greater risk of heart attack than in the general population is reported for persons who have abnormal results of exercise tests.

Nuclear Cardiology. These techniques detect, define, and quantify irradiation that emanates from cardiac structures in order to determine myocardial metabolism, perfusion, and viability [26]. The procedures are basically noninvasive and involve the injection of short-lived radionuclides.

One of the more common procedures uses thallium 201 radionuclide tracer. This substance is able to substitute for ionic potassium so that it rapidly accumulates in viable myocardial cells [26]. The nuclear camera records an image of thallium distribution in the myocardium after injection of the tracer. Thallium may be injected at peak exercise or at rest. With normal myocardial perfusion, the radioisotope is distributed equally throughout the myocardium. If coronary blood flow is significantly decreased, thallium fails to localize in that segment of the myocardium. This is called a *perfusion defect*, or *cold spot*, which is a negative image. Positioning of the individual is crucial in localizing defects, especially if the areas affected are small.

Multigated blood pool imaging supplies information about size, contraction pattern, and ejection fraction of the left ventricle. Stress-induced abnormalities of wall motion can be detected by echocardiography and cardiokymography [16,20]. Cardiokymography is a noninvasive electronic device that shows changes in wall motion by picking up fluctuations of an electromagnetic field induced by the motion [20].

Coronary Arteriography. The coronary arteriogram is the most specific test for diagnosing the presence, location, and extent of coronary artery atherosclerosis. The procedure involves injecting a radiopaque substance into each coronary artery, followed by sequential radiographs of up to 12 per second. In cineangiography, dye is injected and its movement through the vessels is followed. The picture obtained usually is more detailed than that with cinematography, but cinematography provides a dynamic picture. The arteriogram reveals (1) the location of lesions, (2) the degree of obstruction, (3) status of vessels distant to a point of obstruction, and (4) the presence of collateral circulation. The decision to perform coronary artery bypass surgery is usually made on the basis of the results of coronary arteriograms.

Stenosis is commonly graded as (1) normal, (2) less than 50 percent reduction, (3) 50 to 74 percent reduction, (4) 90 percent reduction, (5) greater than 90 percent reduction, and (6) total obstruction [9]. Because of differences in techniques, *cross-sectional reduction* (the measurements indicated above) is not equivalent to the *diameter method* of classification, so that choice of method is crucial in interpreting results of the test.

During coronary arteriography, contrast material can also be injected into the left ventricle. This permits visualization of left ventricular wall motion and chamber size. Pressure readings and oxygen saturations also give valuable information.

Unstable or Preinfarctional Angina

As atherosclerotic disease progresses in the coronary arteries, symptoms of pain may become more severe and occur with increasing frequency. An impending myocardial infarction is often heralded by increasing severity of anginal attacks. The ECG often shows continual signs of ischemia and injury.

Myocardial Infarction

Pathophysiology. Myocardial infarction (MI), or ischemic necrosis of the myocardium, results from prolonged ischemia to the myocardium with irreversible cell damage and muscle death. The time between onset of ischemia and myocardial muscle death is approximately 15 to 20 minutes, although this varies with the individual and the vessel that is occluded. Myocardial infarction almost always occurs in the left ventricle and often significantly depresses left ventricular function. The larger the infarcted area, the greater the loss of contractility. Functionally, myocardial infarction causes (1) reduced contractility with abnormal wall motion, (2) altered left ventricular compliance, (3) reduced stroke volume,

(4) reduced ejection fraction, and (5) elevated left ventricular end-diastolic pressure (LVEDP).

Alterations in function depend not only on the size but on the location of an infarct. An anterior left ventricular infarct often results from occlusion of the left anterior descending coronary artery. Posterior left ventricular infarcts often arise from right coronary artery obstruction, while lateral wall infarcts usually arise from circumflex artery obstruction (Table 21-2). This distribution varies because of individual differences in coronary artery supply. The infarct is also described in terms of where it occurs on the myocardial surface. Figure 21-4 gives the commonly used terms for different types of infarcts based on their location in the ventricular wall. The transmural infarct extends from endocardium to epicardium. The subendocardial type is located on the endocardial surface while the subepicardial occurs on the epicardial surface. Intramural infarction is often seen in patchy areas of the myocardium and is usually associated with long-standing angina pectoris. The relative frequency of different types of myocardial infarctions according to arterial involvement has been documented as follows: left anterior descending artery, 40 to 50 percent; right coronary artery, 30 to 40 percent; and left circumflex artery, 15 to 20 percent [19].

All acute myocardial infarctions have a central area of necrosis or infarction that is surrounded by an area of injury; the area of injury is surrounded by a ring of ischemia (Fig. 21-5). Each of these emits characteristic ECG patterns that help to localize and determine the extent of the infarct on the 12-lead recording.

When myocardial muscle cells die, they liberate the intramyocardial cellular enzymes. These enzymes can be used to date an infarct and partially to judge its severity. Because the affected myocardial muscle is dead, tissue does not regenerate after an infarction. Healing requires the formation of scar tissue that replaces the necrotic myocardial muscle. This involves a series of morphologic changes from no apparent cellular change in the first six hours to total replacement by scar tissue. Table 21-3 outlines these changes.

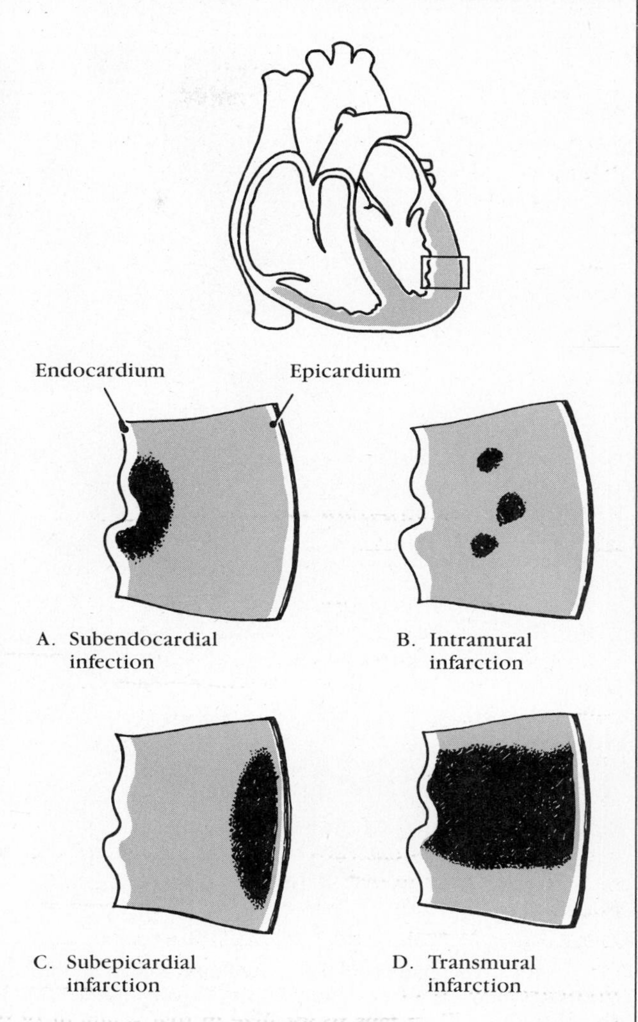

FIGURE 21-4 Names of various types of infarctions based on their location in the ventricular wall. (Adapted from C. Kenner, C. Guzzetta, and B. Dossey, *Critical Care Nursing: Body, Mind, Spirit* (2nd ed.). Boston: Little, Brown, 1985.)

TABLE 21-2 Arterial Myocardial Lesion and Area of Infarction

Coronary Artery Affected	Percentage of Cases	Areas of Infarction
Left anterior descending	40–50	Anterior left ventricle Anterior interventricular septum
Right coronary artery	30–40	Posterior wall of left ventricle Posterior interventricular septum
Left circumflex	15–20	Lateral wall of left ventricle

Source: From S.L. Robbins, R.S. Cotran, and V. Kumar, *Pathologic Basis of Disease* (3rd ed.). Philadelphia: W.B. Saunders Company, 1984. Reprinted by permission.

Scar tissue may inhibit contractility. As contractility fails, the compensatory mechanisms described in Chapter 20 begin to be used in an attempt to maintain cardiac output. Arteriolar vascular constriction, heart rate increase, and renal retention of sodium and water all help to regulate cardiac output. Ventricular dilatation is commonly seen. If a large amount of scar tissue is present, contractility may be greatly compromised and congestive heart failure or cardiogenic shock may ensue.

The clinical manifestations of myocardial infarction depend on the severity of the infarct, the previous physical condition of the individual, and whether earlier infarcts have occurred. They may reflect changes in the autonomic nervous system and in the location of the infarct (Fig. 21-6). The manifestations can range from sudden death due to dysrhythmias or ventricular rupture, to no symptoms whatsoever. Acute, substernal, radiating chest pain is

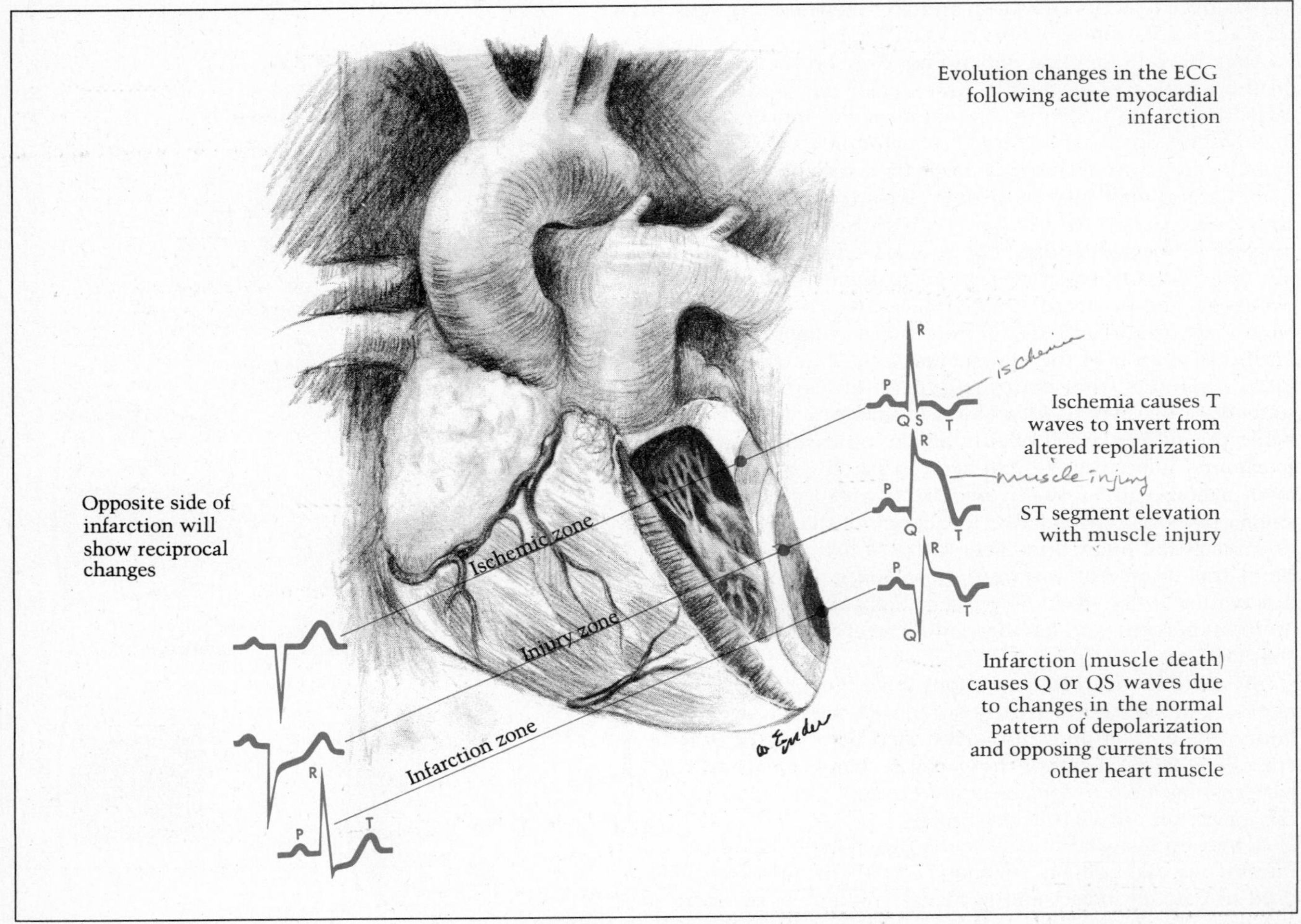

FIGURE 21-5 The effects of cardiac ischemia, injury, and infarction. (From C. Kenner, C. Guzzetta, and B. Dossey, *Critical Care Nursing: Body, Mind, Spirit* (2nd ed.). Boston: Little, Brown, 1985.)

TABLE 21-3 Morphologic Changes of Transmural Myocardial Infarction

Time Postinfarct	Morphologic Appearance
0–6 hours	Usually inapparent
6–12 hours	Pallor of affected area
18–24 hours	Pale, gray-brown
2–4 days	Necrotic focus with hyperemic border, central portion yellow-brown and soft
4–10 days	Yellow-gray to bright yellow (fatty change); central necrotic area, often contains areas of hemorrhage; margins intensely red and highly vascularized
10–14 days	Progressive replacement of necrotic muscle by fibrous, vascularized scar tissue
Up to 6 weeks	Usually total replacement by scar tissue

Source: S. L. Robbins, R. S. Cotran, and V. Kumar, *Pathologic Basis of Disease* (3rd ed.). Philadelphia: W.B. Saunders Company, 1984. Reprinted by permission.

often described. Diaphoresis, dyspnea, nausea and vomiting, extreme anxiety, and any type of dysrhythmia may be noted. Often the clinical features reveal associated complications (see pp. 326–327).

Right ventricular infarction is uncommon but may occur with occlusion of the right coronary artery. The central venous pressure (CVP) may be elevated markedly if acute right ventricular failure develops. Low right ventricular output causing shock often responds well to vigorous fluid therapy. Infusions raise both right and left ventricular filling pressures [10].

Diagnostic Tests. Laboratory studies are often very helpful in the diagnosis of acute myocardial infarction. The complete blood count (CBC) often reveals an elevated leukocyte count; the sedimentation rate and cardiac enzyme levels elevate because of cellular damage. Cardiac enzymes, normally present in myocardial muscle, are available in abnormally large amounts in the blood as a result

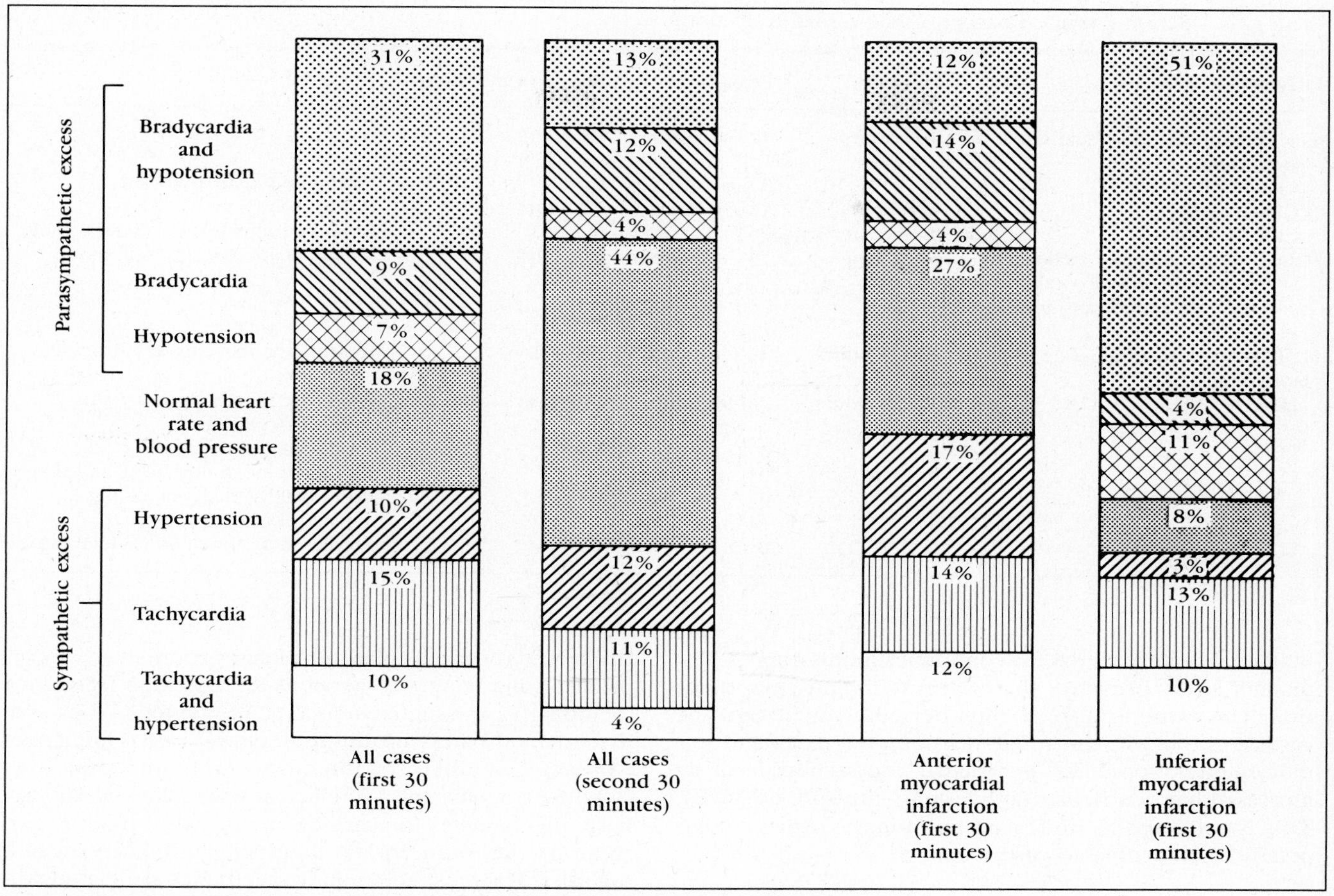

		All cases (first 30 minutes)	All cases (second 30 minutes)	Anterior myocardial infarction (first 30 minutes)	Inferior myocardial infarction (first 30 minutes)
Parasympathetic excess	Bradycardia and hypotension	31%	13%	12%	51%
	Bradycardia	9%	12%	14%	4%
	Hypotension	7%	4%	4%	11%
	Normal heart rate and blood pressure	18%	44%	27%	8%
Sympathetic excess	Hypertension	10%	12%	17%	3%
	Tachycardia	15%	11%	14%	13%
	Tachycardia and hypertension	10%	4%	12%	10%

Figure 21-6 Clinical effects of acute myocardial infarction especially related to autonomic disturbance. (© 1987 Scientific American, Inc. All rights reserved. From *Scientific American Medicine*, Figure 6, Section 1, Subsection X.)

of cellular death. These enzymes include creatinine phosphokinase (CPK), serum glutamic oxaloacetic transaminase (SGOT), and lactic dehydrogenase (LDH) (Fig. 21-7). Their values elevate and return to normal in a characteristic pattern after a myocardial infarction (Table 21-4). Because the enzymes are present in other tissues, coexisting disease can produce misleading enzyme elevations. Isoenzymes provide more specific accuracy. The isoenzyme CPK-MB is usually considered diagnostic of myocardial infarction, especially in the presence of increased levels of LDH_1.

Electrocardiographic changes of acute myocardial infarction consist of pronounced Q waves and ST elevation. These changes are reflected in the leads overlying the area of injury, so that the infarction can be generally localized by the ECG. Over time, the ST segment and T wave changes return to normal, but the Q wave persists as evidence of an old infarction and can be used to localize the defect throughout the person's life.

Bedside techniques to measure pulmonary artery pressures and cardiac output are invaluable in evaluating left ventricular function after MI. Insertion of the Swan-Ganz catheter intravenously through the right heart into the

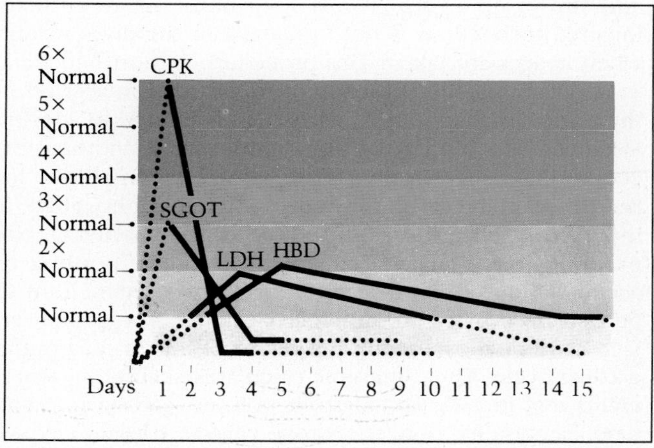

Figure 21-7 Time sequence of serum enzyme elevations in acute myocardial infarction. (From C. Kenner, C. Guzzetta, and B. Dossey, *Critical Care Nursing: Body, Mind, Spirit* (2nd ed.). Boston: Little, Brown, 1985.)

TABLE 21-4 Serum Enzyme Changes in Myocardial Infarction

Enzyme	Elevates	Peaks	Period of Elevation	Site of Formation
CPK (creatinine phosphokinase)	4–8 hours	12–36 hours	72 hours	
Isoenzymes				
CPK I (BB)	0	0	0	Produced mostly by brain
CPK II (MB)	4–8 hours	12–36 hours	72 hours	Produced mostly by heart
CPK III (MM)	0	0	0	Produced mostly by skeletal muscle
SGOT (serum glutamic oxaloacetic transaminase); also called asparate aminotransferase (AST)	6–12 hours	36–48 hours	4–6 days	Mostly heart, liver, muscle tissue
LDH (lactic dehydrogenase)	12–24 hours	24–96 hours	8–14 days	Heart, liver, muscles, erythrocytes
Isoenzymes				
LDH1	12–24 hours	24–96 hours	8–14 days	Produced mostly by heart and erythrocytes
LDH2	0	0	0	Produced mostly by RES
LDH3	0	0	0	Produced mostly by lungs and tissues
LDH4	0	0	0	Produced by placenta, kidneys, pancreas
LDH5	0	0	0	Produced by liver and skeletal muscle

pulmonary artery allows for continuous monitoring of pulmonary artery pressures that reflect left ventricular function. The catheter also permits periodic calculations of cardiac output. A myocardial infarction that results in significant alteration of left ventricular contractility leads to increased left ventricular end-diastolic pressure (LVEDP). This is reflected as increased pulmonary artery wedge pressure and decreased cardiac output.

Myocardial Infarction Imaging. Technetium pyrophosphate myocardial imaging has proved to be a sensitive indicator of acute myocardial damage. After infarction there is an efflux of calcium out of damaged cells. Technetium pyrophosphate combines with the calcium and shows up as a *hot spot*. Normally, intravenously injected technetium is not visualized in the myocardium when images are taken. This procedure is most beneficial in determining the presence of myocardial infarction in the acute situation, but its usefulness is limited to specific instances [26]. Multigated blood pool scan is another procedure that uses pyrophosphate, which has an affinity for red blood cells. Twenty minutes after pyrophosphate is injected, technetium is injected and attaches to the pyrophosphate-tagged red blood cells. The pooling or accumulation of blood in the heart allows technetium to be visualized by a special nuclear camera. The computerized camera allows many images to be taken during the cardiac cycle. The computer calculates several measurements that include end-diastolic volume, end-systolic volume, ejection fraction, and stroke volume. This procedure is of particular benefit in evaluating the effects of infarction on myocardial function. Also, myocardial function can be monitored noninvasively in a variety of situations.

Complications of Myocardial Infarction. *Dysrhythmias*. The most common complication (90%) of acute myocardial infarction is a disturbance in cardiac rhythm. Myocardial infarction itself produces numerous predisposing factors to account for this high frequency, including (1) tissue ischemia, (2) hypoxemia, (3) sympathetic and parasympathetic nervous system influences, (4) lactic acidosis, (5) hemodynamic abnormalities, (6) drug toxicity, and (7) electrolyte imbalance. The two basic mechanisms for cardiac rhythm abnormalities are abnormal *automaticity* and abnormal *conduction*, or both together. The most common dysrhythmias associated with myocardial infarction are listed in Table 21-5. Dysrhythmias may cause a decline in cardiac output, increase in cardiac irritability, and further compromise of myocardial perfusion. The most common cause of death outside of the hospital in individuals with MI is probably ventricular fibrillation.

Congestive Heart Failure and Cardiogenic Shock. Congestive heart failure is a state of circulatory congestion produced by myocardial dysfunction. Myocardial infarction compromises myocardial function by reducing contractility and producing abnormal wall motion. As the ability of the ventricle to empty becomes less effective, stroke volume falls and residual volume increases. The fall in stroke volume elicits compensatory mechanisms to maintain cardiac output (see Chap. 20).

Cardiogenic shock results from profound left ventricular failure, usually from a massive myocardial infarction. This pump failure shock follows myocardial infarction in 10 to 15 percent of cases, and mortality is approximately 80 to 95 percent [19]. The Killip classification of heart failure after acute MI is helpful in determining prognosis and treatment (Table 21-6).

Thromboembolism. Mural thrombi are common in postmortem examinations of individuals who die of myocardial infarction. In a study of 924 fatalities due to acute MI, 44 percent had mural thrombi attached to the endo-

TABLE 21-5 Common Dysrhythmias After Myocardial Infarction

Type of Dysrhythmia	Examples
Ventricular	Premature ventricular contractions (PVCs)
	Ventricular tachycardia
	Ventricular fibrillation
Atrial	Premature atrial contractions
	Atrial flutter
	Atrial fibrillation
Conduction defects	Bundle branch block, right or left
	Second-degree heart block
	Third-degree or complete heart block
Sinus	Sinus tachycardia
	Sinus bradycardia
	Sinus dysrhythmia

TABLE 21-6 The Killip Classification of Heart Failure in Acute Myocardial Infarction

Class	Description
I	No signs of heart failure.
II	Mild or moderate heart failure: rales can be heard over as much as 50 percent of both lung fields.
III	Pulmonary edema: rales can be heard over more than half of both lung fields.
IV	Cardiogenic shock: blood pressure by cuff is less than 90 mm Hg; signs of inadequate peripheral perfusion evident, including reduced urine flow, cold and clammy skin, cyanosis, and mental obtundation.

Source: From *Scientific American Medicine,* Table 1, Section 1, Subsection X.

cardium [19]. These thrombi are usually associated with large infarcts and therefore probably occur more frequently in nonsurvivors than survivors. Mural thrombi adhere to the endocardium overlying an infarcted area. Fragments, however, can produce systemic arterial embolization. Autopsy studies reveal that 10 percent of individuals who die of myocardial infarction also have arterial emboli to the brain, kidneys, spleen, or mesentery.

Almost all pulmonary emboli originate in the veins of the lower extremities. Bedrest and heart failure predispose an individual to venous thrombosis and pulmonary embolism. Both occur in those with acute myocardial infarction. When prolonged bedrest was standard therapy for all cases of MI, the rate of pulmonary embolus was 20 percent. With early mobilization and widespread use of prophylactic anticoagulation therapy, pulmonary embolus has become a rare cause of death as a complication of MI.

Pericarditis. This syndrome associated with MI was first described by Dressler and is often called Dressler's syndrome. It usually occurs after a transmural infarction but may follow subepicardial infarction. It is very common, affecting 50 percent of individuals after transmural infarction. Pericarditis is usually transient, appearing in the first week after infarction. The chest pain of acute pericarditis develops suddenly, being severe and constant over the anterior chest. The pain worsens with inspiration and is usually associated with tachycardia, low-grade fever, and a transient, triphasic, pericardial friction rub [22].

Myocardial Rupture. Rupture of the free wall of the left ventricle accounts for 10 to 15 percent of deaths in the hospital due to acute myocardial infarction [12]. It causes immediate cardiac tamponade and death. Rupture of the interventricular septum is less common, occurs with extensive myocardial damage, and produces a ventricular septal defect.

Ventricular Aneurysm. This event is a late complication of myocardial infarction that involves thinning, ballooning, and hypokinesis of the left ventricular wall after a transmural infarction. The aneurysm often creates a paroxysmal motion of the ventricular wall with ballooning out of the aneurysmal segment on ventricular contraction. The dysfunctional area often becomes filled with necrotic debris and clot, and sometimes is rimmed by a calcium ring. The debris or clot may fragment and travel into the systemic arterial circulation. Occasionally, these aneurysms rupture, causing tamponade and death, but usually the problems that result are due to declining ventricular contractility or embolization.

Valvular Disease

Valvular disease, such as stenosis or insufficiency, may interfere with valve functions and the flow of blood through the heart. In valvular stenosis the valve orifice (opening) narrows and the valve leaflets (cusps) become fused together in such a way that the valve cannot open freely. This narrowing of the opening causes obstruction of blood flow, and as a result, the chamber behind the affected valve must build up more pressure to overcome resistance. The muscle fibers in that chamber must thicken in order to do more work to push the blood through the narrowed opening [13]. Over a period of time, the muscle hypertrophies in response to the added workload. With valvular insufficiency (regurgitation), the valve cannot close completely. The incomplete closure results from scarring and retraction of the valve leaflets. As a result, blood is permitted to flow backward (retrograde) through the opening. The heart chamber, which receives the additional retrograde flow, is then forced to pump the added regurgitant volume together with the volume being received. As a response to the increased volume present in the chamber behind the regurgitant valve, the muscle fibers lengthen or stretch. This dilatation of muscle fiber increases the surface area in order to accommodate the additional volume. Both hypertrophy and dilatation are compensatory mechanisms that occur in the presence of specific valvular defects.

When stenosis and regurgitation occur simultaneously, the defect is called a mixed lesion, and usually is a feature of advanced disease. In the clinical setting, the lesions are classified in terms of the predominant mechanical load that is placed on the heart. This leads to the classification of valvular defects. Stenosis can be predominant or "pure," as can regurgitation, or the lesions can be mixed. In addition to having a mixed lesion on one valve, there may be disease on another valve at the same time. This is known as combined valvular disease, which may present a rather complex clinical picture depending on the number of valves involved and the types of lesions [21].

Diagnostic Tests

Chest Radiography. The chest radiograph (roentgenogram) is used to recognize abnormalities in cardiac size and to identify certain valvular lesions that cause cardiac failure. The cardiac silhouette enlarges, for instance, in the presence of aortic regurgitation (insufficiency) because of the dilatation of the chamber and hypertrophy of the muscle. Cardiac failure as a sequela of mitral stenosis can be seen on chest films as accumulation of fluid in the interlobular spaces of the lung, the result of blood damming back into the pulmonary area.

Electrocardiography. The ECG, which records the electrical current produced by the excitable cells of the myocardium, is useful in diagnosing atrial, ventricular, or biventricular hypertrophy related to valvular disease. Chamber hypertrophy usually causes an increase in amplitude of the QRS complex, and characteristic ST and T wave changes.

The electrocardiogram can also be useful in evaluating acute pericarditis. The ST segments may be elevated or depressed in many leads; T wave inversion may or may not accompany these changes. In addition, if pericardial effusion is present, there may be low voltage in both the QRS complex and T wave in all leads.

Echocardiography. Echocardiography uses sound waves to identify intracardiac structures based on the principle of sonic reflection [8]. When a sound wave passes through a medium such as blood, it is reflected backward, or echoed, when it comes in contact with a medium of different density or elasticity, such as the muscle of the heart. Intracardiac structures have different densities, which are referred to as interfaces. In echocardiography, an ultrasound wave (beam) is transmitted from the transducer to the cardiac interfaces, and these waves are reflected back to the transducer as an echo. The sonic energy is then transformed into electrical energy that can be displayed in graphic form (Fig. 21-8). The recording depends on the transducer's angle and on the intracardiac structures that lie within the beam's pathway [8].

Used as a noninvasive tool at the bedside, echocardiography is employed to assess valvular motion and pumping action of the heart, and to measure cardiac chamber size [4]. Because it assesses valvular motion, the echocardio-

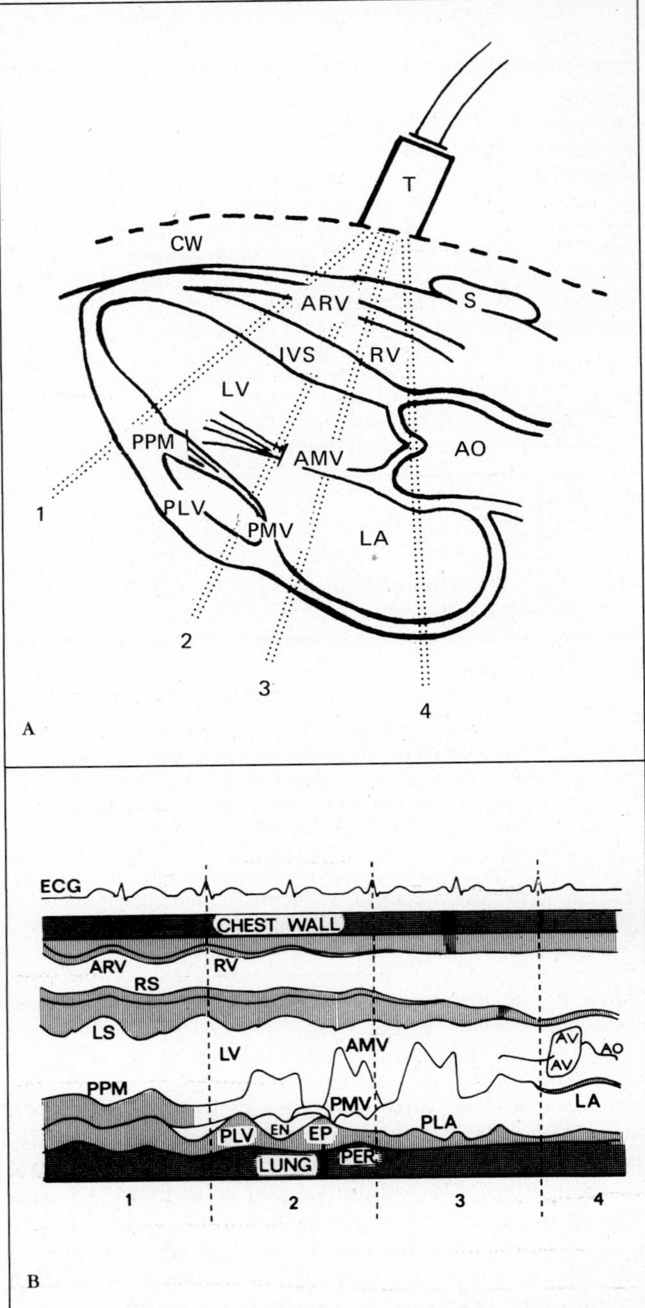

FIGURE 21-8 A. Schematic representation of the course of the ultrasonic beam to achieve the echo represented in B. CW = chest wall; T = transducer; S = sternum; ARV = anterior right ventricular wall; RV = right ventricle; IVS = interventricular septum; LV = left ventricle; PPM = posterior papillary muscle; AMV = anterior mitral valve leaflet; AO = aorta; PLV = posterior left ventricular wall; PMV = posterior mitral valve leaflet; LA = left atrium. B. Schematic representation of an echocardiogram from the four transducer positions. RS = right side of interventricular septum; LS = left side of interventricular septum; En = endocardium; EP = epicardium; PER = pericardium; PLA = posterior left atrial wall; AV = aortic valve cusps. (Reprinted with permission from H. Feigenbaum, Clinical application of echocardiography. *Prog. Cardiovasc. Dis.* 14:531, 1972, Grune and Stratton, Inc., Publishers.)

gram can be used to diagnose such valvular abnormalities as stenosis, regurgitation, mitral valve prolapse, and ruptured chordae tendineae. Fluid inside the pericardial membrane (pericardial effusion) can also be detected. In addition, echocardiography is useful in the assessment of abnormal thickening of the ventricular walls and septum or abnormal dilatation of the cardiac chambers.

Cardiac Catheterization. Cardiac catheterization is an invasive diagnostic procedure that can yield important information regarding the chambers of the heart. A catheter is passed either to the right or left side of the heart; pressure and oxygen are recorded throughout the process. Left heart catheterization assesses the function of the left ventricle and aorta and the mitral and aortic valves. Right heart catheterization assesses the function of the right atrium and ventricle and the tricuspid and pulmonic valves.

In right heart catheterization, the catheter is normally inserted into the antecubital or saphenous vein and guided sequentially into the right atrium, right ventricle, pulmonary artery, and pulmonary arterial wedge position. With left heart catheterization, the catheter is inserted into the femoral or brachial artery and is advanced retrograde through the aorta into the left ventricle. Another method of insertion is the transseptal approach. This is accomplished by inserting a long, curved needle through a catheter positioned in the right atrium in order to puncture the intact interatrial septum. This approach may be employed when mitral disease is suspected [9].

Once a catheter is in place in either the left or right heart, the chambers may be visualized by injecting a radiopaque substance (dye) through the catheter into the specific chamber under investigation. This is known as cardiac angiography. During the injection of the dye, abnormalities in valvular motion such as stenosis or regurgitation may be detected.

Cardiac catheterization is also useful in determining pressure differences between chambers, as in valvular stenosis in which a pressure gradient may be present. This procedure helps to assess the severity of the disease process and to determine whether surgical intervention is necessary. Quantitative measurements of volumes, pressures, ejection fraction, and cardiac output are recorded.

Because it is invasive, the procedure has inherent risks. Right heart catheterization is rarely associated with morbidity or mortality; however, left heart catheterization can produce serious complications [9]. These include cardiac perforation, major dysrhythmias, hypotension, hemorrhage, vascular thrombosis, acute myocardial infarction, and cerebral embolism, as well as death.

Acute Rheumatic Fever: A Major Cause of Valvular Disease

Rheumatic fever is an inflammatory disease that occurs in susceptible persons after untreated pharyngeal infection with group A beta-hemolytic *Streptococcus*. It appears to be an individual immune reaction to the streptococcal organism. The disease causes inflammation of the joints, heart, skin, and nervous system [23]. The attack rate of rheumatic fever is 1 to 3 percent in individuals with untreated streptococcal sore throat. Effective treatment with penicillin virtually eliminates the disease. The most common age of onset is 5 to 15 years, and frequency is greatest in areas of crowded, substandard living conditions. Recurrent attacks of rheumatic fever are common in susceptible, untreated individuals, and carry a greater risk of valvular disease with each recurrence.

Pathophysiology. The joints are affected with an exudative synovitis with associated subcutaneous nodules. A characteristic acute carditis is noted, with the diagnostic lesion, the *Aschoff body*, present in the myocardium. *Verrucae*, which are small, warty vegetations produced by fibrin or ground substance, appear on the valve leaflets. These apparently cause inflammation and exudation, leading to interadherence of the leaflets (Fig. 21-9). These also may develop in a line on the chordae tendineae and produce scarring and shortening of these structures over a long period of time.

During the acute phase of disease the valves and endocardial surface are inflamed and edematous. Nervous system involvement is manifested by chorea, which is rapid, jerky involuntary movements of the arms and legs, and emotional instability [19,23]. No diagnostic central nervous system lesion has been found to explain this manifestation.

Clinical Manifestations. Onset of the disease may be acute or subacute. The acute form causes migratory polyarthritis, which refers to joint inflammation that moves from joint to joint. Fever is characteristic. Tachycardia out of proportion to the level of the fever may be associated with mitral or aortic murmurs, cardiac enlargement, and congestive heart failure. Chorea is uncommon and may begin up to three months after the streptococcal infection.

Erythema marginatum may be noted, and is described as a pink, erythematous rash on the trunk and extremities. It often appears in concentric circles that fade and enlarge in minutes to hours. Rheumatic arteritis, pneumonitis, and pleuritis are other relatively rare manifestations of the disease.

Chronic rheumatic carditis may occur and run a fatal course over a few months. Fortunately, it is rare, and cardiac involvement is subsequently expressed through valvular defects, often years after the initial disease.

Laboratory tests are not diagnostic, but the antistreptolysin O titer (ASO) is increased after streptococcal infection. The erythrocyte sedimentation rate (ESR) is increased, indicating an inflammatory process. Most cases of rheumatic fever abate within 12 weeks. The onset in later years of valvular dysfunction is hard to predict, but treatment of later streptococcal infections, thus preventing rheumatic fever, has led to few reported cases of valvular stenosis or regurgitation in the United States. Significant numbers of cases still are reported from the Middle East, Southeast Asia, and developing countries.

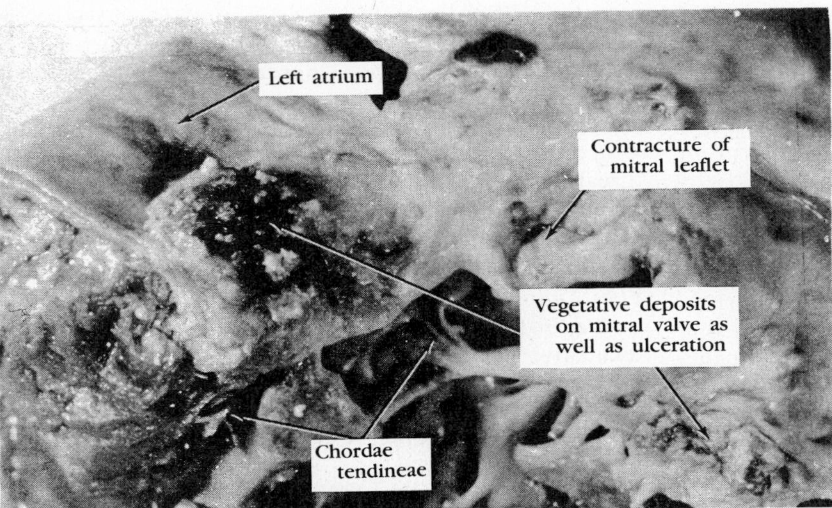

FIGURE 21-9 Mitral valve viewed from above showing vegetative deposits, ulceration of valve leaflets, and fusion of commissures. (From J. Kernicki, B. Bullock, and J. Matthews, *Cardiovascular Nursing*. New York: Putnam, 1971.)

Mitral Stenosis

Stenosis of the mitral valve causes impairment of blood flow from the left atrium to the left ventricle (Fig. 21-10). The impairment is due to an abnormality in the structure of the valve leaflets that prevents the valve from opening completely in diastole. The most common cause of mitral stenosis is rheumatic endocarditis. In pure mitral stenosis (without regurgitation), about one-half of patients describe a history of known rheumatic fever. Mitral stenosis is more common in women than in men [18].

Pathophysiology and Compensatory Mechanisms. The basic alteration in mitral stenosis is decreased blood flow from the left atrium to the left ventricle. As a result of the rheumatic process, the commissures (junctional areas between the leaflets) become fibrous and fused, the chordae become shortened, and the valve becomes funnel-shaped. As the valve becomes more stenotic, the leaflets thicken with scar tissue and become calcified at the valve ring and at the leaflet margins. There are rarely any symptoms until the mitral valve orifice decreases in size from the normal 4 to 6 cm to 1.5 to 2.5 cm [18]. As the orifice further decreases in size, pulmonary symptoms appear. Mitral valve orifice (opening) size correlates relatively well with symptoms. Since the size usually decreases very gradually over a period of years, symptoms are often first noted in the fourth or fifth decade of life.

In the normal heart, there is no functional pressure gradient between the left atrium and left ventricle in diastole. A pressure gradient is the difference in pressure in two chambers when the valve dividing them is open. In mitral stenosis, the gradient is determined by the size of the mitral valve orifice and the flow across the valve. The flow is determined by the duration of diastole (during which filling occurs) and by cardiac output [18]. The stenotic mitral valve does not permit increases in blood flow, so left atrial pressure must increase to discharge its contents into the left ventricle. Because of the constant increase in left atrial volume and pressure, the left atrium dilates and hypertrophies. As the atrium size increases, the risk for developing various atrial dysrhythmias also increases. Atrial fibrillation commonly develops, further compromising the blood flow to the ventricle because of ineffective atrial contraction. Constant increased pressure and volume in the left atrium cause an increase in pressure in the pulmonary veins and capillary bed. If the pressure in the pulmonary capillaries becomes greater than the plasma oncotic pressure, fluid passes into the interstitial spaces and eventually the alveoli.

Chronic elevation of left atrial pressure causes the onset of pulmonary hypertension. Pulmonary hypertension results from chronic elevation of pulmonary capillary pressure. This excessive pulmonary pressure can rise to nearly systemic values, causing an increased pressure load against which the right ventricle must pump. Chronic pulmonary edema (congestion) in the interstitial spaces occurs, and right ventricular failure is the result (see Chap. 20). The classic manifestations of mitral stenosis include pulmonary congestion and all the signs of right heart failure [18].

Clinical Manifestations. Dyspnea as a result of the pulmonary congestion is the most common symptom. Dyspnea is increased by any condition that increases heart rate, such as exercise, stress, fever, or atrial fibrillation with a rapid ventricular response. Paroxysmal nocturnal

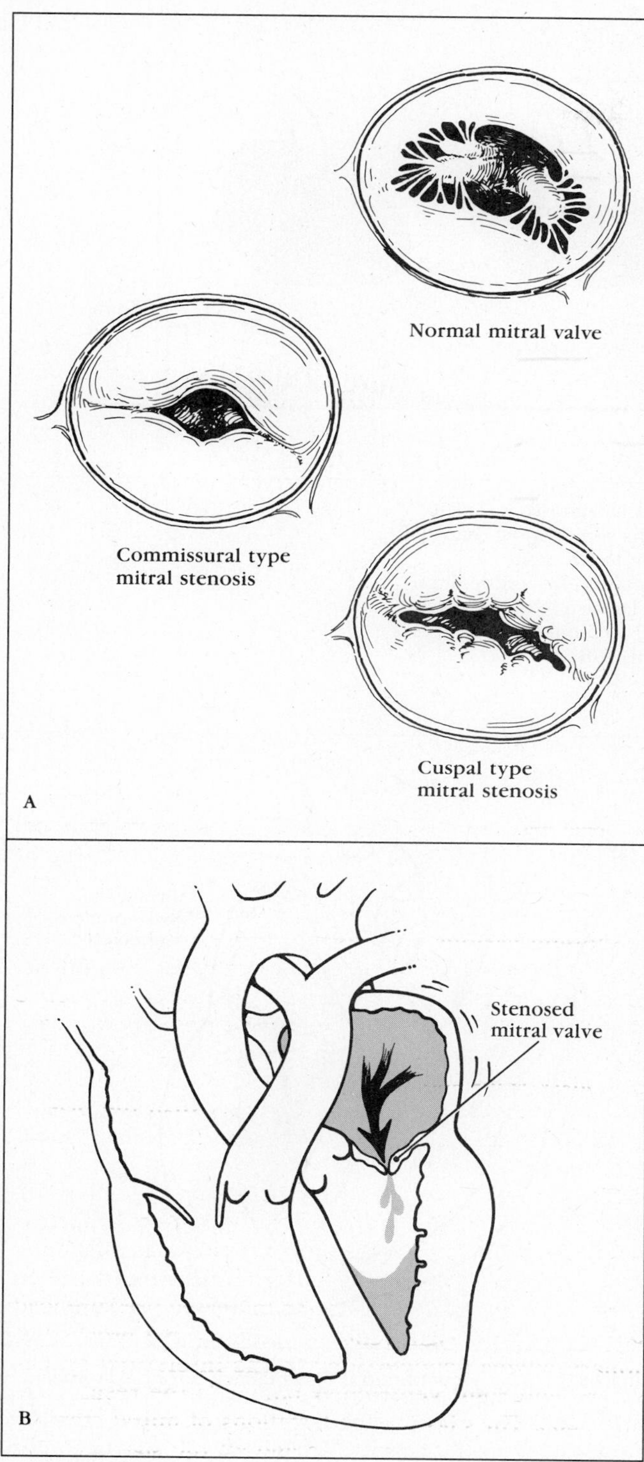

FIGURE 21-10 A. The mitral valve (viewed from the atrium) demonstrating the normal valve in the closed position as well as commissural-type mitral stenosis, in which fusion leads to adherence of leaflets of normal thickness, and cuspal mitral stenosis caused by stiff, fibrocalcific leaflets. (From N.K. Wenger, W. Hurst, and M. McIntyre, *Cardiology for Nurses*. St. Louis: Mosby, 1980.) B. Mitral stenosis as viewed during atrial contraction.

dyspnea may be reported by persons with some degree of right heart failure. Fatigue is also common and is related to both pulmonary hypertension and right ventricular failure. Hemoptysis may occur as the result of (1) frank pulmonary hemorrhage from a ruptured pulmonary vein; (2) pulmonary edema, and seen as frothy pink, blood-tinged sputum; or (3) pulmonary infarction [21]. Palpitations may be reported, especially in the presence of atrial fibrillation. Palpation of the precordium may reveal a parasternal lift with the development of right ventricular hypertrophy [18].

Auscultation reveals (1) a loud first heart sound, (2) an opening snap, and (3) a diastolic rumble (Fig. 21-11). The loud first heart sound is due to closure of the mitral valve apparatus when it remains deep in the left ventricle at the time of contraction. Changes in leaflet mobility also contribute to the production of the loud first heart sound [18]. The opening snap heard on auscultation is thought to result from the sudden snapping of fused commissures of the valve into the ventricle. It also may be due to calcification of the valve leaflets.

The diastolic rumble of mitral stenosis is a loud, long, murmur that begins just after the opening snap and has a decrescendo pattern. It results from the movement of the valve leaflets toward the closed position in middiastole despite the continuing blood flow across the mitral valve produced by the pressure gradient [18].

Diagnostic Tests. The appearance of the cardiac silhouette in mitral stenosis on chest film is characteristic. In the posteroanterior (PA) view, the left heart border is straightened, the pulmonary artery is enlarged, and there is a double density due to left atrial enlargement. In the lateral view the enlarged left atrium and right ventricle are seen.

The electrocardiogram characteristically shows a broad, notched P wave in lead II, called *P mitrale*. This probably reflects atrial enlargement. As many as 40 percent of persons with mitral stenosis develop atrial fibrillation [18]. As pulmonary hypertension develops, right ventricular hypertrophy may be noted.

Loss of posterior leaflet movement, left atrial enlargement, changes suggestive of pulmonary hypertension, and right ventricular enlargement may be seen on the echocardiogram. If mitral stenosis is complicated by the presence of mitral valve incompetence, left ventricular enlargement is also noted on the echocardiogram [18].

Direct measurements of a gradient across the mitral valve cannot be made by conventional means but can be assessed by simultaneous measurement of the pulmonary artery wedge pressure and left ventricular diastolic pressure. Correlation of the pressure gradient with cardiac output, heart rate, and diastolic filling time provides the examiner with data to calculate the mitral valve area [21].

Course and Complications. The uninterrupted course of mitral stenosis is long and progresses toward total disability and death. Atrial fibrillation adds an additional burden to the already compromised hemodynamics.

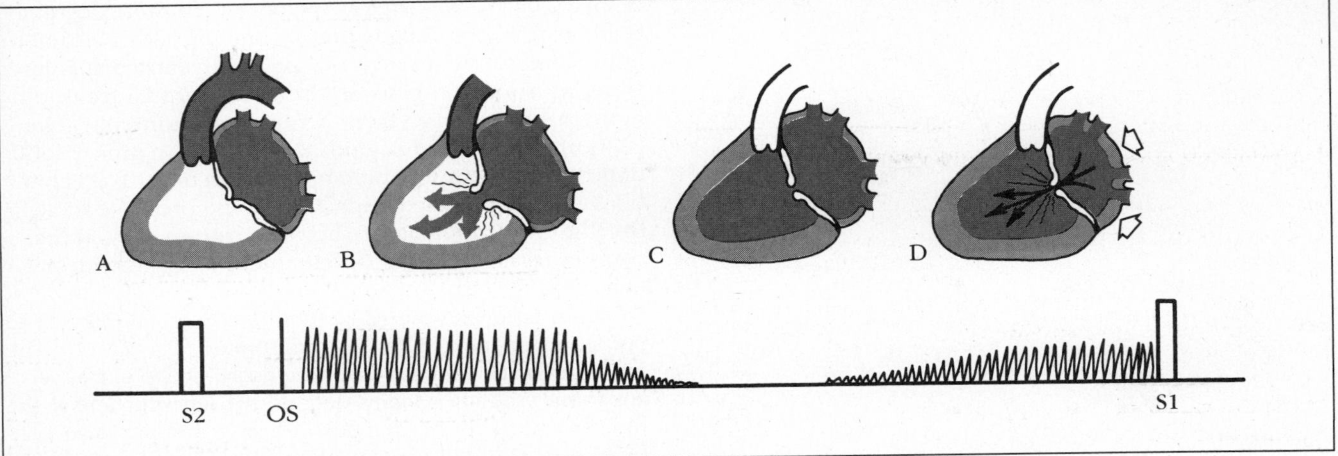

FIGURE 21-11 Hemodynamic basis for the auscultatory findings of mitral stenosis. A. Aortic valve closes; second heart sound (S2) is generated. B. Mitral valve opens and opening snap (OS) occurs; early diastolic component is generated. C. Flow from left atrium to left ventricle diminishes and murmur decreases in middiastole. D. Atrial systole increases flow across mitral valve, resulting in presystolic increase in intensity of murmur. Ventricular systole then causes closure of thickened mitral valve, resulting in loud first heart sound (S1). (From R. Judge, G. Zuidema, and F. Fitzgerald, *Clinical Diagnosis*. Boston: Little, Brown, 1982.)

Systemic emboli complicate the course of mitral stenosis and relate to onset of atrial fibrillation. Pulmonary hypertension is associated with permanent vascular changes. The development of right heart failure from pulmonary hypertension complicates the clinical course of the disease. Fatigue is a major complaint and is often associated with peripheral edema, ascites, liver enlargement, and an enlarged right ventricle.

Mitral Regurgitation or Insufficiency

Mitral regurgitation is described as the backflow of blood from the left ventricle across the mitral valve to the left atrium during ventricular systole. Regurgitation occurs when the mitral valve fails to close completely. The most common cause of mitral regurgitation is rheumatic endocarditis.

Pathophysiology and Compensatory Mechanisms. The same basic processes that lead to mitral stenosis contribute to the production of mitral regurgitation. When changes on the valve leaflets and chordae cause the leaflets to stay in a closed position, stenosis results. When the changes cause the valve to stay in the open position, regurgitation results. The scarring and retraction of the mitral leaflets extend from one leaflet to another, crossing one or more commissures.

In mitral regurgitation, cardiac output is divided into regurgitant and systemic flows (Fig. 21-12). The amount of regurgitant flow is determined by the degree of mitral valve incompetence and the resistance to flow through the aortic valve. Regurgitant flow increases proportionately to mitral valve orifice size. Any factor that increases resistance at the aortic valve, such as aortic stenosis, decreases systemic flow and increases regurgitant flow.

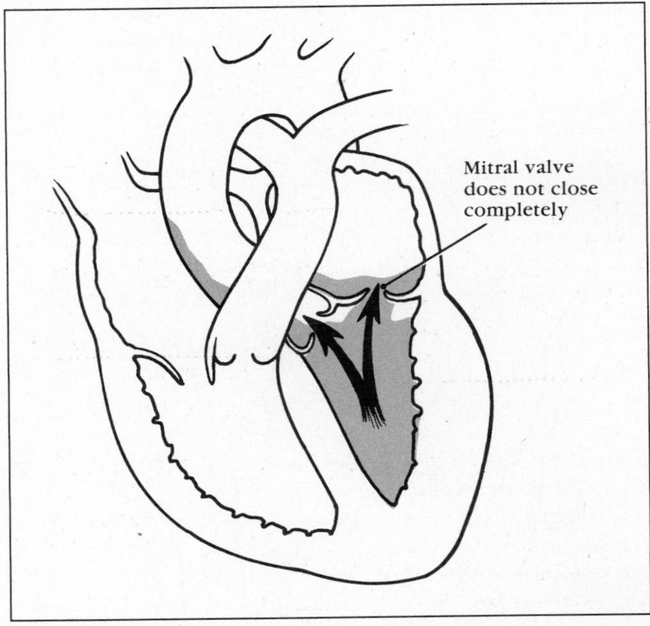

FIGURE 21-12 View of mitral insufficiency during systole.

The left ventricle responds to the increased volume from the left atrium with dilatation and hypertrophy so that sufficient systemic cardiac output is maintained [18]. The regurgitant volume entering the left atrium gradually increases and the left atrium gradually dilates, sometimes to aneurysmal size, to accommodate the increased volume. As a result of left atrial enlargement, the valve anulus stretches and displaces the posterior leaflet of the mitral valve, which leads to further mitral regurgitation. As mitral regurgitation progresses, contractility of the left ventricle decreases, leading to a decrease in systemic flow and onset of left ventricular failure.

Clinical Manifestations. Many people with mitral regurgitation have no symptoms for several years. When symptoms do appear, dyspnea and fatigue are common. They are due to a decreased cardiac output and increased pulmonary venous pressure. Other common symptoms include orthopnea, paroxysmal nocturnal dyspnea, and palpitations.

The person with mitral regurgitation can better tolerate the onset of atrial fibrillation than one with mitral stenosis. Atrial fibrillation occurs in about 75 percent of persons with mitral regurgitation.

The individual's general appearance is normal, but signs of congestive heart failure may be present if the disease is long-standing. In chronic mitral regurgitation the apex impulse is often displaced laterally and is larger than normal. This finding is related to left ventricular dilatation. The systolic murmur characteristic of mitral regurgitation is almost always present [18]. The murmur is loud, high pitched, holosystolic (of constant intensity throughout systole), and heard best at the apex (Fig. 21-13). The murmur may radiate to the axilla or back. The first heart sound is usually diminished in mitral regurgitation. A third heart sound that is associated with the rapid phase of ventricular filling may also be present. If present, the third heart sound indicates some degree of cardiac decompensation.

Diagnostic Tests. Left atrial and ventricular enlargement are frequent findings on chest films in those who have mitral regurgitation. As in mitral stenosis, the left atrium may be greatly enlarged. Pulmonary venous changes may be noted on chest films, but their occurrence is less frequent than in mitral stenosis [18].

The usual ECG findings of chronic mitral regurgitation are atrial and ventricular hypertrophy. Atrial fibrillation is common. Right ventricular hypertrophy, however, is less common in mitral regurgitation than in mitral stenosis [18].

Cardiac catheterization provides data to describe the amount of mitral regurgitation and the pumping ability of the left ventricle. The amount of mitral regurgitation can be measured quantitatively during catheterization. The ejection fraction is measured and is useful in determining the pumping ability of the left ventricle. Cardiac output is usually decreased in symptomatic individuals.

Course and Complications. The course of mitral regurgitation is long and slowly progressive, but the point at which left ventricular contractility is significantly compromised correlates with the time of development of pulmonary congestion [18]. Atrial fibrillation causes a further decrease in cardiac output.

Mixed Mitral Stenosis and Regurgitation

A mitral valve that has both fused commissures and structures that fail to close properly exhibits a mixture of stenosis and regurgitation. The course of these mixed lesions depends on which one is predominant. If the degree of stenosis is greater than the degree of incompetence, there is a smaller amount of backflow of blood across the mitral valve during systole and a smaller amount of forward flow of blood across the valve in diastole. If incompetence is greater than stenosis, there is more backflow of blood across the valve in systole and more forward flow of blood across the valve in diastole [21].

Dyspnea is the most common symptom and may be of acute onset when atrial fibrillation ensues. Palpitations are also common and are frequently related to rapid atrial dysrhythmias. The heart is usually enlarged. The first heart sound may be loud and there may be an opening snap. Often, a third heart sound is present in addition to, or instead of, the opening snap. The characteristic pansystolic murmur of mitral regurgitation and the diastolic murmurs of mitral stenosis are usually present [21]. Pulmonary congestion in mixed stenosis and regurgitation may lead to pulmonary edema, especially with the onset of atrial fibrillation.

Diagnostic Tests. Diagnostic procedures, as with mitral stenosis and insufficiency, are helpful in determining the extent of decompensation from the valvular lesions. The course and complications depend on the extent of the lesions.

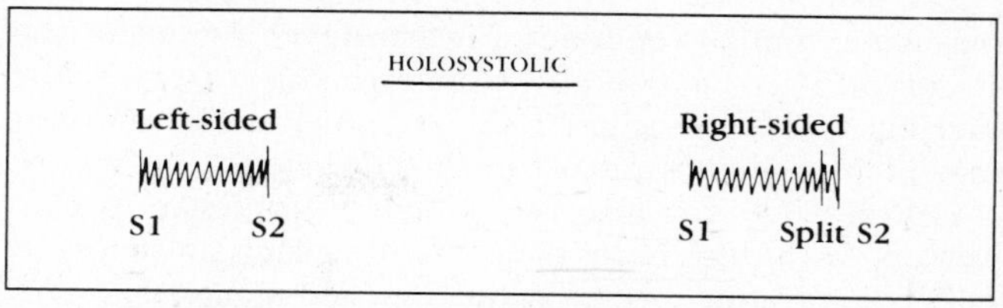

FIGURE 21-13 Holosystolic mitral regurgitation murmur.

Mitral Valve Prolapse

Mitral valve prolapse is a common condition caused by posterior displacement of the posterior cusp of the mitral valve. It is probably a congenital abnormality of the valve tissues in which the large posterior leaflet bulges back into the left atrium during systole [21]. As the ballooning of the leaflet into the left atrium continues, the chordae and papillary muscles become stressed. Contraction of the papillary muscles decreases and mitral regurgitation occurs. The amount of this regurgitation is usually hemodynamically insignificant but may produce symptoms. More frequently, the symptoms produced are the result of an atrial dysrhythmia.

Most persons with mitral valve prolapse are completely free of symptoms. For this reason it is commonly diagnosed during a routine physical examination. A nonanginal type of chest pain may be present together with palpitations, fatigue, and dyspnea.

Mitral valve prolapse is most commonly diagnosed in women in the second to fourth decade of life [18]. There may be a familial tendency toward development of the condition. Auscultation at the apex reveals a late systolic murmur that is crescendo, loud, and musical. The murmur may be preceded by one or more clicks in systole.

Mitral valve prolapse is associated with extracardiac defects, including bony abnormalities such as scoliosis, pectus excavatum, pectus carinatum, and kyphosis.

A normal cardiac shadow is evident on radiographs. The electrocardiogram often reveals several dysrhythmias, especially sinus dysrhythmias, atrial fibrillation, premature ventricular contractions, and ventricular tachycardia. Other ECG changes include ST-T wave abnormalities and prolongation of the QT interval. The echocardiogram is useful in diagnosis and helps to determine the presence and amount of insufficiency.

Complications are rare, but may include bacterial endocarditis or acute mitral insufficiency from chordae rupturing or stretching.

Aortic Stenosis

Among the several causes of aortic stenosis are rheumatic heart disease, congenital aortic stenosis with a bicuspid or a unicuspid valve, degenerative calcific disease of the elderly, and idiopathic hypertrophic subaortic stenosis [18]. The most frequent cause in those under 30 years of age is a congenital stenotic aortic valve. Between 30 and 70 years of age, rheumatic heart disease is the usual underlying cause; in individuals over 70 years of age, the degenerative calcific type is predominant.

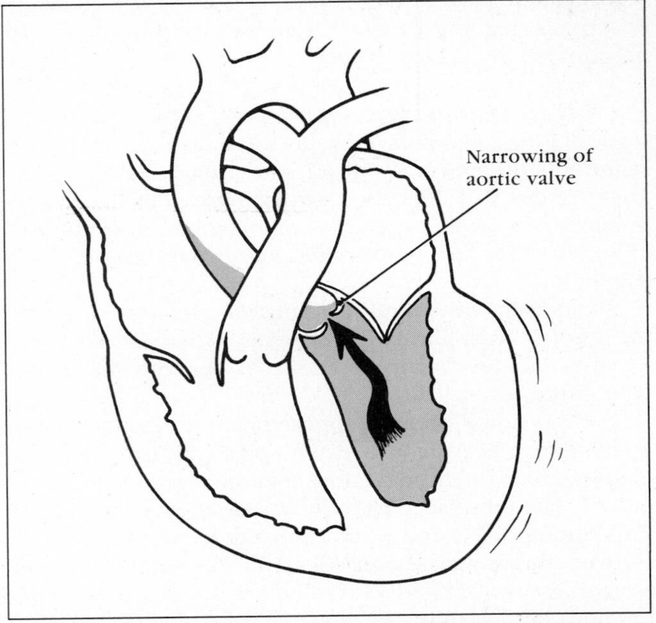

FIGURE 21-14 View of aortic stenosis during systole.

Pathophysiology and Compensatory Mechanisms. Significant narrowing of the valve orifice leads to a decrease in blood flow from the left ventricle to the aorta. The obstruction of outflow from the left ventricle leads also to strain or pressure load on the left ventricle that occurs as the left ventricle tries to push blood through the narrowed opening (Fig. 21-14). This resistance to ejection is reflected by an increase in pressure in the left ventricle to force more blood through the stenotic valve during systole.

A systolic pressure gradient develops between the left ventricle and aorta and is called an *aortic valve gradient*. These hemodynamic consequences are not manifested until the valve orifice, which is normally 2.6 to 3.5 cm^2, has narrowed to approximately one-third of normal. The left ventricle is capable of compensating for increasing pressure demands through hypertrophy for a long period of time (see Chap. 22). This mechanism allows for increasing systolic pressures to maintain an adequate systemic blood pressure. The increased muscle mass requires increased oxygen supply that may or may not be supplied by the coronary arteries. If the stenosis becomes increasingly severe, the persistent pressure overload (strain) leads to myocardial failure.

Clinical Manifestations. The classic clinical manifestations that accompany severe aortic stenosis are chest pain, syncope, and heart failure. Chest pain and syncope are related to reduced cardiac output, increased perfusion needs, and decreased perfusion of the coronary arteries and brain. Congestive heart failure results from chronic strain on the left ventricle.

Chest pain is usually manifested after physical exertion as a result of inability of the heart to increase coronary blood flow [21]. This type of angina can occur in up to 70 percent of persons with severe aortic stenosis [18].

Syncopal episodes, "gray-outs" or periods of confusion associated with severe aortic stenosis, are danger signs. Without surgical intervention, the prognosis is poor.

The chronic strain imposed on the left ventricle eventually leads to heart failure and may terminate in pulmonary edema. Left ventricular failure is the cause of death in over one-half of those who have severe stenosis.

Auscultation may reveal a paradoxic splitting of the second heart sound, which results when the aortic valve closes after the pulmonic valve. In addition, a diamond-shaped (crescendo-decrescendo) systolic ejection murmur begins after the first heart sound, increases in intensity to reach a plateau toward the middle of the ejection period, and fades progressively to end just before the aortic valve closes (Fig. 21-15). An ejection click may also occur during systole as the calcified stiff valve leaflets try to open.

Diagnostic Tests. A chest film may show apical bulging if hypertrophy is present. Calcification of the valve ring may be seen. In the presence of left ventricular failure, pulmonary vascular enlargement may be noted.

Electrocardiographic abnormalities include left ventricular hypertrophy and strain. Left ventricular hypertrophy produces changes in the amplitude of the QRS complex and ST segment displacement (strain pattern) in the precordial leads particularly [18]. Conduction system disturbances such as heart block may be manifested.

x-ray, ECG, echo., cath.

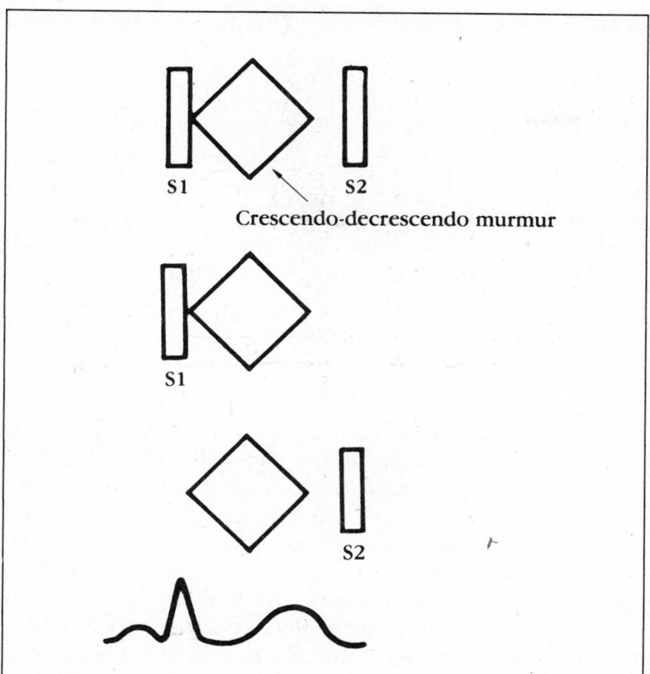

FIGURE 21-15 Diagrammatic depiction of a crescendo-decrescendo murmur. Note the relationship of the sound to the ECG recording below. The examiner should concentrate on each component. The S1 is followed by a sound of increasing intensity that stops just prior to S2.

The echocardiogram is useful in assessing valve structure and motion as well as providing information regarding ventricular function. Changes in the thickness, calcification, and mobility of the aortic valve can be recorded, and ventricular wall thickness can be evaluated.

Cardiac catheterization is useful in determining the systolic gradient across the valve, as well as the valve orifice size. The gradient may be as much as 100 mm Hg, which means, for example, that in order to attain a systemic systolic pressure of 100 mm Hg, the left ventricle must attain a systolic pressure of 200 mm Hg.

Aortic Regurgitation, Insufficiency, or Incompetence

Aortic regurgitation is incomplete closure of the aortic valve. It can occur as a chronic or acute lesion. Causes of chronic lesions include rheumatic fever, syphilis, hypertension, connective tissue disorders, and atherosclerosis [5]. The acute lesion can result from a dissecting aneurysm of the aorta, infectious endocarditis, and occasionally, rheumatic fever.

Pathophysiology and Compensatory Mechanisms. The pathologic process in aortic regurgitation differs with each cause. For example, with rheumatic aortic insufficiency, fibrosis and unequal contracture of the leaflets lead to malalignment of the leaflets [18]. Perforation or destruction of one or more of the leaflets with infectious endocarditis may occur. In syphilitic aortic regurgitation, dilatation of the ascending aorta stretches the individual leaflets, rendering them too short to close completely during diastole. Dissecting aortic aneurysm dilates the valve ring and prevents aortic closure.

The hemodynamic alterations of aortic insufficiency depend on the size of the leak, the diastolic pressure gradient across the valve, and the duration of diastole [18]. During systole, blood is ejected out of the left ventricle through the aortic valve and into the aorta, but some of it flows back into the ventricle during diastole when the pressure in the aorta exceeds that in the left ventricle. Similarly, during diastole, blood flows into the ventricle from the left atrium (Fig. 21-16). The left ventricle then becomes volume-overloaded by receiving blood from the left atrium through the regurgitant valve. An increase in the left ventricular end-diastolic volume results.

If the increase in end-diastolic volume in the left ventricle occurs over a period of time (chronically), the left ventricle gradually dilates as a compensatory mechanism. In other words, the myocardial fibers stretch to increase the surface area to accommodate this extra volume. This dilatation permits the left ventricle to eject a larger stroke volume (Starling's law) in order to maintain the cardiac output.

Long-standing hypertrophy is associated in this case with dilatation and often results in myocardial fibrosis so that cardiac muscle cells become unable to resume their normal shape after surgical replacement of the diseased valve [21]. As a result, left ventricle failure and acute pulmonary edema may ensue.

In *acute aortic regurgitation*, the time factor does not permit the compensatory mechanisms to develop. The

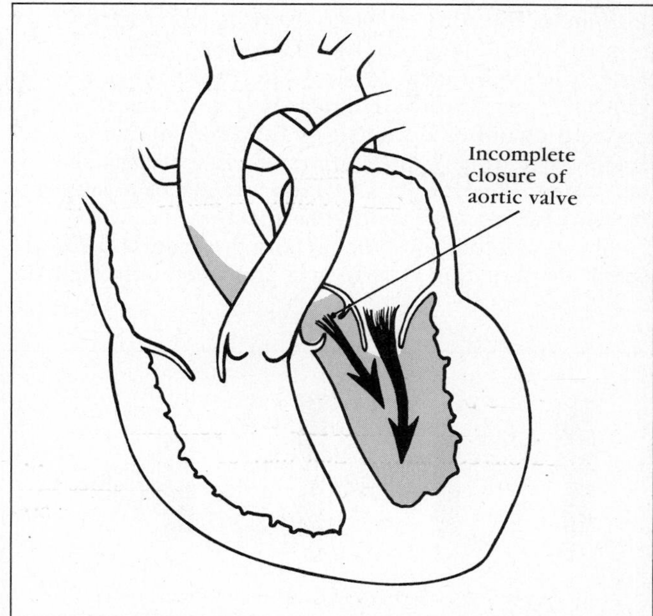

FIGURE 21-16 View of aortic insufficiency during early ventricular diastole.

volume overload in this case is so sudden that acute dilatation occurs and the left ventricle cannot maintain stroke volume and cardiac output. In acute aortic regurgitation there is a sudden increase in the left ventricular end-diastolic pressure. This is reflected to the pulmonary capillary bed, causing pulmonary edema. Death often rapidly ensues unless heroic measures are instituted.

Clinical Manifestations. In chronic aortic insufficiency with the compensatory mechanisms functioning, symptoms may not develop for many years. Palpitations may be described, especially when the person lies on the left side. A prominent apical impulse and an observable left ventricular lift on the precordium are often noted [18]. The onset of heart failure is indicated by increasing fatigue, dyspnea, chest pain, orthopnea, and paroxysmal nocturnal dyspnea.

Auscultatory findings depend on the severity of the regurgitation. In mild regurgitation, a decrescendo diastolic murmur begins shortly after S2 and ends before S1 (Fig. 21-17). With moderate regurgitation, there may be another type of murmur called an *Austin Flint murmur*, which is a diastolic rumble heard at the apex. It is caused by premature closure of the mitral valve during rapid filling of the ventricles and corresponds to the severity of aortic regurgitation.

The diastolic murmur of acute aortic regurgitation differs from those heard in chronic aortic regurgitation. The diastolic murmur can be cooing or coarsely vibrating. The first heart sound may be diminished or absent because of premature closure of the mitral valve [18].

In severe regurgitation the amplitude of the pulse increases markedly when it is palpated. This is noted as a sudden sharp pulse followed by a rapid collapse of the diastolic pulse, and is referred to as a *water-hammer* or *Corrigan's pulse*. A widening of the pulse pressure reflects inability of the aortic valve to exert its influence to maintain the aortic diastolic blood pressure [21]. The ECG reflects left ventricular hypertrophy, especially in the precordial leads, and the echocardiogram reflects the increased chamber dimensions that may occur in later stages [6]. Cardiac catheterization documents the severity and extent of aortic regurgitation and makes quantitative measurements of left ventricular function.

Once symptoms develop, in both the acute and chronic forms, deterioration is fairly swift and, if left untreated, the severe condition eventually leads to heart failure and death.

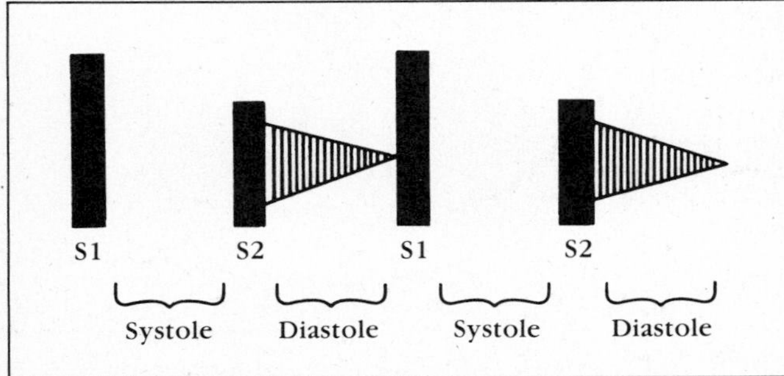

FIGURE 21-17 Diastolic murmur of aortic regurgitation.

Mixed Aortic Stenosis and Regurgitation

When aortic stenosis and regurgitation are both present, the condition is referred to as a mixed lesion. It has been reported that the majority of individuals with aortic valve disease have mixed lesions. Either stenosis or regurgitation usually predominates over the other hemodynamically.

Infective Endocarditis

Infective endocarditis affects the lining of the heart and is caused by an invading microorganism. The causative agents include bacteria, fungi, rickettsiae, and rarely, viruses and parasites [21]. Infective endocarditis has been described by a variety of terms: (1) subacute bacterial endocarditis (SBE), (2) acute bacterial endocarditis (ABE), (3) prosthetic valve endocarditis (PVE), and (4) native valve endocarditis (NVE) and others [5]. Subacute and acute bacterial endocarditis are included in this discussion.

The invading organism of subacute bacterial endocarditis is usually of low virulence and the process can develop gradually over weeks and months [5]. The disease usually affects an already damaged heart, such as one with congenital or rheumatic heart disease. The most common causative organism is *Streptococcus viridans* [2]. Acute bacterial endocarditis often occurs in persons with a normal heart but can affect damaged hearts. Because the organism is of high virulence, the process usually progresses very rapidly. The most common organism is *Staphylococcus aureus*.

The organisms traveling in the bloodstream attach to the endocardial lining of a normal heart or to the area of defect of an abnormal heart. After attaching themselves, the organisms become enmeshed in deposits of fibrin and platelets, with vegetations occurring on the leaflets of the valves. These vegetations vary in size, shape, and color, and may become quite friable depending on the invading organisms (Fig. 21-18) [2]. Acute bacterial endocarditis often produces large friable vegetations that embolize and produce embolic abscesses; SBE produces smaller vegetations that also embolize and lodge in the microcirculation and spleen. Some precipitating factors for ABE are drug abuse and cardiac surgery; SBE often results after dental work or through instrumental manipulation of the upper respiratory tract.

The clinical manifestations of infective endocarditis include fever, hematuria, splenomegaly, petechiae, Osler's nodes, and anemia. Cardiac murmurs are common. The fever and its related symptomatology are dependent on the type of infection. With acute bacterial endocarditis, the fever has a rapid onset with spikes to high elevations that are accompanied by shaking chills [5]. In subacute bacterial endocarditis the fever is usually low-grade, intermittent with elevations, and without chills. In addition, complaints of weakness, fatigue, night sweats, anorexia,

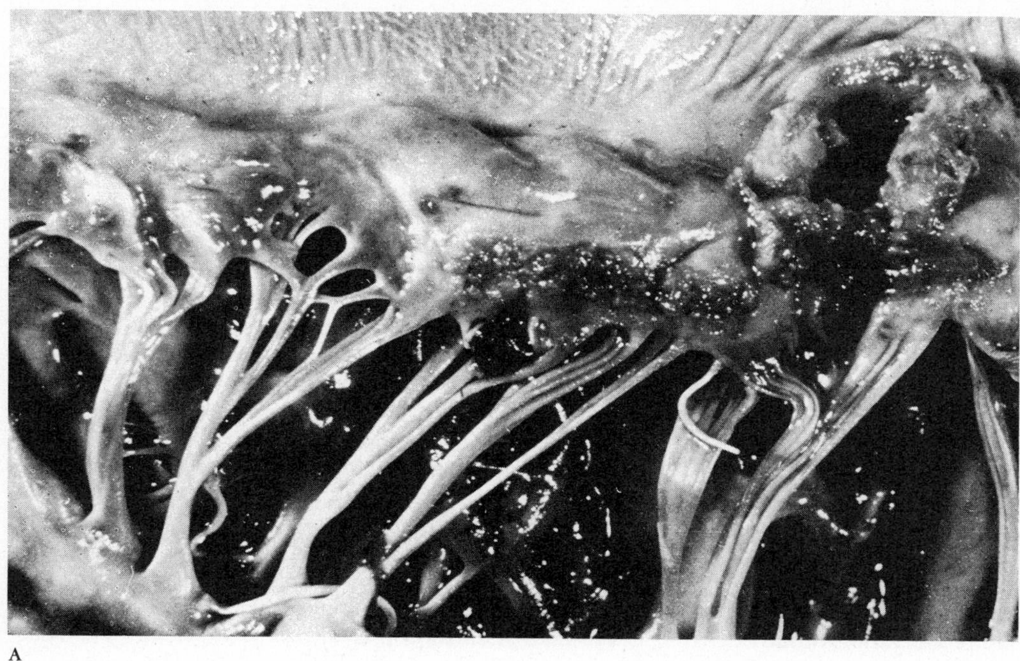

A

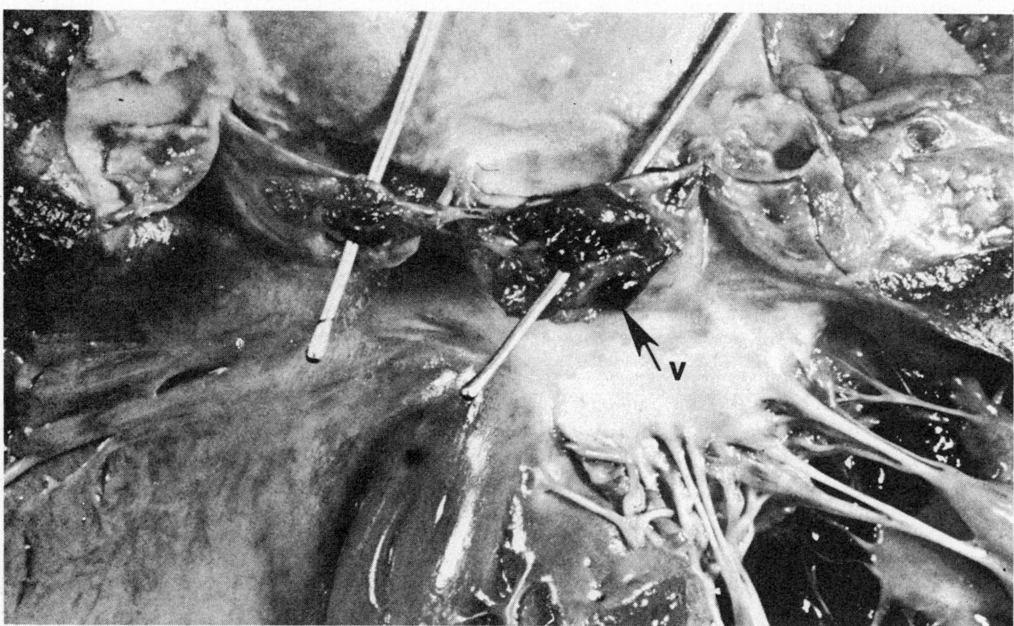

B

FIGURE 21-18 Infective endocarditis. A. The vegetations are massive, crumbly, and hemorrhagic. Top and to the right the valve has been perforated by the infective process. B. The aortic valve cusps are distorted and perforated. Vegetations (V) are present on the ventricular aspect of the valve. (From R. Cawson, A. McCracken, and P. Marcus, *Pathologic Mechanisms and Human Disease*. St. Louis: Mosby, 1982.)

and arthralgias, and exhibition of splenomegaly are common. In both types of infective endocarditis there may be Osler's nodes, which are painful, tender, red subcutaneous nodules in the pads of the fingers; Janeway's lesions, which are flat, small, irregular, nontender red spots on the palms and soles; and Roth's spots, which are retinal hemorrhages that have a white or yellow center surrounded by a red, irregular halo [5].

The vegetations produced by the infectious process settle on the cardiac valves and invade the leaflets. These vegetations prevent normal alignment of the cusps and may therefore cause incomplete closure or regurgitation, leading to cardiac murmurs. The murmurs produced correspond to the affected valve. For example, with mitral insufficiency, a systolic murmur results, and with aortic insufficiency the murmur is an early diastolic murmur.

If the vegetations grow and infiltrate the downstream side of the valve, small fragments may break off as blood is pushed through the valve orifice. These fragments, if located on the left side of the heart, may embolize to the cerebral and systemic circulations and, if on the right side, may embolize to the lungs. In addition, heart failure may ensue with severe hemodynamic alterations that occur from severe valvular regurgitation [5].

The diagnosis of infective endocarditis is based on positive blood cultures, which are present in the majority of cases. Also, a normocytic, normochromic anemia and an elevated sedimentation rate may be noted.

Treatment is aimed at identifying the causative microorganism followed by antibiotic therapy strong enough to penetrate the vegetation and reach the microorganism and kill it. Recovery from untreated infective endocarditis is rare and death often results [5].

Pericarditis

The pericardium is the fibrous sac surrounding the heart that protects the heart and secretes a lubricant for cardiac movement. It also prevents dilatation of the chambers of the heart during exercise and hypervolemia, and contains the heart in a fixed position. In addition, it provides a barrier to infections from the lungs and pleural cavities. Pericarditis is an inflammation of the pericardium that may be caused by open heart surgery (the leading cause), uremia, myocardial infarction, viral or bacterial infections, tumors, anticoagulants, or trauma [22].

As the pericardium becomes inflamed, it may grow thickened and fibrotic. If it does not heal completely after an acute episode, it may calcify over a period of time and form a firm scar surrounding the heart. This interferes with diastolic filling of the ventricles. This condition is then referred to as chronic constrictive pericarditis. Pericarditis may be classified as either acute or chronic (constrictive).

In acute pericarditis some of the clinical manifestations are pain, pericardial friction rub, electrocardiographic changes, pericardial effusion with cardiac tamponade, and a paradoxic pulse. The pain can be described as severe, sharp, and aching; it is usually precordial or substernal; and it may radiate to the left or right shoulder, arm, and elbows. On occasion, pain may spread to the jaw, throat, and ears. It may be intensified by deep breathing, sneezing, coughing, moving, or changing position. The pain may be relieved when the person sits up and leans forward. Acute pericarditis is often confused with the pain of myocardial ischemia, which may lead to misdiagnosis [21].

In addition to pain, one of the most important physical signs of pericarditis is a friction rub that is heard best at the apex and at the lower left sternal border. It is an intermittent, transitory sound that imitates the sound of sandpaper rubbing together. This loud, "to-and-fro," leathery sound may disappear on one day and reappear on the next.

Acute pericarditis can produce the following changes on ECG: (1) ST elevation occurs in two or three standard limb leads and precordial leads V_2 through V_6; (2) reciprocal depressions occur in AV_R and V_1; and (3) several days to weeks after the early stage, the ST segments return to normal and the T waves invert. Low voltage is characteristic and no Q waves develop; this helps to distinguish acute pericarditis from an acute myocardial infarction.

Pericardial effusion may also develop in cases of acute pericarditis. This is fluid that accumulates between the pericardium and myocardium. If the fluid accumulates rapidly, it can cause cardiac compression and tamponade. With pericardial effusion, the heart sounds are faint and apical impulse may disappear. Chest film shows enlargement of the cardiac silhouette. The heart may appear as a "water bottle" configuration (Fig. 21-19). The echocardiogram detects the presence of pericardial fluid.

When fluid accumulates rapidly or in an amount large enough to impair cardiac function, the condition is referred to as *cardiac tamponade*. The amount of fluid that can cause tamponade varies according to the rate of fluid accumulation. In rapid accumulation of fluid, 250 ml may produce significant obstruction. When an effusion develops slowly, 1000 ml or more may accumulate before significant symptoms develop. As fluid collects in the pericardium, the pressure rises in the pericardial cavity to a level equal to the pressures in the heart during diastole. The first structures to be compressed are the right atrium and ventricle because they have the lowest diastolic pressures. This compression causes increased venous pressure with decreased right atrial filling. Systemic venous congestion with edema and hepatomegaly result. There is also a decrease in diastolic filling of the ventricles, which leads to decreases in stroke volume and cardiac output. This can be a life-threatening complication of pericarditis, and death may occur from circulatory collapse [21].

A characteristic sign of cardiac tamponade is *pulsus paradoxus*. This is a large inspiratory reduction in arterial pressure that can be heard with a stethoscope. In pulsus paradoxus the systolic blood pressure drops more than 10 mm Hg during inspiration. If the tamponade is severe, pulsus paradoxus may be palpated as a weakness or disappearance in the arterial pressure during inspiration.

Chronic constrictive pericarditis results from the healing of acute pericarditis and formation of granular tissue that gradually contracts to form a firm scar surrounding

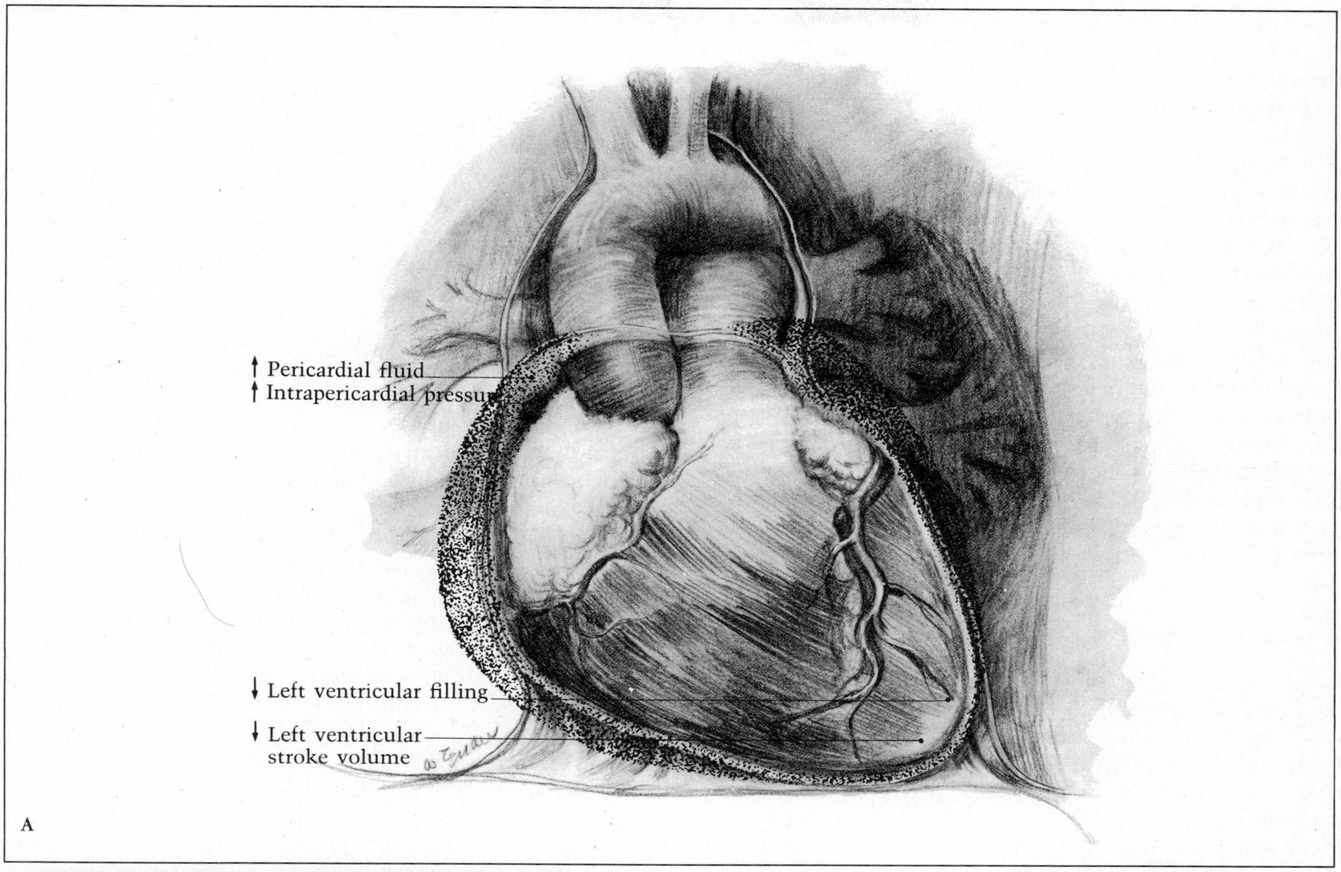

↑ Pericardial fluid
↑ Intrapericardial pressu
↓ Left ventricular filling
↓ Left ventricular stroke volume

A

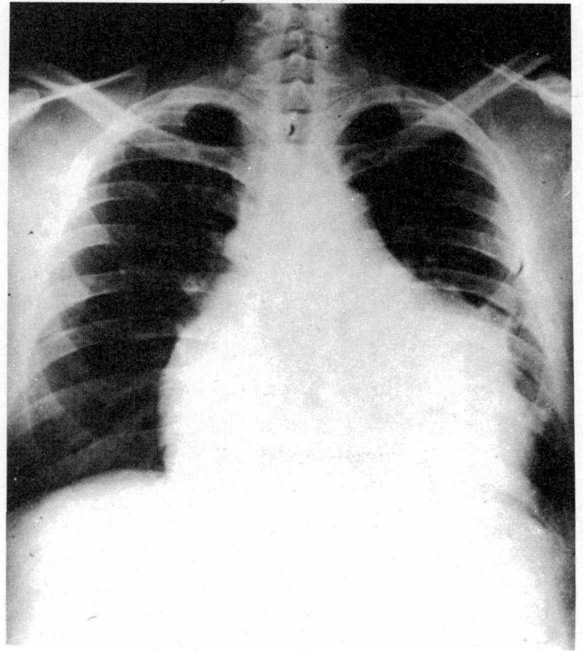

B

FIGURE 21-19 Pericardial effusion and cardiac tamponade. The following hemodynamic effects may result after pericardial effusion: (1) accumulation of pericardial fluid resulting in intrapericardial pressure, (2) elevation of right atrial pressure, (3) elevation of left ventricular end-diastolic pressure, (4) reductions in left ventricular end-diastolic volume and cardiac output, and (5) elevated venous pressure. B. Chest film of an individual with a large pericardial effusion that resulted in pericardial tamponade. (From C. Kenner, C. Guzzetta, and B. Dossey, ***Critical Care Nursing: Body, Mind, Spirit*** (2nd ed.). Boston: Little, Brown, 1985.)

the heart. This scar causes constriction of the heart and therefore interferes with filling of the ventricles; this complication is similar to the physiologic abnormality that results from cardiac tamponade except that it develops slowly.

Clinical manifestations of chronic constrictive pericarditis are weakness, fatigue, weight loss, anorexia, and edema. Individuals may complain of abdominal discomfort due to systemic venous congestion. This discomfort may be related to hepatic congestion and swelling of the abdomen. A characteristic sign of constrictive pericarditis is jugular neck vein distention, which is indicative of elevated venous pressure.

The echocardiogram may show pericardial thickening and paradoxic septal motion in constrictive pericarditis. Also noted on the echocardiogram is that the left ventricular wall moves distinctly outward in early diastole and then remains flat. The chest film may be diagnostic when calcification appears in the pericardium.

Congenital Heart Disease

Congenital cardiovascular disease is an abnormality of structure or function of the heart and/or circulatory system. The abnormalities usually result from an alteration or failure of development of a structure within the heart. The condition causes a shunting or obstructive defect, or both. A cardiovascular shunt refers to blood flow through an abnormal communication between the chambers of the heart or between the pulmonary and systemic circulations. An obstructive defect causes increased intraventricular or interatrial pressures.

The frequency of congenital cardiovascular malformations is difficult to determine because many are asymptomatic and not diagnosed in infancy. Prolapses of the bicuspid aortic and mitral valves are common asymptomatic congenital defects. It is estimated that approximately 0.8 percent of live births are complicated by a cardiovascular malformation [1].

The etiology of congenital heart disease is variable and appears to result from multifactorial interactions between genetic and environmental systems. A causative factor usually cannot be identified. Some environmental insults include viral infection (especially rubella) in the first eight weeks of pregnancy, and drug and alcohol abuse. Maternal lupus erythematosus has been implicated as a major risk factor. Hereditary factors may be involved in such conditions as atrial septal defect, patent ductus arteriosus, and coarctation of the aorta. Some lesions are more prevalent in females (atrial septal defect, patent ductus arteriosus), and some in males (coarctation of the aorta, congenital aortic stenosis). Extracardiac anomalies occur in approximately 25 percent of infants with significant cardiac anomalies [7]. Preterm infants almost all have persistence of the ductus arteriosus, a structure that normally closes at birth. Stillborn infants have a very high frequency of complex cardiac anomalies.

Embryology

To understand the congenital heart defects, one must understand the development of the heart. The heart develops from a straight cardiac tube, which appears in the first month of gestation. This forms the primitive atrium and ventricle, followed rapidly by a large truncus arteriosus. The tube doubles over on itself during the second month of gestation to form two parallel pumping systems, each having two chambers and a great artery (the truncus arteriosus). As a consequence of this doubling, the heart begins to situate in the left side of the chest. An endocardial cushion develops within the common chamber and is the first of the structures to divide the chambers of the heart. From the endocardial cushion, the mitral and tricuspid orifices develop. The large truncus divides into the aorta and pulmonary arteries. Rotation of the truncus coils the aortopulmonary septum and creates the normal spiral relationship between the aorta and pulmonary artery. The truncus arteriosus is connected to the dorsal aorta by six pairs of aortic arches that appear and disappear at different times during the formation of the heart and vessels. Abnormalities of the regression of the arch system in a number of sites can produce a wide variety of arch abnormalities. The major septa of the heart are formed between the twenty-seventh and thirty-seventh days of development [15].

In addition to formation of heart and vessel structures, changes occur in the fetal circulation that enable the newborn to survive in the extrauterine environment. During fetal growth the placenta performs the duties of respiration, excretion, and nourishment for the fetus. There are three essential structures: the *ductus venosus*, a vessel that connects the umbilical vein to the inferior vena cava; the *foramen ovale*, an opening in the interatrial septum; and the *ductus arteriosus*, a vessel that joins the main pulmonary artery and the distal aortic arch.

During fetal life the blood passes from the placenta along the umbilical vein through the ductus venosus and into the inferior vena cava, where it is mixed with venous return from the lower extremities. It enters the right atrium and is mainly channeled through the foramen ovale, a one-way valve, into the left atrium where it is channeled to the rest of the body to provide oxygen and nutrients to all of the tissues. Blood flow from the head and upper extremities returns to the superior vena cava, is channeled into the right ventricle, and is pumped out the pulmonary artery. Because of the nonfunctioning, nonexpanded lungs, the resistance to blood flow into the lungs is higher and blood shunts through the ductus arteriosus into the descending aorta (Fig. 21-20).

Because of the resistance of the lungs, the pressures in the right ventricle and thus those in the right atrium are elevated, causing a right-to-left shunt of blood across the foramen ovale into the left atrium. Birth changes are as follows: the infant cries and expands its lungs, decreasing the resistance in the pulmonary circulation and lowering the pressure in the right side of the heart. With dilatation of the pulmonary vessels and lowered pulmonary arterial

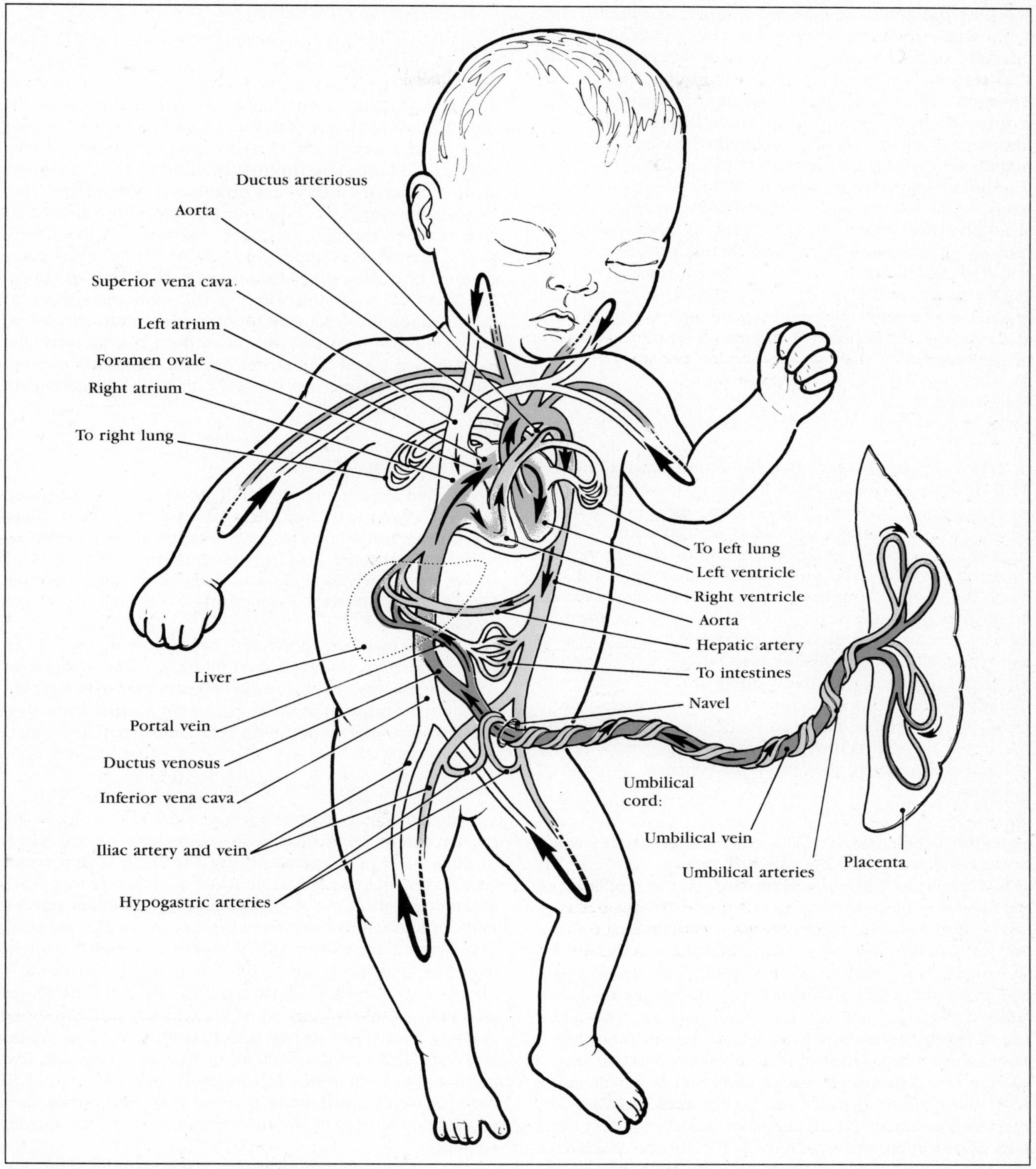

FIGURE 21-20 Diagrammatic illustration of fetal circulation. Arrows show the direction of blood flow.

pressure, the flow is diminished through the ductus arteriosus and it gradually closes, usually becoming a thin ligamentlike structure within six to eight weeks after birth. Clamping the umbilical cord leads to clotting of blood in the umbilical vein and ductus venosus; the latter occludes within one to five days to become a ligament also. The increased systemic resistance created with clamping of the umbilical arteries is transmitted to the left atrium, and this, in conjunction with increased venous return from the lungs, causes the pressure in that chamber to exceed right atrial pressure, thus tending to create a left-to-right flow through the foramen ovale. The foramen ovale acts as a one-way valve, and the tendency toward reversal of flow causes the flap of the valve to close. Closure is followed by gradual, permanent obliteration of the opening by fibrous adherence of the flap to the interatrial septum within six to eight months.

Consequences of Congenital Heart Disease

Left-to-Right Shunt. Because blood flows along the path of least resistance from higher to lower pressures, most congenital defects having an abnormal communication between chambers or vessels end up with a left-to-right shunt. A portion of blood returned to the left heart is diverted back into the pulmonary circuit before it can reach the systemic capillaries. This often causes increased volume in the right heart and subsequently, in the pulmonary circuit. Most atrial and ventricular septal defects and patent ductus arteriosus cause the left-to-right shunt. The result is pulmonary overloading and eventually, pulmonary hypertension and congestion. The systemic circulation may become impaired if the shunt is large. The result may be right ventricular failure due to the continual volume and pressure that the right ventricle is required to pump.

Right-to-Left Shunt. This type of shunt occurs when desaturated, systemic, venous blood is diverted to the left side of the heart without passing through the capillaries of the lungs. For this condition to occur there must be a communication from the right heart to the left heart, and the pressures in the right heart must exceed those of the left.

The common signs and symptoms include cyanosis, polycythemia, clubbing, squatting, and failure to thrive. When cyanosis is present, the shunt is large, with about one-third of the arterial hemoglobin being unsaturated. Polycythemia is the normal reaction of the body to lack of oxygen. The kidneys release erythropoietin, which stimulates the release of more red blood cells (RBCs). The increased numbers of RBCs increase blood viscosity. Clubbing also occurs with long-term polycythemia and cyanosis. The ends of the phalanges become bulbous and the nails curved. The cause of clubbing may be dilatation and engorgement of the local capillaries in an attempt to gain oxygen. The child may assume a squatting position, which may be a way of centralizing the available oxygen. Failure to thrive and growth retardation may be related to tissue hypoxia and poor nutrient absorption.

Patent Ductus Arteriosus

When the embryonic patent ductus arteriosus (PDA) fails to close after birth, it persists as a shunt between the pulmonary artery and the aorta. It often occurs as an isolated defect and is the second most common defect in infants and children [17]. The patent ductus often does not manifest in the early postnatal days, but within about two weeks the blood flow through the ductus from the aorta to the pulmonary artery first produces a systolic and then a continuous machinerylike murmur, indicating a constant flow of blood through the shunt. The result of this condition is increased volume and pressure in the pulmonary system, basically short-circuiting one-fourth to three-fourths of left ventricular output. The signs and symptoms depend upon the volume of the shunt and often are absent. The condition is usually discovered on routine physical examination when the murmur is detected. Other symptoms include pulmonary congestion and manifestations of left heart failure.

Atrial Septal Defects

Congenital atrial septal defects (ASDs) are very common and result from failure of the atrial septum to close. There are various forms: *ostium primum*, *persistent atrioventricular communis*, and *ostium secundum*. Figure 21-21 shows the embryologic development of the atrial septum. Figure 21-22 shows the location of the common types of ASDs.

Clinical manifestations depend upon the size of the defect and the volume of shunted blood. The majority of ASDs are asymptomatic, but right ventricular hypertrophy, frequent respiratory infections, feeding difficulties, dyspnea, fatiguability, and growth retardation may develop.

Ventricular Septal Defects

Ventricular septal defects (VSDs) are considered to be the most common congenital heart lesions and account for 8 to 20 percent of congenital heart disease. The ventricular septum grows in a cephalad (headward) fashion and fuses at the endocardial cushion. It begins as a muscular septum with a membranous portion at the point of closure [14]. The shunt of blood in a VSD is almost always left to right from the high pressure in the left ventricle to the low pressure in the right ventricle (Fig. 21-23). The shunt produces a holosystolic murmur of a high grade, often creating a palpable thrill on the chest wall. In a large shunt there is significant overloading of the right ventricle and pulmonary circulations. In the small defect the shunt of blood is much smaller and may be occluded during part of ventricular systole by the contraction of the muscular septum.

The clinical manifestations of VSDs depend upon the amount of pulmonary overloading and right ventricular strain. In some cases (as many as 10–30%) the defect apparently closes spontaneously and a preexisting murmur then disappears. Pulmonary hypertension and right ventricular failure are signs of poor prognosis without surgical intervention. The defect may progress to a cyanotic

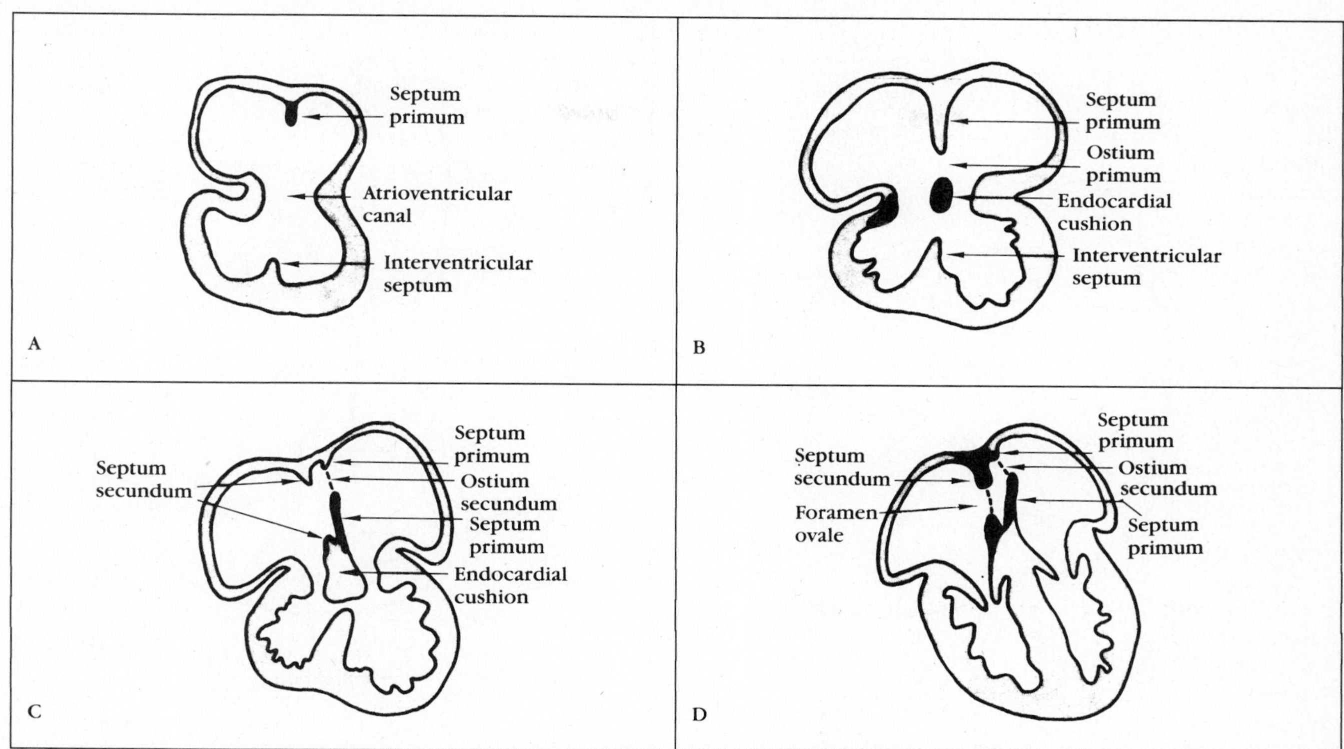

FIGURE 21-21 Schematic illustration of the embryological development of the atrial septum. A. Septum primum beginning to divide the fetal single atrium. B. Development of the endocardial cushion that will form a portion of the atrioventricular valves. C. Two septi, the septum primum and the osteo secundum, basically divide the atria into two chambers. D. The septum secundum forms as an incomplete structure, the septum primum remains as a flap valve. Right-to-left flow of blood in fetal circulation keeps this foramen ovale open. When the flow of blood changes to a left-to-right shunt, the flap valve over the foramen ovale closes, anatomically dividing the chambers. (Reprinted from J. Kernicki, B. Bullock, and J. Matthews, *Cardiovascular Nursing*. New York: G.P. Putnam, 1971.)

condition if the right ventricular pressures become high enough to reverse the shunt to right to left.

Tetralogy of Fallot

This condition was first described by Fallot in 1888. It is the primary cause of cyanotic heart disease and is more common in males than in females. It involves the combination of pulmonary stenosis, ventricular septal defect, dextroposition of the aortic root, and hypertrophy of the right ventricle (Fig. 21-24). The degree of pulmonary stenosis is responsible for the volume and direction of the shunt. It increases right ventricular pressure, causing shunting of blood from the right ventricle to the left through the ventricular septal defect. Pulmonary stenosis also decreases pulmonary blood flow and the available blood for oxygenation. Direct pumping of blood to the aorta from the right ventricle causes direct access of venous blood to the systemic circulation.

Cyanosis is usually severe and deepens during exertion, pulmonary infection, and dyspnea. Clubbing of the fingers also depends upon the degree of cyanosis. The oxygen saturation in the arterial system may be 80 percent or lower, while venous oxygen saturation may be below 60 percent (normal 75–80%) [1]. Polycythemia is compensatory and causes increased blood volume and elevated hematocrit. Cerebral anoxia may cause periods of dizziness and convulsions. Squatting is often a habitual response. Stunting of growth is characteristic. Complications of the condition include cerebral embolism, subacute bacterial endocarditis, and brain damage from hypoxia.

Transposition of the Great Vessels

In the fourth week of gestation the common truncus arteriosus is divided into the pulmonary artery and the aorta. The two vessels rotate so that the pulmonary artery lies anterior and in the right ventricle and the aorta arises posterior and in the left ventricle, thus providing for normal blood flow. In transposition, this rotation does not occur and the aorta arises anteriorly from the right ventricle and the pulmonary artery arises posteriorly from the left ventricle. Blood is pumped from the right ventricle through

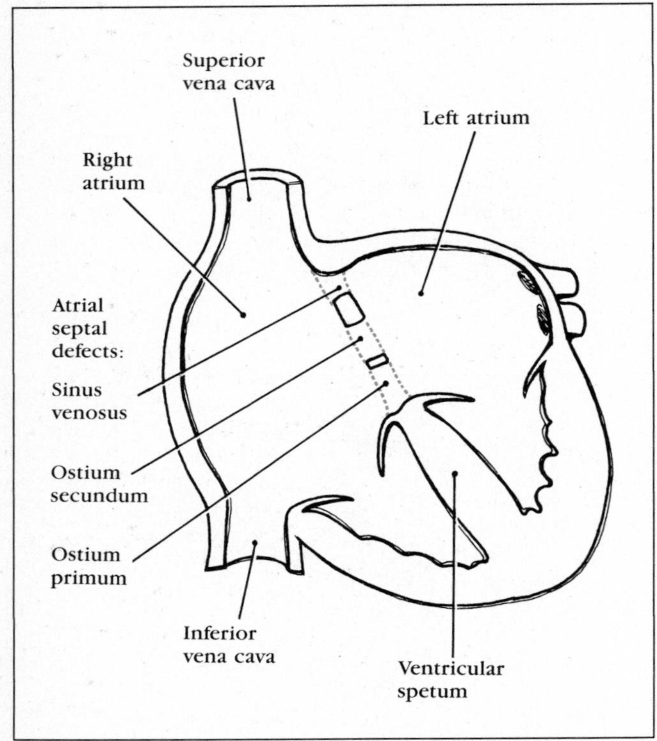

FIGURE 21-22 Location of the common types of atrial septal defects.

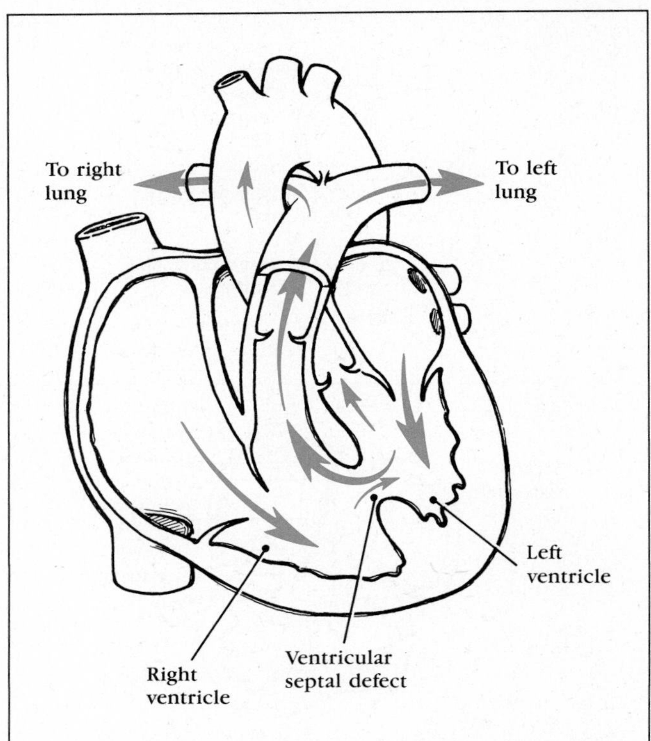

FIGURE 21-23 Blood flow in a ventricular septal defect.

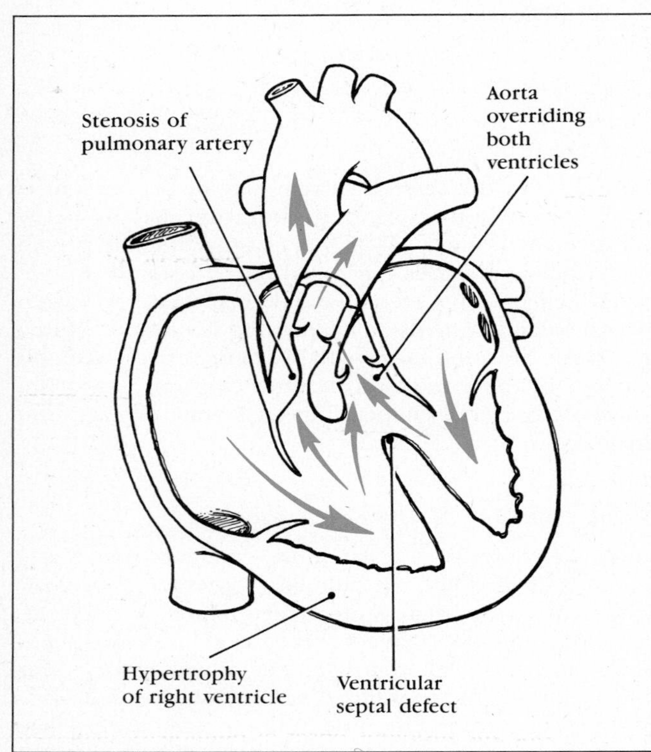

FIGURE 21-24 Blood flow in tetralogy of Fallot.

the aorta to the systemic system, and returns through the cavae to the right atrium. Blood from the left ventricle passes through the pulmonary artery to the lungs and returns through the pulmonary veins to the left atrium (Fig. 21-25). These two closed circuits are obviously incompatible with life.

Other defects usually associated with this condition include atrial septal defects, ventricular septal defects, and enlarged bronchial arteries to carry blood from the aorta to the lungs. In some cases the ductus arteriosus remains patent and the foramen ovale remains open due to the increase in right atrial pressure. The clinical manifestations depend upon the amount of intermixing of blood from the associated life-sustaining defects. Cyanosis may be severe or minimal to absent; it is intensified with exertion. Dyspnea is common, and congestive heart failure frequently occurs in early infancy. Death within the first year is common without surgical intervention.

Coarctation of the Aorta

The aortic arch develops between the fifth and seventh weeks of gestation. The area of the aorta near the ductus arteriosus may develop improperly, leaving a restricted lumen, proximal to, at, or distal to the insertion of the ductus [15]. Postductal coarctation obstructs blood flow beyond the left subclavian artery so that the blood pressure in the upper extremities is much higher than in the

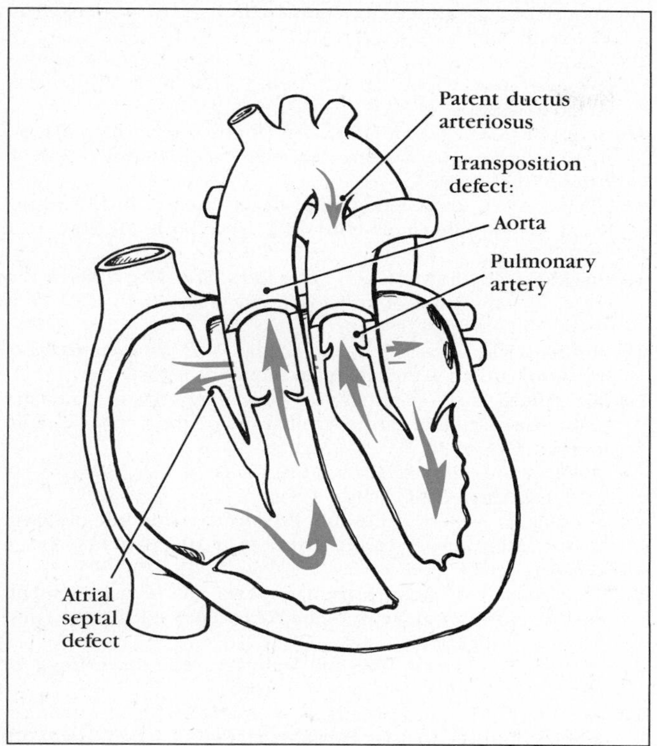

FIGURE 21-25 Blood flow in transposition of the great vessels.

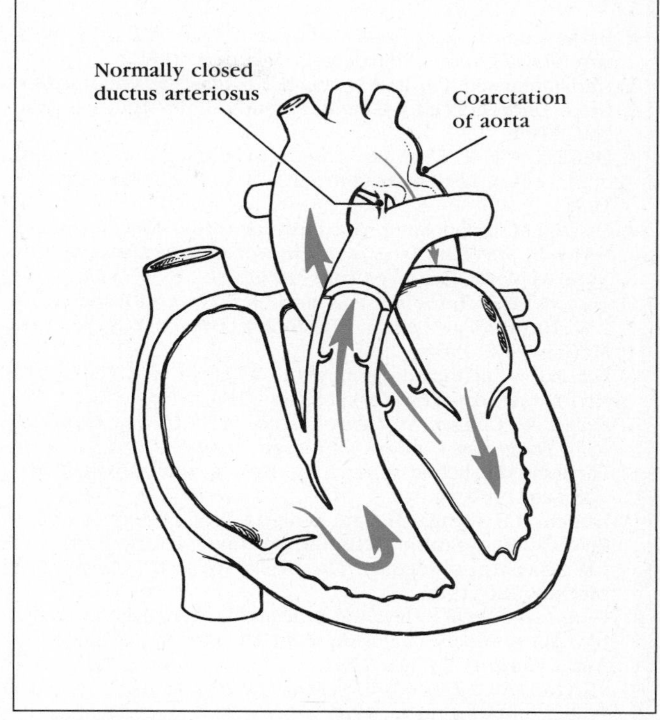

FIGURE 21-26 Postductal coarctation of the aorta.

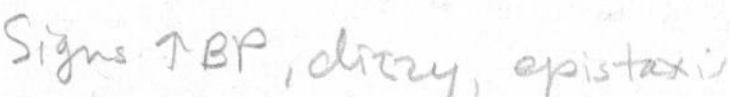

lower extremities (Fig. 21-26). No cyanosis is evident because the ductus closes at birth. The symptoms result from high blood pressure and decreased circulation to the lower extremities. Headaches, dizziness, epistaxis, and intermittent claudication, coolness, or pallor in the lower extremities may be noted. Preductal or ductal coarctation usually results in persistent patency of the ductus with blood shunting from the pulmonary artery to the aorta. The result is cyanosis of the lower extremities. In either case, congestive heart failure may result, especially after 5 years of age [24].

Other Defects

Less common congenital heart diseases include *total anomalous pulmonary venous connection*, with the pulmonary veins connected to the right atrium; *truncus arteriosus*, in which the embryonic truncus fails to divide into the aorta and pulmonary arteries; the *endocardial cushion defect*, in which the valves and septi fail to form adequately and may result in a one-chambered heart; *isolated pulmonary stenosis*, with stricture of the pulmonic valve or pulmonic outlet; and numerous others. *Mitral valve prolapse*, discussed on pages 333–334, results when the posterior leaflet of the mitral valve is abnormally large and inferiorly placed. It causes abnormal cardiac hemodynamics, which can include mitral insufficiency and various cardiac dysrhythmias. This condition is very common, especially in women, and is frequently asymptomatic.

Study Questions

1. Describe the impairments of function in various areas of the heart that may be caused by myocardial infarction.
2. Outline the pathways for radiation of cardiac ischemic pain.
3. Compare the elevation of serum enzymes and ECG changes in immediate and later stages of myocardial infarction.
4. Discuss the predictable complications of myocardial infarction based on the location and extent of the infarct.
5. Compare the hemodynamic consequences of mitral and aortic stenosis and insufficiency.
6. Discriminate among the various heart murmurs produced by acquired and congenital intracardiac defects.
7. Describe the consequences of acute and subacute endocarditis.
8. Compare the defects, hemodynamic features and clinical manifestations of cyanotic and acyanotic congenital cardiac conditions.
9. Why will transposition of the great vessels not sustain life without associated intracardiac defects?
10. Describe the insidious onset of pulmonary hypertension resulting from mitral valve disease and from left-to-right shunts in congenital heart defects.

References

1. Braunwald, E. (ed.). *Heart Disease: A Textbook of Cardiovascular Medicine*. Philadelphia: Saunders, 1980.
2. Christopherson, P.J., and Swarajan, E.S. Infective endocarditis. In S.L. Underhill (ed.), *Cardiac Nursing*. Philadelphia: Lippincott, 1982.
3. DeBusk, R.F. Technique of exercise testing. In J.W. Hurst et al. (eds.), *The Heart* (6th ed.). New York: McGraw-Hill, 1986.
4. Disch, J.M. Diagnostic procedures for cardiovascular disease, Series II. *Surgical Aspects of Cardiovascular Disease*. New York: Appleton-Century-Crofts, 1979.
5. Durack, D.T. Infective and noninfective endocarditis. In J.W. Hurst et al. (eds.), *The Heart* (6th ed.). New York: McGraw-Hill, 1986.
6. Felner, J.M. Echocardiography. In J.W. Hurst et al. (eds.), *The Heart* (6th ed.). New York: McGraw-Hill, 1986.
7. Fink, B.W. *Congenital Heart Disease: A Deductive Approach to Its Diagnosis* (2nd ed.). Chicago: Yearbook, 1985.
8. Fortium, M.J. Echocardiography: How it works. *Med. Times* 108:120, 1980.
9. Franch, R.H., King, S.B., and Douglas, J.S. Techniques of cardiac catheterization including coronary arteriography. In J.W. Hurst et al. (eds.), *The Heart* (6th ed.). New York: McGraw-Hill, 1986.
10. Geft, I.L., et al. ST elevation in leads V_1 to V_5 may be caused by right coronary occlusion and right ventricular infarction. *Am. J. Cardiol.* 53:991, 1984.
11. Guyton, A.C. *Textbook of Medical Physiology* (7th ed.). Philadelphia: Saunders, 1986.
12. Hurst, J.W., et al. Atherosclerotic coronary heart disease, angina pectoris, myocardial infarction, and other manifestations of myocardial ischemia. In J.W. Hurst et al. (eds.), *The Heart* (6th ed.). New York: McGraw-Hill, 1986.
13. Jackle, M., and Halligan, M. *Cardiovascular Problems: A Critical Care Nursing Focus*. Bowie, Md.: Brady, 1980.
14. Kernicki, J., Bullock, B., and Matthew, J. *Cardiovascular Nursing*. New York: Putnam, 1971.
15. Langman, J. *Medical Embryology: Human Development—Normal and Abnormal* (2nd ed.). Baltimore: Williams & Wilkins, 1969.
16. Limacher, M.C., et al. Detection of coronary artery disease with exercise two-dimensional echocardiography. *Circulation* 67:1211, 1983.
17. Plauth, W.H., et al. Congenital heart disease. In J.W. Hurst et al. (eds)., *The Heart* (6th ed.). New York: McGraw-Hill, 1986.
18. Rackley, C.E., Edwards, J.E., and Karp, R.B. Mitral valve disease. In J.W. Hurst et al. (eds.), *The Heart* (6th ed.). New York: McGraw-Hill, 1986.
19. Robbins, S.L., Cotran, R.S., and Kumar, V. *Pathologic Basis of Disease* (3rd ed.). Philadelphia: Saunders, 1984.
20. Silverberg, R.A., et al. Noninvasive diagnosis of coronary artery disease: The cardio-kymographic stress test. *Circulation* 61:579, 1980.
21. Sokolow, M., and McIlroy, M.B. *Clinical Cardiology* (4th ed.). Los Altos, Calif.: Lange, 1986.
22. Spodick, D.H. Pericardial rub: Prospective multiple-observer investigation of pericardial friction in 100 patients. *Am. J. Cardiol.* 35:357, 1975.
23. Stollerman, G.H. Acute rheumatic fever and its management. In J.W. Hurst et al. (eds.), *The Heart* (6th ed.). New York: McGraw-Hill, 1986.
24. Wenger, N.K., Hurst, J.W., and McIntyre, M.C. *Cardiology for Nurses*. New York: McGraw-Hill, 1980.
25. Wenger, N.K., and Sclant, N.C. Prevention of coronary atherosclerosis. In J.W. Hurst et al. (eds.), *The Heart* (6th ed.). New York: McGraw-Hill, 1986.
26. Zaret, B.L., and Berges, H.J. Techniques of nuclear cardiology. In J.W. Hurst et al. (eds.), *The Heart* (6th ed.). New York: McGraw-Hill, 1986.

CHAPTER 22

Hypertension

CHAPTER OUTLINE

Definitions
Etiology of Hypertension

- Age
- Sex
- Race
- Heredity
- Lifestyle
  - *Serum Lipoproteins*
- Diabetes Mellitus
- Secondary Hypertension

Pathophysiology

- Essential Hypertension
- Secondary Hypertension
- Clinical Manifestations of Hypertension
  - *Stroke*
  - *Myocardial Infarction*
  - *Renal Failure*
  - *Encephalopathy*

Diagnosis of Hypertension

LEARNING OBJECTIVES

1. Define *hypertension* as it relates to different age groups.
2. Compare the definitions of *borderline*, *labile*, *benign*, and *malignant hypertension*.
3. List and briefly describe the factors related to the cause of hypertension.
4. Describe briefly the significance of serum lipoproteins in hypertension.
5. Explain how blood pressure levels are normally maintained in the arterial system.
6. Describe the abnormal renin theory in the production of essential hypertension.
7. Compare the pathophysiology of essential and secondary hypertension.
8. List the typical symptoms of hypertension.
9. Explain the four major morbid sequelae of hypertensive disease.
10. List the diagnostic tests used in hypertensive disease.

Hypertension is the most common disease in the United States and is a direct risk factor, contributing to myocardial infarction, congestive heart failure, and cerebrovascular accidents [5]. The etiology of the disorder is poorly understood, treatment is lifelong, and the condition is generally asymptomatic until complications develop. The frequency of sudden death is markedly increased among hypertensive persons.

Table 22-1 Hypertension as It Relates to Different Age Groups

Age Group	Normal	Hypertensive
Infants	80/40	90/60
Children		
7–11 years	100/60	120/80
Teenagers		
12–17 years	115/70	130/80
Adults		
20–45 years	120–125/75–80	135/90
45–65 years	135–140/85	140/90–160/95
Over 65 years	150/85	160/90 (borderline)

Definitions

Hypertension is defined as abnormal elevation of the systolic arterial blood pressure. Levels that are considered to be hypertensive vary with age. Blood pressure (BP) levels fluctuate within certain limits depending on the body position, age, and stress (Table 22-1). *Borderline hypertension* in adults is considered to be consistent readings between 140/90 and 160/95, with readings above 160/95 definitely hypertensive [3]. Hypertension is also frequently classified as mild, moderate, or severe on the basis of the diastolic pressure. Mild hypertension has a diastolic pressure in the range of 95 to 104, moderate 105 to 114, and severe 115 or greater. The diagnosis is made by high readings (>140/90) on three separate occasions after 20 minutes or more of rest [11]. *Sustained hypertension* occurs when the blood pressure remains elevated over hours or days [14]. Persons who have occasional elevation of blood pressure have *labile hypertension*.

The most common feature of hypertension is a mixed elevation of systolic and diastolic blood pressures. Occasionally, the diastolic pressure is elevated without a significant increase in systolic pressure. This indicates an increase in peripheral vascular resistance (PVR) and is most frequent in young persons. Increase in systolic pressure without diastolic elevation may occur in elderly persons, those with hyperdynamic circulation (e.g., hyperthyroidism), or individuals with aortic insufficiency.

Other definitive terms include essential (idiopathic) hypertension, which has no specific etiologic basis and secondary hypertension which is due to a known cause (Table 22-2). *Benign* and *malignant hypertension* refer to the course of the disease, and either may result from essential or secondary hypertension. Benign hypertension is a misnomer because it causes permanent damage, even though it has a gradual onset and begins with blood pressure levels only slightly above normal. Malignant hypertension is rapidly progressive, uncontrollable blood pressure elevation that causes rapid onset of complications, including renal failure, cerebrovascular accident, retinal hemorrhages, congestive heart failure, and encephalopathy.

Etiology of Hypertension

Age

There is a positive relationship between age and the frequency of hypertension; with the prevalence increasing as the individual ages. As much as 50 percent of the population over age 50 years may be hypertensive [10]. Hypertension in those below age 35 years markedly increases the frequency of heart disease (coronary artery disease [CAD]) and premature death [9].

Table 22-2 Causes of Hypertension

Type of Hypertension	Causes
Essential, idiopathic, or primary	Related to obesity, hypercholesterolemia, atherosclerosis, high-sodium diet, diabetes, stress, type A personality, familial history, smoking, and lack of exercise
Secondary	Renovascular
	Parenchymal disease, such as acute and chronic glomerulonephritis
	Narrowing, stenosis of renal artery—due to atherosclerosis or congenital fibroplasia
	Cushing's disease or syndrome
	May be due to increased secretion of glucocorticoids as result of adrenal disease or pituitary dysfunction
	Primary aldosteronism
	Increased aldosterone secretion, often a result of adrenal tumor
	Pheochromocytoma
	Tumor of adrenal medulla causing increased secretion of adrenal catecholamines
	Coarctation of the aorta
	Congenital constriction of aorta usually at the level of the ductus arteriosus with increased blood pressure above the constriction and decreased pressure below the constriction

Sex

Overall, men have a higher frequency than women, but at middle age and beyond, the prevalence begins to change, and disease in women exceeds that in men at the older ages (over age 65 years).

Race

Blacks have at least twice the frequency of hypertension as whites. The consequences of the disease are usually more severe in them. For example, at diastolic levels of 115 or over, mortality for black men is 3.3 times that of similarly hypertensive white men and 5.6 times that of white women [10].

Heredity

Genetic influences play a role in the development of hypertension. Prevalence of the disease is clustered in families. For example, if both parents have essential hypertension, prevalence in offspring is 1 of 2. One hypertensive parent produces a 1 in 3 frequency while normotensive parents produce a 1 in 20 frequency in their children [14].

Lifestyle

The relationship between hypertension and factors such as education, income, diet, and other aspects of lifestyle have been studied with inconclusive results. Low income, low educational levels, and stressful lives or occupations seem to be related to greater frequency of hypertension. Family history of the disease has always been considered a risk factor; however, this relationship may be related more to lifestyle than to a straight genetic link, especially with respect to essential hypertension. Obesity is considered to be a major risk factor. When weight reduction is achieved, blood pressure often returns to the normal range. Cigarette smoking is implicated as a high-risk factor for both hypertension and CAD. Dietary intake of saturated fats is thought to be a major factor in the development of high serum cholesterol levels. Hypercholesterolemia and hyperglycemia are both major factors in the development of atherosclerosis, which is closely associated with hypertension. The lipoproteins responsible for hypercholesterolemia have been studied in terms of atherogenesis.

Serum Lipoproteins. Five families of lipoproteins have been identified: (1) chylomicron, (2) very-low-density lipoprotein (VLDL), (3) intermediate-density lipoprotein, (4) low-density lipoprotein (LDL), and (5) high-density lipoprotein (HDL) [1]. Each group performs different functions in the body. Chylomicrons transport most of the dietary substances, and VLDL carry most of the triglycerides. Much of the plasma cholesterol is carried by LDL; HDL apparently serves as a reservoir for lipoproteins involved in triglyceride transport and in the esterification of cholesterol. The level of HDL is usually higher in women than in men and may encourage the storage of cholesterol in the liver in women [1]. HDL levels are often increased in athletic individuals. Figure 22-1 shows the composition of the major lipoproteins. Research continues into the role of HDL in protection from CAD.

Diabetes Mellitus

The relationship between diabetes mellitus and hypertension is obscure, but the statistics support a definite link

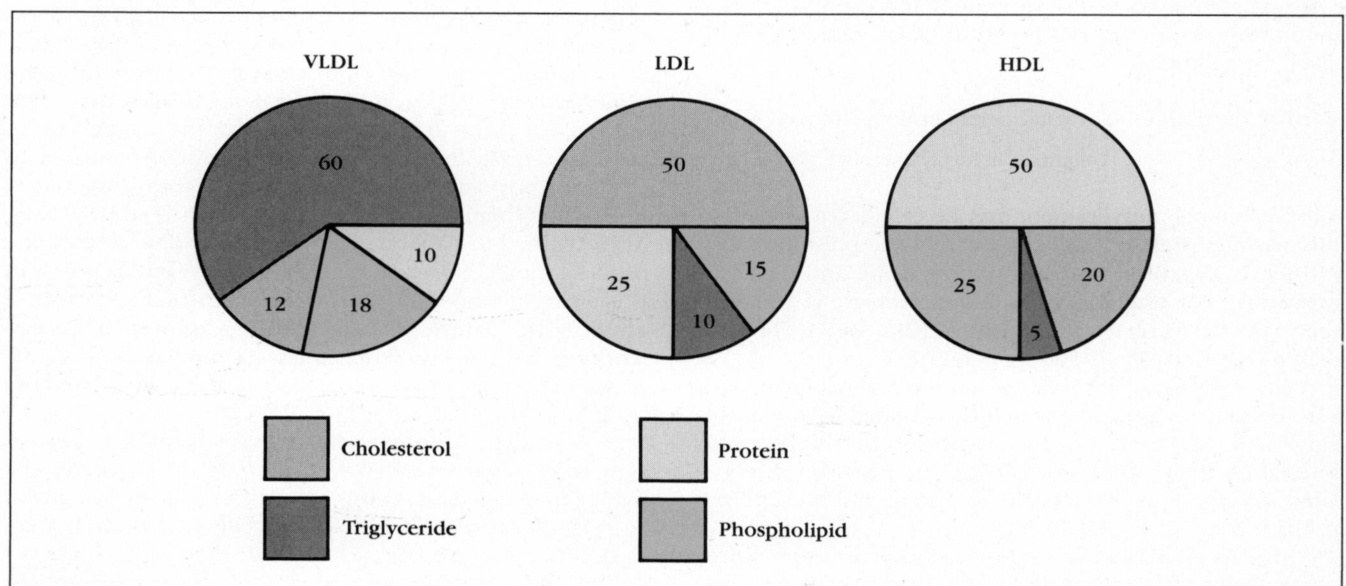

FIGURE 22-1 Contents of the three major lipoproteins in percentages. VLDL = very-low-density lipoprotein; LDL = low-density lipoproteins; HDL = high-density lipoprotein. (From S. Kaufman and S. Papper, *Review of Pathophysiology*. Boston: Little, Brown, 1983.)

between hypertension and CAD. The main cause of death in diabetes mellitus is cardiovascular disease, especially with early onset and poor control of the diabetic condition. Hypertension associated with diabetes causes increased mortality. Mortality in diabetics without hypertension is 2.47 times that of healthy subjects. That of hypertensive diabetics (BP 150/95) is 13.52 times normal. This difference in mortality declines with age, so that at age 50 years, hypertensive diabetics have 2.96 times normal mortality compared to nonhypertensive diabetics, who have 2.21 times normal mortality for age [7,10].

Secondary Hypertension

As is described on pages 351 and 353, hypertension can develop secondary to known diseases (see Table 22-2). When the causative factor is treated, the blood pressure may return to normal.

Pathophysiology

To understand the pathophysiology of hypertension, a review of normal arterial pressure determinants is necessary. Blood pressure is normally maintained within rather narrow limits. During sleep, however, it may fall to 60/40 mm Hg or less, and during exercise, marked increases may be noted that often correspond to changes in heart rate and cardiac output.

Total peripheral resistance is an important factor in the regulation of arterial blood pressure. It is the sum of all resistances offered by the vascular beds of the body. These vary with different organs, but the systemic peripheral resistance has the greatest effect on the mean arterial blood pressure. Very small changes in *arteriolar diameter*, also called the *precapillary sphincter diameter*, cause significant effects on both systemic arterial pressure and blood flow. Mean arterial pressure can be calculated by using the following formula:

$$\text{Cardiac output (CO)} \times \text{total peripheral resistance (TPR)} = \text{mean arterial pressure (MAP)}.$$

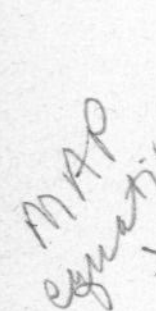

Another simple measurement may be calculated by adding the diastolic pressure and one-third of the pulse pressure (which is the difference between systolic and diastolic pressures). For example, if the blood pressure is 160/100, then $100 + 1/3(60) = 20 + 100 = 120$ (MAP). The normal MAP is from 70 to 100 mm Hg [6].

One other factor that affects systolic and diastolic pressure is aortic impedance, which is regulated by the aortic valve and the elasticity of the aortic wall. The diastolic arterial *volume*, and consequently the pressure, is regulated largely by the tone of the arterioles and precapillary sphincters.

Other factors have an influence on arterial pressure, especially by affecting cardiac output and peripheral resistance. The sympathetic nervous system (SNS) causes increased peripheral vascular resistance and increased cardiac contractility, which, in turn, increase the blood pressure. The SNS also influences the renin-angiotensin-aldosterone (RAA) system, which causes arteriolar constriction through the release of angiotensin II and increased blood volume through the liberation of aldosterone.

The role of the SNS and RAA system in producing hypertension is as follows. In hypertension there is usually an elevation of the afterload, or resistance, against which the ventricle must empty. A higher afterload or resistance requires the ventricle to develop more pressure to empty its contents [4]. Consistent increase in workload requires thicker heart muscle, so the ventricular muscle hypertrophies. This hypertrophy is concentric, with enlargement occurring from the epicardium to the endocardium (Fig. 22-2). The chamber size does not increase so that the heart does not appear enlarged on radiographs, but the increased muscle mass may increase the weight of the heart significantly. Hypertrophy can be demonstrated on ECG by increased amplitude of the R waves of the precordial leads (see Chap. 18). The increased muscle mass increases the myocardial need for oxygen and usually reduces the compliance of the ventricle [4].

Essential Hypertension

There is no real agreement as to the etiology of essential hypertension: 90 percent of all hypertension has no definite identifiable cause. It is known that the arterioles offer abnormally increased resistance to blood flow. This increases peripheral vascular resistance, causes a decreased capillary flow, and results in increased resistance against which the heart must pump. Numerous theories have been offered to explain hypertension, including (1) changes in the arteriolar bed itself, causing chronically increased resistance; (2) abnormally increased tone of the SNS from the vasomotor centers causing increased PVR; (3) increased blood volume resulting from renal or hormonal dysfunction; and (4) a genetic increase in arteriolar thickening causing the abnormal PVR. It is more probably of multifactorial etiology [5,14].

One theory that has been studied extensively is the *abnormal renin theory*. It has been demonstrated that when blood flow to the kidneys is decreased, the juxtaglomerular cells release renin, which reacts with angiotensinogen (a plasma protein formed by the liver) to form angiotensin I, which is then converted to angiotensin II in the lungs. Angiotensin I is elaborated in an intermediate step of the process; it exhibits no physiologic activity, but angiotensin II is a potent vasoconstrictor. The target for angiotensin II effect is the arterioles. Circulating angiotensin II also works in some unknown manner to stimulate aldosterone secretion, which in turn increases blood volume by conserving sodium and water (Fig. 22-3).

Serum renin is not present in every form of hypertension, but it correlates well with some types, especially the malignant form. Classifying hypertension into categories according to plasma renin activity (PRA) is quite helpful in determining the course of the disease. High renin activity (HRA) is often associated with increased aldosterone levels and malignant hypertension. Low renin activity (LRA) accounts for 20 percent of affected persons; 60 percent have normal renin activity (NRA) and 20 percent

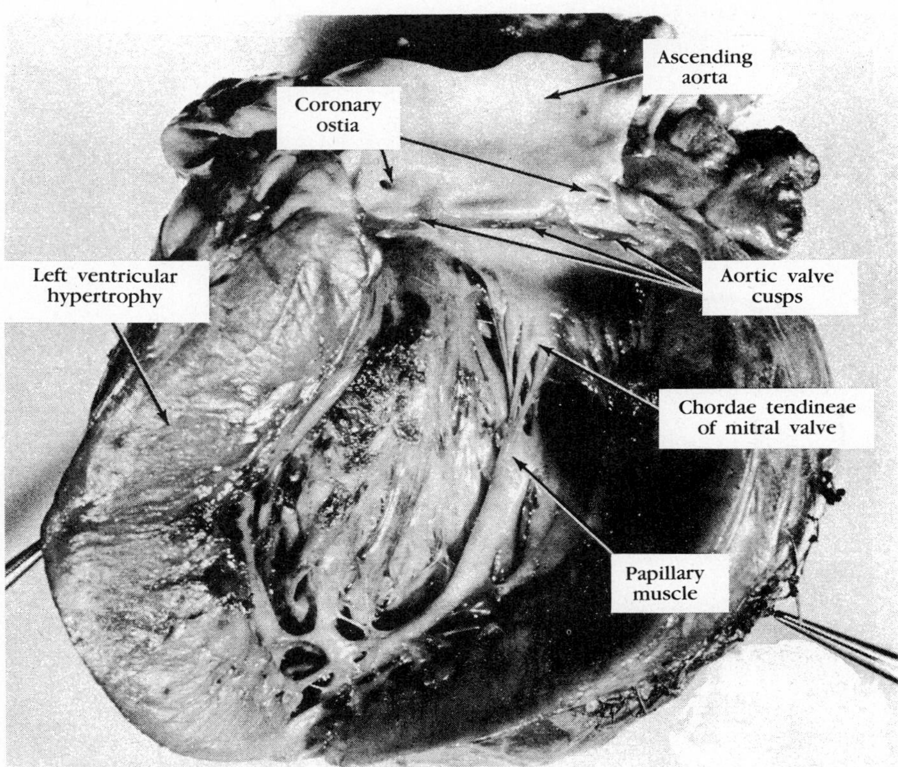

FIGURE 22-2 Marked thickening of the left ventricular myocardium showing a normal aorta and medial leaflet of the mitral valve. (Reprinted from J. Kernicki, B. Bullock, and J. Matthews, *Cardiovascular Nursing*. New York: G.P. Putnam, 1971.)

have HRA [12]. Therapy is now being based on PRA. For example, propranolol (Inderal) is an effective drug for HRA but not LRA. Studies have shown that an absolute or relative excess of renin and angiotensin II is involved with essential hypertension in 50 to 70 percent of identified cases [6,12].

Secondary Hypertension

Secondary hypertension develops from a specific underlying cause (see Table 22-2).

Renovascular hypertension has been studied extensively. It results from atherosclerotic or fibrous dysplastic stenosis of one or both renal arteries [5]. The resultant decrease in renal perfusion causes activation of the RAA system. The degree of hypertension is closely related to the amount of renal ischemia produced by the obstruction. Serum renin levels are usually elevated, but the amount of aldosterone secreted in relation to the amount of angiotensin II present is inappropriately increased for no known reason [3]. The result of this type of hypertension is a marked increase in peripheral vascular resistance and cardiac output, with very high levels of systemic blood pressure.

Renal parenchymal disease, such as glomerulonephritis and renal failure, often causes a renin- or sodium-dependent type of hypertension. The pathophysiology varies depending on the extent of renal insufficiency and type of renal disease. Hypervolemia with normal PVR may appear, or normal or diminished circulation with a very increased PVR or both increased volume and PVR may result.

Cushing's disease is a disease of the adrenal cortex that causes an increase in blood volume and pressure. Excess adrenocorticotropic hormone (ACTH) with bilateral adrenal hyperplasia accounts for about two-thirds of the disease [8].

Primary aldosteronism also is volumic, or salt and water dependent. High blood pressure that results from increased production of aldosterone is a classic example of volume-related hypertension. Although hyperaldosteronism promotes salt and water retention, the ultimate mechanism that sustains the hypertension is unknown [13,15].

Pheochromocytoma is a secreting tumor of chromaffin cells, usually of the adrenal medulla. This tumor causes hypertension as a result of increased secretion of epinephrine and norepinephrine. Epinephrine mainly increases cardiac contractility and rate while norepinephrine mainly increases PVR. The hypertension produced by a pheochromocytoma is usually severe and runs a very malignant course. Surgery offers a potential cure but should be undertaken only when the blood pressure is completely controlled.

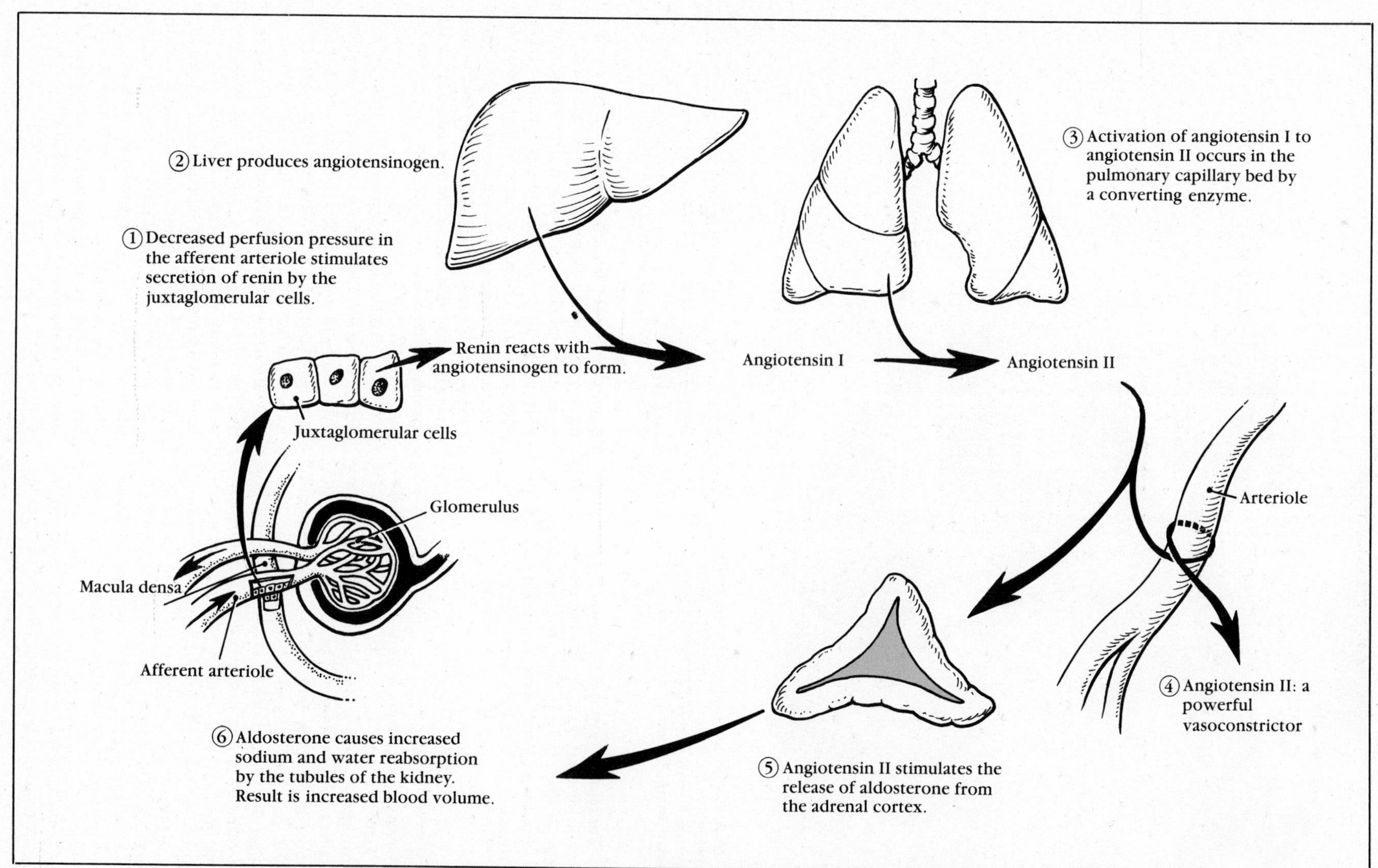

FIGURE 22-3 The renin-angiotensin-aldosterone system.

Coarctation of the aorta is a congenital constriction of the aorta, often at the level of the ductus arteriosus. This produces a syndrome of markedly elevated pressures in the upper extremities and a decrease in perfusion of the lower extremities (see Chap. 21). Sometimes the PRA is increased, but this finding is not consistent and PVR may not be elevated [3].

Clinical Manifestations of Hypertension

When symptoms do occur, hypertension is usually far advanced. The classic symptoms of headache, epistaxis, dizziness, and tinnitus thought to be associated with high blood pressure are no more common in hypertensive than in normotensive individuals. Unsteadiness, waking headache, blurred vision, depression, and nocturia have been shown to be increased in untreated hypertension [2]. Changes in the retina provide some objective clues to the clinical course of the disease. The Keith-Wagener classification indicates a KW1 rating for minimal arteriolar narrowing; KW2 for more significant narrowing and arteriovenous nicking; KW3 for flame-shaped hemorrhages and cotton wool exudates; and KW4 for the above changes with papilledema. Papilledema is always associated with malignant hypertension [11].

The triad of hypertension was first described by Richard Brighton in 1863 and George Johnson in 1873. Brighton described (1) the symmetrically contracted kidneys with fibrotic lesions in the nephrons and (2) concentric hypertrophy of the left ventricle; Johnson described (3) arteriolar hyaline sclerosis of the systemic vessels. These have been accepted as the pathologic sequelae of hypertension, regardless of the cause.

Untreated hypertension damages the small arterioles, which, in turn, causes *target organ dysfunction*. The organs most acutely affected by vascular damage are the brain, eyes, kidneys, and heart. Problems that may result in the target organs are summarized in Table 22-3. The effects on the target organs are the result of prolonged elevation of systemic blood pressure.

The blood pressure remains consistently above the normal level for the age of the person. Many affected persons complain of angina pectoris, especially on exertion or during stressful situations. Headache is occasionally described, especially an occipital type that may be present on waking and may be associated with nausea, vomiting, and mental confusion. Renal dysfunction may be the first sign, with nocturia or hematuria. Symptoms of left ventricular failure are common, especially dyspnea on exertion.

Accelerated (malignant) hypertension is a state in which end-organ damage from the disease occurs rapidly within a short time. It is manifested by a rapid increase in diastolic pressure (130 mm Hg or greater). This is a true emergency, causing symptoms of hypertensive encephalopathy: nausea, vomiting, restlessness, blurred vision, and headache. Renal damage is inevitable. Left ventricular failure, seizures, or coma may develop. Death often ensues without immediate, appropriate treatment.

Four major morbid sequelae are associated with hypertensive disease: (1) stroke, (2) myocardial infarction, (3) renal failure, and (4) encephalopathy [12].

Stroke. Vascular lesions may cause either hemorrhagic or ischemic stroke. The increasing pressures may cause dilatation of the small, sometimes nonelastic, and aged vessels. This, in turn, causes breaks in the vessel and hemorrhage into the brain parenchyma. The dilatations of the smaller intracerebral arteries are called *Charcot-Bouchard Microaneurysms*. These microaneurysms may rupture and cause signs of intracerebral hemorrhage. In the process of aneurysm formation, the vessels undergo some repair, which eventually leads to thickening and tortuosity of the endothelium.

Ischemic infarcts often occur from associated atherosclerosis of the extracranial vessels (carotids and vertebrals). The thickened endothelium of the small vessels decreases or obstructs the blood flow to an area.

Myocardial Infarction. Myocardial infarction may result from atherosclerosis of the coronary arteries or from the same type of hyaline sclerosis previously described in relation to arterioles of the brain. It is believed that hypertension accelerates atherosclerosis because it causes injury to the endothelium, which increases lipid accumulation and atheroma formation [12].

TABLE 22-3 Hypertensive Effects on Target Organs

Organ	Effect	Manifested by
Heart	Myocardial infarction	ECG changes; enzyme elevations
	Congestive failure	Decreased cardiac output S3 or summation gallop auscultated; cardiomegaly on radiograph
	Myocardial hypertrophy	Increased voltage R wave in V_3–V_6; increased frequency of angina; left ventricular strain, manifested by ST and T wave changes
	Dysrhythmias	Usually ventricular dysrhythmias or conduction defects
Eyes	Blurred or impaired vision	Nicking arteries and veins; hemorrhages and exudates on visual examination
	Encephalopathy	Papilledema
Brain	Cerebrovascular accident	Severe occipital headache, paralysis, speech difficulties, coma
	Encephalopathy	Rapid development of confusion, agitation, convulsions, death
Kidneys	Renal insufficiency	Nocturia, proteinuria, elevated BUN, creatinine
	Renal failure	Fluid overload, accumulation of metabolites, metabolic acidosis

Renal Failure. Renal failure from primary hypertension frequently results from progressive damage to the arcuate arteries and the afferent arterioles. Progressive hyaline sclerosis leads to ischemic death of nephrons, and to fibrosis, which leads to contracted kidneys. With significant loss of nephrons, renal failure ensues. This process is markedly accelerated with fibroid necrosis of the larger arteries when it is associated with malignant hypertension.

Encephalopathy. This ominous manifestation results from leakage of water and electrolytes from the brain capillaries into the tissues of the brain. The leakage produces cerebral edema and is often associated with papilledema (optic disk swelling). Encephalopathy is most common in malignant hypertension or when a hypertensive state assumes a malignant pattern. It may be heralded by agitation, convulsions, or coma, and frequently causes death.

Diagnosis of Hypertension

Unlike many other diseases, hypertension is usually asymptomatic and the disease may not be recognized for years unless the person seeks medical attention for another health problem or has a routine blood pressure reading. Correct and accurate measurement of blood pressure is the key element in making the diagnosis. Blood pressure should be measured after at least 5–20 minutes of rest in a quiet, familiar environment. Several positions are usually recommended to attain the most accurate readings: right and left arms with the person sitting, right arm with the person supine, and right leg with the person prone. As noted in Chapter 18, arterial blood pressure is determined by cardiac output and resistance to blood flow. The higher pressure is the systolic pressure and the lower pressure is the diastolic. An error factor of a few millimeters for both systolic and diastolic pressures is accepted, because they are indirect measures.

Examination for vascular insufficiency, including peripheral pulses, is essential. Evidence of cardiac involvement may be revealed by gallop rhythms on auscultation or displacement of the point of maximal impulse (PMI), indicating cardiomegaly. Changes in the vascular bed of the eyes may be noted on ophthalmic examination.

A complete health history should be taken, including family history, age at onset of hypertension, presence of risk factors, diet, symptoms of atherosclerotic disease, and symptoms relating to hypertension. Tests, including an electrocardiogram, intravenous pyelogram, blood urea, and creatinine level, provide supportive objective data. An electroencephalogram may also be indicated. All of the tests are to determine presence and extent of target organ damage.

The prognosis for uncontrolled hypertension is dismal. Statistics of premature death correlate with levels of blood pressure elevation. The risk of cerebrovascular accident, for example, is 5 times higher for hypertensive than for normotensive individuals. Better case finding and proper treatment have improved the outlook for victims of systemic hypertension.

Study Questions

1. Compare the risk factors for hypertension among different populations.
2. Describe the production of elevated blood pressure through an elevated renin mechanism.
3. List and describe the serum lipoproteins and relate their importance in atherogenesis and hypertension.
4. Compare malignant and benign hypertension with regard to course and complications.
5. Discuss the error factor common in blood pressure measurements. How can this be reduced to its lowest level? How can one ascertain the basal blood pressure for an individual?

References

1. Brown, M.S., and Goldstein, J.L. A receptor-mediated pathway for cholesterol homeostasis. *Science* 232:33, 1986.
2. Bullpitt, C.J., Dollery, C.T., and Carne, S. Change in symptoms of hypertensive patients after referral to hospital clinic. *Br. Heart J.* 38:121, 1976.
3. Dustan, H.P. Systemic arterial hypertension. In J.W. Hurst et al. (eds.), *The Heart* (6th ed.). New York: McGraw-Hill, 1986.
4. Ezokowitz, M.D., et al. Cardiovascular diseases. In C.E. Kaufman and S. Papper, *Review of Pathophysiology*. Boston: Little, Brown, 1983.
5. Fishman, M.C., et al. *Medicine* (2nd ed.). Philadelphia: Lippincott, 1985.
6. Ganong, W.F. *Review of Medical Physiology* (12th ed.). Los Altos, Calif.: Lange, 1985.
7. Kannel, W.B. Some lessons in cardiovascular epidemiology from Framingham. *Am. J. Cardiol.* 37:269, 1976.
8. Krieger, D.T. Physiopathology of Cushing's disease. *Endocrine Rev.* 4:22, 1983.
9. McGurn, W.C. *People with Cardiac Problems: Nursing Concepts*. Philadelphia: Lippincott, 1981.
10. Robbins, S.L., Cotran, R.S., and Kumar, V. *Pathologic Basis of Disease* (3rd ed.). Philadelphia: Saunders, 1984.
11. Sokolow, M. Heart and great vessels. In M.A. Krupp, M.J. Chalton, and L.M. Tierney, *Current Medical Diagnosis and Treatment 1986*. Los Altos, Calif.: Lange, 1986.
12. Sokolow, M., and McIlroy, M.B. *Clinical Cardiology* (4th ed.). Los Altos, Calif.: Lange, 1986.
13. Tarazi, R.C., et al. Hemodynamic characteristics of primary aldosteronism. *N. Engl. J. Med.* 289:1330, 1973.
14. Wallace, A.G., Waugh, R.A. Hypertension. In L.H. Smith and S.O. Thier, *Pathophysiology: The Biological Principles of Disease* (2nd ed.). Philadelphia: Saunders, 1985.
15. Weinberger, M.H., et al. Primary aldosteronism: Diagnosis, localization, and treatment. *Ann. Intern. Med.* 90:386, 1979.

CHAPTER 23

Alterations in Systemic Circulation

CHAPTER OUTLINE

Pathologic Processes of Arteries

- Arteritis
- Atherosclerosis
  - *Pathology*
- Arteriosclerosis Obliterans
  - *Pathogenesis*
  - *Pain*
  - *Coldness or Cold Sensitivity*
  - *Impaired Arterial Pulsations*
  - *Color Changes*
  - *Ulceration and Gangrene*
  - *Edema*
  - *Other Trophic Changes*
  - *Superficial Thrombophlebitis*
- Aortic Aneurysms
  - *Abdominal Aortic Aneurysms (AAA)*
  - *Thoracic Aneurysms*
  - *Dissecting Aneurysms*
  - *Saccular Aneurysms*
- Mönckeberg's Sclerosis
- Arteriolosclerosis
- Raynaud's Disease
- Thromboangiitis or Buerger's Disease

Pathologic Processes of Veins

- Obstructive Disease of Veins
  - *Venous Thrombosis*
- Thrombophlebitis and Phlebothrombosis
- Venous Insufficiency and Stasis
- Varicose Veins

Pathologic Processes of the Lymphatic System

Diagnostic Procedures for Vascular Lesions

- Physical Examination
- Doppler Ultrasound
- Angiography
  - *Translumbar Aortography*
  - *Peripheral Arteriography*

LEARNING OBJECTIVES

1. Define *atherosclerosis* and *arteriolosclerosis*.
2. Describe the clinical effects of atherosclerosis in the abdominal aorta; aortoiliac, femoral, carotid, and cerebral arteries; and renal and mesenteric arteries.
3. Explain how a thrombus can become an embolus.
4. Describe the pathologic process of arteriosclerosis obliterans.
5. List the symptoms and signs that are characteristic of arteriosclerosis obliterans.
6. Describe the differences in the pain of intermittent claudication, rest pain, ulceration, and gangrene.
7. Describe the etiology, site, and signs and symptoms of the major types of aneurysms.
8. Differentiate between Raynaud's phenomenon and Raynaud's disease.
9. Explain the mechanism behind the typical color changes in Raynaud's disease.
10. Describe thromboangiitis obliterans (Buerger's disease).
11. Describe the pathology of thromboangiitis.
12. Enumerate the signs and symptoms of arterial insufficiency to a limb.
13. List the three major predisposing factors in venous thrombosis.
14. Differentiate the types of thrombophlebitis.
15. Compare superficial and deep thrombophlebitis with respect to signs, symptoms, and complications.
16. Describe the mechanism that causes chronic venous insufficiency.
17. Describe the etiology of varicose veins.
18. List at least three contributing factors in the development of varicosities.
19. Describe the pathology of venous insufficiency.
20. Identify the skin changes that may be associated with venous insufficiency.
21. Define *lymphedema*, *lymphangitis*, and *lymphadenitis*.
22. Differentiate primary and secondary lymphedema.
23. Describe the following diagnostic procedures that are useful in detecting peripheral vascular disease: arteriography, Doppler ultrasound, translumbar aortography, and peripheral arteriography.

Peripheral vascular disease is a term that, in its broadest sense, applies to disease of any of the blood vessels outside of the heart and to disease of the lymph vessels. It is a general term that usually is used to describe a group of disorders that exhibit thickening and loss of elasticity of the walls of the arteries. Included in this group are atherosclerosis, arteriolosclerosis, and Mönckeberg's medial calcific sclerosis. Many of the changes in the vessels are closely related to advancing age, but the onset of changes is accelerated, probably by diet and other environmental factors.

Pathologic Processes of Arteries

Arteritis

Arteritis is a general term for inflammation of the artery. The process can be infectious or it may be due to some generalized systemic disease. *Takayasu's disease* causes inflammation of the aorta and upper branches, especially in women of the Oriental races [8]. *Polyarteritis nodosa* is a vasculitis of the medium-sized arteries of middle-aged males. It tends to affect the branchings and bifurcations of arteries with an inflammatory process that may lead to weakening of the wall and aneurysms [2]. This condition is often thought to be a connective tissue disorder, but the etiology is unknown. The symptoms vary with the location of the lesions [8].

Atherosclerosis

Atherosclerosis is a disease of the large and medium-sized arteries that begins as a *fibrofatty plaque* on the intimal surface of the vessel (Fig. 23-1). It usually causes no symptoms until the impeded arterial blood flow causes ischemia or infarction of the affected organ.

Many factors have been studied in the development of atherosclerosis. While not totally explanatory for every case, these factors have been correlated statistically to atherosclerotic plaque development (Table 23-1). All of the factors correlate, with many of them usually interact-

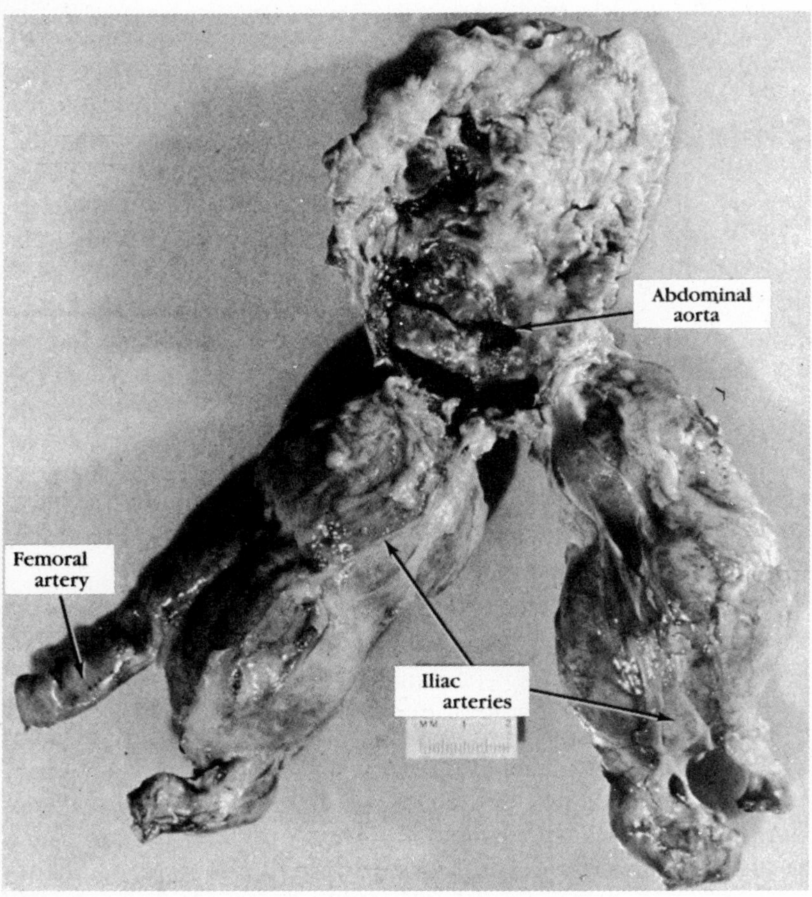

FIGURE 23-1 Opened abdominal aortal showing diffuse atherosclerotic plaques with ulceration. There are aneurysms of both common iliac arteries. (Reprinted from J. Kernicki, B. Bullock, and J. Matthews, *Cardiovascular Nursing*. New York: G.P. Putnam, 1971.)

TABLE 23-1 Factors Implicated in the Development of Atherosclerosis

Factor	Relationship to Disease
Age	Increased frequency with advancing age.
Weight	Probably related to diet; obesity correlates with increased frequency of MI.
Heredity	Increased frequency at early age within certain families points to familial predisposition that also may reflect dietary habits.
Diet	Diet high in saturated fats with frequency of hyperlipidemia increases ischemic heart disease.
Sex	Significantly increased in males until age 75 years or greater, when it approaches equality.
Diabetes	Almost twofold increase as compared to nondiabetics; also relates to obesity.
Cigarette smoking	Correlates with number of cigarettes smoked and decreases when smoking stops.
Hypertension	Correlates with degree of hypertension; diastolic pressure the most important figure.
Occupation or lifestyle	Behavior pattern (type A or B personality) inconclusive but risk appears to be twofold with type A personality.

ing to cause the pathology. Table 23-2 indicates the proposed cellular mechanisms of the atherogenic risk factors. Most of the statistics regarding atherosclerosis are related to myocardial infarction mortality, so that the actual frequency of extracardiac occlusive or nonocclusive atherosclerotic disease can only be surmised.

Pathology. The possible precursor of the lesion of atherosclerosis is the *fatty streak* that often develops within the first decade of life [9]. This streak is composed of lipid material that is deposited on the intima of arteries. When the atherosclerotic lesion forms, it is often referred to as an *atheroma* or an *atheromatous plaque*. It is composed of fatty and fibrofatty material that is white to yellow; it protrudes into the artery and may combine with other localized atheromas to form a large mass [7]. The atherosclerotic plaque contains collagen fibers and connective tissue. The atheroma alone rarely causes arterial obstruction but does so when thrombosis and hemorrhage of the plaque occur (Fig. 23-2). Sometimes the atheromatous lesion causes medial weakening and aneurysmal dilatation of the artery [7]. Calcification of long-standing lesions is common and contributes to stiff, noncompliant vessels.

Because atherosclerosis can be induced in most animals by feeding them a diet high in cholesterol, and because the disease process rarely occurs in humans unless the cholesterol level is greater than 160 mg per dl, hyperlipidemia can be considered as a major causative factor. The lipid in the atheroma is derived from serum lipoproteins [7].

Even though any vessel in the body may be affected by atherosclerosis, the aorta, and coronary, carotid, and iliac arteries are involved with the greatest frequency. A wide range of clinical effects may result from the ischemia and infarction of specific areas. Table 23-3 summarizes some of the common clinical and pathologic effects [9].

Embolization from a thrombosed atheroma causes the characteristic signs of arterial occlusion: (1) diminished or absent pulses, (2) skin pallor and/or cyanosis, (3) pain, and (4) muscle weakness. A large embolus may arise from a thrombosed atheroma in the descending aorta and may travel to the terminal aorta. If the embolus occludes the iliac arteries and terminal aorta, it is known as a *saddle embolus*. Its source is usually the heart, either from a subendocardial infarction or from mitral valve disease.

TABLE 23-2 Proposed Cellular Mechanisms of Atherogenic Risk Factors

Risk Factor	Cellular Mechanism
Elevated serum cholesterol	Increases LDL, which damages endothelium. Increases passage of cholesterol carried by LDL, especially when HDL is low, leading to increased proliferation of smooth muscle cells.
Hypertension	Increases endothelial permeability through increased artery wall tension, endothelial damage from angiotensin, platelet adherence with release of vasoactive agents, and hemodynamic stress.
Cigarette smoking	Damages arterial cell membrane through circulating carbon monoxide, and platelet adherence (vasopressin). Lipid mobilization (catecholamines).

HDL = high-density lipoprotein; LDL = low-density lipoprotein.
Source: C. E. Kaufman and S. Papper, *Review of Pathophysiology.* Boston: Little, Brown, 1983.

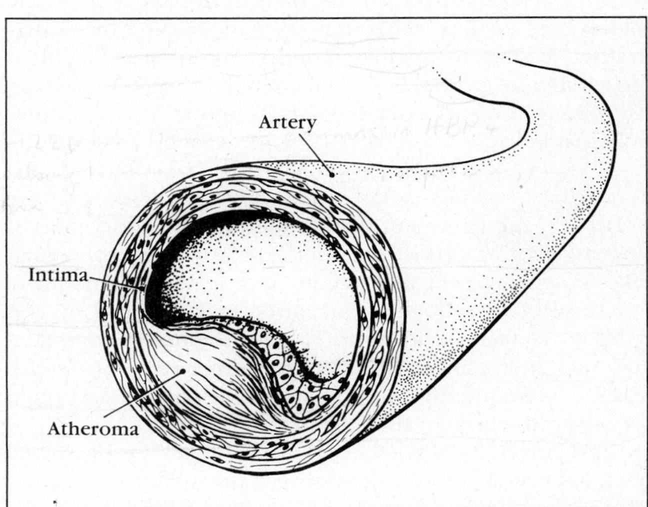

FIGURE 23-2 Schematic of an atheromatous plaque. A central area of necrosis and hemorrhage into the area both impinge on the lumen of the vessels.

TABLE 23-3 Clinical and Pathologic Effects of Atherosclerosis in Different Anatomic Sites

Site	Clinical and Pathologic Effects
Abdominal/terminal aorta	Ischemic effects in lower extremities; gangrene of toes, feet; effects of fusiform abdominal aneurysm; embolism of atherosclerotic debris to smaller arteries
Aortoiliac and femoral arteries	Intermittent claudication; gangrene of toes, feet; aneurysm formation in iliac arteries
Coronary arteries	Angina pectoris; conduction disturbances; myocardial infarction
Carotid and vertebral arteries	Transient ischemic attacks; cerebrovascular accident (CVA) or stroke
Renal artery	Hypertension; renal ischemia (hematuria proteinuria)
Mesenteric arteries	Intestinal ischemia (ileus, bowel performation with peritonitis)

Arteriosclerosis Obliterans

Pathogenesis. Gradual occlusion of an atherosclerotic terminal aorta or of other large vessels can cause symptoms and signs of ischemia to the part supplied. If the terminal aorta is affected, clinical manifestations include intermittent claudication, loss of peripheral hair, shiny skin, and impotence. The term *arteriosclerosis obliterans* is used to describe chronic occlusive arterial disease of the large arteries. It most commonly affects the terminal portion of the aorta and the large and medium arteries, especially those of the lower extremities. Arteriosclerosis obliterans predominantly occurs in men between ages 50 and 70 years. The prevalence and severity of this disorder are increased with concomitant diabetes mellitus.

When a large artery is obstructed, the pressure in the smaller arteries distal to the obstruction decreases and blood flow declines. Thrombosis of the small arteries may follow, leading to occlusion and gangrene if the cellular deprivation of oxygen is critical enough to cause cell death. Gangrene may also occur if an ischemic area becomes infected because of an increased need for blood supply.

Pain. Various types of pain are described that are related to the degree of impairment of circulatory supply. *Intermittent claudication* is an aching, persistent, cramplike, squeezing pain that occurs after a certain amount of exercise of the affected extremity. It is relieved by rest without change of position. This is a common complaint and occurs in almost all persons at some stage of the disease. It is frequently the first symptom noticed and often begins in the arch of the foot or calf of the leg.

Rest pain is usually localized in the digits. It is described as a severe ache or a gnawing pain, often occurring at night and persisting for hours at a time. Rest pain is caused by severe ischemia of tissues and sensory nerve terminals. It may herald the onset of gangrene. It is aggravated by elevation of the extremity and often relieved by dependency.

Pain of ischemic neuropathy usually occurs late in the course of progressive arteriosclerosis obliterans with severe ischemia. This severe pain is often associated with various types of paresthesias. It may be described as a lightning, shocklike sensation that usually occurs in both the foot and leg and follows the distribution of the peripheral sensory nerves. The pain of ulceration and gangrene is usually localized to the areas adjacent to ulcers or gangrenous tissue. It is severe, persistent, and frequently worst at night. The pain is described as an aching sensation and sometimes may be associated with sharp, severe stabs of pain.

Coldness or Cold Sensitivity. Coldness or sensitivity to cold is a frequent symptom of arteriosclerosis obliterans. Complaints of coldness in the digits of the feet with exposure to a cold environment may be associated with color changes such as blanching or cyanosis.

Impaired Arterial Pulsations. Pulsation in the posterior tibial (PT) and dorsalis pedis (DP) arteries is impaired or absent in the majority of lower-extremity occlusions. Impairment of pulsations in the popliteal and femoral arteries is less frequent.

Color Changes. Affected extremities may be of a normal color; but in advanced disease, cyanosis or an abnormal red color, called *rubor*, may be seen, particularly when the extremity is placed in a dependent position. Postural color changes are often asymmetric, and affected extremities or digits become abnormally blanched after being elevated for a few minutes. When the extremity is placed in a dependent position, a delay of 5 to 60 seconds may be required for color to return to the skin. The part first becomes abnormally red, and then gradually the rubor lessens. The rubor is due to maximal dilatation of the arterioles and capillaries of the part [4]. The amount of color change relates to the severity of vascular occlusion.

Ulceration and Gangrene. These lesions may occur spontaneously on an ischemic extremity, or they may result from trauma such as pressure on the toenails from shoes. Gangrene may also result from bruises, nicks, or cuts in the skin; freezing; burning; or application of strong, irritating medicines or chemicals. It is usually confined to one extremity at a time. The lesion may be manifested by small spots on a digit, or it may involve a whole extremity.

Ulcers may develop on the tips of digits, between the toes, or at the base of the flexor surface of the toes. The area around the ulcer is painful and may be swollen or exhibit redness at the margin. Secondary infections are common and lead to abscess formation, cellulitis, and spread of infection.

Edema. In severe cases of arteriosclerosis obliterans, edema of the feet and legs may occur. It is most evident when the legs are in a dependent position. Associated ischemic skin lesions, capillary atony, deep venous thrombosis, and lymphangitis contribute to the edema.

Other Trophic Changes. As a result of moderate to severe chronic ischemia, small scars, depressions, or pitting may form on the tips of the pedal digits. Nail growth is slow and nails may become thickened and deformed; they also may be paper-thin. The digits or an entire foot may appear shrunken and the muscles atrophy; therefore, the calf or thigh may decrease in size.

Superficial Thrombophlebitis. At some stage of the disease, superficial nonvaricose veins are involved in a type of thrombophlebitis. This occurs in approximately 40 percent of persons with arteriosclerosis obliterans. The smaller veins are usually involved with lesions or are red, raised, indurated, tender, cordlike veins that measure approximately 0.5 to 3.0 cm long. The lesions usually cause permanent occlusion of the veins, but the redness and symptoms of thrombophlebitis subside, usually in one to three weeks after onset.

Aortic Aneurysms

An aneurysm is a localized dilation of the wall of an artery. It develops at a site of weakness of the medial layer of the artery. The majority of aneurysms are atherosclerotic, but they may result from congenital defects, infections such as syphilis, and trauma.

Fusiform aneurysms produce circumferential dilatation of the vessel. The wall balloons out on all sides (Fig. 23-3). As the process is occurring, the aneurysmal sac fills with necrotic debris and thrombus. Calcium infiltrates the area. The sac dilates because of a weakened medial layer.

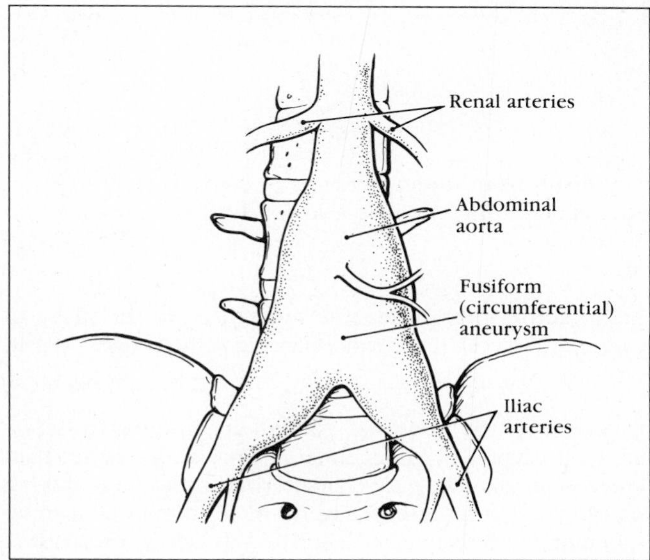

FIGURE 23-3 Fusiform aneurysm of the aorta.

The dangers of this type of aneurysm include rupture, embolization to a peripheral artery, pressure on surrounding structures, and obstruction of blood flow to organs supplied by the tributary arteries.

Abdominal Aortic Aneurysms (AAA). Almost all AAAs are atherosclerotic and occur distal to the branchings of the renal arteries. They often extend to and include the iliac arteries (see Fig. 23-3). Clinical manifestations are usually nonexistent. Occasionally, the person discovers a pulsatile abdominal mass. More frequently, the aneurysm is discovered when a physical examination is performed for some other reason; such as vague abdominal symptoms or poor peripheral circulation.

Rupture may cause the initial symptoms, with bleeding frequently occurring into the retroperitoneal space. In such instances exsanguination is generally prevented due to the location of the hemorrhage. The initial symptoms of this type of hemorrhage include abdominal pain and symptoms of hemorrhagic shock. Pressure from a large or enlarging AAA on surrounding abdominal organs, together with lack of blood supply to the intestines, can precipitate ileus or intestinal obstruction.

Thoracic Aneurysms. Thoracic aneurysms may be caused by atherosclerosis, necrosis of the medial layer, and syphilis. Atherosclerotic aneurysms are usually fusiform and are located in the arch and descending segments (Fig. 23-4). Aneurysms that result from medial necrosis and syphilis are discussed below and on p. 361.

The most common clinical manifestation of thoracic aneurysms is deep, aching pain. This may be associated with erosion of the ribs, or may be an indication that the aneurysm is expanding and that rupture may be imminent [4]. Compression of respiratory structures and of the recurrent laryngeal nerve may cause dyspnea, hoarseness, and coughing. Rupture as the initial manifestation is usually fatal.

Dissecting Aneurysms. These are not true aneurysms and are often called *dissecting hematomas*. An intimal tear and degeneration of the medial layer allow blood to separate the intimal layer from the adventitial layer (Fig. 23-5). Aortic dissection most frequently occurs in the ascending aorta. Eighty percent of individuals with this problem also have systemic hypertension. It also may be associated with the hereditary disorder *Marfan's syndrome*.

Marfan's syndrome is characterized by degeneration of the elastic fibers of the aortic media, usually beginning at the aortic root and spreading segmentally throughout the aorta. Physical examination reveals long arms and legs, thin hands and feet, lax ligaments, and deformities of the thoracic cage [4].

The clinical manifestations of dissection often present a striking change in appearance. External rupture may lead to exsanguination, but more frequently, the process involves dissection from the initial point away from the

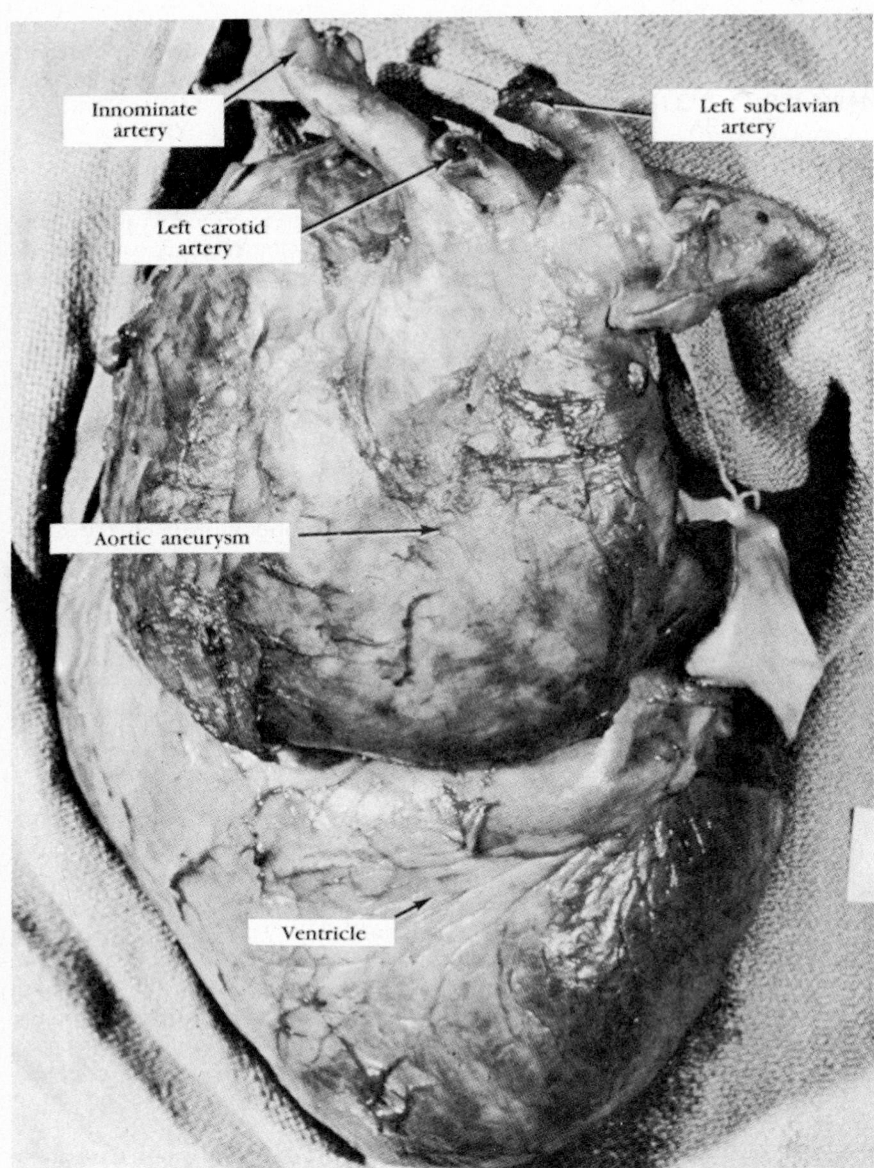

FIGURE 23-4 External view of the heart showing aneurysmal dilation of the ascending aorta and involvement of the arch. (Reprinted from J. Kernicki, B. Bullock, and J. Matthews, *Cardiovascular Nursing*. New York: G.P. Putnam, 1971.)

heart. As it dissects through the aortic segment, it often causes obstruction to vessels branching off the aorta. If it occurs across the arch of the aorta, color changes and cerebral ischemia may be noted suddenly. Aortic regurgitation may result if the dissection occurs through the aortic valve. The affected person usually complains of the sudden onset of severe chest pain that radiates to the back, abdomen, and hips [1].

Mortality of dissecting hematomas is very high. In the initial 24 hours after dissection it is 38 percent, and continues high in the first and second weeks. Two of the main factors that determine mortality are the place of origin of dissection and whether or not the process is self-limiting [4].

Saccular Aneurysms. These are frequently associated with syphilis or congenital malformations rather than atherosclerosis. They are characterized by an outpouching on one side of an artery (Fig. 23-6). Common congenital saccular aneurysms are described as ***berry aneurysms*** when they occur on the arteries of the circle of Willis. The danger of the intracerebral aneurysms is intracranial rup-

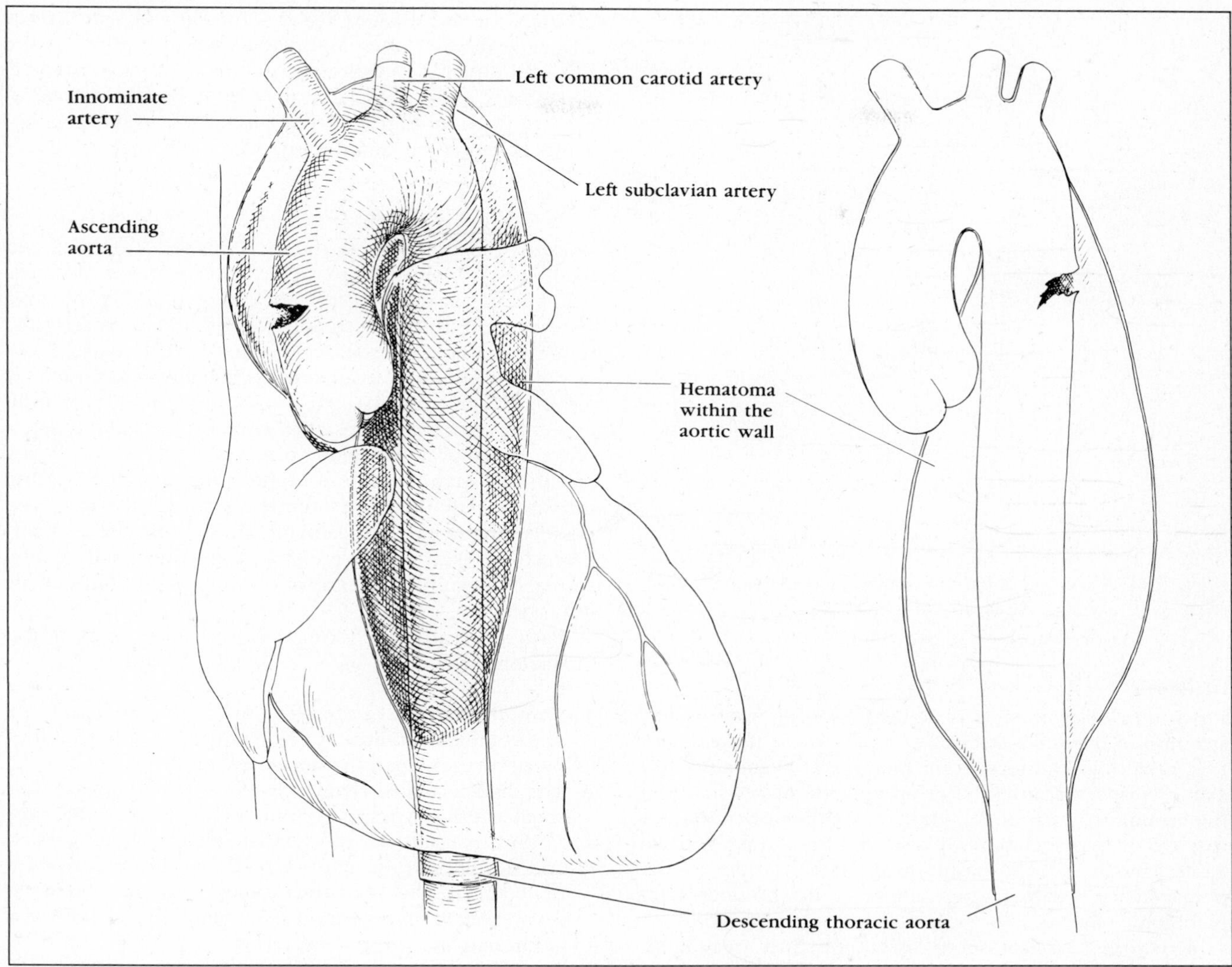

FIGURE 23-5 Aortic dissection most often involves an intimal tear in the proximal ascending aorta or the proximal descending thoracic aorta. The dissection may propagate proximally or distally, or in both directions. Regardless of the site of the tear, aortic dissections are best classified as those that involve the ascending aorta (type A, left) and those that are limited to the descending aorta (type B, right). Type A dissection may or may not also involve the descending aorta. (© 1987 Scientific American, Inc. All rights reserved. From *Scientific American Medicine*, Figure 1, Section 1, Subsection XII.)

ture and bleeding, which often has a fatal outcome (see Chap. 46).

Saccular syphilitic aneurysms most frequently arise on the ascending and descending thoracic aorta. These can compress the mediastinal structures, cause pressure on the surrounding skeletal structures, thrombose, or rupture. Syphilitic or luetic aneurysms are rarely reported in the United States because of improved treatment and measures to control syphilis.

Mönckeberg's Sclerosis

This type of arterial hardening causes focal calcification of the medial layer, especially in the medium-sized arteries. It usually occurs after age 50 years; the vessels become very hard because of the extensive calcification. In some cases atherosclerosis is associated with the calcification process, but the process is not atherosclerotic.

Arteriolosclerosis

Arteriolosclerosis, as its name implies, involves degeneration of the intima and media of small arteries and arterioles. When this affects the kidneys, hypertension results; but hypertension often is the initiator of the condition (see Chap. 22). It also may occur in the peripheral arteries and arterioles of the aged, and is often considered to be a part of the aging process.

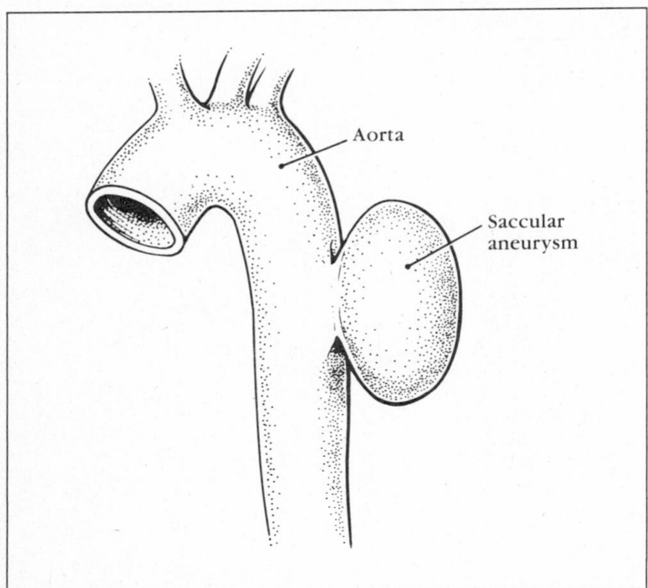

FIGURE 23-6 Saccular aneurysm of the descending aorta.

Raynaud's Disease

Raynaud's phenomenon is defined as an episode of constriction of the small arteries or arterioles of the extremities, resulting in intermittent pallor and cyanosis of the skin of the extremities. After an episode of constriction, hyperemia may produce rubor. Raynaud's phenomenon may occur in association with several conditions and diseases. Thus it is a vasospastic disorder that produces temporary changes in skin color and often has no underlying pathologic basis.

Raynaud's disease occurs predominantly in women, and heredity may play a role in its development. Onset of symptoms usually begins between ages 20 and 40 years. Because investigators rarely are able to examine sections of the blood vessels in cases of early Raynaud's disease, little is known of the pathologic changes in the initial stages. In advanced stages the intima of the digital arteries is thickened.

The typical clinical picture of Raynaud's disease is color changes on exposure to cold. At first only the tips of the fingers are involved, but later the more proximal parts also exhibit color changes. All of the fingers of both hands usually undergo color changes that include pallor, cyanosis, and rubor. The sequential change from pallor to cyanosis and finally to rubor is a characteristic of the disease.

Pallor is caused by spasm of the arterioles and possibly the venules. During this time, blood flow into the capillaries is decreased or absent, causing the affected part to appear dead white. Cyanosis results from capillary dilatation, which occurs later in the course of the disease. Blood flow becomes sluggish with extraction of more oxygen. Rubor indicates excessive hyperemia due to reactive vasodilatation. Exposure to emotional or thermal (cold) stimuli initiate vasoconstriction with subsequent color changes in the digits (Fig. 23-7). Pain characterizes advanced disease, often associated with ulceration on the tips of the digits. Paresthesias such as numbness, tingling, throbbing, and a dull ache may be present. During an actual attack, coldness of the digits is evident, sensory acuity is decreased, and the involved digits may swell.

Thromboangiitis or Buerger's Disease

Buerger's disease affects the medium-sized arteries and medium-sized, mostly superficial, veins of the extremities. It frequently results in arterial occlusion, causing ischemia and gangrene to the extremities. This nonatherosclerotic lesion consists of microabscesses that have a central focus of polymorphonuclear leukocytes usually surrounded by mononuclear cells [10]. Histopathologic evidence indicates that Buerger's disease has some of the characteristics of a collagen or autoimmune disease.

Clinical manifestations include frequent coexisting migratory phlebitis, early tenderness over the involved vessels, upper extremity involvement, absence of heart disease, marked early venospasm, and generally a low serum cholesterol concentration. Invariably, individuals use tobacco.

Pathologically, the disease has certain outstanding characteristics.

1. Thromboangiitis is primarily a disease of the blood vessels of the extremities. It involves the lower extremities more severely than the upper extremities.
2. The disease almost always develops in medium-sized or small arteries. Arteries commonly involved are the posterior tibial, anterior tibial, radial, ulnar, plantar, palmar, and digital. Larger arteries, such as the femoral and brachial, are affected late and only when the disease is severe. Small and medium-sized veins are affected less commonly and large veins rarely.
3. The lesions are focal or segmental and not diffuse.
4. The lesions appear to be of different ages, but in general the disease throughout a single affected segment seems to be of essentially the same age.
5. The disease produces occlusions of the vessels, followed by development of collateral and anastomotic vessels. The secondary anatomic effects of the disease are the result of tissue ischemia [10].

The gross characteristics of the vessels affected by thromboangiitis obliterans vary depending on the age of the lesions at the time they are examined. The vessels appear contracted at the site of destruction. The occluded segments are indurated but not brittle. The arteries are more frequently obliterated than their accompanying veins. In the diseased vessel the occlusion may extend for variable lengths and then stop abruptly. Occlusions may occur at two different levels in the same vessel, and between these sites the vessel may be completely patent.

The most striking physiologic change is the impairment of arterial blood flow. Blood flow through peripheral arteries in the extremities is reduced, particularly in more distal portions. Another factor that contributes to ischemia is

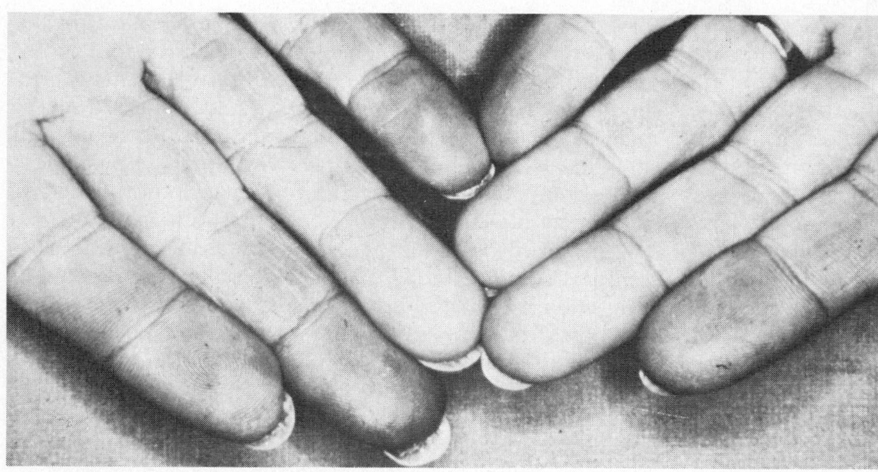

FIGURE 23-7 Cyanosis of the fingers in Raynaud's phenomenon. (From R. Judge, G. Zuidema, and F. Fitzgerald, *Clinical Diagnosis.* Boston: Little, Brown, 1982.)

arteriolar spasm. The degree of spasm varies among individuals and perhaps with the stage of disease.

The degree of arterial insufficiency in the affected extremities depends on two factors: (1) the amount of arterial occlusive disease and (2) the tone of the arterioles, which may vary from normal to moderate or severe spasm.

Venous obstruction, the result of thrombophlebitis, may be an associated factor in the circulatory disturbance in thromboangiitis obliterans. The obstruction is often minor because the venous circulation has a great capacity to develop collateral circulation. In some cases, venous obstruction contributes to malnutrition of capillaries and a tendency to develop edema in the affected extremity if it remains in a dependent position for a long time.

Dependent rubor is caused by the presence in skin of numerous dilated capillaries that contain blood of high oxygen content [3]. Rubor is seen in thromboangiitis that is associated with chronic and moderately severe arterial insufficiency. One explanation, supported by studies of the oxygen content of venous blood, is that capillaries suffer from malnutrition and become atonic, and their capacity to interchange oxygen and other metabolic products is impaired [3,10].

Pathologic Processes of Veins

Obstructive Disease of Veins

Obstructive lesions of the veins may be permanent or temporary, partial or complete. Obstruction to some portion of the main trunk causes the distal large veins to become dilated, with incompetent valves. The small veins and venules may be damaged permanently as a result of pressure, stretching, hypoxemia, and malnutrition. Permanent impairment in interchange of fluid may result from disruption of small vessels. Damaged venous capillaries may function normally when the person is in a recumbent position but show inadequacy in a standing position. This inadequacy is due to increased hydrostatic pressure and sometimes to associated incompetent valves.

Venous Thrombosis. Lesions in veins may produce localized thrombi in small veins or extensive thrombi in the larger veins. Venous thrombosis may develop as a result of an inflammatory or traumatic lesion of the endothelium of the vein wall. In the majority of cases, however, there is no evidence of either. An inflammatory reaction may develop in the wall of the vein as a reaction to primary thrombosis, so that phlebitis may ensue several hours after the thrombus is formed.

Lesions of the endothelium, relative stasis of venous blood flow, and hypercoagulability of blood are the three factors that precipitate venous thrombosis. One or a combination of these factors may produce a thrombus. A thrombus develops as a result of slowed flow in the venous bloodstream and is associated with platelet aggregation. After several days and after development of a secondary reaction in the wall of the thrombosed vein, a sudden proximal extension may protrude from the end of the original organizing thrombus. Emboli may develop at this time from the proximal extension, or the new clot may stick and become organized. Emboli may be small or large, and tend to lodge in the vessels of the pulmonary circulation (see Chap. 27) [6].

A thrombus organizes from its outer margins centrally. In some veins the entire thrombus becomes organized, with complete and permanent occlusion of the lumen. In a large thrombus, involution usually occurs by a process of partial fibrosis and partial lysis, which is probably due to the action of naturally occurring fibrinolysins in the blood. In most cases the center disappears, and a varying portion of the periphery may organize on a fibrous ring. In other instances, bands of fibrous tissue extend across the old lumen of the vein and divide it into many small lumina.

The result is usually some restoration of function of the vein, but the lumen is partially obstructed by the remaining fibrous tissue and decrease of its circular diameter [5].

The degree of inflammatory reaction in the different layers of the veins varies. In some persons the thrombus causes minimal reaction, while in others an intense reaction extends throughout all layers. Inflammatory cells, leukocytes, lymphocytes, and fibroblasts accumulate and cause congestion of capillaries in and around the venous wall. Venous thrombosis causes obstruction to venous blood flow and relates to the size and location of the involved vein. If it occurs in superficial veins and in short segments, collateral circulation will compensate. This may also be true in obstruction of the saphenous vein of the leg or a larger vein of the arm (e.g., median basilic or cephalic), because of the numerous anastomoses that occur. Collateral channels may become evident, even after obstruction of the superior or inferior vena cava [5].

When thrombosis occurs in the iliofemoral or axillary veins, the collateral circulation compensates only partially and venous pressure increases in the veins distal to the thrombosis. This increased pressure results in distention of all veins and even venules of the limb. The increased pressure in the venules and capillaries causes intense congestion of these areas. Pressure changes inhibit normal resorption of fluid and electrolytes from the tissues in the venous end of the capillaries. Edema of the affected limb then develops.

Thrombophlebitis and Phlebothrombosis

Thrombophlebitis refers to an inflamed vein as a result of a thrombus. Phlebothrombosis is probably the same entity but does not exhibit a marked inflammatory component. Thrombosis in a vein ultimately causes inflammatory changes [6].

Idiopathic thrombophlebitis is a recurrent condition that produces segmental lesions in the small and medium-sized veins. The thrombus may be recanalized and the lumen restored, but more frequently the vein becomes completely obliterated. *Suppurative thrombophlebitis* differs in that it usually results from bacterial invasion. The wall of the vein becomes markedly inflamed, and leukocytes infiltrate the area. Bacteria within the thrombus and portions of the endothelium ultimately lead to abscesses. The abscesses may rupture into the bloodstream. *Chemical thrombophlebitis* may result from venous irritation from drugs (e.g., antibiotics or potassium) or other chemicals that gain access to the venous circulation. The thrombus becomes adherent and completely organized, resulting in a vein that is contracted, fibrotic, and cordlike.

The symptoms and signs of thrombophlebitis develop acutely and usually persist for one to three weeks. In small or medium-sized veins, acute thrombophlebitis rarely produces systemic reactions. With involvement of the larger vessels, temperature may rise to as high as 102°F (39°C). Thrombosis of superficial veins often involves redness, pain, tenderness, and localized edema.

Thrombophlebitis of the deep veins of the legs produces calf pain and tenderness in the calf muscles. Enlargement of the calf and a positive Homans' sign may result. Homans' sign refers to pain in the calf muscle when the foot is dorsiflexed. Thrombosis of the iliofemoral vein usually produces a typical, acute, clinical picture. Moderate to severe pain in the thigh and groin with diffuse pain throughout the limb is described. Superficial veins may be prominent and distended in an enlarged limb. The skin of the leg and thigh may be slightly cyanotic. Thrombosis is manifested by impaired or absent pulses from associated arterial spasm. Fever and tachycardia may also be associated. Pitting edema is characteristic, with onset a few days after the obstruction ensues. As the edema becomes chronic, it may be associated with skin changes and brawny edema (thick, hardened skin with nonpitting edema).

Thrombosis of the axillary and subclavian veins produces a clinical picture similar to that of iliofemoral thrombosis. The axillary vein becomes tender, prominent, and enlarged, with pitting edema in the forearm and hand. Superficial veins of the entire arm are prominent and those of the pectoral region on the affected side may be distended.

Venous Insufficiency and Stasis

Chronic venous insufficiency results from stasis of venous blood flow, especially of the iliofemoral veins. Old iliofemoral thrombophlebitis leaves behind a thickened, inelastic vein wall, damaged venous valves, and a partially or sometimes completely obstructed lumen. In the lower extremity the three groups of veins—deep, communicating, and superficial—normally have thin, elastic walls and segmentally spaced valves of the bicuspid type. Venous flow against gravity in the lower limbs is made possible by action of the calf muscle and the competent valves. Muscular compression of the elastic veins forces blood upward and the valves prevent retrograde flow. This mechanism fails in chronic venous insufficiency, usually because of extensive damage from thrombophlebitis.

Ambulatory venous pressure is high, and this upsets the normal equilibrium of capillary fluid exchange, causing congestion and edema. Stasis also results from the high ambulatory pressures, as manifested by changes in the skin and subcutaneous tissues around the distal one-third of the leg and around the ankle. Changes that may occur include edema, hyperpigmentation, dermatitis, induration, stasis cellulitis, and ultimately, venostasis ulcers (Fig. 23-8). Pain may or may not be present. A dull ache in the affected leg may develop after the individual has been standing for variable periods. Pain is usually described as being more severe when standing still rather than when walking. The pain usually disappears within 5 to 30 minutes after assumption of a recumbent position with the leg elevated. Nocturnal muscular cramps may be reported.

Varicose Veins

Varicose veins are dilated, elongated, and tortuous. Varicosity occurs most frequently in the lower extremities where the veins are dilated or become incompetent and superficial (Fig. 23-9). Varicosities probably develop

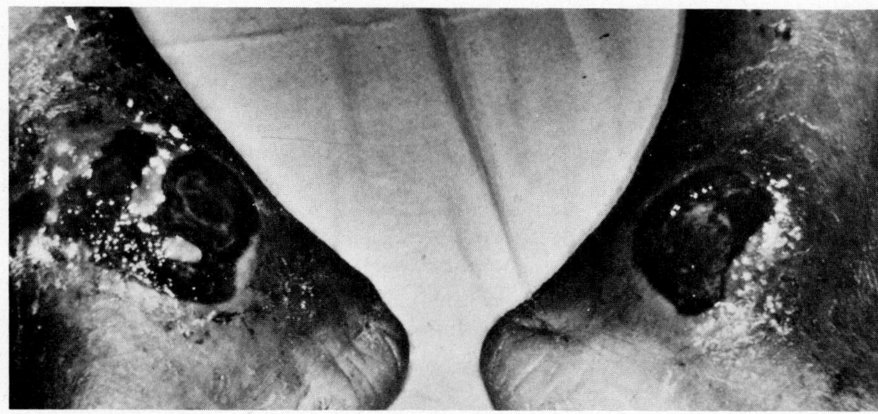

FIGURE 23-8 Bilateral stasis ulcers of the ankles with surrounding dermatitis. (From R. Judge, G. Zuidema, and F. Fitzgerald, *Clinical Diagnosis*. Boston: Little, Brown, 1982.)

because of an inherent weakness in the structure of the veins. Superficial veins dilate when normal resistance against intraluminal pressure is lacking. Primary varicose veins may develop from hereditary predisposition, pregnancy, standing for long periods of time, and marked obesity. Prolonged periods of standing favor development of varicosities because of the high gravitational pressure within the veins. Obesity tends to place external pressure on the veins, especially the iliofemoral veins.

Deep thrombophlebitis often gives rise to secondary varicosities. Loss of valve sufficiency produces unusual strain on the superficial veins. A frequent finding is the presence of localized dilations just distal to the venous valves. Valve incompetency is due primarily to extreme dilatation in the affected veins, which causes separation of the valve cusps. In primary varicose veins the incompetency tends to progress downward in the saphenous main channel as well as in its tributaries. In secondary varicose veins, which arise because of deep vein insufficiency, the incompetency tends to progress upward from incompetent perforating veins in the lower one-third of the leg [3].

Varicose veins can lead to chronic venous insufficiency. In the early stages, localized pain and heat may be noticed after prolonged standing. Persistent edema may develop, together with trophic skin changes and stasis ulcers. The varicose ulcers heal slowly and often become infected.

Diagnosis of venous insufficiency can be made by assessment of physical findings, and occasionally phlebography. *Phlebography* involves injecting radiopaque material into the venous system and taking radiographs of the injected area. It is performed to localize deep vein thrombosis or to evaluate varicosities.

Pathologic Processes of the Lymphatic System

The lymphatic system serves the essential function of draining excess fluids and proteins from the interstitial space. It provides the only means for returning plasma proteins that have leaked into this space to the general circulation. Whenever tissue fluid levels increase, lymphatic drainage also increases. In this way, lymphatic flow is an essential method for control of tissue fluid volume. Venous obstruction and congestive heart failure have been identified as factors that can alter capillary pressure and produce edema. When fluids continually escape into the interstitial spaces, edema may not be noted because of compensation by the lymphatic system.

Obstruction of the lymph vessels interferes with this control mechanism and may precipitate or contribute to edema. Numerous factors may cause lymphedema, and are categorized as inflammatory or noninflammatory. *Lymphangitis* is the word for inflammation of the lymph vessels, usually by bacterial organisms. *Lymphadenitis* refers to inflammation of the lymph nodes. *Lymphedema* specifies edema resulting from lymphatic obstruction.

Primary or idiopathic lymphedema is rare. Milroy's disease, a congenital lymphedema noticeable at birth, is usually caused by faulty development of lymphatic channels. *Lymphedema praecox* affects females predominantly between ages 9 and 25 years. It is characterized by swelling of one or both feet that becomes progressive and unremitting. The lymphatic channels are dilated due to incompetent lymph valves.

Secondary lymphedema is much more common than the primary form. Obstruction of the lymph channels may result from malignant metastatic infiltration of the lymph nodes and channels. Hodgkin's disease, which primarily affects the lymphatic system, also may obstruct the channels. Inflammation or infection of the channels may result in fibrosis and obstruction. A final, very common cause of lymphedema is the surgical removal or irradiation of lymph nodes to prevent the spread of a malignancy.

Lymphedema is essentially the result of stasis. Chronic stasis often leads to *brawny* edema, which describes the appearance of the skin subjected to continual stretch. The skin becomes thick, hardened, infiltrated with plasma proteins, and often "orange-peel" in appearance. The

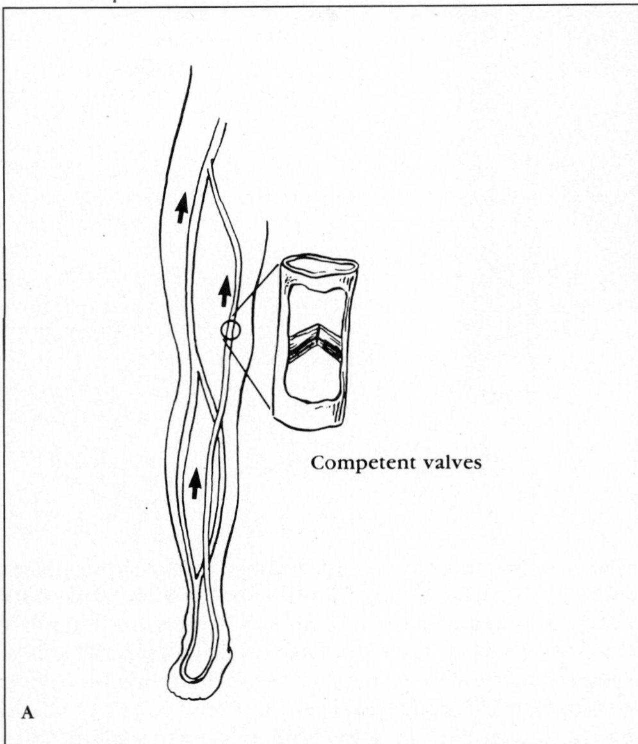

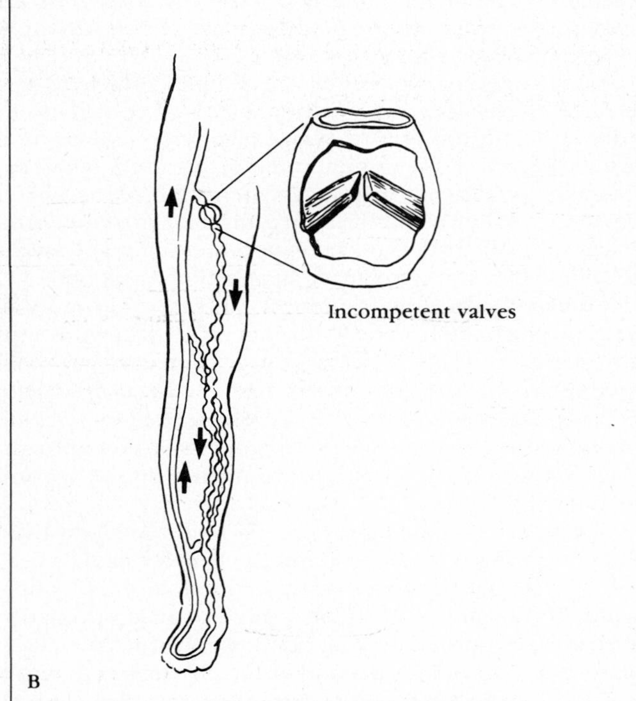

FIGURE 23-9 Chronic venous insufficiency. A. Competent valves, nondilated vessel. B. Incompetent valves, dilated vessel. In the leg varicose veins (B) flow is retrograde due to incomplete closure of valves. (From E.A. Hincker and L. Malasanos [eds.], *The Little, Brown Manual of Medical-Surgical Nursing*. Boston: Little, Brown, 1983.)

edema is different from cardiac edema in that it does not pit on digital pressure.

Inflammatory lymphedema usually occurs after an acute infection of the lymphatic system. Lymphangitis is characterized by painful red streaks following the lymph vessels, which may eventually involve the lymph nodes as well. The agent that most commonly causes lymphangitis is beta-hemolytic *Streptococcus*, but any virulent pathogen may initiate it. Systemic effects include a marked temperature elevation, malaise, and chills. Localized edema occurs and may become progressive if attacks are recurrent. *Chronic lymphangitis* may follow, causing fibrosis of the affected area, further edema, skin changes, and sometimes ulcerations.

Diagnosis of lymphedema is primarily to differentiate it from edema of venous origin. Lymphangiography involves injecting radiopaque dye into the affected lymph vessel and monitoring its passage radiologically. This procedure may localize the source of the obstruction.

Diagnostic Procedures for Vascular Lesions

Physical Examination

Diagnosis of vascular system problems is usually based on the signs and symptoms of arterial occlusion or of venous insufficiency. Palpation of the peripheral pulses is important in estimating blood flow in the peripheral arterial circuit. Systolic bruits over the abdominal area and femoral artery are common, and, in association with other signs, may indicate peripheral arterial disease. Bruits refer to sounds produced in the blood vessels, usually only audible if some factor is obstructing blood flow. Tenderness to palpation or tenderness with the inflation of a blood pressure cuff over the calf or thigh (Lowenberg's cuff sign) gives high suspicion for deep vein thrombosis. Pain on dorsiflexion of the foot with stretching of the gastrocnemius muscle (Homans' sign) also may be present [5]. Ankle edema, especially unilateral, may be seen. Many procedures may be performed to diagnose vascular lesions.

Doppler Ultrasound

This procedure involves the use of a Doppler recorder to hear flow over the larger veins. Flow is normally increased by distal compression of the vein and decreased by the Valsalva maneuver, and varies with respiration. Lack of flow sound may indicate venous thrombosis. Arterial lesions also may be evaluated by Doppler studies. The proximal and distal pressures of the suspected lesion are auscultated to determine the pressure gradient. The Doppler flowmeter is used at the ankle to compare arterial pressure there with brachial systolic pressure.

Angiography

Angiography involves the use of a contrast material of high opacity to outline the great vessels, particularly the aorta and its branches. The contrast material may be injected into an artery, vein, or chamber of the heart.

In individuals with symptoms of obstruction involving the superior vena cava, angiography shows the site and extent of obstruction and may give other important data about it. Angiography also may be of great value in studying known aneurysms of the thoracic aorta.

Specific procedures used to visualize special vessels include (1) translumbar aortography, which is performed mainly to study aortoiliofemoral thromboocclusive disease, (2) renal arteriography, (3) visceral arteriography, and (4) inferior venacavography, especially to identify caval thrombosis.

Translumbar Aortography. In the presence of severe atherosclerosis, the translumbar puncture method of aortography may be preferable because of the hazards of retrograde catheterization from a femoral artery: injuring the arterial wall and embolization from a dislodged thrombus or plaque, perforations, and aggravation of thrombus formation. Because arteriosclerosis obliterans of the lower extremities involves many segments of the vascular system, it is important to evaluate inflow proximal to the diseased artery. Translumbar aortography carries the main risk of retroperitoneal bleeding from direct puncture of the aorta. Careful assessment of blood coagulation and blood pressure are necessary prior to performing this procedure. Aortography can detail the entire peripheral arterial system. Renal arteries can be evaluated for stenosis by injecting dye at the level of these arteries.

Peripheral Arteriography. Femoral arteriography can be performed when aortic visualization is unnecessary and when the lesion is limited to the leg. This approach also may be used to pass a catheter retrograde up the aorta to the desired position for dye injection. The clinical usefulness of this procedure is in the precise localization of atherosclerotic disease, and sometimes in thromboangiitis obliterans and aneurysms.

Study Questions

1. Describe the development of an atherosclerotic plaque and predict the result of obstruction of the peripheral arterial circulation.
2. Differentiate between the clinical pictures of systemic embolization and thrombosis.
3. Compare the clinical manifestations of arterial insufficiency and venous insufficiency.
4. Describe the factors that can lead to varicose veins.
5. Discuss collateral venous circulation.
6. Explain the purposes of lymphatic circulation and the results of total lymph circulation obstruction.

References

1. Erskine, J.M. Blood vessels and lymphatics. In M.A. Krupp, M.J. Chalton, and L.M. Tierney, *Current Medical Diagnosis and Treatment*. Los Altos, Calif.: Lange, 1986.
2. Fishman, M.C. *Medicine* (2nd ed.). Philadelphia: Lippincott, 1985.
3. Juergens, J.L., Fairbairn, J.E., II, and Spittell, J.A., Jr. *Peripheral Vascular Diseases* (5th ed.). Philadelphia: Saunders, 1986.
4. Lindsay, J., DeBakey, M.E., and Beall, A.C. Diseases of the aorta. In J.W. Hurst et al. (eds.), *The Heart* (6th ed.). New York: McGraw-Hill, 1986.
5. Perdue, G.D., and Smith, R.B. Diseases of the peripheral veins and the venae cavae. In J.W. Hurst et al. (eds.), *The Heart* (6th ed.). New York: McGraw-Hill, 1986.
6. Robbins, S.L., Cotran, R.S., and Kumar, V. *Pathologic Basis of Disease* (3rd ed.). Philadelphia: Saunders, 1984.
7. Ross, R. Factors influencing atherogenesis. In J.W. Hurst et al. (eds.), *The Heart* (6th ed.). New York: McGraw-Hill, 1986.
8. Sokolow, M., and McIlroy, M.B. *Clinical Cardiology* (4th ed.). Los Altos, Calif.: Lange, 1986.
9. Wallace, A.G., and Waugh, R.A. Pathophysiology of cardiovascular disease. In L.H. Smith and S.O. Thier, *Pathophysiology: The Biological Principles of Disease* (2nd ed.). Philadelphia: Saunders, 1985.
10. Young, J.R., and de Wolfe, V.G. Diseases of the peripheral arteries. In J.W. Hurst et al. (eds.), *The Heart* (6th ed.). New York: McGraw-Hill, 1986.

Unit Bibliography

Akhtar, M. Management of ventricular tachycardias. *JAMA* 247:671, 1982.

Alboni, P., et al. Intrinsic electrophysiologic properties of reentrant supraventricular tachycardia involving bypass tracts. *Am. J. Cardiol.* 58:226, 1986.

Alpert, M.A., and Flaker, G.C. Arrhythmias associated with sinus node dysfunction. *JAMA* 250:2160, 1983.

Arnsdorf, M.F. Basic understanding of electrophysiologic actions of arrhythmic drugs. *Med. Clin. North Am.* 68:1247, 1984.

Berne, R.M. The role of adenosin in the regulation of coronary blood flow. *Circ. Res.* 47:807, 1980.

Berne, R.M., and Levy, M.D. *Cardiovascular Physiology* (4th ed.). St. Louis: Mosby, 1981.

Boucher, C.A., et al. Determination of cardiac risk by dipyridamole-thallium imaging before peripheral vascular surgery. *N. Engl. J. Med.* 312:389, 1985.

Brandenburg, R.O., et al. *Cardiology: Fundamentals and Practice*. Chicago: Yearbook, 1987.

Braunwald, E. *Heart Disease*. Philadelphia: Saunders, 1980.

Chang, S. *Echocardiography: Techniques and Interpretation*. Philadelphia: Lea & Febiger, 1981.

Chase, K.M. Use vectors to round out an EKG. *RN* 49:18, 1986.

Childers, R. Classification of cardiac dysrhythmias. *Med. Clin. North Am.* 60:3, 1976.

Chung, E.K. *Principles of Cardiac Arrhythmias*. Baltimore: Williams & Wilkins, 1982.

Commerford, P.J., and Lloyd, E.A. Arrhythmias in patients with drug toxicity, electrolyte imbalance, and endocrine disturbances. *Med. Clin. North Am.* 68:1051, 1984.

Conner, R. The electrocardiographic diagnosis of posterior MI. *Crit. Care Nurse* 5:20, 1986.

Conner, R.P. Coronary artery anatomy: The electrographic and clinical correlations. *Crit. Care Nurse* 3:68, 1983.

Davis, M.J. *Pathology of Cardiac Valves*. Woburn, Mass.: Butterworths, 1980.

Dawber, T.R. *The Framingham Study Series: Commonwealth Fund.* Cambridge, Mass.: Harvard University Press, 1980.

deFaire, U., and Theorell, T. *Life Stress and Coronary Heart Disease*. St. Louis: Warren Green, 1982.

Doroghazi, R.M., and Slater, E.E. *Aortic Dissection*. New York: McGraw-Hill, 1983.

Dresdak, R.J. DD and management of cardiogenic shock. *Med. Times* 104:50, 1976.

Dubin, D. *Rapid Interpretation of EKGs* (7th ed.). Tampa: Cover, 1984.

Duke, D.M. Intraventricular conduction block. *Crit. Care Nurse* 4:30, 1982.

Feigenbaum, H. *Echocardiography* (3rd ed.). Philadelphia: Lea & Febiger, 1981.

Fink, B.W. *Congenital Heart Disease: A Deductive Approach to Its Diagnosis* (2nd ed.). Chicago: Yearbook, 1985.

Finklemeier, B.A., and Salinger, M.H. The atrial electrocardiogram: Its diagnostic use following cardiac surgery. *Crit. Care Q.* 4:42, 1984.

Fortuin, N.J. Echocardiography: How it works. *Med. Times* 108:120, 1980.

Foster, S.B. Pump failure following myocardial infarction: An overview. *Heart Lung* 9:293, 1980.

Fowler, N.O. *Cardiac Diagnosis and Treatment* (3rd ed.). Hagerstown, Md.: Harper & Row, 1980. Pp. 186–317.

Friedman, S.A. *Vascular Diseases: A Concise Guide to Diagnosis, Management, Pathogenesis and Prevention*. Littleton, Mass.: Wright-PSG, 1982.

Genest, J., et al. *Hypertension: Physiopathology and Treatment* (2nd ed.). New York: McGraw-Hill, 1983.

Goldberger, E. *Textbook of Clinical Cardiology*. St. Louis: Mosby, 1982.

Gomes, J.C., and El-Sherif, N. Atrioventricular block: Mechanism, clinical presentation, and therapy. *Med. Clin. North Am.* 68:1247, 1984.

Gotto, A.M., et al. *Atherosclerosis: A SCOPE Publication*. Kalamazoo, Mich.: Upjohn, 1977.

Guzzetta, C., and Dossey, B. *Cardiovascular Nursing: Body-Mind-Tapestry*. St. Louis: Mosby, 1984.

Hammond, C. Bundle branch block: When to sound the alarm. *RN* 44:55, 1981.

Holling, H.E. *Peripheral Vascular Diseases: Diagnosis and Management*. Philadelphia: Lippincott, 1972. Pp. 38–56.

Honig, C. *Modern Cardiovascular Physiology*. Boston: Little, Brown, 1981.

Hurst, J.W., et al. (eds.). *The Heart* (6th ed.). New York: McGraw-Hill, 1986.

Jones, R.J. An overview of cardiogenic shock: Approaches. *Primary Cardiol.* 9:38, 1976.

Juergens, J.L., et al. *Peripheral Vascular Disease* (6th ed.). Philadelphia: Saunders, 1986.

Kallenberg, C.G.M., Wouda, A.A., and The, T.H. The systemic involvement and immunologic findings in patients presenting with Raynaud's phenomenon. *Am. J. Med.* 69:675, 1980.

Karassi, A. *Acute Myocardial Infarction*. New York: McGraw-Hill, 1980.

Kernicki, J., Bullock, B., and Matthew, J. *Cardiovascular Nursing*. New York: Putnam, 1971.

Killip, T. Arrhythmias in myocardial infarction. *Med. Clin. North Am.* 60:233, 1976.

Kinney, M.R. (ed.). *AACNs Clinical Reference for Critical Care Nursing*. New York: McGraw-Hill, 1981.

Langman, J. *Medical Embryology: Human Development—Normal and Abnormal* (2nd ed.). Baltimore: Williams & Wilkins, 1969.

Little, R. *Physiology of the Heart and Circulation* (3rd ed.). Chicago: Yearbook, 1986.

MacIver, A.G., et al. The pathology of arterial disease. *Br. J. Anaesth.* 53:675, 694, 1981.

Marcus, M.L. *The Coronary Circulation in Health and Disease*. New York: McGraw-Hill, 1983.

Martin, L.B., and Cohen, L.S. Cardiomyopathy. *D.M.* 28:13, 1981.

Mason, D.T. *Congestive Heart Failure: Mechanisms, Evaluation and Treatment*. New York: Yorke, 1976.

Melstein, S., Sharma, A., and Klein, G. Electrophysiologic profile of asymptomatic Wolff-Parkinson-White pattern. *Am. J. Cardiol.* 57:1097, 1986.

Messen, J.V. Cardiogenic shock: Etiological and pathophysiological considerations, monitoring and management. *Practical Cardiol.* 6:86, 1978.

Moore, H.D., and Rinehart, J.F. Histogenesis of coronary arteriosclerosis. *Circulation* 6:481, 1952.

Phillips, R.E., and Feeney, M.K. *The Cardiac Rhythms: A Systematic Approach to Interpretation* (2nd ed.). Philadelphia: Saunders, 1980.

Plauth, W.H., et al. Congenital heart disease. In J.W. Hurst et al. (eds.), *The Heart* (6th ed.). New York: McGraw-Hill, 1986.

Porterfield, J.G., Porterfield, L., and Brown, S. Sudden cardiac death. *Focus Crit. Care* 13:23, 1986.

Rackley, C.E., et al. Aortic valve disease. In J.W. Hurst et al. (eds.), *The Heart* (6th ed.). New York: McGraw-Hill, 1986.

Robbins, S.L., Cotran, R.S., and Kumar, V. *Pathologic Basis of Disease* (3rd ed.). Philadelphia: Saunders, 1984.

Ross, J.H. Reentrant supraventricular tachycardia. *Crit. Care Nurse* 4:30, 1984.

Scheicht, S. Basic electrocardiography: Leads, axes, arrhythmias. *Clin. Symp.* 35:2, 1983.

Scorde, K.A. Taming the cardiac monitor (Part 1). *Nursing* 12:59, 1982.

Scorde, K.A. Taming the cardiac monitor (Part 2). *Nursing* 12:61, 1982.

Shamroth, L. *The Disorders of Cardiac Rhythm* (2nd ed.). St. Louis: Blackwell/Mosby, 1980.

Shepard, N. A guide to arrhythmia interpretation and management. *Crit. Care Nurse* 2:58, 1982.

Shoenberg, B.S. *Precursors of Stroke: Etiologic, Preventive and Therapeutic Implications*. New York: Oxford University Press, 1982.

Silverman, M.D., et al. *Electrocardiography: Basic Concepts and Clinical Application*. New York: McGraw-Hill, 1983.

Sodeman, W.A., and Sodeman, T.M. *Pathologic Physiology* (2nd ed.). Philadelphia: Saunders, 1986.

Sokolow, M., and McIlroy, M.B. *Clinical Cardiology* (4th ed.). Los Altos, Calif.: Lange, 1986.

Sperelakis, N. Propagation mechanisms in the heart. *Annu. Rev. Physiol.* 41:441, 1979.

Transover, T. A conceptual approach to the electrocardiogram. *Crit. Care Nurse* 66:76, 1982.

Visant, M., and Spence, M. *Common Sense Approach to Coronary Care* (4th ed.). St. Louis: Mosby, 1985.

Winsor, T. The electrocardiogram in myocardial infarction. *Clin. Symp.* 29:3, 1977.

UNIT 9

Respiration

Barbara L. Bullock

This unit is divided into four chapters, each of which deals with aspects of the pulmonary system. Chapter 24 discusses the normal anatomy and physiology of the pulmonary system. It is intended as a review that provides the basis for the material in Chapters 25, 26, and 27, which cover various aspects of pathophysiology of the pulmonary system.

Diseases of the pulmonary system have been categorized as restrictive, obstructive, and other alterations. There is necessarily some overlap among these categories, but an attempt has been made to classify them according to functional impairments. The chapters contain discussion of pathologic, clinical, and diagnostic aspects of pulmonary disease.

The reader is encouraged to use the learning objectives and study questions as study guides and to supplement the material with references listed in the unit bibliography.

CHAPTER 24

Normal Respiratory Function

CHAPTER OUTLINE

Anatomy of the Pulmonary Tree
- Airways
- Anatomy of the Lungs
- Parenchyma of the Lungs

Pulmonary Circulation
Major Muscles of Ventilation
Nervous Control of Respiration
- Nerve Supply
- Respiratory Centers
- Central Chemoreceptors
- Peripheral Chemoreceptors

Compliance and Elastance
The Mechanics of Breathing
- Phases of Ventilation
- Changes in Airway Size
- Airway Resistance
- Tissue Resistance

The Work of Breathing
Substances Important in Alveolar Expansion
- Surfactant
- Alpha$_1$-antitrypsin

Defense of the Airways and Lungs
- Mucociliary Transport, or the Mucociliary Escalator System
- Alveolar Clearance
- Deposition of Particulates in the Airways
- Reflexes of the Airways

Defenses Against Infection
- Defense Against Microbial Agents
- Immunologic Defense
- Interferon

Normal Gas Exchange
- Oxygen Transport to the Tissues
- Oxyhemoglobin Dissociation Curve
- Carbon Dioxide Transport
- Ventilation-Perfusion Relationships

Respiratory Regulation of Acid-Base Equilibrium
Pulmonary Function Testing

LEARNING OBJECTIVES

1. Describe the normal basic pulmonary anatomy.
2. Describe the action of the pulmonary pumping mechanism.
3. Identify the mechanisms of nervous control in the respiratory tract.
4. Compare the concepts of compliance and elastance in the normally functioning pulmonary system.
5. Describe the importance of the anatomic dead space in pulmonary function.
6. Identify the major muscles of respiration and their function.
7. Compare tissue resistance and airway resistance.
8. Relate the concept of work of breathing to oxygen consumption and carbon dioxide production.
9. Describe the major patterns of airway resistance.
10. Describe the anatomy and dynamics of pulmonary perfusion.
11. Compare normal ventilation and perfusion from the apex to the base of the lung.
12. List factors that alter ventilation and perfusion.
13. List the normal pressures in the heart and pulmonary vascular system.
14. Relate the oxyhemoglobin dissociation curve to tissue oxygenation.
15. Outline the pattern of normal gas exchange.
16. Describe the function of surfactant in the alveoli.
17. Describe the function of alpha$_1$-antitrypsin in the lungs.
18. Identify deposition sites of particulates in the airway.
19. List the major protective reflexes of the lungs.
20. Explain the function of the mucociliary transport system in the defense of the lungs.
21. Trace the clearance of particulates from the alveoli.
22. Distinguish between humoral and cell-mediated immunity in the lungs.
23. Describe the role of the macrophages in the lungs.
24. Explain the probable activity of interferon.

To delineate clearly the pathophysiology of respiratory diseases, this chapter reviews the anatomy and physiology of the pulmonary system and includes an in-depth discussion of the following essential concepts: compliance, elastance, resistance, ventilation, perfusion, diffusion, and alveolar airway clearance in health. A description of pulmonary function tests is also included.

To live is to breathe. Between a newborn's first breath and the last expiration is a lifetime of respiration. Breathing is the only bodily function that occurs automatically and can be controlled voluntarily as well. It is also the only bodily function that immediately interacts with the environment, whatever it may be: fresh ocean breeze, stale cigarette smoke, noxious automobile exhaust, damp cellar, or dusty workplace. Normally, breathing occurs below the level of consciousness, rhythmically and inconspicuously, unless some kind of physical stress interferes, such as breathlessness after running, swimming, or climbing a mountain, or when the lungs are impaired by diseases such as asthma, emphysema, bronchitis, pneumonia, or fibrosis.

The human body must adapt itself continually to an unfriendly environment; the lungs especially are constantly attacked by irritants, gases, and microorganisms. Consequently, the respiratory apparatus has developed an elaborate defense system to protect itself and the body from these inhalants.

The main function of the lungs is to take oxygen from the air and deliver it across the alveolar-capillary membrane to the hemoglobin. It is transported on hemoglobin by circulating blood to the tissues. At the tissue line it diffuses across the cellular membrane to the mitochondria to aid in producing energy to support the metabolic processes of life. As a result of these metabolic processes, carbon dioxide is produced that is transported back to the lungs and expelled into the environmental air.

Anatomy of the Pulmonary Tree

Airways

Air normally enters the body through the nose or the mouth. Here and in the pharynx it is warmed, moistened, and filtered. Even though air has been filtered in the upper respiratory tract, it is not sterile when it reaches the lower respiratory tract. Much debris remains, as evidenced by autopsies of the lungs of smokers or those exposed to heavy air pollution.

The air passes through the larynx and into the respiratory tree, which is a series of successively smaller, branching tubes (Fig. 24-1). Immediately below the larynx is the trachea, which divides at a point called the carina into the right and left main stem bronchi. The right main stem bronchus is shorter and wider than the left, coming off the trachea in a nearly straight line (Fig. 24-2). This explains why aspirated objects and fluids lodge more frequently in the right lung than in the left. It also makes suctioning of the left main stem bronchus difficult.

The right and left main stem bronchi divide into the lobar bronchi, which divide into the segmental bronchi. The segmental bronchi then divide into the terminal bronchioles. The diameter of each of these successive segments

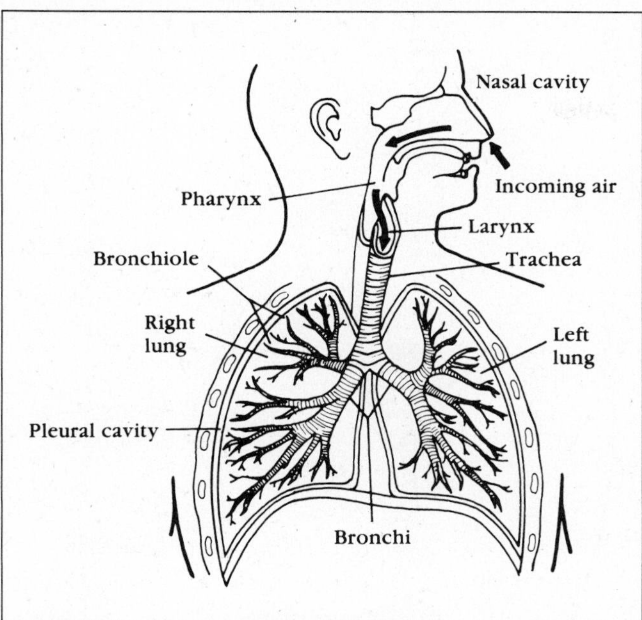

FIGURE 24-1 Respiratory system. (From H.A. Braun, F.W. Cheney, Jr., and C.P. Loehnen, *Introduction to Respiratory Physiology* [2nd ed.]. Boston: Little, Brown, 1980.)

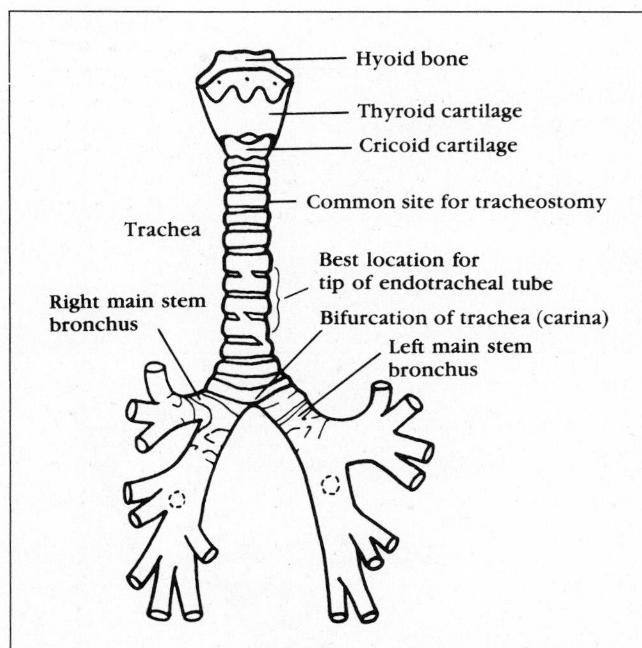

FIGURE 24-2 Tracheobronchial divisions. (From H.A. Braun, F.W. Cheney, Jr., and C.P. Loehnen, *Introduction to Respiratory Physiology* [2nd ed.]. Boston: Little, Brown, 1980.)

is smaller than the last, but the number of airways in the smaller segments is greater than in the larger ones, providing a broader surface area. This anatomic division, called the *generations of bronchi*, ends at approximately the sixteenth generation from the trachea.

The terminal bronchioles branch into the respiratory bronchioles. Occasional alveoli are present in the walls of these latter structures.

Anatomy of the Lungs

The lungs lie in the thoracic cavity, separated from each other by the mediastinum. The lungs are cone-shaped, with the narrow ends, or *apices*, directed upward and the wide *bases* at the lower portion. Each lung is composed of lobes, three on the right and two on the left (Fig. 24-3). The lobes are divided into smaller compartments called *lobules*. The lobules are further divided into smaller segments and terminate finally in the alveolar sacs.

Surrounding the lungs is the pleural membrane, which provides a covering over the lungs and lines the thoracic wall. The layer overlying the lung parenchyma is the *visceral pleura* and the outer layer is the *parietal pleura* (Fig. 24-4). Between these layers is a thin film of serous fluid that allows the visceral layer to move on the parietal layer without friction during normal ventilation. Between the layers is a potential space called the *intrapleural* or *pleural* space.

Parenchyma of the Lungs

The alveolar ducts, the final generation, are totally lined with alveoli (Fig. 24-5). Respiratory exchange of gas takes place only in the alveoli; therefore, these structures are designated collectively as the respiratory zone of the lungs. Because of their tiny size and large numbers, the alveoli have a volume of about 2500 ml in the adult. They have a diffusing area (surface area) about the size of a tennis court, or approximately 70 m^2. Each terminal bronchiole supplies its own unit of several alveoli called the *acinus*. The alveoli in the acinus do not have separate connections with the terminal bronchiole but are of various shapes and are interconnected.

The individual alveolus is one layer of cells thick and is built on a structure of elastin and muscle fibers. Each alveolus communicates with the pulmonary capillary bed to move gases by diffusion across the *alveolocapillary interspace* (Fig. 24-6). Interconnecting the alveoli are tiny openings called the *pores of Kohn* (Fig. 24-7), which allow air to circulate among the alveoli, so that within a second or less after inspiration, all alveoli in an acinus have the same gas concentration. In young children, the pores of Kohn are few in number and poorly developed, but with age these structures increase in number and size.

The pores of Kohn are helpful in the event of obstruction of a small airway. In a process called *collateral ventilation*, if an airway smaller than a lobar bronchiole is obstructed, the alveoli that the airway normally supplies can continue to be ventilated by the pores of Kohn [5]. Collateral ventilation appears to be more effective in adults than in young children.

Pulmonary Circulation

The lung has two blood supplies, the *bronchial* and *pulmonary circulations*. The first consists of the bronchial

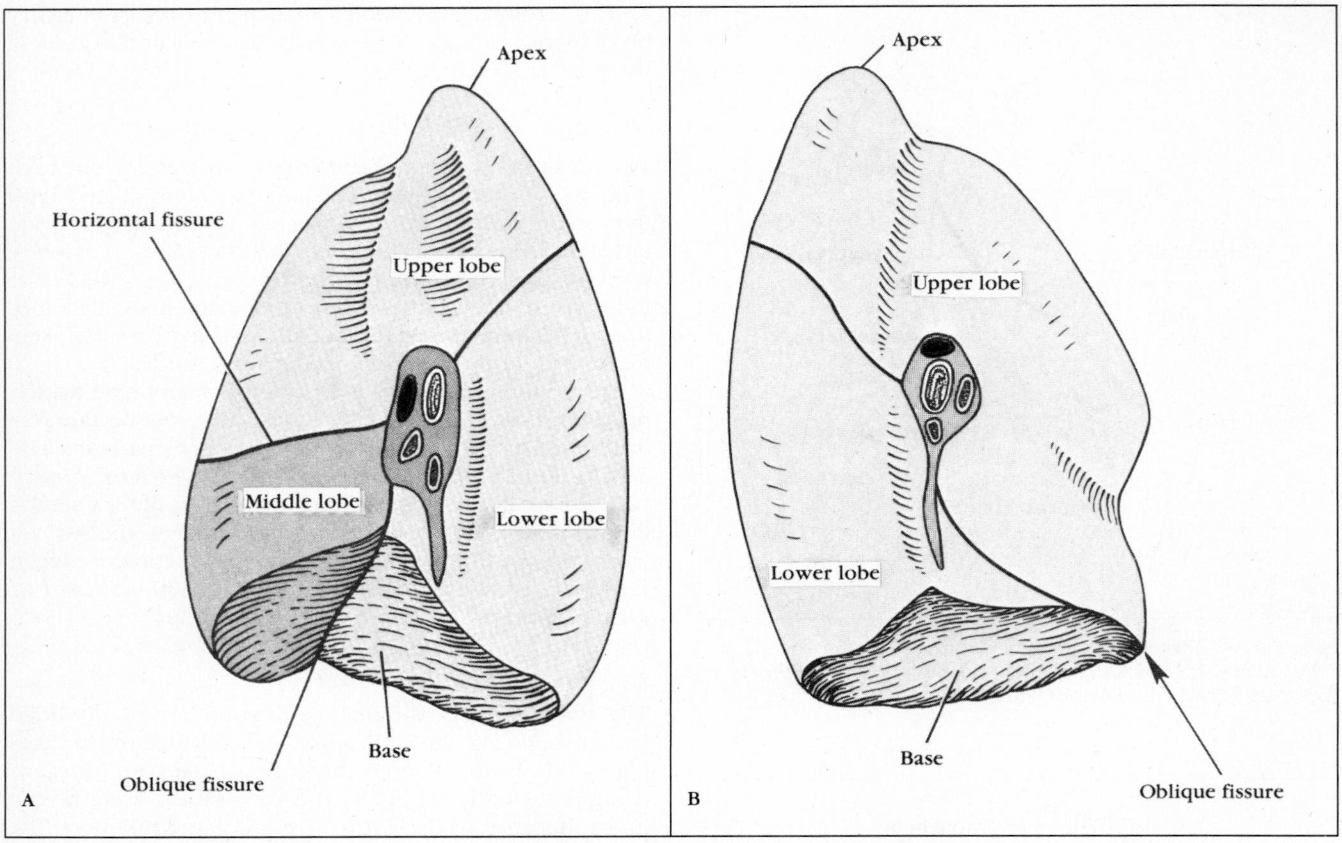

FIGURE 24-3 A. Lateral and medial surfaces of right lung. B. Lateral and medial surfaces of left lung. (From R.S. Snell, *Clinical Anatomy for Medical Students* [2nd ed.]. Boston: Little, Brown, 1981.)

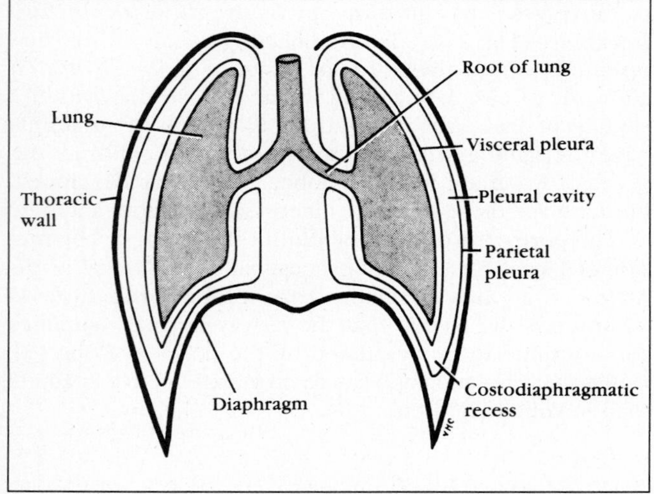

FIGURE 24-4 Position of visceral and parietal pleura with the pleural space. (From R.S. Snell, *Clinical Anatomy for Medical Students* [2nd ed.]. Boston: Little, Brown, 1981.)

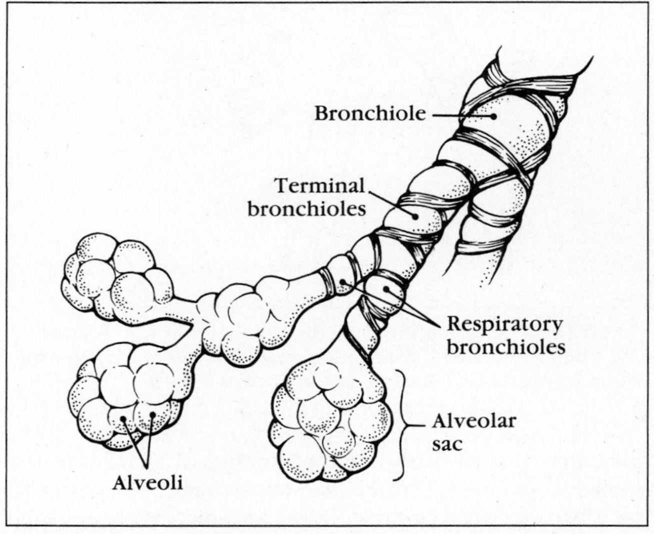

FIGURE 24-5 Termination of the generations of respiratory tubes in alveolar sacs and individual alveoli.

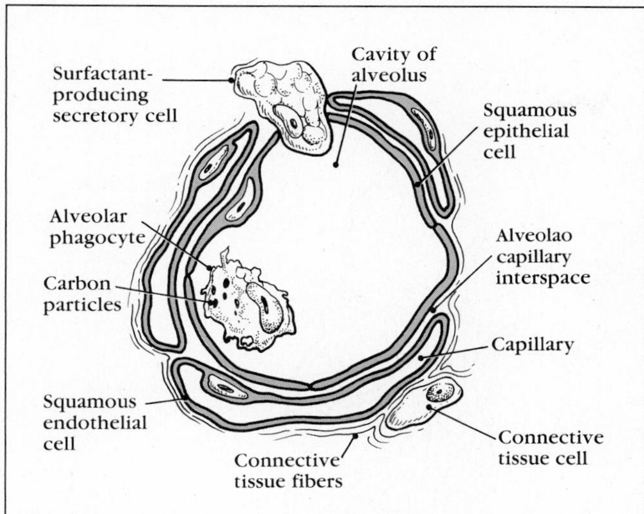

FIGURE 24-6 Representation of single alveolus with surrounding capillaries and other cells. Note alveolocapillary interspace.

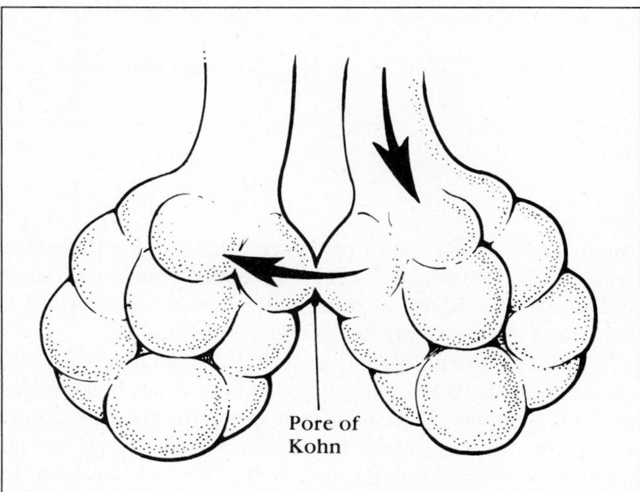

FIGURE 24-7 Schematic demonstration of collateral communication between the alveoli through pores of Kohn.

arteries, which arise in the thoracic aorta and upper intercostal arteries. As a part of the systemic blood supply, these arteries nourish the trachea and bronchi to the level of the respiratory bronchioles. After forming capillary plexuses, some of the bronchial circulation returns through a pulmonary vein to the left atrium, while some empties into the bronchial vein that terminates in the azygous vein which, in turn, empties into the superior vena cava.

The bronchial circulation supplies the lung's supporting tissues, its nerves, and the outer layers of the pulmonary arteries and veins; normally, it supplies neither the alveolar walls and ducts nor the respiratory bronchioles. In the event of interruption of the pulmonary circulation, the bronchial circulation can support the metabolic needs of these tissues, but the tissues lose the ability to participate in gas exchange.

The second blood supply to the lungs is the pulmonary circulation. From the pulmonary artery, the lungs normally receive the entire output of the right ventricle. This blood circulates through the pulmonary capillary bed and then returns to the left heart by way of the pulmonary veins (Fig. 24-8). The pulmonary circulatory system exchanges oxygen and carbon dioxide to maintain the life processes.

Major Muscles of Ventilation

The major muscle of ventilation, which enlarges the chest cavity, is the *diaphragm*. Innervated by the phrenic nerves, this flat, dome-shaped muscle lowers approximately 1 cm in quiet respiration; in forced inspiration it may descend as much as 10 cm. This diaphragmatic movement temporarily compresses the abdominal contents. Consequently, the movement of the diaphragm can be impeded by abnormalities in the abdominal cavity such as ascites and hepatomegaly. If abdominal pain is present, diaphragmatic action is reduced because of the *splinting effect*, a voluntary limitation of ventilatory movements.

The thoracic cavity is further enlarged by an upward and outward motion of the lower ribs accomplished by the *external intercostal muscles*. The upper ribs also move outward. The ribs are attached to the vertebrae in such a way that they rotate on an axis as they are moved by these muscles.

While inspiration normally is an active effort, expiration is a passive one in which the muscles relax and allow the lungs and chest wall structures to return to resting size. The pressure in the thorax gradually rises and air moves out of the lungs.

The *internal intercostal muscles* are used in forced expiration to stiffen the intercostal spaces during straining. The *muscles of the abdominal wall* are also powerful aids to forced expiration. Normally, they are used only to generate the explosive pressure that is necessary for coughing. They also contract at the end of forced inspiration in synchrony with glottic closure to limit and stop the inspiration abruptly. The *accessory muscles*, scalene and sternomastoid, are used during labored breathing to raise the first two ribs and sternum and increase the size of the thoracic cavity.

Nervous Control of Respiration

Nerve Supply

The major nerve supply to the diaphragm is through the two *phrenic nerves*. Each half of the diaphragm is innervated by one of these nerves, which originate mainly from the fourth cervical nerve of the respective side. The eleventh cranial nerve, the accessory, innervates most of the larynx and pharynx.

Bronchial muscle is innervated by both *parasympathetic (vagus) and sympathetic nerve supply*. Increased

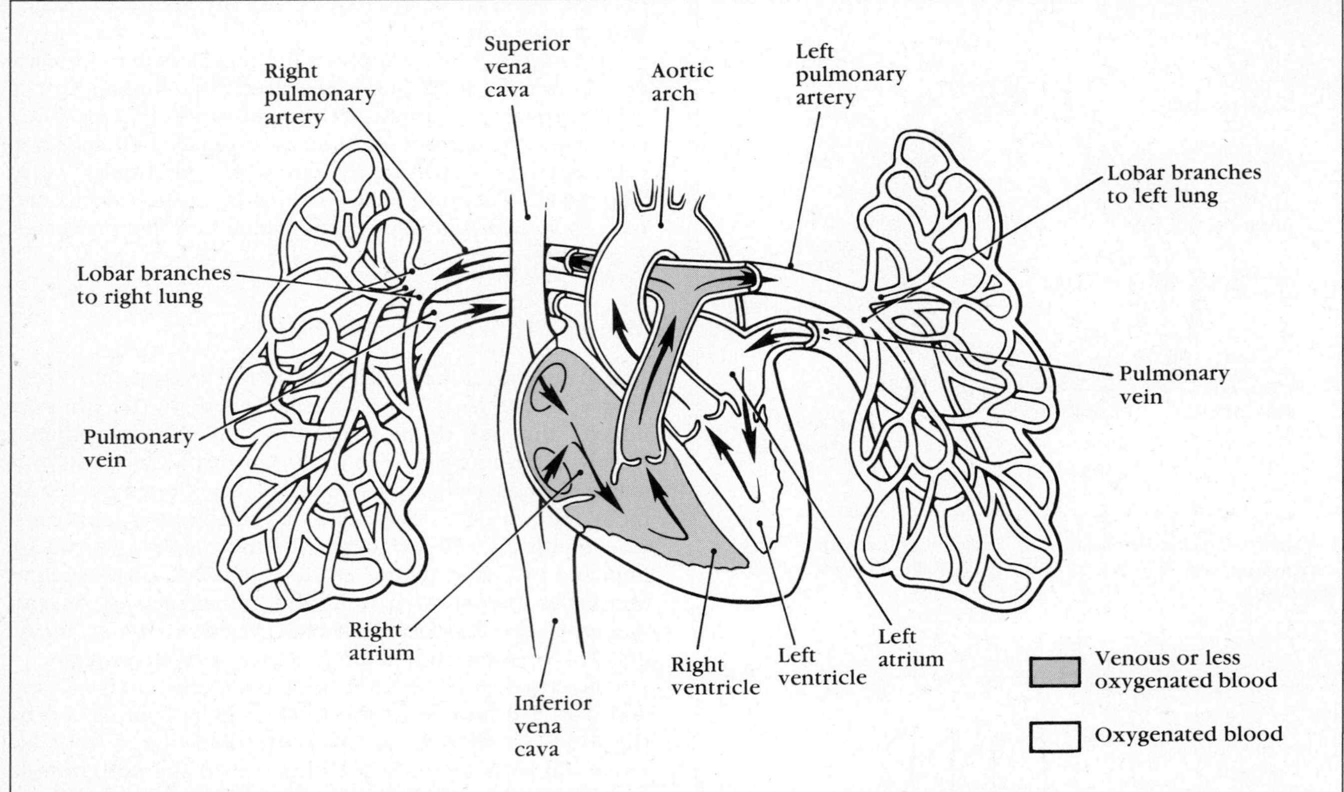

FIGURE 24-8 Circulation from the right heart to the lungs to the left heart.

vagal influence causes bronchoconstriction, while increased sympathetic stimulation causes bronchodilation. Any factor that decreases the caliber of the airway increases resistance and work of breathing, whereas increased caliber of the airway has the opposite effect [18].

The vagus nerve also transmits the appropriate signal to limit inspiration when an overstretch signal is received from the lungs. This reflex, called the *Hering-Breuer reflex*, serves as a protective mechanism to limit lung inflation.

Respiratory Centers

The nervous system adjusts alveolar ventilation to the demands of the body. This occurs through the *respiratory centers* that are located in the medulla oblongata and the pons. Normally, these areas regulate ventilatory rate and depth through the chemical signals of carbon dioxide and hydrogen ion levels.

Central Chemoreceptors

Respiratory neurons located in the medulla oblongata are the major chemosensitive areas (chemoreceptors). Figure 24-9 shows separate areas responsible for inspiration and expiration. The major stimulus for the *inspiratory area* is the carbon dioxide concentration of blood, and this area also transmits input from the peripheral chemoreceptors. The regular rhythm of the ventilatory effort is generated in the inspiratory area. The effort continues below the conscious level, although the conscious control of breathing always overrides the unconscious.

The *expiratory area* is located in a separate part of the medulla but is usually not active unless there is some respiratory distress. When pulmonary ventilation becomes excessive, the expiratory muscles are activated to aid the expiratory effort. How the interaction occurs between the inspiratory and expiratory areas is not known [8].

The *pneumotaxic center* is located in the pons and participates continually in the inspiratory effort through directly limiting the tidal volume of air inspired. Activation of this center increases rate of respiration while decreased stimulation decreases the respiratory rate. Another center in the pons, the *apneustic center*, functions in some brain pathology to cause excessive inflation of the lungs with occasional expiratory efforts.

Peripheral Chemoreceptors

Decreased oxygen tension levels in arterial blood are sensed by the peripheral chemoreceptors of the carotid body and aortic arch (Fig. 24-10). The hypoxic stimulus, described as 30 mm Hg oxygen tension less than normal for the person, is transmitted to the respiratory center. It results primarily in stimulation of inspiratory neurons and effects an increased respiratory rate through the phrenic

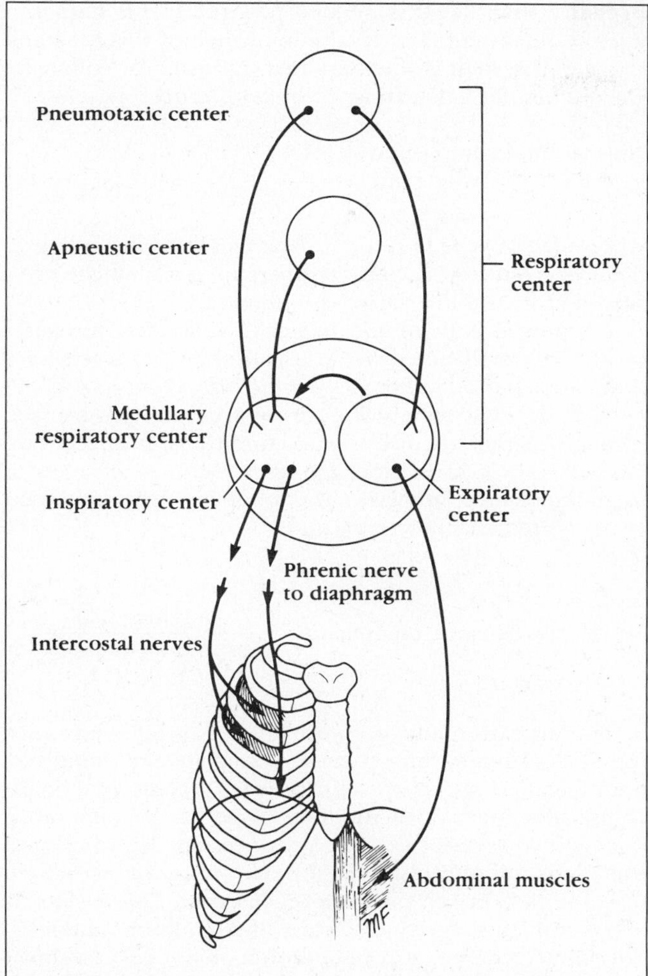

FIGURE 24-9 The medullary inspiratory and expiratory centers. (From R.S. Snell, *Clinical Histology for Medical Students*. Boston: Little, Brown, 1984.)

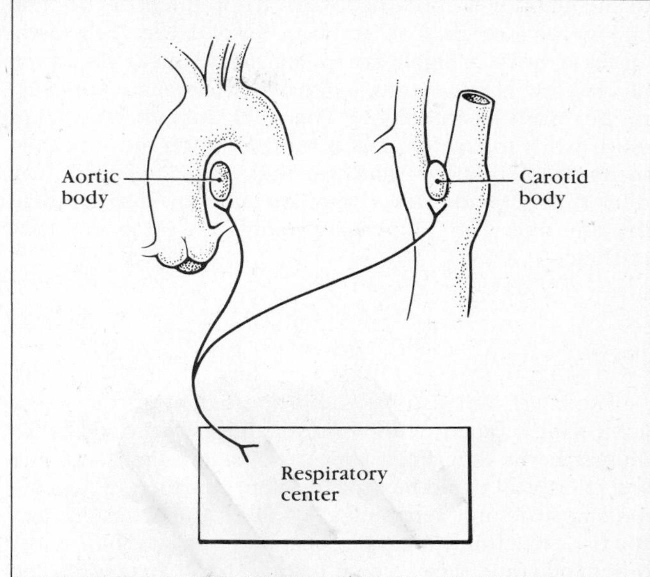

FIGURE 24-10 Decreased oxygen tension causes stimulation of the respiratory center and an increased respiratory rate.

nerve. The peripheral chemoreceptors are also sensitive to changes in carbon dioxide and hydrogen, but the direct effect of the central respiratory center overrides the sensitivity from the peripheral receptors [13].

Compliance and Elastance

To understand pulmonary pathology, it is important to understand the concepts of *compliance* (C) and *elastance* (E), also called *elasticity*. Generally, it can be said that the respiratory system behaves like a pump with a flow-resistive mechanism. The pumping part of the mechanism can be thought of as two separate components: the chest wall with its associated structures and the lungs.

Compliance is a measurement of distensibility, or how easily a tissue is stretched. In other words, the fewer elastic forces to be overcome in order to stretch a substance, the more compliant it is. Compliance is measured and recorded by the amount of volume change that results from pressure applied. Compare the blowing up of an old balloon with that of a new one. Less pressure is needed to make a large volume change in the old balloon while more pressure is required to make a smaller volume change in the new one. Compliance is thus important because the more compliant a tissue is, the less pressure is required to stretch it. Using delta (Δ) as a symbol for change, compliance is expressed as follows:

$$C = \frac{V\ (\text{liters})\ (\Delta\text{volume})}{P\ (\text{cm water})\ (\Delta\text{pressure})}$$

Using the balloon analogy, one can discover which balloon is more compliant if arbitrary numbers are assigned as follows:

Old balloon	*New balloon*
Small pressure needed: 1	Large pressure needed: 10
Large volume change: 10	Small volume change: 3
$C = \frac{10}{1}$	$C = \frac{3}{10}$
$C = 10$	$C = 0.30$

From these figures, one finds that the old balloon is much more compliant, or more easily stretched, than the new one. It thus has fewer elastic forces to oppose the stretch than the new balloon.

Elastance is the opposite of compliance. Whereas compliance refers to the forces promoting expansion of the lung, elastic forces are those promoting the return to the normal resting position or original shape. Compliance and elastance are closely related in pulmonary dynamics. The lungs inherently tend to be elastic, so that without normal aids to expansion they tend to collapse. Compliance refers to the amount of force necessary to produce the volume change or stretch. The amount depends on the elastic forces at work. A highly compliant rubber band, for example, has few elastic forces, while a less compliant (thicker) rubber band has more [3]. The thick rubber band takes more work to stretch it and returns much more readily to its original shape than the thin one. Therefore, the thick rubber band is less compliant and more elastant than the thin one. The following formula is used to calculate elastance:

$$E = \frac{\Delta\text{pressure (P)}}{\Delta\text{volume (V)}}.$$

The chest wall also has the properties of elastance and compliance, but they differ from those of the lungs. To illustrate this difference, one can imagine that the lungs and chest wall could be separated but remain as living and moving structures retaining all of their properties. Each of the two structures could be separated from the pull of the other and could seek its own resting size at an equilibrium between elastance and compliance. In the case of the chest wall freed from the lungs, it would seek a much larger resting size than when it was attached to the lungs. Without the inward pull of the lungs, the chest wall would be abnormally large.

On the other hand, the lungs separated from the chest wall would tend to relax to a much smaller size than when they rested against the chest wall. They have more elastic recoil than might be expected from the amount of elastin and fiber they contain. This is because of a meshlike network, the structure of which itself increases elastic recoil. This arrangement is termed *nylon stocking elasticity*.

Taking the properties of the lungs and chest wall together, it can be seen that elastance of the lungs prevents overdistention of the thorax while chest wall compliance prevents collapse of the lungs. Contraction of the diaphragm, discussed earlier, lowers that muscle and increases the size of the thoracic cage. All of this creates a negative intrapleural pressure, causing air to move from the atmosphere to the lungs. Relaxation of the diaphragm, a passive process, causes the muscle to move to its resting position, intrapleural pressure to increase, and air to move from the lungs to the atmosphere. These properties account for the fact that expiration is normally a passive process, while inspiration is an active process.

Many diseases alter the compliance and elastance of either the lungs or chest wall, but disease need not affect *both* properties of either structure. In general, bronchopulmonary diseases affect lung compliance, while obesity and diseases of the thoracic skeleton or respiratory nerves affect chest wall compliance. Alveolar edema and atelectasis reduce compliance by reducing the number of inflated alveoli. Compliance of the lung is increased by emphysema and is somewhat increased in the aged person. Usually, dynamic measurements of compliance are used rather than estimates of elastance, and changes are referred to as *decreased* or *increased* compliance. In the case of pulmonary fibrosis, where there is increased fibrous tissue and stiffening of the lung tissues, compliance is reduced. More pressure than usual is needed to stretch this lung and chest wall system. The total compliance of this lung and chest wall system is then less than normal. The following is a method for calculating *total compliance*:

$$\text{Normal total compliance} = 0.1 \text{ L (BTPS)/cm } H_2O \quad \text{(during quiet breathing)},$$

where *BTPS/cm* H_2O refers to the fact that the measurement is calculated at body temperature, at ambient pressure, and with water vapor saturation [13].

If a person is being mechanically ventilated, measurements of compliance provide useful objective assessment data over a period of time. *Dynamic lung compliance* calculated in this way is not entirely accurate because the true calculation requires static conditions. It is accurate enough to be a useful tool for assessing gross changes in total compliance, however. The following method is used to calculate dynamic compliance:

$$\text{Effective dynamic compliance} = \frac{\text{expired tidal volume (ml)}}{\text{inspiratory pressure (cm } H_2O)}.$$

The measurement of compliance may be even more useful if related to lung volume. Compliance per lung volume is called *specific compliance*. Decreased specific compliance means that the lung tissue has become more rigid and, in severe cases, the pressures needed to expand the lungs adequately over a period of time are more than the person can produce or maintain. This results in hypoventilation. Many disorders, including obstructions, pulmonary edema, and pneumonia, may decrease both compliance and lung volume. Specific compliance is also related to lung size and may be reduced by 50 percent after pneumonectomy.

The Mechanics of Breathing

As stated previously, a particular pressure is necessary to cause a change in the volume of the lungs. Volume can be changed by either a high pressure from outside the body forcing air in or a negative pressure from inside the body causing air to move into the lungs. Normally, humans breathe by using negative pressure.

Phases of Ventilation

The phases of ventilation involve the movement of the diaphragm and the other respiratory muscles (Fig. 24-11). As the diaphragm descends, it enlarges the intrapleural space, which causes a negative intrapulmonary pressure; the air then flows into the lungs to equalize the pressure. The subatmospheric or negative pressure, which is necessary for air to flow into the lungs, is achieved by enlarging the lung and chest cavity. When the chest and lungs enlarge, the pressure inside the thorax is lower than it was

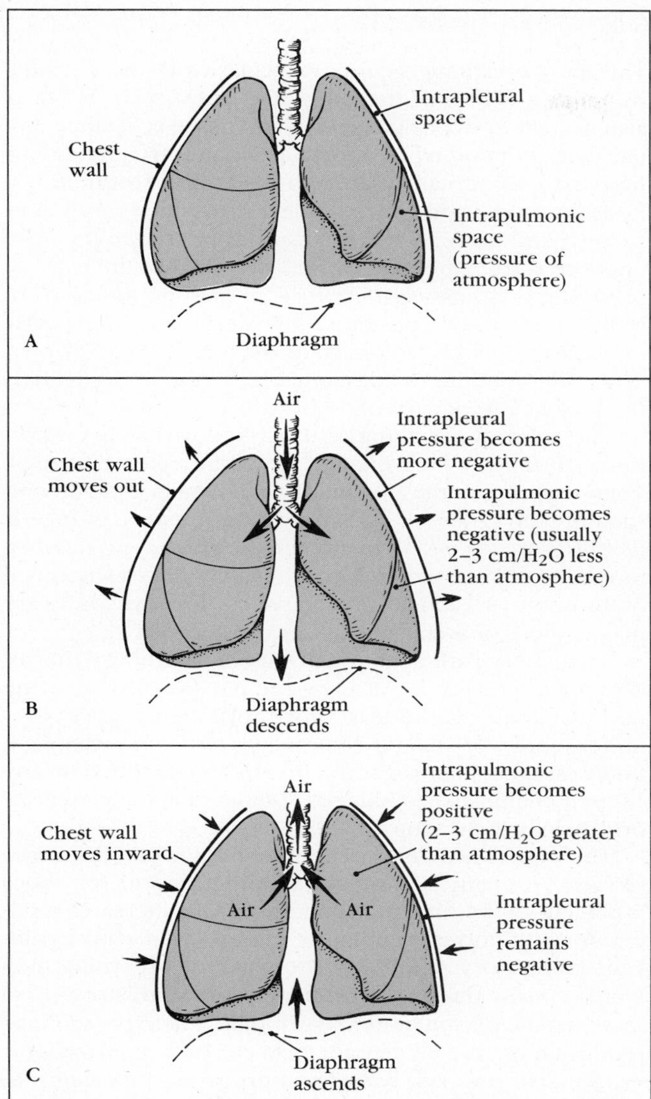

FIGURE 24-11 Phases of ventilation. A. No movement of air. B. Air moves from the environment to the intrapulmonic space. C. Air moves from the intrapulmonic space to the environment.

before the enlargement. At the end of active effort, the diaphragm relaxes and moves upward, which increases intrapulmonary pressure to above atmospheric level. The air moves passively out of the lungs. The elastic recoil of the lung tissue moves the lungs to their resting or unstretched state.

Thus inspiration is an active process initiated by the contraction of the diaphragm and the outward pull by the intercostals. Air moves from greater to less pressure. Expiration is a passive process that occurs when the respiratory muscles relax and the intrapulmonic pressure increases above the atmospheric level. Even when the system is relaxed, the lungs are continually pulling in and attempting to return to their smaller relaxed size. This process creates a negative intrapleural pressure and explains one of the reasons that air is pulled into the chest when the chest wall is punctured.

Changes in Airway Size

The size of the airways is also affected by the process of ventilation. The airways are attached to and supported by the lung parenchyma. Since the lungs expand to fill a larger space on inspiration, all of these structures, including the airways and alveolar ducts, are pulled to a larger size. The size of the airways and alveolar ducts is reduced as lung volume decreases during expiration. During quiet ventilation, some of the smaller airways close during expiration. Because of the effects of gravity, airway closure is more pronounced in the supine position.

Airway Resistance

During respiration, the volume of the thorax and consequently of the airways is changing. Airways offer resistance to airflow, the amount of which directly affects the amount of pressure needed to move air into and out of the lungs.

Pressure-flow relationships may be quite complex even in simple straight tubes. Because the respiratory tree is a series of branching tubes of varying sizes, the relationships become more complex.

The amount of pressure lost because of friction depends on the flow pattern of the air. The two major air flow patterns are *laminar* and *turbulent* (Fig. 24-12). In laminar flow, the gas in the airways is like very thin cylinders moving inside each other. The cylinder on the outside moves slowly and each inner cylinder of air moves progressively faster. Gas density has no influence on the velocity of this type of flow. Basically, the gas flows along a straight line with little friction to the molecules. When airway caliber changes, however, the laminar pattern is altered. Additional pressure may be required to reaccelerate the gas and to reestablish a laminar flow pattern.

When flow rates are high or when airways are partially obstructed or collapsed, airflow becomes turbulent. In normal lungs, turbulent flow occurs in the large central airways because of molecular collision and resistance at

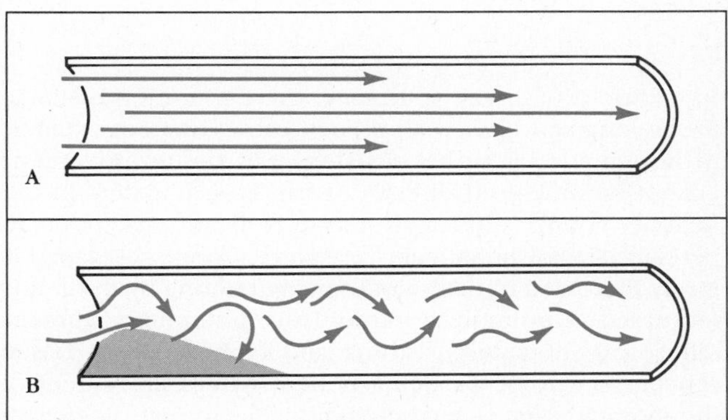

FIGURE 24-12 A. Schematic representation of laminar gas flow. B. Representation of turbulent gas flow.

the sides of the tubes. Laminar flow occurs more readily in the small peripheral airways, which are generally straight and smooth.

Change in airway width greatly alters resistance. When airways widen, resistance is greatly diminished and air flows through easily. When airways narrow, resistance is increased and air moves through them with much more difficulty. It takes more pressure to move air through a narrow airway than a wide one. Studies have shown that if airway radius is reduced by one-half, resistance is increased by 16 times [22]. This fact has great importance for individuals whose airways are narrowed by bronchospasm or pressure from tumors or infectious processes, as increased airway resistance increases the work of breathing.

Since airways normally widen on inspiration and narrow on expiration, resistance is generally greater on expiration than on inspiration. This normal change in resistance helps to explain why air becomes trapped on expiration in asthma or chronic lung disease.

Although there are many extremely small peripheral airways, they are so tiny that they make little difference in the resistance factors that can be measured. It is postulated that the initial changes of chronic lung disease occur in these airways where they cannot be measured [22]. These airways make up areas called *silent zones* where diseases can be present without detection.

In normal respiration in the upright position, the bases of the lungs tend to ventilate better than the apices. This has been demonstrated by having a person inhale radioactive xenon gas and monitoring its diffusion with a radiation camera. During the inspiratory phase the bases undergo a larger change in volume and have a smaller resting volume than the apices. In the supine position this difference disappears and the ventilations become the same. In abnormalities such as pulmonary edema, the apices tend to ventilate better and the smaller airways in the bases often close [22].

Airway resistance can be altered by many factors. A sigh or deep inspiration usually reduces resistance, while forced expiration, even in the healthy individual, increases it. Airway compression is the usual cause of increased resistance during forced expiration, and this factor is markedly enhanced in persons with diseased or weakened airway walls [15].

Tissue Resistance

In addition to airway resistance, there is some resistance in the lung and chest wall tissues, called tissue resistance. Although the frictional resistance of tissue movement cannot be measured directly, it can be calculated. In the healthy, young, adult man, tissue resistance is about 20 percent of total pulmonary resistance. Tissue resistance is rarely increased to the point of being limiting by itself. It is increased in pulmonary sarcoidosis, pulmonary fibrosis, diffuse carcinomatosis, asthma, and kyphoscoliosis. Tissue resistance may be particularly high where movement of the thoracic cage is severely limited, as in neurologic disease, musculoskeletal disease, or deformity of the chest structures.

The Work of Breathing

The act of breathing requires muscular work to overcome the elastic forces of the lungs and chest wall. Work is also needed to overcome airway and tissue resistance. Initial work is minimal at normal breathing frequency but increases significantly at high breathing frequencies. Resistive work is minimized with a slow, deep respiratory pattern and increases with respiratory frequency. The opposite is true of elastic work. Two-thirds of the work of breathing is against elastic forces, prompting the lungs to return to the resting position. Slow, deep breathing greatly increases the work necessary to overcome elastic forces. When the work forces are summarized, respiratory work is the least at a frequency of 14 breaths per minute.

The work of breathing as described earlier is proportional to the pressure change times the volume change. Volume change is the amount of air moved in and out with each breath, called *tidal volume*. The pressure change is that pressure needed to overcome the *elastic* and *resistive* forces [13]. The elastic forces are mainly the elastic recoil of the chest wall and lungs themselves. Resistive forces are mainly those of tissue and airway resistance [13].

Respiratory pathology usually alters breathing patterns. The pattern finally adopted by the individual will be the one that requires the least work, although it always requires more work than the normal pattern. For example, if flow resistance increases, the breathing may be slow and deep. If compliance is reduced, a rapid, shallow pattern of breathing may be adopted.

The work of breathing, as in other body work, consumes oxygen. Normally, at rest, respiration accounts for about 5 percent of the total metabolic rate. This increases moderately with normal ventilatory changes, but with significant respiratory pathology the work of breathing may increase many times [13]. Ultimately, the ventilatory effort may cost the person more oxygen than it delivers and may produce more carbon dioxide than can be eliminated. This progressive process, without appropriate intervention, continues until respiratory failure ensues.

Substances Important in Alveolar Expansion

Surfactant

Surfactant, a phospholipid made up of dipalmitoyl-lecithin, is synthesized in the type II or granular pneumocytes lining the alveolus and is secreted to form a film across the alveolar surface. Surfactant provides surface stability and prevents collapse of the alveolar structures [8].

A deficiency of surfactant results in an increase in the surface tension in the alveolus during expiration that leads to collapse or atelectasis of the alveoli. Amounts of surfactant in the lungs vary according to the diameter of the alveoli. As the alveoli inflate, the surfactant spreads out over the surface of the alveolar membrane. As the alveoli empty, the surfactant layer becomes thicker in relation to the decreased space. Smaller alveoli have a thicker layer while larger alveoli have a thinner layer. This promotes expansion and stability of the alveoli [8].

To be effective, it is necessary that the surfactant layer be replenished continually. The half-life of pulmonary lecithin is 14 hours, which suggests that active synthesis must continually take place in the type II cells of the alveoli. Normal ventilation seems to be the most important factor in the replenishment of surfactant, which probably is due to the need for oxygen in the production of this substance. Hypoventilation may lead to atelectasis due to diminished renewal of surfactant. The underlying problem in this situation is a decreased supply of oxygen with decreased synthesis of surfactant, which leads to decreased surface tension in the alveoli. The result is widespread collapse of the alveoli.

Surfactant may also prevent the transudation of fluid across the alveolar capillary membrane during the respiratory cycle. Fluid exudation from capillary to alveolus has been shown to result from a decrease in the surfactant levels. Therefore, surfactant helps keep the alveoli dry. The absence of surfactant leads to a tendency to pull fluid into the alveoli, causing severe pulmonary edema.

Without surfactant, the surface tension of the alveoli would be fixed. Greater pressure would be necessary to keep an alveolus open, as its volume and radius would decrease on expiration. Atelectasis would regularly occur at low lung volumes due to collapse of small alveoli. Large inspiratory pressures would be required to reopen the alveoli. The point of collapse is referred to as the *critical closing pressure*, and the pressure necessary to open a collapsed alveolus must be enough to overcome surface tension.

Disorders that involve destruction, inactivation, or insufficient production of surfactant cause marked changes in pressure-volume relationships, even without changes in lung or chest wall tissues. Possibly the best known instance of surfactant deficiency is in the infant respiratory distress syndrome (IRDS), also called hyaline membrane disease, although the presence of the membrane seems to be secondary to the pathology rather than the cause of the disease. The condition is closely associated with prematurity and appears to be caused by immaturity of the type II cells and deficiency of surfactant synthesis. Further discussion of a similar problem, adult respiratory distress syndrome (ARDS), appears in Chapter 25.

Alpha$_1$-antitrypsin

In the search for the cause of emphysema, clinicians noted that some families had a high frequency of the disease and that onset was at an early age. The correlation between the absence of alpha$_1$-antitrypsin (a glycoprotein synthesized by the liver) and familial early-onset emphysema was studied and the level of alpha$_1$-antitrypsin was found to be genetically controlled [12]. The homozygous state is linked with early onset of panlobular emphysema. Persons with the heterozygous or intermediate state may have greater susceptibility to emphysema, particularly in the presence of repeated inflammatory reactions.

Exactly how alpha$_1$-antitrypsin protects the lungs is unknown. A widely accepted hypothesis (protease-antiprotease mechanism) states that leukocytes and macrophages release proteases, mainly elastases, in the inflammatory response (Fig. 24-13). That these proteases are capable of producing emphysema has been well established in animal research [11,17]. Proteases are neutralized by alpha$_1$-antitrypsin. Without this inhibitor, these enzymes attack and destroy the alveolar membrane. The protease-antiprotease hypothesis is supported in studies of cigarette smoking [19]. Smokers have increased numbers of neutrophils in the alveoli, and the condensates of smoke stimulate the release of their elastases into the alveoli. Decreased antielastase activity in these individuals results from inhibition of alpha$_1$-antitrypsin activity by oxidants in cigarette smoke and other factors [17].

Until recently, it was thought that the prevalence of some degree of alpha$_1$-antitrypsin deficiency in persons with emphysema was low, accounting for about 1 percent of this population. Studies have shown this percentage to be much greater, on the order of 25 percent. This compares with 5 percent of the healthy population who have some degree of the deficiency [14].

Defense of the Airways and Lungs

Mucociliary Transport, or the Mucociliary Escalator System

The mucociliary escalator system, or *mucous blanket*, provides the major defense of the respiratory tract against disease. The components of this system include the goblet cells, which secrete mucus; the ciliated epithelial cells; and mucus itself.

The *ciliated epithelial cells* of the respiratory tract clear the airways by moving fluid forward (Fig. 24-14A). These cells line the entire respiratory tract with the exception of the anterior one-third of the nose, part of the pharynx, and the alveoli. The surface of each ciliated cell

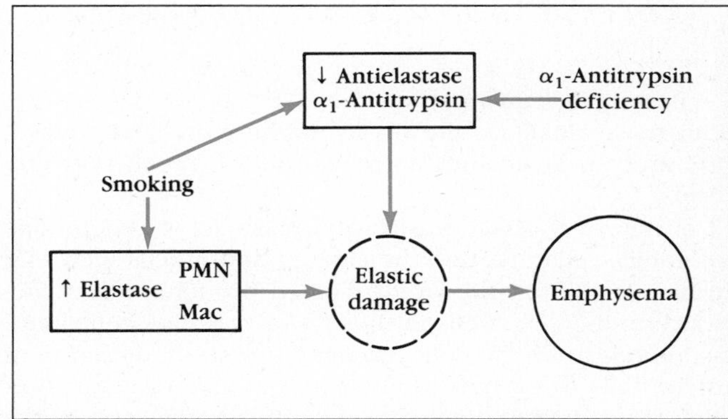

FIGURE 24-13 Protease-antiprotease mechanism of emphysema. PMN = polymorphonuclear leukocytes; Mac = alveolar macrophages. (From S.L. Robbins, R.S. Cotran, and V. Kumar, *Pathologic Basis of Disease* [3rd ed.]. Philadelphia: W.B. Saunders Company, 1984. Reprinted by permission.)

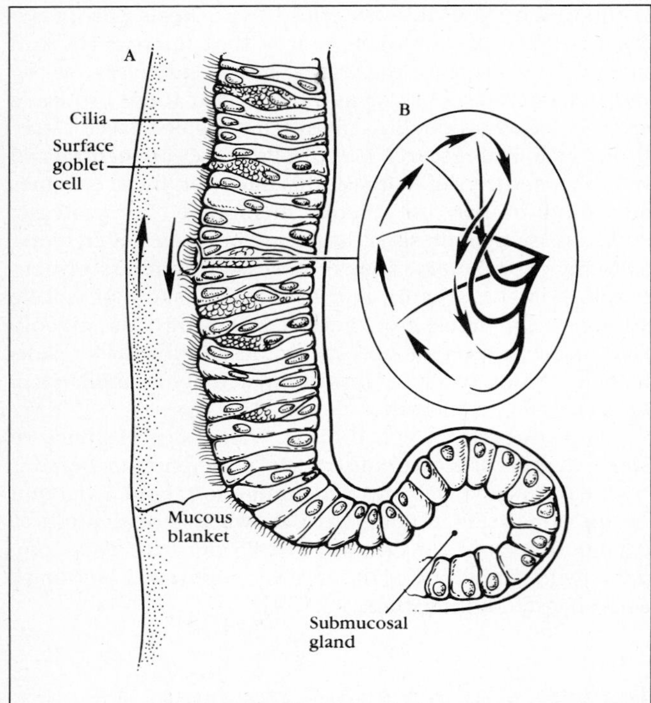

FIGURE 24-14 A. The mucociliary escalator. B. Conceptual scheme of ciliary movement, allowing forward motion to move viscous gel layer and backward motion to take place entirely within more fluid sol layer.

contains about 200 cilia. The cilia move in a continuous wave to carry mucus and debris up the airway to the larynx [16].

From an upright position, the cilia sweep forward about 30 to 35 degrees and then bend to make their recovery (Fig. 24-14B). Comroe [4] likened the movement to strokes of the oars of a boat:

> Each cilium makes a forceful, fast effector stroke forward, followed by a less forceful, slower stroke backward to get in position again. There is precise timing and coordination of the strokes of a row of cilia so that together they move as a wave.

Beating in sequential waves at 1000 cycles per minute, cilia move mucus up the airway. Because the beat is rapid, the mucous layer does not have time to recoil between beats.

A mucous blanket, made up primarily of the secretions of goblet cells that line the airways and mucus-secreting glands located in the larger ciliated bronchi, moves forward on the cilia. Cells in the alveoli may also contribute secretions to the mucous blanket. The rate of secretion of these cells is difficult to estimate because of resorption and expectoration of mucus. The mucous blanket consists of two layers, the *sol layer*, which surrounds the cilia, and the *gel*, or surface, *layer*.

The mucous layers retain a constant depth, and the rate of transport of mucus increases rapidly as mucus moves toward the trachea. Some mucus is resorbed in the large airways to maintain a constant depth, with little removed by evaporation, because inspired air is virtually 100 percent saturated with moisture by the time it reaches the pharynx. Mucociliary transport is known to be altered by depressed ciliary activity, changes in the property of mucus, and injury to the respiratory epithelium cells.

Mucus is produced primarily by the goblet or mucus-secreting cells that lie along the tracheobronchial tree. These cells produce an estimated 100 ml of mucus per day, continually humidifying and protecting the respiratory passages. The mucous covering of the epithelium in the respiratory passages is normally uninterrupted. Adhesive properties of mucus allow particles that bind particulates to adhere so that they can move out of the respiratory tract. Mucus is normally composed of water, electrolytes, and several types of mucopolysaccharides, which accounts for its viscosity.

Alveolar Clearance

Mucociliary transport, lymphatic drainage, blood flow, and phagocytosis all contribute to creating a sterile environment within the alveoli. Macrophage activity is the principal *alveolar* defense against particulates. These alveolar macrophages regularly scavenge the surface of the epithelium, digesting foreign material (represented schematically in Fig. 24-15).

Surface tension may play a part in removing particulates from the lungs. Particulates on the plane move from an area of low surface tension to an area of higher surface tension. Therefore, particulates may move from the environment of alveolar surfactant to the higher surface tension of the respiratory bronchioles and up the mucus escalator to the pharynx [15].

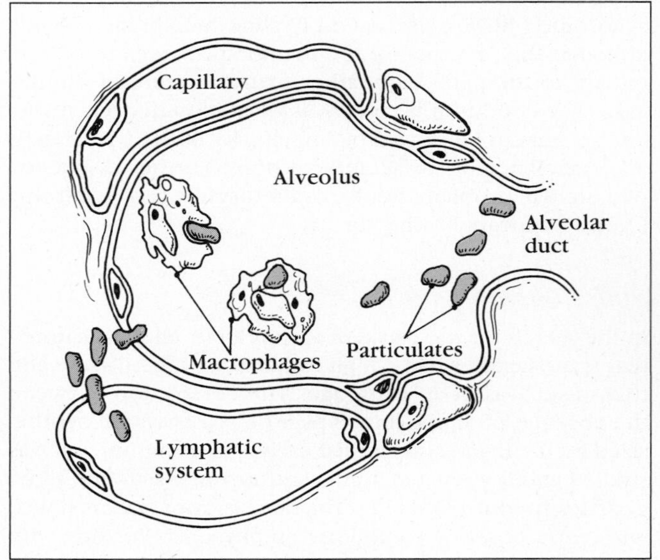

FIGURE 24-15 Alveolar clearance. Macrophage ingestion of particulate matter, particles traveling in the alveolar duct, lymphatic clearance of particulate matter, blood flow clearance, and carriage of particulates within the macrophages.

Some particulates are removed to perivascular, peribronchial, and hilar lymph nodes. The lymphatics probably transport the particulates engulfed in macrophages. It is not clear to what extent blood flow is responsible for alveolar clearance. Kilburn hypothesized that monocytes from the blood enter the air space at the alveolar-bronchial junction where they become lung macrophages, engulfing material left there by other mechanisms [10].

Some particulates remain in the lungs for protracted periods, while others stay for an intermediate period and are cleared. This seems to depend on a number of factors, such as deposition site, nature of the particulate, and host resistance. A small number of particulates remains in the lungs indefinitely. Those such as asbestos, silica, and carbon may stimulate fibroblast proliferation, and, over time, this can create severe restrictive pulmonary disease.

Deposition of Particulates in the Airways

Under normal conditions, an individual inspires 10,000 to 12,000 liters of air daily. Each liter of urban air may have several million particles suspended in it, the majority of which are deposited along the respiratory tract and are cleansed by the defenses of the lungs. Particles smaller than 0.5 μm in diameter usually remain suspended in inhaled air and are expelled from the lungs during expiration.

The first site of deposition of particulates in the airway is the nose (Fig. 24-16). Particulates larger than 10 μm in diameter are filtered out in the nares or trapped in the nasal mucosa. It is the inertia of large particles that determines deposition at these sites. Their large mass and high linear velocity force them to rain out in the nasal mucosa. Together with being filtered, the warming and moistening of air in the nose allows the defense mechanisms of the lower respiratory tract to function more effectively.

As the inhaled air flows over the tonsils and adenoids, particulates are deposited by impaction. These structures are ideally located in the airway to entrap debris that passes over them. In addition to mechanical defense, the tonsils and adenoids may function in the immunologic reaction. Farther along the respiratory tract, linear velocity of air decreases as the surface area increases, which allows particulates in the range of 2 to 10 μm to be deposited on the mucociliary blanket by sedimentation.

Particulates smaller than 2 μm reach the alveoli by gravitational forces and, to a lesser extent, by Brownian movement, which describes the random movement of molecules due to thermal energy. The particulates are removed primarily by mucociliary transport and phagocytosis. Smaller particles may present more of a threat to the lungs than larger ones because they penetrate more deeply and remain longer in the tissue.

Together with size, the aerodynamic properties of particulates and deposition sites must be considered. Asbestos particles, up to 300 μm have been shown to reach the lung periphery where, because of their aerodynamic properties rather than their size, they behave as particles of about 1 μm [18]. This explains why asbestos often severely damages the distal portions of the lungs.

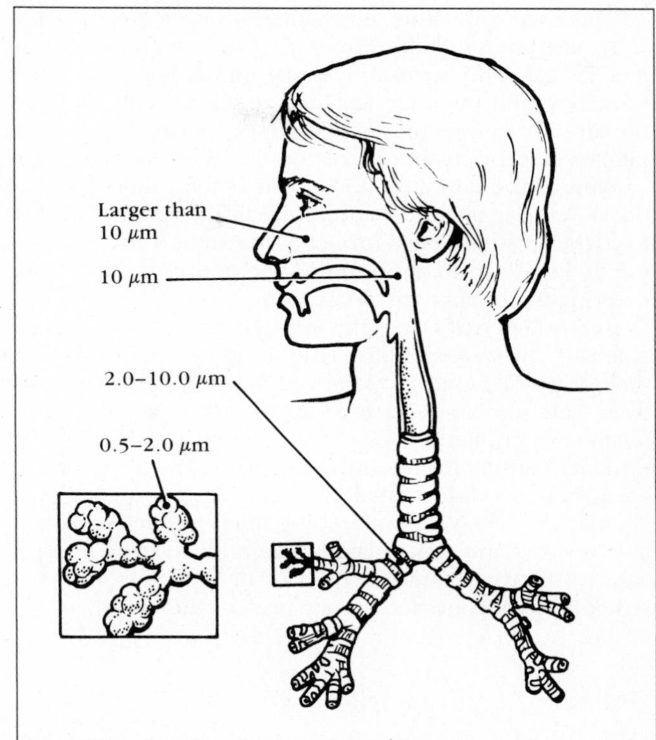

FIGURE 24-16 Deposition of particulates in the airways depends on their size.

Reflexes of the Airways

The respiratory tract is equipped with reflexes that rid it of debris and protect it from inhaled foreign substances. As is true of other mechanisms, hypoactivity or hyperactivity of these reflexes creates conditions that are detrimental to the host.

The *sneeze reflex* is one of the defenses against irritant materials. Particulates or irritants stimulate sensory receptors of the trigeminal nerves, resulting in the sneeze response. The sneeze is characterized by a deep inspiration followed by a violent expiratory blast through the nose.

The *cough reflex* is important in clearing the trachea and large bronchi of foreign matter. Irritants cause different impulses to be carried by the vagus nerve to the medulla. Conscious control can also initiate the cough mechanism. The cough reflex initiates a deep inspiration. The glottis then closes, the diaphragm relaxes, and the muscles contract against the closed glottis. Maximum intrathoracic and interairway pressures are produced that cause the trachea to narrow. When the glottis opens, the large pressure differential between the airways and the atmosphere coupled with tracheal narrowing create airflow through the trachea at velocities as high as 75 to 100 miles an hour [8]. This is very effective in propelling secretions toward the mouth. While the cough is more effective in clearing the major airways, it also may help clear the peripheral airways through a milking action created by the high intrathoracic pressures. This may deliver secretions from the peripheral airways to the main bronchi for expulsion by coughing.

Together with other mechanisms, reflex *bronchoconstriction* protects the upper and lower airways from mechanical and chemical irritants. Both cough and reflex bronchoconstriction are initiated in the subepithelium of the airways by receptors sensitive to irritants. For example, when the receptors are exposed to dust, the reflex narrowing of the airways, along with cough, increases the linear velocity of airflow and assists in the removal of dust from the airways. Reflex bronchoconstriction also protects the alveoli from harmful fumes and prevents gases from entering the pulmonary circulation.

Removal of gases from the inspired air depends on their solubility in water. Highly soluble gases, such as sulfur dioxide and acetone, are removed in the upper respiratory tract. Less soluble gases such as nitrous oxide and ozone reach the peripheral lungs. This accounts for the observation that sulfur dioxide inhalation results in bronchitis while nitrous oxide inhalation may lead to pulmonary edema. The protection offered by reflex bronchoconstriction is dose- and time-related, which means that if exposure to the toxic fumes is brief or of low concentration, reflex bronchoconstriction may protect the lungs.

Defenses Against Infection

Defense Against Microbial Agents

Invasion of the lungs by microbial agents presents special problems in defense. Microorganisms have the ability to replicate themselves, and conceivably, one organism could multiply and completely permeate lung tissue. The defenders against infectious agents must act quickly to kill the organisms before they have sufficient opportunity to multiply, which can be in minutes to hours.

Under normal circumstances, the alveolar macrophage system is the primary bactericidal mechanism for clearing infectious agents from the lungs [11]. The *alveolar macrophages* ingest bacteria at such a rapid rate that the majority are destroyed in situ. The rate of bacterial killing in the lungs exceeds the rate at which the bacteria are transported out of the lungs. This has been demonstrated by radioactive tracer-labeled bacteria. In 24 hours, 30 to 40 percent of the radioactivity is cleared, but nearly all bacteria are killed. This is known as *net bacterial lung clearance*. Three factors contribute to this process: (1) physical transport of bacteria out of the lung, (2) in situ bacterial killing, and (3) bacterial multiplication [9].

The rate of bactericidal activity by the macrophages is influenced by different bacterial strains. For example, *Staphylococcus aureus* is removed at a faster rate than *Proteus mirabilis*. Some organisms are readily inactivated by phagocytosis while others appear resistant to this process.

Conditions in the metabolic environment, such as hypoxia, acidosis, and high levels of cortisol, slow net bacterial lung clearance. Ethyl alcohol and tobacco smoke have been shown to depress clearance, but all organisms are not depressed equally. For example, alcohol completely suppresses the killing of *P. mirabilis* but not of *S. aureus* or *Staphylococcus albus* [9]. This selective action on the alveolar macrophages has important clinical ramifications. In chronic obstructive lung disease, mixed flora are constantly present in the respiratory tract, yet one predominant organism will be responsible for lung infection when it occurs.

Acute viral infections predispose the host to bacterial infections in the lungs. Viruses appear to interfere with alveolar macrophages and suppress their bactericidal ability. The greatest susceptibility appears between the sixth and tenth days after the acute viral infection, during which time superimposed bacterial pneumonias frequently develop.

The dynamics of different responses to bacteria, fluctuations in host resistance, and environmental changes may permit one or another organism to multiply at any given time [1]. All of these factors influence the fate of the microorganism, whether it remains in a localized area or is disseminated throughout the body.

Immunologic Defense

Closely associated with the macrophage system is the *immunologic defense of the lungs*. The cells involved in the specific immune response were described in Chapter 10. These include the T lymphocytes (thymic-dependent) and B lymphocytes (bone marrow-derived), which, in a complex, interacting pattern, provide immunity and defend the body against foreign invasion.

Specialized B lymphocytes become immunoglobulin-secreting plasma cells that assist macrophages in inactivating infectious material. This action is called the *humoral response* and involves five classes of immunoglobulins: IgG, IgM, IgA, IgD, and IgE. The first three classes are important in the control of infectious diseases. Both IgM and IgG provide the primary and secondary antibody responses against pathogens by facilitating opsonization and phagocytosis of bacteria.

Two types of IgA have been identified, *secretory* and *serum*. Secretory IgA is the major immunoglobulin on the surfaces of the mucous membranes. On the respiratory mucosa, IgA protects the lungs against viral and bacterial invasion. It may inhibit the ability of the organisms to adhere to the mucosal surfaces. Persons with chronic bronchitis often have low levels of IgA, which apparently results in a high frequency of recurrent pulmonary infections [20].

The T lymphocytes provide for cell-mediated immunity. They play a major role in attracting macrophages to the site of an infection. Tuberculosis is an excellent prototype for understanding this response. Inhaled tuberculosis bacilli travel from the lungs to the lymph nodes, where the macrophages engulf, process, and concentrate the antigens of the bacilli. A few T lymphocytes bearing receptors for tuberculin antigens react with the bacillus and undergo multiplication. These T cells circulate back to the lungs and release chemical mediators that induce macrophages and other leukocytes to kill the bacteria.

Humoral and cell-mediated immunity function together to protect the body from infection. Both are essential for maximum defense.

Interferon

Interferon is a protein that inhibits viral replication. It appears to be produced and regulated within the cells. Cells react to viruses by producing interferon, which causes unaffected surrounding cells to synthesize another protein that protects the cells by preventing viral replication. All cells seem to produce interferon when exposed to a virus, but viruses differ in their ability to act as interferon inducers. It is thought that lymphocytes assist the host to counteract viruses, and these lymphocytes have the ability to produce interferon. Because of this it has been suggested that interferon may be the mediator of the cellular immune response with certain viruses [1].

Interferon may also be important in protecting the organism against bacteria and tumors. It has been used experimentally in the treatment of cancer and in viral infections in immunosuppressed individuals.

Normal Gas Exchange

Oxygen makes up about 21 percent of the atmospheric air and most of the remaining 79 percent is nitrogen. Carbon dioxide in the atmosphere is only a minute percentage (approximately 0.02%), and miniscule amounts of other trace gases, such as argon, neon, and helium, are present.

Oxygen Transport to the Tissues

The oxygen tension, or partial pressure of oxygen at sea level, is equal to the barometric pressure of 760 mm Hg multiplied by the fraction of oxygen in dry air (20.93%), which equals 159 mm Hg. As the inspired air is warmed and humidified in the upper airways, however, it is diluted by water vapor, and this causes the oxygen tension to fall to 149.3 mm Hg [6]. The inspired air is then further diluted by carbon dioxide in the lower airways and alveoli. Factors that lower inspired oxygen concentration or that raise alveolar carbon dioxide levels also lower alveolar oxygen levels and hence lower arterial blood oxygen tension, which may reduce the delivery of oxygen to the tissues. Table 24-1 displays the blood gas pattern seen when normal arterial blood is drawn for analysis.

Oxygen is delivered by a linked chain of transfers from the atmosphere to the alveoli to the blood and then to the tissues and cells of the body. It diffuses from areas of higher partial pressure to areas of lower pressure. It is transported initially from the air of the atmosphere to the larger airways by movements of the diaphragm and chest wall that cyclically lower the intrathoracic pressure. This results in air moving in and out of the lungs (*ventilation*) and then being delivered by the smaller peripheral airways to the alveoli (*distribution*). Air then crosses the alveolar-capillary membrane (*diffusion*) and is carried in the plasma, bound chemically to hemoglobin. During *perfusion*, blood is delivered through the pulmonary capillary system past the alveoli for the purpose of gas exchange. At the capillary level it diffuses into the tissue fluid surrounding the cells and then to the cells themselves, where it is

TABLE 24-1 Arterial Blood Gas Values

Substance	Values
Oxygen	
Tension	75–100 mm Hg breathing room air
Saturation	96–100% of capacity
Carbon dioxide	
Tension	35–45 mm Hg
Arterial pH	7.35–7.45
Bicarbonate	22–26 mEq/L
H_2CO_3	1.05–1.35 mEq/L (always 3% of PCO_2)

metabolized. Oxygen is essential for cellular metabolism and the cells have no capability to store it. Without constant delivery of oxygen, tissue hypoxia and anaerobic metabolism result. *Tissue hypoxia* is defined as inadequate critical oxygen tension to meet the needs of the cell. *Critical oxygen tension* is that cellular oxygen tension which causes mitochondrial dysfunction [21].

Tissue hypoxia is not synonymous with *arterial hypoxemia*, which refers to decreased oxygen tension in the arterial blood. Tissue hypoxia and arterial hypoxemia may exist simultaneously or independently of each other. Arterial hypoxemia can be measured by measuring arterial blood gas. Tissue hypoxia cannot be directly measured but is assessed on the basis of clinical signs and symptoms.

The relationship between arterial and tissue oxygenation is explained in large part by the relationship between hemoglobin and oxygen. Oxygen and carbon dioxide diffuse across a membrane along a gradient from higher pressure to lower pressure. Most of the oxygen is transported to the body cells in chemical combination with hemoglobin. *Hemoglobin* is a complex spheric molecule that is made up of four heme groups, each of which is enfolded in a chain of amino acids. Each heme group can combine with an oxygen molecule, which gives hemoglobin the capability of carrying four oxygen molecules per hemoglobin molecule. Hemoglobin combined with oxygen is called *oxyhemoglobin* (HbO_2) while oxygen-free hemoglobin is called *reduced hemoglobin* (Hb) (see Chap. 15).

In the adult, normal hemoglobin levels range from 12 to 16 gm per dl of blood. It has been found that 1 gm of hemoglobin fully saturated can carry 1.34 ml of oxygen. Each milliliter of blood with an oxygen tension of 100 mm Hg can carry about 0.03 ml of dissolved oxygen. This means that 100 ml of blood with a hemoglobin of 15 gm and 100 percent saturation has an oxygen content of about 20.4 ml of oxygen, which is expressed as *volumes percent*. A very small percentage of oxygen is carried dissolved in the plasma, but hemoglobin is by far the most important method of oxygen transport in the blood.

Oxyhemoglobin Dissociation Curve

The affinity of hemoglobin for oxygen has been plotted on an oxyhemoglobin dissociation curve (Fig. 24-17). It is

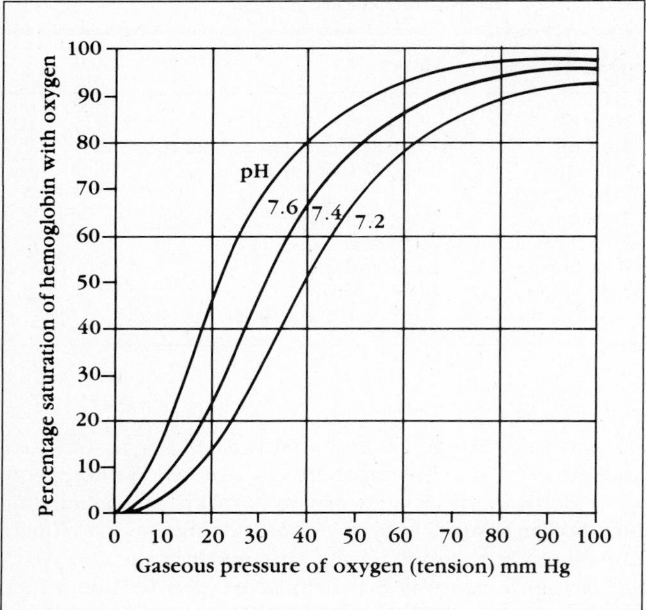

FIGURE 24-17 The oxyhemoglobin dissociation curve.

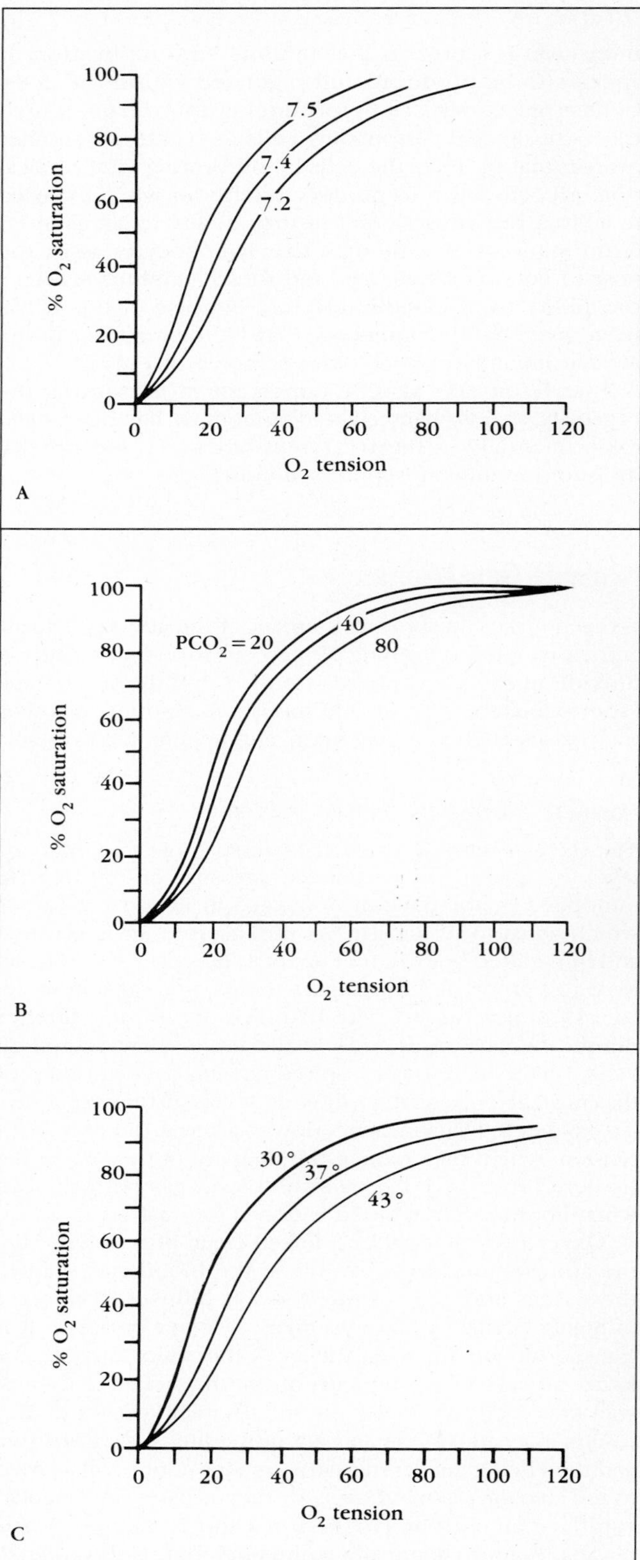

FIGURE 24-18 Effects of (A) pH, (B) PCO_2, and (C) temperature on oxyhemoglobin dissociation curve.

derived by plotting oxyhemoglobin saturation (the percentage of hemoglobin that has combined with oxygen) against the oxygen tension (mm Hg) to which it is exposed. Because oxyhemoglobin dissociation is readily reversible, the curve reflects the ease with which hemoglobin gives up oxygen as well as the ease with which it takes up oxygen. This is important, because, to a large extent, oxygen delivery to the tissues depends on the ease with which hemoglobin gives up its oxygen once it reaches the tissues.

In studying the oxyhemoglobin dissociation curve, it is readily apparent that it is initially very steep and then flattens. The upper portion of the curve is flat, showing that when the oxygen tension (PO_2) is 70 mm Hg or above, hemoglobin becomes nearly fully saturated. When the available oxygen begins to fall below 60 mm Hg, the degree of saturation also falls rapidly. Note in Figure 24-18 that when the PO_2 falls to 40 mm Hg, the saturation of hemoglobin is 75 percent, or approximately the level of venous blood. At 20 mm Hg PO_2 the saturation is 35 percent, which will not sustain life.

Many factors alter the affinity of hemoglobin for oxygen. Some of these are summarized in Figure 24-18. An increase in hemoglobin affinity for oxygen makes the curve shift to the left and oxygen is given up less readily. Alkalemia, hypothermia, and hypocarbia are among factors that can cause a leftward shift. Conversely, acidemia, hypercarbia, and hyperthermia reduce the affinity of hemoglobin for oxygen and cause, by inference, increased oxygen availability to the tissues. Noted on the curve is the ***shift to the right***. Figures 24-18B and C show the effects of pH and body temperature on the affinity of hemoglobin for oxygen.

TABLE 24-2 Factors That Affect Tissue Oxygenation

Oxygen tension arterial blood
Hemoglobin content
Hemoglobin saturation
Blood flow to tissues
Diffusion of oxygen to tissues
Diffusion of carbon dioxide

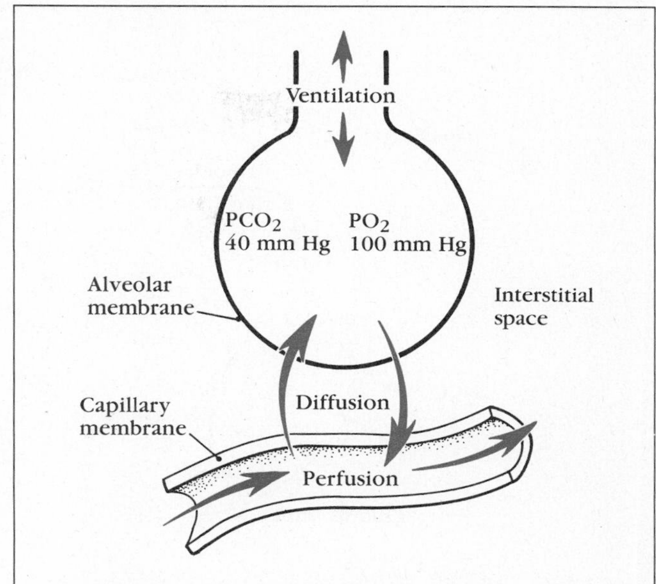

FIGURE 24-19 Movement of gases across the alveolocapillary membrane due to ventilation, diffusion, and perfusion.

Other factors that affect tissue oxygenation are summarized in Table 24-2. Oxygen content of arterial blood is determined by a combination of alveolar oxygenation, hemoglobin level and quality, and hemoglobin affinity for oxygen. Oxygen delivery to the tissues depends on the status of the cardiovascular system and regional perfusion. At the tissue level, oxygenation depends on vascularity, diffusion characteristics, and intracellular mechanisms.

Carbon Dioxide Transport

Carbon dioxide is the product of metabolic combustion and travels the pathway opposite to oxygen's along pressure gradients from tissues to blood to alveoli to airways and then out to the atmosphere. Total amounts of oxygen consumed and carbon dioxide produced are *not* determined by the quantity of ventilation, but rather by the actual *metabolic demands* of the cells. The body at rest requires about 250 cc of oxygen per minute and produces about 200 cc of carbon dioxide per minute as a result of its continuing metabolic cellular requirements. Heavy exercise may increase the production of carbon dioxide up to 20 times this volume.

The normal match between ventilation and perfusion serves the ultimate purpose of supplying oxygen and eliminating carbon dioxide from the cells and eventually from the body. Alveolar ventilation is about 4 liters of air per minute. Cardiac output and resulting tissue perfusion is about 5 liters of blood per minute.

Because carbon dioxide diffuses about 20 times as easily as oxygen, tissue carbon dioxide diffuses rapidly into the venous end of the capillaries with a gradient of less than 1 mm Hg. Venous blood entering the lungs with a PCO_2 of 46 mm Hg readily transfers carbon dioxide into the alveoli (Fig. 24-19). With normal alveolar ventilation, alveolar carbon dioxide ($PaCO_2$) of 40 mm Hg is in equilibrium with the resulting arterial carbon dioxide ($PaCO_2$) of 40 mm Hg. The levels of both alveolar and arterial carbon dioxide are directly and inversely proportional to the volume of alveolar ventilation (Va). Thus, in alveolar hypoventilation, halving the alveolar ventilation from 4 to 2 liters per minute doubles the $PaCO_2$ from 40 to 80 mm Hg. In hyperventilation, doubling the alveolar ventilation from 4 to 8 liters a minute halves the $PaCO_2$ to 20 mm Hg [7,8].

Blood carries carbon dioxide in three different forms: (1) 5 percent or less is transported to the lungs in the *plasma* as *dissolved carbon dioxide*; (2) nearly 70 percent diffuses into the red blood cells and is carried in the form of *bicarbonate*; and (3) approximately 25 percent is carried in the red blood cells bound to hemoglobin.

Figure 24-20 illustrates the reaction of carbon dioxide as it is carried dissolved in the red blood cells. It is important to note that this is a reversible reaction that occurs rapidly at the tissue level where carbon dioxide is picked up and in the lungs where it is released. Most carbon dioxide diffuses into the red blood cells where it is catalyzed in a reaction with carbonic anhydrase and water to form carbonic acid. This carbonic acid immediately dissociates into hydrogen ions (H^+) and bicarbonate ions (HCO_3^-) that can diffuse back into the plasma or may stay in combination with a positive ion in the red blood cells. The excess hydrogen ion formed in this reaction usually binds with the hemoglobin molecule to form hydrogen hemoglobin (HHb). If significant amounts of (HCO_3^-) diffuse into the plasma, a negative ion is drawn into the red blood cells to equalize the electrochemical gradient. This ion is usually chloride and the mechanism of its movement is called the *chloride shift* [8]. This process can provide bicarbonate to the plasma when the pH is decreased. Normally, in the lungs a reverse process occurs very rapidly. Hydrogen is released from hemoglobin and recombines with bicarbonate to form carbonic acid, which dissociates into carbon dioxide and water. Carbon dioxide diffuses out of the red blood cells into the alveoli and is blown off in the exhaled air.

Carbon dioxide may react directly with hemoglobin and be carried in a loose chemical bond on the hemoglobin molecule. This is referred to as *carbaminohemoglobin*

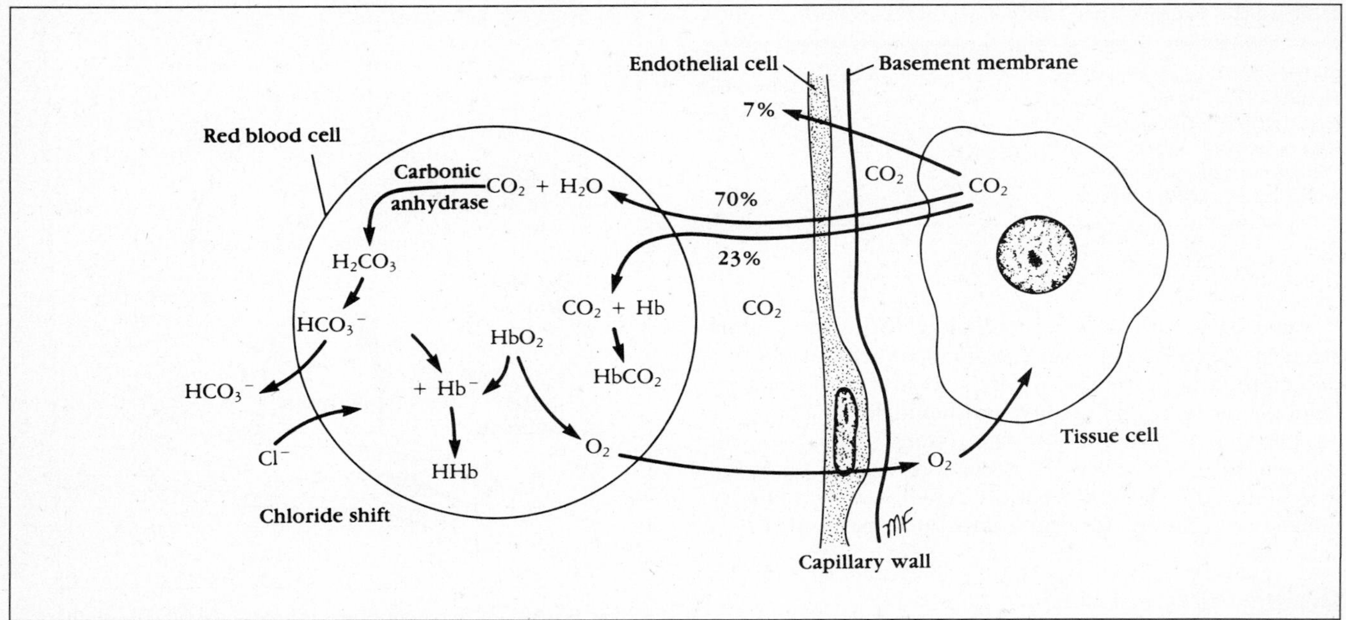

FIGURE 24-20 Methods of carbon dioxide transport in the red blood cell (RBC). Seventy percent of CO_2 is combined with H_2O to form carbonic acid and bicarbonate, 23 percent is carried in combination with Hb, and 7 percent is carried in the plasma. (From R.S. Snell, *Clinical Histology for Medical Students*. Boston: Little, Brown, 1984.)

and accounts for about 25 percent of the carriage of carbon dioxide to the lungs. In the pulmonary capillary bed, carbon dioxide is simply released to the alveoli and blown off in exhaled air.

Ventilation-Perfusion Relationships

Arterial oxygenation is affected not only by ventilation but by the *blood supply to the lungs*. Abnormalities in pulmonary blood flow (perfusion) or in relationships between ventilation and perfusion ($\dot{V}a/\dot{Q}$ ratio) alter arterial oxygen tension and subsequently, oxygenation of body tissues.

Oxygen and carbon dioxide are exchanged as blood circulates through the pulmonary capillary bed. The capillaries are arranged so that each is adjacent to an alveolus. The capillaries are very small, approximating the size of a red blood cell. The capillary wall and alveolar wall are each only one cell thick, so that the diffusing membrane is very thin. Gases, therefore, diffuse across the membrane with little difficulty (Fig. 24-21).

Each red blood cell (RBC) stays in the pulmonary capillary bed about 1 second and exchanges gases with two or three alveoli during this time. Approximately 70 ml of blood is normally exchanging gases at a given moment in the pulmonary capillary bed of an adult, in contrast to the large volume of air that is moved by the alveoli with each breath. This is an important, if temporary, safeguard against oxygen lack. Storing oxygen, even for a few moments, guards against the extra oxygen needs encountered during breath holding [22].

In addition to moving blood to the blood-gas barrier for gas exchange, the pulmonary circulation also provides a reservoir for blood, filters small thrombi from the blood, and traps white blood cells.

Generally, the pulmonary circulation is a low-pressure system with pressures much lower than the systemic circulation. The normal mean pulmonary artery pressure (PAP) is 14 mm Hg. As the mean left atrial pressure of the heart is about 5 mm Hg, the driving pressure across the pulmonary bed is only about 9 mm Hg. Pressure in the pulmonary artery or in the pulmonary capillary bed may be increased by pathology, but an increase in one does not necessarily mean a corresponding increase in the other. The pulmonary and systemic circulations are compared in Table 24-3. Table 24-4 gives the normal pressures in the heart and the pulmonary circulation.

Both acidemia and hypoxemia can stimulate constriction of the pulmonary arteries and thus increase resistance in the pulmonary capillary bed. Either of these conditions causes vasoconstriction alone, and together they provide a synergistic effect. Once this vasoconstriction occurs and persists for some time, it may cause an adverse effect on the right ventricle because of increased work needed to pump blood into the constricted pulmonary vasculature. Over a period of time this may lead to right ventricular hypertrophy (RVH) and subsequent right ventricular failure.

Approximately 10 to 20 percent of the total blood volume is present in the pulmonary vascular bed at any given time. The bed is capable of accepting several times this amount, which allows it to accommodate variations in cardiac output or blood volume. The distensibility of the bed is accomplished both by dilating pulmonary vessels and by opening closed or unused vessels. Distention of the pulmonary vascular bed reduces pulmonary vascular resistance until its capacity is reached. Then as increases in

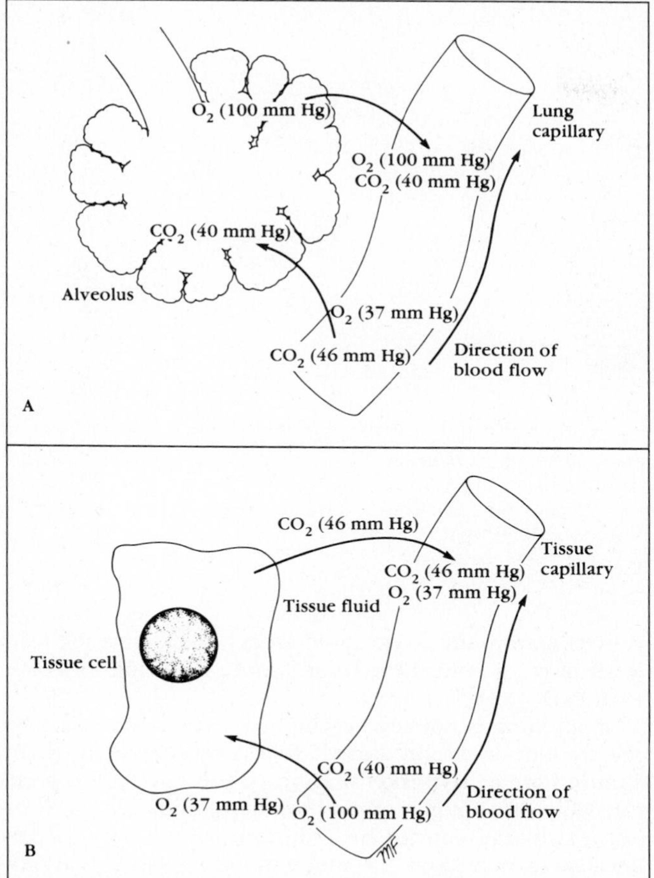

FIGURE 24-21 A. Representation of gas exchange at alveolus. B. Representation of gas exchange at tissue level. (From R.S. Snell, *Clinical Histology for Medical Students*. Boston: Little, Brown, 1984.)

TABLE 24-3 Differences Between Pulmonary and Systemic Circulations

Pulmonary	Systemic
Pressures low 25/8 mm Hg (mean: 14).	Aortic pressure about 100 mm Hg.
Walls very thin with little smooth muscle.	Artery walls thick-walled with much smooth muscle.
System rarely concerned with directing blood between regions (except in case of localized alveolar hypoxia); keeps work of right heart low.	Regulates and distributes blood supply throughout body.
Pressure changes within lungs, symmetric and of low magnitude.	Asymmetric pressure changes of great magnitude throughout body.
Capillaries surrounded by gas have little support; therefore, collapse or distend depending on pressure within and around them.	Surrounded by tissue; less easily changes caliber.
Pressure may be determined by arteriolar/alveolar gradient or arteriolar/venous gradient.	Pressure determined by arteriolar/venous gradient.
Pulmonary vascular resistance is 1/10 that of systemic circulation; able to reduce resistance as pressure in system rises.	Resistance 10 times that of pulmonary circulation; less able to lower resistance when needed.

TABLE 24-4 Approximate Normal Pressures in the Heart and Pulmonary Circuit

Location	Pressure (mm Hg)
Superior vena cava	6–10
Inferior vena cava	6–10
Right atrium	2–5
Right ventricle	25/0–5
Pulmonary artery	25/10
Pulmonary capillary bed	8–12
Left atrium	5–10
Left ventricle	120/0–10
Aorta	120/80
Systemic arteriole	30

blood flow cannot be accommodated, pulmonary vascular resistance increases.

Perfusion changes more rapidly from the top to the bottom of the upright lungs than does ventilation. Therefore, the ventilation-perfusion ratio decreases down the lungs (Fig. 24-22). If the individual is in the upright position, pulmonary blood flow increases linearly from top to bottom due to gravitational forces [15]. At the apex, the pulmonary arterial pressure is just sufficient to raise minimal amounts of blood to the top of the lungs and perfuse the apices. Capillary pressure is very low. If blood volume is reduced for some reason, such as systemic loss or pulmonary capillary destruction, apical perfusion may decrease or cease altogether [22].

Blood flow to the lungs changes with exercise and position. With exercise, all areas of the lung receive increased blood flow. When a person lies down, flow from apices to bases becomes uniform.

The concept of regional differences in ventilation has important ramifications for the person with asymmetric lung pathology. An example might be the person whose left lung appears radiographically to be *whited out* by a process such as pneumonia. To maximize ventilation, perfusion, and gas exchange, the person should not be positioned on the left side. Instead, the person should be turned onto his or her right side or back to capitalize on the abilities of the unaffected lung. Arterial blood gas values can be significantly affected with this type of positioning.

As previously mentioned, the perfusion gradient down the lungs exceeds the ventilation gradient. To state a $\dot{V}_A/\dot{Q}$ ratio, ventilation and perfusion must be expressed in the same units. For example, blood flow of 4 liters per minute and ventilation of 5 liters per minute in the average adult

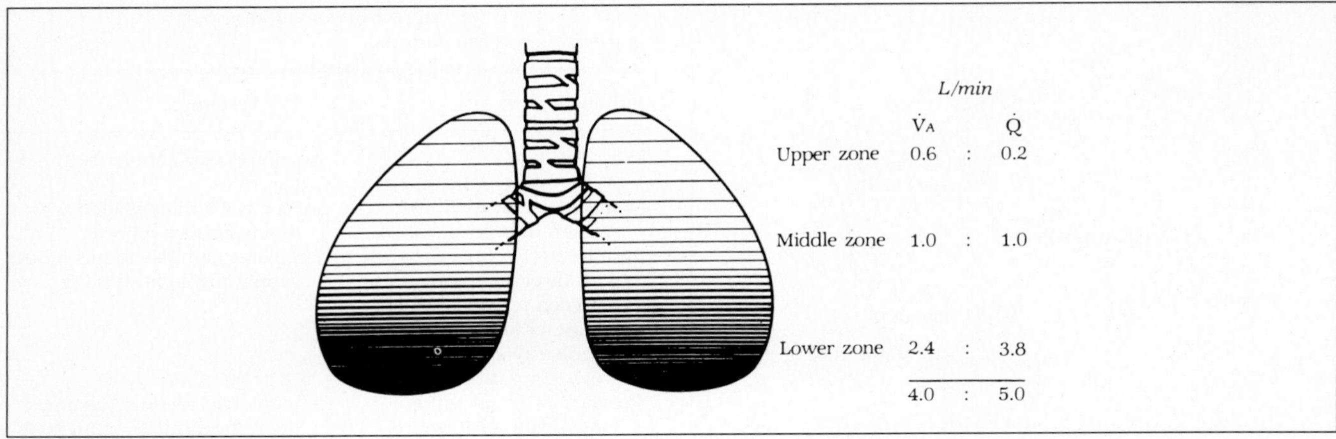

FIGURE 24-22 $\dot{V}/\dot{Q}$ in different zones of the upright lung showing marked variation in values in different areas. In the upright individual upper segments are relatively hypoperfused and $\dot{V}/\dot{Q}$ is high. Lower segments are relatively hypoventilated; $\dot{V}/\dot{Q}$ is low. (From H.A. Braun, F.W. Cheney, and C.P. Loehnen, *Introduction to Respiratory Physiology* [2nd ed.]. Boston: Little, Brown, 1980).

male results in $\dot{V}a/\dot{Q}$ ratio of about 0.8 : 1.0 or 0.8. In the healthy person, the deviation from a ratio of 1 is largely due to anatomic dead space. Normally, a portion of the air inspired does not come in contact with the alveoli and does not participate in gas exchange. This *anatomic dead space* usually remains relatively constant, but *alveolar dead space* (where alveolar gas does not participate in blood-gas exchange) may be significantly altered in pathologic states. The $\dot{V}a/\dot{Q}$ ratio is altered in conditions in which alveolar *dead space ventilation* and thus physiologic dead space ventilation are increased. A higher than normal amount of inspired gas is wasted, with the result that a lower than normal amount of inspired gas is exchanged with the blood. To compensate for this wasted ventilation and to maintain normal PaO_2 and $PaCO_2$, total ventilation must increase. This moves more inspired gas per minute to improve exchange with blood. If the body is incapable of increasing ventilation and blood flow enough to maintain adequate gas exchange, carbon dioxide retention and hypoxemia may result. In any case, the work of breathing is increased. If the body is incapable of altering ventilation and blood flow to meet this need, altered blood gases, decreased cellular oxygenation, and clinical symptoms occur.

The opposite of dead space ventilation is *shunting*. All cardiopulmonary and pulmonary disease leads to problems with dead space ventilation or shunting, or both. Shunting refers to an area that is perfused but not ventilated (Fig. 24-23). A small amount of shunting (less than 2.5% of cardiac output) is normal; it occurs because not all blood is exchanged at the alveolocapillary line. This accounts for the fact that normal oxygen saturation of hemoglobin in arterial blood gases is 96 to 100 percent. Pathologic amounts of shunting may be caused by such problems of nonventilation as atelectasis and pneumonia (see Chap. 25).

In shunting, the $\dot{V}a/\dot{Q}$ is decreased. Blood returning from the affected areas of the lung mixes with blood returning from the oxygenated areas. This lowers the total level of oxygen in the arterial blood, resulting in a lowered PaO_2 [13].

If shunting is not severe, the body can compensate for the amount of carbon dioxide that is not excreted by the shunted areas. Hyperventilation of the unaffected areas can blow off enough carbon dioxide to compensate. Oxygen exchange cannot be compensated for so readily because carbon dioxide is much more diffusible than oxygen. If compensation occurs, it leads to a blood gas pattern of normal $PaCO_2$ with hypoxemia. If the body is unable to compensate adequately for the carbon dioxide exchange, blood gases show acidemia, hypoxemia, and hypercapnia. A compromised pulmonary or cardiovascular system could lead to loss of ability to compensate for the demands of shunting or other abnormalities.

Both shunt and dead space defects are often referred to as $\dot{V}a/\dot{Q}$ mismatching. All other factors being equal, the lung with a $\dot{V}a/\dot{Q}$ mismatch is not able to exchange as much oxygen and carbon dioxide as the lung with a normal $\dot{V}a/\dot{Q}$ ratio.

Respiratory Regulation of Acid-Base Equilibrium

As was described in Chapter 6, the major blood buffers are hemoglobin, the plasma proteins, and the carbonic acid-bicarbonate system. Any increase in carbon dioxide concentration in the blood causes a shift in its pH toward the acidic side and any decrease causes it to shift toward the alkaline side. Therefore, the amount of carbon dioxide present in the blood affects the pH significantly. Carbon dioxide, usually in the form of carbonic acid (H_2CO_3), is closely regulated by the physiologic buffer system of the lungs.

If the metabolic rate increases, the rate of carbon dioxide formation increases and, conversely, if the rate of

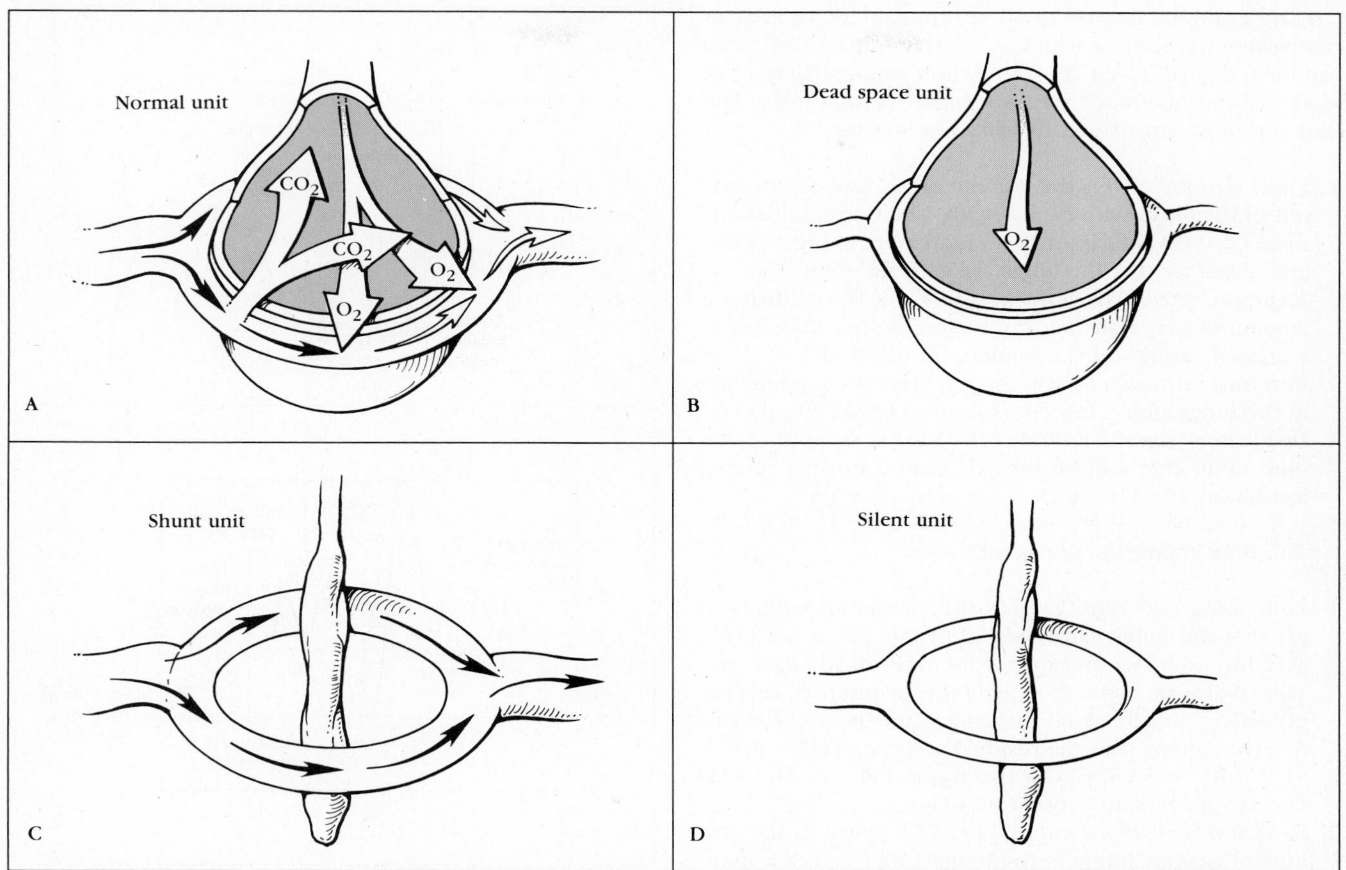

FIGURE 24-23 A. Schematic representation of normal alveolar-capillary unit. B. Representation of ventilation without perfusion. C. Representation of perfusion without ventilation. D. Representation of neither perfusion nor ventilation.

metabolism decreases, the formation of carbon dioxide also decreases. Alveolar ventilation changes according to nervous control of respiration through the *chemoreceptors* in the medulla. These chemoreceptors are extremely sensitive to minute changes in carbon dioxide level and stimulate an increase or decrease in the respiratory rate. If the blood pH declines to 7.0, alveolar ventilation may increase up to 5 times above the resting value. An increase in pH to above 7.4 may decrease alveolar ventilation to one-half the normal value. Thus, the respiratory rate and depth of respiration physiologically can retain or blow off excess carbon dioxide according to the pH of blood.

The two major alterations in acid-base balance related to pulmonary function are *respiratory acidosis* and *alkalosis*. Respiratory acidosis is always due to some factor that compromises ventilation. Thus, hypoventilation leads to retained carbon dioxide and causes an excess of carbonic acid in the blood. The excess carbon dioxide or hydrogen ion is a powerful stimulus for the central chemoreceptor in the medulla oblongata, which initiates a response increasing respiratory rate and depth.

Respiratory alkalosis results from hyperventilation, which blows off carbon dioxide, leading to decreased carbonic acid and a shift of the pH to alkaline.

Pulmonary Function Testing

Pulmonary function tests (PFT) measure many variables, including lung volume. They are important tools in the diagnosis and evaluation of pulmonary status. Spirometric tests have the limitations of recognizing abnormalities only when they are relatively diffuse. Therefore, results of these studies may be normal in early disease states or in localized rather than diffuse conditions. When results of a PFT are abnormal, other clinical data must be collected prior to making an accurate diagnosis [2]. The effectiveness of spirometry also is totally dependent on the ability and cooperation of the person being tested. Pulmonary function study results are evaluated in relation to predicted normals. Tables of norms based on age, sex, and size are used to predict normal values for each person. The tables are not totally reliable because of individual differences among persons.

Pulmonary function tests provide a yardstick in establishing the amount of disability in the course of pulmonary disease. They are used in many settings to diagnose and manage patients with pulmonary or cardiac disability and in epidemiologic surveys for industrial hazards or community disease risks.

Lung contents can be divided into four capacities or compartments, each of which is made up of two or more volumes. Figure 24-24 illustrates how the spirometer is used and the "average" values for the various tests. The *lung volumes* usually are measured as follows:

1. *Tidal volume (Vt)* is the volume of gas moved into and out of the lungs with each breath. The normal tidal volume (± 500 ml) is only a small percentage of the amount of air that the lungs are capable of moving.
2. *Expiratory reserve volume (ERV)* is the additional amount of gas or air that can be forcefully exhaled after a normal expiration is complete (± 1200 ml).
3. *Residual volume (RV)* is the amount of air remaining in the lungs after a forced expiration (± 1200 ml).
4. *Inspiratory reserve volume (IRV)* is the maximum volume of air that can be inhaled after a normal resting inspiration (± 3100 ml).

The *lung capacities* are as follows:

1. *Total lung capacity (TLC)* is the maximum volume of gas that the lungs can hold. All of this gas is not available for exchange because it includes dead space gas. The total lung capacity equals the inspiratory reserve volume plus the tidal volume plus the expiratory reserve volume plus the residual volume (TLC = IRV + Vt + ERV + RV). Given the figures above, the TLC equals approximately 6000 ml of air.
2. *Functional residual capacity (FRC)* refers to the volume of gas remaining in the lungs at the end of a spontaneous expiration, and includes the expiratory reserve volume and the residual volume (FRC = ERV + RV). The functional residual capacity decreases in conditions such as obesity that affect the chest wall mass. With an increased FRC it would take more change in the ventilatory rate or more time to reduce a given high carbon dioxide level than with a normal FRC. The FRC equals approximately 2400 ml of air.
3. *Vital capacity (VC)* can be measured either as expiratory or inspiratory. *Expiratory* vital capacity is the maximum volume of gas that can be exhaled after the deepest possible inspiration. Usually expiratory VC equals *inspiratory VC*, which is the maximum amount of gas that can be inhaled after the fullest possible expiration. *Total vital capacity* therefore equals inspiratory reserve volume plus tidal volume plus expiratory reserve volume (VC = IRV + Vt + ERV). It equals about 5000 cc in men. In severe obstructive pulmonary disease, the inspiratory vital capacity may be much greater than the expiratory. The VC increases with height, usually is greater in men, and is roughly proportional to lean body weight in young adults. It decreases slightly in the supine position due to the splinting of posterior rib movement and reduced diaphragmatic action. On quiet breathing, the lungs are roughly one-third inflated in the supine position and one-half inflated in the upright position.
4. *Inspiratory capacity (IC)* is the maximum volume of air that can be inhaled from a resting position. It equals the tidal volume plus the inspiratory reserve volume (IC = Vt + IRV). A reference value for IC is approximately 3600 ml of air.

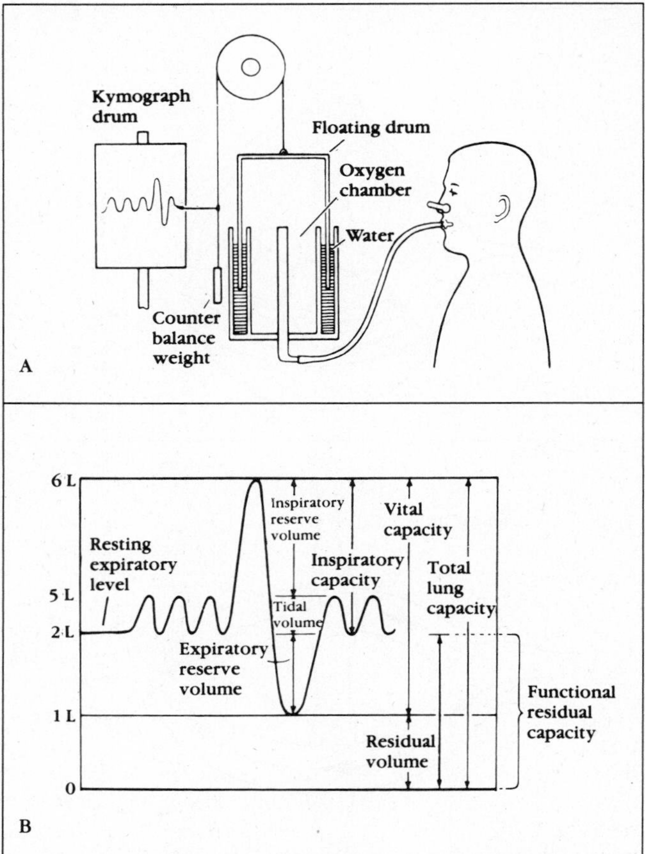

FIGURE 24-24 A. Structure of the spirometer used for direct measurement of lung volumes. B. Components of lung volume. (From E.E. Selkurt, *Basic Physiology for the Health Sciences* [2nd ed.]. Boston: Little, Brown, 1982.)

The residual volume, total lung capacity, vital capacity, and functional residual capacity are not anatomically fixed, but depend on elastic characteristics and muscle forces. Increased age changes all lung volumes and capacities by decreasing the elastic recoil. The resting position (at the end of quiet expiration) shifts in the direction of inspiration, so with age the residual volume and functional residual capacity increase slightly and the vital capacity decreases. This decrease is partially due to stiffening of the thoracic cage and decreased chest mobility.

Besides lung volumes, the *forced expiratory vital capacity* (FVC) can yield much information in persons with chronic obstructive disease. As shown in Figure 24-25A, the amount of air that can be forced out of the lungs on expiration is measured first at 1 second and then the time it takes to complete the expiratory effort. The one-second measurement is called the forced expiratory volume in one second (FEV_1). The shape of the curve is important in indicating abnormalities. Generally, in

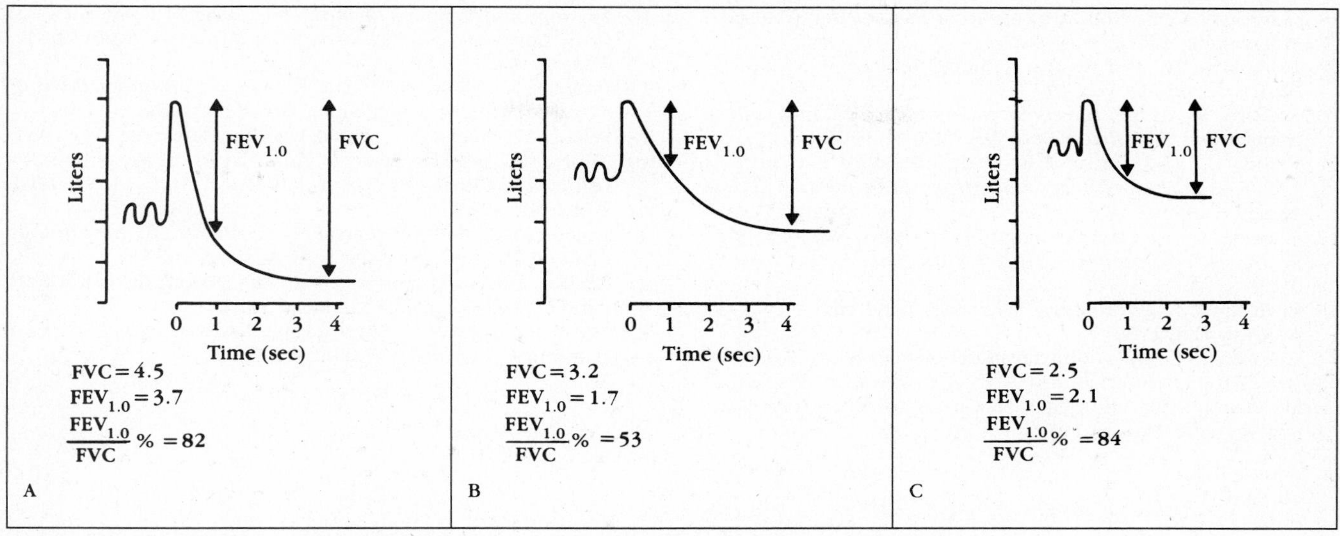

FIGURE 24-25 Patterns of forced expiration. A. Normal B. Obstructive. C. Restrictive. (From H.A. Braun, F.W. Cheney, Jr., and C.P. Loehnen, *Introduction to Respiratory Physiology* [2nd ed.]. Boston: Little, Brown, 1980).

obstructive disease, expiration takes much longer than normal and is less complete because of premature airway closure and subsequent air trapping (Fig. 24-25B). In restrictive disease, the shape of the curve may be normal but compressed due to the smaller chest volume without changes in the actual airflow (Fig. 24-25C). The volume obtained by the FEV_1 is placed over the FVC to get a ratio or percentage. Normally, the FEV_1/FVC is 80 percent, which means that 80 percent of the total volume can be expired in the first second. Generally, in restrictive lung disease, both FVC and FEV_1 are reduced. In contrast, obstructive disease tends to reduce the FEV_1 much more than the FVC (Fig. 24-25B). Mixed restrictive and obstructive patterns are not uncommon, and the FEV_1 may also be affected by changes in airway resistance, elastic recoil, and in lung compliance [15].

Alveolar ventilation, or the amount of gas actually reaching the exchange area, refers to the tidal volume minus the dead space. This is calculated as follows:

$$\dot{V}a = (Vt - Vd) \times f,$$

where *V̇a* is alveolar ventilation in 1 minute; the dot indicates that it is a timed measurement; and *f* equals respiratory frequency. Dead space is usually estimated from standard tables, but it can be approximated to equal an adult's ideal weight in pounds.

Minute ventilation is the total amount of air entering or leaving the body per minute. It is calculated by multiplying the tidal volume by the respiratory rate. It includes the anatomic dead space. The formula for this calculation is as follows:

$$Ve = Vt \times R.$$

Study Questions

1. Explain how the unique structure of the pulmonary system provides for the maximum surface area for gas exchange.
2. Compare compliance and elastance in pulmonary structures and identify which components provide for each.
3. How do the pressures and oxygen saturations within the various chambers of the heart and in the pulmonary system promote maintenance of normal blood gas values?
4. Discuss normal and abnormal ventilation/perfusion relationships.
5. Describe the mechanisms used by the lungs to prevent infection and to protect against foreign material.
6. Relate the oxyhemoglobin dissociation curve to tissue oxygenation.

References

1. Bellanti, J.A. *Immunology III*. Philadelphia: Saunders, 1985.
2. Braun, H.A., Cheney, F.W., Jr., Loehnen, C.P. *Introduction to Respiratory Physiology* (2nd ed.). Boston: Little, Brown, 1980.
3. Burrows, B., Knudson, R., and Kettel, L. *Respiratory Insufficiency* (2nd ed.). Chicago: Yearbook, 1983.
4. Comroe, J.H. *Physiology of Respiration* (2nd ed.). Chicago: Yearbook, 1974.
5. Farzan, S. *A Concise Handbook of Respiratory Diseases* (2nd ed.). Reston, Va.: Reston Pub., 1985.
6. Fitzgerald, M., Carrington, C., and Gaensler, E. Environmental lung disease. *Med. Clin. North Am.* 57:593, 1973.
7. Ganong, W.F. *Review of Medical Physiology* (12th ed.). Los Altos, Calif.: Lange, 1985.

8. Guyton, A.C. *Textbook of Medical Physiology* (7th ed.). Philadelphia: Saunders, 1986.
9. Johansen, W., and Gould, K. Lung defense mechanisms. *Basics Respir. Dis.* 6:2, 1977.
10. Kilburn, K. An hypothesis for pulmonary clearance and its implications. *Am. Rev. Respir. Dis.* 98:449, 1968.
11. Kuhn, C., and Askin, F.B. Lung and mediastinum. In J.M. Kissane, *Anderson's Pathology* (8th ed.). St. Louis: Mosby, 1985.
12. Laurell, C., and Erickson, S. Electrophorphetic alpha$_1$-antitrypsin deficiency. *Scand. J. Clin. Lab. Invest.* 15:132, 1963.
13. Levitsky, M.G. *Pulmonary Physiology* (2nd ed.). New York: McGraw-Hill, 1986.
14. Lieberman, J. Alpha$_1$-antitrypsin deficiency. *Med. Clin. North Am.* 57:691, 1973.
15. MacDonnell, K., and Segal, M. *Current Respiratory Care*. Boston: Little, Brown, 1977.
16. Morrow, P. Dynamics of dust removal from lower airways. In A. Bouhuys (ed.), *Airway Dynamics*. Springfield, Ill.: Thomas, 1970.
17. Robbins, S.L., Cotran, R.S., and Kumar, V. *Pathologic Basis of Disease* (3rd ed.). Philadelphia: Saunders, 1984.
18. Selkurt, E. *Physiology* (5th ed.). Boston: Little, Brown, 1984.
19. Tobin, M.J., and Hutchison, D. An overview of the pulmonary features of alpha$_1$-antitrypsin deficiency. *Arch. Intern. Med.* 142:1342, 1982.
20. Unanue, E.R., and Benacerraf, B. *Textbook of Immunology* (2nd ed.). Baltimore: Williams & Wilkins, 1984.
21. Walter, J.B. *An Introduction to the Principles of Disease* (2nd ed.). Philadelphia: Saunders, 1982.
22. West, J. *Respiratory Physiology: The Essentials* (3rd ed.). Baltimore: Williams & Wilkins, 1985.

CHAPTER 25

Restrictive Alterations in Pulmonary Function

CHAPTER OUTLINE

Atelectasis
Infectious Diseases of the Respiratory Tract
- Upper Respiratory Tract Infection
- Lower Respiratory Tract Infection
  - *Bacterial Pneumonia*
  - *Mycoplasmal Pneumonia*
  - *Viral Pneumonia*
  - *Tuberculosis*

Aspiration Pneumonia
Pulmonary Edema
Traumatic Injuries of the Chest Wall
Pleural Effusion
Pneumothorax
Central Nervous System Depression
Neuromuscular Diseases
- Guillain-Barré Syndrome
- Duchenne Muscular Dystrophy

Respiratory Diseases Caused by Exposure to Organic and Inorganic Dusts
- Silicosis
- Coal Workers' Pneumoconiosis (Black Lung Disease)
- Byssinosis (Brown Lung Disease)
- Asbestosis

Pulmonary Fibrosis
Thoracic Deformity
Obesity
Idiopathic Respiratory Distress Syndrome of the Newborn
Adult Respiratory Distress Syndrome

LEARNING OBJECTIVES

1. Define *restrictive pulmonary disease*.
2. Describe compression and absorption atelectasis.
3. Discuss the role of surfactant in the development of atelectasis.
4. Discuss ventilation-perfusion abnormalities in atelectasis.
5. List the clinical manifestations of this condition.
6. List the organisms and the areas that they affect in upper respiratory tract infections.
7. Describe the etiologic factors in bacterial pneumonia.
8. Discuss the pathophysiology of pneumococcal pneumonia.
9. List the cause of tuberculosis and the role of individual susceptibility in acquiring the disease.
10. Describe the pathophysiology of primary and reinfection tuberculosis.
11. List two causes of aspiration pneumonia and describe the danger of each.
12. Discuss the cardiac and noncardiac causes of pulmonary edema.
13. Describe in detail the pathophysiology of alveolar and interstitial pulmonary edema.
14. Discuss how restrictive pulmonary disease can occur in a person with a simple rib fracture.
15. Describe the hemodynamics of flail chest abnormality.
16. List and describe disease-induced pleural effusions.
17. Outline the clinical manifestations of pleural effusion.
18. Describe tension pneumothorax.
19. Review central nervous system control of respiration.
20. Indicate how a head injury may affect respiration.
21. Define *Guillain-Barré syndrome*.
22. Describe the pulmonary problems that may occur with Guillain-Barré syndrome.
23. Describe the onset of respiratory failure in Duchenne muscular dystrophy.
24. List at least four substances that may cause pneuconiosis.

continued on next page

LEARNING OBJECTIVES continued

25. Outline the ways in which silicosis and asbestosis can cause a restrictive process.
26. Indicate how particulate matter is cleared in coal worker's pneumoconiosis.
27. Relate the development of pulmonary fibrosis to emphysematous changes in the pneumoconioses.
28. Define *byssinosis*.
29. Indicate two chest deformities that may cause restrictive pulmonary disease.
30. Explain why restrictive pulmonary disease can occur in obese individuals, especially those afflicted by the Pickwickian syndrome.
31. Define the role of surfactant in the development of idiopathic respiratory distress syndrome of newborns (IRDS).
32. Describe in detail the pathophysiology of the adult respiratory distress syndrome (ARDS).
33. List at least ten conditions that may lead to ARDS.

Restrictive pulmonary disease is an abnormal condition that causes a decrease in total lung capacity and vital capacity. It involves difficulty in the inspiratory phase of respiration. In this chapter, several conditions are considered, some of which do not precisely fit the above definition but that may lead to significant restriction. Table 25-1 classifies the conditions and their pathogenesis.

Atelectasis

Atelectasis is a very common, acute, restrictive disease that involves the collapse of previously expanded lung tissue or incomplete expansion at birth. It is usually described as a shrunken, airless state of the alveoli.

The two major alterations that occur with atelectasis are compression of lung tissue from a source outside the alveoli and absorption of gas from the alveoli. *Compression atelectasis* may be produced by such conditions as pneumothorax, pleural effusion, and tumors within the thorax (Fig. 25-1A). *Absorption atelectasis* occurs when secretions in the bronchi and bronchioles obstruct these airways and prevent the movement of air into the alveoli (Fig. 25-1B). The air trapped in the alveoli is absorbed and the alveolar sacs collapse. Stasis of secretions in the larger airways provides an excellent medium for bacterial growth and stasis pneumonia.

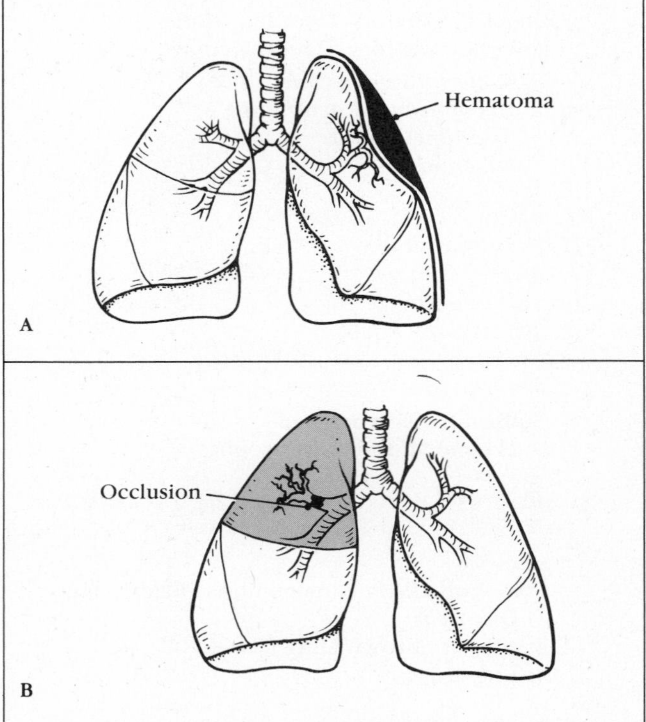

FIGURE 25-1 A. Compression of lung tissue by hematoma. B. Right upper lobe atelectasis caused by bronchial occlusion.

Atelectasis is a common postoperative complication due to retained secretions. After surgery, the patient's protective cough response decreases due to medications and pain. An ineffective cough reflex, which diminishes the tidal volume, and decreased sigh mechanism lead to inadequate alveolar expansion. Increased viscosity of sputum results, with a tendency for secretions to gravitate to the dependent areas.

Adults are susceptible to atelectasis, particularly in the right middle lobe, which is most vulnerable because of the angle of convergence of its bronchus with the right main bronchus. The right middle lobe also seems to have increased susceptibility to bacterial pneumonia, which tends to flourish in copious pooled secretions.

As noted in Chapter 24, the natural tendency of the lungs is to collapse. In other words, elastic forces are constantly trying to force the lung tissue inward. These forces are opposed by the negative intrapleural forces and chest wall expansion. When airflow into the alveoli is obstructed, alveolar sacs collapse and produce little or no surfactant. Surfactant, due to its short half-life, must be constantly replenished and this requires normal ventilation. To offset the tendency to collapse, collateral communication often occurs through the pores of Kohn; the amount of communication partly depends on the overall degree of inflation of the lungs (Fig. 25-2).

Perfusion to the collapsed airways is not affected, so blood shunts by the ineffective alveoli and is not oxygenated. This results in a *perfusion-without-ventilation* shunt, or a direct right-to-left shunt across the lungs

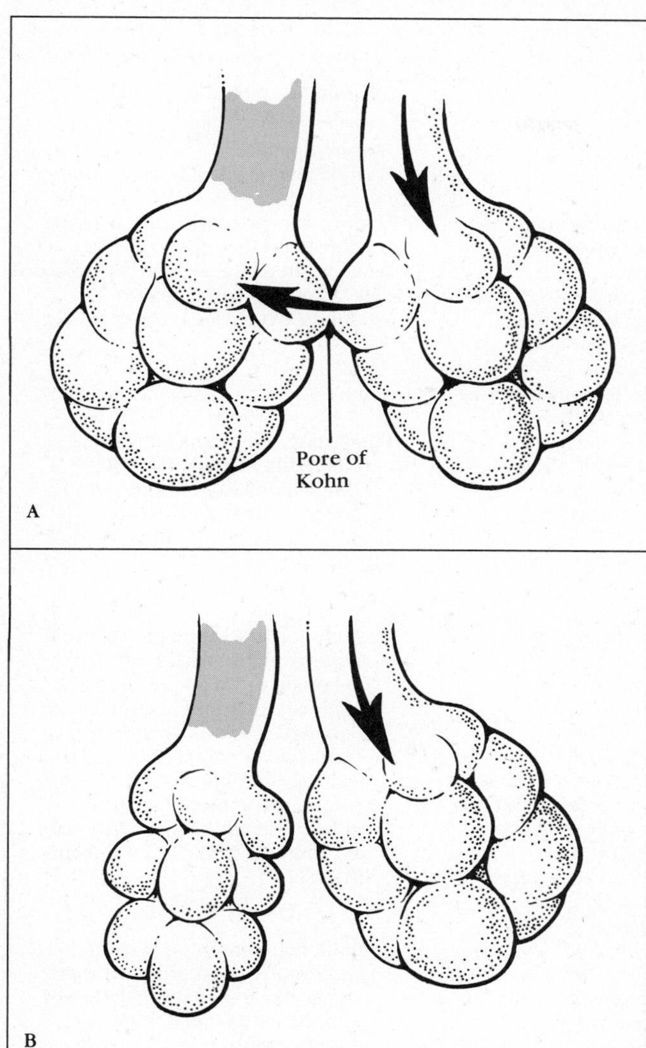

FIGURE 25-2 A. Demonstration of collateral communication between the alveoli through pores of Kohn. B. Atelectasis occurring without this communication.

(Fig. 25-3). Therefore, if atelectasis is significant, hypoxemia will also be significant.

One can readily see that the process of atelectasis may occur in many situations, including the obstructive conditions in which a portion of lung tissue is hyperinflated and adjacent sections are collapsed. Clinical manifestations depend on the amount of atelectasis. Rales in the bases and/or diminished breath sounds are common in postoperative atelectasis. A mild case may produce no symptoms, but as it progresses or becomes more widespread, dyspnea, tachycardia, cough, fever, and disturbances in chest wall expansion may occur. Blood gas analysis shows hypoxemia when significant atelectasis is present. Hypercapnia and decreased pH may herald a progression toward respiratory failure (see Chap. 27).

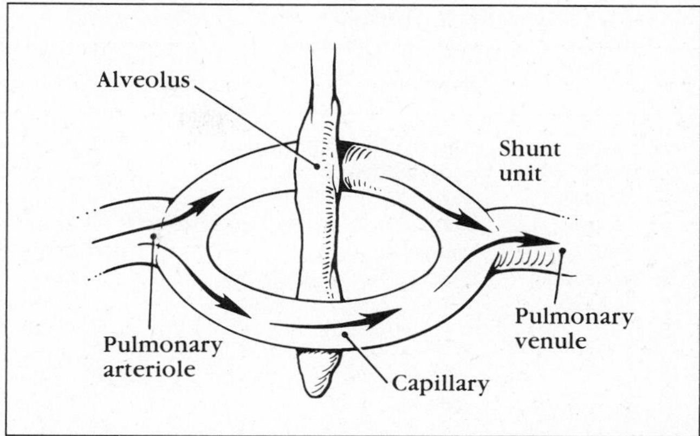

FIGURE 25-3 Demonstration of a right-to-left shunt across the pulmonary bed.

Infectious Diseases of the Respiratory Tract

Infectious processes can involve either the upper or lower respiratory tract, or both. They may be caused by viruses, bacteria, rickettsiae, or fungi, and be mild, self-limited, or very debilitating.

Upper Respiratory Tract Infection

The upper respiratory tract warms, humidifies, and filters the air; in this process it is exposed to a wide variety of pathogens that may lodge and grow in various areas depending on the susceptibility of the host. Pathogens may lodge in the nose, pharynx (particularly the tonsils), larynx, or trachea, and may proliferate if the defenses of the host are depressed. The spread of the infection depends on the resistance mounted by the host and on the virulence of the organism. Figure 25-4 shows the defensive anatomy and physiology of the upper respiratory tract, including the mucociliary blanket, which normally provides a very efficient cleansing mechanism for expelling foreign material.

An example of an upper respiratory tract infection is the sore throat (nasopharyngitis), which, if caused by the bacteria beta-hemolytic streptococci, leads to suppuration in the nasopharynx and tonsils that may spread to the sinuses. Susceptible individuals may later develop a reaction to the organism that is manifested as rheumatic fever (see Chap. 21).

Viruses also cause pathology of the upper respiratory tract. Influenza, for example, is characterized by an acute inflammation of the nasopharynx, trachea, and bronchioles, and leads to edema, congestion, and necrosis of these structures. The common cold is characterized by an acute inflammation of the nasopharynx, pharynx, larynx, and trachea, resulting in swelling of the mucous membranes and mucopurulent serous exudate. The purulence is due to secondary bacterial infection.

TABLE 25-1 Restrictive Diseases

Category	Examples	Pathogenesis	Assessment of Findings
Respiratory center depression	Narcotic and barbiturate dependence	Direct depression of respiratory center.	Respiratory rate: <12/minute; associated signs of hypoventilation
	Central nervous system lesions, head trauma	Injury to or impingement on respiratory centers.	Hyper- or hypoventilation; cerebral edema and its signs
Neuromuscular	Guillain-Barré syndrome	Acute toxic polyneuritis; intercostal paralysis leads to diaphragmatic breathing; vagal and SNS paralysis lead to reduced ability of bronchioles to constrict, dilate, react to irritants.	Reduced negative inspiratory pressure, V_T, V_C, compliance, breath sounds; hypoxemia, hypercapnia
	Duchenne muscular dystrophy	Genetic; thoracoscoliosis; paralysis of intercostals, abdominal muscles, diaphragm, accessory muscles.	Pulmonary symptoms appear late; reduced IC, ERV, V_C, V_T, FRC, compliance PO_2; elevated PCO_2; abnormal respiratory patterns
Restriction of thoracic excursion			
Thoracic deformity	Kyphoscoliosis, pectus excavatum	Deformity of chest compresses lung tissue and limits thoracic excursion.	Reduced breath sounds in affected areas, probably with rales; reduced compliance, TLC, V_C, ERV; signs of hypoventilation, hypoxemia, increased work of breathing
Traumatic chest wall instability	Flail chest	Fracture of a group of ribs leads to unstable chest wall; reduced intrathoracic pressure on inspiration pulls area in and causes pressure on parenchyma; this increases work of breathing and hypoventilation.	Obvious flail, unequal chest excursion, bruising, skin injuries, localized pain on inspiration, dyspnea, reduced breath sounds with rales and rhonchi; reduced compliance, ERV, TLC, V_C, PO_2
Obesity	Pickwickian syndrome	Excess abdominal adipose tissue impinges on thoracic space and diaphragmatic excursion; increased weight of chest restricts thoracic excursion.	Somnolence, twitching, periodic respirations, polycythemia, right ventricular hypertrophy/failure; reduced compliance, ERV, TLC, V_C, PO_2; elevated PCO_2; distant breath sounds

Lower Respiratory Tract Infection

Infectious processes of the lower respiratory tract can be caused by any of the pathogens that affect the upper respiratory tract. These lead to a variety of pathologic and clinical features depending on host resistance and virulence of the organism.

Bacterial Pneumonia. Bacterial pneumonia is a common infection that is a threat to life for many of our population, especially the aged and chronically ill. This threat has been drastically reduced by antimicrobial preparations, which have decreased the death rate, shortened the course of the disease, and prevented many serious complications, such as empyema.

For bacteria to invade the lung successfully, there must be an alteration in net bacterial lung clearance. This alteration may occur as a result of decreased bactericidal ability of the alveolar macrophages or increased susceptibility of the host to infection. Normally, the bactericidal activity of macrophages is extremely important in supplementing the mucociliary escalator system in removing pathogens.

Pneumococcal pneumonia (Streptococcus pneumoniae) is the most common bacterial pneumonia, being responsible for 30 to 80 percent or more of community-acquired pneumonias [5]. It follows an orderly sequence in the lung; its severity depends greatly on host resistance and/or medical intervention. While infection may develop in healthy persons, underlying factors (e.g., malnutrition, alcoholism, aging) seem to increase risk. Pathophysiologically, an initial, acute, inflammatory response occurs that brings excess water and plasma proteins to the dependent areas of the lower lobes. Red blood cells, fibrin, and polymorphonuclear leukocytes infiltrate the alveoli. The bacteria are contained within segments of pulmonary lobes by this cellular recruitment, causing leukocytes and fibrin to consolidate within the involved area.

The inflammatory exudate progresses through stages including *hyperemia* and *red* and *gray hepatization*, and finally terminates in *resolution*. Hyperemia, also called the

TABLE 25-1 (continued)

Category	Examples	Pathogenesis	Assessment of Findings
Pleural disorders	Pleural effusion	Accumulation of fluid in pleural space secondary to altered hydrostatic or oncotic forces.	Unequal chest expansion; dullness and reduced breath sounds in affected area; may be constant chest discomfort; dyspnea if amount of fluid large; if over 250 ml, shows on radiographs; if large, bulging of intercostal spaces
	Pneumothorax	Accumulation of air in pleural space with proportional lung collapse.	Hyperresonance; reduced breath sounds; tracheal deviation away from pneumothorax; tachycardia; unequal chest expansion; breath sounds reduced or absent; shows on radiographs
Disorders of lung parenchyma	Pulmonary fibrosis	Many possible causes: occupational sarcoid, etc.	Reduced compliance, hypoxemia, hypercapnia, and their consequences
	Tuberculosis	Bacterial invasion leads to scarring, reduced compliance, and reduced lung function.	Visible on films; positive skin test, sputum; malaise, weight loss, fatigue, evening fever with night sweats, cough, hemoptysis
	Atelectasis	Obstruction of bronchioles, shrunken airless alveoli; reduced compliance; right-to-left shunting.	Dyspnea, tachycardia, cough, fever, decreased chest wall expansion, hypoxemia, radiologic evidence
Disorders of lung parenchyma	Adult respiratory distress syndrome (ARDS)	Widespread atelectasis; loss of surfactant; interstitial edema, formation of hyaline membrane.	Dyspnea, tachypnea, grunting, labored respirations, hypoxemia, occasional hypercapnia, cyanosis; radiographs show bilateral patchy infiltrates
	Pulmonary edema	Increased pulmonary capillary pressure leads to interstitial and alveolar edema.	Hypoxemia, tachypnea; signs of CHF, radiologic butterfly infiltrates, rales
	Aspiration pneumonia	Chemical irritant from aspirant leads to bronchoconstriction, necrosis, and fibrosis of airways.	Hypoxemia, signs of ARDS, wheezing, tachypnea, tachycardia
	Pneumoconiosis	Inhalation of pollutants, results in scarring, fibrosis, and secondary emphysema.	Slow developing pulmonary signs of dyspnea, hypoxemia, hypercapnia, cor pulmonale

stage of congestion, is characterized by engorgement of the alveolar spaces with fluid and blood. The outpouring of edema fluid provides a rich medium for proliferation and rapid spread of the organism through the lobe [5]. Red hepatization refers to the red appearance of affected lung tissue, which demonstrates the consistency of liver tissue. The stage of gray hepatization occurs when increasing numbers of leukocytes infiltrate the alveoli, causing the tissue to become solid and grayish [5,9]. During resolution, polymorphonuclear leukocytes are replaced by macrophages that are highly phagocytic and destroy the organisms.

The filling of alveoli with exudate, or consolidation, causes them to become airless. Sustained perfusion with poor ventilation occurs in the consolidated area, but this rarely is severe enough to cause a true hypoxemic picture. The infection resolves as exudate is lysed and resorbed by the neutrophils and macrophages. The lymphatics carry exudate away from the site of infection, resulting in restoration of both structure and function of the lung. In some cases, resolution does not occur and the exudate is converted to fibrous tissue, rendering the affected alveoli functionless [5].

The clinical manifestations of pneumococcal pneumonia include fever, cough, pleuritic chest pain, and production of rusty-colored or blood-streaked sputum. Pneumonia in the elderly individual seldom exhibits these classic findings, and the person may experience lethargy, confusion, and deterioration of a preexisting disease [7]. Complications include pleural involvement with empyema and pleuritis, lung abscess, and bacteremia [5].

Bacterial pneumonia also may result from other bacteria, including species of *Staphylococcus*, *Streptococcus*, *Klebsiella*, and *Pseudomonas*. At times, these organisms are opportunistic and lead to additional infection or disease in an already debilitated person. Such imposed conditions often are complicated by abscess formation, empyema, and pleural effusion.

The frequency of gram-negative bacterial pneumonias is increasing at a rapid rate due to antibiotic therapy. It is

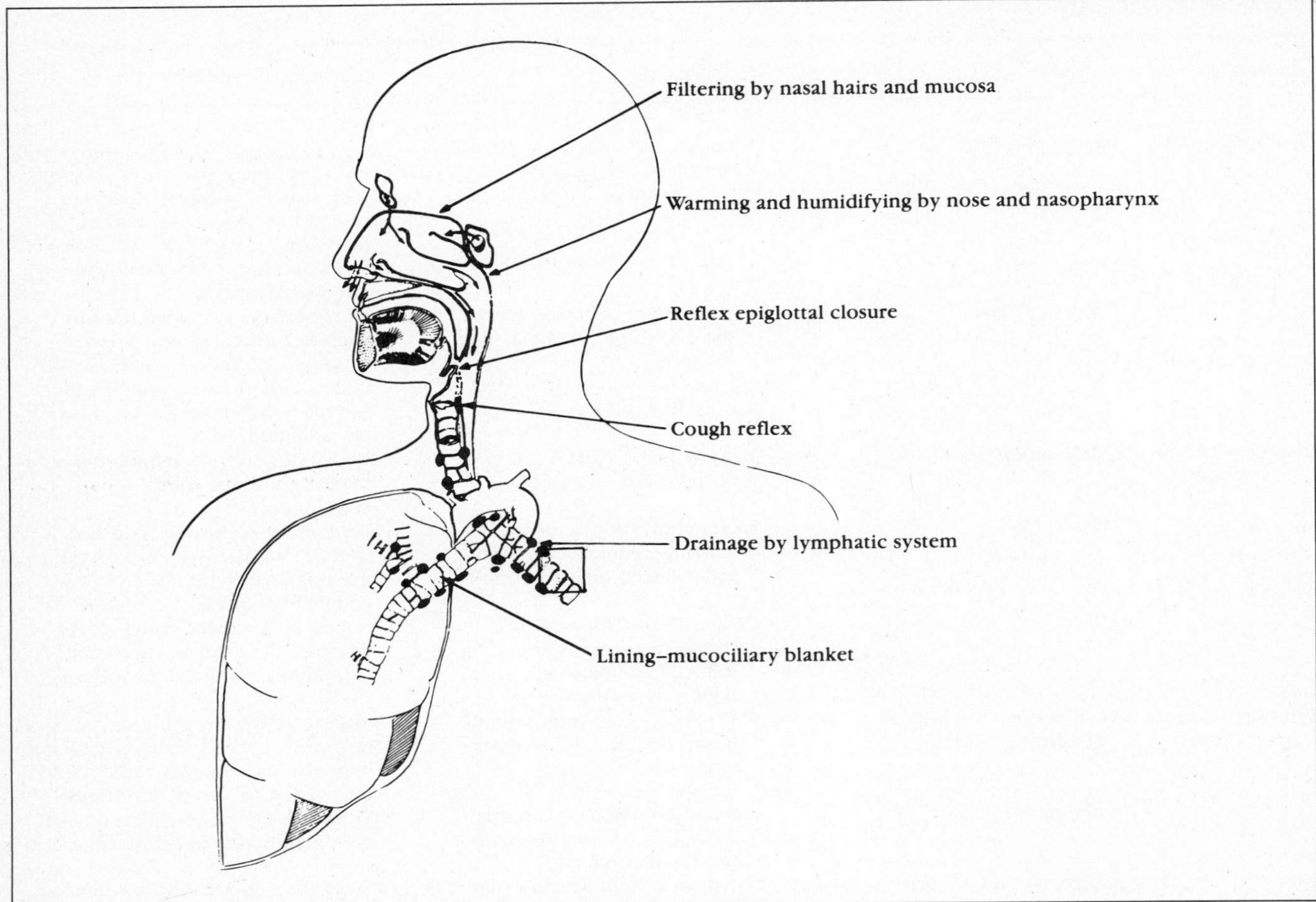

FIGURE 25-4 Defense of the respiratory tract. (Adapted from K. MacDonnell, *Current Respiratory Care*. Boston: Little, Brown, 1977.)

estimated that up to 50 percent of nosocomial bacterial pneumonias are due to gram-negative organisms [5,11]. This type of pneumonia is limited to persons with other debilitating conditions. Diseases included in this group could thus be termed *opportunistic infections* because they are rare in the immunocompetent person.

Mycoplasmal Pneumonia. Mycoplasmal organisms are smaller than bacteria but are not classified as viruses. *Mycoplasma pneumoniae* is a common cause of upper respiratory tract infections, with pneumonia occurring in less than 10 percent of infected subjects [11]. It normally affects younger individuals with fibrinous pleurisy and interstitial pneumonia. The disease tends to be self-limited and is rare after age 45 years [5].

Viral Pneumonia. Viral pneumonias are frequently mild and self-limited in adults but may be rapidly proliferative and fatal in children. The pediatric diseases include bronchiolitis and pneumonia. Epidemics of this viral infection occur in winter and often affect children under 2 years of age [5,12]. In adults, viral pneumonias may affect the alveolar epithelial cells or the bronchioles. The course may be very rapid, causing an acute clinical picture of respiratory distress with or without fever. A major concern with virus infection is that the terminal and respiratory bronchioles may become damaged and then become susceptible to secondary bacterial invasion that spreads to the surrounding alveoli. The common types of viruses are the influenza, adenovirus, and chicken-pox virus.

Tuberculosis. Tuberculosis is caused by *Mycobacterium tuberculosis*, which is classified as an acid-fast bacillus because of its staining property. This disease is most common in malnourished and aged persons, and its spread is closely related to host resistance. It is transmitted by droplets from persons with an active tuberculous process. The portal of entry is usually the respiratory system, but may be the skin or gastrointestinal tract.

Respiratory transmission begins with inhalation of the mycobacteria; because of their small size, the organisms are deposited in the lung periphery, usually in the lower part of the upper lobe or upper part of the lower lobe (Fig. 25-5). In primary infection, the mycobacteria become surrounded by polymorphonuclear leukocytes (PMNs), and inflammation results. After a few days, macrophages replace the PMNs. Some mycobacterial organisms are carried off by the lymphatics to the hilar lymph nodes. The

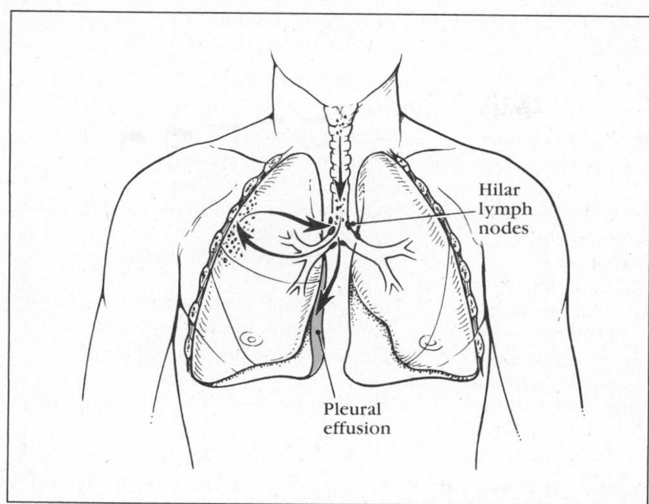

FIGURE 25-5 Tuberculosis organisms are usually deposited in the lung periphery, either in the lower part of the upper lobe or the upper part of the lower lobe. Arrows indicate entrance, deposition, spread to hilar lymph nodes, and pleural effusion.

combination of the initial lesion and lymph node involvement is called the *Ghon complex*, but this rarely results in spread to other body organs.

Macrophages called *epitheloid cells* engulf the mycobacteria. These cells join together to form giant cells that ring the foreign cell. Within the giant cell, caseous necrosis develops, probably a result of acquired hypersensitivity to the organism. Caseous necrosis has a characteristic granular, cheesy appearance. The area surrounding the central core of necrosis is ringed with sensitized T lymphocytes. Fibrosis and calcification develop as the lesion ages, resulting finally in a *granuloma*, which is called a *tubercle*. Collagenous scar tissue encapsulates the tubercle, effectively separating the organisms from the body. The organisms may or may not be killed in the process, but sensitized T lymphocytes develop to enhance the bactericidal activity of the macrophages. This results in cell-mediated immunity that usually lasts throughout life and can be demonstrated by administering purified protein derivative (PPD) of the bacilli. A positive inflammatory wheal response indicates the presence of memory T cells for the mycobacteria.

After initial exposure, 5 percent of individuals who inhale the mycobacteria develop clinical tuberculosis. The clinical manifestations vary, and include night fever, cough, and symptoms of airway obstruction from hilar node involvement. The disease may spread, involving the meninges, kidneys, bones, or other structures. In a small number of individuals, the actual disease develops years after the initial exposure. Mycobacteria that are not destroyed by alveolar defenses lie dormant until a decrease in host resistance allows the original focus to become a source of progressive disease. This *postprimary*, or *reinfection*, *(secondary) tuberculosis* is most frequent in persons who have developed a secondary immunodeficiency, especially from cancer, cirrhosis of the liver, or diabetes mellitus.

Aspiration Pneumonia

Aspiration usually refers to the inhalation of gastric contents, food, water, or blood into the tracheobronchial system. Aspiration pneumonia results when the material is propelled into the alveolar system, and most frequently occurs after vomiting or near-drowning.

Aspiration of gastric contents is relatively common and is especially associated with impaired consciousness, which includes such conditions as cardiac arrest, seizures, strokes, and general anesthesia. The gastric contents are very acidic, having a pH of less than 3. Aspiration of this material results in chemical irritation and destruction of the mucosa of the tracheobronchial tree. In the lungs, areas of hemorrhage and edema occur, especially in dependent portions. The severity of the response depends on the person's physiologic status and the quantity and acidity of the aspirant.

After aspiration, respiratory distress usually begins abruptly with evidence of bronchospasm, dyspnea, tachycardia, and cyanosis. Severe hypoxemia frequently occurs and may precipitate the adult respiratory distress syndrome [2].

Aspirated foodstuffs may be diagnosed by their content or appearance. Lipid-laden macrophages, for example, indicate that fats have been aspirated and have caused an acute or chronic pneumonia [6]. Foods may cause mechanical obstruction of the airway or chemical irritation of the mucosal lining, especially if they are mixed with acid gastric secretions.

In *drowning* or *near-drowning*, aspiration of water usually causes intense laryngospasm, which is not enough to protect the alveoli from fluid. The result of near-drowning is severe hypoxemia and acidosis. Sea water aspiration may lead to secondary pulmonary edema because of the high sodium content of the water [2]. The close relationship between near-drowning and the adult respiratory distress syndrome may, in part, be due to washing out of surfactant from the alveolar linings.

Pulmonary Edema

The pulmonary vascular system has a great capacity to accommodate amounts of blood up to 3 times its normal volume, but at a critical pressure point fluid moves across the alveolocapillary line, and pulmonary edema occurs. Pulmonary edema is simply an accumulation of fluid in the tissues (interstitium and alveoli of the lungs).

Understanding the mechanism by which pulmonary edema occurs is enhanced by the understanding of *Starling's equation* (Fig. 25-6). Hydrostatic and osmotic pressures are the major forces that affect movement of water across the capillary membrane (see Chap. 5). The normal hydrostatic pressure in the pulmonary capillaries is approximately 7 to 10 mm Hg, which is estimated from the pulmonary wedge pressure. The plasma oncotic pressure is approximately 25 mm Hg. Therefore, the alveoli tend to stay "dry" because the pressures oppose fluid movement into the interstitium and alveoli [3].

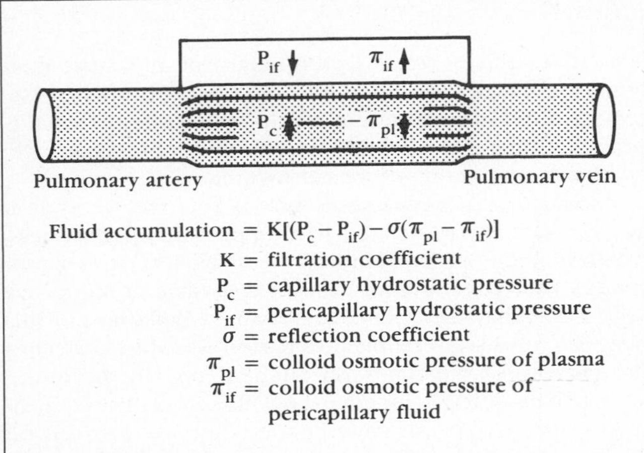

FIGURE 25-6 Starling equation for transcapillary exchange. The reflection coefficient (σ) is a correction factor that relates to the effective difference in the osmotic pressure of proteins that operates across the capillary wall. (Reprinted with permission from A.P. Fishman, *Pulmonary Disease and Disorders*. © 1980 McGraw-Hill. Reprinted with permission of McGraw-Hill Publishers.)

TABLE 25-2 Causes of Pulmonary Edema

Cause	Precipitating Event
Increased capillary hydrostatic pressure	Myocardial infarction, mitral stenosis, fluid overload, pulmonary venoocclusive disease
Increased capillary permeability	Inhaled or circulating toxins, irradiation, oxygen toxicity
Lymphatic insufficiency	Silicosis, lymphangitis, carcinoma
Decreased interstitial pressure	Rapid removal of pleural effusion or pneumothorax, hyperinflation
Decreased colloid osmotic pressure	Overtransfusion, hypoproteinemia
Unknown etiology	High altitude, heroin, neurogenic causes

Source: Reprinted with permission from J.B. West, *Pulmonary Pathophysiology: The Essentials.* (2nd ed) © 1982 The Williams & Wilkins Co., Baltimore.

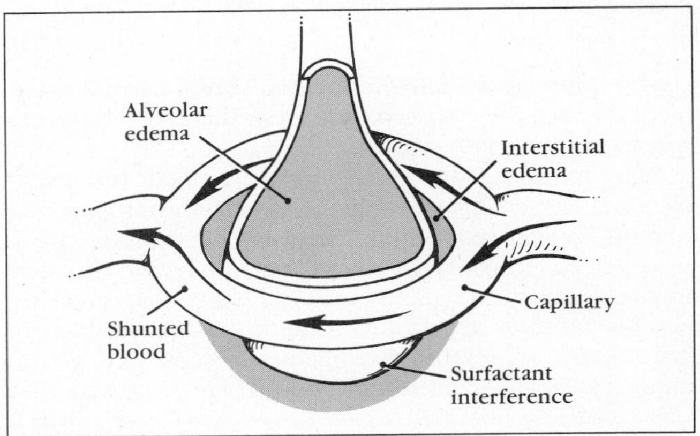

FIGURE 25-7 Schematic representation of interstitial alveolar edema, right-to-left shunting, alveolar edema, and surfactant interference.

Pulmonary edema fluid is distributed positionally. Normally, when a person is in the upright position, the hydrostatic pressures are higher in the lung bases than at the apices [3]. Acute pulmonary edema may show bizarre patterns of distribution because of variations in the transmission of pleural pressures in different areas of the lungs, but in chronic pulmonary edema the fluid tends to accumulate at the lung bases.

Hydrostatic pressure in the pulmonary bed must increase to a level of approximately 25 to 30 mm Hg for pulmonary edema to occur when capillary permeability is normal and the alveolar system is intact. Lymphatic drainage of a few milliliters per hour is usually sufficient to drain any excess protein and fluid that does not move back into the capillary. Lymphatics are probably sparse in the alveolar regions and more plentiful in the peribronchial and perivascular spaces, but these can increase lymph-carrying capacity sixfold to tenfold, so that a sustained increase in hydrostatic pressure can be compensated for by increased lymphatic drainage [15].

The most common cause of pulmonary edema is left ventricular failure (LVF). This is discussed in more detail in Chapter 20. Left ventricular failure may be due to such pathology as acute myocardial infarction, hypertension, or mitral valve disease. Pulmonary edema may also result from acute inflammation, poisoning with certain gases (especially chlorine and nitrogen peroxide), pulmonary aspiration of gastric juice, excessive volume overload, some cases of cerebral damage, and smoke inhalation (Table 25-2). The mechanisms for producing edema are different, but all result in increased interstitial or alveolar fluid (Figure 25-7).

In the case of pulmonary edema from acute inflammation, the result is alveolar damage, which leads to increased permeability and fluid exudation into the alveoli. In cerebral damage, the reaction of the body is to increase sympathetic nervous system stimulation, resulting in diversion of blood to the lungs, which increases the hydrostatic pressure and causes edema. Fluid overloading is rare with a normal heart, but occurs when the fluid volume exceeds the heart's ability to pump it all. Smoke inhalation may be injurious due to chemical pneumonitis from the fumes, gases, and particulate matter [13]. Intraalveolar hemorrhage, congested, edematous alveoli, and interstitial edema may all result from this type of injury.

Pulmonary edema due to heart failure occurs when the left side of the heart is no longer able to accept all of the output sent to it from the right side of the heart. As a result, a small amount of blood is dammed back into the pulmonary circulation with each beat of the heart. Gradually, the amount of accumulated blood exceeds the distensible capacity of the pulmonary vasculature. The excess blood in the pulmonary tree increases pulmonary capillary hydrostatic pressure. This pressure increase is most severe in the dependent areas of the lungs, accounting for increased fluid build-up in the bases.

Pulmonary blood pressure is also raised by reflex vasoconstriction of the pulmonary vessels that occurs in response to hypoxemia, which may result from the decreased cardiac output. As pressure in the pulmonary circulation increases, fluid is forced into the pulmonary interstitial spaces. This phenomenon is known as *transudation*.

Pulmonary edema actually occurs in two stages (Fig. 25-8). The first stage is *interstitial edema*, in which fluid accumulates in the peribronchial and perivascular spaces. The lymphatics attempt to decrease this fluid by widening their lumina and increasing the rate of flow. Some widening of the alveolar walls may also occur at this stage. Interstitial pulmonary edema widens the distance between the alveoli and pulmonary capillaries, but has little effect on gaseous exchange in the early stages.

The second stage occurs when interstitial hydrostatic pressure is so high that it pushes fluid into the alveoli, resulting in *alveolar edema*. The alveoli fill one at a time, diluting surfactant with the incoming fluid. This reduces the surface tension in the alveoli and predisposes them to collapse. Some alveoli may be compressed by surrounding edematous alveoli while others are not aerated because the airways that supply them are filled with fluid. When no oxygen is present in the alveoli, right-to-left shunting occurs; sometimes the shunt may be as large as 50 percent, resulting in severe hypoxemia and later, hypercapnia. This ventilation-perfusion ($\dot{V}/\dot{Q}$) abnormality is called a *shunt unit* (see Fig. 25-7).

The symptoms of pulmonary edema are directly attributable to its pathophysiology. The onset of symptoms may be sudden or gradual. If pulmonary edema is mild and develops slowly, the major symptoms are wheezing, paroxysmal nocturnal dyspnea (PND), and dry cough. When it is fully developed, there is dyspnea, orthopnea, wheezing, and productive cough. The person expectorates profuse amounts of sputum that initially may be white and frothy, but progresses to pink-tinged or bright red.

The elastic work of breathing is greatly increased because the accumulated interstitial fluid causes lung stiffening and loss of compliance. This, together with hypoxemia, leads to a pattern of rapid, shallow breathing. The lungs fill with fluid, which causes moist bubbling, rales, and wheezing. Abnormal heart sounds are common due to heart failure. Chest roentgenograms show cardiomegaly, and the fluid accumulation appears as confluent patchy opacifications that are concentrated centrally in the lungs, having the appearance of a butterfly or bat's wing [14]. Arterial blood gases reflect the degree of hypoxemia and/or hypercapnia.

Traumatic Injuries of the Chest Wall

Traumatic injuries of the chest wall are common results of automobile accidents and other injuries. The injuries may be simple, such as a rib fracture, or as serious as flail chest abnormality.

The most common chest wall injury is *simple rib fracture*. Because it causes inspiratory pain, there is voluntary splinting, which results in restricted tidal volume and an increased respiratory rate. The victim voluntarily inhibits the urge to cough. The young, previously healthy person usually tolerates a fractured rib well, but a person with underlying pulmonary disease or the aged individual may develop impaired clearance of secretions, atelectasis, pneumonia, or even respiratory failure. The condition is further aggravated if the chest is strapped and narcotic analgesics are used. Chest strapping limits the ability to take a deep breath and thus enhances the risk for atelectasis and pneumonia. Compliance and all measurements of lung volume are reduced. The respiratory drive and the cough reflex may be depressed by administration of narcotic analgesics.

If several adjacent ribs in an area are fractured, the sta-

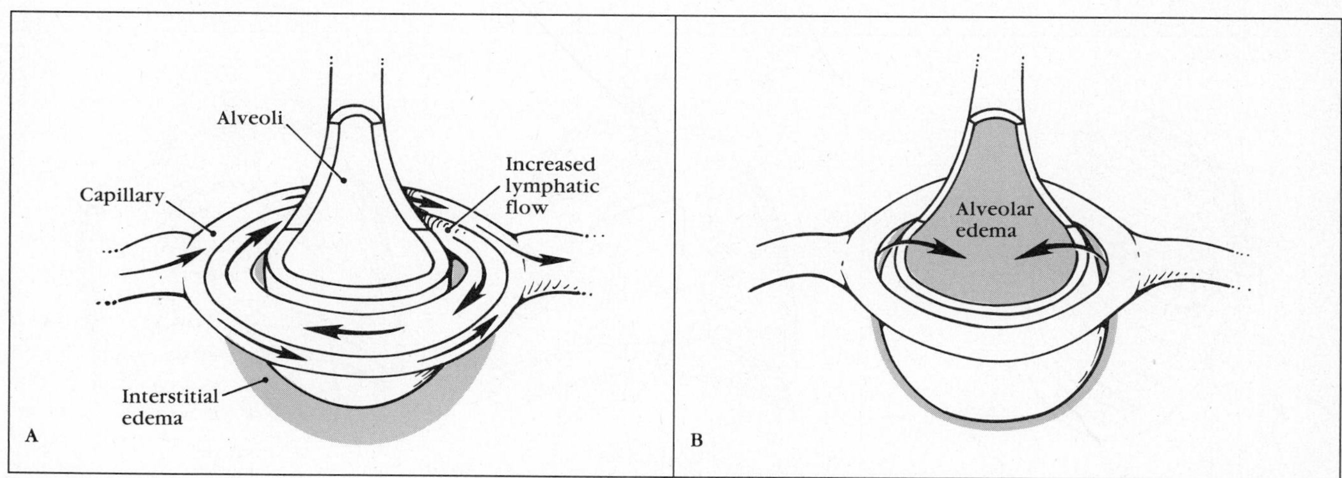

FIGURE 25-8 Illustration of stages of pulmonary edema. A. Interstitial pulmonary edema and increased lymphatic flow. B. Alveolar pulmonary edema.

bility of that area of chest wall may be lost (Fig. 25-9). As a result, on inspiration the intrathoracic pressure is lowered and that area of the chest wall is sucked in. The underlying lung tissue does not expand and gas exchange becomes impaired. Compliance is reduced. When the victim exhales, the affected area of the chest is elevated somewhat because of the increased intrathoracic pressure, creating a paradoxic movement during the ventilatory cycle.

This injury increases the work of breathing and impairs ventilatory efficiency. The more the person works to maintain adequate ventilation, the more paradoxic the respiratory motion. In severe cases, a pendulum movement of the mediastinum may occur with each breath, putting pressure on the otherwise unaffected lung. The paradoxic motion may increase central venous pressure while decreasing venous return to the heart, resulting in decreased blood pressure. Normal breathing is impaired and coughing is impossible, resulting in hypoventilation, hypoxemia, and even respiratory failure. Clinical manifestations of *flail chest* abnormality include the obvious signs of chest wall trauma, "flail" movement with unequal chest excursion, severe dyspnea, pain especially on inspiration, rales, or reduced breath sounds. Chest radiographs show evidence of fractured ribs, and blood gases indicate the degree of hypoxemia.

Pleural Effusion

Pleural fluid is normally produced in quantities just sufficient to lubricate the surfaces of the visceral and parietal pleura so as to provide a smooth sliding surface. This small amount of fluid is continually replenished and resorbed, maintaining a constant amount in the pleural space.

Pleural fluid accumulation or effusion may result from disease or trauma. Conditions that may lead to fluid accumulation include neoplasms, infections, thromboemboli, and cardiovascular and immunologic defects. Thoracic trauma may cause bleeding into the pleural space.

Pleural effusions are frequently categorized as transudates and exudates. Generally, inflammatory diseases and those of tissue destruction produce exudates with a specific gravity above 1.017 and a high concentration of protein and lactic acid dehydrogenase (LDH). Transudates, which are produced by diseases such as congestive heart failure, show lower values for these components, with protein below 3.5 gm per dl and LDH below 200 units [9].

The accumulation of pleural transudates is sometimes referred to as *hydrothorax*. If the effusion contains purulent material, it is called *empyema*. If empyema ultimately leads to fibrous fusing of the lung and chest wall, it is called *fibrothorax*. If the pleural fluid contains blood it is called *hemothorax*.

Fluid in the intrapleural space occupies space and displaces lung tissue by reducing the amount of lung expansion possible by direct pressure on the tissue (Fig. 25-10); it may cause a mediastinal shift, which puts pressure on the opposite lung as well. Compliance decreases, altering ventilation and perfusion on the affected side. When fluid is removed from the pleural space, lung tissue reexpands, allowing ventilation and perfusion to return to normal.

Clinical manifestations depend on the rate of effusion. A hemothorax from a ruptured thoracic aneurysm, for example, causes rapid accumulation of blood, as well as dramatic signs and symptoms of blood loss and a mediastinal shift. In a slower process, 2000 ml of fluid in the pleural space may accumulate before dyspnea is noted. Common symptoms relate to the amount of pulmonary embarrassment, and include dyspnea, blood gas abnormalities, cyanosis, and jugular vein distention.

Pneumothorax

Pneumothorax occurs when air enters the pleural space (Fig. 25-11). Once this takes place, lung tissue is displaced in much the same way as if fluid had entered the space.

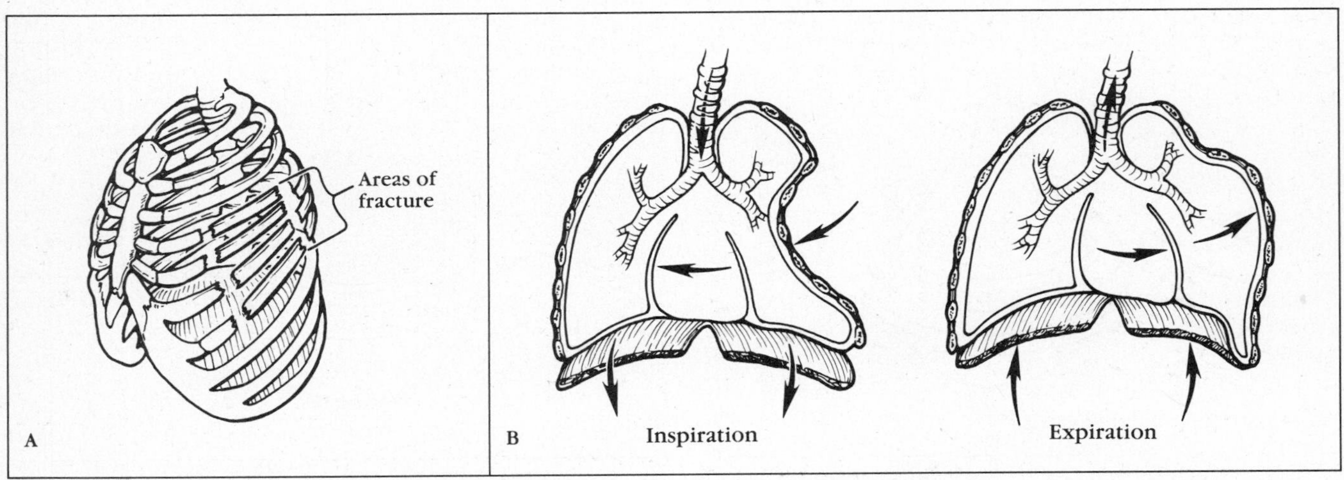

FIGURE 25-9 A. Chest wall injury that can produce flail chest abnormality. B. Physiology of flail chest abnormality.

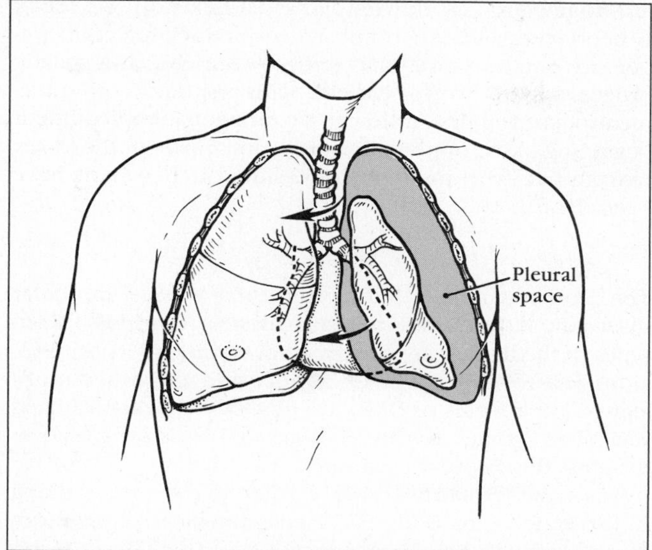

FIGURE 25-10 Pleural effusion. Fluid has collected in the pleural space and displaced lung tissue. Also note shift of fluid into the mediastinum and torsion of the bronchus.

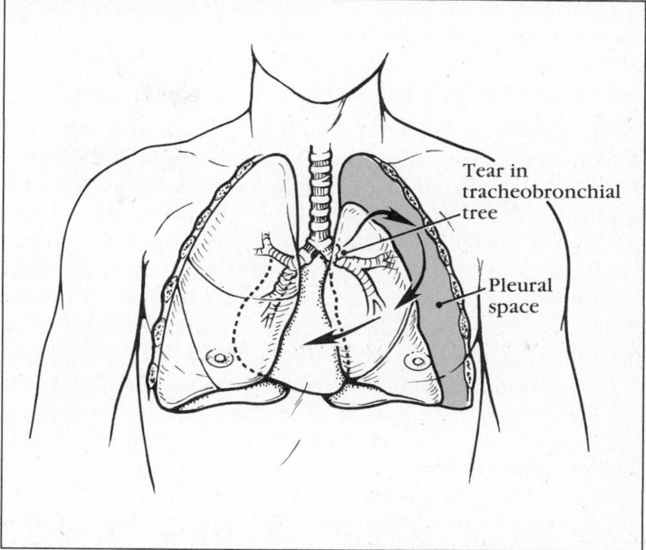

FIGURE 25-11 Pneumothorax. Tear in tracheobronchial tree has caused air to move into the pleural space; the lung collapses, and the mediastinum shifts to the unaffected side.

Air may enter the pleural space from an opening in the chest wall or from the lungs themselves. Some of the causes of pneumothorax from the lungs include puncture by a fractured rib, spontaneous rupture of a superficial bleb, and rupture of a bleb during vigorous mechanical ventilation. Tracheobronchial rupture due to trauma may also cause pneumothorax. Surgical pneumothorax occurs as a part of every thoracotomy. *Spontaneous pneumothorax* may occur in individuals with emphysema when a bleb on the surface of the lung ruptures and releases air into the pleural spaces.

Pressure in the potential intrapleural space is normally lower or more negative than intraalveolar pressure. Therefore, if there is a break in either the integrity of the lung through the visceral pleura or the chest wall through the parietal pleura, air rushes to the area of lowest pressure, the pleural space. This continues as long as the air leak is present. Sometimes air leaks into the pleural space on inspiration, but the tissue seals itself on expiration and outward leakage does not occur. This results in *tension pneumothorax*, which is a life-threatening condition of air build-up in the space, with displacement of and pressure on the structures within the mediastinum. This displacement to the opposite side affects the other lung and may impede the venous return to the heart.

Clinical signs of a significant pneumothorax may include dyspnea and chest pain of sudden onset. The trachea may deviate toward the unaffected side, and vesicular or bronchial breath sounds on the affected side may be reduced. Arterial blood gases may reveal acute hypoxemia at the outset. The degree of all of the clinical signs depends on the extent of the pneumothorax. Symptoms of tension pneumothorax include increasing respiratory distress and cyanosis, bulging sternum, distended neck veins, elevated central venous pressure, and hypotension.

Central Nervous System Depression

The respiratory center is made up of groups of nerve cells that are scattered through the reticular formation in the medulla oblongata. This center is responsible for respiratory rhythm. Although this structure is the major respiratory control, the pons coordinates breathing. The respiratory neural structure in the pons is called the *pneumotaxic center*. Stimulation of this center increases respiratory frequency, while depression slows respiration. The apneustic center also modifies the respiratory pattern. Cranial or cerebral trauma or central nervous system (CNS) lesions, such as malignancies, brain abscesses, and other conditions, may result in injury to or impingement on the mediators of respiration and result in alterations of respiratory patterns.

If head injury affects the pneumotaxic center in the medulla, it may alter the rate, rhythm, and depth of respiration. Apnea may also occur. If CNS depression results because of trauma or disease, it frequently leads to decreased ventilatory drive, decreased responsiveness to ventilatory stimuli, and absence of the sigh mechanism. The result is a restrictive pathology that decreases total lung capacity [10].

Increasing intracranial pressure may lead to pressure on the respiratory center and change in breathing patterns, but more common is hypoxemia in obtunded individuals due to the acute restrictive disease. The airway reflexes are depressed, increasing the risk of obstruction and aspiration.

Neuromuscular Diseases

Many types of neuromuscular diseases may cause impairment of the respiratory system. The most common are summarized in Table 25-3. These can lead to an acute or chronic restrictive pulmonary process.

Guillain-Barré Syndrome

Guillain-Barré syndrome, which is named after the two persons who originally described it, is acute toxic polyneuritis. Typically, in its early stages it is mistaken for a flu syndrome. As it progresses, it is accompanied by varying degrees of muscular weakness and paralysis. This condition appears in some cases to result from an individual hypersensitivity response to a particular type of virus (see Chap. 49). It has been described as occurring after a wide variety of conditions, such as upper respiratory tract infection, mononucleosis, or it may have no antecedent event [9]. The respiratory muscles typically become involved, and death, if it occurs, is most frequently due to respiratory complications.

The pulmonary problems in Guillain-Barré syndrome are threefold. First, paralysis of the internal and external intercostal muscles reduces functional breathing ability. Breathing then becomes entirely diaphragmatic, leading to reduced tidal volume, hypoxemia, and hypercapnia [4]. Second, there is paralysis of the preganglionic fibers of the vagus nerve and of the postganglionic fibers of the sympathetic nervous system. Vagal paralysis causes loss of the normal protective mechanisms that respond to bronchial irritation, foreign bodies, and so on. The reflex bronchoconstriction is also lost. Paralysis of the sympathetic postganglionic fibers causes loss of bronchodilation. Third, the gag reflex is diminished or absent.

Pathologically, segmental loss of myelin sheath in the peripheral nerves may occur. Other body areas are also affected by paralysis, but this is not life-threatening. Even though the syndrome may last for a few weeks, recovery may be complete if respirations are adequately supported during the acute stage.

Clinical manifestations include the rapid onset of symmetric weakness beginning in the legs and moving upward. The muscles are flaccid, and sensory changes may or may not be present. Muscles of the pharynx and larynx may lead to impaired swallowing and gag reflexes. Cough reflex is depressed, and superimposed respiratory infection frequently occurs. Functional return is variable and usually progresses in a reverse pattern, with respiratory improvement occurring first, followed by functional improvement beginning in the upper extremities and finally in the lower extremities. Various types of residual impairment have been described.

TABLE 25-3 Neuromuscular Diseases Exhibiting Respiratory Insufficiency

Disease	Example
Spinal cord disease	Trauma
	Quadriplegia
	Paraplegia
	Poliomyelitis
Motor nerve disease	Acute idiopathic polyneuritis
	Guillain-Barré syndrome
	Landry's ascending paralysis
	Tick-bite paralysis
	Porphyria
Myoneural junction disease	Myasthenia gravis
	Myasthenic syndrome
Muscle-wasting disease	Muscular dystrophy
	Congenital myotonia
Infectious disease	Tetanus

Duchenne Muscular Dystrophy

The most common, rapidly progressive type of muscular dystrophy is Duchenne muscular dystrophy (DMD). Two types of the disease are described according to its progression: one form progresses rapidly and the other more slowly. Both forms of DMD are hereditary, being X-linked recessive. Women are the carriers and their sons tend to manifest the disorder (see Chap. 40).

Muscular weakness results, leading to difficulty walking in the early years of life. Thoracoscoliosis and respiratory muscle weakness then progress rapidly. The muscles seem to weaken in this order: intercostals, abdominals, diaphragm, and accessory muscles of respiration. Despite this respiratory impairment, studies show that alveolar hypoventilation occurs only as an acute or terminal event. As the severity of respiratory involvement increases, many patients are left with the use of only the accessory muscles of respiration. As a result, they may display unusual breathing patterns such as frog breathing, gulping air, head bobbing, and pursed-lip breathing. The final acute respiratory failure is often triggered by an acute respiratory infection [2].

Respiratory Diseases Caused by Exposure to Organic and Inorganic Dusts

Many organic and inorganic dusts have been identified as being injurious to the lungs. The group of diseases caused by these dusts are collectively called the *pneumoconioses*.

Silicosis

Silicosis is probably the best known and most severe of the industrial diseases. It results from inhalation of silicon dioxide. Workers with high silica exposure include masons, potters, sand blasters, and foundry workers.

The main characteristic of silicosis is fibrosis, which is manifested initially as hard nodules of about 1 mm in diameter in lung parenchyma that increase in size and coalesce as the disease progresses. It usually takes 20 years or more of exposure for silicosis to develop interstitial fibrosis and respiratory insufficiency [5].

Silicosis causes defects in the immune response, both humoral and cellular [5]. The reason for the defects is not known. It is believed that the silica particles cause lysis of the macrophages that ingest them [5]. Immune response may then be responsible for the development of the fibrotic lesion. Among the industrial inhalants, silica is particularly dangerous because of its effect on macrophages, allowing the fibrotic lesions to proceed unchecked. This causes a very severe restrictive pulmonary disease.

Coal Workers' Pneumoconiosis (Black Lung Disease)

The efficiency of alveolar clearing of coal dust was demonstrated by Davies [1]. He found that although miners may inhale 100 to 150 gm of dust per year, only 0.5 gm could be recovered at autopsy.

Most coal dust (carbon and silica) is removed by the alveolar macrophages, with the remainder accumulating in the macrophages. Over time, the dust-laden macrophages gather at the perivascular structures and local fibrosis ensues. Early in the disease the process is manifested as a restrictive process with progressive fibrosis. As the disease progresses, the respiratory bronchioles dilate as a result of traction created by the contracting fibrous tissue. Centrilobular emphysema ensues from the dilatation and destruction of the respiratory bronchioles. The walls of the bronchioles break down, forming single spaces. If exposure to coal dust continues, centrilobular emphysema may occur throughout the lungs. Panlobular or primary emphysema characterized by destruction of the alveoli rather than the more central respiratory bronchioles is not observed in relationship to dust inhalation.

A small percentage of those afflicted with simple pneumoconiosis due to silica or coal dust develop a more complicated form of the disease characterized by massive pulmonary fibrosis and chronic restrictive pulmonary disease. While it is generally accepted that simple pneumoconiosis is related to the quantity and composition of dust retained in the lungs, the etiology of complicated pneumoconiosis is not as clear. It has been suggested that the process involves an immunologic mechanism and that it results in the development of massive fibrotic lesions. In the past, the recovery of the tuberculosis bacillus from the lungs of miners with complicated pneumoconiosis led researchers to conclude that the bacillus was the mediator of the immunologic defense. This theory has not been substantiated, and the pathogenesis of the condition remains obscure.

Byssinosis (Brown Lung Disease)

Bronchoconstriction also occurs due to hypersensitivity to inorganic and organic dusts. An example is byssinosis, which results from long-term exposure to cotton dust. Cotton dust extracts have been shown to cause bronchoconstriction, and it is now believed that exposure leads to a discharge of naturally produced histamine, leading to bronchospasm. When histamine stores are depleted, reactivity to cotton dust decreases, which explains the dynamics of byssinosis.

Textile workers experienced chest tightness, low-grade fever, and dyspnea. The symptoms were more pronounced on Monday after a weekend away from the factory. Hence, the syndrome became known as *Monday fever*. Later in the week, the symptoms gradually disappeared. Researchers demonstrated that the textile workers had decreased ventilatory capacities and increased airway resistance during the Monday workday.

Because histamine stores are replenished over the weekend, exposure to the dust on Monday causes the histamine to be released. Histamine stores are depleted as the work week progresses, resulting in disappearance of symptoms and improved ventilatory capacity [16].

Asbestosis

Occupational exposure to asbestos has occurred in the mining, manufacturing, and application occupations. The main use of asbestos is in cement products for construction. The most important health-related effects from asbestos exposure are pulmonary fibrosis and tumors.

Particles of asbestos may be cleared by the mucociliary escalator system or, if deposited deep within the lung parenchyma, may be partially or completely engulfed by alveolar macrophages [3]. Some of the fibers may be removed through lymphatic circulation.

Diffuse pulmonary fibrosis resulting from asbestos exposure is termed *asbestosis*. The fibrosis initially affects the alveolar walls and gradually involves the interstitium. Prominent symptoms include exertional dyspnea, severe nonproductive cough, clubbing of the fingers, and ultimately, symptoms of respiratory failure [3]. Rales and restriction of lung inflation are common clinical findings. Pleural changes may be associated, and include hyaline plaques that undergo calcification. Recurrent exudative pleural effusions may also be associated.

Pulmonary Fibrosis

Pulmonary fibrosis is a chronic restrictive condition that involves diffuse fibrosis of the lung tissue and results in severe loss of compliance with lung stiffness. As indicated above, fibrosis is frequently due to occupational exposure to substances such as glass dusts, coal dusts, and other substances. In cases where the cause is unknown, the disease may be referred to as the *Hamman-Rich syndrome*, or unusual interstitial pneumonitis [11]. *Sarcoidosis* is another disease that includes among its features a severe, diffuse, pulmonary fibrosis. Severely decreased compliance and diffusing capacity may lead to hypoxemia and cor pulmonale.

Thoracic Deformity

Many chest deformities are not severe enough to compromise pulmonary status. Severe deformities do compress lung tissue in one or more areas of the chest, however, and may limit thoracic excursion. Severe *kyphoscoliosis*, in which the body is essentially twisted over to one side, is one example. Another is *pectus excavatum*, or funnel chest, in which the lower end of the sternum is caved in because of attachment to the spine by thick fibrous bands. *Pectus carinatum*, or pigeon breast, causes abnormal prominence of the sternum, and the rib structure may limit respiratory movement. Many other deformities also restrict pulmonary status.

In general, severe thoracic deformities compress portions of lung tissue and limit chest expansion, leading to areas of small lung volume and atelectasis. Compliance, total lung capacity, and other volume measurements are reduced. The pulmonary vascular bed in the affected areas is also reduced, resulting in increased work of breathing, alveolar hypoventilation, and the consequences of hypoxemia.

Because of the wide variety of deformities and their effects on pulmonary status, the pulmonary function of each affected person must be assessed carefully. Generally, the effect of pectus excavatum is not severe, while the effect of kyphoscoliosis varies from mild to very severe.

Obesity

Severe obesity results in restricted ventilation, especially in the supine position. The *Pickwickian syndrome*, or obesity hypoventilation syndrome, is related to morbid obesity and presents a picture of hypoventilation, somnolence, severe hypoxemia, polycythemia, and cor pulmonale [2]. The term comes from Charles Dickens's description of a fat man.

Severe obesity causes pulmonary restriction by two means. First, the extreme excess of adipose tissue in the abdomen tends to force the thoracic contents up into the chest and thus restricts diaphragmatic excursion. Second, the weight of the chest wall greatly increases the amount of work required to move the chest for inspiration. This is especially true for a woman with pendulous breasts. Severe obesity results in reduced compliance, expiratory reserve volume, total lung capacity, and vital capacity, with all of these reductions due to a great increase in the work of breathing and great susceptibility to respiratory infections. Arterial blood gas studies reveal hypercapnia and hypoxemia.

Severely affected individuals have depression of the ventilatory drive and may experience apneic episodes due to upper airway obstruction during sleep. Somnolence is characteristic and may be related to sleep deprivation that occurs as a result of frequent awakenings after the airway-obstruction episodes. Figure 25-12 shows the development of the Pickwickian syndrome.

Idiopathic Respiratory Distress Syndrome of the Newborn

Idiopathic respiratory distress syndrome of the newborn (IRDS) is the most clearly understood abnormality that involves surfactant deficiency. The surfactant layer develops late in fetal life, at about the twenty-eighth to the thirty-second week. Infants born before the twenty-eighth week are at a greater risk for developing acute respiratory distress, and this is still a major cause of death in premature infants. The severity of the respiratory distress and the mortality are related to gestational age at birth.

The pathology of IRDS includes inadequate pulmonary expansion and diffuse atelectasis, which is of a primary type because the lungs have never been expanded. Pul-

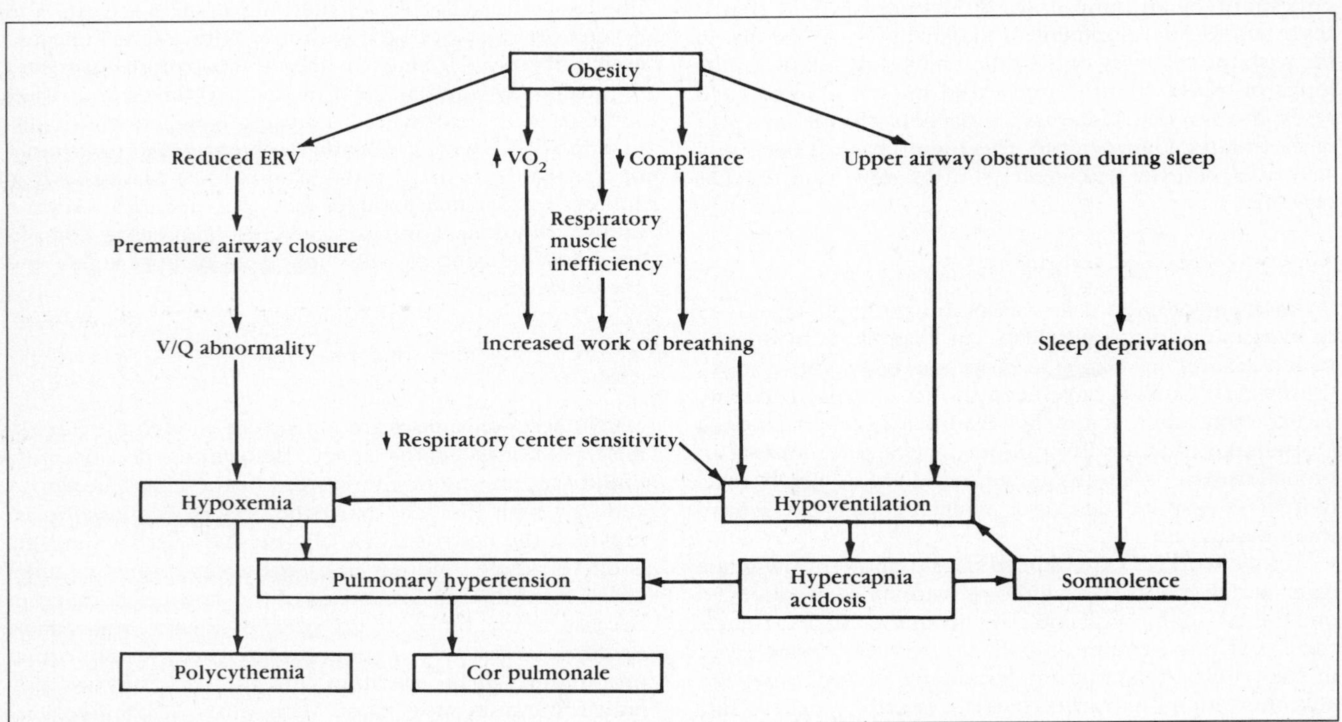

FIGURE 25-12 Pathogenesis and pathophysiology of obesity hypoventilation syndrome. (Reprinted from S. Farzan, *A Concise Handbook of Respiratory Disease,* 1978, Figure 22-4, pp. 223–224. Reprinted with permission of Reston Publishing Co., Simon & Schuster Professional Information Group, 25 Van Zant St., E. Norwalk, CT 06855.)

monary vascular resistance increases because of high pulmonary arterial pressures, presumably due to increased pulmonary arteriolar resistance. The resulting increased pressure creates a higher than normal pressure on the right side of the heart. This high pressure perpetuates fetal circulation by keeping the foramen ovale and the ductus arteriosus patent. The IRDS, or hyaline membrane disease, is characterized by large right-to-left shunting that accentuates hypoxemia and hypercapnia in later stages and is increased by hypoxemia, which leads to increased right heart pressures. Ischemic injury in the lung fields causes fluid to leak into interstitial and alveolar spaces and the hyaline membrane to form. Vascular engorgement occurs, the lymphatics dilate, and cellular debris lines the alveoli, with evidence of degenerating epithelial and endothelial cells in the alveolocapillary membrane. The hyaline membranes are apparently composed of plasma, fibrin, necrotic epithelial cells, and amniotic fluid, and contribute to the respiratory distress [5]. Atelectasis is extensive, with widespread infiltration of the pulmonary tissue [2].

Clinical manifestations include dyspnea from the first moments of life and rapid, shallow respirations. The lower ribs retract on inspiration and an expiratory grunt usually is heard. Hypoxemia is characteristic, and an elevated PCO_2 with respiratory and/or metabolic acidosis may complicate the picture.

Treatment measures are improving the prognosis in this condition. Continuous positive airway pressure (CPAP) is used with good results to improve oxygenation, but the condition still carries about 50 percent mortality.

Table 25-4 Underlying Causes That Can Precipitate Adult Respiratory Distress Syndrome (ARDS)

Reduced perfusion
Cardiogenic shock
Trauma
Major burns
Fat embolus
Hemorrhage
Severe hypovolemia
Increased capillary permeability
Sepsis
Pneumonia
Noxious fume or smoke inhalation
Reactions to drugs
Venoms or toxins
Immune complex diseases
Overtransfusion of crystalloids
Uremia
Direct tissue and capillary insults
Aspiration of GI contents
Rapid decompression
Near-drowning
Oxygen toxicity
Hypoxemia
Fluid overload
Starvation
Other mechanisms, not well understood
High-altitude reactions
Sudden changes in intrathoracic pressure
Central nervous system injuries
Narcotic overdose
Cardiopulmonary bypass

Adult Respiratory Distress Syndrome

The adult respiratory distress syndrome (ARDS) is a condition characterized by severe hypoxemia and progressive loss of lung compliance. It causes severe restrictive disease. It is known by a number of other names, including shock lung, traumatic wet lung, capillary leak syndrome, postperfusion lung, congestive atelectasis, and posttraumatic pulmonary insufficiency.

This syndrome is never a primary disease but occurs secondary to some other insult to the body. General etiologic factors have been identified and classified as to the mechanism of causation (Table 25-4). The following categories are described: (1) reduced perfusion, (2) increased capillary permeability, (3) direct tissue and capillary insults, and (4) others, with obscure mechanisms. The causes of ARDS are many, but all result in essentially the same pathologic process.

The effects of ARDS are similar despite the initiating underlying condition (Fig. 25-13). The insult leads to capillary congestion and consequent alteration of capillary permeability. Endothelial cell damage occurs, as does malfunction of the type II pneumocytes. The activity of these cells decreases, which results in decreased production of surfactant. Fluid leaks into the pulmonary interstitium and eventually into the alveoli. This causes stiffening of the lungs (loss of compliance) and dilution of surfactant. The altered compliance and diluted surfactant work together to lead to widespread atelectasis, which causes hypoxemia. In addition, there may be pulmonary interstitial edema and hemorrhage, the formation of alveolar exudate or hyaline membrane, and a predisposition to secondary pulmonary infection. Widespread atelectasis leads to an increased right-to-left shunt across the pulmonary capillary bed, causing critical hypoxemia.

A special pulmonary pathophysiologic process has been described in individuals exposed to high levels of oxygen for more than 24 to 36 hours. Continuous breathing of high concentrations of oxygen leads to *oxygen toxicity*, with diffuse parenchymal damage resulting in interference with the production of surfactant and formation of hemorrhagic exudate, with fibrin in the alveoli, alveolar ducts, and respiratory bronchioles. The earliest change is thickening of interstitial spaces with fluid containing fibrin, polymorphonuclear leukocytes, and macrophages. Two special processes explain the resulting dysfunction. First, breathing pure oxygen results in absorption of the gas from the alveoli. Nitrogen, normally present in atmospheric gas, is not present under these circumstances and therefore does not exert its function of keeping the alveoli expanded. The result is alveolar collapse. Second, oxygen has a toxic effect on the surfactant-producing cells so that this vital substance is not produced in adequate quantities; without adequate surfactant the alveoli collapse and fluid exudes from the capillaries to the alveolar sacs [8].

The results of ARDS are progressive hypoxemia and reduced lung compliance, despite the administration of

1985

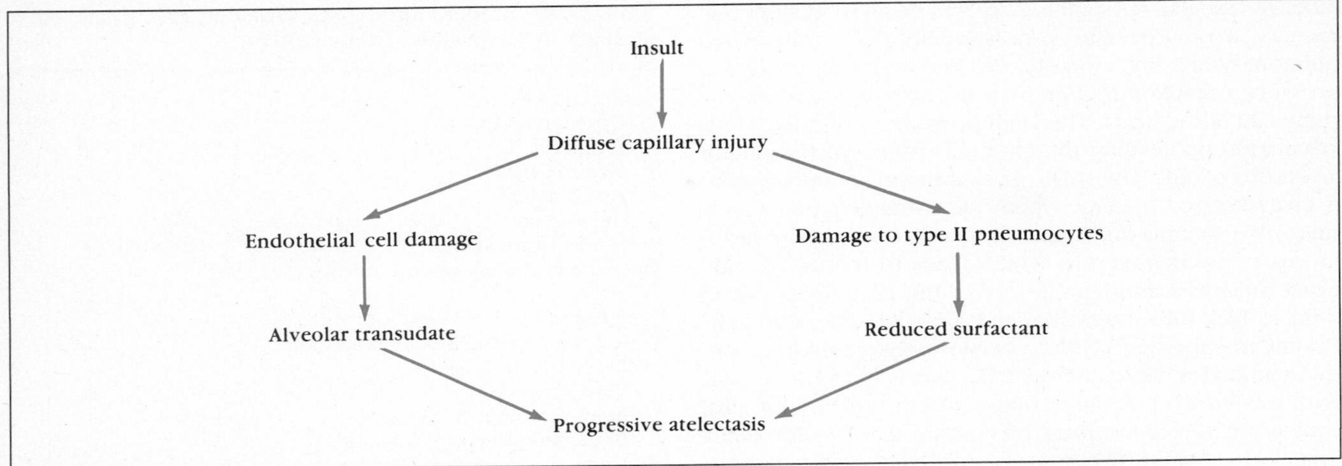

FIGURE 25-13 Simplified pathogenesis of adult respiratory distress syndrome (ARDS).

high levels of oxygen. Any individual whose oxygen tension decreases while receiving high concentrations of oxygen should be considered a prime candidate for ARDS.

Those at a high risk for ARDS should be observed for onset of the condition throughout the first 96 hours after insult. No previous history of lung disease may be obtained, but persons with previous lung pathology are somewhat more susceptible to development of ARDS. Obvious observable symptoms include extreme dyspnea, tachypnea and grunting, and labored respirations that occur late in the phenomenon. Therefore, the arterial blood gases of persons who develop the disease indicate decreasing PO_2 despite oxygen therapy. If the arterial PO_2 is not correctable to above 50 when a person is receiving 100 percent oxygen, there should be a high index of suspicion for this condition. Usually, clinical deterioration is rapid and progressive. Hemoptysis and cyanosis may or may not occur. The hypoxemia and increased work of breathing may initially lead to metabolic acidosis. As respiratory muscles tire, respiratory acidosis occurs. Chest films show progressive, patchy, bilateral infiltrates. The prognosis for affected individuals is improving with the use of positive end-expiratory pressure on volume-cycled ventilators, but it still remains at or above 50 percent [13].

Study Questions

1. Explain the ventilation-perfusion abnormalities in atelectasis. How does a right to left shunt across the pulmonary capillary bed develop?
2. Using pneumococcal pneumonia as an example, describe the pathophysiology of pulmonary infection. How does the inherent defense system in the lungs prevent systemic infection?
3. How does the body react to primary infection with the tuberculosis bacilli?
4. Compare the results of different types of pulmonary aspiration.
5. How do the clinical pictures of interstitial and alveolar pulmonary edema differ?
6. Discuss restrictive pulmonary disease that can be caused by environmental pollution.
7. Describe the process for development of ARDS. List some similarities of precipitating factors.

References

1. Davies, C.N. A comparison between inhaled dust and the dust recovered from human lungs. *Health Phys.* 10:129, 1964.
2. Farzan, S. *A Concise Handbook of Respiratory Diseases* (2nd ed.). Reston, Va.: Reston Pub., 1985.
3. Fishman, A.P. *Pulmonary Diseases and Disorders Update*. New York: McGraw-Hill, 1982.
4. Kealy, S.L. Respiratory care in Guillain-Barré syndrome. *Am. J. Nurs.* 1:59, 1977.
5. Kuhn, C., and Askin, F.B. Lung and mediastinum. In J.M. Kissane, *Anderson's Pathology* (8th ed.). St. Louis: Mosby, 1985.
6. MacDonnell, K., and Segal, M. *Current Respiratory Care*. Boston: Little, Brown, 1977.
7. Niederman, M.S., and Fein, A.M. Pneumonia in the elderly. *Clin. Geriatric Med.* 2:241, 1986.
8. Pierce, A. Oxygen toxicity. *Basics Respir. Dis.* 1:5, 1975.
9. Robbins, S.L., Cotran, R.S., and Kumar, V. *Pathologic Basis of Disease* (3rd ed.). Philadelphia: Saunders, 1984.
10. Shapiro, B., et al. *Clinical Application of Respiratory Care* (3rd ed.). Chicago: Yearbook, 1985.
11. Sodeman, W.A., and Sodeman, T.M. *Sodeman's Pathologic Physiology* (7th ed.). Philadelphia: Saunders, 1985.
12. Stauffer, J.L., and Carbone, J.E. Pulmonary diseases. In M.A. Krupp et al., *Current Medical Diagnosis and Treatment 1986*. Los Altos, Calif.: Lange, 1986.
13. Surveyer, J. Smoke inhalation injuries. *Heart Lung* 9:825, 1980.
14. West, J. *Pulmonary Pathophysiology: The Essentials* (2nd ed.). Baltimore: Williams & Wilkins, 1982.
15. West, J. *Respiratory Physiology: The Essentials* (3rd ed.). Baltimore: Williams & Wilkins, 1985.
16. Ziskind, M. Occupational pulmonary disease. *Clin. Symp.* 30:4, 1978.

CHAPTER 26

Obstructive Alterations in Pulmonary Function

CHAPTER OUTLINE

Acute Obstructive Airway Disease

- Acute Bronchitis
- Asthma
  - *Pathophysiologic Mechanisms*
  - *Clinical Manifestations*

Chronic Obstructive Pulmonary Disease

- Bronchiectasis
- Cystic Fibrosis (Mucoviscidosis)
- Chronic Bronchitis
- Pulmonary Emphysema
  - *Pathophysiology*
  - *Clinical Manifestations*

LEARNING OBJECTIVES

1. Define *obstructive pulmonary disease*.
2. Differentiate between acute and chronic bronchitis.
3. Describe the pathophysiology of an acute asthmatic attack.
4. List two factors that precipitate an asthma attack.
5. List and describe the symptoms that result from bronchoconstriction.
6. Define *pulsus paradoxus*.
7. List the conditions that are classified as chronic obstructive pulmonary disease (COPD).
8. Define the pathology of bronchiectasis.
9. Describe the signs and symptoms of bronchiectasis.
10. Discuss the basis for the development of cystic fibrosis.
11. List the pathologic features of cystic fibrosis.
12. List the criteria used in diagnosing cystic fibrosis.
13. List at least two risk factors in the development of chronic bronchitis.
14. Describe the pathophysiology of chronic bronchitis.
15. Differentiate chronic bronchitis from emphysema on the basis of pathologic and clinical features.
16. Relate similarities of chronic bronchitis and emphysema.
17. Describe the interrelationships of all the obstructive pulmonary diseases.
18. Describe the pathology of the different types of emphysema.
19. Discuss the pathophysiologic course of emphysema.
20. Define *hypoxia*, *hypoxemia*, and *hypercapnia*.
21. Explain why polycythemia occurs with chronic obstructive pulmonary disease.
22. Differentiate between compensated and uncompensated respiratory acidosis.

In general, obstructive pulmonary conditions obstruct airflow within the lungs, leading to less resistance to inspiration and more resistance to expiration. This results in prolongation of the expiratory phase of respiration. Many conditions can obstruct airflow; the more prominent ones are detailed in this chapter.

Acute Obstructive Airway Disease

The classification of an acute obstructive airway disease is dependent on the episodic nature of the condition. The two major entities in this classification are acute bronchitis and asthma. In both, the obstruction is intermittent and reversible.

Acute Bronchitis

Acute bronchitis is a common condition caused by infection and inhalants that results in inflammation of the mucosal lining of the tracheobronchial tree. The most common infectious causes of acute bronchitis include influenza viruses, adenoviruses, rhinoviruses, and the organism *Mycoplasma pneumoniae*. Increased mucus secretion, bronchial swelling, and dysfunction of the cilia lead to increased resistance to expiratory airflow, usually resulting in some air trapping on expiration.

Bronchitis causes cough and production of large amounts of usually purulent mucus with associated wheezing if there is significant air obstruction. Coughing that produces purulent material may indicate a superimposed bacterial infection if the underlying etiology was viral. Once the stimulus for bronchitis is treated or removed, bronchial swelling decreases and the airways return to normal.

Asthma

Asthma is an episodic, acute airway obstruction that results from stimuli that would not elicit such a response in healthy individuals. It has been defined as a disorder characterized by recurrent paroxysms of wheezing and dyspnea that are not attributable to underlying cardiac or other disease. This means that the person with asthma has a tendency toward bronchospasm as a response to a variety of stimuli. The common characteristic of all asthmatic reactions is hyperreactivity of the airways. Between acute attacks, the lungs are usually normal or relatively normal.

While asthma is characterized by wheezing, not all wheezing is asthma. Unilateral localized wheezing may be caused by aspiration of foreign bodies or by a tumor. Other causes include pulmonary emboli, infections, left ventricular failure, cystic fibrosis, immunologic deficiency, and viral respiratory illnesses.

Pathophysiologic Mechanisms. The causes of asthma may be divided into two major categories: extrinsic and intrinsic.

Extrinsic asthma commonly affects the child or young teenager who frequently relates a personal and/or family history of allergy, hives, rashes, and eczema. Results of skin tests are usually positive for specific allergens, indicating the probability that extrinsic asthma is allergic.

Childhood asthma attacks are usually self-limited and frequently are precipitated by exposure to specific antigens. It is not uncommon for the person who "outgrows" asthma in childhood to develop other allergic manifestations in adulthood. Usually, the asthmatic attacks decrease in severity and frequency as the person matures.

The pathophysiology of asthma attacks is related to the release of chemical mediators in an IgE-mast cell interaction (see Chap. 12). This results in constriction of the bronchial smooth muscle, increased bronchial secretion from the goblet cells, and mucosal swelling, all of which lead to significant narrowing of the air passages [2]. It is basically an IgE-associated immune reaction in which the allergen evokes immediate production of histamine and other chemicals by the target organ, which is the lung [11]. The acute respiratory obstruction, resistance to airflow and turbulence of airflow are due to the following three responses: (1) bronchospasm, which involves rhythmic squeezing of the airways by the muscle bands surrounding them; (2) production of abnormally large amounts of thick mucus; and (3) the inflammatory response, including increased capillary permeability and mucosal edema (Fig. 26-1).

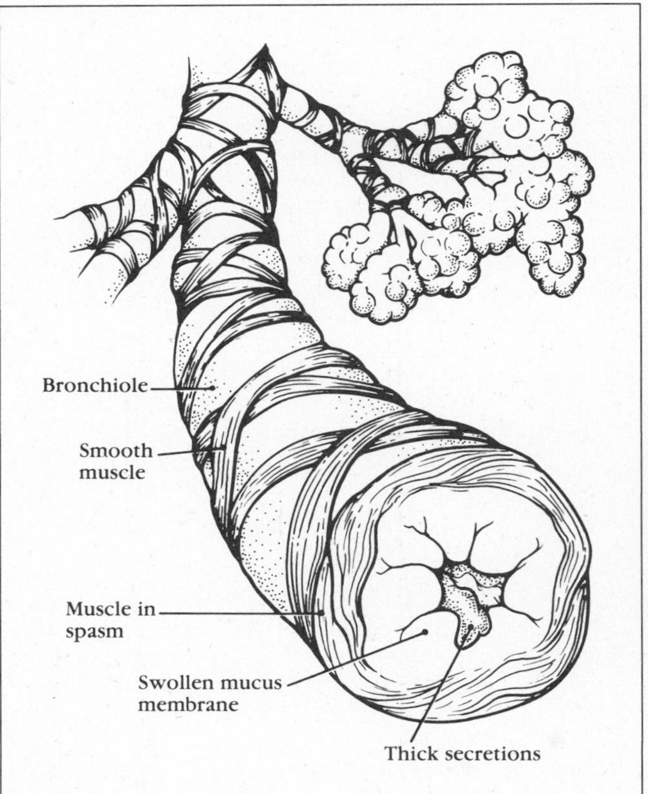

FIGURE 26-1 Bronchial asthma. The bronchiole is obstructed on expiration, particularly by muscle spasm, edema of the mucosa, and thick secretions.

Allergy alone as a basis for the attacks is rare, and many mechanisms may be involved. Whatever the mechanisms, once bronchospasm is induced by one agent, the airway response to superimposed stimuli is greatly enhanced. For example, if a person with a subclinical response to pollen becomes emotionally upset, the airway response to the emotions may be greatly magnified because of the pollen sensitivity already established. It is important to note that, without a tendency toward bronchospasm, emotions, pollen, or other substances do not produce asthma.

Intrinsic asthma usually affects adults, including those who did not have asthma or allergy prior to middle adulthood. The family history for allergy, eczema, hives, and rashes is usually negative. Attacks are most often related to infection of the respiratory tract or to exercise; emotion, allergy, and other factors also may play a part.

In either type, respiratory infection may be a major precipitator of a severe asthma attack. Both bacterial and viral infections may precipitate the attack, but viruses seem to be more important in this respect.

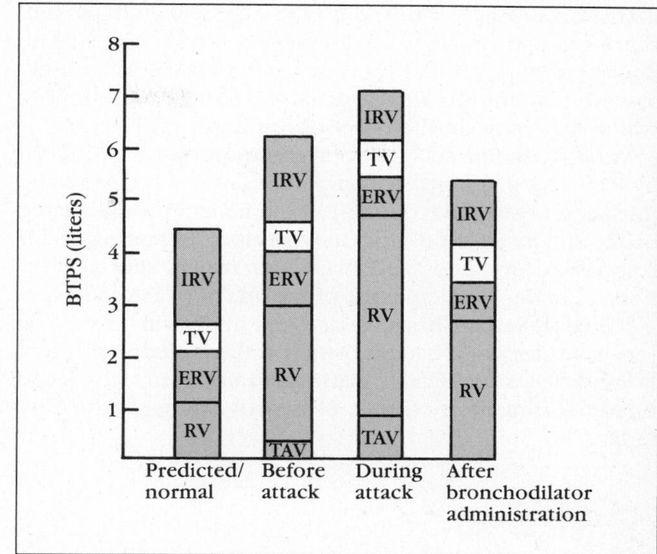

FIGURE 26-2 Pulmonary function before, during, and after an asthma attack. The normal values are indicated as predicted values: inspiratory reserve volume (IRV), tidal volume (TV), expiratory reserve volume (ERV). Before the attack there is a small volume of trapped air (TAV) with a larger than usual residual volume (RV). During the attack the residual volume increases dramatically. After bronchodilator therapy the trapped air volume and residual volume decrease markedly.

Clinical Manifestations. The signs and symptoms of an asthmatic attack are closely related to the status of the airways. Bronchospasm leads to both obstruction of the airways and air trapping. Air trapping is probably due to the acute increase in expiratory flow resistance, which means that the inspired air simply cannot be exhaled in the time available before metabolic demands trigger another inspiration. As a result, a portion of each breath is retained. The hyperinflated alveoli exert lateral traction on the bronchiolar walls so that inspiratory airway diameter is further increased. This may aid slightly in gas exchange, but it requires more inspiratory energy to overcome the tension of the already stretched elastic tissue.

The pressure of the trapped air tends to flatten the diaphragm's ability to function as the major organ of respiration and may oppose expansion of the lower chest. The costal fibers that are attached to the lower ribs are pulled into a horizontal rather than upright position. They can no longer move up and out, so the lower chest cannot expand normally. With the flat, fixed diaphragm, the accessory muscles are called on to enlarge the chest with each inspiration. This increases energy cost and also causes increased inflation of the apices rather than the bases. Figure 26-2 shows characteristic pulmonary function studies before, during, and after therapy for an acute asthmatic attack.

Wheezing, a common sign, can be likened to pulling on the opening of a balloon full of air to make it squeak. The smaller the opening past which the air is rushing, the more squeaking occurs. In the chest, wheezing results from air squeezing past the greatly narrowed airways. Narrowing is caused by bronchospasm plus mucosal edema and obstructive secretions. Since the airways are normally smaller on expiration, expiratory wheezing occurs first. As the attack progresses, wheezing is both inspiratory and expiratory. Wheezes are *adventitious lung sounds*, which are musical, louder than the underlying sounds, and continuous. They are often described as *expiratory* or *inspiratory* to indicate the phase of respiration in which they are loudest [1].

Pulsus paradoxus, or paradoxic pulse, is an objective measurement of bronchospasm. The amplitude of the arterial pulse normally decreases with inspiration and is produced by the pooling of blood in the pulmonary vessels. Due to respiratory distress in the asthmatic attack, the amount of pooling apparently increases.

The paradoxic pulse is an exaggeration of normal, with a fall of arterial blood pressure more than 10 mm Hg on inspiration [9]. It is measured by pumping up the blood pressure cuff to above the systolic pressure and lowering the pressure very slowly while the person breathes quickly. If a paradoxic pulse is present, Korotkoff's sounds become audible first during expiration and then during all phases of respiration [2]. The point at which all beats are equally loud is recorded as the bottom of the paradoxic pulse.

Paradoxic pulse is recorded as follows:

$$\frac{140 - 120}{60}$$

The point at which beats can be heard on expiration = 140; the point at which all beats are equally loud = 120; and the diastolic pressure = 60. Therefore, the example pulsus paradoxus is 20. The normal is less than 8 mm Hg. Assessment of pulsus paradoxus can help to evaluate the severity of airway obstruction [2].

Fatigue is a major problem in an acute asthma attack. The increased work of breathing leads to increased oxygen consumption until a point is reached at which the individual begins to tire and is no longer able to hyperventilate enough to meet the increased oxygen need. The degree of hypoventilation that results can be accurately assessed by monitoring arterial carbon dioxide levels, which may indicate the onset of respiratory failure.

A large amount of yellow or green sputum is produced by the bronchial mucosa in an asthma attack. It tends to be thick and obstructive due to its volume and the associated bronchoconstriction and dehydration. Inflammation is responsible for mucosal edema, which may be due to infection, a common precipitator of the attack (Table 26-1).

Once the attack has subsided and underlying precipitators have cleared, the lungs usually return to normal. There is, however, a significant relationship between asthma and the development of chronic obstructive lung disease later in life.

Chronic Obstructive Pulmonary Disease

Chronic obstructive pulmonary disease (COPD) is the fifth leading cause of death in the United States, with mortality that has nearly tripled in the last 30 years [5]. Chronic obstructive lung diseases (COLD) are similar to asthma in that expiratory airflow is obstructed and exacerbations and remissions are common. The acute and chronic obstructive diseases differ in that the lung tissues do not return to normal between exacerbations in the chronic conditions. Instead, pulmonary damage is a slowly progressive process.

The abbreviations COPD and COLD refer to a group of conditions associated with chronic obstruction to airflow within the lungs. Usually they refer to emphysema or chronic bronchitis, but they may include inflammation of the small bronchi, bronchiectasis, and cystic fibrosis. Asthma, considered in this chapter as an acute obstructive condition, is also often grouped with the chronic conditions. Of these diseases, the obstruction of chronic bronchitis, bronchiectasis, and cystic fibrosis chiefly results from secretions, while that in emphysema is anatomic. Pneumoconiosis is often classified with chronic obstructive diseases, but because of its underlying pathogenesis, it is discussed in Chapter 25.

Bronchiectasis

Bronchiectasis is a chronic disease of the bronchi and bronchioles characterized by irreversible dilatation of the bronchial tree and associated with chronic infection and inflammation of these passageways. It is usually preceded by respiratory infection, especially bronchopneumonia, that causes the bronchial mucosa to be replaced by fibrous scar tissue. This process leads to destruction of the bronchi and permanent dilatation of the bronchi and bronchioles, which allows the areas affected to be targets for a chronic, smoldering infection (Fig. 26-3).

This disease affects all ages and both sexes, often with onset in childhood. Usually the initiating event is an infection, such as pneumonia or bronchitis. It is not known whether the condition begins as an infection or if it is due to abnormal structure of the bronchial walls [2]. It frequently is asymptomatic, but may progress until it is disabling or life-threatening.

The lower lobes are the most vulnerable and usually are filled with a yellow-green, infected material that may spread to the pleural cavity. It may or may not be associated with an acute inflammatory exudate with bronchial ulceration or abscess [7].

The common symptoms are cough and symptoms of infection. The person raises large amounts of mucopurulent sputum and occasionally experiences hemoptysis.

Cystic Fibrosis (Mucoviscidosis)

Cystic fibrosis is a hereditary disorder in which large quantities of viscous material are secreted. It affects the sweat glands, bronchi, pancreas, and mucus-secreting glands of the small intestine (see Chap. 35). It may arise shortly after birth, in childhood, and in early adulthood.

TABLE 26-1 Symptoms of Asthma and Underlying Pathophysiology

Pathophysiology	Symptoms
Bronchospasm Air trapping Diaphragmatic flattening	Dyspnea; orthopnea; coughing; wheezing; chest tightness; elevated paradoxical pulse; tripod position; reduced breath sounds; hyperresonance
Increased work of breathing Fatigue Increased oxygen consumption	Tachycardia; labored breathing; air hunger; intercostal retractions
Increased sputum production Dehydration	Thick, sticky sputum; poor skin turgor; other signs of dehydration
Infection	Thick green or yellow sputum
Inflammation	Bronchospasm, eosinophilia if allergy present
Anxiety	Apprehension/panic

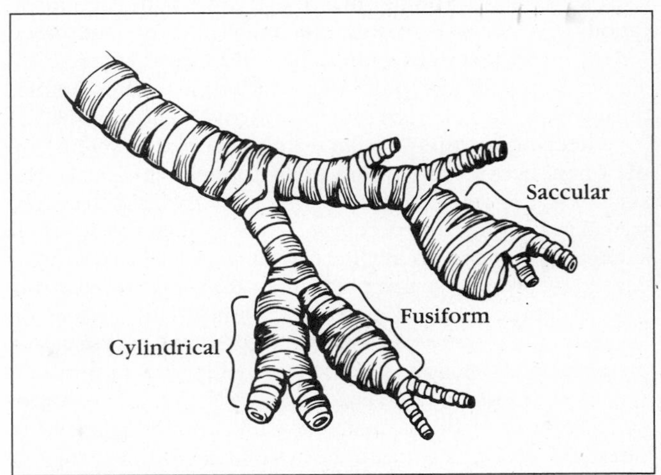

FIGURE 26-3 Various types of bronchiectasis; the morphology varies.

The pathologic features include a high concentration of sodium and chloride in the sweat, and abnormal mucus secretion and elimination. Secretion of tenacious mucus throughout the airways produces airway obstruction that leads to various combinations of atelectasis, pneumonia, bronchitis, emphysema, and other respiratory conditions. Secondary bacterial infection is common.

Associated pancreatic insufficiency causes abnormal stools, malnutrition, and abdominal distention. Intestinal obstruction is common in the neonate.

The clinical manifestations are variable, with some individuals having mainly gastrointestinal symptoms and others developing severe pulmonary problems. All of the manifestations relate to inability to handle excessive secretions. Pulmonary signs and symptoms are very common, and include chronic cough, persistent lung infections, chronic obstructive lung disease, and cor pulmonale.

To diagnose the disease, at least three of the following four criteria are essential [7]:

1. Increased sodium and chloride in the sweat
2. Deficient pancreatic enzymes in the gastrointestinal secretions
3. Chronic pulmonary infections, especially with opportunistic organisms such as *Pseudomonas aeruginosa* and *Staphylococcus aureus*
4. Family history of the problem

The prognosis is variable, with survival past age 20 years increasing. Gastrointestinal and pulmonary problems are encountered throughout life.

Chronic Bronchitis

Continued bronchial inflammation and progressive increase in productive cough and dyspnea not attributable to specific causes are classic features of chronic bronchitis. Usually, the inflammation and cough are responses of the bronchial mucosa to chronic irritation [5].

Pathophysiologically, thickening and rigidity of the bronchial mucosa result from vasodilatation, congestion, and edema. The mucosal areas may be infiltrated with lymphocytes, macrophages, and polymorphonuclear leukocytes. Excessive secretion plus narrowing of the passageways causes obstruction first to maximal expiration and later to maximal inspiratory airflow [8]. Bacteria, especially *Hemophilus influenzae* and *Streptococcus pneumoniae*, are often cultured from the airways [5].

This bronchitis is closely related to emphysema but is usually defined as an abnormality that involves excessive secretion of mucus and bronchial inflammation, while emphysema involves degeneration of the alveolar parenchyma. Bronchitis is closely related to cigarette smoking and/or other environmental pollutants, and may lead to the following: (1) increased airway resistance with or without emphysematous changes, (2) right heart failure (cor pulmonale), and (3) dysplasia of the respiratory epithelial cells, which may undergo malignant change [7,12].

The clinical manifestations include cyanosis, copious production of sputum, mild degrees of hyperinflation, marked hypercapnia, and severe hypoxemia. Heart failure with manifestations of right-sided failure occurs as the disease progresses. These manifestations include jugular venous distention, cardiac enlargement, liver engorgement, and peripheral edema. Bronchitic persons have often been called "blue bloaters" because of the presence of marked cyanosis and edema. The clinical picture varies depending on the amount of associated emphysema. Table 26-2 compares the clinical and physiologic features of the two conditions. Bronchitis and emphysema rarely occur in isolation from each other, and some mixture of clinical signs and symptoms is usually present.

Pulmonary Emphysema

Emphysema is the most common chronic pulmonary disease and is frequently classified with chronic bronchitis

TABLE 26-2 Features That Distinguish Bronchial and Emphysematous Types of Chronic Obstructive Lung Disease

	Bronchial	Emphysematous
Clinical features		
History	Often recurrent chest infections	Often only insidious dyspnea
Chest exam	Noisy chest, slight overdistention	Quiet chest, marked overdistention
Sputum	Frequently copious and purulent	Usually scanty and mucoid
Weight loss	Absent or slight	Often marked
Chronic cor pulmonale	Common	Infrequent
Roentgenogram	Often evidence of old inflammatory disease	Often attenuated vessels and radiolucency
General appearance	"Blue bloater"	"Pink puffer"
Physiologic tests		
Lung volumes		
TLC	Normal or slightly decreased	Increased
RV	Moderately increased	Markedly increased
RV/TLC	High	High
Lung compliance		
Static	Normal or low	High
Dynamic	Very low	Normal or low
Airways resistance		
Expiratory	Very high	High
Inspiratory	High	Normal
Diffusing capacity	Variable	Low
Chronic hypoxemia	Often severe	Usually mild
Chronic hypercapnia	Common	Unusual
Pulmonary hypertension	Often severe	Usually mild
Cardiac output	Normal	Often low

Source: B. Burrows, R.J., et al, *Respiratory Insufficiency.* (2nd ed.) Chicago: Yearbook, 1983.

because of the simultaneous occurrence of the two conditions. In anatomic terms, emphysema involves the portion of lungs distal to a terminal bronchiole (*acinus*) where gas exchange takes place. Emphysema results in permanent, abnormal enlargement of the acinus with associated destructive changes [7]. It may be classified as *vesicular* when it involves the spaces distal to the terminal bronchioles and *interlobular*, or *interstitial*, when it affects the tissue between the air spaces [5]. The common term *pulmonary emphysema* usually designates the vesicular type.

Pathophysiology. Emphysema seems to be due to many separate injuries that occur over a long period of time. Prevalence and severity are greatest in elderly individuals [6]. The elastin and fiber network of the alveoli and airways is broken down. The alveoli enlarge and many of their walls are destroyed. Alveolar destruction leads to the formation of larger than normal air spaces, or pools, which greatly reduce the alveolar diffusing surface. Once the process begins, it progresses slowly and inconsistently. Alveolar destruction also undermines the support structure for the airways, making them more vulnerable to expiratory collapse. There may be associated airway inflammation and consequent increase in mucus production, although many persons with emphysema produce little or no sputum.

The exact mechanism of injury is yet to be determined. Ischemia may cause alveolar breakdown, although specific vascular lesions have not been found [4,10]. Repeated injuries from smoking, infection, and air pollution often lead to emphysema, but the exact mechanism of injury has not been identified.

Specific types of emphysema have been shown to be related to a deficiency in the enzyme *alpha$_1$-antitrypsin*, which inhibits the proteases of elastase and collagenase. These proteases are normally major contributors to tissue destruction during the inflammatory process. Without the inhibition of alpha$_1$-antitrypsin, the destruction or digestion of pulmonary tissue occurs, more at the bases than at the apices of the lungs. This circumstance leads to the onset of severe obstructive lung disease early in adult life, often before age 40 years [10]. The onset of hypoxia and cor pulmonale in these persons heralds a poor prognosis.

The types of emphysema have been classified according to the area of lung affected; that is, classification is anatomic, and may describe lobules or acini (Table 26-3 and Table 26-4). Many types of emphysema can only be classified with certainty by autopsy report. Pulmonary interstitial emphysema is an associated condition that involves overdistention of the alveoli and dissection of air into the perivascular spaces. The dissection may continue into the mediastinum, causing *pneumomediastinum*, or into the pleural cavity, causing *pneumothorax*. Figure 26-4 illustrates the appearance of alveoli in the main types of emphysema.

Emphysema has a major effect on compliance and elasticity. The major abnormality is loss of *elastic recoil* [5]. Because alveolar walls are destroyed, fibrous and muscle tissues are lost, making the lungs more distensible. Even in severe disease, inspiratory airway resistance tends to be normal. Air trapping occurs because of loss of elastic recoil, which increases airway size on inspiration and causes collapse of the small airways on expiration. Thus, a minor obstruction on inspiration is a serious obstruction on expiration. If expiration is forced, a sharp rise in pressure on the airways leads to compression of the bronchi and bronchioles. The resultant distention eventually leads to disruption in the alveolar walls and surrounding musculoelastic tissue around the small airways. Figure 26-5 illustrates the difference between normal alveoli and distended alveoli of emphysema. The loss of gas-exchanging surface with associated vascular changes results in decreased diffusion capacities [5].

TABLE 26-3 Classification of Emphysema

Classification	Description
Diffuse or generalized	Lobules or acini through affected lung
Focal	Associated with focal dust deposition (e.g., coal dust)
Irregular	Associated with shrinkage of fibrotic scars, usually from old disease
Obstructive	Accompanied by demonstrable bronchial obstruction
Bulla	Emphysematous space of more than 1 cm in an inflated lung; may occur in any type of emphysema

TABLE 26-4 Lobular and Acinar Terminology of Emphysema

Lobules	Acini
Panlobular: All lung affected; diffuse throughout lung	Panacinar: Whole acinus affected; diffuse throughout lung
Centrilobular: Spaces around central bronchioles affected; usually affects apices	Centriacinar: Area around alveolar ducts affected; usually affects apices
Periseptal: Occurs at periphery of lobule; less common than above types	Periacinar: Occurs at periphery of acinus; less common than above types
Irregular: Scarring throughout the acinus irregularly	

Clinical Manifestations. The clinical manifestations of emphysema are usually absent in the early stages and very insidious in onset. They may overlap with those of bronchitis. The person with emphysema has often been called the "pink puffer" on the basis of appearance. Dyspnea is characteristic; in the early stages it occurs with exertion and later progresses to dyspnea at rest. Severe hyperinflation of the lungs may lead to increased anteroposterior chest diameter, resulting in the typical barrel chest. Dorsal kyphosis, prominent anterior chest, and elevated ribs all contribute to this appearance (Fig. 26-6). The accessory muscles are used to raise the thorax on

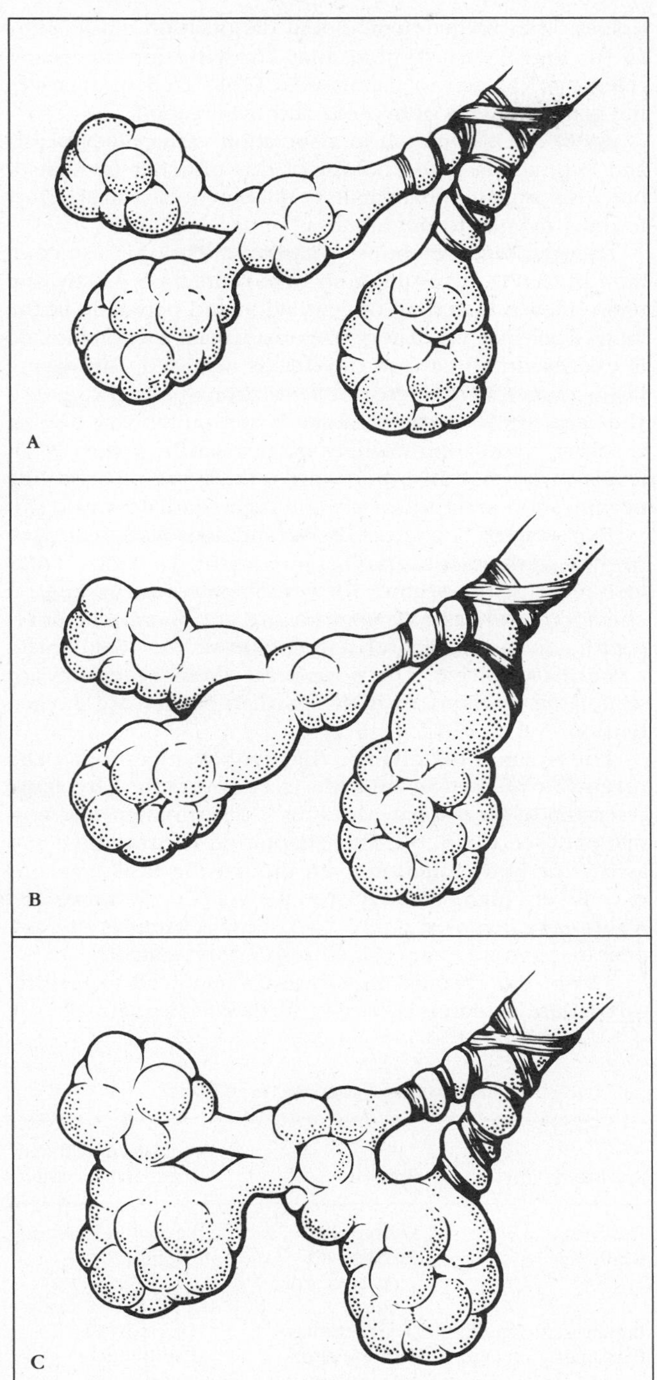

FIGURE 26-4 Alterations in alveolar structure. A. Normal respiratory bronchioles and alveoli. B. Centrilobular emphysema—dilation of the respiratory bronchioles. C. Panlobular emphysemal—destruction of the alveolar walls.

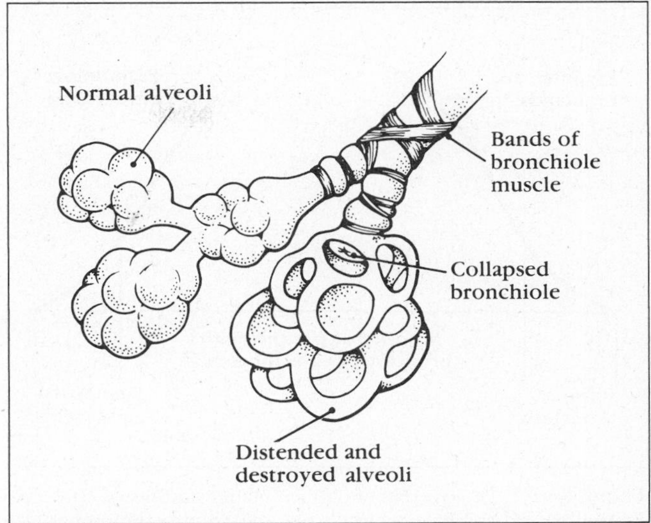

FIGURE 26-5 Distended and destroyed alveoli versus normal ones.

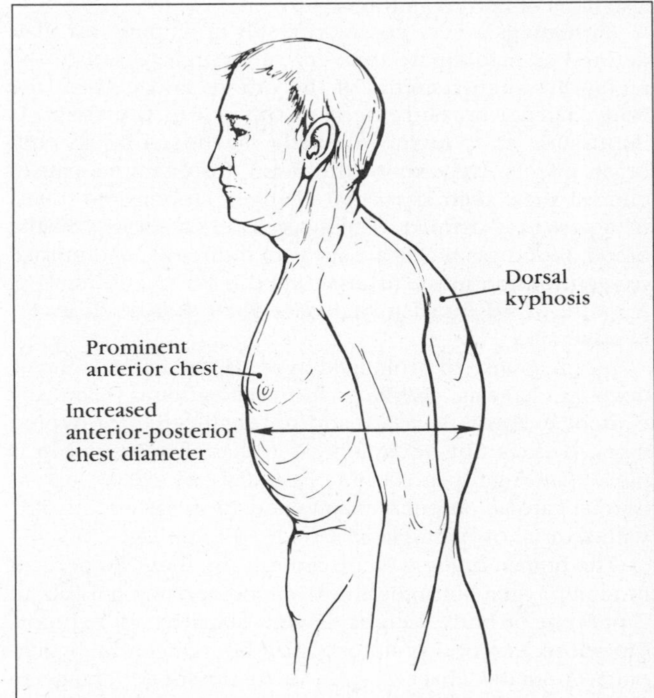

FIGURE 26-6 Barrel chest of emphysema.

inspiration and the abdominal muscles are developed to force air out actively. As a result, the expiratory cycle is prolonged. Pulmonary function tests show a prolonged FEV_1 with decreased vital capacity, despite an increase in total lung capacity. Respiratory sounds are frequently very quiet unless a superimposed infection accounts for expiratory wheezing and rales.

Chronic bronchitis and emphysema coexist in the majority of persons with COPD. Figure 26-7 shows how the clinical manifestations of chronic bronchitis and

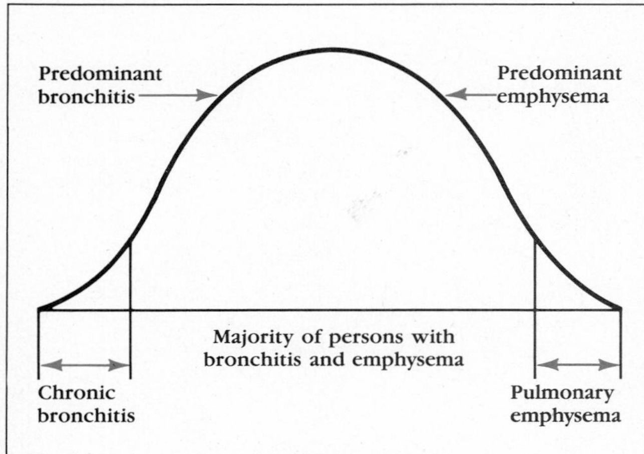

FIGURE 26-7 The overlay of clinical manifestations of chronic bronchitis and emphysema in chronic obstructive pulmonary disease. (From D. Mahler, P. Barlow, and R. Mathay, Chronic Obstructive Pulmonary Diseases. *Clin. Geriatric Med.* 2:2, May 1986. Reprinted by permission.)

emphysema overlap. The majority of persons exhibit manifestations of both conditions [6].

Hypoxia is a very common result of emphysema. It is defined as inadequate delivery of oxygen to satisfy the metabolic requirements of the organs and cells of the body. Direct measurement of oxygen in the tissue is impossible so hypoxia is usually diagnosed by its end-organ effects. Hypoxia of the brain, for example, causes clinical signs such as mental changes, stupor, and coma. *Hypoxemia* is defined as reduced levels of oxygen in the blood. Blood gas levels are measured directly, and normal oxygen tension in the arterial blood is 80 to 100 mm Hg. A value of 40 mm Hg or lower for oxygen indicates hypoxemia.

As a response to prolonged hypoxia, the individual may develop cyanosis, clubbing, and polycythemia. Clinically evident cyanosis is a late and unreliable sign of hypoxemia. It does not occur unless reduced hemoglobin is more than 5 gm per 100 ml of capillary blood. As long as normal cardiac output is maintained, cyanosis occurs only with arterial oxygen levels of under 40 mm Hg.

The human brain, which accounts for about 20 percent of total oxygen consumption while comprising only about 2 percent of body weight, is very sensitive to hypoxia. Therefore, cerebral symptoms may be induced by hypoxemia. A small degree results in restlessness, change in personality, and impaired judgment. Moderately severe hypoxemia causes impaired motor function and confusion. Severe hypoxemia, at levels between 20 and 30 mm Hg, often causes delirium and coma. If persistent and severe, it can cause permanent cortical damage.

Chronic hypoxemia causes a release of renal erythropoietic factor, which reacts with a plasma protein to form erythropoietin. This substance stimulates increased production of red blood cells and blood volume increase (see Chap. 15). The resulting *polycythemia* characteristically develops in patients with COPD and leads to increased blood viscosity, which further impedes oxygenation of the tissues. The oxygen-hemoglobin dissociation curve shifts to the right with hypoxemia, allowing for increased release of oxygen to the tissues. Table 26-5 summarizes the general effects of hypoxia and hypercapnia.

Clubbing is common in association with polycythemia and hypoxemia. The etiology of this disorder is unclear, but it is postulated that capillary dilation occurs in an effort to draw oxygen to the tissues.

Hypercapnia (retention of carbon dioxide) is also common in COPD. It results from hypoventilation mostly due to an uneven match-up of ventilation and perfusion in the lungs. At normal ventilatory rates, inadequate carbon dioxide is excreted and carbon dioxide is retained. Increasing PCO_2 levels leads to increased ventilation due to the central chemoreceptor in the medulla. When pulmonary disease is severe, ventilation changes do not usually return PCO_2 levels to normal. In other words, the work of breathing becomes too great to sustain the high ventilatory rate [3].

Hypercapnia becomes chronic and depresses the receptiveness of the medullary chemoreceptor. The person may lose most of the stimuli for breathing from the central chemoreceptor and depend on the peripheral chemoreceptors on the aortic arch and carotid sinuses to stimulate a ventilatory drive. The peripheral chemoreceptors are stimulated by hypoxemia of less than 60 mm Hg oxygen tension.

The normal pH change that would accompany the retention of carbon dioxide is counteracted by renal retention of bicarbonate, leading to a normal or near normal pH (see Chap. 6). This adaptation is protective and assists the body function even though the PCO_2 remains excessively high. The adjusted pH reflects ***compensated respiratory acidosis***. Table 26-6 shows examples of compensated and uncompensated respiratory acidosis.

Any of the chronic lung diseases may lead to respiratory failure, which is discussed further in Chapter 27.

TABLE 26-5 Diagnosis of Progressive Hypoxia

Symptoms	Signs	Additional Effects from Hypercapnia
Dyspnea	Tachypnea	Severe headache
Restlessness	Tachycardia (bradycardia, late)	Tremor
Impaired judgment	Dysrhythmias	Diaphoresis
Personality change	Hypertension (hypotension, late)	Papilledema
Headache, impaired motor function	Central cyanosis—late (more than 5 gm of reduced hemoglobin per 100 ml of blood)	Asterixis (flapping tremor)
Confusion	Heart and renal failure	Diaphoresis
Delirium	Convulsions	
Coma	Coma	

Source: J. L. Andrews, Jr., Physiology and treatment of hypoxia. *Clin. Notes Respir. Dis.* 13:4, 1974.

TABLE 26-6 Comparative Values for Compensated and Uncompensated Respiratory Acidosis

Arterial Blood Gas Components	Normal Values	Compensated Respiratory Acidosis (an example)	Uncompensated Respiratory Acidosis (an example)
pH	7.35–7.45	7.35	7.22
PCO_2	35–45 mm Hg	54 mm Hg	74 mm Hg
PO_2	80–100 mm Hg	62 mm Hg	40 mm Hg
O_2 saturation	95–100%	83%	69%
HCO_3	22–26 mEq/L	32 mEq/L	28 mEq/L
H_2CO_3	1.05–1.35 mEq/L	1.8 mEq/L	2.9 mEq/L

Study Questions

1. Discuss a typical pattern of onset and result of an acute asthmatic attack. How do asthmatic lungs differ pathologically from emphysematic lungs?
2. Compare the pathologies, etiologies, and clinical courses of bronchiectasis with chronic bronchitis.
3. Describe the pulmonary alterations of cystic fibrosis.
4. Why is it difficult to clearly differentiate the clinical manifestations of chronic bronchitis and emphysema?
5. How does the pathology of emphysema affect the course of the disease?
6. Explain in detail the mechanisms used by the body in reaction to chronic hypoxemia and hypercapnia.

References

1. Braman, S.S., and Davis, S.M. Wheezing in the aged: Asthma and other causes. *Clin. Geriatric Med.* 2:269, 1986.
2. Farzan, S. *A Concise Handbook of Respiratory Diseases* (2nd ed.). Reston, Va.: Reston Pub., 1985.
3. Guyton, A.C. *Textbook of Medical Physiology* (7th ed.). Philadelphia: Saunders, 1985.
4. Hugh-Jones, P., and Whimster, W. The etiology and management of disabling emphysema. *Am. Rev. Respir. Dis.* 117:2, 1978.
5. Kuhn, C., and Askin, F.B. Lung and mediastinum. In J.M. Kissane, *Anderson's Pathology* (8th ed.). St. Louis: Mosby, 1985.
6. Mahler, D.A., Barlow, P.B., and Matthay, R.A. Chronic obstructive pulmonary disease. *Clin. Geriatric Med.* 2:285, 1986.
7. Robbins, S.L., Cotran, R.S., and Kumar, V. *Pathologic Basis of Disease* (3rd ed.). Philadelphia: Saunders, 1984.
8. Sodeman, W.A., and Sodeman, T.M. *Sodeman's Pathologic Physiology* (7th ed.). Philadelphia: Saunders, 1985.
9. Stauffer, J.L., and Carbone, J.E. Pulmonary diseases. In M.A. Krupp et al., *Current Medical Diagnosis and Treatment 1986*. Los Altos, Calif.: Lange, 1986.
10. Tobin, M.J., and Hutchison, D.C.S. An overview of the pulmonary features of $alpha_1$-antitrypsin deficiency. *Arch. Intern. Med.* 142:1342, 1982.
11. Weiss, E. Bronchial asthma. *Ciba Clin. Symp.* 27:1, 1975.
12. West, J.G. *Pulmonary Pathophysiology: The Essentials* (2nd ed.). Baltimore: Williams & Wilkins, 1982.

CHAPTER 27

Other Alterations Affecting the Pulmonary System

CHAPTER OUTLINE

Pulmonary Embolus

- Sequence of Events in Pulmonary Embolization
- Clinical Manifestations
- Fat Embolization

Pulmonary Hypertension
Upper Respiratory Tract Alterations
Carcinoma of the Larynx
Lung Tumors

- Benign Tumors
- Malignant Tumors
  - *Factors Predisposing to Malignancy*
  - *Gross Appearance of Pulmonary Malignancy*
  - *Microscopic Appearance of Pulmonary Malignancy*

Respiratory Failure

- Respiratory Insufficiency
- Respiratory Failure

LEARNING OBJECTIVES

1. Describe the ventilation-perfusion abnormality that occurs with pulmonary embolus.
2. Discuss the underlying risk factors for the development of pulmonary embolus.
3. List and describe three conditions that favor thrombus formation in the deep veins.
4. Describe the clinical manifestations that may occur in the process of pulmonary embolization.
5. Explain briefly how resolution of emboli occurs.
6. Describe the development of pulmonary hypertension.
7. Define *cor pulmonale*.
8. Define *rhinitis*, *pharyngitis*, *sinusitis*, and *laryngitis*.
9. Explain briefly the dangers of laryngeal edema.
10. Classify and briefly describe cancer of the larynx.
11. Define *hamartoma of the lungs*.
12. Discuss some factors that predispose to the onset of malignancy in the lung.
13. Describe the pathology, major clinical manifestations, and prognosis of four major types of intrapulmonary malignancy.
14. List the most common sites of metastasis of lung cancer.
15. Differentiate between respiratory insufficiency and respiratory failure.
16. Explain how adaptation can occur in chronic respiratory insufficiency.
17. List the criteria for diagnosing respiratory failure and the other factors that should be taken into account.
18. Describe the clinical manifestations of respiratory failure.
19. Define *carbon dioxide narcosis*.
20. Discuss the prognoses in acute and chronic respiratory failure.

Several of the pulmonary disease processes do not easily lend themselves to strict classification as restrictive or obstructive. This chapter discusses some of these conditions, including pulmonary embolus, tumors of the lung, and respiratory insufficiency and failure. Respiratory failure may result from many intrapulmonary and extrapulmonary diseases, and it is frequently the cause of death in chronic pulmonary disease.

As discussed in Chapter 24, the normal ratio of alveolar ventilation (4 liters/minute) to volume of blood flow in the pulmonary capillaries ($\dot{V}/\dot{Q}$) is about 0.8 because cardiac output averages about 5 liters per minute. A decrease of alveolar ventilation in relation to perfusion occurs in any part of the lung where airways are obstructed by secretions (bronchitis), expiratory dynamic collapse (emphysema), or muscular spasm (asthma); or where alveoli are collapsed (atelectasis) or are filled with fluid (pulmonary edema). These conditions cause increased venous blood flow past nonventilated alveoli; the oxygen-poor mixture is added to the arterial blood and the result is hypoxemia. As stated previously, hypoxemia resulting from underventilated alveoli is, in essence, a form of right-to-left shunting of venous blood past the alveoli (see pp. 388–390).

Another type of ventilation-perfusion abnormality is the reduction of perfusion in relation to ventilation. This occurs most frequently when pulmonary emboli obliterate arteriolar blood supply, but may occur when cardiac output is reduced because of congestive heart failure. In these examples, ventilated but nonperfused alveoli increase the physiologic dead space because a significant number of alveoli receive inspired air but do not participate in the exchange of oxygen or carbon dioxide.

In conditions in which hypoxemia is the result of a ventilation-perfusion abnormality, the pressure of carbon dioxide (PCO_2) often is normal or low, since compensatory hyperventilation is able to lower the more easily diffusible PCO_2. Thus, the clinical pattern of ventilation-perfusion inequality is often one of hypoxemia with hyperventilation, lowered PCO_2, and even respiratory alkalosis. This picture is directly related to the degree of the ventilation-perfusion defect and eventually may result in hypoxemia, hypercapnia, and respiratory acidosis.

Pulmonary Embolus

A pulmonary embolus is defined as an occlusion of one or more pulmonary vessels by matter that has traveled from a source outside the lung. Any foreign material freely traveling in the systemic venous system must finally terminate in the pulmonary vascular bed. For example, if a clot in a small vein dislodges, it travels through progressively larger vessels until it reaches the right ventricle, where it is pumped by the pulmonary artery to the lungs. The usual cause of pulmonary embolus is a thrombus from the deep veins of the legs or pelvis that dislodges and travels with the flow of blood to the lungs. It may also result from a fat embolus, amniotic fluid embolus, air embolus, particulate matter injected intravenously, or rarely, gas, parasites, or foreign objects.

Pulmonary embolus is probably the third most common acute cause of death in the United States, but the diagnosis is often missed [6]. It is thought that many persons have thrombi in the venous system that may actually embolize but may be diagnosed as a pulmonary infection, pleurisy, or not diagnosed at all. Pulmonary emboli rarely strike the young or healthy but occur in a high-risk group that includes bedridden persons, the obese, elderly, and those with a history of prior emboli or thrombosis. Persons who suffer from congestive heart failure, who undergo abdominal or pelvic surgery, or who have sustained trauma to the legs are also at high risk.

Sequence of Events in Pulmonary Embolization

The right lung is more frequently involved in the embolic process than the left, with the degree of obstruction related to the size of the embolus. It has been shown in some studies that the physiologic consequences of pulmonary embolus are greater than can be explained by the degree of occlusion alone. A large embolus may cause infarction of the lung parenchyma, but this is not directly related to the size of the embolus because the bronchial arteries continue to nourish the lung tissue [3].

As stated before, most pulmonary emboli are the result of thrombi that dislodge from the deep veins of the legs and pelvis. Phlebothrombosis is the most common type of deep vein thrombosis and frequently occurs in immobilized and/or obese persons and in those who have sustained surgical or accidental trauma.

For a thrombus of this nature to form, an abnormality must be present, because clotting rarely occurs when blood flow and vascular integrity are normal. Three conditions have been described that favor clot formation: (1) venostasis, (2) endothelial disruption of the vessel lining, and (3) hypercoagulability.

Local concentration of coagulation factors together with an injury to the venous wall may provide a place for clots to form. As the flow of blood slows or stops over the injured area, the clot begins to form and extends or propagates itself up the vein (Fig. 27-1). It may then retract and pull away from the vessel wall and become a free-floating embolus. Small fragments of the clot may break off and produce several areas of embolization on the lungs. Multiple embolization of the pulmonary capillary bed is more common than occlusion of the main pulmonary artery or its branches.

Once the blood clot lodges in the pulmonary capillary bed, it obstructs blood flow beyond the point of the obstruction. Perfusion in the pulmonary capillary bed stops. If large areas are affected there may be infarction of the lung tissue, which occurs in perhaps 5 to 10 percent of cases with infarcts of various sizes. The newly formed infarct becomes hemorrhagic but later is filled with scar tissue [6].

A wide variety of pathophysiologic responses to a pulmonary embolus occurs, depending on the size of the embolus and the ability of the host to compensate. Small obstructions to the blood supply usually create no hemodynamic changes and are called *silent pulmonary emboli*.

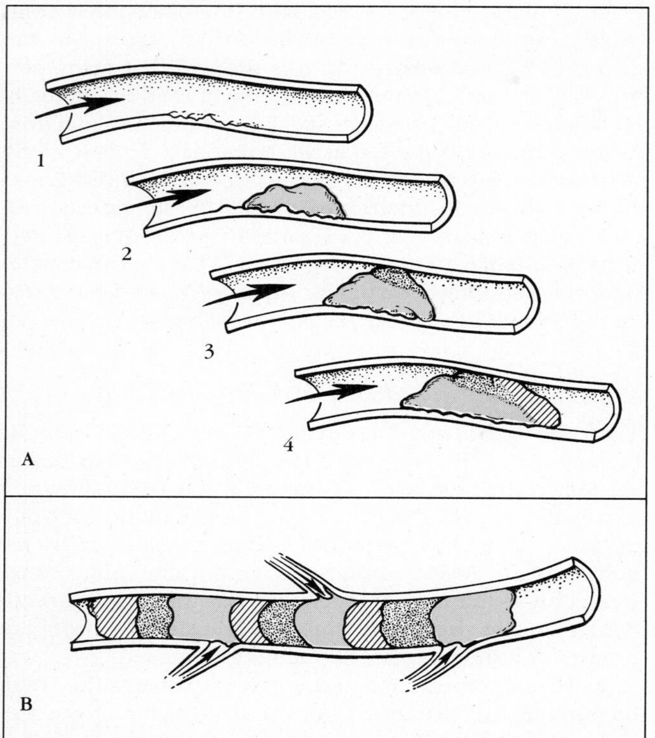

FIGURE 27-1 A. Sequence of clot formation on area of intimal damage. B. Propagation of clot up the length of the vein wall may lead to pulmonary embolus.

Larger obstructions may cause increased resistance to pulmonary blood flow, which may lead to right ventricular failure (cor pulmonale). Studies show that more than 50 percent of the pulmonary vasculature must be obstructed to cause significant increase in pressure in the pulmonary artery [7]. Vasoconstriction in the smaller pulmonary arterial vessels is apparently common and may be due to the liberation of vasoactive substances such as serotonin. Vasoconstriction enhances the risk for pulmonary ischemia and infarction.

The increase in pulmonary artery pressure leads to an increased workload for the right side of the heart in pumping blood into the pulmonary circulation. Tachycardia results and progresses to signs of right ventricular failure, including jugular venous distention, hepatomegaly, and peripheral edema. A large saddle embolus obstructing the main pulmonary artery at its bifurcation to the right and left branches leads to acute cor pulmonale, severe shock, and often, sudden death [3]. Bronchoconstriction due to release of various chemical mediators, such as thromboxanes, prostaglandins, serotonin, and histamine, may produce an asthmalike picture, causing initial misdiagnosis [2].

The process of embolization may be continuous, with small emboli being released from a thrombotic focus over months or years. Often undiagnosed, this process may lead to pulmonary embarrassment.

Resolution of the pulmonary embolus occurs by absorption and fibrosis. Activation of the intrinsic fibrinolytic system may restore the pulmonary circulation within a few hours or days [4]. This may begin as early as a few hours after a small embolic episode. Fibrous replacement converts infarcted lung tissue to scar tissue. Clots are partly or totally dissolved by the fibrinolytic system. Residual material, resistant to fibrinolytic attack, may organize and become small, scarred areas.

Clinical Manifestations

The signs and symptoms of pulmonary embolus vary greatly (Table 27-1). The embolus may be clinically silent with no manifestations at all. The most frequent symptom is the sudden onset of mild, moderate, or severe dyspnea that may occur transiently. Tachypnea that persists is suggestive of pulmonary embolus. Fever and cough, sometimes with associated hemoptysis, often occur. Pain may be absent, mild, or severe, and may be manifested as pleural pain or deep, crushing, substernal pain mimicking that of myocardial infarction. The pain often occurs with pulmonary infarction and may be oppressive and substernal. Anxiety, apprehension, and restlessness are common responses to hypoxemia. Palpitations and weakness associated with profuse perspiration and nausea and vomiting often are present. If embolization is massive, cardiovascular collapse may result, leading to sudden shock, seizures, or cardiopulmonary arrest.

Clinical signs of pulmonary embolus may include splinting of the involved side, cyanosis, distended neck veins, tachycardia with an increased pulmonic sound, or an S3 or

TABLE 27-1 Signs and Symptoms of Pulmonary Embolus

- Initial manifestations
  - May be clinically silent
  - Dyspnea of sudden onset
  - Cough
  - Fever
  - Pain—pleuritic or deep and crushing
  - Hemoptysis
  - Tachypnea
  - Anxiety, apprehension, restlessness
  - Palpitations
  - Weakness
  - Diaphoresis
  - Nausea and vomiting
  - Shock
- Physical examination findings
  - Splinting of involved side
  - Cyanosis
  - Distended neck veins
  - Area of dullness over involved side
  - Tachycardia
  - S3 or S4 gallop
  - Rales
  - Localized decreased breath sounds
  - Localized wheezing
  - Chest film may be normal or show patchy areas of infiltration
- Lung scan and pulmonary arteriogram definitive
- Arterial blood gases frequently show hypoxemia and hypercapnia

S4 gallop. Rales, wheezing, and decreased breath sounds in the affected areas are frequent findings.

Definitive diagnosis is often difficult. Chest radiograph often appears normal, and any abnormalities may be general, such as elevated diaphragm, atelectasis, or pleural effusion. The serum enzyme lactic dehydrogenase (LDH) level is often elevated. Arterial blood gases may show hypoxemia, hypocapnia, and respiratory alkalosis due to the marked tachypnea. Radioisotope lung scan shows perfusion defects in areas of the lung and supports the diagnosis. A pulmonary arteriogram is occasionally performed to provide visualization of the vessels of the pulmonary tree.

Fat Embolization

Fractures of the long bones are the major source of emboli composed of fat particles. The origin appears to be the bone marrow, and the particles enter the bloodstream through the ruptured veins. Fat also may be mobilized from the injured site and may form large globules in the plasma [4]. Alveolar edema often occurs, exhibiting a clinical picture much like the adult respiratory distress syndrome (ARDS). The person begins to exhibit marked respiratory distress, fever, and tachycardia [3].

Pulmonary Hypertension

Pulmonary hypertension can result from heart and/or lung disease. It refers to an increase in pulmonary artery pressure, which increases the workload of the right ventricle. Significant pulmonary vascular obliteration must be present for pulmonary arterial pressure to be elevated, because there is normally a large reserve in the pulmonary capillary bed.

As a rule, pulmonary hypertension involves progressive disease either of the pulmonary vessels or of the lung parenchyma. The medial layer of the pulmonary arteries usually hypertrophies, and the system loses its ability to adapt to stress factors such as increased blood flow or hypoxia. Hypoxic vasoconstriction is a cause and a result of pulmonary hypertension [4].

As the process becomes persistent, end-diastolic pressure in the right ventricle becomes elevated. The right ventricle hypertrophies and further increases its systolic pressure. In the early stages, symptoms of right ventricular failure, or *cor pulmonale* (heart failure resulting from lung disease), occur only during periods of increased stress. As it progresses, cor pulmonale is present all of the time, manifested by jugular venous distention, hepatomegaly, and peripheral edema.

The pulmonary artery pressure, which is normally approximately 25/10 mm Hg, is elevated to above approximately 40/15 mm Hg and may be much higher as the disease progresses. At a certain critical point, the right ventricle cannot compensate for the increased pressure, and intractable cardiac failure occurs.

Death from chronic respiratory disease may be due to heart failure or respiratory failure. Nearly all persons with these diseases exhibit some symptoms of right ventricular failure, also called chronic cor pulmonale.

Other conditions besides chronic obstructive lung disease may cause pulmonary hypertension. Congenital cardiac left-to-right shunts that overload the pulmonary vascular system can eventually cause pulmonary hypertension (see Chap. 21). Also, some valvular conditions, particularly mitral stenosis, cause increased volume and pressure in the pulmonary vascular bed. Any condition in which hypoxia is sustained may cause vasoconstriction and ultimately, pulmonary hypertension. Left-sided heart failure of long-standing duration also may cause this condition.

Upper Respiratory Tract Alterations

Alterations in the upper respiratory tract (URT) are very common, usually self-limiting conditions that include rhinitis, pharyngitis, sinusitis, and laryngitis. Cancer of the larynx is a more serious disease that may affect the URT.

Rhinitis refers to inflammation of the nasal cavities, resulting in a persistent nasal discharge caused by secretory hyperactivity of the submucosal glands of the nasal cavities. The etiology of rhinitis is commonly viral, bacterial, or allergic. The viral form is recognized as the common cold. Allergies or exposure to irritants injure the normal cilia of the nasal mucosa. Bacterial growth often occurs after an initial viral attack.

Pharyngitis usually results from viral or bacterial invasion of the pharynx that causes a sore throat. The appearance of the throat varies depending on the causative agent. Tonsils are often affected and become reddened and swollen, and exude a suppurative discharge. Most pharyngitis is relatively innocuous, but untreated streptococcal infections may have systemic effects in some persons. These effects are manifested as scarlet fever, rheumatic fever, rheumatic heart disease, glomerulonephritis, and so on. Other organisms such as *Corynebacterium diphtheriae* and *Hemophilus influenzae* may cause grave effects.

Sinusitis is an inflammation of the sinus cavities that often spreads from a rhinitis infection to the sinuses. The most common organisms causing this condition are group A *Streptococcus pyogenes*, *Staphylococcus aureus*, and *H. influenzae*. The infection usually causes localized pain in the frontal, maxillary, ethmoid, or sphenoid sinuses (Fig. 27-2). A purulent exudate indicates bacterial infection that, when severe, is associated with the constitutional symptoms of fever, chills, pain in the sinuses, and nasal obstruction. Chronic disease may be indicated by a postnasal discharge and tenderness over the sinus cavity.

Laryngitis often occurs in persons who overuse the voice in singing or other vocal activities. It may also be due to any organism that may affect the URT. It affects both vocal cords and is manifested by cough and hoarseness with loss of the voice. Laryngitis may also be chronic, precipitated by overuse of tobacco, straining the voice, or inhaling toxic gases. Rarely, this condition causes *laryngeal edema* and obstruction to airflow. Complete obstruction causes asphyxia while incomplete obstruction causes laryngeal stridor and acute respiratory distress.

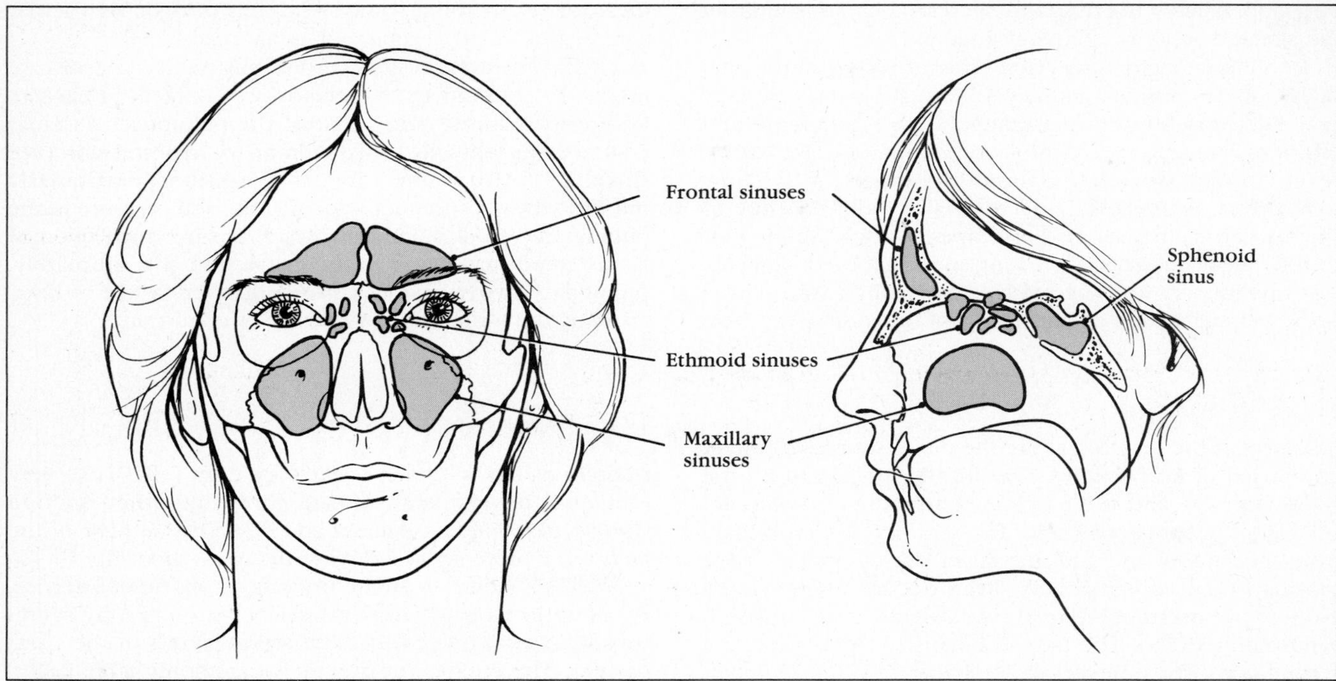

FIGURE 27-2 Location of paranasal sinuses.

Carcinoma of the Larynx

Polyps of the vocal cords are not usually premalignant, but the *laryngeal papilloma* is a true neoplasm that has the potential of undergoing malignant transformation. Most affected persons are, or have been, heavy tobacco smokers.

Most cancers of the larynx arise on the vocal cords and are clinically manifested by hoarseness. This malignancy is closely associated with chronic laryngitis and smoking. Its frequency is greatest in men after the fourth decade.

Clinical manifestations of cancers of the larynx include pain, a palpable lump, dysphagia, and occasionally, respiratory distress. The tumor, being a relatively slow-growing malignancy of the squamous epithelium, is curable in the early stages.

Lung Tumors

Tumors of the lung may be benign or malignant. The majority are malignant and have an unremitting, progressive course leading ultimately to a poor prognosis. The only benign tumor that is discussed in this section is the hamartoma because it is frequently difficult to differentiate it from a malignancy. The malignant tumors are described according to histologic classification and pathogenesis.

Benign Tumors

The *hamartoma* is not a true neoplasm but is a congenital anomaly that frequently leads to tumorlike lesions containing connective tissue, cartilage, and bronchial epithelium in the bronchi or lung tissue [4]. The lesions are encapsulated, firm, and grayish white with a rough, nodular surface; they appear on chest films on the periphery of the lung, in the subpleural area, and endobronchially, making them difficult to distinguish from malignant tumors. These uncommon lung tumors rarely cause any clinical symptoms but must be differentiated from malignancy.

Malignant Tumors

Factors Predisposing to Malignancy. Cigarette smoking, air pollution, and industrial chemicals seem to account for the increasing frequency of bronchogenic carcinoma. Statistical evidence supports the relationship between cigarette smoking and certain types of lung cancer. The death rate from lung cancer is twice as high in urban areas as in rural areas, implicating air pollution as an etiologic factor (see Chaps. 13 and 14). Figure 27-3 shows the phenomenal increase in lung cancer deaths since 1930 [4].

Certain occupations apparently predispose persons to lung cancer. Asbestos workers have about a 10 times greater risk of developing the disease than the general population. More startling, an asbestos worker who smokes has a 90 times greater risk of developing lung cancer than the general population. Other industrial agents that increase risk are uranium, chromate, arsenic, and iron.

Studies suggest a correlation between chronic bronchitis and bronchogenic carcinoma, with the differences in mortality from lung cancer reported among countries being related to varying frequency of chronic bronchitis [5]. The excess mucus secretion characteristic of chronic bronchitis may interfere with the bronchial epithelial cells, making them likely to undergo malignant change.

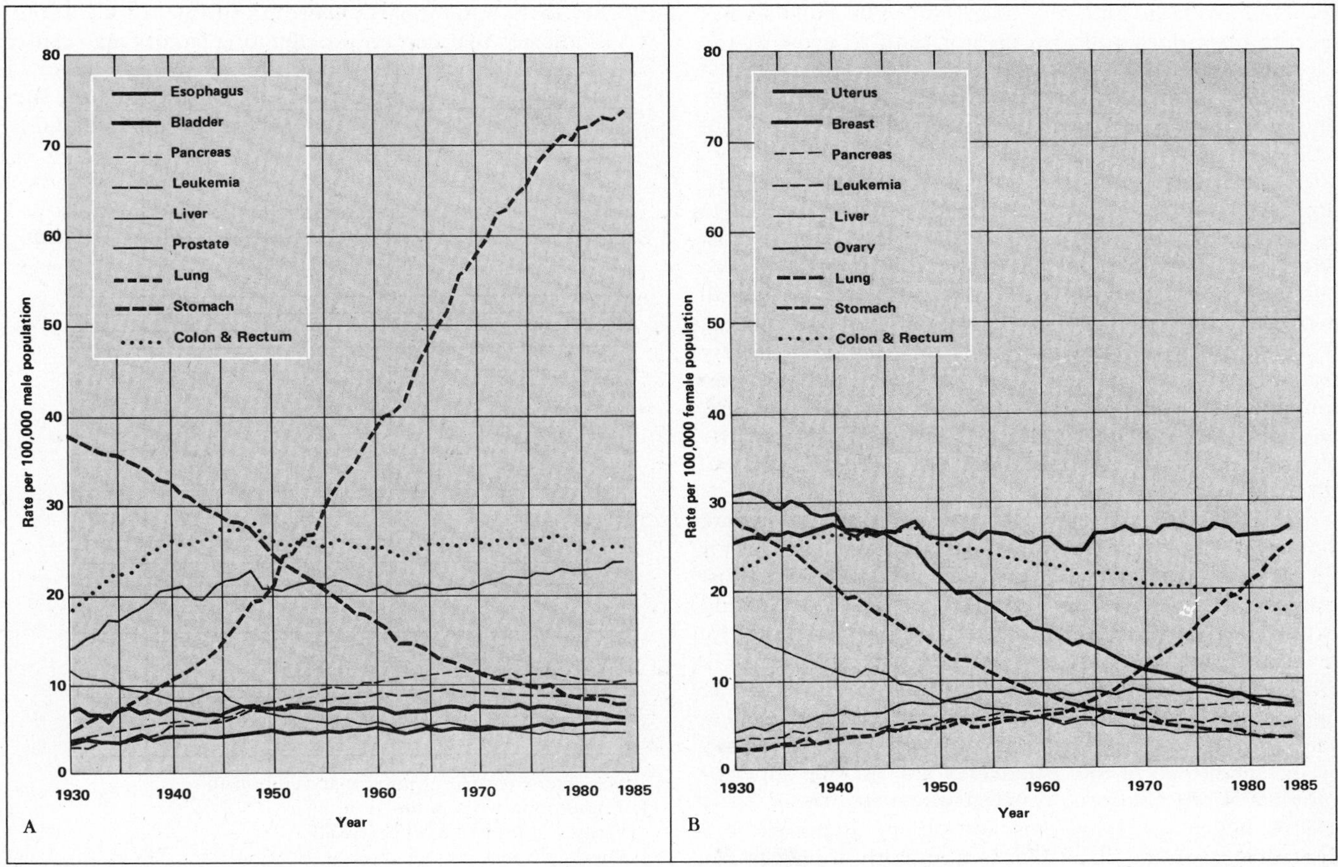

FIGURE 27-3 Cancer death rates for selected sites, adjusted to the age distribution of the 1970 U.S. Census Population. A. Males. B. Females. United States 1930–1984. (Sources of data: U.S. National Center for Health Statistics and the U.S. Bureau of the Census. Reprinted from E. Silverberg, Cancer statistics, Ca-A *Cancer Journal for Clinicians,* Vol. 37, No. 1, Jan./Feb. 1987, pp. 10–11.)

Also, the bronchial mucosa, which is chronically inflamed, exhibits depressed ciliary activity, and airway cleansing is decreased [4].

Gross Appearance of Pulmonary Malignancy. Although variations may occur, the appearance of pulmonary carcinoma may be one of three types: (1) *hilar, infiltrating form*, which causes a large tumor mass that presses on the bronchi; (2) *peripheral* or *nodular form*, which may appear as a single tumor or multiple nodular masses throughout the lung; or (3) *diffuse type*, which looks very much like pneumonia and may be difficult to see grossly [4].

Microscopic Appearance of Pulmonary Malignancy. The *squamous cell carcinoma* is the most common morphologic type of bronchogenic carcinoma. It causes 45 to 60 percent of lung malignancies. The cell type may be well differentiated, but more frequently, it is undifferentiated and quite pleomorphic in appearance. It tends to have large, well-outlined areas of tumor growth arising from the bronchi [6]. These invade surrounding tissue in the early stages of the disease, but later metastasize readily to the lymph nodes, brain, bone, adrenal glands, and liver. This tumor type has a very high correlation with heavy cigarette smoking. The two-year prognosis is poor, with less than 50 percent survival.

The *small-cell (oat-cell) carcinoma* consists of small, dark cells located between the cells of the mucosal surfaces. They are characterized by rapid growth and early metastasis through the lymphatic system and blood. This disease is rare in the peripheral areas and frequently exhibits large, obstructive growths in the main bronchi [4]. These small-cell carcinomas often secrete substances like those normally found in other areas of the body, including ACTH (adrenocorticotropic hormone) and ADH (antidiuretic hormone). The result of ACTH secretion is Cushing's syndrome, leading to obesity, osteoporosis, hypokalemia, alkalosis, and other problems. Secretion of ADH leads to retention of water, hyponatremia, renal sodium loss, anorexia, nausea, and lethargy [1]. The prognosis in this malignancy is very poor, with only 3 to 5 percent survival for two years.

Large-cell, undifferentiated, or giant-cell carcinoma is distinct from the previous two tumors in that the cells involved are large and very anaplastic. The cells do not secrete hormones and also do not tend to grow at the same rate as the small-cell type. The tumor is most frequently located in the peripheral areas of the lungs. The overall prognosis remains very poor, with only about 12 percent survival for 2 years.

Adenocarcinoma of the lungs has no particular relationship to smoking and occurs with equal frequency in men and women. The location of the tumor cells is most often in the periphery of the lungs, with a rapid growth rate and early metastasis to the bloodstream. The overall two-year prognosis is poor, with only 20 percent survival.

The propensity for metastasis, at differing rates, is very common with lung cancer. Over one-half of afflicted persons (perhaps as many as 75%) have metastasis at the time of diagnosis [4]. The spread commonly occurs to the pleura, mediastinum, lymph nodes, liver, bone, brain, and adrenal glands.

The clinical manifestations of carcinoma of the lung are difficult to classify. Most individuals are asymptomatic for a long time or may develop signs of metastasis. The most common symptoms of the primary tumor are cough and expectoration of bloody sputum. Hemoptysis may be severe. Lymph node enlargement may cause encroachment on the superior vena cava, obstruction, and dramatic signs and symptoms. Chest pain, dyspnea, and hoarseness may be present. Often the first symptoms are those caused by distant spread of the malignancy and include superior vena caval obstruction, recurrent nerve paralysis, bone lesions, neurologic symptoms, and others. Radiologic evidence on a routine chest film is frequently the first sign, but by the time a lung tumor is radiologically evident it has usually invaded surrounding structures. Sputum cytology and bronchoscopy help to confirm the diagnosis.

Respiratory Failure

Respiratory Insufficiency

Respiratory insufficiency is said to occur when the lungs are not able to exchange adequate amounts of carbon dioxide and oxygen to carry out the normal activities of daily living. In chronic respiratory insufficiency, the body gradually adapts to the pulmonary dysfunction. This process of adaptation includes hyperventilation, use of accessory muscles to breathe, circulatory changes to adjust the oxygen delivery to vital organs, and renal compensation to maintain the blood pH [3]. In *acute respiratory insufficiency*, hypoxemia and hypercapnia become severe and the compensatory mechanisms instituted by the body do not adjust the oxygen and carbon dioxide levels sufficiently to supply the body's needs. Inadequate tissue oxygen and severe respiratory acidosis occur without immediate treatment.

Respiratory Failure

Respiratory failure is the inability of the lungs to meet the basic demands for tissue oxygenation at rest. Respiratory failure can occur as a result of a wide variety of intrapulmonary or nonpulmonary disorders (Table 27-2). Table 27-3 indicates that certain precipitating factors may cause the exacerbation of preexisting respiratory insufficiency.

The diagnosis of respiratory failure depends on the arterial blood gases. A PO_2 of less than 50 mm Hg and a

TABLE 27-2 Important Disorders Leading to Respiratory Failure, Classified According to Major Areas of Involvement

Intrinsic lung and airway diseases
- Large airway obstruction
  - Congenital deformities
  - Acute laryngitis
  - Foreign bodies
  - Intrinsic tumors
  - Extrinsic pressure
  - Traumatic injury
  - Enlarged tonsils and adenoids
- Bronchial disease
  - Chronic bronchitis
  - Asthma
  - Acute bronchiolitis
- Parenchymal disease
  - Pulmonary emphysema
  - Pulmonary fibrosis of various causes
  - Pulmonary edema, cardiac
  - Severe pneumonia
  - Acute lung injury from various causes
- Vascular disease
  - Massive or recurrent pulmonary embolism

Extrapulmonary disorders
- Diseases of pleura and chest wall
  - Pneumothorax
  - Pleural effusion
  - Fibrothorax
  - Thoracic wall deformity
  - Traumatic injury to the chest wall: flail chest
  - Obesity
- Disorders of respiratory muscles and neuromuscular junction
  - Myasthenia gravis and myasthenialike disorders
  - Muscular dystrophies
  - Polymyositis
  - Botulism
  - Muscle-paralyzing drugs
  - Severe hypokalemia
- Disorders of peripheral nerves and spinal cord
  - Poliomyelitis
  - Guillain-Barré syndrome
  - Spinal cord trauma (quadriplegia)
  - Amyotrophic lateral sclerosis
  - Tetanus
  - Multiple sclerosis
- Disorders of central nervous system
  - Sedative and narcotic drug overdose
  - Head trauma
  - Cerebral hypoxia
  - Cerebrovascular accident
  - Central nervous system inflection
  - Epileptic seizure: status epilepticus
  - Metabolic and endocrine disorders
  - Bulbar poliomyelitis
  - Primary alveolar hyperventilation

Source: Reprinted from S. Farzan, *A Concise Handbook of Respiratory Disease,* 1978, pp. 223–224. Reprinted with permission of Reston Publishing Co., Simon & Schuster Professional Information Group, 25 Van Zant St., E. Norwalk, CT 06855.

TABLE 27-3 Precipitating or Exacerbating Factors of Respiratory Failure

Changes of tracheobronchial secretions
Infection: viral or bacterial
Disturbance of tracheobronchial clearance
Drugs: sedatives, narcotics, anesthetics, oxygen
Inhalation or aspiration of irritants, vomitus, foreign body
Cardiovascular disorders: heart failure, pulmonary embolism, shock
Mechanical factors: pneumothorax, pleural effusion, abdominal distention
Trauma, including surgery
Neuromuscular abnormalities
Allergic disorders: bronchospasm
Increased oxygen demand: fever, infection

Source: Reprinted from S. Farzan, *A Concise Handbook of Respiratory Disease*, 1978, pp. 223–224. Reprinted with permission of Reston Publishing Co., Simon & Schuster Professional Information Group, 25 Van Zant St., E. Norwalk, CT 06855.

PCO_2 of greater than 50 mm Hg often are accepted as determining values [3]. These are related also to the person's age, past history, and overall condition. Acute deterioration of blood gases in the person with chronic lung disease indicates failing compensation and respiratory failure [3]. The disorder may exist with hypoxemia as the predominant problem or with a combination of hypoxemia and hypercapnia.

As respiratory failure ensues, the PCO_2 begins to accumulate and leads to significant respiratory acidosis indicating the inability of the lungs to eliminate the excess carbon dioxide. The normal chemoreceptors for carbon dioxide may become inoperative, and the hypoxic stimulus may be the stimulus for the respiratory effort.

The clinical manifestations are dependent on the underlying cause but especially involve the resulting oxygen-carbon dioxide imbalance [3]. Dyspnea may not occur if there is depression of the respiratory center, so that the respiratory rate may be very rapid or slow. Hypoxemia leads to inadequate tissue perfusion with varying degrees of cyanosis, depending on the amount of right-to-left shunting. This would be seen especially with severe atelectosis or ARDS (see Chap. 25). Hypercapnia refers to PCO_2 levels above 45 mm Hg. It indicates inadequate alveolar ventilation and the inability to release carbon dioxide. The symptoms, which are often associated with hypoxemia, include increased pulse and blood pressure, dizziness, headache, mental clouding and central nervous system depression, muscle twitching, and tremor.

Carbon dioxide narcosis, which occurs as levels of carbon dioxide progressively increase, leads to loss of consciousness, dilation of cerebral blood vessels, increased blood flow to the brain, increased intracranial pressure, and constriction of the pulmonary vessels [3]. Respiratory acidosis is frequent and may develop rapidly or slowly, depending on renal compensation.

The prognosis of acute or chronic respiratory failure depends on the underlying causative mechanisms and whether or not lung function can improve. Respiratory failure is frequently the cause of death in pulmonary conditions.

Study Questions

1. Discuss the clinical manifestations that can develop from pulmonary embolization. Why is the diagnosis of this condition often missed?
2. How can cor pulmonale develop from pulmonary hypertension?
3. Explain the predisposing factors of pulmonary malignancy in relation to the pathology produced.
4. List the favored sites for pulmonary metastasis. Why are these sites chosen by the body?
5. Review the section on COPD in Chapter 26 and describe its progression, through respiratory insufficiency and failure.

References

1. Boyer, M. Treating invasive lung cancer. *Am. J. Nurs.* 77:1916, 1977.
2. Braman, S.S., and Davis, S.M. Wheezing in the aged: Asthma and other causes. *Clin. Geriatric Med.* 2:2:275, May, 1986.
3. Farzan, S. *A Concise Handbook of Respiratory Diseases* (2nd ed.). Reston, Va.: Reston Pub., 1985.
4. Kuhn, C., and Askin, F.B. Lung and mediastinum. In J.M. Kissane, *Anderson's Pathology* (8th ed.). St. Louis: Mosby, 1985.
5. Passey, R. Some problems of lung cancer. *Lancet* 2:107, 1962.
6. Robbins, S.L., Cotran, R.S., and Kumar V. *Pathologic Basis of Disease* (3rd ed.). Philadelphia: Saunders, 1984.
7. Sodeman, W.A., and Sodeman, T.M. *Sodeman's Pathologic Physiology* (7th ed.). Philadelphia: Saunders, 1985.

Unit Bibliography

Andrews, J.L., Jr. Physiology and treatment of hypoxia. *Clin. Notes Respir. Dis.* 13:3, 1974.

Andrews, J.L., Jr. Cor pulmonale: Pathophysiology and management. *Geriatrics* 31:91, 1976.

Andrews, J.L., Jr. The clinical roles of pulmonary function testing. *Med. Clin. North Am.* 63:355, 1979.

Bellanti, J.A. *Immunology III.* Philadelphia: Saunders, 1985.

Bohning, D., et al. Tracheobronchial particle deposition and clearance. *Arch. Environ. Health* 30:457, 1975.

Burrows, B., et al. *Respiratory Insufficiency* (2nd ed.). Chicago: Yearbook, 1983.

Camner, P., et al. Human tracheobronchial clearance studies. *Arch. Environ. Health* 22:444, 1971.

Camner, P., Mossberg, B., and Afzeluis, B. Evidence for congenitally non-functioning cilia in the tracheobronchial tract of two sublets. *Am. Rev. Respir. Dis.* 112:807, 1975.

Cherniack, R., and Cherniack, L. *Respiration in Health and Disease* (3rd ed.). Philadelphia: Saunders, 1983.

Chodash, S. Examination of sputum cells. *N. Engl. J. Med.* 282:854, 1972.

Cohen, A.B., and Gold, W.M. Defense mechanisms of the lung. *Annu. Rev. Physiol.* 37:325, 1975.

Davies, C.N. A comparison between inhaled dust and the dust recovered from human lungs. *Health Phys.* 10:129, 1964.

Dowell, A.R., et al. Lung defense mechanisms: Their importance in respiratory care. *Respir. Care* 22:50, 1977.

Dulfano, M.J., Adler, K., and Phillippoff, W. Sputum viscoelasticity in chronic bronchitis. *Am. Rev. Respir. Dis.* 104:88, 1971.

Farzan, S.A. *A Concise Handbook of Respiratory Diseases* (2nd ed.). Reston, Va.: Reston Pub., 1985.

Fishman, A.P. *Pulmonary Diseases and Disorders: Update.* New York: McGraw-Hill, 1982.

Ganong, W.F. *Review of Medical Physiology* (12th ed.). Los Altos, Calif.: Lange, 1985.

Goldstein, E., Lippert, W., and Warshauer, D. Pulmonary alveolar macrophages: Defender against bacterial infection in the lung. *J. Clin. Invest.* 54:519, 1974.

Gosselin, R.I. Physiological regulators of ciliary motion. *Am. Rev. Respir. Dis.* 93:41, 1966.

Green, G. Pulmonary clearance of infectious agents. *Annu. Rev. Med.* 19:315, 1968.

Green, G. The Amberson lecture: In defense of the lung. *Am. Rev. Respir. Dis.* 102:691, 1970.

Guenter, C.A., and Welch, M.H. (eds.). *Pulmonary Medicine* (2nd ed.). Philadelphia: Lippincott, 1982.

Guyton, A.C. *Textbook of Medical Physiology* (7th ed.). Philadelphia: Saunders, 1986.

Hanson, R., and Dasik, J. The pneumoconioses. *Heart Lung* 6:646, 1977.

Hilding, A. Phagocytosis: Mucus flow and ciliary action. *Arch. Environ. Health* 6:61, 1963.

Hugh-Jones, P., and Whimster, W. The etiology and management of disabling emphysema. *Am. Rev. Respir. Dis.* 117:2, 1978.

Jarstand, C., Camner, P., and Philipson, K. Mycoplasm pneumonia and tracheobronchial clearance. *Am. Rev. Respir. Dis.* 110:415, 1974.

Johansen, W., and Gould, K. Lung defense mechanisms. *Basics Respir. Dis.* 6:2, 1977.

Jones, R., and Weill, H. Occupational lung disease. *Basics Respir. Dis.* 6:3, 1978.

Juers, J., et al. Enhancement of bactericidal capacity of alveolar macrophages. *J. Clin. Invest.* 58:271, 1976.

Kass, E., Green, G., and Goldstein, E. Mechanisms of antibacterial action in the respiratory system. *Bacteriol. Rev.* 30:488, 1966.

Kealy, S.L. Respiratory care in Guillain-Barré syndrome. *Am. J. Nurs.* 1:59, 1977.

Keim, L., Schuldt, S., and Bedell, G. Tuberculosis in the intensive care unit. *Heart Lung* 6:624, 1977.

Kueppers, F., and Black, L.F. Alpha$_1$-antitrypsin and its deficiency. *Am. Rev. Respir. Dis.* 110:178, 1974.

Laurenzi, G. The mucociliary stream. *J. Occup. Med.* 15:175, 1973.

Laurenzi, G., Yin, S., and Guarneri, J. Adverse effects of oxygen on tracheal mucus flow. *N. Engl. J. Med.* 279:333, 1968.

Levitsky, M.G. *Pulmonary Physiology* (2nd ed.). New York: McGraw-Hill, 1986.

Lieberman, J. Alpha$_1$-antitrypsin deficiency. *Med. Clin. North Am.* 59:3, 1973.

MacDonnell, K., and Segal, M. *Current Respiratory Care.* Boston: Little, Brown, 1977.

McKerrow, C., et al. Respiratory function during the day in cotton workers: A study of byssinosis. *Br. J. Ind. Med.* 15:75, 1958.

Miller, D., and Boudrant, S. Effects of cigarette smoke on the surface characteristic of lung extracts. *Am. Rev. Respir. Dis.* 85:692, 1962.

Morgan, T. Pulmonary surfactant. *N. Engl. J. Med.* 284:1185, 1972.

Newhouse, M., Sanchis, J., and Bienstack, J. Lung defense mechanisms. *N. Engl. J. Med.* 295:990, 1976.

Notkins, A., and Oldstone, B.A. *Concepts in Viral Pathogenesis.* New York: Springer-Verlag, 1984.

Passey, R. Some problems of lung cancer. *Lancet* 2:107, 1962.

Pattle, R., Schoch, C., and Battensby, J. Some effects of anesthesia on lung surfactant. *Br. J. Anaesth.* 99:1119, 1972.

Polk, B.V. Cardiopulmonary complications of Guillain-Barré syndrome. *Heart Lung* 5:96, 1976.

Reichel, J. Pulmonary embolism. *Med. Clin. North Am.* 61:1310, 1977.

Robbins, S.L., Cotran, R.S., and Kumar, V. *Pathologic Basis of Disease* (3rd ed.). Philadelphia: Saunders, 1984.

Roitt, I. *Essential Immunology* (5th ed.). Oxford: Blackwell, 1984.

Sade, J., et al. The role of mucus in transport by cilia. *Am. Rev. Respir. Dis.* 102:48, 1970.

Santa Cruz, R., et al. Tracheal mucus velocity in normal man and obstructive lung disease: Effects of terbutaline. *Am. Rev. Respir. Dis.* 109:458, 1974.

Satir, P. How cilia move. *Sci. Am.* 231:44, 1974.

Shapiro, B.A. *Clinical Application of Blood Gases* (3rd ed.). Chicago: Yearbook, 1982.

Shapiro, B.A., et al. *Clinical Application of Respiratory Care* (3rd ed.). Chicago: Yearbook, 1985.

Slonim, N.B., and Hamilton, L.H. *Respiratory Physiology* (4th ed.). St. Louis: Mosby, 1981.

Sodeman, W.A., and Sodeman, T.M. *Sodeman's Pathologic Physiology* (7th ed.). Philadelphia: Saunders, 1985.

Surveyer, J. Smoke inhalation injuries. *Heart Lung* 9:825, 1980.

Wanner, A., et al. Tracheal mucus flow in beagles after chronic exposure to cigarette smoke. *Arch. Environ. Health* 27:370, 1973.

Weiss, E.B. Bronchial asthma. *Ciba Clin. Symp.* 27:1, 1975.

West, J.B. *Ventilation: Blood Flow and Gas Exchange* (3rd ed.). Oxford: Blackwell, 1977.

West, J.G. *Respiratory Physiology: The Essentials* (2nd ed.). Baltimore: Williams & Wilkins, 1985.

West, J.G. *Pulmonary Pathophysiology: The Essentials* (2nd ed.). Baltimore, Williams & Wilkins, 1982.

Wood, R., Wanner, A., and Hirsch, J. Tracheal mucociliary transport in patients with cystic fibrosis and its stimulation effect by terbutalene. *Am. Rev. Respir. Dis.* 111:633, 1975.

Ziskind, M. Occupational pulmonary disease. *Clin. Symp.* 30:4, 1978.

UNIT 10

Urinary Excretion

Barbara L. Bullock

The urinary system maintains the concentration of electrolytes and water in the blood. Chapter 28 explains normal renal function and provides a basis for the subsequent chapters that discuss different forms of renal pathology. Chapter 29 details the immunologic, infectious, and toxic alterations that can affect renal function. Chapter 30 describes the common causes of genitourinary obstruction, with emphasis on the formation of different types of calculi. Benign prostatic hyperplasia and renal tumors are included. Chapter 31 describes renal failure, its causes, and clinical course.

The reader is encouraged to use the learning objectives and study questions to provide a systematic method for study. The extensive bibliography provides a current and historical perspective on theories of renal function and dysfunction.

CHAPTER 28

Normal Renal and Urinary Excretory Function

CHAPTER OUTLINE

Anatomy of the Kidneys

Macroscopic Anatomy
Microscopic Anatomy: The Nephron
Blood Supply to the Kidneys
Innervation of the Kidneys

Physiology of the Kidneys

Glomerular Filtration
Resorption: Tubules
Proximal Convoluted Tubules

Active Transport
Passive Transport

Loop of Henle

Countercurrent Multiplier Effect
Countercurrent Exchanger

Distal Convoluted Tubules and Collecting Tubules

Sodium and Potassium Resorption
Water Resorption

Secretion: Tubules and Collecting Ducts
Substances That Are Secreted

PAH
Hydrogen Ions
Potassium

Accessory Urinary Structures and Bladder

Ureters
Bladder

Micturation Reflex

Urethra

LEARNING OBJECTIVES

1. Describe the location and size of the kidneys.
2. Describe the external structure of the kidneys.
3. Explain the internal structure of the kidneys, including the cortex, medulla, and renal pelvis.
4. Identify Bowman's capsule and the glomerulus.
5. List the main layers of the glomerular membrane, including the epithelial, glomerular basement membrane, and endothelial layers.
6. List the parts of the proximal convoluted tubules, loop of Henle, and distal convoluted tubules.
7. Describe the renal corpuscles and juxtaglomerular apparatus.
8. Identify the collecting tubules, ducts, and papillary duct.
9. Describe the interstitium of the kidneys.
10. Describe the blood supply to the kidneys.
11. Explain the innervation of the kidneys.
12. Explain autoregulation of the kidneys.
13. Describe in detail the mechanisms responsible for urine formation, including glomerular filtration, tubular resorption, and secretion.
14. Define *filtration, filtrate, tubular resorption, transport maximum,* and *secretion.*
15. Describe the pressures responsible for filtration.
16. Calculate the effective net filtration pressure.
17. Describe active transport of glucose ions and protein from the proximal convoluted tubules.
18. Explain the passive transport of water and ions from the proximal convoluted tubules.
19. Describe hypotonic and hypertonic urine formation and explain the countercurrent mechanism in the loop of Henle.
20. Explain renal regulation of the renin-angiotensin-aldosterone system.
21. Discuss antidiuretic hormone and its relationship to water regulation in the distal convoluted tubules and collecting tubules.
22. Discuss the secretion of PAH and potassium.
23. Explain the secretion of hydrogen ions and its relationship to acid-base balance.
24. Describe the structure and purpose of the ureters.
25. Explain the micturation reflex.
26. Differentiate between the female and male urethras.
27. Explain the physical characteristics of urine.

For the body to maintain a steady state, the renal system must function normally. This system not only is important in removing waste products from the blood, it maintains sufficient amounts of water and electrolytes in the blood. Urine is produced by the kidneys and is transported to the ureters, which empty into the bladder. Urine is excreted from the body through the urethra.

Anatomy of the Kidneys

Macroscopic Anatomy

The kidneys are bean-shaped, reddish brown organs that are located retroperitoneally on either side of the vertebral column, extending from the twelfth thoracic vertebra to the third lumbar vertebra. Each kidney is approximately 11.0 cm in length, 5.0 to 7.0 cm in diameter, and 2.5 cm in thickness. The right kidney is slightly lower than the left because the liver is located above it (Fig. 28-1).

Surrounding the kidneys is a layer of adipose tissue, or perirenal fat, that helps protect and support them. A fibrous layer of connective tissue called *renal fascia* encapsulates and anchors the kidneys in place in the abdomen.

Located externally at the concave portion of the kidney is a notch called the *hilus*. The hilus is located in the *renal sinus*, which is a C-shaped cavity. Structures at the hilus of each kidney are the renal artery and vein, lymphatics, nerves, and renal pelvis (Fig. 28-2).

Internally, the kidneys are composed of the *cortex* and the *medulla*. The cortex, the outer portion, lies under the renal fascia and is composed of renal columns called *columns of Bertin*. Originating in the cortex and extending into the medulla are the *uriniferous tubules*, which are made up of the functioning units of the kidneys, the *nephrons*.

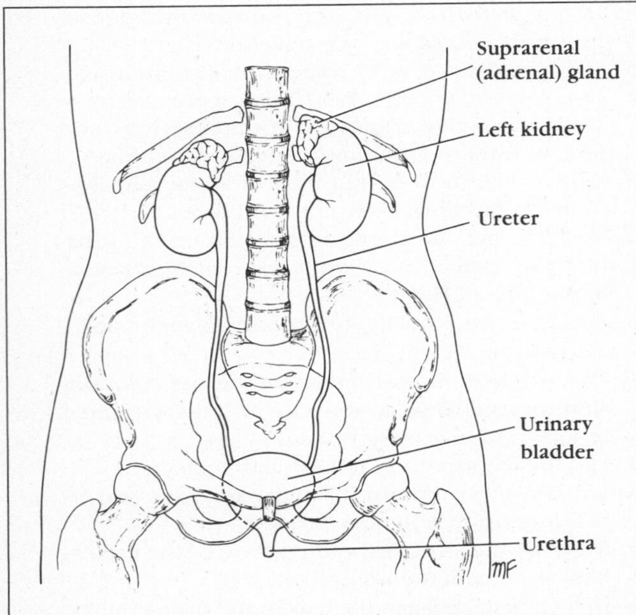

FIGURE 28-1 Posterior abdominal wall showing kidneys and ureters in situ. (From R. Snell, *Clinical Histology for Medical Students*. Boston: Little, Brown, 1984.)

The medulla, the inner portion of the kidney, contains an estimated 8 to 18 *renal pyramids*, so called because they are triangular. They are striated due to the collecting ducts, nephrons, and blood vessels of which they are composed. The apex of each pyramid is called the *papilla*.

Below the papillae is a large cavity called the *renal pelvis*, which is interrupted by cuplike extensions called the *minor* and *major calices*. These structures are lined with transitional epithelium. The minor calices (approximately 10 in number) have openings that collect urine from the *collecting ducts* of the pyramids and empty urine into the major calices (approximately 3 in number) and then into the renal pelvis, where it is excreted from the kidneys to the ureters (see Fig. 28-2).

Microscopic Anatomy: The Nephron

It is estimated that a pair of kidneys contains 2.5 million nephrons. The nephron is a unique and complex structure; it is composed of Bowman's capsule, the proximal convoluted tubule, the loop of Henle, and the distal convoluted tubule. Many distal tubules empty into one collecting duct.

Bowman's capsule is a cuplike structure that surrounds a capillary network called the *glomerulus*; the two together are called the *renal malpighian corpuscle*. The membrane of the glomerular capillaries is composed of three main layers: *epithelial*, *glomerular basement membrane (GBM)*, and endothelial (Figure 28-3) [4]. The main function of the glomerular membrane is to form glomerular filtrate, a solution like plasma but without plasma proteins. This is the initial step in urine formation.

Nephrons are classified as either cortical or juxtamedullary (Fig. 28-4). The glomeruli of the cortical nephrons are in the outer two-thirds of the cortex. The remaining one-third of the cortical area consists of glomeruli of the juxtamedullary nephrons, which contain a long loop of Henle that extends deep into the medulla [6].

Lining the inner layer of Bowman's capsule, adjacent to the glomerulus, is a thin layer of *epithelial cells* called *podocytes*. These podocytes have projections called *pedicles* or *foot processes* that cover the GBM. Between the pedicles are narrow regions called *slit pores*, or *filtration slits*, through which proteins with a molecular weight of less than 50,000 can pass [3]. Because plasma proteins have a slightly higher molecular weight they normally cannot cross the GBM. Because of the location, numbers, and arrangement of slit pores, there is a large surface area that allows for rapid filtration of fluid. Diseases that affect the foot processes allow plasma proteins and sometimes cells to pass into the glomerular filtrate (Chap. 29).

Adjacent to the layer of epithelial cells is the GBM, which consists of a continuous meshwork of fibrillae that contain mucopolysaccharides. This meshwork prevents large proteins and molecules from passing into Bowman's capsule, an extremely important function.

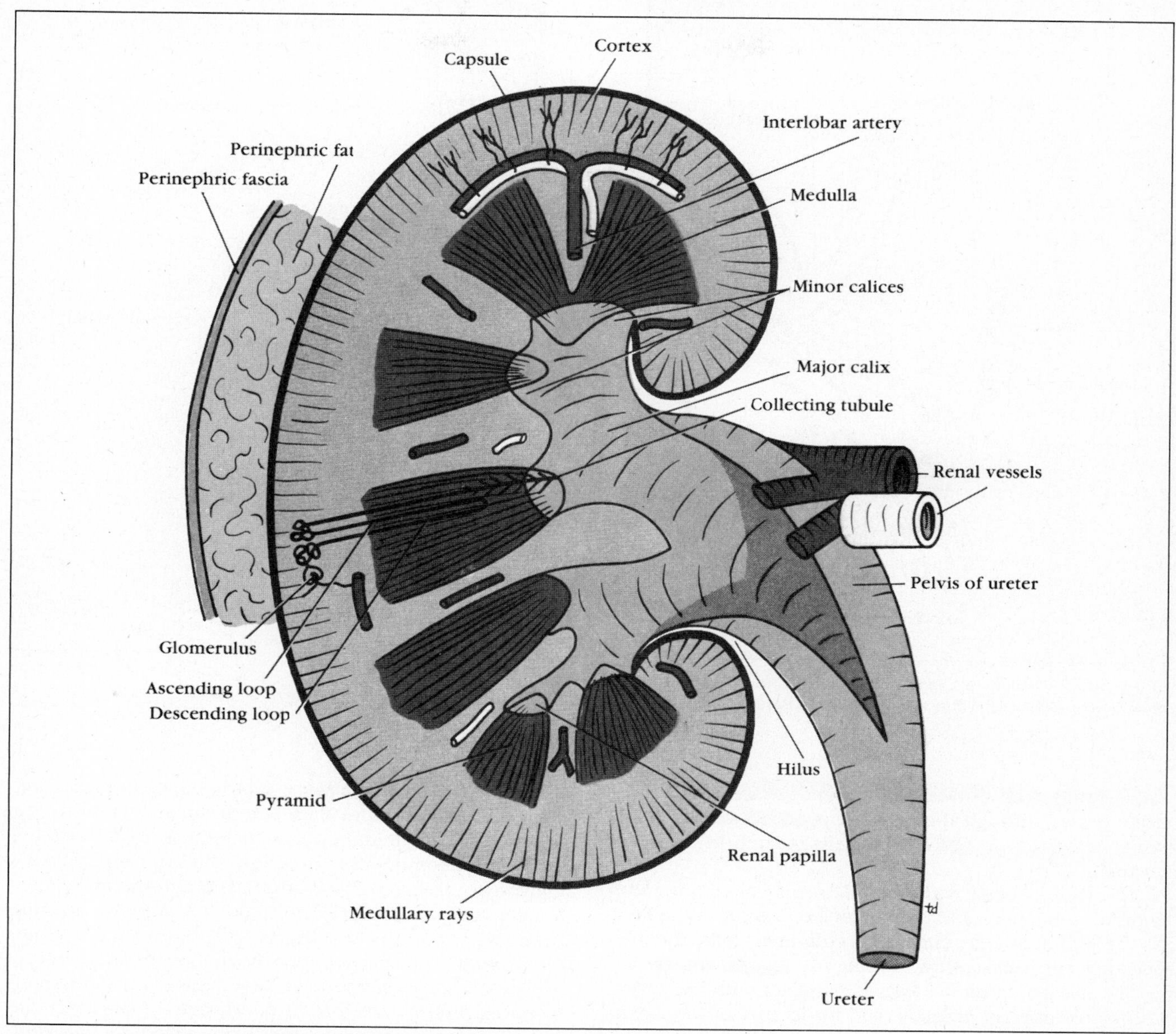

FIGURE 28-2 Longitudinal section through kidney, showing cortex, medulla, pyramids, renal papillae, and calices. Note position of nephron and arrangement of blood vessels within kidney. Note also perinephric fascia and fat and their relation to renal capsule. (From R. Snell, *Clinical Anatomy for Medical Students* [2nd ed.]. Boston: Little, Brown, 1981.)

The inner layer of the glomerular capillary is composed of *endothelial cells*. This layer consists of thousands of pores, of fenestrations, that line the glomerulus and aid in membrane permeability. The glomerular filtrate passes through three layers before it arrives in Bowman's capsule, but each layer is several hundred times more permeable than the usual capillary membrane [4].

Once the glomerular filtrate passes through the glomeruli into Bowman's capsule, it enters the *proximal convoluted tubule (PCT)*, which is located in the cortex and is approximately 14 mm long. Cuboidal epithelial cells line the PCT. On the luminal surface of these cells is a brush border of microvilli that increases the surface area available for secretion and absorption of fluids and solutes. Also located in the PCT cells are mitochondria. More than 65 to 80 percent of the glomerular filtrate is resorbed in the PCT and the remaining 20 to 35 percent proceeds to the loop of Henle.

The two major portions of the *loop of Henle* are the *descending* and *ascending limbs* (see Fig. 28-4). The thickened descending limb begins in the cortex; as it dips into the medulla it becomes thinner and varies in length from 4.5 to 10.0 mm [2].

The descending limb loops and makes a tight hairpin turn upward, where it becomes thin and is called the thin portion of the ascending limb. The main function of both

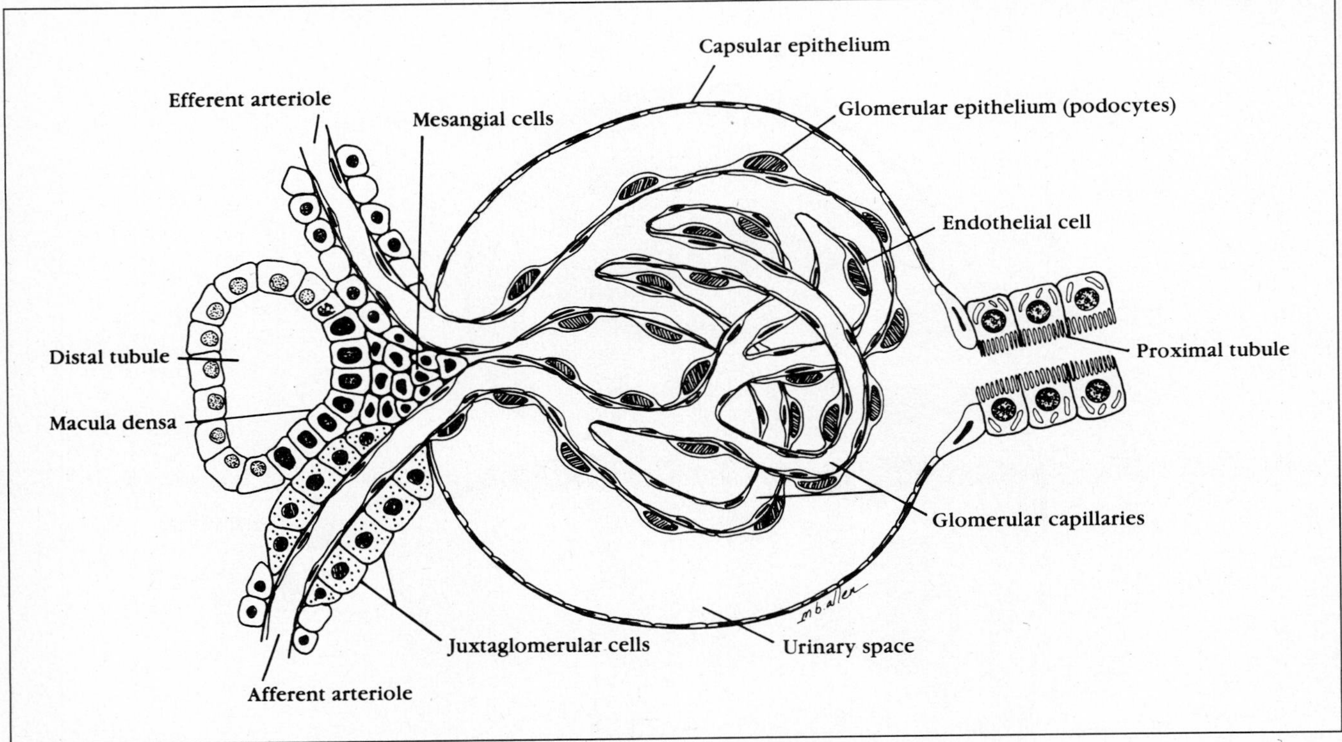

FIGURE 28-3 Bowman's capsule with the glomerulus within. (From M. Borysenko et al., *Functional Histology* [2nd ed.]. Boston: Little, Brown, 1984.)

limbs of the loop of Henle is to concentrate urine. Once urine passes through the limbs, it proceeds to the *distal convoluted tubule (DCT)*, which is located in the renal cortex.

The DCT is lined with cuboidal cells containing mitochondria and fewer microvilli than are present in the PCT. As the cuboidal cells change to columnar cells, the area becomes very dense, thus forming the *macula densa*.

The macula densa lies in close contact with the vascular pole or afferent arteriole and forms part of the *juxtaglomerular apparatus* (Fig. 28-5). Located within the apparatus are juxtaglomerular cells that produce the enzyme *renin*, which transforms angiotensinogen to angiotensin I (see p. 504).

The main function of the DCT is to transport electrolytes and water. Two or more DCTs join together to form the *collecting duct*, which conducts the formed urine. The collecting ducts are lined with cuboidal cells, contain few mitochondria, and terminate in the renal medulla.

Urine is transported from the duct to a *papillary duct (of Bellini)*, which opens into the minor calix. Urine is excreted from the minor and major calices into the *renal pelvis*, *ureters*, *bladder*, and *urethra*.

Blood Supply to the Kidneys

In a resting state, it is estimated, the kidneys receive 20 to 25 percent of cardiac output, which is more than 1000 ml per minute. Thus, by way of the *aorta*, blood enters the hilus of the kidney by a *renal artery*, which branches into segmental arteries and then *interlobar arteries* that run between the pyramids of the medulla (Figs. 28-4 and 28-6). At the corticomedullary junction, the interlobar arteries convert to *arcuate arteries* that penetrate the cortex and branch into smaller arteries called *interlobular arteries*, thus giving rise to the *afferent arterioles (vas afferens glomeruli)*. The afferent arterioles subdivide into a tuft of capillaries called a *glomerulus*. Blood leaves the glomerulus by the *efferent arteriole (vas efferens glomeruli)* and forms a second network of capillaries called the *peritubular capillary network* that mainly encircles the convoluted tubules (proximal and distal). The arrangement of capillaries between the arterioles is unique because it allows a higher pressure to be maintained in the glomerulus. Also, the efferent arterioles are smaller in diameter than the afferent arterioles, again causing higher glomerular pressure due to increased vascular resistance.

The deeper-lying, or juxtamedullary, glomeruli also break up into the peritubular network but have a set of capillaries penetrating the medulla. These thin-walled vessels are in close proximity to the thin ascending and descending loops of Henle and are referred to as the *vasa recta*. The vasa recta aid in concentrating urine.

The *interlobular veins* are formed from the peritubular capillary network and empty into the *arcuate veins* and then the *interlobar veins*, and converge to form the *renal vein*. Blood from the renal vein leaves the kidneys and drains into the *inferior vena cava*.

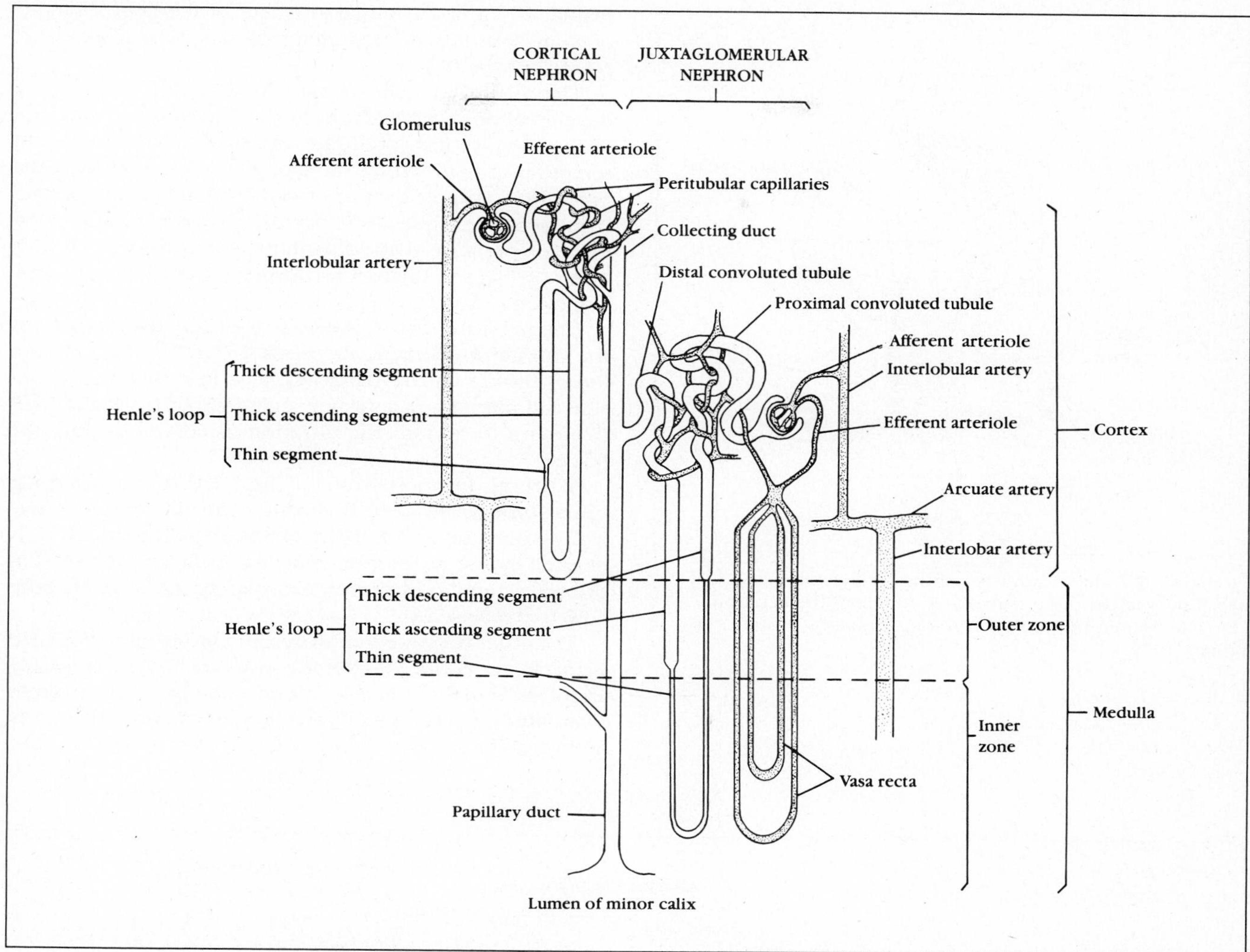

FIGURE 28-4 Structure of cortical and medullary nephrons. Blood supply to the nephron. The vasa recta is shown schematically; this capillary structure normally surrounds Henle's loop. (From M. Borysenko et al., *Functional Histology* [2nd ed.]. Boston: Little, Brown, 1984.)

Innervation of the Kidneys

The kidneys are innervated mostly by the sympathetic division of the autonomic nervous system. The nerve supply generally follows the distribution of the arterial vessels in the renal parenchyma. The nerve supply comes mostly from the celiac plexus, and the mesenteric, upper splanchnic, and thoracic nerves [3]. The sympathetic nerves, when stimulated, constrict the afferent arteriole and cause an increase in blood pressure. The parasympathetic system has important effects on the ureters and urinary bladder but no noted effects on the kidneys per se.

Physiology of the Kidneys

The functions of the kidneys are to maintain a constant plasma concentration of nonelectrolytes and water to ensure the appropriate electrolyte and acid-base balance, and to regulate blood pressure. These maintain the steady state that is essential to sustain life. The kidneys have a large reserve in renal function due to large numbers of nephrons.

The kidneys use three major mechanisms to maintain the steady state that alter the composition of urine to keep the composition of plasma within strict limits. These mechanisms are glomerular filtration, tubular resorption, and tubular secretion.

Glomerular Filtration

Filtration, the initial step in urine formation, is the result of pressures that force fluids and solutes through a membrane. The filtration process occurs between the layers of the glomerulus and Bowman's capsule. The resulting fluid is *glomerular filtrate*, a relatively protein-free solution.

Approximately 125 ml per minute, or 180 liters per day, of glomerular filtrate is produced. Normally, urine output equals approximately 1 to 2 liters per day, which means that the tubules are responsible for resorbing approxi-

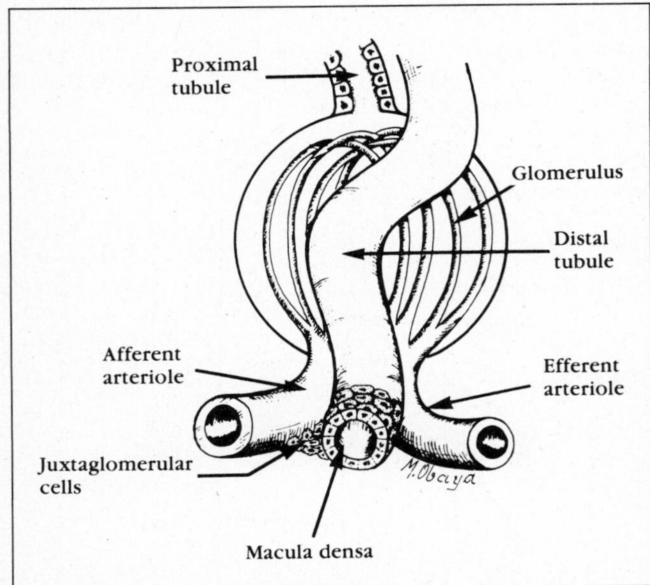

FIGURE 28-5 The relationship of the juxtaglomerular apparatus and the distal convoluted tubule of the nephron. (From S. Papper, *Clinical Nephrology* [2nd ed.]. Boston: Little, Brown, 1978.)

mately 179 liters. The measurement of the large quantity of glomerular filtrate each minute is called the *glomerular filtration rate (GFR)*.

The quantity of filtrate and the filtration process are dependent on several factors. Various pressures contribute to the outward flow of filtrate into Bowman's capsule and retention of fluid within the glomerulus. The *hydrostatic pressure* is a simple outward force created by the systemic blood pressure. The *colloid osmotic pressure* is the inward force or pressure that holds fluid within the glomerulus (Fig. 28-7). (See Chap. 5 for further discussion of colloid osmotic pressure.)

The pressure that is chiefly responsible for filtration is the *glomerular hydrostatic pressure (GHP)*. This pressure forces filtrate out of the glomerulus into Bowman's capsule and normally is approximately 60 mm Hg. If the GHP decreases to 50 mm Hg, filtration usually does not take place.

Working in opposition to the GHP is the *capsular hydrostatic pressure* in Bowman's capsule, which is normally estimated to be about 18 mm Hg. This pressure is exerted by the walls of Bowman's capsule and the fluid in the renal tubule. Increased capsular pressure causes the GFR to decrease [4].

The other pressure that works in opposition to the GHP is the *blood colloidal osmotic pressure (COP)*, normally about 30 mm Hg. Because blood contains more protein than filtrate does, the colloidal property constantly exerts an inward force.

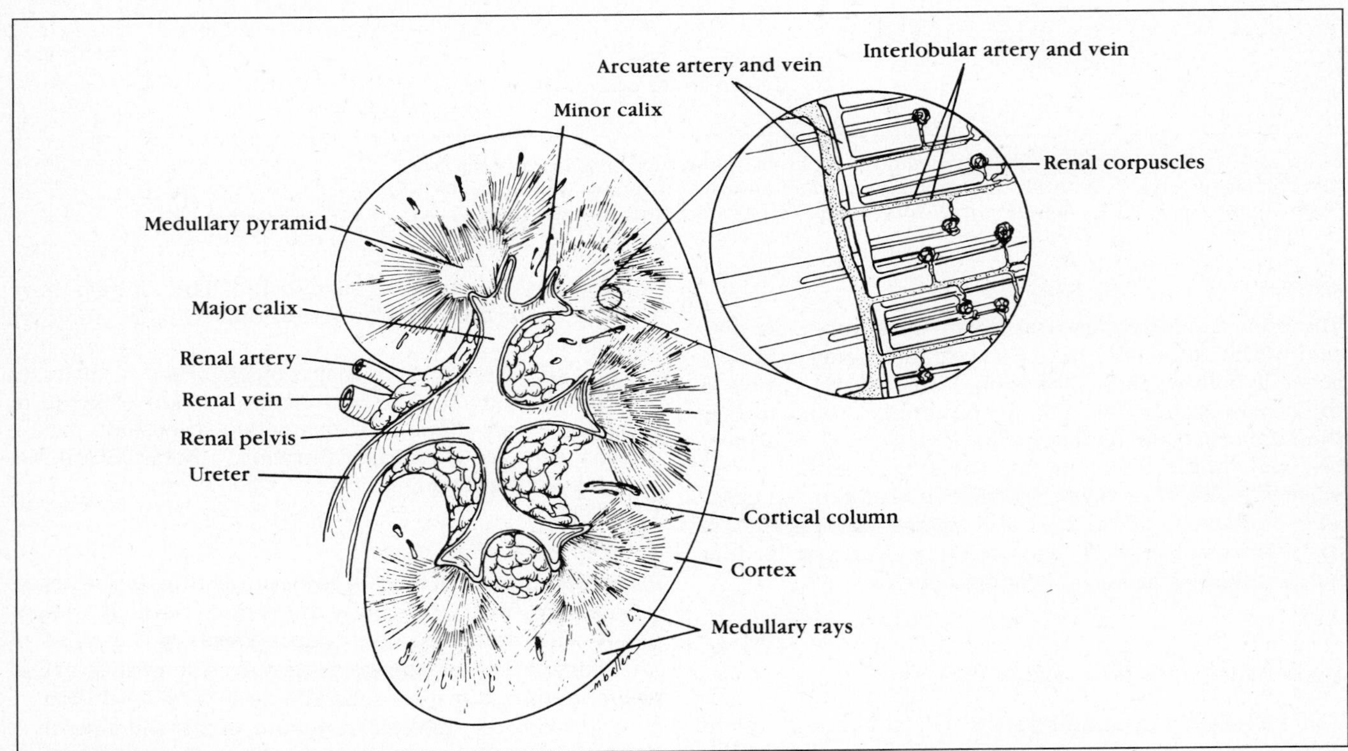

FIGURE 28-6 Hemisected kidney with vascular distribution. (From M. Borysenko et al., *Functional Histology* [2nd ed.]. Boston: Little, Brown, 1984.)

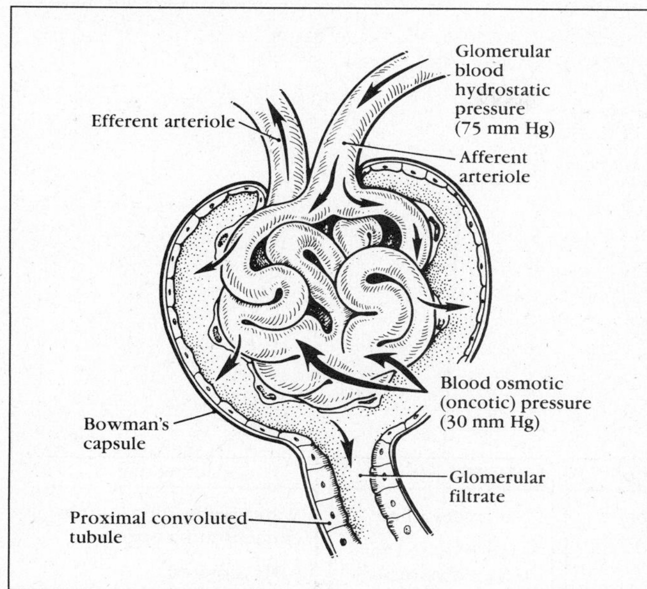

FIGURE 28-7 Schematic representation of the relationship between hydrostatic pressure and colloid osmotic pressure.

The net result of all these pressures—GHP, capsular, and colloidal osmotic—is the *effective filtration pressure* (P_{eff}). To calculate P_{eff}, the following formula can be used:

$$P_{eff} = \text{GHP} - (\text{capsular pressure} + \text{blood colloid osmotic pressure}).$$

For example, if the GHP is 60 mm Hg, the capsular pressure is 18, and the colloid osmotic pressure is 32, the P_{eff} will be 10 mm Hg ($60 - [18 + 32] = 10$). If 1 mm Hg effective filtration pressure produces a GFR of 12.5 ml per minute from both kidneys, then 10 mm Hg produces 125 ml per minute, which is a normal rate. Many factors can change the GFR. Increased hydrostatic pressure or decreased COP can increase the GFR.

Sympathetic nervous system (SNS) stimulation results in vasoconstriction of the afferent and efferent arterioles, which affects the P_{eff}. Because constriction of the afferent arterioles is usually greater than that of the efferent arterioles with sympathetic stimulation, the result is a decrease in GHP, filtration pressure, and GFR.

Resorption: Tubules

As described in the previous section, approximately 179 liters of filtrate of the 180 liters filtered per day are resorbed in the tubules. The kidneys are able to change the composition of urine by excreting different concentrations of substances [4]. This is achieved by resorption and secretion. For example, when a person ingests a large volume of water, the resulting urine is very dilute; in a dehydrated state the urine output is markedly decreased and urine becomes very concentrated. *Tubular resorption*, the second step of urine formation, requires movement of solutes between the filtrate and blood of the surrounding vasa recta and peritubular capillaries.

Proximal Convoluted Tubules

In the *proximal convoluted tubules (PCT)*, tubular resorption is accomplished by active and passive transport (diffusion or osmosis). Approximately 70 percent of glomerular filtrate is resorbed in the PCT. Ions are transported by active and passive transport. Some ions passively follow the active transport of other ions [4].

Active Transport. Active transport is the movement of molecules against a concentration gradient and requires an expenditure of energy. It causes movement of substances from PCT to plasma. The PCT are able to carry on active transport because of their epithelial cells that contain mitochondria. These cells also have a brush border that increases the surface area for resorption and secretion. Some of the substances that are moved actively include glucose, many electrolytes, amino acids, proteins, and vitamins (Fig. 28-8).

Glucose is actively transported from the tubules into the plasma, and normally, none appears in the urine. Glucose apparently binds with the same sodium carrier in the brush border that transports sodium ions through this membrane [4]. This transport is related to a mechanism called *transport maximum (TM)* in which there is a maximum amount of substance that can be resorbed at any time [2]. If the plasma glucose level exceeds approximately 175 mg per dl, glucose appears in the urine (glycosuria) because the transport mechanism has become saturated with glucose and must return it to the tubules where it is excreted in the urine.

Sodium and *potassium* are actively transported from the tubules into the plasma of the peritubular capillaries by way of the basal channels of the epithelial cells. Because sodium and potassium are positive ions, they set up an electronegative cytoplasm in the epithelial cells; this allows negative ions, such as chloride and phosphate, to follow the positive ions [4].

Proteins are resorbed in the PCT through the process of *pinocytosis*. The proteins attach to the membrane of the brush border of the PCT, are ingested by the tubular cells, and are broken down into amino acids, which are transported into the plasma. If permeability of the glomerular membrane increases, large protein molecules can leak into the filtrate, causing proteinuria.

Passive Transport. Passive transport, including osmosis and diffusion, involves the movement of substances across a membrane without the expenditure of energy. It is accomplished by the established electrical gradient of positive ions, mainly sodium, allowing negative ions and water to diffuse across the tubular membrane.

Water is removed from the tubules as the result of the *isosmotic process*, which maintains equal osmotic pressures of fluid inside the tubules and in the plasma. When

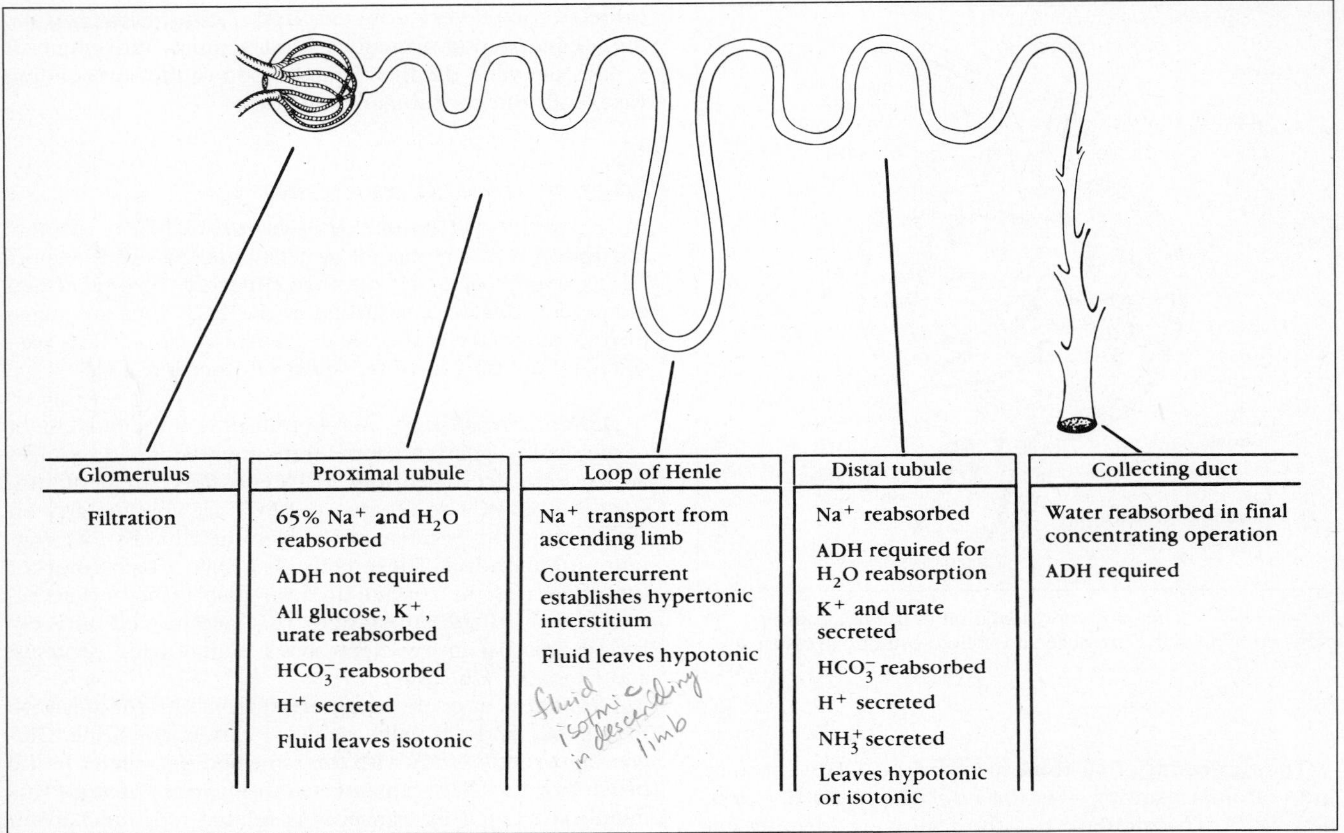

FIGURE 28-8 Major functions of each portion of the nephron. (From S. Papper, *Clinical Nephrology* [2nd ed.]. Boston: Little, Brown, 1978.)

the solutes are actively resorbed into the plasma, the concentration of solute in the tubules decreases and the concentration in the peritubular capillaries increases, causing water to move into the peritubular capillary. Approximately 70 percent of water is resorbed by passive transport in the PCT. The role of the kidneys in controlling osmolality of the plasma through the transport of water is critical in maintaining fluid balance. The excretion of excess water or conservation of water maintains the plasma osmolarity at a fixed specific gravity of 1.010. This regulation is greatly influenced by antidiuretic hormone (ADH) in the distal convoluted and collecting tubules (see p. 440).

Chloride and *bicarbonate* apparently diffuse across the tubular membrane into the peritubular capillaries. In the PCT their diffusion occurs because of an electrochemical gradient created by positive ions.

Loop of Henle

The main function of the loop of Henle is to concentrate urine. For this concentration to occur, the *countercurrent mechanism* is used. The two components of this mechanism are the *countercurrent multiplier* and the *countercurrent exchanger*. The nephrons involved in renal concentration are the juxtamedullary nephrons whose loops of Henle extend into the medulla of the kidney. These loops are surrounded by vessels of the vasa recta. Both the loops of Henle and the juxtamedullary capillary system (vasa recta) work together to concentrate urine. In 20 to 30 percent of the nephrons the loops of Henle extend into the medulla and are surrounded by the vasa recta. Resorption through the vessels of the vasa recta is partly responsible for operating the mechanism that concentrates urine [8].

Countercurrent Multiplier Effect. In the PCT, tubular fluid is neither concentrated nor diluted because resorption is due to water permeability of tubular epithelium [1]. As fluid progresses down the descending limb of the loop of Henle, it is still isotonic to plasma. The excretion of excess solutes (concentrated urine) requires a hyperosmolality of the medullary interstitial fluid. This hyperosmolality is greater in the long segments of the loop of Henle and may increase to as much as 1200 mOsm per liter at the turn of the loop. Sodium and chloride are transported from the thin segment (descending and loop portions) into the medullary interstitium. Current research indicates that this movement occurs when the interstitial concentration of urea is high, causing water to move into the interstitial area. The sodium and chloride concentration then becomes increased in the thin segment, and these ions probably diffuse passively out of this area and into the interstitium [1]. Urea is poorly absorbed by the vasa recta and becomes trapped in the medullary interstitium. It is partly reabsorbed by ascending limbs of the loop of Henle.

As sodium, chloride, potassium, and water move up the ascending limb (thick portion), sodium, chloride, and potassium are transported out of the tubule into the interstitium. Thus, the distal tubule receives a hypotonic fluid [1]. Water is not removed because the ascending limb is nearly impermeable to it. Because this process continuously concentrates the filtrate with sodium chloride and urea in the section of the loop of Henle that is located in the medulla, it is called the *countercurrent multiplier*. As fluid moves up the ascending loop, sodium is transported out and the filtrate becomes more dilute. As the filtrate passes to the distal and collecting tubules, water is resorbed under the influence of antidiuretic hormone, resulting in the final regulation of the specific gravity of the urine. Figure 28-9 summarizes the process for countercurrent multiplication.

Urea is also exchanged by this mechanism and excess is excreted in the urine. Urea is produced through degradation of amino acids, and the amount formed usually depends on the protein intake in the diet and the ability of the liver to convert ammonia to urea. Normally, the body produces 25 to 30 gm of urea each day, but maintains only 8 to 20 mg per dl in the plasma. Approximately half of the urea that is filtered remains in the interstitial fluid of the medulla. The ascending thin limb of the loop of Henle is permeable to urea, but the DCT and collecting ducts are not. Therefore, urea remaining in the tubules at this point is excreted.

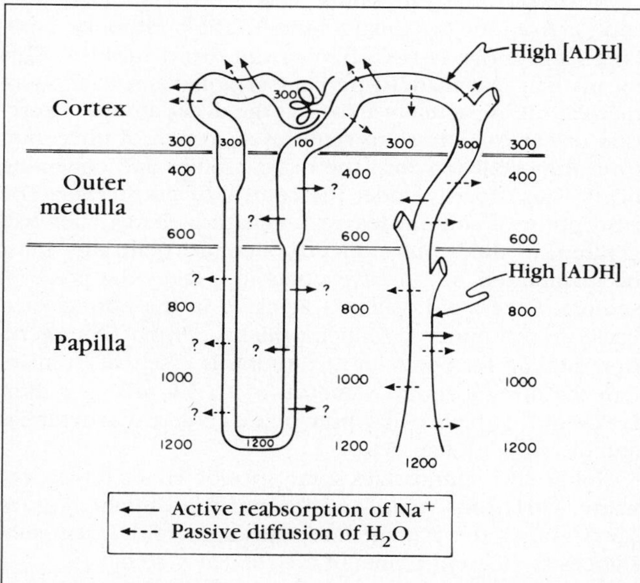

FIGURE 28-9 Operation of the countercurrent mechanism in a normal human during antidiuresis. The numbers refer to the osmolality (mOsm/kg H_2O) of either intratubular or interstitial fluid. Solid arrows denote active resorption of Na^+ (its accompanying anions, mainly Cl^-, being resorbed passively); dashed arrows denote passive resorption of water. The question marks in the loops of Henle indicate that it is not yet known (1) how much H_2O is resorbed from descending limbs, (2) whether soluted transport out of thin ascending limbs is active or passive, and (3) whether Na^+ or Cl^- is actively resorbed from thick ascending limbs. The number of arrows in each nephron segment signifies semiquantitatively the amounts of solute transported relative to water. For example, in ascending limbs of Henle, solute is resorbed to the virtual, but not complete, exclusion of water, since renal membranes are not absolutely impervious to water. (From H. Valtin, *Renal Function: Mechanisms Preserving Fluid and Solute Balance in Health* [2nd ed.]. Boston: Little, Brown, 1983.)

Countercurrent Exchanger. As discussed above, the vasa recta are important in carrying out the countercurrent mechanism. Blood enters the descending limbs of the vasa recta with a solute concentration of 300 mOsm per liter. At this point, sodium, chloride, and urea diffuse from the interstitial fluid into the blood, thus creating a higher osmolality in the blood, which causes water to move back into the blood. At the tip of the U in each of the vasa recta, osmolality can reach 1200 mOsm per liter for a maximum concentration, which is also the concentration of surrounding interstitium.

As blood ascends the vasa recta, water returns to the blood, and sodium, chloride, and urea move back by diffusion into the interstitial fluid. When blood leaves the medulla, its osmolality is slightly higher than that of blood that enters the vasa recta [7]. This mechanism provides a precise balance between the countercurrent systems and prevents sodium from accumulating in the interstitium [8]. This entire action by the vasa recta is called the *countercurrent exchange mechanism*.

Distal Convoluted Tubules and Collecting Tubules

Sodium and Potassium Resorption. The DCT and collecting tubules resorb sodium in smaller amounts than in the loop of Henle, depending on the amount of aldosterone in the blood. The release of aldosterone stimulated by serum potassium concentration and the *renin-angiotensin-aldosterone system* affects sodium resorption at the DCT. Both potassium and angiotensin II apparently are necessary for aldosterone biosynthesis [5].

Located in each kidney are special cells called *juxtaglomerular cells*, which make up the juxtaglomerular apparatus. This apparatus produces *renin*, an enzyme, and secretes it into the blood. The stimulus for this secretion is decreased perfusion pressure in the afferent arteriole. Renin then causes angiotensinogen, a plasma protein, to split and produce *angiotensin I*, a polypeptide that is transformed into *angiotensin II* in the lungs. Angiotensin II causes vasoconstriction throughout the body and stimulates the adrenal cortex to release *aldosterone*. With the release of aldosterone, sodium is transported from the tubules to the blood, passively followed by water; thus, blood volume and blood pressure are increased. Increasing the blood volume causes the renal cells to receive increased amounts of oxygen.

An increase in serum potassium from increased intake provides a direct stimulus for the release of aldosterone. Aldosterone then causes retention of sodium ion and urinary excretion of potassium. This is an important mechanism in maintaining the serum concentration of potassium [5].

Water Resorption. Water is regulated in the DCT and collecting tubules by the production of *antidiuretic hormone (ADH or vasopressin)*. This hormone is produced by the hypothalamus and stored and released by the posterior pituitary gland. It is secreted by the posterior pituitary when the osmoreceptors in the anterior hypothalamus respond to an increase in the osmolarity of the plasma. The hormone directly regulates the permeability of the membranes of the renal epithelial cells. This occurs by binding to receptors in the membranes of the collecting duct.

If amounts of ADH in the blood are increased, water is osmotically moved from the tubules into the capillaries by increasing the permeability of the tubular membrane to water. This results in more concentrated urine and adds water to the plasma. Without ADH, the permeability is decreased, causing water to stay in the tubules and resulting in very dilute urine.

Secretion: Tubules and Collecting Ducts

Secretion, the final step to urine formation, is the movement of fluid and solute from the blood back into the glomerular filtrate, usually requiring an expenditure of energy to cross the electrochemical gradient. Active and a few passive secretory mechanisms are present at various points in the tubules.

Substances That Are Secreted

PAH. Artificially injected organic acids such as para-aminohippurate (PAH) are secreted in the PCT by way of carrier sites. When the plasma PAH concentration is low, almost all of it is secreted into the tubules and very little remains in the blood. The flow of plasma through the kidneys is always slightly greater than the clearance of PAH. Therefore, by knowing the PAH clearance, one can calculate renal plasma flow (RPF) [4]. By knowing the hematocrit and knowing that the average PAH clearance is 630 ml per minute, one can calculate the RPF by the following formula:

$$\text{PAH}\ (1 - \text{Hct}) = \text{RPF}.$$

For example,

$$630\ (1.0 - 0.43) = 1158 \text{ ml per minute}.$$

Hydrogen Ions. Hydrogen ions (H^+) are secreted in the PCT, DCT, and collecting tubules. The number of H^+ secreted is dependent on the pH of the extracellular fluid and the amount of buffer in the glomerular filtrate. The normal pH of urine varies from 4.5 to 8.0 depending on dietary intake and metabolism. If the pH decreases to 4.4, secretion becomes inhibited.

When the hydrogen ion concentration is high in extracellular fluid (plasma), large quantities of hydrogen are secreted. Low concentrations cause small amounts of H^+ secretion.

When ammonia (NH_3^+) is passively secreted by the tubules, it can combine with the actively secreted hydrogen, forming ammonium (NH_4^+). Hence, NH_4 is secreted into the filtrate and sodium (NA^+) is replaced. The exchange of Na^+ and H^+ causes Na^+ to move into the renal capillaries and combine with bicarbonate ion to form sodium bicarbonate. This is one way the renal cells maintain acid-base balance and buffer excess H^+. A special enzyme, carbonic anhydrase, in the renal cells is necessary in this process and causes water and carbon dioxide to combine, resulting in the formation of carbonic acid (H_2CO_3). When H_2CO_3 dissociates, it forms hydrogen and bicarbonate ions ($H^+ + HCO_3^-$). This ammonia-ammonium mechanism is especially important when excess acid loads continually bombard the kidneys, such as with chronic respiratory insufficiency.

Potassium. Potassium ions are transported with sodium from the proximal tubules to the peritubular capillaries and more is resorbed in the distal tubules. This means that less than 10 percent of potassium in the glomerular filtrate actually arrives at the distal tubules. Excretion of excess potassium requires secretion of potassium from the capillaries into the distal tubules and collecting ducts. This is partly under the control of aldosterone. The resorption of sodium leaves a negative electrochemical gradient in the tubules. Electrochemical neutrality must be maintained, so positive potassium takes the place of sodium. Excess potassium is ingested in the normal diet, up to several hundred milliequivalents per day. The secretion method for potassium excretion is essential to maintain the normal serum value of 3.5 to 5.0 mEq per liter. Levels of 7 or higher may precipitate cardiac dysrhythmias and death (see Chap. 5).

Table 28-1 summarizes some specific characteristics of urine. Variations relate to diet and fluid intake. Figure 28-10 shows the average concentrations of different substances at different points of the tubular system.

TABLE 28-1 Physical Characteristics of Urine

pH: 4.6–8.0
Amount: 600–2500 mL/24 hours
Color: Amber or straw-colored and clear
Specific gravity: 1.003–1.030
Protein: 0–0.1 gm/24 hours
Glucose: 0–0.3 gm/24 hours
RBCs: 1–2/microscopic slide
Urobilinogen: 0–4 mg/24 hours

Source: J. Wallach, *Interpretation of Diagnostic Tests* (3rd ed.). Boston: Little, Brown, 1978.

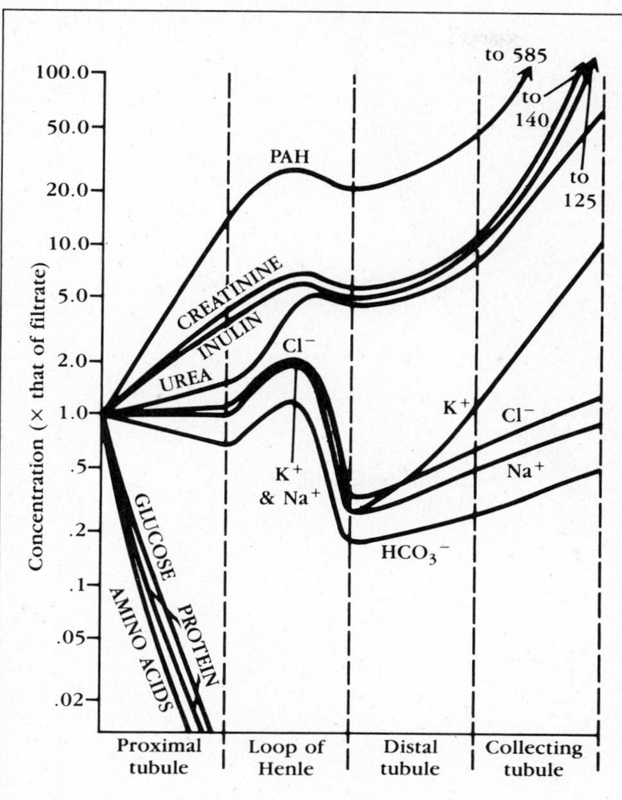

FIGURE 28-10 Composite figure showing average concentrations of different substances at different points in the tubular system. (From A.C. Guyton, *Textbook of Medical Physiology* [7th ed.]. Philadelphia: W.B. Saunders Company, 1986. Reprinted by permission.)

Accessory Urinary Structures and Bladder

When urine is excreted from the kidneys it is transported from the renal pelvis to the ureters by peristaltic wave contractions. It is emptied into the bladder, which releases it into the urethra.

Ureters

The ureters vary in length from 25 to 30 cm and are approximately 1.25 cm wide; they enter the bladder at oblique angles. They are composed of three layers of smooth muscle, including an inner layer of longitudinal muscle, a middle layer of circular muscle, and an outer layer that is a fibrous coat. The ureters also are lined with a layer that is composed of mucous membrane. This layer, because of mucus secretion, cannot be permeated by the constituents of urine (Fig. 28-11).

The peristaltic movement of smooth muscle allows contractions to occur at a rate of 1 to 5 per minute. These cause a spurting action by which urine fills the bladder.

Bladder

When empty, the bladder is like a deflated balloon; when filled with urine, it rises into the abdomen and becomes pear-shaped. The bladder is located behind the symphysis pubis. It is composed of several layers: mucosa, submucosa, detrusor muscle, and serous layer. The mucosal layer, which contains transitional epithelium, in combination with the *rugae* (multiple folds in the mucosa) allows the bladder to stretch during urinary filling. The submucosa contains connective tissue that connects the mucous and muscular layers [6]. The detrusor muscle is composed of longitudinal and circular muscles, allowing for contractility. The serous layer coats the superior portion of the bladder and is formed by the peritoneum.

An area called the ***trigone*** is located at the base of the bladder and is formed by the two ureters and the urethra. Between the bladder and the urethra is an *internal urethral sphincter*; below it is an *external urethral sphincter*. These sphincters are formed by circular muscles and, when stimulated, allow urine to pass from the bladder into the urethra (Fig. 28-12).

Micturation Reflex. Micturation, or voiding, is the result of a spinal reflex from the sacral portion of the spinal cord. Stretch receptors become stimulated when there is 150 to 300 ml of urine in the bladder. The bladder pressure increases with increased filling and the parasympathetic nerves become stimulated. This causes the micturation reflex, which results in contraction of the detrusor muscle and relaxation of the internal sphincter. Urination proceeds unless it is stopped by voluntary contraction of the external sphincter, which is under cerebral control.

Urethra

The urethra, located at the apex of the bladder, is the final excretory passageway for urine. The urethral opening to the exterior is the urinary meatus.

The female urethra is located posteriorly to the symphysis pubis and anteriorly to the vagina. The urethra is approximately 3.75 cm long and is composed of smooth muscle (Fig. 28-13).

When the male urethra leaves the bladder it passes through the prostate gland (*pars prostatica*), then between a membrane portion (*pars memb, anacea*) extending from the prostate to the corpus spongiosum of the penis. Finally, the urethra passes through the corpus spongiosum (*pars spongiosa*) and terminates at the urinary meatus. The male urethra is approximately 20 cm long and transports both urine and semen (Fig. 28-14).

Study Questions

1. Trace the pathway of urine formation from the formation of ultrafiltrate to the final product.
2. Explain how aldosterone and antidiuretic hormone affect the composition of urine.
3. Describe the process utilized by the tubules to concentrate urine.

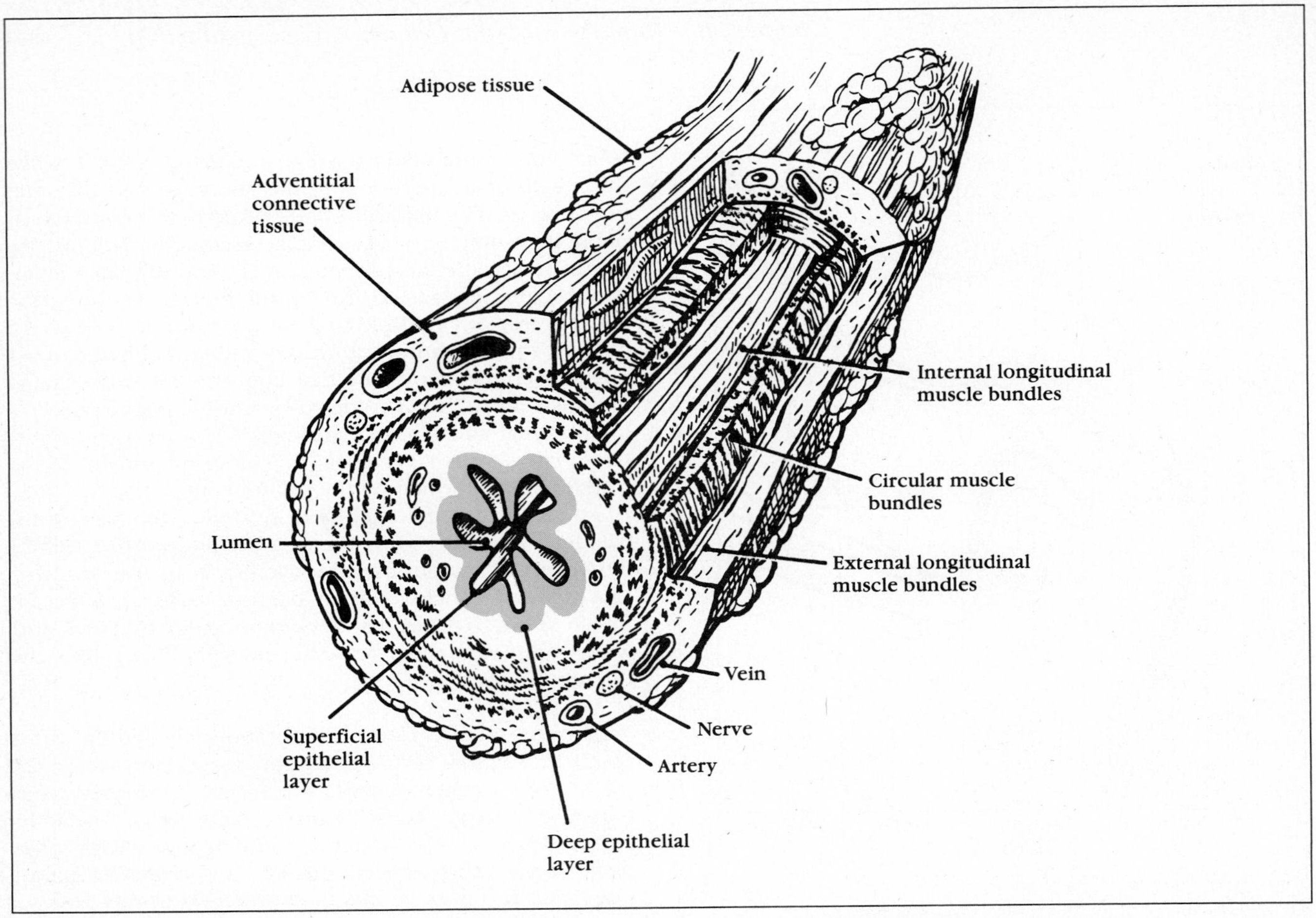

FIGURE 28-11 Structure of the ureter, including smooth muscle layers, outer connective tissue, and blood and nerve supply.

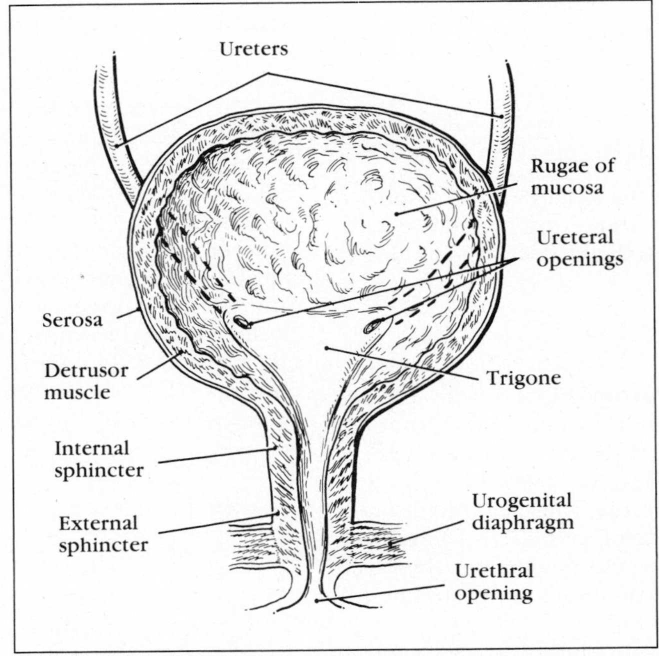

FIGURE 28-12 Structure of the bladder and its internal and external urethral sphincters.

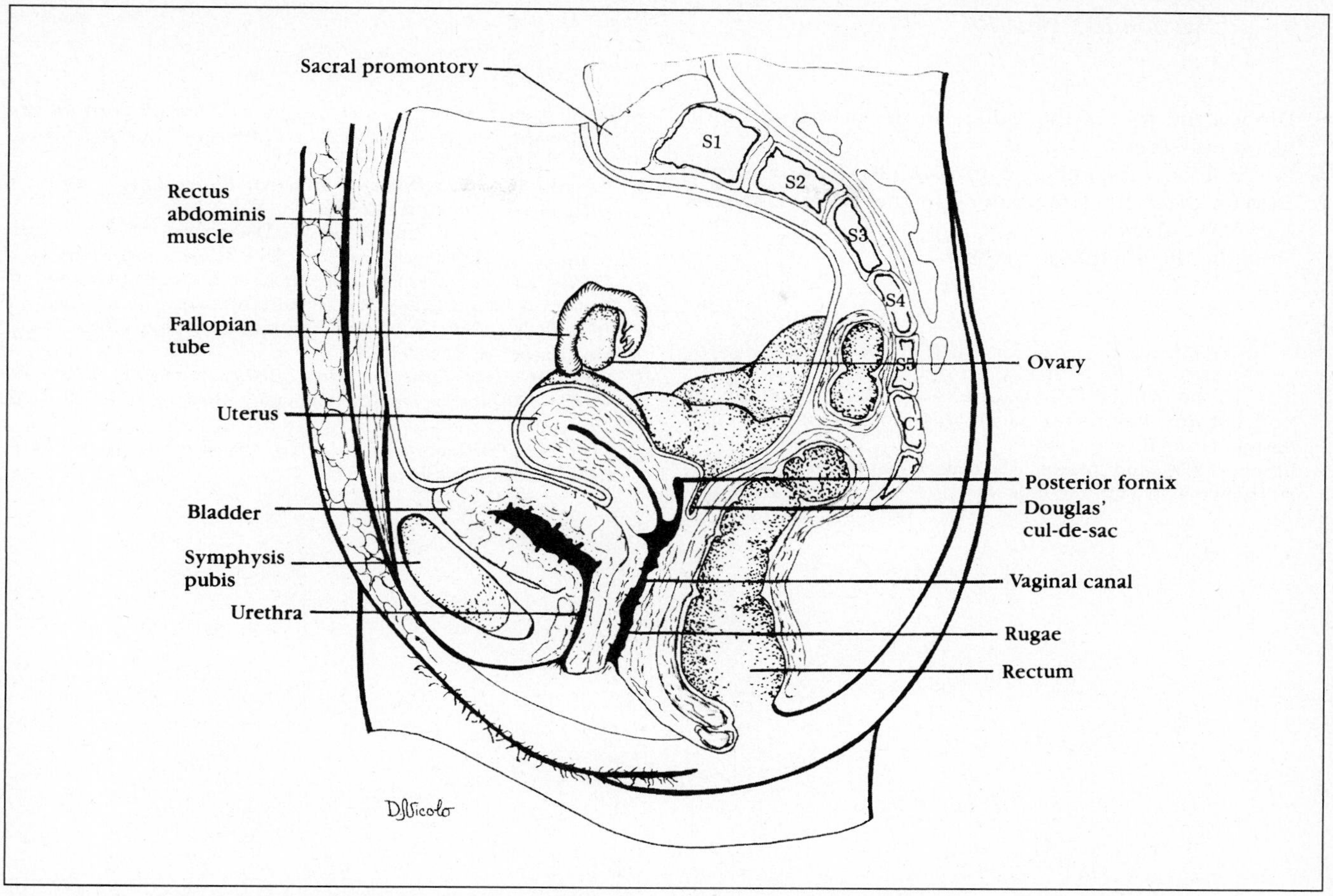

Sacral promontory
S1
S2
S3
S4
S5
C1
Rectus abdominis muscle
Fallopian tube
Uterus
Bladder
Symphysis pubis
Urethra
Ovary
Posterior fornix
Douglas' cul-de-sac
Vaginal canal
Rugae
Rectum
DiNicolo

FIGURE 28-13 Structure of the female genitourinary anatomy. (From M.A. Miller and D.A. Brooten, *The Childbearing Family: A Nursing Perspective* [2nd ed.]. Boston: Little, Brown, 1983.)

Bladder
Pars prostatica
Prostate gland
Pars membraneacae
Membranous portion
Corpus spongiosum
Pars spongiosa
Corpora cavernosum
Urinary meatus

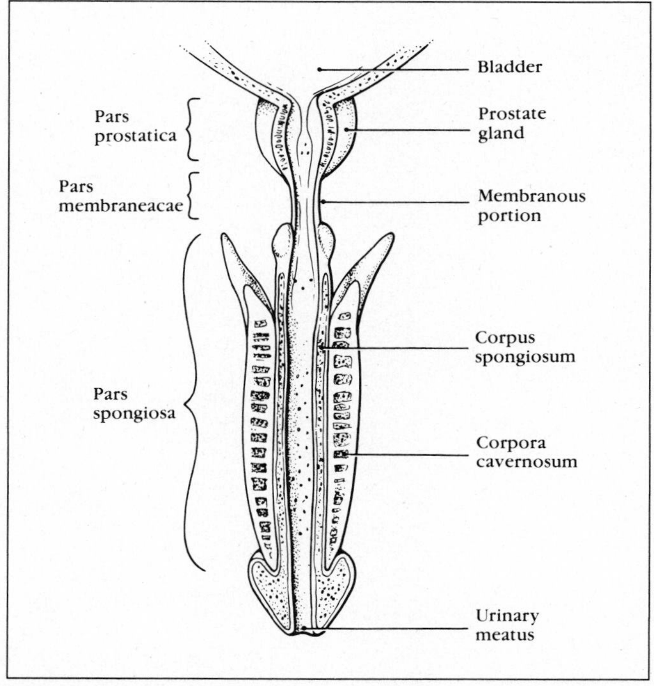

FIGURE 28-14 Structure of the male genitourinary anatomy.

4. Discuss the role of the kidney in the maintenance of blood pressure.
5. Describe how the kidney is involved in erythropoiesis.
6. Explain the role of the kidney in the maintenance of acid-base balance.
7. Describe the micturation reflex.

References

1. Berl, T., and Schrier, R.W. Disorders of water metabolism. In R.W. Schrier, *Renal and Electrolyte Disorders* (3rd ed.). Boston: Little, Brown, 1986.
2. Brenner, B.M., and Rector, F.C. (eds.). *The Kidney* (3rd ed.). Philadelphia: Ardmore, 1986.
3. DeWardener, H.E. *The Kidney: An Outline of Normal and Abnormal Function* (5th ed.). Edinburgh: Churchill Livingstone, 1985.
4. Guyton, A.C. *Textbook of Medical Physiology* (7th ed.). Philadelphia: Saunders, 1986.
5. Linas, S.L., and Schrier, R.W. Disorders of the renin-angiotensin-aldosterone system. In R.W. Schrier, *Renal and Electrolyte Disorders* (3rd ed.). Boston: Little, Brown, 1986.
6. Tortora G.J., and Evans, R.L. Renal Physiology. In G.J. Tortora et al. (eds.), *Principles of Human Physiology*. Hagerstown, Md.: Harper & Row, 1982.
7. Valtin, H. *Renal Function: Mechanisms Preserving Fluid and Solute Balance in Health* (2nd ed.). Boston: Little, Brown, 1983.
8. Vick, R.L. *Contemporary Medical Physiology*. Menlo Park, Calif.: Addison-Wesley, 1984.

CHAPTER 29

Immunologic, Infectious, Toxic, and Other Alterations in Urinary Function

CHAPTER OUTLINE

Infections of the Genitourinary Tract
- Cystitis
- Pyelonephritis
  - *Acute Pyelonephritis (APN)*
  - *Chronic Pyelonephritis (CPN)*

Nephritic Glomerular Disease
- Antiglomerular Basement Membrane Disease
  - *Goodpasture's Syndrome*
- Immune Complex Glomerular Disease
  - *Poststreptococcal Glomerulonephritis (PSGN)*
  - *Nonstreptococcal Glomerulonephritis*
- Rapidly Progressive Glomerulonephritis
- Chronic Glomerulonephritis

Nephrotic Glomerular Disease
- Minimal Change Disease (Lipoid Nephrosis)
- Focal Glomerulosclerosis
- Membranous Nephropathy (Membranous Glomerulonephritis)
- Membranoproliferative Glomerulonephritis (Mesangiocapillary or Tubular GN)

Tubular and Interstitial Diseases
- Toxic Mechanisms
- Metabolic Imbalances
  - *Hyperuricemia*
  - *Hypercalcemia*
  - *Hypokalemia*
- Immune Mechanisms Affecting the Tubulointerstitial Areas
- Renal Tubular Acidosis

Congenital Disorders Leading to Renal Dysfunction

LEARNING OBJECTIVES

1. List the major organisms that can cause cystitis.
2. Differentiate between hemorrhagic and suppurative cystitis.
3. Explain the normal protection against infection in the male and female urinary systems.
4. Describe vesicoureteral reflux.
5. Differentiate between acute and chronic pyelonephritis, pathologically and clinically.
6. State the main causes of end-stage renal disease.
7. Describe antiglomerular basement membrane (anti-GBM) disease, using Goodpasture's syndrome as a model.
8. Explain the significance of crescents in renal pathology.
9. Describe the etiology, pathology, clinical manifestations, and prognosis for poststreptococcal glomerulonephritis.
10. Describe briefly the pathology of rapidly progressive glomerulonephritis.
11. List some etiologic agents of chronic glomerulonephritis.
12. Define *nephrosis*.
13. Explain why persons with nephrotic disease also have hyperlipidemia.
14. Describe the development of edema in nephrotic disease.
15. Describe the relationships among idiopathic nephrotic syndromes, minimal change disease, focal glomerulosclerosis, membranous glomerulopathy, and membrane proliferative glomerulonephritis.
16. Describe how aspirin, phenacetin, codeine, and caffeine can cause nephritis.
17. Outline the mechanisms by which hyperuricemia, hypercalcemia, and hypokalemia can cause tubular or parenchymal alterations.
18. Review the immunologic mechanisms that can cause tubulointerstitial alterations.
19. Describe the mechanisms that can result in renal tubular acidosis (RTA).
20. Explain briefly polycystic disease of the kidneys.

Many factors can affect the genitourinary system and can cause relatively innocuous problems or progressive conditions that lead to renal failure. The most common genitourinary disease is infection of the bladder mucosa that may ascend to the pelvis of the kidney. Other conditions that can cause renal dysfunction include immune complex or antiglomerular basement membrane (anti-GBM) antibody disease, toxic injury, and congenital malformations.

Infections of the Genitourinary Tract

Urinary tract infections (UTI) are diagnosed by culture of the causative microorganism. Active infection is usually considered to be present when more than 100,000 bacteria per ml of urine appear in a clean-voided specimen. The most common cause of UTI is *Escherichia coli*, an aerobic organism present in large numbers in the lower intestinal area. Infections also may be caused by other organisms, such as *Klebsiella*, *Proteus*, and *Staphylococcus* species, especially in the presence of an indwelling catheter.

Cystitis

Inflammation of the bladder is more common in women than men because of the proximity of the urethral opening and vagina to the anal area. Normally, the urethra contains diphtheroids and *Streptococcus* and *Staphylococcus* organisms. Gram-negative organisms may gain access to the bladder during sexual intercourse, after urethral trauma, or as a result of poor hygiene. Normally, these organisms are rapidly expelled by voiding because urine is acidic and flushes away excess bacteria. In men, prostatic secretions have antibacterial properties.

Risk factors for cystitis include intercourse, pregnancy, neurogenic bladder, other kidney disease, obstructive conditions, and diabetes mellitus. The most dangerous sequel of cystitis is pyelonephritis, which is thought to result from organisms in the bladder that have ascended to the renal pelvis (see p. 447). *Vesicoureteral reflux* increases the risk of pyelonephritis from cystitis (Fig. 29-1). This condition occurs in children who have abnormalities of the bladder or urinary tract that allow urine to reflux from the bladder to the renal pelvis.

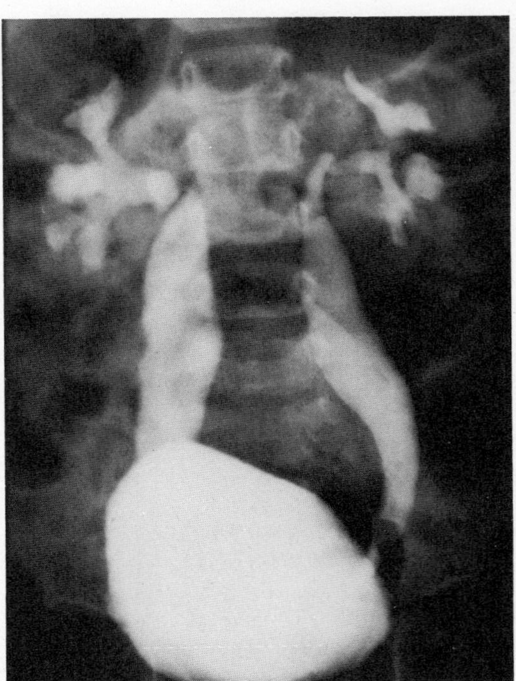

FIGURE 29-1 Grade 4 vesicoureteral reflux in a 2-year-old. (From S. Papper, *Clinical Nephrology* [2nd ed.]. Boston: Little, Brown, 1978.)

The pathology of cystitis varies. If bloody urine is present it is called *hemorrhagic cystitis*; this is a frequent sequel of chemotherapy or radiation therapy over the bladder area. *Suppurative cystitis* occurs when suppurative exudate accumulates on the endothelial lining of the bladder (Fig. 29-2). The exudate is composed of polymorphonuclear leukocytes (PMNs) in early stages, but mononuclear infiltrates appear if the condition progresses to chronic cystitis. Ulcerations may be present in either the acute or chronic stage.

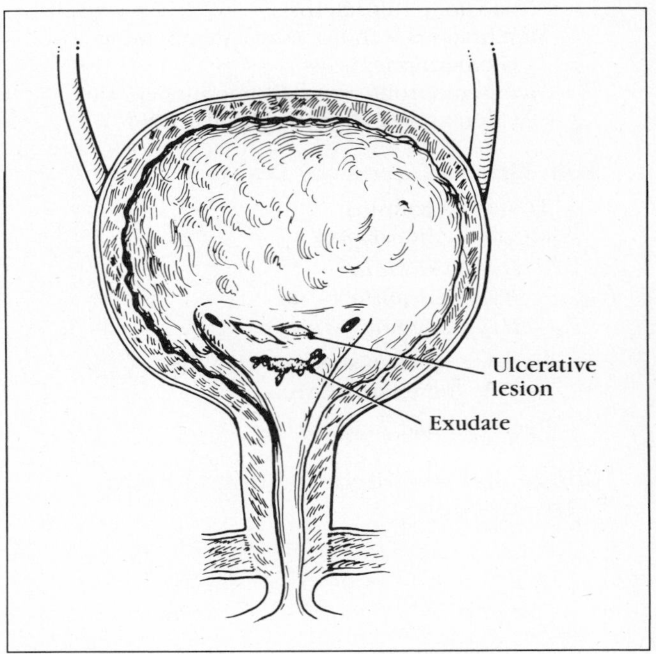

FIGURE 29-2 Suppurative cystitis with ulceration of the bladder mucosa and suppurative exudate on the lining of the bladder.

Clinical manifestations include significant bacteriuria in 60 to 70 percent of cases. Some persons may have symptomatic cystitis that cannot be diagnosed by culture [6]. Dysuria, frequency, urgency, and suprapubic pain are classic symptoms. Any individual who has an indwelling catheter for a long period of time has a high risk for developing cystitis with organisms that become resistant to therapy.

Pyelonephritis

Inflammation of the renal pelvis is called pyelonephritis. It has come to mean *bacterial* kidney infection [7]. Because the genitourinary system is continuous from the urethra to the bladder to the kidneys, ascending infection from the bladder is the most common cause of pyelonephritis [8]. In addition to ascending infection, pyelonephritis may be caused by septicemia (*hematogenous*) or vesicoureteral reflux, or the cause may be unknown. As with cystitis, the infection most frequently is caused by gram-negative bacteria. Two forms of pyelonephritis have been described, acute and chronic.

Acute Pyelonephritis (APN). This disease usually occurs suddenly, with onset of fever, chills, nausea, vomiting, and diarrhea. It may follow a symptomatic or asymptomatic bladder infection or it may result from vesicoureteral reflux. Occasionally, APN is initiated by a bloodborne, virulent organism, but this route of infection almost always signifies the presence of other kidney injury.

Pathologically, APN gives rise to abscesses on the cortical surface of the kidney, which often surround the glomeruli. Glomerular damage is rare but the tubules may rupture. The infection also may follow urinary tract obstruction, with suppurative exudate filling the renal pelvis. Healing usually involves replacement of affected areas of the cortical surface by scar tissue.

Clinical manifestations of APN include the sudden onset of high fever and chills, with marked tenderness on deep pressure of one or both costovertebral areas. Leukocytosis and pyuria with leukocytic casts are common. In the acute phase, some hematuria may be present but it usually does not persist after the acute manifestations have subsided. The symptoms of APN subside with or without treatment, but pyuria may persist for weeks or months. Uncomplicated APN generally responds well to treatment, but a high percentage of recurrence is common [6].

Chronic Pyelonephritis (CPN). This disease is difficult to diagnose except when a history of urinary tract infections, pyuria, and bacteriuria can be elicited. It is a common cause of chronic renal failure, found in 11 to 20% of persons having chronic renal dialysis for endstage renal disease [6].

Pathologically, the kidneys are scarred and irregular, and the calices and renal pelvis are deformed. Gradual atrophy and destruction of the tubules lead to impairment of function that results in chronic renal failure [7]. Chronic pyelonephritis has been reported to follow vascular and hypertensive conditions that affect the glomeruli.

The clinical manifestations of CPN vary, with recurrent episodes of APN or gradual onset of renal insufficiency and failure. Mild proteinuria with lymphocytes and plasma cells is characteristic. While CPN has been linked to bacterial infections, not all affected persons relate a history of UTI. Damage may result from asymptomatic bacterial infection [6].

Nephritic Glomerular Disease

Glomerular injury is the most common cause of chronic renal failure, with immunologically induced glomerulonephritis causing one-half of the cases of end-stage renal failure [6]. Glomerular injury may result from chemicals, irradiation, hypoxemia, and other agents, as well as from immunologically mediated disorders. Two major immunologic mechanisms have been described: (1) antiglomerular basement membrane (anti-GBM) disease and (2) immune complex glomerular disease.

Antiglomerular Basement Membrane Disease

In anti-GBM disease, antibodies form that destroy the GBM and cause a rapidly progressive glomerulonephritis (RPGN) (pp. 448). It may also involve antibodies that form against the alveolar basement membrane (Goodpasture's syndrome).

Goodpasture's Syndrome. This rare autoimmune disorder affects young men more frequently than women and begins abruptly, often preceded by a flulike illness or exposure to hydrocarbon fumes [2]. It may progress rapidly, causing severe and sometimes fatal hemoptysis, or it may exhibit long remissions. More than 90 percent of affected individuals exhibit anti-GBM antibodies, usually of the IgG class [2]. Pathologically, the glomeruli may have nearly normal configuration or they may exhibit focal or necrotizing proliferations called *crescents*. These characteristic lesions of severe renal disease involve massive proliferation of epithelial cells in crescent-shaped masses within the glomeruli (Fig. 29-3). Deposits of fibrin, complement fragments, and immunoglobulins may be present within the crescents. Anti-GBM antibodies may be bound to the alveolar basement membrane. These antibodies can cause alveolar damage and intrapulmonary and extrapulmonary hemorrhage that may be massive and life threatening. Clinical features include hematuria, red cell casts, proteinuria, and nephrosis [2]. Pulmonary bleeding often recurs in episodes and may be fatal even without evidence of renal disease [2]. Rapidly progressive or insidious renal failure may result.

The prognosis for this condition is improving, and depends upon the severity of pulmonary and renal involvement. Treatment with steroids has induced remissions. Renal failure and uremia have been controlled by hemodialysis. Pulmonary hemorrhage usually responds to bilateral nephrectomy.

Immune Complex Glomerular Disease

Many types of glomerular damage are caused by antigen-antibody complexes precipitated in the glomeruli. These complexes have been classified in many ways; Table 29-1 shows exogenous and endogenous mechanisms. Antigen-antibody responses to infectious agents are frequent causes of immune complex disease, but the condition can be

TABLE 29-1 Classification of Immunopathogenetic Mechanisms of Glomerular Disease

Mechanism	Clinical Prototype
Antitissue antibody-mediated disease	
Antibody to "native" glomerular basement membrane glycoprotein antigens	
Exogenous	Antilymphocyte serum treatment
Endogenous	Goodpasture's syndrome and some forms of idiopathic crescentic glomerulonephritis
Antibody to other "native" glomerular antigens (in situ immune complex disease)	
Exogenous	None known
Endogenous	? Membranous glomerulopathy
Antibody to "planted" glomerular antigens	
Exogenous	None known
Endogenous	? Systemic lupus erythematosus ? drugs, ? poststreptococcal, ? glomerulonephritis
Circulating immune complex-mediated disease	
Endogenous antigen	Systemic lupus erythematosus, neoplasia-associated glomerular disease
Exogenous antigen	
Nonreplicating	Serum sickness
Replicating	Bacterial, viral, protozoal glomerulonephritis
Disease associated with activation of alternative complement pathway	Pneumococcal glomerulonephritis, membranoproliferative glomerulonephritis (type II)
Cell-mediated disease	? Minimal change disease (lipoid nephrosis), ? allograft glomerulopathy

Source: R.W. Schrier (ed.), *Renal and Electrolyte Disorders* (3rd ed.). Boston: Little, Brown, 1986.

associated with many types of autoimmune disease, malignancies, and even thyroiditis. The most common exogenous type is poststreptococcal glomerulonephritis, but nonstreptococcal forms are being identified in increasing numbers [6].

Poststreptococcal Glomerulonephritis (PSGN). Group A, beta-hemolytic streptococci have been shown to possess nephrotoxic surface proteins. Glomerulonephritis develops one to two weeks after an infection with this organism. Nasopharyngeal infection is the usual source, but occasionally it may be a streptococcal skin infection. Development of PSGN requires an individual sensitivity to beta-hemolytic streptococci, as is evidenced by the fact that no active infection can be demonstrated by blood or urine cultures. Increased antistreptolysin (ASO) or other streptococcal exoenzyme titers and depressed serum complement level are common.

Pathologically, enlarged hypercellular glomeruli can be demonstrated, with proliferation of cells on the epithelial side of the GBM. Infiltration of the area with PMNs and monocytes is followed by interstitial edema and inflammation. "Humps" can be seen on the epithelial side of the GBM, which probably represent precipitated antigen-antibody complexes. Increased permeability of the GBM results in loss of red blood cells and protein in the urine. A decrease in glomerular filtration rate (GFR) leads to retention of sodium and water. Hypocomplementemia is frequently associated with and results from large amounts of precipitated complement in the complexes.

The clinical manifestations of PSGN include the acute onset of edema, oliguria, proteinuria (usually less than 3 gm/day), anemia, and a characteristic cocoa-colored urine with red blood cell casts. Hypertension is usual and probably results from fluid retention. A markedly elevated ASO titer indicates the presence of circulating antibody to the hemolysin streptolysin O, which is usually elevated within two months after an attack. Other streptococcal exoenzymes include DNAse, beta-hyaluronidase, and NADase. These titers are often increased and are measured by the *streptozyme* test, a combination of tests that is used to screen individuals for recent streptococcal infection. The erythrocyte sedimentation rate (ESR) is usually increased, indicating inflammation.

This disease occurs most frequently in children, most of whom totally recover within a week and then exhibit immunity to further infection. Occasionally, PSGN converts to either a rapidly or slowly progressive form of glomerulonephritis. In either case, renal failure results. Adults who develop PSGN have a higher frequency of persistent proteinuria, hematuria, and renal failure than children. The total recovery rate in adults is 60 percent [1].

Nonstreptococcal Glomerulonephritis. Beside the *Streptococcus* organisms, other bacteria, viruses, and parasites have been implicated in the etiology of acute glomerulonephritis. These also presumably cause the precipitation of immune complexes and lead to a variety of lesions including crescentic GN and proliferative GN [2]. As with PSGN, this type of glomerulonephritis occurs after infection and usually responds well to treatment.

Rapidly Progressive Glomerulonephritis

Rapidly progressive glomerulonephritis (RPGN) leads to renal failure over a period of weeks to months. It may

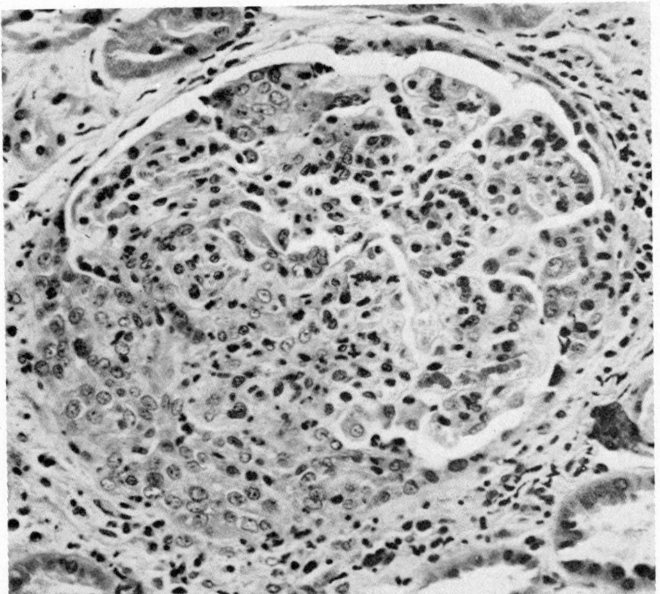

A

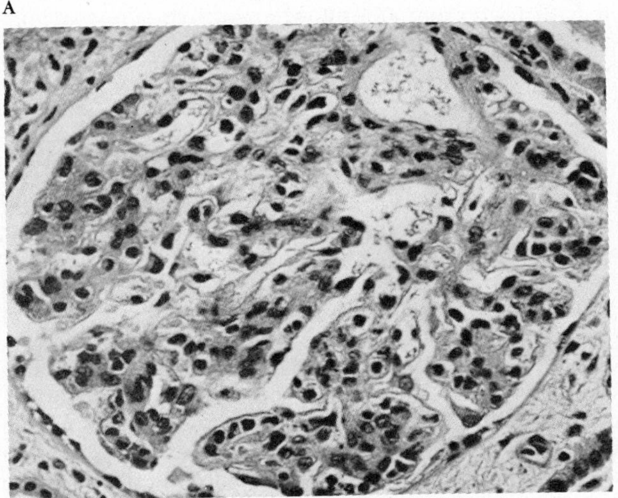

B

FIGURE 29-3 Crescent formation in acute glomerulonephritis. A. Acute exudative glomerulonephritis. Hypercellularity is due to a tremendous increase in the number of polymorphonuclear neutrophils within the capillary loops, together with epithelial cell proliferation (crescents) at the 12, 3, and 7 o'clock positions. B. Acute exudative glomerulonephritis showing a large crescent. (From J. Metcoff, *Acute Glomerulonephritis*. Boston: Little, Brown, 1967.)

occur as a complication of acute or subacute infectious disease, from multisystem disease such as systemic lupus erythematosus, or from Goodpasture's syndrome. It also may occur as an idiopathic or primary condition (Table 29-2).

Pathologically, characteristic capillary proliferation with crescents involves more than 70 percent of the glomeruli. Gaps or discontinuities of the GBM also may be associated with the crescents. Anti-GBM antibodies or deposits of immunoglobulins may be demonstrated on the glomerulus. Circulating antibodies are not usually detected unless the

TABLE 29-2 Causes of Rapidly Progressive Glomerulonephritis

Postacute or subacute infections
Beta-hemolytic streptococci
Bacteria, viruses, parasites
Idiopathic or primary
Multisystem or autoimmune disease

condition is associated with a specific process for which antibody production can be demonstrated.

The idiopathic form of disease is common and may be identified by enlarged, pale kidneys with cellular proliferation in Bowman's space. Crescents form very rapidly, and distort and compress the capillary lumina with fibrin deposition throughout [6]. The GBM is disrupted; interstitial edema with infiltration of leukocytes leads to degenerative changes of the tubules. Crescent formation indicates severe glomerular disease (see Fig. 29-3). Widespread crescent formation indicates a bleak prognosis, with over 90 percent of persons developing chronic renal failure.

Clinical manifestations include a rapid, progressive diminution in renal function, severe oliguria, or anuria with irreversible renal failure in weeks or months [6]. Hypertension, proteinuria, and hematuria are common.

Chronic Glomerulonephritis

Chronic glomerulonephritis (CGN) is an insidiously developing, progressive dysfunction that usually terminates in end-stage renal failure after years of increasing renal insufficiency. It may result from any type of glomerular disease, and exhibits both the nephrotic and nephritic syndromes.

Pathologically, the glomeruli become scarred and may become totally obliterated. The tubules are atrophic. The glomeruli and renal capsule become infiltrated with lymphocytes and plasma cells. Hyalinization of the glomeruli leads to obliteration of the pathology of the original disease. Vascular sclerosis of arteries and arterioles probably contributes to the arterial hypertension that is almost always associated with this disease.

The progression of the condition is related to the underlying disorder but it almost always continues relentlessly to uremia. Proteinuria, hypertension, and azotemia are common, with later manifestations of uremia (see Chap. 31).

Nephrotic Glomerular Disease

Nephrosis refers to the sequelae of albuminuria that is usually greater than 3.5 gm per day. The result of the urinary loss of large amounts of albumin is hypoalbuminemia. A serum albumin level of less than 3 gm per dl results in generalized body edema. Hyperlipidemia results from hepatic lipoprotein synthesis, which is stimulated by the decreased serum protein levels. The excess lipids formed are mostly cholesterol in the early stages, and in late stages triglycerides also become elevated [6].

The loss of protein results from increased permeability of the GBM, which allows plasma proteins to escape into the urine. The resulting hypoalbuminemia causes decreased colloid osmotic pressure and systemic edema (anasarca) (Fig. 29-4). Loss of other proteins may lead to decreased levels of immunoglobulins and anticoagulant factors. The latter is thought to account for an increased incidence of thromboembolic events [6].

Nephrosis may result from glomerulonephritis or from unknown causes (Table 29-3). Several of the more common idiopathic syndromes are discussed in this section.

Minimal Change Disease (Lipoid Nephrosis)

Lipoid nephrosis is the most common nephrosis in children between ages 2 and 8 years. It results in decreased GFR and loss or binding together of adjacent glomerular foot processes. The epithelial cells of the GBM form pedicles or projections called *foot processes*. Normally these structure are involved with preventing large protein and fat molecules from escaping into the urine. Loss and/or binding of these structures allows the leakage of albumin and fat particles into the urine. No antibodies have been demonstrated in this condition, but a relationship with respiratory infections or routine immunization has led to the theory that it is a hypersensitivity reaction. Because it also responds to steroid therapy and is associated with other atopic diseases, it is thought to involve T cells [6].

The disease is named for its pathologic features, which show few changes except that the adjacent glomerular foot processes bind together and allow plasma proteins and fats to pass into the urine. The kidneys appear edematous and pale.

The clinical course is variable, usually including massive proteinuria without hypertension or hematuria. It is characterized by periods of remissions and exacerbations and 90 percent 10-year survival [1]. In a few persons it progresses to focal glomerulosclerosis and then to renal failure.

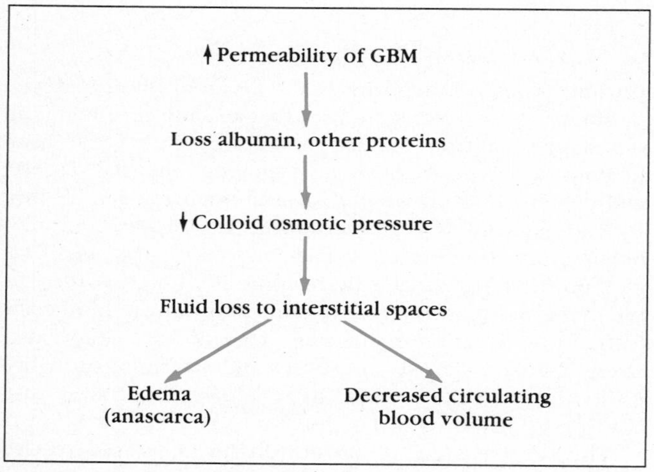

Focal Glomerulosclerosis

This condition involves sclerosis and hyalinization of some of the juxtamedullary glomeruli. Deposits of IgM and C3 fragments are seen on immunofluorescence of the segmental sclerosing lesions [2,6]. A progressive decline in GFR with increasing albuminuria and hypoalbuminemia occur, and renal failure finally results.

Membranous Nephropathy (Membranous Glomerulonephritis)

Membrane nephropathy is most common in young and middle-aged adults. Protein is deposited uniformly in the outer glomerular capillary wall, with the deposits usually containing IgG and complement. Capillary thickening with basement membrane projections account for the loss of protein in urine. The kidneys usually are large, swollen, and pale. If nephrosis with edema and hypoalbuminemia occurs, the disease generally progresses to renal failure. Hematuria and mild hypertension may be present. This disease is usually idiopathic but it may develop in association with systemic lupus erythematosus, exposure to inorganic (gold or mercury) or organic (penicillamine, captopril) drugs, solid tumors, or some infections. It may progress with increasing renal impairment or it may show a spontaneous and complete remission.

Membranoproliferative Glomerulonephritis (Mesangiocapillary or Tubular GN)

In membranoproliferative glomerulonephritis the basement membrane thickens and mesangial cells proliferate. The disease apparently does not occur after a streptococcal infection but does account for 5 to 10 percent of cases of idiopathic nephrosis in children and adults [6]. Abnormalities of the immune system seem to account for circulating immune complexes, and in some persons, *hypocomplementemia*, especially of the C3 component, occurs.

Clinical manifestations include any of the manifestations of the nephrotic syndrome. The disease assumes several forms but tends to be slowly progressive and unremitting.

↑ Permeability of GBM
↓
Loss albumin, other proteins
↓
↓ Colloid osmotic pressure
↓
Fluid loss to interstitial spaces
↙ ↘
Edema (anascarca) | Decreased circulating blood volume

FIGURE 29-4 Development of edema in nephrosis.

TABLE 29-3 Causes of Nephrotic Disease

- Idiopathic or primary
  - Minimal change disease or lipoid nephrosis
  - Focal glomerulosclerosis
  - Membranous glomerulopathy
  - Membranoproliferative, mesangiocapillary, or lobular glomerulonephritis
- Secondary to glomerulonephritis
  - Poststreptococcal
  - Autoimmune diseases
  - Diabetes mellitus
  - Postinfectious: viral, bacterial, parasitic
  - Hypersensitivity reaction to drugs or stings

About 50 percent of affected persons develop chronic renal failure within 10 years [2,6].

Tubular and Interstitial Diseases

Histologic and functional abnormalities of the renal tubules and parenchyma can be caused by many factors. When the etiology is infectious, the term *pyelonephritis* is usually used to describe the process. Nonbacterial factors such as toxins, metabolic imbalances, and immunologic derangements can cause impairment of concentrating ability, metabolic acidosis, and loss of sodium, chloride, potassium, and water. Tables 29-4 and 29-5 describe some of the congenital and acquired tubular disorders.

Toxic Mechanisms

The renal tubules and parenchyma sustain damage from nephrotoxic substances because of the large quantities of renal blood flow and the concentration of the substances in the tubules. The most common toxic substances are pharmaceutic agents, including phenacetin, aspirin, certain antibiotics, and diuretics. *Chronic analgesia nephritis* is a common cause of renal insufficiency in some countries, such as Australia and New Zealand, and occurs most frequently when mixtures of aspirin, caffeine, phenacetin, and codeine are ingested [5]. It is four times more common in females than in males [6]. The mechanism may include inhibition of prostaglandins' vasodilatory effect by aspirin, which may lead to renal ischemia. Phenacetin may

TABLE 29-4 Effects of Congenital Tubular Disorders on Renal Function

Disorder	Altered Function
Single tubular defect	
Nephrogenic diabetes insipidus	↓ Reabsorption of water
Renal glycosuria	↓ Reabsorption of glucose Few tubules (normal Tm_G) Most tubules (↓ Tm_G)
Vitamin D-resistant rickets (familial) (? tubular disorder)	↓ Reabsorption of phosphate
Bartter's syndrome	↓ Reabsorption of potassium, ? ↓ reabsorption of sodium
Cystinuria	↓ Reabsorption of selected amino acids (associated jejunal defect)
Hartnup disease	↓ Reabsorption of amino acids other than those in cystinuria or proline or glycine (associated jejunal defect)
Tubular defects	
Idiopathic Fanconi's syndrome	↓ Reabsorption of glucose, amino acids, and phosphate (and potassium and bicarbonate in some)
Renal tubular acidosis	Proximal tubule ↓ Reabsorption of bicarbonate Distal tubule ↓ Excretion of hydrogen ion

Source: S. Papper, *Clinical Nephrology* (2nd ed.). Boston: Little, Brown, 1978.

TABLE 29-5 Selected Acquired Tubular Disorders

Disorder	Primary Conditions
Single tubular defect	
Acquired nephrogenic diabetes insipidus	Hypercalcemic nephrocalcinosis Hypokalemic nephropathy Sickle cell disease Interstitial nephritis Medullary cystic disease Medullary sponge kidney Multiple myeloma Postobstructive nephropathy Drugs (lithium, demeclocycline, methoxyflurane, glybenclamide, ? isophosphamide, ? propoxyphene, ? colchicine)
Renal salt wasting	Medullary cystic disease Medullary sponge kidney Interstitial nephritis Postobstructive nephropathy
Numerous tubular defects	
Acquired Fanconi's syndrome	Cystinosis Galactosemia Glycogen storage disease Lowe's syndrome Luder-Sheldon syndrome Heavy metals: cadmium, copper (Wilson's disease), mercury, lead Multiple myeloma Light-chain nephropathy Outdated tetracycline
Secondary renal tubular acidosis	
Proximal tubule	Fanconi's syndrome (all causes) Hereditary fructose intolerance Hyperglobulinemia Amyloid Renal transplantation
Distal tubule	Hypercalciuria Hyperglobulinemia Medullary sponge kidney Amyloid Renal transplantation Interstitial nephritis Drugs (amphotericin B, lithium) Toluene "sniffing"

Source: S. Papper, *Clinical Nephrology* (2nd ed.). Boston: Little, Brown, 1978.

CHAPTER 30

Obstruction of the Genitourinary Tract

CHAPTER OUTLINE

Benign Prostatic Hyperplasia

Pathogenesis

The Relationship of Age to Testosterone and Estrogen

Androgen Action in the Prostate

Pathology of the Prostate

Clinical Manifestations

Renal Calculi

Structure and Composition

Factors That May Cause Stone Formation

Alterations in pH

Decrease in Inhibitors

Supersaturation of Urine

Types of Stones

Calcium Stones

Uric Acid Stones

Oxalate Stones

Cystine Stones

Struvite or Magnesium Ammonium Phosphate Stones

Renal Tumors

Benign Tumors

Malignant Tumors

Renal Cell Carcinomas

Wilms' Tumor

Tumors of the Renal Pelvis

LEARNING OBJECTIVES

1. Define *benign prostatic hyperplasia (BPH)*.
2. Locate the urethra in relation to the prostate gland.
3. Discuss the pathogenesis of BPH, including hormonal (testosterone, estrogen, dihydrotestosterone) influences.
4. Discuss the pathology of BPH.
5. List the symptoms and complications of BPH.
6. Define *urolithiasis* and *nephrolithiasis*.
7. Describe the composition of renal calculi.
8. Identify the organic matrix and its function in the formation of stones.
9. List factors that may cause stone formation.
10. Define *staghorn calculi*.
11. Define *hypercalciuria* and *hypercalcemia*.
12. Discuss three classific tions of hypercalciuria.
13. Explain the factors that contribute to the production of uric acid stones.
14. Identify the factors that cause oxalate stones.
15. Identify the major cause of cystine stones.
16. Discuss the formation of struvite stones.
17. List the major benign tumors of the kidneys.
18. Describe the solid and cystic types of cortical adenomas.
19. Identify the malignant tumors of the kidneys.
20. Discuss the pathogenesis of renal cell carcinoma.
21. List the signs and symptoms associated with renal malignancy.
22. Identify the staging mechanism for renal cell carcinoma.
23. Describe the histology of Wilms' tumor.
24. Describe briefly the morphology of tumors of the renal pelvis.

About 50 percent of affected persons develop chronic renal failure within 10 years [2,6].

Tubular and Interstitial Diseases

Histologic and functional abnormalities of the renal tubules and parenchyma can be caused by many factors. When the etiology is infectious, the term *pyelonephritis* is usually used to describe the process. Nonbacterial factors such as toxins, metabolic imbalances, and immunologic derangements can cause impairment of concentrating ability, metabolic acidosis, and loss of sodium, chloride, potassium, and water. Tables 29-4 and 29-5 describe some of the congenital and acquired tubular disorders.

Toxic Mechanisms

The renal tubules and parenchyma sustain damage from nephrotoxic substances because of the large quantities of renal blood flow and the concentration of the substances in the tubules. The most common toxic substances are pharmaceutic agents, including phenacetin, aspirin, certain antibiotics, and diuretics. *Chronic analgesia nephritis* is a common cause of renal insufficiency in some countries, such as Australia and New Zealand, and occurs most frequently when mixtures of aspirin, caffeine, phenacetin, and codeine are ingested [5]. It is four times more common in females than in males [6]. The mechanism may include inhibition of prostaglandins' vasodilatory effect by aspirin, which may lead to renal ischemia. Phenacetin may

TABLE 29-4 Effects of Congenital Tubular Disorders on Renal Function

Disorder	Altered Function
Single tubular defect	
Nephrogenic diabetes insipidus	↓ Reabsorption of water
Renal glycosuria	↓ Reabsorption of glucose Few tubules (normal Tm_G) Most tubules (↓ Tm_G)
Vitamin D-resistant rickets (familial) (? tubular disorder)	↓ Reabsorption of phosphate
Bartter's syndrome	↓ Reabsorption of potassium, ? ↓ reabsorption of sodium
Cystinuria	↓ Reabsorption of selected amino acids (associated jejunal defect)
Hartnup disease	↓ Reabsorption of amino acids other than those in cystinuria or proline or glycine (associated jejunal defect)
Tubular defects	
Idiopathic Fanconi's syndrome	↓ Reabsorption of glucose, amino acids, and phosphate (and potassium and bicarbonate in some)
Renal tubular acidosis	Proximal tubule ↓ Reabsorption of bicarbonate Distal tubule ↓ Excretion of hydrogen ion

Source: S. Papper, *Clinical Nephrology* (2nd ed.). Boston: Little, Brown, 1978.

TABLE 29-5 Selected Acquired Tubular Disorders

Disorder	Primary Conditions
Single tubular defect	
Acquired nephrogenic diabetes insipidus	Hypercalcemic nephrocalcinosis Hypokalemic nephropathy Sickle cell disease Interstitial nephritis Medullary cystic disease Medullary sponge kidney Multiple myeloma Postobstructive nephropathy Drugs (lithium, demeclocycline, methoxyflurane, glybenclamide, ? isophosphamide, ? propoxyphene, ? colchicine)
Renal salt wasting	Medullary cystic disease Medullary sponge kidney Interstitial nephritis Postobstructive nephropathy
Numerous tubular defects	
Acquired Fanconi's syndrome	Cystinosis Galactosemia Glycogen storage disease Lowe's syndrome Luder-Sheldon syndrome Heavy metals: cadmium, copper (Wilson's disease), mercury, lead Multiple myeloma Light-chain nephropathy Outdated tetracycline
Secondary renal tubular acidosis	
Proximal tubule	Fanconi's syndrome (all causes) Hereditary fructose intolerance Hyperglobulinemia Amyloid Renal transplantation
Distal tubule	Hypercalciuria Hyperglobulinemia Medullary sponge kidney Amyloid Renal transplantation Interstitial nephritis Drugs (amphotericin B, lithium) Toluene "sniffing"

Source: S. Papper, *Clinical Nephrology* (2nd ed.). Boston: Little, Brown, 1978.

have a directly toxic effect on the vasa recta or may cause papillary necrosis. The result is fibrosis, necrosis, and calcification of the papillary areas.

The papillae of the kidneys have necrotic areas and calcification fragments. Entire papillae may be sloughed off and excreted in the urine. Headache, anemia, gastrointestinal symptoms, and hypertension also may occur. The kidneys first lose the ability to concentrate urine; severe renal insufficiency leads to azotemia and electrolyte imbalance. If the drugs are discontinued, renal function tends to improve over time.

Hypersensitivity reactions to antibiotics and furosemide or other thiazide diuretics usually begin about 15 days after exposure to the drug. The reactions are characterized by fever, eosinophilia, hematuria, sterile pyuria, proteinuria, and skin rash [6]. Cortical tubulointerstitial nephritis occurs secondary to the papillary necrosis [6]. Oliguria and azotemia develop transiently, or acute renal failure may develop. When the drug is discontinued, recovery usually is complete.

Metabolic Imbalances

Abnormal body metabolism may lead to the production of metabolites that are toxic to the renal tubules. The three imbalances that most frequently cause illness are hyperuricemia, hypercalcemia, and hypokalemia.

Hyperuricemia. The most common cause of hyperuricemia is gout. Gouty nephropathy results from prolonged elevation of the serum uric acid level. Crystalline deposits of uric acid are left in the tubules, especially the distal tubules and collecting ducts. The result is intrarenal obstruction with inflammation and fibrosis of the tubules. Nephropathy is characterized by insidious renal insufficiency, with proteinuria and decreased renal concentrating ability. The precipitated urate bodies induce a *tophus*, which is the urate bodies surrounded by mononuclear giant cells. Tophi commonly occur in the ear, the patellar bursae and around connective tissues. In the kidney, they tend to be deposited in the medulla or pyramids and evoke a typical inflammatory reaction [6].

Acute uric acid nephropathy has been reported after the administration of cytotoxic drugs in the therapy of certain leukemias and lymphomas. Uric acid crystals precipitate in the collecting ducts, leading to partial or total tubule obstruction; the obstruction can result in acute renal failure.

Hypercalcemia. Any condition that causes an increase in circulating calcium can result in increased frequency of calcium stones, obstruction, and nephropathy (see Chap. 30). Deposits of calcium often precipitate in the parenchyma of the kidneys. Intracellular accumulation of calcium can disrupt the cell processes, causing cell death and consequent obstruction of nephrons by cell debris.

Hypokalemia. When moderate or severe hypokalemia persists for several weeks, it can lead to a functional decrease in concentrating ability. Chronic hypokalemia may occur with gastrointestinal diseases and adrenal hyperfunction, and with long-term diuretic therapy. Function usually returns to normal when potassium levels are restored.

Immune Mechanisms Affecting the Tubulointerstitial Areas

Allergic drug reactions may cause acute interstitial nephritis. Antibodies to the tubules have been demonstrated by immunofluorescent studies.

Immune mechanisms may cause a reaction to the renal tubular cells, which frequently occurs in transplant rejections. Also, immune antibodies similar to those causing glomerulonephritis may affect the renal tubules.

Renal Tubular Acidosis

Renal tubular acidosis (RTA) refers to a group of disorders, either primary renal or systemic, characterized by defective secretion of hydrogen ions with normal glomerular filtration. It may be the result of failure to secrete hydrogen ions in the collecting duct or failure to resorb bicarbonate in the proximal tubule [4]. The result is metabolic acidosis. Numerous conditions can produce RTA (Table 29-6). The clinical features relate to the underlying cause, and treatment is directed toward the underlying disorder.

Congenital Disorders Leading to Renal Dysfunction

Renal malformations are very common at birth but may not manifest significant clinical problems until adult life.

TABLE 29-6 Causes of Renal Tubular Acidosis

Distal	Proximal
Hypokalemic or normokalemic	Primary
Primary	Cystinosis
Hypercalcemia	Wilson's disease
Nephrocalcinosis	Lead toxicity
Multiple myeloma	Cadmium toxicity
Hepatic cirrhosis	Mercury toxicity
Lupus erythematosus	Amyloidosis
Amphotericin B	Multiple myeloma
Lithium	Nephrotic syndrome
Toluene	Early renal transplant injury
Renal transplant rejection	Medullary cystic disease
Medullary sponge kidney	Outdated tetracycline
Hyperkalemic	
Hypoaldosteronism	
Obstructive nephropathy	
Sickle cell nephropathy	
Lupus erythematosus	

Source: R.W. Schrier, *Renal and Electrolyte Disorders* (3rd ed.). Boston: Little, Brown, 1986.

Congenital renal disease most frequently results from a developmental defect arising during gestation rather than having a hereditary basis. An exception to this is polycystic disease, which is clearly hereditary.

Renal malformations may result from failure of renal development (renal agenesis or hypoplasia), displacement of the kidneys (abdominal or pelvic), or renal cysts. Developmental malformations account for about 20 percent of chronic renal failure in children. *Adult polycystic disease*, which accounts for 6 to 12 percent renal transplantations, is an inherited condition, autosomal dominant. It affects both kidneys, and renal function deteriorates after the third or fourth decade of life. The kidneys appear to be largely infiltrated with cysts that encroach upon the calices and renal pelvis [6]. Clinical manifestations may include recurrent urinary tract infections, hypertension, abdominal or flank pain, and hematuria [3,9].

Study Questions

1. List the major causative agents for cystitis and discuss how the infection can be prevented.
2. Explain the concept of ascending urinary tract infection.
3. Describe the effects of increased permeability of the glomerular basement membrane.
4. Differentiate between the long-term effects of acute and chronic glomerulonephritis.
5. Describe the development of edema in nephrosis.
6. Explain the concept of nephrotoxicity and what agents can produce this problem.
7. Define renal tubular acidosis.

References

1. Glascock, R.J., and Brenner, B.M. The major glomerulopathies. In E. Braunwald et al. (eds.), *Harrison's Principles of Internal Medicine* (11th ed.). New York: McGraw-Hill, 1987.
2. Glascock, R.J. Clinical, immunologic, and pathologic aspects of human glomerular diseases. In R.W. Schrier (ed.), *Renal and Electrolyte Disorders* (3rd ed.). Boston: Little, Brown, 1986.
3. Fishman, M.C., et al. *Medicine* (2nd ed.). Philadelphia: Lippincott, 1986.
4. Kaehy, W.D., and Gabow, P.A. Pathogenesis and management of metabolic acidosis and alkalosis. In R.W. Schrier (ed.), *Renal and Electrolyte Disorders* (3rd ed.). Boston: Little, Brown, 1986.
5. Kincaid-Smith, P. Analgesic nephropathy. *Kidney Int.* 13:1, 1978.
6. Robbins, S.L., Cotran, R.S., and Kumar, V. *Pathologic Basis of Disease* (3rd ed.). Philadelphia: Saunders, 1984.
7. Rubin, R.H., Tolkoff-Rubin, N.E., and Cotran, R.S. Urinary tract infection, pyelonephritis, and reflux nephropathy. In B.M. Brenner and F.C. Rector (eds.), *The Kidney* (3rd ed.). Philadelphia: Ardmore, 1986.
8. Stam, W., and Turck, M. Urinary tract infection, pyelonephritis, and related conditions. In R.H. Heptinstall, *Pathology of the Kidney* (3rd ed.). Boston: Little, Brown, 1983.
9. Vick, R.L. *Contemporary Medical Physiology*. Menlo Park, Calif.: Addison-Wesley, 1984.

CHAPTER 30

Obstruction of the Genitourinary Tract

CHAPTER OUTLINE

Benign Prostatic Hyperplasia

- Pathogenesis
  - *The Relationship of Age to Testosterone and Estrogen*
  - *Androgen Action in the Prostate*
  - *Pathology of the Prostate*
- Clinical Manifestations

Renal Calculi

- Structure and Composition
- Factors That May Cause Stone Formation
  - *Alterations in pH*
  - *Decrease in Inhibitors*
  - *Supersaturation of Urine*
- Types of Stones
  - *Calcium Stones*
  - *Uric Acid Stones*
  - *Oxalate Stones*
  - *Cystine Stones*
  - *Struvite or Magnesium Ammonium Phosphate Stones*

Renal Tumors

- Benign Tumors
- Malignant Tumors
  - *Renal Cell Carcinomas*
  - *Wilms' Tumor*
  - *Tumors of the Renal Pelvis*

LEARNING OBJECTIVES

1. Define *benign prostatic hyperplasia (BPH)*.
2. Locate the urethra in relation to the prostate gland.
3. Discuss the pathogenesis of BPH, including hormonal (testosterone, estrogen, dihydrotestosterone) influences.
4. Discuss the pathology of BPH.
5. List the symptoms and complications of BPH.
6. Define *urolithiasis* and *nephrolithiasis*.
7. Describe the composition of renal calculi.
8. Identify the organic matrix and its function in the formation of stones.
9. List factors that may cause stone formation.
10. Define *staghorn calculi*.
11. Define *hypercalciuria* and *hypercalcemia*.
12. Discuss three classifications of hypercalciuria.
13. Explain the factors that contribute to the production of uric acid stones.
14. Identify the factors that cause oxalate stones.
15. Identify the major cause of cystine stones.
16. Discuss the formation of struvite stones.
17. List the major benign tumors of the kidneys.
18. Describe the solid and cystic types of cortical adenomas.
19. Identify the malignant tumors of the kidneys.
20. Discuss the pathogenesis of renal cell carcinoma.
21. List the signs and symptoms associated with renal malignancy.
22. Identify the staging mechanism for renal cell carcinoma.
23. Describe the histology of Wilms' tumor.
24. Describe briefly the morphology of tumors of the renal pelvis.

Obstructive disorders may cause considerable renal dysfunction, including hemorrhage and renal failure, if they are left untreated. The principal obstructive conditions are prostatic hyperplasia, renal calculi, and renal tumors.

Benign Prostatic Hyperplasia

Benign prostatic hyperplasia (BPH) affects the majority of men over age 50 years. In years past the word *hypertrophy* was used, which was misleading, because the increase in the size of the prostate gland is due to hyperplastic proliferation of glandular and cellular tissue (Fig. 30-1).

Normally, the prostate gland weighs 20 gm, surrounds the urethra, and consists of four lobes. By age 70 years, the prostate may weigh from 60 to as much as 200 gm [23].

Pathogenesis

The cause of BPH is unknown but it is believed to result from an imbalance between the male and female sex hormones that occurs with advancing age. Normally, testosterone is the main androgen in the blood and forms two metabolites, dihydrotestosterone and 17β-estradiol. Dihydrotestosterone metabolizes to 3α-androstanediol (Fig. 30-2). Dihydrotestosterone is responsible for mediating many of the actions of testosterone. Estradiol is a steroid that possesses estrogenic properties and acts with androgens for many physiologic activities. It can act independently and cause the opposite effect of androgens. Testosterone and its metabolites act together to produce prostatic hyperplasia [28].

The Relationship of Age to Testosterone and Estrogen. In a man older than 60 years, the plasma testosterone level decreases, but BPH can occur 10 to 20 years before decrease is demonstrated [12]. With aging, the estrogen level increases, but does not correlate with the frequency of BPH [2]. The plasma levels of these hormones apparently do not cause BPH; endocrine alterations in the prostate are thought to initiate the process [25].

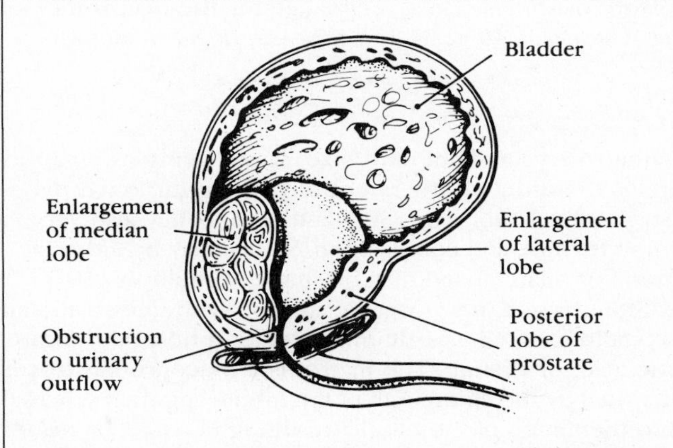

FIGURE 30-1 Enlargement of median and lateral lobes of the prostate gland. Note the obstruction to urinary outflow.

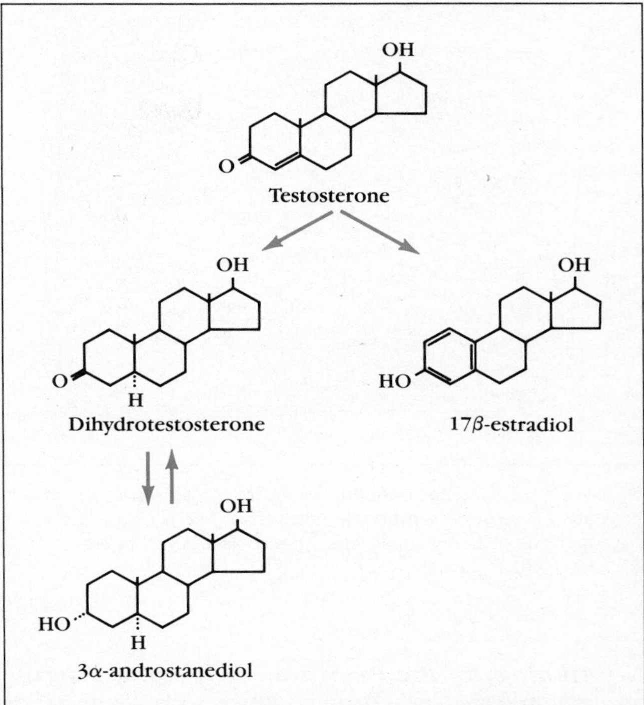

FIGURE 30-2 Plasma testosterone serves as a precursor for two other types of steroid hormones: 5-α-reduced androgens (dihydrotestosterone and 3-α-androstanediol) and 17-β-estradiol. (Reprinted with permission from J.D. Wilson, The pathogenesis of benign prostatic hyperplasia. *Am. J. Med.* 65:745, 1980.)

Androgen Action in the Prostate. In the plasma, testosterone binds to two proteins, globulin and albumin. A small percentage of free hormones is in balance with a protein-bound steroid and is able to enter the cells. Within the cells, testosterone is converted by a 5α-reductase enzyme to dihydrotestosterone. It is then bound to a specific androgen-receptor protein, and the hormone receptor complex changes before entering the nucleus [25]. At this point, interaction of steroid-receptor complexes with acceptor sites on the chromosomes results in increased transcription of specific structural genes [14]. These genes cause the formation of new messenger ribonucleic acid (RNA), resulting in the production of new proteins in the cytoplasm (Fig. 30-3) [28].

Estrogen levels increase in the male with aging and act similarly to androgens [12]. Estrogen binds to specific receptors in the cytoplasm and thus goes into the nucleus as a hormone-receptor complex. This complex interacts with DNA at acceptor sites and results in activation of messenger RNA [8].

Dihydrotestosterone is the hormonal mediator in BPH partly because of decreased catabolism of the molecule and partly because of increased intracellular binding of the molecule. Therefore, the process is accelerated because of increased estrogen, which increases the level of the androgen receptor in the gland and results in prostate growth [27].

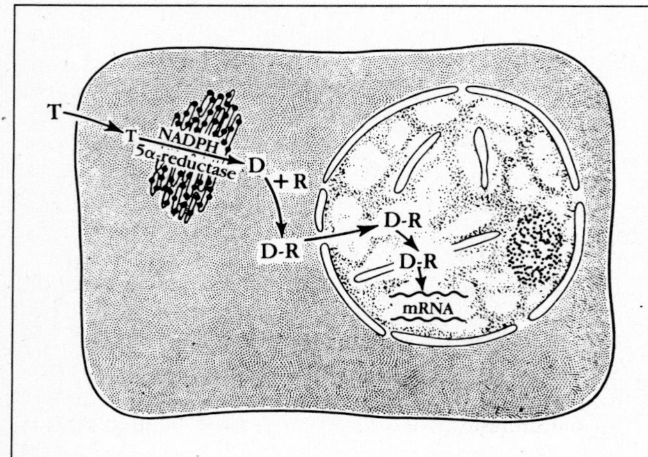

FIGURE 30-3 Current concepts of androgen action in the prostate. (Reprinted with permission from J.D. Wilson, The pathogenesis of benign prostatic hyperplasia. *Am. J. Med.* 65:745. 1980.)

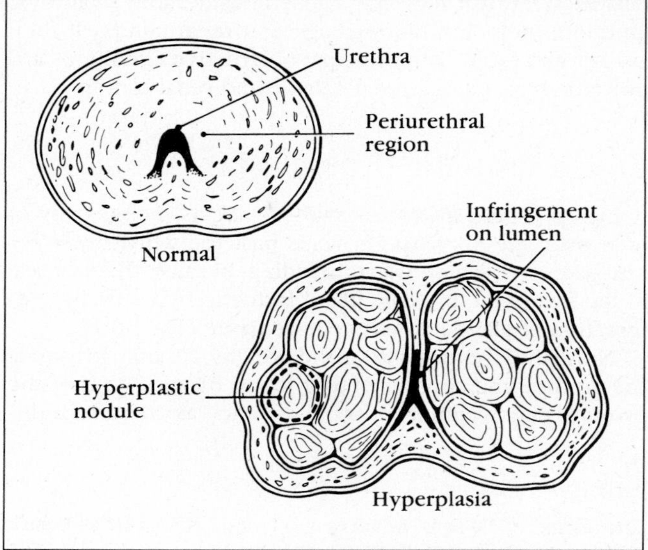

FIGURE 30-4 Relationship to the urethra of normal and hyperplastic prostate. Note infringement on the lumen in the latter.

Pathology of the Prostate. Hyperplasia usually occurs in the median and lateral lobes, with the posterior lobe generally not affected. Seventy-five percent of prostatic carcinomas arise in the posterior lobe [5]. The lobes vary in size and are separated from each other by stroma, including connective tissue and smooth muscle fibers. Enlargement of the lateral lobes compresses the urethra, while enlargement of the medial lobe actually obstructs urine outflow by plugging the urethral orifice (Fig. 30-4) [28].

Hyperplasia, which may be fibromuscular or glandular, results in proliferation of cells, beginning in the periurethral region and causing a smooth and regular appearance of the gland. Located in the adjacent prostatic tissue are areas of ischemia and necrosis encircled by margins of squamous metaplasia. A capsule can be formed surgically between the hyperplastic area and normal tissue. As the periurethral lobes enlarge, the normal tissue and the urethra are compressed.

Clinical Manifestations

When hyperplasia causes significant obstruction, frequency of urination, decrease in force and size of stream, hesitancy, straining to urinate, difficulty in starting and stopping the stream, and inability to empty the bladder are noted. Complications that may arise from BPH include hydroureter, acute urinary retention of sudden onset, acute renal failure, hematuria, calculi, cystitis, reflux, urinary tract infection, and thickening of the bladder muscles.

Renal Calculi

Calculi can form in various areas of the renal system. Crystallization in the renal pelvis or calices is called *nephrolithiasis. Urolithiasis* refers to stones anywhere in the urinary tract. The stones may be composed of calcium salts, uric acid, oxalate, cystine, xanthine, and struvite [6].

Symptoms of urolithiasis may vary from hematuria or oliguria to renal colic. Hematuria results from the damage done by the stone in the urinary tract, and oliguria may result when the stone obstructs the flow of urine [23]. Renal colic results from spasms as calculi are passed, causing flank pain that radiates to the abdomen and groin.

Urinary stones or calculi are common; they are present in approximately 0.9 to 5.4 percent of all autopsies. A review of the literature indicated an average frequency of 7 percent in Scandinavian countries, the United States, and Great Britain [17]. The frequency is higher in men, in persons leading a sedentary lifestyle, and in families with a history of stones. The average age for the occurrence of renal stones is 40 years, but they can occur at any age.

Structure and Composition

Calculi vary in shape and size, some being as small as grains of sand and others entirely filling the renal pelvis (staghorn calculi) (Figs. 30-5 and 30-6). They also vary in color, texture, and composition. Stones may be either unilateral or bilateral and may be single or multiple [19].

Stones contain an organic matrix, or framework, and crystalloids such as calcium, oxalate, phosphate, urate, uric acid, or cystine. The matrix is a mucoprotein that is resorbed by the epithelium of the tubule and then released into the lumen of the tubule, resulting in a site, or *nidus*, for stone propagation [11]. Growth of preformed crystal on a site or nidus is called *metastability*.

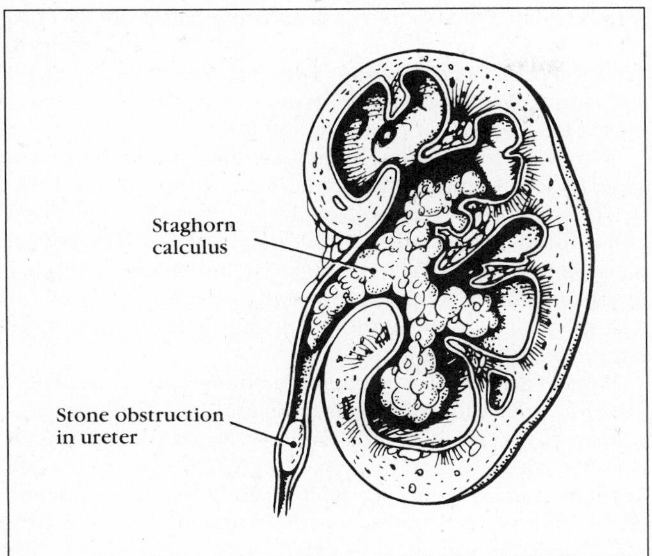

FIGURE 30-5 Staghorn calculus obstructing the entire renal pelvis.

Factors That May Cause Stone Formation

Stone formation may result from alteration in urine pH, decrease in inhibitors, and supersaturation of urine. Not all of these factors have to be present for urolithiasis to occur. The urine almost always shows an increase in concentration of the stones' constituents [23].

Alterations in pH. Crystalloids' solubility is affected by alterations in pH that cause them to leave the urine and attach to the matrix, resulting in crystallization. Stones that form in acid urine contain uric acid, cystine, oxalate, or xanthine. In alkaline urine, most stones contain calcium phosphate or struvite. Persistent use of medications containing aluminum hydroxide, calcium carbonate, ascorbic acid, and sodium bicarbonate affect urinary pH and thus increase the risk of stone formation.

Decrease in Inhibitors. A decrease in inhibitors (magnesium, sodium, pyrophosphate, urea, citrate, amino acids, and trace metals) may cause stone formation. The stone must be stable in order to grow to a size that is clinically significant. Urine contains inhibitors for calcium oxalate and calcium phosphate, but not for uric acid, cystine, or struvite [7]. It was concluded in one study that calculi may result from alterations in several urine components, resulting in abnormal formation or abnormal accumulation of crystals [7].

Supersaturation of Urine. The main cause of stone formation is breakdown of the balance between conservation of water and excretion of materials that are poorly soluble. When urine becomes saturated with certain materials, crystals may form, aggregating to create a stone [6]. As the insoluble material accumulates, urine reaches a critical point at which it can no longer keep the material in solution. This point is called the *upper limit of metastability*, at which time stone growth occurs. Urine pH affects the formation of stones, as some precipitate in acid urine while others require alkaline urine [23].

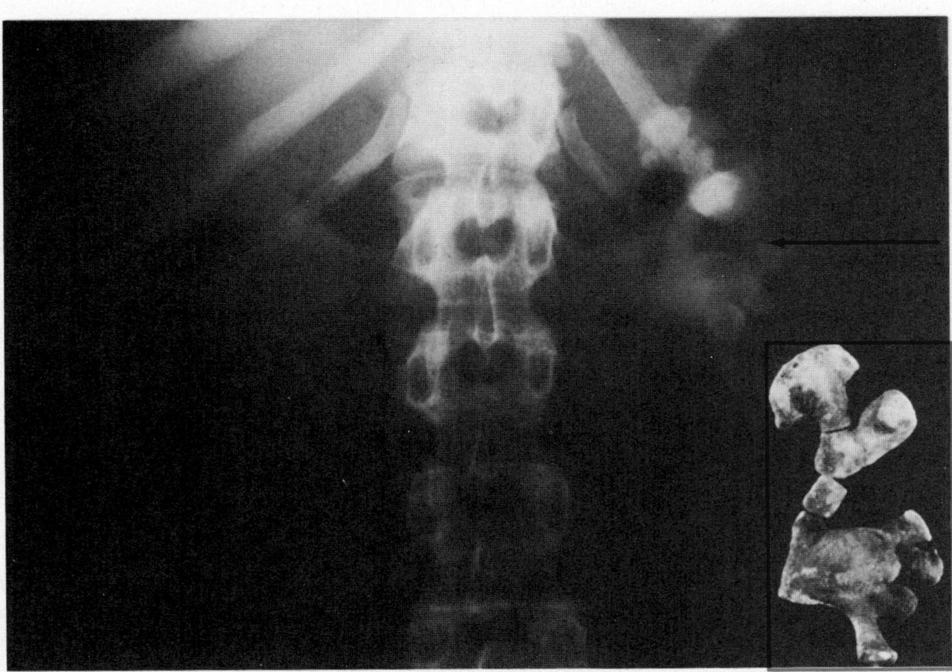

FIGURE 30-6 Radiologic appearance of a large staghorn calculus. Arrow shows location of stone. Insert pictures actual appearance on removal.

Types of Stones

Even though many stones are composed of mixtures of substances, they usually have distinctive characteristics. The majority contain calcium, but uric acid, oxalate, cystine, struvite, and xanthine also may predominate.

Calcium Stones. Calcium stones are often formed in the presence of hypercalciuria and/or hypercalcemia (Table 30-1) [19]. Hypercalciuria occurs with increased excretion of urinary calcium. Calcium stones are white to gray, usually small, and soft. Normally, the calcium level in urine is approximately 75 to 175 mg per 24 hours; hypercalciuria occurs when urinary excretion exceeds 250 mg per 24 hours in women and 300 mg per 24 hours in men [6]. Hypercalcemia occurs when the serum calcium exceeds 5 mEq per liter in adults [26]. Calcium is excreted in the urine in increased amounts or it may precipitate into the kidney substance (nephroçalcinosis).

The three major classifications of hypercalciuria are absorptive, resorptive, and renal [21]. *Absorptive hypercalciuria* results from exaggerated absorption of calcium from the bowel due to an increased rate of conversion of vitamin D that often occurs with hyperparathyroidism. The condition has also been noted with normal levels of serum calcium and phosphorus, normal to low levels of parathyroid hormone, and increased filter loads of calcium (Fig. 30-7) [4,20]. Another explanation for absorptive hypercalciuria is that when the amount of calcium absorption from the gut increases, the serum level increases, thus reducing parathyroid hormone secretion, which leads to an increased filter load of calcium in the glomeruli.

Resorptive hypercalciuria results when calcium is removed or resorbed from the bone. This can occur in persons who are immobilized; for example, after spinal cord injury. Five to ten percent of persons who are immobilized for prolonged periods of time develop renal calculi [6]. Stones resulting from resorption abnormality develop over a long period of time (Fig. 30-8).

A renal defect causing hypercalciuria is the result of a tubular defect causing a calcium leak. An example of this defect is renal tubular acidosis (RTA) in which the distal convoluted tubule and collecting duct are not able to maintain acid urine (see p. 452). Calcium is not as soluble in alkaline urine and may precipitate to form stones. In RTA stones may also be the result of low levels of urinary citrate, an inhibitor of calcium.

Several disorders of calcium metabolism result in hypercalcemia, including Paget's disease, multiple myeloma, and primary hyperparathyroidism. Sixty to eighty percent of persons with primary hyperparathyroidism at some time develop renal calculi and nephrocalcinosis (the presence of calcium deposits in the renal parenchyma) [7,13,20].

TABLE 30-1 Causes of Hypercalcemia and Hypercalciuria

Increased bone resorption
- Hyperparathyroidism—primary and ectopic
- Metastatic tumors
- Multiple myeloma, lymphoma, leukemia (produce bone-resorbing activity)
- Nonmetastatic tumors (produce prostaglandin)
- Immobilization osteoporosis
- Hyperglucocorticoidism
- Hyperthyroidism
- Paget's disease

Increased intestinal absorption of calcium
- Sarcoidosis
- Beryllosis
- Absorptive hypercalciuria
- Vitamin D excess
- Infantile hypercalciuria

Increased calcium intake—milk-alkali syndrome

Renal wasting of calcium
- Fanconi's syndrome
- Renal tubular acidosis
- Hypermineralocorticoidism
- Renal hypercalciuria

Source: From N.A. Kurtzman, *Pathophysiology of the Kidney,* 1st ed., 1977. Table 28-II. Courtesy of Charles C. Thomas, Publisher, Springfield, Illinois.

Uric Acid Stones. Calculi composed of uric acid cause approximately 10 percent of all kidney stones in persons living in the United States [10]. These stones are yellow to brown, smooth and soft, and are formed in acid urine. Both urine supersaturated with uric acid and decreased urinary pH contribute to their formation. The more alkaline the urine, the more soluble the sodium urate, but if urine becomes acid (pH above 5.5) and supersaturated, crystallization may occur [6]. Persons with uric acid stones excrete less urinary ammonia than normal, and acid urine results.

Hypovolemia, due to dehydration or other causes, contributes to stone formation because of the concentrated uric acid and low urinary pH that result. Diseases such as the leukemias cause cell necrosis resulting in hyperuricosuria, because purines convert mostly to uric acids. Massive hyperuricosuria is fairly common after chemotherapy of certain tumors.

Uric acid stones tend to be staghorn and fill the renal pelvis. Their size may be reduced with medical intervention.

Oxalate Stones. Oxalates are present in certain green leafy vegetables, but stones are rarely due to excess consumption of these foods. Stones can be caused from intestinal diseases, increased amounts of ethylene glycol, hereditary disorders, and renal insufficiency [6]. Hyperoxaluria may occur after intestinal bypass surgery and with Crohn's disease. Oxalate stones are hard and gray, and may be smooth or rough. They are usually recurrent, and may be formed in slightly acid or neutral urine. Oxalate, the product of glycine metabolism, is produced from glyoxylate or glycolate.

Cystine Stones. Cystine stones are formed in acid urine and are white or yellow, small, and soft. They are characterized by hexagonal crystals that eventually form staghorn calculi. They usually do not occur in adults unless cystine excretion exceeds 300 mg per day, but affected persons often excrete 600 to 1800 mg per day [23]. Cystinuria is due to an inherited renal tubular defect affecting

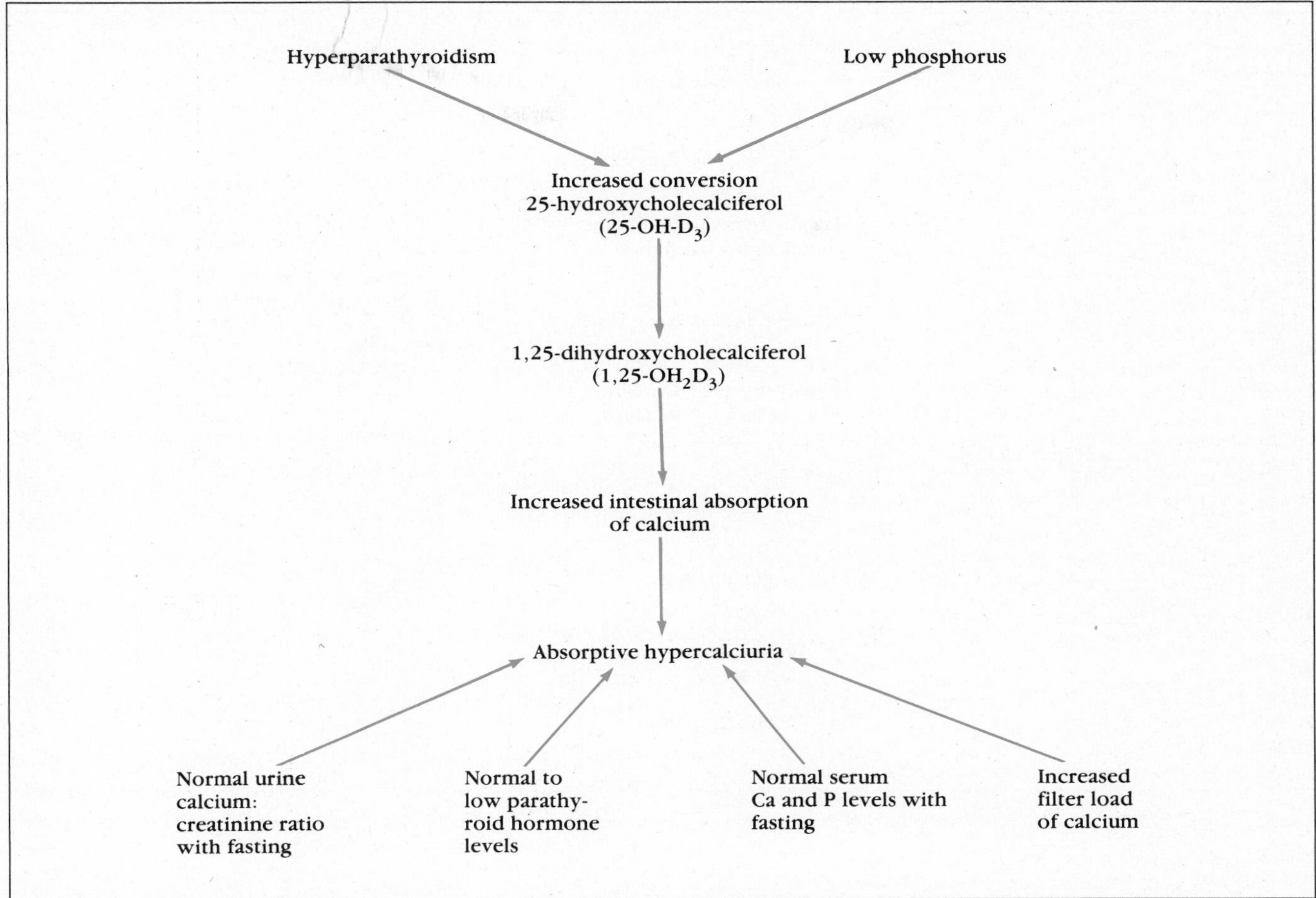

FIGURE 30-7 Absorptive hypercalciuria resulting from hyperparathyroidism or low serum phosphorus level.

the absorption of urine amino acids, including cystine, which is the least soluble [16].

Struvite or Magnesium Ammonium Phosphate Stones. Struvite stones are the result of urinary tract infection, most commonly with bacteria of the *Proteus* species. They may form after bladder catheterization and cystoscopy. Long-term antibiotic therapy may predispose the individual to *Proteus* infection. Struvite stones recur in 27 percent of susceptible persons [7].

The causative bacteria contain the enzyme urease, which splits urea into ammonia and causes elevated urinary pH (Fig. 30-9). The organisms are often called *urea splitters.* Staghorn calculi fill the renal pelvis and are difficult to treat. Sometimes nephrectomy must be performed to relieve the obstruction.

Renal Tumors

Tumors of the renal system can cause damage to the renal parenchyma whether they are benign or malignant. A renal tumor is usually larger when found by palpation than when it is discovered on a routine radiologic examination. Symptoms are usually late in developing and may include complaints of dull pain in the flank area or hematuria. Renal tumors are classified as benign or malignant and also according to their area of involvement (Table 30-2).

Benign Tumors

Cortical adenomas are usually found during postmortem examination of elderly people and are the most prevalent benign tumors of the kidneys. They are usually not larger than 3 cm in diameter and do not produce symptoms unless they enlarge. Two types of cortical adenomas are described [22]:

1. *Solid* tumors, which occur in the subcapsular area and the cortex of the kidney, and are yellow, soft, and round
2. *Cystic* tumors, which occur in the cortex of the kidney and are encapsulated

These adenomas are believed to originate from the tubular epithelium and may be responsible for painless hematuria. They may be difficult to distinguish histo-

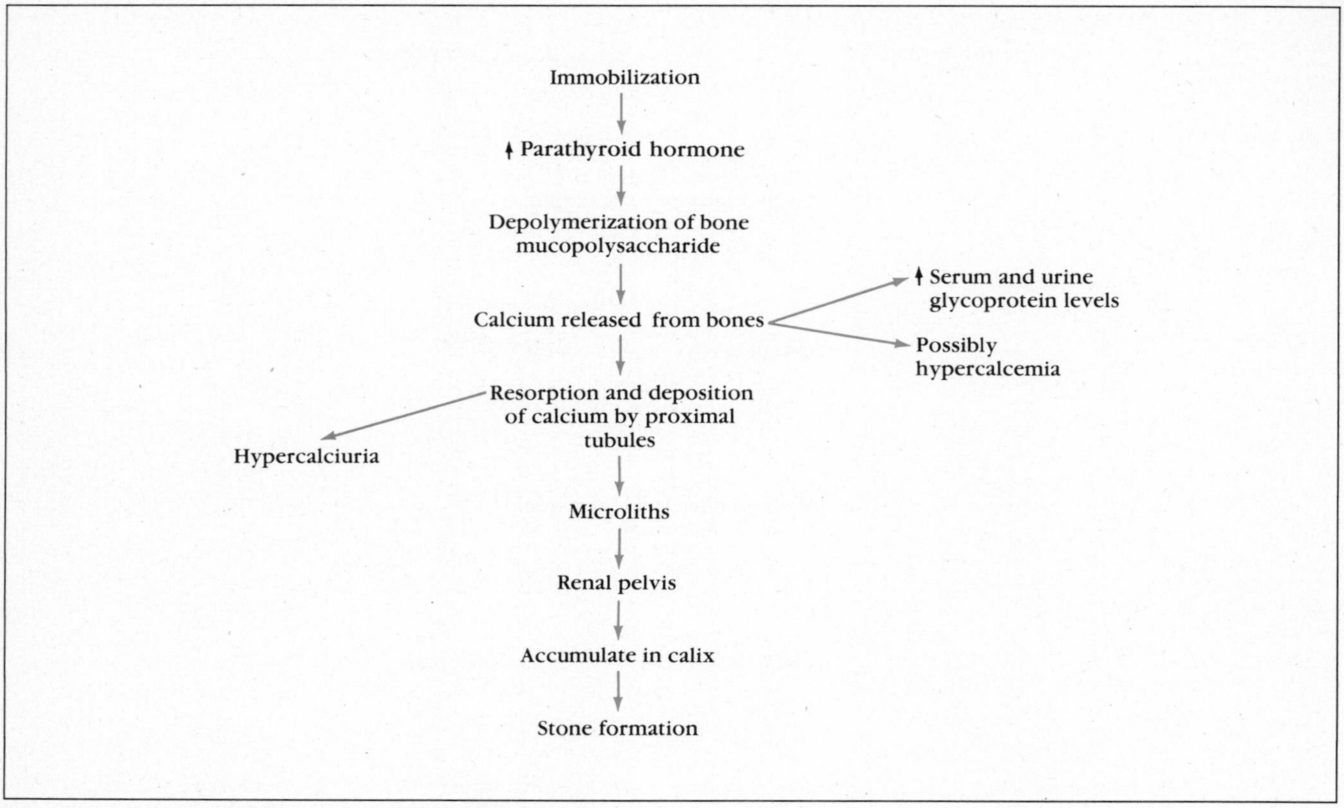

Immobilization
↑ Parathyroid hormone
Depolymerization of bone mucopolysaccharide
Calcium released from bones
↑ Serum and urine glycoprotein levels
Possibly hypercalcemia
Resorption and deposition of calcium by proximal tubules
Hypercalciuria
Microliths
Renal pelvis
Accumulate in calix
Stone formation

FIGURE 30-8 Resorptive alterations causing stone formation.

Urea splitting bacteria
HYDROLYZES
Ammonia
HYDROLYZES
Ammonium hydroxide
↑ pH (alkaline)
Struvite stones
↑ Amounts of deprotonated phosphate

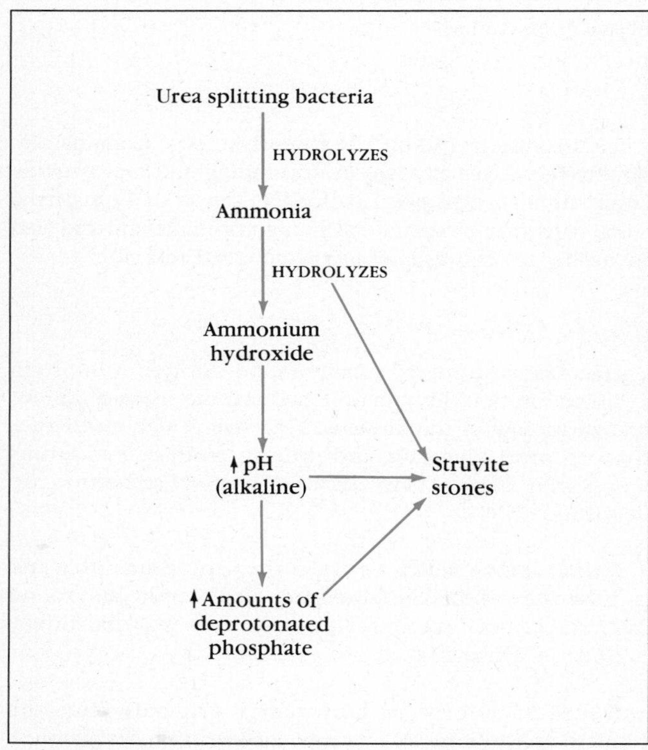

FIGURE 30-9 Formation of struvite stones.

logically from small, well-differentiated renal cell carcinomas [23].

Hemangiomas are rare, and can result in massive hematuria, causing renal colic as blood clots pass through the ureters. These tumors have thin-walled sinuses and are usually present in the renal medulla or pelvis. They generally are single and unilateral.

Lipomas are rare, and originate mainly from the paranephric fat. These tumors, which are usually small in diameter, may develop in the parenchyma, renal capsule, and paranephric tissue.

Juxtaglomerular cell tumors are renin-secreting tumors that originate from the juxtaglomerular apparatus and are associated with high blood pressure. Histologically, various shapes and sizes of granules are seen in the cytoplasm of these tumors [23].

Malignant Tumors

Renal Cell Carcinomas. Renal carcinomas usually occur between ages 50 and 70 years, are most common in males, and account for 85 to 89 percent of tumors of the kidney [8]. A higher percentage of renal adenocarcinomas is reported among users of tobacco products. Renal carcinomas or cysts often occur in association with von Hippel-Lindau disease, which is a hereditary defect involving angiomas of the retinae and cerebellum.

TABLE 30-2 Classification of Renal Tumors

Tumors of the renal parenchyma
- Benign
  - Cortical (tubular) adenoma
    - Solid
    - Cystic
  - Fibroma
  - Lipoma
  - Myxoma
  - Angioma
  - Lymphangioma
  - Hemangiopericytoma
  - Leiomyoma
  - Mixed tumor with combination of above elements (e.g., angiomyolipoma, myxolipoma)
  - Dysontogenetic rests
    - Adrenal cortical rests
    - Chondral and osseous rests
    - Dermoid cysts
    - Endometrioma
- Malignant
  - Adenocarcinoma (tubular) (Grawitz's tumor, hypernephroma)
  - Wilms' tumor
  - Fibrosarcoma
  - Liposarcoma
  - Leiomyosarcoma
  - Angiosarcoma and other compounded sarcomas
  - Metastatic tumors

Tumors of the renal pelvis
- Papilloma
- Papillary transitional cell (epidermoid) or squamous cell carcinoma
- Nonpapillary transitional cell (epidermoid) squamous cell carcinoma
- Mucous adenocarcinoma

Tumors of the renal capsule
- Fibroma
- Lipoma
- Angioma
- Leiomyoma
- Myxoma
- Tumors with combinations of the above elements and their malignant counterpart

Tumors of the paranephric tissue
- Tumors of type found in renal capsule
- Extraosseous osteogenic sarcoma

Source: Reprinted with permission from A. Allen, *The Kidney: Medical and Surgical Diseases* (2nd ed.). New York: Grune & Stratton, 1962.

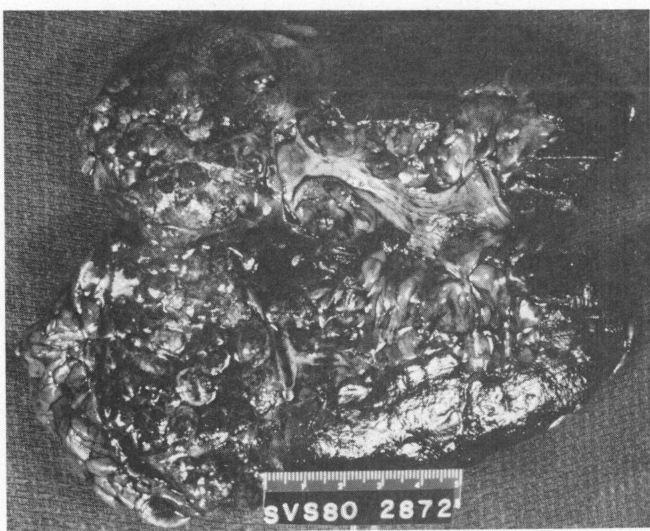

FIGURE 30-10 Renal carcinoma showing enlargement and infiltration of the kidney parenchyma.

Renal carcinomas arise from tubular epithelium and can occur anywhere in the kidney. They vary in size from a few to several centimeters and their weight may be in kilograms (Fig. 30-10). The tumors may proliferate throughout the kidneys to the ureters, invading the hilum, to the renal vein and the inferior vena cava. Their color varies from white to yellow to gray [3].

The tumor margins are usually clearly defined and cause pressure on the renal parenchyma. The tumors often spread or bulge into the renal calices and may extend to the ureter. They characteristically invade the venous system and spread by vascular metastases to the lungs, bone, lymph nodes, liver, and brain. Metastases may occur to almost any organ [15]. Morphologically, the cells may be very anaplastic, giant cells, or clear cells, or they may be more well differentiated.

Another characteristic of renal cell carcinoma is that the abnormal cells produce hormones or hormonelike substances such as erythropoietin, parathyroidlike hormone, renin, gonadotropins, or glucocorticosteroids [23]. The effects of these secretions may lead to diagnosis of the tumor.

The behavior of the tumors is unpredictable, with rapid growth and metastases being followed by years of slow growth. Metastases may resolve after nephrectomy.

Symptoms are variable, with microscopic or macroscopic hematuria being the most consistent feature. Other symptoms include flank pain, fever, weight loss, and tumor mass that may be palpated.

Regardless of type and pattern, there is significant consistency in the staging of renal cell tumors (Table 30-3). Prognosis is based on several factors that include staging, the number of metastases, cell type, and size and weight of the tumor [24].

Wilms' Tumor. Wilms' tumor is a malignant tumor that accounts for 6 to 30 percent of abdominal tumors in children, usually occurring between 2 and 5 years of age [18]. By the time the tumor is discovered, a very large abdominal mass is often palpable. Other symptoms that may develop include microscopic hematuria, pain, fever, vomiting, and hypertension due to renal ischemia. Pulmonary metastasis is often present at the time of diagnosis.

Wilms' tumor is gray to yellow, circular, with a fibrous capsule, and frequently has solid, cystic, and hemorrhagic areas. Histologically, it contains proliferating embryonic connective tissue with dense nuclei. The glomeruli are primitive with a poorly formed Bowman's capsule, and they lack a basement membrane [1]. At first the tumor is

TABLE 30-3 Staging of Renal Carcinomas

TNM Staging			
Clinical	Pathologic	Extent of Disease	Robson Stage
T1	pT1	Tumor within capsule (small)	I
T2	pT2	Tumor within capsule (large)	
T3	pT3	Tumor in perinephric fat	II
T3	V1	Tumor in renal vein	
N1–N3	pN1–pN3	Tumor in regional lymph nodes	III
	V2	Tumors in vena cava	
T4	pT4	Adjacent organ invasion	
M1	pM1	Distant metastases	IV
N4	pN4	Tumor in juxtaregional lymph nodes	

Source: G. Sufrin and G.P. Murphy, Renal adenocarcinoma. *Urol. Surv.* 30:129, 1980.

surrounded by a dense capsule and grows by pushing the renal parenchyma out of its path. When the capsule ruptures, metastasis to the lungs, lymphatic system, liver, and brain occurs rapidly.

Numerous factors determine the prognosis for this tumor, but of great importance is the stage at the time of diagnosis. The National Wilms' Tumor Study has adopted the staging system seen in Table 30-4 [8]. Long-term survival rates have improved to 90 percent with treatment by chemotherapy, radiotherapy, and surgery [23].

Tumors of the Renal Pelvis. Of the malignant tumors of the kidneys, those of the renal pelvis account for 4.5 to 9.0 percent [9]; 85 percent are papillary transitional cell carcinomas, and when diagnosed, more than one-half have invaded the pelvic musculature [9]. Papillary tumors have a cauliflower appearance when in the renal pelvis. Their frequency is increased in persons with analgesia-induced nephropathy, but the precise carcinogen is unknown [23].

TABLE 30-4 Wilms' Tumor Study: Staging of Tumors of the Kidney

Stage	Description
I	Tumor limited to kidney and completely resected
II	Tumor extending beyond kidney but completely resected
III	Residual nonhematogenous tumor confined to abdomen
IV	Hematogenous metastasis
V	Bilateral renal involvement either initially or subsequently

Source: M. Forland, *Nephrology* (2nd ed.). Garden City, N.Y.: Medical Examination, 1983.

Study Questions

1. Differentiate between benign prostatic hyperplasia and carcinoma of the prostate gland on the basis of pathogenesis, pathology, symptoms, and complications.
2. Explain the concept of supersaturation in the production of renal calculi.
3. Discuss how stones can form in the urinary system in the presence of either an acid or an alkaline urine.
4. Describe the pathogenesis of renal cell carcinoma, including presenting signs and symptoms and stages.

References

1. Anderson, W.A.D., and Scotti, T.M. *Synopsis of Pathology* (10th ed.). St. Louis: Mosby, 1980.
2. Bartsch, W., et al. Hormone blood levels and their interrelationships in normal men and men with benign prostatic hyperplasia (BPH). *Acta Endocrinol*. (Copenh.) 90:727, 1979.
3. Bennington, J.L. Histopathology of renal adenocarcinoma. In G. Sufrin and S.A. Beckly (eds.), *Renal Adenocarcinoma* (report no. 10). Geneva: International Union Against Cancer, 1980.
4. Bordier, P., et al. On the pathogenesis of so-called idiopathic hypercalciuria. *Am. J. Med.* 63:398, 1977.
5. Brosign, W. Conservative treatment of benign prostatic hypertrophy. In H. Marberger et al. (eds.), *Prostatic Disease: Proceedings*. New York: Liss, 1976.
6. Coe, F.L. Nephrolithiasis: Causes, classification and management. *Hosp. Pract*. 16:33, 1981.
7. Coe, F.L., and Favus, M.J. Disorders of stone formation. In B.M. Brenner and C.C. Rector (eds.), *The Kidney* (3rd ed.). Philadelphia: Ardmore, 1986.
8. Forland, M. (ed.). *Nephrology*. Garden City, N.Y.: Medical Examinations, 1977.
9. Frayley, E.E. Cancer of the renal pelvis. In D.G. Skinner and J.B. deKernion (eds.), *Genitourinary Cancer*. Philadelphia: Saunders, 1978.
10. Gutman, A.B., and Yii, T.F. Uric acid nephrolithiasis. *Am. J. Med.* 45:756, 1968.
11. Hallson, P.C., and Rose, G.A. Uromucoids and urinary stone formation. *Lancet* 1:100, 1979.
12. Hammond, G.L., et al. Serum steroids in normal males and patients with prostatic disease. *Clin. Endocinol*. (Oxf.) 9:113, 1978.
13. Hellstrom, I. Calcification and calculus formation in a series of seventy cases of primary hyperparathyroidism. *Br. J. Urol.* 27:387, 1955.
14. Higgins, S.I., and Gehring, U. Molecular mechanisms of steroid hormone action. *Adv. Cancer Res.* 28:313, 1978.
15. Karakousis, C.P., and Jennings, E. Renal cell carcinoma metastatic to skeletal muscle mass: A case report. *J. Surg. Oncol.* 17:287, 1982.
16. Kleeman, C.R., et al. Kidney stones: Interdepartmental clinic conference (UCLA School of Medicine). *West. J. Med.* 132:313, 1980.
17. Ljunghall, S., and Hedstrand, H. Epidemiology of renal stones in a middle-age population. *Acta Med. Scand.* 197:439, 1975.
18. Marsden, H.B., and Stewart, J.K. *Wilms' Tumors: Recent Results in Cancer Research. Tumors in Children* (vol. 13). New York: Springer-Verlag, 1968.
19. Melick, R.A., and Henneman, P.H. Clinical laboratory studies of 207 consecutive patients in a kidney-stone clinic. *N. Engl. J. Med.* 259:307, 1958.

20. Pak, C.Y.C., et al. The hypercalciurias: Causes, parathyroid function and diagnostic criteria. *J. Clin. Invest.* 54:387, 1974.
21. Pak, C.Y.C., et al. A simple test for the diagnosis of absorptive, resorptive and renal hypercalciurias. *N. Engl. J. Med.*, 292:497, 1975.
22. Pearse, H.D., and Houghton, D.C. Renal oncocytoma. *Urology* 13:74, 1979.
23. Robbins, S.L., Cotran, R.S., and Kumar, V. *Pathologic Basis of Disease* (3rd ed.). Philadelphia: Saunders, 1984.
24. Sufrin, G., and Murphy, G.P. Renal adenocarcinoma (review article). *Urol. Surv.* 30:129, 1980.
25. Vermeulen, A., and DeSy, W. Androgens in patients with benign prostatic hyperplasia before and after prostatectomy. *J. Clin. Endocrinol. Metab.* 43:1250, 1976.
26. Wallach, J. *Interpretation of Diagnostic Tests* (4th ed.). Boston: Little, Brown, 1986.
27. Walsh, P.C., and Wilson, J.D. The induction of prostatic hypertrophy in the dog with androstanediol. *J. Clin. Invest.* 57:1093, 1976.
28. Wilson, J.D. The pathogenesis of benign prostatic hyperplasia. *Am. J. Med.* 68:745, 1980.

CHAPTER 31

Renal Failure and Uremia

CHAPTER OUTLINE

Acute Renal Failure

- Causes
- Pathogenesis
- Acute Tubular Necrosis
  - *Etiology*
  - *Pathology*
  - *Pathophysiology*
  - *Stages of ARF*
  - *Prognosis*

Chronic Renal Failure

- Pathophysiology
- Physiologic Problems Caused by CRF
  - *Fluid Imbalance*
  - *Sodium Imbalance*
  - *Potassium Imbalance*
  - *Acid-Base Imbalance*
  - *Magnesium Imbalance*
  - *Phosphorus and Calcium Imbalance*
  - *Anemia*
  - *Purpura*
  - *Urea and Creatinine Alterations*
  - *Carbohydrate Intolerance*

Uremic Syndrome

- Neurologic System
- Cardiovascular System
- Respiratory System
- Gastrointestinal System
- Musculoskeletal System
- Hematologic Alterations
- Dermatologic Alterations

LEARNING OBJECTIVES

1. Define *acute renal failure (ARF)*.
2. Define *azotemia* and *oliguria*.
3. List three causes of ARF.
4. Describe prerenal, renal, and postrenal causes of ARF.
5. Discuss the two major causes of acute tubular necrosis (ATN).
6. List some of the drugs that can cause nephrotoxic renal failure.
7. Describe the pathologic features of nephrotoxic and ischemic ATN.
8. Discuss the back-leak theory and tubule obstruction in relationship to oliguria.
9. Discuss the theories concerning the pathogenesis of oliguria.
10. Discuss arterial occlusion and prostaglandins in relationship to oliguria.
11. Identify four stages of ARF including onset and oliguric, diuretic, and postdiuretic stages.
12. Discuss the pathology of water imbalance, hyponatremia, hyperkalemia, metabolic acidosis, anemia, and elevated levels of creatinine, phosphate, and urea during the oliguric stage of ARF.
13. Identify the clinical manifestations characteristic of the diuretic phase of ARF.
14. Define *chronic renal failure (CRF)*.
15. List causes and stages of CRF.
16. Discuss the intact nephron theory and its relationship to CRF.
17. Discuss fluid imbalances in CRF.
18. Define *hypothenuria*, *polyuria*, and *isosthenuria*.
19. Explain how hyponatremia and hypernatremia can occur in CRF.
20. Identify causes of hyperkalemia and hypokalemia in CRF.
21. Discuss three mechanisms that occur in metabolic acidosis in CRF.
22. Explain the relationship of metabolic acidosis and osteodystrophy in CRF.
23. Identify mechanisms that regulate calcium and phosphorus levels.
24. Discuss hyperparathyroidism and vitamin D metabolism in relationship to bone disease.

LEARNING OBJECTIVES continued

25. Explain six factors that lead to anemia in CRF.
26. Identify the etiology of purpura.
27. Discuss urea metabolism and carbohydrate intolerance.
28. Define *uremia*.
29. List symptoms and causes of the altered neurologic system in relationship to uremia.
30. Identify causes of hypertension in relationship to uremia.
31. List and discuss cardiac abnormalities in relationship to uremia.
32. Discuss the effects of uremia on the respiratory system, including uremic lung, uremic pleuritis, pulmonary edema, and infections.
33. Identify gastrointestinal symptoms in relationship to uremia.
34. Discuss gastrointestinal abnormalities in relationship to uremia, including ulcerations, oral changes, bleeding, and constipation.
35. Define *renal osteodystrophy*.
36. List the causes of renal osteodystrophy.
37. Define *osteomalacia*, *osteitis fibrosa*, *soft tissue metastatic calcification*, and *osteosclerosis*.
38. Identify the major hematologic infection in persons with CRF.
39. Discuss dermatologic alterations in relationship to uremia.

Renal failure occurs when the kidneys are unable to remove accumulated metabolites from the blood. The process causes alterations in electrolyte, acid-base, and water balance, as well as the accumulation of substances that normally are totally excreted by the body.

Acute Renal Failure

Acute renal failure (ARF) is a clinical syndrome in which the kidneys are unable to excrete the waste products of metabolism, usually because of renal hypoperfusion. This syndrome may lead to *azotemia*, which is the accumulation of nitrogenous waste products in the blood, and to *oliguria*, in which urine output is less than 400 ml per 24 hours. Approximately 40 percent of ARF is nonoliguric.

Acute renal failure can result from different causes. Research showed that of 2200 cases, 43 percent were related to surgery or trauma, 26 percent to various medical conditions, 13 percent to pregnancy, and 9 percent to nephrotoxins [20]. The causes have been divided into the following major categories: prerenal, renal, and postrenal.

Causes

Acute renal failure is broadly defined as any condition causing sudden suppression of kidney function [5]. It is related to a number of factors, including ischemic disorders, nephrotoxic disorders, diseases of the small blood vessels, diseases of the major blood vessels, and acute interstitial nephritis [30]. The most common causes are ischemia and nephrotoxicity.

Prerenal disease refers to any condition that diminishes renal perfusion pressure, such as hypovolemia and shock. Acute azotemia results due to hypotension, hypovolemia, and decreased renal perfusion. This may be reversed acutely by immediate intervention.

Renal (intrinsic) ARF results from acute parenchymal changes that damage the nephrons. Many conditions can cause parenchymal damage, including acute glomerulonephritis (AGN), vascular diseases, interstitial nephritis, and acute tubular necrosis (ATN). *Acute intrinsic renal failure (AIRF)* can be induced by renal hypoperfusion and ischemia, nephrotoxins, and other mechanisms. It is also called ATN, which is a syndrome of abrupt and sustained decline of glomerular filtration rate (GFR) that is not immediately reversible (see p. 466). Prerenal disease may improve immediately with increased renal perfusion and postrenal conditions may be improved by relieving the obstruction.

The postrenal category includes any condition that obstructs excretion of normally elaborated urine. The most common of these that causes ARF is benign prostatic hyperplasia (BPH). Table 31-1 details the large group of specific disorders that can cause ARF.

The mechanisms of dysfunction vary, but the results are acute inability of the kidneys to excrete waste products and a build-up of nitrogenous waste in the blood.

Pathogenesis

Acute renal failure results in a severe reduction in GFR. Several mechanisms have been proposed in the alteration of GFR, such as the *back-leak theory*, the *tubular obstruction theory*, and the *vascular theories*.

The back-leak theory of increased permeability proposes that the lack of urinary output is caused by disruption of tubular epithelium rather than GFR. Therefore, substances are resorbed from the tubular lumen and inter-

Table 31-1 Specific Disorders That Cause ARF

Ischemic disorders
- Major trauma
- Massive hemorrhage
- Crush syndrome
- Septic shock
- Transfusion reactions
- Myoglobinuria
- Pregnancy: postpartum hemorrhage
- Postoperative, particularly cardiac, aortic, and biliary surgery
- Medical: pancreatitis, gastroenteritis

Nephrotoxins, including hypersensitivity reactions
- Heavy metals: mercury, arsenic, lead, bismuth, uranium, cadmium
- Carbon tetrachloride
- Ethylene glycol
- Other organic solvents
- Radiographic contrast media (particularly in patients with diabetes mellitus)
- Pesticides
- Fungicides
- Antibiotics: aminoglycosides, penicillins, tetracyclines, amphotericin B
- Other drugs and chemical agents: phenytoin, phenylbutazone, uric acid, calcium, nonsteroidal antiinflammatory drugs

Diseases of glomeruli and small blood vessels
- Acute poststreptococcal glomerulonephritis
- Systemic lupus erythematosus
- Polyarteritis nodosa
- Schönlein-Henoch purpura
- Subacute bacterial endocarditis
- Serum sickness
- Goodpasture's syndrome
- Malignant hypertension
- Hemolytic-uremic syndrome
- Drug-related vasculitis
- Pregnancy: abruptio placentae; abortion with and without gram-negative sepsis; postpartum renal failure
- Rapidly progressive glomerulonephritis, unknown etiology

Major blood vessel disease
- Renal artery thrombosis, embolism, or stenosis
- Bilateral renal vein thrombosis

Interstitial nephritis associated with infection
- Streptococcal
- Staphylococcal
- Diptheria
- Leptospirosis
- Brucellosis
- Legionnaires' disease
- Toxoplasmosis
- Infectious mononucleosis

Interstitial nephritis associated with drugs
- Penicillin semisynthetic analogs
- Sulfonamides
- Tetracyclines
- Cephalosporin
- Co-trimoxazole
- Rifampin
- Phenindione
- Warfarin
- Furosemide
- Thiazides
- Azathioprine
- Allopurinol
- Phenytoin

Source: R.W. Schrier, *Renal and Electrolyte Disorders* (3rd ed.). Boston: Little, Brown, 1986.

stitium into the peritubular circulation. In experimental models of ARF, tubular damage was demonstrated anatomically after administration of nephrotoxic substances [7]. The back-leak phenomenon apparently contributes to severe or toxic ARF but probably plays little part in most cases of mild to moderate ARF.

Tubular obstruction by intraluminal casts, debris, and/or interstitial edema may cause a decrease in GFR due to the increased hydrostatic pressure in Bowman's capsule. Demonstration of acute obstruction with casts within one week of onset is usual, but patency usually returns in two weeks. Pressures fall to normal levels at two weeks [7].

Vascular theories relate to decrease in renal blood flow leading to increased renal vascular resistance. This may be due to afferent arteriolar vasoconstriction initially, but later restoration of RBF does not improve the glomerular filtration pressure or renal function. In the initial stage, renal blood flow is definitely decreased. In the established phase, the glomerular filtration rate decreases out of proportion to renal blood flow. Loss of renal autoregulation seems to be the major occurrence and may be related to the renin-angiotensin-aldosterone system or other phenomena.

Acute Tubular Necrosis

Etiology. The two most common causes of ATN are ischemia and exposure to nephrotoxic agents (Table 31-2). Ischemia is the most frequent cause, with its duration determining the extent of damage and the prognosis for return of urinary function. According to one study, ischemia present for 25 minutes or less caused mild and reversible damage [6]. Others showed that two hours of ischemia caused severe and irreversible damage [11].

Nephrotoxic agents destroy tubular cells by direct cellular toxic effects, lysis of RBCs, and intravascular coagulation, precipitation of oxalate and uric acid crystals, and tissue hypoxia [9]. Factors that promote nephrotoxicity of

Table 31-2 Nephrotoxic and Ischemic Mechanisms for the Production of Acute Tubular Necrosis

Nephrotoxins
- Antibiotics: aminoglycosides (e.g., gentamicin), penicillins, tetracyclines, amphotericin B, sulfonamides
- Other drugs and chemicals: phenylbutazone, anesthetic agents, fungicides, pesticides, calcium sodium edetate
- Radiographic contrast materials
- Organic solvents: carbon tetrachloride, ethylene glycol, phenol, methyl alcohol
- Heavy metals: mercury, arsenic, bismuth, cadmium, gold, lead, thallium, uranium
- Heme pigments: hemoglobin, myoglobin

Ischemia
- Hypovolemia (dehydration, hemorrhage, pooling of fluids in burns or ascites)
- Circulatory insufficiency (shock, severe heart failure, dysrhythmias, tamponade)

Source: S. Papper, *Clinical Nephrology* (2nd ed.). Boston: Little, Brown, 1978.

agents include the hydration status, preexisting renal disease, and the person's age.

As one ages, the number of nephrons decreases, so that drugs become more concentrated in the tubules. Persons over 75 years of age exposed to nephrotoxic drugs have a much higher frequency of nephrotoxicity than those between ages 16 and 30 years [18].

Antibiotics, including the aminoglycosides, penicillins, cephalosporins, tetracyclines, amphotericin B, and sulfonamides, are probably the principal causes of renal disruption [27]. Radiographic contrast materials containing iodine, solvents, heavy metals, and pigments of hemoglobin and myoglobin also can cause ATN [27].

Pathology. In the *ischemic type of ATN*, patchy necrosis occurs in the tubules (Fig. 31-1A). The main area of necrosis is in the straight portion of the proximal tubules, but lesions also occur in the distal tubules.

If severe injury has been sustained, injury to the basement membrane occurs and exposes the tubular lumen to the interstitial space. The mitochondria in the epithelium have been noted to be swollen when viewed through the electron microscope [30]. The areas that have no lesions have dilated tubules and flattened epithelium. Damage to the brush border of the proximal tubule cells also results [14,34].

A characteristic finding of ischemic ATN is blockage of tubule lumina by casts. Other abnormalities include leukocytes in the vasa recta, dilation of Bowman's spaces of the glomeruli, interstitial edema, and inflammatory cells in the interstitium. The glomeruli appear to be normal [30].

In the *nephrotoxic type of ATN*, a more uniform appearance is characteristic (Fig. 31-1B). Lesions are located in the proximal tubules, but may occur in the basement membrane and distal tubules when severe injury has been sustained. Usually, less basement membrane disruption occurs with nephrotoxic ATN than with ischemic ATN [16].

Casts, which are debris from cells, obstruct the distal tubules, and necrosis is present in all nephrons. Interstitial edema, leukocytes in the vasa recta, and inflammatory cells in the interstitium are characteristic.

Pathophysiology. *Oliguria* is a cardinal feature of the early stages of ARF with vascular or tubular etiology. Not all forms of ARF exhibit oliguria, but progressive azotemia occurs due to the impaired renal function. The possible mechanisms for the production of oliguria are shown in Figure 31-2 and are described below.

Research suggests that *tubular factors* are the primary sources in the pathogenesis of renal insufficiency (Fig. 31-3) [6]. If oliguria is due to a tubular abnormality, it is believed to be the result either of back-leakage or intratubular obstruction as described previously. The uranyl nitrate model supports the back-leak proposal. When uranyl nitrate is administered to animals it leads to varying degrees of damage to the pars recta; polyuria occurs in

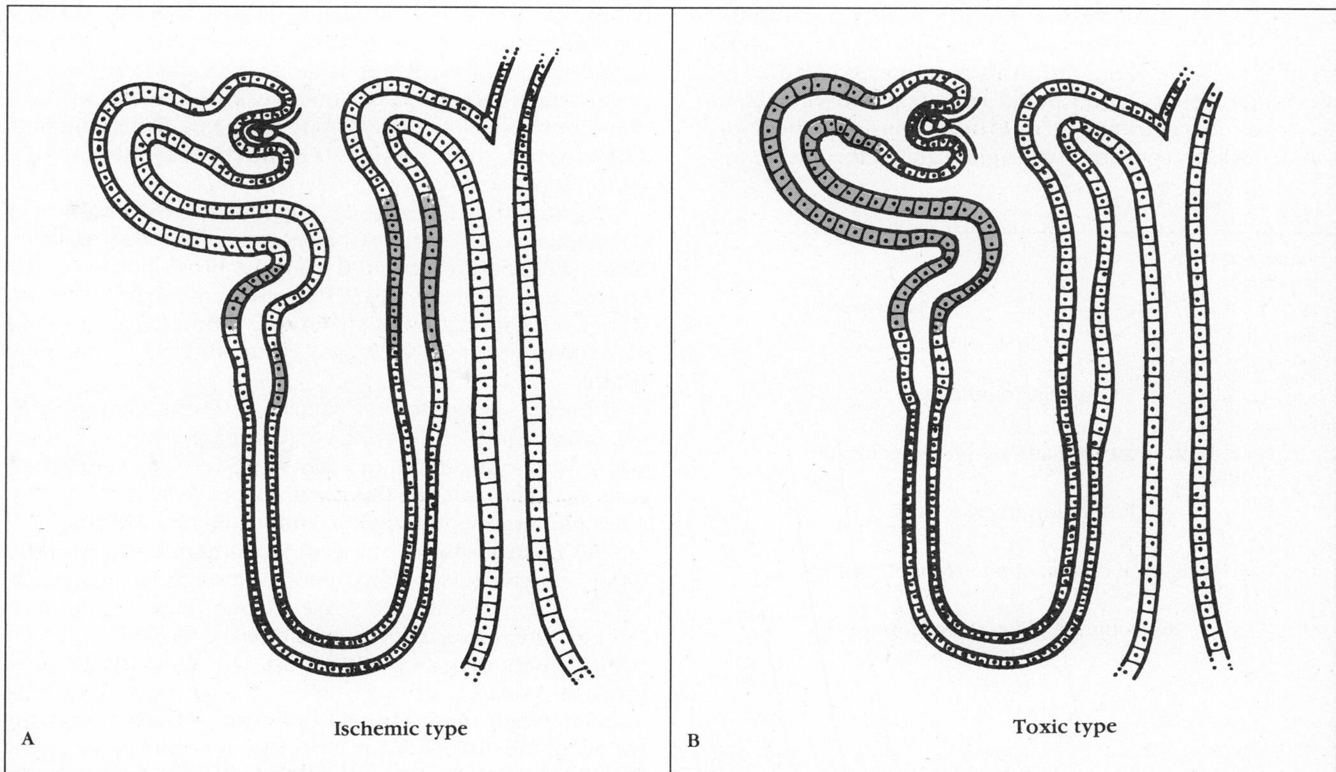

FIGURE 31-1 A. Patchy ischemic necrosis of the proximal tubules. B. Characteristic nephrotoxic injury of large segments of proximal tubule.

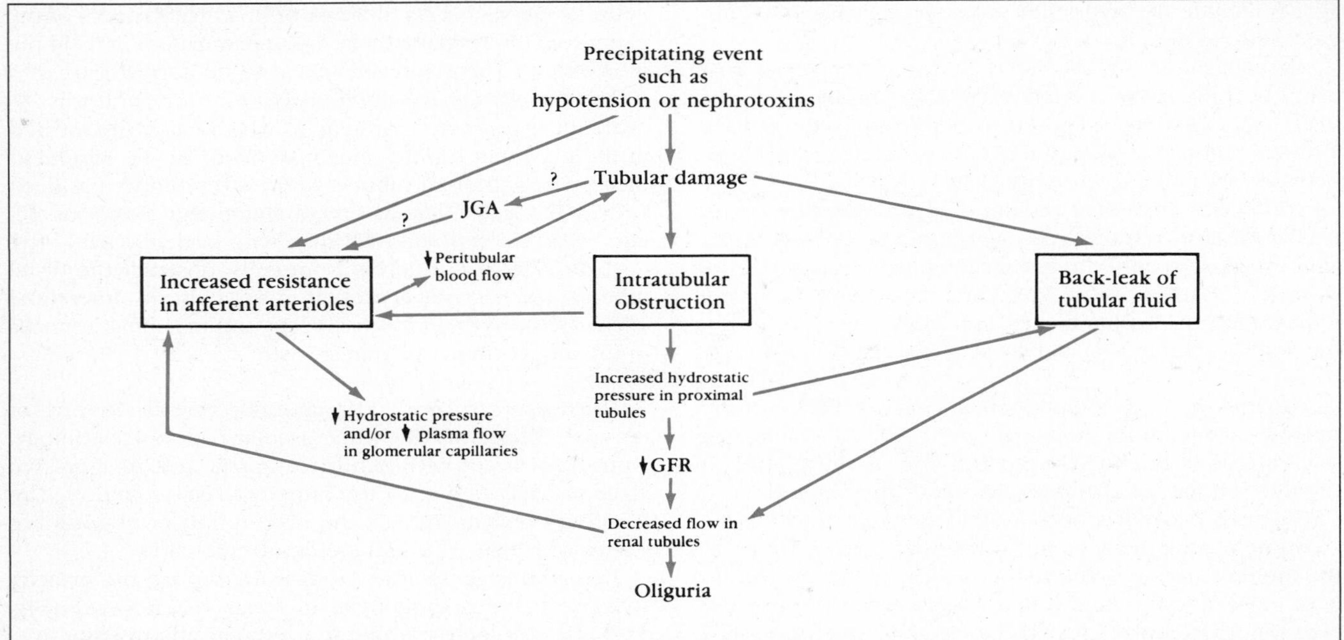

FIGURE 31-2 Schema of possible causes of oliguria in acute renal failure in which the three major theories of its etiology may be reconciled. The theories are stated in the boxes and the arrows indicate the possible interrelationships among them. (From H. Valtin, *Renal Dysfunction*. Boston: Little, Brown, 1979.)

the first 24 to 48 hours, with oliguria occurring later [13,14,22,23]. A decrease in the glomerular ultrafiltration coefficient causes a decrease in the GFR. Electron microscopy has shown a reduction in number and size of glomerular capillary endothelial fenestrae between 2 and 17 hours after uranyl nitrate injection [4]. Therefore, tubule leakage appears to be significant in this mode.

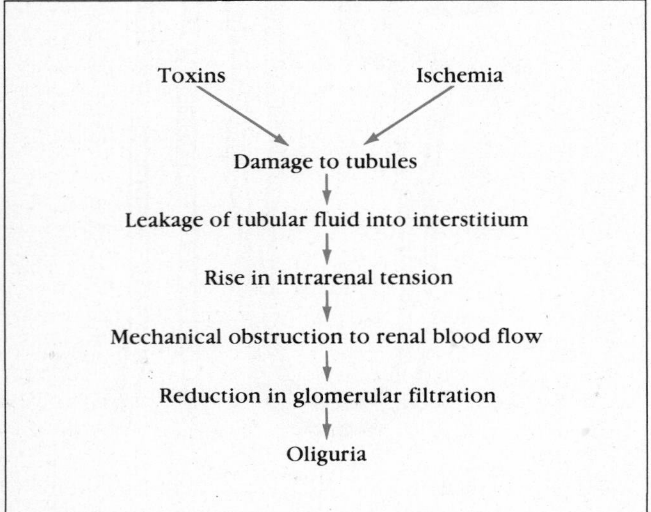

FIGURE 31-3 Chain of events that leads to oliguria in acute renal failure. (From R. Heptinstall, *Pathology of the Kidney* [3rd ed.]. Boston: Little, Brown, 1983.)

Tubular obstruction is believed to be due to casts, debris, and/or interstitial edema. Obstruction may be better understood by examining the *arterial occlusion model*. If arterial occlusion is induced in rats for one hour, oliguria may be present for one week or longer and renal blood flow is reduced about one-half [3,6]. When inulin is administered, the clearance test indicates a reduction by 60 to 90 percent [23].

When the renal arteries are occluded, great numbers of straight proximal tubules become occluded by swollen blebs of microvilli separated from the brush border of the convoluted segments [13]. Therefore, the arterial occlusion model indicates obstruction, tubular leakage, and vasoconstriction, all of which contribute to acute renal failure.

If there is no structural damage to the glomeruli, oliguria may result from *vascular changes*, especially renal artery vasoconstriction. In early stages of ARF, renal vasoconstriction occurs in the renal cortex, resulting in ischemia and a reduction in GFR, and leading to oliguria.

The relationship of the renin-angiotensin-aldosterone (RAA) system to vasoconstriction and oliguria is currently being studied. Renin is released when plasma volume is low. In ARF, experimental studies have shown increased renin levels (Fig. 31-4) [12,30,31]. One hypothesis involves a vasomotor mechanism (Fig. 31-5). It states that initially, when there is renal ischemia, tubular volume is reduced and less sodium chloride is resorbed into the blood. As a result, the sodium chloride concentration in the tubular fluid increases, which is somehow sensed by the juxtaglomerular apparatus (JGA), which then secretes

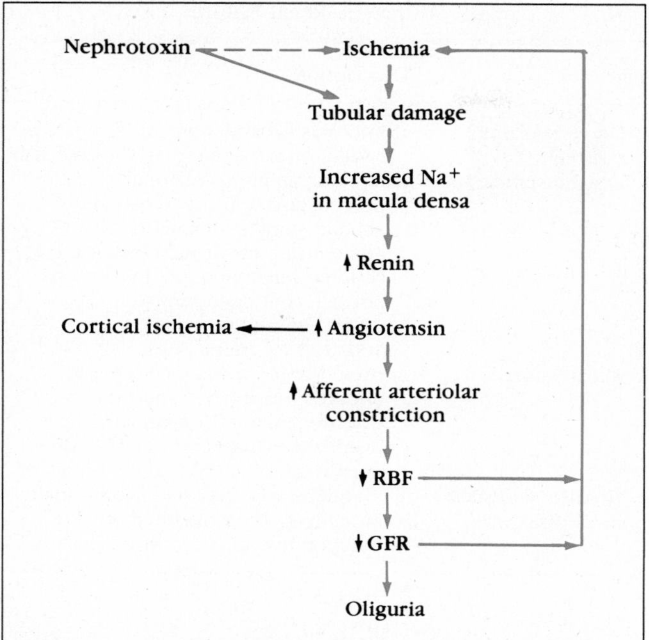

FIGURE 31-4 The possible role of the renin-angiotensin-aldosterone system in the development and maintenance of oliguria (and cortical ischemia) in acute tubular necrosis. (From S. Papper, *Clinical Nephrology* [2nd ed.]. Boston: Little, Brown, 1978.)

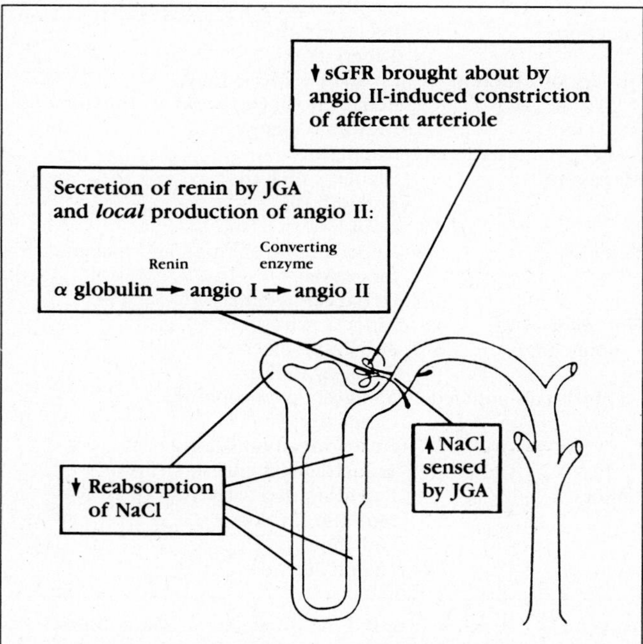

FIGURE 31-5 One theory of the pathogenesis of oliguric acute renal failure. The process is described in the text. JGA = juxtaglomerular apparatus; angio = angiotensin; sGFR = filtration rate of a single glomerulus. (From H. Valtin, *Renal Dysfunction*. Boston: Little, Brown, 1979.)

renin. The secretion of renin causes conversion of angiotensinogen to angiotensin, finally leading to vasoconstriction. Thus, the afferent arteriole constricts, which leads to decreased GFR, increased blood urea nitrogen (BUN), and oliguria. The evidence for this hypothesis is conflicting [34].

Another theory may explain oliguria in relationship to ARF. In studies of arterial occlusion in the rat, renal blood flow is reduced, which leads to swelling of the capillary endothelium with the accumulation of sodium and water [19,30,31].

Increased vascular resistance due to deficient synthesis of a prostaglandin, a renal vasodilator, is being studied [30]. Further research is necessary to determine the significance of prostaglandin deficiency in ARF.

Stages of ARF. The course of ARF can vary tremendously among individuals with different physiologic problems. The four stages of ARF are (1) onset, (2) oliguria, (3) diuresis, and (4) postdiuresis [33].

Onset is the initial or inciting event that causes necrosis of the convoluted tubules. The course of ARF is related to the magnitude of the inciting insult, the period of hypotension, and the length of time the hemodynamics are altered [9].

In *oliguria*, about 50 to 100 ml of urine is formed per 24 hours. If urine production ceases completely, renal obstruction should be investigated. Two major characteristics exhibited during this stage are urine specific gravity of approximately 1.010 and spilling of protein in urine.

Renal blood flow (RBF) is decreased to about one-third of normal, but the GFR falls to less than 1 percent of normal [30]. Because of this, the fluid and electrolyte balance becomes greatly altered.

Water imbalance may occur due to exogenous administration of fluids during the early critical stage. Excess body water may also be related to fat catabolism, with demonstration of mild to moderate hyponatremia. As much as 300 ml of water per day may result from protein and fat catabolism [30]. The hyponatremia that occurs during the oliguric phase is mainly due to the dilution of extracellular fluid, but it may be due to gastrointestinal disturbances, such as vomiting and diarrhea.

Hyperkalemia often occurs during the oliguric stage. This major electrolyte disturbance is due mostly to decreased renal excretion, but may be related to excessive breakdown of muscle protein. Some other factors that may cause excess potassium to be released from the cells include tissue trauma, acidosis, hypercatabolism, and infection. Potassium levels may rise rapidly and lead to fatal cardiac dysrhythmias (see Chaps. 5 and 6).

Metabolic acidosis is sometimes present in the oliguric stage. Because of tubular necrosis, hydrogen is not excreted by the kidneys appropriately and accumulates in the blood.

If ARF persists for two to three days, nearly all individuals develop moderate to severe anemia. Anemia is the result of several factors, including a mild increase of hemolysis, suppressed erythropoiesis (probably due to lack of erythropoietin and uremic toxins), and increased blood loss from uremic coagulation defects (see p. 475). There are no deficits of iron, B_{12}, or folic acid in the anemia.

Elevations of creatinine, phosphate, and urea result from breakdown of muscle protein and inability to excrete metabolites. With the increase of urea and other nitrogenous wastes in the blood, azotemia progresses.

The *diuretic stage* is characterized by output of more than 1000 ml of urine per 24 hours. Diuresis may begin as early as 24 hours after the onset of ARF or it may begin much later. The increased output, as much as 6 liters per day, does not indicate total return of renal function. Tubular function remains altered, which is indicated by large amounts of sodium and potassium lost in urine. Serum urea, creatinine, and other accumulated substances act as osmotic diuretics. They also continue to rise during the first days of diuresis. Dehydration may occur due to the inability to conserve water.

Laboratory values indicate a progression toward normal levels and increased production of red blood cells. Wide fluctuations in fluid and electrolyte balance are common during this stage.

The *postdiuretic, or recovery, stage* begins when urine output returns to normal. Eventually, sometimes for up to 12 months, GFR, RBF, and tubular function return so that the kidneys can again concentrate urine appropriately. Fluid and electrolyte balance improves with alteration in protein intake and prevention of fluid overloading.

Prognosis. The prognosis for ARF depends on the underlying cause, the onset and severity of the disease, and medical intervention. Mortality varies from 30 to 60 percent, with the highest risks being in the traumatized, postoperative, and aged populations [3,9].

Chronic Renal Failure

Chronic renal failure (CRF) is an irreversible condition characterized by diminished functioning of the nephrons, which results in decreased GFR, RBF, tubular function, and resorption ability. Renal impairment is progressive and leads to end-stage renal disease (Table 31-3).

Numerous conditions that cause CRF primarily affect the renal parenchyma (Table 31-4). Regardless of the cause, the result is damage to the nephrons and glomeruli. This damage may be diffused throughout both kidneys or it may be focal. Progressive loss of nephrons leads to greater dysfunction with more difficulty in maintaining an adequate fluid and electrolyte balance. Systemic effects occur in all of the organs of the body. The progression toward *uremia* (urine in the blood) is usually gradual, being controlled by diet and fluid restrictions for long periods of time (Fig. 31-6). When the kidneys can no longer maintain the fluid and electrolyte balance, dialysis becomes necessary.

Pathophysiology

The intact nephron theory aids in explaining the pathophysiology of CRF. Experiments support an *orderliness* of

Table 31-3 Stages of Chronic Renal Failure

Stage	Description
1: Decreased renal reserve	Homeostasis maintained; no symptoms; residual renal reserve 40% of normal
2: Renal insufficiency	Decreased ability to maintain homeostasis; mild azotemia and anemia; may be unable to concentrate urine and conserve H_2O; residual renal function 15–40% of normal; GFR decreases to 20 mL/minute (normal 100–120 mL/min)
3: Renal failure	Azotemia and anemia more severe; nocturia, electrolyte and fluid disorders; difficulty with activities; residual renal function 5–15% of normal
4: Uremia (end-stage renal disease)	No homeostasis; becomes symptomatic in many systems, residual renal function less than 5% of normal

Table 31-4 Causes of Chronic Renal Failure[a]

Type of Disorder	Examples
Immunologic	Glomerulonephritides[b]
	Lupus erythematosus
	Polyarteritis nodosa
	Goodpasture's syndrome
Infectious	Pyelonephritis[b]
	Tuberculosis
Urinary obstruction	Prostatic hypertrophy
	Renal calculi (bilateral or unilateral)
	Urethral constriction
	Neoplasms
Metabolic	Diabetes mellitus[b]
	Amyloidosis
	Gout
Vascular	Hypertension (benign and malignant)[b]
	Infarctions
	Sickle cell anemia
Hereditary and congenital	Alport's syndrome
	Polycystic disease
	Renal hypoplasia
Nephrotoxin-induced	Analgesic nephropathy
	Other drugs
	Heavy metal poisoning
	Industrial solvents
Others	Radiation nephritis
	Multiple myeloma
	Leukemia
	Hypercalcemia

[a]This list is not exhaustive, and the placement of some diseases into one category rather than another is arbitrary.
[b]These are some of the more common causes of chronic renal failure. Although certain other conditions (e.g., prostatic hypertrophy and renal calculi) have a high frequency, they do not often lead to chronic renal failure.
Source: H. Valtin, *Renal Dysfunction.* Boston: Little, Brown, 1979.

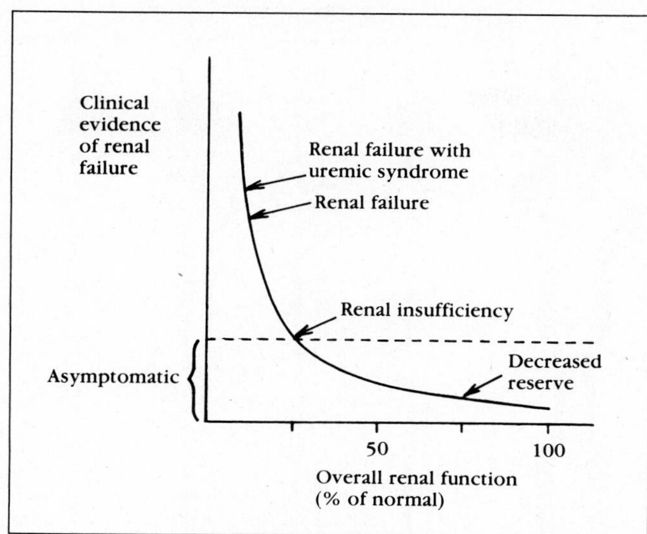

FIGURE 31-6 The relationship of clinical manifestations to renal function. (From S. Papper, *Clinical Nephrology* [2nd ed.]. Boston: Little, Brown, 1978.)

impaired renal function in the diseased kidney, which means that total nephron units are lost [8,17]. This finding lends support to the theory that the manifested net renal function is the result of a decreased number of correctly functioning nephrons, rather than being reflective of the number of diseased nephrons. A crucial feature of this theory is that the balance between the glomeruli and tubules must be maintained. As the nephrons receive more filtrate, they also must be able to resorb more to maintain the steady state [27]. When renal failure occurs it eventually affects all of the body systems.

Physiologic Problems Caused by CRF

Fluid Imbalance. Early in CRF, when the kidneys lose renal function, they are not able to concentrate urine appropriately (*hypothenuria*) and this results in excess water loss (*polyuria*). Hypothenuria is not only related to the diminished number of nephrons, but is due to the increased solute load per nephron. The increased solute (urea) load results because the intact nephrons carrying the solute and water for those nephrons are no longer functioning (Fig. 31-7) [8]. Osmotic diuresis may result, causing the person to become dehydrated.

As greater numbers of nephrons become dysfunctional, an inability to dilute urine (*isosthenuria*) results [15]. At this stage the glomeruli have hyalinized and plasma cannot be filtered easily through the tubules. Fluid overload with water and sodium retention results.

Sodium Imbalance. Maintaining sodium balance is a serious problem in that the nephrons may excrete as little as 20 to 30 mEq of sodium daily or up to 200 mEq daily. The varying amounts of sodium lost are believed to be related to the intact nephron theory. In other words, the damaged nephrons are unable to exchange sodium, so the intact nephrons receive the excess, causing an excess amount to be excreted in the urine. This increased elimination is accompanied by osmotic diuresis, which causes a reduction in blood volume, GFR, and dehydration. Sodium loss may be enhanced by gastrointestinal disturbances, especially vomiting and diarrhea that may aggravate the hyponatremia and dehydration [17].

In severe CRF, sodium balance can be maintained even though flexibility in adjusting to sodium levels is lost. A healthy person can reduce urinary excretion of sodium practically to zero or increase it to above 500 mEq per day when faced with sodium deficit or excess. If the GFR of a person with CRF decreases to less than 25 to 30 ml per minute, obligatory sodium excretion of about 25 mEq per day may occur, with maximum excretion of 150 to 200 mEq [34]. This accounts for dietary sodium restrictions of 1.0 to 1.5 gm per day in CRF.

Potassium Imbalance. Hyperkalemia is rarely a problem in CRF prior to end-stage (stage 4) if water balance is maintained and metabolic acidosis is controlled. Potassium (K^+) balance is believed to be the result of the adaptations made to the increased potassium presented to each functioning nephron. The mechanism for maintaining K^+ balance is not totally understood, but may be related to enhanced aldosterone secretion. As long as urine output is maintained, the potassium level is usually maintained. Hyperkalemia may result, however, from excessive intake of potassium, certain medications, hypercatabolic illness (infection), or hyponatremia. It also is characteristic in uremia or end-stage renal disease (stage 4).

Hypokalemia also can occur in association with vomiting or excessive diarrhea. In tubular renal disease the nephrons may fail to resorb potassium, leading to increased potassium excretion. If hypokalemia persists, the glomerular filtration rate and concentrating ability decrease and the production of ammonia (NH_3) increases. The level of bicarbonate (HCO_3) decreases and sodium (Na^+) is retained. This effect impairs functional ability.

Acid-Base Imbalance. Metabolic acidosis develops because the kidneys are unable to excrete enough hydrogen ion to keep the pH of the blood in a normal range.

Renal tubule dysfunction leads to progressive inability to excrete H^+ ion. In general, the decreased H^+ excretion is proportional to the decreased GFR [28]. Acids, continually being formed by metabolism in the body, are not filtered as effectively through the GBM, the production of NH_3 decreases, and the tubular cell is dysfunctional. Failure to form bicarbonate may also contribute to this imbalance.

Part of the excess serum hydrogen is buffered by the bone salts. As a result, chronic metabolic acidosis increases the possibility of osteodystrophy (Fig. 31-8) [32].

Magnesium Imbalance. The magnesium level is normal in early CRF, but progressive reduction in urinary excretion may cause accumulation. A combination of

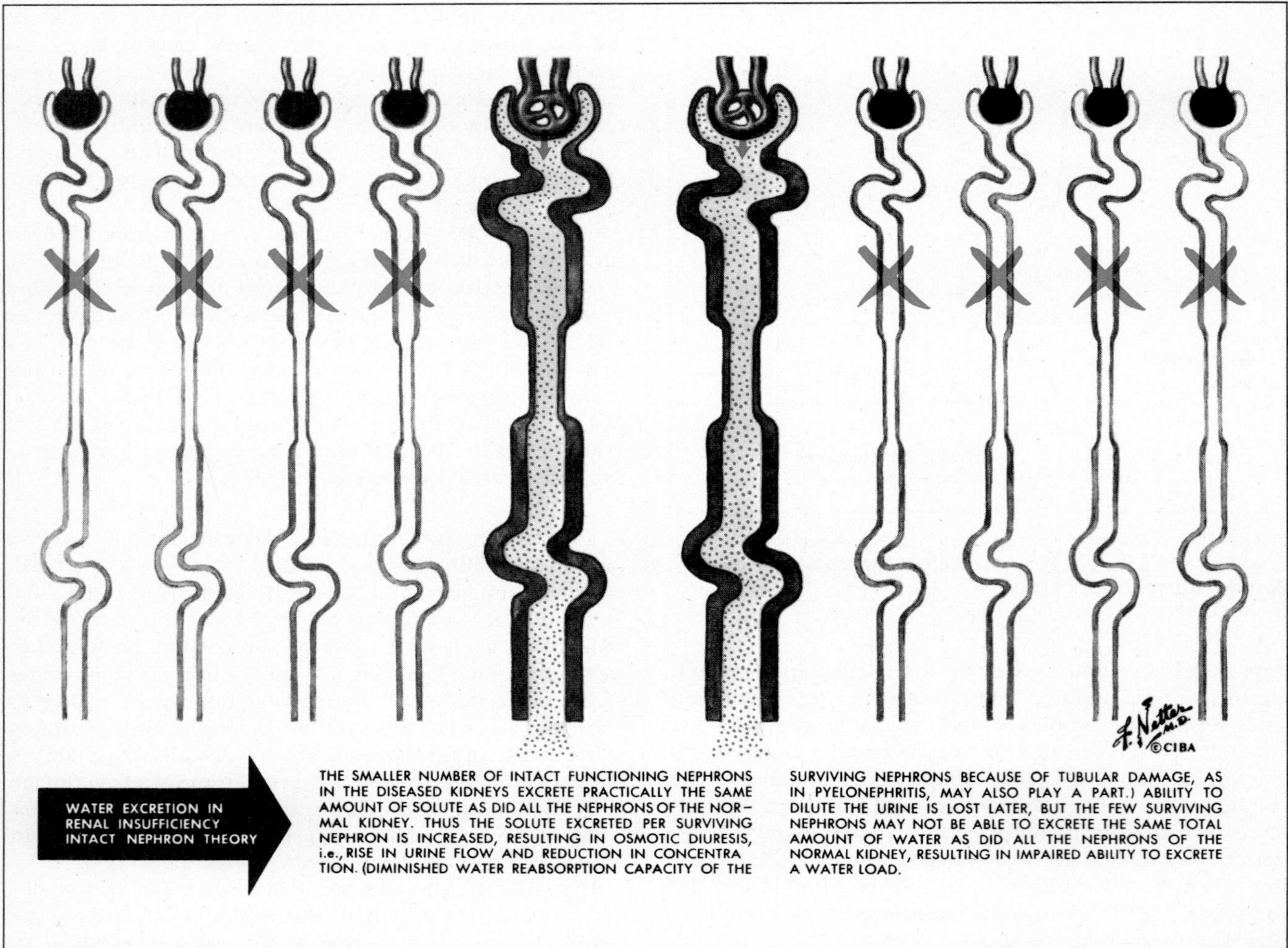

FIGURE 31-7 Water excretion in renal insufficiency. © 1973 CIBA Pharmaceutical Company, Division of CIBA-GEIGY Corp. Reprinted with permission from the CIBA Collection of Medical Illustrations. Illustrated by Frank H. Netter, M.D. All rights reserved.

decreased excretion and high intake of magnesium may result in cardiac or respiratory arrest [24].

Phosphorus and Calcium Imbalance. Normally, calcium and phosphorus levels are maintained by the parathyroid hormone, which causes renal resorption of calcium by the kidneys, mobilization of calcium from bone, and depression of tubular resorption of phosphorus. When renal function deteriorates to 20 to 25 percent of normal, hyperphosphatemia and hypocalcemia occur, leading to secondary hyperparathyroidism [24,32]. This secondary hyperparathyroidism is also associated with altered vitamin D metabolism. When prolonged, it results in renal osteodystrophy (see Chap. 34).

Activated vitamin D normally is responsible for enhancing calcium absorption in the gastrointestinal tract and increasing resorption of calcium from bone. When CRF is present, hypocalcemia develops because of decreased absorption of calcium. Figure 31-8 summarizes the development of renal osteodystrophy in chronic renal failure.

Anemia. A decreased hemoglobin in persons with CRF is the result of several factors: (1) short life span of red blood cells due to altered plasma; (2) increased loss of red blood cells due to gastrointestinal ulceration, dialysis, and blood taken for laboratory analysis; (3) reduced erythropoietin due to decreased renal formation and inhibition from uremia; (4) folate deficiency when the person is undergoing dialysis; (5) iron deficiency; and (6) elevated levels of parathyroid hormone, which stimulates fibrous tissue or osteitis fibrosis, taking up bone marrow space and causing decreased production by the marrow [1]. The normocytic, normochromic anemia, with hematocrit in the range of 15 to 30 percent, is usually proportionate to the degree of azotemia.

Purpura. Purpura may develop that is related to platelet impairment from accumulation of nitrogenous wastes. Purpura is characterized by hemorrhage into the skin and is associated with a general increase in bleeding tendency.

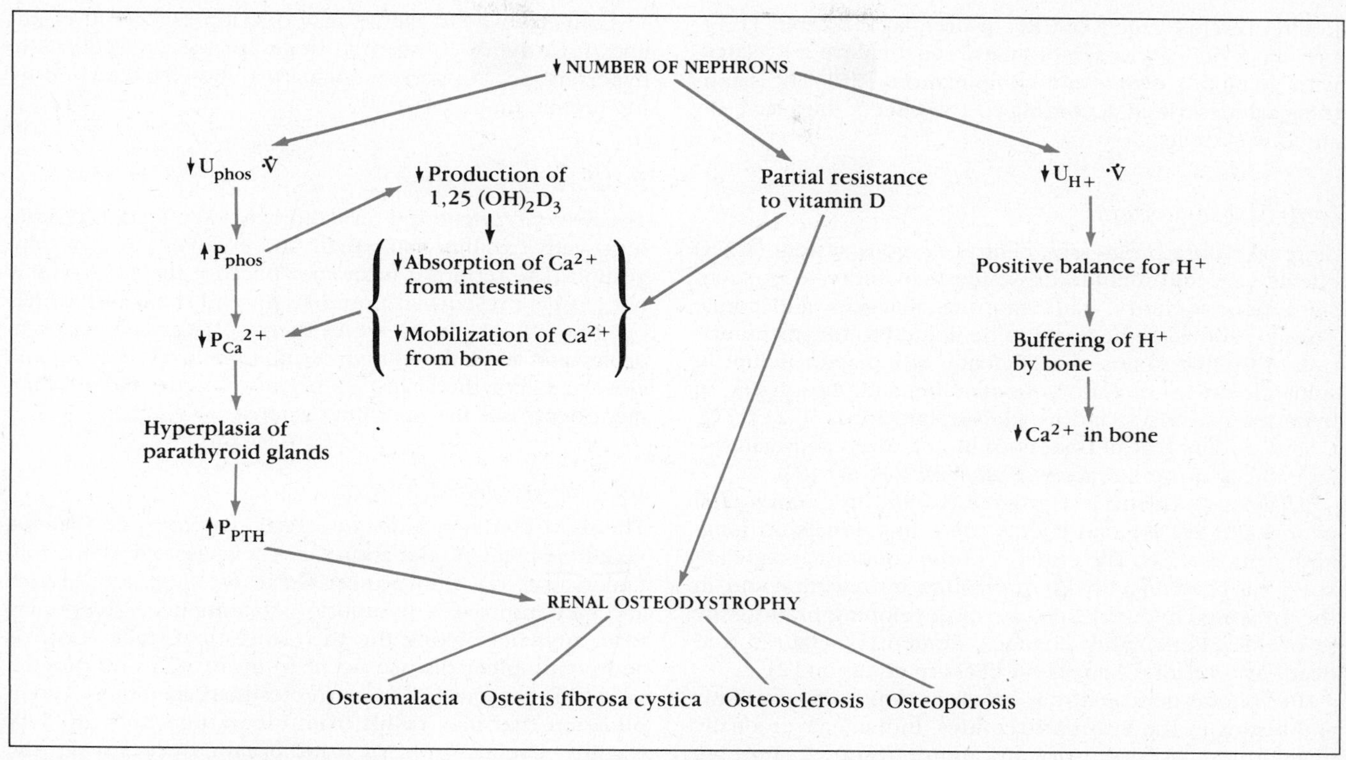

FIGURE 31-8 Possible pathways by which chronic renal failure leads to hyperparathyroidism and osteodystrophy. The various forms of defective bone formation may coexist in the same person. $U_{phos} \cdot \dot{V}$ = urinary excretion of phosphate; $U_h^+ \cdot \dot{V}$ = urinary excretion of hydrogen ions; P_{phos} = plasma concentration of phosphate; $P_{Ca}2^+$ = plasma concentration of calcium; P_{PTH} = plasma concentration of parathyroid hormone; $1,25\ (OH)_2D_3$ = 1,25-dihydroxyvitamin D_3. (From H. Valtin, *Renal Dysfunction*. Boston: Little, Brown, 1979.)

Urea and Creatinine Alterations. Urea is a byproduct of protein metabolism that accumulates as the uremic stage develops. The blood urea nitrogen level is not an adequate indicator of renal disease because it is elevated whenever the GFR decreases and with an increased protein intake. Serum creatinine is a better indicator of renal dysfunction because urinary excretion of creatinine equals the amount produced in the body. Therefore, the GFR can be calculated by changes in serum creatinine (Fig. 31-9). With normal renal function, an increase of serum creatinine from 1.0 to 2.0 mg per dl represents a fall of GFR from 120 to 60 ml per minute. With severe renal failure, plasma creatinine stabilizes at approximately 10 mg per dl [31].

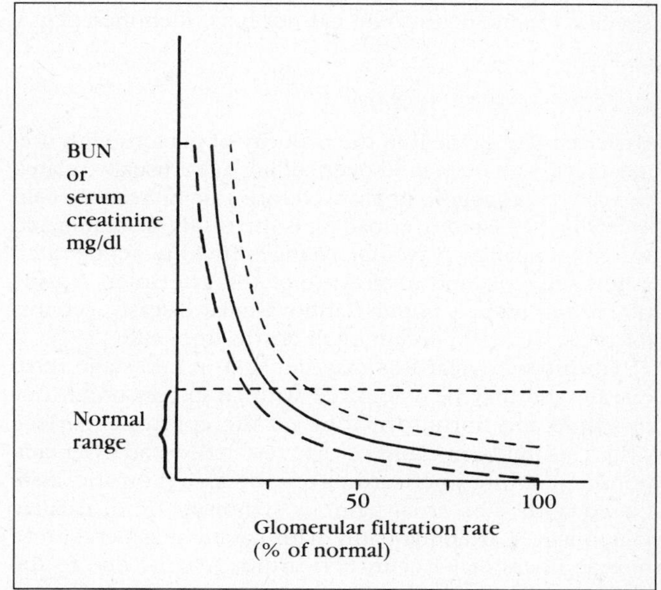

FIGURE 31-9 The relationship of blood urea nitrogen, or serum creatinine concentration, to glomerular filtration rate. The broken lines indicate that there is a family of curves rather than a single one for all persons. (From S. Papper, *Clinical Nephrology* [2nd ed.]. Boston: Little, Brown, 1978.)

Carbohydrate Intolerance. Carbohydrate intolerance can occur in persons with CRF and may be due to impaired degradation of insulin by diseased kidneys and decreased uptake of hepatic glucose. Hyperglycemia correlates with the extent of renal failure.

Uremic Syndrome

As renal failure progresses, it eventually becomes symptomatic and the steady state is not maintained. This condition represents stage 4 of CRF, or uremia (see Table 31-3). Uremia is defined as symptomatic renal failure associated with metabolic events and complications [25]. The symptoms are described according to the effects they have on all body systems.

Neurologic System

As renal failure progresses, central nervous system (CNS) effects vary and include drowsiness, inability to concentrate, poor memory, hallucinations, seizures, and coma. The alterations are believed to be related to the accumulation of uremic toxins, to deficiency of ionized calcium in spinal fluid with retention of potassium and phosphates, to hypertensive crises, and to altered fluid loads [6,21]. The CNS disorders that persist, both in untreated and dialyzed individuals, are called *uremic encephalopathy* [2].

Dialysis dementia is a progressive and frequently fatal neurologic disease that affects some individuals on long-term hemodialysis. The etiology of the condition is unclear but it has been linked with *aluminum* intoxication and, in the growing child, to exposure of developing brain tissue to uremia. Personality changes, dementia, seizures, and death may result. Changes on EEG are common [2].

Peripheral neuropathy is an early symptom of uremia and begins in the lower extremities. Individuals gradually develop a delayed sensory and motor response, burning sensations, and numbness in the feet and legs. Even in the absence of peripheral neuropathy, evidence of autonomic dysfunction, for example, hypotension or impotence, may be present [2]. Peripheral neuropathy may be generalized or in isolated areas, usually manifesting as symmetric and both motor and sensory. Restless leg syndrome or constant leg motion is present in 40 percent of cases. Complaints of crawling, prickling, and pruritus are common. A specific uremic neurotoxin has not been identified [2].

Cardiovascular System

Hypertension, present in the majority of persons with uremia may result from fluid overloading but is usually related to vascular changes (nephrosclerosis) or increased renin secretion [2]. Fluid overloading is the result of sodium and water imbalance. Vascular changes include accelerated atherosclerosis and narrowing of the arterioles. *Hyperreninemia* often is noted. Cardiovascular disease accounts for more than 50 percent of all deaths from CRF [25].

Fibrinous pericarditis may develop in end-stage renal disease and may be associated with an excess of pericardial fluid and fibrin formation on the epicardial surface [21]. This fluid can cause cardiac restriction and even tamponade. Fibrinous pericarditis may be asymptomatic, associated with substernal pain, or symptomatic of cardiac tamponade. Cardiomyopathy with patchy degeneration of muscle fibers may occur. Pericarditis may be due to the uremia and associated with elevated serum urea and creatinine levels. It also may result after dialysis, arising acutely with elevated temperature and pain. Persons who do not comply with routine dialysis therapy tend to have a high frequency of pericarditis [25].

Congestive heart failure may develop as a result of salt and fluid overloading together with the characteristic hypertension. Pulmonary edema may be characterized by the uremic lung.

Respiratory System

The *uremic lung* noted on radiologic examination characteristically exhibits "bat wings" and involves perihilar congestion. The term is a misnomer because the syndrome is not always present with uremia. An end-stage pattern has been noted, which resembles the respiratory distress syndrome and is related to high serum urea levels. Pneumonia also is a major threat in CRF because the uremic environment depresses the immune response.

Gastrointestinal System

The most common gastrointestinal symptoms are nausea, vomiting, hiccups, and anorexia. Their etiology is not well understood, but they are related to the degree of uremia and may improve if hydration is maintained. Ulcers may form anywhere along the gastrointestinal tract. Gastritis and peptic ulcer disease occur in up to 40 to 60 percent of uremic persons [26]. Gastrointestinal bleeding is a complication that may result from ulcerations and capillary fragility. Uremic fetor, or urine breath, occurs when the salivary urea is broken down to ammonia, causing an unpleasant metallic taste. The oral mucosa is often dry and the tongue is yellow-brown. Stomatitis is common, with buccal mucosa ulceration.

Musculoskeletal System

The effects of altered levels of calcium and phosphorus are illustrated in Figure 31-8. The resulting faulty bone metabolism, called renal osteodystrophy, is caused by a combination of hyperparathyroidism, calcium and phosphorus alterations, and decreased synthesis of the active form of vitamin D. Several resulting bone lesions include osteomalacia, osteitis fibrosa, soft tissue calcification, and osteosclerosis.

Hyperparathyroidism is a response to serum containing decreased ionized calcium. The causes of decreased calcium include phosphate retention, altered vitamin D metabolism, altered feedback with calcium and parathyroid hormone (PTH), and other factors. Phosphate retention is a consequence of decreased renal function and higher levels of PTH. Phosphaturia results at the expense of high PTH levels. Phosphate retention also leads to hypocalcemia and increased PTH levels. Calcium feedback is altered, and excessive levels of calcium are required to suppress PTH in uremic persons [10].

Osteomalacia is the result of poor tissue use of vitamin D that causes accumulation of osteoid material after calcification has ceased. *Osteitis fibrosa* occurs when fibrous tissue replaces bone tissue. It may result from secondary hyperparathyroidism. Soft tissue *metastatic calcification* is the deposition of calcium and phosphate crystals in the synovial tissues and soft tissues, especially the eyes, joints,

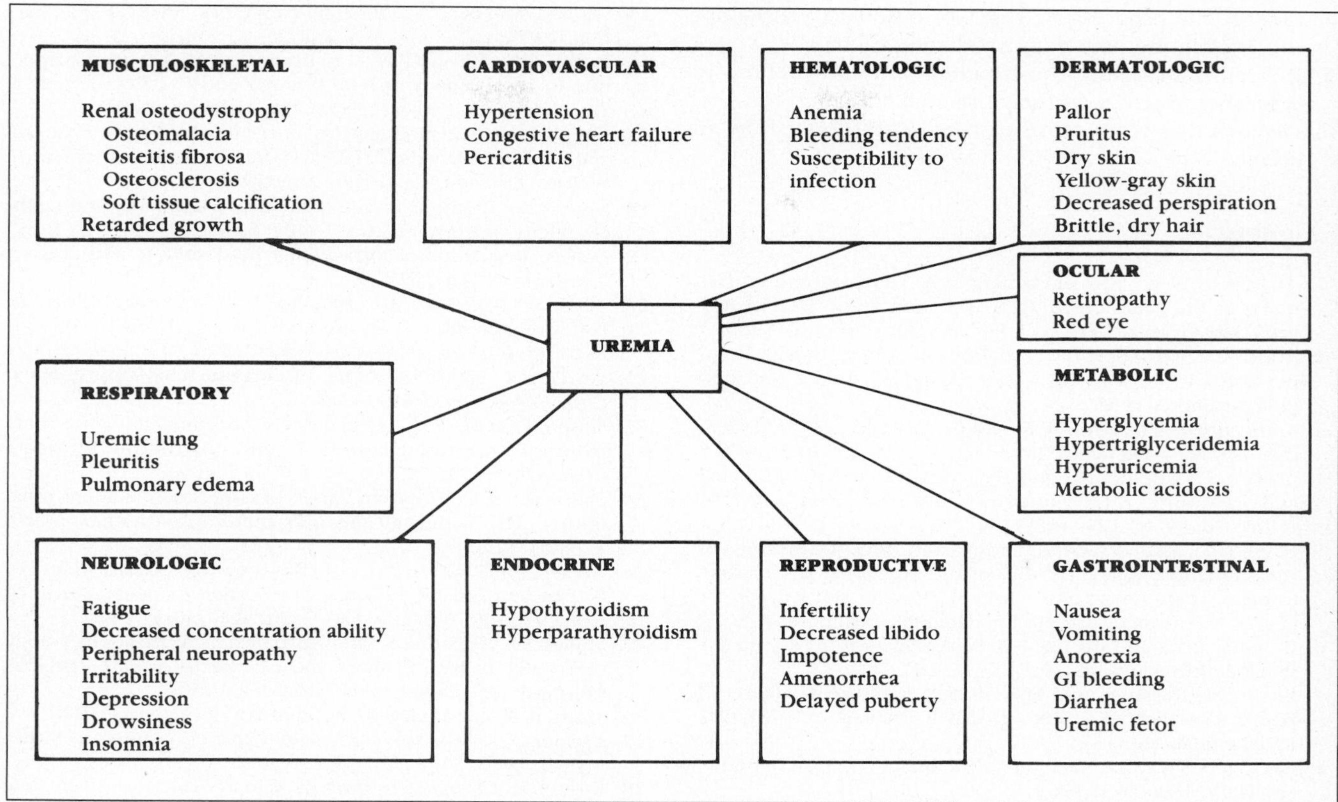

FIGURE 31-10 Systemic effects of uremia. (From S. Lewis, Pathophysiology of chronic renal failure. *Nurs. Clin. North Am.* 16:38, 1981.)

muscles, and lungs. *Osteosclerosis* is believed to be similar to soft tissue calcification and is due to bone redistribution and remodeling. This lesion causes enhanced bone density, mainly affecting the face, skull, and spine.

Renal osteodystrophy causes an enhanced tendency to spontaneous fractures. Many of the complications of this condition can be prevented by using phosphate-binding agents, administering activated vitamin D, and supplementing dietary calcium [24].

Hematologic Alterations

The hematologic effects of uremia include a normocytic, normochromic anemia, and altered hemostasis (see Chaps. 15 and 17). Anemia results from lack of erythropoietin response to hypoxia and obliteration of erythropoietin production sites. Hemolysis of red blood cells is common; it is related to a decreased survival time of erythrocytes in uremic plasma. Uremic plasma interferes with the ability of the erythrocyte membrane to pump sodium out, leading to swelling and hemolysis of red blood cells. Dialysis also may cause hemolysis by mechanical destruction or reaction to the dialysate [6]. Increased frequency of hepatitis is associated with the need for blood transfusions and dialysis therapy. Coagulation defects are caused by platelet defects and occur in most persons with uremia. Abnormal bleeding results, causing a wide range of problems, including epistaxis, purpura, and frank hemorrhage [29]. Depressed immune response leads to a high frequency of infection and inhibition of phagocytosis [1].

Dermatologic Alterations

Skin pallor results from anemia, and there is also a characteristic sallow, yellow pigmentation. Retention of pigmented urochromes results in their deposition in the subcutaneous fat. Dryness of the skin is caused by atrophy of the sweat glands and dehydration. Uremic itching or pruritus is possibly related to excess parathyroid hormone, skin deposits, or peripheral neuropathy [21]. Uremic frost may occur in advanced uremia when the urea deposits are excreted in sweat and crystallize. Soft tissue calcification results from secondary hyperparathyroidism, which leads to chalky plaques being deposited under the skin [25]. Other organ and system alterations also occur, as noted in Figure 31-10.

Study Questions

1. Compare the pathogenesis of nephrotoxic or ischemic acute tubular necrosis.
2. Describe the production of oliguria and anuria in acute renal failure.
3. Explain the significance of the stages of acute renal failure.

4. Identify the progressive stages of chronic renal failure and explain the pathology producing each.
5. Describe, in detail, the biochemical and metabolic imbalances seen in end-stage renal failure.
6. Discuss the production of renal osteodystrophy in uremia.

References

1. Anagnostou, A., and Kurtzman, M.A. Hematologic consequences of renal failure. In B.M. Brenner and F.C. Rector (eds.), *The Kidney* (3rd ed.). Philadelphia: Ardmore, 1986.
2. Arieff, A.I. Neurologic manifestations of uremia. In B.M. Brenner and F.C. Rector (eds.), *The Kidney* (3rd ed.). Philadelphia: Ardmore, 1986.
3. Arendshorst, W.I., Finn, W.F., and Gottschalk, C.W. Pathogenesis of acute renal failure in the rat. *Kidney Int.* 10:5, 1976.
4. Avasthi, P.S., Evan, A.P., and Hay, D. Glomerular endothelial cells in uranyl nitrate-induced acute renal failure in rats. *J. Clin. Invest.* 65:121, 1980.
5. Bastl, C.P., Rudnick, M.R., and Narino, D.G. Assessment of renal function: Characteristics of the functional and organic forms of acute renal failure. In B.M. Brenner and F.C. Rector (eds.), *The Kidney* (3rd ed.). Philadelphia: Ardmore, 1986.
6. Brenner, B.M., and Rector, F.C. (eds.). *The Kidney* (3rd ed.). Philadelphia: Ardmore, 1986.
7. Brezis, M., Rosen, S., and Epstein, F.H. Acute renal failure. In B.M. Brenner and F.C. Rector (eds.), *The Kidney* (3rd ed.). Philadelphia: Ardmore, 1986.
8. Bricker, N.S. On the meaning of the intact nephron hypothesis. *Am. J. Med.* 46:1, 1969.
9. Chapman, A. (ed.). *Acute Renal Failure*. London: Churchill Livingstone, 1980.
10. Coburn, J.W., and Slatopolsky, E. Vitamin D, Parathyroid hormone, and renal osteodystrophy. In B.M. Brenner and F.C. Rector (eds.), *The Kidney* (3rd ed.). Philadelphia: Ardmore, 1986.
11. Cronin, R.E., et al. Norepinephrine-induced acute renal failure. *Kidney Int.* 14:187, 1978.
12. Dibona, G.F., and Saivin, L.L. The renin-angiotensin system in acute renal failure in the rat. *Lab. Invest.* 25:528, 1971.
13. Donohoe, J.F., et al. Tubular leakage and obstruction in acute ischemic renal failure. *Kidney Int.* 13:208, 1978.
14. Dunnell, M.A. A review of the pathology and pathogenesis of acute renal failure due to acute tubular necrosis. *J. Clin. Pathol.* 27:2, 1974.
15. Forland, M. (ed.). *Nephrology*. New York: Medical Examination, 1977.
16. Harris, R.C., Meyer, T.W., and Brenner, B.M. Nephron adaptation to renal injury. In B.M. Brenner and F.C. Rector (eds.), *The Kidney* (3rd ed.). Philadelphia: Ardmore, 1986.
17. Knochel, J.P. The biochemistry of renal failure. In G. Eknoyan and J.P. Knochel (eds.), *The Systemic Consequences of Renal Failure*. Orlando, Fla.: Grune & Stratton, 1984.
18. Lane, A.Z., Wright, G.E., and Blair, D.C. Ototoxicity and nephrotoxicity of amikacin. *Am. J. Med.* 62:911, 1977.
19. Leaf, A. Regulation of intracellular fluid volume and disease. *Am. J. Med.* 49:291, 1970.
20. Levinsky, N.G., and Alexander, E.A. Acute renal failure. In B.M. Brenner and F.C. Rector (eds.), *Renal Failure: The Kidney* (vol. II). Philadelphia: Saunders, 1976.
21. Lewis, S.M. Pathophysiology of chronic renal failure. *Nurs. Clin. North Am.* 16:501, 1981.
22. Mason, J., et al. The early phase of experimental acute renal failure. I. Intratubular pressure and obstruction. *Pflugers Arch.* 370:155, 1977.
23. Mason, J., et al. The early phase of experimental acute renal failure. III. Tubuloglomerular feedback. *Pflugers Arch.* 373:69, 1978.
24. Massry, S.G. Disorders of divalent ion metabolism. In G. Eknoyan and J.P. Knochel, *The Systemic Consequences of Renal Failure*. Orlando, Fla.: Grune & Stratton, 1984.
25. Mujais, S.K., Sabatini, S., and Kurtzman, N.A. Pathophysiology of Uremia. In B.M. Brenner and F.C. Rector (eds.), *The Kidney* (3rd ed.). Philadelphia: Ardmore, 1986.
26. Muth, R. *Renal Medicine*. Springfield, Ill.: Thomas, 1978.
27. Papper, S. *Clinical Nephrology* (2nd ed.). Boston: Little, Brown, 1978.
28. Rose, B.D. *Clinical Physiology of Acid-Base and Electrolyte Disorders*. New York: McGraw-Hill, 1977.
29. Saxton, C.R., and Smith, J.W. The immune system and infections. In G. Eknoyan and J.P. Knochel (eds.), *The Systemic Consequences of Renal Failure*. Orlando, Fla.: Grune & Stratton, 1984.
30. Schrier, R.W. *Renal and Electrolyte Disorders* (3rd ed.). Boston: Little, Brown, 1986.
31. Semple, P.F., et al. Renin, angiotensin II and III in acute renal failure: Note on the measurement of angiotensin II and III in rat blood. *Kidney Int.* 10:5, 1976.
32. Shalhaub, R.J. The medical management of chronic renal failure. *Med. Times*. 107:23, 1979.
33. Solez, K. Acute renal failure. In R.H. Heptinstall, *Pathology of the Kidney* (3rd ed.). Boston: Little, Brown, 1983.
34. Valtin, H., *Renal Dysfunction*. Boston: Little, Brown, 1979.

Unit Bibliography

Andreucci, V.E. *Acute Renal Failure: Pathophysiology, Prevention and Treatment*. Boston: Kluwer, 1984.

Bartsch, W., et al. Hormone block levels and their interrelationships in normal men and men with benign prostatic hyperplasia (BPH). *Acta Endocrinol.* (Copenh.) 90:727, 1979.

Bennett, W.M., Singer, I., and Coggins, C.H. Guide to drug therapy in adult patients with impaired renal function. *JAMA* 223:991, 1974.

Bennington, J.L. Histopathology of renal adenocarcinoma. In G. Sufrin and S.A. Beckley (eds.), *Renal Adenocarcinoma* (report no. 10). Geneva: International Union Against Cancer, 1980. P. 61.

Blagg, C., and Scribner, B.H. Long-term dialysis: Current problems and future prospects. *Am. J. Med.* 68:633, 1980.

Blantz, R.C., and Konnen, K. The mechanism of acute renal failure after uranyl nitrate. *J. Clin. Invest.* 55:621, 1975.

Bordier, P., et al. On the pathogenesis of so-called idiopathic hypercalciuria. *Am. J. Med.* 63:398, 1977.

Brenner, B.M., and Lazarus, J.M. *Acute Renal Failure.* Philadelphia: Saunders, 1983.

Brenner, B.M., and Rector, F.C. (eds.). *The Kidney* (3rd ed.). Philadelphia: Ardmore, 1986.

Bricker, N.S. On the meaning of the intact nephron hypothesis. *Am. J. Med.* 46:1, 1969.

Brooks, D., and Mallick, N. *Renal Medicine and Urology.* Edinburgh, New York: Churchill Livingstone, 1982.

Chapman, A. (ed.). *Acute Renal Failure.* London: Churchill Livingstone, 1980.

Coe, F.L. Nephrolithiasis: Causes, classification and management. *Hosp. Pract.* 16:33, 1981.

Cranston, J.A. Benign enlargement of the prostate gland. *Nurs. Times* 74:789, 1978.

Cronin, R.E., et al. Norepinephrine-induced acute renal failure. *Kidney Int.* 14:187, 1978.

Cummings, N.B. Urolithiasis research: Progress and trends. *Adv. Exp. Med. Biol.* 128:473, 1980.

Dalgaard, O.Z., and Pedersen, K.J. Ultrastructure of the kidney in shock. In G. Ricket (ed.), *Proceedings of the First International Congress of Nephrology.* New York: Karger, 1961.

DeWardener, H.E. *The Kidney: An Outline of Normal and Abnormal Function* (5th ed.). Edinburgh: Churchill Livingstone, 1985.

Donohoe, J.F., et al. Tubular leakage and obstruction in acute ischemic renal failure. *Kidney Int.* 13:208, 1978.

Droller, M.J. Adenocarcinoma of the prostate: An overview. *Urol. Clin. North Am.* 7:578, 1980.

Droller, M.J. Renal cell carcinoma: An overview. *Urol. Clin. North Am.* 7:675, 1980.

Evans, D.B., and Henderson, R.G. *Lecture Notes on Nephrology.* Boston: Blackwell, 1985.

Fearing, M.O. Osteodystrophy in patients with chronic renal failure. *Nurs. Clin. North Am.* 10:461, 1975.

Fine, L.G. Acquired prostaglandin E_2 (medullin) deficiency as the cause of oliguria in acute tubular necrosis: A hypothesis. *Isr. J. Med. Sci.* 6:346, 1970.

Forland, M. *Nephrology.* New Hyde Park, N.Y.: Medical Examination, 1983.

Gabriel, R. *Postgraduate Nephrology* (3rd ed.). Boston: Butterworths, 1985.

Gonick, H.C., and Buckalew, V.M. *Renal Tubular Disorders: Pathophysiology, Diagnosis and Management.* New York: Dekker, 1985.

Hammond, G.L., et al. Serum steroids in normal males and patients with prostatic disease. *Clin. Endocrinol.* 9:113, 1978.

Hautmann, R., Lehmann, A., and Komor, S. Calcium and oxalate concentrations in human renal tissue: The key to the pathogenesis of stone formation? *J. Urol.* 123:317, 1980.

Heptinstall, R.H. Acute renal failure. In R.H. Heptinstall, *Pathology of the Kidney* (3rd ed.). Boston: Little, Brown, 1983.

Higgins, S.J., and Gehring, U. Molecular mechanisms of steroid hormone action. *Adv. Cancer Res.* 28:313, 1978.

Jacobi, H., Moore, R.J., and Wilson, J.D. Studies on the mechanism of 32-androstanediol-induced growth of the dog prostate. *Endocrinology* 102:1748, 1978.

Jensen, D. *The Principles of Physiology* (2nd ed.). New York: Appleton-Century-Crofts, 1980.

Karakousis, C.P., and Jennings, E. Renal cell carcinoma metastatic to skeletal muscle mass: A case report. *J. Surg. Oncol.* 17:287, 1981.

Kinne, R.K. *Renal Biochemistry Cells, Membranes, Molecules.* Amsterdam, N.Y.: Elsevier, 1985.

Kleeman, C.R., et al. Kidney stones: Inter-departmental clinic conference (UCLA School of Medicine). *West. J. Med.* 132:313, 1980.

Lane, A.Z., Wright, G.E., and Blair, D.C. Ototoxicity and nephrotoxicity of amikacin. *Am. J. Med.* 62:911, 1977.

Leaf, A., and Cotran, R. *Renal Pathophysiology* (2nd ed.). New York: Oxford University Press, 1985.

Lewis, S.M. Pathophysiology of chronic renal failure. *Nurs. Clin. North Am.* 16:501, 1981.

Ljunghall, S., and Hedstrand, H. Epidemiology of renal stones in a middle-age population. *Acta Med. Scand.* 197:439, 1975.

Olsen, S. Renal histopathology in various forms of acute anuria in man. *Kidney Int.* 10:5, 1976.

O'Rourke, R.A. *The Heart and Renal Disease.* New York: Churchill Livingstone, 1984.

Pak, C.Y.C., et al. The hypercalciurias: Causes, parathyroid function and diagnostic criteria. *J. Clin. Invest.* 54:387, 1974.

Pak, C.Y.C., et al. A simple test for the diagnosis of absorptive, resorptive and renal hypercalciurias. *N. Engl. J. Med.* 292:497, 1975.

Papper, S. *Clinical Nephrology* (2nd ed.). Boston: Little, Brown, 1978.

Papper, S. The oliguric patient. *Med. Times* 107:70, 1979.

Parks, J., Coe, F., and Favus, M. Hyperparathyroidism in nephrolithiasis. *Arch. Intern. Med.* 140:1479, 1980.

Pearse, H.D., and Houghton, D.C. Renal oncocytoma. *Urology* 13:74, 1979.

Revillard, J.P. Immunologic alterations in chronic renal insufficiency. *Adv. Nephrol.* 8:365, 1979.

Roberts, S.L. Renal assessment: A nursing point of view. *Heart Lung* 8:105, 1979.

Rodman, M., and Smith, D. *Pharmacology and Drug Therapy in Nursing* (2nd ed.). Philadelphia: Lippincott, 1984.

Rose, B.D. *Clinical Physiology of Acid-Base and Electrolyte Disorders* (2nd ed.). New York: McGraw-Hill, 1984.

Rosenow, E.C. Renal calculi: Study of papillary calcification. *J. Urol.* 44:19, 1940.

Seldin, D.W., and Giebisch, G. *The Kidney—Physiology and Pathophysiology.* New York: Raven, 1985.

Shalhaub, R.J. The medical management of chronic renal failure. *Med. Times* 107:23, 1979.

Solez, K., Morel-Maroger, L., and Sraer, J.D. The morphology of "acute tubular necrosis" ("ATN") in man. *Kidney Int.* 12:519, 1977.

Sorkin, M.I. Acute renal failure. *Med. Times* 107:33, 1979.

Stone, W.J., and Rabin, P.L. *End-stage Renal Disease.* New York: Academic, 1983.

Sufrin, G., and Murphy, G.P. Renal adenocarcinoma (review of article). *Urol. Surv.* 10:129, 1980.

Thurau, K., and Boylan, J.W. Acute renal success: The unexpected logic of oliguria in acute renal failure. *Am. J. Med.* 61:308, 1976.

Tichy, A., and Marchuk, J. Watch for this renal time bomb. *RN* 11:41, 1978.

Tobiason, S.J. Benign prostatic hypertrophy. *Am. J. Nurs.* 79:286, 1979.

Tortora, G.J., et al. *Principles of Human Physiology.* Hagerstown, Md.: Harper & Row, 1981.

Vander, A.J. *Renal Physiology* (3rd ed.). New York: McGraw-Hill, 1985.

Venkatachalam, M.A., et al. Ischemic damage and repair in the rat proximal tubule: Differences among the S_1, S_2 and S_3 segments. *Kidney Int.* 14:31, 1978.

Vermeulen, A., and DeSy, W. Androgens in patients with benign prostatic hyperplasia before and after prostatectomy. *J. Clin. Endocrinol. Metab.* 43:1250, 1976.

Walsh, P.C., and Wilson, J.D. The induction of prostatic hypertrophy in the dog with androstanediol. *J. Clin. Invest.* 57:1093, 1976.

Weller, J.M. (ed.). *Fundamentals of Nephrology.* Hagerstown, Md.: Harper & Row, 1979.

Whitmore, W.F. Benign prostatic hyperplasia: Widespread and sometimes worrisome. *Geriatrics* 36:119, 1981.

Wilson, J.D. The pathogenesis of benign prostatic hyperplasia. *Am. J. Med.* 68:745, 1980.

Yu, G.S.M., et al. Renal oncocytoma. *Cancer* 45:1010, 1980.

UNIT 11

Endocrine Regulation

Barbara L. Bullock / *Pituitary Function*

Camille P. Stern / *Adrenal, Thyroid, and Parathyroid Function*

Doris J. Heaman / *Pancreas Function*

The endocrine system is a complex system that coordinates and maintains the steady state through secretion of hormones. The secretion of hormones is generally activated by other hormones and/or neural influences and follows a closely regulated feedback mechanism. Chapter 32 describes pituitary function and explains how alterations can affect other body functions. Chapter 33 details the activity of the adrenal gland, its role in the stress response, and major alterations in function. Chapter 34 follows normal thyroid activity, with discussion of hyperthyroidism, hypothyroidism, and thyroid malignancy. Parathyroid function is also included in this chapter. Chapter 35 discusses the normal endocrine secretion activities of the pancreas (exocrine activities are discussed in Unit 12, Chap. 38). Diabetes mellitus, pancreatitis, carcinoma of the pancreas, and cystic fibrosis are the major pathologies presented in this chapter.

The reader is encouraged to use the learning objectives at the beginning of each chapter to organize the study of this unit. The study questions can be used to test understanding of the content. The unit bibliography is also helpful in providing direction for further study.

CHAPTER 32

Pituitary Regulation and Alterations in Function

CHAPTER OUTLINE

Hormones
Morphology of the Pituitary Gland
Gross Anatomy
Histology
Adenohypophysis
Neurohypophysis
Pars Intermedia

Relationship of the Pituitary to the Hypothalamus
Hypothalamic Secretion of Releasing and Release-Inhibiting Factors
Hypothalamic-Pituitary Neural and Circulatory Structure
Adenohypophysis
Neurohypophysis

Functions of the Anterior Pituitary
Anterior Pituitary Hormonal Function
Thyroid-Stimulating Hormone (Thyrotropin, TSH)
Adrenocorticotropic Hormone (Corticotropin, ACTH)
Follicle-Stimulating Hormone (FSH)
Luteinizing Hormone (LH)
Prolactin (Lactogenic Hormone, PRL)
Growth Hormone (Somatotropin, GH)
Circadian Patterns of Anterior Pituitary Secretions

Functions of the Neurohypophysis
Physiologic Action of Antidiuretic Hormone
Regulation of ADH by the Hypothalamus
Other Factors Regulating ADH Secretion and Release
Oxytocin
Effects on the Uterus
Effects on Lactation
Effects on Fertilization

Introduction to Pituitary Pathology
Pathology of the Anterior Pituitary
Enlargement of the Sella Turcica
Empty Sella Syndrome
Hypopituitarism (Panhypopituitarism)
Deficiency of Single Anterior Pituitary Hormones
Prolactin Deficiency
Gonadotropin Deficiency
Thyrotropin Deficiency
ACTH Deficiency
Growth Hormone Deficiency
Sheehan's Syndrome (Postpartum Pituitary Necrosis)
Hyperpituitarism
Hyperprolactinemia
Hypersecretion of ACTH
Hypersecretion of Growth Hormone (Gigantism, Acromegaly)

Pathology of the Posterior Pituitary
Antidiuretic Hormone Deficiency
Inappropriate ADH Secretion

Tumors of the Pituitary
Adenomas
Malignant Tumors
Primary Lesions
Secondary Lesions

LEARNING OBJECTIVES

1. Describe the basic structure and function of hormones.
2. Indicate the normal structure and location of the pituitary gland.
3. Differentiate the structure and function of the adenohypophysis and the neurohypophysis.
4. Identify the area called the pars intermedia.
5. List and describe the functions of the hormones of the adenohypophysis.
6. Describe the functions of the two hormones of the neurohypophysis.
7. Draw the feedback method of control between the hypothalamus and pituitary.
8. Outline briefly the vascular supply to the pituitary and hypothalamus.
9. List at least four known factors or hormones released by the hypothalamus.
10. Differentiate clearly between specific pituitary hormones and secretions of the target gland.
11. List and describe the effects of growth hormone (GH).
12. Describe the physiologic effects of antidiuretic hormone (ADH).
13. Explain the different factors that cause the release of ADH.
14. Describe briefly the effects of oxytocin on uterine contractility and lactation.
15. Explain the mechanical and hormonal effects of pituitary malfunction.
16. Describe briefly conditions that cause enlargement of the sella turcica and their effects.
17. List some causes of deficiency conditions of the anterior pituitary.
18. Define *panhypopituitarism*.
19. Describe the results of deficiencies in single pituitary hormones.
20. Explain how deficiencies in single pituitary hormones affect the metabolism of the entire organism.
21. Describe Sheehan's syndrome.
22. Describe the results of hypersecretion of single pituitary hormones.
23. Differentiate between gigantism and acromegaly.
24. Define and explain *ADH deficiency* (diabetes insipidus).
25. Explain clearly the syndrome of inappropriate ADH secretion (SIADH).
26. List at least six etiologic factors of SIADH.
27. Relate pituitary tumors to hyperpituitarism and hypopituitarism.
28. List at least three clinical manifestations of pituitary tumors.

The human organism contains complex systems of communication that coordinate and maintain a steady state essential to its functions. Through these systems the body monitors the activities and needs of each of its parts and responds accordingly to maintain normalcy.

Although the nervous system is the dominant controlling influence, secondary mechanisms exist by which one cell can influence the function of other distant cells. The influence is effected through the secretion or inhibition of a variety of elements into the bloodstream. These elements are referred to as hormones, from the Greek root *ormaino*, which means "to excite, arouse, set in motion."

Endocrine cells are so called because they *secrete hormones into the bloodstream*. They may be organized into functional units, as in glands, or may be more diffusely dispersed throughout the tissues. Collectively, these cells and glands make up the endocrine system. They each have specific functions and coordinate with other cells to create an environment conducive to survival of the total organism. Figure 32-1 shows the anatomy and location of the endocrine glands.

Secretion of a given hormone is generally activated by hormonal and/or neural influences on specific target cells by feedback mechanisms. Secreted hormones act selectively on other specific target cells to regulate and maintain normal function. This chapter describes the characteristics of hormones to clarify their effects on target cells. The major focus is on the pituitary gland; its anatomic structure and physiologic function, its role within the complex communication system for maintaining a steady state, its relationship to the overall endocrine system, and pathologic manifestations of functional imbalance.

Hormones

Hormones are chemical substances that exert a physiologic effect on other cells. The capacity to synthesize these substances is not limited to endocrine organs but may be a characteristic of peripheral tissues or even of precursors in the bloodstream. Hormones are classified as local when they affect cells in their immediate vicinity. Local hormones include those of the neurosynapses, such as acetylcholine and the gastrointestinal hormones. General hormones are secretions of the endocrine glands and are carried by the bloodstream to target organs where they exert their effects.

Hormones are also classified according to chemical structure. The basic types are steroids, derivatives of tyrosine (amines), and protein based hormones.

Steroid hormones are derived from a basic precursor, cholesterol. Steroids are lipids and can move through the cell membranes of target tissues to exert their action by affecting the cytoplasm or nucleus. Steroids enter the

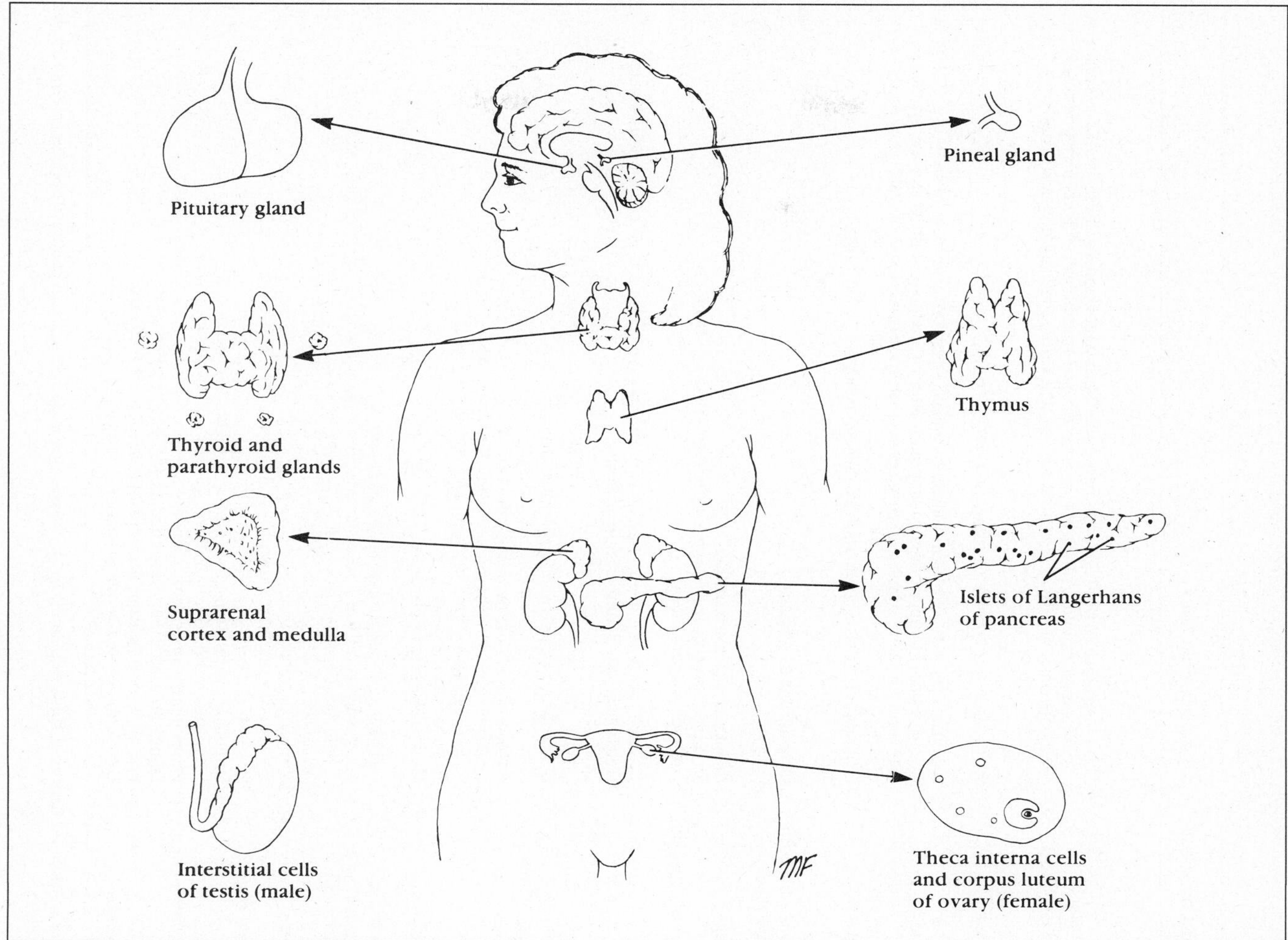

Figure 32-1 Location of the endocrine glands.

cell, bind with a cytoplasmic receptor, and then enter the nucleus to form messenger RNA. This promotes translation at the ribosomes to form new proteins [5].

The amines, or derivatives of the amino acid tyrosine, enter the cell through specific cell membrane receptors and combine with a nuclear receptor. They synthesize proteins, and include the thyroid hormones, and epinephrine and norepinephrine [10].

The proteins, or peptides, are classified according to whether they have long or short chains. The short chains are peptides while the more complex long chains are proteins. Peptide linkage is a major way by which amino acids are joined to form proteins. The average protein has about 400 amino acids [5]. Most protein hormones bind directly with nuclear DNA.

Table 32-1 lists the major endocrine hormones as to type, target tissue, and action. The actions of hormones are highly selective due to binding of specific receptor sites in target tissue. Some, such as epinephrine and glucagon, act on cell membrane receptors, while the lipid-soluble steroids act on intracellular nuclear and cytoplasmic receptors.

All hormone secretion is controlled by an internal system that usually involves negative feedback. Figure 32-2 shows negative feedback in action using hypothalamic control. The regulating factor is apparently the amount of hormone in the blood. If the target organ does not release enough hormone, the controlling gland secretes more until the proper blood level is achieved [5].

Morphology of the Pituitary Gland

Gross Anatomy

The human adult pituitary is approximately 1 cm long, 1.0 to 1.5 cm wide, and 0.5 cm thick. It is round or ovoid and weighs about 0.5 gm. Because of its position beneath the hypothalamus of the diencephalon, it is also called the *hypophysis*, taken from the Greek roots *ypo*, meaning "under," and *phyo*, meaning "to grow." The gland rests in a small depression (hypophyseal fossa) of the sphenoid bone called the *sella turcica*. It is covered by a tough membrane, diaphragma sellae, through which passes the

TABLE 32-1 General Endocrine Glands and Their Hormones

Gland	Hormone (Synonyms)	Target Organ or Tissue	Principal Functions
Pituitary (hypophysis cerebri)			
Adenohypophysis	Somatotropin (growth hormone, somatotropic hormone)	General	Accelerates rate of body growth, particularly growth of bone and muscle. Exerts anabolic effect upon calcium, phosphorus, and nitrogen metabolism. Affects metabolism of carbohydrate and lipid. Elevates skeletal and cardiac muscle glycogen content.
	Thyrotropin (thyrotropic hormone, thyroid-stimulating hormone)	Thyroid	Synthesis and secretion of thyroid hormones.
	Corticotropin (adrenocorticotropin, adrenocorticotropic hormone)	Adrenal cortex	Synthesis and secretion of adrenal cortical steroids.
	Follicle-stimulating hormone	Ovaries, testes	Stimulates growth of ovarian follicle in female, spermatogenesis in male.
	Luteinizing hormone (interstitial cell-stimulating hormone)	Ovaries, testes	Stimulates development of corpus luteum after ovulation and progesterone synthesis therein. In male, stimulates development of interstitial tissue of testes and secretion of androgen.
	Prolactin (luteotropic hormone, luteotropin lactogenic hormone, mammotropin)	Mammary glands	Proliferation of tissue, initiation of milk secretion.
Pars intermedia	α-melanocyte-stimulating hormone and β-melanocyte-stimulating hormone (intermedin)	Expand melanophores in lower vertebrates	Insignificant in humans.
Neurohypophysis	Antidiuretic hormone (vasopressin)	Renal tubules	Facilitates water absorption.
		Arterioles	Produces vasoconstriction, hence exerts a pressor effect.
	Oxytocin	Smooth muscle, especially of uterus	Contraction, parturition.
Thyroid	Thyroxine (T_4)	General	T_3 and T_4 accelerate the metabolic rate and oxygen consumption of all bodily tissues.
	Triidothyronine (T_3)	General	Metabolism of calcium and phosphorus.
	Thyrocalcitonin (same as parathyroid calcitonin)	Skeleton	
Parathyroid	Parathormone	Skeleton, kidneys, gastrointestinal tract	Metabolism of calcium and phosphorus.
	Calcitonin	Skeleton	Metabolism of calcium and phosphorus.
Endocrine pancreas	Insulin	General	Regulates carbohydrate metabolism, stimulates protein synthesis.
	Glucagon, pancreatic	Liver	Stimulates hepatic gluconeogenesis, glucogenolysis.
		Adipose tissue	Stimulates lipogenesis.
Adrenal cortex	Adrenal cortical steroids (e.g., cortisol)	General	Metabolism of carbohydrate.
	Aldosterone	Renal tubules	Metabolism of electrolytes and water.
Adrenal medulla	Epinephrine	Heart muscle, smooth muscle, arterioles	Accelerates heart rate; causes arteriolar vasoconstriction, hence pressor response; stimulates contraction of most smooth muscle.
		Liver, skeletal muscle	Stimulates glycogenolysis.
		Adipose tissue	Stimulates lipolysis.
	Norepinephrine	Arterioles	Causes arteriolar vasoconstriction, hence pressor response.
Testes	Testosterone	Accessory sex organs	Stimulates normal growth, development, and functions.
		General	Stimulates maturation of secondary sex characteristics.
Ovaries	Estrone, estradiol	Accessory sex organs	Stimulates normal growth, development, and cyclic functions.
		Mammary glands	Development of system of ducts.
		General	Stimulates maturation of secondary sex characteristics.
	Progesterone (from corpus luteum)	Uterus	Prepares endometrium for implantation of fertilized ovum.
		Mammary glands	Development of alveolar system.

Source: Adapted from D. Jensen, *The Principles of Physiology* (2nd ed.). New York: Appleton-Century-Crofts. Reprinted by permission of Appleton & Lange, Simon & Schuster Professional Information Group, 25 Van Zant St., E. Norwalk, CT 06855.

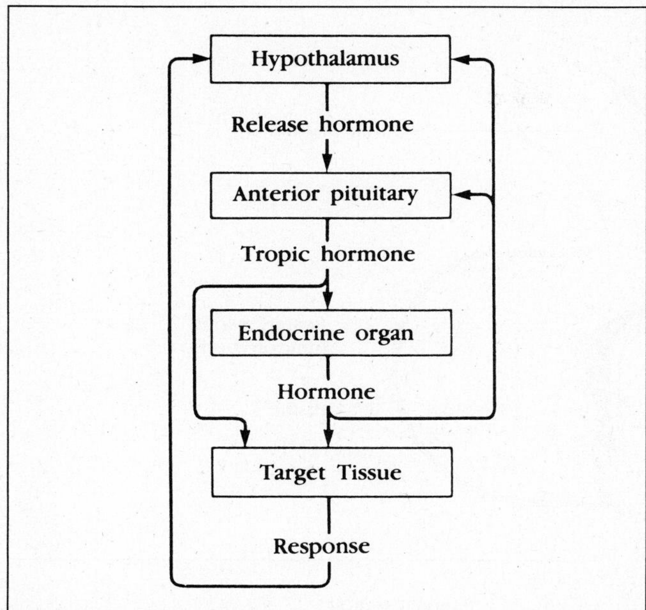

FIGURE 32-2 Possible mechanism of a negative feedback system for maintaining hormone balance. (See text for explanation.)

structure joining the pituitary to the hypothalamus, the hypophyseothalamic stalk. This structure is also called the infundibular stalk. Because disorders of the hypothalamus are often expressed as those of pituitary secretion, one must appreciate the functional and anatomic relationship of the hypothalamus to the pituitary gland [2].

Anatomically and physiologically, the pituitary can be divided into regions that function as distinct and different endocrine organs. The anterior lobe is called the *adenohypophysis*, and is subdivided into two regions: (1) the pars tuberalis, made up of a small mass of tissue running up along the infundibulum and surrounding the stalk; and (2) the pars distalis, which forms the bulk of the anterior lobe. The posterior lobe is called the *neurohypophysis* and includes three regions: (1) neural lobe, (2) infundibular stalk, and (3) median eminence of the tuber cinereum, which forms the attachment with the hypothalamus (Fig. 32-3). The intermediate lobe (pars intermedia) lies between the anterior and posterior lobes and is often considered separate and distinct. Because it is poorly developed in the adult human, its function is questionable. The only known secretion of the intermediate lobe is melanocyte-stimulating hormone (MSH), which is synthesized from a large prohormone that is also a precursor of corticotropin [7]. These hormones do not seem to be of major importance in skin pigmentation in humans.

The pituitary develops from a common germ layer, the ectoderm, but originates from two distinctly different embryologic anatomic sources. The adenohypophysis derives from an upward diverticulum of the ectodermal layer of the roof of the mouth or pharyngeal epithelium known as Rathke's pouch. The neurohypophysis originates as a downward ectodermal diverticulum from the hypothalamic portion of the diencephalon. These two lobes come together to form the hypophysis. Whereas Rathke's pouch loses its connection with the pharyngeal membrane, the neurohypophysis retains neural tract connections with the hypothalamus. These neural fiber connections are crucial in the secretory functions of the neurohypophysis.

The functioning pituitary remains connected to the hypothalamus through the neural tracts of the infundibular stalk and by an elaborate vascular system. These neural and vascular pathways are essential to the function of the pituitary, which is the bridging of the nervous system with the endocrine system [7].

Histology

Adenohypophysis. Traditionally, anterior pituitary cells were classified on the basis of their staining properties. Many of these cells contain secretory granules but some are sparsely granulated or considered to be agranular. This classification has been largely replaced by the development of assays to measure the levels of hormones in the blood. Radioimmunoassays are highly successful in measuring the levels of specific hormones. The ideal test, however, is probably the demonstration of hormone action on target tissues [10].

The following are the recognized anterior pituitary cell types [4]:

1. Somatotropes were originally called acidophilic cells and secrete growth hormone (GH).
2. Lactotropes or mammotropes are also acidophilic and secrete prolactin (PRL).
3. Thyrotropes are basophilic-staining cells that secrete thyroid-stimulating hormone (TSH).
4. Gonadotropes are basophilic-staining cells associated with the lactotropes and secrete luteinizing hormone (LH) and follicle-stimulating hormone (FSH).
5. Corticotropes may exhibit basophilic characteristic or be relatively agranular (chromophobic); they secrete adrenocorticotropic hormone (ACTH).
6. Other cell types include 15 to 20 percent of the anterior pituitary cells, which are either nonsecretory or primitive and whose function is unknown.

Table 32-2 summarizes these cell types with respect to hormones secreted.

The foregoing discussion represents an attempt to simplify cellular-hormonal relationships; however, it is recognized that, in actual fact, no simple one-to-one interaction exists. A review of Table 32-2 shows that in at least two instances, two hormones are secreted by the same type of cell. In other instances, secretion of a given hormone may be stimulated by many factors. Stress, for example, has been shown to increase the secretion of ACTH and TSH.

Neurohypophysis. The neurohypophysis contains neuroglial cells and cells known as *pituicytes*. The pituicytes serve no endocrine function but act as supporting structures for the terminal nerve fibers and tracts of the hypothalamus. The bulk of the posterior lobe consists of

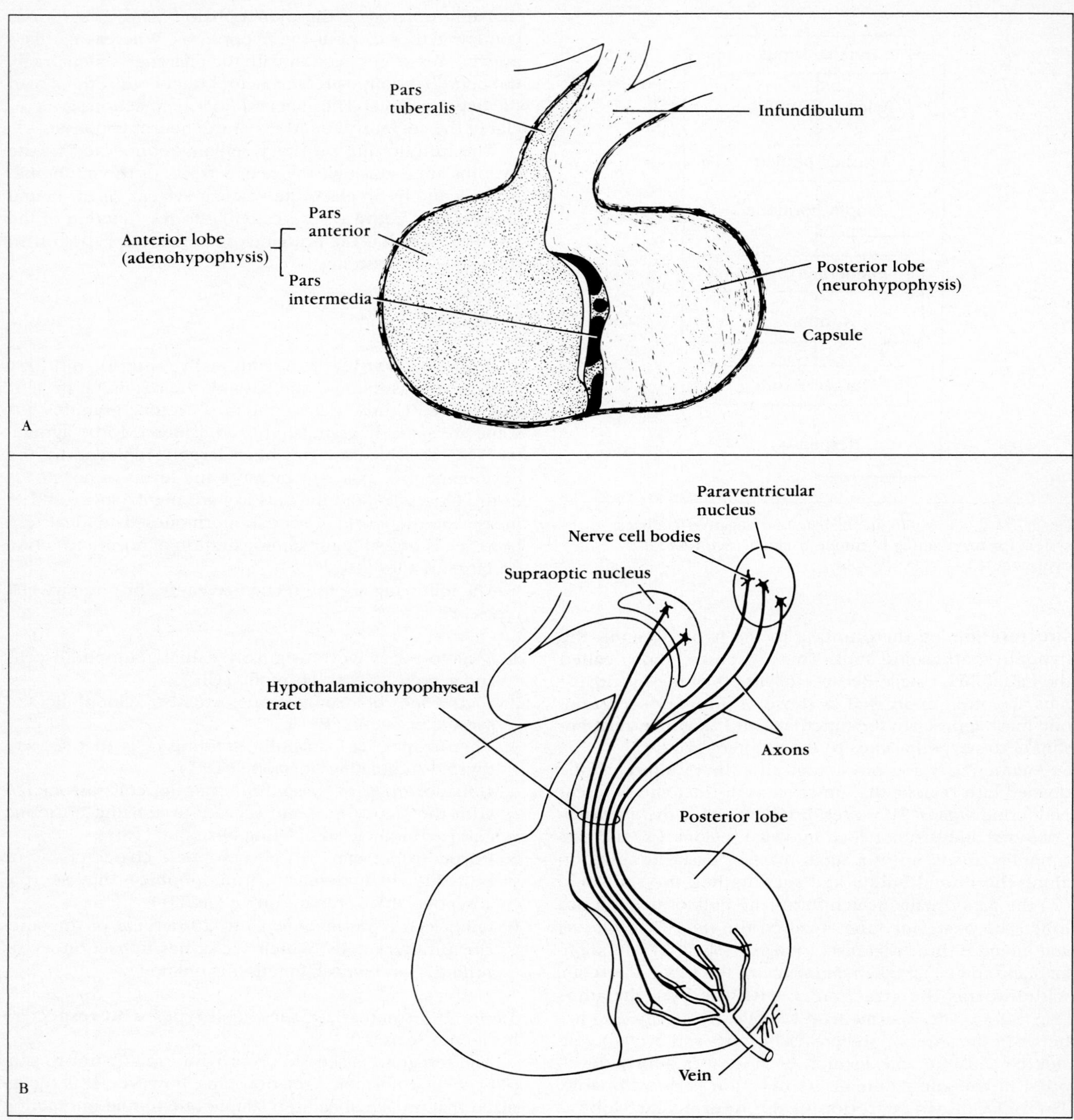

FIGURE 32-3 A. Divisions of the hypophysis. B. The hypothalamohypophyseal tract. C. Diagram showing the target organs of pituitary hormones.

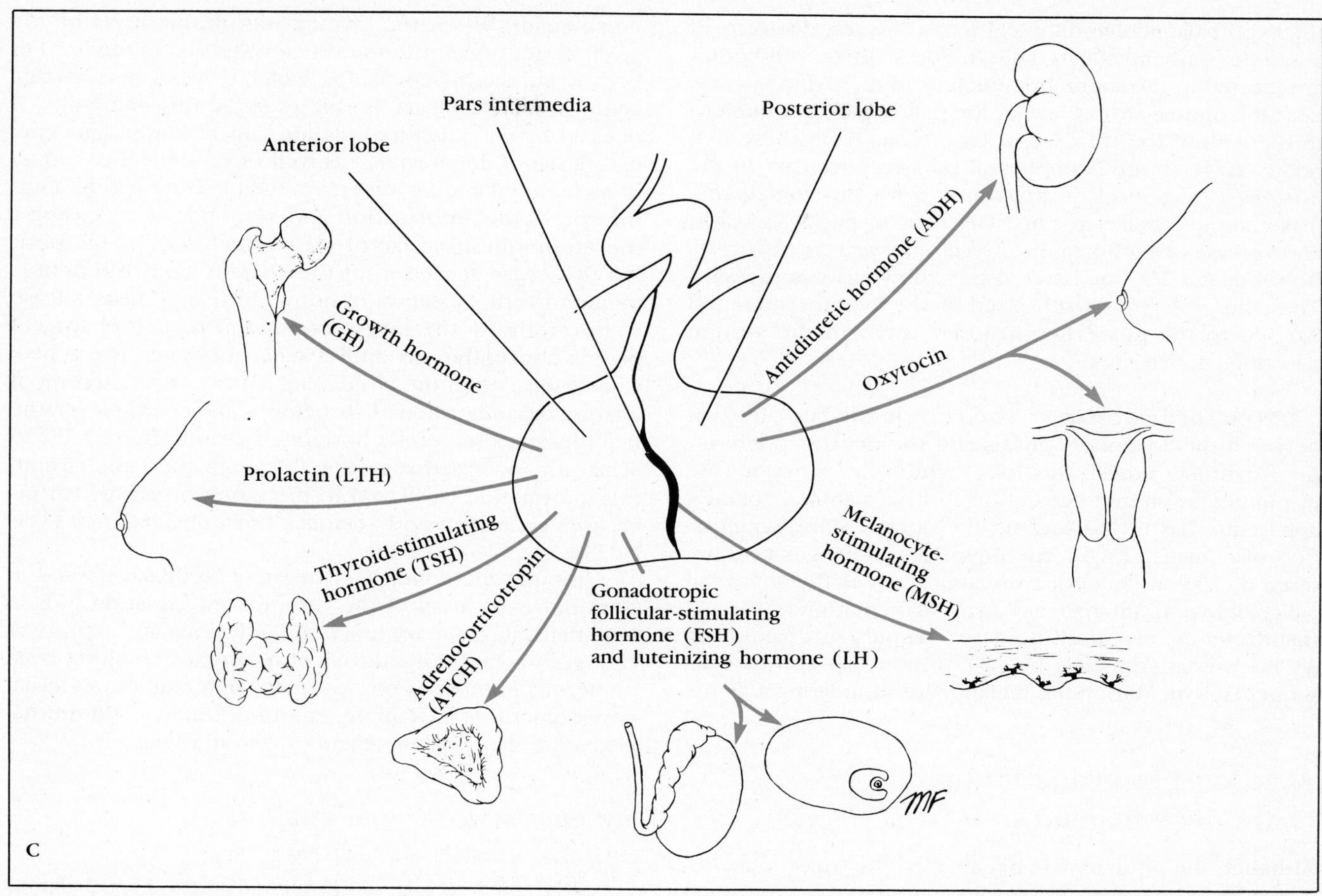

FIGURE 32-3 (continued)

TABLE 32-2 Anterior Pituitary Cell Types

Hormone	Cell Type	Target Organ	Function
Somatotropic hormone, growth hormone	Somatotrope Acidophil	All tissues	Increases rate of protein synthesis in all cells; decreases rate of carbohydrate use throughout body; increases mobilization of fats and use of fats for energy.
Adrenocorticotropic hormone	Corticotrope Basophil, large chromophobe	Adrenal cortex	Regulates secretion of cortisol and corticosteroids; enhances production of adrenal androgens.
Prolactin	Lactotrope Acidophil	Breasts	Produces lactation; stimulates development of alveolar secretory system.
Thyroid-stimulating hormone	Thyrotrope Basophil	Thyroid	Increases all known activities of thyroid glandular cells.
Gonadotropic hormones: follicle-stimulating hormone, luteinizing hormone	Gonadotrope Basophil	Follicles of ovaries, interstitial cells of Leydig in testes, seminiferous tubules of testes	Regulates spermatogenesis; regulates maturation of ovarian follicle and ovulation production of testosterone.

the hypothalamicohypophyseal tract. This tract consists of a bundle of nonmyelinated nerve fibers whose cell bodies are located in the supraoptic nucleus of the hypothalamus near the optic chiasma, and in the paraventricular nucleus in the wall of the third ventricle. Axons from these cell bodies traverse the hypophyseal stalk to terminate in the posterior lobe in close proximity with the vessels that make up the capillary plexus. The neurohypophysis stores and releases two hormones, *oxytocin* and *antidiuretic hormone (ADH)* (the latter also is known as vasopressin). These hormones are synthesized by the hypothalamus and carried to the posterior pituitary through the system described above.

Pars Intermedia. The intermediate lobe lies between the adenohypophysis and the neurohypophysis. As previously noted, this lobe, which has a major role in pigmentation and coloration in lower animal species, apparently has little effect on the normal skin pigmentation of humans [2,3,4]. The pigmentary changes encountered in several endocrine diseases, such as the abnormal pallor of hypopituitarism and hypopigmentation of adrenal insufficiency, are attributed to changes in circulating ACTH. Because ACTH has a common 13-amino acid sequence with MSH, it has melanocyte-stimulating activity.

Relationship of the Pituitary to the Hypothalamus

Although the pituitary has been called the "master gland," it is now known that most of its functions are controlled by the hypothalamus. Secretion of pituitary hormones is activated by signals from the hypothalamus through a complex humoral and neural communication system.

Hypothalamic Secretion of Releasing and Release-Inhibiting Factors

Through feedback and other mechanisms of communication, specialized neurons in the hypothalamus are stimulated to synthesize and secrete substances called releasing and release-inhibiting factors. The function of these factors is to regulate the secretion of pituitary hormones, which, in turn, control the secretion of hormones by target glands of the pituitary; for example, the thyroid, adrenals, and gonads.

The hypothalamus has the capacity to secrete a corresponding releasing factor for each anterior pituitary hormone. For some pituitary hormones, it also secretes a corresponding release-inhibiting factor. For all hormones except prolactin, the releasing factor is of most importance in regulation. For prolactin, however, the inhibiting factor is thought to exercise the most control. Both the releasing and release-inhibiting factors may control the release of GH.

An inverse relationship exists between the blood levels of hormones of the target organs and synthesis and secretion of the related pituitary hormones. Control of secretion through negative feedback occurs by the following mechanism. When the circulating plasma level of any given target organ hormone is elevated above the level of body need, the hypothalamus, which serves as a collecting center for information, is able to sense this imbalance. It does so by encoding information concerning plasma concentration of the hormone as well as various other stimuli in its humoral and neural environment. The hypothalamus interprets this information and responds by releasing a secretion-inhibiting factor (IF), which signals the pituitary to cease secretion of the specific controlling hormone. In turn, cessation of hormone release halts release of hormone by the target organ and therefore lowers plasma concentrations until a state of balance is reached. Conversely, when the circulating plasma concentration of a target organ hormone falls below some critical level, the hypothalamus secretes a hormone-releasing factor (RF) to signal for increased secretion. Through the same circuit, this information is relayed to the target organ, which increases secretion and restores hormone balance (see Fig. 32-2).

Although the concept of negative feedback is valid, it does not explain all of the complex interrelationships of hypothalamic-pituitary functioning. It does not explain all changes in the plasma levels of hormones resulting from numerous influences on the body's internal and external environment. For example, emotion, trauma, and diurnal changes create hormonal and other variations.

Hypothalamic-Pituitary Neural and Circulatory Structures

To understand clearly the influence of the hypothalamus on the pituitary, it is necessary to understand the neural and circulatory structure essential to their interrelationship. It will be remembered from previous discussion that each lobe of the pituitary functions as a distinct and different endocrine gland. Therefore, the structural relationship of each with the hypothalamus is different. The modes of transmission of signals from the hypothalamus are through neural connections for the neurohypophysis and through a complex vascular portal system for the adenohypophysis.

Adenohypophysis. The adenohypophysis secretes or fails to secrete its hormones into the circulation as a result of signals from the hypothalamus that arrive by the hypothalamicohypophyseal portal system. This communication system uses two capillary plexuses organized in series within the structures. Branches of the internal carotid and posterior communicating arteries of the circle of Willis give origin to the superior hypophyseal arteries. These arteries immediately branch to form a network of fenestrated capillaries called the *primary plexus*, located on the ventral side of the hypothalamus (Fig. 32-4). Some capillary loops also penetrate into the median eminence and serve the dual functions of supplying nerve cells around the base of the hypothalamus and of receiving regulating factors secreted by hypothalamic cells.

The primary plexus drains into the sinusoidal hypophyseal portal vessels that carry blood down the infundibular stalk to the anterior pituitary. After reaching the adenohy-

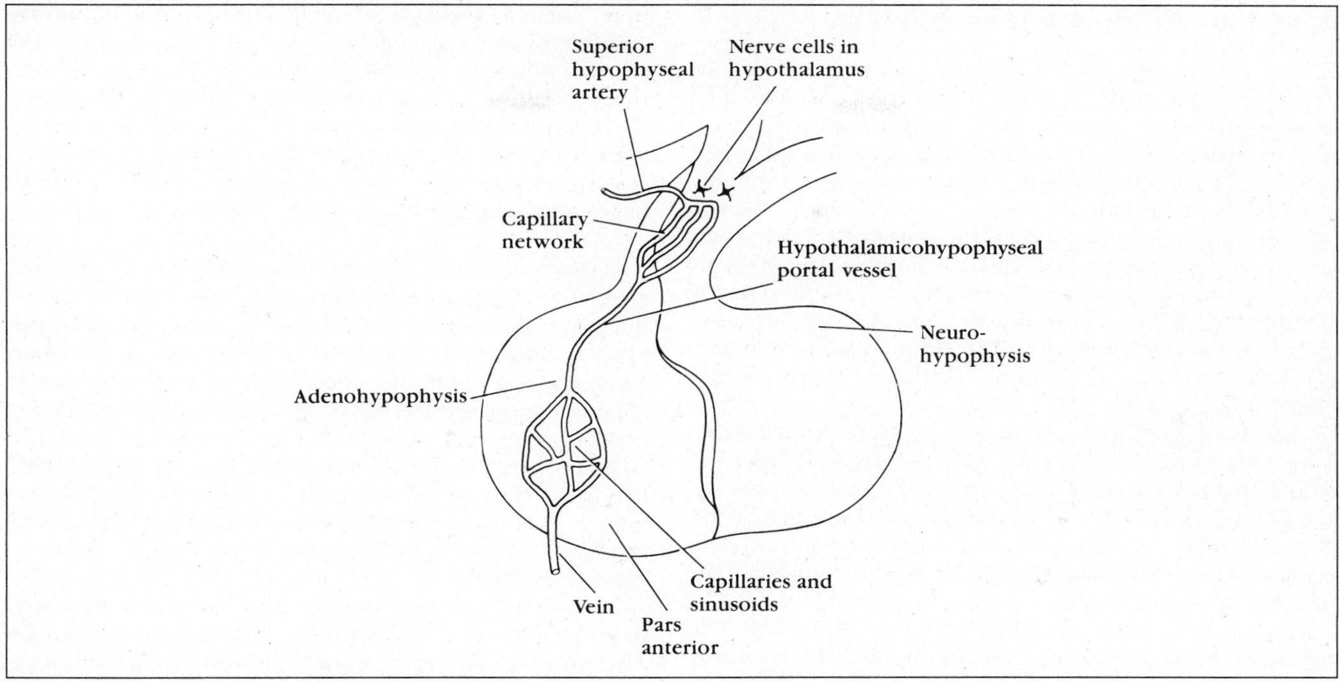

FIGURE 32-4 The hypothalamicohypophyseal portal system.

pophysis, the vessels again form a capillary network called the *secondary plexus*. These vessels maintain the cells of the anterior pituitary and deliver the regulatory factors from the hypothalamus to each cell. Vessels of the secondary plexus drain into the anterior hypophyseal veins. From here, hormones are ultimately transported to their target glands. The system begins and ends in capillaries and is called the *hypothalamicohypophyseal portal system* [5].

Anterior pituitary function is achieved through neural as well as vascular communication. The anterior pituitary, however, is poorly supplied with neural tracts from the hypothalamus. It has no secretomotor nerve fibers and only sparse vasomotor fibers.

The following is a summation of the probable mechanism through which neural transmissions take place. The unusual vascular system of the pituitary facilitates transmission of signals from the central nervous system (CNS) to the adenohypophysis. As discussed previously, before reaching secretory cells of the gland, arterial blood passes through the primary plexus, which extends into the median eminence. Significant numbers of nerve fibers terminate in the vicinity of these capillaries. These nerve fibers release neurosecretory products that are carried through the capillary sinusoids of the anterior lobe through hypophyseal portal vessels to effect release of anterior pituitary hormones [5].

Neural signals may arise from external stimuli such as heat or cold or from internal stimuli such as emotion. Other neural stimuli that exert an influence but are as yet poorly understood include sleep-related and diurnal or circadian rhythms.

Another unique feature of the pituitary gland is that the blood-brain barrier is incomplete in the area where the major plexus of the portal system originates. Endothelial fenestrations provide access for hormone molecules to the hypothalamus and pituitary. This allows for the feedback regulation of pituitary function described on page 483 [2].

Neurohypophysis. The neurohypophysis, unlike the adenohypophysis, contains no cells with secretory granules. It will be remembered that embryologically, the posterior pituitary arises essentially as an invagination from the hypothalamus and retains neural tract connections from this area.

Cell bodies located in the supraoptic nucleus of the hypothalamus synthesize antidiuretic hormone (ADH). Synthesis of oxytocin, the second hormone secreted by the posterior lobe, takes place in the paraventricular nucleus [5].

The neurosecretory process occurs in the following sequence. Hormone biosynthesis takes place within the cell bodies of the supraoptic or paraventricular regions of the hypothalamus in the form of hormonally inactive precursors. The active hormone is thought to be cleaved from the precursors during the one to two hours in which they are transported down the axons of the neuron fibers to the posterior pituitary. By-products of this cleavage are the proteins *neurophysins*. The posterior pituitary contains two distinct neurophysins that provide specific carriers essential for the transport of ADH and oxytocin [2]. Hormones are stored in the posterior pituitary until release is triggered by the hypothalamus. Because neurosecretory cells retain their capacity to conduct electrical impulses, stimuli from the cell bodies in the hypothalamus are conducted down the axons of the neurosecretory fibers to trigger hormone release.

Functions of the Anterior Pituitary

It is known that the adenohypophysis secretes at least six hormones, four of which directly control the functioning of specific target glands—the thyroid, adrenals, and gonads. Hormones that control the functioning of target glands are called *trophic* from the Greek *trophos*, meaning "to nourish," or *tropos*, meaning "to turn toward." The six peptide hormones secreted by the anterior pituitary are (1) growth hormone, also called somatotropin (GH or STH); (2) adrenocorticotropic hormone, also called corticotropin (ACTH); (3) thyroid-stimulating hormone, also called thyrotropin (TSH); (4) follicle-stimulating hormone (FSH); (5) luteinizing hormone (LH); and (6) prolactin (PRL) (Fig. 32-5; see Table 32-1).

All except growth hormone and prolactin regulate the functions of other endocrine glands and are therefore trophic hormones. Growth hormone, ACTH, and prolactin are polypeptides, while TSH, LH, and FSH are glycoproteins. Growth hormone stimulates the secretion of the somatomedins from the liver. These small proteins act as intermediaries in the action of GH itself.

As discussed earlier, secretion of pituitary hormones is regulated by hypothalamic release or release-inhibiting factors or hormones. These include thyrotropin-releasing hormone (TRH), growth hormone-releasing hormone (GHRH), corticotropin-releasing factor (CRF), and luteinizing hormone-releasing hormone (LRH), also called gonadotropin-releasing hormone (GnRH). In addition, two release-inhibiting substances are liberated by the hypothalamus. These are growth hormone release-inhibiting hormone (GHRIH), also called *somatostatin*, and prolactin-inhibiting factor (PIF). A *factor* is a substance that has the actions of a hormone but has not been identified as a distinct chemical compound. A *hormone* has been so identified [5].

Release factors are liberated by neurosecretion, which is the release of a substance from nerve endings directly into the bloodstream. Liberated release factors or release-inhibiting factors are carried to the sinuses of the anterior pituitary. Within the adenohypophysis, the release and release-inhibiting factors act on the gland's cells to control their secretions. The mechanisms that trigger synthesis and release of the factors include feedback as well as various other stimuli in the internal and external environments.

Anterior Pituitary Hormonal Function

Thyroid-Stimulating Hormone (Thyrotropin, TSH). The physiologic role of thyroid-stimulating hormone is to activate synthesis and secretion of the hormones of the thyroid to maintain the size of the gland and its rate of blood flow (see Chap. 34). The pathologic problems that result from derangements in TSH secretion are the same as those of hypersecretion and hyposecretion of the thyroid hormones.

Adrenocorticotropic Hormone (Corticotropin, ACTH). The physiologic role of adrenocorticotropic hormone is to regulate synthesis and secretion of adrenal steroids by adrenal cortical tissue. It also maintains the size and blood flow of the adrenal cortex. Excessive secretions of the cortex result in enlargement of the gland, and absence or marked diminution results in atrophy. Pathologic problems that stem from imbalance in ACTH secretion are equivalent to those caused by hypersecretion or hyposecretion of adrenal hormones (see Chap. 33).

Follicle-Stimulating Hormone (FSH). In men, the target organs for FSH are the testes, where the hormone directly stimulates the germinal epithelium of the seminiferous tubules to activate and facilitate the rate of spermatogenesis. For optimal effects, it appears to require the concomitant presence of LH. These hormones are sometimes used to treat infertility in both men and women.

In women, the target organs for FSH are the ovaries; FSH is essential for the normal cyclic growth of the ovarian follicle. It is responsible for the development and growth of a large number of Graafian follicles and for an increased ovarian weight.

The gonadotropins stimulate the synthesis of testosterone in men and estradiol and progesterone in women. As with other anterior-lobe hormones, secretion is triggered from the hypothalamus and is mediated by feedback mechanisms. Therefore, increased circulation levels of androgens and estrogens inhibit FSH secretions (see Unit 16) [4].

Luteinizing Hormone (LH). Target organs for LH in the male are the testes, where it stimulates the growth and secretory activity of the testicular interstitial cells (Leydig's cells). This action stimulates the synthesis and secretions of the male androgen, testosterone.

The female target organs are the ovaries, where LH is essential for ovulation. Action of the hormone readies the ovarian follicle and forms the corpus luteum from the ruptured follicle. As noted previously, the presence of FSH is required to accomplish these functions [3].

Prolactin (Lactogenic Hormone, PRL). The predominant physiologic roles for prolactin are in breast development and lactation. The hormone acts in synergy with estrogen to promote growth and development of the female mammary glands; therefore, it is said to have a dual role in lactation. It acts with estrogen to prepare the mammary glands for lactation and then initiates secretion of the nutrients of these glands. Prolactin secretion increases during pregnancy, reaching a peak with delivery. The secretion is regulated by a release-inhibiting factor. Release may also be initiated by suckling. The initiation and adequacy of secretion show physiologic variations associated with sleep, stress, and other stimuli, similar to other pituitary hormones.

Growth Hormone (Somatotropin, GH). Growth hormone is the only hormone secreted by the anterior pituitary that has no specific target organ. All cells of the human body may be considered target cells for this hormone.

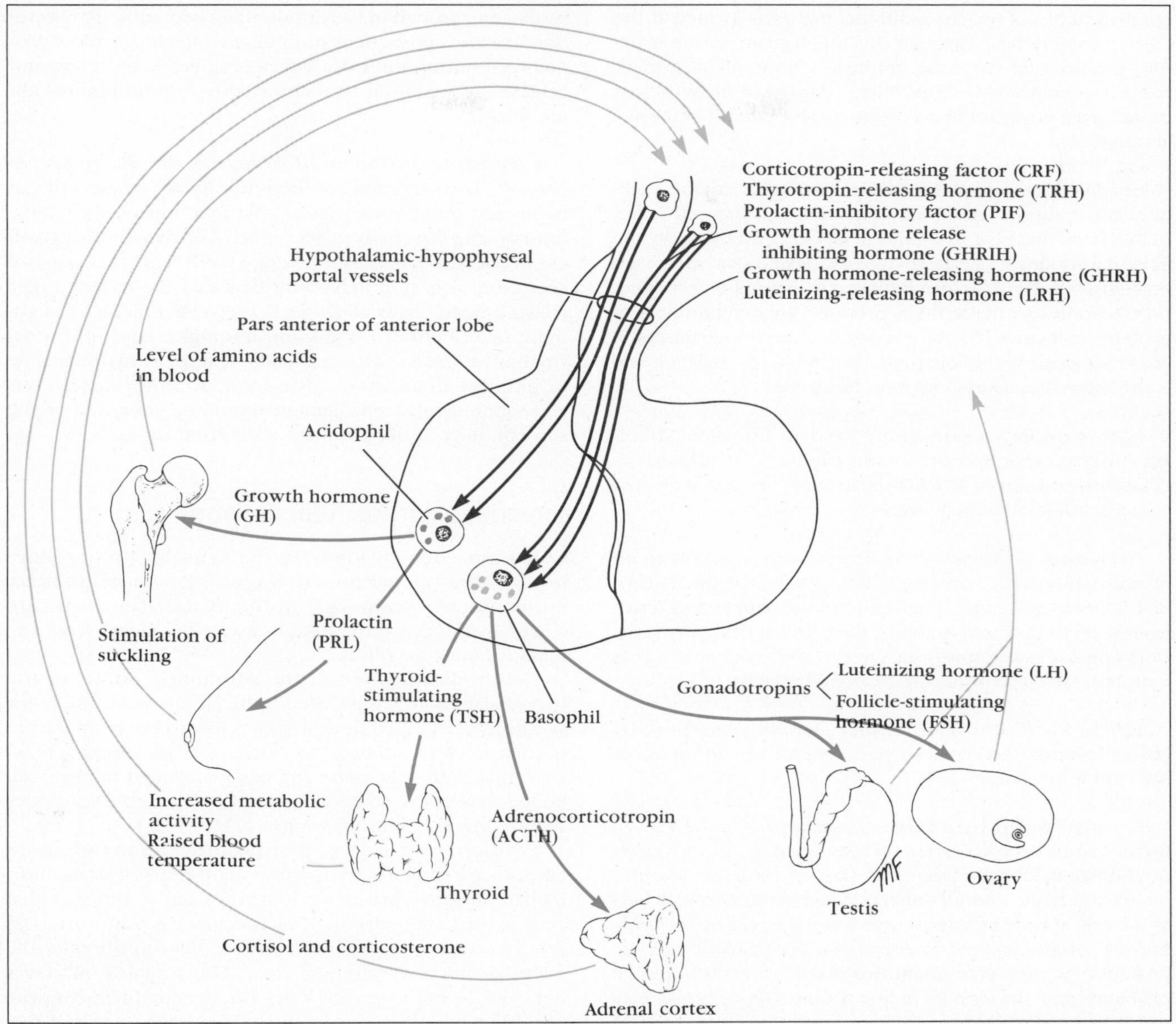

FIGURE 32-5 The mechanisms involved in controlling the activities of the pars anterior of the anterior lobe of the pituitary gland. Note the important feedback mechanisms.

Somatotropin is regulated by release factors from the hypothalamus and by somatomedin, a substance synthesized in the liver. As growth is a complex phenomenon, many other factors play a role in the rate and mode of growth. Action of GH is influenced by other hormones such as thyroid hormone, insulin, the steroids, and androgens. It is also influenced by nutritional status, exercise, stress, diurnal variations, and sleep. Secretion of GH is suppressed by an inhibiting factor (somatostatin). The growth hormone varies from the other hormones in that it is species specific. In recent years it has been synthesized from *Escherichia coli* bacteria through recombinant DNA technology. This type of GH can be used to treat deficiency [2]. Effects of growth hormone may be summarized as follows.

Effects on Growth of Bone and Cartilage. Growth hormone exerts an indirect rather than direct effect on the growth of bone and cartilage. It stimulates growth of these structures by promoting the synthesis of several proteins that are collectively called somatomedin. These proteins are known to be formed in the liver and probably in the muscle and kidneys also. Somatomedin acts directly on the bone and cartilage to promote growth. It is essential to the depositing of chondroid sulfate and collagen [5]. Because the formation of cartilage is accelerated and the epiphyseal plates widen, additional matrix is formed at the ends of long bones. Through this mechanism, linear structure is increased. After the epiphyses close, linear growth is no longer possible. Therefore, excessive growth hormone after adolescence results in thickening of bones and tissues.

Effects on Protein Metabolism. Growth hormone facilitates the transport of amino acids through the cell membrane. This increase in amino acid concentrations in the cells is thought to be partially responsible for increased protein synthesis. It is also believed to exert a direct effect on ribosomes to make them produce greater numbers of protein molecules [5]. As a result of these mechanisms, it creates a positive nitrogen and phosphorous balance and is therefore an anabolic protein hormone.

Effects on RNA Formation. Growth hormone stimulates the transcription process in the nucleus, causing increased formation of RNA. This, in turn, promotes growth by promoting protein synthesis.

Decreased Catabolism of Protein. In addition to an increase in protein synthesis, a decrease in the breakdown of cell proteins occurs. The reduction is believed to result from growth hormone's ability to mobilize free fatty acids from adipose tissue to supply energy. This response acts as a protein sparer as well as a carbohydrate sparer [5].

Effects on Electrolyte Balance. Growth hormone increases gastrointestinal absorption of calcium and reduces Na^+ and K^+ excretion [3].

Effects on Fat and Glucose Metabolism. Growth hormone exerts a strong influence in stimulating fat catabolism in adipose tissue. This action results in the production of large amounts of acetylcoenzyme A, which acts as a ready source of energy and has the effect of reducing the use of glucose for energy (glucose sparing). In the presence of excessive quantities of GH, several potential problems may develop from this action. The response may result in increased ketone levels in the blood (ketogenic effect) or in increased concentration of liver lipids (fatty liver). The glucose-sparing effect of fat catabolism results in storage of increased amounts of glucose in the cells as glycogen. When cellular capacity becomes saturated, circulating blood levels of glucose are elevated (diabetogenic effect), resulting in increased demand for insulin. If this effect persists long enough, the beta cells of the islets of Langerhans are exhausted and diabetes mellitus results [4]. Growth hormone is not the only anterior pituitary hormone that increases blood glucose levels, however; ACTH, TSH, and PRL all have this capacity.

Two additional facts seem important to the understanding of growth hormone. First, GH fails to cause growth if carbohydrate is lacking. Second, secretion of GH is increased during episodes of hypoglycemia *except* those that occur in adult hypopituitarism.

All of this information indicates that growth hormone has many functions other than those of stimulating and supporting growth in the developing child. Although secretion and the subsequent physiologic effects are most pronounced during the early developing years, secretion and release are essential to many bodily functions throughout life.

Circadian Patterns of Anterior Pituitary Secretions. The secretions of the pituitary are cyclic and can be demonstrated on a regular rhythmic basis called *circadian* or *diurnal rhythm*: Secretion of GH and PRL is greatest in the early hours of sleep; ACTH regulates cortisol secretion, reaching maximum between 2 A.M. and 4 A.M., causing peak levels at about 8 A.M.; TSH reaches a maximum level between 8 P.M. and midnight. Loss of diurnal rhythm can be an early diagnostic feature of hypothalamic or pituitary dysfunction. Measurement of hormone levels and supplemental replacement should be governed by the susceptibility of the pituitary at different times [3,7].

Functions of the Neurohypophysis

Unlike the adenohypophysis, the neurohypophysis does not function as an endocrine gland. Posterior pituitary hormones are synthesized in the hypothalamus and are stored in the posterior lobe to await the signal from the hypothalamus for release.

Cell bodies located in the supraoptic nuclei of the hypothalamus are considered to be largely responsible for synthesis of ADH, while cell bodies located in the paraventricular nuclei synthesize oxytocin. It is recognized, however, that both supraoptic and paraventricular nuclear cell bodies synthesize some amount of both of the hormones secreted by the neurohypophysis (Fig. 32-6).

Synthesis and secretion of posterior lobe hormones take place in a two-step process [7]. In the first step, a hormonally inactive precursor is synthesized in the specified cells of the hypothalamus. This precursor is transported by way of secretory granules down the neuron fibers of the hypothalamicohypophyseal tract. The actual hormone is believed to be separated from the precursor during the period in which the granules traverse the axons of this tract to reach the posterior lobe. Hormones are then stored in the posterior pituitary until appropriate stimulus for secretion is initiated by the hypothalamus. Because neurosecretory cells and fibers also have the capacity to conduct electrical impulses, action potentials initiated by stimulus to cell bodies of the hypothalamus are conducted down the axons of the neuron fibers to stimulate release of the hormones.

Physiologic Action of Antidiuretic Hormone

The kidneys are the specific target organs of ADH. In the presence of ADH, the distal tubules and collecting ducts of the nephrons become more permeable to water, causing increased water resorption. This results in decreased concentration (osmotic pressure) of the extracellular fluid (plasma). It is known that in the absence of ADH, tubules and collecting ducts of the nephrons are almost com-

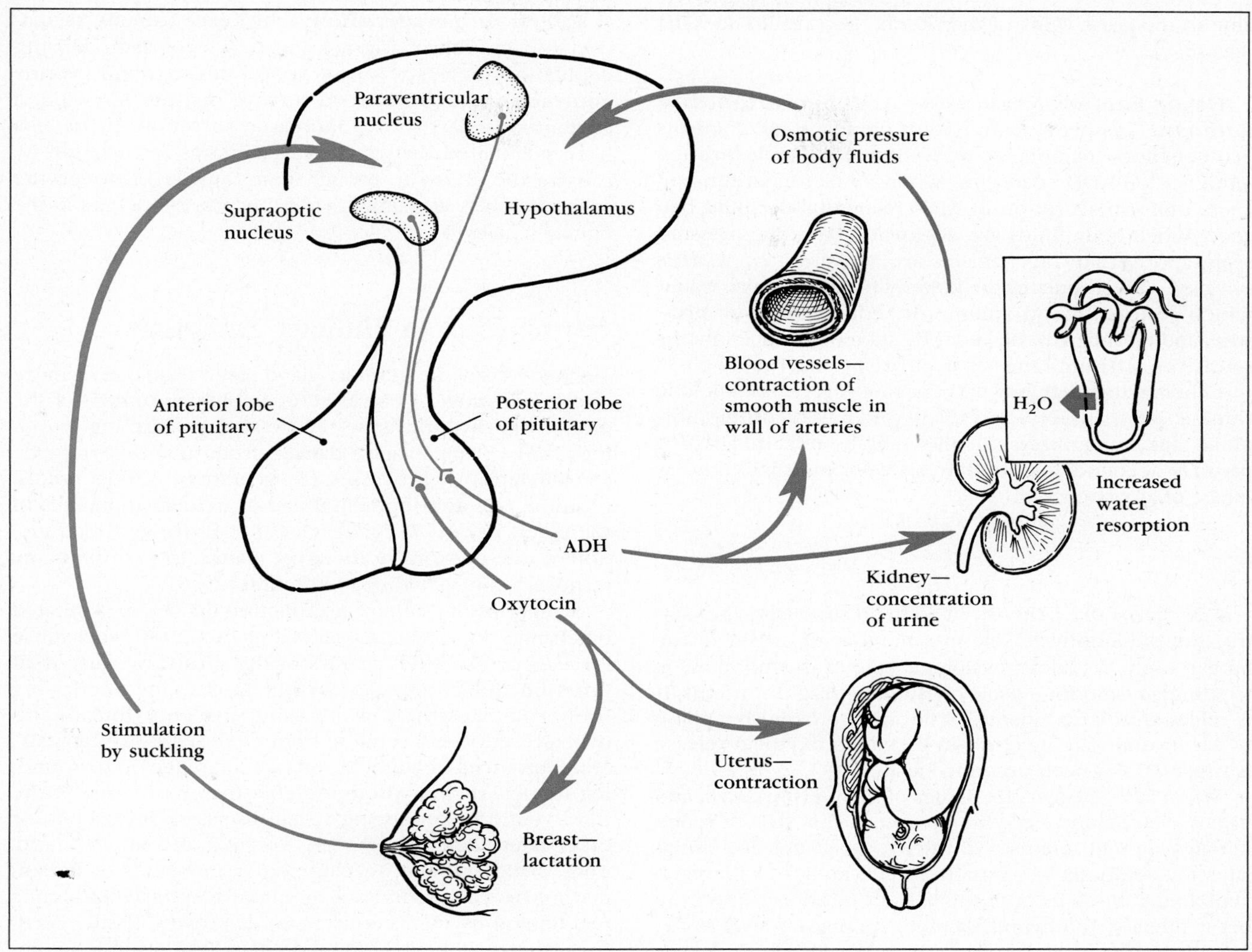

FIGURE 32-6 Schematic drawing of the mechanisms involved in controlling the activities of the posterior lobe of the pituitary gland.

pletely impermeable and little or no water is resorbed [5].

In addition, ADH has a vasopressor effect when administered in large doses and may cause hypertension. The effect is caused by direct action of ADH on smooth muscles in the vascular wall. It may improve systemic fluid volume by reducing the size of the vascular bed.

Regulation of ADH by the Hypothalamus. Increased osmolarity of plasma and decreased circulating vascular volume are the major physiologic stimuli for initiating ADH secretion. Both osmoreceptors and volume receptors influence the hypothalamus to initiate the signal for release of ADH [5].

Osmoreceptors located in the hypothalamus consist of small vesicles surrounded by a semipermeable membrane in which nerve endings are embedded. Increased osmolarity of plasma in the vicinity of the hypothalamus causes water to move out of these osmoreceptors, decreases their volume, and reduces the degree of stretch sensed by neurons. This response presumably stimulates the hypothalamus and initiates the electrical impulse that signals for pituitary release of ADH.

Although the exact location of *volume receptors* is not known, they are generally thought to be outside the CNS, probably predominantly in the thoracic cavity. Apparently, the circulating vascular volume sensed in the thoracic region, rather than the vascular volume of the total body, is the crucial factor in ADH release. For example, a shift in blood volume, caused by pooling of blood in the periphery, is accompanied by ADH release, as is change from a supine to a sitting or standing position. Exposure to high temperatures, which shifts blood from deeper to more superficial regions, increases ADH secretion, while exposure to cold temperatures, which shifts blood from superficial to deeper regions, reduces its secretions. Positive-pressure respiration, which decreases blood volume in the great veins of the thorax, also results in ADH release.

Other Factors Regulating ADH Secretion and Release. As previously noted, feedback mechanisms protect blood osmolarity and volume balance through influence on ADH secretion. When all factors are in balance, uniform secretion of ADH maintains the fluid balance. When body fluids are depleted or osmotic pressure rises, appropriate mechanisms are activated and ADH is released. This stimulates the kidneys to resorb more water, which restores blood volume or reduces osmotic pressure, and balance is achieved. The state of balance inhibits release of ADH until further need arises (see Fig. 32-6).

Other factors that may influence ADH secretion include trauma, pain, anxiety, and drugs such as nicotine, morphine, and tranquilizers. Alcohol inhibits secretion, which partially accounts for the diuresis associated with excess intake of alcohol.

Oxytocin

Effects on the Uterus. Oxytocin stimulates the contraction of smooth muscle in a number of organs in the human body. A major physiologic role of this hormone is to stimulate smooth muscle cells in the pregnant uterus. It is released in large quantities during the expulsive phase of parturition. The mechanism by which oxytocin release is triggered has been described as follows.

When labor begins, the tissues of the uterine cervix and vagina distend and become stretched. This stretch reflex initiates afferent impulses to the hypothalamus and stimulates the synthesis of oxytocin in cell bodies of the paraventricular nucleus. Oxytocin then migrates down the nerve fibers of the hypothalamicohypophyseal stalk to the neurohypophysis. From there it is released into the circulation and is carried by the blood to the uterus, where it acts on smooth muscle cells to reinforce uterine contraction. Since greatest amounts of oxytocin are present in the blood during the expulsive stage of labor, it appears that the quantity released depends on the forcefulness of uterine contractions and the degree of stretch of cervical and vaginal tissues. It is recognized that oxytocin may be one of the factors that precipitate labor [7].

Effects on Lactation. A second major role of oxytocin is to eject milk from lactating breasts. Milk formed by cells of the breasts is stored until suckling begins. For approximately 30 seconds to 1 minute after suckling is initiated, no milk is ejected. This is called the latent period. During this period, suckling stimuli to the nipple initiate signals that are transmitted to neuron cell bodies in the paraventricular and supraoptic nuclei to initiate posterior pituitary release of oxytocin. Circulating blood transports oxytocin to the breasts where it initiates contraction of myoepithelial cells to force milk out of the alveoli into the ducts and lacteal sinuses opening to the nipple [5]. Because epinephrine inhibits oxytocin secretion, emotion, anxiety, and pain can inhibit oxytocin release and thus, lactation.

Effects on Fertilization. In lower animals, distention and stretch of vaginal and cervical tissues during copulation increases the secretion of oxytocin. Uterine contractions experienced during orgasm have been attributed in part to this increased secretion. It has also been postulated that oxytocin facilitates fertilization by causing the uterus to propel semen upward through the fallopian tubes. It is unknown if this process occurs in the human female [5].

Introduction to Pituitary Pathology

Malfunctions of the pituitary gland result from one or more of the following: (1) invasive or impinging tumors of the pituitary or hypothalamus, (2) vascular infarction within the gland, (3) mechanical damage from trauma or surgery, (4) inflammatory processes, (5) genetic or familial predisposition, (6) developmental and structural anomalies of the gland itself, (7) feedback from prolonged malfunction of one or more of its target glands, (8) autoimmune responses, and (9) idiopathic origin [2,3,8].

Symptoms of pituitary malfunction may be precipitated by changes in hormonal balance or by purely mechanical forces. For example, tumors of the pituitary cause malfunction due to pressure from their space-occupying properties, destruction of tissue, and contributions to hypersecretion as a result of tumor cell secretory capacity. More advanced or larger lesions may impinge on surrounding tissues, such as the optic chiasma or the area of the third ventricle, producing visual disorders, headaches, or other neurologic changes [3]. Vascular and tumor infarctions, structural and developmental anomalies or inflammatory processes, and autoimmune responses influence functioning by compromising or destroying tissue. Feedback from malfunction of a target gland can result in hyperplasia of the pituitary gland.

Since the pituitary is a crucial link in the production of several hormones, abnormalities of the gland often alter normal hormone secretion. Pressure or tissue destruction may compromise function and result in problems associated with hyposecretion. Conversely, because many tumors of the pituitary secrete hormones, the presence of these lesions may result in symptoms stemming from hypersecretion.

Factors that influence hormone secretions of the pituitary inevitably influence functions of the specific endocrine gland(s) depending on the hormone(s). For example, conditions that stimulate hyperfunctioning of the pituitary initiate excessive activation of the target organ(s), while suppression or destruction of pituitary tissue with loss of hormone secretions results in hypofunction of target organs.

For convenience, pituitary pathology may be categorized as disorders of the adenohypophysis or of the neurohypophysis. These may be subdivided further as disorders of hyperfunctioning or of hypofunctioning. Because the anterior and posterior lobes of the pituitary operate in general as distinct and separate functional units, malfunctions of each differ characteristically.

Pathology of the Anterior Pituitary

Four types of anterior pituitary disorders are usually described: (1) enlargement of the sella turcica with or without evidence of a space-occupying lesion, (2) visual disorders, (3) hypopituitary hormone secretion, and (4) hyperpituitary hormone secretion [2]. Hormone deficiencies resulting in malfunction may be classified as primary, secondary, or tertiary: primary deficiencies are the result of disease of the target gland; secondary deficiencies result from pituitary lesions or disorders; tertiary deficiencies result from hypothalamic disorders [2].

Evaluation of persons with pituitary diseases may include physical examination and radiologic, neuroophthalmic, and/or endocrine diagnostic studies. The types of tests used and the extent of testing are dependent on the symptoms. Radiologic studies include plain skull films, computerized axial tomography (CT) scans, pneumoencephalography, and arteriography. Neuroophthalmic evaluation is done by formal visual field examination using tangent screening. Endocrine studies include plasma and urinary excretion levels of each of the pituitary and target gland hormones. Radioimmunoassay is an important advance in diagnosing endocrine problems; using antibodies that are specific for certain chemical groups. The accuracy of assay results depends on the specificity of the antibody and its ability to bind the hormone [1]. Other assays include protein binding and radioreceptor assays that use proteins to bind to the hormones.

Chemical assays and free hormone levels are other methods of determining certain hormone concentrations. Free hormone can be assessed directly or by measuring bound hormone and calculating the free level. Plasma or urinary levels indicate marked excess or deficiency. To evaluate the results, the normal circadian pattern, stress reaction, and other factors must be taken into consideration. Urine measurements are much more effective for steroid hormones than for protein-derived hormones because the metabolites of the former are excreted in urine. Dynamic testing assesses the ability of the gland to respond to stimulation. Hormones that stimulate a response may be administered, or suppressive drugs or substances may be given. Many other tests provide indirect information, including levels of blood sugar, serum calcium, and serum potassium [1].

Enlargement of the Sella Turcica

An increase in the size of the sella turcica often results from erosion of this structure caused by pressure from lesions in the pituitary region. Enlargement may be caused by pituitary adenomas, craniopharyngiomas, meningiomas, epithelial cysts, granulomas, malignant tumors of primary origin, or metastasis from carcinoma of the breast. Enlargement may result from nontumorous enlargement of the sella, called *empty sella syndrome.* Sella enlargement may also result from primary hypothyroidism or hypogonadism, which may be attributed to hyperplasia of the thyrotropes or gonadotropes, as it is accompanied by elevated thyrotropin or gonadotropin levels [2]. This is most frequent in children.

Endocrine evaluation for an enlarged sella turcica should include assessment of thyroid and adrenal hormone levels together with basal gonadotropin levels. Basal prolactin levels are important since more than one-half of pituitary tumors secrete prolactin.

Empty Sella Syndrome. This condition is classified as primary or secondary according to its underlying cause. Primary, or idiopathic, sella syndrome results from an abnormally large opening through which the hypophyseal stalk passes. This is often a developmental defect. With increased intracranial pressure, the arachnoid membrane tends to herniate through the opening, creating a sac filled with cerebrospinal fluid. This compresses the pituitary gland against the wall of the sella turcica, creating the appearance of an empty sella (Fig. 32-7). The condition may also occur as a consequence of necrosis of a pituitary adenoma or of Sheehan's syndrome, which are discussed on pages 497 and 500. Empty sella can develop secondary to spontaneous infarctions or regression of a tumor. The secondary variant of the syndrome results from ablation of the gland by irradiation or surgery.

Radiographically, the sella may appear enlarged or normal in size. The primary disease is rarely manifested as pituitary hypofunction. When hypofunction occurs, it is usually evidenced by depressed growth hormone and gonadotropin secretion.

Approximately 90 percent of persons with primary sella syndrome are female. It is diagnosed most often in obese, hypertensive, middle-aged women who have borne many children. The tendency for the pituitary to enlarge during pregnancy and regress afterward may be the basis of pathogenesis. Headache is a common symptom. Visual field defects are rare but do occur in persons who have infarction of a pituitary tumor with subsequent development of empty sella or when the optic chiasma prolapses into the sella.

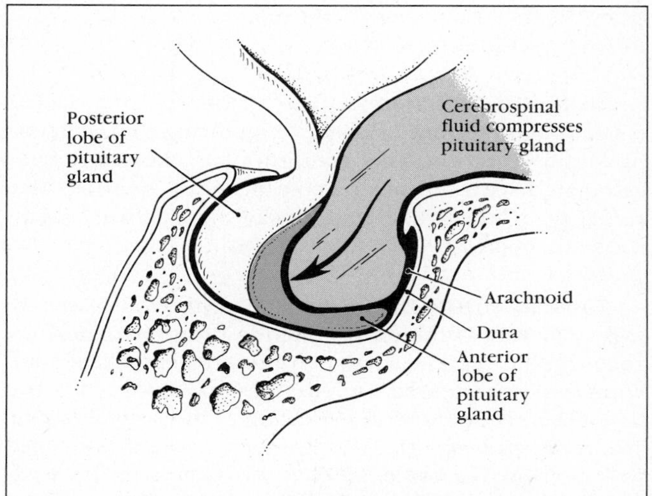

FIGURE 32-7 Empty sella syndrome.

Hypopituitarism (Panhypopituitarism)

Hypopituitarism may be initiated by any destructive process or lesion of the pituitary gland. Surgical hypophysectomy (removal of the pituitary) causes dramatic clinical features of both anterior and posterior hormone deficiency [4]. The most common processes are Sheehan's pituitary necrosis, nonsecreting adenomas, and craniopharyngioma [9]. Other causes include cysts, inflammation of the pituitary as a result of diabetes, meningitis, sarcoidosis, tuberculosis, syphilis, metastatic malignancy, and granulomas that may be nonspecific. Anterior pituitary hormone deficit may occur singly or in various combinations of several deficits. The speed of onset and extent of hormone deficiency depend on the nature and size of the precipitating cause. Onset may be acute and life threatening as in acute adrenocortical insufficiency. More often, however, onset is slow and may occur over a period of months or years. Clinical signs and symptoms rarely manifest until at least 75 percent of the anterior lobe is destroyed [8].

In adults, the clinical features of panhypopituitarism may include absence of axillary and pubic hair, genital and breast atrophy, skin pallor, pallor of nipples, fine skin wrinkling (especially of the face), intolerance to cold, premature aging, poor muscle development, amenorrhea in premenopausal women, loss of previously normal libido and potency in men, and several endocrine deficiencies. Shortness of stature may be evident if onset occurs before puberty. If hypothyroidism is marked, overweight is common. Reduced visual acuity, optic atrophy, and hemianopsia may occur if there is suprasellar expansion of a lesion or mass.

Diagnosis is made on the basis of history and physical examination, neuroophthalmic examination, and plasma immunoassay. Treatment consists of hormone replacement to reestablish function. Thyroid replacement, cortisone, or hydrocortisone may be used as indicated. In women, diethylstilbestrol or premarin helps to maintain secondary sex characteristics, while androgens or testosterone can restore libido and potency in men.

Deficiency of Single Anterior Pituitary Hormones

Prolactin Deficiency. Postpartum failure to lactate is the only symptom of clinical significance in deficient prolactin secretion. This condition has classically been associated with the postpartum pituitary necrosis that results from hemorrhage and shock during delivery (Sheehan's syndrome).

Gonadotropin Deficiency. As previously stated, hypogonadism is the most common pituitary deficiency among adults. Its occurrence in the premenopausal adult woman is manifested by amenorrhea, atrophy of the breasts and uterus, and cornification of the vaginal orifice. The adult man experiences testicular atrophy associated with decreases in libido, potency, beard growth, and muscle tone. When onset of the deficiency occurs prior to puberty, the manifestations include eunuchoid appearance, lack of development of secondary sex characteristics, and infertility. Men fail to develop facial hair, an adult male voice, and normal genitalia. Women fail to manifest normal breast development and onset of menses. Both sexes may exhibit absence of axillary and pubic hair. The most common tumors responsible for the syndrome are the craniopharyngioma and chromophobe adenoma [2,4].

Frölich's syndrome is a severe gonadotropin deficiency that usually affects prepubertal boys. It includes obesity and hypogonadism associated with diabetes insipidus, retardation, and visual problems, all of which are related to hypothalamic rather than pituitary dysfunction. The obesity is probably the result of hypothalamus-induced over-eating [6].

Thyrotropin Deficiency. Hypothalamic or pituitary hypothyroidism exhibits some symptoms in common with primary hypothyroidism but is usually less severe. Isolated TSH deficiency is rare, however, and symptoms of other anterior lobe hormone deficiency are usually present concomitantly. This factor distinguishes pituitary from primary hypothyroidism. In pituitary hypothyroidism, fine wrinkling of the skin and loss of secondary sex characteristics, which are related to gonadal insufficiency, are distinguishing characteristics. Menstrual history is significant since menorrhagia is common in primary hypothyroidism, while amenorrhea is expected in the pituitary form [3].

ACTH Deficiency. Deficiency of ACTH is the most serious of the endocrine deficiencies in persons with pituitary disease [3]. Like pituitary hypothyroidism, ACTH deficiency is usually associated with deficiency of other pituitary hormones; this can be a characteristic, distinguishing pituitary origin from adrenal origin of disease. Symptoms include poor response to stress, nausea, vomiting, hyperthermia, and collapse. Decreased skin and nipple pigmentation is exhibited, which also distinguishes pituitary hypoadrenalism from primary adrenal disease (see Chap. 33).

Growth Hormone Deficiency. This condition results from pituitary insufficiency of growth hormone that affects children in the formative years. It is generally caused by a suprasellar cyst or craniopharyngioma, resulting in hypothalamic or pituitary hypofunction. Genetic transmission of GH deficiency accounts for about 10 percent of pituitary dwarfism and results from an autosomal recessive trait [3]. It is often associated with evidence of sella turcica destruction seen radiographically. It can also be caused by ischemic necrosis and inflammatory changes.

Deficiency of GH is considered in children whose proportional short stature (below the third percentile) is far below that of their healthy counterparts (Fig. 32-8) [3]. Other characteristics include delayed sexual development associated with bright rather than dull mentality. Most children with this condition exhibit excess subcutaneous fat, poorly developed muscles, thin hair, and underdeveloped nails. In some cases an appearance of premature aging is evident, with dry, wrinkled skin.

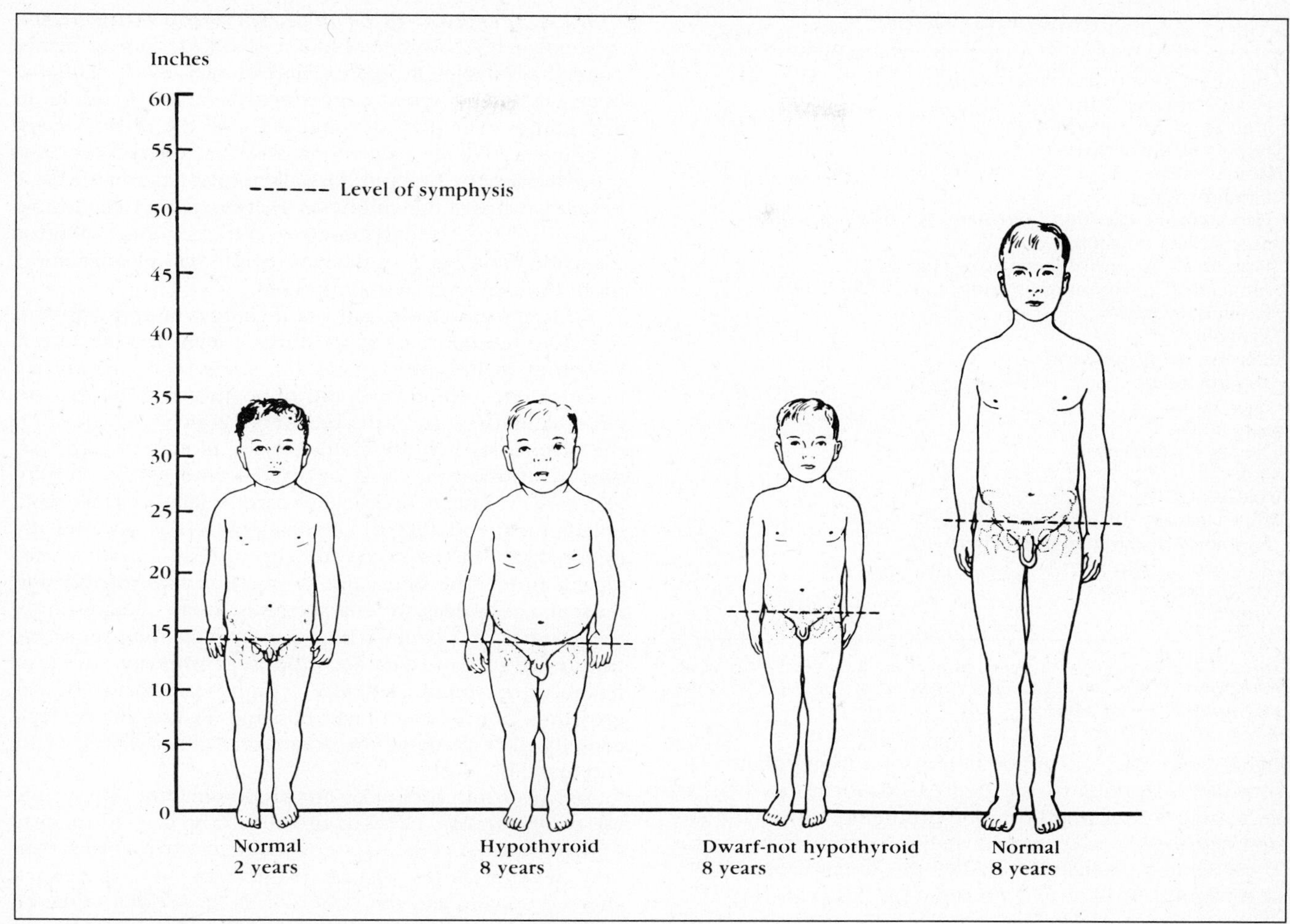

FIGURE 32-8 Normal and abnormal growth. Hypothyroid dwarfs retain their infantile proportions, whereas dwarfs of the constitutional type and, to a lesser extent, of the hypopituitary type have proportions characteristic of their chronologic age. (From L. Wilkins, *The Diagnosis and Treatment of Endocrine Disorders in Childhood and Adolescence* [3rd ed.], 1966. Courtesy of Charles C. Thomas, Publisher, Springfield, Illinois.)

The characteristics of anatomic symmetry without gross deformity and normal mentality distinguish the person with GH deficiency from one with *cretinism* due to thyroid deficiency [8].

Sheehan's Syndrome (Postpartum Pituitary Necrosis). This manifestation of depressed pituitary function was first described as pituitary necrosis occurring postpartally after a delivery complicated by hemorrhage and shock. In the course of pregnancy, the pituitary gland enlarges and develops increased circulation. In the event of acute blood loss, which sometimes accompanies labor and delivery, sudden systematic hypotension can precipitate ischemia and destruction of the anterior lobe [8]. The result is hypofunction of the gland. There may be a lag of months or years between the intrapartum incident and full development of symptoms. Characteristic symptoms are common to a variety of pathologic processes that destroy a significant proportion of pituitary function. Therefore, the syndrome may be produced by any destructive lesion of the pituitary.

Symptoms depend on the degree of impairment of pituitary function relative to the extent of tissue destruction. These initially include evidence of increased intracranial pressure (ICP), headache, visual deficits, stiff neck, papilledema, and convulsions, later followed by symptoms of hormone deficiency including gonadal, thyroid, or adrenal effects [2].

Table 32-3 depicts the etiologies of pituitary disease. Evaluation and diagnosis are by physical examination, neuroophthalmic evaluation, and measurement of baseline hormone levels.

Hyperpituitarism

Pituitary hypersecretion generally involves overproduction of only a single hormone except in certain hormone-secreting tumors [3]. It is often due to a decreased feedback

TABLE 32-3 Etiology of Pituitary Disease

Congenital or hereditary conditions
  Single hormone deficiency
  Multiple hormone deficiency
  Hypothalamic deficiency
Neoplasms
  Pituitary tumors
  Hypothalamic disorders: metastatic or other neoplasms
Vascular malformations
  Postpartum necrosis (Sheehan's syndrome)
  Intracranial aneurysm or arteriovenous malformation
  Pituitary infarction
  Vasculitis
Infections or granulomas
  Tuberculosis
  Meningitis
  Sarcoidosis
Trauma: head injury
Surgery
Irradiation
Miscellaneous
  Emotional deprivation in children
  Tay-Sachs disease
  Hemochromatosis
  Others

Source: Reproduced with permission from R.G. Petersdorf et al., *Principles of Internal Medicine* (10th ed.). Copyright © 1983, McGraw-Hill Book Company.

signal when there is hypofunction of a target gland. The pituitary responds to the decreased hormone level by increasing stimulating hormone production. Pituitary adenomas also may secrete primarily one type of hormone. These almost exclusively involve the somatotropic (GH), lactotropic (PRL), or corticotropic (ACTH) cells [3].

Hyperprolactinemia. Women with prolactin-secreting adenomas may exhibit galactorrhea, amenorrhea, or depressed libido. Some exhibit evidence of decreased estrogens and hirsutism (excessive hair growth in inappropriate places), which are believed to be the result of depression of ovarian function or stimulation of adrenal androgen function. Men with prolactin-secreting adenomas do not exhibit galactorrhea because of lack of development of acini in the male breasts. These lesions in men usually occur only as space-occupying lesions with hypogonadism. The hypogonadism apparently occurs because of a defect in endogenous gonadotropin-releasing hormone (GnRH) [4]. Diagnosis and evaluation are by radiologic studies and studies of basal prolactin levels.

Hypersecretion of ACTH. Excess secretion of ACTH by the pituitary gland results in *Cushing's disease*. Excess ACTH stimulates excess cortisol, which alters the distribution of fat, blood glucose, and many other conditions. When the excess cortisol is due to adrenal overproduction, the condition is called *Cushing's syndrome*. Manifestations of Cushing's syndrome are detailed in Chapter 33. Cushing's disease of pituitary origin is most frequently due to a basophil ACTH-secreting adenoma of the gland. Excess ACTH causes hyperplasia and hyperfunction of the adrenal cortex.

Hypersecretion of Growth Hormone (Gigantism, Acromegaly). Hypersecretion of GH occurring before puberty results in gigantism. This pituitary abnormality has been defined as height exceeding 80 inches in adults or exceeding 3 standard deviations above the mean for age in children. The disorder is the result of oversecretion of growth hormone by a pituitary adenoma in a growing child before closure of the epiphyses. Before epiphyseal closure, growth is linear and symmetric. Hypogonadism is often associated and leads to delayed epiphyseal closure and a more prolonged growth period [4].

Clinical features of gigantism include symmetric growth of stature to enormous proportions, sometimes reaching 8 to 9 feet in height (Fig. 32-9). Growth is symmetric because both epiphyseal and oppositional bone growth occur concurrently. Affected persons may also develop the distortions that are characteristic of acromegaly. Cardiac hypertrophy is often associated with mild hypertension that eventually may lead to cardiac failure [4]. Thyroid enlargement and adrenal cortical hyperplasia occasionally occur. Early in the course of the disease, persons with gigantism may be unusually strong, but osteoporosis and muscular weakness are characteristic in later stages [2,4].

Acromegaly occurs when growth hormone-secreting tumors of the pituitary develop after puberty and after fusion of the epiphyses. After epiphyseal closure, linear growth of bones is no longer possible. Tissues thicken and growth takes place in the acral areas (hands, feet, nose, and mandible) [2].

Somatotropic adenomas are predominantly responsible for these tumors. Growth of the tumor may ultimately destroy normal cells. As a consequence, hypopituitarism may develop as the disease progresses. Both sexes are affected equally and the condition is most often detected in the third or fourth decade of life. The disease progresses slowly and insidiously and often goes undetected for years. Persons may first notice progressive increase in ring, shoe, hat, and glove sizes. The skull and head increase in size and the fingers and hands become broad and spade-like. Increased growth of subcutaneous connective tissue of the face leads to coarsening of the features (Fig. 32-10). The face assumes a thick, fleshy appearance. The lips are thickened and enlarged, and have accentuated skin folds. The ears and nose become enlarged because of hypertrophy of the cartilages. There is overgrowth of the supraorbital ridge and the cheeks become prominent. Overgrowth of the maxilla results in lengthening of the face, and alveolar bone growth results in separations of the teeth. Overgrowth of the mandible results in prognathism (jaw projection). Hypertrophy of the costal cartilage leads to in increased circumference of the chest. Absorption of bone is rapid and osteoporosis occurs. Acromegalic arthritis develops from proliferation of joint cartilage and affects joints of the long bones and the spine. Long bones thicken and become massive. There is often bowing of the legs. The skin becomes thickened, and hirsutism occurs in females. The tongue enlarges and may protrude from the mouth. The lungs, liver, spleen, kidneys, and intestines enlarge twofold to fivefold. Hypertension, coronary artery atherosclerosis, and marked cardiomegaly occur. Conges-

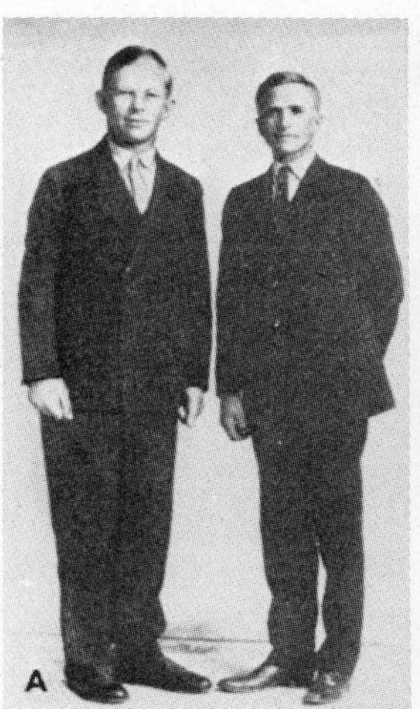

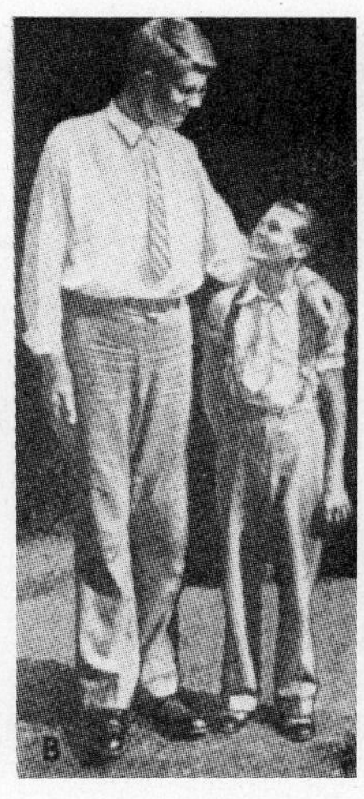

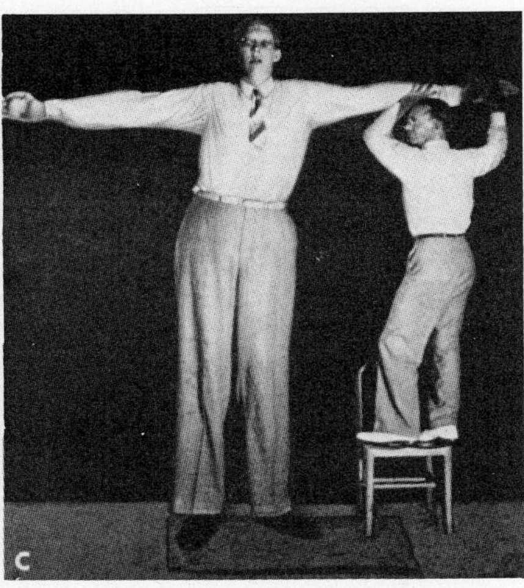

FIGURE 32-9 One of the most notable examples of growth hormone excess in the human was Robert Wadlow, later known as the "Alton giant." Although he weighed only 9 pounds at birth, he soon began to grow excessively, and by 6 months of age weighed 30 pounds. At 1 year he had reached a weight of 62 pounds. Growth continued throughout his life. Shortly before his death at age 22 from cellulitis of the feet, he was 8 feet, 11 inches tall and weighed 475 pounds, according to the careful measurements of Dr. C.M. Charles. A. Age 9 years; height 6 ft., 1 in. (shown with his father). B. Age 13 years; height 7 ft., 2 in. (shown with a friend of the same age). C. Age 20 years; height 8 ft., 6 in.; weight 430 lb. (A and B from F. Fadner, *Biography of Robert Wadlow,* 1944. Courtesy of Bruce Humphries, Publishers. Courtesy of Drs. C. M. Charles and C. M. MacBryde.)

tive heart failure often develops. The gonads enlarge but their function is subnormal. The adrenals, thyroid, and parathyroid become enlarged [2].

The typical physical picture is one of a big, burly person with forward carriage of the head, prognathism, kyphosis, bowlegs, prominent forehead, thickened chest, and husky, cavernous voice. Many men develop impotence and women develop amenorrhea. Apparently, growth of the adenoma impinges on the normal cells and induces insufficiency of other hormones.

Diagnosis is by assessment of physical characteristics, and serial radiographs and photographs. Laboratory immunoassay of plasma growth hormone levels and response to glucose stimulation during a glucose tolerance test can help in diagnosis. Persons normally suppress GH after ingestion of 100 gm glucose, but the acromegalic may show increased levels [2].

Pathology of the Posterior Pituitary

Pathologic conditions stemming from lesions of the neurohypothesis are rare. Posterior lobe pathology is almost always related to primary disease or other processes outside the gland itself. The posterior lobe releases two hormones, ADH and oxytocin, which are synthesized and secreted by the hypothalamus.

Antidiuretic Hormone Deficiency

A deficiency in ADH release causes the condition known as *diabetes insipidus*. The underlying causes of ADH deficiency have been categorized as follows: (1) neoplastic or inflammatory processes impinging on the hypothalamoneurohypophyseal axis, such as adenomas, metastatic carcinoma, abscesses, meningitis, tuberculosis, or sarcoidosis; (2) surgical or irradiation injury to the hypothalamoneuralhypophyseal axis, such as hypophysectomy; (3) severe head injuries; and (4) idiopathic influences. Rarely, the syndrome is familial and inherited as a Mendelian dominant [8,9].

Lack of ADH causes a failure of the distal and collecting ducts of the nephrons to resorb water. The resulting clinical features of diabetes insipidus include polyuria, excessive thirst, and polydipsia. Polyuria causes a slight rise in serum osmolarity that stimulates the thirst center. Normal function of the thirst center ensures that polydipsia will replace water lost through polyuria [9]. Symptoms are usually sudden in onset and are pronounced, with urine output reaching 10 or more liters in a 24-hour period. Urine is pale, and its concentration is very dilute.

Diagnosis is on the basis of clinical manifestations, dehydration tests, and response to vasopressin administration. Treatment is administration of ADH (vasopressin), usually by nasal spray.

Inappropriate ADH Secretion

The syndrome of inappropriate ADH secretion (SIADH) is defined as persistent release of ADH unrelated to plasma osmolarity or volume deficit. The normal feedback inhibition of the posterior pituitary is hypoactive or inactive, causing continued release of ADH. The result is excessive resorption of water in the renal system and excessive

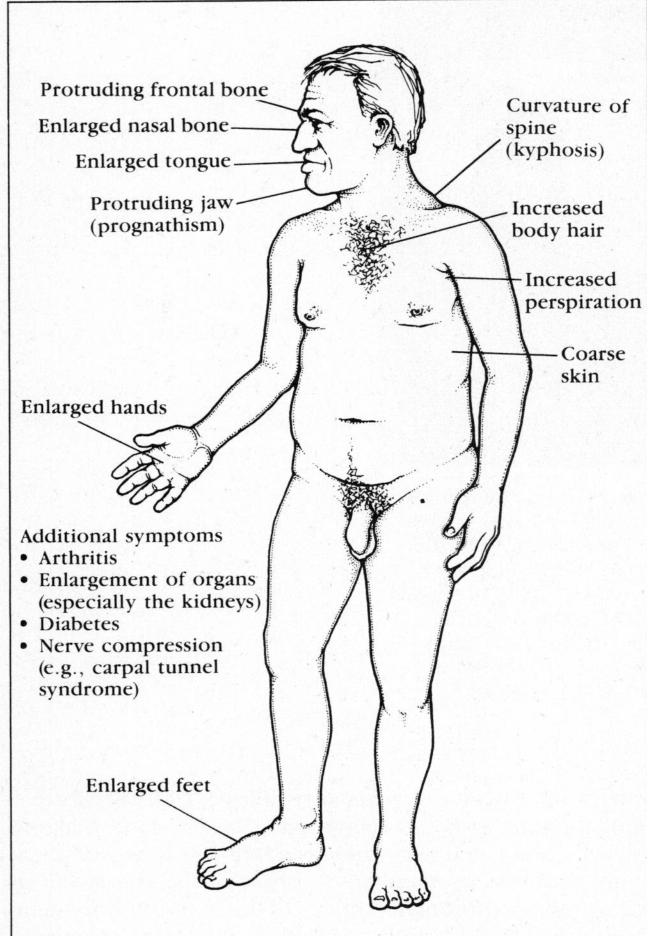

FIGURE 32-10 Composite of all symptoms of acromegaly. (From M. Beyers and S. Dudas [eds.], *The Clinical Practice of Medical-Surgical Nursing* [2nd ed.]. Boston: Little, Brown, 1984.)

TABLE 32-4 Causes of SIADH

Malignancy
Oat-cell carcinoma of lung
Carcinoma of pancreas
Lymphosarcoma, reticulum-cell sarcoma, Hodgkin's disease
Carcinoma of duodenum
Thymoma
Nonmalignant pulmonary disease
Tuberculosis
Lung abscess
Pneumonia
Central nervous system disorders
Skull fracture
Subdural hematoma
Subarachnoid hemorrhage
Cerebrovascular thrombosis
Cerebral atrophy
Acute encephalitis
Tuberculous meningitis
Purulent meningitis
Guillain-Barré syndrome
Lupus erythematosus
Acute intermittent porphyria
Physical or emotional stress
Pain
Drugs
Chlorpropamide
Vincristine
Cyclophosphamide
Carbamazepine
Oxytocin
General anesthetics
Narcotics
Barbiturates
Thiazide antidepressants
Tricyclic antidepressants
Miscellaneous
Hypothyroidism
Positive-pressure respiration

Source: Reproduced with permission from R.G. Petersdorf et al., *Principles of Internal Medicine* (10th ed.). Copyright © 1983, McGraw-Hill Book Company.

retention of water with expansion of fluid volume. Fluid overload, hyponatremia, and hemodilution result.

The syndrome may occur from a stimulus inside the hypothalamohypophyseal system or one from an outside source (Table 32-4). It may occur as a result of a tumor of the hypothalamus or hypophysis that impinges on tissues that control secretions. More often it is the result of secretions of ADH by nonendocrine tumors. Oat-cell bronchogenic carcinoma is the most common ADH-secreting lesion causing SIADH. Other conditions capable of this ectopic secretion include carcinoma of the pancreas, lymphoma, bronchogenic tuberculosis, Hodgkin's disease, and thymoma. Disorders and trauma of the central nervous system (CNS) such as subdural hematoma and infection may be the basis of malfunction. Conditions such as stress, pain, and hypovolemia may cause the physiologic release of ADH in the absence of hypertonic plasma [9]. Diagnosis is made on the basis of serum sodium levels and the clinical picture of hypervolemia. It should be suspected in any person with hyponatremia who has hypertonic urine.

Management includes fluid restriction, diuretics, assessment of sodium balance, assessment for evidence of congestive heart failure, and treatment for the underlying cause of the syndrome. No drugs are currently available that effectively suppress ADH.

Tumors of the Pituitary

Adenomas

More than 90 percent of all pituitary neoplasms are adenomas. Pituitary tumors account for 6 to 18 percent of all brain tumors, only 10 to 20 percent of which are nonfunctioning [4]. Pituitary adenomas may be classified according to predominant cell type. They may also be classified according to their secretory qualities. They may interfere with pituitary functions by virtue of their space-occupying properties or by secretions of various hormones. In general, problems stemming from the space-occupying factor are the result of destruction or suppression of surrounding tissue. Those stemming from secretory properties result in hypersecretion or hyperfunction. All lesions may produce CNS symptoms or visual problems because of their space-occupying properties, depending on the size and location of the lesion.

The growth pattern of adenomas is variable and unrelated to hormone secretion. The tumors often become apparent clinically because of their compressive effect or impingement on adjoining structures. Pituitary adenomas are almost always benign but may exhibit aggressive growth so that surgical removal is impossible [4].

Pituitary adenomas may cause neurologic and/or endocrinologic clinical signs and symptoms, including visual or neurologic deficits, headaches, or impaired gonadal function. The tumors may be discovered accidentally on review of skull films [4]. Growth disturbances such as acromegaly or giantism may be the major sign of a GH-secreting adenoma. Prolactin-secreting hormones cause gonadal dysfunction while ACTH-secreting adenomas may produce Cushing's disease.

Craniopharyngiomas (Rathke's pouch tumors) are tumors of congenital origin derived from remnants of Rathke's pouch. These lesions commonly occur in young children and are generally cystic, although some are solid. They are usually well encapsulated and are generally benign, although some develop malignancy. Many contain sufficient calcification to be visualized on radiographs. They may reach considerable size (8–10 cm in diameter). Because of location, they frequently compress the optic nerve, leading to visual impairment [3,4].

Malignant Tumors

Primary Lesions. Although they are rare, primary malignant lesions do occur in the anterior lobe of the pituitary. They occasionally arise in preexisting benign adenomas or craniopharyngiomas. Characteristically, they are fast-growing and rapidly exhibit clinical manifestations. They are also massive and extensively invade nearby structures; distant metastasis may occur, especially to the liver. The histologic distinction between rapidly growing adenoma and carcinoma is often difficult [8].

Secondary Lesions. Neoplastic metastasis to the pituitary is rare. It may occur with carcinoma of the breast, lung, or thyroid.

Study Questions

1. Briefly explain the differences in structure and action of steroid and protein-based hormones.
2. Draw a feedback system for each of the major hormones of the anterior and posterior pituitary, including the known stimulating and inhibiting factors. What happens if any one of these factors malfunctions?
3. Describe the concept of target organ response to these hormones.
4. How does gigantism differ from acromegaly?
5. Identify the factors related to SIADH and explain the physiologic results of this condition.
6. What are the most common manifestations of pituitary tumors? Explain the pathology causing these manifestations.

References

1. Baxter, J.D. Principles of endocrinology. In J.B. Wyngaarden and L.H. Smith (eds.), *Cecil's Textbook of Medicine* (17th ed.). Philadelphia: Saunders, 1985.
2. Daniels, G.H., and Martin, J.B. Neuroendocrine regulation of the anterior pituitary and hypothalamus. In E. Braunwald, et al. (eds.), *Harrison's Principles of Internal Medicine* (11th ed.). New York: McGraw-Hill, 1987.
3. Daughaday, W.H. The anterior pituitary. In J.D. Wilson and D.W. Foster (eds.), *Williams' Textbook of Endocrinology* (7th ed.). Philadelphia: Saunders, 1985.
4. Frohman, L.A. The anterior pituitary. In J.B. Wyngaarden and L.H. Smith (eds.), *Cecil's Textbook of Medicine* (17th ed.). Philadelphia: Saunders, 1985.
5. Guyton, A. C. *Textbook of Medical Physiology* (7th ed.). Philadelphia: Saunders, 1986.
6. Olefsky, J.M. Obesity. In E. Braunwald et al. (eds.), *Harrison's Principles of Internal Medicine* (11th ed.). New York: McGraw-Hill, 1987.
7. Reichlin, S. Neuroendocrinology. In J.D. Wilson and D.W. Foster (eds.), *Williams' Textbook of Endocrinology* (7th ed.). Philadelphia: Saunder, 1985.
8. Robbins, S.L., Cotran, R.S., and Kumar, V. *Pathologic Basis of Disease* (3rd ed.). Philadelphia: Saunders, 1984.
9. Streeten, D.H.P., Moses, A.M., and Miller, M. Disorders of the neurohypophysis. In E. Braunwald et al. (eds.), *Harrison's Principles of Internal Medicine* (11th ed.). New York: McGraw-Hill, 1987.
10. Wilson, J.D. Principles of endocrinology. In E. Braunwald et al. (eds.), *Harrison's Principles of Internal Medicine* (11th ed.). New York: McGraw-Hill, 1987.

CHAPTER 33

Adrenal Mechanisms and Alterations

CHAPTER OUTLINE

Anatomy of the Adrenal Glands
The Adrenal Cortex

- Adrenocortical Hormones
  - *Control of Secretion*
- Adrenocorticotropic Hormone (ACTH)
- Feedback System of Cortisol-ACTH Levels
- Biorhythms: Effects on ACTH Secretion
- Effects of Stress on ACTH Secretion
- Renin-Angiotensin-Aldosterone System
- Effect of Electrolytes on Aldosterone Secretion
- Adrenocortical Hormone Biosynthesis
- Transport of Steroid Hormones
- Physiologic Actions of Mineralocorticoids
- Physiologic Actions of Glucocorticoids
- Physiologic Actions of Androgens

Altered Adrenocortical Function

- Adrenocortical Hyperfunction
  - *Cushing's Syndrome*
  - *Primary Aldosteronism*
  - *Secondary Aldosteronism*
  - *Adrenogenital Syndromes*
  - *Congenital Adrenal Hyperplasia*
- Adrenocortical Hypofunction
  - *Primary Adrenocortical Insufficiency*
  - *Adrenal Crisis*
  - *Secondary Adrenocortical Insufficiency*

The Adrenal Medulla

- Catecholamines
  - *Catecholamine Biosynthesis and Storage*
  - *Catecholamine Secretion*
- Altered Function of the Adrenal Medulla
  - *Pheochromocytoma*
  - *Multiple Endocrine Neoplasia*

LEARNING OBJECTIVES

1. Discuss the normal anatomy of the adrenal gland.
2. Describe the mechanisms of regulating adrenocortical hormone secretions.
3. Identify the pattern of synthesis of each of the major hormones of the adrenal cortex.
4. Outline the physiologic effects of mineralocorticoids, glucocorticoids, and androgen hormones.
5. Identify the process that results in Cushing's syndrome.
6. Define *Cushing's syndrome* and its major clinical manifestations.
7. Differentiate between primary and secondary aldosteronism.
8. Describe the pathologic process and resulting physical changes of the adrenogenital syndromes.
9. Outline the clinical manifestations of primary adrenocortical insufficiency.
10. Compare primary and secondary adrenocortical insufficiency.
11. Discuss the clinical features of adrenal crisis.
12. Describe catecholamine biosynthesis and storage.
13. Describe the etiology of pheochromocytoma.
14. Outline the major clinical features of pheochromocytoma.
15. Discuss multiple endocrine neoplasia syndrome (MEN) and its relationship to pheochromocytoma.

The adrenal cortex and the adrenal medulla share adjacent sites but have no similar functions. The hormonal anatomy and physiology of both of these structures are discussed in this chapter. Altered states of function are also included.

Anatomy of the Adrenal Glands

The adrenal, or suprarenal, glands are located retroperitoneally at the superior pole of each kidney. Although structurally connected, the adrenal cortex and adrenal medulla are separate organs in both tissue origin and physiologic function.

The adrenals are rather flat, with the right gland having a pyramidal appearance and the left a curved, semilunar shape (Fig. 33-1). A thick, fibrous capsule surrounds the glands, and peritoneal fasciae, independent of the kidneys, provide support. The usual weight of each gland in a healthy adult is between 3 and 6 gm and, in general, the adrenals tend to be slightly heavier in males [2].

Arterial blood supply is from the renal, or inferior, phrenic arteries or directly from the abdominal aorta. Once inside the glands, the vessels break up into sinusoids and drain medially into the glands. Venous drainage is different for the right and left glands. The right adrenal empties venous blood directly into the vena cava, while the left empties into the left renal vein (Fig. 33-1). Nervous innervation is both sympathetic and parasympathetic. Nerves enter through the cortex and progress to the medulla.

The golden yellow adrenal cortex encompasses the medulla, which is more medially located. Three distinct layers compose the cortex. The first is the *zona glomerulosa*, composed of a thin layer of irregularly shaped cuboidal cells. Immediately beneath is the second layer, the *zona fasciculata*. Cuboidal cells of this layer run in long strands and are separated by the sinusoidal spaces. During periods of adrenal inactivity, the cells of this layer become filled with vacuoles, but during periods of active function the cells become very compact. The third layer

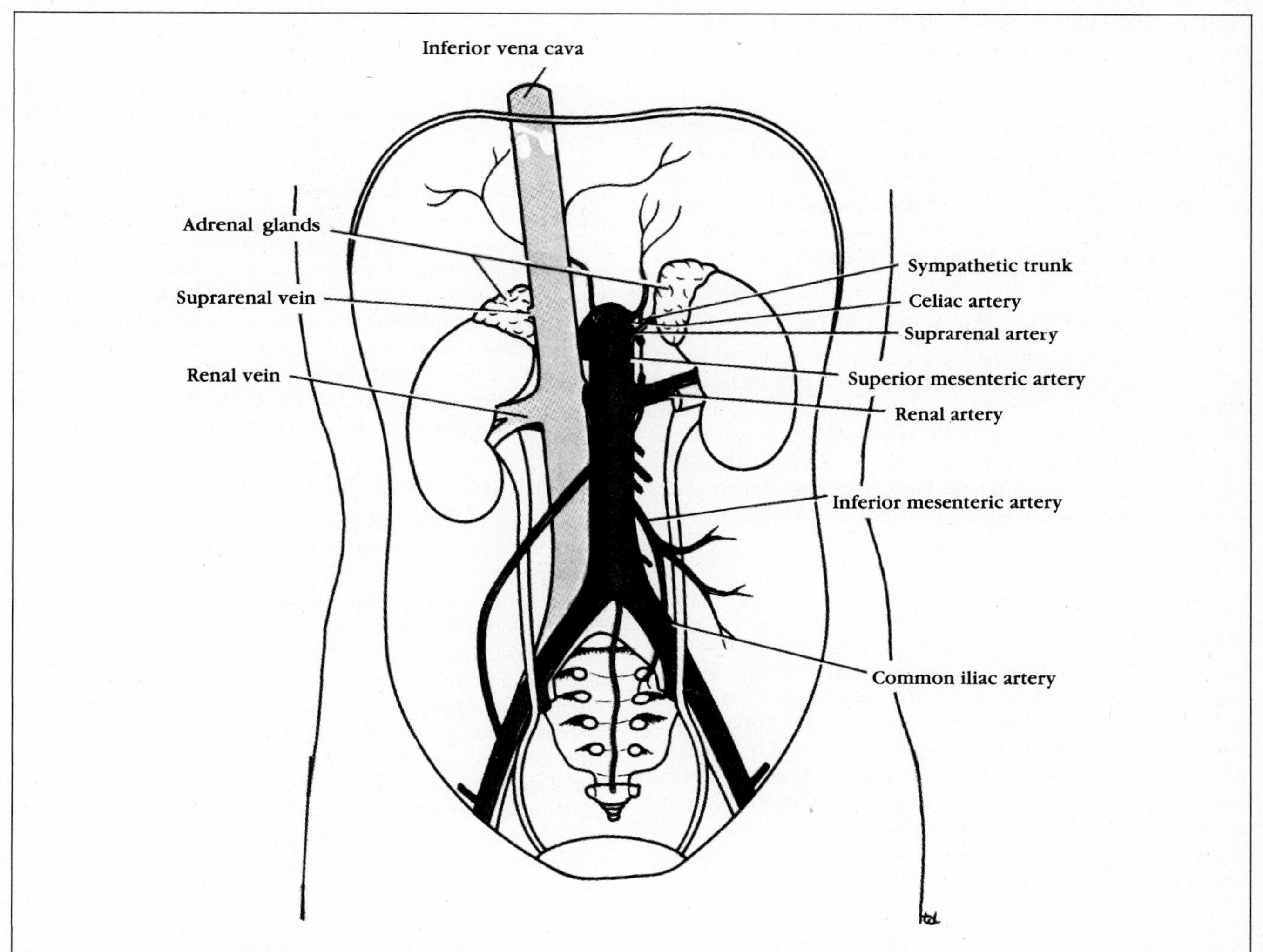

FIGURE 33-1 Position of the adrenal glands on the kidneys. (From R. Snell, *Clinical Anatomy for Medical Students* [2nd ed.]. Boston: Little, Brown, 1981.)

of the cortex, the *zona reticularis*, is composed of groups of cells of very irregular shape (see Fig. 33-2).

The adrenal medulla lies central to, and is surrounded by, the adrenal cortex. It is flat and gray and it is composed of sheets of irregularly shaped masses of cells with small nuclei [2]. The cells are surrounded by sinusoidal blood vessels.

The Adrenal Cortex

Adrenocortical Hormones

The adrenal cortex is responsible for secreting three major groups of steroid hormones. The *mineralocorticoids* and *glucocorticoids* are the two most important of these, with the third and less significant being the *androgens*. The major glucocorticoid is *cortisol*, which is secreted mostly by the zona fasciculata. The major mineralocorticoid is *aldosterone*, which is secreted by the zona glomerulosa almost independently of adrenocorticotropic hormone (ACTH) influence; ACTH is necessary only to maintain the viability of the glomerulosa cells. Androgens are produced by the cells of the zona fasciculata and probably the zona reticularis.

Control of Secretion. Regulation of adrenocortical hormone secretion is accomplished mainly through ACTH, which exerts direct control over the glucocorticoids and sex steroids. Aldosterone secretion is primarily controlled by the renin-angiotensin-aldosterone system, and by serum potassium and serum sodium levels (Fig. 33-2).

Adrenocorticotropic Hormone (ACTH)

This hormone is produced by the anterior pituitary gland. Its release is controlled by corticotropin-releasing factor (CRF), which is produced by the hypothalamus. Normally, the amount of circulating ACTH is controlled by three factors: (1) circulating levels of cortisol, (2) individual biorhythms, and (3) stress. These factors, together with states of dysfunction, stimulate CRF to release ACTH into the bloodstream.

Feedback System of Cortisol-ACTH Levels

When circulating levels of cortisol (the principal glucocorticoid) decrease, ACTH acts directly on the adrenal cortex to stimulate production. Increased secretion of cortisol occurs within a few minutes after ACTH initiates production of the hormone. Low levels of ACTH result in decreased hormone biosynthesis and in decreased renal blood flow. Thus, circulating levels of cortisol respond directly to a feedback system with ACTH. Decreased cortisol levels result in stimulation of ACTH, while elevated levels cause decreased release of ACTH (see Chap. 32).

Biorhythms: Effects on ACTH Secretion

Individual biorhythms, or *circadian* or *diurnal rhythms*, affect the normal circulating levels of ACTH. The pattern is related to sleep periods and may be altered by changes in daily activity [21]. In the hours prior to and just after waking, ACTH levels reach the highest peak of the 24-hour day. The levels decrease continually during the remainder of the day. In relation to this, cortisol levels rise at approximately the same times as the ACTH levels and also decline as the day progresses. Usually, the plasma cortisol concentration is highest on awakening in the morning, falls later during the day, and reaches the lowest levels during the first two hours of sleep [21]. From this point, cortisol gradually returns to its maximum level prior to the period of waking. While the basic pattern of biorhythms is similar for all humans, wide variations can occur in any individual.

Effects of Stress on ACTH Secretion

Any physical or emotional stress increases the secretion of ACTH, resulting in increased production and secretion of cortisol (see Chap. 4). Stresses that may initiate this reaction include illness, hypotension, and exposure to extreme cold. The mechanism behind this is thought to be related to the ability of glucocorticoids to provide the body with the materials needed for energy. These materials include amino acids, protein, fatty acids, glucose, sodium, and water, levels of all of which increase in a stressful situation [1].

Specific stress responses of the body occur with the stages of the general adaptation syndrome as defined by Selye [9]. During the initial stages of the alarm phase, acute release of epinephrine produces characteristic catecholamine effects. This is followed by changes that resemble adrenocortical hormone insufficiency, such as decreased blood pressure, decreased serum glucose, and serum sodium levels, and increased serum potassium levels. The period of insufficiency is followed by a period of active adrenocortical function that continues until a stable baseline has been reestablished. Stable levels of hormone production occur during the resistance phase. If the stage of exhaustion is reached, adrenocortical hormone insufficiency may once again be encountered.

Renin-Angiotensin-Aldosterone System

The renin-angiotensin-aldosterone (RAA) system is the major influence over the production of aldosterone by the zona glomerulosa. Initially, the enzymelike substance renin is released from the juxtaglomerular apparatus in the nephrons of the kidneys in response to changes in perfusion pressure and solute delivery in the renal distal tubules. Through a complex process of hydrolysis, renin undergoes chemical changes to become angiotensin II, which exerts a strong control over the regulation of aldosterone secretion (see Fig. 33-2). The mechanism by which this is accomplished is not completely understood. It is known that the action is rapid and that the production of aldosterone stops when angiotensin II is removed. The RAA system does not influence production or secretion of cortisol.

Effect of Electrolytes on Aldosterone Secretion

The electrolyte with the major influence on aldosterone secretion is potassium. When serum potassium levels are

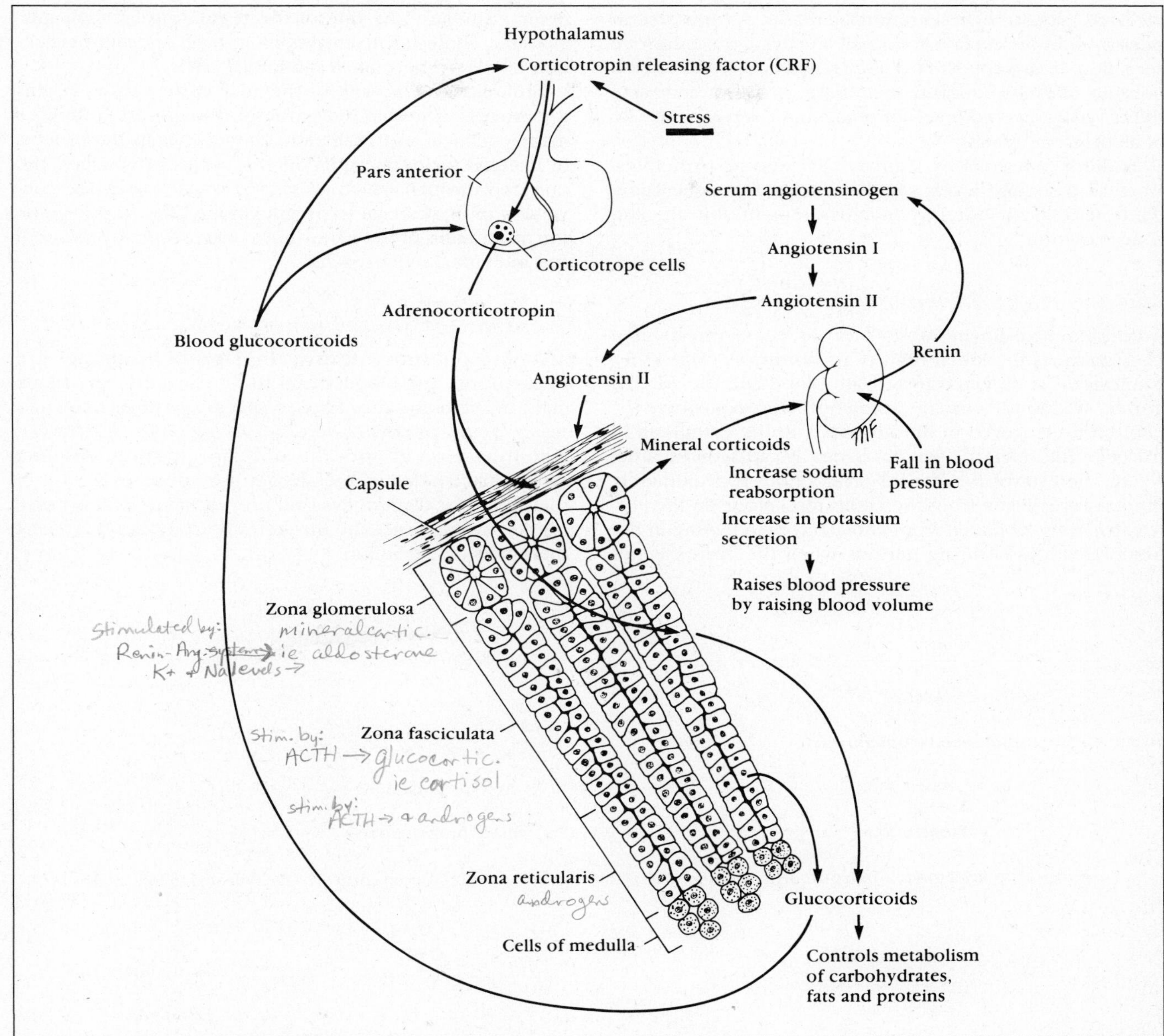

FIGURE 33-2 Mechanisms involved in the control of mineralocorticoid secretion and glucocorticoid secretion of the suprarenal (adrenal) cortex.

elevated, aldosterone secretion increases. An increase in potassium of less than 1 mEq per liter triples aldosterone secretion. It also appears that potassium affects the release of renin, exerting an indirect stimulus on aldosterone synthesis [20]. Lowered levels of potassium decrease the rate of aldosterone release.

Sodium functions by similar, but reverse, principles. Decreased sodium levels stimulate aldosterone secretion, while increased sodium concentrations inhibit aldosterone secretion.

Adrenocortical Hormone Biosynthesis

Adrenocortical hormone, or steroid, biosynthesis uses cholesterol as the initial basis of its hormones (Fig. 33-3). Cholesterol is obtained from both blood and the adrenal cortex. Within the cortex, during normal states of activity, cholesterol is stored in lipid droplets in the cytoplasm of the cells. Although the adrenal cortex is capable of synthesizing cholesterol for steroid production, approximately 80 percent is taken from the cholesterol stores in the cortex that were obtained from cholesterol circulating in the bloodstream [4]. During periods when the cortex is not being stimulated by one of the regulating mechanisms, available cholesterol remains in storage, and the production of steroid hormones is minimal [20].

Stimulation from any of the adrenal regulators begins the process of steroid biosynthesis. Cholesterol undergoes many chemical and enzymatic conversions in the process of manufacturing steroids. In this series of changes, the one step through which all steroids must pass is the conversion of cholesterol to pregnenolone [20]. At this point, the production of the major hormones occurs by different and individual mechanisms.

Transport of Steroid Hormones

After steroid biosynthesis, the steroid hormones are released into the bloodstream to be carried to the tissue cells. In the blood they bind to specific proteins known as *transcortins*, or *corticosteroid-binding globulins (CBG)*, which have an affinity for all major steroids. Binding causes inactivation of the steroid hormones, excretion of the steroid by the kidneys, and prevention of excess tissue uptake. At the target site the steroids are released to exert their physiologic action.

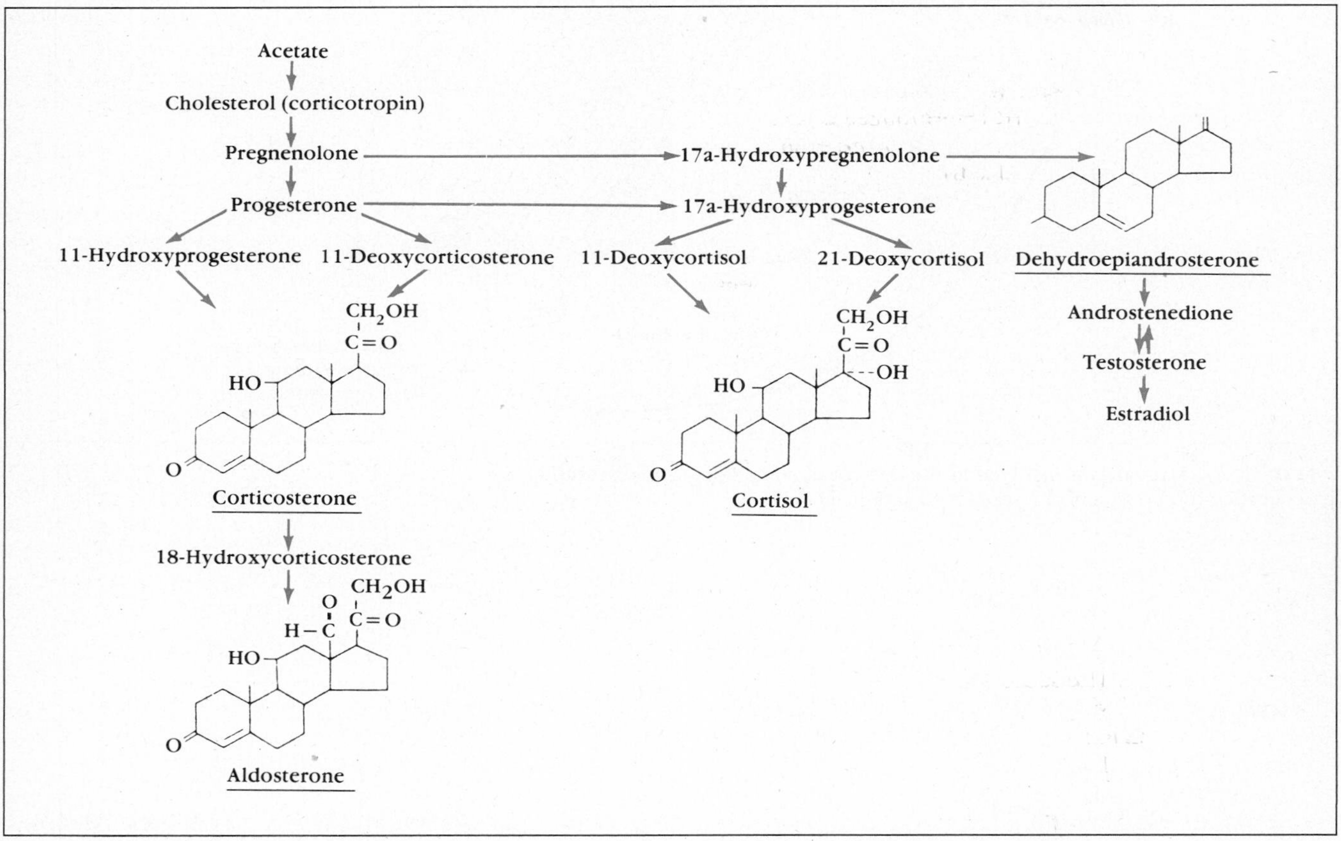

FIGURE 33-3 Formation of adrenocortical hormones. (Reprinted from D. Jensen, *The Principles of Physiology* [2nd ed.]. New York: Appleton-Century-Crofts. Reprinted by permission of Appleton & Lange, Simon & Schuster Professional Information Group, 25 Van Zant St., E. Norwalk, CT 06855.)

Physiologic Actions of Mineralocorticoids

The principal mineralocorticoid that exerts a physiologic action is aldosterone. Almost all mineralocorticoid activity is produced by this steroid, but cortisol contributes slightly. The single most important action of aldosterone is sodium retention. Because of this action and its resultant effect on intracellular and extracellular fluid volume, aldosterone has a profound effect on fluid balance.

Sodium retention results in a simultaneous loss of potassium by excretion in the urine. This exchange of ions takes place in the distal renal tubules. Together with sodium, water is also retained [7]. Thus, higher circulating levels of aldosterone cause sodium retention, increased plasma volume, and higher blood pressure, while decreased circulating levels have opposite effects. Any excess or deficit in normal circulating aldosterone can lead to a variety of basic electrolyte disturbances with resultant effects on body functions.

In addition to the tubules, aldosterone acts on other tissues to retain sodium. Salivary and sweat glands are influenced to conserve sodium in extreme heat. Absorption of sodium by the intestinal mucosa prevents excess loss in fecal waste. Aldosterone also conserves sodium by influencing the exchange of intracellular and extracellular water.

Physiologic Actions of Glucocorticoids

Glucocorticoids are named for their ability to regulate serum glucose levels by several mechanisms. Their effect, however, is not as pronounced or prolonged as that of the regulating ability of insulin. In looking at the total picture of the effects of glucocorticoid activity, the primary action in the tissues is *catabolic*, with increased breakdown of proteins and increased excretion of nitrogen. In the liver, however, *anabolic* actions occur, such as increased amino acid uptake and increased synthesis of RNA and protein.

The activities generated by the glucocorticoids are accomplished by the production and secretion of cortisol. Cortisol is important in the control and metabolism of carbohydrates, lipids, and proteins; also, it assists in metabolic reactions to stress. In greater than physiologic amounts, the effect of cortisol in inflammation and allergies is vital.

The action of cortisol on carbohydrate metabolism may be primarily viewed by its two major effects on glucose production and use. The first major effect of cortisol is to increase the amount of glucose released by enhancing the ability of the liver for gluconeogenesis (glucose production). This is accomplished by stimulating adipose tissue to release free fatty acids, the gluconeogenic substrate needed by the liver. The second major action of cortisol is to decrease the use of glucose by the tissues. In muscle, adipose, and lymphatic tissues, uptake and metabolism are reduced. Through these actions — increased gluconeogenesis and the inhibition of glucose use by tissues — serum glucose concentrations are increased.

By stimulating the release of fatty acids from tissue stores into the plasma, lipids in the form of free fatty acids are made available for energy use. This ability to mobilize fat stores is one of the factors that cause a metabolic alteration in times of stress or deprivation from the use of glucose to the use of fatty acids for energy [6]. It is not understood how cortisol initiates the mobilization of fatty acids, or why fat deposits are removed from one area of the body and deposited in another, as may easily be seen in adrenocortical dysfunction.

The effects of cortisol on protein are twofold. First, it decreases protein stores in all tissues of the body except the liver. This is carried out by preventing the synthesis of protein and by breaking down protein stores in the cells into amino acids. Second, protein synthesis in the liver is stimulated. Amino acids are released into the liver from cell protein catabolism, thereby increasing the amount of amino acids available to the liver for protein synthesis.

The exact mechanism by which cortisol responds to stress is not completely understood, yet it is recognized as being almost essential for survival of the human organism. Any extreme physical or emotional stress may initiate the response, including severe trauma, emotional upset, chronic or debilitating diseases, infection, or extreme temperatures (Fig. 33-4).

Administration of glucocorticoids, specifically cortisol, in larger than normal amounts decreases the inflammatory response to infection or injury. Each step of the process of inflammation is blocked by steroids. Cortisol reduces the passage of water into and out of the cell and decreases the amount of fibrous tissue formation [7]. Also, allergic processes are stopped with the administration of cortisol, which alters the inflammatory process that occurs in response to any allergen. The exact mechanism by which the components of the inflammatory process are blocked is not completely understood, but it is believed to be related to the ability of the glucocorticoids to stabilize cell membranes and prevent rupture of the lysosomes [2].

Cortisol affects the blood cells in a variable manner. The circulating levels of eosinophils and lymphocytes are decreased, while red blood cell and platelet production is increased. Because of the decreased lymphocytes, humoral immunity is decreased and infection may occur [6].

Physiologic Actions of Androgens

Adrenal androgens, or male sex hormones, produced in the adrenal cortex have little physiologic significance in the healthy adult. Some of the androgens produced are converted to testosterone, the major male sex hormone; however, hypersecretion of the cortex can cause the appearance of dramatic masculizing changes as a result of the androgens.

Altered Adrenocortical Function

Adrenocortical Hyperfunction

Cushing's Syndrome. The term *Cushing's syndrome* refers to the clinical manifestations that result from excess glucose production caused by hypersecretion of cortisol from the adrenal cortex. Although clinically similar, three separate factors may cause Cushing's syndrome: (1) adrenal

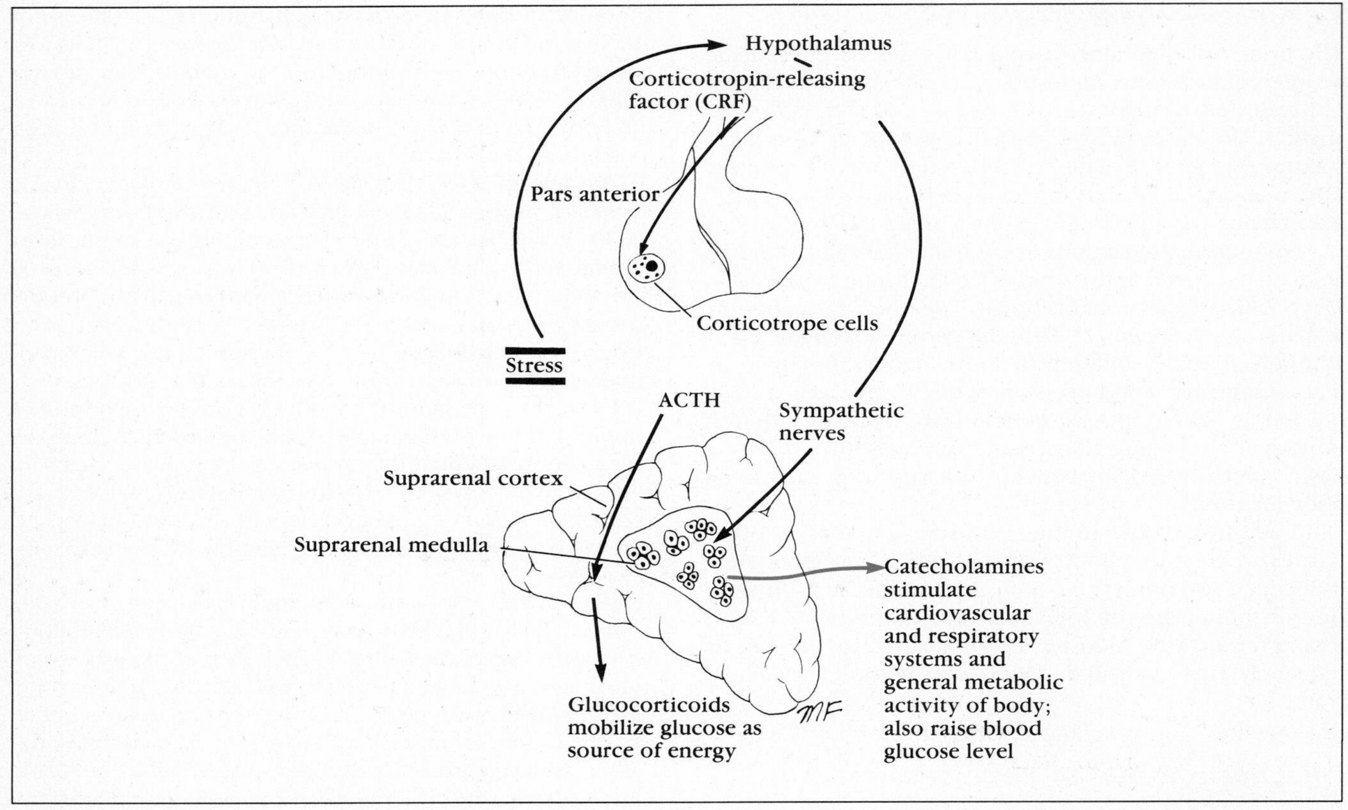

FIGURE 33-4 The effects of stress on the activities of the suprarenal gland.

neoplasms, (2) hypersecretion of ACTH by the anterior pituitary (this condition is called *Cushing's disease*), and (3) ectopic ACTH syndrome [21].

The growth of adrenocortical cells into a tumor that secretes cortisol causes cellular growth and additional secretion of cortisol. As cortisol secretion increases, it is no longer controlled by ACTH. Eventually, cortisol secretion by the neoplasm exceeds that of normal adrenocortical cells, at which point the normal cells may cease producing cortisol altogether. Cortisol-secreting tumors of the adrenal glands rarely secrete excessive androgenic hormones.

In pituitary-dependent Cushing's disease, cortisol oversecretion is caused by excessive release of ACTH from the anterior pituitary gland [11]. This causes increased secretion and release of both cortisol and androgenic hormones. Some authors classify all forms of conditions involving excessive cortisol secretion as Cushing's syndrome [10,15,16].

The third form of Cushing's syndrome occurs from excess production of ACTH by a neoplasm not located in the adrenal gland. This particular form often occurs in persons with oat-cell carcinoma of the lung [19]. Other malignant neoplasms may secrete ACTH, causing this peculiar paraneoplastic syndrome.

In addition to hypersecretion of cortisol, two other factors are apparent in Cushing's syndrome, regardless of etiology. These are the absence of circadian rhythm changes in the release of ACTH and cortisol, and lack of increased ACTH and cortisol secretion in response to stress [5].

With increased cortisol secretion there is an increased rate of gluconeogenesis, resulting in elevated serum glucose levels. Eventually, the islet cells of the pancreas are no longer able to produce sufficient amounts of insulin, and diabetes mellitus results [6]. Loss of protein occurs almost everywhere in the body except the liver. In the muscular system, protein loss results in decreased strength and muscle wasting. Humoral immunity is reduced, decreasing the threshold to infection. Skin tissues lose collagen and become very thin, tearing and bruising easily. In the bones, osteoporosis can cause weakness and actual fractures. Hyperpigmentation may be seen and is due to the melanostimulating properties of ACTH.

In general, the clinical signs and symptoms vary only slightly with the etiology of the disease. Although scattered in the population, Cushing's syndrome is four times more frequent in women than in men; the peak ages affected are 35 to 50 years [7]. Androgens are responsible for a few of the bodily changes, but most of the abnormalities are direct results of hypercortisolism. The three classic manifestations are truncal obesity, purple striae, and round facial features. The frequency of different clinical effects is noted in Table 33-1.

Truncal obesity results from the mobilization of fat in the lower parts of the body to the trunk, causing the abdomen to be greatly protuberant, even as the extremi-

TABLE 33-1 Clinical Effects of Cushing's Syndrome and Their Frequency

Effects	Frequency (%)
Obesity	94
Facial plethora	84
Hirsutism	82
Menstrual disorders	76
Hypertension	72
Muscular weakness	58
Back pain	58
Striae	52
Acne	40
Psychologic symptoms	40
Bruising	36
Congestive heart failure	22
Edema	18
Renal calculi	16
Headache	14
Polyuria/polydipsia	10
Hyperpigmentation	6

Source: Reproduced with permission from P. Felig et al. *Endocrinology and Metabolism* (1st ed.). Copyright © 1981, McGraw-Hill Book Company.

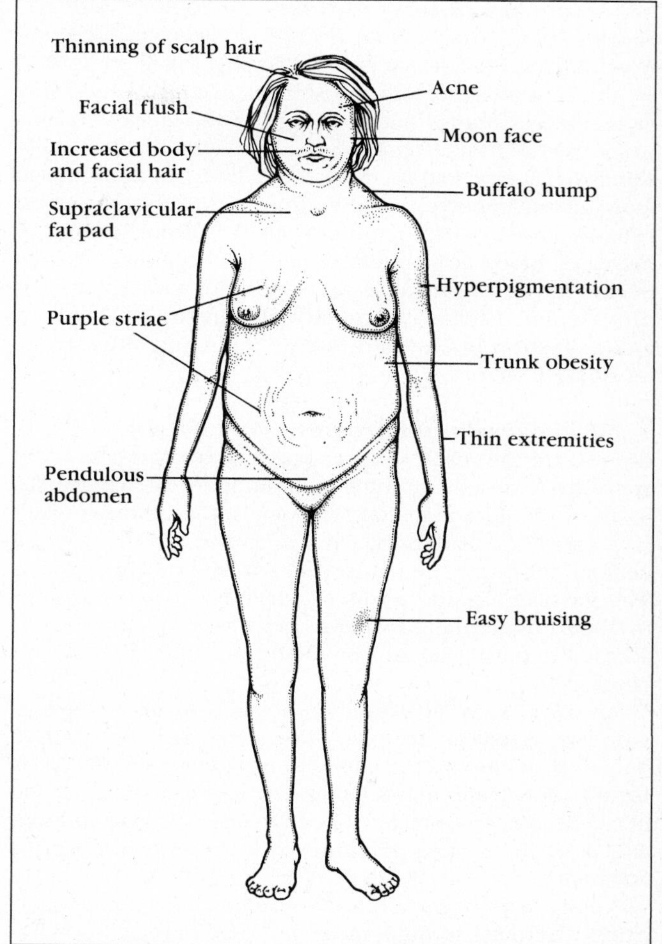

FIGURE 33-5 A composite of symptoms in Cushing's disease. (From M. Beyers and S. Dudas [eds.], *The Clinical Practice of Medical-Surgical Nursing* [2nd ed.]. Boston: Little, Brown, 1984.)

ties become thin and wasted. Often, persons affected with Cushing's syndrome are unable to rise from a squatting position without assistance. The enlarged abdomen is characteristic and may be an extension of thoracic accumulation of fat, the buffalo torso. Fat accumulation around the neck and cervical area is termed the *buffalo hump*. Purple striae appear on the abdomen as a result of the stretching of the abdominal skin when the fat cells are being deposited. They are purple as a result of the collagen deficit in the skin tissues. Round and full facial features, often called moon facies, also result from the hypercortisolism (Fig. 33-5).

Other manifestations also often occur. Excessive androgen secretion results in excess hair growth, often on the face, which is especially prominent in women. Androgen hormones may cause the appearance of acne and oligomenorrhea. Extreme androgen excess may result in coarsening of the voice, recession of the hairline, and hypertrophy of the clitoris. Psychiatric disturbances may surface, with personality alterations or more severe changes. Polyuria may result from hyperglycemia. Varying degrees of hypertension are exhibited, often with the development of left ventricular hypertrophy. The mortality of Cushing's syndrome is 50 percent or greater unless treatment is initiated. Death usually results from severe infection.

When Cushing's syndrome occurs in children, growth ceases. If treatment is not begun before the epiphyses of the bones have sealed, short stature is permanent [21].

Primary Aldosteronism. Primary aldosteronism, also known as *Conn's syndrome*, is the result of excessive and uncontrolled secretion of the mineralocorticoid aldosterone. The usual cause is an adrenocorticol adenoma; rarely, it results from adrenal hyperplasia. Because aldosterone conserves sodium and wastes potassium, the clinical features of this disorder are a direct result of those functions.

The principal features of primary aldosteronism are hypernatremia and hypokalemia. Therefore, this condition may be suspected in any hypertensive patient who concurrently exhibits hypokalemia (less than 3.5 mEq/L). Conservation of sodium leads to retention of water, resulting in increased volume in the extracellular and vascular compartments, which in turn results in arterial hypertension. This condition may resemble hypertension originating from cardiovascular disease.

Loss of potassium may result in a variety of manifestations, depending on the severity of the depletion. The most common result is muscle cramps and weakness. Occasionally, it may progress to tetany and even muscle paralysis as a result of hypokalemia. Changes in the pattern of cardiac conduction may develop.

Alterations in renal function are apparent, as this is the primary site of sodium conservation. Polydipsia, polyuria, and nocturia occur in response to the sodium-induced increased fluid volume and volume-dependent hypertension.

Secondary Aldosteronism. Secondary aldosteronism results from stimulation of aldosterone secretion from outside the adrenal cortex. Usually, this is stimulated by the renin-angiotensin-aldosterone system. Almost any factor decreasing the blood supply to the kidneys results in increased plasma renin levels. Thus, the mechanism is somewhat compensatory: increased renin leads to increased aldosterone secretion and sodium conservation; water retention results from sodium conservation, leading to increased blood flow to vital organs. Edema, however, only occurs in the presence of preexisting or underlying cardiovascular disease. Secondary aldosteronism leads to a combination of elevated plasma renin and aldosterone levels [18].

Adrenogenital Syndromes. The adrenogenital syndromes are the result of adrenocortical overproduction of androgens, caused by tumor or adrenocortical hyperplasia. In all of the adrenogenital syndromes, the ultimate result is the same—virilization. The age and sex of the affected person determine the nature and severity of the disorder. The most common causes of adrenogenital syndromes include congenital adrenal hyperplasia, "postpubertal" adrenal hyperplasia, adrenal adenoma, and adrenal carcinomas [13].

Androgens are ultimately converted to the male hormone testosterone. Testosterone is extremely potent, and only small amounts are required to produce bodily changes. In the adult male, masculizing effects are masked by the production of testosterone from the testes. It is in children and in adult females that the virilization becomes most apparent.

Young boys begin to develop secondary sex characteristics, regardless of their age at the time of onset. Females respond to androgen stimulation with hirsutism, clitoral hypertrophy, and other masculizing effects (Fig. 33-6).

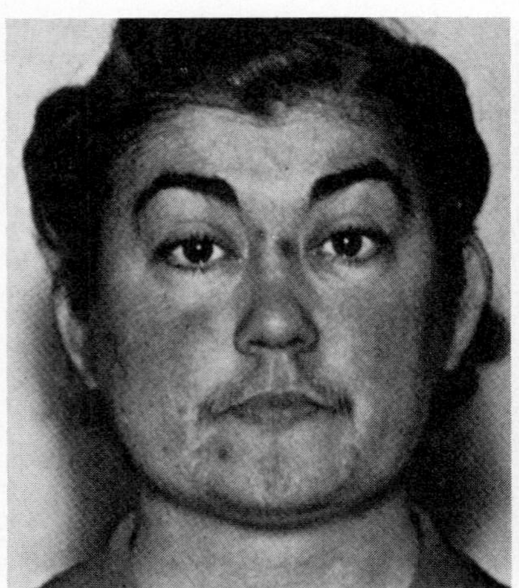

A

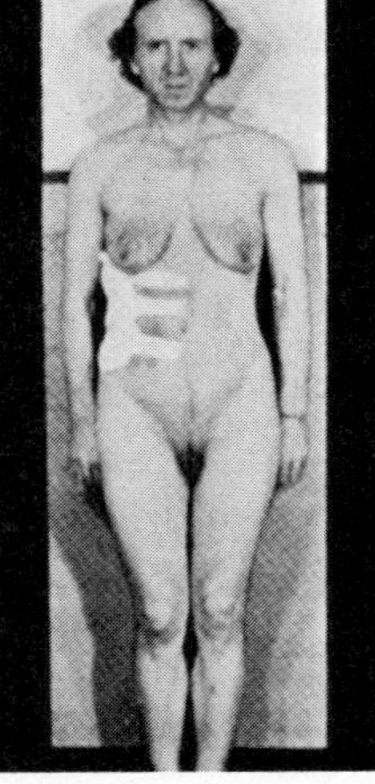

B

FIGURE 33-6 Adrenogenital syndromes of the female. (From J.D. Wilson and D.W. Foster, *Williams' Textbook of Endocrinology* [7th ed.]. Philadelphia: W.B. Saunders Company, 1985. Reprinted by permission.)

Congenital Adrenal Hyperplasia. This is one of the most common adrenogenital syndromes and results from a congenital deficiency in the enzymes causing adrenocortical biosynthesis. Its incidence is estimated to be 1 in 50,000 births in the United States [3]. There is not an absence of the enzymes, but an error in metabolism pathways of steroid production. The appearance of clinical manifestations is dependent on the point at which synthesis of cortisol, aldosterone, and androgens is blocked. There may be clinical signs and symptoms either of glucocorticoid or mineralocorticoid deficiency or excess. Also, androgen excess and virilization, or sexual ambiguity and infantism may occur. For example, in the most frequently encountered of these conditions, a defect in 21-hydroxylase, excessive androgen production in the female fetus may cause the external genitalia to resemble those of a male, while internal structures—uterus, ovaries, and fallopian tubes—are normal and functional. Male children have the infant Hercules appearance [14].

Adrenocortical Hypofunction

Primary Adrenocortical Insufficiency. Also known as Addison's disease, primary adrenocortical hypofunction results from insufficient secretion of adrenocortical hormones due to insidious and profound destruction in the adrenal glands. It is not a common disorder and becomes evident only if 90 percent of the functioning adrenocortical cells have been destroyed [18]. The two major causes of adrenal destruction resulting in this condition are idiopathic atrophy (80%) and tuberculosis (20%) [5]. Idiopathic atrophy has been attributed to an autoimmune disorder, with adrenal autoantibodies present in many affected persons [4]. In areas where tuberculosis is poorly controlled, the frequency of Addison's disease is high. It is interesting to note that in disease of tubercular origin, men are usually affected, whereas in idiopathic atrophy women are affected more frequently [5].

Clinical manifestations depend on the degree of hormonal deficiency. Changes in the skin are usually the most dramatic; they occur in about 98 percent of affected persons and help to diagnose the primary (adrenocortical) insufficiency [18]. Skin color changes result from increased ACTH, which is uninhibited by steroid response from the adrenal cortex. Areas of hyperpigmentation become visible because the pituitary increases the production of ACTH in an attempt to compensate, and ACTH also has melanostimulating properties. These darkened areas are especially visible in the body areas most exposed to light, pressure areas, hand creases, and buccal mucosa [14]. Areas of vitiligo (pale patches surrounded by excess pigmentation) are also apparent. Muscular weakness and fatigue commonly occur.

Many individuals experience hypotension as a result of volume depletion. Sodium and potassium retention results in depletion of extracellular volume, which in turn causes decreased cardiac output and decreased blood pressure [12]. Hypoglycemia can also result from the decrease in gluconeogenesis caused by the reduction in cortisol levels. Nausea, vomiting, weight loss, and diarrhea are the most common gastrointestinal disturbances. Other body changes include loss of hair, decreased sexual function, and mental disturbances ranging from mild neuroses to deep depressions [12]. Because the symptoms are often vague, and the disease onset insidious, the potential for adrenocortical insufficiency should be evaluated in any person who is seriously ill without a specific identifiable cause [20].

It has been reported with increasing frequency that other physiologic disorders may be associated with primary adrenocortical insufficiency. This association has been called *Schmidt's syndrome*, which refers to autoimmune endocrine failure together with polyglandular failure [5,21]. Disorders that may be associated include gonadal failure, thyroid dysfunction, diabetes mellitus, hypoparathyroidism, and pernicious anemia.

Adrenal Crisis. Adrenal crisis (Addisonian crisis, acute adrenal insufficiency) usually occurs because of a sudden decrease or absence of adrenocortical hormones. It may affect persons with both treated and undiagnosed Addison's disease in which the individuals are exposed to major stresses, such as trauma, infection, surgery, or severe illness. Affected persons may develop severe dehydration due to nausea and vomiting. Weakness, confusion, and hypovolemic shock are also associated [21]. Immediate intervention is necessary or death will ensue rapidly. The cause of the crisis is not completely understood, but it may be due to primary disease in the adrenal gland itself, such as hemorrhage, infection, or infarction [17].

Secondary Adrenocortical Insufficiency. Secondary adrenocortical insufficiency results from decreased cortisol secretion due to atrophy of the adrenal cortex. The disorder is a result of decreased ACTH secretion caused by pituitary or hypothalamic disease or by therapeutic pharmacologic doses of glucocorticoids. Mineralocorticoid secretion is usually not affected. Clinically, the features may resemble those of primary insufficiency, except for the absence of hyperpigmentation. The most common cause of secondary adrenocortical insufficiency is acute withdrawal of exogenous steroid therapy [16]. When a person is receiving steroid therapy, slow tapering off is required to allow the adrenal glands to return to active production of their own corticosteroids.

The Adrenal Medulla

Catecholamines

The most important human catecholamines are epinephrine, norepinephrine, and dopamine, which are synthesized in the brain, sympathetic nerve endings, and chromaffin tissues. The adrenal medulla produces and secretes the catecholamines epinephrine (adrenalin) and norepinephrine (noradrenalin) from the chromaffin cells of the medulla. As related to these two catecholamines, the adrenal medulla functions as a part of the autonomic nervous system [14]. These cells stain readily with chromium salts and secrete adrenalin. Adrenal medullary secretion is approximately 80 percent epinephrine and 20 percent norepinephrine [6].

Epinephrine exerts its greatest effect on the heart, increasing both rate and contractility. It is a potent mediator of the metabolic rate. Norepinephrine, on the other hand, is secreted both by the adrenal medulla and the sympathetic nerve terminals. It exerts its greatest influence on the arterioles, causing vasoconstriction that leads to increased blood pressure. Stimulation of the sympathetic nervous system (SNS) causes both direct SNS effects and release of the adrenal medullary hormones.

Catecholamine Biosynthesis and Storage. The precursor for catecholamine biosynthesis is tyrosine. Through the processes of hydroxylation, decarboxylation, and methylation, tyrosine yields norepinephrine and, ultimately, epinephrine (Fig. 33-7). The sequence of the process is as follows [5,20]:

tyrosine → dihydroxyphenylaline (dopa)
→ dopamine (DA)
→ norepinephrine (NE) → epinephrine (E).

It is thought that the tyrosine hydroxylase reaction is the slowest enzymatic conversion, and that this is probably the factor that controls the rate of catecholamine production [4].

Catecholamine is stored by subcellular particles, called granules, which are present in most adrenomedullary cells in the chromaffin granules.

Catecholamine Secretion. Catecholamines may be released with acetylcholine stimulation of calcium passage into the chromaffin granules and subsequent liberation into the extracellular fluid [4,5]. As the adrenal medulla produces the major portion of circulating epinephrine, a small amount is released into the bloodstream almost continuously. Norepinephrine is primarily produced by the sympathetic ganglion cells. Release of large amounts of catecholamines occurs after SNS stimulation. Other substances and conditions that may stimulate the release of epinephrine and norepinephrine include serotonin, bradykinin, exercise, hypovolemia, glucagon, and hypoglycemia [10]. Catecholamines participate in metabolic processes together with insulin and glucagon [21]. The action of the catecholamines is opposite that of insulin and similar to that of glucagon, such that it is the interaction that is important.

Extremely stressful situations cause a massive release of epinephrine and norepinephrine, which results in the fight-or-flight syndrome. This enables the body to react effectively to any severe hazard or threat to survival. Physiologic response to this massive release of epinephrine includes increased blood pressure and heart rate, pupil dilatation, decreased peristalsis, and circulatory constriction in all major organ systems except the muscular and cardiovascular. The response to norepinephrine stimulation is similar, but with the major action being increased arterial blood pressure, a result of vigorous vasoconstric-

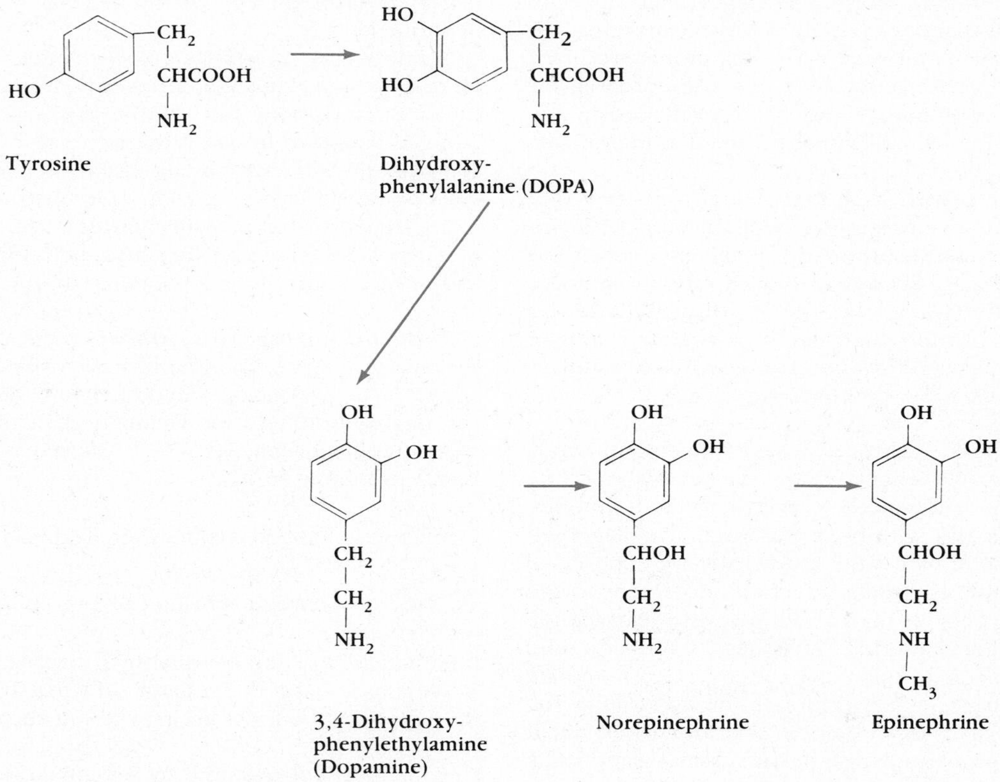

Tyrosine → Dihydroxyphenylalanine (DOPA) → 3,4-Dihydroxyphenylethylamine (Dopamine) → Norepinephrine → Epinephrine

FIGURE 33-7 Steps in the synthesis of norepinephrine and epinephrine from tyrosine. (From I. Danishefsky, *Biochemistry for Medical Sciences*. Boston: Little, Brown, 1980.)

tion. These responses are apparently normal catecholamine actions that are accelerated to meet the unusual and immediate cellular demands [20].

Altered Function of the Adrenal Medulla

The only significant disorders of altered function of the adrenal medulla are neoplasms. The gland itself is not considered necessary for life, as the body has other sources of catecholamines. The presence of a *pheochromocytoma* in the adrenal medulla produces apparent states of hyperfunction of the adrenomedullary catecholamines.

Pheochromocytoma. Pheochromocytomas are rare tumors of the adrenal medulla whose primary clinical manifestation is hypertension. Pheochromocytomas originate in the chromaffin cells of the medulla.

During fetal life, the chromaffin cells are widespread in the developing body, and their function is associated with the sympathetic ganglia. After birth, most of these cells disappear. Those remaining cluster in the adrenal medulla. While 95 percent of all functioning chromaffin tumors are located in the adrenal medulla, others have been found in chromaffin cells in the chest, neck, and abdomen [4].

Pheochromocytomas occur in either sex, usually between ages 25 and 50 years. Children are rarely affected. It is not uncommon for this disorder to affect more than one member of the same family. The tumors are usually benign and bilateral, but a small percentage are malignant with metastasis. Tumors are usually well encapsulated and extremely vascular. Because of their high vascularity, rupture can cause massive hemorrhage that can be fatal [8]. In a few afflicted persons the actual tumors may be palpable.

The pheochromocytoma produces and secretes excessive quantities of epinephrine and norepinephrine into the bloodstream, resulting in clinical manifestations of catecholamine excess. Therefore, the individual remains in an accelerated state of response similar to the fight-or-flight response. Symptoms may occur spontaneously or may be induced with increased physical or emotional activity or stress [10].

The primary finding is systemic arterial hypertension. Elevated blood pressure may be sustained or intermittent, mild or malignant, depending on the rate and amount of catecholamine secreted. Most pheochromocytomas secrete a greater amount of norepinephrine, which is then responsible for the hypertension [8]. Together with this, the smaller amounts of epinephrine produced are responsible for the myocardial side effects. Sustained elevation of catecholamine secretion can lead to cardiomegaly, left ventricular failure, cardiomyopathy, and ultimately, death due to heart failure. Cardiac dysrhythmias may also be observed.

Other metabolic effects include excessive perspiration, palpitations, headaches, hyperventilation, and flushing. Increased frequency of neurofibromatosis, a familial disorder, has been associated with pheochromocytoma.

Multiple Endocrine Neoplasia. Pheochromocytomas may also be associated with a disorder known as multiple endocrine neoplasia syndrome (MEN) (see Chap. 35). This complicated group of disorders is termed multiple because of the multicentricity and bilateral growth of the tumors, as well as the involvement of several glands [10]. One of the important aspects concerning the association of symptoms is that 85 percent of persons with either familial or sporadic pheochromocytomas who also have medullarthyroid carcinomas are normotensive, whereas over 60 percent of persons with familial or sporadic pheochromocytomas not associated with medullary carcinoma have chronic hypertension [21].

Study Questions

1. Outline the normal feedback system for the regulation of glucocorticoids and mineralocorticoids from the adrenal glands.
2. Describe the systemic effects of Cushing's syndrome.
3. How does long-term administration of corticosteroids cause adrenocortical insufficiency?
4. Why is the adrenal gland essential to life?
5. How are catecholamines synthesized and regulated?
6. Describe the main manifestations of pheochromocytoma.

References

1. Carrieri, V.K., Lindsey, A.M., and West, C.M. *Pathophysiological Phenomena in Nursing: Human Responses to Illness*. Philadelphia: Saunders, 1986.
2. Chaffee, E.E., and Lytle, I.M. *Basic Physiology and Anatomy* (4th ed.). Philadelphia: Lippincott, 1980.
3. Dillon, R.S. *Handbook of Endocrinology* (2nd ed.). Philadelphia: Lea & Febiger, 1980.
4. Ezrin, C., Godden, J.O., and Volpe, R. *Systematic Endocrinology* (2nd ed.). Hagerstown, Md.: Harper & Row, 1979.
5. Felig, P., et al. *Endocrinology and Metabolism*. New York: McGraw-Hill, 1981.
6. Guyton, A.C. *Textbook of Medical Physiology* (7th ed.). Philadelphia: Saunders, 1986.
7. Hall, R., Anderson, J., and Besser, M. *Fundamentals of Clinical Endocrinology*. Chicago: Yearbook, 1980.
8. Harris, R.B., and Dela Roca, R.R. Pheochromocytoma: A medical review. *Heart Lung* 13(1):73, 1984.
9. Jeffries, W.M. *Safe Uses of Cortisone*. Springfield, Ill.: Thomas, 1981.
10. Jubiz, W. *Endocrinology: A Logical Approach for Clinicians* (2nd ed.). New York: McGraw-Hill, 1985.
11. Kohler, P. O. Diseases of the hypothalamus and anterior pituitary. In R. G. Petersdorf et al. (eds.), *Harrison's Principles of Internal Medicine* (10th ed.). New York: McGraw-Hill, 1983.
12. Larson, C.A. The critical path of adrenocortical insufficiency. *Nurs. 84* 14(10): 66, 1984.
13. Longcope, C. Adrenogenital syndrome. *Hospital Medicine* 20:4, 1984.
14. Marsden, P., and McCullagh, A.G. *Endocrinology*. Littleton, Mass.: PSG Publishing Co., 1985.
15. Mazzaferri, E.L. *Textbook of Endocrinology* (3rd ed.). New Hyde Park, N.Y.: Medical Examination, 1986.
16. Metz, R., and Larson, E.B. *Blue Book of Endocrinology*. Philadelphia: Saunders, 1985.
17. Richelin, S.D. Neuroendocrinology. In J.D. Wilson and D.W. Foster (eds.), *Williams' Textbook of Endocrinology* (7th ed.). Philadelphia: Saunders, 1985.
18. Robbins, S.L., Cotran, R.S., and Kumar, V. *Pathologic Basis of Disease* (3rd ed.). Philadelphia: Saunders, 1984.
19. Sodeman, W.A., and Sodeman, T.M. *Sodeman's Pathologic Physiology: Mechanisms of Disease* (7th ed.). Philadelphia: Saunders, 1985.
20. Williams, G.H., and Dluhy, R.G. Diseases of the adrenal cortex. In E. Braunwald et al. (eds.), *Harrison's Principles of Internal Medicine* (11th ed.). New York: McGraw-Hill, 1987.
21. Wilson, J.D., and D.W. Foster (eds.). *Williams' Textbook of Endocrinology* (7th ed.). Philadelphia: Saunders, 1985.

CHAPTER 34

Thyroid and Parathyroid Functions and Alterations

CHAPTER OUTLINE

Anatomy of the Thyroid Gland
Physiology of the Thyroid Gland
- Thyroid Iodide Pump
- Structure and Storage of Thyroid Hormones
- Release and Transport of Thyroid Hormones

Calcitonin: Formation and Function
Functions of the Thyroid Hormones
- Physiologic Effects on Metabolic Processes
- Physiologic Effects on Protein Metabolism
- Physiologic Effects on Carbohydrate Metabolism
- Physiologic Effects on Lipid Metabolism
- Physiologic Effects on Vitamin Metabolism

Altered Thyroid Function
- Goiter
- Hyperthyroidism
  - *Clinical Manifestations of Hyperthyroidism*
  - *Thyroid Storm*
  - *Graves' Disease*
  - *Toxic Multinodular Goiter*
  - *Toxic Adenoma*
- Hypothyroidism
  - *Clinical Manifestations*
  - *Cretinism*
  - *Endemic Goiter*
  - *Adult Hypothyroidism*
  - *Sick Euthyroid Syndrome*
  - *Myxedema Coma*
  - *Chronic Autoimmune Thyroiditis*
  - *Nontoxic Goiter*
- Malignant Thyroid Tumors
  - *Papillary Carcinoma*
  - *Follicular Carcinoma*
  - *Anaplastic Carcinoma*
  - *Parafollicular Carcinoma*

The Parathyroid Glands
- Anatomy
- Function
  - *Effect of Parathyroid Hormone on Bone Resorption*
  - *Effect of Parathyroid Hormone on Kidney Resorption*
  - *Effect of Parathyroid Hormone on Intestinal Resorption*

Altered Function of the Parathyroid Glands
- Hypoparathyroidism
  - *Clinical Manifestations*
  - *Idiopathic Hypoparathyroidism*
  - *Postoperative Hypoparathyroidism*
  - *Pseudohypoparathyroidism*
- Hyperparathyroidism
  - *Primary Hyperparathyroidism*
  - *Secondary Hyperparathyroidism*
  - *Tertiary Hyperparathyroidism*

LEARNING OBJECTIVES

1. Describe the normal anatomy of the thyroid gland.
2. Explain the process by which the thyroid hormones are formed.
3. Identify the function of the iodide pump.
4. Describe the mechanism for releasing and transporting the thyroid hormones.
5. Describe the function of calcitonin.
6. Describe the effects of the thyroid hormones on metabolic processes, carbohydrate metabolism, and vitamin metabolism.
7. Define *goiter*.
8. Identify the clinical manifestations of hyperthyroidism.
9. Outline the autoimmune component of Graves' disease.
10. Relate the signs and symptoms of Graves' disease to underlying pathophysiology.
11. Differentiate between toxic multinodular goiter and toxic adenoma.
12. Identify the clinical manifestations of hypothyroidism.
13. Identify the cause of cretinism.
14. Describe the physical changes and underlying causes of adult hypothyroidism.
15. Differentiate adult hypothyroidism and sick euthyroid syndrome.
16. Compare thyrotoxic crisis and myxedema coma.
17. Identify the common element in chronic autoimmune thyroiditis.
18. Differentiate the etiology and symptoms of each of the thyroid carcinomas.
19. Describe the normal anatomy of the parathyroid glands.
20. List the effects of parathyroid hormone.
21. Explain the importance of thyrocalcitonin to the parathyroid glands.
22. Describe hypoparathyroidism.
23. Identify the two major causes of hyperparathyroidism.
24. Differentiate between pseudohypoparathyroidism and pseudopseudohypoparathyroidism.
25. Compare the effects of primary, secondary, and tertiary hyperparathyroidism.

The thyroid gland is primarily responsible for controlling the rate of metabolic processes in the body. The parathyroid glands control calcium levels and bone resorption. These two glands are related by proximity and, as recently discovered, by function. In this chapter normal structure and physiology are explored and the major disorders of these glands examined.

Anatomy of the Thyroid Gland

The thyroid gland is the second largest endocrine gland in the human body and its primary function is to regulate and control the rate of metabolism. The thyroid is located in the anterior neck, between the larynx and the trachea (Fig. 34-1). In the normal thyroid, two lobes lie slightly lateral to the trachea, one on either side, and are connected by a thin band of tissue known as an isthmus. Generally, the isthmus lies just below the cricoid cartilage of the trachea. Characteristically, the superior portion of each lobe is somewhat pointed, while the inferior portion is rounded and blunt.

The thyroid is reddish and beefy in appearance and has a rubbery texture on palpation. In the average adult, the gland weighs 20 to 30 gm. It is enclosed in two layers of connective tissue, with the outer layer being continuous with the cervical fascia of the neck and the inner layer of connective tissue closely adhering to the gland itself [7].

Thyroid tissue originally develops from the oral epithelium. In an adult, the foramen cecum, a depression on the dorsum of the tongue, points to the location from which

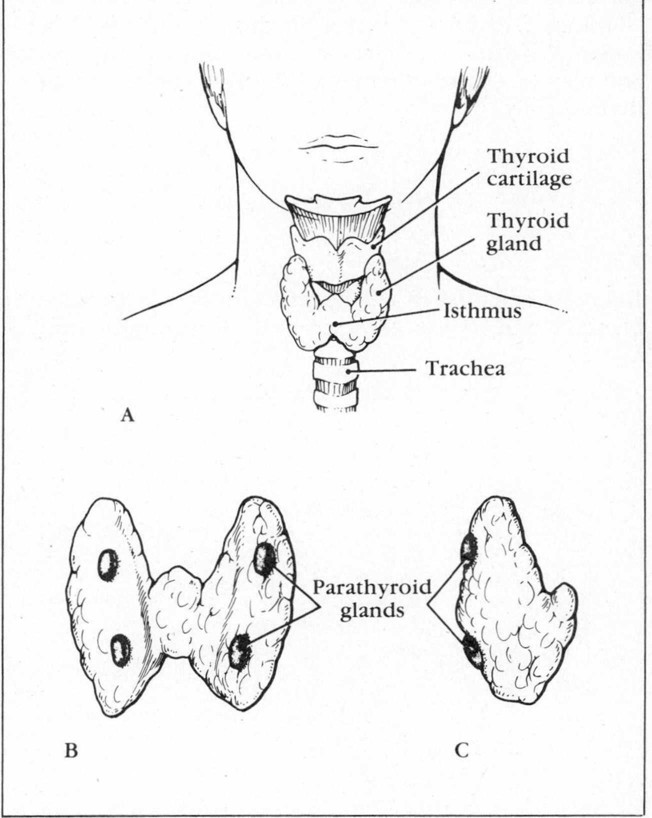

FIGURE 34-1 The thyroid gland. A. Anterior view. B. Posterior view showing parathyroid glands. C. Lateral view.

thyroid tissue evolved. Rarely, a connecting duct that connects the thyroid and the foramen cecum may remain. This is known as the *thyroglossal duct*.

Blood supply to the thyroid arises from two main pairs of arteries. Branching from the external carotid arteries, the superior thyroid arteries enter and supply the upper portions of the lobes. The inferior thyroid arteries, arising from the subclavian arteries, supply the lower portion of the lobes. It is estimated that 4 to 6 liters of blood per hour circulate through the thyroid.

Nervous system control is accomplished primarily from the second to fifth thoracic spinal nerves and through the superior and middle ganglia of the thoracolumbar nervous system controls. Cervical ganglia provide the thyroid with adrenergic stimulation, while the vagus nerve provides cholinergic stimulation.

The body of the thyroid is composed of a mass of tiny follicles that are all approximately of equal size (Fig. 34-2). These follicles, or sacs, are each in effect separately functioning glands the size of a pinhead. The iodine-accumulating function of each follicle is directly proportional to its individual surface area [19]. Although the sacs do not have outside openings, rich vascular, lymph, and nervous networks surround them, exchanging iodine for hormones. The follicles have a single-layer epithelial lining, and an amorphous, secretory fluid, colloid, fills each sac. The primary component of colloid is a large protein molecule called *thyroglobulin*, from which the thyroid hormones are released.

Another distinct cell type in the thyroid gland is the *parafollicular* cell. It has an ovoid and irregular shape and may be scattered among the other, more numerous thyroid cells.

Physiology of the Thyroid Gland

Thyroid Iodide Pump

Iodide is essential to the normal function of the thyroid gland. When iodide enters the body through eating or drinking, it is rapidly absorbed into the bloodstream from the gastrointestinal tract within about an hour. Circulating in the blood, iodide is competed for by the thyroid and the kidneys. Approximately two-thirds of the iodide circulating in the bloodstream is excreted in urine, and the remaining one-third is selectively removed from the blood by the thyroid.

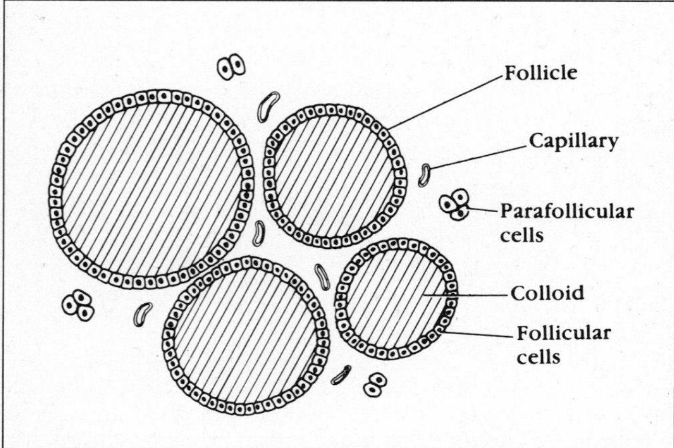

FIGURE 34-2 Follicles of thyroid gland showing colloid filling each sac.

Removal of iodide from the circulation is accomplished by means of an iodide pump or trap. Thyroid-stimulating hormone enhances and is most influential in iodide transport, although other factors also affect the mechanism [19]. Normally, the iodide pump is able to concentrate iodide to about 25 times greater than the concentration in the blood, but at those times when the thyroid gland becomes maximally active, the concentration can increase to as high as 350 times greater than blood concentration [5]. Once iodide is taken into the thyroid cell, it is oxidized to iodine [13].

To prevent a basic iodine deficiency, sufficient intake is necessary. Ingested quantities of iodine vary, depending on the natural content in the soil and water in any given environment, and on the intake of iodine-enriched salt and foods. Ordinary table salt contains 1 part sodium iodide to 100,000 parts of sodium chloride.

Structure and Storage of Thyroid Hormones

The thyroid iodide trap is an active, energy-requiring mechanism. At the beginning of this process, iodine is removed from the circulation in the form of sodium or potassium iodide. It then passes through the follicular cells and into the colloid. The thyroglobulin molecules in the colloid contain an active amino acid, tyrosine, which combines with the iodine in the process of forming the thyroid hormones.

Iodine ions must first undergo a change to an active, elemental form of iodine. This occurs under the influence of the enzyme *perioxidase*. Once iodine is in a simple form, it is able to combine with the tyrosine ring. Active iodine attaches itself to the 3 position of the tyrosine ring to form the molecule *monoiodotyrosine* (MIT). After the formation of MIT, the 5 position of the tyrosine ring becomes iodized. This structure becomes diiodotyrosine (DIT) (Fig. 34-3).

Two separate combinations of these molecules form the two main thyroid hormones. When two DIT molecules fuse in a coupling reaction, thyroxine (T_4) is formed. The fusion of molecules of MIT and DIT form triiodothyronine (T_3). Nearly 10 times more thyroxine than triiodothyronine is secreted from the thyroid gland but, as it circulates, some of the thyroxine deiodinates, making 2 to 3 times as much available to the tissues. Triiodothyronine is 3 to 5 times more active than thyroxine, but the duration of thyroxine is 3 to 5 times longer. Thus, the overall effect of both hormones is similar, and their functions appear to be identical [13].

These thyroid hormones are stored in the follicular colloid as a part of the thyroglobulin molecule. The thyroid gland is unique in its ability to store hormones in the thyroglobulin molecule. Colloid in the normal thyroid is pri-

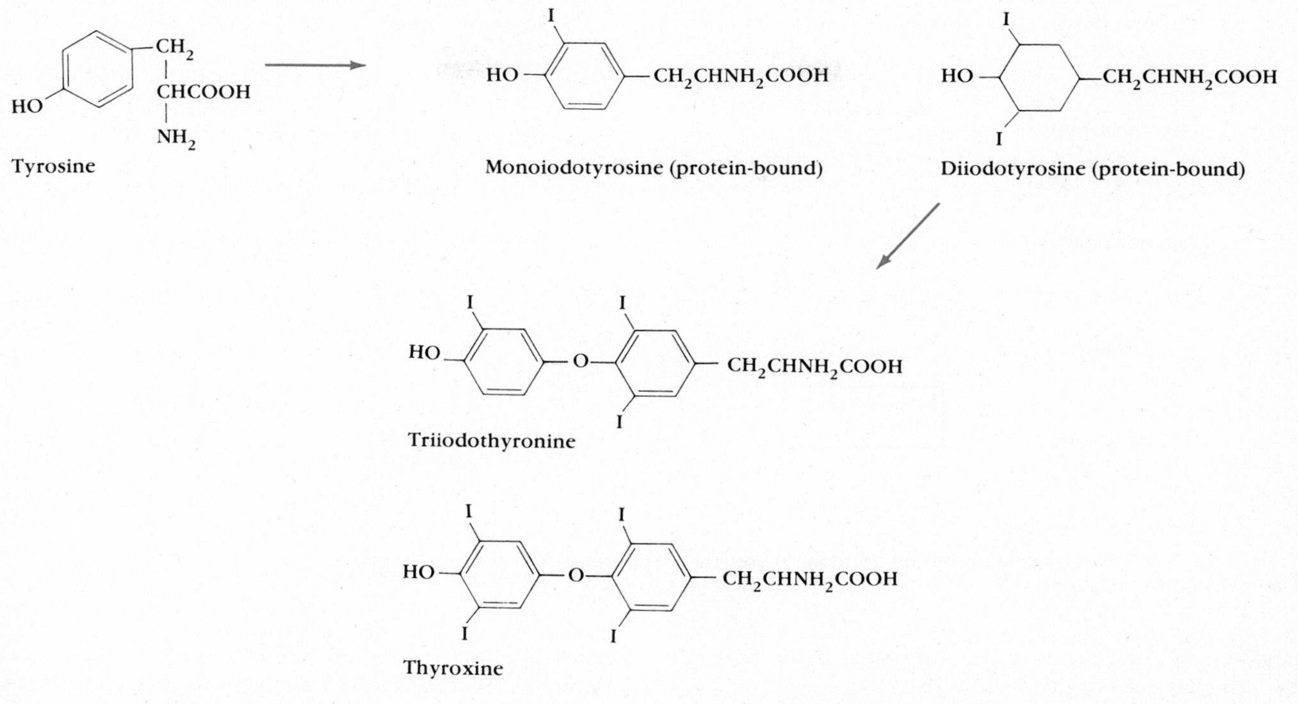

FIGURE 34-3 Tyrosine, and compounds formed by its iodination in the thyroid gland, including the thyroid hormones triiodothyronine and thyroxine.

marily composed of thyroglobulin molecules. In effect, this is a storage mechanism, which functions if synthesis of the thyroid hormones should cease.

Release and Transport of Thyroid Hormones

The thyroid hormones are regulated through an extremely complex interaction. The hypothalamus, pituitary, and thyroid glands are a part of the interaction, which is further controlled by higher centers in the brain. The major regulator of thyroid hormone secretion is thyroid-stimulating hormone (TSH or thyrotropin), which is a glycoprotein hormone secreted by the anterior pituitary gland. It is thought to be responsive to very slight changes in thyroid hormone levels [16]. The release of TSH is mediated by the thyroid-releasing factor (TRH) from the hypothalamus. This factor stimulates the synthesis and release of TSH. Thyroid hormones inhibit these functions, thereby exerting influence on the feedback regulation of TSH secretion. The relationship of TRH, TSH, and the thyroid hormones exists as a feedback system (Fig. 34-4). Whenever T_3 and T_4 levels become too low in the circulating bloodstream, TRH triggers the release of TSH to increase the secretion of T_3 and T_4. It accomplishes this by increasing all of the known activities of the thyroid gland cells [5]. As the blood levels of T_3 and T_4 begin to rise, the anterior pituitary decreases secretion of TSH, thereby decreasing the rate of thyroid hormone production. Thyroid-stimulating hormone stimulates an increase in the size and number of the follicular cells, thereby increasing their ability to absorb iodide [8]. It also increases the breakdown of thyroglobulin, releasing thyroxine and triiodothyronine hormones from the thyroid gland. Through these mechanisms, adequate levels of hormones are maintained in the bloodstream at all times.

When the hormones are needed, an enzymatic reaction splits the thyroglobulin molecule and frees the hormones for entry into the bloodstream. In the blood, thyroxine and triiodothyronine immediately combine with circulating plasma proteins. The affinity of circulating hormones and proteins is so great that the hormones are released to the tissue cells very slowly. As the hormones enter the cells, both thyroxine and triiodothyronine bind with intracellular proteins where they are again stored. They are then inside tissue cells and are available to nourish those cells. The hormones have a direct effect on the mitochondria of the cells, resulting in an increased total number and an increased concentration of oxidative enzymes [8,13]. Through these actions, the hormones directly influence cell metabolism and metabolic rate. The thyroid hormones are used within several days to several weeks.

Calcitonin: Formation and Function

In the 1960s another thyroid hormone, ***calcitonin***, was discovered. Its formation and mechanisms of action are so different that it must be considered separately from thyroxine and triiodothyronine. Calcitonin is a large polypeptide containing 32 amino acids. It is synthesized in the

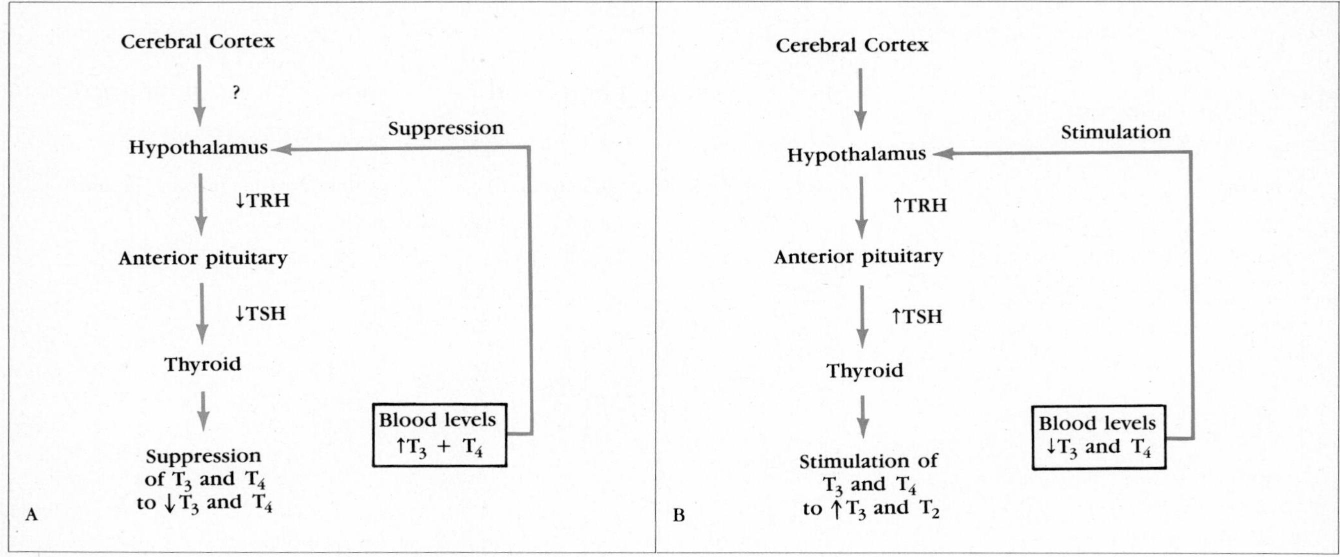

FIGURE 34-4 Feedback system of thyroid hormone secretion. A. Suppression to decrease levels. B. Stimulation to increase levels.

parafollicular, or C, cells of the interstitial tissue between the follicular cells of the thyroid [5].

Calcitonin has a direct effect on bone tissue by counteracting hypercalcemia. Increased serum calcium levels stimulate the release of this hormone from the thyroid gland. Once released, it inhibits bone resorption, thus inhibiting the rate of release of calcium from bone tissue to plasma. This process causes a reduction in blood calcium levels. The action of calcitonin is essentially the reverse action of the parathyroid hormone (see p. 525). Whereas the action of parathyroid hormone is long-acting and continually maintains constant levels of circulating calcium, calcitonin only begins to act when there is excess calcium in the blood. It does not block parathyroid hormone or prevent its release. Calcitonin merely exerts an opposite action on both bone and kidneys. Bone resorption by osteoclasts is inhibited, and in response to calcitonin, the loop of Henle allows calcium to be filtered out and excreted in urine.

Functions of the Thyroid Hormones

Physiologic Effects on Metabolic Processes

Because the thyroid hormones are carried to all body tissues, their effects are widespread and varied. They exert influence over all major body systems, as well as the most intricate of cell functions. Their major influence is to increase basal metabolic rate (BMR), which is heat production and energy expenditure in the body. A test to measure BMR is actually a measurement of oxygen consumption. Several nonthyroid factors can affect the usefulness of this test.

The basal metabolic rate rises during periods of increased hormone production and secretion, thus increasing energy expenditure and heat production. When this occurs, the effect of *calorigenesis*, the use of food for energy, is also increased. The process of calorigenesis increases the consumption of oxygen by the body.

Physiologic Effects on Protein Metabolism

The thyroid hormones increase protein synthesis and thus are essential for normal growth and development in children and young adults. When fat and carbohydrate stores have been depleted, proteins may be used for energy. This protein depletion results in a negative nitrogen balance. It is not clear whether this is a direct result of the thyroid hormone or due to a negative caloric balance [19]. Releasing proteins also releases amino acids, making them available for energy, and increases the rate of gluconeogenesis.

Physiologic Effects on Carbohydrate Metabolism

Thyroid hormones affect virtually every function of carbohydrate metabolism. They are responsible for increasing the rate of gluconeogenesis, rapid cellular uptake of glucose, increasing intestinal absorption of glucose and galactose, and increasing the rate of glucose uptake by adipose tissue.

Especially in carbohydrate metabolism, thyroid hormones are interactive with, or dependent on, other hormones. Insulin secretion is increased, which also enhances carbohydrate metabolism.

Physiologic Effects on Lipid Metabolism

Thyroid hormones essentially stimulate all aspects of lipid or fatty metabolism. The major result of their influence is depletion of fat storage, especially of lipids. This leads to increased plasma concentration levels of free fatty acids. Serum cholesterol, however, is lowered by the action of thyroid hormones, probably due to increased intestinal excretion and conversion of cholesterol into bile acids.

Physiologic Effects on Vitamin Metabolism

Because thyroid hormones increase the rate of metabolic processes, they increase the physiologic need for vitamins. As many vitamins contain enzymes or coenzymes, increased secretion of thyroid hormones causes depletion of vitamins due to the liberation of enzymes, unless the intake of vitamins by ingestion is increased.

Altered Thyroid Function

Goiter

The presence of a goiter, or enlarged thyroid gland, is not necessarily indicative of thyroid dysfunction, but may demonstrate insufficient iodine intake [13]. Goiters may appear in states of hypofunction as well as hyperfunction [13]. The gland enlarges in an attempt to produce sufficient amounts of thyroid hormones. Various types of disorders can alter the size and state of the thyroid (Fig. 34-5). Without the presence of identifiable clinical manifestations, an enlarged thyroid gland is referred to as a *nontoxic goiter*.

Hyperthyroidism

Hyperthyroidism, also known as *thyrotoxicosis*, is characterized by increased T_3 and T_4 production, often 5 to 15 times normal rates, resulting in an excess amount of thyroid hormones that are circulated to the tissues. Hyperthyroidism may be related entirely to disease of the thyroid, or it may originate from outside the thyroid. It may be permanent or temporary, mild or severe. The severity of the disease may be affected by the person's age, duration of hyperthyroid function, and presence of other disease processes in any other organ system. Thirty to 40 percent of all cases of thyrotoxicosis occur in persons over age 60 years [10].

Because of the increased amount of thyroid hormones reaching the cells, all metabolic activities are accelerated. Thus, basal metabolic rate rises, energy expenditure is increased, and heat production rises.

Clinical Manifestations of Hyperthyroidism. The clinical manifestations of hyperthyroidism are varied and may arise in any major organ system (Fig. 34-6). One of the primary features is a palpable goiter or growth of a preexisting goiter. The skin becomes flushed, warm, and moist. Hair tends to be very fine and break easily; in some instances hair is lost. Nails of the fingers and toes break easily and often separate from the beds.

Hyperthyroidism often causes a stare. This is due to upper eyelid retraction and frequently occurs with thyrotoxicosis. Movements of the eyelids are jerky and irregular. Most persons with hyperthyroidism develop some *exophthalmos*, protrusion of the eyeballs that may cause difficulty in closing eyelids. The causes of exophthalmos are edematous swelling of the retroorbital tissues and degenerative changes in the muscles that control the eyes [5].

Cardiovascular system changes are pronounced due to the increased metabolic demands on the heart. Pronounced tachycardia is always present, even during sleep. Often, systolic blood pressure rises [14]. Palpitations occur due to the increased force of cardiac contractions. Atrial or supraventricular dysrhythmias are not uncommon. Generally, persons who have no underlying or preexisting cardiac failure are able to maintain the increased rate of cardiovascular function required. Hyperthyroidism may eventually precipitate congestive heart failure, however.

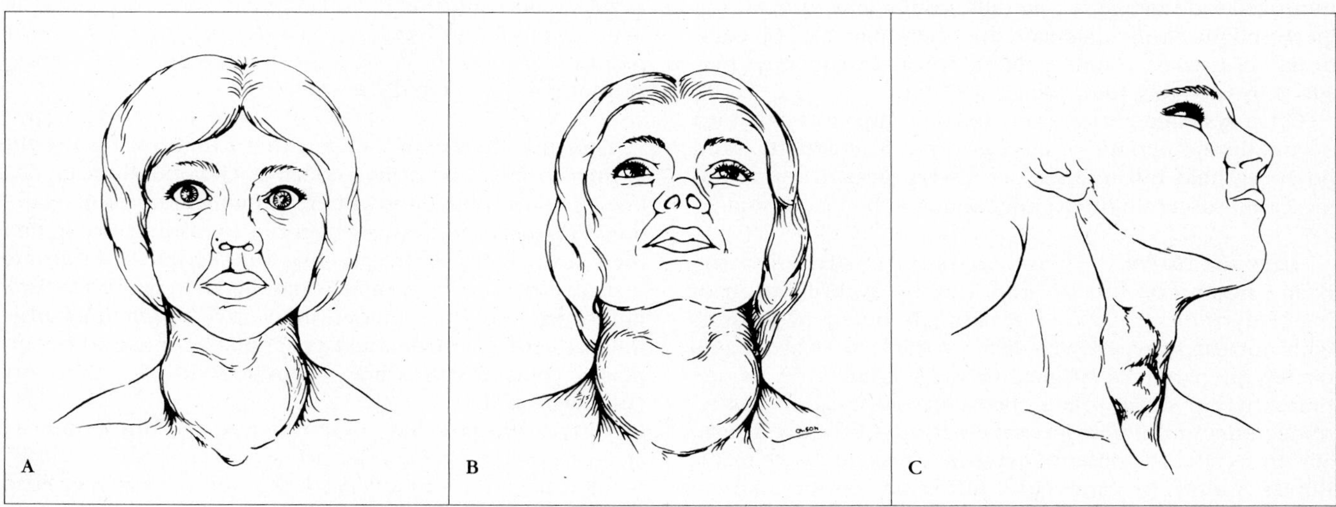

FIGURE 34-5 Thyroid abnormalities. A. Diffuse toxic goiter (Graves' disease) with exophthalmos. B. Diffuse nontoxic goiter. C. Nodular goiter. (From R.D. Judge, G.D. Zuidema, and F.T. Fitzgerald [eds.], *Clinical Diagnosis* [4th ed.]. Boston: Little, Brown, 1982.)

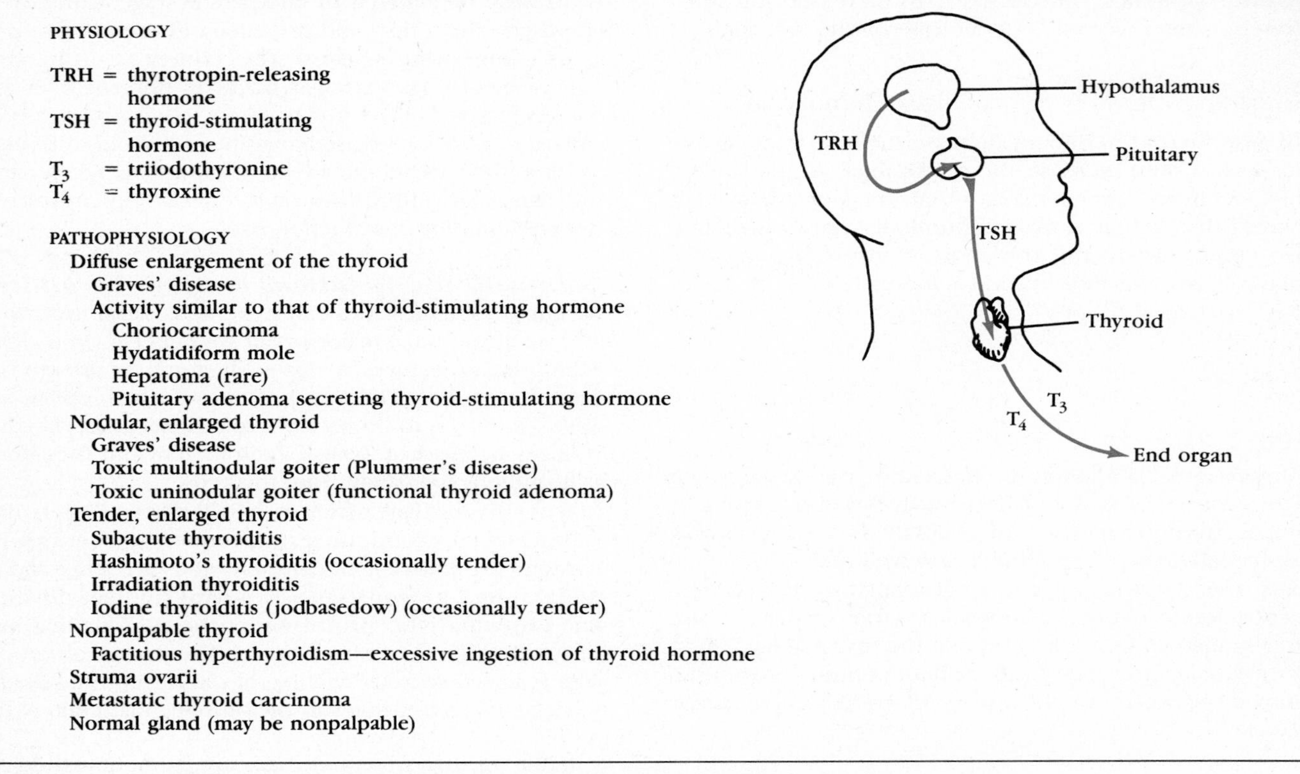

FIGURE 34-6 Hyperthyroidism: physiology and pathophysiology (From R.D. Judge, G.D. Zuidema, and F.T. Fitzgerald [eds.], *Clinical Diagnosis* [4th ed.]. Boston: Little, Brown, 1982.)

Changes in nervous system function are indicated by increasing restlessness and nervousness, decreased attention span, and the need to be almost constantly in motion, even though fatigue occurs rapidly. Afflicted persons also become emotionally labile, having bursts of temper and rapid mood changes.

In the gastrointestinal system, increased appetite is apparent, but there is usually associated weight loss. Increased food intake is generally insufficient to meet the increased metabolic demands, and there may also be complaints of nausea, vomiting, or diarrhea. The affected person is usually very thin, even emaciated.

Other systemic changes may become apparent. Dyspnea occurs during periods of increased physical activity. Mild polyuria, heat intolerance, excessive perspiration, and increased susceptibility to infection may be manifested.

Thyroid Storm. Thyrotoxic crisis, or thyroid storm, is an uncommon but life-threatening complication of hyperthyroidism. It may occasionally occur in persons with untreated hyperthyroidism or those who are inadequately prepared for surgical thyroidectomy [15]. At one time, thyroid storm was a common complication of thyroidectomy in the postoperative period. Currently, it usually arises after the onset of extreme stress, such as a major illness, injury, or especially, infection. Other medical causes include trauma, diabetic ketoacidosis, toxemia of pregnancy or labor, and premature discontinuation of antithyroid therapy [9].

The symptoms of thyroid storm result from a sudden increase in thyroid hormone levels in the bloodstream, resulting in a marked increase in all of the clinical manifestations of hyperthyroidism. The hallmark is considered to be uncontrolled fever of 100°F to 106°F. Other hypermetabolic symptoms include profuse diaphoresis, shock, vomiting, and dehydration. Central nervous system symptoms may also be exacerbated, including hyperkinesis, anxiety, and confusion [15]. The physiologic effects of the hypermetabolic processes are so devastating to the body tissues that those in crisis must receive immediate intervention, or death rapidly ensues.

Graves' Disease. The most common and well-known form of hyperthyroidism is Graves' disease, also known as exophthalmic goiter, diffuse toxic goiter, Basedow's disease, and primary hyperthyroidism. It is not simply a disease of the thyroid, but a multisystem syndrome that may include major manifestations of hyperthyroidism, diffuse thyroid enlargement, infiltrative ophthalmopathy, infiltrative dermopathy, and generalized lymphoid hyperplasia. These features may occur individually or in any combination.

Graves' disease may occur at any age but primarily strikes those between age 30 and 50 years. Generally, women have the disease more frequently than men, and more than one member of the same family is often affected.

It is now accepted that there is an autoimmune component to this disease. In the 1950s, a substance was discovered in the serum of many individuals with Graves' disease. It was an immunoglobulin G1, later called *long-acting thyroid stimulator (LATS)*. It has all of the functions of TSH but the effects are longer lasting and are not subject to the control of rising levels of thyroid hormones in the blood. In nearly every person with untreated Graves' disease, LATS is detected [4]. More recently, a thyroid-stimulating autoantibody (TSAb) has been found to be the functional analog to TSH, binding so strongly to TSH-receptor sites that it can actually prevent the binding of TSH [18]. Because the autoantibody is not under feedback control, thyroid hypersecretion results. The exact mechanism is not clearly understood.

Hereditary and genetic factors are also accepted contributors to the development of Graves' disease. This form of hyperthyroidism frequently occurs in more than one family member and may affect several generations of the same family. Thus, genetic and autoimmune components are of major influence. It has also been suggested that severe emotional stress may be a factor, as the disease frequently arises after a severe emotional or physical trauma [1].

The outstanding clinical features of Graves' disease are diffuse and palpable goiter, unilateral or bilateral exophthalmos, pretibial myxedema, and signs of hypermetabolism, or thyrotoxicosis [13,19]. The onset of symptoms is usually gradual. Complaints of nervousness, irritability, fatigue, heat intolerance, and weight loss are common. These symptoms are a result of the increased metabolic rate.

The thyroid gland is enlarged to 2 to 3 times the normal size in most cases. It may, however, be massively enlarged or remain near normal size. Enlargement is usually symmetric and the surface is smooth.

Exophthalmos, the most common ocular change, is usually accompanied by periorbital edema. The individual has a characteristic bulging, wide-eyed stare. Often, the eye musculature is so affected that the cornea and sclera are damaged due to inability to close the eyes. Exophthalmos usually gradually disappears with treatment of the hyperthyroidism. Infiltrative ophthalmopathy is a more serious and extensive involvement and may cause permanent changes in eye function. It also may cause especially difficult problems in treatment.

Infiltrative dermopathy, commonly called *pretibial myxedema*, is a dramatic manifestation that generally affects the pretibial area of one or both legs, causing a bark-like appearance of the skin. Localized edema and swelling of the skin and subcutaneous tissues occur. Hyaluronic acid accumulates in the interstitial spaces and, combining with water, forms edema that is boggy and nonpitting. Individuals with pretibial myxedema have a profound immunologic disruption, and it is thought that these dermatologic changes are a direct result of that immunologic reaction [13].

Toxic Multinodular Goiter. In some persons with a long-standing history of nontoxic goiter, hyperthyroidism may appear insidiously. This disorder is known as toxic multinodular goiter, or *Plummer's disease*. Women over age 50 are most frequently affected. The origin of the mechanism that causes nontoxic goiter to become toxic is not known.

The clinical manifestations are mild in comparison to Graves' disease. Thyrotoxicosis signs are less prominent, and serum thyroxine levels are only marginally elevated. Cardiovascular symptoms are the most pronounced. Individuals may develop atrial fibrillation, tachycardia, and congestive heart failure; also apparent are muscle weakening and fatigue. It is often difficult to diagnose toxic multinodular goiter because of its slow onset. The signs and symptoms may be attributed to lethargy and aging.

Toxic Adenoma. Toxic adenoma is a less common form of hyperthyroidism. It usually results from the development of a follicular adenoma. These adenomas are subdivided according to the size of the follicles into macrofollicular, microfollicular, and embryonal varieties [19]. It may occur in pairs or triplets. The function of the adenoma may be more or less than that of normal thyroid gland tissue, but it is capable of functioning without the stimulation of LATS or TSH.

As the adenoma grows, it begins to take over the function of normal thyroid tissue. Eventually, without intervention, complete atrophy and suppression of the remainder of the thyroid gland occurs [19]. The adenoma must reach the size of 2 to 3 cm before it is capable of producing a state of hyperthyroidism. The lesion may undergo necrosis and hemorrhage of its center. If this occurs, symptoms of thyrotoxicosis recede, and the remainder of the thyroid gland tissue resumes normal functioning.

Individuals usually affected with toxic adenoma are in the 30- to 40-year age range and generally have a history of a lump in the neck that has been growing slowly for many years. Clinical features are not pronounced; cardiovascular symptoms are likely to be the most prominent.

Hypothyroidism

Hypothyroidism is the result of a deficiency of thyroid hormone, leading to a decreased rate of body metabolism and a general slowing down of body processes. Any of the following factors may contribute to the onset of hypothyroidism: hypothalamic dysfunction, TRH or TSH deficiency, pituitary disorders, specific idiopathies, thyroid deficiencies, and thyroid destruction [2]. The degree of dysfunction is related to the relative amount of hormone deficiency in the tissues. Hypothyroidism is fairly common and is recognized as an underdiagnosed health problem, particularly in the elderly [12].

Clinical Manifestations. Changes in the skin occur with hypothyroidism when hyaluronic acid binds with water. The combination produces the characteristic baggy, full, edematous skin. Edema is most apparent in the face, hands, and feet. The skin is pale, cool, and very dry. Wounds or breaks in the skin heal very slowly.

Cardiovascular symptoms may closely resemble those of congestive heart failure. Cardiac output is decreased, as are heart rate and circulating blood volume. Peripheral vascular resistance is increased, ultimately resulting in decreased flow of blood to the tissues. The term *myxedema heart* refers to the clinical picture of an enlarged heart, with electrocardiographic (ECG) and serum enzyme changes.

The gastrointestinal tract, together with other body functions, slows down under the influence of a hypothyroid state. Most persons have a decreased appetite and, contrary to popular belief, only a slight increase in weight. Decreased peristalsis leads to accumulation of gas and complaints of constipation.

Hypothyroid effect on the nervous system also decreases function. Thinking and movement begin to slow down. Mental dullness is often apparent. Personality changes may occur, resulting in severe depression or extreme agitation and anxiety. Movements are slow and disorganized, causing the appearance of clumsiness.

Other body system changes also result from hypothyroidism. Muscular pains are common and strength decreases. Reduced renal blood flow and glomerular filtration contribute to the cardiovascular changes. Anemia and changes in clotting factors occur. In both sexes hypothyroidism decreases sexual drive.

Exactly the opposite of hyperthyroidism, hypothyroidism causes decreased thyroid function and reduced energy metabolism, resulting in a lower metabolic rate. Protein synthesis and degradation are reduced, resulting in retarded growth of bone and muscle tissue. Glucose absorption from the stomach and intestines is delayed, resulting in delayed insulin time. As with protein, the synthesis and degradation of lipids are decreased. The net result is a decreased rate of energy metabolism.

Cretinism. Thyroid hormone deficiency during embryonic and neonatal life results in a state known as cretinism in infants and young children. It is not readily apparent at birth and it may take several weeks to several months before hypothyroidism is discovered. The infant becomes sluggish and falls behind the normal rate of growth and development. Mental retardation and delayed growth patterns are characteristic.

Cretins are dwarflike in stature. Their arms and legs are short in relationship to the trunk of the body (Fig. 34-7). The face of a cretin is broad and puffy, and the teeth are usually malformed; the skin is coarse and dry with sparse hair. The abdomen is protuberant, which often results in umbilical hernias. Early recognition and treatment reverse the effects of hypothyroidism in an infant, preventing the onset and development of cretinism.

Endemic Goiter. In some areas of the world, an iodine deficiency exists in the environment to the degree that goiters may be common among the people dwelling in that region. The term *endemic goiter* refers to such an area and population. The Great Lakes region of the United States and mountainous areas of other countries, such as the Swiss Alps, are noted for iodine deficiency of their soil and water (Fig. 34-8).

Because of the lack of iodine, the thyroid is unable to synthesize thyroxine and triiodothyronine, resulting in decreased serum levels of thyroid hormones. Secretion of TSH is increased, and the thyroid becomes very hyperplastic, leading to the formation of a goiter that is the attempt by the gland to produce thyroid hormones.

Adult Hypothyroidism. Severe hypothyroidism in the adult is often called *myxedema*. Its onset is slow and may not be recognized for many years. Primary adult hypothyroidism results from the loss or destruction of thyroid gland tissue. This may be caused by an autoimmune or disease process within the thyroid or removal of the gland or may occur after treatment for Graves' disease. Secondary hypothyroidism results from pituitary TSH insufficiency, usually due to a lesion in the pituitary gland.

Early symptoms of adult hypothyroidism are fatigue and lethargy. A goiter may be present, which indicates an attempt to compensate for the deficiency [13]. Marked sensitivity to cold temperatures occurs as well as gradual slowing of mental and physical function. These progress through the course of the disease. The skin, hair, and nails become very dry, with the hair and nails becoming brittle and breaking very easily. The muscles and joints are stiff and aching, especially in the morning after waking. Slight weight gain is often noted despite decreased appetite.

As the clinical signs and symptoms continue to develop, the full picture of myxedema may appear (Fig. 34-9). Thickness, especially in the face, hands, and feet, becomes apparent, caused by the same process that results in pretibial myxedema in the person with Graves' disease. The voice becomes hoarse and the tongue thickens. The body temperature is lower than normal, resulting in mild hypothermia. Finally, mental and physical lethargy progress to extremes. If untreated, this process will continue for many years.

Sick Euthyroid Syndrome. A clinical condition that may occur in acutely or chronically ill persons has been called the sick euthyroid syndrome [16,19]. The most common finding is depressed T_3 and T_4 levels, deficient enough to be well within the definition of hypothyroidism. Sick euthyroid syndrome is distinct from primary hypothyroidism, however, in that the TSH levels are not elevated. The TSH response to TRH may be slightly elevated but not above the normal range [16].

Sick euthyroid syndrome is rather common in intensive care units after a variety of illnesses and disorders such as surgery, myocardial infarction, renal insufficiency, ketoacidosis, cirrhosis, thermal injury, and other critical conditions [16]. Therefore, it is important that this problem be differentiated from true thyroid disease as quickly as possible.

Myxedema Coma. Myxedema coma is a medical emergency in persons with hypothyroidism. The comatose state is the most severe expression of profound hypothyroid function [14,17]. It usually occurs during the winter months and affects mostly elderly myxedematous persons. Any stress, such as extreme cold, trauma, infection, central nervous system depressants, or physical stress, may precipitate this crisis. Lethargy progresses to coma, with hypotension and hypothermia on examination. Hypo-

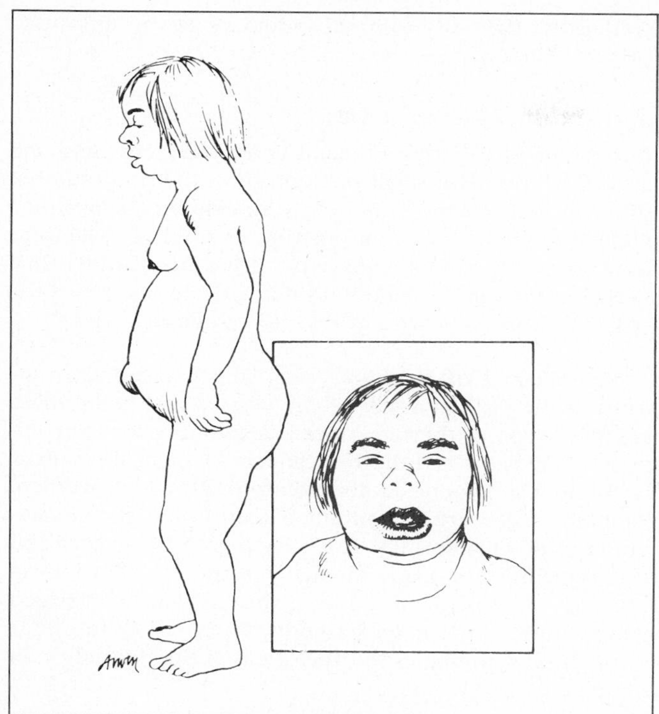

FIGURE 34-7 Hypothyroidism (cretinism). (From R.D. Judge, G.D. Zuidema, and F.T. Fitzgerald [eds.], *Clinical Diagnosis* [4th ed.]. Boston: Little, Brown, 1982.)

thermia is considered to be the most characteristic symptom. The coma results from a continuous slowing of the vital centers; the respiratory center becomes more depressed, cardiac output continues to drop, and cerebral hypoxia increases as a result. Other changes include hypotension, bradycardia, hypoventilation with respiratory acidosis, and carbon dioxide narcosis, together with a variety of fluid and electrolyte disorders [9]. Without intervention, mortality is as much as 50 percent [3].

Chronic Autoimmune Thyroiditis. This form of thyroiditis, also known as *Hashimoto's disease*, primarily occurs in women aged 30 to 50 years, but it may occur at any age and is thought to be a major cause of hypothyroidism in children [19]. The two most characteristic findings are a large, palpable goiter and high levels of circulating autoantibodies.

The goiter results from defects of hormone biosynthesis in the thyroid. Because of the failure to produce adequate hormone levels, the pituitary produces TSH abundantly. The result is a goiter without clinical evidence of thyrotoxicosis. Chronic autoimmune thyroiditis may lead to hyperthyroidism, but usually results in thyroid hypofunction.

The thyroid gland enlarges very gradually. The goiter becomes firm and rubbery, and usually is minimally tender, although extreme pain can occur. When left untreated, the gland will continue to enlarge over the years.

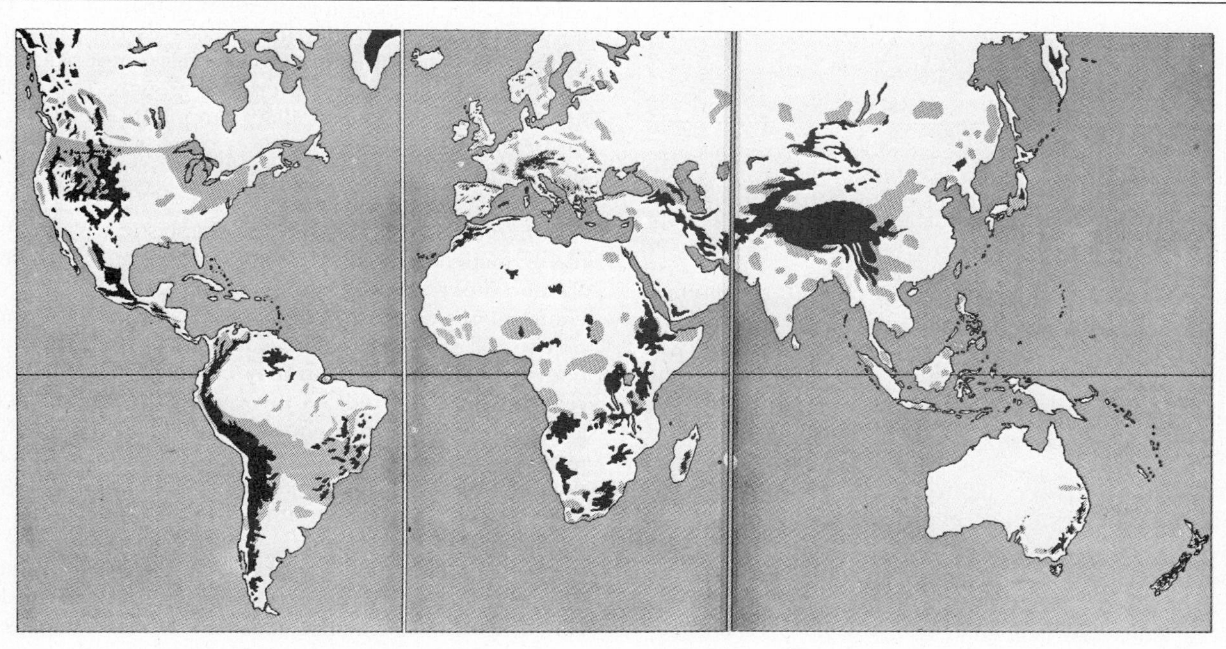

FIGURE 34-8 Regions of endemic goiter and the mountainous terrain with which it is often associated were mapped by the World Health Organization. Areas where iodine-deficiency goiter is endemic are shown in gray. Populations near sea coasts are seldom affected due to the iodine content of seafood. Not all inland areas are equally affected; the geology and remoteness of mountainous regions (solid black) make them most susceptible. (Illustration by Robin Ingle from "Endemic Goiter" by R. Bruce Gillie. Copyright © 1971 by Scientific American, Inc. All rights reserved. *Scientific American,* June 1971, Vol. 224:6.)

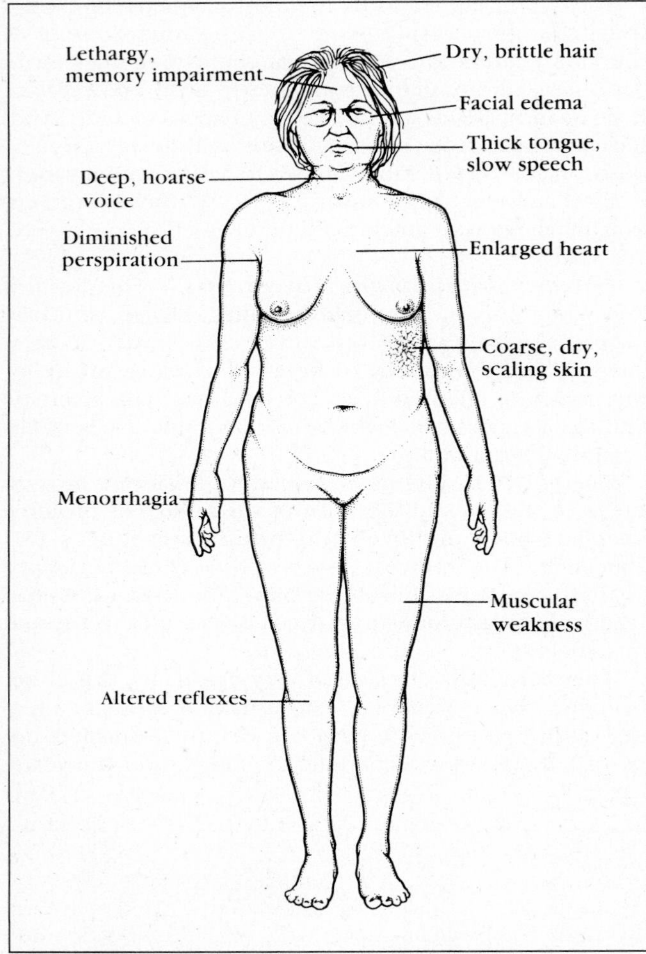

FIGURE 34-9 A composite of the symptoms of myxedema. (From M. Beyers and S. Dudas, *The Clinical Practice of Medical-Surgical Nursing* [2nd ed.]. Boston: Little, Brown, 1984.)

There is often a family history of chronic autoimmune thyroiditis, or a history of family members with Graves' disease, nontoxic goiter, or primary hypothyroidism. Also, families may show an increased frequency for other autoimmune disorders, such as rheumatoid arthritis or pernicious anemia.

Nontoxic Goiter. Sometimes the thyroid gland enlarges without evidence of alterations in rate of body metabolism. This is termed a *nontoxic*, or simple, goiter. It commonly occurs at puberty, during adolescence, or during pregnancy. This disorder occurs in 10 percent of all North American women [13].

Several causes may be responsible for the goiter, such as iodine deficiency or genetic enzymatic defects. They result in a decreased rate of production of thyroid hormones, which in turn results in increased secretion of TSH from the pituitary. Hyperplasia of thyroid tissue occurs in compensation and, in mild cases, there is usually no clinical evidence of alteration in function. If thyroid hypertrophy is severe, there may be signs of hyperthyroidism. Generally, the only clinical evidence is the enlarged, palpable thyroid.

Malignant Thyroid Tumors

Carcinoma of the thyroid gland is not very common and accounts for only a small percentage of the total number of diagnoses of cancer. No existing evidence supports a familial tendency or predisposition to thyroid carcinoma other than the parafollicular type. It has been shown that radiation therapy in childhood dramatically increases the risk of at least two forms of thyroid carcinoma [6].

Papillary Carcinoma. Papillary carcinoma originates in the papillary cells of the thyroid and is the most common type of thyroid cancer, accounting for approximately one-half of all thyroid cancers. It is most frequent in children and young adults and especially affects women. Radiation exposure in childhood contributes to the causation of this malignancy. It is a slow-growing cancer and may remain in the gland for many years. The first indication may be a palpable node in the thyroid or enlarged lymph nodes in the neck region. Metastasis can occur through the lymphatics to other areas of the thyroid or, in some cases, to the lungs.

Follicular Carcinoma. Follicular carcinoma, as the name implies, originates in the follicular cells and accounts for 20 to 25 percent of thyroid carcinomas. It affects an older population, usually over 40 years of age; it occurs in women 2 to 3 times more frequently than in men. Childhood exposure to radiation increases the risk of this malignancy. The initial feature is an asymptomatic thyroid nodule exhibiting slow patterns of growth. This tumor is more invasive than the papillary carcinoma and may spread through the area blood vessels. Common sites of metastasis are the lungs and bones.

Anaplastic Carcinoma. Anaplastic carcinoma is a highly malignant form of thyroid cancer and accounts for about 10 percent of thyroid cancers. It is slightly more common in women than in men. Metastasis occurs rapidly, first to the surrounding areas and then to all parts of the body. Initially, the person may complain of a mass in the region of the thyroid. As the cancer involves structures adjacent to the thyroid, hoarseness, stridor, and difficulty swallowing may occur. Tracheal deviation and tumor ulceration may develop [8]. Life expectancy after diagnosis usually is only several months.

Parafollicular Carcinoma. Parafollicular, or medullary, carcinoma is unique among the thyroid cancers. Only a small number of cases are related to this type. It generally affects women more than men and most often in those past 50 years of age. Parafollicular carcinoma also metastasizes quickly, often to distant sites of the body, such as the lungs, bones, and liver. Its distinctive feature is its ability to secrete calcitonin because of its origin in the parafollicular cells. This carcinoma frequently has familial tendencies and may be associated with multiple endocrine neoplasia (MEN) (see pp. 550 and 551).

The Parathyroid Glands

Anatomy

The parathyroid glands, four in number, lie posterior and adjacent to the thyroid gland. There is one parathyroid gland in each superior and inferior lateral area of the thyroid. Each gland is small, about the size of a pea, and their combined total weight is approximately 120 mg. The glands are reddish brown or yellowish brown and each is enclosed in a small fibrous capsule (see Fig. 34-1).

The parathyroid glands secrete *parathyroid hormone* (*parathormone*, or *PTH*). Secretion of this hormone is not under the control of the pituitary gland but is directly regulated by a negative feedback system of the circulating blood levels of calcium. Therefore as calcium levels fall, more parathyroid hormone is secreted; as calcium levels rise, hormone secretion is reduced. Almost any factor reducing serum calcium levels stimulates the release of parathyroid hormone [13].

There are two cell types in the parathyroid gland—the oxyphil cell and the chief, or principal, cell. Oxyphil cells are slightly larger but are not actually engaged in the secretion of hormones and do not have a known function [7]. Chief cells are responsible for producing and secreting parathyroid hormone (Fig. 34-10).

Function

The parathyroid glands regulate the serum levels of calcium in the body and control the rate of bone metabolism. Vitamin D and calcitonin also affect calcium metabolism. Vitamin D is obtained through dietary ingestion of foods with a high content of the vitamin and through synthesis in the skin. Foods containing vitamin D include milk products and fish-liver oils. Many vitamin D-enriched foods are also available. Vitamin D synthesized in the skin is known as calciferol and is activated on direct exposure to sunlight.

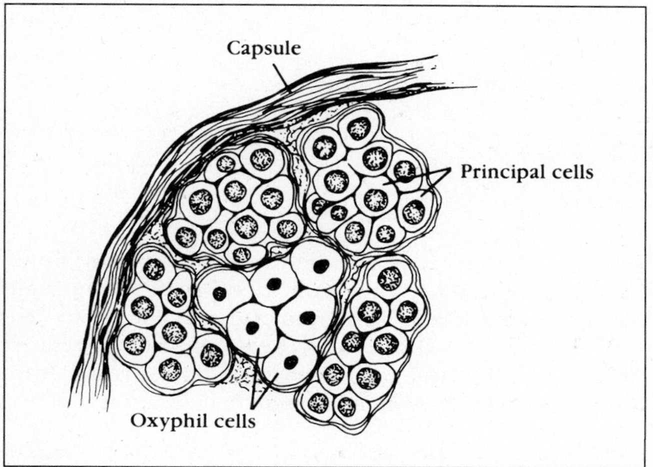

FIGURE 34-10 Parathyroid glands. The cells are arranged in cords by loose connective tissue. The principal cells are predominant in number. Oxyphil cells are recognized by their smaller, more condensed nuclei and larger relative cytoplasmic volume. (From M. Borysenko et al., *Functional Histology* [2nd ed.]. Boston: Little, Brown, 1984.)

Vitamin D is essential for calcium absorption from the intestinal tract into the bloodstream. It also increases retention of calcium and phosphorus, and controls the mineralization of bone matrix. Thus, it is important in controlling and maintaining circulating levels of calcium [13].

Calcitonin, or thyrocalcitonin, which is produced and secreted by the parafollicular cells of the thyroid gland, opposes the action of the parathyroid hormone and lowers blood calcium levels. Serum calcium levels are decreased when calcium circulating in the blood is transferred back to the bones (Fig. 34-11).

To maintain calcium levels, parathyroid hormone acts on bones, kidneys, and intestines to resorb calcium. Some of calcium's most important effects are (1) to increase plasma calcium concentration and decrease plasma phosphate concentration, (2) to increase urinary excretion of phosphate but decrease urinary excretion of calcium, (3) to increase the rate of skeletal remodeling and the net rate of bone resorption, (4) to increase the number of osteoblasts and osteoclasts on bone surfaces, (5) to cause an initial increase in calcium entry into the cells of its target tissues, (6) to alter the acid-base balance of the body, and (7) to increase gastrointestinal absorption of calcium [19].

Effect of Parathyroid Hormone on Bone Resorption. Because the greatest storage of calcium in the body is in bone, it is here that parathyroid hormone has its greatest effect on increasing the rate of metabolic breakdown of bone tissue. Primarily, this action is exerted on osteoclasts, which are large cells with several nuclei that participate in the resorption of bone [5]. After the release of parathyroid hormone, osteoclasts resorb an area of mineralized bone to release calcium. Parathyroid hormone also stimulates the formation of new osteoclasts and delays the conversion of osteoclasts into osteoblasts, which are the principal cells of bone formation. The overall strength of bone is not substantially altered by this process in a healthy person with normally functioning parathyroids.

Effect of Parathyroid Hormone on Kidney Resorption. The action of parathyroid hormone on the kidneys involves increased resorption of calcium ions and decreased resorption of phosphate ions. These actions occur at different sites in the kidneys and by different mechanisms. Decreased resorption of phosphate is due to the effect of parathyroid hormone directly on tubular absorption, and the increase in calcium resorption is due to a direct effect on the distal convoluted tubule. In early research, the effect of parathyroid hormone on the tubular absorption of phosphate was considered to be the primary and most important role. Now, however, it is recognized that this action is secondary to the hormone's role in bone resorption of calcium.

Effect of Parathyroid Hormone on Intestinal Resorption. Parathyroid hormone also influences the resorption of calcium from the small intestine. It is necessary for activated vitamin D to be present for this process

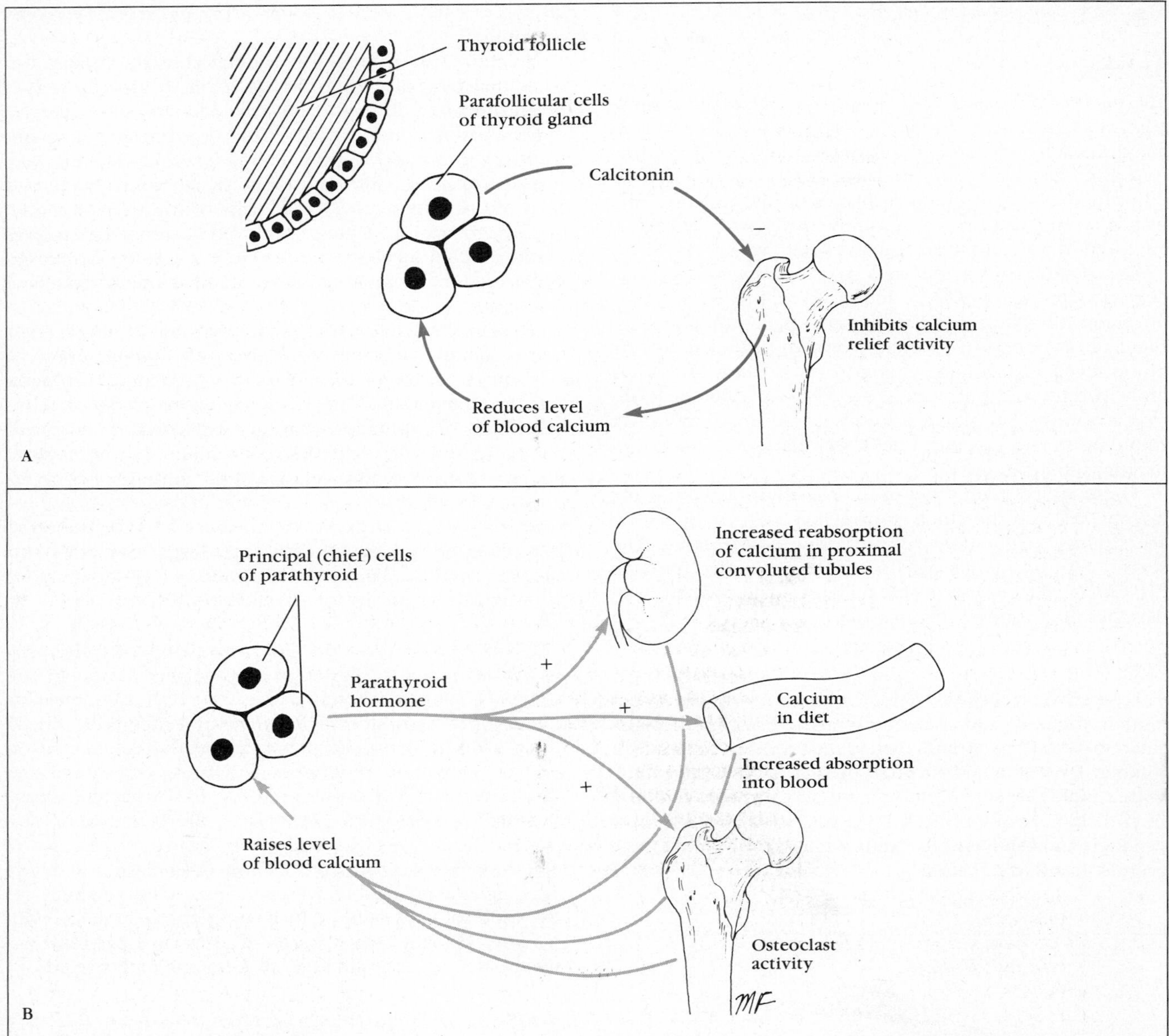

FIGURE 34-11 A. Regulation of calcitonin secretion by the parafollicular cells of the thyroid gland. B. Regulation of the parathyroid gland.

to occur. Resorption of calcium from the intestines also increases absorption of calcium phosphate, thus decreasing the amount of phosphate elimination.

Altered Function of the Parathyroid Glands

Hypoparathyroidism

Hypoparathyroidism results when insufficient amounts of parathyroid hormone are secreted, or when the hormone fails to act at the tissue level. Without circulating parathyroid hormone, calcium is not resorbed from bone, kidneys, or intestines. The result is a decreased serum concentration of calcium. This, in turn, causes increased neuromuscular excitability and the symptoms of tetany. Therefore, all of the clinical manifestations result from decreased levels of serum calcium concentration.

Clinical Manifestations. In 70 percent of cases of hypoparathyroidism, tetany becomes the major clinical manifestation [19]. It begins with numbness and tingling of the extremities and progresses to stiffness, cramps, and spasms. Carpal spasms are common and are the most prominent symptoms. If serum calcium levels continue to fall, the neuromuscular manifestations become more severe and pronounced [7]. Laryngeal muscles are very susceptible to spasms, and death by asphyxiation can result if intervention is not immediate. At the very least, wheezing due to bronchospasm occurs.

When hypoparathyroidism exists for several months to several years, other physical changes may become apparent. Nails become brittle and may atrophy, and horizontal ridges are apparent on the surface. Persons often experience alopecia in patches on the head and almost complete loss of eyebrows. The skin becomes coarse and dry with patches of brownish pigment. Papilledema is often present and may occur with increased intracranial pressure. The electrocardiogram of hypocalcemia may show a lengthening of the Q–T interval. Serum calcium levels fall and remain subnormal. Sometimes, personality changes and psychiatric symptoms occur, such as emotional lability, extreme irritability and anxiety, depression, and delirium. Convulsions and grand mal seizures may occur.

Three clinical signs are used to diagnose tetany and hypoparathyroidism. (1) The first test is for a positive Chvostek's sign. A quick tap or light blow over the parotid gland near the ear produces twitching of the facial muscles, especially the upper lip, nose, and eye. (2) Trousseau's sign is elicited by occluding blood supply to the arm for three minutes. The result is positive when carpopedal spasms occur (Fig. 34-12). (3) Erb's sign is considered positive when a 6-mV current produces a motor response. Specific positive responses to any of these clinical signs is usually considered diagnostic.

Idiopathic Hypoparathyroidism. Idiopathic hypoparathyroidism is relatively uncommon. The course of dysfunction is variable. It may be congenital or acquired, mild or severe, transient or lifelong. Generally, the congenital form is related to defective or absent parathyroid glands. Children are most commonly diagnosed, with females being affected twice as often as males. It is widely suspected that an autoimmune state may be related to the idiopathic form. The symptoms, including tetany, are usually quite severe.

Postoperative Hypoparathyroidism. More common than the idiopathic form, hypoparathyroidism may be related to damage or removal of the parathyroid glands during thyroid surgery. Removing the thyroid without detaching the parathyroids is the most frequent cause. Any surgery that involves manipulation of the structures of the throat, such as a radical neck dissection, however, can result in clinical features of hypoparathyroidism.

With damage or partial removal, the remaining parathyroid tissue is usually able to compensate. Thus, the loss of parathyroid hormone is transient. Complete removal of the glands would result in total loss of parathyroid function, and severe hypocalcemia would rapidly follow.

Pseudohypoparathyroidism. Pseudohypoparathyroidism, also known as *Albright's hereditary osteodystrophy*, is a form of hypoactive functioning that is familial in origin. It is widely believed to be transmitted by an X-linked dominant gene. Hypocalcemia and hypophosphatemia are characteristic of this disorder. The parathyroid glands are normal in size or slightly enlarged, and there is no deficit in circulating levels of parathyroid hormone. Women are affected twice as frequently as men.

These persons have developmental skeletal abnormalities and usually exhibit a mild to moderate degree of mental retardation. They are short and stocky, often less than 5 feet tall, and are often obese. The face is very round

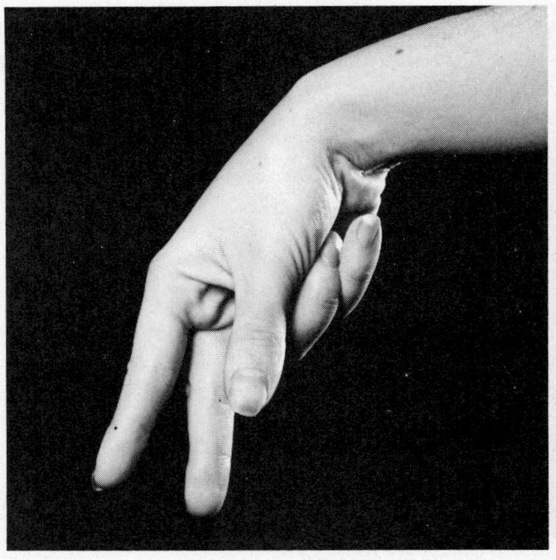

A

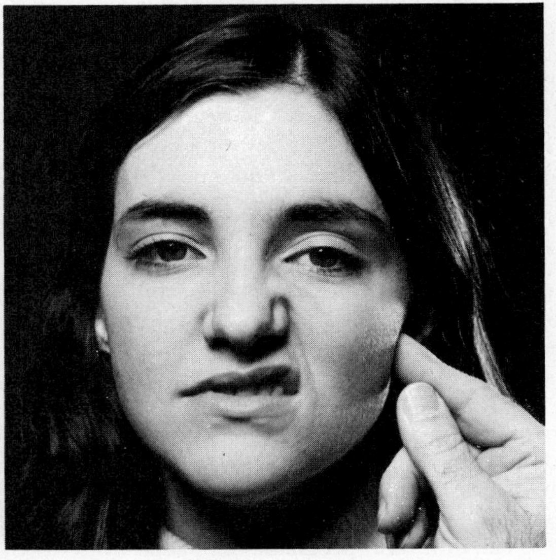

B

FIGURE 34-12 Diagnostic signs of hypoparathyroidism. A. Carpopedal spasm in Trousseau's sign. B. Facial muscle contraction in Chvostek's sign. (From M. Beyers and S. Dudas, *The Clinical Practice of Medical-Surgical Nursing* [2nd ed.]. Boston: Little, Brown, 1984.)

due to structural abnormalities in the development of the facial and cranial bones. The metacarpal bones are short and stubby. Usually, there is some degree of widespread subcutaneous soft tissue ossification and calcification.

Pseudopseudohypoparathyroidism is very similar to pseudohypoparathyroidism. The major difference between it and pseudohypoparathyroidism is that levels of serum calcium and phosphates are normal. Familial tendencies also exist with this disorder.

Hyperparathyroidism

Much more common than hypoparathyroidism, the frequency of hyperparathyroidism appears to be continually increasing. The specific etiology of any form of hyperparathyroid function is not well understood. Hypersecretion of parathyroid hormone results in elevated serum calcium levels and excessive secretion of phosphorus by the kidneys. In most cases, a single benign adenoma is the cause. It is also thought that a history of long-standing hypocalcemia may contribute to the predisposition to hyperparathyroidism. The three forms of hyperfunction of the parathyroid glands are usually recognized as primary, secondary, and tertiary.

Primary Hyperparathyroidism. Primary hyperparathyroidism is usually characterized by hypercalcemia that results from failure of the normal feedback mechanism to decrease secretion of parathyroid hormone. The three most common causes are parathyroid adenomas, hyperplasia of all four parathyroid glands, or some form of parathyroid carcinoma [12]. As the serum calcium concentrations rise, parathyroid secretion is no longer reduced and calcium levels continue to increase.

The clinical manifestations are variable and nonspecific. Some persons experience mild symptoms, while others have severe symptoms. The most common manifestation is from renal calculi in the genitourinary system, which probably result from precipitation of calcium and phosphate in the kidneys [6].

Other variable symptoms include renal symptoms, skeletal changes, and hypercalcemia. In addition to the formation of renal stones, hematuria may be noted. Gastrointestinal complaints include anorexia, nausea, vomiting, and constipation, as well as generalized abdominal pain [14]. Changes within the skeletal system are diverse. Sometimes new bone is laid as quickly as calcium is resorbed, and the person has only mild complaints of vague skeletal pains. At other times various bone diseases such as osteoporosis or osteomalacia may result.

Secondary Hyperparathyroidism. In secondary hyperparathyroidism levels of circulating parathyroid hormones are high, perhaps initiated by a variety of causes that result in a low serum calcium concentration. Such causes may include low-calcium diet, pregnancy or lactation, rickets, and osteomalacia. In the Western world the usual cause is renal failure. Low calcium levels cause the parathyroid glands to become hyperplastic in order to compensate for the condition that initially caused the low calcium levels. After compensation attempts, calcium may remain low or may attain normal levels (see Chap. 31).

Tertiary Hyperparathyroidism. Tertiary hyperparathyroidism results from previously developed, long-standing secondary hyperparathyroidism. Autonomous secretion of parathyroid hormone continues without regard for serum calcium levels. In most instances, adenomas have developed in the already-hyperplastic parathyroid glands after the onset of secondary hyperparathyroidism [12]. This condition is accompanied by abnormally high calcium levels. Tertiary hyperparathyroidism is often described in persons with renal failure who develop hypercalcemia.

Renal osteodystrophy, which may occur with tertiary hyperparathyroidism, arises in persons with chronic renal failure who develop hyperphosphatemia [6]. Parathyroid hyperfunction then occurs and increases serum calcium concentrations (see Chap. 31). Metastatic calcifications in the soft tissues, such as the eyes, lungs, or joints, may occur [11].

Study Questions

1. Describe the synthesis, release, and action of thyroid hormones.
2. How does calcitonin differ from the other thyroid hormones?
3. How can a goiter develop in both hyper- and hypothyroidism?
4. Relate the manifestations of hyperthyroidism to the actions of the thyroid hormones.
5. Describe exophthalamus.
6. Explain the clinical manifestations of hypothyroidism on the basis of its pathophysiology.
7. Differentiate thyrotoxic crisis and myxedema coma.
8. What are the main purposes of the parathyroid glands? How are they controlled?
9. How does hyperparathyroidism result from renal failure?

References

1. Chaffee, E.E., and Lytle, I.M. *Basic Physiology and Anatomy* (4th ed.). Philadelphia: Lippincott, 1980.
2. Clinical highlights: Causes of hypothyroidism. *Hosp. Med.* 20(1):163, 1984.
3. Dillon, R.S. *Handbook of Endocrinology* (2nd ed.). Philadelphia: Lea & Febiger, 1980.
4. Felig, P., et al. *Endocrinology and Metabolism*. New York: McGraw-Hill, 1981.
5. Guyton, A.C. *Textbook of Medical Physiology* (7th ed.). Philadelphia: Saunders, 1986.
6. Hall, R., Anderson, J., and Besser, M. *Fundamentals of Clinical Endocrinology*. Chicago: Yearbook, 1980.

7. Jacob, S.W., et al. *Structure and Function in Man*. Philadelphia: Saunders, 1981.
8. Jubiz, W. *Endocrinology: A Logical Approach for Clinicians* (2nd ed.). New York: McGraw-Hill, 1985.
9. Klein, I.L., and Levey, G.S. Thyroid storm and myxedema coma. *Emergency Med.* 5(4):33, 1984.
10. Leebaw, W.F., and Morley, J.E. Effects of aging on normal and abnormal function. *Consultant* 24(7):165, 171, 1984.
11. Lewis, S.M. Pathophysiology of chronic renal failure. *Nurs. Clin. North Am.* 16:501, 1981.
12. Marsden, P., and McCullagh, A.G. *Endocrinology*. Littleton, Mass.: PSG, 1985.
13. Mazzaferri, E.L. *Textbook of Endocrinology* (3rd ed.). New Hyde Park, N.Y.: Medical Examination, 1986.
14. Metz, R., and Larson, E.B. *Blue Book of Endocrinology*. Philadelphia: Saunders, 1985.
15. Patient Care Highlights. Is your patient in thyroid storm? *Patient Care* 18(5):191, 195, 1984.
16. Streck, W.F., and Lockwood, D.H. *Endocrine Diagnosis: Clinical and Laboratory Approach*. Boston: Little, Brown, 1983.
17. Urbanic, R.C., and Mazzaferri, E.L. Thyrotoxic crisis and myxedema. *Heart Lung* 7:435, 1978.
18. Volpe, R. Autoimmune thyroid disease. *Hosp. Pract.* 19(1):141, 148, 151, 1984.
19. Wilson, J.D., and Foster, D.W. (eds.). *Williams' Textbook of Endocrinology* (7th ed.). Philadelphia: Saunders, 1985.

CHAPTER 35

Normal and Altered Functions of the Pancreas

CHAPTER OUTLINE

Anatomy and Physiology

Physiologic Regulation of Insulin Secretion
Effect of Insulin on Facilitated Diffusion
Metabolic Effects of Insulin

Liver
Adipose Tissue
Muscle

Physiology of Glucagon
Somatostatin
Regulation of Blood Glucose

Diabetes Mellitus

History
Classification
Stages
Frequency and Etiology
Insulin-Dependent Diabetes

Infection and Autoimmunity

Noninsulin-Dependent Diabetes

Alteration of Insulin Secretion
Bihormonal Theory
Insulin Resistance
Heredity
Age
Body Weight
Sex
Diet
Pregnancy
Stress

Introduction to the Pathology of Diabetes

Pathology of the Pancreas
Vascular System Pathology
Pathology of the Kidneys
Pathology of the Eyes
Nervous System Pathology
Skin Changes
Hepatic Fatty Changes
Muscle Changes

Clinical Manifestations and Complications

Diabetic Ketoacidosis
Hyperglycemic, Hyperosmolar, Nonketotic (HHNK) Coma
Lactic Acidosis
Insulin Reactions

Clinical Course
Laboratory Findings

Fasting Blood Sugar (FBS)
Two-Hour Postprandial Blood Sugar
Glucose Tolerance Test (GTT)
Glycosylated Hemoglobin (HbA_{1c})
Urine Glucose
Urine Ketones
Volume of Urine in a 24-Hour Period

Pancreatic Islet-Cell Disease

Hyperinsulinism
Zollinger-Ellison Syndrome (Gastrinoma, Ulcerogenic Tumor)
Werner's Syndrome (Multiple Endocrine Neoplasia)

Pancreatitis

Acute Pancreatitis

Frequency and Etiology
Pathology
Clinical Manifestations
Complications
Diagnostic Tests

Chronic Pancreatitis

Carcinoma of the Pancreas

Carcinoma of the Head of the Pancreas
Carcinoma of the Body and Tail of the Pancreas
Clinical Manifestations
Clinical Course

Cystic Fibrosis (Mucoviscidosis, Fibrocystic Disease of the Pancreas)

Frequency
Pathogenesis

Gastrointestinal Tract
Respiratory System
Reproductive System
Sweat Glands

Clinical Manifestations
Laboratory and Diagnostic Findings

LEARNING OBJECTIVES

1. Describe the anatomy of the pancreas, its size, shape, parts, ducts, and cells.
2. Explain the physiologic regulation of insulin secretion.
3. Describe the metabolic effects of insulin.
4. Explain the actions of glucagon and somatostatin, and their effects on metabolism.
5. Discuss the frequency and etiology of diabetes mellitus.
6. Differentiate between the types of diabetes.
7. Relate the stages or degrees of abnormality of diabetes.
8. Explain the pathophysiology of diabetes.
9. Relate the clinical manifestations of diabetes to the pathophysiologic changes.
10. Explain the pathophysiology of complications of diabetes mellitus.
11. Differentiate ketoacidosis; hyperglycemic, hyperosmolar, nonketotic coma; and lactic acidosis.
12. Outline the physiologic responses to hypoglycemia.
13. Identify tests used in the diagnosis and evaluation of diabetes mellitus.
14. Explain the pathophysiology of pancreatic islet-cell diseases; hyperinsulinism, Zollinger-Ellison syndrome (gastrinoma), and multiple endocrine neoplasia (Werner's syndrome).
15. Discuss the frequency and etiology of acute pancreatitis.
16. Describe the chemical and pathologic changes characteristic of pancreatitis.
17. Relate the clinical manifestations of acute pancreatitis to the histologic alterations.
18. Discuss the complications of acute pancreatitis.
19. Relate laboratory findings of acute pancreatitis.
20. Compare clinical manifestations and complications of acute and chronic pancreatitis.
21. Discuss the frequency, etiology, types, and clinical course of carcinoma of the pancreas.
22. Discuss the frequency and genetics of cystic fibrosis.
23. Describe the pathophysiologic changes that occur in various body systems in cystic fibrosis.
24. Relate the clinical manifestations of cystic fibrosis to the pathophysiologic changes.
25. Discuss laboratory and diagnostic findings related to cystic fibrosis.

This chapter describes the anatomy, physiology, pathology, and alterations in function of the pancreas. The pancreas is important in the digestion and metabolism of food. Much of its anatomic structure serves gastrointestinal function, but special cells in the islets of Langerhans influence metabolism through the secretion of insulin and glucagon. Too much insulin causes hypoglycemia and too little causes diabetes mellitus. Conversely, too much glucagon causes diabetes and too little leads to hypoglycemia. Diabetes mellitus is the most common disease associated with pancreatic islet dysfunction and is a leading cause of death in the United States.

Anatomy and Physiology

The pancreas is an elongated retroperitoneal gland that lies in the upper portion of the posterior abdominal wall. It resembles a fish, with its head and neck lying in the C-shaped curve of the duodenum, its body extending horizontally behind the stomach, and its tail touching the spleen (Fig. 35-1). The head is at the level of the second lumbar vertebra, makes up about 30 percent of the gland, and lies within the concavity of the duodenum. The neck, the narrowed portion between the head and body, joins to the body, which accounts for the largest portion of the gland. The tail tapers off from the body. The pancreas is of firm consistency and has a characteristic lobular appearance with a light yellow and slightly pink coloration.

In the adult, the total length of the pancreas varies between 12 and 20 cm, with a width of 3 to 5 cm and maximal thickness of 2 to 3 cm. Its weight is between 70 and 120 gm.

The pancreas is composed of both exocrine and endocrine tissue. The exocrine portion forms the largest mass of the gland and is composed of small groups of *acini* (grapelike formations) in which digestive enzymes and large volumes of sodium bicarbonate are synthesized and transported. The acini form a network of larger ducts that eventually drain into the major secretory ducts of Wirsung and Santorini. The duct of Wirsung extends from the surface of the tail of the pancreas to the duodenum at the ampulla of Vater, usually alongside the common bile duct. It empties into the duodenum at the same place as the common bile duct, the duodenal papilla. In most cases, the sphincter of Oddi surrounds both ducts. In one-third of cases, the duct of Wirsung and the common bile duct form a common channel before terminating at the ampulla of Vater. The accessory duct of Santorini exits from the main duct near the neck of the pancreas and enters the duodenum approximately 2 cm above the main duct.

The endocrine portion of the pancreas, the islets of Langerhans, are embedded between exocrine units like small islands. The islets contain four types of cells, *alpha*,

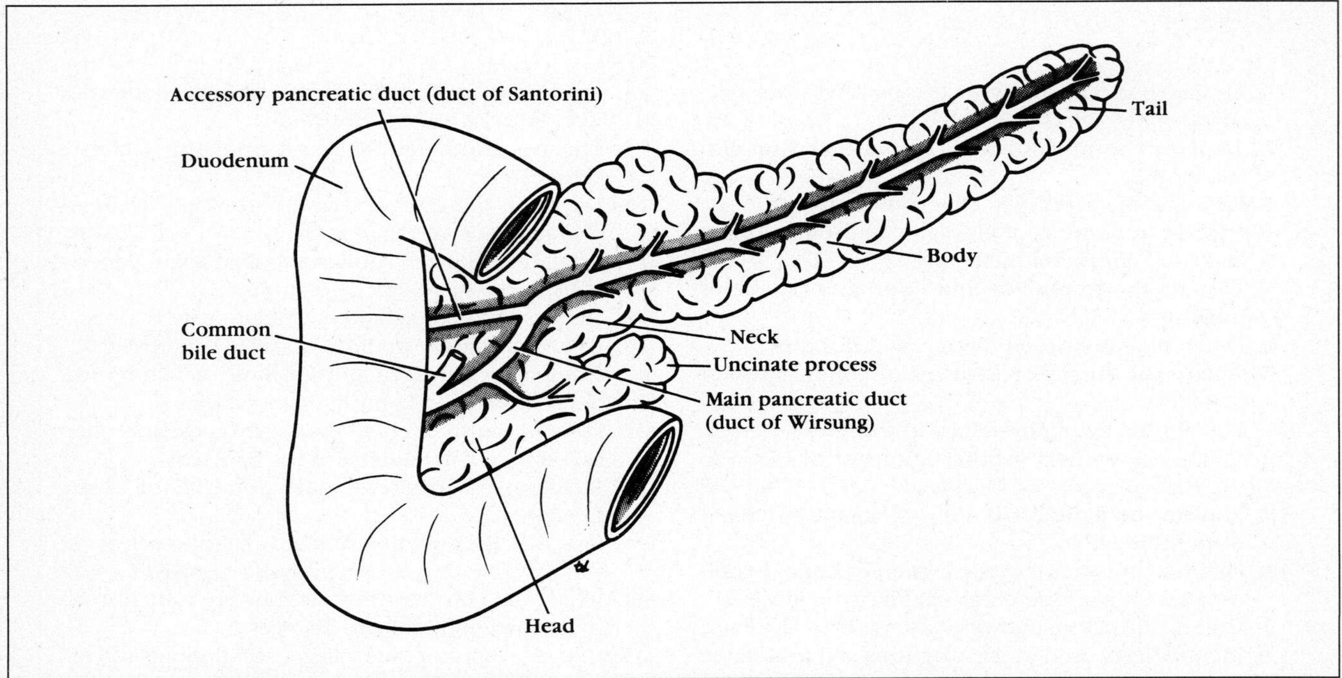

FIGURE 35-1 Parts of the pancreas. (From R. Snell, *Clinical Anatomy for Medical Students* [2nd ed.]. Boston: Little, Brown, 1981.)

beta, *delta*, and the recently described *PP (pancreatic polypeptide)* cells (Figs. 35-2 and 35-3). These types comprise 20, 70, 5 to 10, and 1 to 2 percent of islet cell population, respectively. All of these cells empty their secretions into the bloodstream. Alpha cells secrete *glucagon*, beta cells secrete *insulin*, and delta cells contain secretory granules that secrete *somatostatin*. The PP cells have small dark granules and are present on the islets and on the exocrine pancreas. The PP cells secrete a unique *pancreatic polypeptide* that causes gastrointestinal effects of gallbladder contraction and inhibition of pancreatic enzyme secretion. No metabolic effects by pancreatic polypeptide on glucose, fat, or amino acids have been established. Studies have revealed elevated basal and postprandial PP in lean persons who have noninsulin-dependent diabetes mellitus [21]. Although there are as many as 2 million islets, 20 to 300μ in diameter, the endocrine portion composes only about 1 percent of the weight of the pancreas.

Physiologic Regulation of Insulin Secretion

The main function of the endocrine portion of the pancreas is to secrete *insulin*, a hormone essential for normal carbohydrate metabolism. Insulin also influences the metabolism of fats and proteins. Therefore, it is a prime anabolic hormone and integrates the major metabolic fuels (see Fig. 35-3).

Insulin consists of two amino acid chains and is synthesized from a biologically inactive precursor, *proinsulin*, by the beta cells. Study indicates that proinsulin itself is derived from an even larger polypeptide, *preproinsulin* [16]. The average adult pancreas secretes an estimated 35 to 50 units of insulin daily.

Carbohydrate (primarily glucose), fats, and proteins, influence insulin output during meals. Insulin is the only known hormone that reduces the circulating glucose levels. Although numerous physiologic factors may alter insulin secretion, output is regulated mainly by blood glucose level through a negative feedback mechanism (Fig. 35-4). When glucose in the blood that is perfusing the pancreas exceeds approximately 100 mg per dl, an immediate beta cell response extrudes the granule's contents from the beta cell. When blood glucose levels fall, the rate of insulin secretion also decreases. The release of insulin is biphasic. Glucose prompts both an immediate and a sustained release as more insulin is synthesized. The feedback mechanism is very rapid acting, with insulin levels reaching 10 to 20 times the basal rate with blood glucose levels of 300 to 400 mg per dl. The cessation of secretion is equally rapid, occurring within minutes after restoration of blood glucose to fasting level [10].

Amino acids can also stimulate insulin secretion in varying degrees. The most potent stimulants are arginine, lysine, and phenylalanine. Insulin, in turn, promotes transport of the amino acids into the tissue cells.

Fats, although weak stimulators of insulin release, promote sufficient amounts to prevent ketoacidosis. Oral ingestion of fat triggers release of gastrointestinal hormones that augment insulin secretion.

While insulin secretion is mostly considered in terms of response to nutrients, measurable amounts are secreted at a low basal rate between meals and during prolonged fasting. The gastrointestinal hormones secretin, cholecystoki-

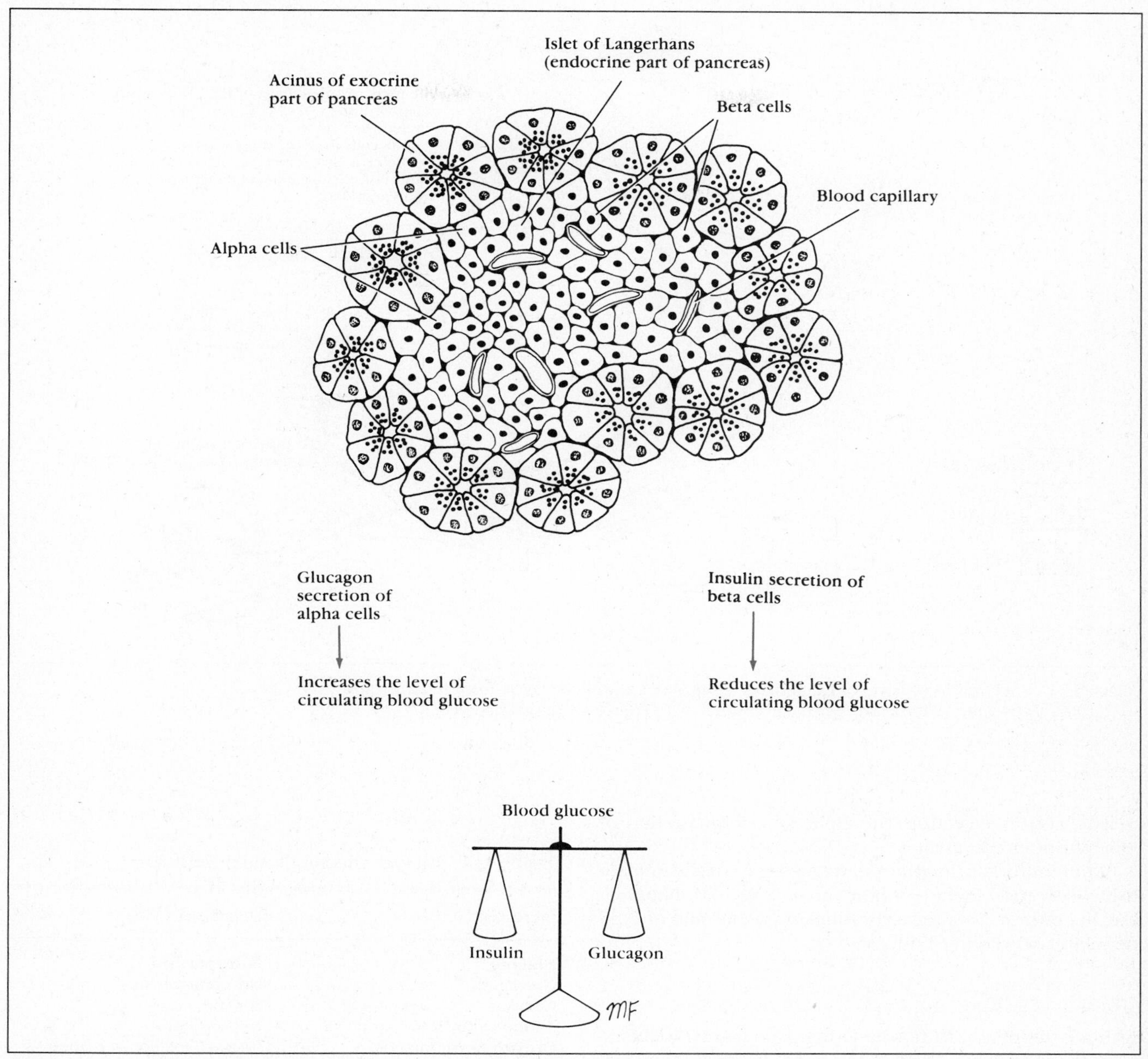

FIGURE 35-2 Regulation of the secretion of insulin and glucagon from the cells of the islets of Langerhans.

nin (CCK), gastrin, and gastric-inhibiting peptide (GIP), which are released by the gastrointestinal tract after a meal, stimulate pancreatic insulin release. These hormones, released during digestion, cause an "anticipatory" increase in blood insulin preparatory for the glucose and amino acids absorbed from the meal.

Other hormones that either directly increase the secretion of insulin or potentiate glucose stimulation of insulin are glucagon, cortisol, growth hormone progesterone, and estrogen. Prolonged increased amounts of these hormones can lead to exhaustion of the beta cells and diabetes. High pharmacologic doses of corticosteroids may also induce diabetes, especially in persons with a tendency toward diabetes.

The autonomic nervous system also plays a major role in modulating insulin secretion between meals, during times when there is no intake, and in response to stressors. Norepinephrine and acetylcholine, transmitters of the autonomic nervous system, and the adrenal medulla hormone epinephrine influence secretions of alpha, beta, and delta cells of the islets of Langerhans. The alpha-adrenergic activities of the sympathomimetic amines (epinephrine and norepinephrine) inhibit insulin secretion. Although catecholamine stimulation of beta-adrenergic sites in-

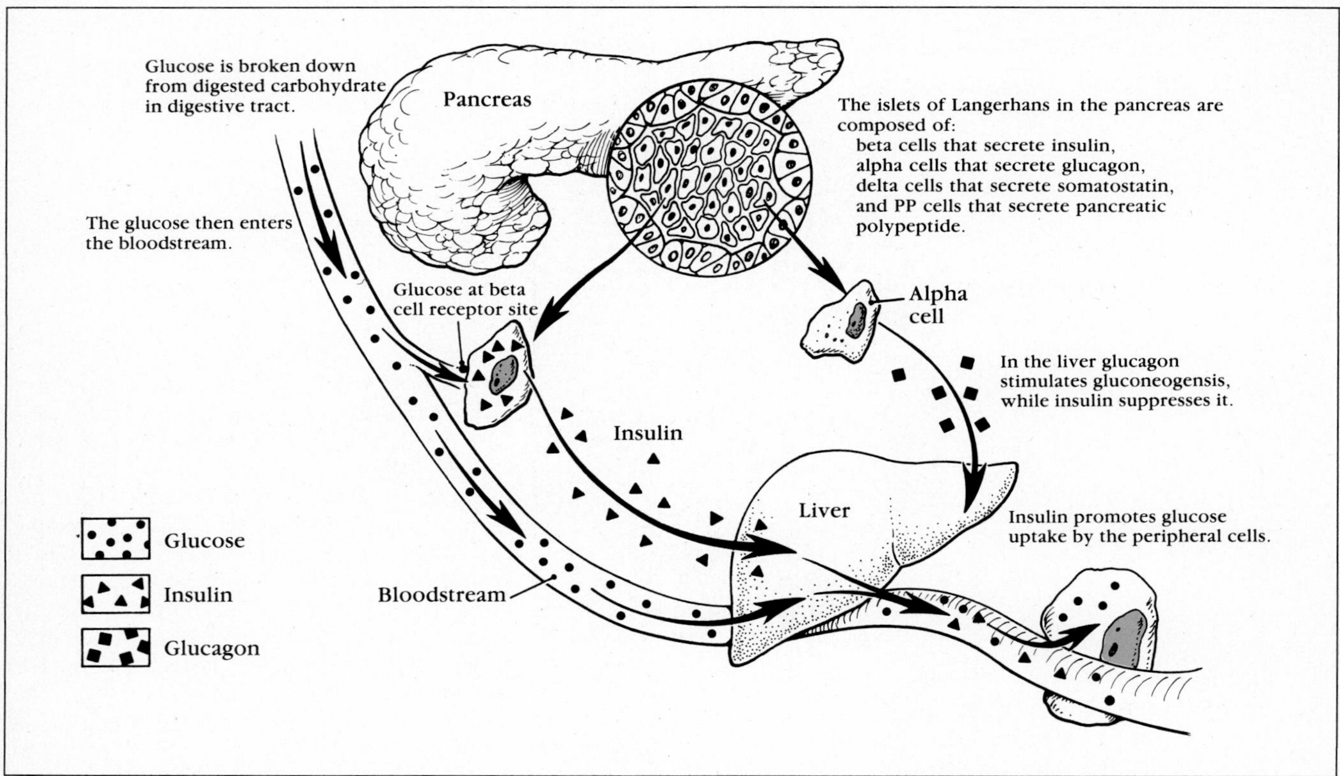

FIGURE 35-3 Secretions of islets of Langerhans. (Reprinted with permission from *Patient Care* 3:17, 1982. Copyright © 1982, *Patient Care,* Oradell, N.J. 07649. All rights reserved.)

creases insulin secretion, the alpha-adrenergic action of epinephrine predominates.

Other factors, primarily pharmacologic, that stimulate insulin secretion include sulfonylurea drugs and theophylline. In contrast, beta-receptor-blocking agents and diazoxide inhibit secretion (Table 35-1).

TABLE 35-1 Factors Affecting Insulin Secretion

Increases	Decreases
Glucose	Epinephrine
Glucagon	Norepinephrine
Cortisol	Somatostatin
Amino acids	Hypokalemia
Growth hormone (GH)	Fasting (except in diabetes)
Secretin, gastric-inhibitory peptide (GIP), possibly other hormones of small intestine	Nervous impulses by way of sympathetic nervous system
Nervous impulses—especially oral and pharyngeal mucosa by way of vagus nerve	Diazoxide[a]
Sulonylureas[a]	Beta-receptor-blocking agents[a]
Alpha-receptor-blocking agents[a]	
Beta-receptor-stimulating agents[a]	
Theophylline[a]	

[a]Pharmacologic agents.

Source: Reprinted with permission from J. O'Hara and C. Warfield, The diabetic neuropathies. *Hosp. Prac.* November 1984, Vol. 19, No. 11, p. 436.

Effect of Insulin on Facilitated Diffusion

Insulin is an influential hormone that affects the biochemical function of every organ in the body. Its most important action is to accelerate the transport of glucose across most cell membranes in the body. In the absence of insulin, the rate of transport of glucose into body cells is about one-fourth normal; when an excess is secreted, the rate may increase to 5 times normal. Figure 35-5 illustrates the carrier-mediated transport of the inside of the membrane and its release transport by means of a carrier mechanism called *facilitated diffusion*, or carrier transport. Insulin influences this transport of glucose into the cell by combining with a receptor protein in the cell membrane. A direct action on the cell membrane is implied because glucose transport occurs within seconds or minutes. Once the glucose concentration inside the cell is equal to that on the outside, additional glucose is not transferred into the cell. Insulin is especially effective in facilitating transport of glucose in skeletal and adipose tissue, the liver,

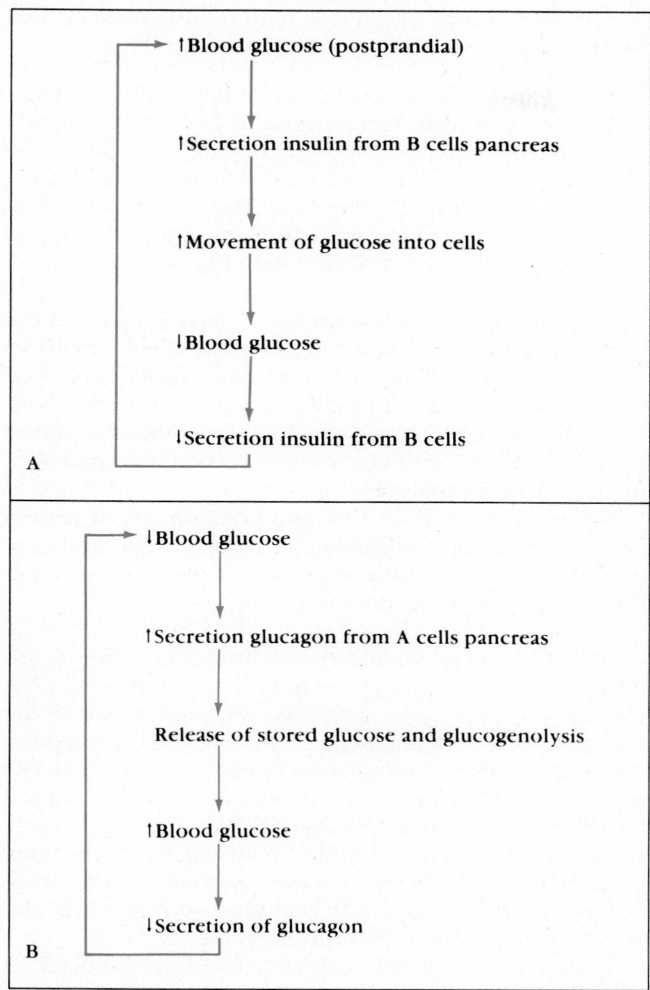

FIGURE 35-4 Negative feedback system of (A) insulin and (B) glucagon.

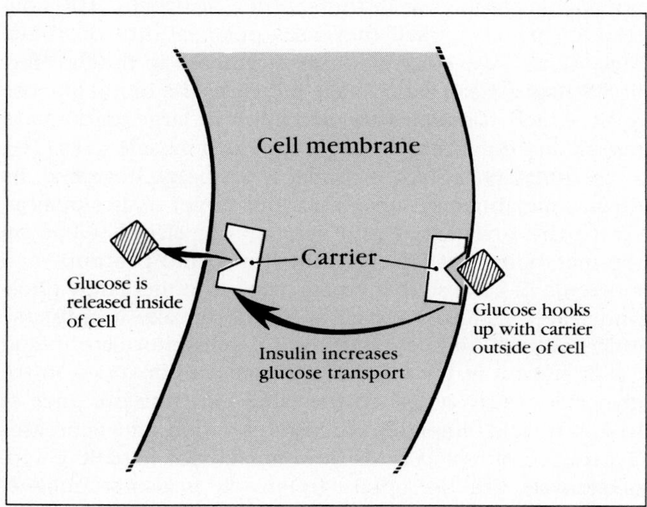

FIGURE 35-5 Insulin increases glucose transport.

and the heart. Adipose and skeletal tissues alone make up 65 percent of body weight.

Insulin does not enhance glucose transport into the brain, erythrocytes, leukocytes, intestinal mucosa, or epithelium of the kidneys. The brain continues to function normally when insulin deficiency causes hyperglycemia. In erythrocytes and leukocytes, the level of free glucose is close to that in plasma. These cells do not suffer from insulin deficiency, but they cannot survive glucose deficiency.

Metabolic Effects of Insulin

Insulin stimulates reactions that involve fats, carbohydrates, and proteins. Insulin affects *carbohydrate* metabolism by increasing the rate of glucose metabolism, decreasing blood glucose concentration, and increasing glycogen stores in the muscle and liver. Insulin affects *fat metabolism* by increasing the rate of glucose transport into fat cells, forming lipids from fatty acids, and promoting storage in adipose tissue. Insulin affects *protein metabolism* and increases the quantity of protein by increasing translation of the messenger ribonucleic acid (RNA) code in the ribosomes to form more protein, and by enhancing transcription of deoxyribonucleic acid (DNA) to form more RNA, thereby resulting in additional protein synthesis.

Insulin's diverse effects are integrated so that it is the prime synthesis and storage hormone in metabolism. Its actions are focused on three metabolically important target tissues—*liver*, *adipose tissue*, and *muscle*; they are summarized in Table 35-2 and in the following discussion.

Liver. The liver is the major site for synthesis of glycogen, lipids, and protein, and is the major endogenous source of glucose. Insulin is secreted by the pancreas into the portal system and enters the systemic circulation through the liver. The role of the liver with respect to

TABLE 35-2 Target Sites and Metabolic Actions of Insulin

Substance	Liver	Adipose Cell	Muscle
Carbohydrate	Glycogen synthesis Gluconeogenesis Glycogenolysis	Glucose transport Glycerol synthesis	Glucose transport Glycolysis Glycogen synthesis
Fat	Lipogenesis	Triglycerides Fatty acid synthesis Promotes storage	
Protein	Proteolysis for gluconeogenesis		Amino acid uptake Protein synthesis Protein anabolism

insulin and carbohydrate homeostasis is unique because of the following aspects:

1. Insulin promotes glycogen storage by inhibiting the action of an enzyme, phosphorylase, responsible for breakdown of liver glycogen and release of glucose into circulation.
2. Insulin also promotes glycogen synthesis by increasing the action of enzymes necessary for formation of glycogen.
3. Insulin is not necessary for transport of glucose into the liver, as the liver cells are freely permeable to glucose. The uptake is increased by glucokinase, an enzyme that is responsible for "trapping" glucose inside liver cells so that the intracellular concentration is roughly equal to the plasma concentration.
4. In the basal state, glucose is continuously released from the liver at a rate of 2.0 to 3.5 mg per kg per minute (200–350 gm/day) [23]. The ability of the liver to release free glucose derives from its capability for glycogenolysis and gluconeogenesis, and its possession of an enzyme that promotes further breakdown of glycogen into glucose. This process is critical during prolonged fasting when glucose is oxidized minimally in most tissues and is used almost exclusively by the brain. Once glucose is in the free form, it readily diffuses into the circulating blood and the liver cell membrane.
5. In the basal state, between meals when the blood glucose level falls and the pancreas secretes less insulin, glycogen synthesis and storage are halted.
6. The concentration of insulin in portal blood is over 2 times greater than that in peripheral blood. This concentration is due to the secretion of insulin by the pancreas directly into the portal system [25].
7. Absorbed hexoses have direct access to the liver through the portal vein prior to circulating to peripheral tissues. Because of the previously mentioned characteristics, the liver is important in buffering blood glucose. When there is an excess of insulin and/or glucose, the hepatic cells take up large quantities of glucose, which are deposited as glycogen as well as being converted to fat. Approximately 60 percent of glucose ingested in a meal is stored in this manner [10]. When there is an absence of insulin or the blood glucose concentration falls too low, the hepatic cells release quantities of glucose into the blood by breaking down stored glycogen (glycogenolysis) and forming new glucose (gluconeogenesis). Thus, insulin enables the organism to maintain a stable blood glucose balance.

Adipose Tissue. Maintenance of energy balance is a major role of adipose tissue. It is the only tissue that can store a variable amount of "fuel" in the form of fat. The oxidation of 1 gm of fat yields 9 calories. Unlike the liver cell, the fat cell (adipocyte) membrane is capable of excluding glucose. Adipose tissue does not release glucose but can release free fatty acids (FFA) and certain amino acids. Insulin greatly enhances the transport of glucose into fat cells and promotes fat storage in adipose tissue.

The metabolism of glucose within fat cells occurs in several steps:

1. Glucose is rapidly phosphorylated within the fat cell.
2. Glucose is further metabolized to 2-carbon fragments (acetylcoenzyme A), which are converted to fatty acids.
3. A larger portion is degraded by the process of glycolysis into alpha-glycerophosphate. The latter readily combines with free fatty acids to form triglycerides, the primary storage form of fat within the adipose cell.

Insulin promotes fat storage by (1) inhibiting the action of the enzyme lipase within the fat cell, which results in inhibition of both lipolysis and release of fatty acids into the circulation; and (2) promoting glucose transport into the cell. Through its action on glucose metabolism, insulin provides the precursors necessary for combining and storing fatty acids as triglycerides.

Fatty acids and all of the lipid components of plasma greatly increase in the absence of insulin. High lipid concentrations in the plasma, especially cholesterol, increase the risk of developing atherosclerosis.

Muscle. As in adipose tissue, insulin increases transport of glucose across the membrane into muscle cells through the process of facilitated diffusion. Once in the cell, the glucose is metabolized completely to carbon dioxide or, if oxygen is limited, to lactic acid. After the glucose molecule that enters the cell is phosphorylated, it is used for energy or stored as glycogen. Unlike the liver, muscle cannot release glucose from stored glycogen into the body fluids because it lacks the necessary enzyme, glucose phosphatase, to convert glycogen into glucose. Very little glucose is stored in the form of triglyceride.

Quantitatively, muscle cell consumption of glucose is small during a resting state. Muscle tissue uses mostly fatty acids for energy because the normal resting muscle membrane is almost impermeable to glucose except in the presence of insulin. During exercise, however, glucose use increases greatly. This usage of glucose requires smaller amounts of insulin, as exercising muscle fibers are more permeable to glucose in the absence of insulin. The contraction process itself increases permeability of fibers. Muscles also use large amounts of glucose in the first few hours after a meal. Food intake increases the blood glucose level, which stimulates the secretion of large amounts of insulin and the transport of glucose into muscle cells [10].

In summary, insulin is primarily a storage hormone. Its diverse metabolic actions on various target tissues demonstrate the integrated and synergistic effect it has on the metabolism of fats, carbohydrates, and protein. Each molecule of glucose that enters a cell is immediately phosphorylated. Adipose tissue and muscle take up glucose only under the influence of insulin, phosphorylate it, and either store it in the form of glycogen or convert it to triglycerides (fatty acids). At the same time, the presence of free fatty acids impedes glucose oxidation and decreases the release of amino acids from muscle for hepatic gluconeogenesis. Glucose uptake by muscle is also stimulated, providing fuel to replace fatty acids whose release from adipose tissue is inhibited by insulin. Fat accumulation is also increased by release of fatty acids at the adipose cell from lipoproteins that arrive by way of the circulation from the liver and gastrointestinal tract. The antilipolytic action of insulin on the adipose cell increases fat storage, and thereby inhibits gluconeogenesis in the liver by depriving the liver of fatty acids and cofactors used in gluconeogenesis.

Physiology of Glucagon

Glucagon, a hormone secreted by the alpha cells of the islets of Langerhans, is important in regulating carbohydrate metabolism. Its secretion results in an increase in blood glucose concentration. The major effects of glucagon are stimulation of *glycogenolysis* and *gluconeogenesis* (see Fig. 35-3). It also promotes proteolysis and ketogenesis.

Glucagon is very potent and causes glycogenolysis in the liver, which quickly increases blood glucose. Only 1 gm per kg of glucagon can elevate the blood sugar approximately 20 percent within minutes. The hormone can continue to increase blood glucose levels, even after the glycogen level in cells has been exhausted, by increasing gluconeogenesis in liver cells [5].

Glucagon secretion is regulated by blood glucose concentration. Changes in blood glucose levels have the opposite effect on glucagon secretion from that on insulin secretion. A decrease in the level of blood glucose increases glucagon secretion. In almost every instance, glucagon has a metabolic effect directly opposite that of insulin: insulin promotes storage of glycogen in liver and muscle, glucagon inhibits it; insulin inhibits glycogenolysis, glucagon promotes it; insulin inhibits lipolysis, glucagon stimulates it. Thus, a negative feedback system with opposing action of insulin and glucagon maintains blood glucose levels (see Fig. 35-4). Glucagon secretion is increased by exercise, starvation, insulin lack, and amino acid ingestion. It is important in maintaining glucose levels during fasting, exercise, and stressful situations. It helps to protect the body against hypoglycemia.

Somatostatin

Somatostatin, a hormone excreted by the delta (D) cells of the pancreas, acts as a neural agent by inhibiting secretions of insulin and glucagon and other nonislet hormones. Although not a neurotransmitter, its actions are opposite to those of acetylcholine. The release of somatostatin is stimulated by epinephrine. Somatostatin is also widely present in the central nervous system, primarily the hypothalamus. Smaller amounts have been noted in the cells of the thyroid and gastrointestinal tract. The precise mechanism of somatostatin in metabolic processes is not clearly defined, but it is postulated that it may be important in regulating insulin and glucagon secretion [25].

Regulation of Blood Glucose

In the healthy person the blood glucose ranges between 80 and 90 mg per dl in the fasting state. This concentration rises to 120 to 140 mg per dl after a meal. The feedback system returns the concentration to normal within about two hours after the last absorption of carbohydrates.

Blood glucose level is vital in maintaining nutritional balance in the brain, retinae, and germinal epithelium of the gonads, because glucose is the only nutrient that can be used to supply adequate energy. More than one-half of all glucose formed by gluconeogenesis during the interdigesting period is used by the brain [5].

The liver acts as a reservoir and buffering system for glucose. The liver stores sufficient glycogen to maintain a normal blood sugar for 12 to 24 hours. When blood glucose levels are high, almost two-thirds of the glucose is stored, and when blood glucose concentration falls below normal, the stored glucose is released to maintain the blood level. When the blood glucose level is high (e.g., after meals), insulin secretion is increased to return the concentration to normal.

The glucagon feedback system assists in maintaining the range of glucose concentration by stimulating glycogenolysis and gluconeogenesis. Under normal circumstances, the insulin feedback mechanism is the most important, but in starvation states or excessive use of glucose during stress and exercise, the glucagon system becomes very important.

Stimulation of the sympathetic nervous system causes a rise in blood glucose level. The release of catecholamines epinephrine and norepinephrine stimulates glycogenolysis in the liver, resulting in rapid release of glucose into the circulation.

Growth hormone and cortisol increase blood glucose levels less rapidly than the insulin-glucagon system. Both hormones decrease use of glucose in peripheral cells. Cortisol also stimulates gluconeogenesis, thereby resulting in an increased blood glucose level. Growth hormone and glucocorticoids are secreted during periods of hypoglycemia and decrease the rate of glucose use by most cells of the body. These hormones are less powerful in regulating blood glucose than insulin and glucagon, and require hours rather than minutes to effect a change in the serum glucose.

Diabetes Mellitus

Diabetes is a metabolic disorder characterized by a relative or absolute lack of the hormone insulin, which results in impaired use of carbohydrates and altered metabolism of fats and protein. The word *diabetes,* from the Greek meaning “a siphon,” suggests excessive urine formation; the word *mellitus,* from the Greek meaning “honey,” suggests sweetness.

History

Writings about diabetes go back more than 3000 years to the Ebers papyrus, in which afflicted persons were described as passing frequent and large amounts of urine. Ayur Veda described the sweetness of the urine and noted that ants were attracted to it. He wrote of weakness, emaciation, polyuria, and carbuncles in affected persons. Aretaeus, a first-century Greek physician, is credited with naming the disorder. He described the disease as a "melting down of the flesh and limbs into urine." Lipemia of diabetic blood was noted by Helmunt sometime between 1573 and 1664 A.D. The first diagnostic sign of the disease was established by Thomas Willis in the seventeenth century, when he tasted the urine of his patients and noted its sweetness. A French physician, Michel Chevreul, discovered that the sweetness was caused by sugar. In 1869 Langerhans, still a medical student, described the group of cells in the pancreas that produce insulin. Elliot Joslin was prescribing dietary restrictions long before the discovery of insulin. In 1921 Banting and Best were able to purify islet cell tissues from dogs and obtained a drop in blood sugar when the tissue was injected into diabetic animals. Within six months, insulin was administered to humans and the "rapid melting" and "speedy death" described by Aretaeus were alleviated.

In 1936 long-acting insulins were introduced, protamine being added to prolong the action and zinc being added for stability. In 1942 Hagedorn modified the PZI (protamine zinc insulin) and produced the first intermediate-acting insulin, NPH (neutral protamine Hagedorn). Globin and lente insulins soon followed. In 1955 oral hypoglycemic agents were introduced. Insulin has been further purified and biosynthetic human insulin has been developed through recombinant DNA techniques.

TABLE 35-3 Classification of Diabetes Mellitus and Other Types of Glucose Intolerance

Clinical types
Diabetes mellitus
Insulin-dependent (IDDM), type I
Noninsulin-dependent (NIDDM), type II
Nonobese NIDDM
Obese NIDDM
Other types including diabetes melliltus associated with certain conditions and syndromes that may be (1) pancreatic disease, (2) hormonal, (3) drug- or chemical-induced, (4) insulin receptor abnormalities, (5) certain genetic syndromes, (6) or other
Impaired glucose tolerance (IGT)
Nonobese IGT
Obese IGT
Impaired glucose tolerance associated with certain conditions and syndromes that may be (1) pancreatic disease, (2) hormonal, (drug- or chemical-induced), (4) insulin-receptor abnormalities, (5) certain genetic syndromes
Gestational diabetes (GDM)
Normal glucose tolerance but risk classes
Previous abnormality of glucose tolerance (PrevAGT)
Potential abnormality of glucose tolerance (PotAGT)

Source: Reprinted with permission from *Diabetes,* Vol. 28, December 1979, pp. 1042–1043.

Classification

In 1979 the National Diabetes Data Group and National Institutes of Health endorsed by the World Health Organization and the American Diabetes Association outlined a classification of diabetes (Table 35-3) [14]. The majority of cases consist of one of two variants: *type I, insulin-dependent diabetes mellitus (IDDM)* and *type II, noninsulin-dependent diabetes mellitus (NIDDM)* (Table 35-4).

Type I diabetes, previously called juvenile-onset diabetes, has an onset generally before age 30 years in persons who are not obese. Only 10 percent of these individuals have a positive family history of a diabetic parent or sibling, although there may be a family history of the disease. Plasma insulin levels are low and respond very little or not at all to insulin stimulators such as glucose or oral hypoglycemics. These persons are ketosis prone and require exogenous insulin. The pancreas contains little or no extractable insulin, and the overall beta cell mass is reduced. Ability to synthesize insulin is evident at birth, but the level falls with time. About one-third experience a "honeymoon" period, a remission characterized by temporary restoration of insulin secretion, which is reflected in C-peptide release (measure of residual beta cell secretory capacity). This period is followed by a relapse within weeks or months.

Type II diabetes, previously called adult-onset diabetes, usually occurs after age 30 years, and about 70 to 80 percent of affected persons are obese. This type accounts for approximately 80 percent of total cases of diabetes. In contrast to IDDM, individuals with NIDDM have a positive history of diabetes in the immediate family. At birth these persons synthesize insulin, but the level falls as they age and beta cell function deteriorates. Insulin resistance may also occur, together with relative insulin deficiency. These persons are not ketosis prone. *Maturity-onset diabetes in young people (MODY)*, has been included in the type II classification. In these persons, diabetes is mild, ketosis resistant, noninsulin dependent, and occurs before age 25 years. It affects children as young as 10 years, and there may be a pattern of inheritance.

Types I and II disease comprise the majority of diabetic persons. Diabetes can also occur in association with other conditions and syndromes such as pancreatic disease, Cushing's syndrome, insulin-receptor abnormalities, genetic syndromes, and hormone- or drug-induced disorders. Gestational diabetes occurs only during pregnancy. Pregnancy may be a diabetogenic condition. Women demonstrate varying degrees of glucose intolerance related to metabolic effects of hormones secreted during pregnancy. Clinical manifestations may be evident in persons with a predisposition for diabetes. Impaired glucose tolerance (IGT) is a clinical class that includes those whose glucose tolerance tests are abnormal. They are asymptomatic but are recognized at higher risk for diabetes than the general population (Tables 35-3 and 35-4).

Stages

Diabetes can also be classified by degree or stage of abnormality based on measurable carbohydrate tolerance and presence or absence of hyperglycemia. Classifications are outlined in Table 35-5 using the American Diabetes Asso-

TABLE 35-4 Comparison of Types I and II Diabetes

Variables	Type I	Type II
Age of onset	Frequently before age 20; most commonly preadolescence; can occur after age 30	Usually after age 30; can occur before age 30
Onset	Abrupt	Insidious
Body Weight	Thin	Usually obese (80%)
Symptoms	Polyuria, polydipsia, polyphagia, weight loss, weakness, fatigue	Polyuria, polydipsia, polyphagia, vulvovaginitis, often asymptomatic
Control	Wide fluctuations of blood sugar in relation to growth, diet, insulin, and exercise	Stable, usually easily controlled
Exogenous insulin	Needed by all	May be needed during stress or initial management
Oral hypoglycemics	Not useful	May be useful in 30–40% of cases
Beta cells of pancreas	Destruction or inability of cells to secrete insulin	Secrete inadequate or varying amounts of insulin
Ketoacidosis	Most prevalent first 5 years of known diabetes and in teenage years	Uncommon except with stress, infection
Insulin reactions	Frequent	Uncommon

ciation terminology. The separation of stages is arbitrary. An individual may remain in one stage, progress to another, or revert to a prior one. Progression or regression of carbohydrate intolerance may occur slowly, never occur, or occur rapidly.

Frequency and Etiology

Diabetes is a common disorder of the endocrine system, with over 2 million affected individuals in the United States alone. Because carbohydrate tolerance is decreased in the elderly, disease frequently increases in later years. Various theories have been offered to explain the genesis of diabetes. Multifactorial causes such as genetic, metabolic, microbiologic, and immunologic etiologies have been cited for the variants of the disease [8]. Abnormalities may occur in the *beta cell* (inadequate insulin secretion, abnormal insulin), *plasma* (abnormal binding, destruction), and *target cell* (cell membrane or intracellular abnormalities).

Insulin-Dependent Diabetes

Current thinking leans toward beta cell destruction and absence or severe lack of insulin in the causation of IDDM. Genetic predisposition to beta cell destruction, infection, autoimmunity, and environmental factors have been postulated as causative mechanisms [5,23].

Infection and Autoimmunity. No specific environmental factor has been identified in the pathogenesis, but viral agents are highly suspected. Many types of infections have been reported to precede the onset of diabetes mellitus. These include mumps, rubella, varicella, measles, influenza, coxsackie virus, cytomegalovirus (CMV), and viral and occasionally bacterial pneumonias. In addition, the number of cases diagnosed increases during autumn and winter when viral infections are most frequent [13]. This temporal association of onset of IDDM with an infection may be related to genetic susceptibility of beta cells to viruses and other toxic agents.

The exact role of viruses is not established, but investigations have implicated either (1) virus-induced injury of the beta cell and autoimmunity against the islet cell, or (2) breakdown of beta cell mass due to prior autoimmune reactions of unknown cause [24]. Specific human leukocyte antigen (HLA) types are more common in IDDM, especially in children. These children tend to have high levels of islet cell antibodies (ICAs), lymphocytes, monocytes, and eosinophils. The ICAs have been found in the islets of recent-onset IDDM. In addition, sensitized T cells reactive against beta cells have been identified [5]. These

TABLE 35-5 Stages of Diabetes

Determinant	Prediabetes	Subclinical Diabetes	Latent	Overt
Fasting blood sugar	Normal	Normal	Normal or abnormal	Abnormal
Glucose tolerance test	Normal	Normal; abnormal during pregnancy stress	Abnormal	Abnormal
Delayed and/or decreased response to glucose	+	++	+++	++++
Symptoms	None	None	None	Present
Vascular changes	+	+	++	+++

findings are strengthened by the association of other autoimmune disorders (e.g., Addison's disease, pernicious anemia, and thyroid disease) with IDDM. The person with NIDDM lacks this antigenic tendency.

In summary, the pathogenesis of IDDM is most frequently related to a combination of environmental (probably viral), genetic (HLA-linked), and immunologic factors, with viral-induced injury occasionally being a component of autoimmunity.

Noninsulin-Dependent Diabetes

The pathogenesis of noninsulin-dependent diabetes mellitus, in which the lack of insulin is not severe has been explained as a consequence of various etiologic factors. The following is a summary of several theories that have been offered.

Alteration of Insulin Secretion. The changes of NIDDM may not be due to an actual reduction in beta cell mass and insulin production but to either inadequate or a delayed initial-phase response to the glucose load. Second-phase responses are within normal ranges or elevated. Even though second-phase secretion reverts plasma glucose to basal levels, postprandial hyperglycemia results. This alteration is demonstrated in NIDDM when the rise in plasma insulin is delayed after oral glucose intake, when peak insulin level is reached after the glucose peak, and when diabetic blood glucose curves in healthy, nondiabetic persons (simulated by computer-programmed glucose infusions) are compared with those of persons with NIDDM. The latter secrete less insulin than age-, sex-, and weight-matched healthy subjects. Similar findings of impaired insulin secretion have been noted in prediabetics [19].

Bihormonal Theory. Normally, a rise in blood glucose level depresses glucagon secretion, and a fall in glucose is followed by a rise in glucagon. A relative or absolute hyperglucagonemia has been demonstrated in both forms of diabetes after the ingestion of food. Infusion with somatostatin lowers glucose levels. It is postulated that there is inappropriate control not only of the beta cell but of the alpha cell, the source of glucagon, as a causative factor in the disease [19].

Insulin Resistance. Insulin resistance, a common characteristic in NIDDM, is a major factor in pathogenesis. It exists when a specific quantity of insulin produces less than the normal anticipated biologic effect at target sites. Insulin resistance and hyperinsulinemia are associated with obesity. Insulin resistance can be attributed to three principal causes: (1) an *abnormal beta cell secretory product*, such as abnormal insulin molecule or incomplete conversion of proinsulin to insulin; (2) *circulating insulin antagonists* such as antiinsulin antibodies, antiinsulin receptor antibodies, or elevated levels of opposing regulatory hormones (e.g., growth hormone, cortisol, glucagon, or catecholamines); and (3) *receptor defects in target tissues* (decrease in receptors in a variety of cells) [16]. Alterations are demonstrated when the insulin requirements are increased during infection, stress, or endocrine disorders.

Heredity. For centuries it has been noted that diabetes "runs in families," because approximately 40 percent of persons who develop the disease have a positive family history. In general, a genetic component is accepted in the etiology. Family histories, twin studies, and studies of histocompatibility of antigens confirm this [2,18]. Although evidence supports the role of genetic factors in both IDDM and NIDDM, the pattern of inheritance has not been established. The *recessive gene theory* holds that diabetes is transmitted as a recessive genetic characteristic that is present in about 20 percent of the population. The theory of *multifactorial inheritance* holds that diabetes results from an interaction between several different genes and environmental factors [18]. Both IDDM and NIDDM exhibit genetic differences. Studies of identical twins and first-generation relatives of diabetics reflect a concordance rate (both twins affected) in IDDM of less than 50 percent, but a concordance rate approaching 100 percent for twins with NIDDM [2,18]. Therefore, genetic factors play a greater role in the occurrence of NIDDM than of IDDM.

Age. Except for IDDM, increasing age is related to an increased prevalence of diabetes. The frequency rises sharply after age 40 years, probably reflecting a general change in glucose tolerance. The blood glucose level is low in childhood and rises progressively; after age 70, about 15 percent of the population may show a mild abnormal glucose tolerance. The separation between diabetes and nondiabetes may present a problem if tolerance is not adjusted for age. This increasing frequency has been explained as a decrease in body function occurring in all body cells with senescence.

Body Weight. About 80 percent of individuals with NIDDM are obese, and the frequency of diabetes in obese individuals is greater than in the general population. The interrelationship occurs because obesity is associated with insulin insensitivity in target tissues (muscle, liver, and adipose cells). It is well known that blood levels of insulin are higher in the obese individual and take longer to return to the fasting state. Obesity acts as a diabetogenic factor because the accompanying insulin resistance increases the need for insulin. As the obese are resistant to the effects of insulin, in practice, the obese diabetic responds poorly to treatment with insulin. Weight loss increases glucose tolerance.

Sex. Diabetes is more frequent in women than in men. Between ages 40 and 60 years, women diabetics outnumber men almost 2:1. In Japan, Malaya, and India, diabetes is 50 to 100 percent more common in men. In the West Indies, the sex distribution is equal, but black women with the disease outnumber men. The reason for increased occurrence in women may be related to the late effects of high parity, which may not be manifested until after age 45 years.

Diet. Certain factors implicate diet as a possible causative factor in the onset of diabetes. The frequency is great in wealthier communities in the United States. The effects of high-carbohydrate and high-fat diets in the causation of NIDDM have been studied extensively. Modification of dietary intake of carbohydrates minimizes hyperglycemia in these individuals, and limitation of saturated fat intake may delay the onset of atherosclerosis.

Numerous theories, none mutually exclusive, explain the variants of diabetes. In many cases, there is no single biochemical cause of the disorder, and it can be described only in terms of impairment of insulin secretory response due to multifactorial causes. Similarly, it is difficult to separate factors that are the result of disease and those that cause disease.

Pregnancy. During pregnancy, alterations in carbohydrate metabolism occur. To provide for the energy requirements of the fetus, fasting hypoglycemia and increased lypolysis occur. The workload of the pancreas and tissue insensitivity to insulin increases. The clinical picture may resemble that of NIDDM.

Stress. Any form of stress with the neuroendocrine response increases gluconeogenesis and glycogenolysis. Infection, life changes, and various environmental factors can be stressors that induce or worsen a diabetic state.

Introduction to the Pathology of Diabetes

Few diseases have as many widespread and systemic lesions as diabetes. Changes occur in the pancreas, blood vessels, kidneys, and eyes. In classic insulin-dependent diabetes mellitus the number of islet cells is reduced, degranulation of beta cells and fibrosis of the islets may occur, and there may be lymphocytic infiltration. In noninsulin-dependent diabetes mellitus the number of islets is usually normal, the degree of beta cell granulation is somewhat reduced or may be normal, and hyaline deposits may be observed.

Pathology of the Pancreas. *Hyalin.* A frequent pancreatic lesion is hyalinization of the islets. Hyalin, an eosinophilic, glassy, translucent material, may infiltrate small areas or the entire islet. It may have the fibrillar structure characteristic of amyloid [19]. Progressive accumulation of the deposits reduces beta cell mass. Hyalinization occurs in IDDM, but is more common in NIDDM and correlates with the duration of the disease. It may occur in nondiabetics.

Fibrosis. Thickening of the capsule and islets by fibrous connective tissue is a common change, and the islet cells may be completely replaced by collagen tissue. This change is correlated with the duration of diabetes, and it also occurs in nondiabetics who have pronounced atherosclerotic changes and in persons with other types of pancreatic lesions.

Degranulation of Beta Cells. A reduction in beta cells is a consistent finding and is most frequent in IDDM. The amount of beta cell granulation correlates with the amount of extractable pancreatic insulin.

Vacuolation. Beta granules are replaced by distended, foamy, watery, vacuolated beta cells. Glycogen accumulation is related to the level and duration of hyperglycemia, and is reversible.

Leukocytic Infiltrations. Eosinophils and lymphocytes infiltrate the islets in an inflammatory type of reaction that is referred to as insulitis. The inflammatory infiltrates are considered a type of immunologic reaction.

Hypertrophy and Hyperplasia of Islets. These processes occur infrequently except in the children of diabetic mothers and mothers with a latent diabetic tendency. The mother's hyperglycemia causes fetal hyperglycemia and compensatory fetal islet hyperplasia.

Vascular System Pathology. Vascular lesions are a hallmark of diabetes and are probably related to hyperlipidemia. Electron microscopic studies have revealed microangiopathy (thickening of the walls of the arterioles, capillaries, and venules) in the kidneys, retinae, and neural and epidermal vascular beds. Atherosclerosis, characterized by fatty intimal plaque and intimal fibrosis, appears mostly in the large vessels. Lipid deposits, called *atheromas* or *plaque,* are laid down on the intimal surfaces. Lipids (cholesterol, triglycerides, phospholipids) circulate in plasma as large molecules combined with proteins and are called lipoproteins. Low-density lipoprotein (LDL) carries about 75 percent of circulating cholesterol while high-density lipoprotein (HDL) carries about 15 to 20 percent. Investigations have revealed an inverse correlation of high-density lipoprotein with atherosclerosis [7] (See Chap. 21). Fibroblasts and calcium may be deposited, and calcified plaques develop in the vessels. The hyperlipidemia characteristic of diabetes also relates to the high frequency of hypertension in diabetes.

The atherosclerosis is the major factor in the high frequency of myocardial infarction, cerebral vascular accidents, and gangrene of the extremities in diabetes. Coronary atherosclerosis is up to 5 times more prevalent than in the general population, and myocardial infarction is the most common cause of death [17]. Atherosclerosis is most prevalent in diabetic women, including those who are premenopausal. Atherosclerosis develops within a few years of the onset of the disease. Persons who have had diabetes for 10 to 15 years, whatever the age of onset, usually have significant atherosclerosis [19].

The principal clinical manifestations of peripheral arterial disease are ischemic lesions of the feet and of the lower extremities. In addition, neurotrophic changes cause loss of sensation, which may decrease attention to small injuries that become infected. A small break may lead to cellulitis, lymphangitis, infection, and necrosis of tissue (Figs. 35-6 and 35-7). The arterioles also become thickened and microcirculation is impaired.

Pathology of the Kidneys. The kidneys are usually affected in diabetes. The predominant renal changes are

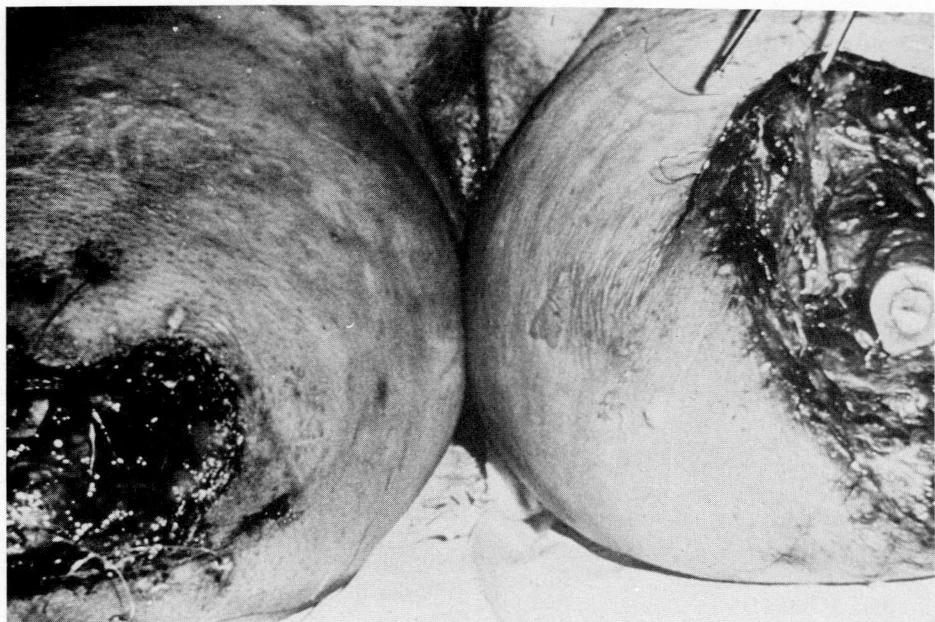

FIGURE 35-6 Necrosis and gangrene of stumps. (Courtesy of Dr. Walter C. Grundy, pathologist.)

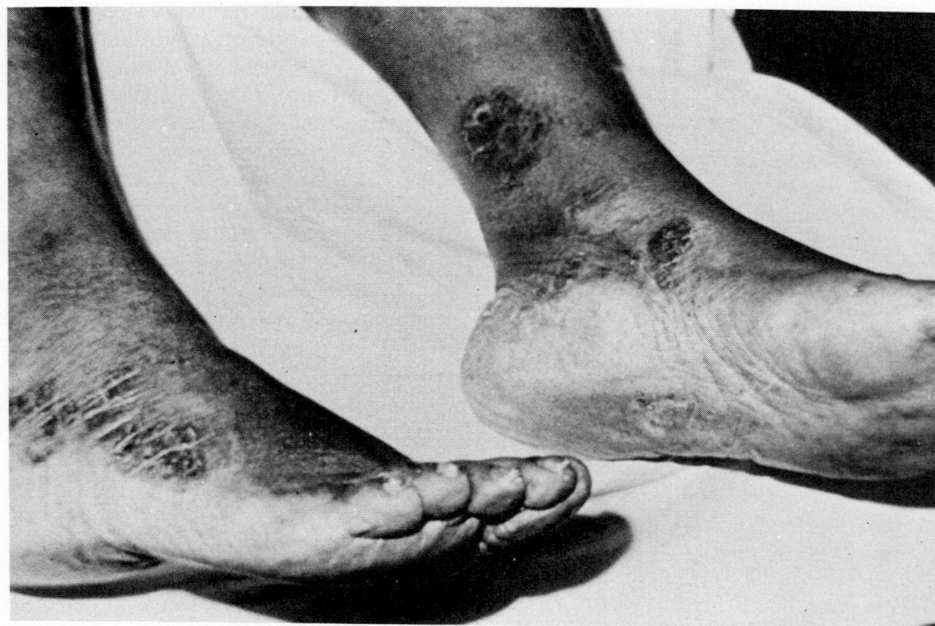

FIGURE 35-7 Atherosclerosis and venostasis of lower legs. (Courtesy of Dr. Walter C. Grundy, pathologist.)

three lesions of the glomeruli: *nodular glomerulosclerosis*, *diffuse glomerulosclerosis*, and *exudative lesions*. Approximately 20 percent of deaths in diabetes under age 40 years can be related to kidney failure.

Nodular Glomerulosclerosis. Nodular glomerulosclerosis (Kimmelstiel-Wilson lesion, a specific lesion of diabetes) appears as a round hyalin mass in the glomerulus and results in focal thickening of the basement membrane. The mass is located in the periphery of the glomerulus and is often surrounded by capillary loops. It occurs in 25 percent of those with long-term diabetes [19].

Diffuse Glomerulosclerosis. Diffuse glomerulosclerosis involves overall thickening of the basement membrane of the glomerular capillaries, together with increased deposits of matrix in the mesangial portion. This condition is the most common form of nephropathy and leads to proteinuria, which is initially intermittent, then persistent. Eventually, sclerosis may involve the entire glomerular bed and cause renal failure [19].

Exudative Lesions. Exudative lesions in the kidneys take two forms. Glassy, brightly eosinophilic, crescentic deposits that hang into the uriniferous space are called capsular drops. Similar deposits are called fibrin caps when they occur on the outer surface of the glomerular capillaries. The capsular drops are diagnostic of diabetes [19].

Other Lesions. Other common renal lesions affect the vascular supply, renal pelvis, and medulla. Atherosclerosis and arteriolosclerosis of the renal artery or arterioles are common and may be related to hypertension. Pyelonephritis is usually a bacterial ascending infection of the kidneys, which occurs most frequently in diabetics. *Necrotizing renal papillitis* or renal medullary necrosis involves unilateral or bilateral necrosis of the renal pyramids, which may result in sloughing of necrotic papillae in urine.

Pathology of the Eyes. *Retinopathy.* Diabetic retinopathy, the inclusive term for several retinal changes related to diabetes, is the fourth leading cause of blindness in the United States. Duration of disease is a variable in its development. Whether visual handicap occurs depends on whether the macula are involved. This condition is rare before the growth-spurt years and develops slowly, corresponding to the duration of the disease. Retinopathy follows alterations in blood flow through the retinae and has various manifestations: thickening of retinal capillaries, microangiopathies, and microaneurysms, which are discrete saccular dilatations or outpouchings of vessels (Fig. 35-8). The microaneurysms are asymptomatic; they are seen as discrete, dark red, circular spots near retinal vessels and are diagnostic of diabetes mellitus.

Hemorrhages are usually present in the macular area between the superior and inferior temporal vessels and resemble red blotches. If located in the area of the fovea, they can destroy central vision. Exudates occur due to abnormal porosity of the retinal vessels and seepage of fluid into the retinae. Soft exudates, called cotton wool spots, are large, fluffy, and gray-white, and may resolve in several weeks. More commonly, hard exudates are yellow, with discrete sharp edges that may coalesce, take longer to develop, and produce retinal degeneration. Venous changes include enlarged, irregular veins, sometimes resembling strings of sausages.

Lesions of the Vitreous. Lesions of the vitreous are a most serious complication and include neovascularization, or formation of new vessels, and fibrous tissue in the fundus. In time, atrophy of new vessels and contraction of fibrous tissue affect central and peripheral vision. Changes between fibrovascular tissue and the vitreous may lead to hemorrhage and retinal detachment.

Cataracts. Accumulation of sorbital (polyhydroxy alcohol formed from glucose) causes cataracts by accumulating in the lens. Opacities of the lens are common in diabetics, are usually of gradual onset, and are similar to senile cataracts. Transitory lens changes due to dehydration also occur in diabetics.

Nervous System Pathology. Neurons are vulnerable to the ketoacidosis of uncontrolled diabetes and the hypoglycemia of insulin reactions. Neuropathy may involve the peripheral nerves, brain, spinal cord, cranial nerves, or the autonomic nervous system. The relationship between metabolic aspects of disease and diabetic neuropathy remains unknown. Failure of affected persons to improve with management of hyperglycemia supports the proposed relationship between peripheral neuropathy and a process independent of glucose and insulin metabolism. A correlation has been found, however, between duration of disease and diabetic control [12]. Earlier research focused on abnormalities of myelinated nerve fibers due to a metabolic defect affecting Schwann cells and myelin. More recently, *myo*-inositol, an alcohol sugar present in normal nerves and essential in axonal function, has been implicated. Experimental studies reflect a correlation between nerve *myo*-inositol and metabolic control. Glycosylation of nerve myelin may also be a factor in neuropathy [15,19].

Polyneuropathy, characterized by myelin degeneration and eventual irreversible injury to axons, is caused by an accumulation of abnormal metabolites and by depletion of substances necessary for nerve cell conduction. The associated sensory loss and motor weakness usually occur first and most severely in the feet.

Mononeuropathy is probably related to ischemia and infarction of the vessels that supply the nerves. Manifestations of nervous system involvement include pain, paresthesia, decreased proprioceptive sensations, motor impairment, and muscle weakness and atrophy.

Alterations in the autonomic nervous system may lead to nocturia and atony of the bladder, postural hypotension, and delayed gastric emptying. Disturbances in neural innervation of the pelvic organs lead to sexual impotence in men and orgasmic difficulties in women.

Because of peripheral arterial ischemic disease and neurotrophic changes, the feet of diabetics are more

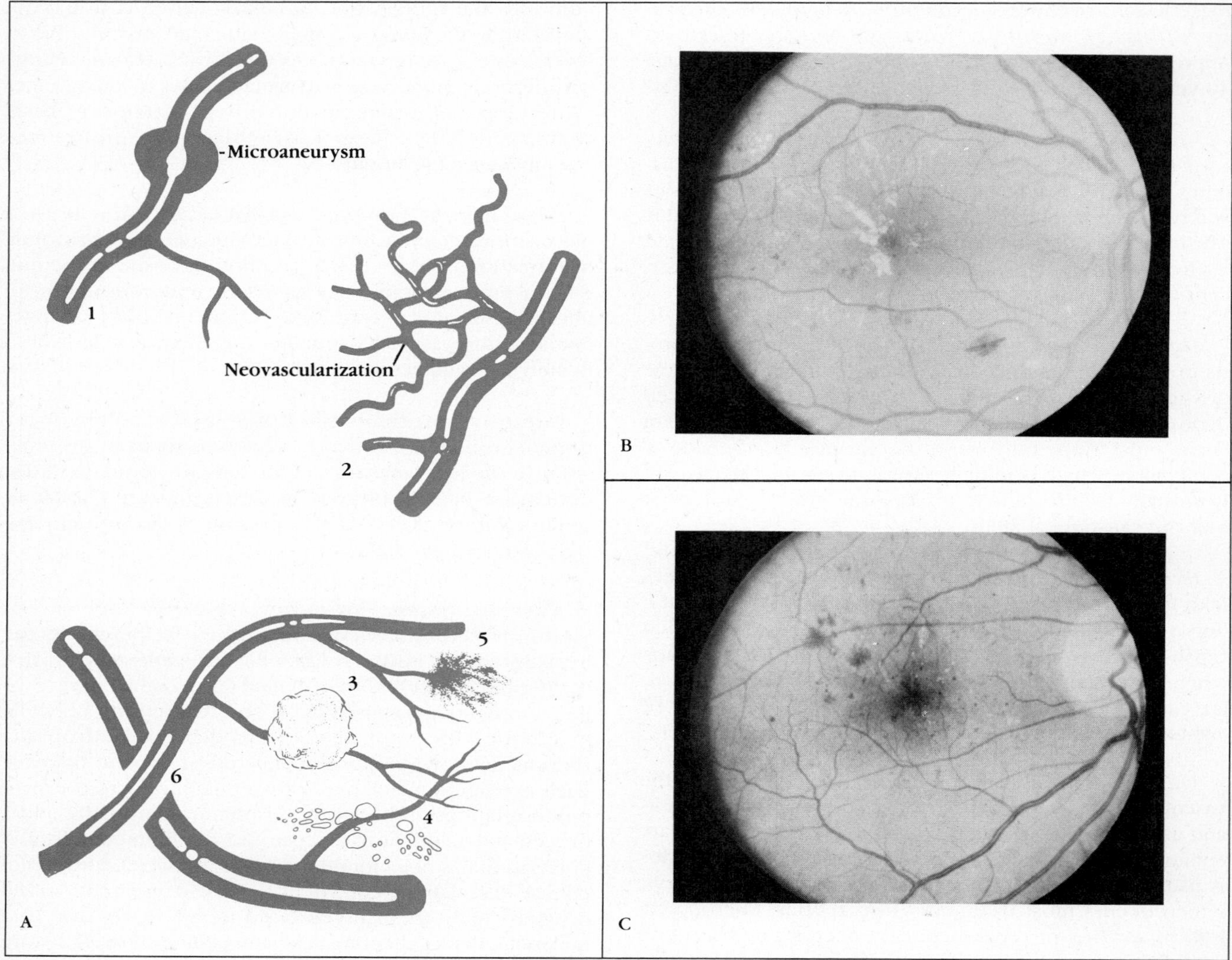

FIGURE 35-8 Characteristic diabetic changes in the retina. A. Blood vessels of the fundus shown with (1) microaneurysms, (2) new vessel formation (neovascularization), (3) soft exudates, (4) hard exudates, (5) hemorrhages, and (6) arteriovenous nicking. B. Diabetic retinopathy with hard exudates. C. Deep retinal hemorrhage. (From R. Judge, G. Zuidema, and F. Fitzgerald [eds.], *Clinical Diagnosis* [4th ed.]. Boston: Little, Brown, 1982.)

susceptible to infection because of loss of sensation. A pathologic condition may not be noticed and may progress rapidly.

Charcot's joint, or neuropathic joint disease, develops because of the trauma and stress of joint motion. Relaxation of supporting structures of the joint leads to cartilage degeneration, disorganization, and collapse of bones. Neuropathic joint disease usually involves the feet.

Various classifications of neuropathies have been proposed. These are often based on anatomic and clinical features (Tables 35-6 and 35-7).

Skin Changes. The skin is frequently an indicator of diabetes and is structurally different from that of the nondiabetic. Dryness is due to dehydration and occurs in poorly controlled diabetes. Poor skin turgor may be related to protein wasting and dehydration. Impaired granulocyte function and decreased circulation lead to skin changes and may also contribute to infection.

Necrobiosis Lipoidica Epidermis. This lesion is most frequent on the shins and usually develops after diabetes has been present for years. The skin lesion begins as a papule that progresses to a soft, yellow, ulcerated plaque. Histologically, the lesion consists of collagen surrounded by an inflammatory infiltrate composed of lipid-laden macrophages [11].

Diabetic Dermopathy (Shin Spots). Dermopathy is seen microscopically as atrophy of the epidermis and fibrosis of the dermis. These hemorrhagelike areas are brown, scaly, round patches and look as though the per-

TABLE 35-6 Classification of Diabetic Neuropathies on Anatomic Basis

Structure	Lesion	Clinical Features
Nerve terminals	Polyneuropathy	Glove and stocking sensory loss, distal painless ulceration, mild peripheral weakness, edema of Charcot's joints, distal reflex loss
Mixed spinal or cranial nerve	Mononeuropathies	Pain, weakness, sensory loss; may be spinal or cranial
Nerve root	Radiculopathy	Pain or sensory loss in root distribution
Nerve terminal(?) or muscle?	Amyotrophy	Pain in anterior thigh, buttocks, or hips; muscle weakness
Sympathetic ganglion	Automatic	Postural hypotension, impotence, gastropathy, bladder atony

Source: Reprinted with permission from S. Locke, "The peripheral nervous system in diabetes mellitus," *Diabetes* 13:307, 1964.

TABLE 35-7 Distribution and Clinical Features of Diabetic Autonomic Neuropathies

System	Features
Cardiovascular	Diminished cardiac beat-to-beat variation; orthostatic hypotension; diminished sympathetic cardiac drive
Genitourinary	Erectile impotence; retrograde ejaculation; neurogenic bladder; female sexual dysfunction
Gastrointestinal	Decreased gastric motility, gastroparesis; nocturnal (diabetic) diarrhea; constipation; fecal incontinence
Miscellaneous	Abnormal pupil reactivity; sweating disturbances; impaired adrenergic glucose counterregulation; vasomotor instability

Source: Reprinted with permission from J. O'Hara and C. Warfield, The diabetic neuropathies. *Hosp. Pract.* November 1984, Vol. 19, No. 40.

son has been struck time and time again in the shins. There is no associated pain or ulceration [11].

Infections. Bacterial infections are more frequent in diabetics than in nondiabetics. Infections arising from acne may expand and progress into cellulitis. Furuncles and carbuncles are of serious concern. Dermatophytosis (athlete's foot) is common, and although relatively harmless in the nondiabetic, may lead to serious infection and loss of a foot in the diabetic. Monilial infections occur in the diabetic, often in the genitalia, groin, and under the breasts. The high moisture, the glucose content of the skin, and chafing support the growth of *Candida albicans*, especially in the obese person. Severity of infections may be worsened by reduction of circulation and nerve degeneration.

Lipodystrophy (Lipohypertrophy and Lipoatrophy). These skin lesions are caused by insulin injections. Scar and fatty tissue accumulations beneath the skin, similar to a lipoma, form large bumps (lipodystrophy) with repeated injection of insulin. These sites tend to become fibrous and insensitive, and insulin is absorbed poorly from the areas. Long-term administration of insulin can also cause lipoatrophy, the disappearance of adipose tissue at the site of injections. Atrophy is not accompanied by significant fibrosis. There may be a combination of atrophy and dystrophy or an area of atrophy surrounded by hypertrophy.

The use of single-peak insulin, a chemically pure form of insulin, is thought to decrease the extent of lipodystrophy. Rotating injection sites, and administering insulin in the deep subcutaneous tissue at room temperature also helps to prevent lipodystrophy.

Xanthomas. Firm, yellowish pink nodules develop under the epidermis of knees and elbows, on the periorbital areas, and buttocks as a result of the hyperlipemia of diabetes. The lesions may be as large as 5 mm and the papule is surrounded by an inflammatory-type halo. Although these nodules are not limited to persons with diabetes, they signify high serum triglyceride levels and disappear with return of triglycerides to normal.

Hepatic Fatty Changes. In long-standing diabetes, fatty changes develop and the size of the liver increases. Infiltration of fat causes it to appear yellowish, and glycogen vacuoles may be present in nuclei of the cells. These liver changes are related to elevated serum lipid levels.

Muscle Changes. Degenerative changes occur in striated muscle in persons who have long-standing, poorly controlled diabetes. The pathology is probably related to microangiopathy and neuronal degeneration. Diabetic amyotrophy, a syndrome of muscle weakness, pain, and atrophy, occurs in the elderly, especially males. The disorder is usually limited to the psoas and quadriceps muscles.

Clinical Manifestations and Complications

Persons with diabetes generally have polydipsia, polyuria, polyphagia, weight loss, and weakness. Many also have infections, particularly with *Staphylococcus aureus* and *Candida monilia* organisms.

The predominant pathophysiology of diabetes is due to (1) impaired use of glucose by cells; (2) increased mobilization, abnormal metabolism, and deposition of fats; and

(3) depletion of protein in body tissues. The manifestations occur from insulin deprivation, which results in *hyperglycemia* (blood glucose as high as 200–1000 mg/dl) due to the impaired uptake of glucose, especially into muscle and adipose tissue, and increased gluconeogenesis and glycogenolysis by the liver. These factors, together with increased dietary intake of carbohydrate, result in an increased blood sugar level.

With hyperglycemia, osmotic pressure of the plasma increases, fluid shifts to the intravascular compartment, and cells become dehydrated. When the blood glucose level reaches approximately 160 to 180 mg per ml, the renal tubules are unable to resorb all of the glucose filtered by the glomeruli, and glycosuria occurs. When the blood glucose level reaches 300 to 400 mg per ml, a common occurrence in untreated diabetes, the person may lose as much as 100 gm of glucose into the urine each day. The renal excretion of glucose requires accompanying water and produces osmotic diuresis, *polyuria*. Excessive urination also increases loss of water, potassium, sodium, and chloride, resulting in extracellular fluid depletion and compensatory intracellular dehydration. As sodium and potassium are lost, electrolyte imbalance, weakness, fatigue, and malaise occur. Loss of water causes an increase in serum osmolality, which stimulates the thirst center in the hypothalamus and the body's response of *polydipsia*. With the loss of large quantities of glucose and semistarvation of the cells, there is a compensatory increase in hunger, *polyphagia*. As the level of insulin, an anabolic hormone, decreases, protein and fat catabolism increases, resulting in the release of ketones, nitrogen, and potassium into the circulation. Weight loss is common, especially in IDDM.

Diabetic Ketoacidosis. The metabolic result of lack of insulin and severe dehydration is ketoacidosis. The signs and symptoms are pronounced manifestations of uncontrolled diabetes. Polyuria, polydipsia, polyphagia, weakness, and anorexia, plus nausea, vomiting, and abdominal pain occur in increasing severity. Ketonemia, gastric dilatation, and decreased peristalsis from potassium loss contribute to nausea and vomiting. The gastrointestinal symptoms and tender abdomen may mimic a surgical emergency. Ketonuria increases electrolyte loss. Ketoacidosis may be considered intracellular starvation. It is the metabolic consequence of lack of insulin and severe dehydration.

The most important pathogenic element in ketoacidosis is marked decrease in insulin production that leads to hyperglycemia, glycosuria, and progressive metabolic acidosis. Without insulin, glucose cannot enter the cells and accumulates in the blood, increasing osmolality and pulling water from the cells into the intravascular compartment. The body enters a catabolic state and there is a shift from carbohydrate to protein and fat metabolism. Fats are broken down (lipolysis) for energy faster than they can be metabolized. The ketone acids (acetoacetic and beta-hydroxybutyric acids) are strong and dissociate to yield hydrogen ions, consequently causing a drop in pH. At a plasma pH of 7.2, the individual's respiratory center is stimulated to prevent further decline in pH, and breathing becomes deep and rapid (Kussmaul respiration). The acetone formed during ketosis is volatile and is blown off during expiration, giving the breath a sweet or fruity odor. When acidosis depresses their action, ketones are not well metabolized, so that acidosis and catabolism are enhanced. Hypovolemia and increased blood viscosity may also cause thrombi or emboli, myocardial infarction, or cerebrovascular accidents.

Protein catabolism results in the breakdown of amino acids and electrolytes from muscle tissue. The liver, the primary site for glucose synthesis, converts amino acids to glucose, perpetuating the hyperglycemic and acidotic states. The metabolic derangement is also increased by the presence of glucoregulatory hormones during diabetic ketoacidosis. The antagonistic activity exhibited by these hormones promotes gluconeogenesis and worsens the hyperglycemia.

When the lungs are no longer able to maintain pH by blowing off carbon dioxide, plasma carbonic acid levels rise and acidosis progresses. Further decrease in pH, accompanied by hyperosmolality, dehydration, hypotension, and tissue breakdown, contribute to depression of cerebral function and eventually, lead to coma and death (Fig. 35-9). Individuals with NIDDM rarely develop ketoacidosis.

Hyperglycemic, Hyperosmolar, Nonketotic (HHNK) Coma. This variation in hyperglycemic diabetic coma has been recognized with increasing frequency. It is characterized by extreme hyperglycemia (800–2000 mg/dl) and hyperosmolality (greater than 350 mOsm/kg), mild or undetectable ketonuria, and absence of acidosis. The syndrome occurs almost exclusively in older persons and in individuals with mild diabetes that does not require insulin.

The mechanism of HHNK is best understood by considering the principles of osmolality. Without insulin to lower blood glucose, the blood becomes more concentrated, as glucose is a large molecule that does not pass cell walls easily and draws large amounts of water. The profound hyperglycemia is largely responsible for the increased plasma osmolality that causes an osmotic diuresis. The intracellular fluid is drawn out to help equalize the increasing osmotic pressure of blood hypertonic with sugar. Water in the intracellular fluid moves from cells into the bloodstream, leaving cells dehydrated and shrunken. Dehydration stimulates secretion of the glucoregulatory hormones glucagon, cortisol, and epinephrine. If hypokalemia also occurs, it decreases insulin secretion. These two events cause further hyperglycemia.

Initially, fluid intake balances the fluid lost to glycosuria. Later, however, intake is not sufficient and dehydration ensues. Gradually, the person becomes more obtunded and unable to respond to thirst. Without treatment with insulin and fluids, the process becomes self-perpetuating. Hyperosmolality leads to hemoconcentration and is conducive to thrombus formation. Fluid losses lead to hypovolemia and shock. If these are not corrected, death may result.

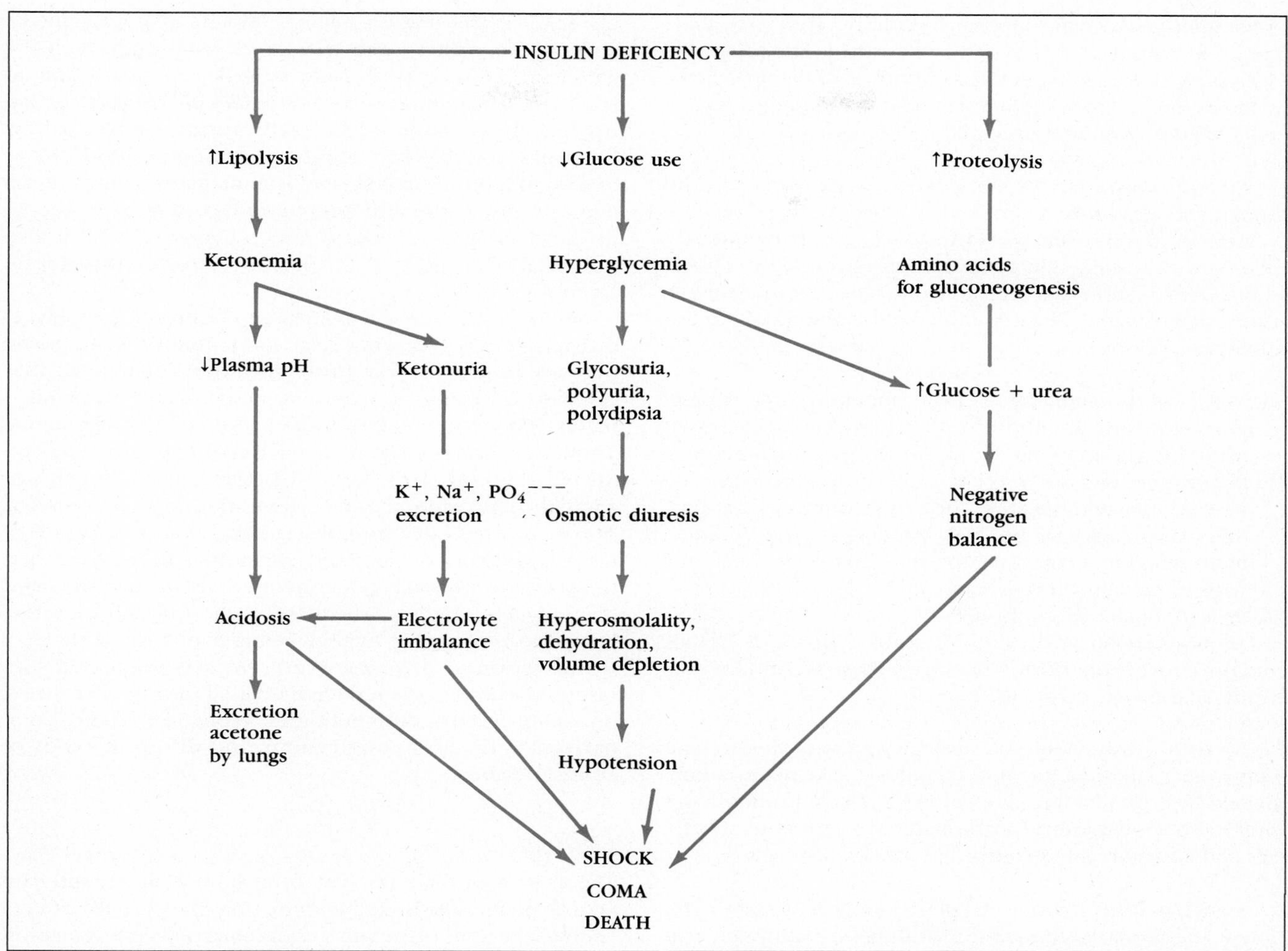

FIGURE 35-9 Pathogenesis of ketoacidosis.

Similarities exist between HHNK and ketotic coma. In both, a shortage of insulin and a defect in use of glucose result in hyperglycemia, osmotic diuresis, and dehydration. Elevation of urea nitrogen levels usually occurs in both, although the causes may be different. Metabolic acidosis occurs in both, but less frequently in the hyperosmolar disorder.

The major difference is that large quantities of ketone bodies are produced in ketotic coma but not in hyperosmolar coma. No insulin is secreted in ketotic coma, but some residual ability to secrete insulin remains in hyperosmolar coma (HHNK). The small quantities of circulating insulin probably prevent the mobilization of fat from tissues and release of ketone bodies. The lesser elevation of plasma growth hormone and cortisol in hyperosmolar coma also account for decreased ketone bodies.

The signs and symptoms of HHNK are polyphagia, polydipsia, polyuria, glycosuria, dehydration, abdominal discomfort, hyperpyrexia, hyperventilation, electrolyte imbalance, central nervous system (CNS) dysfunction, postural hypotension, and shock. Impaired mental status is related to dehydration and/or electrolyte imbalance. The skin has decreased turgor, mucous membranes are dry, and the eyes are sunken and soft. Some degree of renal impairment occurs in many affected persons.

An acute illness or surgery may trigger the onset of HHNK as well as stressful events, for example, pancreatic disease, myocardial infarction, hemodialysis, severe myocardial infarction, renal dialysis, severe burns, and hyperalimentation. A number of drugs (corticosteroids, diuretics, diphenylhydantoin, and immunosuppressive agents) may also induce the syndrome.

The laboratory results are similar to those of ketoacidosis except that glucose levels are usually higher (often greater than 1000 mg/dl), and serum osmolalities are also more elevated (greater than 350 mOsm/kg H_2O). Bicarbonate concentrations and pH are often normal but may decrease as the syndrome progresses. There is usually no ketoacidosis in classic cases, but lactic acidosis may result from hypovolemic shock. Plasma acetone is absent or slightly elevated; creatinine and blood urea nitrogen levels become elevated with renal impairment. Compared with ketoacidosis, there is less elevation of the plasma free fatty acids (FFA), growth hormone (GH), and cortisol. The prognosis in hyperosmolar coma is not as good as in diabetic ketoacidosis, and death is often attributed to the underlying or associated disease that precipitated the coma.

Lactic Acidosis. When anaerobic glycolysis in the body produces more lactic acid than can be used or converted to glucose, lactic acidosis occurs. It frequently occurs with sustained hypoxia or hypotension (e.g., shock, septicemia, hemorrhage, renal insufficiency, or starvation). Lactic acidosis may develop in diabetic patients in the following situations:

1. Those with complications from phenformin (a hepatic gluconeogenesis inhibitor that has been withdrawn from the market by the Food and Drug Administration). Phenformin and some related biguanides are still used outside the United States. The drug alone does not produce lactic acidosis but may precipitate the derangement when it accumulates in toxic amounts in patients with unrecognized renal failure.
2. As a spontaneous syndrome.
3. In association with diabetic ketoacidosis or HHNK coma. As hypoperfusion occurs in these conditions, lactic acid may accumulate.

Lactic acidosis should be suspected in any stuporous or comatose patient in metabolic acidosis. Diagnosis is confirmed by a plasma lactate level in excess of 7 mmole per liter, with a low plasma bicarbonate level, absence of ketosis, and an anion gap produced by the excess lactate.

Insulin Reactions. Hypoglycemia is a rather frequent metabolic complication of diabetes, although it is largely a consequence of insulin therapy. Most diabetic individuals who take insulin experience a hypoglycemic reaction at some time. Reactions result from (1) an overdose of insulin, (2) inadequate food intake, (3) increased amounts of exercise, and (4) nutritional and fluid imbalances due to nausea and vomiting.

The symptoms of hypoglycemia reflect glucose deprivation to the brain. The following physiologic responses occur: (1) epinephrine release (sweating, shakiness, nervousness, headache, palpitations, increased blood pressure, heart rate, and respirations); (2) parasympathetic nervous system response (hunger, nausea, eructation); and (3) cerebral function decline (bizarre behavior, dulled sensorium, lethargy, convulsions, coma). Clinical signs and symptoms may not correlate with blood glucose level. They may occur when the glucose level drops very rapidly from a very high to a still-elevated level.

The adrenergic response results in increased liver glycogenolysis to raise blood glucose concentration and stimulation of the reticular activating system to a state of wakefulness and alertness. If the liver glycogen supply is exhausted and glucose is not replaced, convulsions and permanent brain damage result.

Hypoglycemia can also occur independently of insulin. The following conditions can cause low blood glucose levels: severe *liver disease*, which impairs glycogen uptake and release; *adrenocortical insufficiency*, in which the glucocorticoids (cortisol and cortisone) are unavailable to stimulate gluconeogenesis; and *islet-cell tumors*, which overproduce insulin. Some medications, such as salicylates, oral antidiabetic agents, propranolol, monoamine oxidase inhibitors, and certain sulfonamides, contribute to hypoglycemia. Alcohol (ethanol) has long been recognized as an agent that can induce hypoglycemia. It also potentiates the effects of insulin and oral antidiabetic agents.

Somogyi described a syndrome of chronic hypoglycemia in persons receiving large amounts of insulin. Some persons have wide variations in blood sugar level that occur when insulin dosage is increased to control elevated levels. The exogenous insulin produces hypoglycemia. These individuals often have nocturnal hypoglycemia, followed by hormone-mediated hyperglycemia. Epinephrine, adrenal corticosteroids, and growth hormone are secreted as part of the body's response to the excessive action of insulin. Epinephrine spurs glycogenolysis in the liver, corticosteroids stimulate gluconeogenesis in the liver, and hyperglycemia occurs. The blood sugar is usually elevated, but periods of severe hypoglycemia may be experienced. If this *rebound hypo-hyperglycemia* is suspected, the insulin dose is slowly reduced, divided into smaller doses, or administered at different times. Table 35-8 offers a comparison between hypoglycemia and different types of coma in diabetes.

Clinical Course

The course of diabetes may be insidious or abrupt. The ketosis-prone insulin-dependent type that usually affects younger persons sometimes undergoes transient remission after onset, called a honeymoon period, which may last a few weeks to a few months; then glucose intolerance becomes unstable or brittle. The person is very sensitive to changes in exogenous insulin, dietary deviations, growth spurts, unusual physical activity, infection, and stress, and is vulnerable to hypoglycemia and ketoacidosis.

Maturity-onset, nonketosis-prone diabetes may have few if any symptoms and follows an insidious course. Thus, the person with nonketosis-prone, noninsulin-dependent diabetes usually does not experience the acute metabolic syndrome, but suffers from other complications.

Laboratory Findings

Numerous laboratory tests are performed to diagnose and follow the course of diabetes mellitus.

Fasting Blood Sugar (FBS). Normal test values rule out significant diabetic problems but do not completely exclude diabetes, since only approximately 30 to 40 percent of cases can be diagnosed with a FBS. The fasting blood sugar should be measured in the early morning at least eight hours after a meal. Normal values are 65 to 100 mg per dl using a method specific for glucose, or 80 to 120 mg per dl using a method that measures all blood

TABLE 35-8 Comparison of Hypoglycemia, Diabetic Ketoacidosis (DKA), Lactic Acidosis, and Hyperglycemic Nonketotic Coma (HHNK)

Variables	Hypoglycemia	DKA	Lactic Acidosis	HHNK
Physical response	Trembly, weak; difficulty talking	Nausea, vomiting; polyuria; polyphagia; polydipsia; headache	Similar to DKA (varied, depending on factors contributing to development)	Similar to DKA
Mental status	Anxious, confused; behavior changes	Irritable; comatose	Acute changes in state of consciousness; stuporous; comatose	Similar to DKA; stuporous; focal motor seizures
Blood pressure	Normal	Low	Low	Low
Skin	Cold, moist, pale	Hot, flushed, dry	Pallid, dry	Very dry
Mucous membranes	Normal	Very dry	Dry	Extremely dry
Respiration	Normal	Hyperventilation	Hyperventilation	Normal
Urine sugar	0–2+	4+	0–2+	4+
Urine acetone	0	4+	0–2+	0–1+
Blood sugar	40 mg or less	300–800+ mg	80–200 mg	800–2000 mg
Serum ketones	0	4+	0–2+	0–2+
Blood CO_2	24–30	5–16 or less	5–16	18–24
Plasma lactic acid	Normal	Normal	High	Normal
Plasma pH	7.4	7.1–7.3	6.8–7.2	7.4

sugars and reducing substances. A fasting blood sugar above 120 mg per dl should be further investigated with a glucose tolerance test.

Two-Hour Postprandial Blood Sugar. Values may range from 200 to 2000 mg per dl depending on duration and severity of the diabetes. Glucose levels are rarely elevated two hours after carbohydrate intake in nondiabetics.

Glucose Tolerance Test (GTT). The GTT is based on the principle that a nondiabetic person can absorb a test amount of glucose from circulation at a faster rate than a diabetic. As demonstrated in Figure 35-10, when a nondiabetic fasting person ingests 1 gm glucose per kg of body weight, the blood glucose rises to peak levels of 150 to 160 mg per dl and falls to normal within two to three hours. The urine usually remains free of glucose.

In the diabetic, the blood sugar peak levels are much higher, and the return to fasting levels is delayed five to six hours because of a lack of insulin response to the glucose.

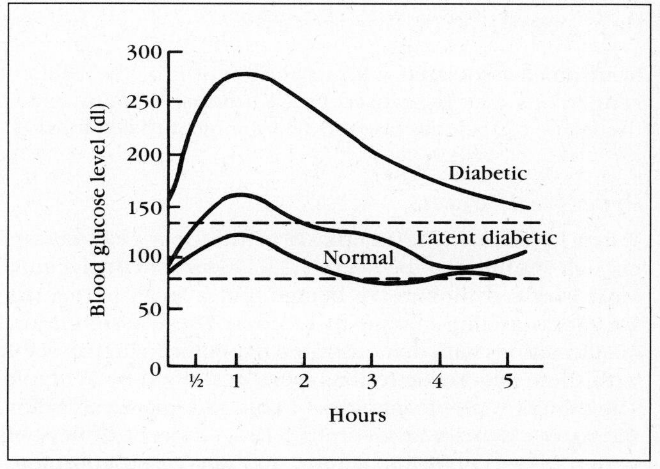

FIGURE 35-10 Glucose tolerance curves.

Glycosylated Hemoglobin (HbA_{1c}). About 5 percent of hemoglobin in the red cells is usually a variety called hemoglobin A_{1c}. Glycosylated hemoglobin (HbA_{1c}) is formed slowly and irreversibly from glucose and hemoglobin throughout the 120-day life span of the red blood cell. The process occurs through a nonenzymatic process that results in attachment of glucose to protein hemoglobin. The higher the blood glucose level, the more hemoglobin A_{1c} is present in the red cell. In nondiabetic adults the level of HbA_{1c} is 2.2 to 4.8; in children, 1.8 to 4.0. Good diabetic control should maintain a level of 2.5 to 6.0. A value above 8.0 reflects poor control.

This test decreases the problem of spurious results for blood glucose, because it depends little on cooperation, stress, exercise, food intake, and renal threshold. Also, HbA_{1c} is useful in monitoring how well diabetic individuals control blood glucose at home and in differentiating noncompliance from an acute illness that results in elevated blood glucose. As a diagnostic tool, it is not as discriminating in identifying borderline diabetes as glucose tolerance or fasting blood sugar. Glycosylation of a large number of proteins is being investigated in various laboratories [25].

Urine Glucose. In normal kidneys, the glucose filtered through the glomeruli from the blood is resorbed in the proximal tubules. The renal tubules have a maximum absorptive capacity (renal threshold) of approximately 160 to 180 mg per dl of blood. At blood levels greater than this, sugar is spilled into the urine and can be detected by screening methods. Glucose may appear in the urine at normal blood levels in persons without diabetes if the ability of the renal tubules to absorb glucose is impaired. Many diabetics, especially those with a history of atherosclerosis, may have a higher renal threshold, which prevents the appearance of glucose in urine until the blood level is quite high.

Urine Ketones. Ketonuria refers to the loss of ketone bodies, such as acetone, beta-hydroxybutyric acid, and acetoacetic acid, in the urine. This reflects the abnormal oxidation of fats and may occur in diabetes, glycogen storage disease, starvation, and high-fat diets. Occasionally, ketones are present with fever or other conditions that increase metabolic requirements. Accumulation of acidic ketones in the blood leads to metabolic acidosis and an acetone smell to the breath.

Volume of Urine in a 24-Hour Period. A nondiabetic person secretes an average of 1200 to 1800 ml of urine in 24 hours, while the uncontrolled diabetic excretes 2000 ml or more in 24 hours.

Pancreatic Islet-Cell Disease

Syndromes associated with hyperfunction of the islets of Langerhans may be caused by (1) diffuse hyperplasia of the islets, (2) adenomas, and (3) malignant islet tumors.

Hyperinsulinism

When hyperplasia or neoplasia of the beta cells occurs, enough insulin may be secreted to induce hypoglycemia. Most islet cell tumors are benign, but a small percentage are metastasizing malignant tumors. The classic clinical manifestations with demonstrated hypoglycemia that occur with these pancreatic lesions were described by Whipple. The triad of Whipple includes (1) blood sugar levels below 50 mg per dl after an overnight fast; (2) central nervous symptoms of confusion, stupor, and decreased consciousness related to fasting or exercise; and (3) prompt relief of signs and symptoms by administration of glucose [19]. The triad is not specific for persons with hyperinsulinism due to islet-cell disease, and may occur in other types of hypoglycemia.

The insulin-producing adenomas, or insulinomas, vary in diameter from 0.15 to 15.0 cm and may weigh over 1500 gm. They occur singly or scattered throughout the pancreas and usually appear as encapsulated firm nodules that are distributed throughout the pancreas and compress the surrounding tissue. Histologically, they do not differ from the normal islet cell [19].

Hyperinsulinism may also be caused by hyperplasia of the pancreatic islets, an alteration that occurs in infants born of diabetic mothers. The infant responds to the elevated blood sugar levels of the mother by producing increased numbers of cells and an increase in size of the cells. After delivery, the increased secretion causes serious episodes of hypoglycemia.

Zollinger-Ellison Syndrome (Gastrinoma, Ulcerogenic Tumor)

A syndrome described by Zollinger and Ellison is a clinical condition of peptic ulceration associated with a nonbeta-cell islet tumor. It is characterized by large amounts of gastric secretion of hydrochloric acid and pepsin. The stimulus for the hypersecretion is attributed to gastrin; hence the tumor is also known as a gastrinoma. Although most of the tumors occur in the pancreas, approximately one-tenth are located in the duodenum or duodenal wall.

Various types of islet cells have been implicated as the causative agents. Gastrin-producing delta cells have been found in tumors and hyperplastic tissue, but it is still unclear whether these cells are the distinct agents responsible for gastrinomas [19].

Microscopically, the tumors resemble islet cells or cancerous tumors. Approximately 50 percent of individuals have metastases located in regional lymph nodes. There may be metastasis to bones, mediastinum, and skin. Morbidity and mortality are usually attributed to the effects of the secretion of gastrin from the tumor and its metastases, and complications of ulcer disease such as bleeding and perforation. The tremendous gastric hypersecretion leads to intractable ulcers. The high acidity of the small intestine causes inactivation of pancreatic lipase, and this precipitates bile salts and causes fluid and electrolyte imbalance. Large volumes of acid gastric juices promote diarrhea. As a result, many persons develop malsorption syndromes. Alteration in the intestinal mucosa from acidity affects absorption of nutrients. *Steatorrhea* (excessive excretion of sebum or fat in feces) may occur from the mucosal defects that interfere with transport of fats and other nutrients across the mucosa. Also, acid inactivates pancreatic lipase and decreases bile acids, which contribute to fat malsorption. Calcitonin levels are also elevated. This elevation is attributed to stimulation of calcitonin release from the thyroid by gastrin.

Approximately one-fourth of persons with Zollinger-Ellison syndrome have a hereditary form of peptic ulcer disease. The syndrome occurs most frequently between ages 30 and 65 years and affects men more than women.

Werner's Syndrome (Multiple Endocrine Neoplasia)

Werner's syndrome is familial with an autosomal dominant pattern of transmission. Numerous adenomas are present in the parathyroid glands, pituitary, and pancreas. Involving several glands, the disorder is often associated with peptic ulcer and gastric hypersecretion (Zollinger-Ellison syndrome). Both Zollinger-Ellison and Werner's syndromes have been found in some families, implying that the syndromes are variants of the same mutant gene. Some of the tumors are malignant, and the newer term *multiple endocrine neoplasia (MEN)* has replaced the term *multiple endocrine adenomatosis* previously used.

The major syndromes that are caused by multiple endocrine hyperfunction are multiple endocrine neoplasia

(MEN). Several of the conditions are familial with an autosomal dominant pattern. There are three types of MEN syndromes:

1. Type I (MEN I, Werner's syndrome) includes tumors or hyperplasia of the parathyroids, thyroid, pancreatic islet cells, pituitary, and adrenal cortex. The clinical manifestations vary depending upon the systems involved. More than one-half of those affected have adenomas of two or more different endocrine glands, and three or more different glands are involved in one-fifth of these persons.
2. Type II (MEN II, Whipple's syndrome) includes pheochromocytoma, medullary thyroid carcinoma, and parathyroid hyperplasia (see Chaps. 33 and 34).
3. Type III (MEN III, mucosal neuroma syndrome) includes medullary thyroid carcinoma and pheochromocytoma, but may be accompanied by distinct dysmorphic features such as neuromas of the lips, buccal mucosa, tongue, and gastrointestinal tract.

Clinical manifestations of MEN include intractable peptic ulcers, hyperparathyroidism, hyperinsulinism, Cushing's syndrome, and hypertension related to pheochromocytoma [19].

Table 35-9 Factors in the Etiology of Pancreatitis

Alcoholism
Biliary tract disease
Postoperative (abdominal, nonabdominal)
Postendoscopic retrograde cholangiopancreatography (ERCP)
Trauma (abdominal injury)
Metabolic (hyperlipidemia, uremia, renal failure, after renal transplantation, hypercalcemia, pregnancy, cystic fibrosis, kwashiorkor)
Vascular (shock, lupus erythematosus, thrombocytopenic purpura, polyarteritis, athermatous embolism)
Drugs
- Association
  - Immunosuppressive—corticosteroids, L-asparaginase, azathioprine
  - Diuretics—thiazides, furosemide, ethacrynic acid
  - Estrogens, oral contraceptives
  - Antibiotics—tetracyclines, sulfonamides
- Possible association
  - Acetaminophen
  - Isoniazid, rifampin,
  - Propoxyphene,
  - Valproic acid, procainamide
  - Anticoagulants

Infections (mumps, viral hepatitus, coxsackievirus, echovirus, *Ascaris, Mycoplasma*)
Mechanical (ampulla of Vater tumor, Crohn's disease, diverticula, pancreas divisum)
Penetrating duodenal ulcer
Hereditary pancreatitis
Idiopathic

Pancreatitis

Acute Pancreatitis

Pancreatitis, or inflammation of the pancreas, is characterized by hemorrhage, necrosis, and suppuration of pancreatic parenchyma. Pathologic changes occur in varying degrees of severity and are caused by escape of active lytic pancreatic enzymes into the glandular parenchyma.

Frequency and Etiology. This condition accounts for approximately 1 out of every 500 medical and surgical hospital admissions. Acute pancreatitis occurs most frequently in middle life and more in women than in men. Two major causes, *alcoholism* and *gallstones*, are responsible for 50 to 90 percent of cases. Factors in the etiology of pancreatitis are listed in Table 35-9. In men, pancreatitis is often associated with high consumption of alcohol, but the condition develops only after years of alcohol abuse. Gallstones have been demonstrated in the feces of 40 to 60 percent of persons with acute pancreatitis [19].

Pancreatitis may also occur as a result of surgical trauma, particularly that involving the pancreas and adjoining organs. Other possible causes are metabolic (hyperparathyroidism, pregnancy, uremia, and kidney transplantation), certain drugs (opiates, thiazides, steroids, oral contraceptives, and sulfonamides), vascular disease, infection, and nutritional and hereditary factors.

Pathology. The chemical and pathologic changes characteristic of pancreatitis reflect the pancreatic enzymes. What triggers the activation of enzymes and the exact role of the pancreatic enzymes is speculated to be autodigestion [1].

The major histologic alterations in pancreatitis are (1) *necrosis of fat (lipolysis)*, (2) *proteolytic destruction of pancreatic parenchyma (proteolysis)*, (3) necrosis of blood vessels with *hemorrhage*, and (4) *inflammation*.

The exocrine pancreas secretes over 20 enzymes. The proteolytic enzymes are secreted in a proenzyme or inactive form that prevents autodigestion of the pancreas. Trypsin plays a major role, as it activates the major proteolytic enzymes involved in autodigestion (Fig. 35-11). Trypsin is normally secreted from the pancreas in the form of trypsinogen and is activated in the duodenum (see Chap. 38). The major initiating pathology is premature activation of trypsinogen in the pancreas. Significant amounts of trypsin, chymotrypsin, and elastase have been detected in the diseased pancreas.

Elastase exists in high concentrations in granules of acinous cells and is present in pancreatic secretions as an inactive precursor. When activated by trypsin, it causes elastic fibers of blood vessels and ducts to dissolve. Hemorrhage due to breakdown of elastic fibers of the vessels may be minor or extreme, varying from red blood cells and fibrin clots to large masses of blood over large areas. Prekallikrein is converted to kallikrein by trypsin. Kallikrein leads to the release of bradykinin and kallidin (a plasma kinin), which further increase vasodilatation and vascular permeability. Phospholipase A acts on phospholipids, with

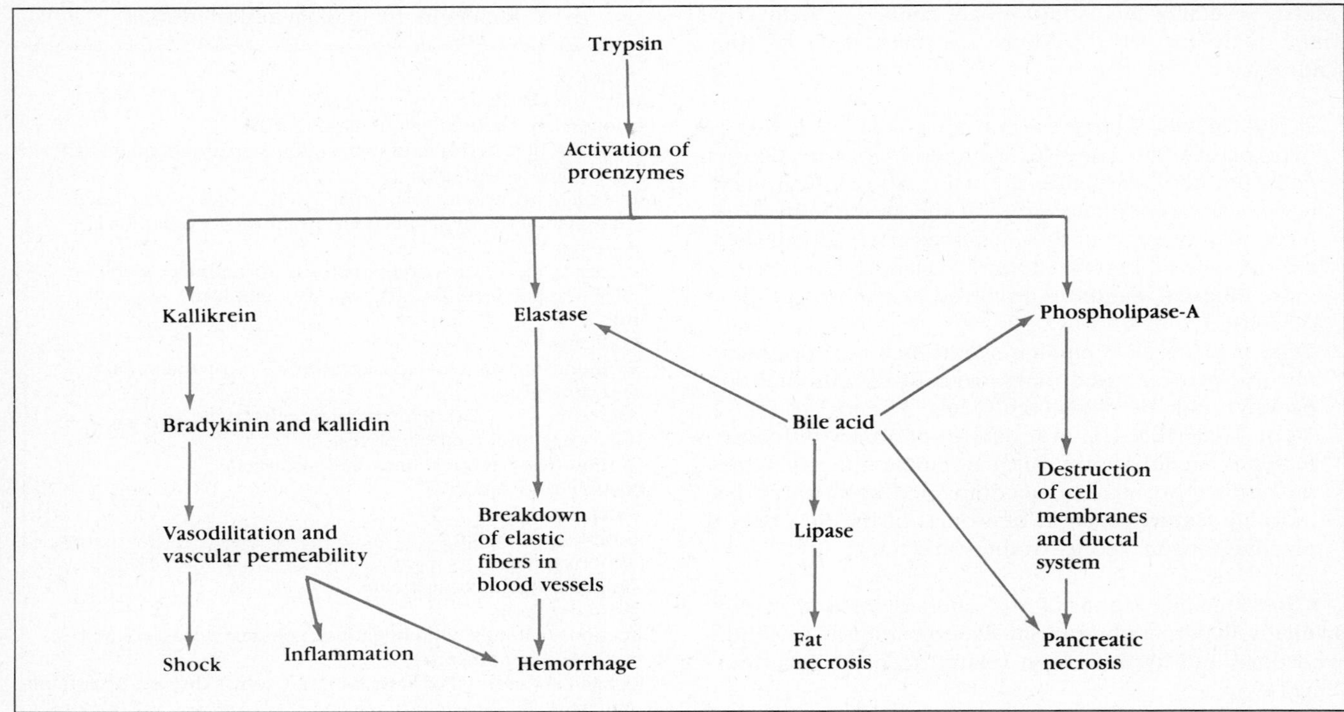

FIGURE 35-11 Pathogenesis of acute pancreatitis. (Adapted from L.H. Smith and S.O. Thier *Pathophysiology: The Biologic Principle of Disease*. Philadelphia: W.B. Saunders Company, 1981. Reprinted by permission.)

a resultant release of compounds that have strong cytotoxic effects and damage cell membranes and the ductal system, leading to necrosis. There are inhibitors in the plasma or in the pancreas itself that can quickly inactivate the proteolytic enzymes. Whether deficiencies in the inhibitors are factors in pancreatic disease is unknown.

A leukocytic reaction appears around the areas of hemorrhage and necrosis. Secondary bacterial invasion may produce a suppurative necrosis or abscess. Milder lesions may be absorbed, or they may calcify or become fibrotic when they are more severe. When fluid is walled off by fibrous tissue during the inflammatory process, a pancreatic cyst known as a pseudocyst is formed.

Several theories are offered to explain the mechanisms and sequence of events leading to activation of enzymes within the pancreas rather than the intestinal lumen.

According to the *duct obstruction theory*, obstruction of the common channel causes a reflux of bile that results in activation of pancreatic enzymes. The main pancreatic duct joins the common bile duct in two-thirds of individuals [19]. Many persons with pancreatitis have no common channel, and the respective ducts join the duodenum separately. Bile reflux occurs frequently with pancreatitis, however, and it is believed to be active in the inflammatory process. Duodenal reflux may occur if the sphincter of Oddi is damaged by disease. Impacted gallstones in the common duct or duodenal papilla could also dilate and obstruct the sphincter. Rupture of the ducts occurs from active pancreatic secretion in the presence of ductal obstruction of any cause and consequent tearing of cell membranes, permitting activated enzymes to leak back into the gland [1].

Alcohol-induced changes are major factors in the pathogenesis of pancreatitis. Alcohol is a stimulator of pancreatic secretions and also causes duodenal edema of the ampulla of Vater, obstructing flow of secretions. Long-term alcohol ingestion increases the protein concentration of secretions, which leads to formation of protein plugs in the ducts and subsequent obstruction by the precipitates. Alcohol may decrease the tone of the sphincter of Oddi and cause duodenal reflux. Another factor predisposing alcoholics to pancreatitis may be the elevated serum triglyceride levels that occur after a meal [9].

Hyperlipidemia is known to be associated with pancreatitis. Experimental studies indicate that lipolysis of triglycerides by pancreatic lipase in the pancreas leads to high concentration of free fatty acids in tissues [19]. Animal studies indicate that these free fatty acids can initiate pancreatic injury [20].

Hypercalcemia is believed to be a factor in activating trypsinogen and in the subsequent development of acute pancreatitis. An association of pancreatitis with parathyroid adenomas and carcinomas has been noted.

Acinar cell injury caused by viruses, endotoxins, toxic chemicals, ischemia, or trauma may precipitate activation and release of pancreatic enzymes. This theory is postulated for pancreatitis not caused by alcoholism or biliary disease [19].

Clinical Manifestations. There are no precise clinical features that distinguish pancreatitis from other disorders. *Abdominal pain* and tenderness are present in almost all cases of acute pancreatitis and frequently occur in chronic pancreatitis. The pain is usually severe and may reach full intensity in a matter of minutes or gradually over several hours. It is frequently localized in the epigastrium, becoming more severe to the right or left of the epigastrium or generalized throughout the upper abdomen. Pancreatic pain is usually steady, boring, and penetrating. Unlike the pain of biliary colic, it radiates straight through to the back in approximately one-half of affected persons. Individuals are restless and may seek relief by flexing the spine, by bending forward and flexing the knees against the chest, or by lying on one side with knees flexed. Characteristically, the pain of acute pancreatitis lasts for hours and days rather than a few minutes or a few hours.

The pain of pancreatitis is related to ductal swelling, extravasation of plasma and red cells, and release of digested proteins and lipids into surrounding tissue. The pancreatic capsule is stretched by the edema, exudate, red cells, and digestive products. These substances seep out of the gland into the mesentery, causing a peritonitis that stimulates the sensory nerves and causes intense pain in back and flanks when the gland is damaged extensively. During an acute attack, the pain is generalized over the abdomen because of peritoneal irritation and release of kinins. Large doses of narcotics are avoided because they may induce spasm of the sphincter of Oddi, which aggravates the pancreatitis and increases pain. As pain increases with the spread of intraperitoneal and retroperitoneal inflammation, local or diffuse paralytic ileus may occur. Peripheral vascular collapse and shock may develop rapidly. The stretching of the gland may also cause nausea and vomiting. Vomiting and abdominal distention are also related to intestinal hypomotility and chemical peritonitis.

Other nonspecific findings include hypotension, tachycardia, and shock. Bowel sounds are usually diminished. A pancreatic pseudocyst may be palpable in the upper abdomen. In severe necrotizing pancreatitis, discoloration of the flanks (Grey Turner's sign) or around the umbilicus (Cullen's sign) may be noted. A history of a prior attack of pancreatitis may be a valuable indicator if clinical manifestations are related to pancreatitis.

The extensive injury to tissue, necrosis, and inflammation produce fever in approximately two-thirds of individuals with acute pancreatitis. Fever is due to absorption of pyrogens into the circulation, but persistent high fever or temperature spikes imply pancreatic abscess or other septic complications [23].

Complications. *Cardiovascular Complications*. With massive exudation of plasma into the retroperitoneal space and, in cases of hemorrhage, there is a drop in blood pressure and rise in pulse. Activation of the proteolytic enzyme kallikrein liberates bradykinin and kallidin, which are vasoactive peptides. The result is marked peripheral vasodilatation, which further reduces blood pressure. Accumulation of fluid in the small bowel, a third-space shift, causes additional loss of fluid and leads to systemic hypotension and shock.

The decrease in intravascular volume together with hypotension diminishes urinary output, and acute tubular necrosis (ATN) of the kidneys may result. Myocardial and cerebral ischemia may also occur [23].

Coagulation Defects. Although not a frequent feature of the disease, hypercoagulability of blood due to elevations in levels of platelets, factor VIII, fibrinogen, and possible factor V may occur.

Ileus. The large and small bowel may dilate in a general response to inflammation of the peritoneum. The gut may contain air and fluid, contributing to hypovolemia.

Pulmonary-Pleural Complications. Acute pancreatitis is frequently accompanied by a pleural effusion. The fluid may be hemorrhagic. This pleural effusion apparently is caused by the retroperitoneal transudation of fluid, with markedly elevated secretion of amylase into the pleural cavity from the inflamed, swollen pancreas.

Gastrointestinal bleeding. This may occur in association with a pseudocyst or abscess, mucosal bleeding of the duodenum caused by adjacent inflammation of the pancreas, or esophageal or gastric varices related to splenic or portal vein thrombosis [2,9]. Gastritis and esophagitis in alcoholics may be a source of hemorrhage in pancreatitis.

Hypocalcemia. Sharp falls in serum calcium levels may occur in acute pancreatitis, related to extensive lipolysis of peripancreatic mesenteric and fatty tissues, releasing free fatty acids that combine with calcium to form soaps. The parathyroids do not rapidly compensate for the abrupt lowering of calcium by the mechanism of soap formation. Neuromuscular irritability and tetany result from severe hypocalcemia.

Acidosis. Lactic acidosis may result from the central hypovolemia, or occasionally ketosis occurs when there is extensive destruction of the gland.

Hyperlipidemia. High levels of serum lipids are often noted during attacks of pancreatitis, especially alcoholic pancreatitis and in persons with preexisting elevated triglyceride levels. The plasma may have a creamy appearance.

Pseudocysts. Inflammatory pseudocysts are a frequent complication during recovery from an episode of severe acute pancreatitis. The cysts are nonepithelium-lined cavities that contain plasma, blood, pancreatic products, and inflammatory exudate. They are solitary and measure 5 to 10 cm in diameter. They occur as a result of destruction of tissue and obstruction in the ductal system. Pancreatic juice may collect in them and leak into the peritoneal cavity. If large, pseudocysts may impinge on neighboring structures such as the portal vein, causing *acute portal hypertension*, and on the bile duct, causing *jaundice*. Occasionally, the cysts rupture and cause generalized peritonitis [23].

The formation of inflammatory pseudocysts may be associated with pancreatic ascites, which develops from a direct communication between the pseudocyst and the peritoneal cavity.

Pancreatic Abscess. One of the most serious complications of acute pancreatitis is pancreatic abscess, a collection of purulent and necrotic tissue. It occurs if an episode of pancreatitis is severe enough to cause parenchymal necrosis and if the pancreatic and retroperitoneal tissues become secondarily infected. There are usually several foci of infection rather than a discrete abscess that can be easily drained. Pancreatic abscesses may develop in pancreatitis of various etiologies; however, most occur in association with alcohol abuse. They account for about 3 to 4 percent of all cases of pancreatitis. Fistulization into an adjacent structure with massive bleeding may occur.

Jaundice. Mild jaundice is common in acute pancreatitis. The swelling of the head of the pancreas impinges on the common bile duct that passes through it. If the bile duct is compressed by pseudocysts, or stones, jaundice may be more severe.

Diagnostic Tests. The cardinal findings of acute pancreatitis are *increases in serum amylase* and *lipase* activities. Serum amylase values usually exceed 200 Somogyi units; normal levels are 60 to 180 Somogyi units per dl. The amylase : creatinine clearance ratio is increased and isoamylase determination reflects increased *p*-isoamylase. There does not appear to be a correlation between elevation of amylase and severity of disease.

Serum lipase activity parallels that of serum amylase and abnormal levels persist for a longer time. Normal serum lipase values depend on the laboratory procedure used, but are generally below 1.5 units per ml. The increased activities occur shortly after onset of disease, almost always within the first 24 hours, and may remain high for weeks.

Leukocytosis with increased polymorphonuclear leukocytes and a shift to the left is frequent. The white blood counts range from 9000 to 20,000 but occasionally rise to 50,000. The *hematocrit* may be elevated from loss of serum into the peritoneal spaces with resultant hemoconcentration.

Hyperglycemia is related to various factors such as increased glucagon, decreased insulin, and increased glucocorticoid and catecholamine levels. *Hyperlipidemia* often occurs and may predate the onset of overt pancreatitis. *Levels of serum calcium and magnesium* decrease, especially in persons with fat necrosis. Blood calcium levels may fall and remain down for 7 to 10 days. Hypocalcemia is an indicator of severe pancreatitis.

Ultrasonic examination of the pancreas in severe pancreatitis may help to confirm a clinical impression, assess degree of resolution of inflammation, and reveal dilatation of common bile duct secondary to obstruction and presence of gallstones. *Computerized axial tomographic* (CT) scan may be performed if unexplained abdominal pain suggests either pancreatitis or pancreatic carcinoma. Scans may also be used in prolonged pancreatitis or recurrent pancreatitis to rule out a pseudocyst or interductal calculi. *Roentgenograms* may be obtained to rule out a perforation and exclude other diagnoses.

Chronic Pancreatitis

Manifestations of chronic pancreatitis are similar to those of acute pancreatitis except for their chronicity and recurrence. If bouts recur, pancreatic insufficiency may result, even though the pancreas has considerable functional reserve.

In chronic pancreatitis, histologic changes persist even after the etiologic agent has been removed. In the United States, the most common cause of chronic pancreatitis is alcohol abuse. The pathologic changes are characterized by the deposition of protein plugs in the pancreatic ductules. An inflammatory process is set up and fibrous tissue is deposited. Eventually, there is intraductal calcification and marked parenchymal destruction, with only a few islet cells and some acinar tissue remaining.

Exocrine pancreatic insufficiency is manifested by steatorrhea (excess fat in the stools), azotorrhea (excess nitrogenous material in the feces), and weight loss. Microscopically, the stool exhibits fat globules and striated meat fibers that indicate impaired digestion of fats and proteins. Endocrine pancreatic insufficiency may lead to diabetes mellitus. Abdominal pain is a serious problem in chronic pancreatitis and may be responsible for severe weight loss, malnutrition, and general dibility. During early stages of the disease, the person may be asymptomatic between attacks.

The predominant complications of chronic pancreatitis that are associated with abdominal pain are pancreatic pseudocyst, stricture and obstruction of the common bile duct or pancreatic duct, and occasionally, carcinoma of the pancreas.

Carcinoma of the Pancreas

Carcinoma of the pancreas occurs mainly in the exocrine portion of the gland in the ductal epithelium. Pancreatic cancers have a poor prognosis, causing about 6 percent of all neoplastic deaths in the United States. A significant increase in frequency has been attributed to smoking, consumption of alcoholic beverages, and consumption of fat. Increased risk has also been associated with disease of the gallbladder and bile duct (extrahepatic). Most tumors occur in individuals over 60 years of age; they rarely occur before age 40 years.

Clinical symptoms of cancer of the pancreas depend on its site of origin and manifestations of metastasis. Tumors of the head of the pancreas tend to obstruct the bile duct and duodenum, and lead to early symptoms of obstructive jaundice; carcinoma of the body and tail are less easily recognized clinically, and become apparent only when adjacent structures are involved or when metastatic dissemination produces symptoms.

Most carcinomas of the pancreas grow in well-differentiated glandular patterns and are *adenocarcinomas*. About 10 percent assume an *adenosquamous* pattern or an uncommon pattern of extreme anaplasia with *giant-cell* formation. About 0.5 percent arise in cysts and are called *cystadenocarcinoma*. An *acinar cell carcinoma* occasionally occurs in children [3,19].

Carcinoma of the Head of the Pancreas

Tumors of the head of the pancreas are fairly small lesions with poorly defined margins. They often impinge on the common bile duct and pancreatic duct, causing atrophy of the pancreas. The tumors usually extend to the duodenum and cause compression and crowding of the common bile duct and ampulla of Vater, with distention of the gallbladder.

Carcinoma of the head of the pancreas is usually not a widely disseminated lesion because it produces biliary duct obstruction and jaundice at an early date. Individuals usually die of hepatobiliary dysfunction before the tumor has become widely disseminated.

Carcinoma of the Body and Tail of the Pancreas

These tumors are usually large and invade the entire tail and body of the pancreas; they may even be palpable in the thin individual. They spread more extensively than tumors of the head. They crowd the vertebral column, spread into the retroperitoneal spaces, and may even invade the spleen, adrenals, colon, or stomach. Metastases spread by way of the splenic vein, which lies on the margins of the organ, to surrounding nodes and the liver. The liver may be enlarged 2 to 3 times its normal size [19].

Clinical Manifestations

The clinical manifestations are those that relate to the encroachment of the pancreas on surrounding organs. Dull epigastric abdominal pain, which may radiate to the back; insidious weight loss with anorexia; and jaundice are among the few characteristic signs or symptoms that point to a diagnosis of pancreatic cancer. Occasionally, anorexia is accompanied by a curious aversion to meats and a metallic taste in the mouth [3]. Jaundice occurs in 80 to 90 percent of persons with carcinoma of the head of the pancreas, and occurs in 10 to 40 percent of those with tumors of the body and tail [9]. Often, large tumors that arise from the head of the pancreas encase the common bile duct. Jaundice is accompanied by pruritus. Weight loss and jaundice are often accompanied by a distended gallbladder.

Nausea, vomiting, weakness, fatigue, diarrhea, and dyspepsia are also fairly common. Vomiting may indicate gastric or duodenal encroachment or peritoneal metastasis. Hematemesis and melena indicate invasion of the tumor into duodenal or gastric organs that are very vascular. Approximately one-fourth of persons with pancreatic malignancy have a palpable abdominal mass when examined and often complain of both constipation and diarrhea. Emotional disturbances may be noted. Thrombophlebitis and diabetes mellitus are other clinical features. An abdominal bruit may be auscultated in the periumbilical area and left upper quadrant due to compression of the splenic artery by a tumor.

Clinical Course

Carcinomas of the pancreas progress insidiously, and are most likely present for months and perhaps years before symptoms appear. Major symptoms include weight loss, abdominal pain, back pain, anorexia, nausea, vomiting, generalized malaise, and weakness. Pain occurs in advanced stages of disease. Jaundice is present in about one-half of those with carcinoma of the head of the pancreas [3].

Laboratory procedures are important in providing clues to the presence of these cancers in their early stages. Approximately 80 to 90 percent have elevated levels of carcinoembryonic antigen (CEA). Measurement of this antigen may be helpful in following the course of pancreatic malignancy, with titers of greater than 20 mg per ml usually being associated with metastases. As with obstructive jaundice, serum bilirubin levels increase, stools become clay colored, and urine urobilinogen levels fall. Alkaline phosphatase levels are elevated [3].

Radiologic procedures can assist in localizating tumors and differentiating them from cysts. A CT scan of the pancreas is helpful in confirming presence of tumor.

Spontaneously appearing phlebothrombosis, also called migratory thrombophlebitis, is noted in carcinoma of the pancreas (Trousseau's sign). Trousseau diagnosed his own fatal disease when he developed migratory thrombophlebitis. Thromboses appear and disappear in other forms of cancer, but the two highest correlations are in pancreatic and pulmonary neoplasms. The thromboses are attributed to confinement to bed and surgical treatment. Thromboplastic factors have been identified in the serum that lead to a hypercoagulable state due to thromboplastic properties of the necrotic products of the tumor [19].

Cystic Fibrosis (Mucoviscidosis, Fibrocystic Disease of the Pancreas)

Cystic fibrosis, formerly referred to as mucoviscidosis or fibrocystic disease of the pancreas, is a systemic disease of infancy or childhood. Alterations in the secretory process of the exocrine (mucus-producing) glands result in several complications, especially in the pulmonary system and gastrointestinal tract.

Frequency

Cystic fibrosis (CF) has been recognized clearly as a disease entity only since the late 1930s. It is now considered to be a common inherited condition and the most fatal genetic disease in whites. The incidence is between 1 in 1800 and 1 in 1850 in white populations. Black and Oriental races are rarely affected.

Cystic fibrosis is transmitted by the autosomal recessive mode of inheritance. There is no difference in sex distribution. Chromosome number and structure are normal, and carriers of the gene (heterozygotes) show no symptoms of the disease. Approximately 5 percent of the population carry the CF gene. More children with this disease are surviving to adulthood, marrying, and reproducing, so genetic risks are now being considered. Affected persons transmit the gene to all of their offspring, but the children cannot develop the disease (homozygote) unless both parents are carriers.

Pathogenesis

The exact cause of cystic fibrosis remains unknown. Much research and study have been devoted to the condition, but a single hypothesis has not evolved to explain the alterations in mucous and sweat glands and the basic metabolic defect. Mucus abnormalities are apparent, but the glands themselves are normal until cellular changes related to the disease process occur. Elevation in sweat chloride levels seems to be the only consistent biochemical alteration (Fig. 35-12).

The anatomic changes of CF are thought to result from obstruction of exocrine ducts by glycoproteins that affect epithelial tissue. Abnormalities have been reported in autonomic nervous system function, related to reduction of cell membrane beta-adrenergic receptors on leukocytes [4,6]. Higher levels of calcium have been found in cells and certain mucous glands of persons with CF, particularly the salivary glands [22]. Both intracellular calcium and autonomic nervous system activity influence secretory processes of glands and have been cited as factors in the pathogenesis of CF. Abnormalities in serum that inhibit ciliary activity have been found in vitro. It is speculated that these mucociliary inhibitors in serum are low-molecular-weight glycoproteins [19].

The organs most frequently involved in CF are the lungs, pancreas, intestine, liver, reproductive tract, and sweat and tear glands (Fig. 35-12).

Gastrointestinal Tract. The extent of changes is related to whether secretions are carried to the gastrointestinal tract from cells with narrow necks, such as the goblet cells; from wide-mouthed ducts, such as glands in the duodenum; or from narrow ducts, such as those in the pancreas, liver, and salivary glands. The thick, tenacious secretions tend to cause more problems in longer, narrow ducts, with resultant changes in tissues and alterations of function. The greatest alterations in structure and function occur in the pancreas.

Structural Changes in the Pancreas. Abnormalities in the pancreas occur in approximately 85 percent of affected persons. These changes are evident microscopically and macroscopically as early as the neonatal period. The changes are variable and depend on the age of onset and severity of disease. They may consist of accumulation of mucus or, as the disease progresses, to blockage of the collecting ducts, damage to acinar tissue, fibrosis and duct dilatation, and degeneration of the parenchyma. The ducts may be replaced by fat and fibrous tissue and converted into cysts. These changes in appearance are the bases for the designation fibrocystic disease of the pancreas.

Pathologic changes begin during fetal life and are frequently severe enough by birth to prevent exocrine secretions from reaching the duodenum. The development of diabetes mellitus in some older persons is suggestive of impairment of the blood supply by progressive fibrosis.

Functional changes occur as a result of structural alterations. There is a lack of enzymes (trypsin, amylase, lipase) in the duodenum, and as a result, proteins are not completely digested and nitrogen is excreted in the stools; starch is not completely broken down and appears as granules; fats are largely undigested and are excreted in the stools in excessive amounts. The stools are large and oily, and have a pungent odor caused in part by breakdown products of protein produced by bacteria in the intestine.

Liver. Blockage of the bile duct by mucus and mononuclear periportal cell infiltration leads to cirrhosis and portal hypertension. Esophageal varicies and splenomegaly may result.

Intestine. Absence of pancreatic enzymes and altered gastrointestinal mucous secretions produce thick tenacious plugs of viscid mucus that obstruct the lumen of the small intestine, causing meconium ileus.

Salivary Glands. The salivary glands frequently undergo histologic changes such as dilatation of ducts and glandular atrophy and fibrosis.

Pathologic changes also occur in other glands. Plugging occurs in the bile ducts leading to fibrosis and liver dysfunction. Cystic fibrosis is an important cause of hepatic cirrhosis and portal hypertension in adolescents and young adults.

Respiratory System. Pulmonary changes occur in almost all persons and usually are the primary determinants of the ultimate outcome of the disease. Both upper and lower respiratory tracts are involved because of the presence of mucus-secreting glands and cells. The lungs are structurally normal at birth, but problems begin in the small bronchioles, where the thick, tenacious mucus collects and provides a medium for bacterial growth. The most common organisms are *Staphylococcus aureus*, *Hemophilus influenzae*, and *Pseudomonas aeruginosa*. The mucoid form of the last is especially troublesome.

Infection alters the integrity of the bronchial epithelium and invades the peribronchial tissues. Bronchiectasis develops in the terminal bronchioles. Trapping of air produces an overinflated barrel-shaped chest. Mucopurulent exudates are also present in the upper respiratory tract. Nasal polyps occur with increased frequency and are often associated with sinus infections. Pulmonary hypertension

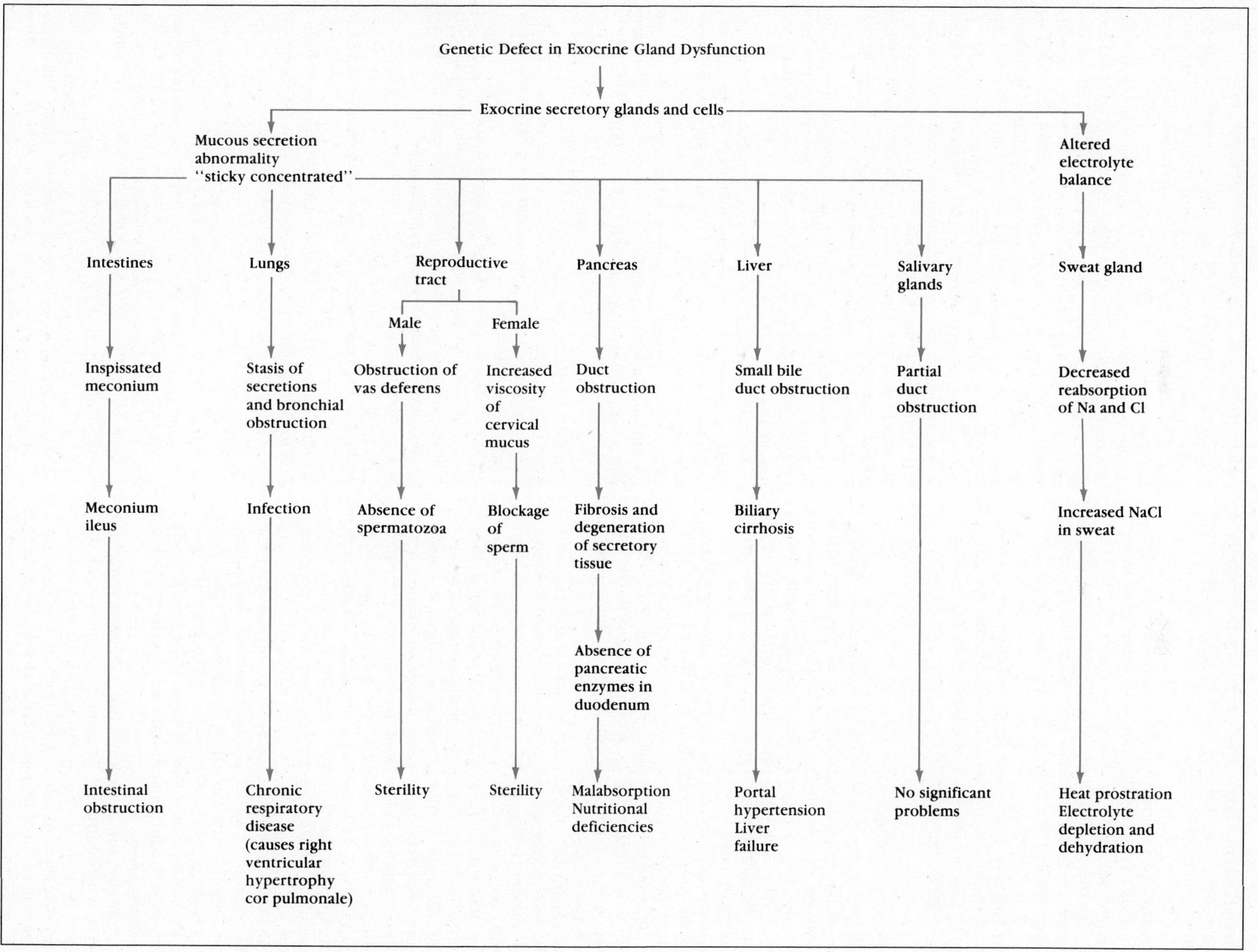

FIGURE 35-12 Pathogenesis of cystic fibrosis.

results from thickened arterioles, which together with the obstructive bronchial disease, leads to right ventricular hypertrophy and cor pulmonale.

Reproductive System. Abnormalities include atresia or obstruction of the vas deferens and epididymis in the male. Spermatogenesis is decreased or absent.

In the female, mucus-producing glands of the cervix may also produce viscid mucus that blocks the entry of sperm. The frequency of cervical polyps is increased.

Sweat Glands. Although there is a high electrolyte content of the sweat and an alteration in resorption of sodium chloride in the sweat ducts, no structural abnormalities are noted in the ducts.

Clinical Manifestations

Because CF affects several organ systems in varying degrees, it is sometimes difficult to recognize. Most individuals are diagnosed in early childhood because of symptoms related to the respiratory and gastrointestinal systems. A very early manifestation of cystic fibrosis is meconium ileus in the newborn, which blocks the small intestine with thick, tenacious, puttylike meconium. The degree varies from a delay in passing meconium (meconium-plug syndrome) to an obvious intestinal obstruction, usually in the area of the ileocecal valve, that may be accompanied by atresia, volvulus, or perforation and peritonitis. Prolapse of the rectum related to chronic constipation is a common complication in children with untreated CF.

In the classic case, the child is examined after 1 month of life because of respiratory symptoms, failure to thrive, and foul-smelling, bulky, greasy stools. Any one or all characteristics may be noted. In some cases, symptoms are not apparent until several years have passed. Infants often have a dry, repetitive cough that occurs in an attempt to remove the sticky secretion. Vomiting may follow a bout of coughing. Classic progression of chest infection occurs, with increased coughing and sputum, development of barrel chest, finger clubbing, dyspnea, and cyanosis. Sputum is thick, sticky, and difficult to expectorate. In the early stages it is yellow, particularly if due to *S. aureus*. With the mucoid strain, *P. aeruginosa*, sputum is greenish and slimy.

Microscopic examination of the stool reveals the presence of numerous fat globules. Children often compensate for stool losses with a voracious appetite, but they lose weight, exhibit tissue wasting, and fail to grow. In geographic areas where humidity is high, babies with cystic fibrosis may develop dehydration and electrolyte imbalance due to salt loss.

Uncommonly, the disorder may be diagnosed during adolescence or adulthood. Diagnosis is difficult, as the sweat test is less reliable in these age groups than in younger ones. Persons with cystic fibrosis who have not had severe chest infection may have abdominal problems, diabetes, or liver disease.

Laboratory and Diagnostic Findings

Criteria for diagnosis of CF include increased electrolyte concentration of sweat, absence of pancreatic enzymes, impaired fat absorption, chronic pulmonary involvement, and family history of the disorder.

The *sweat test* is the simplest and most reliable method to confirm the diagnosis. Up to age 20 years, a level of more than 60 mEq per liter of sweat chloride is diagnostic of cystic fibrosis. Values between 50 and 60 mEq per liter are highly suggestive. The sweat test is repeated if results are questionable or if they are negative and clinical manifestations are strongly suggestive of CF. Reliable sweat tests are difficult to obtain in the first three to four weeks of life, as the sweat glands are not yet well developed functionally.

Roentgenograms reveal changes in respiratory and gastrointestinal systems. Chest films reveal slightly increased diameter of upper chest, with overaerated lungs, widespread consolidation, and fibrotic changes. There may be areas of lobar or segmental collapse.

Changes in radiologic patterns of the small intestine are noted in cystic fibrosis as in other malsorptive diseases. Fibrosis abnormalities are also evident in barium studies of the duodenum.

Pancreatic deficiency is noted on examination of duodenal contents for pancreatic enzyme (trypsin and chymotrypsin) activity. Trypsin is absent in approximately 80 percent of affected persons. Chemical examination of feces reveals marked steatorrhea. Normal stools should not contain more than 4 gm of fat per day. Stools of children with cystic fibrosis often contain 15 to 30 gm per day.

Study Questions

1. List the pancreatic hormones and describe their effect on glucose metabolism.
2. Why is insulin called the fat-storage hormone?
3. Compare insulin-dependent and noninsulin-dependent diabetes mellitus according to pathology, course of disease, clinical manifestations, and complications.
4. Describe the process by which dehydration and shock can develop from hyperglycemia.
5. What is the relationship between alcoholism and pancreatitis?
6. Discuss the pathology of acute and chronic pancreatitis.
7. Why do the clinical manifestations of cystic fibrosis occur?

References

1. Banks, P.A. *Pancreatitis*. New York: Plenum Press, 1979.
2. Barnett, A.H. Diabetes in identical twins: A study of 200 pairs. *Diabetologia* 20:57, 1981.
3. Cello, J.P. Carcinoma of the pancreas. In J.B. Wyngaarden and L.H. Smith (eds.), *Cecil's Textbook of Medicine*. Philadelphia: Saunders, 1985.
4. Davis, P.B., et al. Abnormal adrenergic and cholinergic sensitivity in cystic fibrosis. *N. Engl. J. Med.* 302:1453, 1980.
5. Doniach, D. Etiology of type I diabetes mellitus: Heterogeneity and immunologic events leading to clinical onset. *Annu. Rev. Med.* 23:13, 1983.

6. Galant, S.P. et al. Impaired beta-adrenergic receptor binding and function in CF neutrophils. *J. Clin. Invest.* 68:253, 1981.
7. Ganda, O.P. Pathogenesis of Macrovascular Disease Including the Influence of Lipids. In A. Marble et al. (eds.), *Joslin's Diabetes Mellitus* (12th ed.). Philadelphia: Lea & Febiger, 1985.
8. Granda, O.P., and Soeldner, S.S. Genetic, acquired and related factors in the etiology of diabetes mellitus. *Arch. Intern. Med.* 137:461, 1977.
9. Greenberger, N.J., and Toskes, P.P. Diseases of the pancreas. In E. Braunwald et al. (eds.), *Harrison's Principles of Internal Medicine* (11th ed.). New York: McGraw-Hill, 1987.
10. Guyton, A.C. *Textbook of Medical Physiology* (7th ed.). Philadelphia: Saunders, 1986.
11. Kozak, G.P., and Krall, L.P. Disorders of the skin. In A. Marble et al. (eds.), *Joslin's Diabetes Mellitus* (12th ed.). Philadelphia: Lea & Febiger, 1985.
12. Locke, S., and Tarsy, D. The nervous system and diabetes. In A. Marble et al. (eds.), *Joslin's Diabetes Mellitus* (12th ed.). Philadelphia: Lea & Febiger, 1985.
13. MacMillan, D.R., et al. Seasonal variation in the onset of diabetes in children. *Pediatrics* 59:133, 1977.
14. National Diabetes Data Group. Classification and diagnosis of diabetes mellitus and other categories of glucose intolerance. *Diabetes* 28:1039, 1979.
15. O'Hare, J.A., and Warfield, C.A. The diabetic neuropathies. *Hosp. Pract.* 19:40, 1984.
16. Olefsky, J.M. Insulin resistance and insulin action. *Diabetes* 30:148, 1981.
17. Osterby, R. Basement membrane morphology in diabetes mellitus. In M. Ellenberg and H. Rifkin (eds.), *Diabetes Mellitus: Theory and Practice* (3rd ed.). New Hyde Park, N.Y.: Medical Examination, 1983.
18. Pyke, D.A. Genetics of diabetes. *Clin. Endocrinol. Metab.* 6:1, 1977.
19. Robbins, S.L., Cotran, R.S., and Kumar, V. *Pathologic Basis of Disease* (3rd ed.). Philadelphia: Saunders, 1984.
20. Saharia, P., et al. Acute pancreatitis with hyperlipemia: Studies with an isolated perfused canine pancreas. *Surgery* 82:60, 1977.
21. Service, J., et al. Pancreatic polypeptide: A for lean non-insulin-dependent diabetes mellitus? *Diabetes Care* 8, July-August, 1985.
22. Shapiro, B.L., and Larn, L.F. Calcium and age in fibroblasts from control subjects and patients with cystic fibrosis. *Science* 216:417, 1982.
23. Smith, L.H., and Thier, S.O. (eds.). *Pathophysiology: The Biological Principles of Disease* (2nd ed.). Philadelphia: Saunders, 1985.
24. Srikanta, S. Type I diabetes mellitus in monozygotic twins: Chronic progressive beta cell dysfunction. *Ann. Intern. Med.* 99:320, 1983.
25. Unger, R.H., and Foster, D.W. Diabetes mellitus. In J.D. Wilson and D.W. Foster (eds.), *Williams' Textbook of Endocrinology* (7th ed.). Philadelphia: Saunders, 1985.

Unit Bibliography

Anderson, J.R. *Muir's Textbook of Pathology*. London: Edward Arnold, 1985.

Anderson, R.A., et al. Effect of exercise (running) on serum glucose, insulin, glucagon and chromium excretion. *Diabetes* 31:212, 1982.

Barrett, E.J., and Defronzo, R.A. Diabetic ketoacidosis: Diagnosis and treatment. *Hosp. Pract.* 19:89, 1984.

Biesbroeck, J.J., et al. Abnormal composition of high density lipoproteins in non-insulin-dependent diabetes. *Diabetes* 31:126, 1982.

Bogardus, C., et al. Effects of physical training and diet therapy on carbohydrate metabolism in patients with glucose intolerance and non-insulin-dependent diabetes mellitus. *Diabetes* 33:311, 1984.

Braunwald, E., et al. *Harrison's Principles of Internal Medicine* (11th ed.). New York: McGraw-Hill, 1987.

Cahill, G.F., and McDevitt, H.O. Insulin-dependent diabetes mellitus: The initial lesion. *N. Engl. J. of Med.* 304:1454, 1981.

Carter Center of Emory University. Closing the gap: The problem of diabetes mellitus in the United States. *Diabetes Care* 8:391, 1985.

Dillon, R.S. *Handbook of Endocrinology* (2nd ed.). Philadelphia: Lea & Febiger, 1980.

DiMagno, E.P. Answers to questions on acute pancreatitis. *Hosp. Med.* 19:91, 1983.

Felig, P., et al. *Endocrinology and Metabolism*. New York: McGraw-Hill, 1981.

Gann, D.S., and Lilly, M.P. The neuroendocrine response to multiple trauma. *World J. Surgery* 7:101–118, 1983.

Geelhoed, G.B., and Chernow, B. *Endocrine Aspects of Acute Illness*. New York: Churchill Livingstone, 1985.

Ginsberg-Fellner, F., et al. HLA antigens, cytoplasmic islet cell antibodies and carbohydrate tolerance in families of children with insulin-dependent diabetes mellitus. *Diabetes* 31:292, 1982.

Gorbman, A. *Comparative Endocrinology*. New York: Wiley, 1983.

Guthrie, D.W., and Guthrie, R.A. The disease process of diabetes mellitus. *Nurs. Clin. North Am.* 18:617, 1983.

Hall, R., Anderson, J., and Besser, M. *Fundamentals of Clinical Endocrinology*. Chicago: Yearbook, 1980.

Hall, R., and Kobberling, J. *Thyroid Disorders Associated with Iodine Deficiency and Excess*. New York: Raven Press, 1984.

Ham, A.W., and Cormack, D.W. *Histology* (8th ed.). Philadelphia: Lippincott, 1979.

Jubiz, W. *Endocrinology: A Logical Approach for Clinicians* (2nd ed.). New York: McGraw-Hill, 1985.

Laycock, J.F., and Wise, P.H. *Essential Endocrinology*. New York: Oxford University Press, 1983.

Longcope, C. Adrenogenital syndrome. *Hosp. Med.* 20(4):79-85, 1985.

Marsden, P., and McCullagh, A.G. *Endocrinology*. Littleton, Mass.: PSG Publishing Co., 1985.

Martin, C.R. *Endocrine Physiology*. New York: Oxford University Press, 1985.

Mazzaferri, E.L. *Textbook of Endocrinology* (3rd ed.). New Hyde Park, N.Y.: Medical Examination, 1986.

Metz, R., and Larson, E.B. *Blue Book of Endocrinology*. Philadelphia: Saunders, 1985.

Mishell, D.R., and Davajon, V. *Infertility, Contraception, and Reproductive Endocrinology*. Oradell, N.J.: Medical Economics Books, 1986.

Mohan, V., et al. High prevalence of maturity-onset diabetes of the young (MODY) among Indians. *Diabetes Care* 8:171, 1985.

Moore-Ede, M.C., Sulzman, F.M., and Fuller, C.A. *The Clocks That Time Us: Physiology of the Circadian Timing System*. Cambridge, Mass.: Harvard University Press, 1982.

Robbins, S.L., Cotran, R.S., and Kumar, V. *Pathologic Basis of Disease* (3rd ed.). Philadelphia: Saunders, 1984.

Shearman, R.P. *Clinical Reproductive Endocrinology*. New York: Churchill Livingstone, 1985.

Skelton, C.W. Use of glycosylated hemoglobins in the long-term management of diabetes. *Nurse Prac.* 11:42, 1986.

Smith, L.E., and Thier, S.O. (eds.). *Pathophysiology, the Biological Principles of Disease* (2nd ed.). Philadelphia: Saunders, 1985.

Sodeman, W.A., and Sodeman, T.M. *Sodeman's Pathologic Physiology: Mechanisms of Disease* (7th ed.). Philadelphia: Saunders, 1985.

Srikanta, S., et al. Autoimmunity to insulin, beta cell dysfunction, and development of insulin-dependent diabetes mellitus. *Diabetes* 35:139, 1986.

Streck, W.F., and Lockwood, D.H. *Endocrine Diagnosis: Clinical and Laboratory Approach*. Boston: Little, Brown, 1983.

Urbanic, R.C., and Mazzaferri, E.L. Thyrotoxic crisis and myxedema. *Heart Lung* 7:435, 1978.

Ward, W.K., et al. Pathophysiology of insulin secretion in non-insulin-dependent diabetes mellitus. *Diabetes Care* 7:491, 1984.

Wilson, J.D., and Foster, D.W. (eds.). *Williams' Textbook of Endocrinology* (7th ed.). Philadelphia: Saunders, 1985.

Wyngaarden, J.B., and Smith, L.H. (eds.). *Cecil Textbook of Medicine* (17th ed.). Philadelphia: Saunders, 1985.

UNIT 12

Digestion, Absorption, and Use of Food

Barbara L. Bullock

Knowledge of the anatomic and functional activities of the entire gastrointestinal system is essential for the understanding of the pathologies of part or all of the system. Digestion, absorption, and use of food require the participation of all of the gastrointestinal organs, including the liver and pancreas. Alterations can occur at any point in the system and affect the entire system. Chapter 36 describes the normal activities of the gastrointestinal system, including the oral tract, stomach, intestines, and other components. Chapter 38 includes the normal liver and pancreatic exocrine functions. Chapter 37 details alterations in the gastrointestinal system, while Chapter 39 explains alterations in hepatobiliary function. Included in Chapter 39 is a discussion of obesity as a disorder of nutritional balance. Pancreatic alterations were considered in Chapter 35 (Unit 11).

The reader is encouraged to use the learning objectives as study guides for chapter content. Study questions at the end of each chapter can be answered by synthesis of the material presented in each chapter. The unit bibliography also gives resources for further study.

CHAPTER 36

Normal Function of the Gastrointestinal System

CHAPTER OUTLINE

Appetite, Hunger, and Satiety
Anatomy of the Gastrointestinal Tract

- Oral Cavity
- Pharynx
- Esophagus
- Stomach
- Small Intestine
- Large Intestine

Physiology of the Digestive System

- Oral Secretions and Movement of Food to the Stomach
- Gastric Motility and Secretion
- Secretion and Absorption in the Small Intestine
  - *Carbohydrate Absorption*
  - *Protein Absorption*
  - *Fat Absorption*
  - *Water Absorption*
  - *Electrolyte Absorption*
- Secretion, Absorption, and Excretion in the Large Intestine

LEARNING OBJECTIVES

1. Differentiate appetite, hunger, and satiety.
2. Locate the hunger and the appetite centers in the brain.
3. Identify the oral structures that prepare food for later absorption.
4. Describe the function of salivary ptyalin.
5. Define briefly *functional syncytium* as applied to the gastrointestinal system.
6. Locate the gastroesophageal or lower esophageal sphincter and briefly describe its functional significance.
7. Locate and describe clearly the function of the gastric glands.
8. Define *chyme*.
9. Identify the four layers of the intestinal wall.
10. Describe the appearance and function of the microvilli.
11. Identify the blood supply, nerve supply, and lymphatic drainage of the gastrointestinal system.
12. Locate the subdivisions of the large intestine.
13. Relate the importance of oral secretions to the process of digestion.
14. Describe the process of swallowing.
15. Delineate clearly the purposes of gastric secretions in digestion.
16. Describe the relationship of nervous and hormonal mechanisms in the process of digestion.
17. Outline briefly the neurogenic, gastric, and intestinal phases of gastric secretions.
18. Define and list examples of *secretagogues*.
19. Describe how the intestines inhibit gastric secretions.
20. Describe specifically where nutrients are absorbed in the small intestine.
21. Relate the mechanisms necessary for the absorption of carbohydrates, proteins, and fats.
22. List briefly the form and mechanism for the absorption of nutrients, vitamins, and minerals.
23. Describe the process of defecation.
24. Explain briefly the role of the large intestine in regulating water balance.

Normal functioning of the human body is dependent on an intact digestive system. In the broadest sense, the gastrointestinal tract is a tubular structure called the *alimentary canal*, which extends from the pharynx to the anus. Throughout this tubular structure ingested food is processed, digested, and absorbed. The nutrients absorbed may be further processed by accessory organs, used for energy, or stored for later energy.

For digestion to occur, the vital functions of motility, secretion, and absorption must proceed in a regulated fashion. Finally, by participating in the excretion of waste products, the gastrointestinal system helps to keep the host in a balanced state. In the adult, the steady state normally provides for a balanced body weight so that ingested nutrients are used and weight remains stable.

TABLE 36-1 Participation of the Oral Structures in Process of Digestion

Structure	Process
Teeth	Reduce food to sizes appropriate for swallowing; break down dense particles.
Tongue	Places food in proper position for swallowing; mixes secretions to moisten food.
Salivary glands	Moisten and lubricate foods in the mouth; add ptyalin enzyme for digestion of starches.
Muscles of mastication, or chewing	Provide movement for the grinding of food to smaller particles; provide more surface area for the digestive enzymes to act.

Appetite, Hunger, and Satiety

Appetite refers to a desire for specific types of food [2]. Learned patterns of behavior alter the appetite, creating a desire for food beyond the needs of the body. Hunger refers to the desire for food that results from the manifest need for energy. Satisfaction of hunger is called satiety.

The hunger center is in the *hypothalamus*, as is the *satiety center*, but the two have been shown to be in separate locations [2]. The feeling of hunger is frequently generated by rhythmic contractions of the stomach, which may cause a painful sensation called hunger pangs. Stimulation from the hunger center is related to the nutritional status of the body. Especially important in this process is the concentration of glucose in the blood. A decreased concentration of blood glucose intensifies the hunger response. Serum fat levels and amino acids also affect satiety. Distention of the gastrointestinal tract suppresses the hunger center through inhibitory signals, probably from sensory signals by the vagal nerves [2].

The *appetite center* is more subtly controlled by the cortical areas and is stimulated by the senses of sight, touch, and smell. Even thoughts of food can stimulate the appetite center. Alterations of appetite for specific foods are conditioned by culture, environment, and socioeconomic circumstances.

Anatomy of the Gastrointestinal Tract

The activity of the gastrointestinal tract is carried out through a continuous structure that begins with the oral cavity and terminates with the anal sphincter (Fig. 36-1).

Oral Cavity

The lips, tongue, cheeks, teeth, taste buds, and salivary glands are associated with the oral cavity and contribute to the process of preparing food for eventual absorption. This preparation includes reducing food particles to manageable size, stimulating salivary glands to increase saliva secretion, and moving food to the appropriate position for swallowing. Table 36-1 summarizes the oral structures and their participation in the process of preparing food for digestion.

The submandibular, parotid, and sublingual salivary glands continuously secrete *saliva*, which contains large amounts of water and small amounts of sodium, chloride, bicarbonate, urea, and a few other solutes (Fig. 36-2). Saliva also contains *ptyalin* (salivary amylase), an enzyme that digests starches. The average amounts of salivary secretion range from 1000 to 1500 ml per day. Stimulation for this secretion is relayed to the medulla by the parasympathetic fibers of the facial, trigeminal, glossopharyngeal, and vagus nerves. Efferent parasympathetic stimulation leads to increased secretion of saliva. Stimulation of the sympathetic system causes localized vasoconstriction and a decrease in salivary secretion.

Pharynx

The pharynx is an important structure for the process of swallowing. It actively moves food into the esophagus, while closing and sealing off the trachea. Once the swallowing reflex is initiated by voluntary movement of food to the back of the mouth, swallowing continues as a reflex activity.

Esophagus

The esophagus provides a passageway for food from the pharynx to the stomach. It is a muscular, pliable tube that is easily affected by intrathoracic and intraabdominal pressures or volumes. The esophagus is lined with a mucosal layer composed of squamous epithelium [6]. Glands along its length secrete mucus to lubricate the bolus of food passing through.

The construction of the smooth muscle of the esophagus and other structures in the alimentary canal has been described as a *functional syncytium* because the smooth muscle fibers lie very close to each other. This construction allows for waves of muscular contraction called *peristalsis* [2].

Approximately 5 cm above the esophageal entry to the stomach is a narrowed area called the *gastroesophageal*,

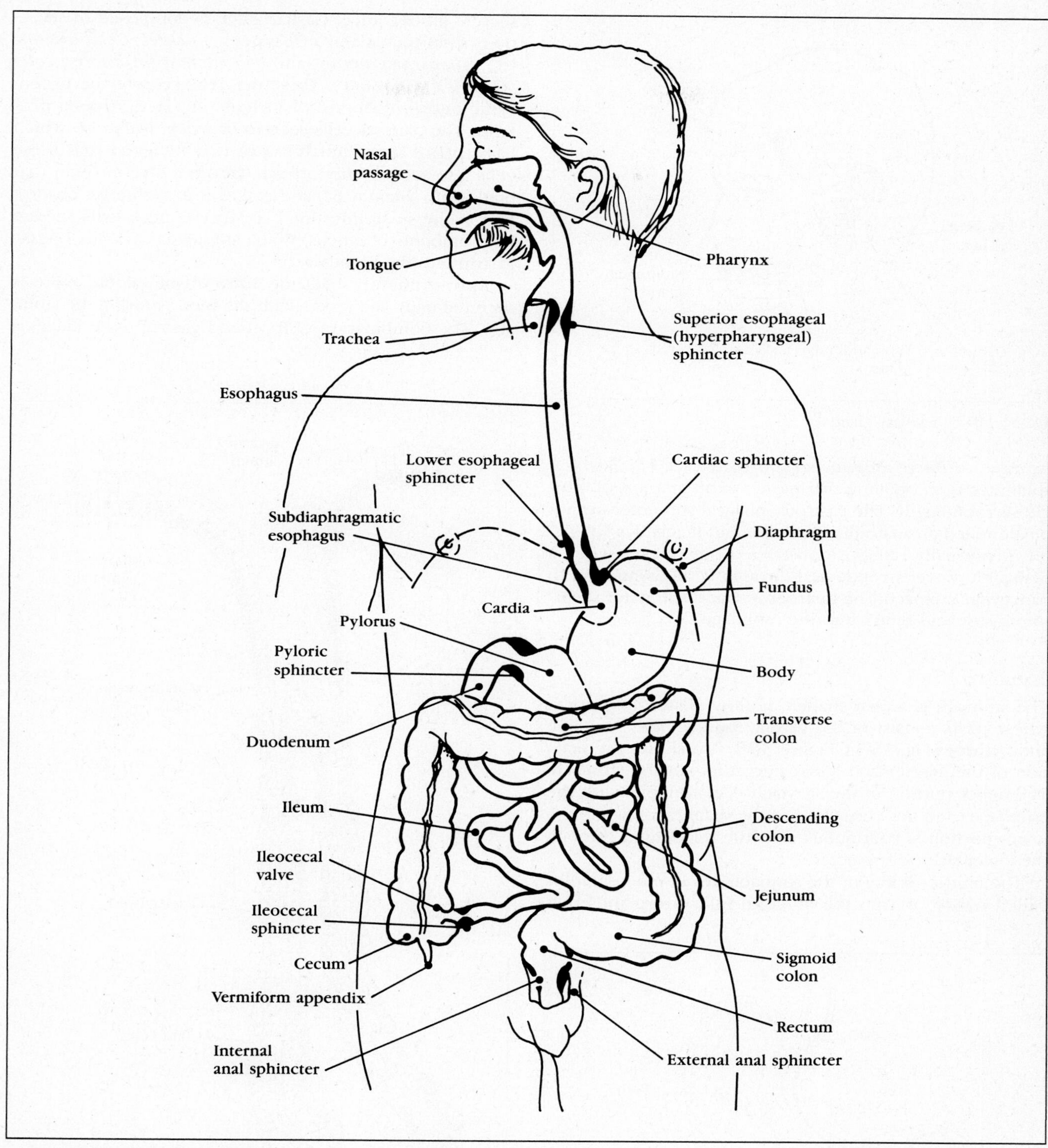

FIGURE 36-1 The digestive system.

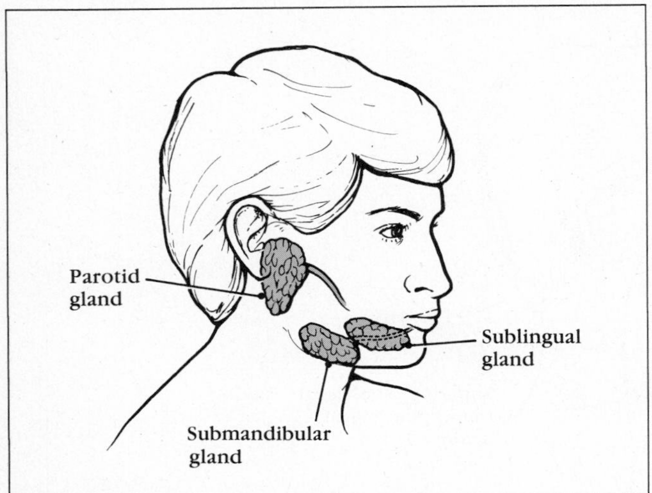

FIGURE 36-2 Salivary glands.

cardiac, or *lower esophageal sphincter* (see Fig. 36-1). A sphincter is an opening that has an extra amount of muscle surrounding it. The gastroesophageal sphincter cannot be identified on anatomic dissection but it acts as a sphincter. It normally remains constricted but relaxes when a peristaltic wave is conducted through it, allowing food to pass to the stomach. The gastroesophageal sphincter seems to prevent acid reflux into the esophagus.

Stomach

The stomach is a pear-shaped, hollow, distensible organ whose parts consist of the cardia, fundus, body, antrum, and pylorus (Fig. 36-3). Figure 36-3 also shows the position of the greater and lesser curvatures of the stomach. The upper portion of the stomach is continuous with the esophagus and lies very close to the diaphragm, while the lower portion is continuous with the duodenum through the lower pyloric sphincter.

The interior lining of the stomach lies in mucosal folds called *rugae*. Within the mucosal folds are glands that secrete gastric juice. Gastric juice is composed of secretions from four major cell types: (1) *chief*, (2) *parietal*, (3) *mucus-producing*, and (4) *gastrin-producing cells (G cells)* (Fig. 36-4). The chief cells secrete the proenzyme *pepsinogen*, which, when activated, digests proteins. The parietal cells secrete *hydrochloric acid*, which has a pH of approximately 0.8. It is believed that these cells also secrete the intrinsic factor, a glycoprotein that binds with vitamin B_{12} and makes it available for absorption in the small intestine [2]. Mucous neck cells secrete large amounts of mucus. When stimulated, G cells release gastrin into the bloodstream [5].

Approximately 1500 to 3000 ml of gastric juice is secreted daily and mixes with the food entering the stomach. The combination of food and gastric juice makes a

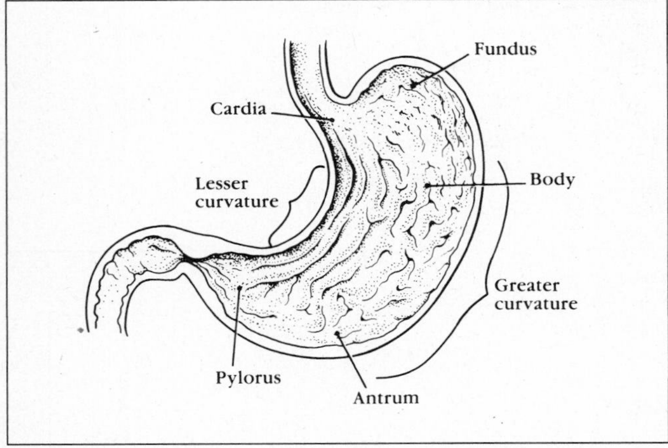

FIGURE 36-3 Segments of the stomach. Note the greater and lesser curvatures.

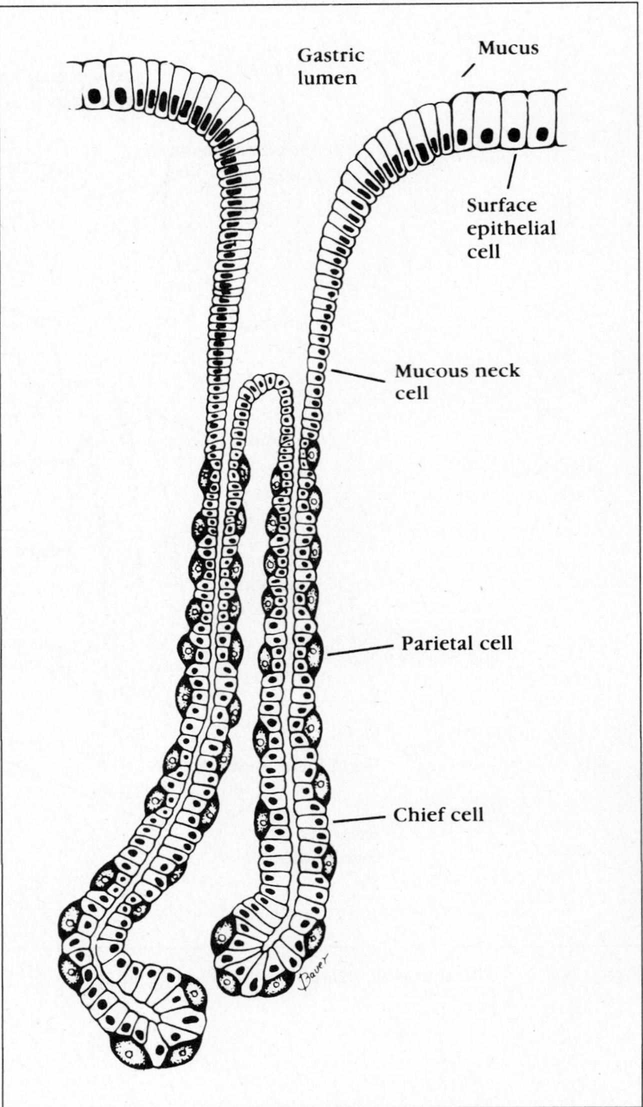

FIGURE 36-4 Glands from the body of the stomach that produce gastric secretions. (From E.E. Selkurt, *Basic Physiology for the Health Sciences* [2nd ed.]. Boston: Little, Brown, 1982.)

semiliquid mass called *chyme*, which is propelled into the small intestine through the pyloric sphincter (Fig. 36-5).

The nervous supply to the stomach is through the intrinsic and the autonomic nervous systems. The intrinsic system begins in the esophagus and continues all the way to the anus. The layers involved in this system include the *myenteric* and the *submucosal plexuses*. These control the tone of the bowel, rhythmic contractions, and the velocity of excitation of the gut. The autonomic nervous system (ANS) increases excitation through the parasympathetic branches, especially in the esophagus, stomach, large intestine, and anal region. The main function of the sympathetic portion of the ANS is to inhibit activity of the gastrointestinal system.

The arterial blood supply to the stomach comes mainly from the celiac artery. Venous blood is drained through the gastric veins, which connect to and terminate in the portal vein (Fig. 36-6). The stomach has profuse lymphatic drainage through lymphatic vessels and nodes (Fig. 36-7).

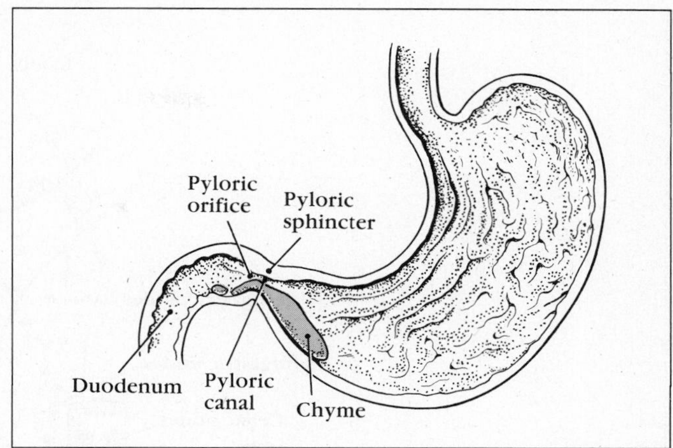

FIGURE 36-5 Movement of chyme through the pyloric sphincter.

Small Intestine

The small intestine extends from the pylorus to the ileocecal valve. It is approximately 12 feet long in the living human. In the cadaver it is longer because the muscles of the intestinal wall are relaxed [9]. The small intestine is divided into sections: ***duodenum***, ***jejunum***, and ***ileum*** (see Fig. 36-2). Absorption and secretion occur throughout the length of the small intestine (see Table 36-2).

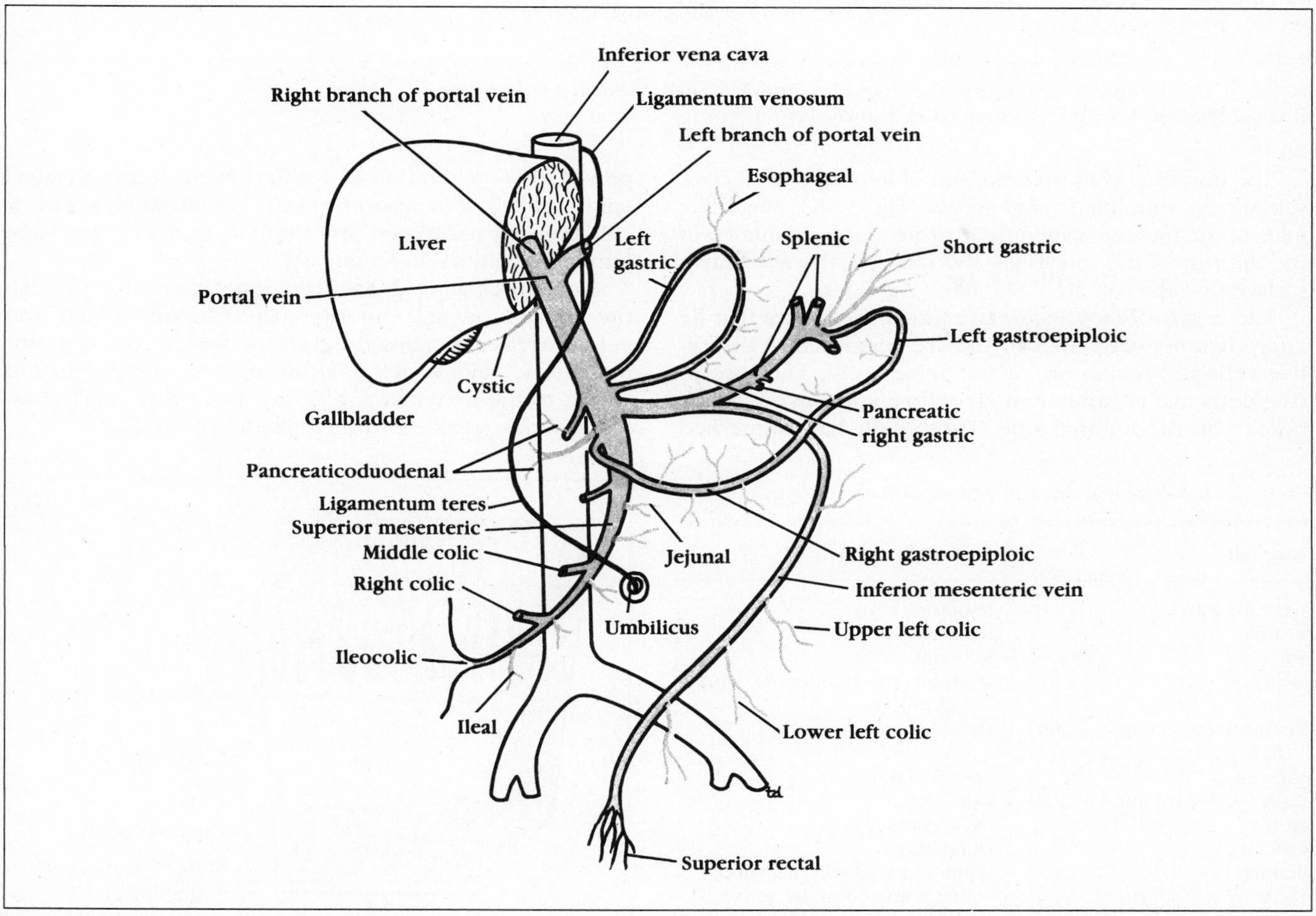

FIGURE 36-6 Venous drainage of the stomach and small intestine. (From R.S. Snell, *Clinical Anatomy for Medical Students* [2nd ed.]. Boston: Little, Brown, 1981.)

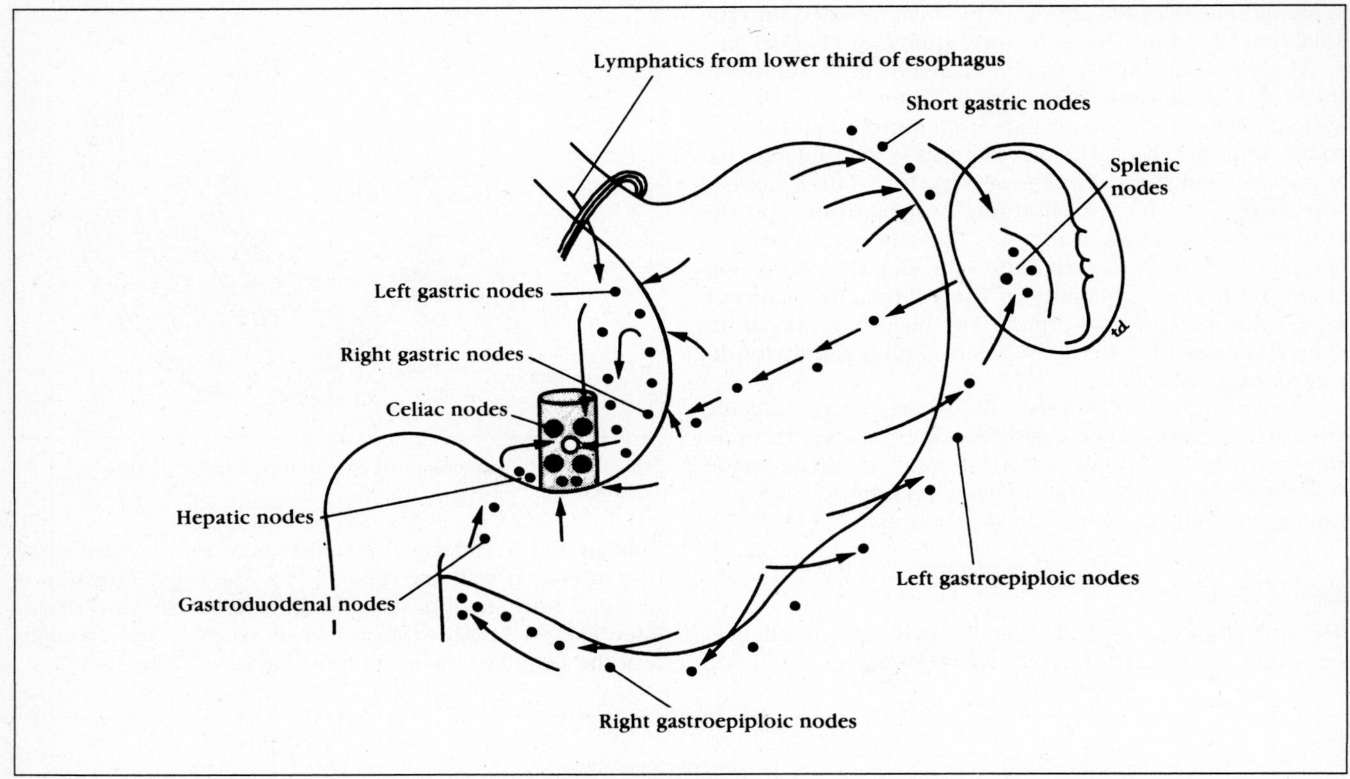

FIGURE 36-7 Lymphatic drainage of the stomach. (From R.S. Snell, *Clinical Anatomy for Medical Students* [2nd ed.]. Boston: Little, Brown, 1981.)

The intestinal wall is composed of four layers: mucosa, submucosa, muscularis, and serosa (Fig. 36-8). Fingerlike folds of the mucosa, called *villi*, project into the lumen of the interior of the intestines and increase the absorptive surface by approximately 600-fold (Fig. 36-9).

The *crypts of Lieberkühn* are pitlike structures that lie in grooves between the villi and are composed of absorptive cells and mucus-producing goblet cells. The absorptive cells are columnar in structure and have a brush border on the luminal side. These cells have a marked power for regeneration and differentiate from intestinal epithelial cells into absorptive cells. An intestinal epithelial cell lives approximately five days, after which it is shed into the intestinal secretions [9].

Blood circulation to the small intestine occurs through the gastroduodenal, superior pancreaticoduodenal, and celiac arteries. Venous drainage is through the superior mesenteric vein, which empties into the portal vein and travels to the liver (see Fig. 36-6). The entire small intestine is richly supplied with lymphatic vessels.

TABLE 36-2 Principal Sites of Absorption

Nutrient	Absorptive Site
Carbohydrates	Jejunum
Protein	Jejunum
Fat	Jejunum
Water	Jejunum; also duodenum, ileum, and colon
Fat-soluble vitamins—A, D, E, K	Duodenum
Vitamin B_{12}	Terminal ileum
Other water-soluble vitamins	Duodenum
Iron	Duodenum
Calcium	Duodenum
Sodium	Jejunum by passive diffusion; ileum and colon by active transport
Potassium	Jejunum and ileum

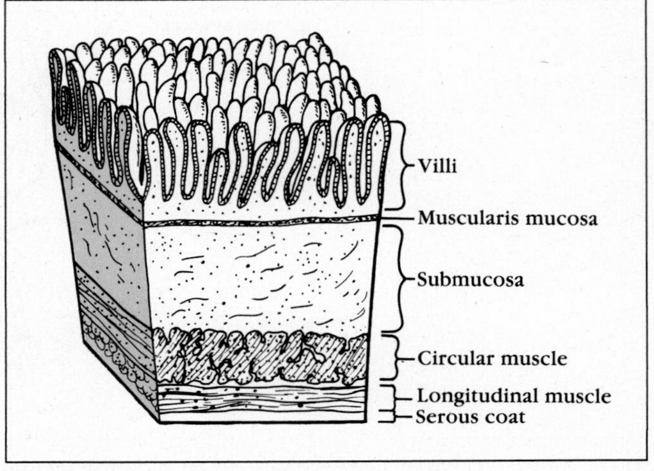

FIGURE 36-8 Layers of the intestinal wall.

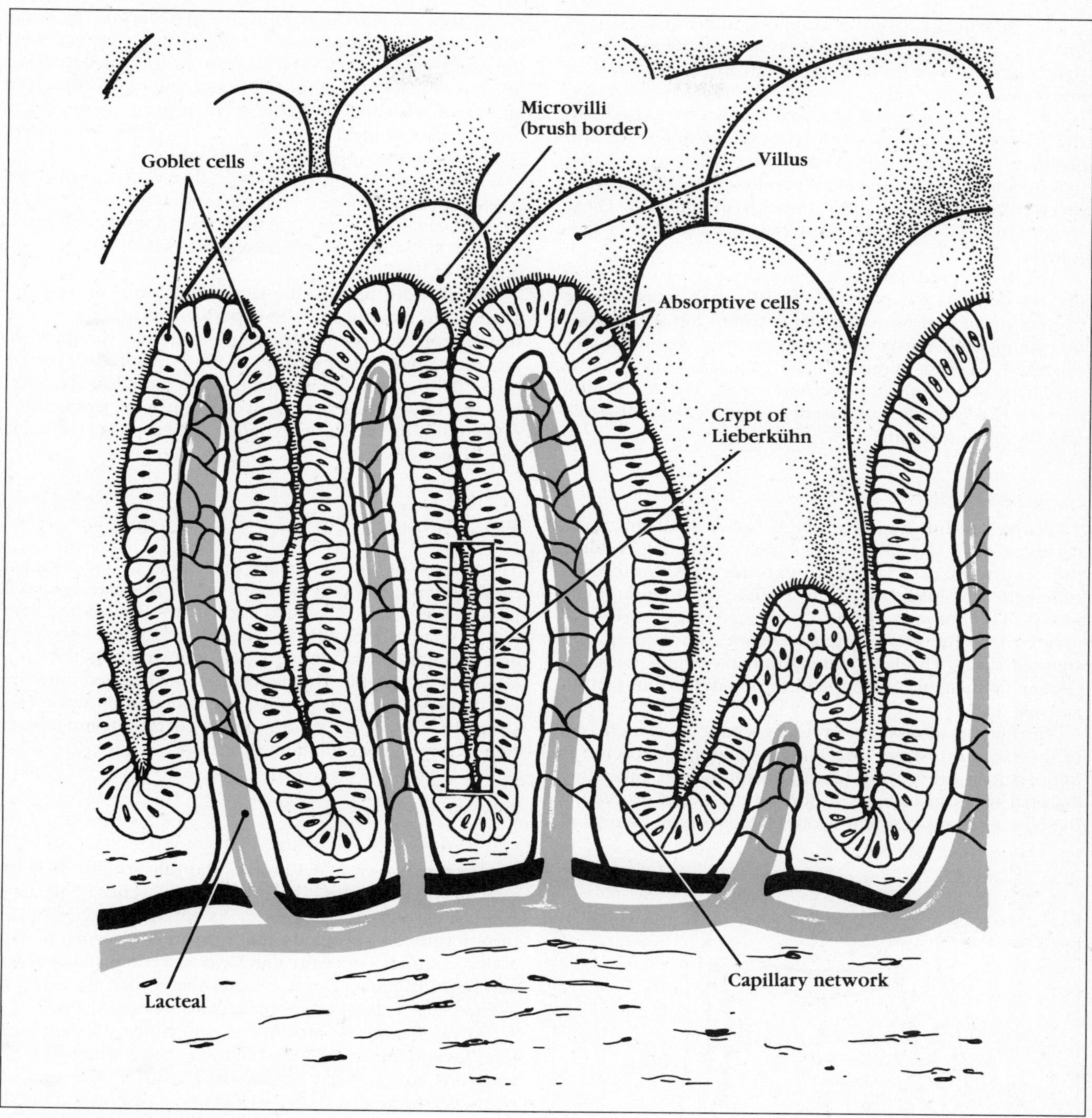

FIGURE 36-9 Structure of the intestinal villi.

The intestinal cells form large quantities of secretions that have a neutral pH. These secretions contain enzymes that function to a limited extent in the breakdown of nutrients. Another important secretion is *cholecystokinin (CCK)*, which is secreted from the mucosa, absorbed into the bloodstream, and stimulates the gallbladder and pancreas (see Chap. 38). At one time it was believed that two hormones, cholecystokinin and pancreozymin, were secreted by the mucosa of the upper small intestine. These were found to be the same hormone, now called cholecystokinin.

The liver, gallbladder, and pancreas, considered in greater detail in Chapter 38, are essential organs in the promotion of digestion. Chyme entering the small intestine stimulates CCK by distending the small intestine. This hormone, in turn, stimulates the pancreas to release its enzymatic secretions into the duodenum. The stimulation from CCK causes the gallbladder to contract and push bile into the small intestine.

Large Intestine

The large intestine begins with the end of the ileum at the ileocecal valve (Fig. 36-10). The area of meeting is called the cecum. A small structure extends from the cecum called the *appendix*, which is a relatively nonfunctional pouch. The colon portion of the large intestine is subdivided into the ascending, transverse, descending, and sigmoid areas. The large intestine itself begins with the cecum, contains the colon, and terminates in the rectum and anal canal.

The number of mucus-secreting goblet cells is increased in the large intestine. The mucous material secreted is important in preventing trauma to the bowel, providing material that causes feces to form a mass, and protecting the bowel against resident bacteria. Most of the liquid and electrolytes from the semiliquid material of the small intestine are absorbed in the large intestine, especially in the ascending and transverse colon. Feces usually consist of approximately three-fourths water and one-fourth solid matter, of which about 30 percent is dead bacteria. The brown color of fecal material is produced by breakdown products (simpler pigments) of bilirubin.

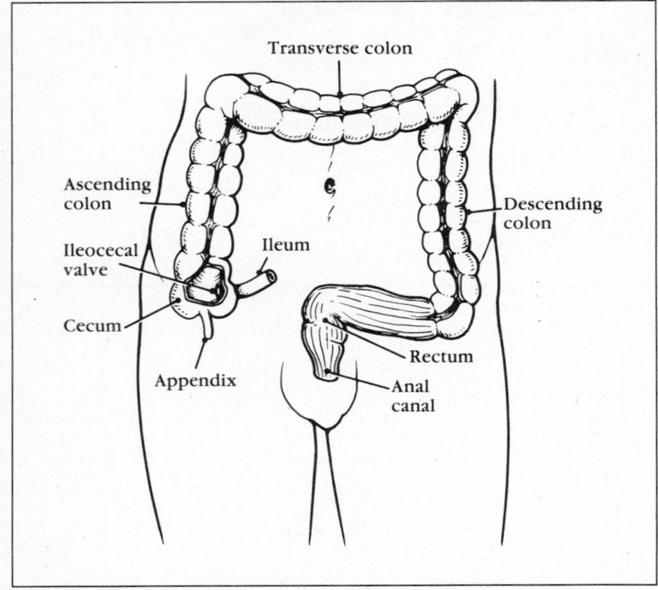

FIGURE 36-10 Segments of the large intestine.

The rectum is approximately 20 cm of the final descending portion of the large intestine and terminates in the anal canal. It is separated from the sigmoid colon by an external sphincter, the *sphincter ani*, which opens to the outside of the body.

The blood supply to the large intestine is profuse and arises from branches of the superior and inferior mesenteric arteries. Venous drainage is mainly through the mesenteric veins, terminating in the portal veins (see Fig. 36-6). This system is important in the pathology of portal hypertension, because increased portal pressure is reflected in the veins surrounding the esophagus and anal canal (see Chap. 39).

Physiology of the Digestive System

The process of digestion takes substances in one form and breaks them down into molecules that are small enough to pass through the intestinal wall to the blood and lymphatic system. This activity requires chemical secretions and mechanical movements, all working together in a coordinated fashion. The molecules may be moved by simple diffusion, active transport, or facilitated diffusion (see Chap. 1). The processes of motility, secretion, and absorption work together to effect digestion.

Oral Secretions and Movement of Food to the Stomach

The major digestive secretion of the salivary glands is the enzyme ptyalin, which breaks down starches. This amylase, or carbohydrate digester, is active not only in the mouth, but continues its function in the stomach. The action continues until the digestive secretions of the stomach begin to alter chyme. It is estimated that up to 30 to 40 percent of starches are broken down by ptyalin.

Saliva contains water, mucus, and other substances. It liquifies and lubricates ingested food. The amount of saliva secreted is regulated by the parasympathetic nervous pathways. Increased secretion occurs in response to irritation of stomach mucosa, which initiates a reflex increase in salivation.

The movements of the tongue are important to position the *bolus* of ingested food, which has been reduced to smaller sizes by the teeth, into proper alignment for swallowing. The taste buds, scattered over the mucous membrane of the tongue surface, carry sensory input through the seventh and ninth cranial nerves to the brain where taste is interpreted. Perception of taste is a complex process, with various areas of the tongue being sensitive to different tastes. Figure 36-11 illustrates the areas of the tongue that respond to sweet, sour, salty, and bitter tastes.

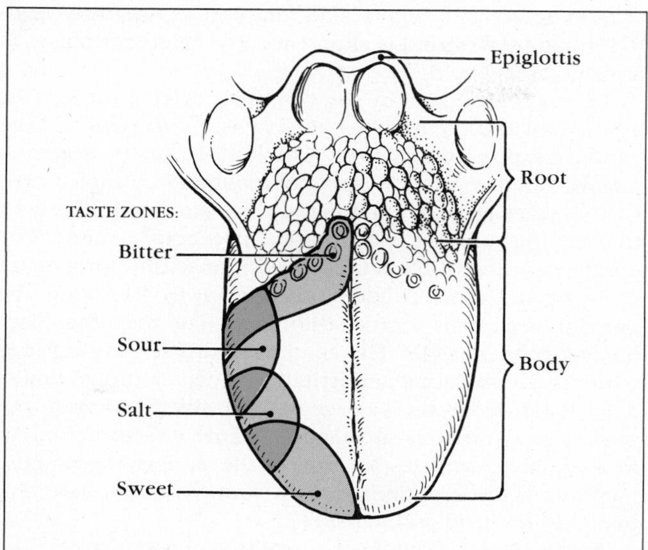

FIGURE 36-11 The tongue and areas of taste.

The major motor nerve of the tongue is the hypoglossal, which is closely aligned with the vagus nerve. It innervates the extrinsic and intrinsic muscles to move the tongue into various positions.

Swallowing is the key event in the initiation of digestion because it increases esophageal peristaltic motion, decreases pressure in the lower esophagus, and initiates the gastroenteric reflex. This reflex increases small bowel motility and assists in moving nutrients along the alimentary canal.

The act of swallowing, or deglutition, is initiated when the tongue moves a bolus of food to the pharynx. The cricopharyngeal sphincter relaxes for 1 second or less and the *primary peristaltic wave* is initiated. This wave begins in the pharynx and spreads to the esophagus [2]. The respiratory passages are closed to prevent food from moving into them. The bolus of food then passes through the pharynx to the esophagus in approximately 1 second (Fig. 36-12). The respiratory passages reopen and breathing resumes.

As food passes into the esophagus, peristalsis and pressure changes move it toward the stomach. Peristalsis, which occurs throughout the gastrointestinal tract, is a series of sequential muscular movements. The primary wave moves down the esophagus and *secondary peristalsis* continues until all of the food is in the stomach [2]. The syncytium of the entire system allows for wavelike movements of the smooth muscle. As the food moves toward the lower esophageal or gastroesophageal sphincter, the wave of peristalsis causes the normally constricted area to relax, and the food moves into the stomach. The peristaltic waves are initiated by vagal reflexes from the esophagus to the medulla oblongata back to the esophagus [2]. These are termed *vagal central* and *local pathways* [4].

Gastric Motility and Secretion

The fundus of the stomach increases its volume as it fills with food, and by its distensibility maintains a low intragastric pressure. The antrum is responsible for mixing food through contraction waves that push the food (now chyme) toward the pylorus. Solids must be broken down to less than a millimeter in size before they can pass through the pyloric sphincter. Gastric motility patterns occur in phases: phase I occurs 1.5 to 2 hours after meals when gastric contractions decrease to one every 4 to 5 minutes; phase II is a 30-minute span of irregular contractions; this is followed by phase III which is 5 to 15 minutes of sweeping contractions [4]. Hunger pangs may be experienced during phases II or III. Contractile movements in the full stomach are of three types: (1) peristaltic waves, (2) contractions of the antrum, and (3) contractions of the fundus and body.

Peristaltic activity in the stomach arises from a pacemaker located high on the greater curvature of the stomach. Electrical slow waves are propagated through the longitudinal muscle layer to the pyloris. This cyclic wave of partial depolarization and repolarization occurs in humans about three times per minute [4].

The glands of the stomach secrete 1500 to 3000 ml of gastric juice per day. Secretory activity follows a regular daily pattern, with the least secretion occurring in the early mornings. The amount of gastric secretion also varies

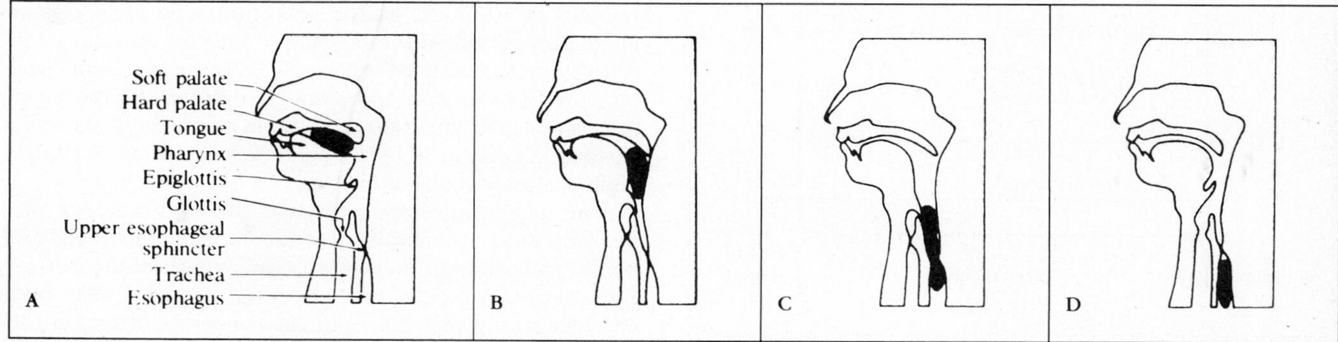

FIGURE 36-12 Passage of a food bolus from the mouth through the pharynx and upper esophagus during swallowing. (From E.E. Selkurt, *Physiology* [5th ed.]. Boston: Little, Brown, 1984.)

with individual dietary habits, other stimuli that provoke secretions, and the strength of the inhibitory mechanisms.

Gastric juice contains mucus, intrinsic factor, hydrochloric acid, pepsinogen, and the electrolytes sodium, potassium, chloride, and bicarbonate. Certain other enzymes such as gastric lipase, urease, lysozyme, and carbonic anhydrase are also present in the secretions. The three types of cells that make up the gastric glands secrete mucus, pepsinogen, and hydrochloric acid (see Fig. 36-4).

The parietal cells in the fundus and body of the stomach secrete hydrochloric acid as a highly concentrated juice with a pH of approximately 0.8. A suggested mechanism for the formation of hydrochloric acid (HCl) is illustrated in Figure 36-13. The theory relating hydrochloric acid secretion to bicarbonate replenishment in the blood is supported by the observation that each hydrogen (H^+) ion secreted is matched by bicarbonate (HCO_3^-) that is returned to the blood. This means that the amount of bicarbonate entering the blood during the gastric secretory phase is directly proportional to the amount of acid secreted. Carbon dioxide enters the cell or is formed in the cell during metabolism, reacts with water catalyst by using carbonic anhydrase, and forms carbonic acid. This carbonic acid then dissociates to bicarbonate and hydrogen. The hydrogen ion enters the parietal cell canaliculi by active transport, while bicarbonate is diffused back into the blood. The chloride ion is also actively transported from blood to the canaliculi [8]. Only during periods of relative gastric inactivity is adequate carbon dioxide produced to make a small amount of hydrochloric acid. During digestion, the parietal cell takes its needed carbon dioxide from the circulating blood. This elevates the venous pH after eating, which has been called the *postprandial alkaline tide*. The urine also becomes more alkaline [3,4].

Pepsin is the main proteolytic enzyme of gastric juice. It is secreted by the chief cells of the gastric glands in the form of pepsinogen. It has no digestive activity until it is activated into pepsin, which occurs in the presence of hydrochloric acid and previously activated pepsin. Pepsin is most active in a highly acid medium. It functions optimally in a pH of 2 and is almost inactive in secretions with a pH greater than 5.

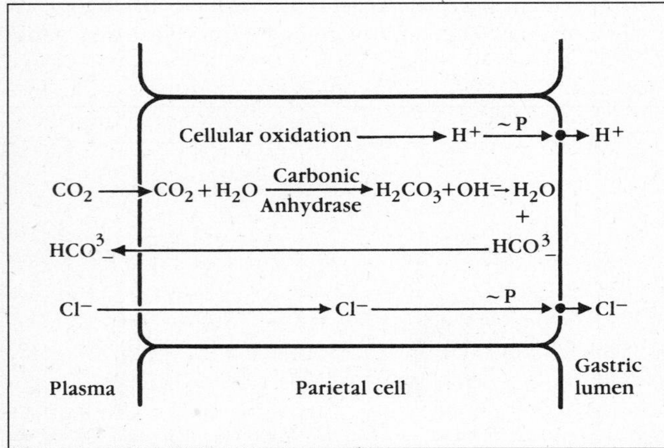

FIGURE 36-13 A possible mechanism for the gastric secretion of HCl. (From E.E. Selkurt, *Basic Physiology for the Health Sciences* [2nd ed.]. Boston: Little, Brown, 1982.)

Mucus is produced by the columnar cells of the surface epithelium and the mucous neck cells of the glands of the cardia, corpus, and pylorus. The surface of the stomach mucosa has a continuous layer of columnar epithelial cells that secretes large amounts of viscous and alkaline mucus to coat the mucosa and create a protective sheet. The epithelial lining of the stomach has remarkable properties of repair and can reproduce itself in 36 to 48 hours. The mucous neck cells secrete thinner mucus than the other mucus-secreting cells. The amount of this secretion varies with vagal stimulation and irritation. This additional line of defense lubricates the passage of food, absorbs pepsin, and washes away noxious substances. Failure to secrete mucus in adequate quantities to protect the underlying mucosa increases the susceptibility of the mucosa to the action of hydrochloric acid and pepsin [2].

Gastric juices contain the enzymes gastric lipase, gastric amylase, gastric urease, carbonic anhydrase, and lysozyme. Gastric lipase acts primarily on butterfat, and has little effect on other fats, which require bile for their digestion. Gastric amylase has a minor role in digesting starch. Gastric urease, formed by the bacteria that contaminate the gastric mucosa, splits urea to produce ammonia. Carbonic anhydrase, present in the epithelial cells and in high concentrations in parietal cells, is thought to be produced by the disintegration of desquamated epithelial cells and is essential in forming hydrochloric acid. Lysozyme is a carbohydrate-splitting enzyme present in small amounts in the gastric juice. Its cellular origin is not known.

Gastric motility is governed by the peristaltic waves that occur every 15 to 25 seconds and mix ingested food with gastric secretions. The result of this movement and mixing is the thin, highly acidic liquid, chyme. Chyme is moved into the small intestine mostly because of the higher pressure gradients in the stomach that exceed the duodenal pressure. The acidity and amount of chyme entering the duodenum help to regulate the duodenal and pancreatic secretions.

Digestion is regulated by both nervous and hormonal mechanisms. Innervation through the vagus nerve excites stomach excretion directly by stimulating the gastric glands. Distention of the stomach wall activates local reflexes to stimulate gastric secretion. The local reflexes elicit autonomic nervous system activity and cause the release of the hormone gastrin. This hormone is absorbed into the bloodstream and stimulates the gastric secretory glands to cause a marked increase in gastric acid secretion. Gastric secretion is believed to occur in three phases: cephalic, gastric, and intestinal.

The cephalic phase prepares the stomach for food and digestion. It is under nervous control, and is initiated by stimuli such as the sight, smell, or thought of food. Impulses from receptors such as the retinaes, taste buds, and olfactory glands travel to the cerebral cortex, and the motor fibers of the vagi of the stomach stimulate the glands of the stomach to secrete juice rich in hydrochloric acid and gastrin [4].

The gastric phase is initiated when food enters the stomach. Gastrin is released by acetylcholine stimulation of the gastrin-producing cells. The process is triggered by distention of the stomach caused by food and by exposure of the mucosa to substances called *secretagogues*. Examples of secretagogues are caffeine and alcohol. Gastrin is absorbed in the blood and stimulates acid and pepsin secretion from parietal and chief cells, which produce about two-thirds of the total gastric secretions [4]. Food in the stomach initiates local reflexes in the intramural plexus of the stomach, and vasovagal reflexes stimulate parasympathetic stimulation to increase the secretion. The rate of secretion in response to gastrin continues for several hours while food remains in the stomach. Both the gastrin and vagal mechanisms are important in gastric secretion. Gastrin also has extragastric action, including the stimulation of insulin and release of calcitonin. It causes muscle contraction of the lower esophageal sphincter, small intestine, colon, and gallbladder. It inhibits smooth muscle contraction of the pyloric, ileocecal, and Oddi sphincters [4].

The intestinal phase of gastric secretion is less active than the cephalic or gastric phases, but once initiated it may last for 8 to 10 hours while food remains in the duodenum. This phase is not well understood but it begins with the entrance of acidic chyme into the small intestine, which leads to an increase in gastrin secretion [4].

The intestines also inhibit gastric secretion when there are partially digested proteins, acid, fat, or hypertonic solutions in the duodenum. Distention, caused by the presence of food, initiates the *enterogastric reflex*, which slows the influence of the vagus nerve. The purpose of the enterogastric reflex appears to be to delay stomach emptying until some emptying can occur in the small intestine. Intestinal hormones, especially secretin and CCK, oppose the stimulatory effects of gastrin and slow the movement of chyme from the stomach to the small intestine [2]. This inhibitory feedback prevents excessive acid secretion and protects the intestinal mucosa from injury. During the interdigestive phase, while no digestion is occurring in the gastrointestinal tract, the stomach secretes only a few milliliters of gastric juice per hour. Normally, secretions in the stomach follow a steady, dynamic course regulated by both nervous and hormonal factors that foster structural and functional integrity in the mucosa. Pathologic conditions, drugs and chemicals, or surgery can disrupt the balance between secretion and inhibition.

The best-known chemical stimulant of gastric secretion is *histamine*, which is released from surface mast cells during an antigen-antibody reaction. Although less potent than gastrin, histamine causes the parietal cells to secrete large amounts of gastric juice. Large amounts of endogenous histamine may be present in the gastric mucosa, and during active secretion small amounts are present in gastric juice and urine. Physical or emotional stress increases the release of histamine.

Caffeine and nicotine are secretagogues that increase the amount and acidity of gastric secretion. Alcohol has been found to stimulate only the amount of gastrin secretion. Aspirin, alcohol, and bile salts alter the permeability of the epithelial barrier and allow back-diffusion of hydrochloric acid, which may result in injury to tissue and blood vessels. Aspirin produces changes in the gastric mucosa and decreases the total output of mucus, which reduces its protective effect on the gastric mucosa. It has been observed that prolonged administration of large quantities of corticotropic and adrenal steroids increases gastric secretion, which favors the development or recurrence of peptic ulcers [8]. The frequency may not be quite as significant as previously reported. A number of studies have reported a slight increase in frequency of peptic ulcers in persons treated with adrenocortical steroid drugs [1]. Parasympathetic agents such as acetylcholine, reserpine, and pilocarpine are also secretory stimulants. Insulin, through its hypoglycemic effects, excites the vagus nerve and increases gastric gland activity [3].

Belladonna and its alkaloids atropine and hyoscine depress secretions by reducing vagal stimulation. Synthetic anticholinergic drugs, such as propantheline bromide (Probanthine), are used to control gastric activity and secretion.

Emotional disruptions have long been recognized as exerting an important influence on the secretory and motor functions of the stomach. Studies seem to indicate that prolonged anxiety, guilt, conflict, hostility, and resentment lead to engorgement of the gastric mucosa and increased secretion (see Chap. 4). The significant decrease in gastric secretion after complete vagotomy suggests that hypersecretion is caused by excessive stimulation of the vagus nerve.

Secretion and Absorption in the Small Intestine

The major nutrients are absorbed mostly in the small intestine, with the simpler substances generally being absorbed in the first portion of the small bowel. Substances requiring greater hydrolysis and simplification are absorbed at later points in the small intestine. Table 36-2 shows the specific absorption sites of major nutrients. The anatomic structure, previously detailed on pages 564–570, provides the mechanism for this to occur. In the small intestine, secretions are received from the pancreas and liver and are supplemented by intestinal secretions. *Secretions of the small intestine* include enzymes, hormones, and mucus. These substances, listed in Tables 36-3 and 36-4, include secretions from the pancreas and liver. The major effects of all of the enzymes and hormones are detailed in the tables.

All of the secretions work together to digest carbohydrates, proteins, and fats. Absorption depends on the proper hydrolysis of nutrients by secretions that increase the movement from the intestinal lumen to the bloodstream. Biliary secretions include bile salts, lipids, water, electrolytes, and bilirubin. Of these, bilirubin is a waste product that gives color to feces. Bile salts exert a detergentlike effect on fat and emulsify it. The pancreatic secretions contain enzymes and large amounts of bicarbonate and water. Formation of pancreatic and biliary secretions is detailed in Chapter 38.

TABLE 36-3 Digestive Enzymes

Enzyme	Source	Substrate	Products	Remarks
Ptyalin	Salivary glands	Starch	Smaller carbohydrates	
Pepsin	Chief cells of stomach mucosa	Protein (nonspecific)	Polypeptides	
Gastric lipase	Stomach mucosa	Triglycerides (lipids)	Glycerides and FAs	
Enterokinase	Duodenal mucosa	Trypsinogen	Trypsin	Activates or converts trypsinogen to trypsin; trypsinogen hydrolyzed to expose active site.
Trypsin	Pancreas	Protein and polypeptides	Smaller polypeptides	Converts chymotrypsinogen to chymotrypsin.
Chymotrypsin	Pancreas	Proteins and polypeptides (different specificity than trypsin)	Smaller polypeptides	
Nuclease	Pancreas	Nucleic acids	Nucleotides (base + sugar + PO_4)	
Carboxypeptidase	Pancreas	Polypeptides	Smaller polypeptides	Cleaves carboxy terminal end.
Pancreatic lipase	Pancreas	Lipids, especially triglycerides	Glycerides, free FAs, glycerol	Very potent.
Pancreatic amylase	Pancreas	Starch	2 disaccharide units = maltose	Very potent.
Aminopeptidase	Intestinal glands	Polypeptides	Smaller peptides	
Dipeptidase	Intestine	Dipeptides	2 amino acids	
Maltase	Intestine	Maltose	2 glucose	
Lactase	Intestine	Lactose	1 glucose, 1 galactose	
Sucrase	Intestine	Sucrose	1 glucose, 1 fructose	
Nucleotidase	Intestine	Nucleotides	Nucleosides and phosphates (base + sugar)	
Nucleosidase	Intestine	Nucleosides	Base and sugar	
Intestinal lipase	Intestine	Fats	Glycerides, FAs, glycerol	

Note: Enzymes act on each other during and after digestion, but it is only after digestion (after their substrates are removed) that they have any marked effect on each other.

TABLE 36-4 Hormones of Digestion

Hormone	Source	Agents That Stimulate Production	Action
Gastrin	Gastric mucosa (primarily pylorus)	Distention of stomach and some protein derivatives	Stimulates production of HCl.
Enterogastrone	Mucosa of small intestine and duodenum	Fats, sugars, or acids in intestine	Inhibits gastric secretion and mobility.
Secretin	Duodenal mucosa	Polypeptides, acids, etc., in intestine (duodenum)	Stimulates pancreas to produce a watery, enzyme-poor juice, with high HCO_3^- content.
Cholecystokinin	Duodenal mucosa	Fats in duodenum	Stimulates pancreas to produce enzyme-rich juice and stimulates gallbladder to contract and release bile.

The chyme that enters the duodenum is highly acidic because it was mixed with large amounts of hydrochloric acid in the stomach. All of the intestinal enzymes work best in an alkaline medium, which requires chyme to be neutralized and alkalinized. The amount of the alkaline pancreatic secretion has been shown to be closely correlated with the pH of the chyme entering the small intestine.

Chemical and mechanical digestion requires that food be changed into the forms that can be moved by the process of absorption through the mucosal lining cells to the blood and lymph vessels. The diffusible forms include monosaccharides, amino acids, fatty acids, glycerol, and glycerides [2]. Figure 36-14 shows schematically where materials are absorbed in the entire gastrointestinal system. Nearly all of the nutrients are absorbed in the small intestine and 90 percent of all absorption occurs here.

Carbohydrate Absorption. Carbohydrates are ingested primarily as disaccharides, starches, and polysaccharides. Polysaccharides are hydrolyzed into their component disaccharides by the action of ptyalin and the gastric, intestinal, and pancreatic amylases. Intact disaccharides can be passively absorbed by the small intestine, but relatively few are absorbed in this manner. Most are first split into monosaccharides by enzymes located in the intestinal microvilli. These monosaccharides are then actively absorbed into the blood capillaries of the villi. Absorption occurs against a concentration gradient and apparently requires active transport, although the method by which this occurs is obscure. It is known that sodium increases cellular permeability to glucose, so that glucose transport is related to sodium transport.

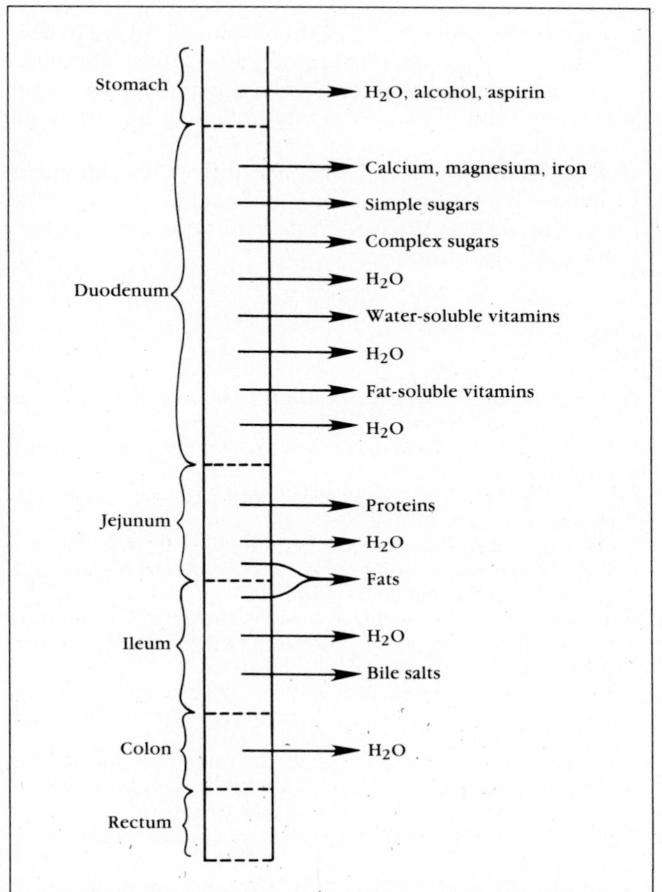

FIGURE 36-14 Absorption of nutrients in the digestive tract.

Protein Absorption. Protein absorption occurs mostly in the duodenum and jejunum. As a result of gastric pepsin and pancreatic enzymes, 70 percent of protein ingested in the diet is presented to the intestinal absorptive membrane in the form of small peptides, and 30 percent is in the form of amino acids. The amino acids are immediately absorbed, but only a small amount of peptide is absorbed intact. The majority of the peptides are reduced by peptidases in the microvilli to amino acids, and absorption rapidly follows. The sodium transport mechanism also probably provides for amino acid transport. Many amino acids apparently need pyridoxine, a component of vitamin B_6, to aid in transport.

Fat Absorption. Dietary fat consists mainly of long-chain triglycerides, which are hydrolyzed intraluminally into fatty acids and monoglycerides. Hydrolysis occurs in the jejunum through the action of lipase. The most important lipase is secreted from the pancreas [2]. Bile salts and fatty acids aggregate to form *micelles*, which are water-soluble structures. A major function of bile salts is to make fat globules fragmentable by agitating them in the small bowel [2]. These fragments attach themselves to the surface of the epithelial cells. The fatty acids leave the micelles and enter the cell by diffusion, while the bile salts are released to return to chyme to aid in the absorption of more fats. When the fats in the duodenum and upper jejunum have been removed, bile salts are resorbed and eventually returned to the liver. Lipids are resynthesized into tryglycerides in the endoplasmic reticulum of intestinal epithelial cells. Molecules of triglycerides then organize into minute fat droplets, which contain small amounts of phospholipid and cholesterol and protein-coated surface. These droplets, called *chylomicrons*, then pass out of the base of the epithelial cells and enter either the bloodstream or the lymphatic system. Approximately 80 to 90 percent of all fatty acids enter the bloodstream in the form of chylomicrons. Small amounts of fats are not digested and are excreted in the feces.

Water Absorption. Approximately 8 liters of water per day are absorbed from the small intestine into the portal blood, entirely by the process of diffusion [2]. The greatest amount of this absorption occurs in the jejunum. Water crosses the intestinal cell membrane by passing through the pores of this membrane. The rate of absorption is very great and probably is enhanced by glucose and oxygen. Therefore, active transport may increase water absorption through shifting of other ions.

Electrolyte Absorption. Additional water is absorbed in the large intestine. Electrolytes, like water, must cross the intestinal cell membrane by passing through its pores or by using a membrane carrier. Like water, electrolytes are absorbed primarily into the portal blood rather than into the lymphatic system, and the absorption rate is greater in the proximal than in the distal portion of the small bowel. Monovalent electrolytes such as sodium, chloride, potassium, nitrate, and bicarbonate are more easily absorbed than polyvalent electrolytes such as calcium, magnesium, and sulfate.

Most of the *sodium* is absorbed in the jejunum, with less being absorbed in the ileum and the colon. The mechanism for this is active transport of sodium from the epithelial cells into the intercellular spaces. This requires a carrier and energy. Increased sodium concentration in the intercellular spaces creates an osmotic gradient for water, which follows the sodium passively. Both sodium and water are finally absorbed into the capillaries of the villi [2].

Chloride passively moves through the membranes of the duodenum and jejunum. It is actively transported in the large bowel, where it is exchanged in close relationship to bicarbonate ions, which are used to neutralize any acid products in the large intestine.

Potassium can be passively or actively absorbed through the intestinal mucosa [2,3]. Most absorption occurs in the jejunum and ileum through a system not clearly identified [3].

Calcium is absorbed by active transport throughout the small intestine, but most actively in the duodenum. The solubility of calcium salts is increased in duodenal acid, rather than in the more alkaline medium lower in the intestines. The rate of calcium absorption is altered by the level of parathyroid hormone in the blood (see Chap. 34). Vitamin D is important in stimulating the rate of intestinal absorption; it is activated by a specific process in the kidneys and then increases calcium absorption.

Most *iron* is absorbed in its ferrous form in the duodenum. An acid medium facilitates iron absorption. Iron uptake is an active process and is facilitated by *ascorbic acid*, which reduces the ferric to the ferrous form. The rate of absorption is extremely slow, but increases with iron deficiency and decreases with excessive dietary intake of iron.

The *vitamins* are absorbed primarily in the proximal intestine, except for vitamin B_{12}, which is absorbed in the ileum. Most vitamins are passively absorbed. Some are stored in the body and some have to be replenished on a regular basis. Vitamin B_{12} forms a complex with the intrinsic factor that, in the ileum, is bound to a specific, unknown receptor in the mucosa and, finally, is absorbed into the blood.

Secretion, Absorption, and Excretion in the Large Intestine

The function of the large intestine is mainly to absorb water, but it also is vital in synthesizing vitamin K and some B-complex vitamins and in forming and excreting feces [7].

The movements of the large intestine are a part of the peristaltic activity initiated by the ingestion of food. The final movement of the large intestine is *mass peristalsis*, which drives digested waste material into the rectum. This usually occurs three to four times a day. The glands of the lining of the large intestine secrete mucus that lubricates the material and protects the lining of the bowel.

Active bacteria in the bowel ferment any remaining carbohydrate and release hydrogen, carbon dioxide, and methane gas, and break proteins down into amino acids. This activity gives fecal material its odor.

Water (1800–3000 ml) is absorbed daily in the large intestine, together with a few electrolytes. This absorption regulates the consistency of the feces and provides for final water balance in the gastrointestinal system.

Defecation is the process of emptying the rectum and is initiated by distention of rectal walls. The external sphincter is under voluntary control and relaxes when intraabdominal and intrathoracic pressures increase, pushing the fecal material out of the body. Increased rectal and intraabdominal pressures may increase the vagal tone and reflexively decrease the heart rate.

Study Questions

1. What is the difference between appetite and hunger? Give some examples and indicate factors that can affect each.
2. Explain the process of digestion from the intake of basic nutrients to the elimination of wastes. How and where are each of the nutrients broken down for absorption?
3. Describe the peristaltic wave, including initiation and perpetuation.
4. What factors enhance gastric motility? What inhibits it?
5. Where are the major electrolytes, minerals, and vitamins absorbed? What special conditions are necessary for their absorption?

References

1. Greenberger, N.J. *Gastrointestinal Disorders: A Pathophysiologic Approach* (3rd ed.). Chicago: Yearbook, 1986.
2. Guyton, A.C. *Textbook of Medical Physiology* (7th ed.). Philadelphia: Saunders, 1986.
3. Jensen, D. *The Principles of Physiology* (2nd ed.). New York: Appleton-Century-Crofts, 1980.
4. Nord, H.A., and Sodeman, W.A. The Stomach. In W.A. Sodeman and T.M. Sodeman, *Sodeman's Pathologic Physiology* (7th ed.). Philadelphia: Saunders, 1985.
5. Rankin, R.A., and Welsh, J.D. Gastroenterology. In C.E. Kaufman and S. Papper, *Review of Pathophysiology*. Boston: Little, Brown, 1983.
6. Skinner, D.B. The Esophagus. In W.A. Sodeman and T.M. Sodeman, *Sodeman's Pathologic Physiology* (7th ed.). Philadelphia: Saunders, 1985.
7. Sodeman, W.A., and Watson, D.W. The Large Intestine. In W.A. Sodeman and T.M. Sodeman, *Sodeman's Pathologic Physiology* (7th ed.). Philadelphia: Saunders, 1985.
8. Spiro, H.M. *Clinical Gastroenterology* (3rd ed.). New York: Macmillan, 1986.
9. Watson, D.W., and Sodeman, W.A. The Small Intestine. In W.A. Sodeman and T.M. Sodeman, *Sodeman's Pathologic Physiology* (7th ed.). Philadelphia: Saunders, 1985.

CHAPTER 37

Alterations in Gastrointestinal Function

CHAPTER OUTLINE

Diseases of the Oral Cavity

Alterations in the Gums and Teeth
Changes in the Oral Mucosa

Esophageal Alterations

Achalasia
Gastroesophageal Reflux and Esophagitis
Hiatal Hernia
Esophageal Varices
Carcinoma of the Esophagus

Alterations in the Stomach and Duodenum

Gastritis
Acute Gastritis
Stress Ulcers
Peptic Ulcer Disease (PUD)
Gastric Ulcers
Duodenal Ulcers
Complications of PUD
Gastric Carcinoma

Alterations in the Small Intestine

Celiac Disease
Celiac Enteropathy (Nontropical Sprue)
Tropical Sprue
Regional Enteritis: Crohn's Disease
Enteritis

Alterations in the Large Intestine

Adynamic or Paralytic Ileus
Intestinal Obstruction
Hernias
Congenital Megacolon or Hirschsprung's Disease
Diverticula
Hemorrhoids
Ulcerative Colitis
Polyps
Carcinoma of the Colon

LEARNING OBJECTIVES

1. List the major sources of inflammation of the gums.
2. Describe the anatomic and functional changes occurring with achalasia.
3. Outline the mechanism for mucosal damage that occurs with esophagitis.
4. List at least two diagnostic procedures that demonstrate reflux.
5. Describe pathophysiologically a rolling hiatal hernia and a sliding hiatal hernia.
6. Trace the development of esophageal varices.
7. Classify the most common morphologic form of carcinoma of the esophagus.
8. Differentiate between acute and chronic gastritis.
9. Differentiate the types of peptic ulcerations according to underlying etiology, symptomatology, and relationship to malignancy.
10. Describe briefly the pathology of gastric carcinoma.
11. Describe the pathologic changes that result in malsorption in celiac enteropathy and tropical sprue.
12. Differentiate regional enteritis and ulcerative colitis on the basis of etiology, pathology, symptomatology, and course of the disease.
13. Define *adynamic* or *paralytic ileus*.
14. Distinguish between paralytic ileus and bowel obstruction.
15. Define *reducible*, *incarcerated*, and *strangulated hernias*.
16. Describe Hirschsprung's disease.
17. Explain why diverticula are common in elderly persons.
18. List some common conditions that can cause hemorrhoids.
19. List some ways that the American diet may cause carcinoma of the colon.
20. Differentiate the pathology and symptomatology of carcinomas arising in different areas of the colon.

Diseases of the Oral Cavity

Alterations in the Gums and Teeth

The gums, or *gingiva*, are subject to localized inflammatory diseases, or they may react to other systemic diseases or drug therapy. *Gingivitis*, inflammation of the borders surrounding the teeth, may result in pain, bleeding, and destruction of gingival tissue. When this inflammation spreads to the underlying tissues, bones, or roots of the teeth, it is called *peridontitis*. This destructive disease may result in purulent drainage and loss of teeth.

Overgrowth of the gingiva occurs in persons having long-term treatment with phenytoin (Dilantin). Hormonal and metabolic conditions may cause an increased inflammatory response, with enlarged gingiva noted especially at puberty, during pregnancy, and with such conditions as leukemia and thrombocytopenia.

Changes in the Oral Mucosa

Changes in the oral mucosa often reflect systemic changes in the body. A variety of conditions may cause these mucosal changes and the manifestations vary. For example, in scarlet fever the tongue becomes bright red (strawberry tongue), while in *Candida albicans* (thrush), localized white lesions of the oral mucosa occur.

Tumors of the oral mucosa are uncommon but are much like skin tumors, except that many of the oral growths are benign, so-called hamartomas, rather than true, growing lesions [7]. The salivary glands may also develop tumorous growths of a benign or malignant nature.

Esophageal Alterations

Although many conditions affect esophageal motility and secretion, only the major alterations are reviewed in this section.

Achalasia

Achalasia is an uncommon disorder of esophageal motility (Fig. 37-1A). The combination of decreased peristalsis plus constriction of the lower esophageal sphincter characterizes the condition. Degeneration of the myenteric ganglion cells in the esophagus and alterations in vagal tone apparently are the precipitating causes. The esophagus becomes distended and may retain several liters of fluid.

This condition becomes chronic and slowly progressive, causing dysphagia, vomiting, nausea, and weight loss. Lung changes, related to repeated episodes of nocturnal aspiration, may be associated. The degree of swallowing difficulty in the early stages is increased by stress and anxiety. Increasing dysphagia results, and finally even liquids become difficult to swallow.

Diagnostic tests usually include barium swallow, which reflects a normally functioning pharynx and cricoesophageal sphincter, but after a few centimeters, peristaltic action stops or decreases to ineffectual motions. The distended, nonemptying lower esophagus is easily visualized as a pouch that narrows into the esophagogastric junction (Fig. 37-1B). Although the lower esophageal sphincter does not open in response to swallowing, it may open slightly as food moves into the area and allow some contents to pass through.

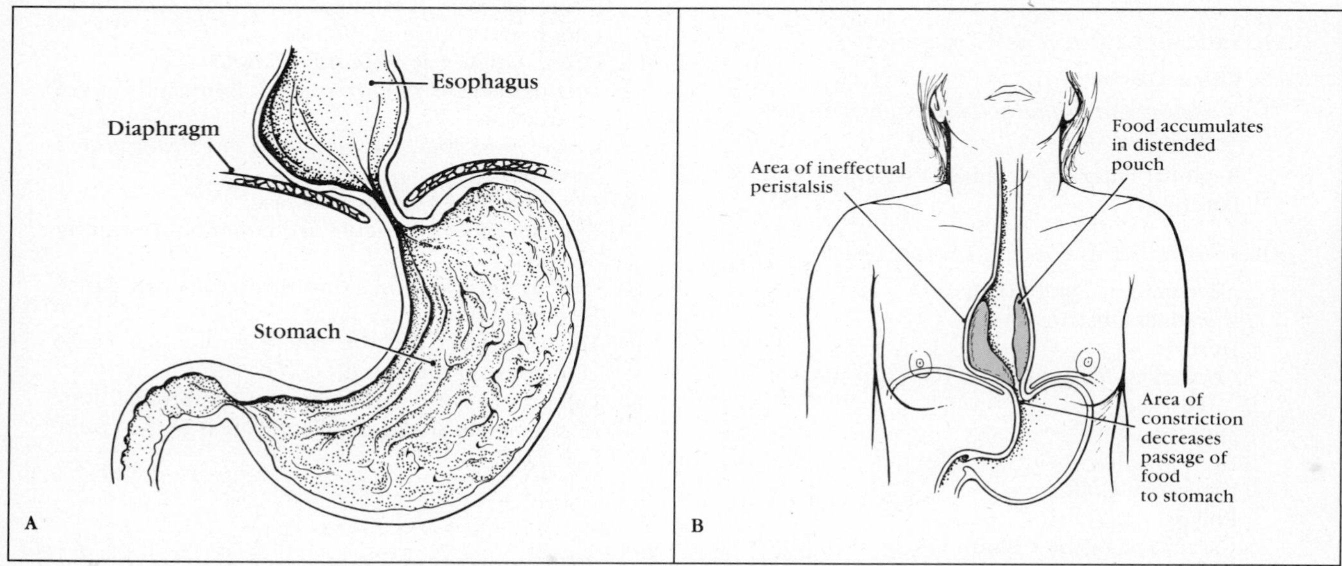

FIGURE 37-1 A. Schematic representation of location and appearance of achalatic esophagus. B. Nonemptying or poorly emptying lower esophagus resulting from achalasia.

Frequent follow-up examinations are required because these persons have a statistical increase in frequency of esophageal carcinoma. Surgical intervention may be required to decrease the amount of obstruction.

Gastroesophageal Reflux and Esophagitis

Gastroesophageal reflux is the movement of gastric contents into the esophagus. Normally, pressure on the lower esophageal sphincter prevents backflow, or secondary peristalsis moves gastric contents from the esophageal mucosa before damage occurs. An incompetent lower esophageal sphincter is believed to be the primary cause of reflux esophagitis. Other causes include prolonged gastric intubation, ingestion of corrosive chemicals, uremia, infections, mucosal alterations, and systemic diseases such as systemic lupus erythematosus [7]. Frequent regurgitation through the gastroesophageal junction causes substernal pain. The reflux may be accentuated by postural changes, such as assuming a supine position. Pulmonary aspiration is a common complication when the condition is severe [4].

Esophagitis, inflammation of the esophageal mucosa, most frequently results from gastroesophageal reflux that may be due to prolonged vomiting or an incompetent lower esophageal sphincter. Mucosal damage is related to the contact time between the esophageal mucosa and gastric contents, as well as the acidity and quantity of gastric secretions.

Gastric hydrochloric acid alters the pH of the esophagus and permits mucosal protein to be denatured. The pepsin in the gastric secretion has proteolytic properties that are enhanced when the pH is around 2. The combination of pepsin and hydrochloric acid increases the capacity for damage. Often increased bile salts are associated with gastroesophageal reflux and enhance the effect of the hydrogen ion on the mucosa. This reflux has been shown to cause an inflammation that penetrates to the muscularis layer, resulting in motor dysfunction and decreased esophageal clearance. The results are increased esophageal contact time, more muscle damage, and increased amounts of reflux (Fig. 37-2) [2,6].

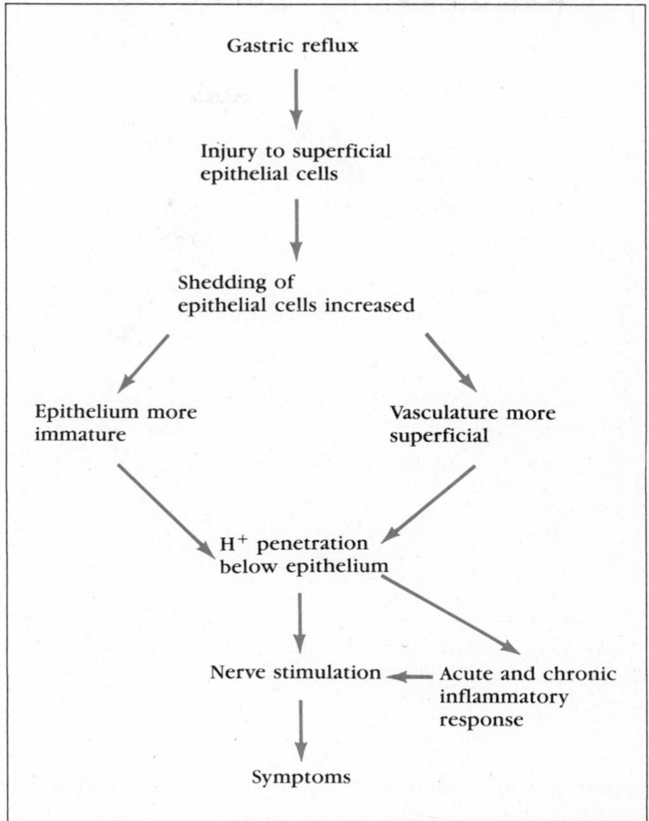

FIGURE 37-2 Possible mechanism for symptoms of reflux esophagitis. (From C.E. Kaufman and S. Papper, *Review of Pathophysiology*. Boston: Little, Brown, 1983.)

The most common symptoms of esophageal inflammation include heartburn, retrosternal discomfort, and the regurgitation of sour, bitter material. These symptoms are frequently precipitated by ingestion of large amounts of fatty, spiced foods and alcohol. Symptoms correlate with the amount and acidity of reflux. Dysphagia for both solids and liquids increases when severe obstruction occurs. Permanent strictures may develop that make food passage difficult. Irritation of the mucosa may cause bleeding and eventually produce an iron-deficiency anemia. Nocturnal reflux of material into the pharynx may lead to aspiration into the lungs. Reflux may occur in the upright or supine positions, or both [6].

Diagnosis is difficult but may be based on clinical, radiographic, and endoscopic appearances. The most effective tests are measurement of pH in the esophagus and biopsy to demonstrate inflammatory changes [6]. Scintiscanning, which involves swallowing a radionucleotide, can demonstrate reflux by measuring radioactivity of the esophagus in serial scans.

Hiatal Hernia

A hiatal hernia is a condition in which part of the stomach protrudes through the opening of the diaphragm (Fig. 37-3). This condition may be continuous or occur sporadically. The continuous type is called a *rolling hernia* and occurs in fewer than 10 percent of persons with this condition. The sporadic type, or *sliding hernia*, accounts for 80 to 90 percent of hiatal hernias and occurs with changes in position or with increased peristalsis. The stomach is forced through the opening of the diaphragm when the person lies down and moves back to its normal position when the subject stands upright. This type of hernia may be associated with a congenitally short esophagus or may be secondary to postgastritis scarring.

Many persons with hiatal hernia exhibit no symptoms. Symptoms such as heartburn, gastric regurgitation, dysphagia, and indigestion are accentuated by assuming the

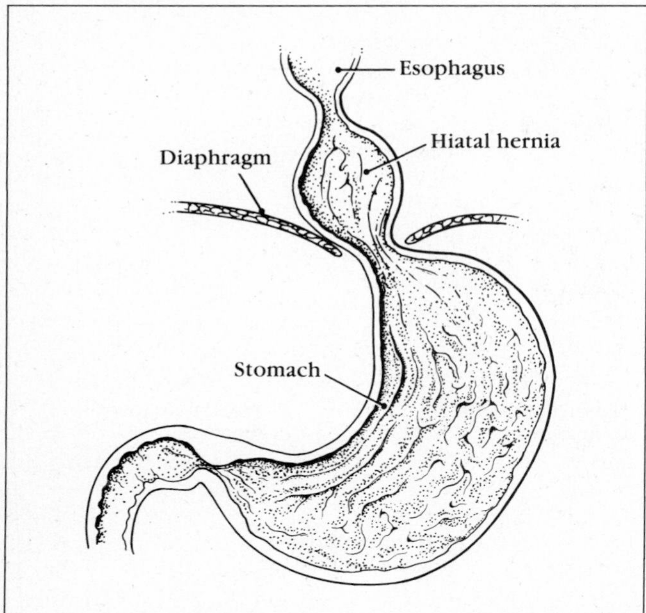

FIGURE 37-3. Schematic representation of location and appearance of hiatal hernia.

supine position postprandially, with overeating, physical exertion, or sudden changes of posture.

Radiographs reveal a hernia. A test to determine the presence of gastroesophageal reflux, the acid-perfusion study, includes instilling hydrochloric acid into the stomach. When reflux does not occur, the hiatal hernia is considered to be of little clinical importance, and the person usually remains asymptomatic.

Esophageal Varices

This condition (presented in greater detail on p. 608) is closely related to portal hypertension and involves protrusion of the esophageal veins into the esophageal lumen (Fig. 37-4). The distended, thin-walled veins become subject to rupture, a catastrophic event that may occur spontaneously or after vomiting.

Rupture of these vessels creates a very large amount of bleeding into the gastrointestinal system and usually leads to large-volume hematemesis. The first bleeding event results in 40 percent mortality; subsequent episodes are equally catastrophic [6,7].

Carcinoma of the Esophagus

About 10 percent of malignancies of the gastrointestinal tract arise in the esophagus; they usually remain asymptomatic until they become surgically unresectable. This type of malignancy usually occurs after age 50 years and more than 80 percent occurs in males. A strong correlation among heavy alcohol intake, cigarette smoking, and esophageal carcinoma has been recorded in the literature [5].

The squamous cell carcinoma is the most common morphologic form. The malignancy may grow around the esophagus at the level of the diaphragm, impinging on the lumen or the tube, or it may cause a bulky, ulcerating tumor mass. The greatest percentage of tumors are located in the middle and lower one-third of the esophagus.

This disease is usually asymptomatic for long periods, with the earliest complaint being mild dysphagia that becomes progressive. Postprandial regurgitation may motivate the person to seek medical assistance. Weight loss is a common complaint; hematemesis and guaiac-positive stools are relatively uncommon. Invasion of surrounding structures may result in back pain, and pressure

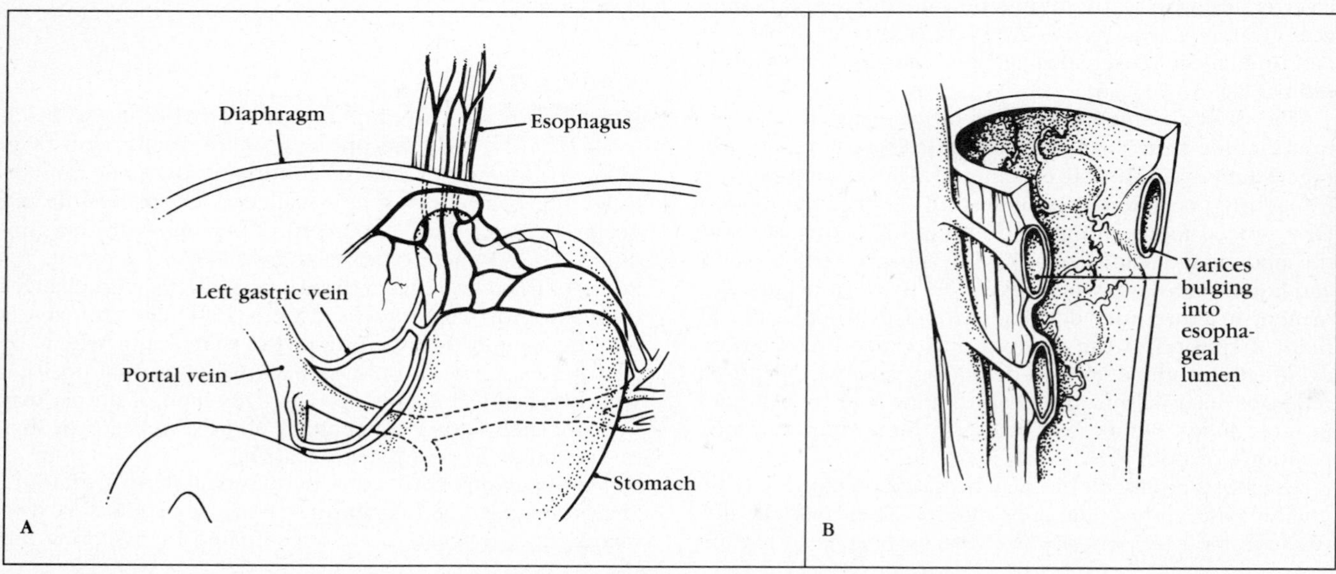

FIGURE 37-4 A. Venous plexus around the esophagus. B. Dilated venous channels from portal hypertension. These varices bulge into the lumen of the esophagus and rupture easily.

on respiratory structures may cause varying degrees of respiratory distress.

Definitive diagnosis is through esophagoscopy with biopsy of the tumor mass. Other diagnostic measures such as barium swallow, chest film, and blood tests give additional information.

Alterations in the Stomach and Duodenum

Gastritis

Gastritis is a general term that refers to inflammation of the gastric mucosa that may occur in the presence of an excess or complete absence of gastric acid secretion. The classifications acute and chronic describe the onset and course of the disease. Chronic gastritis may be associated with gastric mucosal atrophy, achlorhydria, and peptic ulceration.

Acute Gastritis. Acute gastritis causes transient inflammation of the gastric mucosa, mucosal hemorrhages, and erosion into the mucosal lining. It is frequently associated with alcoholism, aspirin ingestion, smoking, and severely stressful conditions such as trauma, burns, central nervous system damage, chemotherapy, and radiation therapy. Hydrochloric acid is present in gastritis, but its secretion does not have to be excessive [6]. Erosion of the gastric mucosa can result in a massive gastric hemorrhage. Therefore, acute gastritis may be associated with discomfort or serious outcome.

Stress Ulcers

Stress erosion or ulceration occurs after a major insult to the body. Causes include hypovolemic or septic shock, peritonitis, and serious brain injury. Gastric ulcerations after brain damage are called *Cushing's ulcers*; those after burn injury are called *Curling's ulcers*. Ulceration can usually be attributed to ischemia.

When gastric erosions occur, they are multiple and superficial, and are present in large areas of the gastric mucosa. Superficial erosions form, as well as discrete ulcers, especially in the fundus. Such injury potentiates damage by continual activation of pepsinogen. Gastric acid secretion is sometimes increased, and the erosions often localize in the acid-secreting portion of the stomach. Two mechanisms for production of stress ulcers have been proposed: (1) mucosal ischemia, which relates to lack of blood supply to the gastric mucosa in the poststress period and results from a sympathetic vasoconstrictive action; and (2) enhanced back-diffusion of hydrogen ions due to increased sensitivity of the disrupted gastric mucosa to hydrochloric acid and pepsin. The surface mucosal cells are disrupted, and stimulation of the myenteric plexus leads to hypersecretion of gastric acid and pepsinogen [4]. Histamine is also released from damaged cells and its effects increase the damage (Fig. 37-5) [4].

The major clinical manifestation of stress ulcers is massive, painless, gastric bleeding with onset 2 to 10 days after the original insult. This bleeding, from multiple sites in the gastric mucosa, is very difficult to control. Because of the danger of bleeding after acute stress, preventive measures are routinely used to decrease hydrogen ion secretion and to neutralize gastric acid.

Peptic Ulcer Disease (PUD)

Peptic ulcers (peptic ulcer disease, or PUD) are ulcerative conditions of the gastrointestinal tract that result from acid-pepsin imbalance. They are thought to develop when the aggressive proteolytic activities of the gastric secretions are greater than their normal protective abilities. An increase in acid and pepsin from any cause may produce ulcerations if the protective mechanisms are not adequate. Major factors that alter the mucosal barrier are failure to regenerate the mucous epithelium at a sufficient rate, decrease in quantity and quality of mucus, and poor local mucosal blood flow. It has been suggested that vascular occlusion of small nutrient vessels in the mucosa or submucosa causes localized necrosis and subsequent ulcer formation. Peptic activity alone is not responsible for ulcerations; individual susceptibility is essential.

The most frequent site for peptic ulcers is the pyloric region of the duodenum, but lesions also occur in other areas of the stomach (Fig. 37-6). Duodenal ulcers comprise 80 percent of all peptic ulcers. They are 4 times more common than gastric ulcers. Ulcerative conditions are very common, affecting approximately 10 to 15 percent of the general population. Table 37-1 provides an explanation of differential features of PUD.

Gastric Ulcers. The primary problem with gastric ulcers appears to be decreased resistance of the gastric mucosa to ingested substances. The level of hydrochloric acid secretion is usually normal or reduced. True *achlorhydria*, or lack of hydrochloric acid secretion, is rare with these ulcers, and when present, usually signifies the presence of a gastric carcinoma. Because gastric ulcers often occur in conjunction with gastric atrophy, the secretions may contain mostly water and small amounts of mucus. The intrinsic factor may not be secreted, causing decreased absorption of vitamin B_{12} and *pernicious anemia*.

Pathologically, gastric ulcers are often associated with atrophy of the gastric glands. Gastritis always surrounds the ulcerated area, which supports the theory that this is an inflammatory disease. The classic ulcer has a sharply punched-out appearance with a smooth, clean base. The mucosa surrounding it is often edematous. Bleeding may occur if the ulceration erodes through a vessel. Gastric ulcers may be malignant and exhibit a shaggy, necrotic base, as opposed to the smooth base of nonmalignant ulcers. Gastric ulcers transform into malignancy frequently enough to call them premalignant and to encourage frequent follow-up in this condition.

Gastric ulcers can be diagnosed by barium swallow (upper gastrointestinal series) and direct endoscopy. Biopsy and routine cytology studies can be performed with endoscopy. Gastric analysis usually reveals lower than normal output of hydrochloric acid, but the large overlap of values makes this an obsolete test for gastric

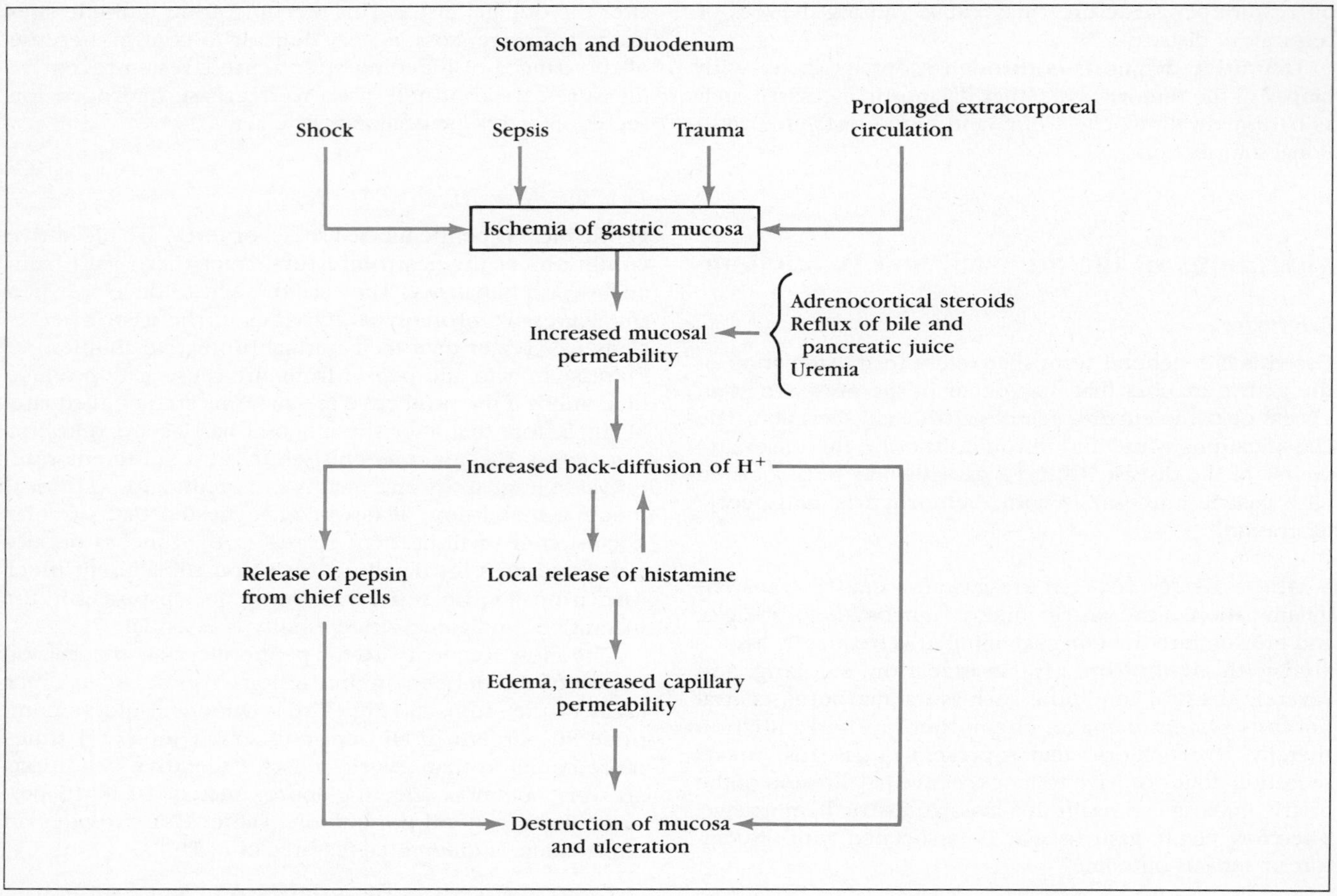

Stomach and Duodenum
Shock
Sepsis
Trauma
Prolonged extracorporeal circulation
Ischemia of gastric mucosa
Increased mucosal permeability
Adrenocortical steroids
Reflux of bile and pancreatic juice
Uremia
Increased back-diffusion of H+
Release of pepsin from chief cells
Local release of histamine
Edema, increased capillary permeability
Destruction of mucosa and ulceration

FIGURE 37-5 Diagram of events postulated to occur in the production of stress ulcers. (Reproduced with permission from N.J. Greenberger, *Gastrointestinal Disorders: A Pathophysiologic Approach* [3rd ed.]. Copyright © 1986 by Yearbook Medical Publishers, Inc., Chicago. Adapted from W. Silen and J.J. Skillman. In G.H. Stollerman [ed.], *Advances in Internal Medicine*, Vol. 19. Chicago: Yearbook Medical Publishers, 1974.)

Gastric ulcer
Lesser curvature
Duodenal ulcer
Pyloric valve
Greater curvature
Pyloric antrum

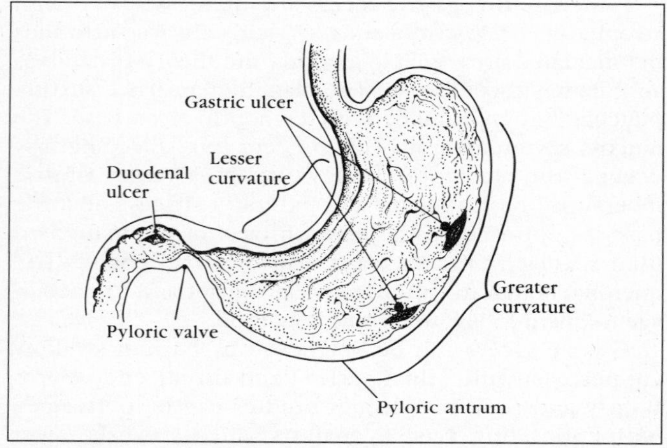

FIGURE 37-6 Common locations of gastric and duodenal ulcers.

ulcers [4]. Benign ulcers frequently localize on the greater curvature of the stomach and are usually smaller than malignant lesions. If there is associated achlorhydria, the ulcers are almost always malignant.

The most common symptom with gastric ulcer disease is epigastric pain. The pain may or may not be relieved by eating or it may be precipitated when food is ingested. Gastric ulcers that localize in the pyloric area often relay symptoms of duodenal ulcers. Nausea, vomiting, and weight loss are common. Hemorrhage occurs in approximately 25 percent of these persons and is often profound. Perforation of the ulcer into the peritoneal cavity is less frequent than with duodenal ulcer. Healing and recurrence are common, with lack of healing or failure to decrease in size suggesting gastric malignancy. Healing, with a decrease in the size of the ulcer by 50 percent, should occur in three months or less after initiation of therapy [4,6].

TABLE 37-1 Differential Features of Peptic Ulcer

Type of Lesion	Frequency	Pathophysiology	Clinical Features	Course
Duodenal ulcer	Men: women, 3:1 Peak frequency 5th–6th decades Prevalence 10–12%	Normal to increased parietal cell mass Normal to increased gastric acid secretion Normal to mildly elevated circulating gastrin levels Excessive gastrin response to meals, excessive parietal cell sensitivity Genetic factors—familial tendency, frequent blood group O, nonsecretor Positive associations—chronic obstructive lung disease, hepatic cirrhosis, pancreatic insufficiency, hyperparathyroidism Located in duodenal bulb, pyloric channel, postbulbar area	Pain: rhythmicity, periodicity, chronicity Pain-food-relief-pain pattern	Remissions and exacerbations for 10–25 years after onset. "Once an ulcer, always an ulcer." Seasonal trend (spring and fall).
Gastric ulcer	Men: women, 3–4:1 Peak frequency 6th–7th decades Duodenal ulcer: gastric ulcer 4:1	Normal to decreased parietal cell mass Normal to decreased gastric acid secretion (not achlorhydria) Normal to elevated circulating gastrin level Presence of gastritis Abnormal gastric mucosal barrier Abnormal pyloric function, bile reflux Ulcerogenic drugs	Pain-food-relief-pain pattern, or food-pain pattern Weight loss, anorexia	Remissions and exacerbations less than in duodenal ulcer; high recurrence rate. No seasonal trend.
Gastric erosions or stress ulcer	No sex difference Related to severe stress, sepsis, burns, trauma, head injuries	Head injuries—marked gastric acid hypersecretion Others—gastric mucosal ischemia, acid back-diffusion, acute gastritis	Bleeding frequent in recognized cases; may be severe, persistent (actual frequency unknown)	Half of those who bleed require surgery.

Source: Reproduced with permission from N.J. Greenberger, *Gastrointestinal Disorders: A Pathophysiologic Approach* [3rd ed.]. Copyright ©1986 by Yearbook Medical Publishers, Inc., Chicago.

Duodenal Ulcers. Numerous causes and predisposing factors in combination upset the balance between the protective mechanism and the acid-pepsin proteolytic action in the duodenal wall. Duodenal ulcers occur in the presence of acid, but hyperacidity is not always a significant component. Persons with excess acid secretion may also have excess secretion of gastrin or gastrinlike substances from the duodenal wall, as well as from the parietal cells. Strong family history of the disease and type O blood group support a theory of genetic weakness in this disease [4]. Elevated serum pepsinogen level is under study as a significant indicator of predisposition to duodenal ulcer. Hyperpepsinogenemia is inherited as an autosomal dominant trait and may account for as much as 50 percent of simple duodenal ulcers [4].

The emotional factors that increase gastric secretions and influence the pathogenesis of duodenal ulcerations often precipitate the onset or recurrence of symptoms. Studies have been conducted to identify a so-called ulcer personality, but the findings have not been conclusive [9]. Endocrine factors, such as estrogen and the adrenal steroids, also may contribute to the formation of ulcerations.

Duodenal ulcers are usually deep, with a sharp line of demarcation from uninvolved tissue. Most of these ulcerations occur in the first portion of the duodenum, close to the pylorus. Disruption of the integrity of the mucosal wall caused by the acid-pepsin imbalance penetrates the entire thickness of the mucosal membrane, including the muscularis mucosa. Healing requires the formation of granulation tissue and scar. Secretory cellular functions are lost in the area of scarring.

A typical duodenal ulcer is a round or oval-shaped, indurated, funnellike lesion that extends into the muscularis layer. It is frequently located within 1 to 3 cm of the pyloric junction, on either the anterior or posterior wall.

Acute ulcerations may develop on chronic ulcers, and perforations through the duodenal wall in active ulcers result in spilling of gastric or duodenal contents into the peritoneum and peritonitis. Erosion of an artery or a vein at the base of the lesion may cause a hemorrhage. The amount of bleeding depends on the vessel involved, and the effects are related to the rapidity and amount of blood loss.

Scar formation may cause deformity, shortening, and stiffening of the duodenum, which may interfere with normal emptying of the stomach. Actual obstruction may result from stenosis, spasm, or edema, and/or inflammation.

Clinical manifestations of duodenal ulcerations include a documented pattern of remissions and exacerbations over varying periods of time. An attack is frequently triggered by stress, and exacerbations have been observed to occur most frequently in the fall and spring seasons.

A definite pain-food-relief pattern is characteristic of duodenal ulcer. Pain usually develops 90 minutes to 3 hours after eating, often waking the person at night. This pain is immediately relieved by food or antacids. Pain on awakening in the early morning is rare, which is thought to be due to decreased gastric secretions [4]. The pain is usually described as steady, boring, burning, aching, or hungerlike, and is localized in the midepigastrium, the right epigastric area, or sometimes in the back. Its mechanism in duodenal ulcers is thought to be related to irritation of exposed sensory nerve endings by hydrochloric acid. It may result from increased motility or spasm of the muscles at the ulcer site. Rarely, pain is not described, and the ulcer is discovered when complications arise.

Other gastrointestinal symptoms include heartburn and regurgitation of sour juice into the back of the mouth. Anorexia is not a usual complaint because the individual seeks relief of pain through eating. A duodenal ulcer may rupture because of erosion through the duodenal wall, and this leads to contamination of the peritoneal cavity. As in gastric ulcer disease, hemorrhage may lead to profound blood loss and hypovolemic shock; a slowly bleeding ulcer may be detected by guaiac-positive stools. Localized tenderness around the epigastric area is the only common finding on physical examination.

Diagnosis of duodenal ulcer requires a reliable and accurate history of the characteristic pain. Radiologic and fluoroscopic examinations with barium swallow demonstrate ulcer craters and niches as well as outlet deformities. Gastric endoscopy, direct visualization of the gastric mucosa through a lighted scope, is useful in revealing lesions too small or superficial to be seen on radiographs. Tissue for histologic studies may also be taken during the procedure. Gastric juice analysis may be helpful in persons who do not have typical duodenal ulcer disease to determine the cycle of hydrochloric acid and pepsin secretion. Basal acid output and maximal histamine stimulation analysis may be performed. Basal acid output measures the acidity of gastric secretions without a known or intentional stimulation. Achlorhydria after histamine stimulation demonstrates loss of secretory function and almost never occurs with duodenal ulcerations.

A 12-hour nocturnal test provides information regarding secretion during a prolonged basal state. Nocturnal levels of hydrochloric acid and pepsin are frequently higher in persons with duodenal ulcers than in those with gastric ulcers. Zollinger-Ellison syndrome exhibits very high measurements of gastric acid secretion (see Chap. 35).

All of the therapeutic approaches for duodenal ulcer disease are directed toward relieving pain, promoting healing, and preventing complications. Helping the person recognize lifestyle and personal factors that precipitate symptoms may enhance compliance with therapy and thus help prevent recurrence of the disease.

Complications of PUD. Hemorrhage occurs in 15 to 20 percent of cases of PUD. It may be manifested by melena (occult blood in the stools) or hematemesis and hemorrhagic shock [4]. Other complications include perforation of the wall, which is most common with duodenal ulcer disease and causes abdominal pain and peritonitis. Penetration of the ulcer into surrounding structures is relatively uncommon, but may affect the pancreas, liver, and abdominal wall. Symptoms of penetration are those of damage to the affected area.

The inlet and outlet of the stomach may become obstructed; this is most common in the pyloric area. Obstruction may cause severe pain, vomiting, weight loss, and anorexia. The ulcer may be intractable, with frequent recurrences and/or lack of response to therapy. Other complications, especially obstruction and penetration, may lead to intractable ulcers. When ulcers continue despite therapy, Zollinger-Ellison syndrome must be ruled out (see Chap. 35).

Gastric Carcinoma

Ninety to 95 percent of all malignancies of the stomach are classified as carcinomas. The frequency of gastric carcinoma has been declining steadily over the past few decades in the United States, but in several countries, especially Japan, Iceland, and Finland, it is high. Apparently, however, its occurrence is declining as well in the high-risk countries [7]. Survival rates are poor, with less than 5 to 15 percent surviving for five years after diagnosis. Early diagnosis has improved the mortality figures, so that if the lesion is confined to the mucosa and submucosa, five-year survival is 60 to 90 percent [7].

Environmental factors evidently play a large part in the origin of gastric cancer. These include a number of associated factors, the significance of which generally is not known. They include diet, socioeconomic class, occupation, urban residence, and others [7].

Diet has been implicated in the causation of gastric carcinoma, especially with regard to the nitrates that are used as food preservatives. These convert to nitrites, which convert to nitrosamine, a well-known carcinogen [9].

Genetic or hereditary linkage is supported by an increased risk among families and the preponderance of occurrence in persons with blood group A. Gastric carcinoma also affects an older population and is associated with atrophic gastritis or polyps of the stomach.

Pathologically, these carcinomas may arise anywhere on the mucosal surface. They begin as in situ (localized) lesions that progress to lesions called early gastric carcinoma (EGC). These are limited to the mucosa and submucosa. Early spread to regional lymph nodes may occur. As the lesions progress, they may infiltrate the wall and/or protrude as bulky masses into the outlet of the stomach [6]. Ulceration may occur, with a shaggy, necrotic-appearing base. A diffuse form of carcinoma has been identified that causes thickening of the entire stomach wall, the so-called leather-bottle stomach. Distant metastasis is frequent, most often to the liver, lungs, ovaries, and peritoneum. These metastases are often already established at the time of diagnosis.

The clinical manifestations are often vague and nonspecific, including early satiety, loss of appetite, weight loss, abdominal pain, vomiting, and change in bowel habits. Anemia and guaiac-positive stools may be discovered. Bleeding may result from vascular erosion as the tumor ulcerates [6]. Pain in gastric carcinoma is rare but may imitate ulcer pain or be related to partial outlet obstruction. Massive hemorrhage may cause hemorrhagic shock.

The only definitive diagnostic test is gastric biopsy, usually obtained through gastric endoscopy. Other studies may be helpful, such as barium swallow, blood work, and additional tests to demonstrate a mass in the gastric area.

Alterations in the Small Intestine

Most nutrient absorption occurs in the small intestine. Any alteration of the integrity of the small bowel can result in malsorption, whether the source is motor or mucosal.

Malsorption refers to inadequate absorption of ingested nutrients and water. *Maldigestion* is the inability to absorb foodstuffs because they have been broken down inadequately. Table 37-2 outlines some of the major causes of malsorption. It can be seen that it may be caused by many mechanisms and that the categories are not entirely separate. In other words, many disorders can cause malsorption through several mechanisms. Some of the more common disease conditions are discussed in this section; other related conditions are presented in Chapter 39. Table 37-3 summarizes the major laboratory tests commonly used to detect malsorption [11].

Celiac Disease

Celiac Enteropathy (Nontropical Sprue). This disease has many names and is thought to be related to a genetic defect that results in gluten intolerance. Its frequency is greater in women than in men and onset of symptoms usually is in young adulthood.

Histopathologic changes in the absorptive surface in response to exposure to the protein gluten or its breakdown products, found mostly in wheat, are responsible for the manifestations of a general malsorption syndrome. The mechanism underlying this reaction is not known, but it is theorized that an enzyme deficiency or autoimmune reaction occurs. The hypothesis of enzyme deficiency, or toxic theory, suggests that specific peptidases are missing either from the brush border or from the cytoplasm of the epithelial cells of the intestinal mucosa, and as a result, gluten is not effectively hydrolyzed to smaller peptides and amino acids. Studies have not demonstrated specific deficiencies, and have, in fact, shown that although levels

TABLE 37-2 Causes of Malsorption

- Incomplete digestion of nutrients
  - Pancreatic insufficiency
  - Primary — deficient production of pancreatic enzymes
    - Chronic relapsing pancreatic enzymes
    - Cancer of the pancreas
    - Cystic fibrosis
    - Extensive pancreatic resection
  - Secondary — defective use of pancreatic enzymes
    - Post–Billroth II
    - Zollinger-Ellison syndrome
  - Deficiency of conjugated bile salts
  - Impaired synthesis or release
    - Severe liver disease
    - Extrahepatic biliary tract obstruction
  - Abnormal loss
    - Ileal resection
    - Ileectomy
    - Ileal bypass
    - Severe disease of the terminal ileum
  - Accelerated deconjugation by bacterial overgrowth
    - Surgically created blind loops
    - Fistulas — enteroenteric, enterocolic, gastrojejunocolic
    - Chronic intestinal obstruction due to adhesions or strictures
    - Small bowel diverticula
    - Motor abnormalities except scleroderma
  - Drug-induced precipitation or sequestration
    - Neomycin
    - Calcium carbonate
    - Cholestyramine
  - Inadequate mechanical mixing of chyme with digestive enzymes
  - Post–Billroth II
  - Post–total gastrectomy
- Abnormalities of the absorptive surface
  - Biochemical or genetic
    - Disaccharidase deficiency
    - Abetalipoproteinemia
    - Primary vitamin B_{12} malsorption
    - Cystinuria
    - Hartnup disease
    - Celiac sprue
  - Inflammatory or infective disorders
    - Tropical sprue
    - Regional enteritis
    - Eosinophilic enteritis
    - Infectious enteritis
- Lack of absorptive surface
  - Intestinal resection
  - Gastroileostomy
- Lymphatic obstruction
  - Whipple's disease
  - Intestinal lymphangiectasia
  - Lymphoma
- Cardiovascular disorders
  - Mesenteric vascular insufficiency
  - Congestive heart failure
  - Constrictive pericarditis
- Endocrine and metabolic disorders
  - Diabetes mellitus
  - Hypoparathyroidism
  - Adrenal insufficiency
  - Hyperthyroidism
  - Carcinoid syndrome

TABLE 37-3 Laboratory Tests Specific to the Detection of Malsorption

Test	Normal Finding	Meaning of Abnormal Findings
Fecal fat balance: quantitative determination of stool fat	6 gm (or fewer) of fatty acids extracted from stool in 24 hours	More than 6 gm/24 hours—clinically significant steatorrhea
D-xylose tolerance test	4 gm (or more) D-xylose excreted by kidneys in 5 hours; or 20 mg (or more) D-xylose/dl of blood in 1–2 hours	Decreased values in diseases of intestinal mucosa and in intestinal stasis; values normal in pancreatic insufficiency
Schilling test	Greater than 7% of radioactive vitamin B_{12} excreted in urine/24 hours	Decreased value can indicate (1) lack of intrinsic factor, (2) competition by bacteria, (3) disease of ileum
With administration of intrinsic factor		Decreased—(2) or (3) above
After 2 weeks of antimicrobial therapy		Decreased—(1) or (3) above
Serum carotene	70 IU/dl of serum	Decreased with malsorption and also perhaps due to dietary insufficiency or hepatic disease
^{14}C triolein absorption (break test)	More than 3.5% of $^{14}CO_2$ appears in breath/hour (6 hr)	Correlates with chemical stool fat

of peptic hydrolases and other brush border enzymes are depressed in untreated cases, they return to normal after treatment with a gluten-free diet [13].

The proposal that gluten or its metabolites initiate a hypersensitivity reaction in the intestinal mucosa is supported by the majority of evidence. Gluten proteins have been shown to have antigenic properties, and circulating antibodies to dietary gluten have been demonstrated in persons with active celiac enteropathy. The lamina propria of affected mucosa contains mononuclear leukocytes and plasma cells. Serum levels of immunoglobulin A are elevated and levels of IgM are depressed. Corticosteroid therapy has been shown to improve both intestinal absorption and histologic appearance.

Regardless of cause, the mucosal changes are characteristic. The villi are flattened or absent; the epithelium is disorganized and consists of cuboidal rather than the normal columnar cells. The brush border is thickened and the lamina propria is infiltrated with inflammatory cells. Cytoplasmic changes include membrane disruption and rounded mitochondria. All of these changes result in malsorption, with impairment of uptake and transport of nutrients.

Clinical features include frequent, foul-smelling, steatorrheic stools (i.e., the stools have a fatty or greasy appearance). Loss of body weight and malsorption of fat-soluble vitamins are common. Severe muscle wasting and hypoproteinemia may occur.

Treatment measures support gluten hypersensitivity in that a dramatic or delayed remission of symptoms occurs when barley, wheat, rye, and oats are removed from the diet. Restoration of the normal mucosal epithelium occurs and malsorption decreases.

Tropical Sprue. This disease differs in etiology from celiac enteropathy but is usually characterized by identical mucosal changes in the small intestine. It probably results from nutritional and bacterial alterations and has greatest frequency in certain tropical areas. It may be caused by *Escherichia coli* bacteria. Symptoms may not arise for months or years after exposure [7]. Because the mucosal lesions result in malsorption, the clinical picture closely resembles that of celiac enteropathy. Treatment with folic acid is restorative in some cases, and antibiotics may be helpful.

Regional Enteritis: Crohn's Disease

Crohn's disease most commonly affects the terminal ileum, but any portion of the gastrointestinal tract may become involved. The frequency of this chronic inflammatory disease is equal in males and females, is slightly higher in members of the Jewish race, and exhibits a familial predisposition. Onset is most common between ages 15 and 20 years, with a secondary peak between ages 55 and 60 years. It is much more frequent in the United States, Britain, and Scandinavia than in Japan, Russia, and South America [7]. Crohn's disease and ulcerative colitis have many etiologic similarities and commonly are grouped as ***inflammatory bowel disease (IBD)***. The origins may be infectious, immunologic, psychosomatic, dietary, hormonal, or unknown [7]. Viruses continue to be studied as major possible causative factors [7]. The immunologic features of the disease may be primary or secondary responses to the viral organism [7].

Gross inspection of the affected bowel discloses shallow, longitudinal, mucosal ulcers; long or short areas of stricture; and a cobblestone appearance of the mucosa (Fig. 37-7). The last results from interconnecting fissures that cut deeply into the intestinal wall and create islands of mucosa elevated by the existing transmural (full-wall thickness) inflammation and its accompanying edema. The bowel wall becomes congested, thickened, and rigid, with adhesions involving the periintestinal fat [5]. Areas of involvement are localized and interrupted by areas of normal gut. Sometimes, several segments of bowel are affected and are separated by normal bowel. These segments are called ***skip lesions*** and produce chronic partial intestinal obstruction [8]. Fistulas to other parts of the

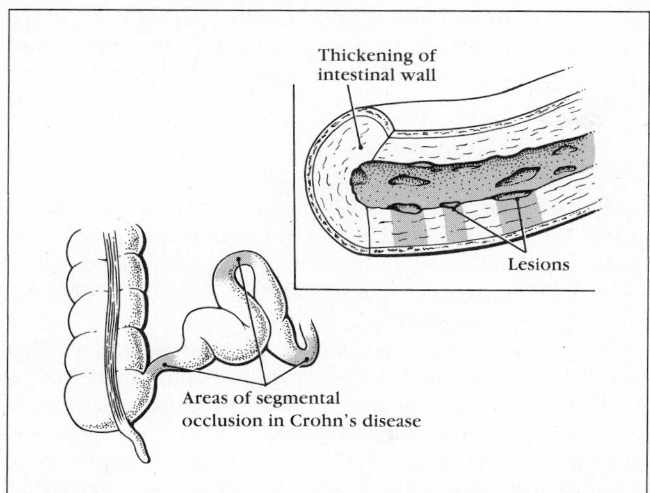

FIGURE 37-7 Schematic appearance of Crohn's disease showing segmental areas of occlusion and transmural involvement of intestinal wall.

gastrointestinal tract or other adjacent structures may be present.

Microscopically, all layers of the intestinal wall, particularly the submucosa, are edematous and infiltrated with aggregations of lymphocytes and macrophages [7]. Characteristic noncaseating granulomas, which have large mononuclear phagocytes and multinucleated giant cells, form in the bowel wall and often are present in the regional lymph nodes. Dilated lymphatic channels and lymphoid deposits occur at all levels of bowel involvement.

The inflammatory changes cause functional disruption of the mucosa, producing malsorption, especially of bile salts and vitamin B_{12}, which are normally absorbed in the jejunum and ileum. Fluid imbalances occur when large segments of ileum are affected.

The strictures and fistulas that occur with this disease predispose the intestine to bacterial overgrowth and abscess formation. Bowel obstruction and peritonitis may be the results of strictures and abscesses.

The clinical manifestations of Crohn's disease vary, with diarrhea being a dominant symptom, often accompanied by fever and right lower quadrant or abdominal pain. The apparent linkage with stress and personality factors have been studied extensively with inconclusive results, except that depression and dependency are typical personality patterns. The clinical manifestations are variable, usually beginning with insidious onset of malaise and diarrhea. As the disease progresses, weight loss, occult blood in the feces, and nausea and vomiting occur. Obstruction and ileus may occur. Fistulas develop in 10 to 15 percent of cases and peritonitis may result from rupture of the fistulous connection.

A significant correlation of this disease with several autoimmune diseases and with adenocarcinoma of the small bowel exists. Chronic debilitation may finally require bowel resection.

Diagnosis of regional enteritis is based on the clinical history, physical examination (which may reveal a right lower quadrant mass), and characteristic radiograph. The string sign is commonly noted on radiologic studies (Fig. 37-8).

Enteritis

Enteritis, or gastroenteritis, is an inflammatory process that may affect the stomach or small intestine. It may be caused by viruses, bacteria, or allergic reactions. When it is due to an organism, it may occur with the ingestion of contaminated food, especially contamination by staphylococci, which produce a toxin that reacts with the small intestine mucosa. Dysentery caused by bacteria affects the colon. The pathologic process has varying manifestations that result in abdominal cramping, diarrhea, and vomiting.

Fluid-electrolyte imbalance often results. Parasites may localize in the gastrointestinal tract or invade the circulation. Eosinophilic enteritis is uncommon but may result from an allergy. It is manifested by the accumulation of eosinophils in the gut wall. In general, enteritis causes inflammatory changes in the intestinal mucosa that return to normal when the precipitator is removed.

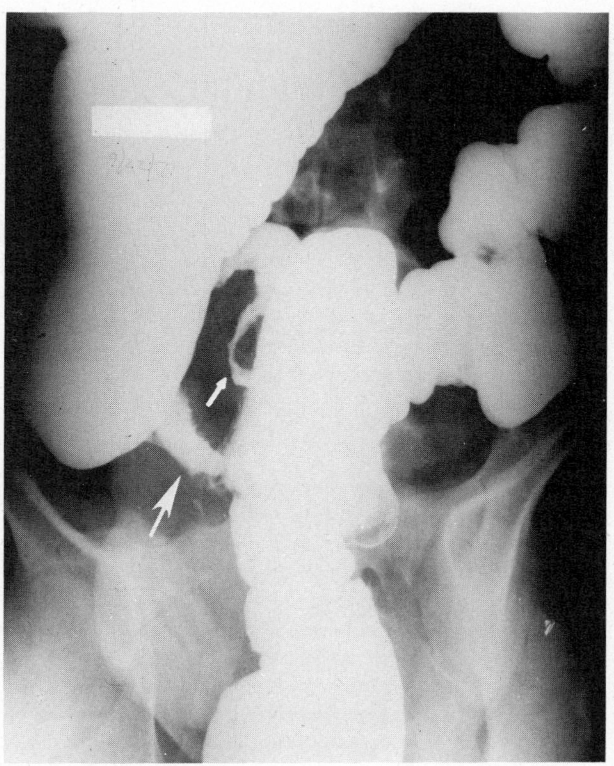

FIGURE 37-8 Crohn's disease. Radiograph of colon showing wide fistula (*large arrow*) between cecum and sigmoid colon and irregularly narrowed distal ileum (*small arrow*). (From J.H. Stein [ed.], *Internal Medicine*. Boston: Little, Brown, 1983.)

Alterations in the Large Intestine

Adynamic or Paralytic Ileus

The word *ileus* has come to refer to a functional obstruction of the bowel. It may occur in the small or large intestine and is often classified as physiologic or paralytic. Lack of propulsive peristalsis creates an inability to move bowel contents downward, which leads to absence of bowel sounds and bowel distention. Physiologic ileus may be the result of anesthesia, interruption of nerve supply to the bowel, or abdominal operation. Paralytic ileus may result from intestinal ischemia, abdominal wound infections, electrolyte disturbances, or certain metabolic diseases. All true ileus can be described as *adynamic*, having absent propulsive motor activity [12].

The result of ileus is distention of the bowel with gas and fluid. The process is similar to actual bowel obstruction. Colonic bacteria may contribute to the abdominal distention and cause marked alterations of fluid and electrolyte balance. Loss of potassium leads to further intestinal atony. Vomiting and hypotension can result in metabolic acidosis. As fluid shifts to the intestinal area, central blood volume decreases and distention increases [12]. If there is associated mesenteric ischemia, necrosis and rupture of the bowel may occur, causing peritonitis. Clinical findings include abdominal distention, decreased or absent bowel sounds, and signs of dehydration and shock.

Intestinal Obstruction

Intestinal obstruction is blockage of the lumen of the bowel by an actual mechanical obstruction. Figure 37-9 illustrates some causes, which include foreign bodies, volvulus, adhesions, intussusception, hernias, ischemia, infarction, and neoplasms.

Initially after blockage occurs, gas and air are the primary bowel distenders and distention occurs proximal to the area of blockage. As the process continues, gastric, biliary, and pancreatic secretions pool. Water, electrolytes, and serum proteins also begin to accumulate in the area. Pooling and bowel distention decrease the circulating blood volume due to a so-called third-space shift that moves water into the area proximal to the obstruction and thus decreases plasma volume. Bowel wall edema also interferes with the blood supply to the bowel tissue and depresses normal sodium transport in the mucosa (Fig. 37-10).

Strangulation of a bowel segment may cause necrosis, perforation, and loss of fluid and blood into the inactive

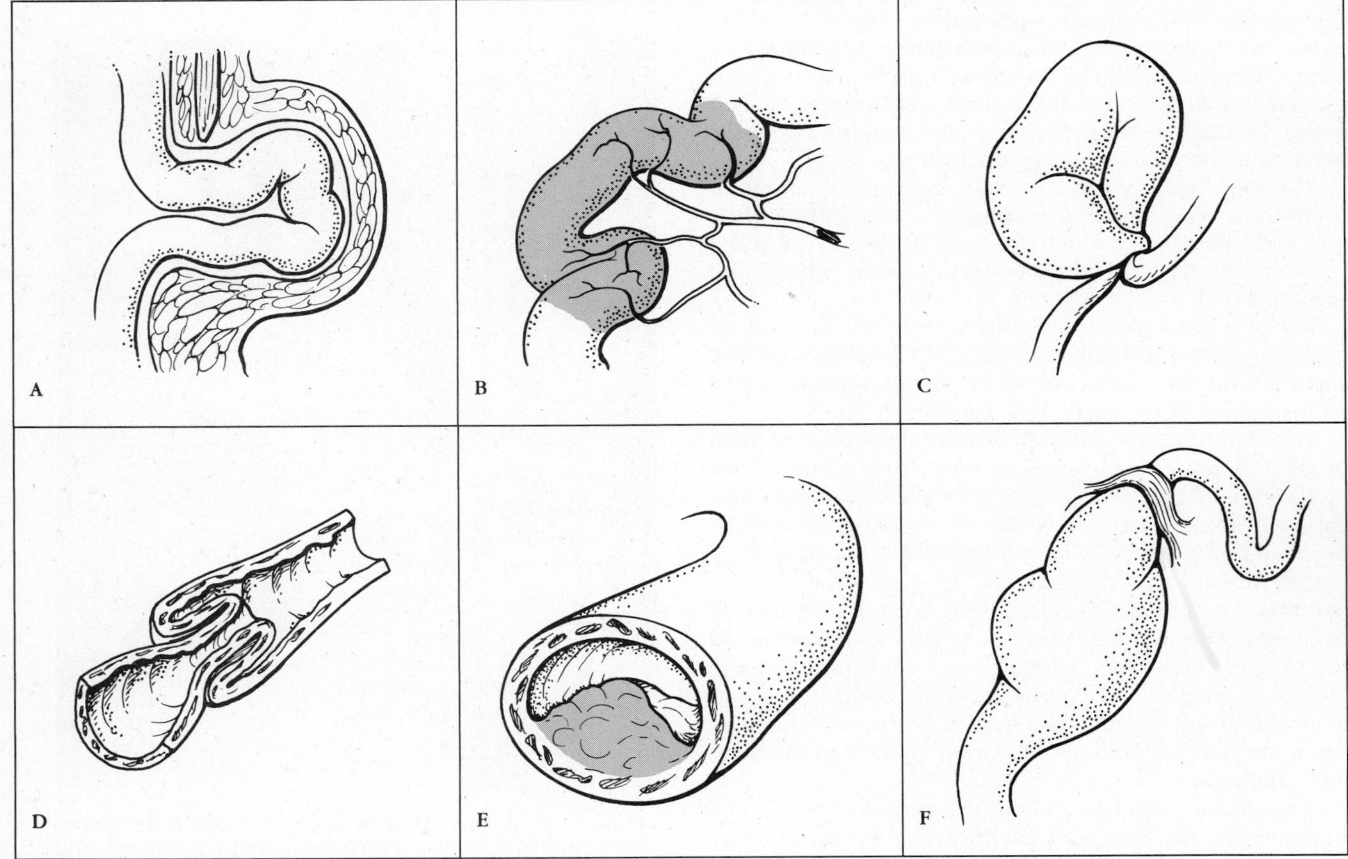

FIGURE 37-9 Illustration of major causes of actual intestinal obstruction. A. Hernia. B. Mesenteric occlusion. C. Volvulus. D. Intussusception. E. Neoplasm. F. Adhesions.

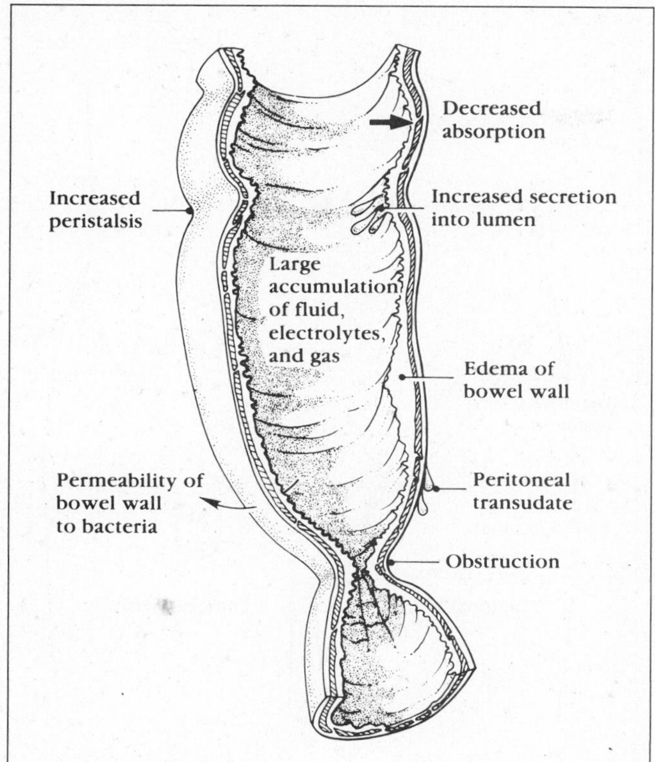

FIGURE 37-10 Pathophysiology of intestinal obstruction and peritonitis. (From P.A. Jones, C.F. Dunbar, and M.M. Jirovec, *Medical-Surgical Nursing*. New York: McGraw-Hill, 1978.)

bowel. Impairment of blood supply leads at first to increased peristalsis and bacterial invasion of the tissue, and finally causes necrosis and peritonitis when intestinal contents are released into the peritoneal cavity. Stasis of the intestinal contents provides an area for increased growth of organisms, with toxins being released into the tissues further disrupting the intestinal cellular dynamics. Loss of fluids and electrolytes is a major problem and results in decreased systemic circulating fluid volume due to the shift from the vascular to the intestinal lumen.

Clinical manifestations include the acute onset of severe, cramping pain that correlates roughly to the area or level of obstruction. Pain may decrease in severity as the distention of the bowel and abdomen increases, which is probably due to impaired motility in the edematous intestine. Increases in rate and force of peristalsis cause loud, high-pitched bowel sounds (*borborygmi*) in the early period, but these may progress to a silent bowel as the condition persists. Vomiting is almost always present and may be bilious or feculent (having the appearance of feces) depending on the level of the obstruction. Diarrhea may occur if obstruction is not complete.

Hypovolemic shock is the result of a shift of fluid greater than 10 percent of body weight. This has been calculated to be about 700 ml in a person weighing 70 kg [10]. Septicemic shock may also result from contamination of the peritoneum when the bowel ruptures. Sepsis and/or hypovolemic shock produce a life-threatening clinical picture that must be treated aggressively.

Tenderness, rigidity, and fever are usually indicative of peritonitis. Leukocytosis and elevation of serum amylase level are also common. Distention of the bowel may be noted radiologically, but this does not give conclusive evidence of the cause or exact level of obstruction.

Hernias

A hernia is a defect in the abdominal wall. It may occur in the scrotal or inguinal area or in the abdominal wall or diaphragm (Fig. 37-11). Incisional hernias occur in an area weakened by surgical incision. Whatever the cause, the defect allows abdominal structures (e.g., peritoneum, fat, bowel, or bladder) to fill the area, producing a sac filled with the material. Abdominal contents usually move into the defect when abdominal pressure increases. If the bulging of the sac is intermittent, the hernia is called *reducible*. *Incarcerated hernias* contain abdominal contents all the time, and *strangulated hernias* cause necrosis of the abdominal contents due to lack of blood supply. Necrosis of the bowel then leads to all the clinical manifestations of intestinal obstruction.

Congenital Megacolon or Hirschsprung's Disease

Hirschsprung's disease is usually manifested in early infancy and is caused by congenital absence of parasympathetic ganglion cells in the submucosal and intramuscular plexuses. Consequently, the bowel becomes greatly dilated, with no peristaltic action in the aganglionic area. The aganglionic region remains contracted without reciprocal relaxation, and this produces a functional obstruction. The area most frequently affected is the rectosigmoid.

Hirschsprung's disease is a congenital disorder with much higher frequency in males than in females. When manifested in early infancy, abdominal distention, constipation, and vomiting occur. Occasionally, this condition is diagnosed in young adults who describe a lifelong problem with constipation.

Megacolon, or enlargement of the colon, may also be produced by any process that inhibits bowel evacuation. Among such processes are psychogenic megacolon, which results from ignoring the urge to defecate, some neurologic disorders, fecal impaction, and chronic depression.

The clinical manifestations depend on the degree of aganglionosis or bowel distention. The person is often poorly nourished and anemic, and rarely produces fecal material. The congenital type is often associated with other anomalies such as Down syndrome.

Diverticula

Diverticula are multiple saclike protrusions of the mucosa along the gastrointestinal tract. Although the terms are loosely used, a *true diverticulum* has all layers of the bowel in its walls, while a *false diverticulum* occurs in a weak area of the muscularis of the bowel.

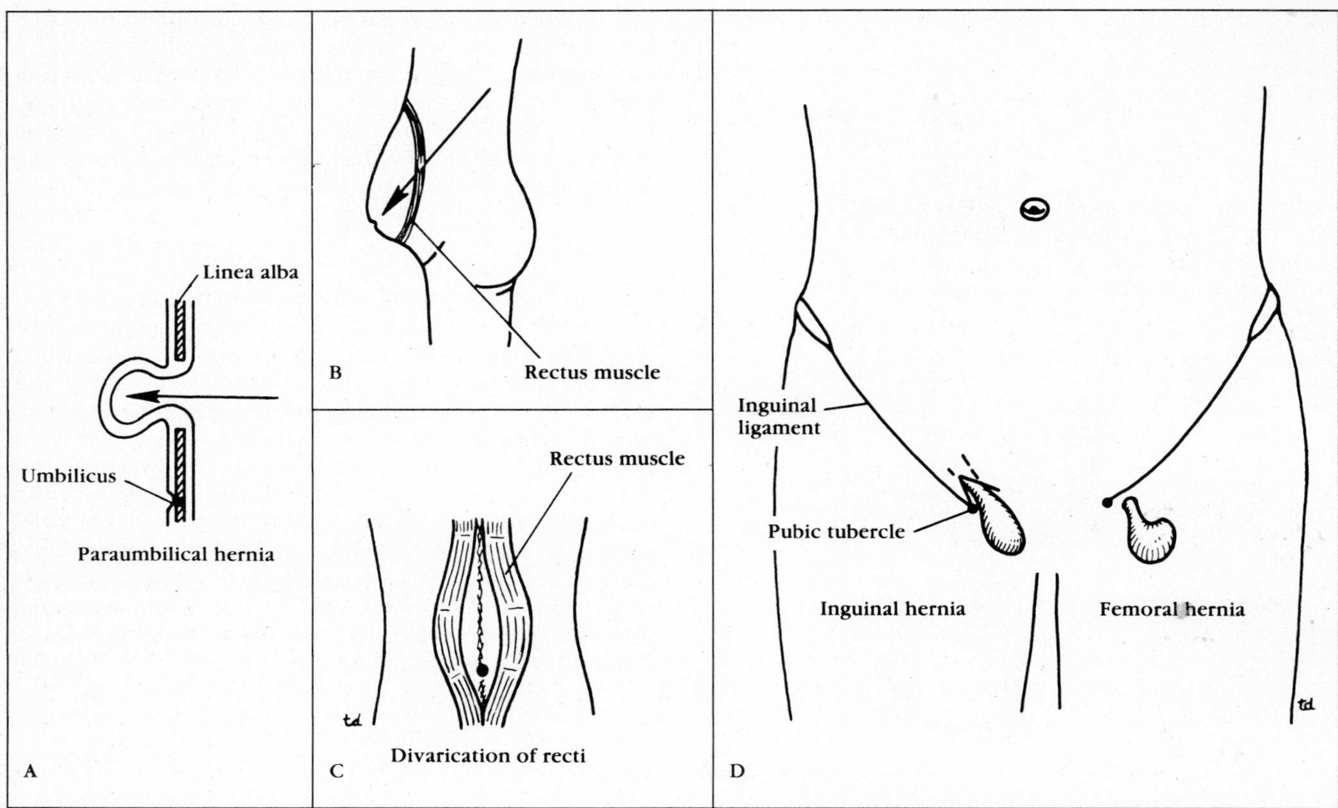

FIGURE 37-11 Types of hernias. A. Paraumbilical. B. Epigastric. C. Divarication of rectus abdominus. D. Inguinal and femoral. (From R.S. Snell, *Clinical Anatomy for Medical Students* [2nd ed.]. Boston: Little, Brown, 1981.)

An example of true diverticular disease is ***Meckel's diverticulum***, occurring in 1 to 2 percent of the population. This sac, located 1 to 3 feet proximal to the ileocecal junction, is formed by persistence of a mesenteric structure that normally closes in fetal life. It may be lined with ileal mucosa or contain other types of gastrointestinal mucosal cells. Complications include gastrointestinal bleeding and inflammation [5]. False colonic diverticula are common and usually occur in the sigmoid colon.

Because of their frequency in elderly persons, it is thought that these weaknesses are related to the blood supply or nutrition of the bowel in the elderly [3]. Lack of dietary fiber or roughage and decreased fecal bulk also have been correlated with this process.

Diverticulosis refers to the presence of diverticula in the colon that are rarely symptomatic. ***Diverticulitis*** is inflammation in or around a diverticular sac that results in retention of undigested food and bacteria in the sac. This forms a hard mass called a *fecalith* [3]. Colonic obstruction, fistulae, and abscesses can result. Rupture of the infected material into the peritoneal cavity may lead to peritonitis.

The clinical manifestations of symptomatic diverticular disease vary. Constipation is frequently reported. Fibrosis in the area may develop and cause obstruction by adhesions. The complaint of lower, left-sided abdominal pain may be associated with the signs of peritonitis; including guarding, fever, abdominal rigidity, and rebound tenderness.

Radiographs and sigmoidoscopy may not indicate the extent of the problem. Surgery may be performed if the process causes obstruction or perforation.

Hemorrhoids

Hemorrhoids are dilatations of the venous plexus that surrounds the rectal and anal areas. These dilatations are very common and develop in susceptible persons due to increased pressure in the venous plexus. Hemorrhoids are often related to other types of abnormalities, especially varicose veins. Predisposition may result from constipation or pregnancy; bleeding hemorrhoids may be a dangerous outcome of portal hypertension (see Chap. 39).

The dilated venous sacs protrude into the anal and rectal canals where they become exposed; thromboses, ulcerations, and bleeding develop. Hemorrhoids may be painful and irritating. Bright red bleeding during defecation or with increased intraabdominal pressure is common. Usually blood loss is insignificant, but chronic anemia may be an outcome. Bleeding in association with portal hypertension may be profound and even life threatening.

Ulcerative Colitis

Ulcerative colitis is primarily an inflammatory disease of the mucous membrane of the colon. Purulent exudate and blood are common, and the chronic inflammation may cause bleeding throughout the mucosa. The disease may be confined to the rectum, or it may affect segments of the colon or even the entire colon. The bowel fills with a bloody, mucoid secretion that produces a characteristic cramping pain, rectal urgency, and diarrhea. The colon wall becomes thickened and edematous. The process is usually confined to the mucosal layer and rarely affects the muscularis.

Complications of ulcerative colitis include intestinal obstruction, dehydration, and major fluid and electrolyte imbalances. Malsorption is common, and loss of blood in the stools may cause chronic iron-deficiency anemia.

There is a significant relationship between ulcerative colitis and cancer of the colon. Ten to 15 percent of persons with ulcerative colitis for more than 10 years develop colon carcinoma.

The etiology of ulcerative colitis is unknown, but a genetic basis has been suggested because the disease occurs with increased frequency in some families. Other agents such as viruses and microorganisms may be implicated, and the disease is associated with autoimmunity. The plasma serum in some persons with the disease has been shown to have an antibody to the colonic epithelial cells. These factors have led to research into a possible autoimmune nature of this condition. Many of the etiologic factors of Crohn's disease are also common to ulcerative colitis.

Clinical manifestations are variable and the disease has periods of remissions and exacerbations. The major classic symptoms include cramping abdominal pain, bloody diarrhea, fever, and weight loss. The person usually becomes debilitated. Laboratory findings include anemia, leukocytosis, hypoalbuminemia, electrolyte imbalance, and increased serum alkaline phosphatase. Despite their evident pathologic differences, ulcerative colitis and regional enteritis may be confused clinically. Table 37-4 shows the major differences between them. Diagnosis of ulcerative colitis is on the basis of clinical features; results of barium enema, and sigmoidoscopic appearance of the mucosa. Biopsy and cultures are essential to exclude carcinoma and bacterial diarrhea [3].

Table 37-4 Major Differences Between Ulcerative Colitis and Crohn's Disease

Variable	Ulcerative Colitis	Crohn's Disease
Extent of disease	Mucosa	Entire wall
Ulceration	Extensive, superficial	Patchy, deep
Mesentery	Normal	Thickened
Lymph nodes	Normal	Diseased
Granulomata	Absent	Present (25–75%)
Distribution[a]	Symmetric	Eccentric
Skip areas	Never[b]	Common
Diseased rectum	Always[b]	10–20%
Small intestine disease	Never[b]	Usual
Results of surgery	Cure	Frequent recurrence

[a]Radiologically, the entire circumference of the colon is involved in ulcerative colitis, whereas in Crohn's disease only one side may be diseased.
[b]The words "always" and "never" should not be used to describe biological processes, but here they are probably appropriate.
Source: From B. N. Brooke et al., *Crohn's Disease Aetiology, Clinical Manifestations and Management*, 1977. Reprinted by permission of Macmillan, England.

Polyps

A polyp in the large intestine is a benign growth that protrudes into the lumen. Polyps are divided into two major categories, *adenomatous* and *hyperplastic*.

Adenomatous polyps are true neoplasms. The growths begin in the mucosa deep within the crypts of the colonic mucosal glands [9]. The polypoidal cells continue to divide and become hyperplastic growths. When reproductive control is lost throughout the mucosal crypt, a neoplasm results. Polyps are very common in the general population. They rarely exceed 5 mm in diameter. These growths may be discovered by routine sigmoidoscopy or barium enema. They may bleed, causing bright red feces. The major clinical significance of hyperplastic polyps is that they have potential for becoming neoplastic or adenomatous.

Adenomatous polyps may be benign or malignant, and it is difficult to determine the difference unless they have obviously invaded the surrounding mucosa. Smaller growths are called *tubular* or *glandular polyps*, and the larger ones are called *villous adenomas*. Twenty-five to 50 percent of villous adenomas harbor carcinomas. Some researchers see their development as a sequence of events from controlled hyperplasia through a series of stages to terminate in carcinoma [7]. Polyps are usually surgically excised because they have such a close relationship with carcinoma of the colon. In general, the larger the polyp, the greater the risk for malignancy [7].

Carcinoma of the Colon

This disease is second only to lung cancer in causing death from cancer in the United States. When colon and rectal cancer is detected and treated in early localized stages, five-year survival is 80 to 90 percent [1]. Frequently associated with polyposis of the colon, carcinoma of the colon has a familial tendency and may be associated with dietary factors. It is common in both men and women; it occurs at all ages, but frequency is greatest in the fifth, sixth, and seventh decades. Prevalence is greatest in northwest Europe and North America and lowest in South America, Africa, and Asia.

Investigations have led to the study of animal fat in the diet, anaerobic bacteria of the large bowel, and fiber content of the diet [7]. Each of these factors may partially explain the disease's geographic distribution. The fiber aspect is interesting in that increased bulk in the diet decreases the transit time and also the time of contact between food and bowel. In the average American diet, the transit time may be as much as 4 to 5 days compared to 30 to 35 hours in African blacks. Since the American diet is much lower in fiber than the black African diet, colonic cancer is much more prevalent in America [7].

About 70 to 75 percent of these carcinomas arise in the rectum, rectosigmoid area, or sigmoid colon [7]. The type of the growth depends on the area of origin. Left-sided carcinoma tends to grow around the bowel, encircling it and leading to early obstruction. On the right side, the tumors tend to be bulky, polypoid, fungating masses. Either type may penetrate the bowel and cause abscess, peritonitis, invasion of surrounding organs, or bleeding. These tumors do tend to grow slowly, and they remain asymptomatic for long periods of time. Ninety-five percent of carcinomas of the colon are adenocarcinomas that secrete mucin, a substance that aids in extending the malignancy [7]. Metastasis may occur to the liver, lungs, bone, or lymphatic system.

Clinical manifestations depend on the location of the tumor. The person may have melena, diarrhea, and constipation; these are the most frequent manifestations of left-sided lesions. Right-sided tumors often cause weakness, malaise, and weight loss. Pain is rare with either type and, if present, may result from contractions of the bowel related to partial obstruction of the colon or nerve involvement [6]. The tumor mass often is palpated on physical examination. Obstruction of the bowel may be the first sign of the disease. Often at the time of diagnosis some extension of the tumor has occurred, but as this malignancy grows slowly, it is considered to be highly curable with early diagnosis.

Diagnosis requires the standard procedures of proctoscopy, barium enema, radionucleotide scanning, and determination of levels of tumor antigens. Colon cancers produce a wide variety of tumor antigens, carcinoembryonic antigen (CEA) being the most well known. The CEA is positive in nearly 100 percent of cases with widespread metastases. The usefulness of the CEA test is being evaluated because normal levels do not rule out malignancy; however it can gauge the effectiveness of therapy. "Normal" levels of CEA are less than 2.5 ng per ml, but they may be elevated in nonmalignant inflammatory disease, especially of the gastrointestinal tract [11].

Prognosis with colorectal carcinoma depends on the extent of bowel involvement, the presence or absence of spread, differentiation of the lesion, and the location of the lesion within the colon. It is frequently staged by the TNM system as follows [7]:

TIS: carcinoma in situ
T_1: no involvement of the muscle wall, may be polypoid or papillary
T_2: involvement of the muscle wall
T_3: all layers of wall involved with extension to adjacent structures
T_4: same as T_3 with evidence of fistulas
T_5: tumor spread beyond the immediate adjacent area
N: refers to the number of lymphatic nodes involved
M: refers to the evidence of metastasis

Study Questions

1. How can esophagitis be precipitated by chronic vomiting? Describe the pathophysiologic process altering the esophageal mucosa.
2. Discriminate among the causes of peptic ulcerations using precipitating factors, symptoms, and complications as criteria.
3. Support or reject the autoimmune basis theory for regional enteritis and/or ulcerative colitis (it may be helpful to refer to Unit 5).
4. Describe the sequence of events that occurs with paralytic ileus and bowel obstruction. Why is this condition devastating to the individual if it continues for more than 48 hours?
5. Discuss the pathology of carcinoma of the colon. How can this condition be detected in its early stages? What are the indications of metastasis of the tumor?

References

1. *Cancer Facts and Figures, 1986*. New York: American Cancer Society, 1985.
2. Fisher, R.S., and Cohen, S. Gastroesophageal reflux. *Med. Clin. North Am.* 62:3, 1978.
3. Fishman, M.C., et al. *Medicine* (2nd ed.). Philadelphia: Lippincott, 1985.
4. Greenberger, N.J. *Gastrointestinal Disorders: A Pathophysiologic Approach* (3rd ed.). Chicago: Yearbook, 1986.
5. Kissane, J.M. *Anderson's Pathology* (8th ed.). St. Louis: Mosby, 1985.
6. Rankin, R.A., and Welsh, J.D. Gastroenterology. In C.E. Kaufman and S. Papper, *Review of Pathophysiology*. Boston: Little, Brown, 1983.
7. Robbins, S.L., Cotran, R.S., and Kumar, V. *Pathologic Basis of Disease* (3rd ed.). Philadelphia: Saunders, 1984.
8. Sodeman, W.A., and Watson, D.W. The large intestine. In W.A. Sodeman and T.M. Sodeman, *Sodeman's Pathologic Physiology* (7th ed.). Philadelphia: Saunders, 1985.
9. Spiro, H.M. *Clinical Gastroenterology* (3rd ed.). New York: Macmillan, 1985.
10. Stahlgren, L., and Morris, N. Intestinal obstruction. *Am. J. Nurs.* 77:999, 1977.
11. Wallach, J. *Interpretation of Diagnostic Tests* (4th ed.). Boston: Little, Brown, 1986.
12. Watson, D.W., and Sodeman, W.A. The small intestine. In W.A. Sodeman and T.M. Sodeman, *Sodeman's Pathologic Physiology* (7th ed.). Philadelphia: Saunders, 1985.
13. Westergaard, H., and Dietschy, J.M. Normal mechanisms of fat absorption and derangements induced by various diseases. *Med. Clin. North Am.* 58:6, 1974.

CHAPTER 38

Normal Hepatobiliary and Pancreatic Exocrine Function

CHAPTER OUTLINE

Anatomy of the Liver

Physiology of the Liver

- General Information
- Protein Synthesis and Metabolism
  - *Synthesis of Amino Acids*
  - *Amino Acid Metabolism*
  - *Plasma Proteins*
- Fat or Lipid Metabolism
- Carbohydrate Metabolism
- Phagocytosis
- Biotransformation of Foreign Substances
- Bile Synthesis
  - *Bilirubin*
  - *Bile Salts*
  - *Electrolytes*

Major Liver Function Tests

- Serum Enzymes
- Bilirubin
- Plasma Proteins
- Urine Urobilinogen
- Bromsulphalein Excretion
- Liver Scanning (Scintiscans)
- Liver Biopsy
- Computerized Tomography

The Galbladder

Exocrine Pancreatic Function

- Exocrine Pancreatic Secretion
- Nervous and Hormonal Regulation of Pancreatic Secretions
- Protein Digestion
- Fat Digestion
- Carbohydrate Digestion

LEARNING OBJECTIVES

1. Locate the anatomic structures vital to the function of the liver lobule.
2. Describe the structure of the liver sinusoids.
3. Identify the cells of the mononuclear phagocyte system in the sinusoids of the liver.
4. Explain the purpose of the dual blood supply to the liver.
5. Describe the role of the liver in protein synthesis and metabolism.
6. Review the relationship of albumin to the colloid osmotic pressure.
7. Identify the factors necessary for capillary fluid dynamics.
8. State the relationship of protein, ammonia, and urea in the liver.
9. List and describe the purpose of the plasma proteins produced by the liver.
10. Explain why the lymphatic system is important in plasma protein absorption.
11. Outline the role of the liver in fat synthesis and metabolism.
12. Describe how the liver functions in carbohydrate metabolism.
13. Define *proteolysis*, *deamination*, and *transamination*.
14. Describe the oxidative and conjugative reactions that affect drug and hormone metabolism.
15. Explain specifically the effect of alcohol on liver function.
16. Define *hepatotoxin*.
17. Describe the process for the conjugation of bilirubin.
18. List and briefly describe the activities of each of the components of bile.
19. List and describe the major liver function tests.
20. Differentiate briefly between the constituents of liver and gallbladder bile.
21. Describe the hormonal and nervous factors that cause the emptying of the gallbladder.
22. Differentiate between endocrine and exocrine secretions of the pancreas.
23. Delineate specifically the actions of the major enzymes in pancreatic secretions.

Knowledge of the anatomic and functional activities of the liver is essential to understanding the alterations exhibited by the liver in pathologic states. Liver function involves the secretion of bile and the formation of many essential substances. The effects of these activities on all the metabolic processes of other organs are crucial to maintaining a steady balance in the body. Basic reviews of liver anatomy and physiology and the accessory function of the gallbladder and pancreas are included in this chapter. The reader is referred to the comprehensive materials listed in the unit bibliography for additional information.

Anatomy of the Liver

The liver is a large, glandular organ weighing approximately 1.5 kg in the adult. It is composed of two major divisions, the right and left lobes. The right lobe contains two lobes, called the quadrate and caudate lobes. The many units within the lobes that perform the functions of the liver are called the *lobules*. The structure of the liver and blood flow through the lobules are illustrated in Figure 38-1. An admixture of venous and arterial blood within the *sinusoids*, or capillaries, of the lobules provides both oxygen and nutrients to the liver.

The lobules process many substances in the *hepatocytes*, or liver cells. The venous blood supply, carried by a branch of the portal vein, moves highly concentrated foodstuffs, including fats, carbohydrates, and proteins that have been absorbed from the small intestine. The arterial blood supply contains high concentrations of oxygen. The lobules are composed of sinusoids, rows of cuboidal hepatocytes, bile capillaries, and branches of the hepatic artery and portal vein (Fig. 38-2). The sinusoids and surrounding hepatocytes provide a processing plant for the raw materials delivered to the liver from the small intestine.

The sinusoids are lined with cells of the mononuclear phagocyte system, which are called *Kupffer cells*. These cells trap foreign material and function mainly in phagocytosis. The porous endothelial lining allows plasma proteins to pass from the sinusoid to a narrow space around the hepatocyte, which is called the space of Disse [3]. This space connects with the lymphatic system and allows drainage of plasma proteins and excess fluid (Fig. 38-3).

Within the liver lobules are *canaliculi*, which are the receptacles for bile produced by the hepatocytes (see Fig. 38-2). A meshwork of bile ducts forms from the canaliculi and terminates eventually in the common bile duct, which empties into the duodenum during digestion. The gallbladder receives bile from the liver and then stores, concentrates, and releases it into the common bile duct under appropriate stimulation (see p. 601).

The blood supply to the liver is through divisions of the hepatic artery and portal vein, which pass through the complex sinusoidal network to form venules and veins. These finally terminate in the hepatic vein, which empties into the inferior vena cava (see Fig. 38-1). The physiologic tasks that must be performed by the liver require access to a large quantity of the circulation. About 30 percent of cardiac output flows through the liver each minute, making this organ a large reservoir for blood. Even with its large volume and flow, the pressure in the portal system remains low. The liver can distend and increase its volume by a great margin before portal pressure increases [7].

Physiology of the Liver

General Information

The liver performs a wide variety of vital, life-sustaining functions. The hepatocyte is responsible for maintaining these functions through its numerous organelles [4]. It is important in the synthesis and metabolism of protein, carbohydrates, and fats, and also performs the essential function of phagocytosis, which occurs constantly while blood passes through the liver. Many foreign substances, such as pharmacologic agents, are biotransformed as they pass through the liver. Producing and excreting bile, together with processing bilirubin into a form that can be excreted, are essential liver functions. Enzymes are necessary to carry out many activities and these are also synthesized by this organ. Many hormones are biotransformed or inactivated by the liver, which also stores many vitamins and minerals. The major functions of the liver are discussed in the following section.

Protein Synthesis and Metabolism

Proteins are nitrogen-containing constituents of all cells and tissues in the body and are present in all body fluids except bile and urine. Proteins are essential to the formation of the cells, as well as to synthesis of enzymes, hormones, immunoglobulins, and blood cells. All proteins are in a state of constant turnover, making the task of maintaining body functions an awesome one.

The primary function of protein metabolism is to synthesize proteins. Unlike fats and carbohydrates, proteins are not stored, and the size of the amino acid pool is the result of the actual turnover of body proteins and amino acids from exogenous or dietary sources. Protein synthesis depends on the availability of amino acids in the pool at any given time. The ratio of available amino acids is of extreme importance in that every protein is made up of specific amino acids in absolute sequences. If one of these amino acids is absent, synthesis of a specific protein is not possible.

Synthesis of Amino Acids. Of the many amino acids making up human proteins, 10 cannot be synthesized in adequate amounts to meet the body's metabolic needs. These have been termed *essential amino acids (EAAs)* and are available through dietary intake. The EAAs are not all required in the same amounts; rather a ratio is used. Foods that contain proteins with the correct proportion of EAAs have high biologic value. Egg albumin is considered to have a nearly perfect mixture; therefore, all other proteins are compared to that mixture. If one EAA is lacking in the diet, *negative nitrogen balance* results. That is, when one or more essential amino acids are missing

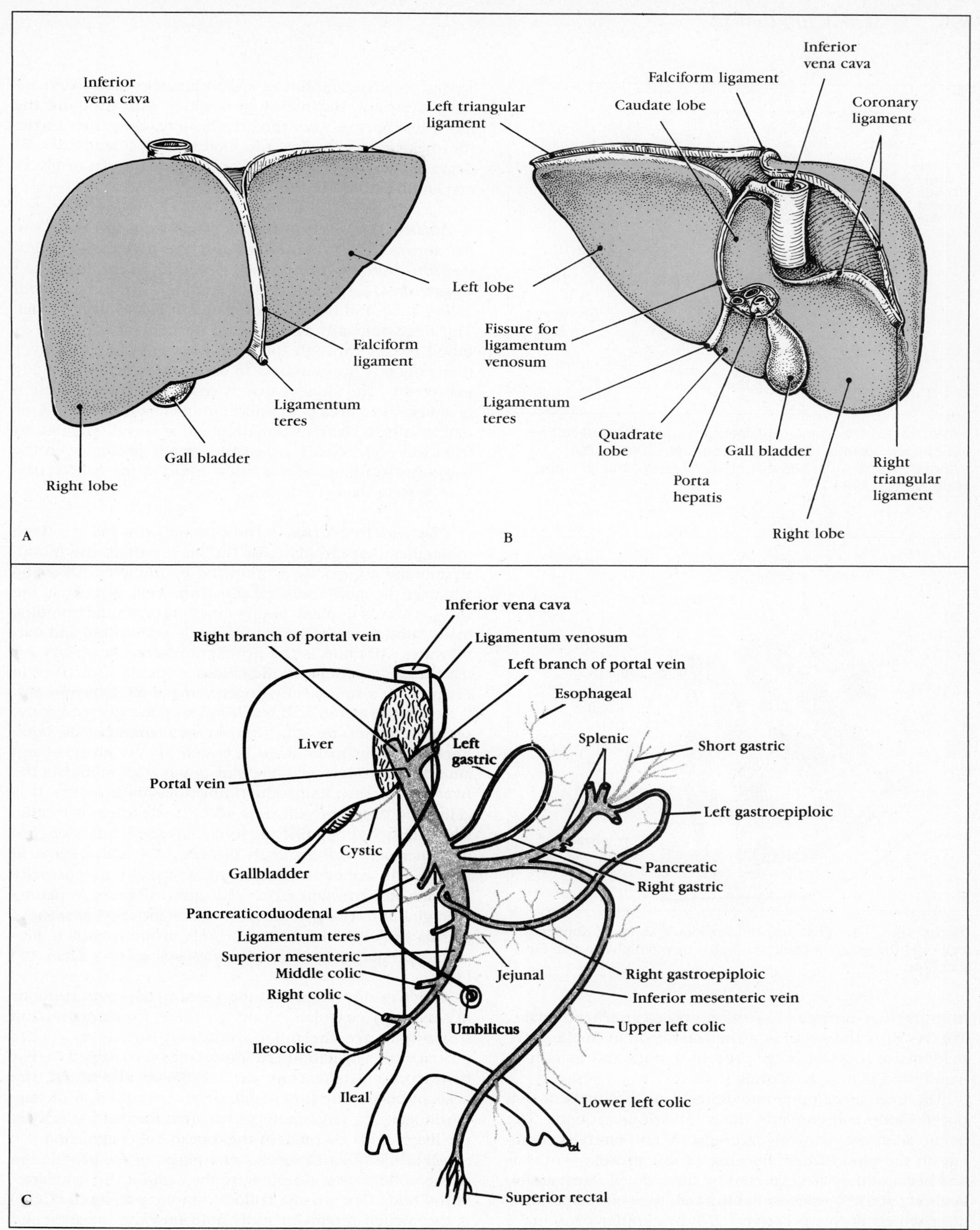

FIGURE 38-1 Macroscopic appearance of the liver. A. Lobes of the liver. B. Posterior surface showing gallbladder and inferior vena cava. C. Blood flow to the liver from the portal vein. (From R.S. Snell, *Clinical Anatomy for Medical Students* [2nd ed.]. Boston: Little, Brown, 1981.)

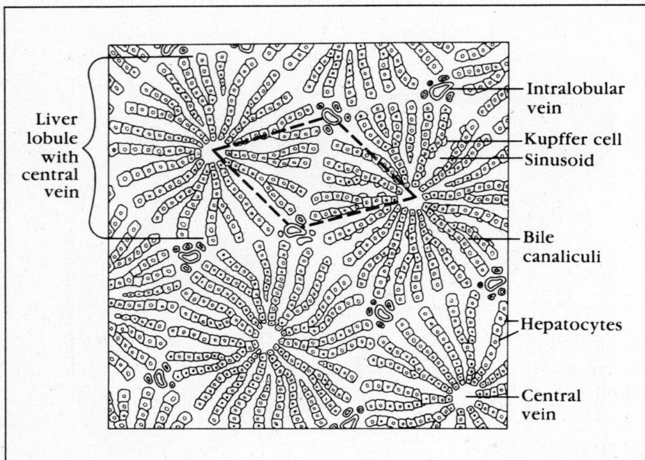

FIGURE 38-2 Schematic diagram of liver lobules. Broken lines indicate liver acinus. (From M. Beyers and S. Dudas, *The Clinical Practice of Medical-Surgical Nursing* [2nd ed.]. Boston: Little, Brown, 1984.)

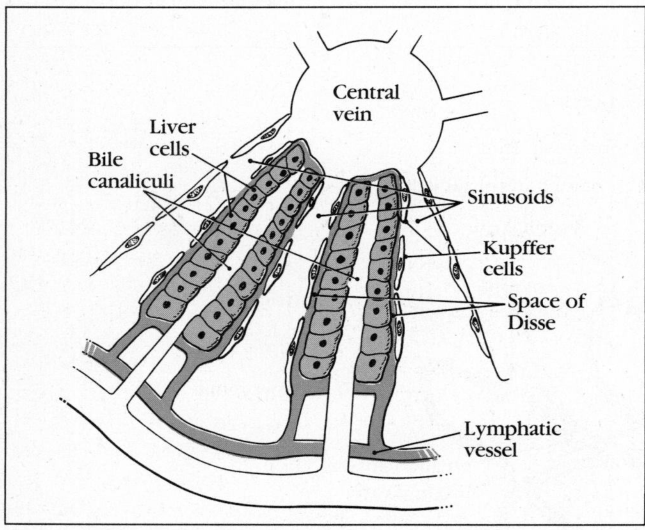

FIGURE 38-3 Another view of liver lobule showing Kupffer cells and the space of Disse through which lymphatic material can flow.

from the diet, nitrogen excretion exceeds nitrogen intake. The result is the same as if the total protein intake were inadequate. Loss of body protein occurs and usually is manifested as muscle wasting [11].

The liver takes up amino acids from the nutrient-rich portal blood and converts them to various proteins. The amino acids are relatively strong acids and rarely accumulate in the bloodstream because of this protein synthesis and because they are excreted by the kidneys. Most amino acids are actively transported through the cell membranes, after which they are converted into cellular proteins, a reaction that requires an enzymatic reaction. These cellular proteins can be broken down rapidly to form amino acids that can be transported out of the cells to the bloodstream [5]. The amount of amino acids in blood remains fairly constant, but may vary slightly with diet and the individual person. After the cells have reached their capacity for storing proteins, the excess amino acids can be degraded and used as energy, or changed into fat or glycogen and be stored in this form [9].

Amino Acid Metabolism. The liver is the major site for amino acid metabolism and the process—called *deamination of amino acids*—results in the formation of ammonia. Large amounts of ammonia are formed from amino acids and from bacterial action in the large bowel. The liver normally removes 80 percent of ammonia as blood passes through the portal system [12]. The liver then converts the ammonia to urea, which is more readily excreted by the kidneys than is ammonia. The conversion of ammonia to urea is an important mechanism of the liver that results in biotransformation and removal of ammonia from the body. Nearly all of the urea is produced in the liver; this substance is much less toxic to the central nervous system than is ammonia.

Plasma Proteins. The plasma proteins are large molecules that circulate for the most part in the bloodstream and are mainly synthesized by the liver. All of the albumin, the most abundant plasma protein, is made in the liver. It serves in many bodily functions, including binding many substances in the plasma; such as bilirubin and barbiturates. Albumin is the principal protein necessary for maintaining colloid osmotic pressure (COP) (described in Chap. 5). It also binds hydrogen ion and alters serum pH.

When the amino acid levels in blood are decreased, the plasma proteins are split to make new amino acids. Equilibrium is thus maintained between plasma proteins and amino acids. Decreased levels of amino acids stimulate the liver to increase its production of plasma proteins. It is estimated that approximately 400 gm of protein is synthesized daily [3]. Significant liver damage leads to hypoproteinemia, which markedly disrupts COP and amino acid levels. The concentration of plasma proteins normally remains at a constant ratio, with more albumin in plasma than globulin. The globulins consist of about 15 percent of plasma proteins and are the protein group to which antibodies produced by B lymphocytes belong (see Chap. 10) [3].

The liver also synthesizes the majority of plasma proteins necessary to coagulate blood. Of these, prothrombin and fibrinogen are the most abundant; however, all the proteins of coagulation are important (see Chap. 17). For prothrombin formation, the liver uses vitamin K, the absorption of which depends on the production of bile. Fibrinogen is a large-molecule protein formed entirely by the liver and is essential in the cascade of coagulation.

All of the plasma proteins participate in the production of the colloid osmotic pressure throughout the capillaries of the body. The plasma colloid osmotic pressure (PCOP) is that which retains or pulls fluid into the intravascular area. Because the plasma proteins are too large to cross the capillary membrane, they remain in increased concentrations at the capillary line and produce an osmotic pressure or pull. This has been described as an inward pressure or force. The level of the PCOP remains constant at the arteriolar, capillary, and venular sections of the capillary, and provides the major force encouraging fluid to return to the capillary and the intravascular area.

Plasma proteins are not easily lost into the interstitial spaces because of their size. When some are leaked into the interstitial area, the only route for return to the bloodstream is through the profuse lymphatic drainage in the interstitial compartment. The lymphatic vessels empty into the lymphatic and thoracic ducts, which empty directly into the superior vena cava.

Fat or Lipid Metabolism

The liver forms almost all of the lipoproteins, which contain mixtures of triglycerides, phospholipids, and cholesterol, as well as protein. These are in the form of high-density lipoproteins (HDL) and very low-density lipoproteins (VLDL), which are discussed on page 616. Cholesterol is used to form bile salts, which are important in the absorption of fats in the small intestine. It is also used to form the steroid hormones.

Ninety-five percent of the fat ingested daily in the American diet is in the form of triglycerides, which contain both saturated and unsaturated fatty acids. The liver can convert carbohydrates or proteins to fat. Insulin causes the movement of glucose into the cell and promotes fat storage if the glucose is not used for energy (see Chap. 35).

Carbohydrate Metabolism

Carbohydrate may be released by the liver in its usable form, glucose, after it has been stored in the form of glycogen. About 5 to 7 percent of normal liver weight is stored glycogen. When blood glucose increases above normal, glycogenesis is stimulated. Glycogenesis is the formation of glycogen from carbohydrate sources, especially glucose. Conversely, when the blood sugar level falls below normal, glycogenolysis is stimulated. Glycogenolysis is the breakdown of glycogen into glucose.

The liver maintains normal blood glucose levels. After a high-carbohydrate meal, an increased amount of carbohydrate is delivered to the liver, where it is stored and released when the blood glucose level begins to drop. The pancreatic hormone *glucagon* is very important in initiating the release of glucose by the liver.

In the process called *gluconeogenesis*, the liver synthesizes glucose from noncarbohydrate substances, especially proteins. Glucose needs that cannot be met from glycogen stores or exogenous sources must be met through this process. This is critically important for the cells that cannot use fat for metabolism—the blood cells and the cells of the kidney medulla. The cells of the central nervous system use glucose preferentially but can adapt to fatty acid oxidation in the form of ketones in two to four days. During fasting, such as between meals and during sleep, the carbon skeleton of amino acids is converted to glucose for energy.

Phagocytosis

The sinusoids of the liver are lined with Kupffer cells, which pick up and destroy foreign material circulating through the liver. The portal vein, which circulates the venous blood from the intestine to the liver, carries a higher concentration of toxins and bacteria than other venous blood because these substances are absorbed when nutrients are absorbed from the intestine.

If the level of bacteria or foreign material in the sinusoids increases, the Kupffer cells become active, proliferate, and destroy the foreign material. This activity is crucial in preventing the spread of pathogens to the systemic circulation.

Biotransformation of Foreign Substances

Destruction, biotransformation, and inactivation of foreign substances are carried out in the hepatocytes, and substances are changed to acceptable forms for excretion. Many of the endocrine secretions are inactivated in the liver, and many pharmacologic agents are biotransformed there. Some substances are *conjugated* in the same way as bilirubin, with glucuronic acid, while others may be inactivated by proteolysis, deamination, or oxidation. *Proteolysis* refers to the breakdown of proteins into simpler substances. *Deamination* means the removal of the amino acids and may involve *transamination* or transfer of this group to another acceptor substance. *Oxidative deamination* causes the release of the amino radical [6].

The oxidative and conjugative reactions promote the biodegradation and/or excretion of foreign substances. It has been found that many drugs affect the reactions of other drugs or hormones and that these interactions, whether they involve speeding up or slowing down the reactions, occur in hepatocytes. An example is the metabolism of warfarin (Coumadin), the effects of which can be potentiated by aspirin. Phenobarbital increases the activity of drug-metabolizing enzymes and hastens the inactivation of warfarin and other agents. Many endogenous hormones, especially corticosterone and aldosterone, are inactivated and conjugated for excretion by the liver. Estrogens impair the secretory activity of the hepatocytes and may alter the results of liver function tests.

Acute alcohol intoxication inhibits drug metabolism by the liver. The chronic alcoholic, however, metabolizes drugs quickly and has an increased tolerance to them, unless there is associated liver failure, which appears to cause decreased drug tolerance. Many drug interactions with alcohol vary according to whether the person is acutely intoxicated or sober. Acute intoxication often potentiates the activity of central nervous system depressants, antihypertensives, antidiabetics, anticoagulants, and antiinflammatory agents [8].

Substances that are directly toxic to liver cells are called *hepatotoxins*. One drug that is a known hepatotoxin in excessive dosages is acetaminophen (Tylenol), which causes centrilobular necrosis due to the exhaustion of the glutathione to which it is normally conjugated. If, in response to an overdose, a glutathione precursor is given, the subject will be protected from permanent liver injury. If no treatment is given, the rate of liver failure after overdose is very high and often fatal.

Most liver damage resulting from foreign substances is due to hypersensitivity reactions by hepatic cells after exposure to drugs. Some drugs cause jaundice; a notable example is chlorpromazine, which causes cholestasis within the liver. Several other drugs can cause parenchymal necrosis; isoniazid and halothane anesthetic are typical examples [8].

Bile Synthesis

Bile is formed by the liver and stored and concentrated by the gallbladder. The liver secretes 250 to 1500 ml of bile per day [1]. The hepatocytes make bile, which is a liquid material normally composed of bilirubin, plasma electrolytes, water, bile salts, bicarbonate, cholesterol, fatty acids, and lecithin.

Bilirubin. Bilirubin is excreted from the body only in the form of *conjugated bilirubin*. Most of the bilirubin is released in the breakdown of red blood cells. The red blood cells give off hemoglobin, which further breaks into its component parts, *heme* and *globin*. The globin portion is a protein that probably returns to the intracellular amino acid pool. The heme portion is broken down further into bilirubin and iron. The iron is either stored in the form of *ferritin* (a combination of a liver protein called apoferritin and iron), or it is used to produce new hemoglobin (Fig. 38-4).

Bilirubin undergoes several reactions and ends up being bound to albumin, on which it travels to the liver. It is called *unconjugated*, *fat-soluble*, or *indirect* bilirubin because it cannot be excreted in bile or through the kidneys. In the liver it is converted on the smooth endoplasmic reticulum to a water-soluble form when it combines with *glucuronic acid* through the intervention of the enzyme *glucuronyl transferase* [4]. In this water-soluble or conjugated form it can be secreted into bile and excreted by the intestine or, in special circumstances, by the kidneys. In the intestine, the intestinal bacteria change the excreted bilirubin to *urobilinogen*. Some of this material is resorbed and reexcreted by the liver. Most of the bilirubin is converted to *stercobilinogen*, which is oxidized to *stercobilin* before being excreted in the feces [3]. Stercobilin and other bile pigments impart the brown color to feces.

In summary, bilirubin must be converted to a conjugated, water-soluble form in order to cross the cell membrane of the hepatocytes and be excreted in bile. In bile duct obstruction, conjugated bilirubin can cross the membrane of the glomeruli and be excreted by the kidneys. Excess bilirubin leads to the condition called jaundice, which is described in detail on pages 606–607.

Bile Salts. The bile salts function as detergents and break fat particles into smaller sizes. They aid in making fat more soluble by forming special complexes called

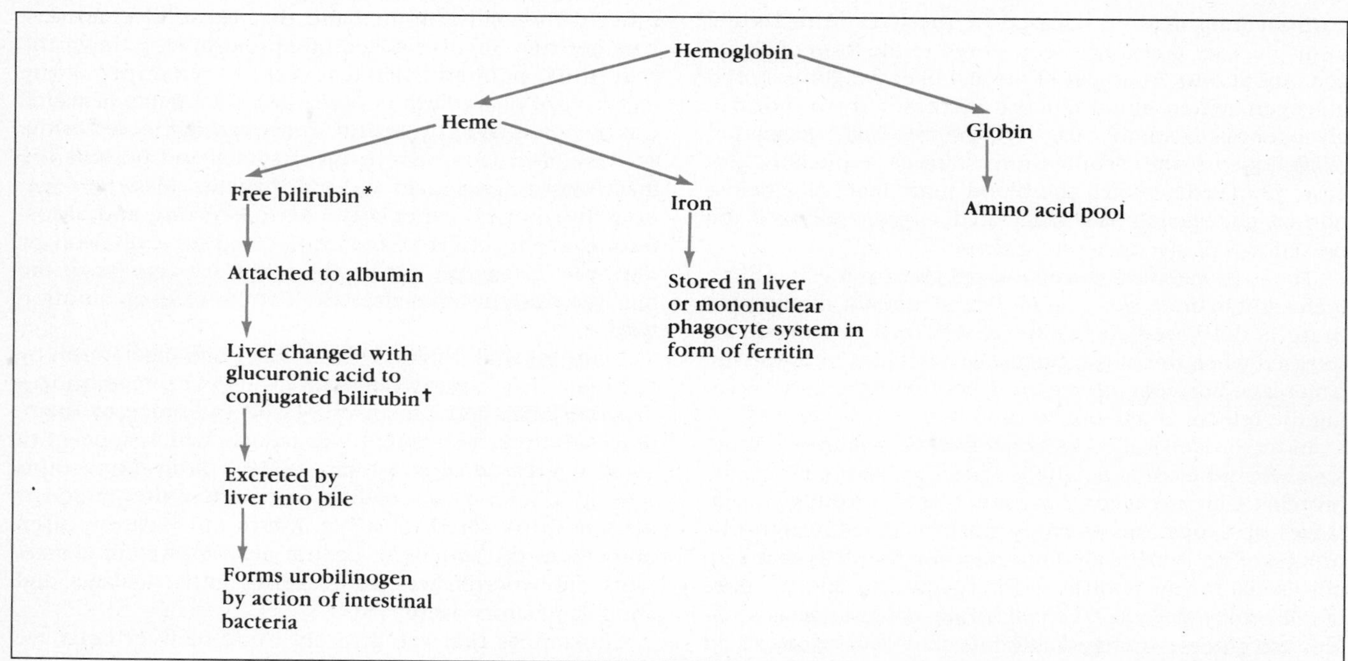

FIGURE 38-4 Fate of hemoglobin. *Free unconjugated, indirect bilirubin persists until the liver changes its form. It is lipid soluble, water insoluble, and nonexcretable. †Conjugated, direct, or bilirubin glucuronide is the form after conjugation with glucuronic acid. It is water soluble, fat insoluble, and excretable.

micelles, which are soluble in the intestinal mucosa. Bile salts are formed by the liver with cholesterol precursors; large amounts can be formed and secreted during periods of increased need. The bile salts are also essential for the absorption of the fat-soluble vitamins A, D, E, and K.

Electrolytes. The electrolytes in bile are to some extent resorbed through the gallbladder mucosa because of the concentrating process that occurs in that organ (see p. 601). Substances that are not absorbed become highly concentrated in the gallbladder bile. For example, liver bile contains about 0.04 gm per dl of bilirubin, while gallbladder bile contains about 0.3 gm per dl. Resorption of water, electrolytes, and free cholesterol in secreted bile occurs in the small intestine. Cholesterol is excreted through the formation of bile salts and directly in the bile. Imbalance can cause excessive cholesterol in bile and may predispose a person to gallstone formation (see p. 615).

Major Liver Function Tests

The major liver function tests provide an index of hepatic function and are helpful in establishing a differential diagnosis in intrahepatic and extrahepatic pathology. The tests are summarized in Table 38-1.

Serum Enzymes

Alkaline phosphatase of the serum is an enzyme that is produced in the liver, kidneys, bone, and other areas, and is excreted in bile. Serum levels are elevated in conditions that increase calcium deposits in bone—viral hepatitis, obstructive jaundice, malignancies, and many other conditions. Serum levels may be decreased in hypoparathyroidism, pernicious anemia, hypothyroidism, and a few other conditions.

Serum glutamic oxaloacetic transaminase (SGOT) is an enzyme that is produced and concentrated in skeletal muscle, cardiac muscle, and liver. It catalyzes certain deamination processes. The SGOT level is increased in acute myocardial infarction, liver disease, muscular diseases, pancreatitis, and other conditions.

Serum glutamic pyruvic transaminase (SGPT) is present in high concentrations in the liver and to a lesser extent, the heart and skeletal muscle. Levels increase with all types of hepatic injury.

Lactic dehydrogenase (LDH) is present in large quantities in liver tissue. Its level is elevated significantly in liver damage and also with cardiac and muscular damage. The level is increased with pulmonary embolus, certain malignancies, pernicious anemia, and others. The LDH isoenzymes are isolated into concentrations of isoenzymes 1 through 5, specific isoenzymes are concentrated in different organs. Isoenzyme LDH-5 is the most specific to liver disease, especially hepatitis.

Serum isocitrate dehydrogenase (ICD) is concentrated in liver tissue. It is elevated in viral hepatitis, infectious mononucleosis, liver poisons, and to some extent, metastatic carcinoma. It is not elevated in acute myocardial infarction, and may be used to differentiate between liver and myocardial disease.

Bilirubin

Bilirubin is measured as a total value and in its conjugated and unconjugated fractions. These evaluations measure the ability of the liver to conjugate and excrete bilirubin in the intestine. A high level of unconjugated bilirubin with a normal or high level of conjugated bilirubin usually indicates significant intrahepatic cellular damage, but this may also occur with hemolytic jaundice. An increase in conjugated bilirubin and a normal or slight increase in unconjugated bilirubin level, especially in the presence of dark urine and light stools, are almost conclusive evidence of biliary obstruction.

Plasma Proteins

Albumin, the most abundant plasma protein, maintains the plasma colloid osmotic pressure, synthesizes specific amino acids, and binds certain molecules for transport from one area to another. Albumin levels are evaluated by a process called electrophoresis. Decreased serum albumin, or hypoalbuminemia, results from severe hepatocellular dysfunction. The result of albumin depression is alteration of COP, leading to systemic edema.

Fibrinogen levels are important in determining the potential for normal blood coagulation. Depletion of this protein occurs in *disseminated intravascular coagulation*, in which precipitation of fibrin in the small vessels and rapid depletion of the clotting factors result (see Chap. 17). Deficiency also is noted in conditions that can cause fibrinolysis, such as hemorrhage, burns, poisoning, and cirrhosis.

The *globulins* are important in the production of antibodies (see Chap. 10). They also act with albumin to maintain intravascular colloid osmotic pressure. Alterations of globulin levels occur with immunosuppression and with chronic inflammations. Elevation or suppression of globulin levels is not a specific sign of liver disease.

Another protein that is measured in liver function screening is *prothrombin*. The prothrombin time reflects the presence of prothrombin, fibrinogen, and other factors. A prolonged prothrombin time (PT) indicates a deficiency of prothrombin and the other clotting factors or impaired uptake of vitamin K. The test measures the factors of the extrinsic system and the common pathway of both extrinsic and intrinsic systems (see Chap. 17). The *partial thromboplastin time (PTT)* measures factors concerned in the intrinsic clotting pathway and the common pathway, and is a good screening test for bleeding disorders. The other clotting factors can be separately measured, and their levels may be altered in liver dysfunction.

Urine Urobilinogen

Small amounts of bilirubin are usually excreted in the urine in the form of urobilirubin. Conjugated bilirubin may be present in urine when an excessive amount is not

TABLE 38-1 Major Liver Function Tests

Test	Normal Level	Abnormalities
Alkaline phosphatase	2–5 BU/ml	↑ Biliary obstruction ↑ Early drug toxicity ↑ Cholestatic hepatitis ↑ Extrahepatic inflammatory condition
Serum glutamic oxaloacetic transaminase (SGOT)	5–40 U/ml	↑ Acute myocardial infarction ↑ Liver damage and most liver disease ↑ Muscle, pancreas, brain, lung, bowel damage ↓ Some severe liver disease ↓ Diabetic ketoacidosis
Serum glutamic pyruvic transaminase (SGPT)	5–35 U/ml	↑ Markedly in liver necrosis and acute hepatitis ↑ Slightly in myocardial infarction ↑ Pulmonary, renal, pancreatic injury ↑ Slightly in cirrhosis and chronic liver disease
Lactic dehydrogenase (LDH)	200–680 U/ml	↑ Cardiac injury ↑ Hepatitis, especially LDH isoenzyme 5 ↑ Malignant tumors ↑ Muscle, pulmonary, and renal disease
Serum isocitrate dehydrogenase (ICD)	50–180 Sigma U/ml	↑ Markedly in liver disease
Bilirubin		
Total	0.2–0.9 mg/dl	↑ Hepatocellular necrosis or damage
Direct	0.1–0.4 mg/dl	↑ Cholestasis due to obstruction
Indirect	0.1–0.5 mg/dl	↑ Hemolytic anemia
Plasma proteins		
Total	6–8 gm/dl	↓ Severe liver disease
Albumin	3.5–5.5 gm/dl	↓ Pyelonephritis and nephrosis
Globulin	1.5–3.0 gm/dl	↓ Malnutrition and protein lack ↓ Chronic inflammation
Fibrinogen	0.2–0.4 gm/dl	↓ Disseminated intravascular coagulation ↓ Congenital afibrinogenemia ↓ With depletion of other coagulation factors ↓ With major alteration of hemodynamics in body, e.g., circulatory shock

Note: ↑ = test results are increased in these conditions; ↓ = test results are decreased in these conditions.

being cleared from the plasma. This finding is common in obstructive biliary tract disease and severe cirrhosis of the liver.

Bromsulphalein Excretion

This test measures the ability of the liver to remove a dye from the circulation. Liver injury is probable when more than 10 percent of injected dye remains in circulation after 45 minutes.

Liver Scanning (Scintiscans)

Scans are performed to visualize the position, shape, size, and structure of the liver. They involve injecting radiopharmaceutical isotopes, which are taken up by hepatocytes, Kupffer cells, or neoplasms. Several scanning procedures are used, with some isotopes concentrating in neoplasms or in areas of inflammation, and others concentrating in the hepatocytes; areas of abscess or tumor produce a void in the scan.

In reading the liver scan, one looks for areas of increased or no uptake, depending on the isotope used. Agents that are excreted in the bile can be followed for bile duct obstruction, while those having affinity for mononuclear phagocytes are concentrated in the spleen. Changes in the liver scan can also assist in following the course of cirrhosis. Persons with early hepatomegaly have even distribution of the radiopharmaceutical agent. As the disease progresses, the left lobe of the liver enlarges, the right lobe becomes smaller, and the spleen takes up increased amounts. As liver failure progresses there may be a spotty appearance due to the fibrosis dividing the lobules.

Liver Biopsy

Liver biopsy is performed to make a precise diagnosis of liver disease. It can be beneficial in the diagnosis of hepatitis, cirrhosis, and sometimes, primary neoplasms. It may be performed as open biopsy during a surgical procedure or as a needle biopsy using a percutaneous intercostal approach. In the latter, the material aspirated from the

TABLE 38-1 continued

Test	Normal Level	Abnormalities
Prothrombin time	11–16 seconds (control); 80–100% of control	↑ (Prolonged) severe liver disease, especially cirrhosis ↑ Fibrinogen deficiency ↑ Warfarin therapy ↑ Biliary destruction
Partial thromboplastin time	22–37 seconds	↑ (Prolonged) in bleeding disorders, especially of the intrinsic pathway ↑ Heparin therapy ↑ Cirrhosis and severe liver disease
Urine bilirubin	0 mg/24°	↑ Biliary obstruction ↑ Cirrhosis ↑ Hepatitis
Urine urobilinogen	0–4 mg/24°	↓ Biliary obstruction Normal or ↑ cirrhosis
Bromsulphalein (BSP) excretion	5% retention after 45 minutes	↑ Fever ↑ All types liver disease ↑ Specific drugs, e.g., morphine ↑ Acute cholecystitis ↑ GI bleeding
Liver scans		
Colloidal	Uptake of colloid by Kupffer cells	Demonstrates large defects; false negative result with small defects
Rose bengal	Uptake of dye by hepatocytes	Area of reduced intake, "hole" in neoplastic or inflammatory cells
Gallium	Little uptake of dye by normal cells	Uptake by neoplastic and inflammatory cells
Liver biopsy	Normal hepatocytes	Specific pathology of any material sampled; diagnostic of cirrhosis, malignancy, hepatitis, etc.
Computerized tomography	Normal integrity on image of intraabdominal organs	Fluid collections in liver differentiated from tumors; gallbladder or duct enlargement visualized

needle is examined histologically for abnormalities. Accurate placement of the needle is imperative for precise diagnosis. Care must be exerted to prevent laceration of the liver and consequent hemorrhage.

Computerized Tomography

This popular procedure provides a radiologic image of the abdominal organs without the need to inject dyes or isotopes. It helps in initial evaluation of liver disease in differentiating fluid-filled from tumor-filled lesions. The appearance of the surrounding organs and ducts can also be assessed. It is a sensitive scan for determining metastases of primary malignancies, but less so for fluid-filled bile ducts [4].

The Gallbladder

The gallbladder is a saclike organ that is attached to the inferior portion of the liver. It receives bile from the liver that has been diverted from the common bile duct (Fig. 38-5). The liver secretes about 700 ml of bile, which flows continuously through the bile duct to the intestine. This flow, called *choleresis*, is increased after meals [1]. The gallbladder's maximum volume is 40 to 70 ml, but its bile is 5 to 10 times more concentrated than that of the liver. Approximately 90 percent of the water content of gallbladder bile is continually absorbed by the mucosa. Its electrolyte composition includes an increased concentration of potassium and calcium and a decreased amount of chloride and bicarbonate as compared to liver bile [2,3]. The gallbladder is composed of folds and rugae and can increase its size to accommodate incoming bile.

The gallbladder empties its bile into the common bile duct when a stimulus is received. The major stimulus for this is cholecystokinin (CCK), a hormone secreted from the duodenal mucosa when fat-containing foods arrive in that area. The CCK causes bile to move into the intestine by causing contractions of the gallbladder and relaxation of the sphincter of Oddi [1]. The gallbladder also receives stimulation from the autonomic nervous system. The parasympathetic division is the major mediator for con-

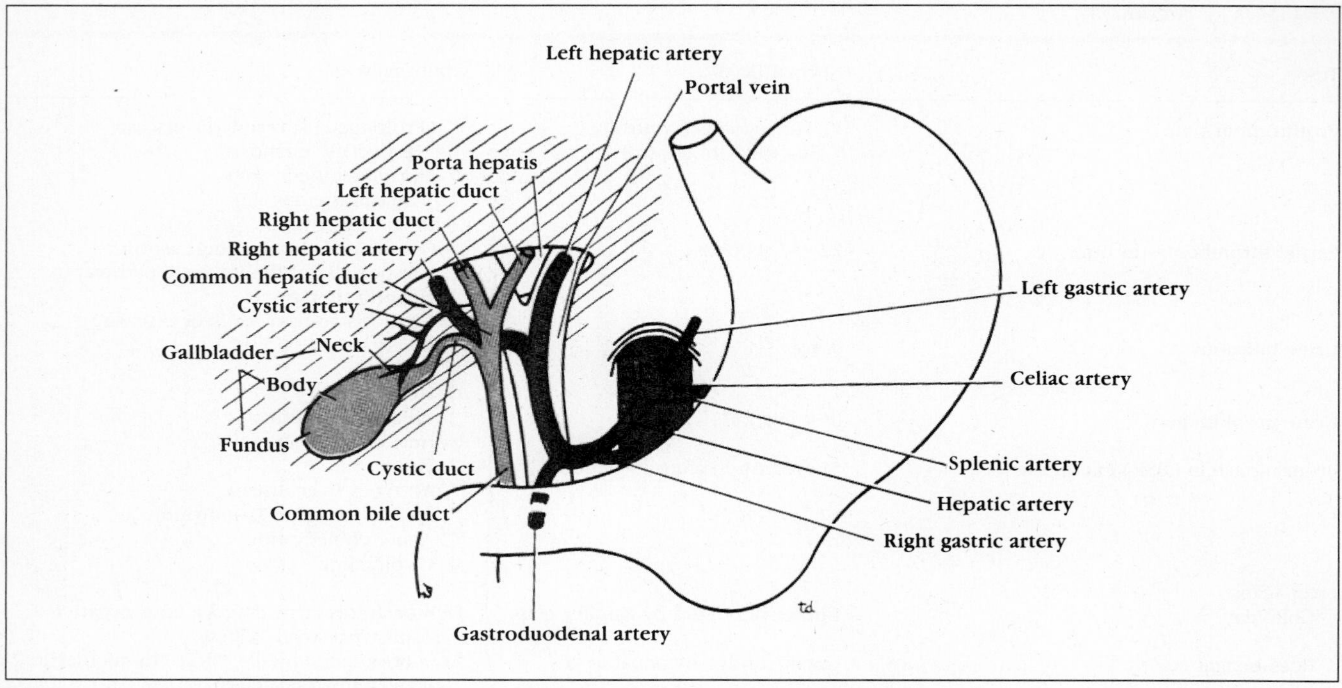

FIGURE 38-5 Appearance and location of gallbladder. (From R.S. Snell, *Clinical Anatomy for Medical Students* [2nd ed.]. Boston: Little, Brown, 1981.)

traction of the gallbladder, while stimulation of the sympathetic division causes relaxation of the organ.

Alterations in function of the gallbladder are discussed in Chapter 39. Gallstones and inflammation of the gallbladder are common causes of abdominal pain.

Exocrine Pancreatic Function

The pancreas is a large organ that lies behind the stomach and extends between the spleen and the duodenum. It is composed of a head, a body, and a tail, which contain the acinar cells and the cells of the islets of Langerhans (Fig. 38-6). The exocrine acinar cells secrete digestive juices, while the endocrine islet cells secrete hormones that are essential in glucose metabolism. The exocrine functions, or those related to digestion, involve the secretion of pancreatic juice into a system of ducts that empty into the pancreatic duct and, in turn, the ampulla of Vater. Pathologic alterations in the pancreas are discussed in Chapter 35.

Exocrine Pancreatic Secretion

The cells of the pancreas that secrete pancreatic juice are *acinar cells*. The secretion is composed of an alkaline component and enzymes necessary for digesting proteins, fats, and carbohydrates. The alkaline component contains sufficient bicarbonate ion to give the pancreatic juice a pH of about 8. The pancreas can secrete up to 4000 ml of fluid daily [7]. The enzymes are made by the acinar cells and stored until stimulated for release. The enzymes contained in the secretion are (1) *amylase*, which hydrolyses carbohydrates to disaccharides; (2) *pancreatic lipase*, which hydrolyses fats to yield glycerol and fatty acids; and (3) the *preproteolytic enzymes*, mainly trypsinogen and chymotrypsinogen, which, when activated, hydrolyze

TABLE 38-2 Enzymes of Mammalian Pancreatic Secretion

Zymogen	Enzyme	Activator
Trypsinogen	Trypsin	Enterokinase, Ca^{++}, trypsin
Chymotrypsinogen	Chymotrypsin	Trypsin
Procarboxypeptidase A	Carboxypeptidase A	Trypsin
Procarboxypeptidase B	Carboxypeptidase B	Trypsin
Proelastase	Elastase	Trypsin
Proelastomucase	Elastomucase	Trypsin
	Amylase	Chloride
	Lipase	Emulsifying agents
	Esterase	Bile salts
Prophospholipase A	Phospholipase A	Bile salts Trypsin
	Cholesterol esterase	Bile salts

Source: Reprinted from *Sophomore Introduction to Medicine* by J.R. Meadows. Gastroenterology Section, Department of Medicine, Indiana University School of Medicine, 1978, p. 74. Reprinted by permission of the author.

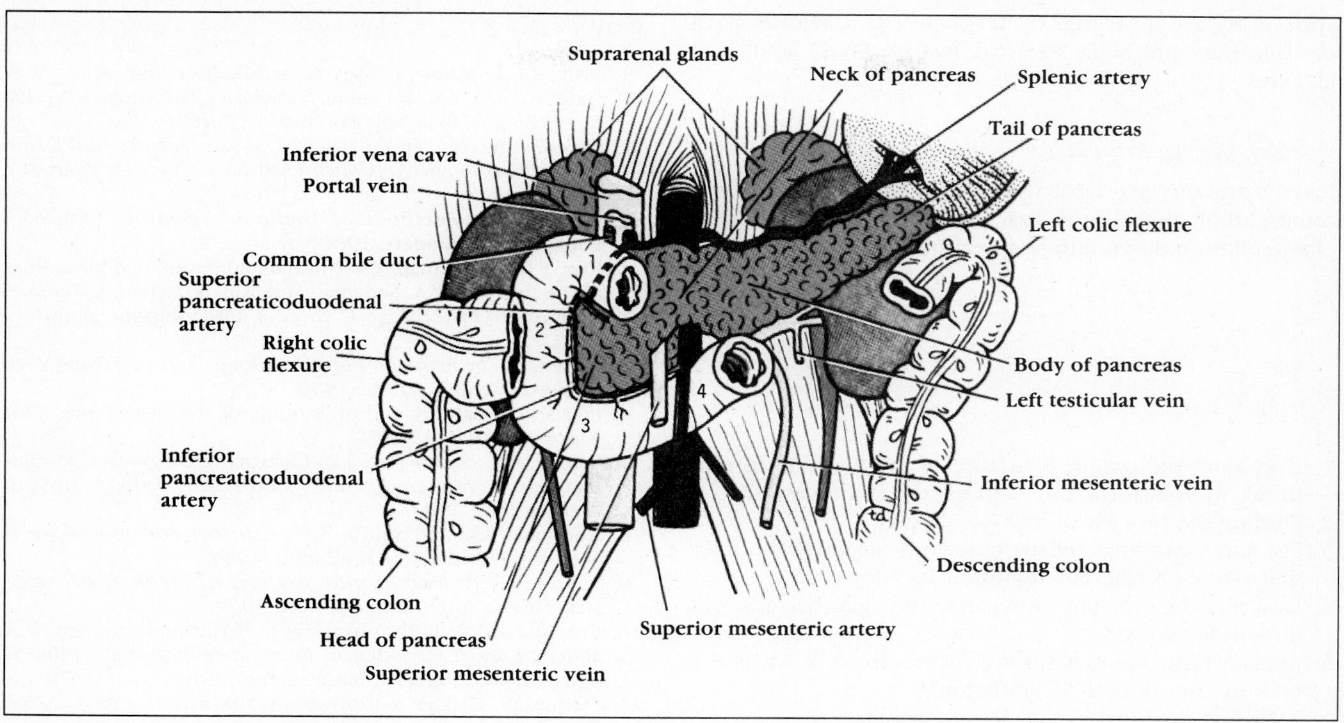

FIGURE 38-6 Appearance and location of the pancreas. (From R.S. Snell, *Clinical Anatomy for Medical Students* [2nd ed.]. Boston: Little, Brown, 1981.)

proteins to amino acids. Table 38-2 summarizes the enzymes and proenzymes of pancreatic secretions.

Nervous and Hormonal Regulation of Pancreatic Secretions

Nervous stimulation of the pancreas is mainly through the vagus nerve, which transmits impulses to the pancreas during the cephalic and gastric phases of digestion. This results in the secretion of enzymes by the acinar cells. The nervous influences also affect the secretion of the endocrine islet cells.

The hormonal mechanisms are mainly mediated through *secretin* and *cholecystokinin*. When chyme containing fat and/or amino acids comes into contact with the mucosal cells of the duodenum, the hormone is released, causing the pancreas to secrete large amounts of fluids with large amounts of bicarbonate and few or no enzymes. This alkaline secretion neutralizes the highly acid gastric juice emptied into the duodenum from the stomach, stops the activity of gastrin, and provides an alkalinity of about pH 7, which is optimal for pancreatic enzyme activity. Cholecystokinin also is released from the intestinal mucosa in the presence of food, and increases the secretion of pancreatic enzymes from the acinar cells. Distention of the intestinal wall by food is the apparent stimulus for the release of CCK.

Protein Digestion

Trypsinogen is converted to the active enzyme trypsin in an alkaline medium through the action of *enterokinase*, which is released by the intestinal mucosa when it comes into contact with chyme. Trypsin then activates other trypsinogen molecules and triggers the conversion of chymotrypsinogen into chymotrypsin. These proteolytic enzymes can split proteins into amino acids for absorption in the intestine.

The most important protective mechanisms to prevent digestion of the pancreas by the enzymes it secretes are synthesis of enzymes in an inactive form and the presence of a *trypsin inhibitor* that is secreted by the same cells that secrete the pancreatic enzymes. This trypsin inhibitor is stored in the cytoplasm of the cells surrounding the enzyme granules and prevents the activation of trypsin, thus preventing activation of the other proteolytic enzymes. When the pancreas becomes damaged or when a duct is blocked, pancreatic secretions accumulate. It is hypothesized that the trypsin inhibitor is overwhelmed and the pancreatic enzymes become activated to cause acute pancreatitis [3].

Fat Digestion

Pancreatic lipase is an important ingredient for fat breakdown. There are several forms of pancreatic lipase that apparently are activated by trypsin [10]. It works with the bile salts and helps to break fats into fatty acids and glycerol.

Carbohydrate Digestion

Pancreatic amylase hydrolyzes starches, glycogen, and other carbohydrates into disaccharides. It does not break plant cellulose down into simpler substances.

Study Questions

1. How does the unique structure of the liver aid in synthesis, biotransformation, and excretion of wastes?
2. Outline the process of bile formation.
3. List some essential substances synthesized by the liver that are not formed in any other location.
4. Describe the concept of negative nitrogen balance and how it develops.
5. Explain how amino acids are metabolized. What is the end product of their degradation?
6. What are the purposes of plasma proteins?
7. What are the functions of bile salts?
8. Discuss the role of bile and pancreatic secretions in digestion.

References

1. Bolt, R.J. Pathophysiology of gallbladder disease. In W.A. Sodeman and T.M. Sodeman, *Sodeman's Pathologic Physiology* (7th ed.). Philadelphia: Saunders, 1985.
2. Greenberger, N.J., and Wenship, D.H. *Gastrointestinal Disorders: A Pathologic Approach* (3rd ed.). Chicago: Yearbook, 1986.
3. Guyton, A.C. *Textbook of Medical Physiology* (7th ed.). Philadelphia: Saunders, 1986.
4. Iber, F.L., and Lathan, P.S. Normal and pathologic physiology of the liver. In W.A. Sodeman and T.M. Sodeman, *Sodeman's Pathologic Physiology* (7th ed.). Philadelphia: Saunders, 1985.
5. Jensen, D. *The Principles of Physiology* (2nd ed.). New York: Appleton-Century-Crofts, 1980.
6. Pierce, L. Anatomy and physiology of the liver. *Nurs. Clin. North Am.* 12:259, 1977.
7. Rankin, R.A., and Welsh, J.D. Gastroenterology. In C.E. Kaufman and S. Papper, *Review of Pathophysiology*. Boston: Little, Brown, 1983.
8. Rodman, M.J., and Smith, R.W. *Clinical Pharmacology in Nursing*. Philadelphia: Lippincott, 1984.
9. Schneider, H. *Nutritional Support of Medical Practice*. Hagerstown, Md.: Harper & Row, 1977.
10. Snodgrass, P.J. Pathophysiology of the pancreas. In W.A. Sodeman and T.M. Sodeman, *Sodeman's Pathologic Physiology* (7th ed.). Philadelphia: Saunders, 1985.
11. Steffee, W. Cancer and protein malnutrition. *Compr. Ther.* 3:30, 1977.
12. Zakim, D. Pathophysiology of liver disease. In L.H. Smith and S.O. Thier (eds.), *Pathophysiology: The Biological Principles of Disease* (2nd ed.). Philadelphia: Saunders, 1985.

CHAPTER 39

Alterations in Hepatobiliary Function

CHAPTER OUTLINE

General Considerations in Liver Dysfunction

- Jaundice
  - *Impairment of Uptake, Conjugation, or Secretion of Bilirubin*
  - *Excessive Destruction of Red Blood Cells*
  - *Obstructive Jaundice*
- Ascites
- Fatty Liver
- Clotting Disturbances
- Portal Hypertension and Esophageal Varices
- Hepatorenal Syndrome
- Liver Failure
- Hepatic Encephalopathy and Coma
- Drug-Related Liver Damage

Cirrhosis of the Liver

- Biliary Cirrhosis
- Postnecrotic Cirrhosis
- Alcoholic (Laennec's) Cirrhosis

Cancer of the Liver

- Primary Malignancies
- Metastatic Carcinoma

Viral Hepatitis

- Hepatitis A
- Hepatitis B
- Immunologic Features
- Pathologic Features
- Clinical Course
- Delta Hepatitis
- Non-A, Non-B Hepatitis

Gallbladder Disease

- Cholecystitis and Cholelithiasis
  - *Clinical Manifestations*
  - *Diagnosis*

Obesity: A Major Disturbance in Nutritional Balance

- Lipid Transport
- Problems with Excess Fat Production and Storage

LEARNING OBJECTIVES

1. Define and describe *jaundice* and its etiology and physiologic effects.
2. Explain how ascites can result from liver failure.
3. Describe the pathologic appearance of fatty liver.
4. Define *portal hypertension*.
5. Relate esophageal varices to portal hypertension.
6. Define *hepatorenal syndrome*.
7. List the physiologic changes of liver failure.
8. Describe how hepatic encephalopathy and coma can result from liver failure.
9. Explain the major pathologic features of cirrhosis of the liver.
10. Define *alcoholic hepatitis*.
11. Differentiate between primary and metastatic carcinoma of the liver.
12. Discuss the etiology, incubation, pathology, and clinical features of hepatitis A and B.
13. Define *cholelithiasis* and *cholecystitis*.
14. List the major constituents of biliary tract stones.
15. Describe the clinical manifestations of biliary obstruction.
16. Define *obesity*.
17. Differentiate between adult-onset and juvenile obesity in relationship to accumulation of fat cells.
18. Describe the major source of lipids and how lipids are transported and metabolized.
19. List at least five chronic health problems that are associated with obesity.

As described in Chapter 38, the liver has a wide range of intricate metabolic functions. Its large reserve accounts for the lack of clinical signs of dysfunction until large portions of the organ are greatly diseased or damaged. It is estimated that 10 percent of liver function is necessary to sustain life.

This chapter organizes liver and gallbladder dysfunction into general effects of alterations and how these effects apply to specific diseases. Common alterations in liver and gallbladder function are included, as is obesity resulting from excessive fat metabolism.

General Considerations in Liver Dysfunction

Jaundice

Jaundice (icterus) refers to the yellowish or greenish hue imparted to a person's skin by something that disturbs the flow of bile or bilirubin (bile pigment). Bilirubin may accumulate in its unconjugated or conjugated form, staining the skin, sclerae, and all the tissues of the body. The four major types of jaundice result from impairment of uptake, conjugation, or secretion of bilirubin; excessive destruction of red blood cells; and obstructive conditions [9]. The two most common causes are lysis of red blood cells and obstruction of the bile ducts or liver cells.

Impairment of Uptake, Conjugation, or Secretion of Bilirubin. Neonatal jaundice may occur when there is a deficiency of *glucuronyl transferase*, an enzyme necessary for the conjugation of bilirubin with glucuronic acid. Frequently occurring in premature infants, this impairment has been successfully treated with phenobarbital, which stimulates the essential enzymatic reaction. Improvement in the degree of jaundice usually occurs within days to weeks. In a related condition, the *Crigler-Najjar syndrome*, glucuronal transferase activity is congenitally absent and unconjugated bilirubin accumulates and crosses the blood-brain barrier. The result is *kernicterus*, which is the deposition of pigment in the basal ganglia of the brain, causing brain damage. Kernicterus only occurs in premature or newborn infants, because the blood-brain barrier develops impermeability to bilirubin during early infancy.

Impaired uptake of bilirubin that interferes with its conjugation may cause jaundice. Decreased uptake by the hepatic cells is probably due to lack of sufficient glucuronyl transferase to effect the release of the unconjugated bilirubin from the albumin on which it has been carried. This is usually a benign, familial condition, called *Gilbert's syndrome*, and occurs in up to 5 percent of the male population [7]. It creates significant jaundice when stress increases both the metabolism of bilirubin and the need for conjugation. Two types of Gilbert's syndrome have been described, one that involves decreased bilirubin clearance, especially with fasting, and one in which hemolysis can be demonstrated. The first type is more common and has few clinical side effects except for transient jaundice.

Excessive Destruction of Red Blood Cells. Excessive destruction of red blood cells causes jaundice through hemolysis. The red blood cells break down into hemoglobin and red cell fragments. Hemoglobin is processed further to heme and globin, as described on page 220, releasing free, unconjugated bilirubin into the plasma. Hemolysis can occur with blood transfusion reactions, after cardiopulmonary bypass, in sickle cell anemia, in marrow destruction of red blood cells, and with some pharmacologic agents. The blood transfusion reaction involves an antigen-antibody reaction to the donor red cells. The red cells are destroyed in an acute hemolytic reaction.

In *sickle cell anemia*, abnormal hemoglobin and a fragile cell membrane lead to hemolysis and an increase in the amount of free unconjugated bilirubin in plasma. The precipitating cause of hemolysis is usually hypoxemia, leading to sickling of the red cell and fragmentation as it passes through tight spaces (see Chap. 15). The liver retains the capability to conjugate bilirubin but it becomes overwhelmed with the free bilirubin and cannot conjugate all that is sent to it.

Bone marrow disease leads to destruction of red blood cells before they leave the marrow. This can be caused by thalassemia and by some pharmacologic agents. Levels of either or both unconjugated and conjugated bilirubin may be elevated. Generally classified as bone marrow developmental problems, or *defective erythropoiesis*, are conditions in which the erythrocytes, poorly manufactured, are fragile and have a short life span. These cells hemolyze as they pass through the pulp of the spleen and other tight spaces. The result is that an excess of unconjugated bilirubin reaches the liver for conjugation.

Many drugs can cause hemolysis from drug-induced, defective erythropoiesis or as a side effect of the drug. Hemolysis usually results from a hypersensitivity reaction to the drug. Some examples of implicated drugs include chlorpromazine (Thorazine), quinidine, phenacetin (acetophenetidin), sulfonamides, penicillins, cephalosporins, and insulin. Thalassemias are a group of congenital diseases in which defective synthesis of hemoglobin leads to an increased propensity for hemolysis.

Obstructive Jaundice. Three types of obstructive jaundice have been described: (1) intrahepatic block, or failure of the hepatocytes to function; (2) prehepatic block, in which unconjugated bilirubin is not being circulated through the liver because of obstruction in the extrahepatic circulation; and (3) posthepatic block, which commonly results from cholestasis as a result of cholecystitis or cholelithiasis.

Intrahepatic obstruction frequently occurs with hepatitis and hepatocellular failure from cirrhotic fibrosis or hepatic scarring. Some pharmaceutic agents, such as the oral contraceptives and chlorpropamide (Diabenase), have been shown to cause intracellular damage and blockage in certain persons.

Extrahepatic obstructive conditions in adults include gallstones, malignancies of intrahepatic or extrahepatic source, surgical obstruction of the ampulla of Vater, and others. Obstruction in infancy most commonly results from congenital atresia of the biliary tree [7]. The obstruction limits the excretion of bilirubin in the bile, and an excess of conjugated bilirubin accumulates [9].

The physiologic effects of obstruction depend on the ability of the liver to conjugate and excrete bilirubin. When the source of jaundice is hepatocellular failure, increased serum levels of unconjugated bilirubin often result due to failure of hepatocytes to produce conjugated bilirubin. Extrahepatic obstruction causes increased levels of conjugated bilirubin with excretion of bilirubin in the urine. As the liver becomes engorged with bilirubin, the activity of the hepatocytes diminishes and the serum unconjugated and conjugated bilirubin levels increase.

Jaundice, caused by conjugated or unconjugated bilirubin, is important in establishing the source and sometimes the severity of the causative condition. Deposition of pigments in the skin lead to the yellowish or greenish discoloration, which may be most noticeable in the sclerae of the eyes. In neonates, increased bilirubin levels may lead to kernicterus and neurologic impairment. In adults, the degree of jaundice often correlates with the severity of liver dysfunction. Assessment of the degree of jaundice is difficult in dark skinned individuals, but intense yellowish discoloration can be seen in the sclerae.

Ascites

Ascites is the accumulation of fluid in the peritoneal cavity, which usually results directly from increasing portal pressure and/or decreasing plasma protein levels. Sodium retention as a result of aldosterone retention and excessive lymphatic flow may add to the amount of ascitic fluid. Figure 39-1 illustrates the factors that can contribute to the development of ascites.

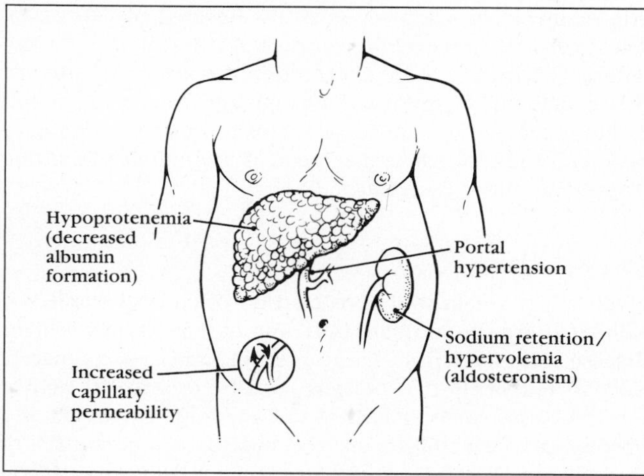

FIGURE 39-1 Factors contributing to the development of ascites.

Portal hypertension, or increased pressure in the portal venous system, can occur because of an intrahepatic block to blood flow through the liver. The resultant increase in capillary pressure leads to disruption of the normal osmotic force at the capillary line, pushing fluid into the peritoneal cavity.

Decreased plasma proteins, especially albumin, lead to a reduction in the plasma colloid pressure, which decreases the inward forces, or in the resorption pressures, further encouraging fluid to pass into the peritoneal space. Albumin synthesis is depressed in conditions of liver failure.

The ascitic fluid, or transudate, contains large quantities of albumin, the loss of which results in further hypoalbuminemia. Complicating this process is a decrease or depletion of central blood volume as the amount of ascitic fluid increases. As a compensatory mechanism, the body increases the secretion of aldosterone from the adrenal cortex, which leads to retention of sodium and water. The retention indirectly provides more available fluid and increased ascites.

Antidiuretic hormone (ADH), which is synthesized by the hypothalamus and released by the posterior pituitary, also is secreted in greater quantities when the central blood volume is depleted. Increases in renal tubular water resorption and blood volume result.

It is probable that elevated intrasinusoidal pressure within the liver associated with cirrhosis leads to an increase in the lymphatic flow, which, by oozing lymph fluid from the hepatic surface, causes increases in the ascitic fluid and in its protein concentration [9].

Other factors may potentiate this condition, but positive feedback results; the compensatory efforts of the body end up being self-defeating and lead away from the steady state. Without intervention, the course progressively degenerates, leading to greater ascites.

Ascites causes abdominal swelling that is noted as increased girth. The extra intraabdominal fluid may cause pressure on the diaphragm and respiratory difficulties. Ascitic fluid may be removed by peritoneal tapping, but it frequently reaccumulates rapidly. The associated hypoproteinemia may lead to further ascites together with production of generalized edema, or *anasarca*. It results mostly from a decrease in the plasma colloid osmotic pressure generated from the decreased albumin levels, encouraging fluid exudation into all of the interstitial compartments.

Fatty Liver

Fatty liver refers to infiltration of hepatocytes by fat or lipid material. This infiltration by itself usually does not significantly disrupt the physiologic processes of the cells, but over time the fatty cells become surrounded by fibrous tissue that separates the liver lobules. The pathologic appearance may be either micronodular or macronodular. Micronodular infiltration can only be seen with a high-intensity microscope, but macronodular lobules have fat infiltration and fibrosis that are visible grossly.

Several factors influence the deposition of fat. A diet high in fat may overwhelm the metabolic activity of the liver, leading to increased triglyceride stores. A diet with too little protein, such as with starvation, leads to mobilization of fatty acids from adipose tissue. Fatty acids then travel to the liver and infiltrate the hepatocytes. Alcoholism leads to fat accumulation in the parenchymal cells of the liver and distention of the cytoplasm with fat. In certain areas, the infiltrated cells undergo fibrosis, which increases the likelihood of portal hypertension.

Whether alcohol is a direct hepatotoxin or a producer of nutritional inadequacy has been studied. The weight of the evidence supports the claim that it is hepatotoxic (see Chap. 3). Large amounts of alcohol have been demonstrated to increase accumulation of lipids within the cells, resulting in a liver that weighs 2.0 to 2.5 kg (normal weight is about 1.5 kg) and appears soft and greasy when cut [9]. Alcohol may affect the conversion of fatty acids to lipoproteins in the liver, but the mechanism for its induction is not precisely known.

Clotting Disturbances

Because the liver produces many of the major clotting factors, liver dysfunction of 60 percent or more leads to depletion of these factors and a tendency to bleed. A decrease in the uptake of vitamin K into hepatocytes leads to defective synthesis of factors II (prothrombin), VII (proconvertin), IX (Christmas factor), and X (Stuart-Prower factor) [10]. Vitamin K deficiency may result from fat malsorption when bile amounts are inadequate. The major clotting dysfunction results from depressed production of prothrombin, and other clotting factors may also be depressed.

Deficiency in clotting factors is noted in laboratory tests because these factors have a short half-life in blood. Albumin synthesis may be depressed for a period of time before it is noted in laboratory values because it has a long half-life [10]. The platelet count may be inadequate as a result of hypersplenism, which is a frequent companion of liver failure. The hypersplenism results from congestion caused by the portal hypertension [9]. In liver failure an increased risk of hemorrhage is always present, especially when it is associated with esophageal varices and portal hypertension.

Portal Hypertension and Esophageal Varices

Obstruction of blood flow through the liver results in increased pressure in the portal venous system. The term *portal hypertension* refers to high pressures in the portal vein and its tributaries. Meeting resistance in the portal vein, blood seeks collateral channels around the high pressure areas or through the obstructed liver. In the portal system, the vessels most susceptible to the high pressure are the esophageal and the hemorrhoidal veins (Fig. 39-2). The esophageal veins protrude into the lumen of the esophagus and become thin-walled varices that look like bulging bags on the inner surface of the esophagus.

Esophageal varices can become irritated by gastric acidity or by spasmotic vomiting. Alcohol and other irritants can cause chemical breakdown of the walls of the varices. Any of these situations can result in rupture and massive upper gastrointestinal hemorrhage. The two main factors that encourage hemorrhage are depressed formation of clotting factors and high portal pressures. Continued vomiting after the first bleeding event usually results in additional bleeding. Rupture of esophageal varices may result in exsanguination and death if it is not treated immediately. Rectal hemorrhoids also may rupture and bleed under pressure, causing a massive amount of bright red bleeding from the rectum. Anything that can cause increased motility of the lower gastrointestinal tract can increase the risk for hemorrhage from this area.

Collateral channels develop because of the high portal pressure and provide a route for direct shunting of blood from the portal veins to the inferior vena cava, thus bypassing the liver. The shunted blood contains large amounts of ammonia that may precipitate onset of hepatic encephalopathy. The bloodborne bacteria absorbed from the small intestine and normally processed and biotransformed in the liver also are shunted directly into the systemic circulation. Toxic substances may bypass the liver without being metabolized and may accumulate in the body with deleterious effects on the nervous system.

Bleeding from esophageal varices, duodenal ulcers, or other sources may precipitate jaundice and production of ammonia due to the processing and absorption of products of the red blood cell in the intestine. These developments may lead to increased risk of encephalopathy, which, with the bleeding event, may be life threatening.

Hepatorenal Syndrome

In liver failure, the development of associated renal failure indicates a very poor prognosis. The hepatorenal syndrome seems to leave the kidneys almost normal morphologically but functionally impaired. It is diagnosed in persons developing acute renal failure in the presence of significant hepatic disease; frequently it is precipitated by clinical deterioration such as a gastrointestinal bleeding episode or the onset of hepatic coma [9].

Hepatorenal syndrome begins suddenly, with decreased urinary output and elevated serum urea nitrogen and creatinine levels. It is accompanied by elevated blood ammonia level and increasing jaundice, probably due to the failure of bilirubin to be excreted in the urine. At autopsy, no permanent morphologic change can be demonstrated in the kidneys. The syndrome seems to be an evolutionary process of functional impairment of the kidneys resulting from liver failure (see Chap. 31).

Liver Failure

Liver failure refers to a constellation of clinical manifestations that are the ultimate outcome of many types of liver disease. The liver has a large reserve, and approximately 80 percent of its parenchyma can be destroyed before clinical signs of liver failure are evident. Cirrhosis and chronic active hepatitis are the most common causes of liver failure. Chemicals and drugs, such as carbon tetrachloride and halothane, can cause massive liver necrosis. Reye's syndrome, fatty liver of alcoholism, and antibiotics

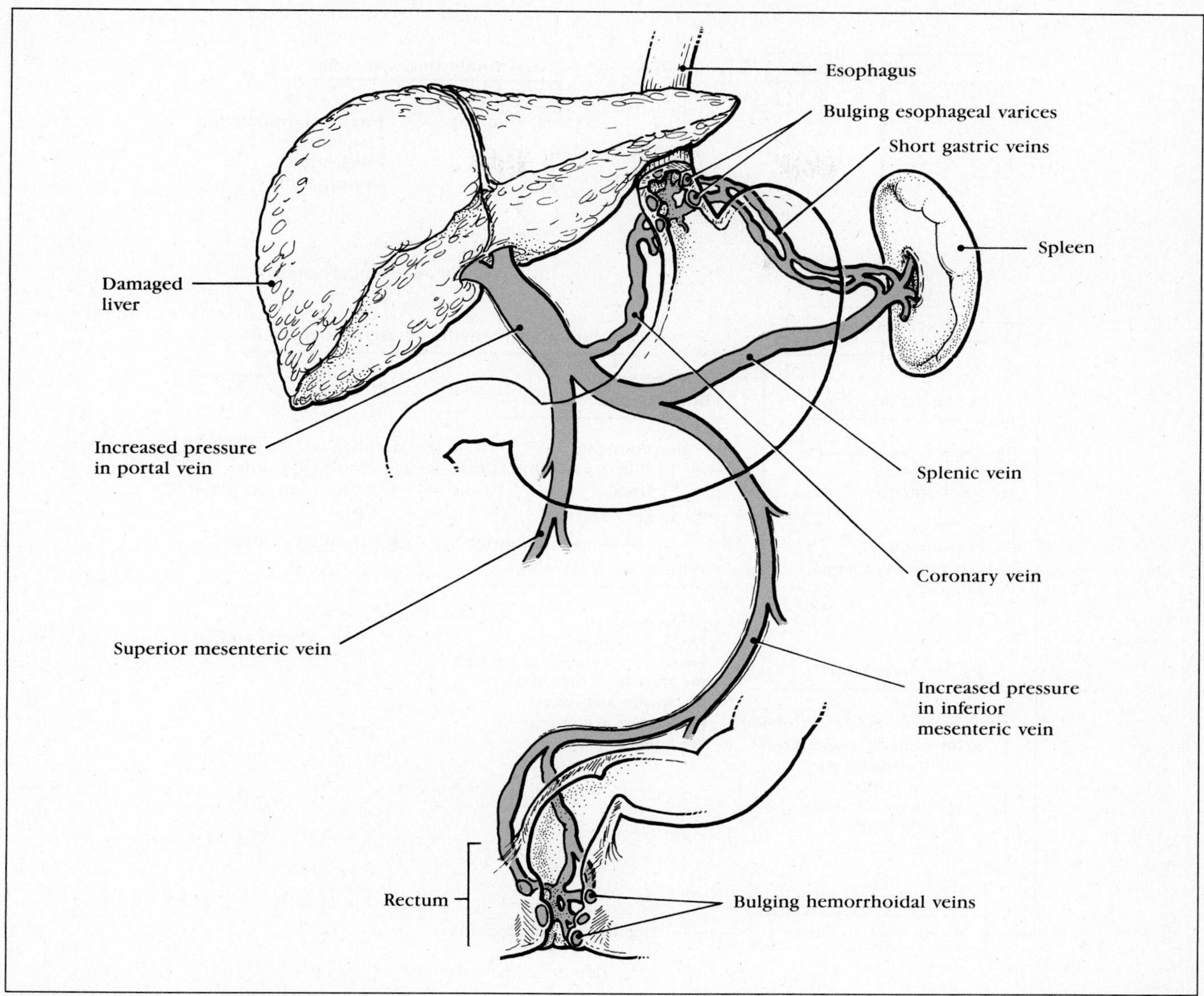

FIGURE 39-2 Appearance of esophageal varices and dilated hemorrhoidal veins resulting from portal hypertension.

such as tetracycline can cause functional insufficiency [9]. These conditions cause liver damage that leads to a number of characteristic physiologic changes, including (1) jaundice, with increased conjugated and unconjugated bilirubin levels; (2) changes in neurologic status with hepatic encephalopathy and coma; (3) hypogonadism and gynecomastia due to imbalance of androgen-estrogen levels; (4) palmar erythema with vasodilation in the palms of the hands and feet; (5) spider angiomas of the skin, probably related to clotting disturbances and/or increased portal pressure; (6) fetor hepaticus, a peculiar musty odor of the breath often associated with high serum ammonia levels; and (7) ascites and edema related to portal hypertension and hypoalbuminemia (Fig. 39-3).

The characteristic wasting of liver disease is manifested by muscular atrophy, weight loss, and loss of plasma proteins and clotting factors. Liver failure frequently causes death from cirrhosis; recovery depends on the amount of liver damage sustained.

Hepatic Encephalopathy and Coma

Hepatic encephalopathy refers to an alteration in the neurologic status in persons with significant liver disease. Its onset may be gradual but more frequently it is precipitated by a major hemodynamic insult in the marginally compensated individual suffering from cirrhosis of the liver. Conditions that may precipitate encephalopathy include bleeding from esophageal varices, ingestion of narcotics or barbiturates, anesthetics, excessive protein intake, electrolyte imbalance, and hemodynamic alterations such as hypovolemia or shock. Anything that can increase the

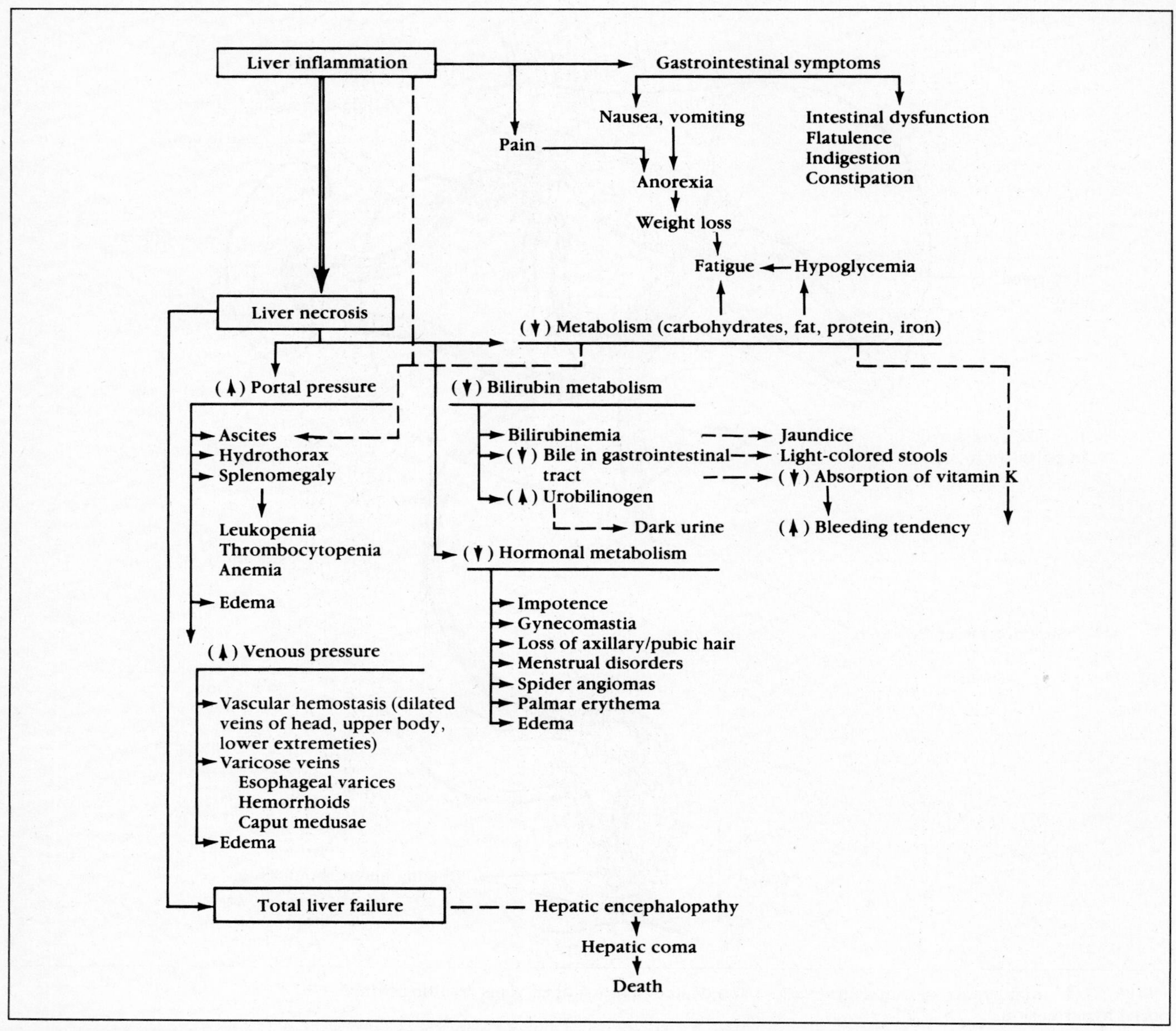

FIGURE 39-3 Progression of liver cell failure. (From W.J. Phipps, B.C. Long, and N.F. Woods, ***Medical-Surgical Nursing*** [2nd ed.]. St. Louis: Mosby, 1983.)

metabolic demands placed on the borderline liver can precipitate liver failure with resultant encephalopathy and coma [5].

Onset of the neurologic condition is related to the inability of the liver to metabolize nitrogenous products absorbed from the intestine. These nitrogenous products may include dietary protein or proteins released in gastrointestinal bleeding episodes. Serum ammonia levels are often elevated in encephalopathy, and other substances probably produce the clinical syndrome as well [6]. The liver is believed to produce some substances that are important in normal brain metabolism, and these substances may be depressed in liver damage.

Hepatic encephalopathy has been described in terms of phases that vary in length and may progress insidiously from one level to the next. Advanced hepatic disease is invariably present, frequently complicated by portal hypertension. The onset phase of encephalopathy is heralded by personality changes, including disturbances of awareness, forgetfulness, increased irritability, and confusion. As the condition progresses, a phase having the distinct neurologic patterns of hyperreflexia and asterixis occurs. *Asterixis* is a peculiar "flapping tremor" that can be elicited by dorsiflexion of the hands. Violent, abusive behavior, accompanied by changes on the electroencephalogram (EEG) are frequent. The EEG changes of characteristic, symmetric, high-voltage, slow-wave patterns occur 1 to 3 times per second and are imposed on a relatively normal reading.

Progression of encephalopathy to coma results in absence of the flapping tremor and depression or decline of the wave forms on the EEG. A positive Babinski's sign and hyperactive reflexes occur with the onset of the comatose phase. Persons exhibiting recurrent or progressive forms of this condition have been found to have distinctive changes in the brain tissue, with proliferation of the astrocytes and patchy cortical necrosis. When these changes occur, areas of permanent damage result [9].

Drug-Related Liver Damage

Drug reactions are responsible for a number of toxic effects on the human body. Table 39-1 lists several drugs that can cause hepatotoxic effects. Hepatotoxicity can result from formation of toxic metabolites as the liver is biotransforming the drug, or from a drug metabolite converting an intracellular protein into an immunogenic molecule. The damage sustained depends on dosage and individual hypersensitivity. Some drugs affect a significant number of persons and the damage occurs in a relatively short period of time. Many drugs cause problems only due to hypersensitivity reactions, and these may not be manifested for weeks to months after initiating therapy (Table 39-2). The pathology depends on the amount and location of injury [9].

TABLE 39-1 Drug-Induced Hepatic Disease

Pattern of Reaction	Drug Implicated
"Pure" cholestatis	^{17}C alkylated steroids (anabolic, contraceptive)
	Estrogens
Cholestasis with hepatocyte injury	Chlorpromazine
	Erythromycin
	Some oral antidiabetics
	Some antithyroid drugs
	6-Mercaptopurine
	? Azathioprine
	Para-aminosalicylic acid
	Sulfonamides
Fatty change (steatosis)	Tetracycline
	Methotrexate (usually with hepatocyte necrosis)
Zonal (centrilobular) necrosis	Halothane
	Acetaminophen
	Salicylates
	Phenacetin
	Isoniazid
Submassive to massive necrosis	Halothane
	Isoniazid
	α-Methyldopa
	Acetaminophen
	Iproniazid
Acute hepatitis	Halothane
	Isoniazid
	Iproniazid
	Phenytoin
	Salicylates
Chronic, persistent hepatitis	α-Methyldopa
	Oxyphenisatin
	Isoniazid
	Salicylates
Chronic, active hepatitis	α-Methyldopa
Cirrhosis	Drugs causing acute or chronic active hepatitis
	Methotrexate
Budd-Chiari syndrome	? Oral contraceptives
	Pyrrolizidine alkaloids (bush tea)
	Urethane
Peliosis hepatis	^{17}C alkylated steroids (anabolic, contraceptive)
Granulomas	Phenylbutazone
	Sulfanomides
	α-Methyldopa
Adenoma of liver	^{17}C alkylated steroids (anabolic, contraceptive)
Focal, nodular hyperplasia	Oral contraceptives
Hepatocellular carcinoma	^{17}C alkylated steroids (anabolic, contraceptive)

Source: S. L. Robbins, R. S. Cotran, and V. Kumar, *Pathologic Basis of Disease* (3rd ed.). Philadelphia: W.B. Saunders Company, 1984. Reprinted by permission.

Cirrhosis of the Liver

The word *cirrhosis* is a general term for a condition that destroys the normal architecture of the liver lobules. It has the following three important structural features: (1) destruction of liver parenchyma, (2) separation of the lobules by fibrous tissue, and (3) formation of regenerative nodules [8]. Cirrhosis is classified according to its causative agent and the resultant pathologic configurations. The major classifications are biliary, postnecrotic, and alcoholic.

Biliary Cirrhosis

Biliary cirrhosis may be due to an intrahepatic block that obstructs the excretion of bile or it may occur secondary to obstruction of the bile ducts. The ultimate outcome differs with each type.

Intrahepatic biliary stasis is considered to result from two major mechanisms. *Primary intrahepatic stasis* is caused by autoimmune destruction of interlobular bile ducts. This type is most frequent in women over age 40 years, suggesting an endocrine contribution. Specific and nonspecific immunologic abnormalities have been implicated based on the demonstration of antibodies and impaired T lymphocyte function [3]. *Secondary biliary cirrhosis* results from obstruction of the hepatic or common bile duct and produces stasis of bile in the liver. This excess bile may lead to progressive fibrosis, parenchymal cell destruction, and regenerative nodules. The last is an apparent reaction of the interlobular bile ducts to the increased amounts of bile within them. Injury, inflammation, and scarring result from stasis of bile in the lobular compartments [9].

Both intrahepatic and extrahepatic biliary cirrhosis show evidence of fibrosis that surrounds hepatocytes and

TABLE 39-2 Mechanisms of Drug-Induced Hepatotoxicity

	Direct	Indirect
Mechanism of liver injury	Protoplasmic poison	Interference with hepatic secretory or excretory processes without parenchymal damage Hepatic necrosis produced by competition or binding with essential metabolites, inhibition of specific enzyme functions
Time interval between exposure and liver damage	Brief	Latent period (1–4 weeks) to sensitization
Toxicity	Dose dependent	Independent of dose
Reproducible in experimental animals	Common	Infrequent
Frequency	High	Low
Hepatic lesions	Distinct liver cell necrosis	Variable; hepatitislike; cholestasis; mixed
Rash, fever, eosinophilia, arthralgia	Unusual	High frequency
Examples	CCl_4, $CHCl_3$, phosphorus	Chlorpromazine, chlorpropamide, chlorothiazide

Source: Reproduced with permission from N.J. Greenberger, *Gastrointestinal Disorders: A Pathophysiologic Approach* (3rd ed.).

separates the lobules. Scarring and injury are located in close proximity to the interlobular bile ducts.

The clinical course is usually more severe in the primary than the secondary type because surgical intervention usually relieves the biliary stasis with the latter. Jaundice may be severe with either type and is associated with bilirubinemia and clay-colored stools. Results of liver function tests are abnormal, with alkaline phosphatase and cholesterol levels often becoming markedly elevated. When the serum cholesterol exceeds 450 mg per dl, *cutaneous xanthomas* (nodular swellings filled with cholesterol and tissue macrophages) may develop. Levels of both conjugated and unconjugated bilirubin may rise. With increasing liver damage, all the signs of hepatocellular failure may appear.

Postnecrotic Cirrhosis

Postnecrotic cirrhosis follows massive liver necrosis and involves the destruction of lobules and even lobes of the liver. It may occur after hepatitis or after exposure to hepatotoxins such as carbon tetrachloride and certain drugs. A period of time after the onset of disease or injury passes during which the liver attempts to regenerate. The liver may become small and composed of large nodules separated by fibrous bands or scars. The nodules become infiltrated with lymphocytes. The liver architecture is distorted due to cell loss and attempts at parenchymal regeneration [10].

Early clinical manifestations include an enlarged, tender liver that later becomes shrunken and nodular. Signs of portal hypertension are often present, and many problems of liver dysfunction complicate the condition. This type of cirrhosis is suspected in persons who have no history of excessive alcohol ingestion but who have signs of chronic liver disease. Abnormal results of liver function tests are the rule and liver biopsy determines the underlying pathology. This condition is also associated with an altered immune system, often with increased immunoglobulins, positive antinuclear antigen tests, and positive LE (lupus erythematosus) cell preparations.

Alcoholic (Laennec's) Cirrhosis

This disease entity has been shown to be caused by chronic alcoholism, often following a pattern of fatty liver, alcoholic hepatitis, and finally, alcoholic cirrhosis [9]. At least 10 to 20 percent of persons who are chronic alcoholics have clinical or morphologic evidence of cirrhosis. Significant frequency of the disease is noted in highly civilized countries, among all economic classes, and in all races.

Alcohol has been shown to be a hepatotoxin and induces metabolic changes within the liver, leading to fat infiltration of the hepatocytes and scarring between the lobules (see Chap. 3). There is usually a close association between poor diet and long-term alcohol abuse.

The liver becomes enlarged, and hepatocytes degenerate and become infiltrated by leukocytes and lymphocytes. Intracellular inclusions called *Mallory's bodies*, or alcoholic hyalin, produce sclerosing hyaline necrosis [6,9]. The early disease has an inflammatory character that decreases as the cirrhotic process progresses to the destruction of hepatocytes. Infiltrating fibroblasts and collagen formation lead to early scar formation. Acute exacerbations of alcoholic hepatitis cause inflammation and further damage to the liver parenchyma. As cirrhosis ensues, the liver capsule becomes firm to the touch, and regenerative nodules form, resulting in a hobnail appearance. As the pathology progresses, the liver shrinks in size and becomes finely nodular in appearance. The nodules are surrounded by evenly spaced, grayish connective tissue [9]. The liver pathology is usually associated with enlargement of the spleen.

The physiologic results of Laennec's cirrhosis depend on the amount of inflammation, degeneration, infiltration of the cells by fat, and scarring. Liver cell degeneration may lead to portal hypertension and ascites. Jaundice and esophageal varices often occur later in the disease. All of the complications associated with liver dysfunction may occur depending on the degree of parenchymal damage. Some of the more common ones are clotting disorders, hypoproteinemia, signs of biliary obstruction, and gastrointestinal bleeding.

Clinically, cirrhosis of this type is an insidious condition causing abnormal liver function tests, fluid retention, ascites, and esophageal varices (Fig. 39-4). With abstinence from alcohol, results of liver function tests may return nearly to normal, but excessive ingestion of alcohol or continued poor diet may lead to decompensation. Alcoholic hepatitis occurs, leading to bouts of decompensation and finally to liver failure.

It has been shown that 50 percent of persons with significant cirrhosis of the liver die of the disease within five years. Disease progression can be markedly altered by abstinence from alcohol. Death may be due to liver failure, infection, gastrointestinal bleeding, or hepatocellular carcinoma, which occurs in 5 to 10 percent of cases [9].

Cancer of the Liver

Tumors of the liver that cause functional impairment and hepatomegaly are almost always malignant. The rare benign tumors are often classed as angiomas or adenomas.

Primary Malignancies

Primary carcinoma of the liver is relatively rare and may arise within hepatocytes, from the canaliculi or small biliary ducts, or it may be of mixed type. Hepatocellular carcinoma (HCC) accounts for 80 to 90 percent of primary malignancies of the liver [9].

A study of the epidemiology of primary liver tumors shows that they may be related to diet and other types of liver disease, especially hepatitis. In the United States, the prevalence of primary liver carcinoma is less than 3 percent, while in some parts of Africa this malignancy may represent 50 percent of all cancers in men and 20 percent in women. Some of the influences that may contribute to its occurrence include (1) carcinogenic agents in food, (2) cirrhosis of the liver, (3) viral infections of the liver,

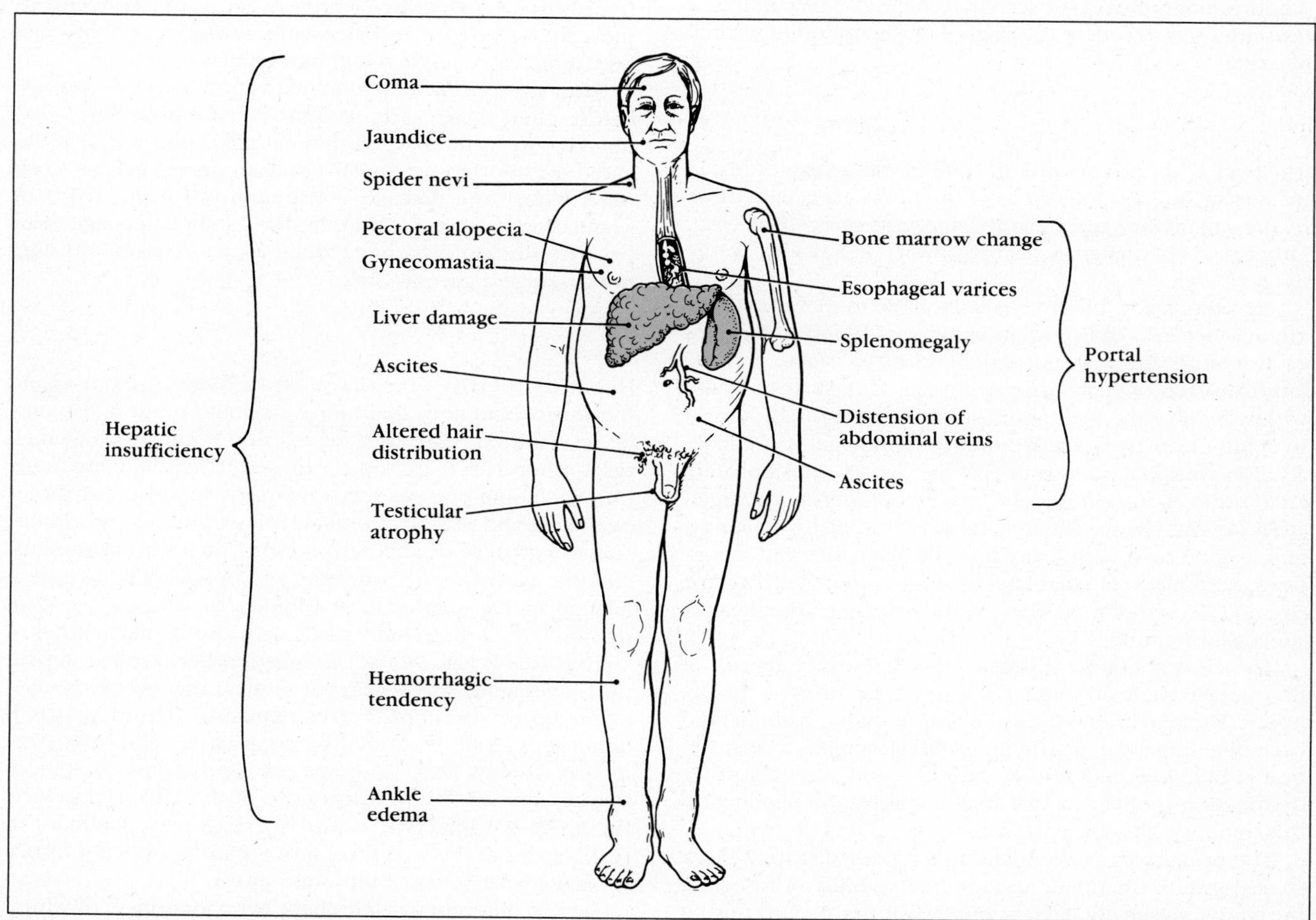

FIGURE 39-4 Clinical effects of cirrhosis of the liver.

and (4) parasitic liver infections [9]. Viruses, especially hepatitis B (HBV), can account for the difference in frequency of liver cancers in the United States and Africa. Markers for the HBV in the latter country are almost invariably present [9].

Pathologically, the growth may be limited to one area, occur in numerous nodules, or occur as infiltrates on the surface of the liver [6]. The tumors may secrete different substances, especially bile products. Usually the growth rate is very rapid and terminates in gastrointestinal hemorrhaging, liver failure, and death.

Physiologically, these tumors interfere with the normal function of the hepatocytes, but they often create no difficulty until they are far advanced. Biliary obstruction with jaundice, portal hypertension with ascites, and different sorts of metabolic disturbances related to the functional impairment of hepatocytes result. Metabolic disturbances include hypoalbuminemia, hypoglycemia, and bleeding problems.

Clinically, the affected person exhibits signs of debilitation, weight loss, and cachexia. Jaundice, ascites, and other signs of liver failure are often related to progression of the condition and frequently are seen in the terminal state [8]. Tumors of the liver are rarely considered to be resectable. Precise diagnosis is made by biopsy, but liver and computed tomography (CT) scans are helpful. Liver function tests are used to reflect the degree of disruption of normal function.

Metastatic Carcinoma

The liver is very frequently the site of metastases of malignancies arising in other areas of the body, especially those of the pulmonary tract, breast, and gastrointestinal tract. Other types of malignancies metastasize less readily to the liver.

Physiologically, the liver is vulnerable to metastatic carcinoma because of the large volume of blood it receives each minute, the high nutrient level of its blood, and the large reserve of lymphatic drainage. Metastases usually widely involve the liver and disrupt its function. Results of liver function tests are frequently abnormal, especially alkaline phosphatase, serum enzymes, and Bromsulphalein (BSP) retention. The level of carcinoembryonic antigen (CEA) in the serum, which is increased in many malignancies, is increased with many liver malignancies and metastases. Serum levels correlate to some extent with tumor size and degree of metastasis, and decrease markedly after successful treatment.

The clinical course relates to the rapidity of growth of the metastatic lesion and the site of the primary malignancy. The nutritional status declines rapidly, with marked cachexia, muscular wasting, and hepatomegaly. Obstruction of bile flow may lead to jaundice, and all of the other dysfunctions of liver disease may be present depending on the amount of liver involvement.

The prognosis of liver metastasis is poor due to the lack of response to treatment and the impossibility of resecting the tumor surgically. Five-year survival has been reported to be less than 5 percent.

Viral Hepatitis

Hepatitis is inflammation and injury of the liver. It is a reaction of the liver to a variety of conditions, specifically viruses, drugs, and alcohol. This section details acute hepatitis resulting from viral infection.

Acute viral hepatitis is an infectious disease that is caused by at least two strains of viruses, hepatitis A and hepatitis B. These organisms are distinguished by their antigenic properties, but both types are transmissible; and the complications that may result can inflict permanent liver damage. Non-A, non-B hepatitis and delta agent hepatitis have been identified. There is no clear distinction in the clinical features caused by each virus.

Hepatitis A

Hepatitis A (HAV) infection results most frequently from fecal-oral contamination by the hepatitis A virus, but may result from the infusion of infected blood. It frequently occurs in crowded, unsanitary living conditions, has no sex predilection, and is often epidemic in children or young adults. It has been called the "dormitory disease," as epidemics may break out and infect large numbers of students living close together. This infection may also be transmitted by shellfish, which process and concentrate the contaminated material. Contaminated water has also been implicated as carrying the organism.

After exposure, incubation takes about two to six weeks before clinical signs are evident. The antibody level rises quickly after the onset of clinical signs and remains elevated for approximately 10 years. In areas such as Costa Rica, where the disease is endemic, 90 percent of the population have anti-HA antibodies by their teenage years [9]. The disease does not induce a carrier state and does not produce a chronic state.

Hepatitis B

Hepatitis B (HBV) results most frequently from blood transfusion and needle virus contamination but it also may be transmitted orally and venereally. Populations at high risk for hepatitis B are those exposed to needle contamination, including persons receiving many blood transfusions, personnel and persons in renal dialysis units, drug addicts, sexual partners of affected persons, male homosexuals, children with Down syndrome, and persons taking immunosuppressive medications. Families or other close contacts of any of these individuals may also be at high risk.

Hepatitis B has a longer incubation period than hepatitis A, averaging six weeks, but clinical manifestations can occur up to six months after exposure. The hepatitis B organism can be identified by an antigen called the *Australian antigen (AA)*. This antigen is present in the bloodstream and lacks the critical core of the HBV. Therefore, the AA is not infective, but it is a diagnostic hallmark of HBV. Levels of this and several other antigens begin to rise several weeks before symptoms appear.

Several different particles have been identified, of which the *Dane particle* has been called the hepatitis B particle.

It is composed of two coats, or shells, and probably is the intact hepatitis B virus. The particle core is synthesized within the nucleus of the hepatocyte and is composed of HBV core, DNA, and antigen [9]. An associated antigen, the *hepatitis B surface antigen (HBsAg)*, may contain several related antigens that may be used to differentiate hepatitis B from other hepatitis. Through laboratory studies, the hepatitis B virus has been classified as a DNA virus, which means that it uses deoxyribonucleic acid for replication [9].

Immunologic Features

With both hepatitis A and B strains, a nonspecific increase in levels of immunoglobulins gamma (IgG) and macroglobulin (IgM) occurs. Type-specific IgG antibodies form after the infection and may persist for years in the sera. This accounts for the probable lifetime immunity exhibited by patients after hepatitis A infections [1]. Specific antibody to HBsAg has been noted to persist for 6 to 12 months after infection. These antibodies are present in 20 to 30 percent of the general population in the United States and probably serve as a protection against infection with the hepatitis B virus [9].

Pathologic Features

Pathologically, HAV and HBV infections are difficult to distinguish, and the pathology may be mild or extensive depending on the severity of the disease. The following three major features are evident: (1) liver cell injury, necrosis, and scarring; (2) regeneration of liver cells with an increased number of mitotic figures, sometimes with crowded, disorganized cells; and (3) mononuclear phagocyte system reaction with swelling and reduplication or proliferation of Kupffer cells. The degree of any of the pathologic changes differs depending on the severity of the disease and the resolution. In HAV, parenchymal recovery is usually complete within six months. In HBV, parenchymal recovery may not occur at all.

Clinical Course

The clinical course is commonly described in three phases: *prodromal*, *icteric*, and *recovery*. The development, duration, and severity of the phases depend on the amount of hepatocellular damage. The prodromal phase is the period of time when the person first becomes symptomatic with complaints of anorexia, nausea and vomiting, and many flulike symptoms. It usually precedes jaundice by one to two weeks. A low-grade fever characteristically occurs with hepatitis A. Dark, bilirubin-positive urine and clay-colored stools may occur one to five days prior to the onset of jaundice.

The icteric phase is heralded by the onset of jaundice and a total bilirubin level of 2.5 mg per dl or greater. The liver becomes enlarged and tender. Laboratory findings may be grossly abnormal. The recovery phase is the period of time when symptoms resolve. Liver enlargement decreases, but not to normal, and results of liver function tests remain abnormal but recede toward normal. This period lasts 2 to 12 weeks and total recovery usually occurs in 3 to 4 months. The course of HBV is usually more severe than that of HAV and leads to a variety of clinical syndromes. These can encompass an asymptomatic carrier state to a fulminant progressive hepatitis [9].

The major sequela to hepatitis B is chronic active hepatitis that may lead to liver failure and death. Rare complications may be pancreatitis, pneumonia, peripheral neuropathy, and an increased risk of carcinoma of the liver [3]. The person usually recovers completely.

Delta Hepatitis

This disease is produced by an RNA virus distinct from all others. It has abrupt onset with similar symptoms as hepatitis B. The delta agent and B virus often coinfect, or the delta may be opportunistic when the HBV is present [1]. It is transmitted by blood, serous body fluids, contaminated needles, and blood transfusions.

The diagnosis is often missed or is called an exacerbation of chronic hepatitis B. Delta hepatitis is a common and serious cause of fulminant hepatitis, with 25 to 50 percent of fulminant HBV thought to relate to the delta agent. Delta agent is a defective virus that requires HBV to multiply [1].

Non-A, Non-B Hepatitis

This disease is caused by at least two unidentified agents distinct from the HAV and HBV. These viruses can produce an infection similar to HAV or HBV, but they can induce an active, carrier, chronic, or fulminant state [9]. The incubation period varies from 14 to 180 days, with epidemics being reported in India and Africa [1]. It is most common in young adult males [1,9].

Chronicity in non-A, non-B hepatitis may result and symptoms may progress to cirrhosis. The usual pattern is one of improvement within two to three years.

Gallbladder Disease

Cholecystitis and Cholelithiasis

The most common disorders of the gallbladder are cholecystitis (inflammation) and cholelithiasis (gallstones). Inflammation of the gallbladder is the second most frequent cause of abdominal pain that requires abdominal surgery, the first being appendicitis. Dietary factors, including high fat intake, have long been associated with cholecystitis.

Cholelithiasis refers to biliary tract stones, most of which form in the gallbladder itself. Their major constituents are *cholesterol* and *pigment*. The stones often contain mixtures of components of bile. Those composed primarily of cholesterol account for 80 percent of gallstones in the United States. Gallstones occur in an estimated 20 million Americans per year, with considerable differences based on race and socioeconomics. Ten to 15 percent of adults in the United States have cholelithiasis, of which 50 percent are asymptomatic. There is a dramatic increase in frequency among American Indians and Swedish individuals. Some predisposing factors include middle age, female sex, obesity, and possibly multiparity. Pregnancy, oral contraceptives, and estrogen therapy may be contributors.

Clinical Manifestations. The clinical manifestations of gallstones arise when the stones migrate to and obstruct the common bile duct. The obstruction causes pain and blocks bile excretion. Visceral pain is precipitated by biliary contractions and is termed *biliary colic*. This pain is not colicky, but is usually perceived as a steady, severe aching or pressure in the epigastrium [2].

Obstruction of the bile duct is followed by acute cholecystitis that may be due to increased pressure and ischemia in the gallbladder or to chemical irritation of the organ caused by prolonged exposure to concentrated bile. Primary bacterial infection may cause cholecystitis, but in up to 80 percent of cases, obstructive stones in the bile duct are present. Therefore, it is thought that bacterial contamination may either be secondary to the stasis or may result from severe infection such as septicemia. Pancreatic reflux may occur and cause irritation by contact of pancreatic enzymes with the mucosa of the bile duct.

Acute cholecystitis may cause complications with abscesses and/or perforation of the gallbladder. Chronic cholecystitis usually is associated with stones in the biliary ducts and is manifested by intolerance to fatty food, nausea and vomiting, and pain after eating.

Diagnosis. The simplest diagnostic sign is nonvisualization of the gallbladder on oral or intravenous cholecystogram. The white blood cell count may be elevated to 10,000 to 15,000. Bilirubin level is often increased, causing jaundice. The pain of cholecystitis may mimic myocardial infarction, peptic ulcer, or intestinal obstruction, among other conditions.

Obesity: A Major Disturbance in Nutritional Balance

The major nutritional problem in the developed world is the excessive ingestion of sugars, fats, and protein, leading to obesity [9]. Obesity is defined as a 20 percent increase over ideal body weight. This excess is due to adipose tissue deposition [4]. Twenty to 30 percent of the male population and 30 to 40 percent of the female population in the United States suffer from obesity [4].

Eating patterns and appetite are considered on page 568. Obesity results when the appetite induces caloric intake above the metabolic expenditure of these calories. Other less common causes are Cushing's disease, several rare hypothalamic disorders, hyperinsulinemia, and hypothyroidism.

Subcutaneous fat tissue may accumulate through increased numbers of fat cells or through the enlargement of individual adipocytes (fat cells). Studies indicate that the number of fat cells in the body are laid down during three phases of life: (1) during the last three months of gestation, (2) during early childhood, and (3) immediately after puberty [4]. In the adult, an increase in adiposity is primarily due to an increased size of the adipocyte. Studies have also shown that persons with severe obesity have a combination of increased size and numbers of adipocytes. When the onset of obesity is in the adult years, it is due to fat cell enlargement, and mild to moderate obesity results [4].

Obesity has been linked to the etiology of many diseases; however, it seems to be a contributory factor rather than a causative one. The major diseases of association are hypertension, cardiovascular atherosclerotic disease, diabetes mellitus, pancreatitis, and kidney diseases. Many of these conditions also demonstrate hyperlipoproteinemia, especially in the form of hypercholesterolemia.

Lipid Transport

Knowledge of how lipids are transported and the significance of lipoprotein types enhances the understanding of fat deposition in the obese individual. The largest source of lipids is dietary fats. These are carried in the forms of chylomicrons, very-low-density lipoproteins (VLDLs), remnants of cholestryl esters and triglycerides, low-density lipoproteins (LDLs), and high-density lipoproteins (HDLs) (see Chap. 22). The VLDLs interact with the lipoprotein lipase enzyme, which contributes to the formation of LDLs and eventually establishes a cycle by which LDLs deliver cholesterol to extrahepatic cells [3,9]. The VLDLs are produced when the liver converts excess carbohydrate to fatty acids and, through another conversion process, forms triglycerides that are the core of the VLDLs. The LDL is the form of most of the total cholesterol of the plasma [3]. This is important in the pathway for the synthesis of steroid hormones as well as in supplying cholesterol to other cells of the body. The HDLs pick up cholesterol, which then reacts with a plasma enzyme, leading again to the formation of LDLs (Fig. 39-5).

In the obese person, when an excess of carbohydrate, fat, or protein reaches the cells, it can be converted to energy, fat stores, and cholesterol. Fat is broken down to acetate, which, when not needed for energy, is metabolized into fat or adipose stores. Energy production for the most part requires oxygen, while synthesis of fat does not. Apparently, many individuals supply their cells with too many calories; at the same time these cells do not get enough oxygen, which results in formation of fat within the adipose tissue [9].

Problems with Excess Fat Production and Storage

Other factors that favor fat production are a decreased thyroid secretion and increased levels of circulating insulin. Thyroid hormones increase the oxidative capability in the Krebs cycle. Excessive insulin leads to fat synthesis and storage.

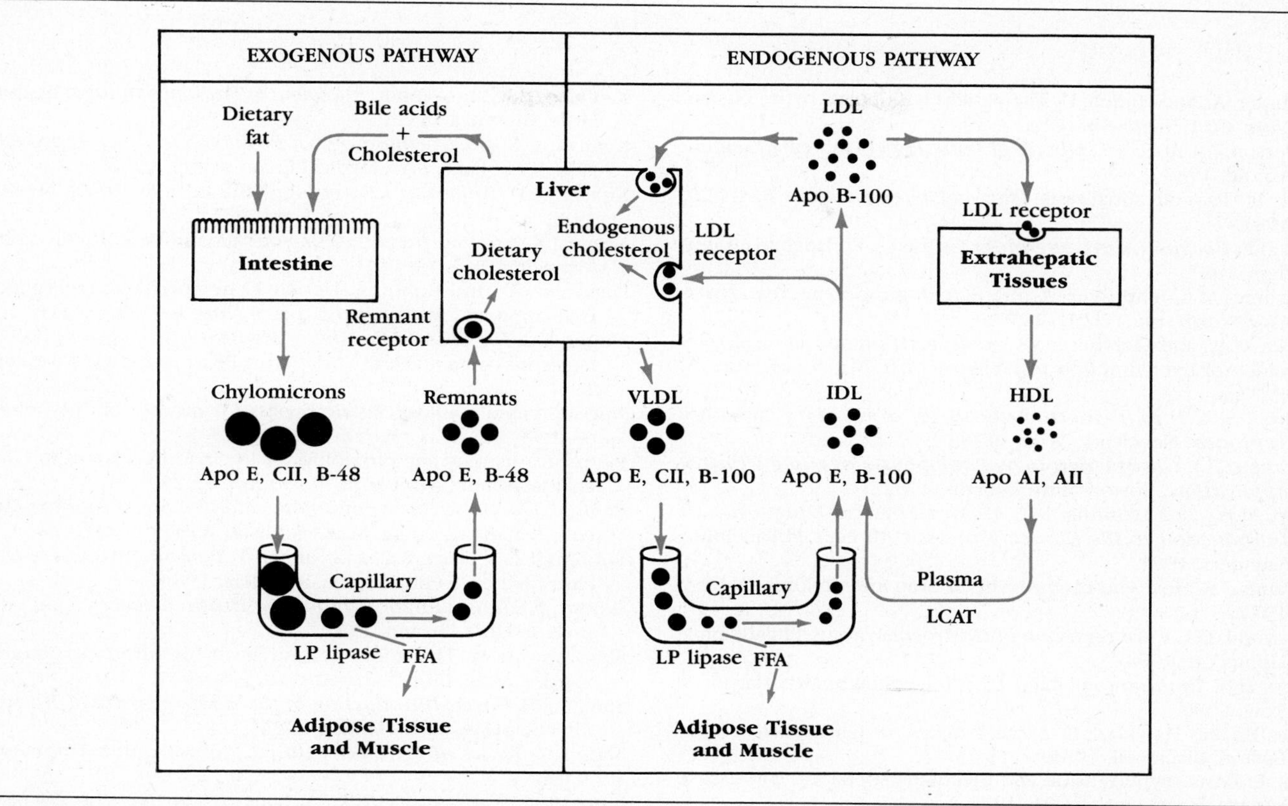

FIGURE 39-5 Model for plasma triglyceride and cholesterol transport in humans. VLDL = very low-density lipoprotein; IDL = intermediate density lipoprotein; LDL = low-density lipoprotein; HDL = high-density lipoprotein; and LCAT = lecithin cholesterol acyltransferase (catalyzes reaction). (From E. Braunwald et al. [eds.], *Harrison's Principles of Internal Medicine* [11th ed.]. New York: McGraw-Hill, 1987.)

Besides being associated with many diseases, obesity increases cardiac workload, can interfere with respiratory excursion, aggravates arthritis and back ailments, and precipitates and aggravates varicose veins. Gallbladder disease is associated with obesity, and the mortality from cancer has been shown to be increased in persons who are 25 percent or more overweight, especially in breast, colon, and endometrial cancers [9]. In general, obesity is a serious risk factor for many diseases. It can be controlled if the appetite is decreased through behavior modification.

Study Questions

1. Explain the development of cirrhosis of the liver. Relate the manifestations of liver failure to the pathology described.
2. Describe the concept of portal hypertension, including the development of esophageal varices, hemorrhoids, and ascites.
3. Discuss the similarities and differences among the different types of hepatitis.
4. What factors predispose a person to gallstones? How do gallstones manifest clinically?
5. Discriminate among the various sources of lipids and indicate how they are transported and metabolized.

References

1. Benenson, A.S. *Control of Communicable Diseases in Man* (14th ed.). Washington, D.C.: American Public Health Association, 1985.
2. Bolt, R.J. Pathophysiology of gallbladder disease. In W.A. Sodeman and T.M. Sodeman, *Sodeman's Pathologic Physiology* (7th ed.). Philadelphia: Saunders, 1985.
3. Brown, M.S., and Goldstein, J.L. A receptor-mediated pathway for cholesterol homeostasis. *Science* 232(4): 34, 1986.
4. Felig, P., Hanel, R.J., and Smith, L.H. Metabolism. In L.H. Smith and S.O. Thier, *Pathophysiology: The Biological Principles of Disease* (2nd ed.). Philadelphia: Saunders, 1985.
5. Fishman, M.C., et al. *Medicine* (2nd ed.). Philadelphia: Lippincott, 1985.
6. Greenberger, N.J., and Winship, D.H. *Gastrointestinal Disorders: A Pathophysiologic Approach* (3rd ed.). Chicago: Yearbook, 1986.
7. Iber, F.L., and Lathan, P.S. Normal and pathologic physiology of the liver. In W.A. Sodeman and T.M. Sodeman, *Sodeman's Pathologic Physiology* (7th ed.). Philadelphia: Saunders, 1985.
8. Rankin, R.A., and Welsh, J.D. Gastroenterology. In C.E. Kaufman and S. Papper, *Review of Pathophysiology*. Boston: Little, Brown, 1983.
9. Robbins, S.L., Cotran, R.S., and Kumar, V. *Pathologic Basis of Disease* (3rd ed.). Philadelphia: Saunders, 1984.
10. Zakim, D. Pathophysiology of liver disease. In L.H. Smith and S.O. Thier, *Pathophysiology: The Biological Principles of Disease* (2nd ed.). Philadelphia: Saunders, 1985.

Unit Bibliography

Altshuler, A., and Hilden, D. The patient with portal hypertension. *Nurs. Clin. North Am.* 12:317, 1977.

Anderson, J.R. *Muir's Textbook of Pathology* (12th ed.). London: Arnold, 1985.

Beck, M. Two intestinal tests: One oral, one anal. *Nurs. 81* 11:20, 1981.

Berk, J.E. *Bockus' Gastroenterology* (4th ed.). Philadelphia: Saunders, 1985.

Bossome, M.C. The liver: A pharmacologic perspective. *Nurs. Clin. North Am.* 12:291, 1977.

Boyer, C.A., and Oehlberg, S.A. Interpretation and clinical relevance of liver function tests. *Nurs. Clin. North Am.* 12:275, 1977.

Cohen, S. *Clinical Gastroenterology, a Problem-Oriented Approach*. New York: Wiley, 1983.

Daorken, H.J. *Gastroenterology, Pathophysiology and Clinical Application*. Boston: Butterworths, 1982.

Delp, M.H., and Manning, R.T. *Major's Physical Diagnosis: An Introduction to the Clinical Process* (9th ed.). Philadelphia: Saunders, 1981.

DiPalma, J.R. How you can prevent GI drug interactions. *RN* 7:63, 1977.

Eastwood, G.L. *Core Textbook of Gastroenterology*. Philadelphia: Lippincott, 1984.

Eisen, H.N. *Immunology* (2nd ed.). Hagerstown, Md.: Harper & Row, 1980.

Elias, E., and Hawkins, C. *Lecture Notes on Gastroenterology*. Boston: Blackwell, 1985.

Ellis, P. Portal hypertension and bleeding esophageal and gastric varices. *Heart Lung* 6:791, 1977.

Farmer, R.G., Achkar, E., and Fleshler, B. *Clinical Gastroenterology*. New York: Raven Press, 1983.

Ferguson, G.C. *Pathophysiology, Mechanisms and Expressions*. Philadelphia: Saunders, 1984.

Flint, L.M. Trauma: The University of Louisville School of Medicine symposium. *Heart Lung* 7:247, 1978.

Golden, A., Powell, D., and Jennings, C.D. *Pathology: Understanding Human Disease* (2nd ed.). Baltimore: Williams & Wilkins, 1985.

Greenberger, N.J., and Winship, D.H. *Gastrointestinal Disorders: A Pathophysiologic Approach* (3rd ed.). Chicago: Yearbook, 1986.

Groer, M., and Pierce, M. Guarding against cancer's hidden killer: Anorexia-cachexia. *Nurs. 81* 2:6, 1981.

Guyton, A.C. *Textbook of Medical Physiology* (7th ed.). Philadelphia: Saunders, 1986.

Haughey, C. What to say . . . and do . . . when your patient asks about CT scans. *Nurs. 81* 2:72, 1981.

Hegner, B. *Pathophysiology*. Long Beach, Calif.: ELOT, 1980.

Hurst, J.W. *The Heart* (6th ed.). New York: McGraw-Hill, 1986.

Jenson, D. *The Principles of Physiology* (2nd ed.). New York: Appleton-Century-Crofts, 1980.

Junquiera, L.C., and Carneiro, J. *Basic Histology* (3rd ed.). Los Altos, Calif.: Lange, 1980.

Katz, J. Gastrointestinal hormones. *Med. Clin. North Am.* 57:175, 1973.

Kaufman, C.E., and Papper, S. *Review of Pathophysiology*. Boston: Little, Brown, 1983.

Kennan, C.R. *Gastroenterology, a Problem-Oriented Approach*. New Hyde Park, N.Y.: Medical Examination, 1986.

Kissane, J.M. *Anderson's Pathology* (8th ed.). St. Louis: Mosby, 1985.

Kroner, K. Are you prepared for your ulcerative colitis patient? *Nurs. 80* 10:43, 1980.

Lamphter, T., and Robin, A. Upper GI hemorrhage: Emergency evaluation and management. *Am. J. Nurs.* 81:1814, 1981.

Netter, F.H. *The CIBA Collection of Medical Illustrations (Vol. 3) Digestive System*. New York: CIBA Pharmaceutical Products, 1957.

Nursing grand rounds. Gastric bypass for morbid obesity. *Nurs. 81* 2:54, 1981.

Pierce, L. Anatomy and physiology of the liver in relation to clinical assessment. *Nurs. Clin. North Am.* 12:259, 1977.

Ramsey, J.M. *Basic Pathophysiology: Modern Stress and the Disease Process*. Reading, Mass.: Addison-Wesley, 1982.

Robbins, S.L., Cotran, R.S., and Kumar, V. *Pathologic Basis of Disease* (3rd ed.). Philadelphia: Saunders, 1984.

Selkurt, E.E. *Basic Physiology for the Health Sciences* (2nd ed.). Boston: Little, Brown, 1982.

Shaninpour, N. The adult patient with bleeding esophageal varices. *Nurs. Clin. North Am.* 12:331, 1977.

Sheldon, H. *Boyd's Introduction to the Study of Disease* (9th ed.). Philadelphia: Lea & Febiger, 1984.

Shiff, L. *Diseases of the Liver* (4th ed.). Philadelphia: Lippincott, 1975.

Sleisenger, M.H., and Fordtran, J.S. *Gastrointestinal Disease: Pathophysiology, Diagnosis and Management* (3rd ed.). Philadelphia: Saunders, 1983.

Smith, C. Abdominal assessment. *Nurs. 81* 2:42, 1981.

Smith, L.E., and Thier, S.O. (eds.). *Pathophysiology: The Biological Principles of Disease* (2nd ed.). Philadelphia: Saunders, 1985.

Snell, R.S. *Clinical Anatomy for Medical Students* (2nd ed.). Boston: Little, Brown, 1981.

Sodeman, W., Jr., and Sodeman, W.A. *Pathologic Physiology: Mechanisms of Disease* (7th ed.). Philadelphia: Saunders, 1986.

Sodeman, W.A., and Sodeman, T.M. *Sodeman's Pathologic Physiology* (7th ed.). Philadelphia: Saunders, 1985.

Spiro, H.M. *Clinical Gastroenterology* (3rd ed.). New York: Macmillan, 1983.

Sugar, E. Hirschsprung's disease. *Am. J. Nurs.* 81:2065, 1981.

Taylor, P.D. Organ transplantation series: Liver transplantation. *Am. J. Nurs.* 81:1672, 1981.

Thompson, M. Managing the patient with liver dysfunction. *Nurs. 81* 11:100, 1981.

Thorpe, C., and Caprins, J. Gallbladder disease: Current trends and treatments. *Am. J. Nurs.* 80:2181, 1980.

Wallach, J. *Interpretation of Diagnostic Tests* (4th ed.). Boston: Little, Brown, 1986.

Worthington, B. Nutrition symposium. *Nurs. Clin. North Am.* 14:197, 1979.

UNIT 13

Musculoskeletal Function

Barbara L. Bullock / *Muscular System Function*

Joan Williamson and Thomas Fender / *Skeletal System*

The musculoskeletal system provides for the framework and for voluntary movement of the body. The muscular system is described in Chapter 40, beginning with the appearance of the muscle cell and progressing to the process of muscle contraction. Smooth muscle physiology is contrasted to that of skeletal muscle, and cardiac muscle structure is reviewed. Common primary muscle abnormalities are described. Chapter 41 describes the architectural framework of the body, especially in relationship to the formation and composition of bone. No attempt has been made to list all of the bones of the body; the reader is referred to the anatomy texts listed in the unit bibliography for this information. The important disease processes of bone are covered, as are traumatic bone and joint injuries. Pathophysiology of the disease processes and wound healing is discussed.

As with each unit, the reader is encouraged to use the learning objectives as study guides for chapter content. The study questions at the end of each chapter help to test synthesis of the content. The bibliography lists a number of excellent resources for further research.

CHAPTER 40

Normal and Altered Functions of the Muscular System

CHAPTER OUTLINE

Anatomy of Striated Muscle
- Description of Muscle Cell
- Myofibrils, Actin, and Myosin
- Organelles of the Muscle Cell
- Neuromuscular or Myoneural Junction

Physiology of Striated Muscle
- Generation of an Action Potential
- Sliding Filament Theory
- The "Walk-Along" Mechanism
- Return to Muscle Relaxation
- Energy Requirements of Muscle Contraction
  - *Stored ATP*
  - *Phosphocreatine (Creatine Phosphate)*
  - *Anaerobic Metabolism*
  - *Aerobic Production of ATP*
- Circulatory Adjustments to Exercise

Anatomy of Smooth Muscle
- Visceral (Unitary) Smooth Muscle
- Multiunit Smooth Muscle

Physiology of Smooth Muscle
- Action Potentials in Smooth Muscle
  - *Spike Potential*
  - *Slow-Wave Potential*
- Smooth Muscle Tone
- Neuromuscular Junctions of Smooth Muscle

Anatomy of Cardiac Muscle

Alterations in Muscles of the Body
- Common Problems in Muscles
  - *Cramps*
  - *Strain*
  - *Twitches, Fasciculations, and Fibrillations*
  - *Tetany*
  - *Myoclonus*
  - *Tics*
  - *Other Motor Disorders*
- Hypertrophy
- Atrophy
- Rigor Mortis

Pathologic Processes Affecting the Skeletal Muscles
- Muscular Dystrophies
  - *Duchenne Muscular Dystrophy*
  - *Adult Forms of Muscular Dystrophy*
  - *Laboratory and Diagnostic Tests*
- Myasthenia Gravis
- Rhabdomyosarcoma

LEARNING OBJECTIVES

1. Describe the anatomic components of striated muscle tissue.
2. Define *actin* and *myosin* and their interactions.
3. Discuss the functions of the organelles of the muscle cell.
4. Briefly describe the neuromuscular or myoneural junction.
5. Explain the sliding filament theory.
6. Explain the contraction of a muscle from the generation of an action potential to the return to the resting stage.
7. Describe four ways by which energy is provided to the muscle cell.
8. List and briefly describe the circulatory adjustments to exercise.
9. Compare the anatomy of smooth muscle to that of striated muscle.
10. Differentiate the two types of action potential in smooth muscle.
11. Describe the functional difference between visceral and multiunit smooth muscle.
12. Differentiate briefly the anatomy of cardiac muscle and that of striated muscle.
13. Define common problems in muscles: *cramps*, *twitches*, *fasciculations*, *fibrillation*, *tetany*, *myoclonus*, and *tics*.
14. Differentiate between adaptive and maladaptive muscular hypertrophy.
15. Describe at least four causes of muscular atrophy.
16. Classify the major types of muscular dystrophy.
17. Describe the pathology and clinical course of Duchenne muscular dystrophy.
18. List the laboratory and diagnostic findings that are helpful in the diagnosis of muscular dystrophy.

The muscles of the body are well adapted to the work they must perform. Coordination of skeletal muscle provides the human being with functions ranging from gross motor activities to fine, precise mobility. Involuntary muscle coordination includes the regular contractions of the heart muscle, gastrointestinal peristalsis, and other essential functions. From the moment of conception, the human body is programmed to perform with coordination for many years. When alterations in muscular function occur, the entire body is affected.

Anatomy of Striated Muscle

Striated muscle forms the voluntary or skeletal muscular system. Cardiac muscle, which is involuntary, is also striated muscle. Skeletal striated muscle is the predominant type of muscle in the human body. The muscles are arranged in regular bundles that are surrounded by a sheath of connective tissue called *epimysium*. This structure provides the connective tissue arrangement that binds muscles together and to other structures, while still allowing some freedom of movement.

Description of Muscle Cells

A single muscle is composed of hundreds to thousands of muscle fibers [4]. The muscle fibers are bundles of long, multinucleated cells in which the oval-shaped nuclei are close to the cell membrane [3]. Bundles of fibers called *fascicles* are embedded in a web of connective tissue called the *perimysium* (Fig. 40-1). Each of the individual muscle fibers is bounded by a network of delicate tissue called *endomysium*. This tissue contains an extensive supply of capillaries and nerve fibers, and provides support for the blood vessels and nerves that are adjacent to the muscle fibers [3].

Muscle cells have a reddish appearance that is due to the presence of the *myoglobin* pigment, an oxygen depot in muscles. The muscles that must maintain activity for periods of time usually contain more myoglobin than others.

Skeletal muscle fibers, whose diameter ranges between 10 and 100 μ, may extend the entire length of the muscle unit or may be joined by connective tissue. Muscle is termed *striated* when it has characteristic markings of regularly appearing bands around the muscle fibers. These bands appear as alternating light and dark areas along the muscle fiber. These areas occur due to interface of actin and myosin that projects a gridlike appearance.

The muscle cell contains sarcoplasm, which has many myofibrils, numerous mitochondria, sarcoplasmic reticulum, a T tubule system, numerous sarcoplasmic inclusions, and nuclei very close to the cell membrane. The cell membrane is called the *sarcolemma* (see Fig. 40-1).

Myofibrils, Actin, and Myosin

The myofibrils are the contractile units of the muscle. Each myofibril is composed of repeating units called *sarcomeres*, which are composed of contractile proteins *actin* and *myosin* (Fig. 40-2). This structure is the functional unit of skeletal and cardiac muscle. Actin is a thin filament and has two proteins—*troponin* and *tropomyosin*—associated with it [2]. The myosin filaments, about 1500 per fibril, are thicker and have projections known as crossbridges that extend outward toward the actin molecule.

Actin and myosin, lying beside each other, partially overlap, causing the myofibril to have alternate light and dark bands that can be seen only under polarized light in unstained preparations. The light bands containing only

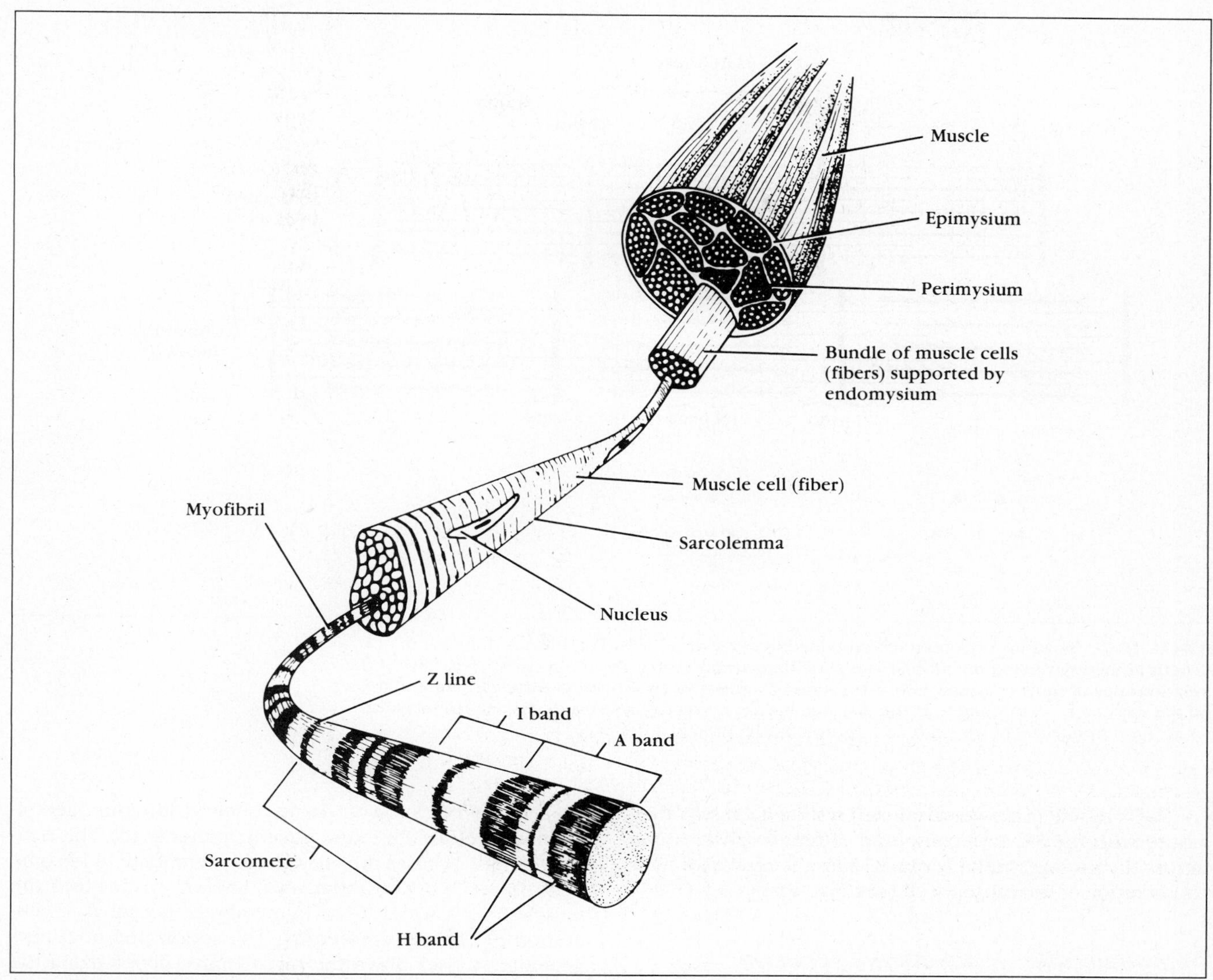

FIGURE 40-1 Structure of striated muscle. (From R.S. Snell, *Clinical Histology for Medical Students*. Boston: Little, Brown, 1984.)

actin filaments are called *I bands*, while the dark bands containing myosin filaments and part of the actin filaments are called *A bands*. In the middle of the light band is a dark line called the *Z line*. Between the Z lines is the smallest contractile apparatus, the *sarcomere* (see Fig. 40-2) [9].

Organelles of the Muscle Cell

The inside of the cell contains *sarcoplasm*, which is the cytoplasm of the muscle cell. In addition to myofibrils, the cell contains structural and chemical parts common to all cells (Fig. 40-3). Especially important are the mitochondria, sarcoplasmic reticulum, T tubules, electrolytes, and water. Large quantities of potassium, magnesium, and phosphates are present, together with enzymatic proteins, bicarbonate, sulfate, and small amounts of sodium, chloride, and calcium.

Mitochondria, present in enormous numbers, provide a major source of energy for contraction. Energy is produced through a supply of adenosine triphosphate (ATP), which is mostly formed by the extraction of energy from nutrients and oxygen (see pp. 8–10).

The sarcoplasmic reticulum (SR) is similar to the endoplasmic reticulum of other cells. Its major function appears to be to transport calcium into the sarcomere unit to initiate muscle contraction. The SR is composed of tubules running longitudinally and parallel to the myofibrils. The tubules terminate in closed sacs at the end of each sarcomere (terminal cisternae). This allows for communication during depolarization and contraction. The SR is highly developed in skeletal muscle but is less well developed in cardiac muscle cells. That in smooth muscle is poorly developed with narrow tubules of reticulum beneath which are many vesicles called *caveolae* [3,6].

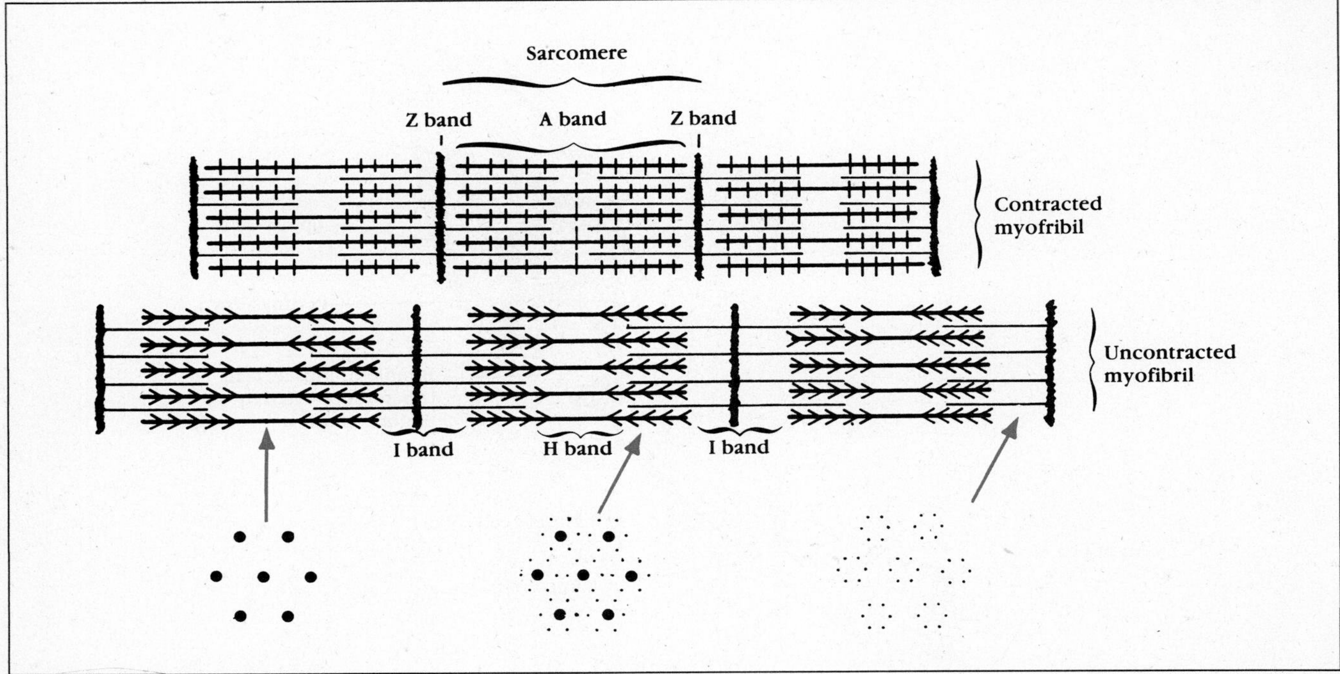

FIGURE 40-2 Portions of contracted and uncontracted myofibrils. The I bands diminish in length in the contracted myofibrils. The punctuate arrays represent an ultrastructural view of the relationships of thick (myosin) and thin (actin) filaments in cross section through different areas of the sarcomere. A sarcomere is the distance between successive Z bands. (From M. Borysenko et al., *Functional Histology* [2nd ed.]. Boston: Little, Brown, 1984.)

The T tubule (transverse tubule) system is closely associated with the SR. It is composed of tubules that extend across the sarcoplasm but open to and communicate with the exterior of the muscle cell (see Fig. 40-3).

Neuromuscular or Myoneural Junction

Each skeletal muscle fiber normally receives innervation from a motor nerve. The nerve fiber branches at its end to form a motor end plate or myoneural junction that indents the surface of the muscle fiber membrane (Fig. 40-4). The junction of the axon terminal with the muscle fiber includes the following two important structures: (1) the synaptic gutter, the indentation of the fiber membrane where the axon terminal comes in close contact with the fiber; and (2) the synaptic cleft, the small space between the axon and the muscle. Within the axon terminal are synaptic vesicles that contain *acetylcholine*, the excitatory chemical transmitter. *Cholinesterase* is present on the surface of the folds of the synaptic gutter and destroys acetylcholine immediately after the response is initiated.

Physiology of Striated Muscle

Generation of an Action Potential

For a skeletal muscle to contract, a stimulus from the nervous system must be present. When this stimulus arrives from the nerve axon to the myoneural junction, acetylcholine is released into the synaptic gutter space. This neurotransmitter causes the muscle cell membrane to become very permeable to sodium ions. Sodium rushes into the muscle fiber, causing a rise in membrane potential or generation of end plate potential. The action potential thus generated passes down the sarcolemma, depolarizing the T tubule system and causing the release of calcium ions from the SR. Calcium ions, thus released, strongly bind with troponin-tropomyosin, and the sliding of actin on myosin occurs. This initiates the contractile phase.

Sliding Filament Theory

The basis of muscular contraction is the movement or sliding of actin on myosin, which results in shortening of the entire sarcomere unit. Actin and myosin have been shown to have a strong affinity for each other that is inhibited by the proteins troponin and tropomyosin. The structure of myosin facilitates cross-linkages with actin, completing the system needed to perform the muscular contraction.

Pure actin filaments bind strongly with myosin when they are in the presence of magnesium ions and ATP, which exist in abundance in the myofibrils. When troponin and tropomyosin are added to the thin filaments, binding between actin and myosin is inhibited. When the muscle is at rest, troponin and tropomyosin cover the actin filaments so that they cannot bind with myosin. Initiation of the contractile process requires that troponin

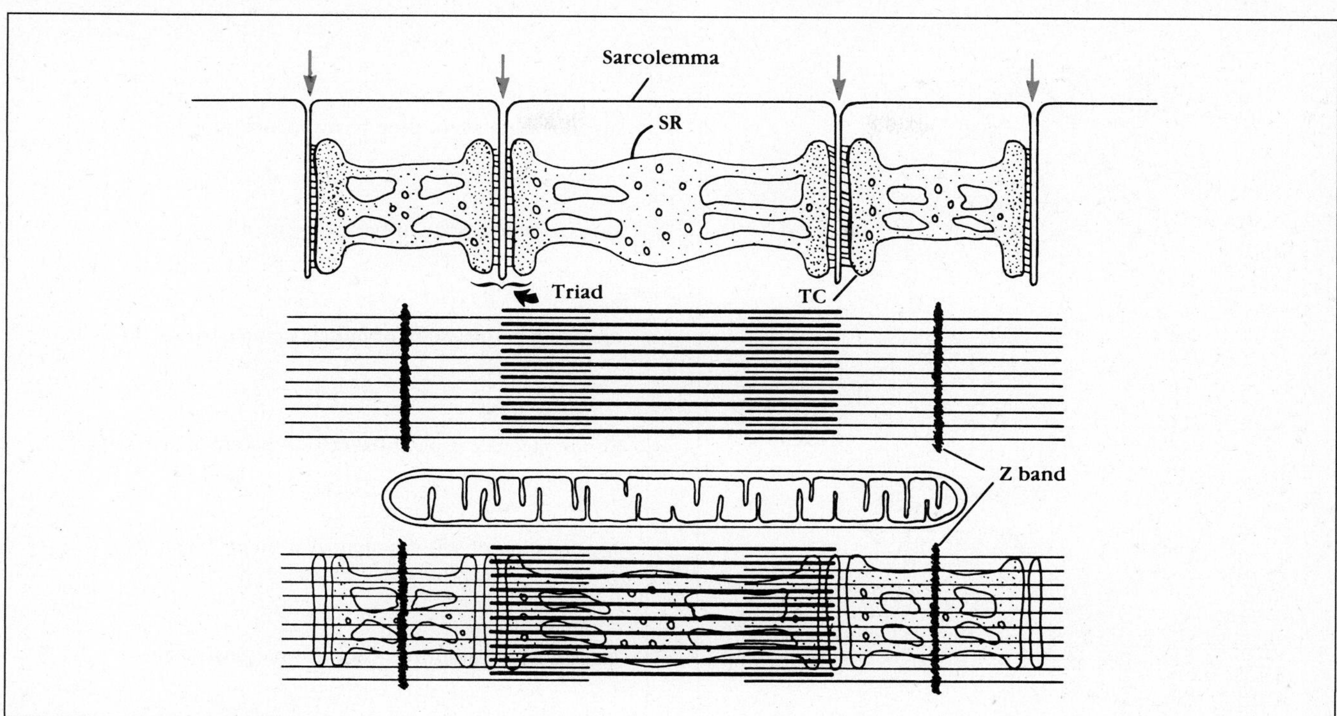

FIGURE 40-3 Thin section of skeletal muscle as it might appear on electron microscopy. Proceeding from the plasmalemma (sarcolemma) inward are the sarcoplasmic reticulum (SR), the sarcomere of a myofibril, a mitochondrion separating adjacent myofibrils, and a sarcomere with its associated sarcoplasmic reticulum. The arrows indicate points along the plasmalemma where T tubules invaginate the fiber at the A–I junction of sarcomeres. The terminal cisterns (TC) of the SR are associated with the T tubules by short junctional feet, forming the triad where excitation-contraction coupling occurs. (From M. Borysenko et al., *Functional Histology* [2nd ed.]. Boston: Little, Brown, 1984.)

and tropomyosin be inhibited. Calcium ions, released from the SR, bind to sites on troponin molecules. This binding causes the troponin molecule to change shape, which pulls on the tropomyosin strands, moving them to the side and uncovering the cross-bridge binding sites on the actin molecules [6]. Adenosine triphosphate interacts at the site, splits, and activates myosin. Myosin binds to actin creating a cross-bridge that moves the thin (actin) filaments toward the center. The cross-bridge is broken by the binding on a new ATP molecule. Splitting of this molecule causes the binding to reform at a different place on the actin molecule. This *power stroke* pulls the actin on the myosin in a step-by-step process described as a ratchetlike movement by Huxley in 1954 [4]. The ATP is essential to provide energy through splitting for the cross-bridge movement and to break the myosin-actin connection, which allows the cross-bridge on myosin to return to its original position.

The "Walk-Along" Mechanism

The exact way by which the cross-bridges on myosin interact with actin is not totally understood. The cross-bridges attach to and disengage from active sites on the actin filament in a "walk-along" fashion (Fig. 40-5) [2]. The attachment causes dragging of the actin filament (sliding of actin on myosin). After this power stroke, the sites are disengaged and attach to the next active site, pulling the actin filament step by step toward the center of the myosin filament. The cross-bridges theoretically operate independently of each other, so that if more cross-bridges are in contact with the actin filament, the force of the contraction is greater [2].

Return to Muscle Relaxation

Calcium must be returned to the tubules of the SR so that troponin and tropomyosin can resume their inhibitory function. This is accomplished by an active *calcium pump* in the walls of the SR. This pump also can concentrate calcium within the tubules, which creates a low level of calcium in the myofibrils. As calcium leaves troponin, it returns to its original configuration, which then allows tropomyosin strands to recover the actin-binding sites [6]. Without a communication between actin and myosin, the sarcomere unit extends and the muscle relaxes. Figure 40-6 summarizes the process.

The sodium pump also is required to restore sodium-potassium balance and water balance within the cell. This active process is described in Chapter 1.

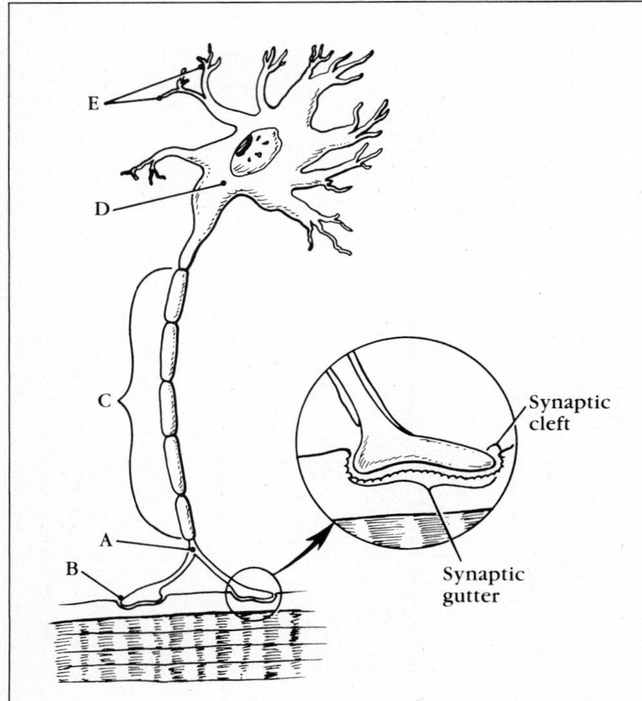

FIGURE 40-4 Myoneural or neuromuscular junction. A. Terminal branching of nerve fibers for the end plates. B. Junction of axon terminal and muscle cell membrane. C. Axon. D. Nerve cell. E. Dendrites.

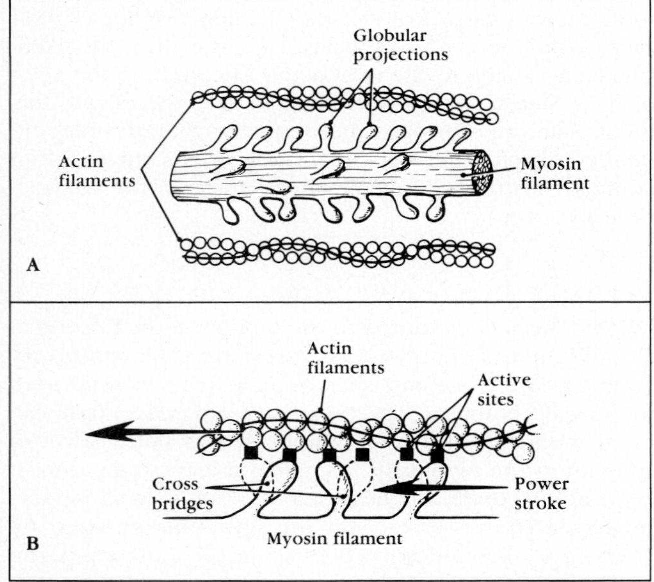

FIGURE 40-5 Walk-along mechanism for muscle contraction. A. The relationship between the myosin filament with its globular projections and the actin filaments. B. The hinges of the myosin filament attach to successive active sites on the actin filaments.

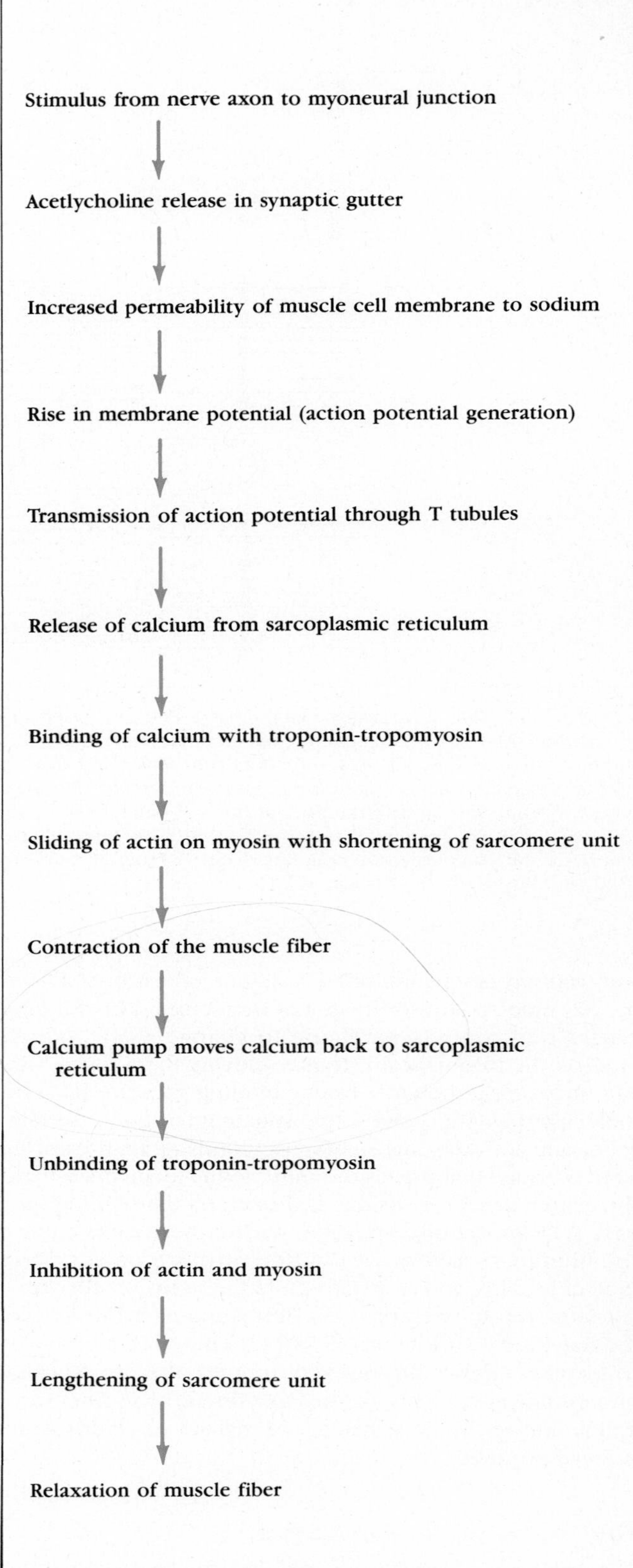

FIGURE 40-6 Summary of the processes of muscle contraction and relaxation.

Energy Requirements of Muscle Contraction

Four physiologic reactions are available to provide energy (ATP) for muscle contraction: (1) use of the limited supply of ATP stores within the cell; (2) conversion of high-energy stores from phosphocreatine (creatine phosphate); (3) generation of ATP through anaerobic glycolysis; and (4) oxidative metabolism of acetyl CoA.

Stored ATP. Adenosine triphosphate is a high-energy compound that is supplied mostly through an oxidative process. The ATP existing in the resting muscle cell is rapidly depleted during muscular contraction. Continued demand for energy is met by donation of phosphate from phosphocreatine stores and by anaerobic production of ATP. As exercise is sustained the increased blood flow to muscle allows for the aerobic production of more ATP.

Phosphocreatine (Creatine Phosphate). Muscle has a small store of creatine phosphate that can rapidly donate its phosphate to produce ATP and energy. This process occurs very rapidly, but the stores of creatine phosphate are rapidly depleted. Resynthesis in the resting muscle occurs from metabolism of food.

Anaerobic Metabolism. Anaerobic metabolism provides ATP when the cellular supply of oxygen is insufficient to produce enough to meet the energy requirements of the cell. In the muscular system, it is often used when the skeletal muscles are taxed, as in athletic exertion. Without the adequate oxygen supply, pyruvate does not enter the citric acid cycle to yield carbon dioxide and water, but rather is reduced to lactic acid. The net ATP formed is much less than with oxygen, but it allows the muscle cells to continue their activity for a short period of time.

Aerobic Production of ATP. As exercise is sustained, blood flow to the area is increased and a new steady state of muscle metabolism is achieved through the initiation of aerobic production of needed ATP.

Once the intense level of activity has stopped, the body consumes excess amounts of oxygen, as evidenced by the labored breathing of runners after a long-distance race. The intake of oxygen oxidizes the excess lactic acid and also aids in the metabolism that replenishes supplies of ATP and creatine phosphate. The amount of excess oxygen that is required to recover from the intense activity is in direct relationship to the energy demands of the body. The amount of oxygen needed is called the *oxygen debt*.

At rest the skeletal muscle uses mostly fatty acids for energy production. During exercise the uptake of glucose and fat increases. It is estimated that 90 percent of carbon dioxide is produced through the use of fat [2].

Circulatory Adjustments to Exercise

Exercise performance depends on the ability of the circulatory system to compensate for increased needs. Blood flow to the muscles is increased by opening capillary beds not open at rest. The stimuli for this phenomenon are probably tissue hypoxia and release of local vasodilator agents. Exercise increases cardiac output and heart rate, while vasodilation decreases systemic vascular resistance.

Dynamic exercise (isotonic) results in increases in systolic blood pressure, heart rate, and stroke volume, and normal or depressed diastolic pressure. This type of exercise is exemplified by jogging, running, walking, and playing tennis, among other activities. Sympathetic nervous system stimulation produces vasoconstriction in other vascular beds such as the kidneys, gastrointestinal tract, and others. Increased metabolic activity increases the body temperature so that heat loss is initiated. The two main methods of heat loss are through cutaneous vasodilation with radiation from the skin and sweating with evaporation [11].

Exercise may also be static or isometric; that is muscle contractions create tension but do not move a load. Isometric exercise results in elevation of both systolic and diastolic blood pressures, increased systemic vascular resistance, and a modest increase in cardiac output and heart rate.

Therefore, static exercise principally increases cardiac afterload stress by increasing systemic vascular resistance, while dynamic exercise increases the preload stress by increasing venous return and cardiac output [11].

Muscles vary according to the work required of them. It should be noted that the speed of contraction is matched to the function endowed on the corresponding muscle. Eye muscles, for example, which provide fine, precise movement, react swiftly, while large muscles, such as those necessary to maintain posture, react slowly. The larger, slower muscles have smaller fibers and more capillaries and mitochondria than do faster-moving muscles [2]. They are often called *red* muscles because they contain large quantities of myoglobin.

Muscle tone is the term applied to the tautness of healthy muscle tissue at rest. This tone is probably maintained by spinal cord impulses.

Exercise training over a period of weeks to months increases the number and size of mitochondria in the muscle cells; the level of mitochondrial enzyme activity; the capacity of muscle to oxidize fat, carbohydrate, and ketones; myoglobin levels; and the capacity to generate ATP [11]. The net effect is to increase the capability of muscles to extract oxygen and to increase aerobic capability at any given workload. The results on the cardiovascular system are decreases in heart rate, blood pressure, and systemic vascular resistance, and increased stroke volume at any submaximal workload [11].

Anatomy of Smooth Muscle

The anatomy of smooth muscle differs somewhat from that of striated muscle, but the greatest difference between the two is functional. The smooth muscle cell is long and spindle-shaped, and has a single nucleus near the center of the cell. A sarcolemma surrounds the fiber, beneath which are many vesicles called *caveolae*. These may function like SR in storing calcium [6]. Smooth muscle fibers lack the characteristic striations of skeletal fibers and vary markedly in length. The lack of striations probably is due to poorly developed SR and T tubule system. Two distinct groups of smooth muscle have been identified: visceral and multiunit (Fig. 40-7). The three different filaments are described for smooth muscle are the thin (actin), thick (myosin), and intermediate (dense bodies) filaments that are neither actin nor myosin and run continuously through the fiber [2].

Visceral (Unitary) Smooth Muscle

Visceral smooth muscle is present in the walls of the hollow visceral organs, such as the uterus, gut, and bile ducts. The cells are closely aligned and form large sheets of tissue. Because of the close proximity of cells, an action potential spreads cell to cell along the muscle until the entire muscle mass is stimulated. These muscles respond to innervation from the autonomic nervous system to increase or decrease the rate of activity, but it is a slow response to this stimulation.

Multiunit Smooth Muscle

Multiunit smooth muscle is present in the ciliary muscles of the eyes and in the piloerector muscles of the skin that cause goose flesh. The arrangement of cells is similar to that of striated muscle. Multiunit smooth muscles are individually innervated. They contract more rapidly than the visceral smooth muscle.

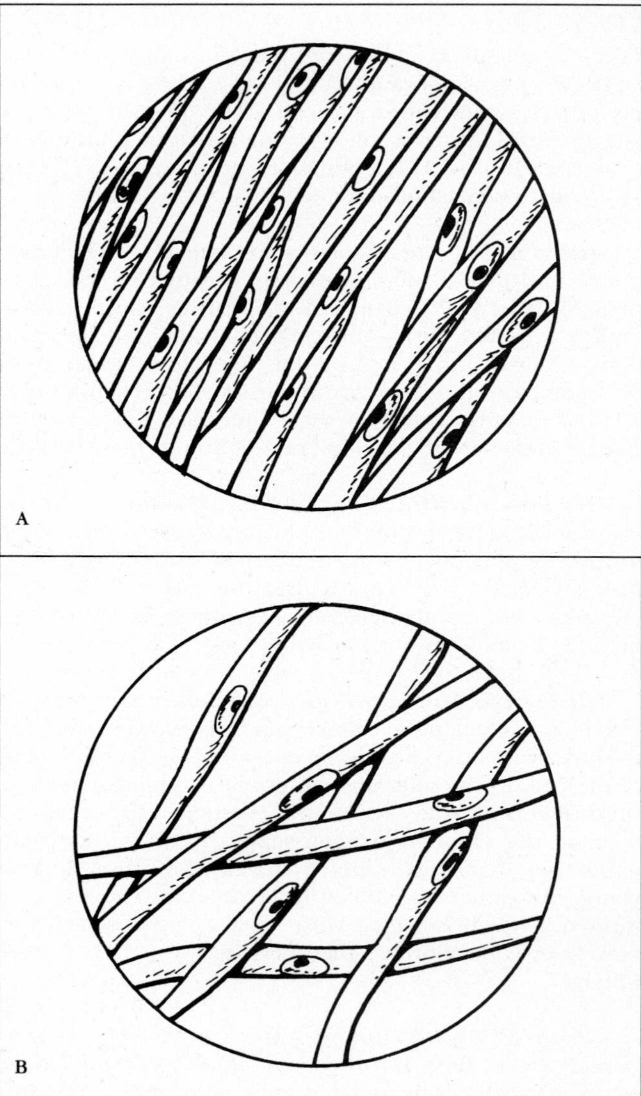

FIGURE 40-7 A. Visceral smooth muscle as present in the walls of hollow visceral organs. Note close arrangement of fibers. B. Multiunit cells as present in cillary muscles of the eyes, for example. Note loose arrangement of fibers.

Physiology of Smooth Muscle

Four properties distinguish smooth muscle contractions from other types: (1) the contractile process is relatively slow, with contractions lasting for long periods of time; (2) energy expended during the long contractions is far less than that of striated muscle; (3) in certain circumstances, such as childbirth, the strength of contractions can be very forceful; and (4) slow relaxation follows the slow contraction.

In visceral smooth muscle, electrical excitation proceeds from one muscle fiber to the next due to tight junctions that allow the impulse to pass from muscle cell to muscle cell, a syncytial effect.

Action Potentials in Smooth Muscle

Spike Potential. Action potentials develop differently in visceral smooth muscle tissue. The spike potential, similar to that of striated muscle, can be elicited by (1) electrical stimulation, (2) hormone action, (3) nerve fibers, and (4) spontaneous generation in the muscle fiber itself [2]. A typical spike action potential can be recorded much like that in skeletal muscle.

Slow-Wave Potential. The second type of action potential is the slow-wave potential. Some smooth muscle is self-excitatory, needing no apparent external stimulation. This is evidenced by rhythmic peristaltic waves. The slow waves apparently contribute to the action potential, a type of pacemaker wave.

Action potentials also may involve *plateaus*, long periods of depolarization, prolonged contraction, and slow repolarization. Prolonged contractions occur in the ureters, vascular system, and uterus [2]. Waves of contraction, called *peristalsis*, occur along the gastrointestinal tract. These are inhibited by stimulation of the sympathetic nervous system (SNS) and augmented by stimulation of the parasympathetic nervous system [3].

Smooth Muscle Tone

Smooth muscle tone relates to the ability of fibers to maintain long-term contraction, which occurs in the peristaltic type of contraction. The smooth muscles of the arterioles exhibit continuous variable degrees of contraction that respond to changing autonomic nervous stimulation. These may also be responsive to local tissue factors or circulating hormones.

Neuromuscular Junctions of Smooth Muscle

Two types of neuromuscular junctions are present in the innervation of smooth muscle: (1) the *contact type*, in which the nerve fibers come into direct contact with the muscle cells, and (2) the *diffuse type*, which occurs when nerve fibers never come into direct contact with the smooth muscle fibers. The contraction may be initiated by nerve impulses (through transmitter substances), chemical agents, changes in the muscle itself, and even local stretch or distention.

Smooth muscle has a nerve supply for inhibition and one for excitation. The transmitters for this, acetylcholine and epinephrine, are secreted by the autonomic nervous system. The response to the chemical transmitters varies, but generally, if acetylcholine excites an organ, norepinephrine acts as an inhibitor and vice versa (see p. 717).

Anatomy of Cardiac Muscle

Prior to advancements in microscopic technology, cardiac muscle cells were thought to form a morphologic syncytium. *Syn* refers to being together, *cyte* means cell. Light microscopy reveals cardiac tissue to have cross-striations with unique dark bands encircling the fibers at random sites. Seemingly, the cells are incomplete and branch into one another, forming a continuous mass of protoplasm. Electron microscopy, however, reveals that cardiac muscle cells are netlike in appearance, with fibers running together, spreading apart, and again running together in no apparent pattern. The dark bands that can be seen with the light microscope are abutting bands of tissue encircling the cardiac fibers (Fig. 40-8). They are called *intercalated disks* and are located at the sites of the Z bands. The disks represent areas where membranes of adjacent cells' ends approach each other. Functionally, these disks allow a wave of depolarization to pass unhindered from one cell to the next. Although each cardiac fiber branches and anastomoses with other fibers, a plasma membrane actually encases each fiber. Each cell has a single, centrally located nucleus. An abundance of elongated mitochondria are present close to the myofibrils in cardiac tissue. As in skeletal cells, myofibrils and the contractile proteins (actin and myosin) are present.

Structural differences between skeletal and cardiac tissue are apparent. A sarcoplasmic reticulum is present in

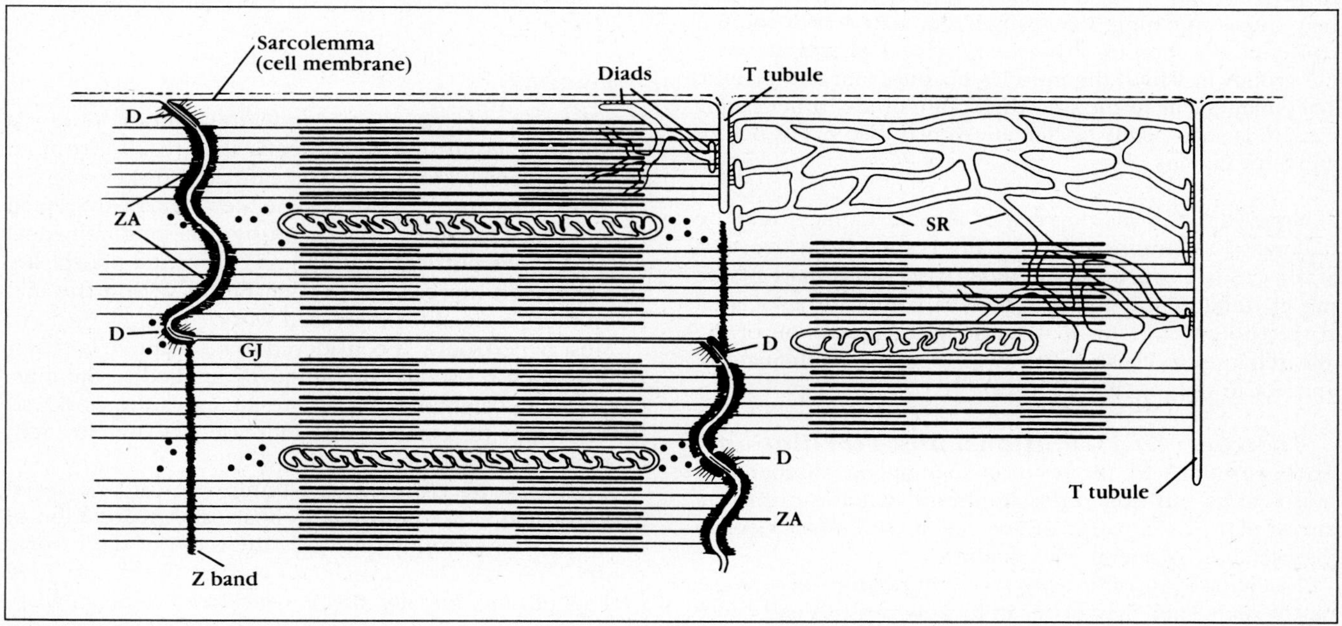

FIGURE 40-8 A thin section through cardiac muscle as it might appear on electron microscopy. Portions of two cardiac muscle fibers are depicted in the area where their plasmalemmas associate to form the intercalated disk. Desmosomes (D) provide structural integrity to the disk. Thin filaments insert into the fascia adherens (ZA) of the disk. The gap junctions (GJ) are located in the horizontal part of the disk. The disk occurs where a Z band would have been. The T tubules occur at the Z lines. The sarcoplasmic reticulum (SR) forms a sleeve around the myofibrils, but here it is depicted alone to show its pattern more clearly. (From M. Borysenko et al., *Functional Histology* [2nd ed.]. Boston: Little, Brown, 1984.)

cardiac muscle, but it is very rudimentary in comparison to that of skeletal muscle. The T tubules are 5 times larger in cardiac tissue than in skeletal tissue and are lined with mucopolysaccharide filaments. These filaments seem to trap calcium ions that are used by the sarcoplasm once an action potential has been initiated. Because the *terminal cisternae* of skeletal tissue are missing in cardiac tissue, scientists believe that the T tubules act as reservoirs for calcium in cardiac muscle, as the terminal cisternae do in skeletal tissue.

Myocardial muscle fibers are structured in such a way that the atria and ventricles, when normal and intact, react individually as syncytial units. The specialized conductive units—the sinoatrial (SA) node, atrioventricular (AV) node, bundle of His, and Purkinje fibers—work in concert to cause cardiac contraction. The physiology of cardiac contraction is described in detail in Chapter 18.

Alterations in Muscles of the Body

Common Problems in Muscles

Cramps. Cramps, or spasms, are frequent occurrences in the skeletal muscles. They may be idiopathic or associated with motor system disease, metabolic disease such as uremia, tetanus, and electrolyte depletion, especially of sodium, potassium, and calcium. Muscle cramps are often reported at night or during rest and may be due to lowered blood sugar levels at night. Dehydration also may cause cramping, especially if associated with sodium depletion. Cramps are involuntary spasms of specific muscle groups in which the muscles become taut and painful. They may occur in the calf, thigh, hip, or any other major muscle group. Visible fasciculations may also occur before and after cramps [5].

Strain. Various degrees of muscle damage may be diagnosed as strain, which usually results from overuse. Strains usually occur at the most susceptible part of the muscle-tendon unit and may be very painful or associated with tendinitis. Strains may cause an inflammation of the affected muscle, causing it to swell, become erythematous, and hot to the touch.

Twitches, Fasciculations, and Fibrillations. These reactions are the result of spontaneous discharge of motor units and single muscle fibers. Twitches occurring at rest may be idiopathic or associated with motor neuron disease and peripheral neuropathies.

Fasciculations are involuntary contractions of a single motor unit. They may occur in healthy persons and cause visible dimpling or twitching of the skin. Fasciculations may occur rhythmically, starting and stopping for no apparent reason. Those during contraction of a muscle indicate excessive irritation and may occur years after poliomyelitis or a degenerative nervous system disease. The molecular pathogenesis is not fully understood but apparently involves hypersensitivity of the neuronal membrane to acetylcholine [7]. Continuous fasciculations, called *myokymia*, of unknown etiology may involve all of the voluntary muscles. They may be abolished or alleviated by curare, succinylcholine, and diphenylhydantoin [7].

Fasciculation is often confused with fibrillation, which results from the contraction of single muscle fibers. It occurs when the motor unit of the axon is destroyed [7].

Tetany. Tetany, a spasmotic condition, most frequently results from hypocalcemia and hypomagnesemia. It is probably due to unstable depolarization of the distal segments of the motor nerves [2]. Hyperventilation may precipitate tetany by lowering serum carbon dioxide level, which reduces the level of ionized calcium.

Myoclonus. A sudden, unexpected contraction of a single muscle or group of muscles that involves the limbs more than the trunk is called myoclonus. This disorder has many causes, from idiopathic benign (sleep) jerks to central nervous system disease [7].

Tics. Tics differ from myoclonus in that they are sudden, behavior-related, repetitive movements that may be a form of learned behavior or occur as a part of Tourette's syndrome. In the latter, tics may be accompanied by involuntary vocalizations [7].

Other Motor Disorders. Many motor disorders and disturbances are as benign, such as fatigue of the muscles, or are representative of severe central nervous system dysfunction, such as convulsions. Those related to central nervous system dysfunction are described in Unit 15.

Hypertrophy

Hypertrophy, enlargement of individual muscle fibers, is an adaptive condition of the cells that results from an increased demand for work. The cardiac and skeletal muscle cells apparently cannot regenerate to adapt to a need for increased function. They adapt by enlarging individual fibers. Various nutrients such as ATP, creatine phosphate, and glycogen increase in concentration within the cell when there is need for increased work.

Most hypertrophy is considered to be adaptive in that it results when resistance is continually applied to the muscle walls. A weightlifter or athlete increases the workload through specific muscles that increase size and strength up to a physiologic limit.

Cardiac hypertrophy is a common result of arterial hypertension, aortic valvular stenosis, and coarctation of the aorta. Hypertrophy increases the force of the cardiac contraction, which can maintain cardiac output for long periods of time. Initially, this is considered to be an adaptive mechanism, but it may become maladaptive if the nutritional needs of the hypertrophied ventricle outstrip the blood supply from the coronary arteries.

Atrophy

Atrophy refers to the decrease in muscle mass due to diminution in size of the myofibrils. Atrophic muscles can result from such diverse factors as aging, immobilization, chronic ischemia, malnutrition, and denervation [8]. *Disuse atrophy* describes wasting of muscle tissue due to lack of muscle stress; an example is atrophic changes occurring after a bone fracture and treatment with casting.

Ischemia causes an inadequate blood supply, so that the oxygen and nutrients required for cellular maintenance are diminished. Eventually, ischemic changes may result in infarction of the tissue.

Denervation causes atrophic muscular changes that become irreversible. Loss of normal neural stimulation and reduction of muscle tone seem to be the major factors in these changes, rather than lack of weight bearing. If a muscle cell is reinnervated within three to four months, full function can be restored. After this time, some of the muscle fibers become permanently atrophied, and after two years muscle function is rarely restored.

Atrophy of muscle tissue may also occur in malnutrition or wasting diseases such as cancer, cirrhosis of the liver, and so forth. The muscle does not receive adequate nutrition and consequently protein wasting occurs.

Rigor Mortis

Rigor mortis is a state of muscular contraction that occurs approximately two to four hours after somatic death. It results from nonproduction of ATP, which is necessary to break the cross-bridges and promote lengthening of the sarcomere unit [6]. The contracture becomes intense and the joints become fixed into immovable positions. This state continues for approximately 15 to 25 hours, after which gradual autolysis of muscle protein causes the onset of muscle and tissue flaccidity [2].

Pathologic Processes Affecting the Skeletal Muscles

Myopathies is the general term given to diseases intrinsic to muscles. The category includes inherited muscular dystrophies, inherited and acquired metabolic myopathies, and inflammatory myopathies. Following is a brief review of the muscular dystrophies.

Muscular Dystrophies

The muscular dystrophies are genetically determined, progressive diseases of specific muscle groups. The syndromes are classified mainly by the distribution of involved muscles. Classification may also be based on pattern of inheritance, age of onset, and speed of progression [8]. Several members of the same family may be affected, with males predominating and females carrying the genetic abnormality. Muscle fiber necrosis is a major pathologic finding in muscular dystrophy. Studies imply that intracellular calcium overload is an essential factor because it activates proteases and impairs mitochondrial function [1,10].

Duchenne Muscular Dystrophy. This genetic recessive disorder occurs almost exclusively in males. It is characterized by early development of motor difficulties, inability to walk, symmetric weakness of the arms, and enlargement of the muscles of the calves. Intellectual impairment is common.

Pathologically, calcium accumulates in muscle fibers. Associated with this is activation of the *complement* cascade demonstrated in muscle fibers undergoing necrosis [1]. Nonnecrotic fibers do not demonstrate a positive reaction for complement, but excess calcium has been demonstrated in nonnecrotic muscle fibers [1].

The progression of the disease usually is characteristic, with lower extremity weakness progressing upward and finally affecting the head and chest muscles. The characteristic pseudohypertrophy of calf muscles is due to infiltration of the fibers with fatty deposits. The muscle becomes significantly weakened. Weakness of the back muscles results in lordosis. Respiratory or cardiac failure often causes death.

Prognosis in this disease is very poor, with death usually occurring before age 20 years. Prior to that time, increasing disabilities require much medical assistance.

Adult Forms of Muscular Dystrophy. Adult forms of muscular dystrophy such as Becker's, limb-girdle, facioscapulohumeral, and myotonic forms have a later onset and differ somewhat by the pattern of muscle involvement, heredity, and rate of progression.

Laboratory and Diagnostic Tests. Most persons with any form of muscular dystrophy have elevated levels of enzymes normally present in the muscles. These include creatine phosphokinase (CPK), lactic dehydrogenase (LDH), glutamic transaminase, and glucose phosphate isomerase. All of the findings indicate abnormal muscle plasma membranes [8]. Lymphocyte abnormalities also have been described.

Electromyography reveals weak electrical currents present in the muscle cell. Muscle biopsies are abnormal due to the presence of fatty tissue deposits in the cells.

Myasthenia Gravis

Myasthenia gravis is a disease related to the inability of the neuromuscular junctions to transmit nerve impulses to the muscle cells effectively. It is discussed in more depth on pages 856–857.

Rhabdomyosarcoma

The rhabdomyosarcoma is a malignant tumor of striated muscle. It occurs most commonly in children and adolescents, and may affect the striated muscles of the extremities, head, or neck. This type of sarcoma is very invasive with extremely anaplastic cells [8]. Five-year survival is 30 to 40 percent; treatment includes resection, radiation therapy, and chemotherapy.

Study Questions

1. Explain the process of skeletal muscle contraction.
2. Compare smooth muscle contraction and cardiac muscle contraction to skeletal muscle contraction.
3. Differentiate between action potentials in skeletal, smooth, and cardiac muscles.
4. Describe how the large skeletal muscles adapt to stress, such as is caused by running.
5. How does muscular atrophy result from disuse or spinal cord injury?
6. Describe the pathologic features and results of muscular dystrophy.

References

1. Cornelia, F. Muscle fiber degeneration and necrosis in muscular dystrophy and other muscle disease: Cytochemical and immunocytochemical data. *Ann. Neurol.* 12:694, 1984.
2. Guyton, A.C. *Textbook of Medical Physiology* (7th ed.). Philadelphia: Saunders, 1986.
3. Ham, A.W., and Cormack, D.H. *Histology* (8th ed.). Philadelphia: Lippincott, 1979.
4. Huxley, H.E. The double array of filaments in cross-striated muscle. *J. Biophys. Biochem. Cytol.* 3:631, 1957.
5. Kaufman, C.E., and Solomon, P. *Review of Pathophysiology*. Boston: Little, Brown, 1983.
6. McClintic, J.R. *Physiology of the Human Body* (3rd ed.). New York: Wiley, 1985.
7. Plum, F., and Posner, J. Neurology. In L.H. Smith and S.O. Thier (eds.), *Pathophysiology: The Biological Principles of Disease* (2nd ed.). Philadelphia: Saunders, 1985.
8. Robbins, S.L., Cotran, R.S., and Kumar, V. *Pathologic Basis of Disease* (3rd ed.). Philadelphia: Saunders, 1984.
9. Tortora, G.J., Evans, R.L., and Anagnostakos, N.P. *Principles of Human Physiology*. New York: Harper & Row, 1982.
10. Uchino, M., et al. Structural proteins of the opaque muscle fibers in Duchenne muscular dystrophy. *Neurology* 35(9), 1364, 1985.
11. Wallace, A.G., and Waugh, R.A. Pathophysiology of cardiovascular diseases. In L.H. Smith and S.O. Thier (eds.), *Pathophysiology: The Biological Principles of Disease* (2nd ed.). Philadelphia: Saunders, 1985.

CHAPTER 41

Normal and Altered Structure and Function of the Skeletal System

CHAPTER OUTLINE

Normal Structure and Function of Bone

- Bone Formation
  - *Cellular Components*
  - *Intramembranous Ossification*
  - *Endochondral Ossification*
- Bone Structure
  - *Microscopic Structure*
  - *Cancellous and Medullary Bone*
  - *Nerve and Blood Supply*
- Types of Bones
  - *Long Bones*
  - *Short Bones*
  - *Flat Bones*
  - *Irregular Bones*
- Bone Growth and Factors Affecting Bone Growth
  - *Location of Bone Growth*
  - *Calcium and Phosphorus*
  - *Vitamin D*
  - *Calcitonin*
  - *Sex Hormones*
  - *Growth Hormone*
  - *Weight Bearing*
  - *Other Factors*

Normal Structure and Function of Joints

- Types of Joints
- Classification of Synovial Joints
  - *Ball-and-Socket Joints*
  - *Condyloid Joints*
  - *Hinge Joints*
  - *Pivot Joints*
  - *Saddle Joints*
  - *Gliding Joints*
- Bursae
- Ligaments and Tendons

Fractures and Associated Soft Tissue Injuries

- Classification of Fractures
- Signs and Symptoms of Fractures
- Fracture Healing
  - *Conditions That Modify Healing*
  - *Alterations in Nerve Function Due to Bone Trauma*
- Compartmental Syndromes
- Other Associated Soft Tissue Traumas

Alterations in Bone Development

- Osteogenesis Imperfecta
- Osteopetrosis (Marble Bones, or Albers-Schönberg's Disease)
- Fibrous Dysplasia of Bone
  - *Albright's Syndrome*
- Paget's Disease
- von Recklinghausen's Disease
- Osteoporosis
- Rickets/Osteomalacia
- Scurvy
- Avascular Necrosis

Infectious Diseases of Bone

- Osteomyelitis
- Tuberculosis
- Syphilis

Alterations in Skeletal Structure

- Scoliosis
- Clubfoot (Talipes)
- Congenital Dislocation of the Hip

Alterations in Joints and Tendons

- Arthritis
  - *Rheumatoid Arthritis (RA)*
  - *Osteoarthritis*
- Gout
- Bursitis
- Baker's Cyst
- Tumors of Joints
  - *Synovial Sarcoma*
- Tenosynovitis
- Fibromatosis

Bone Tumors

- Classification of Tumors
  - *Bone-Forming Tumors*
  - *Tumors of Cartilaginous Origin*
  - *Tumors of Marrow Origin*
  - *Tumors of Undetermined Origin*
- Hematogenic Tumors

LEARNING OBJECTIVES

1. Name the three types of bone cells and their functions.
2. Differentiate between intramembranous and endochondral ossification in bone formation.
3. Describe the gross anatomy of the femur as a typical long bone of the body.
4. Describe the blood supply to a bone, including the nutrient and periosteal arteries.
5. Give examples of long, short, flat, and irregular bones.
6. Describe epiphyseal growth.
7. Name the factors that retard and the factors that accelerate bone growth.
8. Explain the calcium-parathyroid feedback mechanism.
9. Relate calcium and parathyroid levels to vitamin D absorption and production.
10. Discuss the feedback mechanism for calcitonin and calcium.
11. Explore the relationship among the level of sex hormones, age, and bone formation.
12. Discuss the effects of weight bearing on bone formation.
13. State the three classifications of joints and give examples of each.
14. Describe the structures of tendons, ligaments, and bursae.
15. Define *complete*, *comminuted*, *compression*, *depressed*, *stress*, and *avulsion fractures*.
16. Describe the process of fracture healing.
17. List five factors that modify the healing of fractures.
18. Differentiate among delayed union, nonunion, and malunion.
19. Relate the symptoms of anterior compartmental syndrome.
20. Describe the clinical syndrome of osteogenesis imperfecta.
21. Describe the polyostotic form of fibrous dysplasia (Albright's syndrome).
22. Describe Paget's disease of bone.
23. Discuss the skeletal manifestations of the hormone condition in von Recklinghausen's disease.
24. Name five types of persons at high risk for developing osteoporosis.
25. Identify the usual pathogenesis of rickets or osteomalacia.
26. Compare rickets and scurvy with regard to etiology and physical findings.
27. Describe the pathology of avascular necrosis of the head of the femur.
28. Describe the course of osteomyelitis from beginning infection to the chronic stage.
29. Describe the bone alterations that may occur with tuberculosis and syphilis.
30. Describe the physical changes of scoliosis.
31. List some causes of a congenitally dislocated hip.
32. Explore theories of causation of rheumatoid arthritis.
33. Describe the joint pathology of rheumatoid arthritis.
34. Discuss how rheumatoid arthritis affects other systems such as heart, lungs, eyes, and nerves.
35. Name the joints most commonly affected with degenerative changes.
36. Describe the metabolic disorder responsible for gout.
37. List the most commonly inflamed bursae and relate the principal causes.
38. Describe basic differences between benign and malignant bone tumors.
39. Name three benign tumors arising from cartilage tissue and three from bony tissue.
40. Compare and contrast the sarcomas of cartilaginous origin with those of osteogenic origin with respect to symptoms, gross pathology, survival, and frequency.
41. Define *Ewing's sarcoma*, including frequency and survival.
42. Discuss the skeletal involvement and symptoms of multiple myeloma.

Normal Structure and Function of Bone

The framework of the human body is the skeletal system. This system of more than 206 bones protects internal organs, provides for support and movement through its muscle attachments, serves as a storehouse for mineral supply, and produces blood cells. A living, dynamic tissue, bone contains blood, nerves, and lymph supplies, and provides for the constant movement of calcium, phosphorus, and other minerals into and out of the bloodstream.

Bone is a collagenous protein that is partially composed of complex calcium salts. The organic matrix of bone, called *osteoid*, is made up primarily of collagen (protein), some polysaccharides, and lipids. The salts, which consist of calcium carbonate ($CaCO_3$), and calcium phosphate ($Ca_3[PO_4]_2$), form a substance that is a hard crystalline salt. The matrix supplies *tensile strength* (resistance to being pulled apart), while the mineral deposits provide *compressive strength* (resistance to being crumbled). This combination gives bone the tensile strength of white oak and compressive strength greater than granite [9].

Bone Formation

Cellular Components. Bone tissue is constantly being formed and reformed. This modeling is facilitated by three types of cells. *Osteoblasts* are formed from osteogenic cells present in the endosteum, periosteum, and epiphyseal plates of long bones. These are bone-forming cells that synthesize the collagenous matrix osteoid in the process of *ossification*. This protein substance becomes calcified to produce hard bone. Osteoblasts also help control the calcification of bone. Alkaline phosphatase, which is thought to aid in the mineralization process, is produced by osteoblasts [8]. Osteoblasts synthesize osteocalcin and osteonectin, both of which bind to calcium and have a local effect on calcification of bone [11]. When the matrix surrounding the osteoblasts becomes calcified, the cells are called *osteocytes*. *Osteoclasts* are cells of mesenchymal origin whose primary function is the resorption of bone. These cells actually phagocytize bone by producing acids that make the bone salts soluble and then digesting the organic matrix [14].

Intramembranous Ossification. Bone formation begins in early fetal life. The fetal skeleton is composed mostly of hyaline cartilage that undergoes ossification. The swapping of the cartilaginous material with bone, begun in utero, continues until after puberty. There are two main types of bone formation: intramembranous and endochondral. The more simple and direct type is *intramembranous ossification*, which occurs in the flat bones of the face and skull. In the cartilaginous fetal structure, osteoblasts secrete organic material that calcifies; from this center of ossification, small bone spicules build up an interlacing network on which more bone is developed. Eventually, the osteoblasts are trapped in small spaces called *lacunae* and become osteocytes. The spongy bone developed is then covered by layers of compact bone.

Endochondral Ossification. This is the process by which the long bones of the body are formed (Fig. 41-1). The "baby skeleton," which is cartilage, is transformed into bone by ossification, which begins in the center of the shaft, the *diaphysis*, and in each end, the *epiphysis*, of the bone. This formation spreads, and with it the destruction of cartilage, until only two thin strips are left at either end of the bone (the epiphyseal plate), which remain until bone growth and maturation are completed. As spongy bone is formed within, marrow is formed in the spaces and the marrow cavity develops in the center of the bone. The osteoblasts on the outside form layers of hard, compact bone. The perichondrium, which is the layer surrounding the early cartilage, becomes the periosteum, and as more layers of compact bone are laid circumferentially, osteoclasts make the marrow, or medullary cavity, larger in order to support the larger bone.

Bone Structure

Microscopic Structure. Bone has three structural forms: cortical or compact (hard surface area), cancellous or spongy, and medullary (inner core). Whenever bone matrix is laid down rapidly and haphazardly, as occurs after fractures and in fetal growth, the resultant immature form is termed *woven bone*. The microscopic structure of

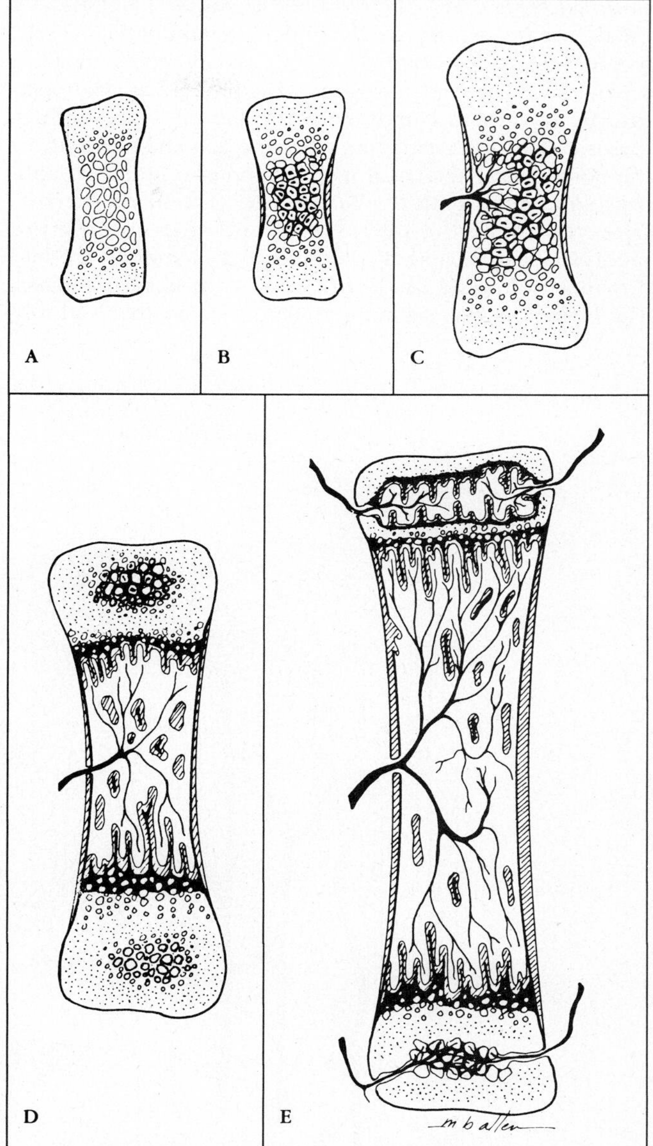

FIGURE 41-1 Some major events in the formation of a long bone by endochondral ossification. A. Hyaline cartilage model; hypertrophy of central chondrocytes. B. Hypertrophied chondrocytes begin to die due to initiation of matrix calcification; formation of the bone collar. C. Invasion of blood vessels and pluripotential osteoprogenitor cells; resorption of calcified cartilage matrix to form exposed surfaces for bone tissue apposition in primary center of ossification. D. Growth of bone and formation of marrow cavity by cartilage proliferation at epiphyseal ends, bone tissue apposition at calcified cartilage surfaces, and resorption in diaphyseal cavity; initiation of secondary center of ossification above; elongation of bone collar. E. Further growth of bone; formation and development of secondary center of ossification above, leaving cartilaginous epiphyseal plate separating epiphysis from diaphysis; appearance of additional secondary center of ossification below; growth in girth of bone by concomitant bone tissue apposition on outer diaphyseal surface and resorption from inner surface. Black = calcified cartilage; black arborizations = blood vessels; parallel diagonal lines = bone tissue. (From M. Borysenko et al., *Functional Histology* [2nd ed.]. Boston: Little, Brown, 1984.)

compact bone consists of numerous, parallel, longitudinal canals, the ***haversian canals***, which contain blood vessels, lymphatics, and nerves (Fig. 41-2). Around each canal are several layers, or rings, of bone called *lamellae*. Connecting the haversian canals with the lamellae are minute canals called *canaliculi* that carry oxygen and nutrients to the bone cells. Each canal with its contents and surrounding lamellae is called a ***haversian system*** or *osteon*. Directly under the periosteum and surrounding the medullary canal, several thicknesses of lamellae are laid down surrounding the entire shaft with hard thickness. The haversian systems run parallel to each other and longitudinally from metaphysis to metaphysis, and are connected transversely by tubes called *Volkmann's canals*. Blood vessels from the periosteum enter the bone and pass through these canals to enter and leave the haversian system.

Cancellous and Medullary Bone. Cancellous bone is present in flat bones and in the ends of long bones. It is a collection of *trabeculae*, or beams of bone, which gives it a spongy appearance and adds strength due to the many interlacing parts (Fig. 41-3). The spaces in between these trabeculae are filled with bone marrow. The red

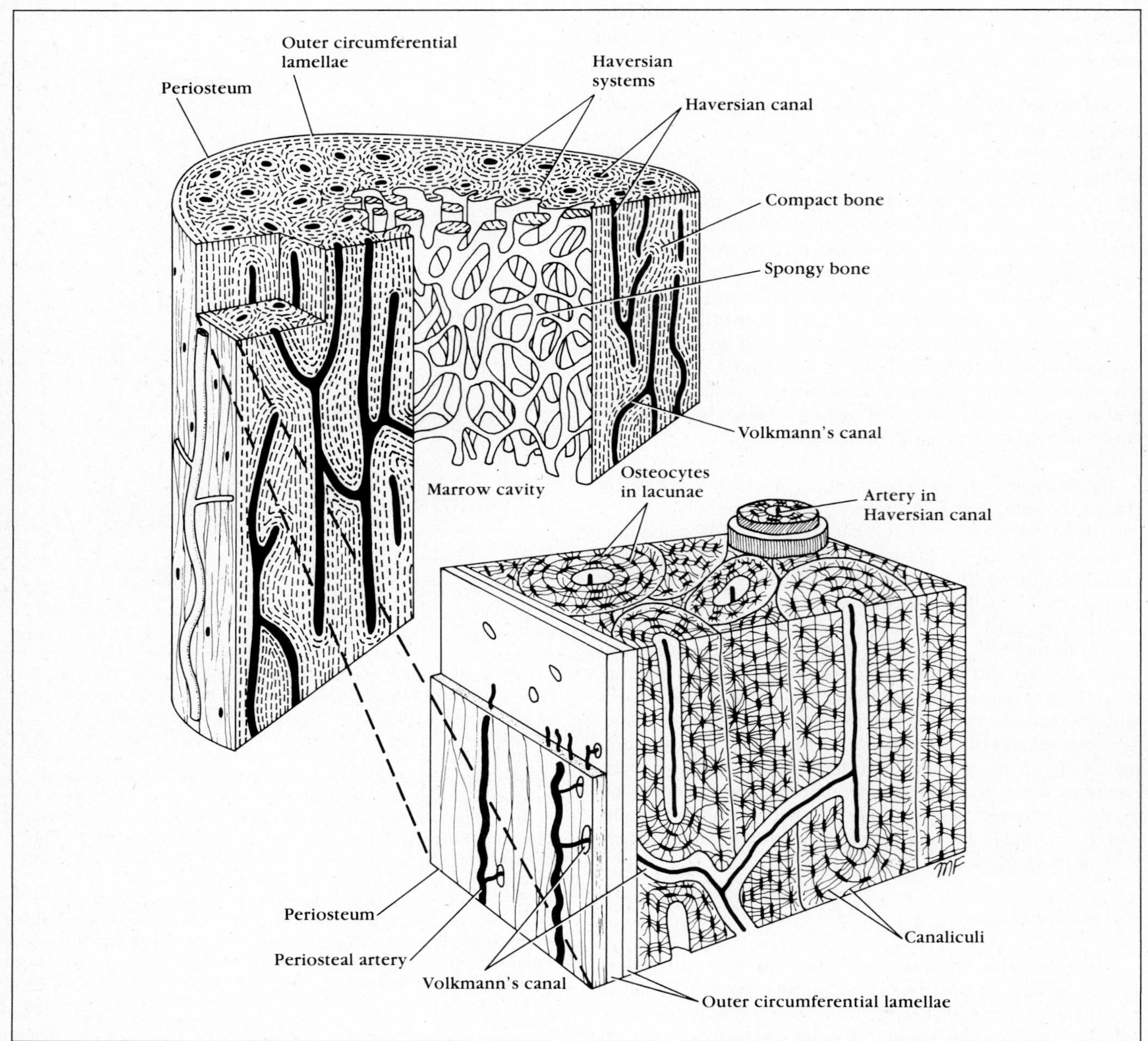

FIGURE 41-2 Compact bone tissue in histologic section. (From R.S. Snell, *Clinical Histology for Medical Students*. Boston: Little, Brown, 1984.)

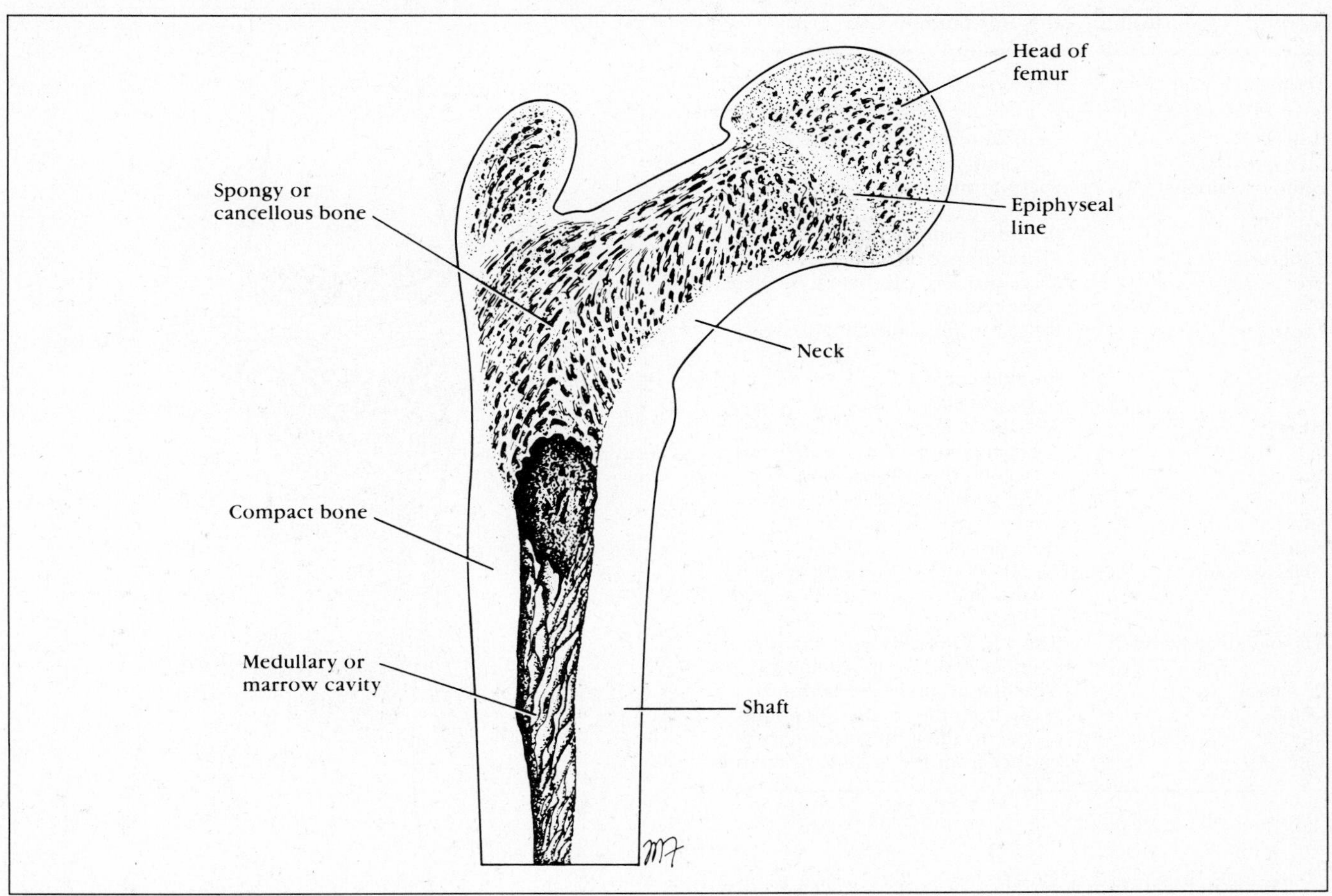

FIGURE 41-3 Bone structure. Note the differences in the three forms of bone structure: spongy, compact, and medullary. (From R.S. Snell, *Clinical Histology for Medical Students*. Boston: Little, Brown, 1984.)

marrow actively participates in the formation of red blood cells, and in the adult is present in the cancellous bone of the ribs, sternum, vertebrae, and pelvis. Red marrow is present in many bones in infants and is gradually converted to yellow marrow, so-named because it is composed of fat cells. Most long bones of the adult contain yellow marrow rather than red. Medullary bone is simply a continuation of cancellous bone and is the central area filled with marrow, blood, and lymph vessels.

Nerve and Blood Supply. Because bone is living tissue, nutrients must be supplied and waste material removed. Total bone blood flow has been estimated at from 200 to 400 ml per minute [7]. Small bones usually have a single artery and vein entering them, with large bones having several. The chief artery, which enters near the middle of the shaft of long bones, is called the *principal nutrient artery* (see Fig. 41-1E). After piercing the shaft and reaching the medullary canal, it branches into ascending and descending branches and ends in sinusoidal capillaries. The artery and its branches supply the marrow and cortex, as well as the haversian systems.

Nerve supply to bone is sparse and present mainly in the periosteum. It consists of both afferent (sensory) and sympathetic fibers, with the autonomic ones accompanying and controlling the dilatation of bone blood vessels. Pain of bone tumors is thought to arise from the afferent fibers, and that of fractures is largely due to pain fibers in the surrounding soft tissue and periosteum [9].

Types of Bones

Most commonly, bones are classified as long, short, flat, and irregular. Table 41-1 provides common anatomic terms.

Long Bones. Long bones are the bones of the extremities and have an elongated shape. Each one consists of two *epiphyses*, or ends, which are knobby areas containing cancellous bone, the *diaphysis*, which composes the shaft or long portion, and the *metaphysis*, which contains the epiphyseal plate and newly formed bone. In the adult, the metaphysis and epiphysis are continuous.

TABLE 41-1 Anatomic Terms in Common Use

Term	Definition
Process	General term for any bony prominence
Spine or spinous process	Sharp prominence
Tubercle	Rounded prominence on a bone
Tuberosity	Protuberance on a bone
Trochanter	Large process, e.g., below the neck of the femur
Crest	Ridge, or linear prominence, e.g., iliac crest
Condyle	Rounded protruding mass that carries an articular surface, e.g., knuckle
Head	The top or beginning, the most prominent part, e.g., enlargement beyond the constricted part as in the femoral head
Sinus	Cavity within a bone
Foramen	Hole or opening in a bone
Axial skeleton	The 80 bones composing the skull, vertebral column, sternum, and ribs
Appendicular skeleton	The 126 lower bones composing the upper and lower extremities
Proximal	Near the origin of the limb
Distal	Away from the origin of the limb
Medial	Nearer to the midline of the body
Lateral	Farther from the midline of the body

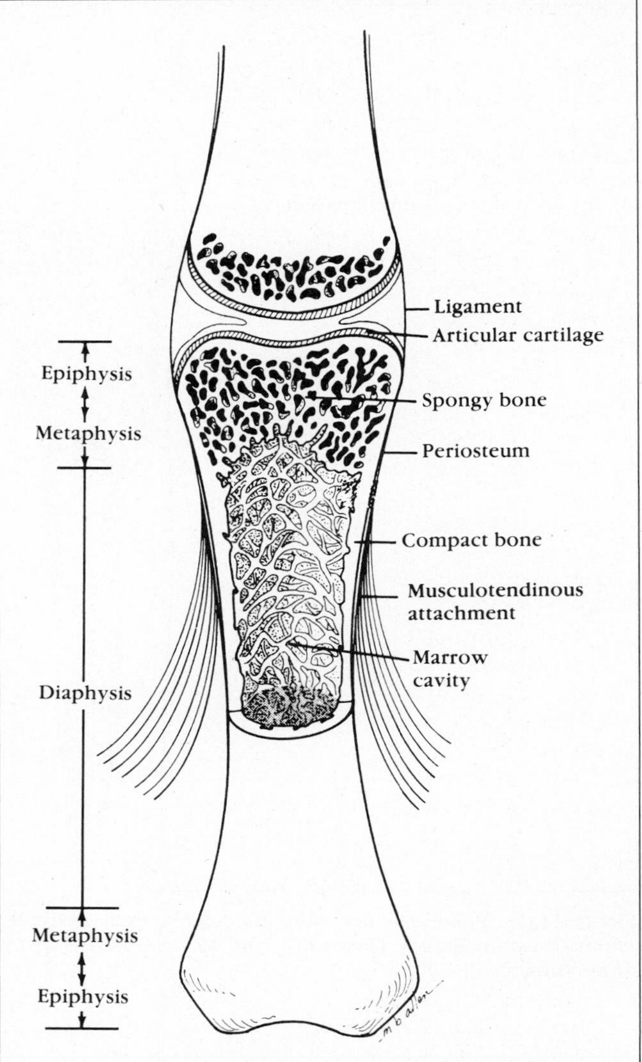

FIGURE 41-4 A long bone and some of its relationships. (From M. Borysenko et al., *Functional Histology* [2nd ed.]. Boston: Little, Brown, 1984.)

The outer and inner surfaces of bone are covered with specialized connective tissue. The dense, white, fibrous membrane wrapping the outside is called the *periosteum* and is composed of two layers. The outer, or *fibrous layer*, has relatively few cells and is made up of fibrous tissue. The inner layer of the periosteum is very vascular and has an osteogenic function. Lining the marrow and haversian cavities as well as the spaces of spongy bone is a membrane called the *endosteum*. In addition to supplying a site of attachment for tendons and ligaments, the periosteum is richly supplied with nerves and blood vessels that are important in nourishing the bone. Long bones form most of the appendicular skeleton, such as the femur, humerus, and phalanges (Fig. 41-4).

Short Bones. Short bones, such as those in the wrist, are cube-shaped and consist of cancellous bone enclosed in a thin case of compact bone. These often are combined with other short bones.

Flat Bones. The bones of the skull, ribs, scapulae, and sternum are examples of flat bones. Their function is largely protective. They consist of two plates of hard compact bone covering a thin layer of cancellous bone. These bones, especially the ribs and sternum, are important sites for blood formation.

Irregular Bones. The other bones are classified as irregular because they are irregular in shape; they are similar in composition to the short bones. The vertebrae and the ossicles of the ears are examples.

Bone Growth and Factors Affecting Bone Growth

Location of Bone Growth. The epiphyses of a long bone are separated from the shaft by the epiphyseal plate, which is responsible for the longitudinal growth of bone. On the distal side of this plate, osteoblasts are constantly secreting the bone matrix, which immediately becomes ossified, increasing the length of the bone. At the same time, on the proximal side of the epiphyseal plate, new cartilage is being formed. During puberty, ossification exceeds cartilage formation; gradually the cartilaginous epiphyseal plate becomes completely ossified and linear bone growth ceases. Epiphyseal closure occurs about three years earlier in women than it does in men, in whom bone length ceases to increase at about age 20 years [7].

As bones grow longitudinally, they also increase in circumference. Osteoblasts on the inner surface of the periosteum deposit layers of new bone, while osteoclasts in the area next to the medullary cavity make the canal larger to fit the larger bone. Bone growth does not stop when a person reaches puberty. Throughout life, bone continues to form and resorb, a process called *remodeling*. In the young adult, approximately one-sixth of total skeletal calcium is turned over every year, yet when a person reaches the fourth or fifth decade of life, resorption begins to outpace formation. Thus, with advancing age, 0.7 percent of the total skeletal mass is lost yearly [14]. Remodeling is influenced by many factors, including calcium and phosphorus metabolism, hormones, and the environment.

Calcium and Phosphorus. The exact mechanism that causes calcium to deposit and new bone to form remains a mystery. Certain nutritional, endocrine, and environmental states must exist, however, for the process to occur in an orderly fashion.

Adequate amounts of calcium and phosphorus must be present in the plasma and interstitial fluid that bathes the osteoblasts for new bone to be formed. These critical amounts are thought to be maintained in part by a partial membrane formed by osteoblasts. This membrane acts as a barrier between bone fluid and the extracellular fluid of the body (Fig. 41-5) [7]. The osteoblasts connect with other osteocytes deep in the bone where calcium can move into and out of the cell. Calcium salts precipitate on the surface of collagen fibers at periodic intervals. The initial calcium salts are a mixture of calcium and phosphate that become *hydroxyapatite crystals* through a process of resorption and reprecipitation, or substitution and addition of atoms [8]. Hydroxyapatite crystals (chemical formula $Ca_{10}[PO_4]_6[OH]_2$) provide the crystalline structure of bone mineralization.

With a normal diet, a person takes in approximately 1000 mg of calcium, of which 300 mg is absorbed in the intestines. From there it goes to the extracellular fluid and some of it is returned to the intestinal tract through bile and pancreatic enzymes. A large amount of the daily intake is excreted in the feces, with the kidneys excreting the rest [22]. In spite of this large amount of calcium movement into and out of the body, the serum calcium level remains constant at about 10 mg per dl. The serum pH and albumin levels affect the amount of calcium in the blood [22]. The constancy of this extracellular fluid calcium is maintained by vitamin D, parathyroid hormone, and calcitonin.

Calcium and phosphate are supplied in the diet mainly in milk and meats. Phosphate is absorbed with calcium. When calcium is absorbed in abundance, so is phosphate. Excess phosphate is excreted along with excess calcium in the feces and urine.

When the serum calcium ion concentration is high, production of *parathyroid hormone (PTH)* is severely curtailed. This results in a lowered serum calcium level

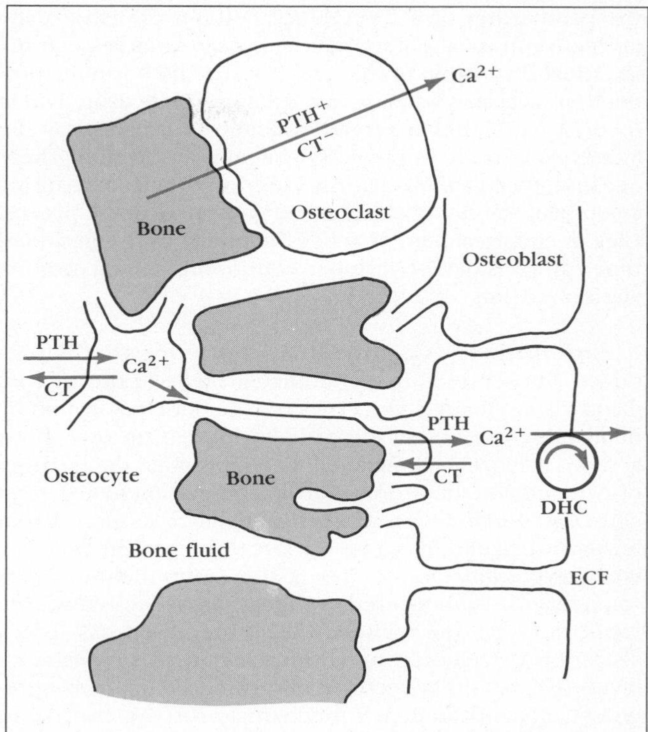

FIGURE 41-5 Parathyroid hormone (PTH) increases and calcitonin (CT) decreases the permeability of bone cells to calcium, whereas 1,25-dihydroxycholecalciferol (DHC) facilitates the active transport of calcium from osteoblasts into extracellular fluid (ECF). (From W.F. Ganong, *Review of Medical Physiology* [12th ed.]. Copyright © 1985. Lange Medical Publishers. Reprinted by permission.)

(see Chap. 34). Conversely, when serum calcium levels are lowered, parathyroid hormone secretion increases, which expands vitamin D activity and absorption of calcium in the intestinal tract. Parathyroid hormone promotes the formation of osteoclasts and retards the production of osteoblasts. The net result is increased resorption of bone, which causes the short-term effect of elevating serum calcium levels. Parathyroid hormone increases renal tubular resorption of calcium and decreases the resorption of phosphate ions.

Vitamin D. Vitamin D is a steroid hormone that is taken in the diet and is formed in the skin by the action of the ultraviolet rays of the sun. For dietary vitamin D to be absorbed, bile must be present. Through a series of events in the liver and kidneys, vitamin D_2 and D_3 are converted to 1,25-dihydroxycholecalciferol (1,25-[OH]2D), which is the active form of the vitamin. It controls serum calcium levels principally by controlling the absorption of calcium by the gut [15]. When the dietary intake of calcium is low, the kidneys increase their production of activated vitamin D, which increases the amount of calcium absorbed by the ileum. Vitamin D increases calcium resorption in the distal nephrons of the kidneys [15]. Renal failure depresses the resorption of calcium by the kidneys as well as curtailing the production of 1,25-(OH)2D. Vitamin D is virtually ineffective in renal failure, which causes a decrease in the intestinal absorption of calcium. Parathyroid hormone production increases when serum calcium levels drop, which increases 1,25-dihydroxycholecalciferol formation by the kidneys and leads to increased calcium absorption. These negative feedback mechanisms are important in ensuring an optimal amount of calcium and phosphate in the plasma. Lack of either calcium or active vitamin D over a period of time can considerably hamper continuing bone formation and remodeling.

Calcitonin. Calcitonin is a hormone that is produced and secreted by parafollicular cells of the thyroid gland. Its immediate effect is to reduce bone resorption by decreasing osteoclast activity and increasing osteoblast activity. A more prolonged effect is to reduce the quantity of osteoclasts being formed from the mesenchymal stem cells. Calcitonin does not significantly alter serum calcium levels in the adult; its effect is more significant in children, who have a more rapid rate of bone remodeling. Calcitonin may be administered in Paget's disease to reduce the rapid rate of bone turnover [22]. Increased calcitonin secretion is triggered by an increase in plasma calcium levels. The resulting decrease in serum calcium levels provides a second feedback mechanism for the control of blood calcium.

Sex Hormones. *Estrogen* has osteoblastic-stimulating activity. At puberty, a young girl has a rapid growth spurt before the epiphyseal plates close, which is attributed to estrogen. Therefore, girls stop growing a few years before their male counterparts. Throughout the premenopausal period, estrogen promotes bone formation by increasing intestinal absorption of calcium and phosphorus and increasing calcitonin production. In the postmenopausal woman, osteoporosis can be caused by the lack of estrogen.

Testosterone in the male increases bone length and thickness, and at the same time enhances epiphyseal closure. A decline in testosterone in the elderly man can cause osteoporosis.

Growth Hormone. The anterior lobe of the pituitary gland secretes the growth hormone (somatotropin), which causes a linear increase in long bones by increasing cartilage formation, widening the epiphyseal plates, and increasing the amount of matrix laid down in the ends of the long bones (see Chap. 32).

An excess of growth hormone in the growing person can cause gigantism. In the adult, whose epiphyseal plates are closed, the characteristic bone and soft tissue deformities of acromegaly result. Pituitary insufficiency can result in dwarfism in the child.

Weight Bearing. It has long been observed that muscles atrophy and bones demineralize when a limb is immobilized. Weightlessness experienced by astronauts was noted to cause loss of bone calcium and bone weakness [18]. Physical compression stimulates osteoblastic deposition, probably by generating an electrical potential. This potential at the compression site stimulates osteoblastic activity and increases bone formation. Electrical signals can also stimulate epiphyseal growth [20]. Studies in animals show that increased activity leads to an increase in bone mass, while inactivity, especially in growing animals, leads to a decrease in bone mass, decrease in the length and thickness of bones, and irregular articular surfaces and epiphyseal lines [20]. Local skeletal mass increases in the bones most used in physical exertion, such as playing tennis, weightlifting, and dancing.

Other Factors. *Glucocorticoids* cause an increase in protein breakdown in all tissues of the body. Because bone matrix is a protein product, an increase in steroids, as in Cushing's disease, can decrease matrix formation and weaken the bones, causing osteoporosis. Steroids also have the specific effect of depressing osteoblastic activity [8].

As was described earlier, two-thirds of the volume of bone is made up of osteoid organic material. Because all living tissues contain protein, anything that causes a decrease in protein in the body, such as starvation, retards bone formation.

Lack of vitamins A and C also decreases the ground substance in bone and leads to decreased bone formation. Persons having long-term heparin therapy develop osteoporosis, because heparin apparently speeds up the breakdown of collagen [21].

Thyroid hormone increases bone loss by increasing the activity of the osteoblasts [14]. Insulin increases the ability of the collagen matrix to produce osteoblasts. A summary of factors affecting bone growth is given in Table 41-2.

Normal Structure and Function of Joints

Types of Joints

Even though individual bones are hard and inflexible, the human body can have graceful flowing movements. Any motion, whether writing a letter or playing football, is brought about by the simultaneous movement of several *articulations*, or joints. Almost all of the bones of the body are joined to each other in one way or another. Some permit a range of motion and some allow none at all. Joints are classified in several ways, but the most common grouping is according to the degree of movement they

TABLE 41-2 Factors That Affect Bone Formation

Facilitate	Retard
Calcium	Hyperthyroidism
Phosphorus	Vitamin deficiency
Estrogen	Starvation
Calcitonin	Diabetes
Vitamins D, A, and C	Steroids
Growth hormone	Inactivity/immobility
Exercise	Heparin
Insulin	Thyroid

permit, as follows: *synarthroses*, immovable; *amphiarthroses*, somewhat movable; and *diarthroses*, freely movable. Joints may also be classified according to the material that connects them; for example, cartilaginous, fibrous, and synovial [9].

Using the degree of movement classification, the subgroups and their types are described in this section (Fig. 41-6). Synarthroses provide little movement, have a rigid surface, and include the bones of the skull. The sutures of the cranial bones are joined together by fibrous tissue and interlocking projections and indentations. These joints are not completed at birth and an infant has six gaps, or *fontanelles*, between bones. *Synchondrosis*, another type of immovable joint, is cartilage joining two bony surfaces. An example of synchrondrosis is the "joint" between the epiphysis and diaphysis of long bones that disappears after puberty. A third type of synarthrosis is a *gomphosis* (nail), which resembles a peg in a hole; an example is a tooth in the jaw.

Amphiarthroses are joints that permit very limited motion. A symphysis is a joint in which the bones are connected by disks of fibrocartilage. Examples are the symphysis pubis and the intervertebral disks between the vertebrae. One can see the benefits of such flexibility of the pelvis in childbirth and in the backbone with any movement. A *syndesmosis* is a slightly movable joint in which the bones are connected by ligaments permitting some bending and twisting; an example is the articulation between the tibia and fibula.

Diarthroses are often called *synovial* joints. They are freely movable and require lubrication to reduce the friction and abrasion that occur when one surface moves on another. The articulating surfaces of the bone are covered by a white, slick hyaline cartilage, and the entire joint is surrounded by an articular capsule that is filled with viscous synovial fluid. The inner layer of this capsule is a slippery, smooth membrane, while the outer layer is a tough, fibrous membrane. This inner, or *synovial*, membrane is rich in capillaries and cells, and is composed of secreting and phagocytic cells. The secretory cells produce synovial fluid, which contains water and protein [18]. The glucose level of the fluid is similar to that of serum. The chief function of this fluid is to lubricate and supply nutrients to the cartilage. The excess protein it contains is returned to the blood by way of the lymphatic system that drains the area. Synovial joints are supplied with sensory nerves that cause pain when there is an accumulation of inflammatory cells in the synovial tissues.

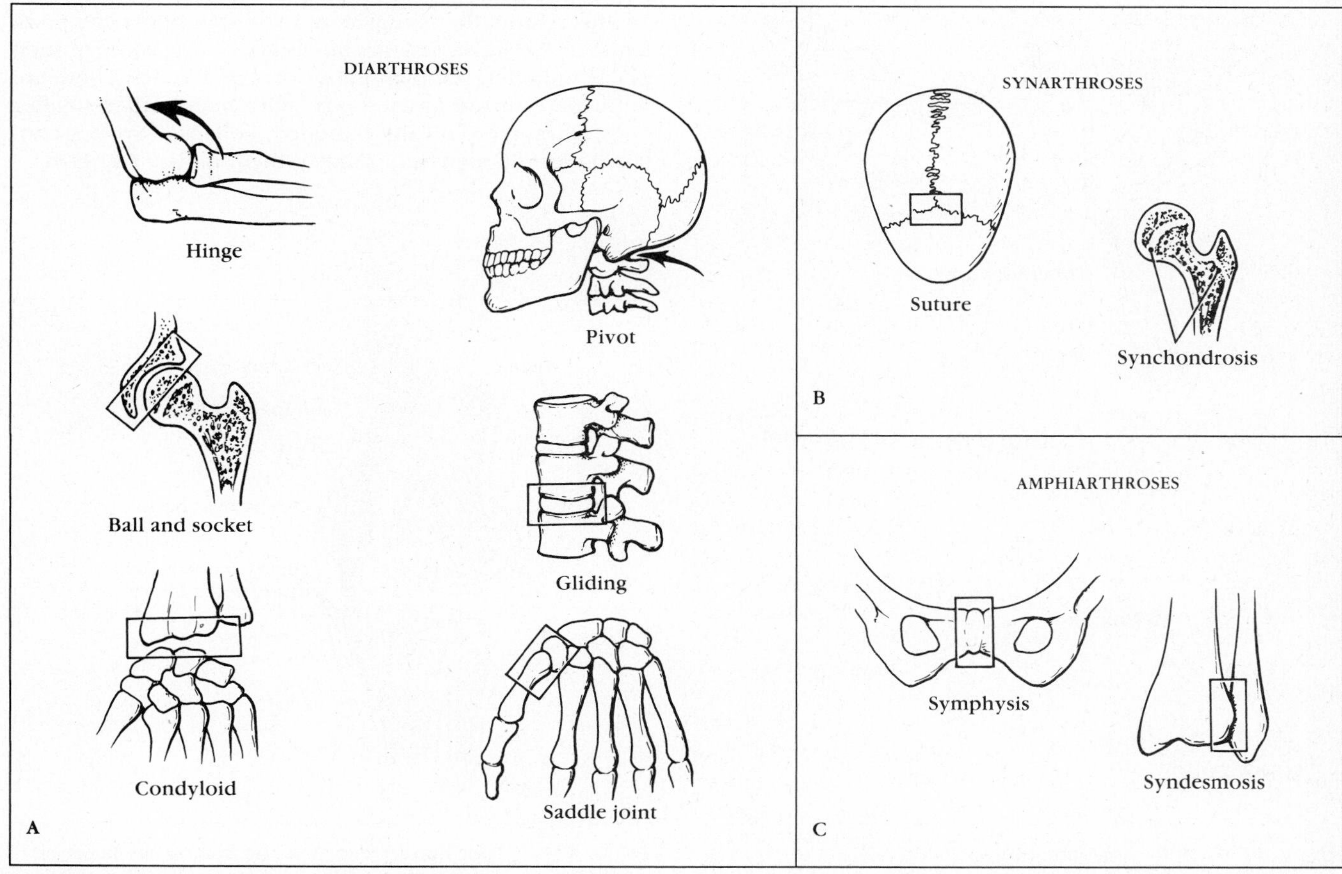

FIGURE 41-6 Types of joints based on degree of movement.

Classification of Synovial Joints

The synovial joints permit a variety of motion and are classified according to the shape of the articulation and the motion it facilitates (Fig. 41-7).

Ball-and-Socket Joints. These joints allow the greatest degree of motion and are formed by a bone fitting into a cup-shaped cavity of another bone. Examples are the hip and shoulder joints.

Condyloid Joints. An oval-shaped articular surface fits into an elliptical cavity. These joints allow much movement, similar to the ball-and-socket, but abduction and adduction are limited. An example is the wrist between the radius and carpal bones.

Hinge Joints. This type of joint permits movement in one plane only. The surface of one bone is convex, the other concave, and they fit together smoothly. Examples are the knee, elbow, and finger joints.

Pivot Joints. Pivot joints allow for rotation and supination and pronation. Examples are the atlas and axis joints of the head and the juncture between the head of the radius and the radial notch of the ulna.

Saddle Joints. The articular surface of one bone is concave in one direction and convex in another, while the other bone is just the opposite, so that the two sides fit together smoothly. An example is the carpometacarpal joint at the base of the thumb.

Gliding Joints. The bone surfaces are flat or only slightly curved, thus permitting sliding movement in all directions. Examples of this type of joint are the carpal bones of wrist and the intervertebral joints.

All movements of joints may be classified as (1) gliding, producing some bone displacement; (2) angular, in which the angle between bones is changed; and (3) rotation, a twisting of a body part [18]. Table 41-3 summarizes the movements of the joints and how they can be altered.

Bursae

Bursae are small, flat cavities that are lined with synovial membrane and filled with synovial fluid [18]. It is questionable whether or not bursae are present in normal tissue, but rather are an alteration in response to increased mobility and pressure. Unless there is superimposed inflammation, symptoms do not occur [14]. The chief function of bursae is to reduce friction between moving parts; for this reason, they are generally located between bones, tendons, and ligaments that move against one another, such as the shoulders, elbows, hips, heels, and knees. There are 50 named bursae in the body, with many other smaller ones. They are typically flattened, collapsed spaces containing just enough fluid to keep them moist (Fig. 41-8).

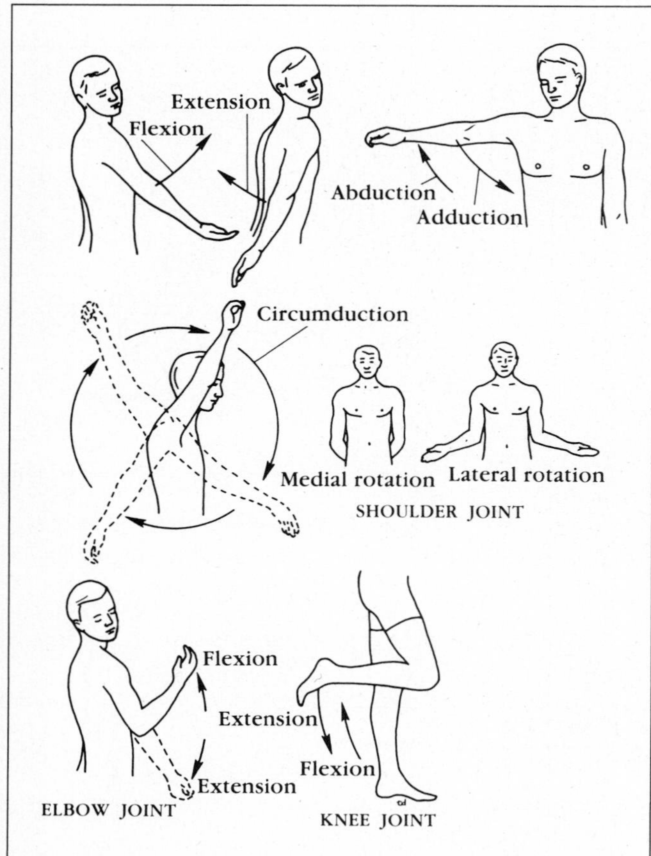

FIGURE 41-7 Some anatomic terms used in relation to movement. (From R.S. Snell, *Clinical Anatomy for Medical Students* [2nd ed.]. Boston: Little, Brown, 1981.)

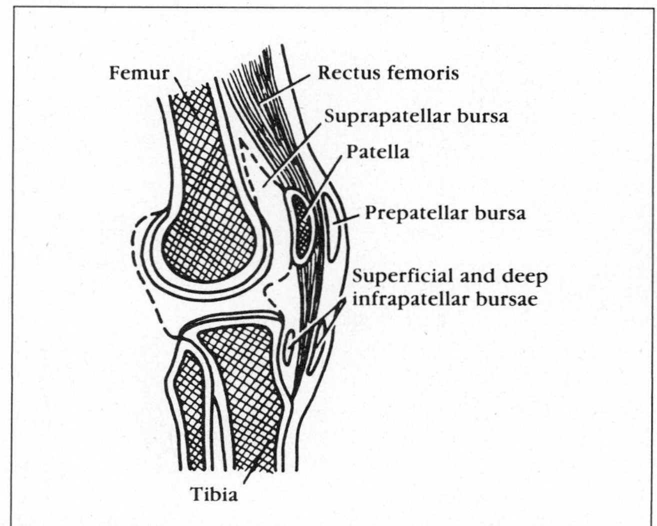

FIGURE 41-8 Four bursae related to the front of the knee joint. (From R.S. Snell, *Clinical Anatomy for Medical Students* [2nd ed.]. Boston: Little, Brown, 1981.)

TABLE 41-3 Movements of Joints

Name of Joint	Type of Movement	Normal Movements	Effects of Alterations
Vertebral	Diarthrotic (may be classified as synarthrotic, cartilaginous, amphiarthrotic)	Bending, stretching, twisting of entire column; slight movement between vertebrae	Pain when moving or lifting; stiffness; low back pain
Clavicular	Diarthrotic	Elevating, protracting, retracting	Pain; inability to move shoulder forward or backward; inability to lift shoulder
Shoulder	Diarthrotic (ball and socket)	Flexion, extension, abduction; rotation; circumduction of upper arm	Pain; stiffness; immobility; heat; inability to lift objects; cannot bring arm in toward body; range of activity curtailed
Elbow	Diarthrotic (hinge and pivot joint)	Flexion, extension; supination of lower arm and hand; pronation of lower arm and hand	Immobility; pain; stiffness; heat; activities of daily living greatly diminished; swelling
Wrist	Diarthrotic	Flexion, extension; abduction of hand; adduction of hand	Pain; stiffness; swelling; common complaints of inability to do common activities of daily living such as cooking, opening lids, various grooming activities; may complain of dropping things
Hand	Diarthrotic	Flexion, extension, abduction, adduction, circumduction of thumb; thumb and finger apposition; flexion, extension, limited abduction and adduction of fingers; flexion, extension of fingers	Pain; swelling; stiffness; drops objects; deteriorating writing; ability to perform activities of daily living greatly diminished (buttoning clothes, tying knots or bows, combing hair, etc.)
Hip	Diarthrotic (ball and socket)	Flexion; extension; abduction; adduction; rotation; circumduction	Pain; stiffness; immobility; heat; limping; loss of range of motion; inability to put on garments that require lifting the legs; cannot climb stairs
Knee	Diarthrotic (hinge)	Flexion; extension; slight tibial rotation	Pain; stiffness; swelling; immobility; limping, falling; redness, swelling; heat
Ankle	Diarthrotic (hinge)	Dorsiflexion; plantar flexion	Pain; stiffness; immobility; limping; unusual discomfort with shoes; foot drop
Foot	Diarthrotic	Flexion; extension; gliding; inversion; slight abduction, adduction	Pain; stiffness; immobility; avoidance of standing and walking; shoes ill-fitting

Source: Reprinted by permission of J. Moore.

Ligaments and Tendons

Ligaments and tendons are structures composed of connective tissue that hold the body together. There are two types of ligaments, those that connect viscera to each other and those that connect one bone to another [9]. Tendons always connect voluntary muscle to another structure.

Ligaments are composed of distinct bands of connective tissue. The yellow ones are elastic (vertebral column) and allow for stretching. The white ligaments, such as at the knee, do not stretch, and provide stability.

Tendons are actual extensions of muscles and attach muscles to bones or to other tissues. The thick, collagenous tissue has fibers that run in one direction so it can withstand a great deal of pull. These parallel bundles give tendons a glistening, shiny, white appearance. As a part of broad and flat muscles, they have the same general appearance, and similarly, when they are part of a long slender muscle, they are cordlike. The long, hard, cordlike tendons running into the hands and feet have been termed *leaders*. Tendons that cross bones or other tendons are lubricated by nearby bursae or the tendon sheath that surrounds them. Tendons receive sensory fibers from muscle nerves, nearby deep nerves, and overlying superficial nerves. Blood supply to tendons is scarce and it is for this reason that injured tendons heal slowly.

Fractures and Associated Soft Tissue Injuries

Fractures are most commonly defined as breaks in continuity of bone. They are ruptures of living tissue and normally are the result of trauma, but may be caused by repeated stress and fatigue (*stress fracture*) or an underlying disease (*pathologic fracture*). They may have associated extensive soft tissue damage with hemorrhage into muscles and joints, dislocation and rupture of tendons, nerve damage, and disruption of blood supply.

Fractures occur when a force (energy) is imposed on a bone that is greater than it can absorb. They are described in terms of types and directions of fracture lines (Fig. 41-9).

Classification of Fractures

Simple fractures do not disrupt the skin overlying the bone. *Compound fractures* disrupt the overlying skin.

Fractures are either *complete*, in which there is complete interruption in the continuity of bone, or *incomplete*, with some part of the bone intact (Figs. 41-10 and 41-11). If a bone is broken in such a manner as to produce three or more fragments, it is called *comminuted* (Fig. 41-12). An *impacted fracture* is one in which one fragment of bone is embedded in the substance of the other. A fracture characterized by crushed bone is called a *compression* fracture and usually involves the spinal column (Fig. 41-13). A *depressed* fracture, frequently seen in skull fractures, occurs when the bone is driven inward. Repeated mechanical stress and strain can result in a *stress* fracture (Fig. 41-14). *Pathologic fractures* occur in diseased bone with little external force or with trivial trauma. Severe twisting or straining may cause a tendon or ligament to pull its bony attachment completely off the main part of the bone, producing an *avulsion* fracture.

Fracture lines may be described as longitudinal, transverse, oblique, or spiral (Fig. 41-15). Other descriptive terms include overriding, angulation, and displacement (Fig. 41-16).

In general, soft tissue damage is greatest when a direct force is applied over the area, but is usually decreased when the force that breaks the bone is applied distal to the fracture. Table 41-4 lists mechanical forces and types of fractures that may be associated with them. These relate primarily to the long bones.

Signs and Symptoms of Fractures

Common signs associated with fractures include local swelling, loss of function or abnormal movement of the affected part, and various deformities, which include angulation, shortening, or rotation of the part. A *crepitation*, or grating sound, may be produced by bone fragments rubbing together. Pain or local tenderness is normally present. It is not uncommon, however, for a period of a few minutes to a half-hour after a fracture, for local shock to occur with complete anesthesia and flaccidity of the area. This is due to a temporary loss of nerve function at the site of the fracture [1]. Associated vascular injury causes swelling, pallor, pain and/or numbness, and pulselessness. When the sharp burning pain becomes a deep throbbing sensation, tissue anoxia is suspected [16].

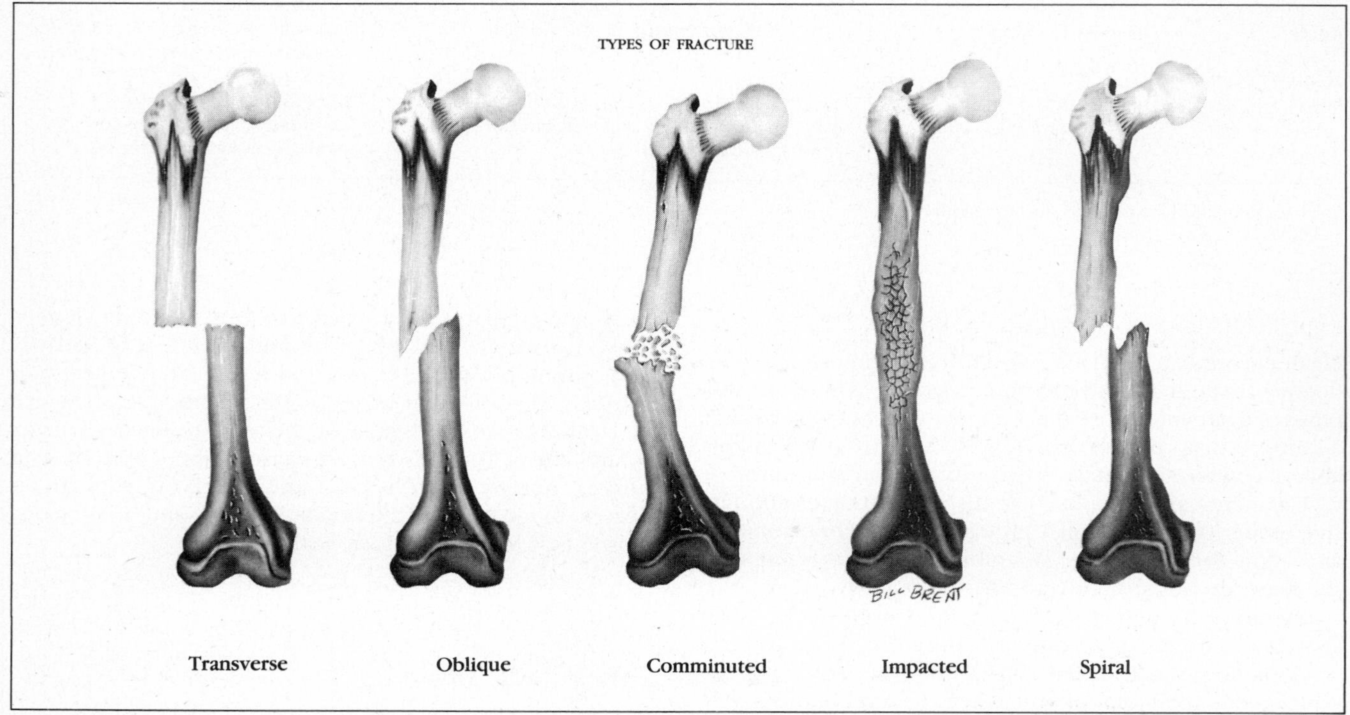

FIGURE 41-9 Some terms used for different types of fractures. (From N. Caroline, *Emergency Care in the Streets* [2nd ed.]. Boston: Little, Brown, 1983.)

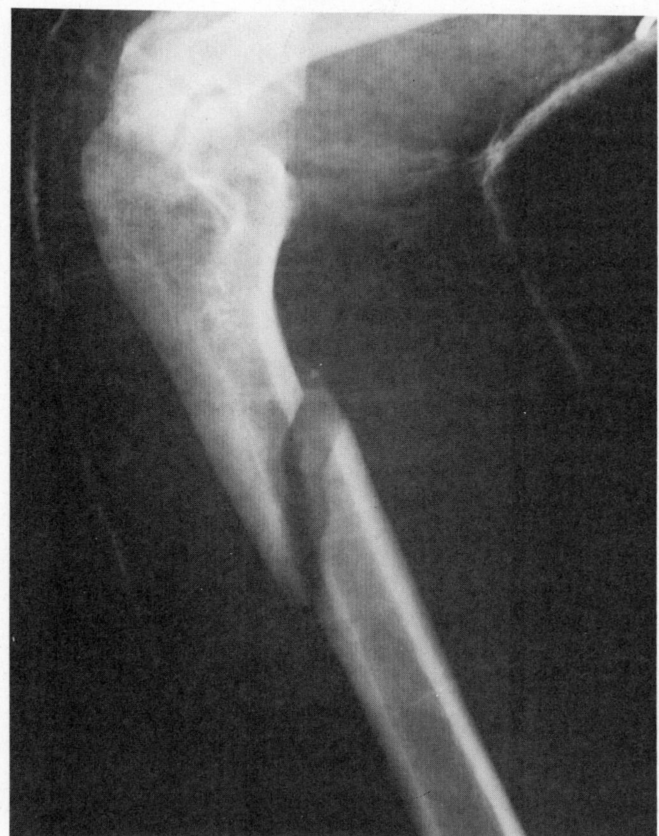

FIGURE 41-10 Complete fracture of the humerus.

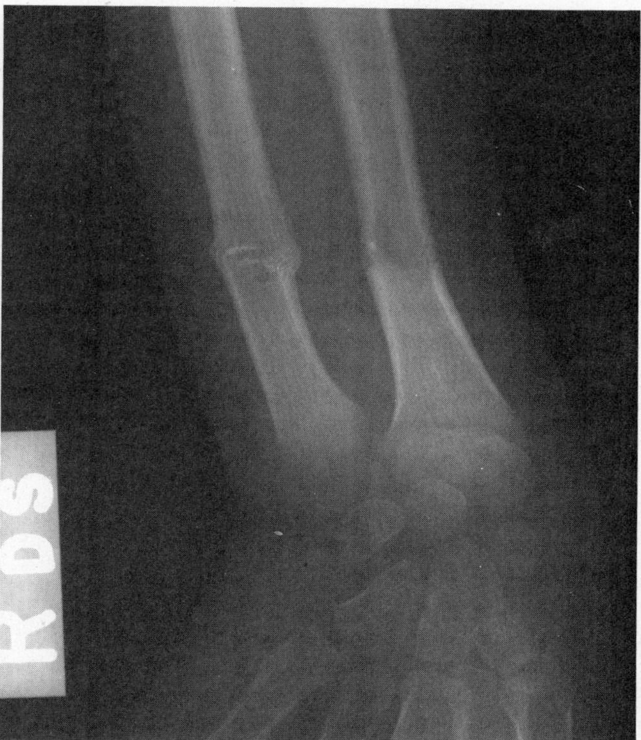

FIGURE 41-11 Greenstick fracture of the radius and ulna. Usually occurs in children.

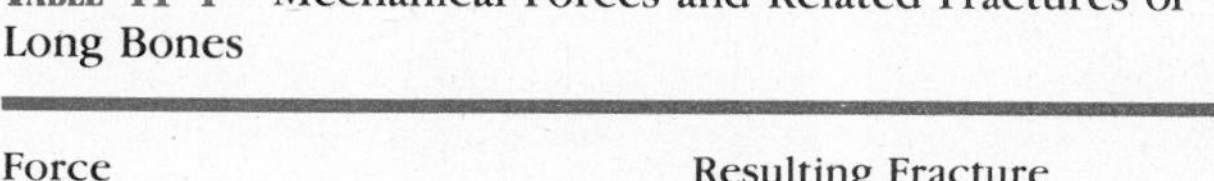

TABLE 41-4 Mechanical Forces and Related Fractures of Long Bones

Force	Resulting Fracture
Twisting	Spiral
Angulation	Transverse
Angulation with axial compression	Transverse with separate triangular piece (butterfly)
Twisting, angulation, and axial compression	Short oblique
Direct blow	Transverse
Crushing blow	Comminuted

Fracture Healing

It normally takes a good deal of force to break a bone, and there is often associated soft tissue damage. Once a fracture has occurred, blood vessels and periosteum rupture, and blood seeps into the fracture site from the fragments. This is called the *fracture hematoma*, which develops within 48 to 72 hours after injury. This hematoma surrounding the fracture site provides a loose fibrin mesh in which fibroblasts and capillary buds form a granulation tissue that replaces the blood clot. Osteoblasts and chondroblasts become active in forming new bone and cartilage,

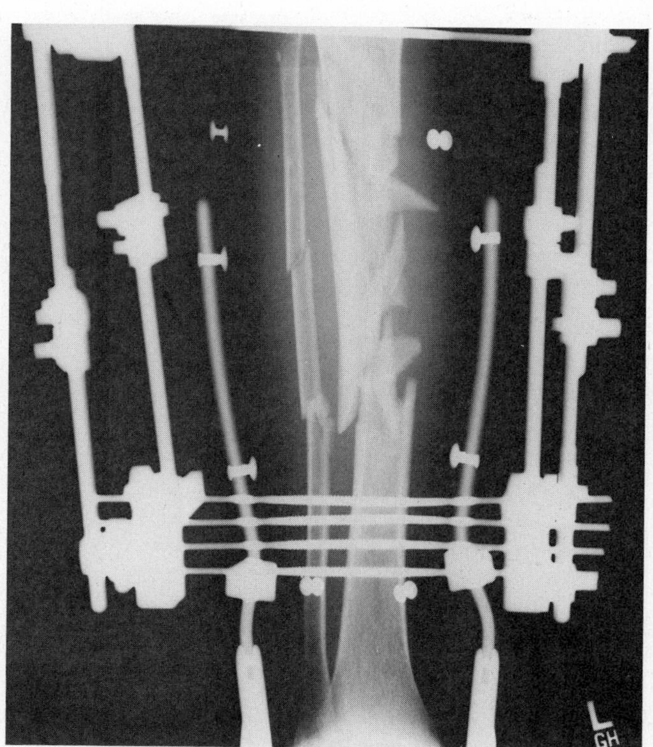

FIGURE 41-12 Comminuted fracture of the tibia and fibula that resulted from a direct blow from a car bumper. Radiograph shows the Hoffman apparatus used for treatment.

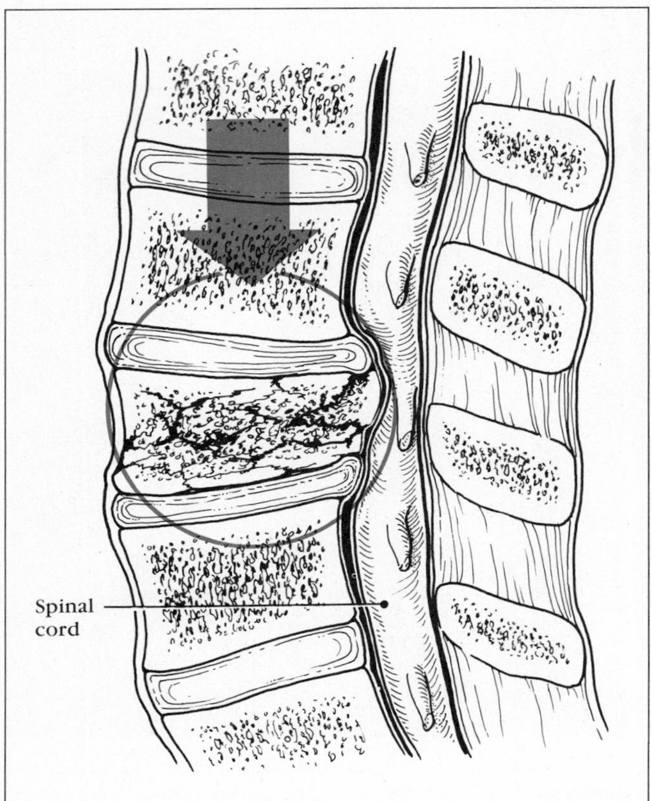

FIGURE 41-13 Compression fracture in the lumbar vertebrae.

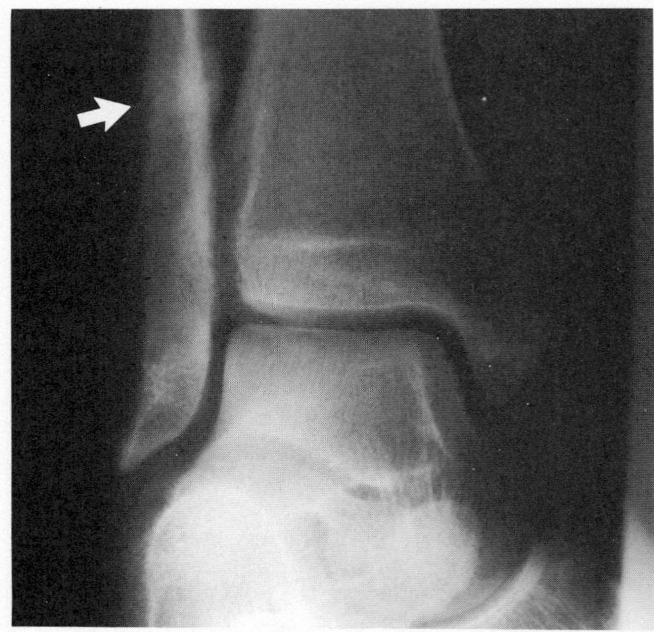

FIGURE 41-14 Stress fracture of the fibula in a distance runner.

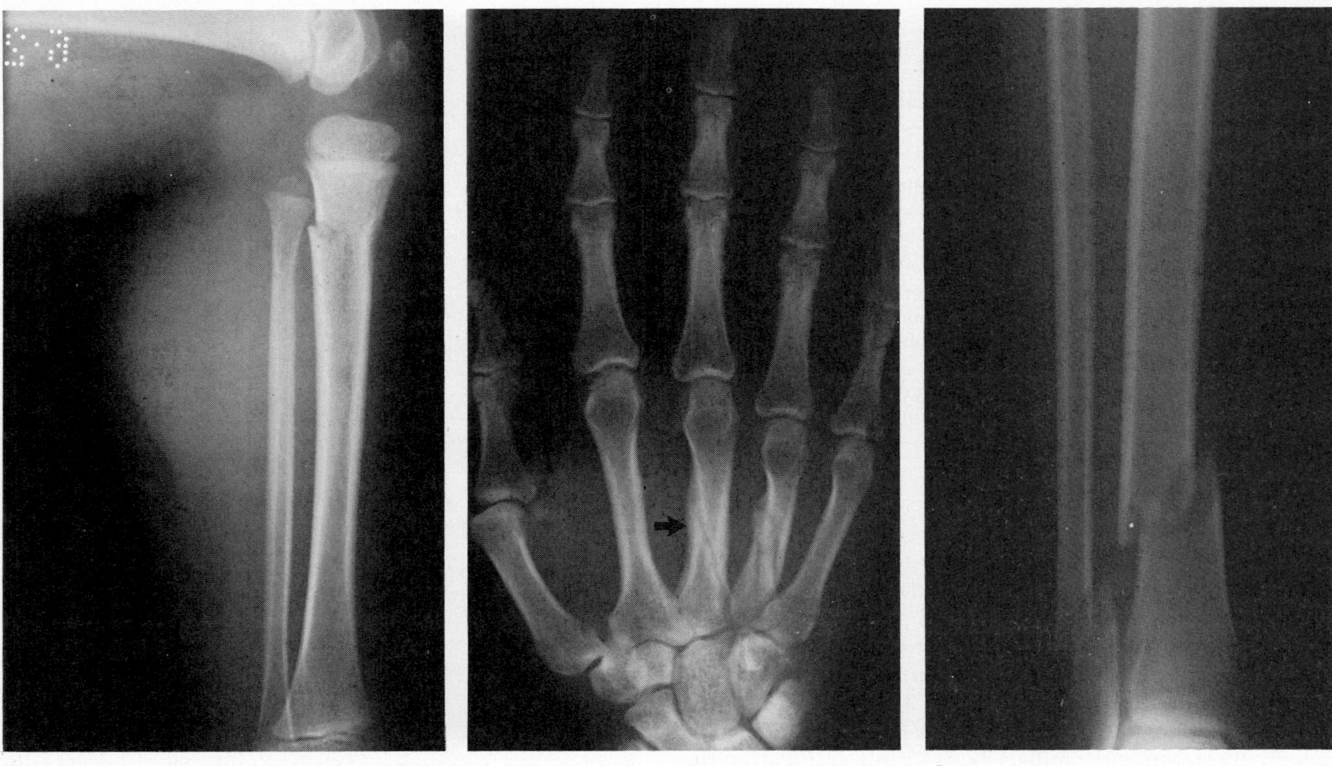

FIGURE 41-15 A. Transverse fracture of the tibia. B. Oblique fracture of the third and fourth metacarpals. C. Spiral fracture of the tibia and fibula.

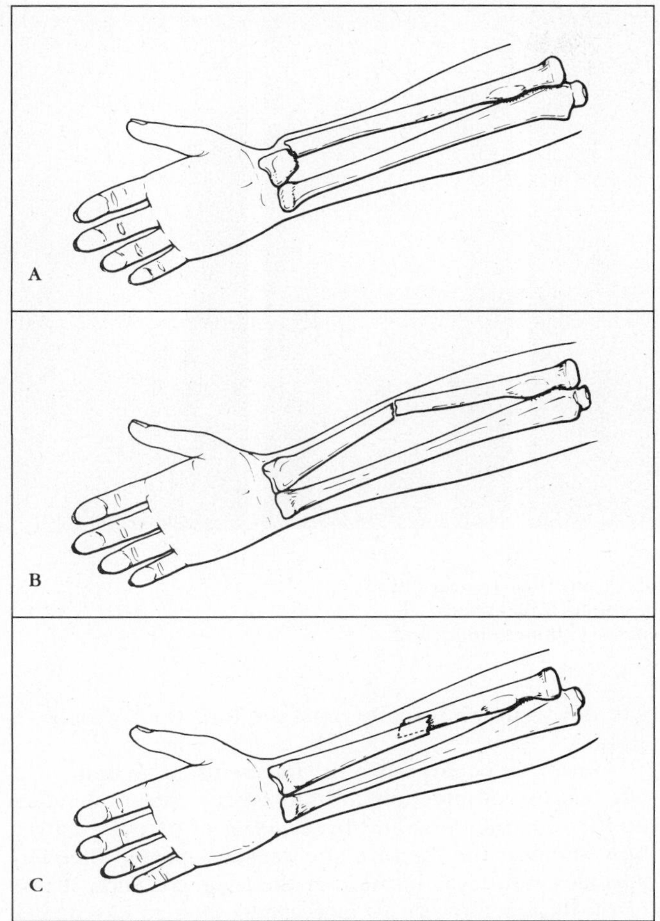

FIGURE 41-16 Descriptive terms indicating types of fractures. A. Displacement. B. Angulation. C. Overriding.

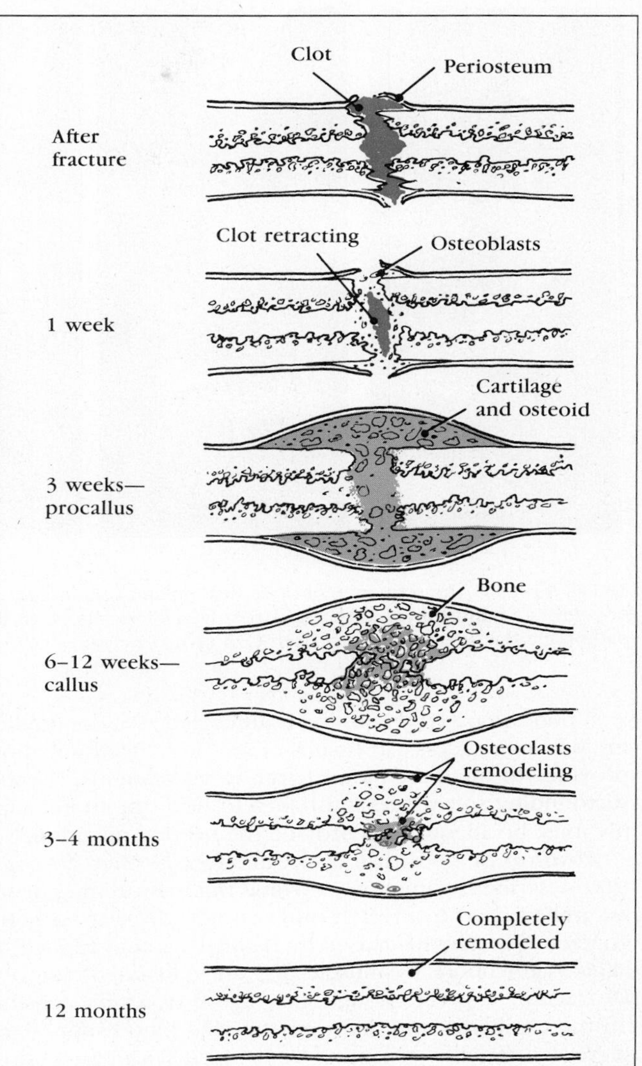

FIGURE 41-17 Healing of a fracture. (From T. Duckworth, *Lecture Notes on Orthopedics and Fractures* [2nd ed.]. London: Blackwell Scientific Publications Limited. Reprinted by permission.)

which within a week are dispersed throughout the soft tissue callus. This temporary bony union is called a provisional or primary union or *procallus* [5,14]. The procallus creates a balloon or collar over the fracture site and extends well past it. As healing continues, a *bridging external callus* is formed. New bone spicules proliferate as mineral salts are laid down. The late medullary callus appears to be responsible for the slow growth of new bone across a fracture gap [5].

As the gap in fractured bone is bridged and fracture fragments become united, mature bone begins to replace the callus [5]. The excess callus already laid down is reabsorbed by the osteoclasts. The fracture site becomes firm in about three to four months and radiographs show united bone (Fig. 41-17).

The remodeling process is controlled by the weight-bearing and muscle stresses put on the bone. That is, through the process of formation and resorption, bone returns to an architecturally sound state. *Wolff's law* describes this as a feedback system in which local instability stimulates bone formation and lack of stress stimulates bone resorption [1,15]. In a period of a year, a simple bone fracture resumes an almost normal appearance if aligned correctly (Fig. 41-18).

Conditions That Modify Healing. Because fracture healing is a continuous, sequential process, any interruption may modify the final result. This may be due to inadequate immobilization, poor blood supply, distraction of fragments, interposition of soft tissue, or infection.

When the bone is completely transected, *immobilization* is required to hold the fracture fragments rigidly in place. Any movement of the fragments could rupture the fracture hematoma. This reverses and thus prolongs the healing process because bleeding into the fracture site recurs. Immobilization is the first line of defense in ensuring a solid union.

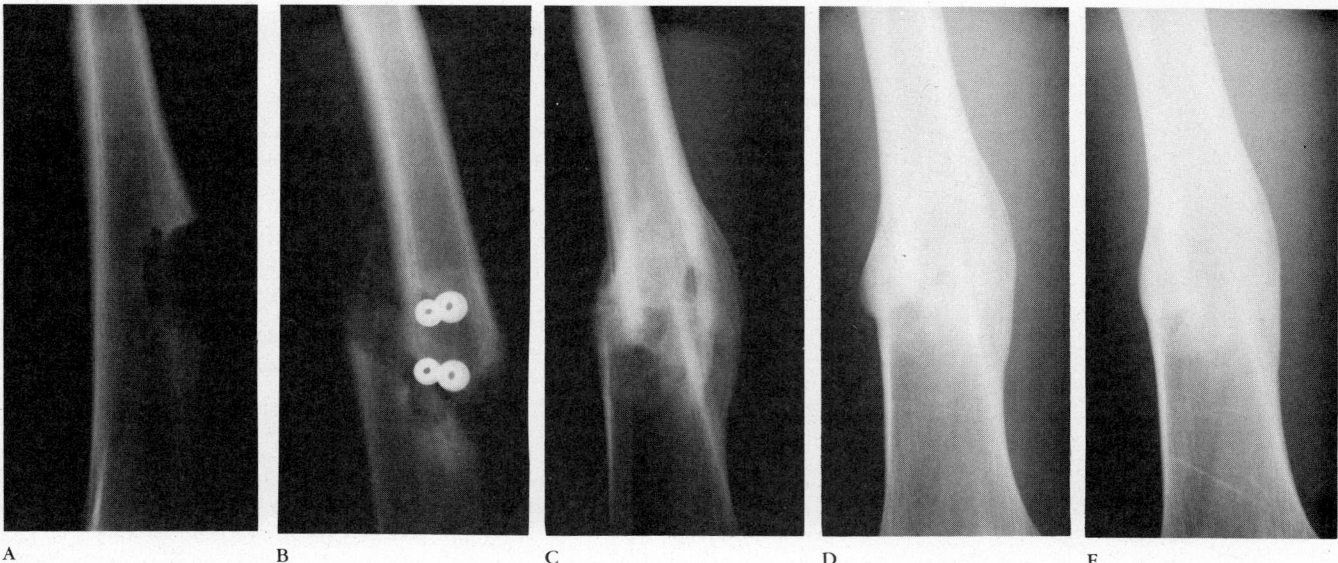

FIGURE 41-18 The sequence of bone healing and remodeling is demonstrated in a 13-year-old boy with a chondromyxoid that was removed surgically. A. Initial appearance. B. Repaired pathologic fracture one month later. C. A procallus forms. D. Osteogenesis. E. Bone remodeling.

A poor *blood supply* to the traumatized area can modify the healing process. All tissues of the body need nutrition provided through the bloodstream to maintain life. For the surrounding soft tissue and bones to heal, the blood supply must be adequate to provide the needed nutrition.

Position or *aposition* also can affect healing. *Distraction* describes a situation in which the fracture fragments are pulled apart from each other so that there is no bony contact. This may be caused by skeletal traction applied to align fragments or by muscle pull on individual fractures. Distraction, if great enough, may cause excessive tension on the capillaries and decrease the vital blood supply. An increased fracture gap must be bridged with granulation tissue, which increases healing time. When the healing time is increased, the chance of nonunion also increases. Distraction also is associated with the complication of separation of the fracture fragments by soft tissue that seals off the surface of one or both bones. This is known as *interposition of soft tissue*. If one or both of the fragments become covered with soft tissue, the hematoma is unable to form, and growth of granulation tissue is inhibited. This leads to a poor osseous union (Fig. 41-19A).

Compound fractures open internal structures to various microorganisms; therefore, *infection* becomes the major complication of bone healing. The open area is a rich culture medium for infection in the tissues and also for osteomyelitis (Fig. 41-20). Osteomyelitis retards healing by destroying newly forming bone and interrupting its blood supply.

Delayed union is a term used to denote increased healing time. Although each person heals at a different pace, the average time needed to completely heal a fracture is generally consistent. A delayed union normally results from a breakdown in the early stages of healing; that is, inadequate immobilization, breakdown in hematoma formation, and/or poor alignment. Infection at the fracture site delays union, usually until the infectious process is stopped.

Nonunion occurs when the fragments fail to unite, usually because of infection and movement. Infection causes continuous bleeding and breakdown of osteoid matrix. Movement at the fracture site causes repeated bleeding episodes and decalcification at the fragment ends; it may cause the fracture gap to increase to such an extent that the ends no longer touch, leading to a permanent nonunion.

Malunion is union of the fragments in a position that modifies function. The wrist fracture in Figure 41-19B was allowed to heal in poor alignment and resulted in shortening of the extremity and alteration of function.

After a fracture of a long bone or the pelvis, a person may experience a *fat embolus*. This is frequently associated with hypovolemic shock after a major trauma in which the fracture was sustained. The mechanical theory of fat embolus holds that with the damage to adipose tissue and the release of fat globules from the marrow of the fractured bone, globules enter the ruptured blood vessels in the area of trauma.

Because fat emboli also occur in persons with other conditions, other theories have emerged as to their causation. With any stress, catecholamines are released that mobilize fatty acids and neutral fats into the bloodstream. These become coated with platelets to form larger emboli. Thrombocytopenia often results and a specialized form of disseminated intravascular coagulation (DIC) may ensue. Free fatty acids in the bloodstream have been noted to have a toxic effect on the capillaries, causing them to become blocked [14]. Whatever the cause, fat emboli in the bloodstream travel to the lungs where they may lodge, causing damage to the alveolar membrane, and lead to the adult respiratory distress syndrome. Microemboli that pass through the lungs enter the systemic circulation and often lodge in the brain, causing neurologic symptoms. Fat

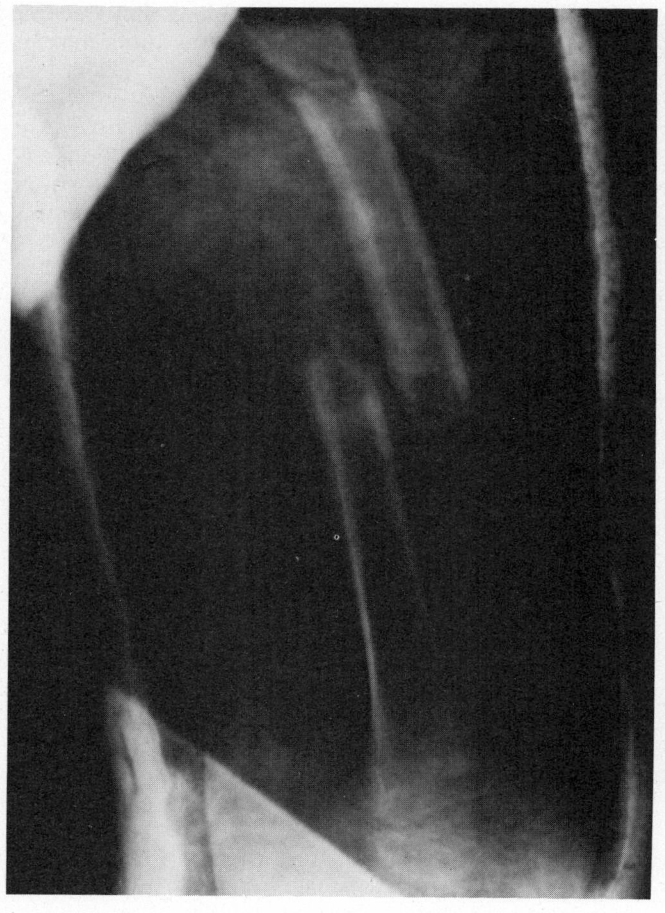

A

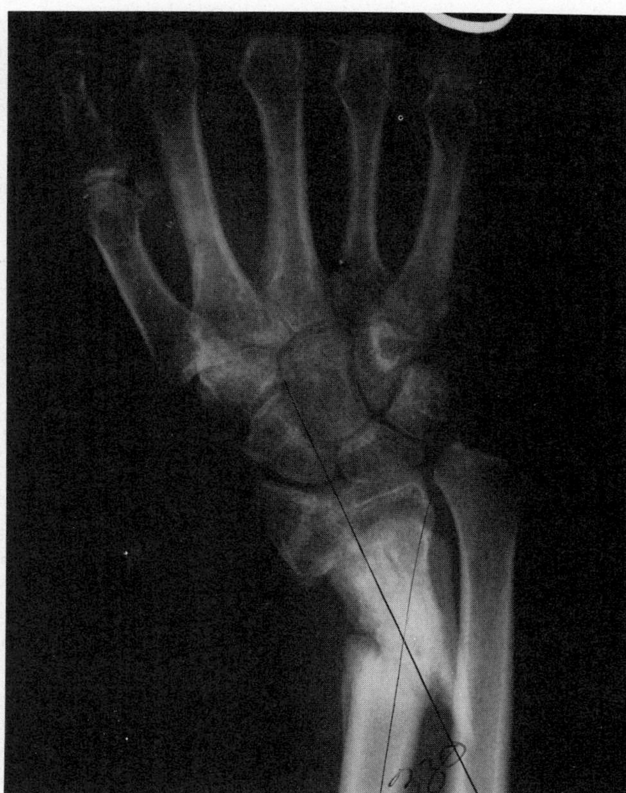

B

FIGURE 41-19 A. Loss of apposition in this fractured femur increases the likelihood of soft tissue interposition and delayed union or nonunion. B. Malunion of the radius due to poor alignment during healing.

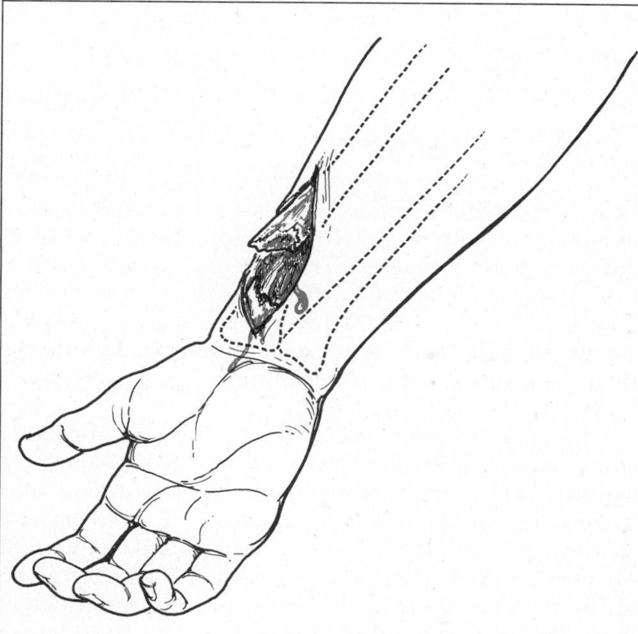

FIGURE 41-20 Compound fracture of radius with surrounding soft tissue damage.

emboli occur from 24 to 72 hours after injury. The person experiences chest pain and sudden respiratory difficulty. A low-grade fever, mental confusion, petechiae, and fat globules in the urine support the diagnosis [5,14].

Alterations in Nerve Function Due to Bone Trauma. Soft tissue injuries such as laceration of a major artery, the insidious compartmental syndrome, disabling tendon avulsion, and serious visceral injury are associated with fractures. If left untreated, they lead to alteration of function.

Sometimes a fracture causes an injury to adjacent structures. The fragments may rupture and compress nerves that may also be damaged by dislocation or direct trauma. Injuries of the axillary, radial, and peroneal nerves are described as compartmental syndromes.

The axillary nerve may be damaged by fractures or dislocations around the shoulder or by penetrating wounds and direct blows. The axillary nerve is composed of C5 and C6 fibers and is a branch of the posterior cord of the brachial plexus. It emerges at the level of the humerus head and winds around the neck of the humerus. It supplies the deltoid and teres minor muscles. The deltoid muscle is used as an abductor for the shoulder; therefore, inability to abduct the shoulder indicates damage to the axillary nerve.

The radial nerve is commonly injured in spiral fractures of the humerus. It may be completely severed, impaled on a fractured fragment, or entrapped between the fragments. Lacerations of the arm and proximal forearm, and gunshot wounds are also common causes of radial nerve injury. Temporary nerve damage may also result from direct pressure from using crutches or hanging an arm on the back of a chair. The radial nerve is composed of the fibers from some of the cervical spinal nerves (C5, C6, C7, and C8) and, sometimes, the thoracic spinal nerve, T1. It is primarily a motor nerve that innervates the biceps, supinates the forearm, and extends the wrist, fingers, and thumb. Therefore, it can be assumed that injury would result in inability to extend the elbow or supinate the forearm. A typical wrist drop occurs that includes inability to extend the fingers. Complete return of function can be expected in most persons with temporary nerve damage. In others, function may not return for as long as three months to a year. When function does not return, surgery is usually indicated; but it should be noted that the radial nerve has a greater ability to regenerate than all other large nerves. This is probably because the radial nerve is primarily a motor nerve that is involved mainly in gross muscle movements.

Peroneal nerves are classified as common, superficial, and deep. The common peroneal nerve emerges from the popliteal fossa and encircles the fibula neck. Damage may be the result of a direct blow, for example, a baseball bat hitting the fibula head with or without the presence of fractures. The result is a foot drop deformity, in which the foot returns to normal in a few hours if the nerve is not ruptured.

Compartmental Syndromes

Compartmental syndromes are uncommon complications of fractures and affect primarily the forearm and tibia. They are generally referred to as Volkmann's ischemia and anterior tibial compartmental syndromes. *Volkmann's ischemia* (volar compartmental syndrome) usually is related to the common supracondylar fracture of the humerus in children. Fracture of the tibia is common in anterior compartmental syndrome. Compartmental syndromes may result from a cast placed too tight, from intercompartmental bleeding, burns, and snake or spider bites.

The compartments of the leg and forearm are composed of bones, muscles, nerves, and other associated structures encapsulated by the fascia and the skin, thus making a closed space (Fig. 41-21). When injury occurs, the pressure builds within the compartment due to bleeding and soft tissue reaction. When the swelling reaches a point at which the fascia permits no further outward enlargement, the increasing pressure is directed inward and compresses blood vessels and other components of the compartment. When tissue pressure increases to equal the diastolic pressure, the microcirculation ceases, although the peripheral pulse is unchanged. Within 30 minutes, damage to nerves begins that results in irreversible functional loss if allowed to persist for 12 hours. Muscles require an abundant blood supply, and when the microcirculation is severely compromised they become ischemic, with onset of necrosis in 2 to 4 hours that becomes irreversible in 12 hours.

Anterior compartmental syndrome is heralded by pain in the anterior aspect of the tibia, paresthesia over the distribution of the deep peroneal nerve, and pain on passive dorsiflexion of the toes. The area appears swollen and blisters may develop on the skin. If the syndrome is allowed to proceed unchecked, paralysis, anesthesia, contractures, foot drop, and gangrene may develop, which in turn may lead to loss of the limb.

Volkmann's ischemia produces a disturbing contracture if untreated. Pain is the predominant symptom; it is referred to the palmar area and is exacerbated on passive extension of fingers. Some degree of sensory loss in the fingers occurs in the early stages. Formation of contractures described as clawlike deformities of the hand, wrist drop, and paralysis then result.

Other Associated Soft Tissue Traumas

Tendons may also be damaged due to fractures. When ligaments and tendons are involved in fractures, avulsion fractures may result. Damage to the extensor tendon of the distal phalanx can serve as an example. When a fracture occurs, it avulses (pulls apart) a small piece of bone to which the tendon is attached, leading to inability to extend the distal phalanx. If left untreated, a mallet deformity may result. If tendon damage caused by fractures is left untreated, it may lead to dysfunction of its bony attachment.

Visceral damage, or damage to internal organs, may also occur from fractures. Examples include fracture of the pelvis in which the bladder is ruptured, and rib fractures causing perforation of the lung.

Alterations in Bone Development

Osteogenesis Imperfecta

Osteogenesis imperfecta is a group of hereditary disorders in which defective connective tissue formation leads to extremely fragile bones. Homozygous infants with the recessive trait are most severely affected and mortality is high in the first year of life. The bones of the skull and face are poorly ossified, with numerous fractures occurring in the long bones. Death of the infant during childbirth may occur due to trauma to the brain, which is relatively unprotected by the soft, membranous skull.

The dominant trait produces a less severe type called *osteogenesis imperfecta tarda* (Fig. 41-22). This clinical syndrome is characterized by brittle, thin bones with deformities caused by numerous fractures, dwarfism with deformed extremities, and slow physical development. Mental development is usually normal. Associated features are relaxed ligaments, a high frequency of hernias, fragile skin, and hearing disorders. Blue sclerae are characteristic and thought to be due to defective fibrous tissue of the sclerae enabling the color of the vitreous to show through.

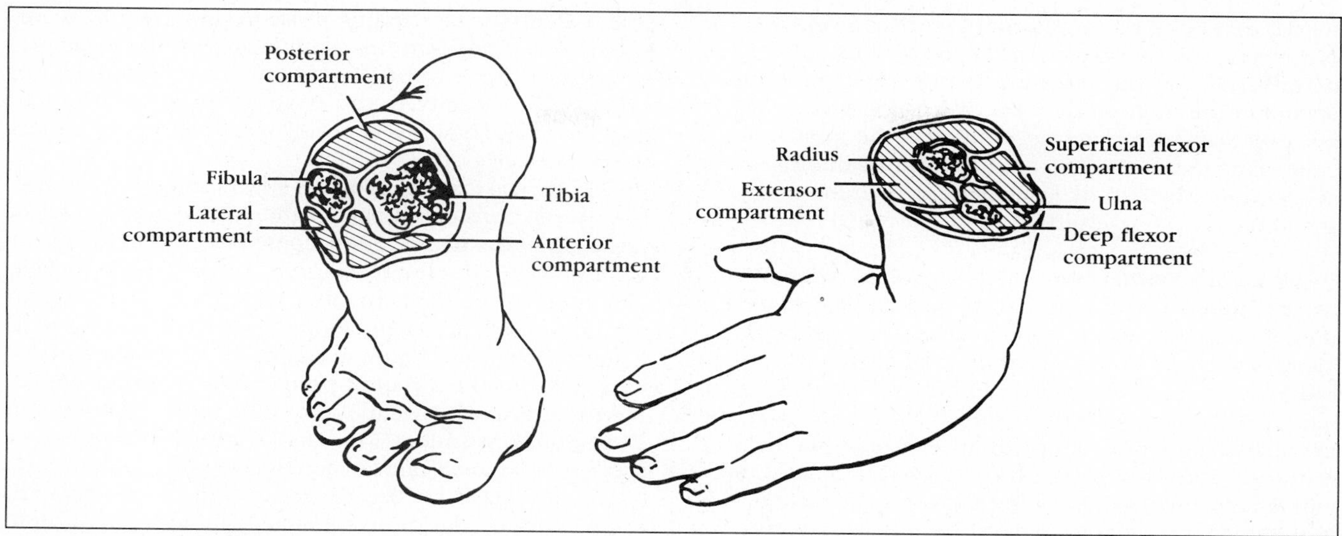

FIGURE 41-21 Compartments of the lower leg and forearm. (From E.A. Hincker, and L. Malasanos, *The Little, Brown Manual of Medical-Surgical Nursing*. Boston: Little, Brown, 1983.)

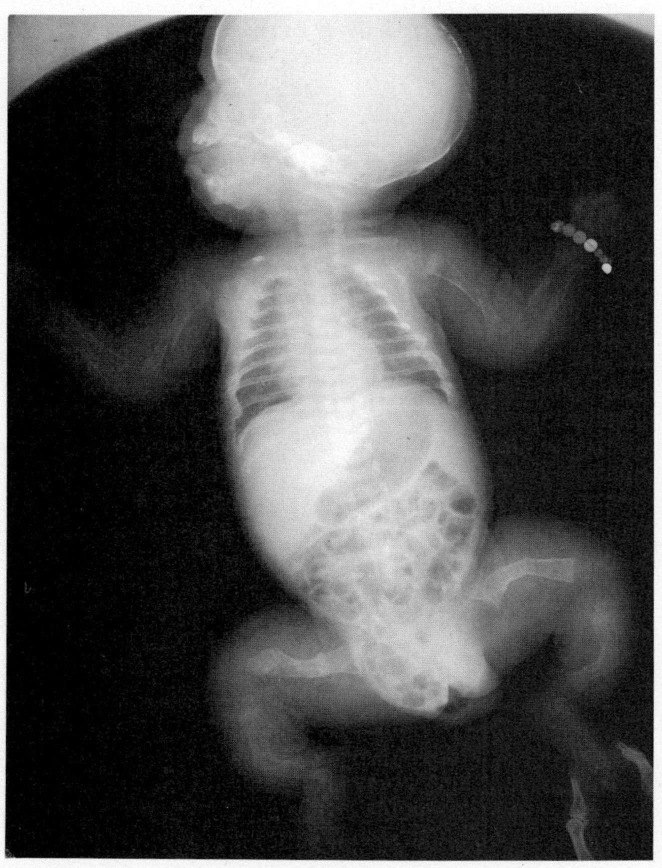

FIGURE 41-22 Classic example of osteogenesis imperfecta in an infant. Diffuse osteoporosis with bone deformities of the extremities and pathologic fractures of the humeri, femori, and ribs.

Osteopetrosis (Marble Bones, or Albers-Schönberg's Disease)

Osteopetrosis is a familial disease characterized by overgrowth and sclerosing of bone. Although the bones are heavy and thick, they tend to break rather than bend, and many fractures often occur. When this disease is due to a recessive trait, it is called ***malignant osteopetrosis*** and can cause death in utero or in early life. The autosomal dominant trait causes less severe problems that may not be diagnosed until adulthood.

Pathologic changes include an increase in cortical bone to nearly twice its normal density, with the growth being almost exclusively endochrondral; crowding of the marrow cavity, often with complete marrow obliteration, results. Signs and symptoms of the disease relate to the skeletal malformations and the defects in hematopoiesis. Optic nerve impingement due to failure of modeling of the skull can result in blindness. Deafness can occur due to overgrowth of bone in the middle and inner ear. Cranial nerve palsies, nystagmus, and hydrocephalus may also be present. The teeth usually erupt late and develop cavities early; osteomyelitis of the jaw often develops. Anemia can be profound due to the small marrow spaces, and the enlarged liver and spleen are sources of extramedullary hematopoiesis. As in osteogenesis imperfecta, treatment is only palliative, but children who reach adulthood can look forward to a relatively normal life span.

Fibrous Dysplasia of Bone

Fibrous dysplasia, which is characterized by replacement of cancellous bone by fibrous tissue, can affect one bone (monostotic) or many (polyostotic). The fibrous lesion begins in the medullary canal and spreads to the cortex, with cancellous bone and marrow being replaced by yellow-gray, fibrous tissue. The cortex is thin, and bowing deformities and fractures are common. If this disease occurs in the monostotic form, the lesion grows slowly, but eventually deformity occurs unless the mass is surgically removed. If the polyostotic form of the disease is accompanied by extraskeletal signs, it is called Albright's syndrome.

Albright's Syndrome. This disease is differentiated by precocious puberty in females, café au lait pigmentation of the skin over the bone involvement, and predominantly unilateral bone deformity, especially of the skull and long bones. When the facial bones are affected, asymmetry of the face with distortions of the nose, jaw, and even severe displacement of an eye may occur [15]. Although fibrous dysplasia has no proved genetic links, multisystem involvement of the polyostotic form does suggest some basic genetic defect. Hypothalamus involvement with increased secretion of pituitary hormones is being investigated [14].

Paget's Disease

As early as 1877 Sir James Paget described a disease of chronic bone inflammation that caused softening and bowing of the long bones. Paget's disease existed in ancient times as proved by the study of bones in archaeologic collections. Evidence of the disease has been found in the skulls of American Indians and even Neanderthals.

The disease is rare in persons under 40 years of age, with men and women being equally affected. The frequency of the disease has ranged statistically from 0.1 to 3.0 percent. The latter figure includes subclinical cases in which the disease was discovered microscopically on autopsy. The possible causes are many but no exact etiology has been defined. Paget himself thought it was due to a chronic infection, and he called the disease "osteitis deformans." Other etiologic possibilities include hormonal dysfunction, autoimmune states, vascular disorders, and neoplastic disease. The most recent speculation is that the cause is a latent virus. Nuclear inclusions, characteristic of a long-standing virus, have been found in the osteoclasts of individuals with Paget's disease [19]. The disease occurs late in life, which allows time for a long period of latency.

Pathologically, Paget's disease is characterized by resorption of bone followed by rapid overgrowth, a phenomenon that can occur in different stages in the same person and even in the same bone. The histologic features are usually described in phases. The initial, osteolytic or destructive, phase is marked by extensive resorption of existing bone, with the presence of numerous multinucleated osteoclasts [10]. The mixed or active phase occurs when the osteoclasts destroy the ordered lamellar bone and osteoblasts respond to the destruction by rapid disposition of vascular connective tissue and remodeled lamellar bone. At this time, the area appears to be highly vascular, with cement lines forming at sites where the lamellae are erratically joined, giving a mosaic appearance that may completely replace the preexisting bone [19]. The osteoblastic or sclerotic phase occurs when bone formation outstrips resorption, with lamellar bone as the predominant ingredient. Bone size and thickness are increased primarily in the head, femurs, humeri, and scapulae. This bone is soft, poorly mineralized, and subject to fractures (Fig. 41-23).

The clinical features progress slowly and bone deformities can be considered part of the normal aging process. The long bones of the legs become bowed and the pelvis is misshapen. The thorax shortens, causing loss of height. The bones of the skull are often affected, leading to symptoms of vertigo, headache, and progressive deafness due to compression of the eighth nerve. In the early stages of disease, pain in the affected bones may be experienced. Increased vascularity of the rebuilding bone, together with cutaneous vasodilatation, can produce warmth over affected bone, requiring an increase in cardiac output [10].

No cure exists for Paget's disease, but newer therapies use calcitonin and diphosphates to inhibit osteoclastic activity [13]. Mithramycin, a drug used in cancer therapy, may also be effective, which suggests that the etiology is a virus-induced neoplastic process [16].

von Recklinghausen's Disease

Osteitis fibrosa cystica, or von Recklinghausen's disease of bone, is characterized by progressive resorption and destruction of bone brought about by long-standing hyper-

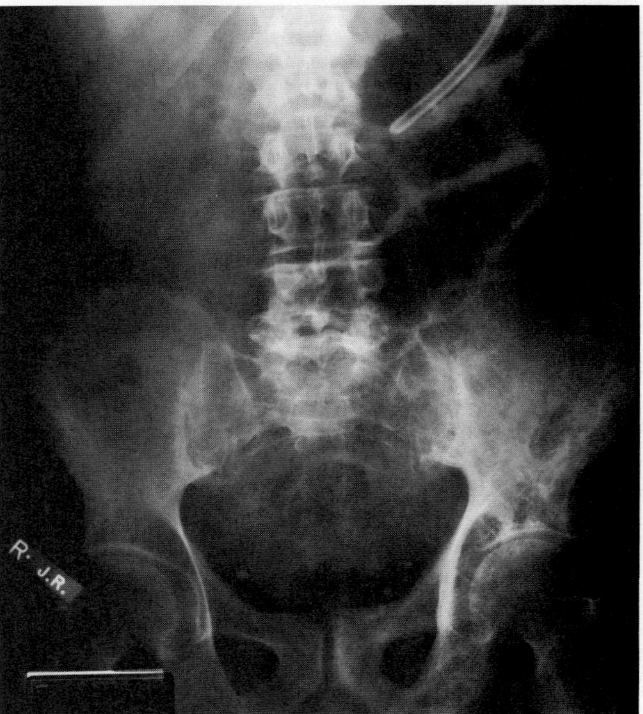

FIGURE 41-23 Paget's disease of bone. Punched-out areas in the acetabular cavity, iliac wing, and ischial and pubic rami represent areas of resorption and remodeling that occur simultaneously.

parathyroidism. Parathyroid hormone (PTH) excretion causes calcium and phosphorus to be removed from bone (see p. 639). Hyperplasia or neoplasia of the parathyroid glands may cause a hypersecretion of this hormone and thus demineralization of bone. Secondary hyperparathyroidism, as in chronic renal insufficiency, leads to decreased conversion of vitamin D to its active form in the kidneys and decreased absorption of calcium in the intestine. The low serum calcium level stimulates PTH secretion.

In the early stages of both primary and secondary hyperparathyroidism, changes in bone resemble osteomalacia or osteoporosis. With advanced disease, there is osteoclastic resorption of bone, which is replaced by fibrous tissue in the marrow spaces. The cancellous and cortical bones undergo thinning with resultant deformities. In focal areas of bone resorption, large fibrous scars develop, yielding minute to very large cysts, called *brown tumors*. These nonmalignant granulomas receive their brownish color from degeneration and hemorrhage into the site. Fractures and joint pains result that can be reversed if the levels of PTH are reduced.

Osteoporosis

Osteoporosis is a metabolic bone disease due to reduction in both bone matrix and mineralization. It results in brittle bones that fracture quite easily. Because bone remodeling, with resorption being balanced by formation, normally occurs throughout life, anything that either increases resorption or decreases formation causes loss of bone mass. The rate of resorption follows the surface-volume mass of bones. Therefore, because the trabeculae are composed of sheets of bone and have more surface volume than cortical bone, they are lost more rapidly. This loss leads to increased frequency of fractures in the weight-bearing bones where trabecular bone predominates. The vertebral bodies, radial head, and femoral neck are examples of this type of bone. Similarly, resorption is accelerated on the endosteal surfaces of trabecular bone while formation is occurring at the periosteal surfaces, thus leading to wider bones with a thinner, more porous cortex. The ratio of bone mineral to matrix formation is constant, but there is simply a reduction in both. This contrasts with osteomalacia, in which the matrix is normal but the mineralization is deficient.

Osteoporosis may be caused by genetic, nutritional, mobility, drug-related, hormonal, and age factors. Deficiencies in protein, vitamins C, D, and A, and calcium can lead to reduced matrix and mineralization [17]. Estrogen and testosterone stimulate osteoblastic activity so that with menopause, the frequency of osteoporosis increases. Current theory suggests that estrogen may antagonize parathyroid hormone, which has a bone-resorption effect. Estrogen may also affect the absorption and excretion of calcium and phosphorus by direct action on the gastrointestinal tract, possibly through enhancing the metabolism of vitamin D [1]. Women with artificially induced menopause seem to develop the disease faster than those with normal, more slowly declining hormone levels. Other endocrine changes such as diabetes mellitus and thyrotoxicosis, wherein protein synthesis is decreased and catabolism increased, respectively, also cause osteoporosis. Cushing's disease, with its protein catabolic loss, has the same bone results as prolonged steroid therapy. Prolonged therapy with heparin and certain cancer drugs, may lead to osteoporosis. X-ray irradiation, as well as that resulting from radioactive materials, may affect bone by damage to the osteoblasts. Immobility of a limb and prolonged bedrest can also cause bone loss.

It has been estimated that osteoporosis affects one in four women over age 60 years. Bone loss begins in women at about age 45 and in men between 50 and 60 years of age [14]. Complications of the disorder, especially hip fractures, make it the twelfth leading cause of death in the United States [2]. The decline of estrogen after menopause combines with low bone mass to make certain groups of women more prone to the disease. White women tend to have less bone mass than black women and thin women have less than obese women. Smokers seem to have less bone mass and tend to undergo menopause earlier than nonsmokers. In general, osteoporosis is most frequent in thin, small-built, fair-complexion, freckled, blond women with a sedentary lifestyle [1].

Hip fractures account for more morbidity than all of the other osteoporotic fractures combined. More than 200,000 women suffer hip fractures in the United States each year [3]. In men hip fractures are often related to long-term immobility such as after a stroke or head injury. Fractures of the distal forearm are common but rarely cause death. Vertebral fractures, either complete or compression, can occur with a minimal amount of trauma and may cause few symptoms. These vertebrae never regain their normal shape and account for the loss of height and the so-called dowager's hump seen in older women and men.

The prevention and treatment of osteoporosis have brought about much study and controversy. Studies suggest that various combinations of estrogen, calcium, vitamin D, and sodium fluoride seem to retard bone loss. These treatments are most effective when begun in the perimenopausal or early postmenopausal woman [1]. Estrogen appears to stop postmenopausal bone loss for as long as it is taken, although it is not without its side effects. Calcium intake of 1.5 gm per day is recommended either in the diet or as a supplement. In those with vertebral fractures, sodium fluoride induces the formation of new bone and decreases the frequency of other fractures. Vitamin D supplements may retard osteomalacia in the elderly who have deficient diets and minimal sunlight exposure. Studies suggest that regular exercise retards bone loss [3].

Rickets/Osteomalacia

Rickets is a disease in the infant or growing child that usually is caused by a lack of vitamin D. Osteomalacia in the adult results from a calcium and/or a phosphorus deficiency. Vitamin D deficiency alone is rare in the United States in adults.

The mineral deficiency can result either from a decrease in calcium absorption or an increase in phosphorus loss by the kidneys. In chronic renal failure the kidneys are unable to activate vitamin D and excrete phosphate. The accompanying hyperparathyroidism increases bone resorption. In the aged individual, low dietary intake of calcium and vitamin D combined with intestinal malsorption can decrease bone mineralization.

The primary pathology consists of lack of mineralization of bone with a relative increase in uncalcified osteoid. The normal time for osteoid to become calcified is about 12 to 15 days, but in osteomalacia, the time interval lengthens to several months [14]. Due to the lack of mineralization, the bones are soft, and bow and break easily. Because bone formation in the growing child is most accelerated at the ends of the long bones, the epiphyseal tissue in rickets is soft, with the normally sharp, narrow line of ossification being replaced by a wide, irregular zone of soft, gray tissue. Bowed legs and deformities of the costochondral junction (rachitic rosary) and thorax (pigeon breast) together with defective tooth enamel are evidence of rickets. In the adult, osteomalacia is displayed by mineral changes and pain in the lumbar vertebrae, pelvic girdle, and long bones of the lower limbs. Fractures occur with only minor trauma. Deformities can also occur in adults when the muscles and tendons change the shape of the softened bone [14].

Scurvy

Vitamin C (ascorbic acid) is necessary for the production of the collagen of fibrous tissue and bone matrix. A deficiency of vitamin C leads to scurvy, which is characterized by hemorrhages, anemia, and bone and teeth changes. Hemorrhages can occur in any organ and can vary from tiny petechiae to large hematomas. Bone disturbances are evidenced by a defective osteoid and a relative increase in resorption over formation. This leads to a decreased density of bone. Bleeding, spongy gums, and loose teeth are common. Scurvy in infants usually does not appear until after 6 months of age, and it takes from three months to a year of severe vitamin C deficiency to produce scurvy in an adult.

Avascular Necrosis

The word *osteochondrosis* refers to a set of conditions affecting the epiphyseal region of bone in children during the growth period. The pathology is brought about by avascular necrosis in the area that causes the bone of the epiphysis to soften and die (Fig. 41-24). Various names have been ascribed to avascular necrosis occurring in specific areas, but *Legg-Calvé-Perthes disease* is the most familiar [5].

The onset of the condition appears to be growth related. Until ages 3 and 4 years, the predominant blood supply to the femoral head comes across the growth plate from the metaphysis of the femur with other supply from the lateral epiphyseal vessels. At about 4 years of age the growth plate begins to block the metaphyseal blood supply, and full development of the ligament artery supply to the femoral head is reached when the child is age 7 or 8 years. This leaves a period of time when the blood supply to the femoral head is dependent on the lateral epiphyseal vessels.

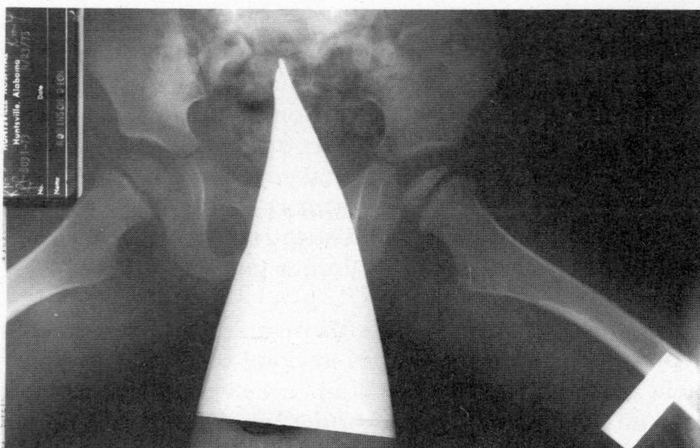

FIGURE 41-24 Legg-Calvé-Perthes disease. Flattened right femoral head is result of necrosis. Left femoral head is normal.

Precipitating causes of avascular necrosis may be trauma, infections, or inflammation. In the two- to four-year course of the disease, three stages occur. (1) Avascular necrosis causes the bone of the femoral head to soften and die, but the cartilage surrounding it, nourished by synovial fluid, remains viable. (2) Blood vessels from adjacent viable tissue grow in through the neck of the femur and begin the slow process of removing dead bone a little at a time, a process called creeping substitution. (3) Areas of resorbed bone are filled with new bone and ossification occurs. All three of these stages—necrosis, removal of dead bone, and reossification—may occur simultaneously within the same bone. Children may complain of aching pain and limited motion early in the disease, but later processes remain painless.

Osgood-Schlatter disease usually occurs in boys from 10 to 15 years of age and is characterized by a painful, tender, and enlarged tibial tubercle. It is caused by a pull of the patellar tendon on the tibial tubercle epiphysis, caused by sudden or continuous strain during growth. The condition may not be a true osteochondrosis but may be due to injury [5]. Serial films show changes due to aseptic necrosis that results from avascular changes. Like Legg-Calvé-Perthes disease, pain disappears shortly after onset but the tibial tubercle may remain enlarged.

Infectious Diseases of Bone

Osteomyelitis

Osteomyelitis occurs when the bone and bone marrow are invaded by pyogenic organisms. Infection of bone can come about in three ways: (1) by direct expansion from a neighboring focus; (2) by direct contamination, as with compound fractures or open wounds; and (3) by hematogenous spread from distant sites of infection (infected tonsils, boils, upper respiratory infections) [14]. The last occurs most frequently in children and young persons under age 21 years.

The causative organism in 60 to 70 percent of cases is hemolytic *Staphylococcus* [14]. Streptococci, coliform bacteria, pneumococci, gonococci, or any bacterial or fungal agent may be involved. The infecting organism enters the bone through the nutrient or metaphyseal vessels and moves into the medullary canal. Vascularity increases, causing edema. Polymorphonuclear leukocytes accumulate in the area. In a few days, thrombosis of local vessels occurs and ischemia results. Portions of bone tissue die. Pus in this confined space is under pressure and is pushed out through Volkmann's canals to the surface of the bone. It then spreads subperiosteally and can enter the bone at another level, or burst out into the surrounding tissue. In infants, before the epiphyseal cartilage seals off the metaphysis, spread can go directly to the joint and cause a suppurative arthritis. In older individuals, if joint involvement does occur, it does so through subperiosteal spread. The dead bone is separated from viable tissue and granulation tissue forms beneath the area of dead bone and infection. The necrotic bone, isolated from viable tissue, is termed *sequestrum* [14]. New bone forms from the elevated periosteum. This bone, called the *involucrum*, envelopes the granulation tissue and sequestrum. Small sinuses permit the pus to escape.

In chronic osteomyelitis, the granulation tissue becomes scar tissue and forms an impenetrable area around the infection. New area of bone develops to isolate the area further. The process is characterized by chronically draining sinuses with organisms that are resistant to antibiotic therapy.

The person with acute osteomyelitis appears acutely ill with fever, chills, and leukocytosis. The affected limb becomes very painful; the pain is often described as a constant throbbing. Redness and swelling usually occur over the site and sensitivity to the touch is characteristic. Radiologic evidence is noted after about 10 days and reflects bone destruction. Blood cultures are usually positive for the causative organism; massive antibiotic therapy usually arrests the disease.

Tuberculosis

Tuberculosis is a systemic disease caused by the tubercle bacillus, which spreads through the body through lymphatic or hematogenous route (see Chap. 25). Skeletal involvement is rare now due to adequate therapy, but when it occurs it is often caused by seeding of the bacillus in the marrow cavity. The infection causes destruction of bone tissue and caseous necrosis that may enter the joint cavities or occur under the skin as an abscess with draining sinuses. Tubercular skeletal lesions usually do not wall themselves off, so invasion of joints and intervertebral disks may cause many deformities. Tuberculosis of the spine, called *Pott's disease*, most frequently occurs in children and can lead to kyphosis, scoliosis, or the hunchback deformity.

The onset of skeletal tuberculosis, in contrast to acute pyogenic osteomyelitis, is insidious, beginning with vague description of pain. Complications of tuberculosis of the spine include paraplegia and meningitis. Tuberculosis of the hip and knee joint has greatest frequency in children.

Syphilis

Congenital or acquired syphilis of the bone is rare in the United States. In congenital syphilis, the spirochetes are delivered through the fetal bloodstream to the bones, where they inhibit osteogenesis. The epiphyseal plate is severely damaged and may actually be separated from the metaphysis. Bone syphilis is marked by endarteritis and periarteritis, and reactive bone forms from viable surrounding periosteum. Granulation tissue between the periosteum and cortical bone is laid down. In the tibia, a resulting saber shin deformity gives a curved appearance to the anterior portion of the bone.

Acquired syphilis may also cause osteochondritis or periosteitis; there is a possibility that frank syphilitic lesions will appear within the medullary canal. The skull and vertebrae, as well as the long bones, can be affected in acquired syphilis.

Alterations in Skeletal Structure

Scoliosis

Scoliosis is a lateral curvature of the spine that can result from another disease such as polio or cerebral palsy. Most commonly it is as an idiopathic disorder. It is estimated that over 1 million Americans have some degree of scoliosis, with girls being affected 8 times more than boys. It is most frequent in the early adolescent years.

The curvatures are classified according to location and consist of a primary, fixed curve with compensatory curves above and below it (Fig. 41-25). The deformity occurs slowly and is accelerated by the preadolescent growth spurt. The shoulder blade protrudes, the level of the iliac crests becomes unequal, and the curvature appears to be exaggerated when the individual bends over. In general, the younger the age when the curvature is noticed and the higher up in the thorax it occurs, the poorer the prognosis [5]. Severe scoliosis can affect the heart and lungs by restrictive action. It may be markedly improved by surgical procedures.

Clubfoot (Talipes)

Clubfoot deformities, the most frequent of the orthopedic congenital deformities of the lower extremities, occur with greatest frequency in boys. Two-thirds of cases are unilateral. Clubfoot may be caused by genetic and environmental factors. Generally, the talus points downward and the foot is adducted. The clinical varieties are termed *easy* and *resistant*, with the easy cases responding to strapping and stretching alone and the resistant cases requiring surgical intervention.

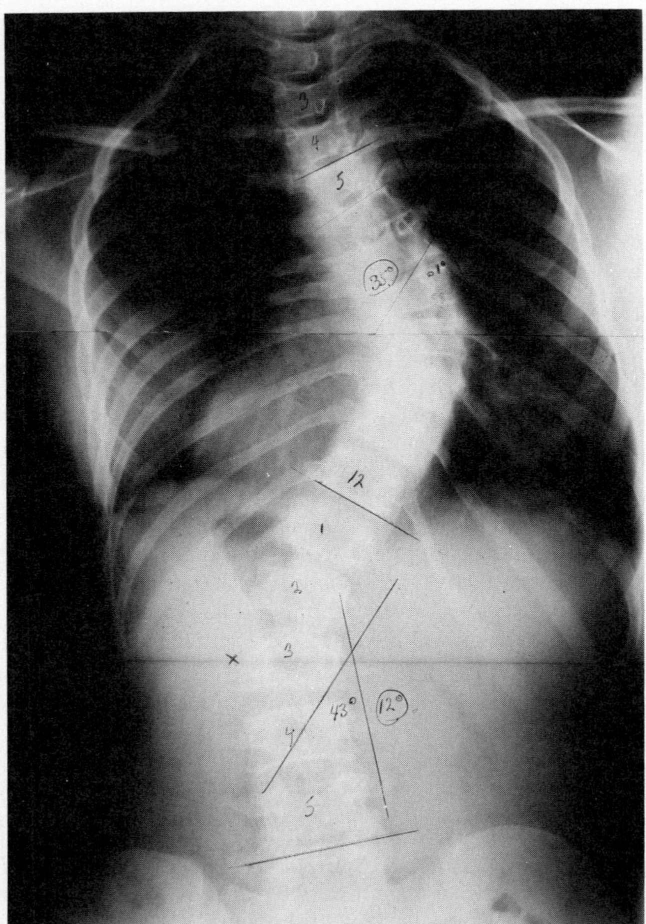

FIGURE 41-25 Scoliosis of the spine with a thoracic primary curve and compensatory curve in the lumbar spine. Vertebral bodies are marked at the approximate beginning and end of each curve and are used to measure the degree of curvature.

Congenital Dislocation of the Hip

Congenital dislocation of the hip is probably caused by a combination of genetic and environmental factors. Genetic factors are linked to both joint laxity and acetabular dysplasia. Also, just prior to delivery of a full-term infant, the pregnant woman secretes a ligament-relaxing hormone that crosses the placental barrier and enhances joint laxity. This fact accounts for the relative rarity of hip dislocation in premature infants. Other environmental factors include intrauterine malposition, breech presentation during delivery, and swaddling of neonates in some cultures.

Pathologically, the acetabulum is defective and the femoral head is completely out of the joint, being posterior and superior to the acetabulum. Most frequently, this is a unilateral occurrence. On examination, one sees asymmetric groin skin creases, with the affected leg being shorter than the other. The leg cannot abduct completely; when it is extended and flexed at the hip, a click called *Ortolani's click* may be felt or heard. Because the femoral head must be in correct alignment with the acetabulum for the bones and joint to grow and develop normally, early detection is necessary. Reduction after age 6 years is almost impossible, and secondary bone changes occur that cause the child to walk with a typical lurching gait. The younger the age of treatment, the more likely that complete hip function will be restored.

Alterations in Joints and Tendons

As discussed earlier, the joints allow the body to be mobile. The synovial joints are most affected by alterations. Studies have shown that this type of articular cartilage, which is lubricated and nourished by synovial fluid, has many microscopic spaces filled with water, causing it to be elastic and able to bounce back despite daily subjection to compression [12].

Arthritis

The most frequent joint diseases are the arthritides, which affect 1 out of every 20 to 30 Americans and constitute a financial and health problem of considerable magnitude. Arthritis simply means inflammation of a joint, and it occurs in many forms. *Suppurative* arthritis implies an infection of the joint with pyogenic organisms; *tuberculous arthritis* is inflammation secondary to tuberculosis. The most crippling of the arthritis group is *rheumatoid arthritis*, which has many forms.

Rheumatoid Arthritis (RA). This chronic inflammatory disease has been studied extensively in attempts to uncover an etiologic agent. In recent years, theories have supported an infectious cause or an autoimmune response. Many bacteria and viruses have been studied without success with respect to their causing RA. The Epstein-Barr virus has been found to react with lymphocytes, transforming them into immunogens [14]. A significant body of knowledge seems to back the immune response theory.

Antibodies known as *rheumatoid factor (RF)* have been demonstrated in the sera of almost all individuals with RA. Synovial lymphocytes produce IgG, which is targeted as being foreign, and production of IgG and IgM antiimmunoglobulins result. These antiimmunoglobulins are actually the rheumatoid factor. By binding with IgG, the antigenic target, the resulting complex activates the complement system in the joint. The RF titer is in direct relationship to the severity of the disease, although the actual stimulus for the formation of RF is unknown. The numerous T lymphocytes in the joint may become sensitized to the joint collagens, causing an immunologic response that is enhanced by the release of lymphokines and presence of prostaglandins [6,14]. Increased physical or emotional stress has always been recognized as a precipitator of acute exacerbations, but the mechanisms for the stress interaction are unknown.

Joint destruction is the primary pathology of RA and may affect any synovial membrane in the body. Joint inflammation with effusion is accompanied by capsular and periarticular soft tissue inflammation, causing swelling, redness, and painful motion of the joint. Proliferative synovitis persists and the synovium becomes a thickened, hyperemic, densely cellular membrane called a *pannus*, which invades and erodes surrounding cartilage and bone. Joint motion causes bleeding within the cavity. Clots of fibrin and newly formed granulation tissue fill the joint space. Pannus destroys the articular cartilage and underlying bone, resulting in loss of motion. The muscles that pull across the joint give rise to flexion and extension and subluxation deformities. Subcutaneous rheumatoid nodules, which are areas of necrosis surrounded by lymphocytes and plasma cells, are present in about one-fourth of persons affected. Figure 41-26 shows articular cortical resorption in the feet.

The fluid aspirated from the joint is thin and cloudy, and has an elevated white cell level. The lysosomal enzymes released from these neutrophils may be a factor in cartilage destruction. As the acute inflammatory process subsides, granulation tissue becomes scar tissue and eventually bone, causing a true ankylosis (fixed, stiff joint). Local degenerative muscle is gradually replaced by fibrous tissue and the involved bones show osteoporosis.

Rheumatoid arthritis is a systemic disease, but it less frequently affects other areas of the body. Small and large arteries anywhere in the system can develop acute necrotizing vasculitis with thrombosis. The vasculitis can cause the vascular insufficiency of Raynaud's phenomenon or obliterative vasculitis from intimal proliferation. The manifestations of cardiac disease include conduction disturbances, myocarditis, and valvular impingement [6]. In the lungs, the person may exhibit pleuritis or interstitial pneumonitis. The eyes may show uveitis, keratoconjunctivitis, or chronic inflammation. Neuropathies, skeletal muscle inflammations, and spleen and liver enlargement may result.

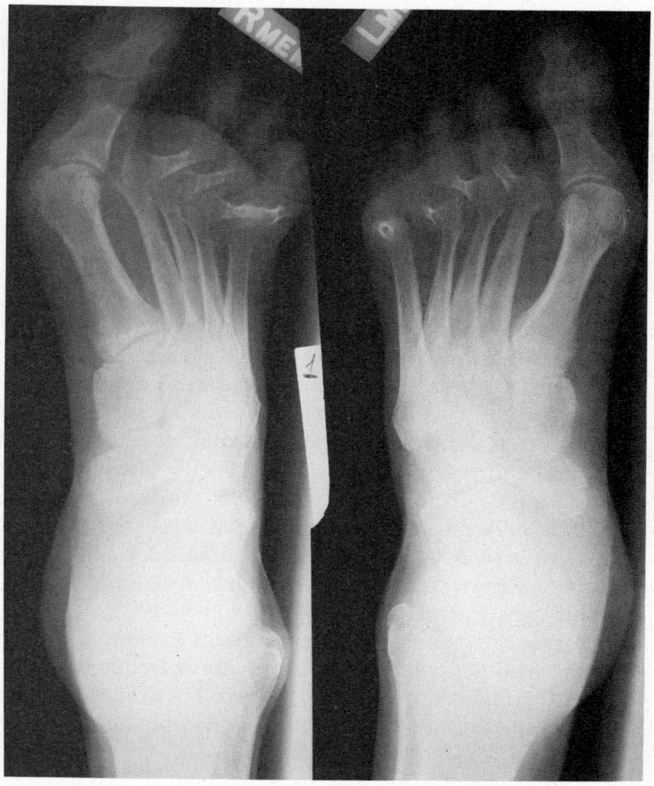

FIGURE 41-26 Rheumatoid arthritis in the feet with ulnar deviation of the phalanges. Articular cortical resorption is noted, which is common with RA.

The disease affects females in a ratio of 3 : 1 over males, with most individuals being between 20 and 50 years of age. The onset can be vague or acute. Fatigue, fever, and malaise may precede actual joint pain, or high fever and aching joints may herald the onset of the disease. Joint stiffness is more noticeable in the morning or after rest. The erythrocyte sedimentation rate is elevated. Exacerbations are common and often cause increasing damage with greater stiffness and deformities. Surgical procedures to replace dysfunctioning joints are often required (Figs. 41-27 and 41-28).

Variants of rheumatoid arthritis include ***juvenile rheumatoid arthritis*** and ***ankylosing spondylitis***. The onset of juvenile RA in persons age 16 years or less is usually abrupt, with chills and high fever, or it may appear insidiously with typical stiffness of one or more joints. The joint pathology is like the adult form, and subcutaneous lesions may also be present. RF is present infrequently. Fortunately, over one-half of these young persons have a complete remission. Permanent deformities are more common in those with acute febrile onset, multiple joint involvement and a positive RF [14].

Ankylosing spondylitis, or Marie-Strümpell disease, is a variant of RA with a genetic linkage that involves the

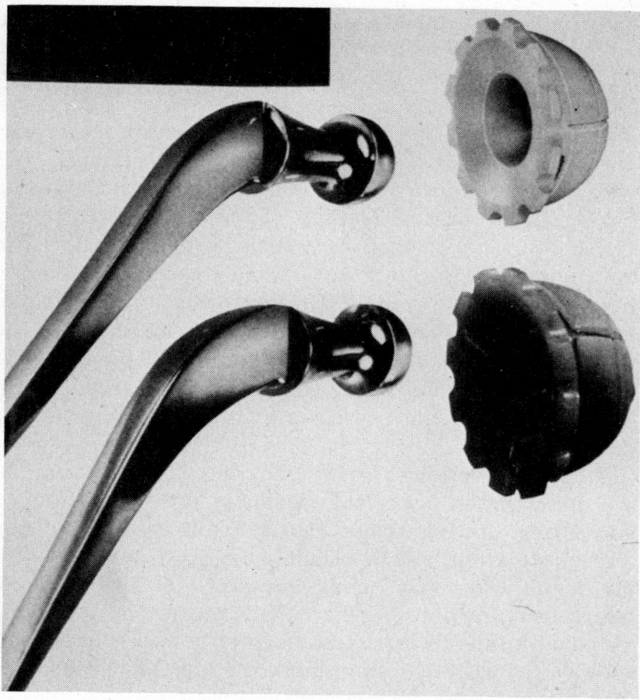

FIGURE 41-27 Stainless steel femoral head and shaft fits into the artificial acetabulum, which is glued into correct placement.

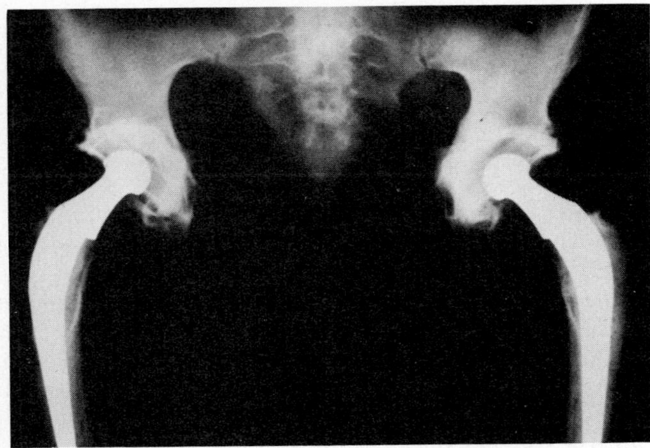

FIGURE 41-28 Total hip replacement with ball and socket.

sacroiliac joints, spine, and adjacent soft tissue. Destruction of cartilage and bone results in fibrous and bony ankylosing of the spine, giving the patient the typical stiff or "poker" spine. The disease is only slightly more prevalent in men than in women, and the symptoms in men are more severe. The peak age range is from 20 to 40 years [14]. An elevated erythrocyte sedimentation rate (ESR) is characteristic, and evidence of IgG, IgA, and immune complex formation indicates that it is an immunologic disease [5].

Osteoarthritis. The term *osteoarthritis* is misleading because inflammation is not a usual component of this condition. *Degenerative joint disease* more clearly defines the disease. The frequency usually is age related, with most of those affected being over 50 years old. Joints have a limited way in which to respond to the compressive forces in day-to-day living. In osteoarthritis, it has been found that the matrix in the articular cartilage is depleted, thus "unmasking" the basic collagen structure. Normally, the matrix spreads compression stress hydrostatically, but with its depletion the collagen fibers may rupture, causing flaking, fissuring, and eroding of the articular cartilage. These alterations are characteristic of the disorder. The bone immediately under the affected area shows proliferation of fibroblasts and new bone formation. Periosteal bone growth also increases at the joint margins and at the site of ligament or tendon attachments, which causes the development of bone spurs or ridges, called *osteophytes*. The synovial capsule decreases in size, and movement is limited.

Degenerative joint disease generally affects joints that are under much pressure, especially the spine, fingers, knees, hips, and shoulders. Pain and stiffness after resting are generally relieved by walking, but permanent ankylosing of the joints may occur. Persons who have occupational stress, are obese, or have faulty posture have greatest frequency of the disease. Trauma, such as sports injuries to a joint at an early age, can render the individual more susceptible to osteoarthritis with advancing years. Studies have shown a *wear-and-tear* process, with increased frequency in joints under stress.

Gout

Gout is caused by the presence of monosodium urate crystals in the joints, which causes acute arthritis. These crystals precipitate in the joints when body fluids are supersaturated with uric acid. Gout is generally classified as primary or secondary. Primary gout is a genetic disorder in which the exact defect of uric acid metabolism is unknown in the vast majority of cases. Ninety percent of all gout is primary, with men being most frequently affected. Secondary gout occurs whenever some superimposed condition either increases the production of uric acid or decreases its excretion. Diseases characterized by rapid breakdown of cells (e.g., leukemia), hemolytic anemia, cytolytic agents, and drugs that decrease excretion of urates (e.g., thiazides and mercurial diuretics) have all been implicated in secondary gout.

In the body uric acid is made by the enzymatic breakdown of tissue and dietary purines. Gout, a hyperurisemic syndrome, can result from overproduction of uric acid, retention of uric acid due to renal malfunction, or both [14]. Normal purine metabolism is complicated, involving numerous enzymes and two pathways. Although the exact error of metabolism is unknown in most cases, the result is an abnormally large amount of uric acid in the blood. At an excessive point, uric acid crystals precipitate into the joint fluids, the kidneys, heart, earlobes, and toes. The mass of urate crystals surrounded by inflammation with lymphocytes, plasma cells, and macrophages is called a *tophus*. Tophi may clump together and form large plaque-like encrustations that invade the articular surface and underlying bone causing deformities. Gout is described in three stages:

Stage 1: high blood uric acid concentration is noted but the individual is usually asymptomatic.
Stage 2: bouts of acute gouty arthritis occur, with attacks and remissions common for many years.
Stage 3: the disabling joint disease is compounded by renal changes, with renal stones, colic, and hypertension being common.

Acute gouty arthritis is heralded by the sudden onset of acute pain, usually in one joint in the lower extremity. Fifty percent of the time attacks occur in the metatarsophalangeal joint of the great toe. Redness, swelling, and exquisite tenderness over the joint may be accompanied by chills and fever. Persons often relate unusual stress preceding an attack, which could include overeating, overindulgence in alcohol, emotional stress, or physical exertion. A person may be asymptomatic for months or even years between attacks. Over many years, disabling, chronic, gouty arthritis may develop.

Atherosclerosis becomes a problem in almost half of persons with gout, and death occurs most frequently from myocardial infarction or renal failure. Treatment consists of a variety of drugs that inhibit uric acid production.

Bursitis

Bursae are classically described as enclosed sacs containing a small amount of fluid that lubricates and cushions joints. Inflammation of a bursa is common and may be caused by unusual use of a part, by trauma, infection, or rheumatoid arthritis. The inflammation results in an excess production of fluid in the sac, causing distention of the sac and pain. Commonly affected bursae are (1) the prepatellar bursae, of which the cause is kneeling (housemaid's knee or nun's knee); (2) the olecranon bursae, subject to the repeated trauma of leaning on one's elbows (bartender's elbow); (3) the bursa located on the plantar aspect of the heel, which is subjected to repeated pressure (postman's heel); and (4) the bursa of the metatarsophalangeal joint of the great toe (bunion).

Baker's Cyst

Baker's cyst is a firm, cystic mass along the medial border of the popliteal space. It occurs mostly in children, and is believed to be caused by fluid distention of the bursal sac associated with local muscles. Some cysts communicate directly with the joint cavity. Swelling is usually the only symptom, and surgical excision, although possible, is not often necessary.

Tumors of Joints

Synovial Sarcoma. Tumors of joints are uncommon, but may occur on the tendon sheath, the bursae, and around the joints. Primitive mesenchymal cells, rather than synovial membrane cells, form the primary tumor. A gray-white mass invades along muscle and fascial planes, and although the tumor is slow-growing, it can metastasize to the lungs, bones, and brain.

Tenosynovitis

Tenosynovitis is an inflammation of the tendon sheath and the enclosed tendon that primarily affects the wrists, shoulders, and ankles. This condition is thought to be use related, and occupational stresses, such as typing and heavy labor, may precipitate it. Synovial fluid and fibrin constituents within the tendon sheath may cause adhesions. These inflammations cause extreme pain on movement and may exhibit heat and redness or inflammation. Bacterial invasion of pyrogens and tuberculosis also have been implicated as causes of tenosynovitis.

Fibromatosis

Palmar fibromatosis denotes chronic hyperplasia of the fascia in the palm of the hand, leading to fibrosis and a deformity called Dupuytren's contracture. The fingers, most often the ring and little fingers, contract into a fixed, flexed position. Usually bilateral, this condition is most frequent in middle-aged men. Heredity is believed to be a major factor in causation.

Plantar fibromatosis is similar to palmar fibromatosis, but it usually does not cause contractures. Nodular masses of fibrocytes arise from the plantar fascia, usually on the medial side of the foot. Trauma is thought to be the cause.

Bone Tumors

Tumors in the skeletal system can be either primary or secondary. Primary lesions can be benign or malignant. Of these, benign tumors are much more common and usually are self-limiting. Malignant tumors of the bone, although rare, are devastating and often fatal. Diagnosis is based on careful history, tumor location, and radiographic appearance.

Benign bone tumors are usually slow-growing, noninvasive, and well localized. Adolescents or young adults are usually affected most frequently and the tumor growth stops when the skeletal system reaches maturity. Because of their noninvasive characteristics, benign tumors cause little or no pain and are often discovered secondary to another complaint or pathologic fracture.

Malignant neoplasms grow rapidly, spread and invade irregularly, and cause pain. Classic signs are constant or intermittent pain, usually worse at night; an unexplained swelling over a bone; a feeling of warmth of the skin over the bone, with prominent veins. Adolescents and young adults are most commonly affected. These tumors metastasize to other parts of the body and are usually fatal without early diagnosis and treatment.

Secondary tumors of the skeletal system are usually from primary sites in the breasts, lungs, kidneys, or other body systems. As the primary lesion grows and invades surrounding tissue, clumps of cancerous tissues are carried by the blood and lymphatic system to the bone, where they continue to grow and cause destruction.

The growth of tumors in the bone often causes increased radiodensities due to increased osteoblastic activity within the tumor. This can be seen on radiographs, which is helpful in diagnosis. Some tumors cause the bone to appear translucent, indicating increased osteoclast activity.

Classification of Tumors

Primary bone neoplasm may be classified according to the skeletal tissue from which it arises: osseous, cartilage, or marrow. Tumors in each of these categories may be benign or malignant. Other bone tumors, such as giant-cell tumors, do not have these origins. This section discusses only the more common tumors, benign and malignant; that is, osteoblastic (bone-forming) and chrondrogenic tumors, tumors of marrow origin, and those of unknown origin.

Bone-Forming Tumors. Benign osteoblastic tumors include *osteomas* and *osteoblastomas*. *Compact osteoma* is a benign tumor composed of dense bone with a well-circumscribed edge. It frequently arises in the cortical surface of bone of the skull and paranasal sinuses. Symptoms are caused from impingement of the tumor on the brain or sinuses. The tumors cause the face to become unfortunately distorted.

Osteoid osteoma most commonly affects the femur and tibia, but can grow in any bone in the body except the skull. It is usually located in the diaphyses of long bones. It occurs predominantly in males between ages 5 and 25 years. The tumor consists of a well-rounded, central nidus that is sharply demarcated from a surrounding zone of bone. The nidus may range from a few millimeters to a centimeter and consists of osteoid tissue and trabeculae (Fig. 41-29). The tissue is reddish gray and is granular to the touch. It may be removed surgically because it causes localized pain, especially at night.

Benign osteoblastoma is a rare tumor that is sometimes confused with osteoid osteoma or even giant-cell tumor. It occurs most frequently in males in the first three decades of life. Its most common site is the spinal cord. Pain is a cardinal symptom, usually due to the pressure on adjacent structures, such as the spinal cord or nerve roots. It seems to be less severe than that caused by an osteoid osteoma and may be referred to a site distant from the tumor. Other symptoms depend upon the location of the tumor and include weakness or even paraplegia. There is no characteristic radiographic appearance. In some cases, one may see bone destruction that is more or less demarcated from normal bone. When the tumor is in a long bone, it may take on the appearance of an osteoid osteoma with a sclerotic border, except that the nidus may be many times longer. Surgical removal usually relieves compression on the spinal column and nerve root.

The most prevalent malignant tumor of osteoid origin is the *osteogenic sarcoma* or *osteosarcoma*. Within this tumor the tumor cells proliferate osteoid or immature bone. Osteosarcoma is the most common and most fatal primary bone tumor, often affecting people between ages 10 and 20 years [15]. It occurs more often in males than in females and usually during periods of rapid skeletal growth. Irradiation and oncogenic viruses have been explored in its etiology [14]. When this lesion does occur in later years of life, it is usually related to Paget's disease. Radiation treatment for other tumors has also been indicated in the causation of osteogenic sarcoma in later life.

To be classified as a true osteogenic sarcoma, an osteoid substance must be produced. The tumor may show a predominance of elements, with osteoid, chondroid, or fibromatoid differentiation [4].

Osteosarcomas usually occur in long tubular bones, but the skull, maxilla, spinal column, and clavicles, as well as other bones, are also affected. The femurs, tibias, and ulnae are the most frequent sites (Fig. 41-30). Over age 25 years, its frequency in flat and long bones is nearly equal [14]. The tumor usually is a localized swelling with tenderness associated with a large mass. Pain may or may not be present. Sometimes the tumor is found on incidental radiographic examination of an injury. It tends to recur within one to two years.

The survival rate with osteosarcoma was dismal when resection or amputation alone was employed. Three-year survival of 65 to 75 percent has been achieved using the combination of aggressive chemotherapy and surgery [14]. Interferon and other immunotherapy is still experimental.

Tumors of Cartilaginous Origin. *Benign chondrogenic tumors* include *osteochondroma* and *chondroblastoma*. Many of these tumors are asymptomatic and are only discovered accidentally because of an injury to the area. Osteochondromas form a long mass produced by progressive endochondral ossification of a growing cartilaginous cap. The tumor is basically osseous and protrudes from the cortex of the bone with or without a stalk. The caps are usually cauliflower-shaped and occur mainly in persons between the first and second decades of life (Fig. 41-31). The growth of the tumor parallels that of the

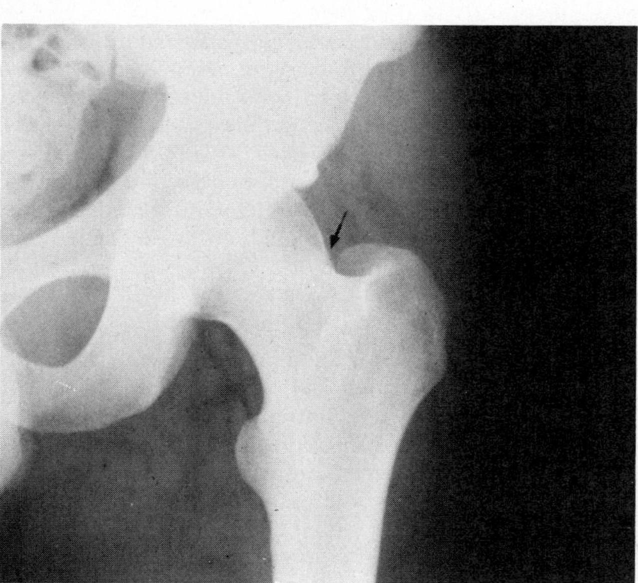

FIGURE 41-29 Osteoid osteoma. Small transport area indicated by arrow represents the central nidus.

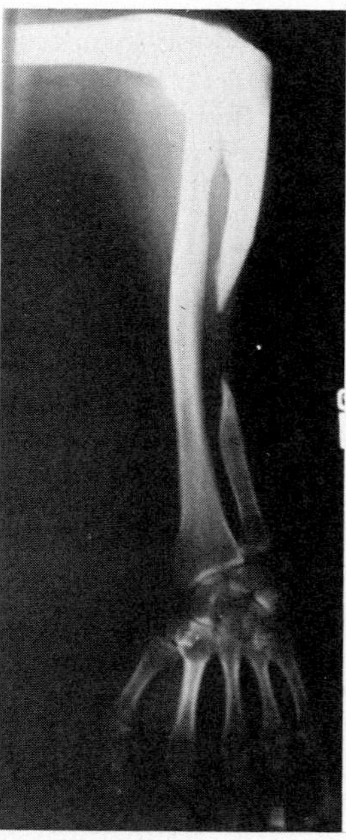

FIGURE 41-30 Osteogenic sarcoma. Note the complete destruction of the ulna.

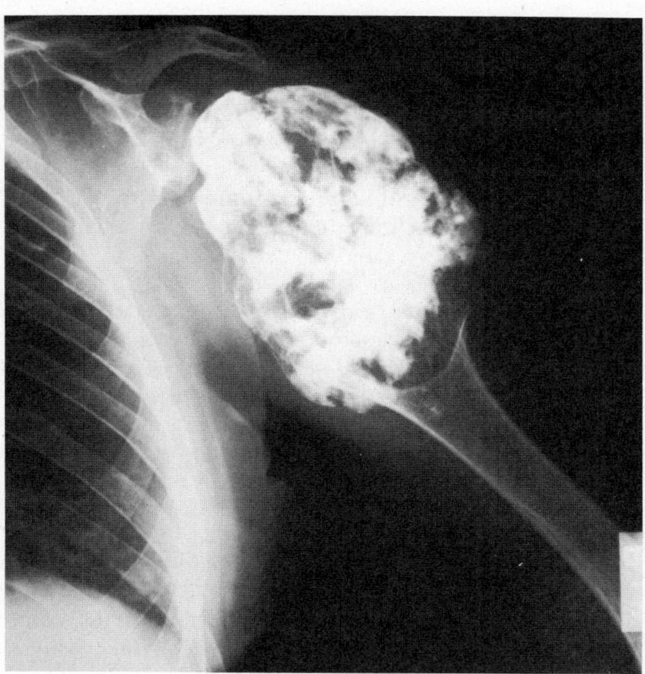

FIGURE 41-31 Osteochondroma of the proximal right humerus is unusually large. Shows cartilaginous and osteoid matrix being laid down.

adolescent, and once the epiphyses have closed, it normally stops. Multiple osteochondromas may occur when more than one bone is affected, with each growth having the same characteristics as the single osteochondroma.

Osteochondromas rarely undergo malignant change to osteosarcomas. This transformation occurs most frequently with multiple tumors and occasionally after surgical removal of an osteochondroma. The most common site for the tumorous mass is the metaphyseal region of long bones, specifically the femur and tibia, but it can affect any bone that develops by endochondral ossification.

Endochondroma is the term used to describe a tumor when it only involves the medulla and is encapsulated by an intact cortex. It commonly affects the small bones of the hands and feet but may affect ribs, sternum, spine, and long bones of persons between ages 20 and 30 years. The tumor usually affects the phalanges of the hand, producing a central area of rarefaction (decreasing density and weight) (Fig. 41-32). Normally discovered during treatment of a fracture after a trivial injury, the tumor appears radiographically as a well-defined, translucent area with the cortex intact and areas of calcification.

Benign chondroblastoma closely resembles giant-cell tumors and affects mainly persons under age 20 years or before epiphyseal closure, whereas giant-cell tumors are rare under age 20 years. Histologically, chondroblastomas differ from giant-cell tumors in that they contain foci of calcification, trabeculae of osteoid tissue, and well-developed bone, as well as more or less well-defined areas of cartilaginous matrix, features that are not usually present in giant-cell tumors. Chondroblastomas are virtually always benign, localized lesions that do not recur and do not invade.

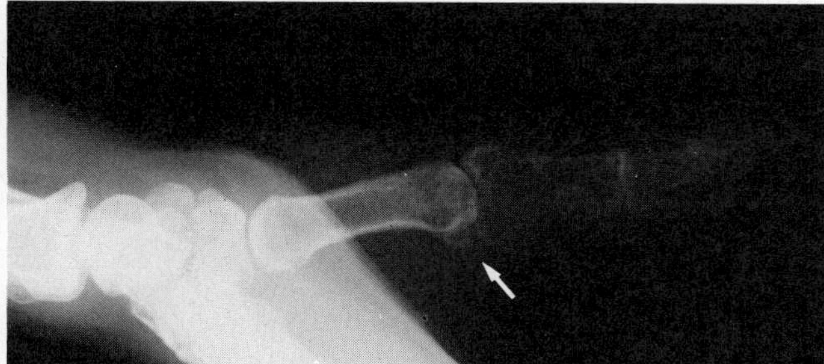

FIGURE 41-32 Endochondroma of the thumb.

Localized pain may be experienced and is often referred to the adjacent joint region. Wasting of muscle mass due to disuse caused by pain and limping may also be observed.

Radiographically, an area of central bone destruction is clearly demarcated by surrounding normal bone. There may be margins of increased bone density with mottled areas of calcification within the lesion. The tumor almost always involves the epiphyses and frequently the adjacent metaphyses, which are also seen on the films [4].

Chondrosarcoma is a malignant bone tumor of cartilaginous origin. It can arise from benign chondrogenic origins, as described earlier, or may develop spontaneously. The tumor is rare; it occurs more frequently in men than in women [14]. It is primarily a condition of adulthood and old age, and rarely metastasizes until it has grown to a large size [15].

Chondrosarcomas usually originate in the trunk and the upper ends of the femur and humerus, with points of attachments of muscle to bone at the knee, pelvis, shoulder, and hip being prevalent. Virtually any bone of the body can be affected.

Physical symptoms may include pain, swelling, and a palpable mass due to the active invasive growth of the tumor. Tumors located in the trunk and long bones may be evidenced only by pain, which makes radiographic findings important. These usually include mottled areas of calcification and areas of osseous destruction (Fig. 41-33). Even when treated with wide resection, recurrence has been encountered even after 10 years. Metastases may occur many years after initial diagnosis and treatment.

Tumors of Marrow Origin. *Ewing's sarcoma*, although rare, is one of the most lethal bone tumors. Approximately 90 percent of individuals affected are under age 30 years; the greatest number of tumors occur in the second decade of life. They affect slightly more males than females [14]. The long tubular bones are most commonly involved, with the innominate bones—the pelvis, ischium, ribs, scapula, and sternum—following in that order, and then virtually any other bone in the body (Fig. 41-34).

Ewing's sarcoma, like many other invasive tumors, results in pain, a tender mass, and venous distention. Some

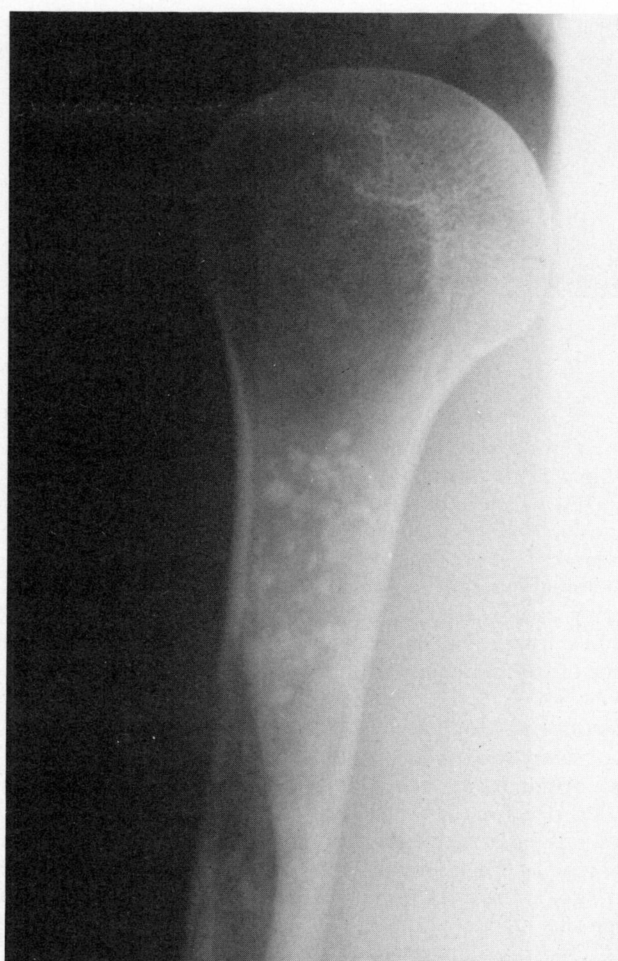

FIGURE 41-33 Chondrosarcoma of the humerus. Mixed lytic and sclerotic areas give patchy appearance to bone.

individuals may have anemia, temperature elevation, and sometimes leukocytosis that supports an inflammatory etiology [4]. This tumor generally has its origin in the medullary canal, growing outward and creating a lytic area on radiographs. Some spicules of bone may be seen, but this is reactive bone and not part of the neoplasm. Elevation of the periosteum is typical, followed by periosteal bone formation, which creates what is known as an onion-skin appearance, seen radiologically.

Tumors of Undetermined Origin. *Giant-cell tumors* are poorly understood, apparently malignant, distinct neoplasms. Cases of seemingly benign giant-cell tumors have been reported to undergo malignant transformation. For this reason, a histomorphic grading system has been developed, with grade I benign and grade II malignant [14]. Unfortunately, this system is not always accurate, as one part of the tumor may appear benign while another part may appear malignant [15].

Giant-cell tumors generally affect individuals between ages 20 and 55 years. Peak occurrence is in the third decade of life. It affects females somewhat more frequently than males. Most giant-cell tumors arise in the epiphyses of long bones, with over one-half of the lesions close to the knee in the distal femur and proximal tibia; other sites are the sacrum, vertebrae, humerus, and radius, as well as other bones [4].

Giant-cell tumors usually begin forming within cancellous bone. As they grow and invade, the cortex may be thinned or even broken, but new reactive bone generally preserves the cortex. The expansion of the tumor in the epiphyses classically forms a clublike deformity. Radiographs reveal a somewhat translucent area at the ends of the long bones, with a thin cortex (Fig. 41-35).

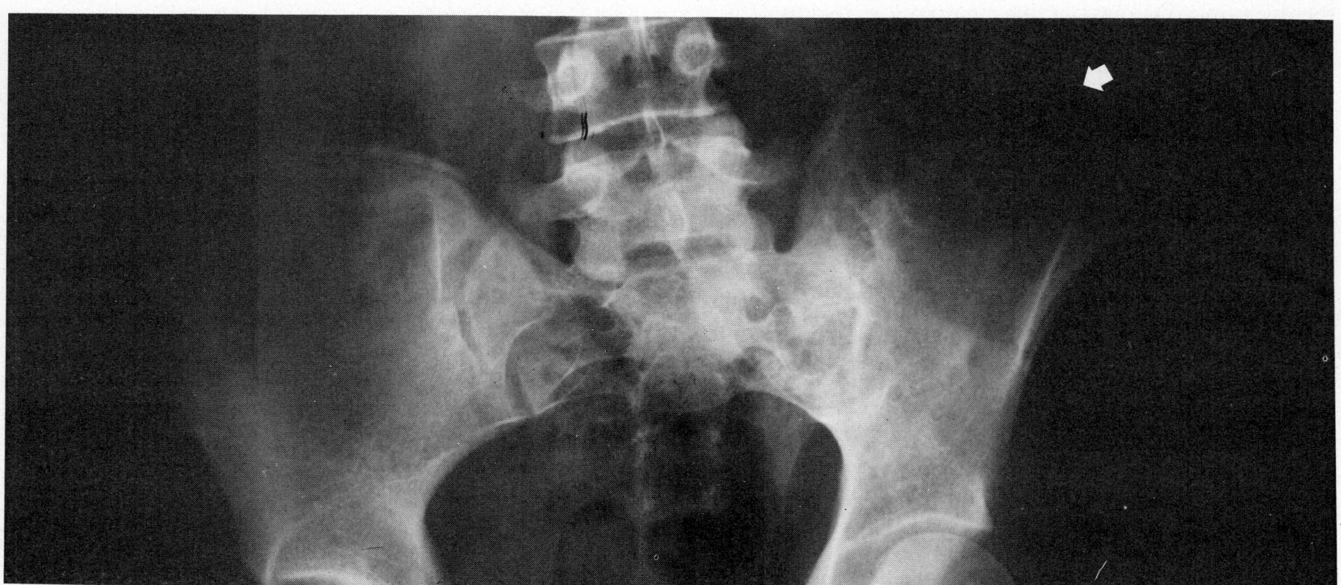

FIGURE 41-34 Ewing's sarcoma. Note that the top of the ischium has been carved out by tumor.

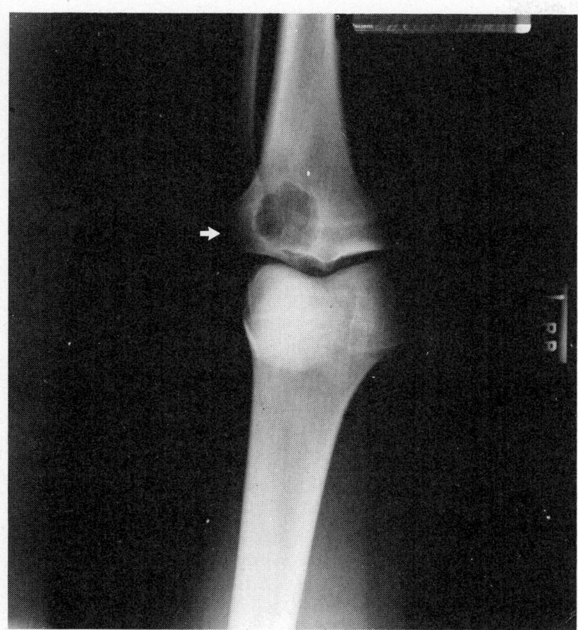

FIGURE 41-35 Giant-cell tumor of the tibia (*arrow*).

Hematogenic Tumors

Multiple myeloma is the most common neoplasm of the bone. It is composed of plasma cells showing variable degrees of differentiation. This condition is further described in Chapter 15, but the skeletal effects are discussed here.

Multiple myeloma affects women and men equally, rarely occurs before age 50 years, and has its peak frequency in the fifth and sixth decades. It has a predilection for the vertebral column, but ribs, skull, pelvis, and virtually any bone in the body may be affected. Multiple myeloma appears radiographically as multifocal destructive bone lesions throughout the skeletal system, producing what appear to be rounded, punched-out areas (Fig. 41-36) [14]. These areas may measure up to 5 cm with no surrounding zone of sclerosis. Pathologic fractures of the vertebrae are common.

The individual has a history of pain that is often referred to the spinal column. Neurologic symptoms occur because of compression of vertebral bodies or nerve roots

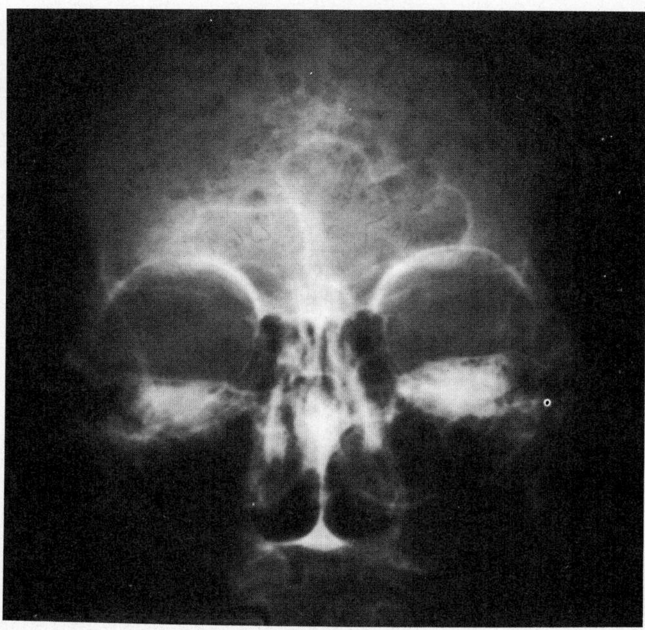

A

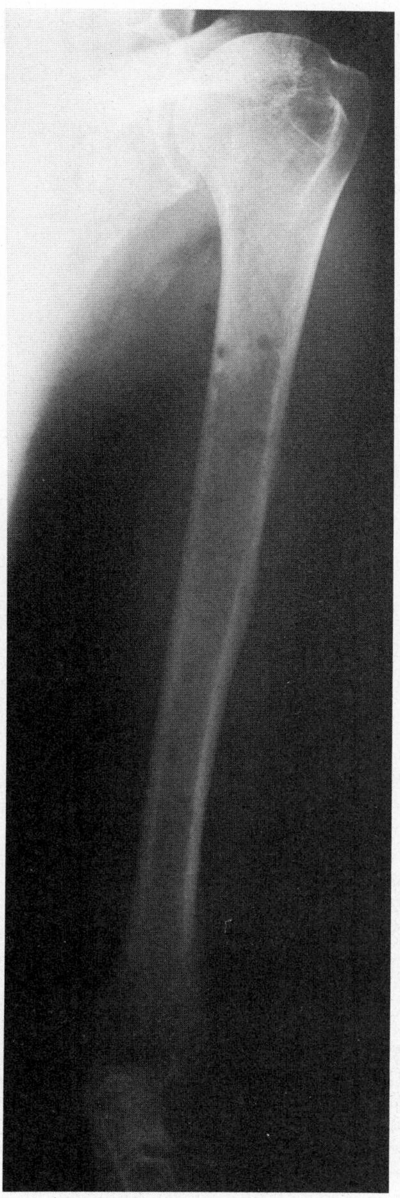

B

FIGURE 41-36 Multiple myeloma (A) of the skull, (B) of the humerus. Note numerous lytic defects and diffuse osteoporosis characteristic of multiple myeloma.

due to extension of the neoplasm. Weakness, loss of weight, hemorrhagic disorders, and renal involvement are also associated with multiple myeloma. Hypercalcemia, hyperuricemia, and presence of Bence Jones protein in the urine are frequently noted.

Study Questions

1. Explain the formation and growth of bone.
2. What factors are essential in promoting healthy bone tissue?
3. What are the effects of weight bearing and exercise on bone formation?
4. Discuss fracture healing. How does it vary with different types of fractures?
5. Explain how osteoporosis occurs and what might be done to prevent it.
6. Describe rheumatoid arthritis, using this chapter and Chapter 12.
7. Compare the pathology of rheumatoid arthritis with osteoarthritis.
8. Discuss the different types of tumors that can affect bone. How do their etiologies, pathologies and clinical courses differ?

References

1. Apley, A. *System of Orthopedics and Fractures* (5th ed.). London: Butterworths, 1977.
2. *Calcium Currents.* (National Dairy Promotion and Research Board), 1, 1986.
3. Cummings, S.R., Nevitt, M.C., and Haber, R.J. Prevention of osteoporotic fractures. *West. J. Med.* 134:5, 1985.
4. Dahlin, D. *Bone Tumors*. Springfield, Ill.: Thomas, 1967.
5. Duckworth, T. Lecture notes on orthopedics and fractures (2nd ed.). Boston: Blackwell, 1984.
6. Fudenberg, H., et al. *Basic and Clinical Immunology* (3rd ed.). Los Altos, Calif.: Lange, 1980.
7. Ganong, W. *Review of Medical Physiology* (12th ed.). Los Altos, Calif.: Lange, 1985.
8. Guyton, A.C. *Textbook of Medical Physiology* (7th ed.). Philadelphia: Saunders, 1986.
9. Hollingshead, W. *Textbook of Anatomy* (3rd ed.). Hagerstown, Md.: Harper & Row, 1974.
10. Krane, S. Paget's disease of bone. *Clin. Orthop.* 127:124, 1977.
11. Lane, J., and Vigorita, V. Osteoporosis. *Orthop. Clin. North Am.* 151:4, 1984.
12. Mankin, H. The reaction of articular cartilage to injury and osteoarthritis. *N. Engl. J. Med.* 291:1285, 1974.
13. Markow, R., and Lane, J. Current concepts of Paget's disease of bone. *Orthop. Clin. North Am.* 15:4, 1984.
14. Robbins, S.L., Cotran, R.S., and Kumar, V. *Pathologic Basis of Disease* (3rd ed.). Philadelphia: Saunders, 1984.
15. Rodrigo, J.J. *Orthopaedic Surgery: Basic Science and Clinical Science*. Boston: Little, Brown, 1986.
16. Ryan, W. Treatment of Paget's disease of bone with mithramycin. *Clin. Orthop.* 127:106, 1977.
17. Sharpe, L. Disorders of the musculoskeletal system. In E.A. Hincker and L. Malasanos (eds.), *The Little, Brown Manual of Medical-Surgical Nursing.* Boston: Little, Brown, 1983.
18. Silverstein, *A. Human Anatomy and Physiology*. New York: Wiley, 1980.
19. Singer, F. The etiology of Paget's disease of bone. *Clin. Orthop.* 127:37, 1977.
20. Steinberg, M., and Trueta, J. Effects of activity in rat bone growth. *Clin. Orthop.* 156:59, 1981.
21. Vaughan, J. *The Physiology of Bone*. London: Oxford, 1975.
22. West, J. (ed.). *Best and Taylor's Physiological Basis of Medical Practice* (11th ed.). Baltimore: Williams & Wilkins, 1985.

Unit Bibliography

Albright, J., and Miller, E. (eds.). Osteogenesis imperfecta. *Clin. Orthop.* 159:1, 1981.

Aloia, J.F. Estrogen and exercise in prevention and treatment of osteoporosis. *Geriatrics* 37(6):81, 1982.

Apley, A.G. *System of Orthopaedics and Fractures* (5th ed.). London: Butterworths, 1977.

Arnstein, A.R. Recent progress in osteomalacia and rickets. *Ann. Intern. Med.* 67:1296, 1967.

Aroncheck, J.M., and Haddad, J.G. Paget's disease. *Orthop. Clin. North Am.* 14:1–3, 1983.

Berne, R.M., and Levy, M.M. *Physiology*. St. Louis: Mosby, 1983.

Bowen, J.R., Foster, B.K., and Hartzell, C.R. Legg-Calvé-Perthes disease. *Clin. Orthop.* 185:97, 1984.

Brown, A.M., and Stubb, D.W. *Medical Physiology*. New York: Wiley, 1983.

Clawson, D.K., and Frederick, A.M. Compartmental syndromes. *Clin. Orthop.* 113:2, 1975.

Cohen, A.S. *Progress in Clinical Rheumatology*, Vol. 1. Orlando, Fla.: Grune & Stratton, 1984.

Dahlin, D.C. *Bone Tumors: General Aspects and Data on 3,987 Cases* (2nd ed.). Springfield, Ill.: Thomas, 1967.

Downie, P.A. *Cash's Textbook of Orthopaedics and Rheumatology for Physiotherapists*. Philadelphia: Lippincott, 1984.

Duckworth, T. *Lecture Notes on Orthopaedics and Fractures* (2nd ed.). Boston: Blackwell, 1984.

Ferguson, A. Segmental vascular changes in the femoral head in children and adults. *Clin. Orthop.* 200:291, 1985.

Fox, J.H., and Kelly, W.N. Management of gout. *JAMA* 242:4, 1979.

Fraumeni, J.F., Jr. Stature and malignant tumors of bone in childhood and adolescence. *Cancer* 20:967, 1967.

Frost, H.M. *Orthopaedic Biomechanics*. Springfield, Ill.: Thomas, 1976.

Gould, J.A., and Davies, C.J. *Orthopaedic and Sports Physical Therapy*. St. Louis: Mosby, 1985.

Harrison, M., and Burwell, R. Perthes' disease: A concept of pathogenesis. *Clin. Orthop.* 156:115, 1981.

Ibsen, K.H. Distinct varieties of osteogenic imperfecta. *Clin. Orthop.* 50:279, 1967.

Jaffe, H. The classic Paget's disease of bone. *Clin. Orthop.* 127:4, 1977.

Kessler, R.M., and Hertling, D. *Management of Common Musculoskeletal Disorders*. Philadelphia: Harper & Row, 1983.

Kleerehoper, M., Talia, K., and Parfitt, A. Nutritional endocrine and demographic aspects of osteoporosis. *Orthop. Clin. North Am.* 3:550, 1981.

Kuska, B. Acute onset compartment syndrome. *J. Emerg. Nurs.* 8:75, 1982.

Macnab, I., and Rorabeck, C.H. The pathophysiology of the anterior tibial compartmental syndrome. *Clin. Orthop.* 113:52, 1975.

Mankin, H.J., and Gebhardt, M. Advances in the management of bone tumors. *Clin. Orthop.* 200:73, 1985.

Marieb, E.N. *Essentials of Human Anatomy and Physiology*. Menlo Park, Calif.: Addison-Wesley, 1984.

Milgram, J.W. Radiographical and pathological assessment of the activity of Paget's disease of bone. *Clin. Orthop.* 127:43, 1977.

Morizumi, H. Comparative study of alterations in skeletal muscle in Duchenne muscular dystrophy and polymyositis. *Acta. Pathol. Jpn.* 34(6):1221, 1984.

Mountcastle, V.B. *Medical Physiology* (14th ed.). St. Louis: Mosby, 1980.

Nachemson, A. Advances in low back pain. *Clin. Orthop.* 200:266, 1985.

Narakas, A. Surgical treatment of traction injuries of the brachial plexus. *Clin. Orthop.* 133:71, 1978.

Nordin, B., et al. New approaches to the problem of osteoporosis. *Clin. Orthop.* 200:181, 1985.

Oh, W.H., and Mitral, M.A. Fat embolism: Current concepts of pathogenesis, diagnosis, and treatment. *Orthop. Clin. North Am.* 9:767, 1976.

Posner, A. The mineral of bone. *Clin. Orthop.* 200:87, 1985.

Rodman, G.P., and Shumaker, H.R. (eds.). *Primer on Rheumatic Disorders*. Atlanta: Arthritis Foundation, 1983.

Rodrigo, J.J. *Orthopaedic Surgery, Basic Science, and Clinical Science*. Boston: Little, Brown, 1986.

Russell, W.D. A clinical and pathological staging system for soft tissue sarcomas. *Cancer* 40:1562, 1977.

Ryan, W. Treatment of Paget's disease of bone with mithramycin. *Clin. Orthop.* 127:106, 1977.

Salter, R.B. *Textbook of Disorders and Injuries to the Musculoskeletal System* (2nd ed.). Baltimore: Williams & Wilkins, 1983.

Silverstein, A. *Human Anatomy and Physiology*. New York: Wiley, 1980.

Simmons, D. Fracture healing perspectives. *Clin. Orthop.* 200:100, 1985.

Singer, F., and Mills, B. The etiology of Paget's disease of bone. *Clin. Orthop.* 127:37, 1977.

Turek, S.L. *Orthopaedics, Principles, and Their Application* (4th ed.). Philadelphia: Lippincott, 1984.

Turner, R.A., and Wise, C.M. *Textbook of Rheumatology*. Winston Salem, N.C.: Medical Examination, 1986.

Vander, A.J., Sherman, J.H., and Luciano, D.S. *Human Physiology: The Mechanisms of Body Function*. New York: McGraw-Hill, 1985.

UNIT 14

Protective Coverings of the Body

Marcia Hill

The skin is the largest and one of the most metabolically active organs of the body, but its function is often underestimated. It is a dynamic organ that regulates body temperature and fluid balance, and prevents microbial invasion. Hair and nails can also be considered as protective coverings to the body.

Chapter 42 discusses the protective and complex metabolic activities of skin. Chapter 43 describes common inflammatory processes, tumors, and traumatic alterations in skin integrity.

The reader is encouraged to use the learning objectives as guides to facilitate the study of this important organ. Study questions at the end of each chapter help to test learning of major concepts. The bibliography at the end of the unit provides sources for further study of these topics.

CHAPTER 42

Normal Structure and Function of the Skin

CHAPTER OUTLINE

Anatomy and Physiology

- Epidermis
  - *Layers of the Epidermis*
  - *Life Cycle of Epidermal Cells*
  - *Nonkeratinocytes*
  - *Skin Pigmentation*
  - *Chemical Properties of the Epidermis*
- Dermis
  - *Layers of the Dermis*
  - *Components of the Dermis*
  - *Cellular Components of the Dermis*
  - *Functions of the Dermis*
- Subcutaneous Tissues
- Epidermal Appendages
  - *Sweat Glands*
  - *Sebaceous Glands*
  - *Hair*
  - *Nails*
- Blood Supply
- Nervous Control
- Vitamin D Synthesis in the Skin

LEARNING OBJECTIVES

1. Discuss the embryonic development of the skin.
2. Describe the characteristics of the layers of the epidermis.
3. Describe the life cycle of the epidermal cell.
4. Discuss the chemical properties of the epidermis.
5. Describe the production of melanin.
6. List the layers of the dermis.
7. State the components of the dermis.
8. Discuss the function of the dermis.
9. Describe the structure and function of the subcutaneous tissues.
10. List the epidermal appendages.
11. Describe the process of sweat production and its function in regulating heat.
12. Compare the structure and function of sweat and sebaceous glands.
13. Discuss the growth and development of hair.
14. Describe the blood and nerve supply to the skin.
15. Explain the role of the skin in vitamin D production.

The skin is the largest organ of the body, with a surface area of 1.8 sq meters and comprising 15 percent of total body weight in the average adult [9]. This surface area increases 7 times from birth to maturity. The skin's consistency ranges from the thick (0.25 in.), tough, yet pliable covering of the body to the thin (0.007 in.), delicate, mucous membranes of the mouth, nose, and eyelids. The skin, having the characteristics of being both pliable and durable, allows for mobility and protection. At the same time it is one of the most sensitive organs of the body, capable of transmitting a variety of sensations, such as fine touch, pain, temperature, and pressure [9].

Anatomy and Physiology

The skin is composed of three major layers that are, from the surface inward, the epidermis, dermis, and subcutaneous tissues (Fig. 42-1). These layers have the following functions: (1) they protect against the external environment, (2) maintain and regenerate layers, (3) participate in defending the body against foreign substances, (4) preserve the internal fluid environment, (5) participate in excreting wastes, (6) assist in regulating body temperature, (7) produce vitamin D, and (8) affect psychosocial aspects of daily living (Table 42-1).

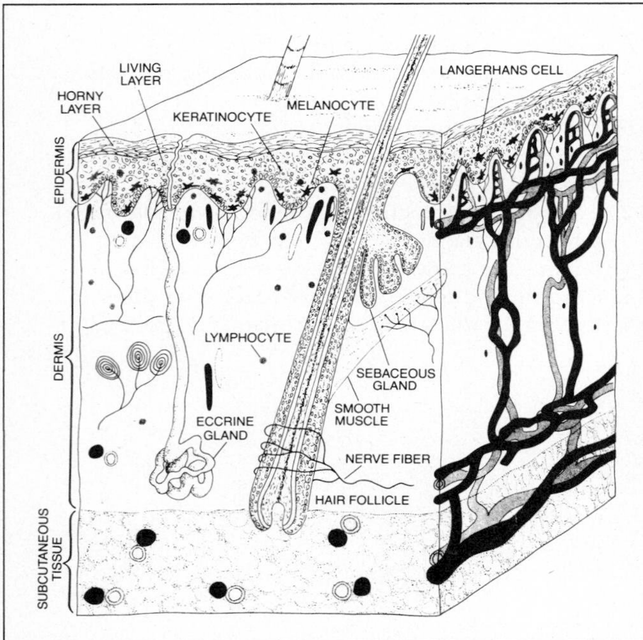

FIGURE 42-1 Complex anatomy of the skin is suggested in an idealized drawing. The surface is covered by a horny layer of dead keratinocytes filled with the protein keratin. Living keratinocytes dominate the epidermis and proliferate as dead cells are lost from the surface. Melanocytes, which secrete pigment granules responsible for skin color, are at the base of the epidermis. Langerhans' cells, dendritic cells that process antigens applied to the surface of the skin, lie above the basal layer of keratinocytes. The dermis is largely a network of connective tissue and is underlaid by fatty subcutaneous tissue. The specialized keratinocytes of the hair follicles form hair. The dermis is richly supplied with nerve fibers, some of which innervate sensory nerve endings, and with blood vessels. T lymphocytes are scattered through the skin, primarily in the epidermis and the upper dermis. (From R.L. Edelson and J.M. Fink, The immunologic function of the skin. *Sci. Am.*, June 1985, illustration on p. 48 by Ilil Arbel. Copyright © by Scientific American, Inc. All rights reserved.)

Epidermis

The epidermis consists of stratified epithelium, hair follicles, and sweat and sebaceous glands [3].

Layers of the Epidermis. The main layers, or strata, of the epidermis, from the dermis to the surface, are the stratum germinativum, stratum spinosum, stratum granulosum, stratum lucidum (present only on the palms and soles), and stratum corneum (Fig. 42-2).

The deepest layer, the stratum germinativum, or *basal layer*, is one cell thick and lies in contact with the dermis. Within the basal layer are basal cells, which are cuboidal or columnar, have oval nuclei, and are united to each other by desmosomes, or bridges. These cells are attached to a basement membrane by tonofibrils, or half-desmosomes. The epidermis is also attached to the dermis by interlocking, irregularly shaped processes of basal cells with corresponding dermal processes that extend different depths into the dermis (dermoepidermal junction). Processes are present in varying numbers throughout the skin. For example, eyelids have few processes, while nipples have a complex system of ridges, and fingertips have parallel ridges that form cavernous valleys and tunnels [4]. The highly individualized patterns of fingertips are the results of these valleys. In the normal epidermis, mitosis of new basal cells is limited to the basal layer. During regeneration, mitosis continues upward into the squamous layer.

Throughout the basal layer are dispersed melanocytes, which form melanin and are responsible for pigmentation of the skin. These cells are wedged between the basal cells. When stained, melanocytes have clear cytoplasm and small, dark nuclei [5].

The stratum spinosum, or prickle cell layer, contains cells with a polygonal shape. Bridges hold the cells together. As these cells move toward the surface they begin to flatten. Within the cells, fibril or keratin precursors make a three-dimensional framework throughout the cytoplasm [3].

The stratum granulosum, or granular cell layer, is from two to four cells thick and lies directly above the stratum spinosum. The cells become diamond-shaped and are filled with keratohyalin (hematoxylin) granules [4]. During keratinization, these granules form the interfibrillary substance that cements keratin fibers together [10].

The stratum lucidum is not present in all skin sections but is in the thick epidermis, such as the palms of the hands and soles of the feet. This layer provides a friction surface.

The horny stratum corneum varies in thickness from 0.02 mm on the forearm to 0.5 mm or more on the soles of the feet (see Fig. 42-2). The cells of this layer are flat,

TABLE 42-1 Functions of the Skin

Function	Epidermis	Dermis	Subcutaneous Tissue
Protection	Keratin provides protection from injury by corrosive materials. Inhibits proliferation of microorganisms because of dry external surface. Mechanical strength through intracellular bonds.	Provides fibroblasts for wound healing. Provides mechanical strength through collagen fibers, elastic fibers, ground substance. Lymphatic and vascular tissues respond to inflammation, injury, and infection.	Absorbs mechanical shock.
Water balance	Low permeability to water and electrolytes prevents systemic dehydration and electrolyte loss.		
Temperature regulation	Eccrine sweat glands allow dissipation of heat through evaporation of sweat secreted onto skin surface.	Cutaneous vasculature, through dilation or constriction, promotes or inhibits heat conduction from skin surface.	
Sensory organ	Transmits a variety of sensations through neuroreceptor system.	Encloses extensive network of free and encapsulated nerve endings for relaying sensations to the brain.	Contains large pressure receptors.
Vitamin synthesis	7-Dehydrocholesterol present in large concentrations in malpighian cells; photoconversion to vitamin D takes place.		
Psychosocial	Body image alterations result with many epidermal diseases, such as generalized psoriasis.	Body image alterations occur with many dermal diseases, such as scleroderma.	

Source: T. Rosen, M. Lanning, and M. Hill, *Nurse's Atlas of Dermatology*. Boston: Little, Brown, 1983.

have no nuclei, and constitute the keratin layer. Keratin is a tough, fibrous protein that resists chemical change. The stratum corneum shields the body from environmental damage and maintains the internal milieu. The skin has the lowest water permeability of any biologic membrane. This low permeability retards water loss and prevents most toxic agents from entering the body. The horny cells are shed continuously, making way for new cells.

Life Cycle of Epidermal Cells. The life cycle of epidermal cells involves three phases: mitosis, keratinization, and exfoliation. Epidermal cells, the major ones being keratinocytes, are continuously formed in the basal or germinative layer at a rate commensurate with the constant loss. New cells move from the basal layer to the stratum corneum in a random fashion that is influenced by the rate of keratinization and by the time that each cell left the basal layer. Transit time from basal layer to surface is anywhere from 12 to 25 days. An increase in mitotic rate occurs within 24 to 36 hours after an injury.

Mitosis is affected by two major factors: the diurnal cycle and hormones. Mitosis seems to occur at a greater rate during periods when the body is at rest or asleep. Hormonal influences include androgens, which cause the growth of hair in the typical masculine locations: over the pubis, on the face, on the chest, and on other locations of the body. Androgens aid in the formation of hair follicles and sebaceous glands. Estrogen hormones aid in the formation of the vaginal epithelium and provide for skin softness. Mitosis may be inhibited by adrenalin, levels of which are increased during times of wakefulness.

The second phase in the epidermal cell life cycle is keratinization. As the epidermal cell from the basal layer moves toward the surface, it loses its ability to undergo mitosis. Instead, it begins to synthesize fibrillar and amorphous proteins, keratin, and membrane-coating granules. The cell finally loses its nucleus and cellular organelles, becomes part of the stratum corneum, and is shed. The fibrillar proteins make up the fibrils in the epidermal cell and give the stratum corneum strength and chemical inertness. As the cell moves toward the surface, more and more fibrils form, until they make up 50 percent of the protein in stratum corneum cells. Amorphous proteins that make up the other 50 percent are embedded in a matrix and have no definite structure. Membrane-coating granules are formed and align near the apical part of the cell membrane. They fuse with the membrane, break it, and discharge their contents into the intercellular spaces

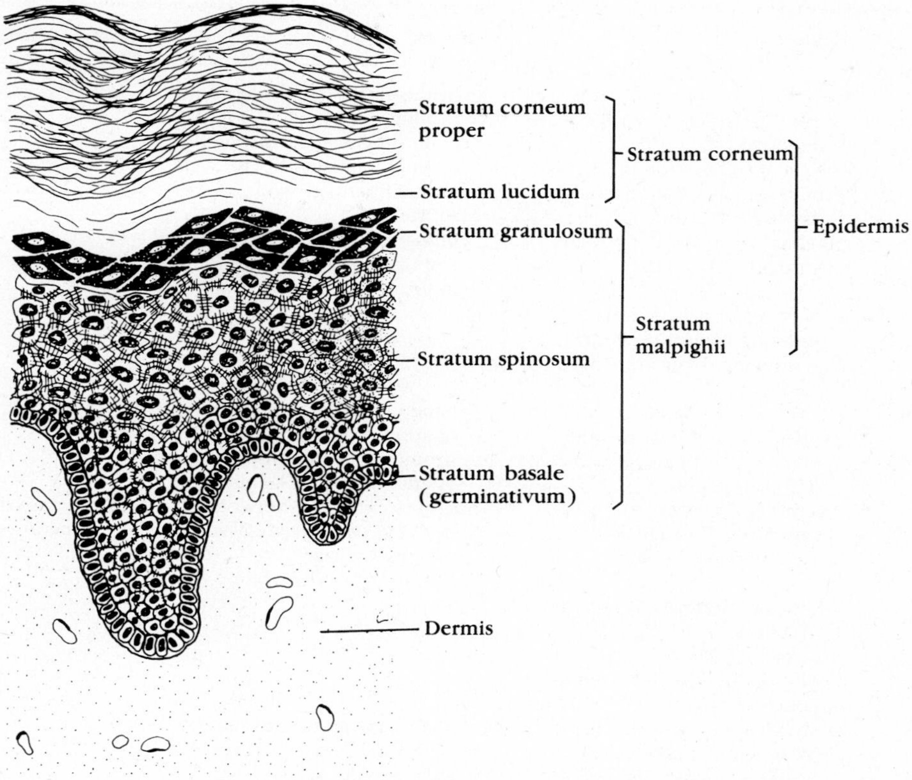

FIGURE 42-2 The epidermis of thick skin in vertical histologic section, with its various layers. (From M. Borysenko et al., *Functional Histology* [2nd ed.]. Boston: Little, Brown, 1984.)

in the granular layer of the stratum malpighii. The function of membrane-coating granules is not clear, but they may bind cells together.

As the epidermal cell moves closer to the surface, keratohyalin granules form. These granules are present in cells immediately below the horny layer. When a cell reaches the horny layer, its membrane thickens. The nucleus and organelles disintegrate and are eliminated from the cell.

At the end of keratinization, cornified cells are cemented together in varying thicknesses. Those at the surface are shed, resulting in exfoliation, which is the last phase in the life of an epidermal cell (Fig. 42-3).

Keratinocytes provide an environment for other cell types, including nonkeratinocytes such as melanocytes, Langerhans cells, Merkel cells, and possibly, lymphocytes [3].

Nonkeratinocytes. *Langerhans cells* are dendritic nonkeratinocytes that are thought to function as a part of the immune system. They are present in the basal and suprabasal layers of the dermis and occasionally in the dermis [3]. *Merkel cells* are present in the undersurface of the epidermis and oral mucosa. They probably function as touch receptors [6]. *Lymphocytes*, especially T lymphocytes, have been reported to be part of normal epidermis [2]. Other cells of the immune defense system are present in the dermis and subcutaneous tissues.

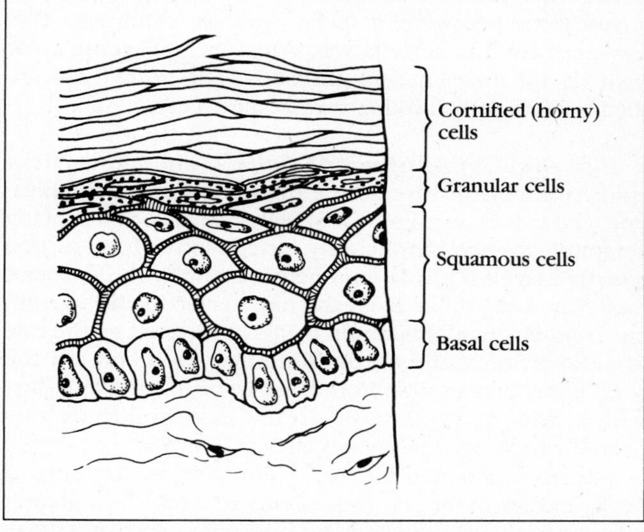

FIGURE 42-3 Life cycle of the epidermal cell.

Skin Pigmentation. The color of the skin is determined by melanocytes, which originate in the germinative layer of the epidermis and in hair follicles. The main function of melanocytes is to synthesize pigment granules, or melanosomes. The main component of melanosomes is melanin, which ranges in color from light yellow to black. The melanocytes are classified as connective tissue cells [6]. They appear in the basal layer of the epidermis as *clear cells* before they begin to produce melanin.

Melanocytes produce and disperse melanin to keratinocytes (keratinizing basal cells) and hair cells. Melanin is a biochrome of high molecular weight and is produced by oxidation of the amino acid tyrosine with tyrosinase. It forms with a protein matrix in the melanosome to make a melanoprotein. As more melanoprotein is formed, the melanosome grows to become a melanin granule and eventually loses the activity of the enzyme tyrosinase.

Formed melanin is transferred to keratinocytes by active phagocytosis of the distal end of the dendritic processes of the melanocyte. The amount of melanin in these melanocyte dendrites determines skin color (Fig. 42-4). In light-skinned individuals, melanin is present primarily in the basal layer of the epidermis. In dark- or black-skinned individuals, it is present throughout the epidermis, including the outermost horny layer. Melanogenesis increases after exposure to ultraviolet light or x-rays. After exposure, the melanocytes in the basal layer increase activity, become larger, develop longer dendrites, and produce more melanin. They may increase in number after exposure to ultraviolet light [5,6]. Melanin acts as a screen to protect the deep layers of the epidermis and the dermis from too much solar ultraviolet radiation [5].

Skin pigmentation is controlled by genes and hormones. Genes regulate the number and shape of melanocytes in the epidermis and hair follicles. Hormonal influences have been shown through the study of hyperpigmentation, as noted in hyperpituitarism and Addison's disease. Estrogen, progesterone, and melanocyte-stimulating hormone (MSH) contribute to increased pigmentation in various areas of the body during pregnancy. Apparently MSH does not play a major role in pigmentation in the human [4]. Excess amounts of MSH, however, produce a bronzed discoloration of the skin (see Chap. 31). The exact hormonal mechanism for increasing pigmentation is not known.

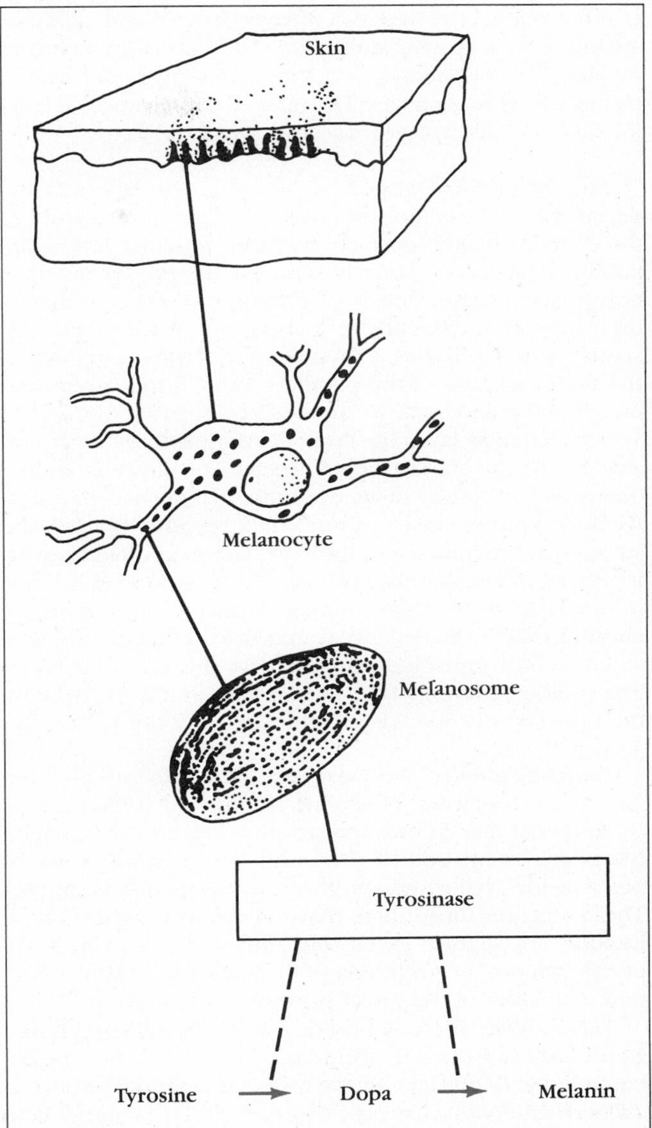

FIGURE 42-4 Melanogenesis in human skin as seen in the light and electron microscopes and at the molecular level. (From E. Braunwald, *Harrison's Principles of Internal Medicine* [11th ed.]. Copyright © 1987. McGraw-Hill Book Company. Reproduced with permission.)

Chemical Properties of the Epidermis. The epidermis contains carbohydrates and various enzymes that influence skin cell activity. In normal skin, small amounts of glycogen are present, scattered in various areas of the body, such as the scrotum and scalp, and in cells surrounding pilosebaceous and sweat gland openings. After the skin has been traumatized, the amount of glycogen in the epidermis increases.

The epidermis also contains glucose, which diffuses easily into the cells, the amount depending on the serum glucose levels. Eighty to 90 percent of the energy in epidermal cells is derived from adenosine triphosphate (ATP), which is generated through respiration and glycolysis. Intense glycolytic activity in the presence of oxygen is a specific feature of the epidermis that is especially important during wound healing and skin regeneration.

Enzymes in the epidermis that influence all activity include alkaline phosphatase, acid phosphatase, and esterases. Alkaline phosphatase is not present in normal epidermal cells but is present in a damaged epidermis and disappears after healing. Acid phosphatase is a component of the normal epidermis. Esterases seem to facilitate cell migration [4].

Dermis

The dermis, or *corium*, lies between the epidermis and subcutaneous tissues (see Fig. 42-1). It consists of a matrix of loose connective tissue, a fibrous protein embedded in an amorphous ground substance. The dermis is traversed by blood vessels, nerves, and lymphatics and is penetrated by epidermal appendages. The mass of the dermis accounts for 15 to 20 percent of total body weight [3].

Layers of the Dermis. The two main layers in the dermis are (1) the finely textured papillary dermis and (2) the deeper, thicker, coarsely textured reticular layer. The papillary layer lies directly beneath the epidermis. It is composed of thin fibers of collagen, reticular fibers, branching elastic fibers, fibroblasts, abundant ground substance, and capillaries. When the epidermis is removed, the upper surface of the papillary layer forms a negative image of the underside of the epidermis.

The reticular layer lies beneath the papillary layer and extends to the subcutaneous tissue. This layer is mainly composed of thick collagen bundles enmeshed in a network of coarse elastic fibers. It is responsible for the strength and toughness of the skin. There are fewer reticular fibers, blood vessels, fibroblasts, and ground substance in this layer than in the papillary layer [3]. Sensory nerve endings, hair follicles, sweat and sebaceous glands, and some smooth muscle are present in the reticular layer. The combined layers of the dermis vary in thickness, being thinnest over the eyelids and thickest over the back [3].

Components of the Dermis. The two layers of the dermis are composed of varying amounts of collagen, elastic and reticular fibers, and ground substance. Collagen fibers are composed of tropocollagen, a triple helix of polypeptide chains, which makes up most of the dermis. The molecules form fibers that unite into bundles. These bundles are slightly extensible and wavy, allowing for a certain amount of stretching of the skin. The collagen content is thickest in the lower portion of the dermis.

Elastic fibers are composed of microfibrils and elastin. The elastic fibers are abundant in human skin, being entwined with collagen in the reticular layer of the dermis and extending into the papillary dermis. These fibers help secure the epidermis to the dermis and, with arrectores pilorum muscles, anchor blood vessels. They can be deformed by small force and recover their original dimensions [4].

Reticular fibers are young, finely formed fibers of collagen. They are present within and under the epidermal basement membrane and also help to secure the epidermis to the dermis.

Ground substance is present in small amounts in normal skin. It is the structureless portion of connective tissue lying outside of cells, fibers, vessels, and nerves that holds all these components together. Ground substance consists of water, electrolytes, glucose, plasma proteins, neutral and acid mucopolysaccharides, and mucoproteins [4].

Cellular Components of the Dermis. The three major cells that are present in the dermis are (1) fibroblasts, (2) macrophages, and (3) mast cells. *Fibroblasts* are the most abundant of these cells; they secrete procollagen, proelastin, microfibrillar proteins, elastin, and components of ground substance [3]. *Macrophages* probably develop from the blood monocytes and can be fixed or ameboid cells that help rid the dermis of foreign substances and cell residue. Macrophages participate in the immune response and are vital to wound healing, inflammation, tissue resorption, and recycling of tissue components (see Chap. 9). *Mast cells* are present in perivascular connective tissue and their microscopic appearance shows the cytoplasm to be filled with large metachromatic granules. Under certain physical and chemical conditions, these cells degranulate. Such conditions include exposure to cold, heat, x-rays, ultraviolet light, toxins, certain peptides, and protamine sulfate. When degranulation occurs, the substances of heparin and histamine are released. Heparin prevents blood clotting and, in small amounts, accelerates lipid transportation. Histamine increases capillary permeability, contracts smooth muscle, increases chemotaxis, produces an itching sensation, and increases gastric secretion [4].

Functions of the Dermis. The dermis provides the main protection of the body from external injury. Its flexibility allows joint movement and localized stretching, but resists tearing, shearing, and local pressure. When skin is at rest, the protective collagen network is slack. When exposed to tension, the skin "gives" until the slack is taken up. Skin kept taut for long periods of time becomes fatigued, and stretching results. This is exhibited by the stretch marks or striae gravidarum (a pinkish-white or gray line seen where skin has been stretched by pregnancy, obesity, tumor, etc.), which are irreversible. The skin also becomes thinner when compressed under force and wells up around the surface of compression. Pressure damage may occur from long duration of pressure and distribution of force. Most damage is done as a result of long pressure, but severe point pressure can injure underlying and cutaneous tissues.

The dermis also provides the necessary substratum on which the epidermis receives nutrients and grows. It serves as a barrier to infection by way of hyaluronic acid in the ground substance, which prevents bacterial penetration [3]. Hyaluronic acid also binds water and helps maintain dermal turgor. The skin may also store water and electrolytes. Dermal concentrations of cations are slightly above those in blood, so that cations stored in the dermis may be tapped to maintain normal levels in blood.

Subcutaneous Tissues

The third major layer of skin is the subcutaneous tissue. It is loose-textured, white, and fibrous. Fat and slender elastic fibers are intermingled. Subcutaneous papillae jut into the dermis. These are larger and more dispersed than dermal papillae. It is through these that blood vessels and nerves enter the upper layers of skin.

The subcutaneous tissue layer contains blood and lymph vessels, roots of hair follicles, secretory portions of sweat glands, cutaneous and sensory nerve endings, and fat. Subcutaneous fat varies in amount throughout the body and is absent in the eyelids, penis, scrotum, nipples, and areolae. The unequal fat distribution between males and females is partially a result of hormonal influence. Strands or sheets of white, fibrous, connective tissue support the fat tissue.

The subcutaneous tissue contains voluntary and involuntary muscles. Voluntary muscle is present on the scalp, face, and neck. Involuntary smooth muscle is present in the dartos muscle of the scrotum and in the muscle tissue of the areolae and nipples. Subcutaneous tissue is a heat insulator, shock absorber, and calorie-reserve depot.

Epidermal Appendages

The sweat glands, sebaceous glands, hair, and nails compose the epidermal appendages. These extend through layers of the skin (Fig. 42-5).

Sweat Glands. There are two types of sweat glands: eccrine and apocrine. The *eccrine* sweat glands are present all over the body and are most numerous in thick skin. They open to the surface epidermis and descend through the dermis to just above the subcutaneous layer of the skin. These glands are especially prominent on the soles of the feet, palms of the hands, and axillae.

Eccrine glands are simple, coiled, tubular glands that may be divided into four segments. The lowermost, or secretory, portion has two layers of cells. Of these, myoepithelial cells make up the outer layer and contract to facilitate sweat release. The inner layer is composed of clear large cells and dark small cells, which contain glycogen and polysaccharides, respectively. The secretory layer is one cell layer thick. In ascending order, the remaining portion of the eccrine unit includes the coiled dermal duct and a straight dermal duct, which opens on the surface of the epidermis through the spiraled intraepidermal duct (see Fig. 42-5). The coiled and straight dermal ducts are two cell layers thick and are composed of cuboidal basophilic epithelium. The duct narrows as it ascends to the surface and widens again as it becomes the intraepidermal spiral duct. The cells lining the spiraling duct are keratinized but have no melanin [3,4].

Eccrine glands produce sweat to aid in regulating body temperature. Control of sweating is located in the hypothalamus (see following discussion), which responds to changes in body temperature [4]. Sweat is formed in the secretory coil of the eccrine unit. The solution here is isotonic or slightly hypertonic and contains lactate with small amounts of bicarbonate. In the dermal duct, sodium, chloride, and water are resorbed. As sweat exits onto the epidermis it is hypotonic. As the rate of sweating increases, sodium and chloride concentrations in the sweat also increase, whereas potassium, lactate, and urea concentrations decrease. Not all eccrine glands function all of the time, but they respond promptly to heat stress. The amount

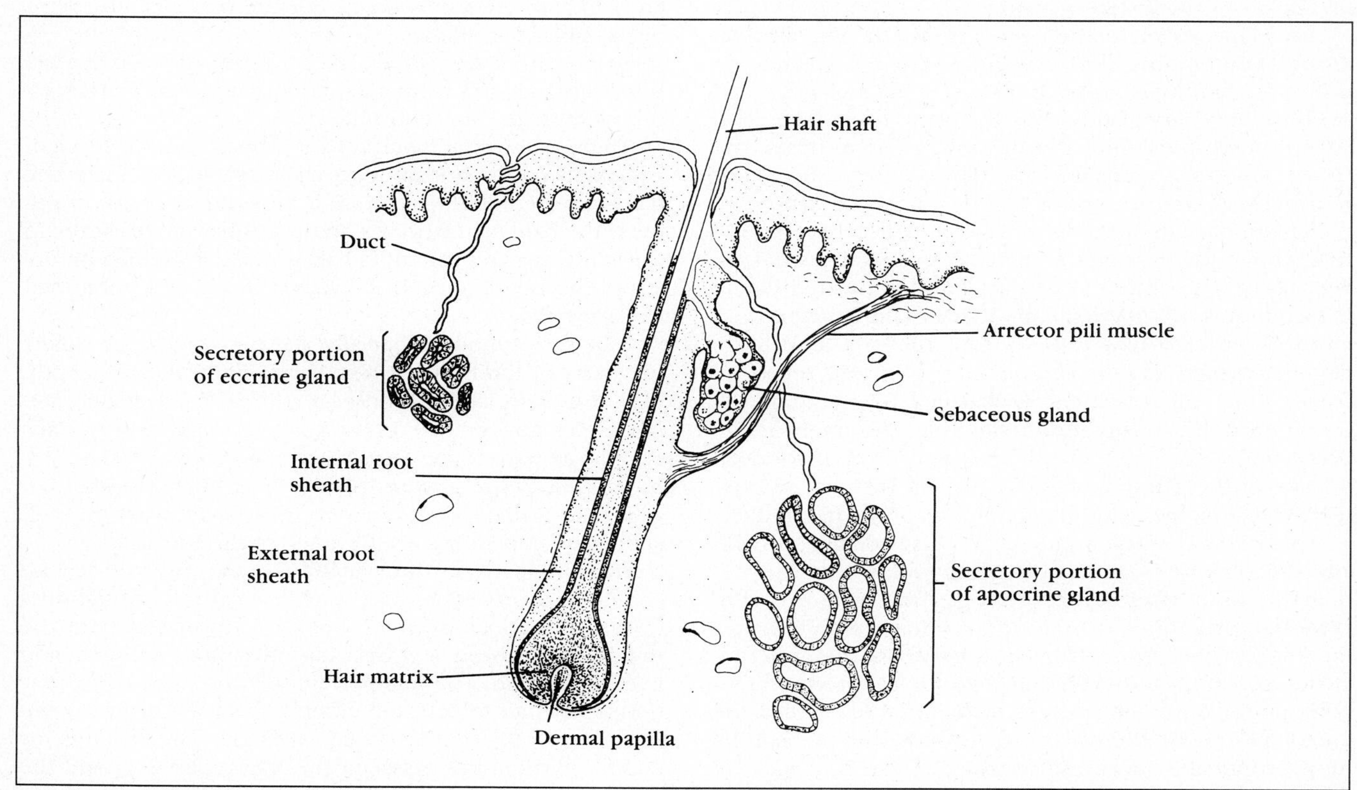

FIGURE 42-5 Some cutaneous appendages. (From M. Borysenko et al., *Functional Histology* [2nd ed.]. Boston: Little, Brown, 1984.)

of sweat produced depends on the amount of heat to which the person is exposed. Two to three liters of sweat per hour may be produced in an adult exposed to extreme heat conditions. Eccrine sweat is a colorless and odorless hypotonic solution that is 99 percent water and 1 percent solutes, such as sodium chloride, potassium, urea, protein, lipids, amino acids, calcium, phosphorus, and iron. The specific gravity is 1.005, and the pH ranges from 4.5 to 7.0.

The skin plays passive and active roles in controlling body temperature. Passively, skin is a barrier to the external environment. Actively, the eccrine units, together with the cutaneous blood vessel network, participate in regulatory heat exchange. The sweat glands cool the surface of the skin with the liquid sweat, which evaporates, causing further cooling. The cutaneous vessels dilate or constrict to dissipate or conserve body heat. The control of this process is in the hypothalamus, the neural thermostat.

The hypothalamus is stimulated by changes in surface and blood temperatures. An increase in body temperature of 0.5°C causes the hypothalamus to send a message by way of cholinergic fibers of the sympathetic nervous system to the sweat glands, which pour sweat onto the body surface, causing cooling when it evaporates [4].

Heat is the primary stimulus to eccrine sweat production, but other physiologic stimuli can stimulate sweating. Gustatory sweating occurs on the face and scalp after eating spicy foods. Emotional stress causes sweating on palms, soles, axillae, and forehead that may extend to the whole body. Pain, nausea, or vomiting also may cause localized or generalized sweating.

Apocrine sweat glands are present in the axillae, around the nipples, the anogenital region, external ear canals (ceruminous glands), eyelids (Moll's glands), and breasts (mammary glands). These glands make a secretion with an unknown function in humans. In animals, the secretion attracts animals of the opposite sex. The glands remain small until puberty, when they begin secreting [4].

Apocrine gland ducts empty into the pilosebaceous follicle above the entrance of sebaceous gland ducts (see Fig. 42-5). The coiled secretory gland is located in the lower dermis or subcutaneous tissues. The straight duct empties into the hair follicle. The apocrine coil has a larger diameter than the eccrine coil. The inner secretory layer of the coil is one cell layer thick. Surrounding the secretory cells are myoepithelial cells, basement membrane, and elastic and reticular fibers. The straight ductal portion of the gland has two cell layers with no myoepithelium and merges with the epithelium of the hair follicle.

Apocrine sweat has a milky color and contains protein and carbohydrates. In the duct, the sweat is sterile and odorless. Only after reaching the surface, where it contacts bacteria, does it take on an odor. Two steps are involved in the production of sweat from the apocrine glands, secretion and excretion. Sweat is secreted continuously and fills the duct before being excreted. When the duct is full, peristaltic waves produced by the myoepithelium propel the secretion outward. Excretion may be stimulated by emotional stress and hormones such as epinephrine.

Sebaceous Glands. Sebaceous glands arise as epithelial buds from the outer root sheath of the hair follicle. The glands are present throughout the body, except in the palms of the hands and soles and dorsa of the feet. Because these glands develop as buds from the root sheath, they are almost always associated with hair follicles, but are found in some hairless skin, such as that of the nipples, prepuce, labia, and glans penis. The size of sebaceous glands is inversely proportional with the diameter of hair in the follicles. They are largest where hair is sparse or absent, such as on the forehead, nose, chest, and back.

Several lobules compose the glands. The lobules are surrounded by a thin, vascular, fibrous, tissue capsule in the dermis. The cells next to the capsule provide the germinative layer and correspond to the germinative cells of the basal layer of epidermis (see Fig. 42-5). The germ cells change, taking up and filling with lipid, become bloated and disintegrate, and their contents of lipid and cell debris is discharged into the sebaceous duct as sebum. Other components of sebum include phospholipid, esterified cholesterol, triglycerides, and waxes. Sebum is then evacuated to the follicle and to the surface. Sebum is what produces oily skin; it lubricates the hair and skin and prevents drying. Sebaceous glands are holocrine glands, because they have no lumen and form secretions from decomposition of cells.

Hair. Human beings are covered with hair in all areas except the palms, soles, dorsum of digits, lips, glans penis, labia, and nipples.

Hair is needed to screen the nasal passages and protect the scalp and eyes from sun and sweat; it also provides a means of sexual attraction [8].

There are several types of hair. Primary hair, or *lanugo*, is present on the human fetus and infant. These same fine hairs may be noted on the adult as *vellus* hairs. An example is the bald man who has fine vellus hair on his scalp. In the adult, coarse pigmented hair is most developed on the scalp, the beard and chest areas in men, and pubic and axillary areas.

Hair varies morphologically and biologically on different parts of the body. It also varies in structure, length, rate of growth, and response to stimuli. For instance, sex hormones govern hair growth in the pubic and axillary regions as part of the secondary sex characteristics. Sex hormones do not govern other hair growth. Morphologically, hair is divided into four types: straight, wavy, helical, and spiral, depending on the angle of the hair follicles.

Hair originates in the hair follicle, and the two may be considered one structure, with the follicle developing from the fetal epidermis. The hair and follicle can be divided into three sections: infundibulum, isthmus, and inferior portion. The infundibulum is the uppermost portion of the hair follicle and extends from the orifice down to the opening of the sebaceous gland. The isthmus, or middle portion, lies between the sebaceous duct and the erector muscle. The inferior portion is the section from the muscle to the base of the follicle.

The hair bulb lies at the lower end of the follicle and encloses an ovoid, vascular papilla of connective tissue. The matrix cells of the bulb surround the papilla as it juts upward into the bulb (Fig. 42-6). At an outlet at the distal end of the bulb, the papilla emerges and is continuous with the connective tissue sheath that surrounds the follicle. The hair bulb is covered with concentric layers of tissue and enclosed by a thin outer root sheath. A basement membrane of reticular fibers and neutral mucopolysaccharides lies against the outer root sheath. A fibrous sheath lies next to the basement membrane and is composed of collagen and fibroblasts. Melanocytes are present in the bulb and in the outer root sheath. The color of hair depends on the amount and distribution of melanin within it.

The hair matrix cells differentiate into six layers. The single-cell outer layer cornifies first and lies next to the outer root sheath. Outer layers from the outside include a two-cell-thick layer of Huxley, cuticle of the inner root sheath, cuticle of the hair, hair cortex, and hair medulla [8].

The mitotic activity of the matrix cells is very great, with hair matrix being replaced every 12 to 24 hours. The hair and inner root sheath are joined, so that they grow at the same rate. When the hair and inner sheath reach the level of the isthmus, the inner sheath disintegrates and the outer sheath begins to cornify. As the hair reaches the surface opening of the follicle, it is called a hair shaft, and is a dead cornified structure extending out from the follicle. The hair shaft now has three components left over from

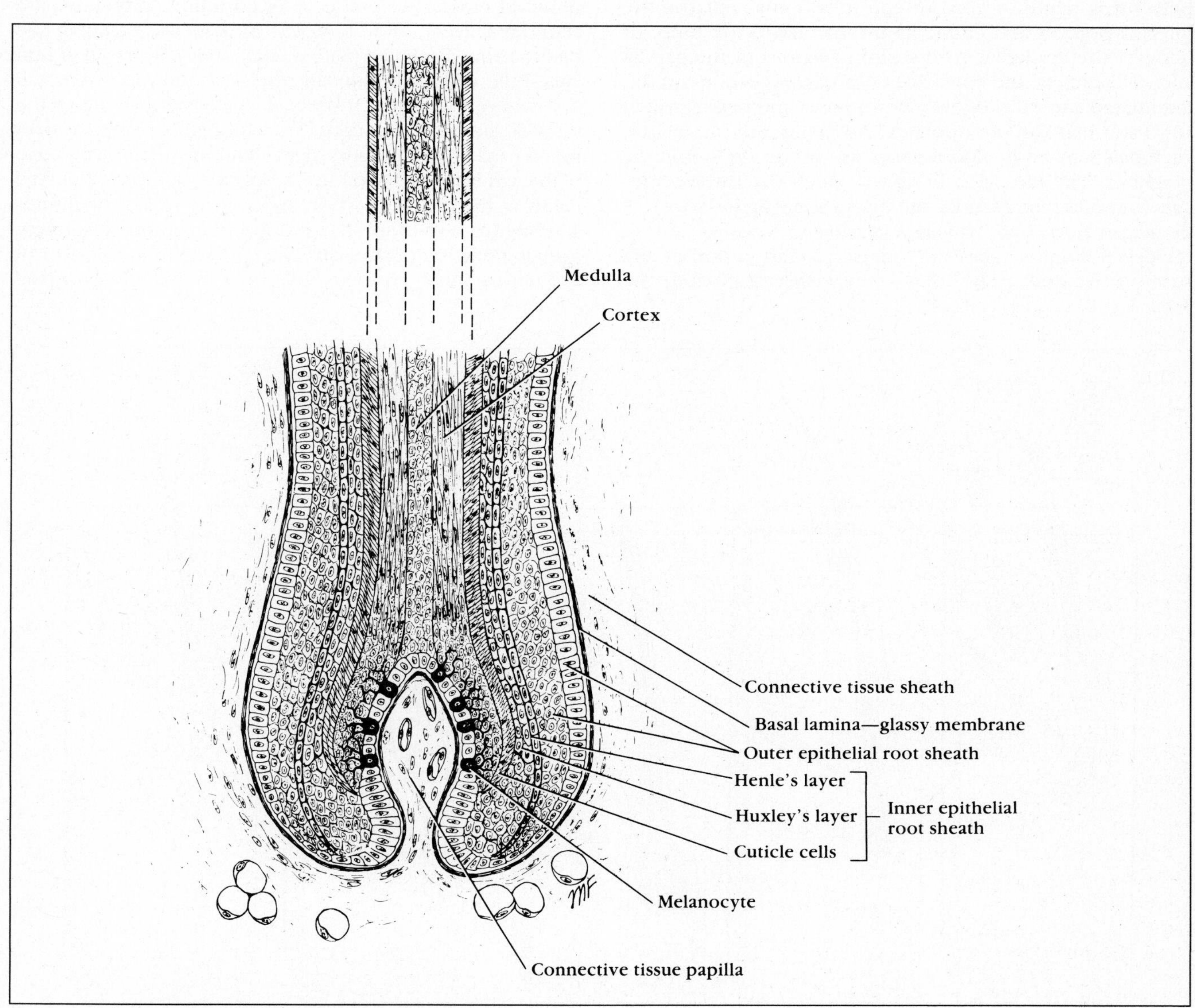

FIGURE 42-6 Detailed structure of a hair shaft and a hair follicle in longitudinal and cross sections. (From R.S. Snell, *Clinical Histology for Medical Students*. Boston: Little, Brown, 1984.)

the original six of the matrix: the outer cuticle, cortex, and inner medulla. The medulla is sometimes absent in human hair. The cortex is composed of tightly packed keratinocytes lying parallel along the length of hair. The cuticle surrounds the hair in overlapping squames.

The growth of hair occurs in cycles: *anagen*, growing; *catagen*, involuting; and *telogen*, resting (Fig. 42-7). Anagen begins when a papilla joins with cells that enclose it. The papilla juts into the hair bulb, and new matrix cells in the bulb begin to form a hair and push toward the surface. As it pushes to the surface, the old hair in the follicle is loosened, pushed out, and lost. At the end of anagen, the hair follicle contains the infundibulum, the isthmus, and the inferior portion. In catagen, the inferior portion disappears, the outer root sheath cornifies around the bulbous end of the hair shaft, melanin synthesis ceases, and the bulb turns white. A cord of epithelial cells replaces the inferior portion and connects the papilla to the bulb. In telogen, the epithelial cord shrinks away from the papilla and disconnects; the epithelial cells of the cord are undifferentiated and wait to join a new papilla and begin anagen [8]. Each hair follicle operates independently; therefore each hair may be in a different phase of the cycle from its neighbor. The life cycle of hair through the three stages varies in different parts of the body. Scalp hair—which is in anagen from 3 to 10 years, in catagen 3 weeks, and in telogen 3 months—has the longest growth period of any hair on the body. The longer the growing period, the longer the hair. Scalp hair grows 0.35 mm daily and is influenced by factors such as nutrition, light, hormones, and temperature [8]. The phases of the hair cycle may be influenced by illness, which may place growing-phase hairs into resting-phase hairs that can be more easily lost or shed.

Attached to the hair follicle is the arrectores pilorum, a smooth muscle attached to connective tissue hair sheath and inserted in the dermal papilla. Contraction of this muscle erects hair, squeezes out sebum, and creates goose flesh during the spasm.

Nails. The nails are composed of specialized layers of epithelial cells and are protective coverings at the ends of fingers and toes (Fig. 42-8). The rectangular nail plates on the dorsal surfaces of the ends of fingers and toes are composed of closely welded cells of cornified epithelium, are semitransparent, and allow the pink of the vascular nail bed to show. Each nail plate is surrounded by a fold of skin called the nail wall. The nail plate rests on top of the nail bed where fibers attach the nail to the periosteum of the distal phalanx of each digit. The nail bed is abundant with blood vessels and sensory nerve endings. The distal edge of the nail is freely movable. The proximal edge is attached firmly at the nail root. At the base of the nail is the lunula. This white half-moon-shaped area is the most actively growing portion of the nail. The epithelium in this area of the nail is thick, and the cells here become keratinized

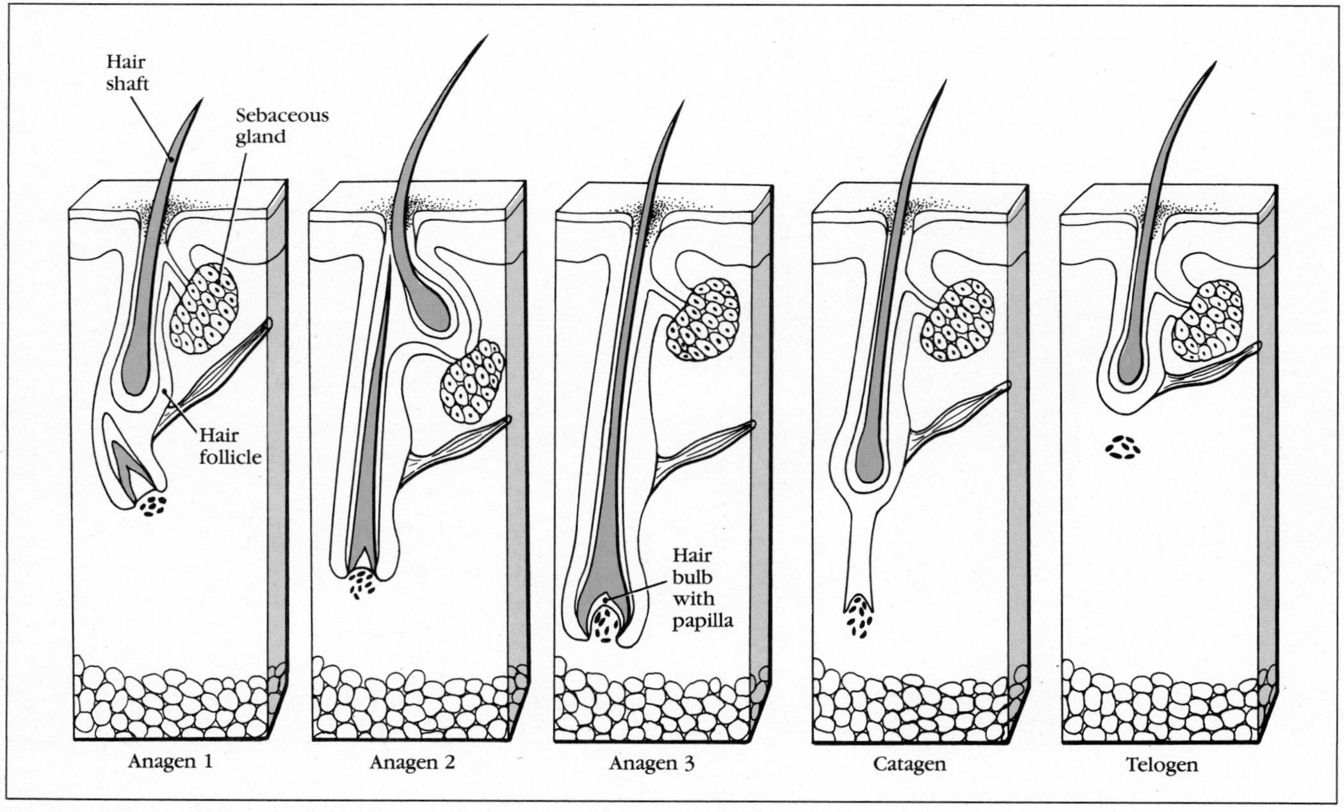

FIGURE 42-7 Growth cycle of hair.

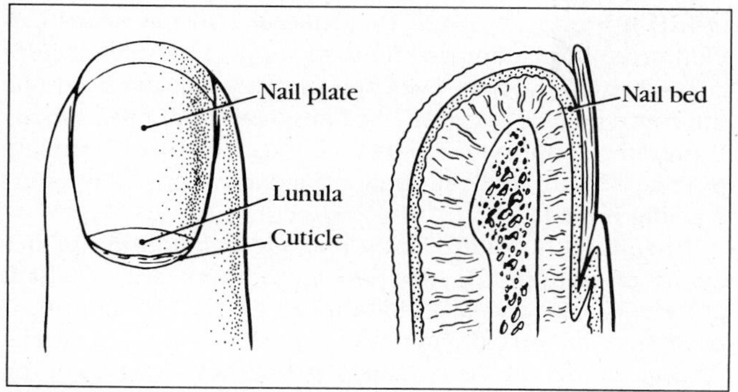

FIGURE 42-8 Structure of the nail in cross section of a finger.

with harder keratin than that present in the hair or the epidermis. From the lunula the nail grows longitudinally over dermal ridges of the nail bed at a rate of about 1 mm per week [7].

Blood Supply

Blood supply to the skin varies in different parts of the body, depending on factors such as the type of skin perfused, thickness of the skin's layers, and types and numbers of skin appendages. Common to skin throughout the body are deep subdermal arterial plexus and a superficial subpapillary plexus. The vascular structures arise from the mesenchyma. Endothelial cells line all parts of the vasculature. In the small capillaries, one endothelial cell surrounds the lumen. Collagen or reticular fibers ensheath the capillaries. Arterioles have an intima, a smooth muscle layer, and an adventitia of collagen and elastic fibers. Venules consist of epithelium and collagen. In larger veins, smooth muscle and elastic fibers are present.

The number of blood vessels is greater than necessary to meet the biologic needs of the skin tissues. The vessels have two functions: (1) to provide oxygen and nutrients to skin cells, together with moving wastes, and (2) to aid in thermal regulation.

The vessels are arranged in a three-dimensional network consisting of the two plexuses (deep and superficial) and the vessels that connect them (Fig. 42-9). The deep plexus is joined to larger vessels in the subcutaneous layer. The deep plexus lies in the lower portion of the dermis. The superficial plexus lies beneath the papillary dermis. A network of capillaries reaches up into the dermal papilla to nourish the upper layers of skin.

A second route of blood flow is through arteriovenous shunts located in the upper part of the reticular dermis (Fig. 42-10). These shunts, known as *glomi*, are important in regulating heat. They are present throughout the skin but are particularly prevalent in the pads and nail beds of fingers and toes, soles and palms, ears, and center of the face. The shunts enable blood to bypass the capillaries and increase blood flow. The plexuses and arteriovenous shunts are controlled by the sympathetic nervous system and respond to various chemical agents such as epinephrine and histamine.

Nervous Control

The skin is a major sensory organ. Dermal nerve endings receive stimuli from touch, pressure, temperature, pain,

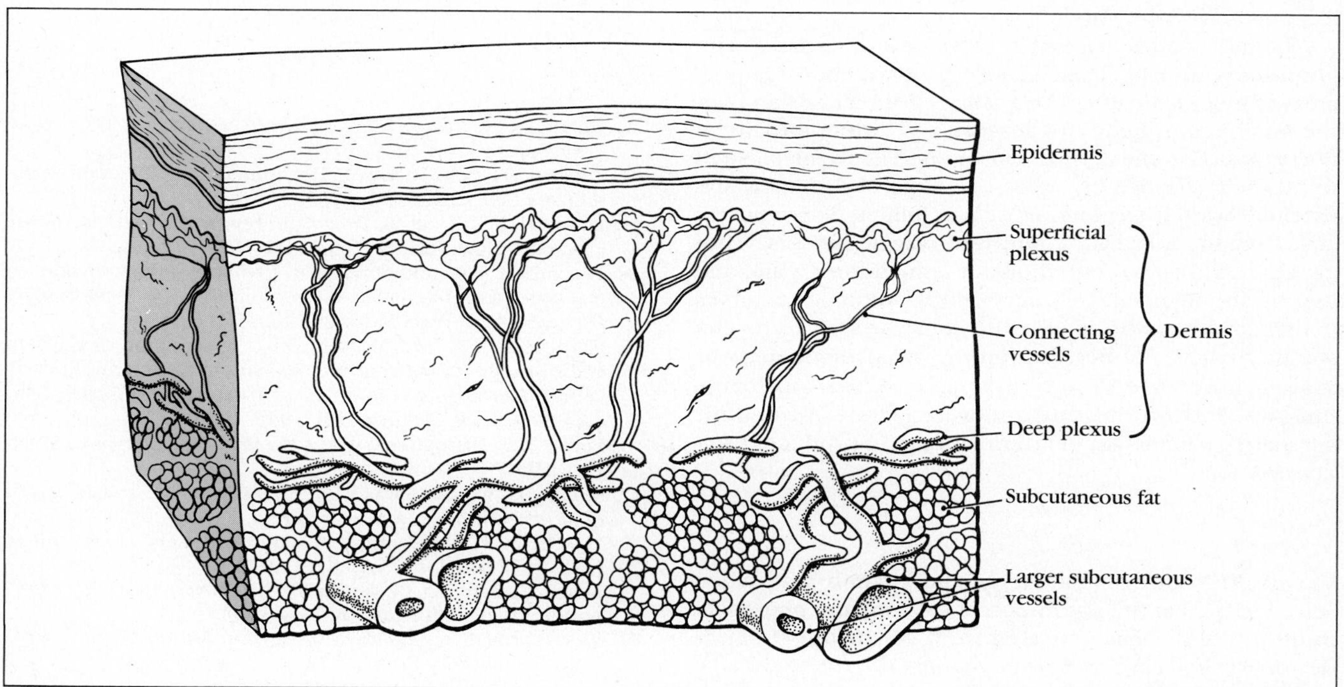

FIGURE 42-9 Blood vessels of the subcutaneous tissue.

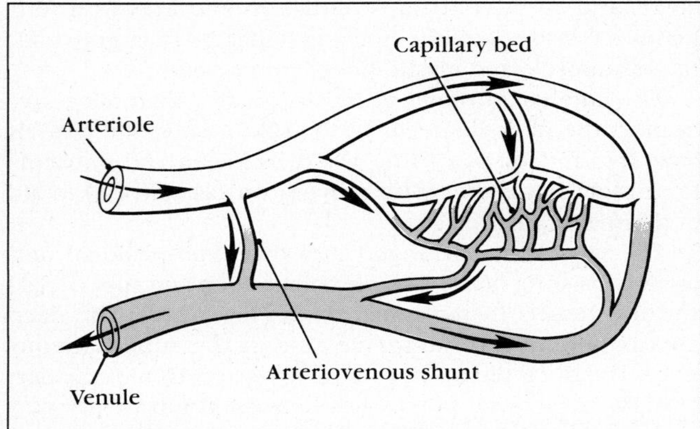

FIGURE 42-10 Blood flow through arteriovenous shunts.

and itch. Nerve endings are most numerous on palms, soles, fingers, and mucocutaneous areas of lips, glans penis, and clitoris.

Temperature, pain, and itch are perceived by unmyelinated nerves ending in the dermal papilla and surrounding hair follicles. Meissner's corpuscles receive touch stimuli. They lie in the papillary derma on the palms and soles and consist of myelinated and unmyelinated nerve fibers. Pacini's corpuscles sense pressure and are located on the soles, palms, nipples, and genital and perianal regions. These encapsulated end organs of myelinated and unmyelinated fibers swiftly send messages to the central nervous system. Mucocutaneous end organs are present in regions such as lips, tongue, gums, eyelids, genitalia, and perianal area. These organs probably perceive general sensory stimuli and are present in the subpapillary dermis. Myelinated nerves enter the end organ, lose their myelin, and form numerous networks.

The mucocutaneous end organs, Meissner's and Pacini corpuscles, are specialized sensory nerve end organs in areas of modified hairless skin. The remainder of skin over the body is supplied with sensory and autonomic nerve fibers located in the dermis. Sensory nerves are myelinated up to their terminal branches, are large in diameter, and extend toward the epidermis or hair follicle. These nerves arise from the spinal cord, return by way of the dorsal root ganglia, and receive sensations of temperature, pain, and itch on the unmyelinated nerve ends. Autonomic nerves to the skin are motor, and they do not always have a myelin sheath. Branches of nerves from the sympathetic nervous system innervate blood vessels, arrectores pilorum muscles, and eccrine and apocrine glands. Autonomic adrenergic stimulation of arteriolar muscle produces vasoconstriction.

Vitamin D Synthesis in the Skin

Vitamin D is an essential fat-soluble vitamin that, when activated, aids in the absorption of calcium and phosphate in the intestine. The activated form of vitamin D (1,25-dihydroxycholecalciferol) is commonly referred to as vitamin D hormone. Vitamin D hormone also mobilizes calcium from bone compartments to support plasma calcium concentration. Current evidence suggests that the hormone improves renal absorption of calcium but not of phosphate. It therefore improves mineralization of bone by increasing plasma calcium and phosphate concentrations to support forming bone [1].

Vitamin D hormone is not a single compound but is a family of compounds, the two most important of which are vitamin D_2 and D_3. Vitamin D_3, or cholecalciferol, is produced in the skin when it is exposed to ultraviolet irradiation. The skin cells contain 7-dehydrocholesterol in the epidermis. Ultraviolet light penetrates the epidermis and causes 7-dehydrocholesterol to undergo photolysis to form previtamin D, which over a period of a few hours isomerizes to form vitamin D_3. Vitamin D_3 is then transported in the blood bound to serum protein. It is converted in two steps to vitamin D hormone and may then be stored in the liver and in body fat [1]. Vitamin D_2, or ergocalciferol, is the therapeutic form of vitamin D and is transported to the liver and kidneys, where it is converted to vitamin D hormone [3] (see Chap. 41).

Study Questions

1. Explain the process of skin development from the dermis through the epidermis.
2. What are the functions of skin?
3. Discuss heat regulation by the skin.
4. How is melanin formed? How does it function to protect the skin?
5. How is hair formed? What factors determine its texture and color?

References

1. DeLuca, H.F. *Vitamin D: Metabolism and Function*. New York: Springer-Verlag, 1979.
2. Edelson, R.L., and Fink, J.M. The immunologic function of the skin. *Sci. Am.* 252(6):46, 1985.
3. Fitzpatrick, T.B., et al. *Dermatology in General Medicine* (3rd ed.). New York: McGraw-Hill, 1984.
4. Fitzpatrick, T.B., and Soter, N.A. Pathophysiology of skin. In N.A. Soter and H.R. Baden, *Pathophysiology of Dermatologic Diseases*. New York: McGraw-Hill, 1984.
5. Fitzpatrick, T.B., and Mosher, D.B. Pigmentation of the skin and disorders of melanin metabolism. In E. Braunwald et al. (eds.), *Harrison's Principles of Internal Medicine* (11th ed.). New York: McGraw-Hill, 1987.
6. Lever, W.F. *Histopathology of the Skin.* Philadelphia: Lippincott, 1967.
7. Montagna, W., and Parakhal, P.F. *The Structure and Function of Skin*. New York: Academic Press, 1974.
8. Moschella, S.L., Pillsbury, D.M., and Hurley, H.J. *Dermatology* (vol. 1). Philadelphia: Saunders, 1975.
9. Rosen, K., Lanning, M., and Hill, M. *The Nurse's Atlas of Dermatology*. Boston: Little, Brown, 1983.
10. Woodburne, R.T. *Essentials of Human Anatomy*. New York: Oxford University Press, 1978.

CHAPTER 43

Alterations in Skin Integrity

CHAPTER OUTLINE

Inflammation
- Skin Sensitivity
  - *Urticaria*
  - *Angioedema*

Common Inflammatory Diseases of the Skin
- Dry Skin
- Acne
- Hidradenitis Suppurativa
- Dermatitis/Eczema
  - *Contact Dermatitis*
  - *Atopic Dermatitis*
  - *Seborrheic Dermatitis*

Viral Infections of the Skin
- Herpes Simplex
- Varicella
- Herpes Zoster
- Warts (Verrucae)
- Rubeola (Measles)
- Rubella

Bacterial Infections of the Skin
- Impetigo
- Folliculitis
- Furuncles and Carbuncles

Fungal Diseases of the Skin

Scaling Disorders of the Skin
- Psoriasis
- Pityriasis Rosea

Skin Tumors
- Benign Tumors
  - *Seborrheic Keratosis*
  - *Hemangioma*
  - *Keratoacanthoma*
  - *Actinic Keratosis*
- Malignant Tumors
  - *Basal Cell Carcinoma*
  - *Squamous Cell Carcinoma*
  - *Malignant Melanoma*

Traumatic Alterations in the Skin
- Burns
  - *Partial-Thickness Burns*
  - *Full-Thickness Burns*
  - *Localized Changes Due to Burn Injury*
  - *Systemic Changes Due to Burn Injury*
  - *Electrical Burn Injuries*
  - *Chemical Burn Injuries*
- Decubitus Ulcers (Pressure Sores)
  - *Classification and Treatment of Decubitus Ulcers*
- Other Traumas

LEARNING OBJECTIVES

1. List the types of information on elicited when questioning the individual to obtain history of the skin.
2. Describe the pathophysiology of the inflammatory response.
3. State the two types of skin sensitivity responses.
4. Explain the pathophysiologic process that results in acne.
5. List and describe the three types of dermatitis/eczema disease.
6. List the complications of atopic dermatitis.
7. State the cause and precipitating factors of herpes simplex.
8. Describe the features and course of varicella virus disease.
9. Discuss the mechanism of activation of herpes zoster, its target population, and persons at greatest risk of infection.
10. Discuss the cause and treatment of warts (verrucae).
11. Describe the features of rubeola.
12. State the instance in which rubella has serious complications.
13. Review the common characteristics of impetigo.
14. List the common organism causing folliculitis.
15. Explain the use of systemic antibiotics in treatment of furuncles and carbuncles.
16. Give examples of fungal diseases of the skin.
17. List the predisposing factors for superficial fungus of the skin.
18. Compare the two examples of scaling disorders of the skin and their treatments.
19. State and discuss briefly the types of benign skin tumors.
20. List two premalignant skin lesions.
21. Differentiate the three types of malignant skin tumors.
22. Compare and contrast the differences between partial- and full-thickness burns.
23. Describe the changes that occur in the skin as a result of thermal injury.
24. Discuss the systemic changes that occur as a result of burn injury.
25. State the causes, types of injuries, and effects of electrical and chemical burns.
26. Discuss the critical factors in the formation of decubitus ulcers.
27. Describe the various stages of decubitus ulcer formation.
28. Discuss the skin changes resulting from abrasions, incisions, puncture wounds, and lacerations.

To understand the pathophysiology of the skin and its diseases, one must know the descriptive terms used to characterize skin lesions and comprehend the inflammatory processes that herald the diseases. A systematic approach to the lesions prepares one to assess the extent of disease.

The approach to identifying skin lesions begins with a simple but specific investigative process. To obtain a history, the individual is questioned with regard to the following: (1) characteristics of the lesion, (2) distribution of many lesions, (3) length of time present and recurrence, (4) medications taken, both systemic and topical, (5) family history of disease, and (6) environmental or personal exposure to hazardous material. Once the history is obtained, the lesion is assessed. Visible body areas must be inspected, together with areas frequently overlooked, such as skin folds, scalp, hands, and feet.

Table 43-1 lists the basic nomenclature used to describe lesions. Figure 43-1 shows the appearance of various lesions. Description of a lesion may require a combination of these terms.

Inflammation

The body's response to injury is to generate inflammation. Sources of injury to the skin include bacteria, viruses, temperature extremes, and chemical or mechanical irritants.

Inflammation causes alterations in the surrounding blood vessels and adjacent tissues. Redness or erythema is the hallmark of inflammation. An irritant causes injury to the site, which results in a vascular reaction with fluid exudation, and edema. Pressure from the edema or chemical irritation from the release of various mediator substances causes pain due to irritation of the nerve fibers in that area. The duration of the inflammatory response varies.

Skin Sensitivity

Urticaria and angioedema can be classified as diseases or as reactions to injury or an allergen.

Urticaria. This vascular reaction, commonly called hives, is manifested by transient erythema or whitish swellings (wheals) of the skin or mucous membranes [1]. Skin changes or lesions are the result of increased vascular permeability and local release of histamine or other vasoactive substances [16]. These may result in localized edema. Edema may begin to resolve within several hours. These lesions often cause pruritus and a stinging sensation. *Acute urticaria* can be defined as a cutaneous vascular reaction that evolves over a short period, from days to several weeks, and usually has a detectable cause. It resolves completely. Urticaria lasting longer than six weeks is clas-

TABLE 43-1 Skin Lesions

Lesion	Description
Primary lesions	
Macula	Flat (nonelevated) discoloration of the skin, less than 5 mm in diameter.
Patch	Similar to a macula, but more than 5 mm in diameter.
Papule	Solid, circumscribed, elevated lesion, less than 5 mm in diameter; often caused by accumulation of inflammatory cells, proliferation of neoplastic cells, or deposit of metabolic by-products.
Nodule	Similar to a papule, but 5 mm to 5 cm in diameter.
Tumor	Solid mass, more than 5 cm in diameter, usually extends deeper into the skin.
Plaque	A flattened, raised lesion with more lateral dimension (surface area) greater than height (elevation above the skin); sometimes the result of clustering of papules; has the feel of a thickened area of skin.
Vesicle	Small, circumscribed, elevated lesion containing fluid; diameter less than 5 mm.
Bulla	Larger version of a vesicle, more than 5 mm in diameter; alternatively called a blister.
Pustule	Yellow-white vesicle filled with pus.
Cyst	Semisolid or fluid-filled mass surrounded by a capsule; usually located in the deeper portions of the skin.
Wheal	Transient, round, irregularly shaped, faint pink elevation; caused by edema fluid in the dermis.
Comedo	Plugged, dilated pore, often called blackhead or whitehead.
Hemorrhagic flat lesions	
Petechia	Hemorrhagic macula less than 5 mm.
Purpura	Hemorrhagic patch 5 mm to 5 cm.
Ecchymosis	Large hemorrhagic mark; black-and-blue spot.
Secondary lesions	
Scale	Excessive accumulation of loosely adherent keratin; usually seen in papules and plaques.
Erosion	Superficial loss of epidermis; not associated with scarring; often accompanies vesicles, bullae, or pustules.
Excoriation	Linear erosion caused by scratching.
Ulcer	Deep erosion resulting from loss of epidermis and part of dermis; often heals with a scar.
Crust	Accumulation of dried sebum, serum, cellular and bacterial debris over a damaged epidermis; often overlies erosion and is seen in vesicles, bullae, and pustules.
Lichenification	Thickened skin with accentuated markings; caused by chronic rubbing and scratching.
Fissure	Crack in the epidermis.
Atrophy	Thinning of the skin at site of disorder; appreciated best by palpation.

Source: T. Rosen, M. Lanning, and M. Hill, *The Nurse's Atlas of Dermatology*. Boston: Little, Brown, 1983.

sified as *chronic urticaria*. It may persist for years; it also may go away and then recur. The underlying cause is usually unknown.

The etiologies of urticaria are numerous and can include such components as foods, inhalants, drugs, injectants (e.g., blood, vaccines), chemicals, mechanical and environmental irritants, and psychogenic factors.

Treatment involves removing the causative agent. Antihistamines are often used. Alleviating irritation factors, instituting elimination diets, and preventing and treating dry skin may be of benefit.

Angioedema. Angioedema is a reaction that involves edema not only of the superficial skin but of the subcutaneous tissues. The differences between urticaria and angioedema are degree and location. Angioedema can be described as giant wheals, often involving the mucous membranes. It can cause many physical symptoms including severe respiratory distress, especially when it affects the larynx; this complication constitutes a medical emergency.

Common Inflammatory Diseases of the Skin

Dry Skin

Dry skin in itself is a noninflammatory condition, but it can become reddened at a late stage. It is extremely common and consists of roughened, flaky skin with or without pruritus [3].

The defect, which occurs commonly in the aging process, involves loss of water, electrolytes, and skin lipids. It is frequent in dry and/or cold climates, and environmental conditions aggravate the condition if it previously existed. Dehydration after sweating dries out the surface keratin, and itching and inflammatory changes can be superimposed [3]. Treatment of dry skin involves rehydration with a moisturizer and water, together with barrier creams used consistently.

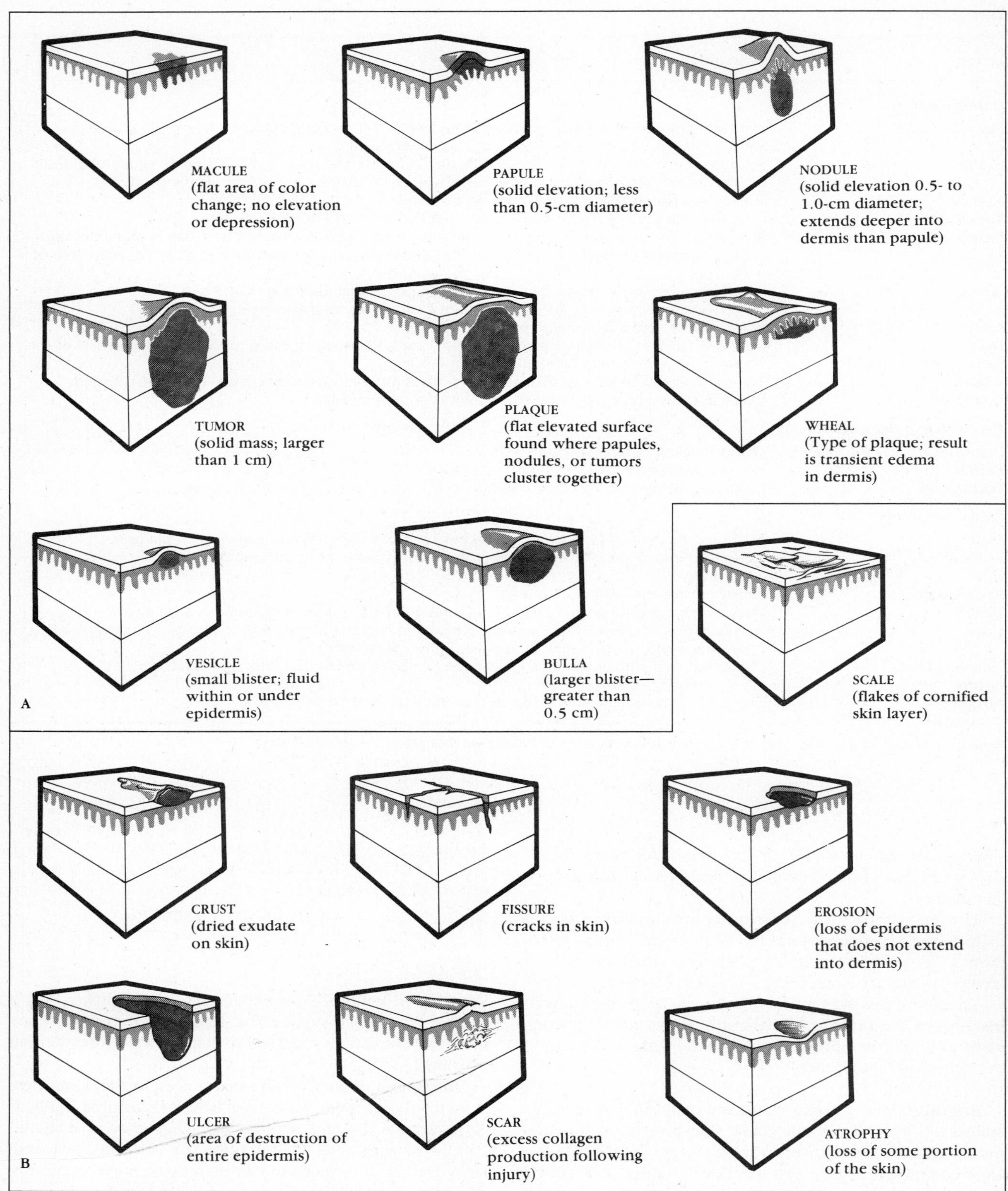

FIGURE 43-1 A. Primary skin lesions and their characteristics. B. Secondary skin lesions and their characteristics. (From J. Sana and R. Judge, *Physical Assessment Skills for Nursing Practice* [2nd ed.]. Boston: Little, Brown, 1982.)

Acne

Acne vulgaris is a common, chronic, inflammatory disease of the sebaceous glands and hair follicles of the skin, also known as the pilosebaceous ducts (Fig. 43-2). Its occurrence is based on two factors: (1) accumulation of sebum, which is the fatty secretion liberated by the breakdown of sebaceous cells, and (2) irritation of the area around the hair follicle, leading to a perifolliculitis.

The exact etiology of acne is unknown, but it may be due to either increased activity of the sebaceous glands or inability of the material secreted to escape through a narrow opening. The resulting inflammation is precipitated by the combination of sebum, bacteria, and subsequent release of fatty acids. The last is caused by the hydrolytic action of the lipases, which are furnished by the bacteria on the sebum itself. The inflammatory reaction, with resulting edema, probably causes the sebaceous follicle to perforate its wall and develop perifolliculitis.

The development of acne is dependent on several factors: heredity, use of oil-based cosmetics or skin treatments, ingestion of drugs (e.g., steroids, androgens), and the presence of bacteria. Sebaceous glands are hormonally controlled, and the androgenic hormones may increase the development and secretion of sebaceous glands.

The lesions are located in the areas of predominant pilosebaceous glands—face, chest, back, neck, and upper arms.

The early noninflammatory lesions are of two types, white (closed) and black comedones. The white comedo occurs in a closed excretory duct that has a very small, possibly microscopic, opening that prevents drainage. This lesion may lead to an inflammatory process and give rise to a papule or pustule. The black comedo (blackhead) is a widely dilated follicle filled with discolored, horny material that plugs an excretory duct of the skin. Both types of lesions obstruct the emptying of sebum to the surface, and may develop into small papules, pustules, nodules, or cysts. With time, most pustules and cysts open, drain, and heal. If severe, these lesions may result in scarring. The prevalence of acne is increased during adolescence and early adulthood, but it is usually self-limited. The central theme of medical treatment involves reducing the inflammation of the pilosebaceous glands by fostering their free drainage, avoiding rupture, and limiting bacterial growth.

Hidradenitis Suppurativa

Although not a common disease, hidradenitis suppurativa is a severe, chronic inflammation of the apocrine glands. It usually affects the axillae, but can occur in the anogenital area. It begins as a reddened, tender subcutaneous nodule. The lesion may suppurate and drain or resolve spontaneously. If the condition recurs, sinuses can develop that can result in extensive scarring.

Treatment ranges from topical antibiotics for mild cases to systemic antibiotics for more advanced lesions. Surgical incision and drainage may be required for acutely inflamed nodules.

Dermatitis/Eczema

Dermatitis and eczema are words that are used interchangeably. They constitute the superficial inflammatory diseases of the skin. Morphologically, the changes of acute and chronic dermatitis are specific and recognizable.

Contact Dermatitis. This classification includes inflammations that are the result of contact with external agents, either chemical allergens or mechanical irritants.

The lesion begins in the area of contact. Its shape stimulates the area of local exposure (Fig. 43-3). The irritant removes some of the protective mechanisms of the skin, such as lipids and other hydrophilic material, and causes varying degrees of dryness. When contact is with strong compounds or is prolonged, lesions may evolve. If exposure is continued, acute dermatitis can progress to the chronic form. In most circumstances, complete tissue repair is possible if the irritant is removed and permanent changes in the skin have not taken place.

Contact dermatitis can be subdivided into two types: primary irritant and allergic.

Primary irritant contact dermatitis causes a nonallergic skin reaction. Repeated or extended contact by a mild irritant such as detergent is necessary to cause skin dam-

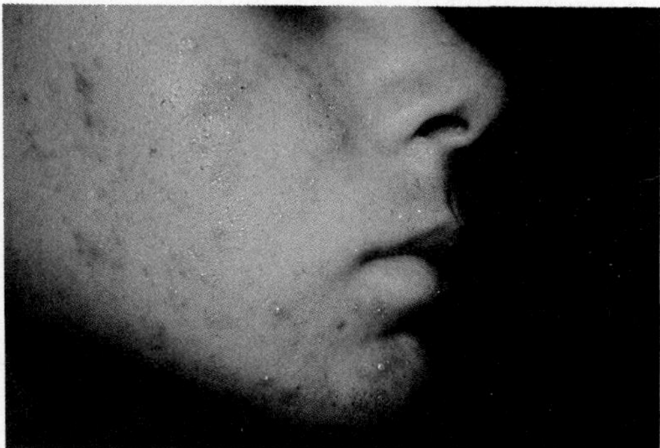

FIGURE 43-2 Acne: papules, pustules, and scarring. (From K. Arndt, *Manual of Dermatologic Therapeutics* [3rd ed.]. Boston: Little, Brown, 1983.)

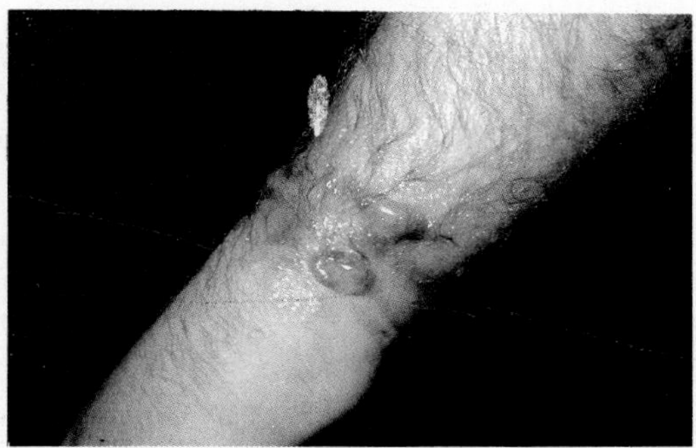

FIGURE 43-3 Contact dermatitis from leather watchband. (From K. Arndt, *Manual of Dermatologic Therapeutics* [3rd ed.]. Boston: Little, Brown, 1983.)

age. Strong irritants cause immediate damage on initial contact.

Mechanical irritation is due to inflammation from mechanical factors such as large-size particles of certain materials that cause pruritus. One example is wool, resulting in dermatitis that is due to the mechanical scratchiness of the irritant itself, not the mediation of a chemical substance.

The frequency of chemically caused contact dermatitis has increased. A basic substance, such as water, can indirectly be a chemical irritant through prolonged exposure and removal of the skin's protective barriers. Soaps and detergents increase the drying and facilitate the irritating action of water. Other chemicals and medications may cause an irritant dermatitis. Various biologic irritants, including human excrement, saliva, and tears, result in dermatitis after prolonged contact. Biologic irritants can also cause a predisposition to the development of yeast and bacterial infections, compounding the problem.

Allergic contact dermatitis is a delayed-hypersensitivity dermatitis. It results from exposure of a previously sensitized individual to contact allergens. Some of the causes include poison ivy antigens, many industrial chemicals, some drugs, and some metals.

Removal of the sensitizer is necessary for treatment. The causative agent can be identified by a history, patch testing, or a use test. Unless the condition is severe, medical treatment includes soaks and corticosteroid creams. When dermatitis becomes severe and frequent, systemic steroids may be required.

Atopic Dermatitis. This is a highly specific disease that results from a genetically determined lowered threshold to pruritus and is characterized by intense itching [1]. It may appear as a small papule, but there is evidence that scratching is the major factor producing the lesion. The intense scratching leads to erythema, weeping, scaling, and lichenification. The histology is that of a nonspecific dermatitis. The dermatitis occurs in areas of flexion and extension, such as the popliteal spaces, antecubital fossae, and neck area. The list of exacerbating factors includes sudden changes in weather, psychologic stress, contact with wool or furs, and primary irritant chemicals.

Many complications can develop with atopic dermatitis, including an increase in the severity of viral infections. Affected persons should not be vaccinated against smallpox, as disseminated vaccinia can develop and cause a generalized infection of the skin. These persons are also prone to bacterial and fungal infections, ocular complications, and allergic contact dermatitis.

Treatment involves palliation by reducing or controlling precipitating events and providing symptomatic relief of pruritus. Topical agents afford some relief. The prognosis is difficult to determine, but studies have demonstrated that the duration of disease is long, although the frequency of attacks is less after adolescence.

Seborrheic Dermatitis. This inflammatory, erythematous, and scaling disease predominates in areas of the body that have numerous seborrheic glands. Often it is compared to dandruff, which is the noninflammatory counterpart, or mild form. It occurs as an accelerated epidermal, immature growth. This entity involves not only the scalp, but the eyebrows, portions of the forehead, bridge of nose, and trunk. Treatment includes antiseborrheic shampoos and topical agents.

Viral Infections of the Skin

Herpes Simplex

Categorized as a virus, herpes simplex is also known as a fever blister or "cold sore." It is caused by type I herpes simplex virus. Initially, it is an acute condition with groups of vesicles on an erythematous base, which later become purulent and crusting. Distribution may occur to any area of the body, but the most frequently affected are the lips and perioral and genital areas; the lesions may be painful and pruritic (Fig. 43-4). They resolve usually within two weeks.

It is believed that first exposure to infection occurs by the fifth year of life, but is not often observed. Nevertheless, the person has developed antibodies to the virus. A small percentage of children have primary gingivostomatitis or vulvovaginitis as a result. Recurrence throughout life may result from either reactivation of the virus or reinoculation, and may be precipitated by stress-producing factors such as fever, excessive sun exposure, common cold, illness, and injury.

Herpes progenitalis has become a frequent infection of the genital area and is believed to be caused by the type II herpes virus. Studies are currently investigating a relationship of this virus to cervical cancer.

Because no cure has been discovered, treatment of herpes simplex is basically symptomatic relief. Acyclovir (Zovirax) has been shown to be effective in shortening the duration of episodes; it may possibly decrease the number of recurrences, but the drug is too new for its long-term effects to be known. Prevention can only be aimed at avoiding the identified precipitating factors.

Varicella

Otherwise known as chickenpox, varicella is caused by the herpes zoster virus. An airborne, highly contagious virus in the prodromal and vesicular stages, it affects children more frequently than adults.

The varicella has an incubation period of 10 to 20 days. The prodromal stage often begins with moderate fever and malaise. Pink papules 2 to 4 mm in size are surrounded by a reddened halo (dew drop on a rose petal) that later dries and crusts. Lesions usually occur in groups; their distribution on the face, scalp, trunk, and arms is common. Generalized symptoms of headache, moderate fever, anorexia, and malaise may continue after the lesions erupt. Varicella in adults is much more severe than in children.

The usual treatment for varicella in children is aimed at keeping the skin lesions dry and relieving pruritus with lotion as necessary.

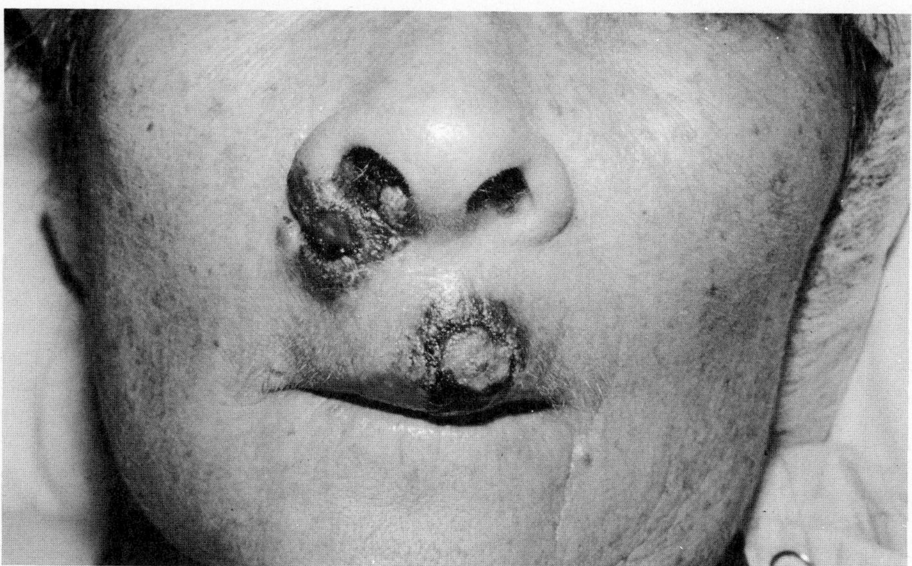

FIGURE 43-4 Lesions caused by the herpes simplex virus. (From K. Rosen, M. Lanning, and M. Hill, *The Nurse's Atlas of Dermatology*. Boston: Little, Brown, 1983.)

Herpes Zoster

Herpes zoster is also produced by a varicella virus and it is often referred to as shingles. This acute inflammatory disease occurs when the dormant varicella virus is activated. It is most frequent in the elderly population, but it can occur in any age group. In the older person, pain usually precedes the lesion by one to two days.

The initial features are erythema and discomfort, followed in one to seven days by grouped vesicles along a unilateral dermatome (Fig. 43-5). These vesicles later crust and clear in approximately two and one-half weeks.

Severe pain can result, and persistence is a feared complication. Although uncommon, generalized herpes zoster can result, a condition usually associated with a systemic malignancy of the lymphoma group [16]. A susceptible individual may develop chickenpox after exposure to this varicella virus.

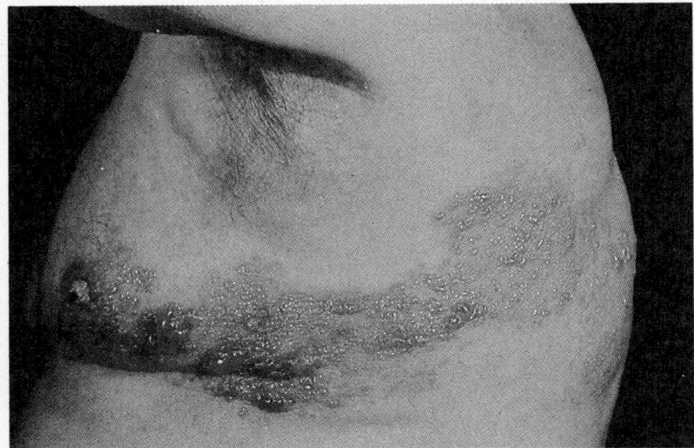

FIGURE 43-5 Herpes zoster. (From K. Arndt, *Manual of Dermatologic Therapeutics* [3rd ed.]. Boston: Little, Brown, 1983.)

Warts (Verrucae)

Verrucae, or warts, are viral infections of the skin. There are three main types: verruca vulgaris (common wart), verruca plantaris (plantar wart), and condyloma acuminatum (venereal wart). It is believed that these are variations of the same virus.

The etiology of warts is not clearly understood, but they can be transmitted by contact from person to person. They are benign lesions and frequently occur at sites of injury or along a break in the skin.

Verruca vulgaris is a raised, well-circumscribed growth with an irregular gray surface, frequently present on the hands. Although treatment is often unsatisfactory, surgical removal, electrosurgery, and cryosurgery have been used. Many warts resolve without treatment.

Verruca plantaris differs from the common wart by its location and the effect that pressure has on the lesion. The wart tends to grow on the soles of the feet, and pain is frequent due to the irritation of walking. As a result, the wart tends to grow inward.

Condylomata acuminata are lesions established primarily in warm, moist anogenital areas. Although known as venereal warts, they do not necessarily stem from sexual contact. They are large, pinkish or purplish projections with a rough surface.

Rubeola (Measles)

Rubeola is a highly contagious infection caused by a myxovirus. The incubation period is approximately 10 to 14 days. Its course usually begins with fever and symptoms of upper respiratory infection that occur six to seven days after inoculation and last 24 hours. The disease then enters what is known as the invasion phase, with development of high fever, chills, malaise, headache, photophobia, and dry cough. These symptoms last for four to seven days. Lesions begin as inflammation or petechiae of the soft palate, followed by Koplik's spots, which are blue-white spots surrounded by a bright halo over the buccal mucosa. A macular eruption appears on the face, upper extremities, and trunk.

Rubella

Also known as German measles, this common, acute, infectious disease is caused by a myxovirus. The incubation period ranges from 12 to 25 days and begins with malaise and mild fever approximately 4 to 5 days before lesions appear. Lesions are small, irregular, pink macules and papules that appear initially on the face, spreading to the entire body. They fade rapidly within two to three days. Adenopathy of the superficial cervical and posterior auricular glands is common.

Rubella is serious in pregnant women, especially in the first trimester, when transmission to a fetus results in fetal anomalies. A titer is available to assess immunity. Vaccination is given to school-aged children and, with caution, to women of child-bearing age with low rubella titers.

Bacterial Infections of the Skin

Impetigo

Impetigo is an acute bacterial infection that occurs superficially on the skin as serous and purulent vesicles that later rupture and form a golden crust (Fig. 43-6). It frequently occurs in children, but persons in ill health are also predisposed to it. A common location for lesions is the face, but they may involve the extremities.

Causative organisms include β-hemolytic streptococci and coagulase-positive staphylococci. Impetigo is autoinoculous and can be transmitted among humans. Influencing factors include poor hygiene, tropical climates, and improper sanitation. A serious complication is glomerulonephritis, which may not be prevented by antibiotic treatment.

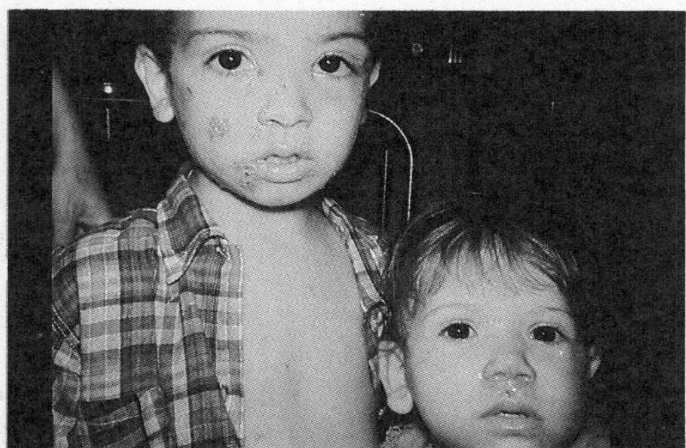

FIGURE 43-6 Impetigo. (From K. Arndt, *Manual of Dermatologic Therapeutics* [3rd ed.]. Boston: Little, Brown, 1983.)

Folliculitis

This bacterial infection of the skin originates within the hair follicle. Staphylococci are the usual causative organisms. Folliculitis appears as a pustule located at the opening of the hair follicle, predominantly on the scalp and extremities. The basic lesion is a reddened macule or papule surrounding the hair follicle. Predisposing factors include poor hygiene and maceration. Folliculitis can extend into the deeper skin layers if not treated promptly, and systemic antibiotics may be necessary.

Furuncles and Carbuncles

Furuncles, also known as boils, frequently develop from a preceding staphylococcal folliculitis and are usually located in body areas containing hair follicles. Irritation, maceration, and lack of good hygiene are predisposing factors in their development. The lesions are nodules that are usually tender and red. They frequently remain tense for two to four days, become fluctuant, and later drain purulent material [1].

Carbuncles are larger staphylococcal abscesses that drain through various points. Some cases of furuncles and almost every case of carbuncles requires systemic antibiotic therapy.

Fungal Diseases of the Skin

Fungal diseases of the skin can be classified into three groups: superficial, intermediate, and deep. Some are *opportunistic* and affect a susceptible host while some are truly *pathogenic* and can infect a healthy person [16]. The superficial diseases result in what is commonly known as ringworm (tinea capitis), athlete's foot (tinea pedis), "jock itch" (tinea cruris), and tinea versicolor. These fungal diseases are primarily caused by dermatophytes that invade the superficial layers of the epidermis, hair, and nails. They are characterized by areas of scaling and erythema, and frequently exhibit vesicles and fissures [20]. Moisture, heat, and maceration are predisposing factors for growth; consequently, lesions appear in areas between toes, the axillae, nails, and groin. Treatment involves local therapy. With certain resistant fungi, griseofulvin, a fungicidal and fungostatic antibiotic, is used.

Intermediate fungal diseases invade both the superficial and deeper tissues. Moniliasis caused by *Candida albicans* is an example. This organism can also produce deep invasion when the host's resistance declines [16].

Deep fungal infections invade deeper structures of living tissue and include diseases such as sporotrichosis, candidiasis, histoplasmosis, and aspergillosis (see Chap. 8). A much higher incidence of opportunistic deep fungal infections is being seen because of medical progress with the use of immunosuppressive drugs and invasive procedures [16].

Scaling Disorders of the Skin

Psoriasis

Psoriasis is a chronic, genetically determined disease of epidermal proliferation (Fig. 43-7). The increased cell turnover rate and production of immature cells result in the classic features of sharply defined erythematous plaques covered by silvery white, loosely adherent scales.

The precise etiology is not known, but genetic and environmental factors are of significance in its development. It is viewed as a chronic disease with much diversity in its location, severity, and frequency. Exacerbating factors include local trauma, overexposure to the sun, infection, stress, and physical illness [18].

It can occur in all ages and is often distributed over the knees, elbows, scalp, and lumbosacral skin. When involved, the nails show pitting and dimpling. Psoriasis may be associated with arthritis. A serious but rare condition known as pustular psoriasis also can occur, which causes high fever, elevated white blood cell count, electrolyte imbalance, and malaise. This condition can be fatal [21].

Psoriasis usually can be controlled, and remission is possible. Avoiding local skin injury, infection, and stress, maintaining good nutrition, and avoiding excessive weight gain improve the control of this disease.

Pityriasis Rosea

This is a common, acute disease of the skin, usually affecting the adolescent and young adult. Its course is self-limited and it is thought to be infectious, possibly caused by a virus.

Clinical manifestations often arise after a prodrome of malaise, fatigue, and headache. The first lesion, known as the herald patch, is a single, oval, ringlike plaque that is later followed by lesions that are usually flat, erythematous patches covered by a fine scale; they resemble the primary plaque, but are smaller (Fig. 43-8). Lesions are often pruritic. Distribution is most frequently on the neck, trunk, and arms.

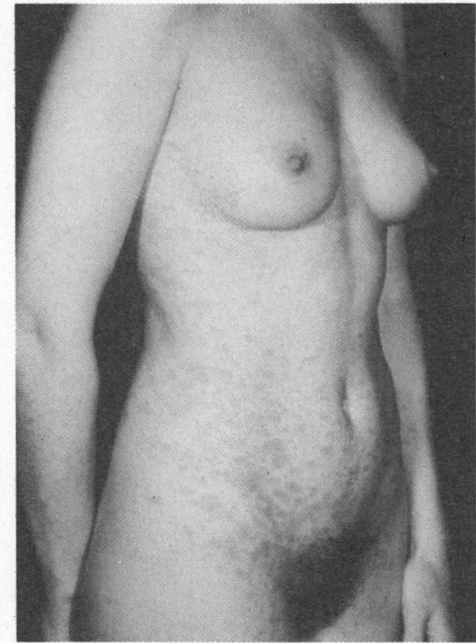

FIGURE 43-8 Pityriasis rosea. (From K. Arndt, *Manual of Dermatologic Therapeutics* [3rd ed.]. Boston: Little, Brown, 1983.)

Skin Tumors

Tumors of the skin can be divided into two basic categories, benign and malignant. Characteristics of benign tumors include structural differentiation, and they are usually composed of well-differentiated cells. These lesions are slow-growing, and growth may stop entirely [12]. Malignant lesions show disorganization and abnormalities. They frequently grow rapidly and infiltrate surrounding tissues. Metastasis is common, depending on the origin of the tumor.

Benign Tumors

Seborrheic Keratosis. Seborrheic keratosis is the most common tumor in the elderly. A strong predisposing factor is prolonged exposure to the sun. The skin lesion is slightly raised, light brown, and sharply demarcated; pigmentation may deepen and the skin become thick (Fig. 43-9).

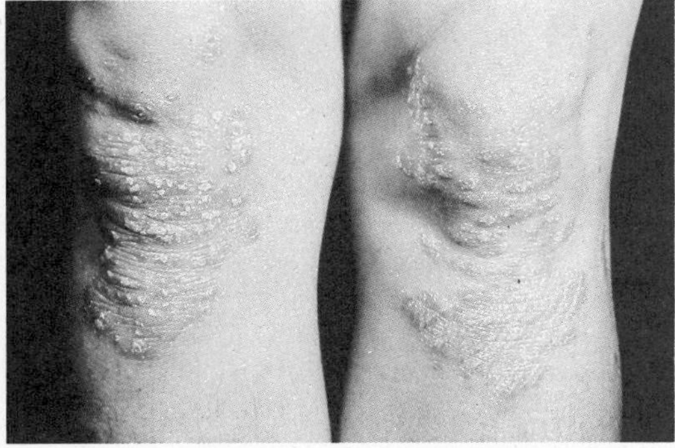

FIGURE 43-7 Psoriasis of the knees. (From K. Arndt, *Manual of Dermatologic Therapeutics* [3rd ed.]. Boston: Little, Brown, 1983.)

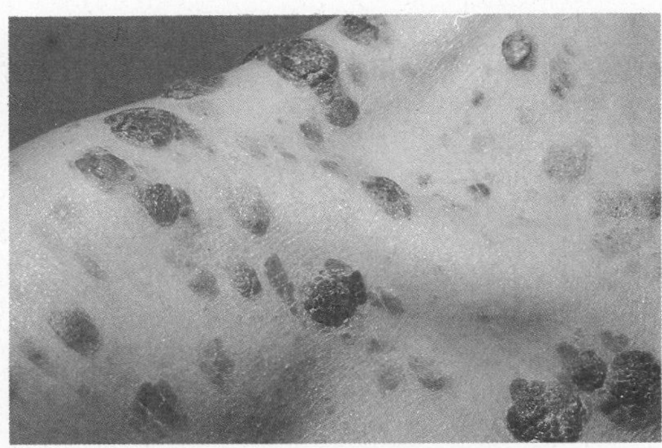

FIGURE 43-9 Seborrheic keratoses of the shoulder and clavicle. (From K. Arndt, *Manual of Dermatologic Therapeutics* [3rd ed.]. Boston: Little, Brown, 1983.)

The lesion is covered with a greasy crust that is loosely attached. Locations include the trunk, shoulders, face, and scalp. Malignant transformation is quite uncommon and most lesions do not require treatment unless they pose cosmetic difficulties or raise suspicions of malignancy.

Hemangioma. Hemangioma is a benign tumor of newly formed blood vessels. There are many different types. A strawberry hemangioma frequently appears as a dome-shaped, fully red, soft lesion with sharply demarcated edges. It has a tendency to grow slowly and usually regresses completely.

The *port-wine stain*, or nevus flammeus, is a congenital vascular malformation [11]. It is usually unilateral and located on the face and neck. It appears as a flat, red patch. Unfortunately, it is present at birth and grows as the child grows.

Cavernous hemangiomas are usually not congenital. The location includes both the skin and subcutaneous tissues, and features of the lesions depend on their extent, varying from round to flat and from bright red to deep purple.

Keratoacanthoma. Keratoacanthoma is a benign, cutaneous tumor with a central crater. Because it resembles squamous cell carcinoma, lesions are removed and examined histologically.

Actinic Keratosis. Actinic keratosis is a premalignant lesion. Common names include "senile" or "solar" keratosis. Lesions are sharply demarcated, rough, red to brown or gray. At high risk to develop the condition are fair-skinned persons whose skin easily burns with sun exposure. Age of onset is related to the amount of sun exposure. Treatment is necessary, since a number of these lesions progress to squamous cell carcinoma. A variety of methods can be used to destroy them, including curettage, electrodesiccation, cryotherapy, topical chemotherapy, and excisional biopsy.

Leukoplakia is the most common premalignant lesion, occurring as a whitish patch on the mucosa of the oral cavity [20]. It occurs most frequently in elderly women.

Malignant Tumors

Basal Cell Carcinoma. Basal cell carcinoma is also known as basal cell epithelioma and is the most frequent type of skin cancer. Most basal cell carcinomas arise from the epidermis and hair follicles [10]. They tend to occur mainly in older persons, and the majority of lesions appear with cumulative, prolonged exposure to the sun. Persons who have had radiation therapy for breast, lung, or other types of internal malignancy have an increased risk. Although they rarely metastasize, treatment is necessary, for they may become locally destructive and can erode into a vital area. Studies of T lymphocyte depression in the cutaneous tissues of these individuals supports the theory that ultraviolet light impairs host defense mechanisms and allows the tumor to escape immune surveillance [10].

Characteristically, the carcinoma has a smooth surface with a pearly border, often with ulceration of its center (Fig. 43-10). Usually, numerous telangiectasias (localized groups of dilated, small blood vessels) are visible [16]. Treatments include cryotherapy, curettage, electrodesiccation, and topical chemotherapy.

Squamous Cell Carcinoma. Squamous cell carcinoma is a malignant lesion that can affect both the skin and mucous membranes. It most frequently occurs in sun-damaged areas or areas exposed to irradiation or burns. The squamous cell carcinoma may also arise in scars, chronic ulcers, fistulas, and sinuses [10]. The burn scar may serve as an initiator, or cocarcinogen, in the production of these malignancies [10]. Immune alterations have been described that include elevated levels of circulating T lymphocytes. These may be suppressor or killer cells, but their importance has not been delineated [10]. Langerhans cells are reported to be decreased in squamous cell, but not basal cell, carcinoma [10]. These cells are thought to function as a part of the mononuclear phagocyte system in antigen processing [16].

Characteristically, the carcinoma appears as a rough, hyperkeratotic nodule with an indurated base (Fig. 43-11). It may ulcerate and can metastasize. Surgical excision is the treatment of choice. In some instances, curettage and electrodesiccation, irradiation, and chemotherapy can be used.

Malignant Melanoma. Malignant melanoma is a cancer arising from the melanin-producing cells. It is associated with increased risk of invasion and metastasis. Risk of developing some forms of the disease is increased with exposure to the sun. Recognizing the lesion early is important, since prognosis is dependent on such factors as early removal, size, type, and extension. Five-year survival improved 12.3 percent to 70 percent between 1930 and 1980 [7]. All nevi should be inspected regularly, and self-examination should be taught.

Melanoma occurs most frequently in young and middle-aged adults. The most common location in men is the

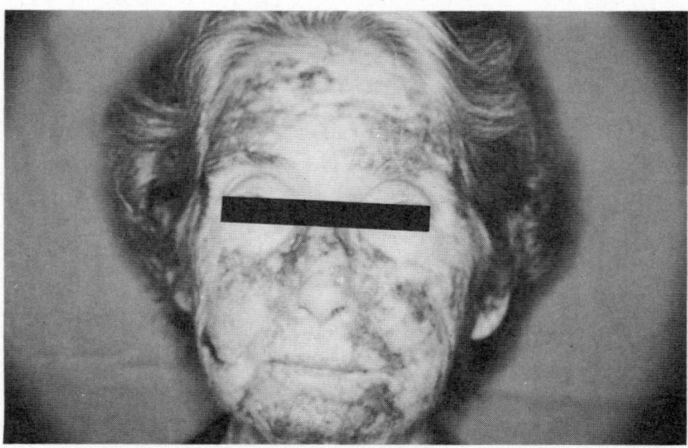

FIGURE 43-10 The smooth surface and pearly border of basal cell carcinoma. (From K. Rosen, M. Lanning, and M. Hill, *The Nurse's Atlas of Dermatology*. Boston: Little, Brown, 1983.)

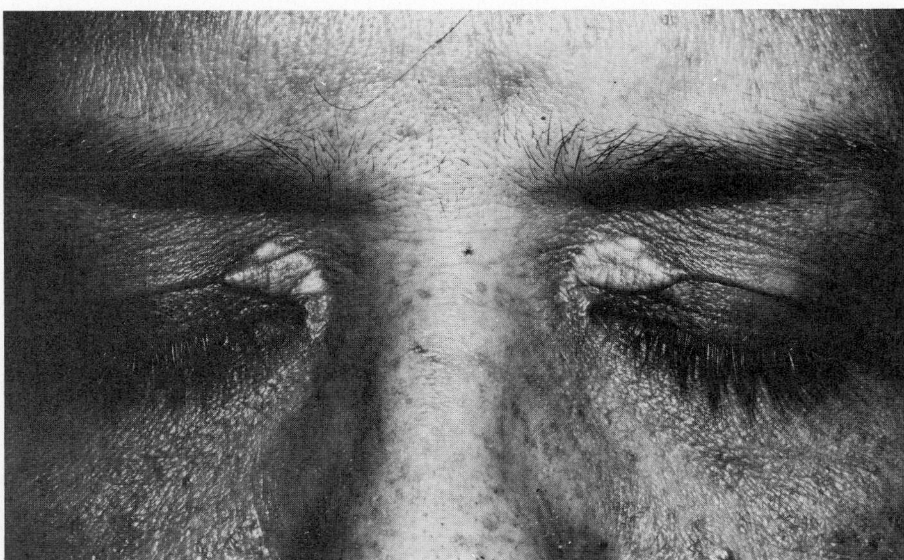

FIGURE 43-11 The characteristic look of squamous cell carcinoma. (From K. Rosen, M. Lanning, and M. Hill, *The Nurse's Atlas of Dermatology*. Boston: Little, Brown, 1983.)

trunk and in women the legs [7]. The significant characteristics are variable colors and irregular borders and surfaces. Nevi may have brown or black pigmentation with shades of red, white, or blue. Small satellite lesions 1 to 2 cm away from the primary lesion may be seen.

Melanomas acquire new antigens, some of which are the oncofetal and histocompatibility antigens. The nevi often undergo several morphologic changes before exhibiting invasive, cancerous properties. Study of the relationship of melanomas to viral carcinogens is intriguing but not conclusive at this point [7]. Only a small percentage (20%) of these malignancies occur in nevi that have been present for a period of time. A new nevus that rapidly undergoes malignant changes is often described. The malignant melanoma is highly invasive and spreads rapidly to the lymphatic system, with metastasis to any organ of the body.

Traumatic Alterations in the Skin

Burns

Burns are suffered by approximately 2 million persons annually, of which 130,000 require hospitalization and 10,000 die [2]. In a large five-year study of adult burn patients, the average age was 44 years, 78 percent were black, and 62 percent were men. Major causes of burns included flames (44.8%), scalds (28.5%), and chemicals (9.7%). The injuries resulted from direct assault, cooking, smoking, explosion, house fire, contact with hot objects, bathtub accidents, house chores, and a variety of other factors, in that order. Individuals considered to be predisposed to burn injury were the elderly, those living alone, alcohol and drug abusers, and the physically and mentally ill [2].

Burn injuries occur in every age group and both sexes. When they occur, they involve not only the skin tissue but all of the systems of the body. The depth of thermal injuries depends on the burning agent, temperature, and length of exposure to the heat [13]. The equilibrium point for skin is approximately 44°C (111.2°F). This temperature can be tolerated up to six hours without burning. The rate of skin destruction doubles with each degree rise, so that at 70°C (158°F), fleeting exposure will produce total epidermal necrosis [13].

Burns are classified as first-, second-, and third-degree. A more precise classification may be made on the basis of partial-thickness, deep dermal, or full-thickness injury. It is often difficult to ascertain the depth of injury in the initial postburn period. To complicate matters further, a partial-thickness injury may convert to a deep dermal or full-thickness injury as a result of wound sepsis and microcirculatory insufficiency with delayed degeneration of deep epithelial appendages. As time progresses, the depth and extent of the burn become more apparent.

Partial-Thickness Burns. Each degree of burn wound depth has various characteristics. Partial-thickness burns include first- and second-degree and deep dermal injuries (Table 43-2). The first-degree burn involves the epidermis (Fig. 43-12). It may be caused by exposure to sunlight, brief exposures to a heat source, splashed hot liquid, high-intensity short-duration explosions, and chemical and electrical injury. A first-degree burn is pink to red, painful, and slightly edematous. The epidermis peels in three to six days, with itching and redness persisting a week or more. The wound leaves no scar when healed [13].

TABLE 43-2 Classification of Burns

Degree	Tissue	Appearance	Symptoms	Resolution
First				
Partial-thickness	Epidermis	Red, pink, slight edema	Pain	Epidermis peels in 3–6 days; itch, redness in a week or so; no scar
Second				
Partial-thickness				
Superficial	Epidermis and upper dermis	Mottled pink to red; blistering; edema; moist	Sensitive	Heals in 10–14 days without grafting; no scar if no infection or trauma to wound
Deep dermal	Epidermis, dermis to subcutaneous tissue	Varies: white, tan, cherry red; red area blanches; dark, coagulated capillary streaks; blister and moist, or dry	May or may not be sensitive; if hair follicle present, hair does not pull out	Has potential to heal spontaneously over several months; may be excised or grafted
Third				
Full-thickness	Epidermis; dermis; subcutaneous layer; no viable epithelial cells remain	White, tan, brown, black, deep cherry red; red areas do not blanch; wet or dry; sunken; eschar; coagulated capillaries	Anesthetic; hair pulls out	Grafting required after debridement
Fourth				
Full-thickness	Epidermis, dermis; subcutaneous layer; fascia; muscle; bone	Blackened; depressed; bone is dull and dry	Anesthetic; hair pulls out	Grafting required

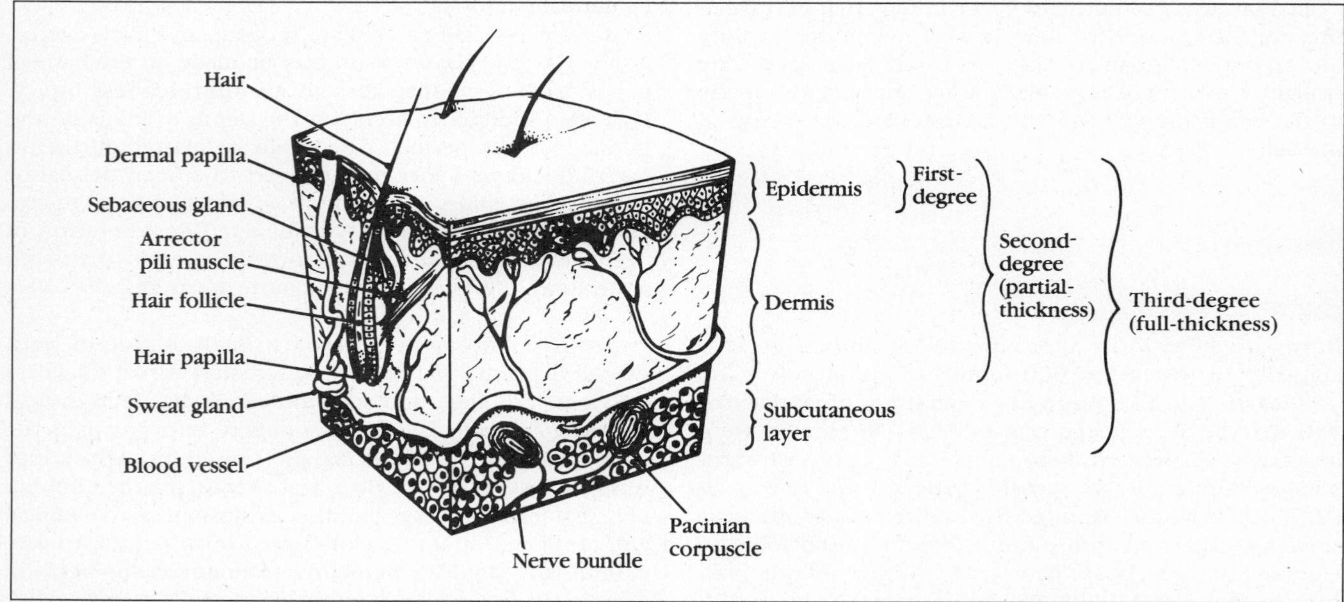

FIGURE 43-12 Areas affected by first-, second-, and third-degree burns.

The second-degree partial-thickness burn may be superficial or deep dermal. It results from intense flash heat, hot liquid, contact with hot objects, chemicals, or electrical injury.

The superficial burn involves the epidermis and dermis. It has a mottled pink to red color (Fig. 43-13). It exhibits blistering and subcutaneous edema, is moist and very sensitive. This burn heals in 10 to 14 days without grafting. If it does not become infected or traumatized, usually no scar forms.

The deep dermal burn varies in color, being mottled with more white than red, a dull white, tan, or cherry red. The red areas blanch and refill. Dark streaks of coagulated capillaries may be seen. The burn extends down to the subcutaneous tissue. If epidermal appendages are intact, it has the potential to heal spontaneously without grafting, as viable skin cells are present in the appendages. It takes several months for a deep dermal burn to heal spontaneously. The wound may be blistered and moist, or it may be dry; it may or may not be sensitive; if a hair follicle remains, the hair will not pull out. The epithelium produced is extremely thin and may break down easily; the burn may convert to a full-thickness burn if it becomes infected. Many deep dermal burns are excised and grafted [13].

Full-Thickness Burns. These are full-thickness injuries that have no viable epithelial cells. The causes may be the same as for first- and second-degree burns. The wound appearance may vary, being white, tan, brown, black, and/or deep cherry red. The red areas do not blanch. The burn is usually dry and has a sunken, leathery appearance. The leathery covering is called *eschar*. A black network of coagulated capillaries may be seen. This wound itself is anesthetic and hair pulls out easily. Grafting is required to close the wound (Fig. 43-14) [13].

The third-degree burn may also involve the subcutaneous fat layer, fascia, muscle, and bone. Some authors call this type a fourth-degree burn. It appears black and depressed. If bone shows through, it appears dry and dull. Grafting is necessary to close this wound. If a graft is required over bone, small perforations are made in the bone to the marrow. Granulation buds grow from these holes, coalesce, and form a bed to accept the graft [13].

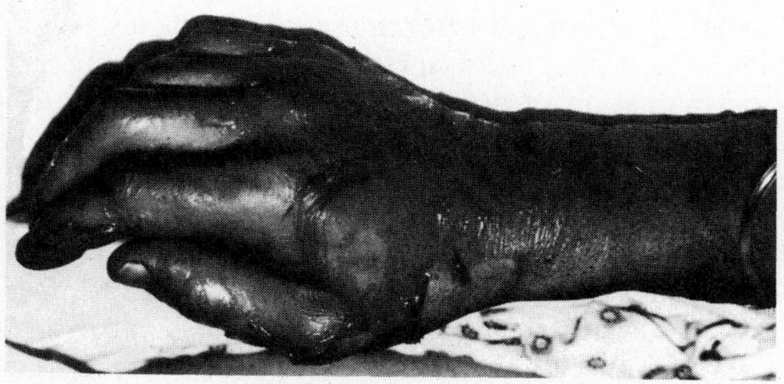

FIGURE 43-13 Partial-thickness burn injury. (From C.V. Kenner, C.E. Guzzetta, and B.M. Dossey, *Critical Care Nursing* [2nd ed]. Boston: Little, Brown, 1985.)

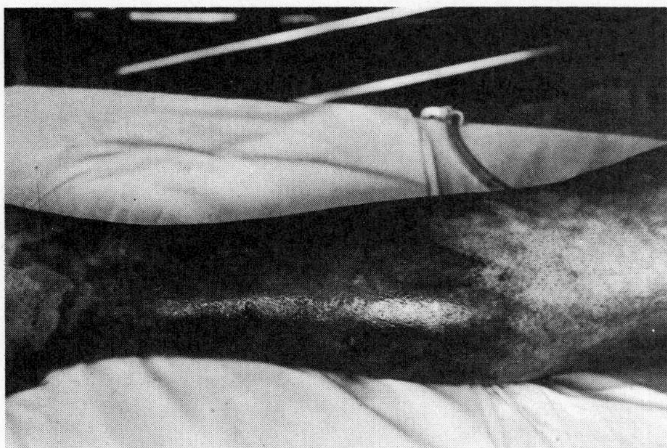

FIGURE 43-14 Full-thickness burn injury of the right leg. (From C.V. Kenner, C.E. Guzzetta, and B.M. Dossey, *Critical Care Nursing* [2nd ed.]. Boston: Little, Brown, 1985.)

This degree of burn depends on the temperature of and duration of exposure to the heat source. The severity of the injury is dependent on the size of the burned area, its depth and location, the age of the victim, the presence of concomitant illness or injury, and the psychologic status of the victim. In assessing the burn situation further, it is helpful to know the circumstances surrounding the injury. Important information includes such things as place of injury, exposure to electricity, exposure to fumes, and other factors that may complicate the recovery.

Estimating the percentage of total body surface area that has been burned is critical in determining fluid and nutritional requirements. The classic rule of nines has been a standard for estimating burn area (Fig. 43-15) [14]. This helpful method has some limitations, depending upon the age of the burned patient (a child's head represents a greater percentage of body area than an adult's) and the extent of actual third-degree injury [13].

Localized Changes Due to Burn Injury. When skin is burned, many localized changes occur. Protein in cells is denatured and enzymes are inactivated. The tissue becomes coagulated, desiccated, or carbonized, depending on the temperature of the heat source and the length of exposure to it. Even with mild heat, the normal metabolic activity of a cell is altered. Burns caused by long exposure to low-intensity heat are characterized by major changes in deeper tissues.

The stratum corneum is the water vapor barrier in the body. When it is destroyed, large amounts of fluid are lost. In a deep wound, the fluid loss is greater and often continues until the wound finally is closed, usually by grafting.

Burns extending down to and damaging the stratum germinativum do not regenerate if all parts of this layer are destroyed. Heat extending to the "cement" that binds the epidermis to the dermis causes the epidermis to loosen; lost fluid fills in the space and a blister develops. When new epidermis is formed beneath the blister, the blister dries and peels off.

The dermis, composed of collagen fibers, elastin, and mast cells, is damaged when exposed to high degrees of

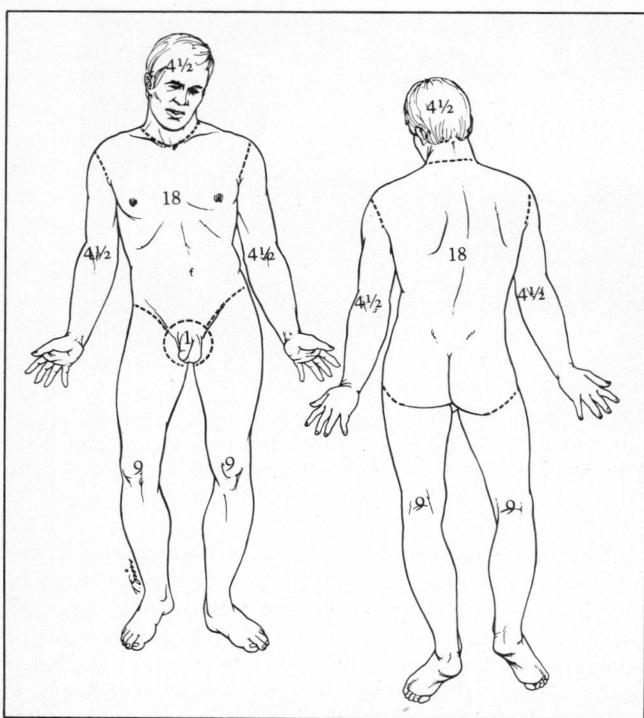

FIGURE 43-15 The rule of nines. Each arm is 9 percent, the head 9 percent, the torso and abdomen 18 percent, the back 18 percent, and each leg 18 percent. (From C.V. Kenner, C.E. Guzzetta, and B.M. Dossey, *Critical Care Nursing* [2nd ed.]. Boston: Little, Brown, 1985.)

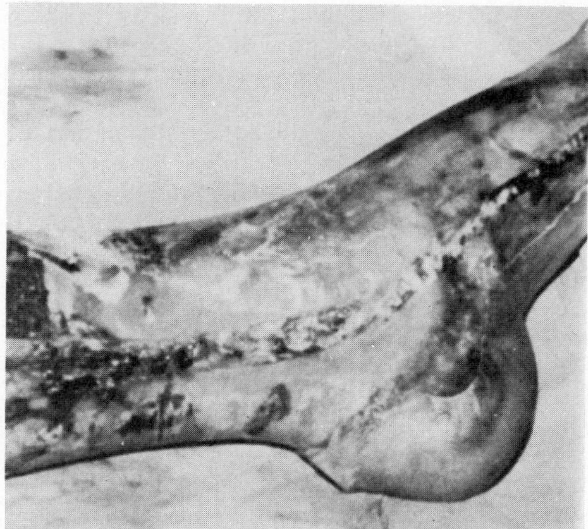

FIGURE 43-16 Escharotomy site. (From C.V. Kenner, C.E. Guzzetta, and B.M. Dossey, *Critical Care Nursing* [2nd ed.]. Boston: Little, Brown, 1985.)

heat. The epidermal appendages, if intact, contain epidermal cells in the external sheaths of hair follicles. Glands can grow out and form new epithelium. When the burn extends to the subcutaneous tissues, the collagen fibers that normally anchor the dermis to the subcutaneous layer now hold the leathery burn eschar in place. Bacteria that form under the eschar release enzymes that lyse the collagen fibers, making it easier to remove eschar.

The melanocytes in the epidermis do not regenerate well, and in deep burns, the skin color usually does not return. As blood vessels are damaged from the thermal injury, color changes occur in the burn. In sunburn, the vessels in the subpapillary and papillary plexuses dilate, causing reddening. In a severe burn, coagulation of vessels causes the area to lose redness and be whiter, with the vessels themselves coagulating into blackened lines in the wound.

Plasma leaks from damaged blood vessels and provides the fluid for blisters. Lymph vessels, compressed by edema from the wound, cannot drain the affected area. Escharotomy may become necessary if tissue swelling compromises the venous return and arterial blood supply, which can cause ischemic changes in the involved area (Fig. 43-16) [13].

Systemic Changes Due to Burn Injury. Many changes occur throughout the body as a result of burn injury. Responses in the circulatory system account for color changes and the edema of burns. Contraction of the skin capillaries causes blanching. The wound appears white if the superficial dermis is coagulated. Later, when arterioles and capillaries dilate, it appears red. The capillaries lose protein-rich fluid through their abnormally permeable walls into the surrounding tissues, creating the most characteristic feature of the burn wound, *edema*.

Normally, plasma and interstitial fluid are chemically similar, except for blood cells and large plasma proteins, which elevate the colloid osmotic pressure in the blood. After burn injury, plasma proteins such as albumins and globulins leak out of the damaged capillaries and into the interstitial spaces. The loss of protein-rich fluid decreases the intracapillary colloid osmotic pressure causing fluid to shift into the tissues (see Chap. 5). There is also an accompanying rise in intracapillary pressure as a result of capillary dilatation and increased blood flow of the inflammatory process. The loss of protein from capillaries is termed *capillary sieving* [1]. The amount of sieving is correlated with the severity of the burn. The more severe the burn, the more protein is lost. Capillary permeability also increases in tissues around the burn and other areas of the body [13].

The permeability of tissue cells in and around the burn seems to allow abnormal interchange of fluids and electrolytes between cells and interstitial fluid. A limiting factor for extravasation of fluid is increased tissue pressure. Tissue pressure increases as fluid loss increases, and reaches a point at which the tissue can hold no more fluid.

The depth of the burn affects the volume and composition of edema fluid. In first-degree burns, protein loss is insignificant and edema slight, because vasodilatation is the only circulatory change. A second-degree burn has more severe capillary damage and more tissue damage. At first assessment, the surface area of burn is easily seen, but the depth is not always immediately apparent. Large volumes of fluid can escape beneath the wound before swelling is noted. The third-degree burn has large injury to skin and area beneath and around it, which accounts for extensive fluid losses.

Edema can be displaced by pressure, move to dependent areas, and spread beyond the burn. The rate of edema formation depends on temperature of the heat source, duration of exposure, area of the burn, and the time since injury. It is difficult to ascertain fluid loss by the amount of visible edema, because such loss occurs deep in the wound beneath it and in the vulnerable third spaces, such as the peritoneal cavity and even the lungs [13]. The leathery eschar does not expand with edema pressure, and large amounts of fluid collect beneath it, putting pressure on underlying tissues. The pressure may be relieved by escharotomy.

Studies show that fluid losses occur rapidly in the period immediately after the burn and decline in about 48 hours. The rate of loss slows when the capillary endothelium returns to its normal state, when the tissue pressure is in balance with capillary hydrostatic pressure, or when capillary stasis occurs. In minor uncomplicated burns, edema is chiefly resorbed by the lymphatic system and takes approximately as long as it took the edema to form. Lymphatics also drain larger burns, but this process may take weeks.

The amount of protein lost from plasma varies. Albumin and globulin are lost, with greater amounts of albumin lost than globulin owing to the smaller size of the albumin molecule. Immediately after the burn, the concentration of protein in plasma increases, because there is greater loss of water and electrolytes together with the protein loss. The following compensatory mechanisms exist to counteract fluid loss: interstitial fluid in unburned areas is absorbed by the blood; blood vessels in the spleen and unburned skin constrict, reducing the space the remaining blood volume must fill; and fluid is absorbed by the gut. Thirst may be intense. In minor burns, these mechanisms suffice. In major large burns, fluids and proteins must be replaced [13].

Hemoconcentration is a sequel to capillary fluid loss. The fluid portion of blood is lost to the tissues, allowing the cellular elements to concentrate. The hematocrit rises; blood flow becomes sluggish, compromising tissue nutrition and oxygenation. Thrombosis sometimes develops in these affected areas.

Water and electrolytes shift back and forth across normal capillary walls. Burn injury alters the shifts by increasing capillary permeability, causing protein loss and altered colloid osmotic pressure. Potassium is released from severely injured cells, causing elevated serum potassium levels and cardiac dysrhythmias (see Chap. 5). Sodium may increase in burn tissue, taking water with it. When the victim begins diuresis after 48 hours or so, potassium and sodium are excreted. Careful monitoring of electrolyte levels is important, so that replacement therapy may be initiated and electrolyte concentrations in replacement fluids, for example, sodium, may be reduced.

In some burns, there is a substantial loss of red blood cells, intensifying the effects of plasma loss. This usually occurs in deep burns and seems to be a gradual process. The loss of red blood cells is due in part to hemolysis in the burned area, which results in hemoglobinemia and hemoglobinuria soon after the burn occurs [16]. Free hemoglobin in the plasma indicates a severe burn. For 24 to 48 hours, delayed hemolysis of partially damaged red blood cells occurs. Further decrease in red blood cells results from thrombosis and sludging. Anemia develops as a result of red cell loss as well as with bleeding during debridement and other causes.

Additional fluid is lost as insensible water loss from evaporation from the burn wound surface and through the respiratory system. Respiratory loss is greatest when a tracheostomy is required. Pulmonary dysfunction requiring tracheostomy is common in third-degree burns involving 25 to 70 percent of total body surface [6].

Signs and symptoms of fluid deficiency include thirst, restlessness, and disorientation. Plain water given to relieve thirst may lead to water intoxication. Solutions with balanced electrolytes must be administered to avoid this. Fluids are usually given intravenously because of the frequency of vomiting after burn injury. Changes in the central nervous system are useful in following the progress of therapy. Restlessness is an early indication that fluid replacement therapy is ineffective. Disorientation in the first 24 hours usually means that more intensive treatment is needed.

The depletion of fluid to edema and insensible loss reduce circulatory blood volume and can result in reduced cardiac output and inadequate tissue perfusion. Tissue hypoxia may result, causing a shift to anaerobic cellular metabolism. Acidosis and irreversible burn shock can occur. The acid-base balance is disrupted because the buffering mechanism is upset by fluid shift in the body compartments, hyperventilation, and reduced renal function. Blood urea levels may rise if protein catabolism is excessive or large amounts of nitrogen are released from burned tissue in the presence of oliguria.

The respiratory system is often altered by burn injury, by inhalation injury, and by therapy. Heat exposure and irritants cause swelling and tissue breakdown. Respiratory tissues are irritated by gases from burning materials, such as carbon monoxide. Altered circulation may lead to inadequate pulmonary circulation. Hypoxia may result from the decreased amount of oxygen circulating. Aspiration pneumonia may develop from vomiting episodes. Tracheal or laryngeal obstruction may result from edema in the head and neck region, causing pressure against the trachea and larynx. Also, inflamed linings of trachea and larynx swell and block the airway. Edema under tight eschar in burns of the torso restricts chest movements, which also may lead to respiratory problems. The adult respiratory distress syndrome (ARDS) is an ominous complication of burn injury and may result after shock or severe hypoxia [6]. Finally, pulmonary emboli are always a danger as a result of changes in the vasculature, sepsis, and immobilization.

Physical findings in the respiratory system include singed nasal hairs and reddened or dark pharynx. Irritation and heat damage to respiratory tissue may lead to respiratory stridor, dyspnea, and copious secretions, often carbonaceous. Deep full-thickness burns of the face also cause burning of pharyngeal tissues. Laryngeal edema, focal erosion, focal laryngitis, and necrosis may be evident. Edema may be exhibited by hoarseness. Respiratory disorders that may occur during the course of therapy include pneumonia, atelectasis, obstruction from mucus plugs, ARDS, and septic emboli from infected venosections.

The gastrointestinal tract is also affected. Changes there include acute stress (Curling's) ulcers, gastric dilatation, paralytic ileus, and bleeding.

Acute gastric and duodenal ulcers in burn victims are morphologically identical to acute stress ulcers in people without burns. Acute stress ulcers in individuals with and without burns are mostly gastric [16]. They occur in 20 to 30 percent of persons with total body surface burns. Ulcers may occur in the stomach, duodenum, or both. The anatomic location of stress ulcers differs from that of peptic and duodenal ulcers not caused by stress. Stress gastric ulcers are present in the fundic mucosa as opposed to the pyloric mucosa of other gastric ulcers. Stress duodenal ulcers are located in the posterior, rather than the anterior duodenum. They have several foci when they occur in the stomach and a single focus when they occur in the duodenum [16].

Gastric ulcers are generally smaller than duodenal ulcers. Those of 2 to 3 mm are difficult to see during gastroscopy, or even autopsy, but they are deep enough to cause significant bleeding. Many ulcers are hidden in the rugal folds. Stress ulcers exhibit a relative lack of inflammatory response, which may be due to the fact that many occur in the terminal stages of burn illness. Many of these stress ulcers are colonized with gram-negative bacilli. Vascular congestion and submucosal edema are often present. No single theory is held concerning pathogenesis of Curling's stress ulcers. They are similar morphologically to steroid-induced ulcers, but their pathogenesis is different from that of peptic ulcers. Bleeding and perforation are common complications.

Gastric dilatation and paralytic ileus may appear early after burn injury. These conditions are neurologic in origin, may be secondary to fear or pain, or may occur as a result of hypovolemia or sepsis.

Liver dysfunction often occurs with burn injury. Factors that contribute to liver dysfunction include bacterial infection, lack of proper nutrition, drugs, anesthesia, blood transfusions leading to viral or serum hepatitis, and hepatic hypoxemia. Hepatic hypoxemia seems to be a result of a decrease in circulating fluid volume. The necrosis that results is usually minimal and focal, of a fatty nature, and reversible.

The kidney changes that occur may be permanent or temporary. Temporary kidney changes are manifested by oliguria, which results from a decreased glomerular filtration rate from the decreased circulatory volume. Blood urea nitrogen (BUN) and creatinine levels are elevated, and the level of antidiuretic hormone may be increased. Tubular damage may occur when the kidneys are presented with an increased amount of protein breakdown products from the burn. If there is a history of prior kidney disorder, or if the person does not receive adequate treatment, permanent damage may occur. Hematuria may be present as a result of damaged red blood cells. Death may result from acute renal insufficiency despite adequate treatment.

Stress also enhances the secretion of adrenocortical hormones. The adrenal medulla secretes large amounts of epinephrine and norepinephrine (see Chap. 4).

Problems in coagulation may occur after severe burn injury and may result from the burn, from complications secondary to the injury, or from therapy. Abnormalities include decreases in platelet count, clot retraction time, and partial thromboplastin and prothrombin times, along with elevated fibrinogen levels. A circulating heparinlike material that prolongs clotting times and depresses the prothrombin level is also present. These defects seem to occur in large burns involving large body surface areas, as well as in smaller burns. Consumption or use of clotting factors plays a role in coagulopathies. Coagulopathies, such as disseminated intravascular coagulation (DIC) frequently occur and are treated with transfusions of platelets, fresh-frozen plasma, whole blood, fibrinogen concentrations, and other clotting factors.

Wound infections are a major problem in burns and may lead to sepsis, which is the most common cause of death [9,16]. The frequency of infection is correlated with the extent and depth of the injury and with the success of treatment measures [9]. Bacteria, both gram-positive and gram-negative, invade the wound surface and eventually reach the viable surrounding tissue. Products liberated by the bacteria can produce septic shock [16]. Major burn injury also produces immune suppression, which can affect T lymphocytes and macrophages [16]. In a large study of burn wound colonization and treatment, numerous strains of bacteria colonized the wounds within the first 24 hours. If treatment measures were not effective, penetration into the deeper tissues occurred and sepsis was a frequent result [9]. The study demonstrated the importance of decreasing the size of open, full-thickness wounds to prevent infection.

Electrical Burn Injuries. Various lesions occur as a result of electrical burns. Six factors determine the extent of these injuries: (1) type of current (direct or alternating), (2) voltage of current, (3) resistance of body tissues, (4) value of current flowing through the tissues, (5) pathway of the current through the body, and (6) duration of contact with the electrical source.

Direct current does not produce the same contraction of muscle and low-voltage direct current is not as dangerous as alternating current. High-voltage direct current, however, is often fatal.

Alternating current produces tetanic muscle contraction at low voltages which prevents the victim from releasing contact with the circuit. These low-voltage currents often result in ventricular fibrillation [23]. Low voltage means less than 500 volts, and high voltage is greater than 500 volts. Low-tension injuries most often occur in the home and are likely to involve children and infants [8]. The usual source of current is a household plug; a curious child may stick a small object into the outlet. High-tension injury commonly occurs in adults working with electric lines or equipment. These injuries have a high mortality, often due to cardiac asystole.

The body tissues offer varying degrees of resistance to electrical current. The resistance of tissues, in order of least to greatest, is as follows: nerves, blood, muscles, skin, tendons, fat, and bone. Skin resistance varies from person to person. The epidermis is nonvascular and offers high resistance when it is dry but, when wet, moisture decreases resistance and enhances the flow of current. The dermis offers low resistance because it is highly vascular.

Thin skin is less resistant than thick skin, making the palms and soles most resistant. Usually, the greater the skin resistance, the greater the local burn, and the less the skin resistance, the more the internal injury. Current in contact with the skin eventually causes blistering. Blisters are moist and conduct current through the skin along the tissues of least resistance—blood vessels and nerves. Vessel walls are damaged and thrombi occur, often at a site far from the site of the electrical injury, making it difficult to evaluate the full extent of damage at the initial evaluation. Progressive tissue necrosis can occur for 12 to 14 days after the injury [13].

Electric current may flow through the heart, producing ventricular fibrillation and often immediate death. High-voltage current often travels to the respiratory center of the brain, causing respiratory arrest and death [13].

The value of the alternating current flowing through the body determines the resulting injury. Contact with a circuit produces muscle contraction, which may be severe enough to prevent the victim from releasing himself or herself from the source of current. If cardiac or respiratory arrest does not occur and the victim remains conscious, he or she may complain of ringing in the ears and deafness for a time, or visual disturbances such as flashes and brilliant luminous spots.

The pathway through the body is also important in determining the extent of injury. The longer the contact, the greater amount of damage.

The injury in electrical burns may be one or more of three types: (1) entry and exit wounds, (2) electrothermal burns (flash or arc burns), and (3) flame burns. The entry wound occurs at the contact site. It may be small or large and usually appears as an ischemic, yellow-white, coagulated area, or it may be charred. It is dry and painless, and the edges are well defined [17]; however, the extent of damage may be far greater than is evident on the surface. Necrosis of subcutaneous tissues and muscle from arterial thrombi may occur, or lack of thrombosis may cause hemorrhaging. Damage may be due to heat from the passage of current or due to the action of the current itself [17].

The exit wound appears as a blow-out type of injury caused by arcing current between victim and a nearby ground [13]. It is a dry area with depressed edges. The exit wound is usually more severe than the entry wound [13].

Electrothermal burns are from the heat of the current passing near, but not through, the skin. The depth of the wound depends on the closeness to the electrical source. These are mainly associated with high-tension current. The electricity arc leaping from the high current has a temperature of 2500°C.

Flame burns occur when heat from an electrical current ignites clothing. They may cause more serious injury than the electrical injury itself.

The tetanic contractions that lock the victim to the electric source may cause fractures and dislocations of joints. Cataracts often develop months to years after an electrical injury involving the head area.

Abdominal injury may occur as a result of electrical trauma to the abdomen. The extent of injury is difficult to determine at first. Abdominal symptoms may not arise until days after the injury.

Renal involvement seems to be more prevalent in electrical than in thermal injury. The damage may be caused by the initial electric shock, direct current damage to the kidneys and/or kidney vessels, abnormal protein breakdown in the damaged tissue, or a combination of all three.

Chemical Burn Injuries. Chemical burns result from exposure to acid and/or alkaline chemicals (Table 43-3). Most lethal burns result from military conflict and industrial accidents. Domestic and laboratory accidents and criminal assaults usually result in smaller areas of damage [13]. The injury may result from chemical changes as well as from thermal injury to the tissues, depending on the nature of the chemical.

Tissue damage is dependent upon five factors: (1) pH or concentration of the chemical, (2) amount of agent contacting the skin, (3) duration of contact, (4) amount of tissue penetration, and (5) mechanism of action of the chemical [13]. Chemical changes in tissues include denaturation, precipitation, alkalization, edema, separation of the epidermis from the dermis, disorganization of epidermal appendages, and widening and coalescence of collagen bundles.

Chemical agents are often classified by the way in which they affect protein. Oxidizing agents are corrosive and cause extensive protein denaturation. Some agents are desiccants and cause cellular dehydration. Others cause anoxic tissue damage [13]. The depth of chemical burns is often difficult to evaluate.

Acid burns most frequently occur in industrial plants as immersion injuries. They are often a result of splattering or spilling of an acid substance. The wound is painful and persists because of the chemical action. Its depth and appearance vary, depending on the amount of acid and length of exposure. Systemic changes are rare, but acid fumes may be inhaled. Treatment is best accomplished by initial dilution of the acid.

Alkali burns result from chemical irritation from a highly alkaline substance. One example is phosphorus burns, which are painful and often occur as a result of warfare. Phosphorus melts at body temperature and penetrates into tissue. When exposed to air, the wound smokes; in the dark, it glows bluish-green. Copper sulfate is used to treat these burns by inactivating the phosphorus. The chemical is then removed surgically. Caution must be used in working with copper, as its use may result in copper toxicity with massive hemolysis of red blood cells and acute renal tubular necrosis.

TABLE 43-3 Chemical Burns: Pathophysiology and Treatment

Type	Mechanism	Appearance	Treatment: Cleanse	Treatment: Neutralize	Treatment: Debride
Acid burns					
Sulfuric Nitric Hydrochloric Trichloroacetic	Exothermic reaction; cell dehydration; protein precipitation	Gray, yellow; brown, black; soft to leathery eschar	Water	Sodium bicarbonate	Debride
Phenol			Ethyl alchohol	Sodium bicarbonate	Debride
Hydrofluoric			Water	Sodium bicarbonate; magnesium oxide; glycerin paste; calcium gluconate	Debride
Alkali burns					
Potassium hydroxide Sodium hydroxide	Exothermic reaction; cellular dehydration; saponification of fat; protein precipitation	Erythema and blister; soapy, thick eschar; painful	Water	Acetic acid or ammonium chloride	Debride
Lime			Brush off lime powder	Acetic acid or ammonium chloride	Debride
Ammonia	Same as above, plus laryngeal and pulmonary edema	Gray, yellow; brown, black; deep; soft leathery texture	Water	Acetic acid or ammonium chloride	Debride
Phosphorous	Thermal effect; melts at body temperature; runs and ignites at 34°C	Gray blue green; glows in dark; depressed, leathery eschar	Water	Copper sulfate	Debride and remove phosphorous particles

Source: K. Arndt, *Manual of Dermatologic Therapeutics* (3rd ed.). Boston: Little, Brown, 1983.

Complications of all types of burn wounds include infection, contractures from scarring, renal failure, ulcers, liver failure, pneumonia, urinary tract infection, and acidosis. The frequency of complications increases with the severity of the burn.

Decubitis Ulcers (Pressure Sores)

The word *decubitis* derives from the Latin *decumbo*, meaning "lying down" [22]. During the late nineteenth and early twentieth centuries, persons with decubitus ulcers generally had wasting diseases, such as tuberculosis, osteomyelitis, and chronic renal failure. Now, those at risk have conditions that alter mobility, such as individuals with spinal cord injuries, the ill elderly who are incontinent, and persons who are bed- or wheelchair-bound. Decubitus ulcers create significant health problems because they increase the length of hospitilization, increase health care costs, and increase the chances of death.

Four critical factors play a role in decubitus formation: (1) pressure, (2) shearing forces, (3) friction, and (4) moisture. Pressure is the most critical, and these ulcers are accurately called *pressure sores*. Pressure is defined as the exertion of force on a surface by an object in contact with the surface [22]. The force is the weight of the individual applied onto the object upon which he or she is lying. Pressure is not evenly distributed over the body when lying or sitting. It is greatest over bony prominences, and it is over these areas that decubitus ulcers develop.

A balance exists between interstitial pressure and solid tissue pressure to make a total tissue pressure of zero. With an increase in external pressure over an area, the interstitial fluid pressure increases, elevating total tissue pressure. As a result, capillary and arteriolar pressures rise, causing fluid to filter from capillaries. Edema and autolysis of cells follow. As the pressure continues, lymph vessels are occluded, resulting in accumulation of anaerobic metabolic wastes and tissue necrosis [15]. The duration and magnitude of pressure are key factors in the amount of tissue damage. With high pressure, it takes less time for tissue necrosis to occur. Constant pressure of 70 mm Hg for more than 1 to 6 hours produces irreversible tissue damage, depending upon the condition of the skin and the person's nutritional status [22]. If pressure is intermittently relieved, tissue change is minimal.

As a pressure sore develops, the first sign is skin erythema from reactive hyperemia. Continuous pressure causes necrosis of tissue, and initially an eschar forms that covers and protects the wound. Loss of eschar allows bacterial invasion, and infection results [22].

The sliding of adjacent tissue layers provides a progressive relative displacement of tissues. These shearing forces may be accentuated when the head of the bed is raised and the torso of the person slides down, exerting pressure to the sacrum and deep fascia while the posterior sacral skin is fixed. The shearing force in the deep superficial fascia stretches and angulates blood and lymph vessels, causes thrombosis, and undermines the dermis. The subcutaneous fat layer lacks tensile strength and is vulnerable to the mechanical shearing force. The two surfaces that are in contact move across each other, causing friction. This action removes the outer protective stratum corneum and hastens the onset of ulceration. Friction occurs when a person is dragged across bed sheets, so-called sheet burn. The sacral ulcer commonly is formed in this way [4].

Fecal matter, urine, and perspiration irritate and macerate the skin, softening it and making it more vulnerable to pressure sore formation.

Classification and Treatment of Decubitus Ulcers. Decubitus ulcers may develop in stages and in categories (Table 43-4). In stage 1, the sore is reversible. It resembles an abrasion where the epidermis is abraded, exposing the underlying dermis. An acute inflammatory response occurs; the wound is irregular in shape, is red, warm, and indurated, and is painful in a normally innervated person. Relief of pressure and local cleansing usually resolve the ulcer in 5 to 10 days.

A stage 2 decubitus ulcer is also reversible. As pressure continues, the entire dermis is affected. The wound appears as a shallow, full-thickness ulcer with distinct edges, early fibrosis, and skin color changes. The inflammatory response is present. Relief of pressure and local cleansing allow the wound to heal.

In stage 3, the decubitus is extended downward, and the epidermis, dermis, and subcutaneous tissues are involved. This full-thickness skin defect spreads peripherally, because the fascia underlying the subcutaneous layer is resistant to pressure. A small broken area may appear on the surface, with a larger area beneath. The epidermis thickens and rolls over the wound edge toward the ulcer base. The ulcer has a dark-light pigmentation. The skin layers are completely distorted, and the wound begins to drain foul-smelling fluid (Fig. 43-17). Systemic problems begin to occur in a stage 3 decubitus ulcer. As in a full-thickness burn injury, fluid and protein are lost [15]. The person may experience fever, dehydration, anemia, and leukocytosis.

In a stage 4 wound, the fascia underlying the subcutaneous tissue is penetrated and the wound is rapidly undermined. Complications include osteomyelitis of bone, sepsis, joint dislocations, and release of toxins. The condition may be fatal [15].

A closed decubitus has no external opening but, inside, may act and appear as a stage 3 or 4 lesion. These ulcers occur after long pressure insults with shear stress. A bursalike cavity forms and is filled with debris from the necrosis

TABLE 43-4 Classification of Decubitus Ulcers

Stage	Layers of Skin	Wound Appearance	Systemic Changes	Resolution
1	Partial-thickness	Irregular; warm; erythema; pain; edematous	None	Reversible with relief of pressure and local cleansing
2	Partial-thickness Epidermis Dermis	Shallow skin ulcer; edges distinct; fibrosis; skin color changes	None	Reversible with relief of pressure and local cleansing
3	Full-thickness Epidermis Dermis Subcutaneous layer	Thick epidermal ulcer margin; light and dark pigmentation; skin layers distorted; drains foul-smelling fluid	Infection; fat necrosis; loss of fluid and protein; fever; dehydration; anemia; leukocytosis	Relief of pressure; systemic treatment with IV fluids; diet; medications; debridement and wound graft
4	Full-thickness Epidermis Dermis Subcutaneous fat Fascia Muscle Bone	Large open area; bone shows through	Osteomyelitis; sepsis; joint dislocation; toxic; fatal	Radical surgery to remove necrotic areas; general support measures (IV's; diet; medications)
Closed	Subcutaneous tissue and deeper	No external sign until later, when skin ruptures; inside appears as a stage 3 or 4 wound; bursalike cavity with necrotic debris	Infrequent infection	Wide excision; removal of bursa sac; flap graft with muscle

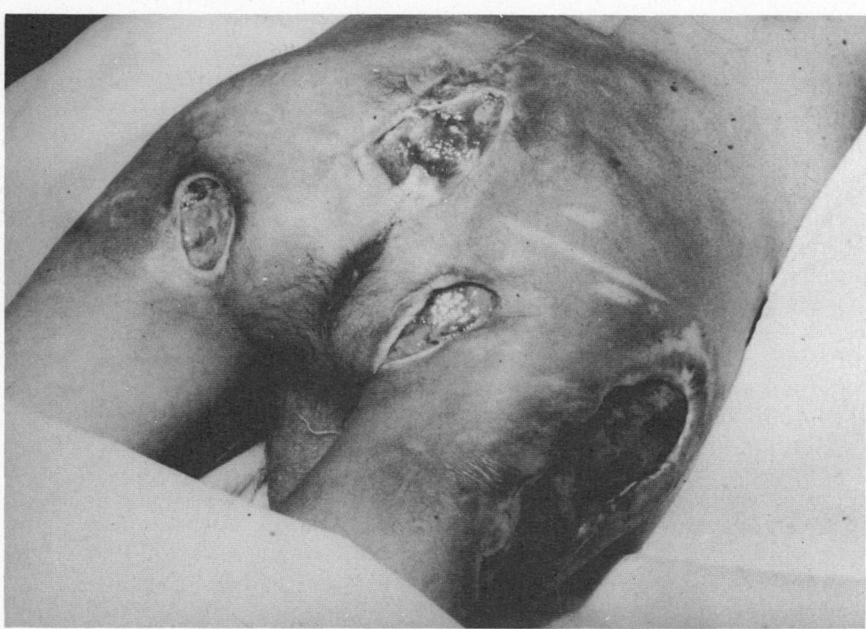

FIGURE 43-17 Because of widely undermined edges produced by shearing forces, this sacral ulcer communicates with ischial and trochangeric ulcers bilaterally. (From M.B. Constantian, *Pressure Ulcers*. Boston: Little, Brown, 1980.)

of subcutaneous and deeper areas. This type of decubitus ulcer often occurs over ischial tuberosities. Eventually, the overlying skin ruptures.

Other Traumas

Other traumas to the skin include blunt wounds, abrasions (scrapes), incised wounds (as in incision), puncture wounds, and lacerations (cuts). An abrasion is a superficial open wound in which the outer surface layers of skin are scraped off. Nerve endings are exposed and bleeding is minimal. The wound often contains foreign matter that may initiate an inflammatory response. This type of wound normally heals spontaneously. An incision is a clean, straight-edged wound that goes through all layers of skin; it bleeds freely and heals cleanly when sutured. Puncture or stab wounds are deeper than they are wide and are caused by knives, pins, needles, spikes, and so forth. Underlying structures may be damaged, with concealed blood loss. A laceration is a cut or tear of tissues and is unlikely to heal without treatment [21].

In all traumatic skin wounds, tissue viability is critical and is dependent upon circulation of blood to the area. All open traumatic wounds are contaminated and host resistance must be supported [19]. The stages of wound healing, discussed in Chapter 9, involve a characteristic inflammatory response initiated by vasoconstriction that decreases bleeding. This is followed by vasodilatation and increased vascular permeability leaking plasma proteins into the wound. The final stage involves neutrophilic leukocytes that destroy bacteria [5]. This produces pus and suppuration of surrounding tissues. If the affected tissue can totally regenerate, it replaces the necrotic tissue. Scar formation may become necessary to bridge an area of tissue destruction.

Study Questions

1. How do the manifestations of viruses in the skin differ from those of bacteria?
2. Compare the cause, course of disease, and prognosis of the three types of malignant skin lesions.
3. Discuss the manifestations of burn injury as related to location, extent, and complications that can develop.
4. How does edema result from burn injury? How can this produce burn shock?
5. Describe the pathophysiology of electrical shock with direct and alternating currents.
6. What are the major factors that precipitate the formation of decubitus ulcers?
7. Describe the process of skin healing from trauma or burns. (Hint: Use Chapter 9 to clarify the process.)

References

1. Arndt, K. *Manual of Dermatologic Therapeutics* (3rd ed.). Boston: Little, Brown, 1983.
2. Brodzka, W., Thornhill, H.L., and Howard, S. Burns: Causes and risk factors. *Arch. Phys. Med. Rehabil.* 66(11):746, 1985.
3. *Bermuda Symposium on the Diagnosis and Management of Dry Skin*. New York: Chesebrough-Ponds, 1984.
4. Constantian, M.B. *Pressure Ulcers: Principles and Techniques of Management*. Boston: Little, Brown, 1980.
5. Cuono, C.B. Physiology of wound healing. In F.J. Daghar (ed.), *Cutaneous Wounds*. Mt. Kisco, N.Y.: Futura, 1985.

6. Demling, R.H., et al. Early lung dysfunction after major burns: Role of edema and vasoactive mediators. *J. Trauma* 25(10):959, 1985.
7. Elder, D.E., and Clark, W.H. Malignant melanoma. In B.H. Thiers and R.L. Dobson (eds.), *Pathogenesis of Skin Disease*. New York: Churchill Livingstone, 1986.
8. Hunt, J.L. Electrical injuries of the upper extremity. In R. Salisbury and B. Pruitt (eds.), *Burns of the Upper Extremity*. Philadelphia: Saunders, 1976.
9. Kagan, R.J., et al. Serious wound infections in burned patients. *Surgery* 98(4)10:640, 1985.
10. Lang, P.C. Nonmelanoma skin cancer. In B.H. Thiers and R.L. Dobson (eds.), *Pathogenesis of Skin Disease*. New York: Churchill Livingstone, 1986.
11. Levene, G.M., and Calnan, D.C. *Color Atlas of Dermatology*. Chicago: Yearbook, 1974.
12. Moschella, S.L., Pillsbury, D.M., and Hurley, H.J. *Dermatology* (2nd ed.). Philadelphia: Saunders, 1985.
13. Munster, A.M., and Ciccone, T.G. Burns. In F.J. Daghar (ed.), *Cutaneous Wounds*. Mt. Kisco, N.Y.: Futura, 1985.
14. Nicher, L.S., et al. Improving the accuracy of burn-surface estimation. *Plastic Reconstr. Surg.* 76(3)9:425, 1985.
15. Reuler, J., and Cooney, T.G. The pressure sore: Pathophysiology and principles of management. *Ann. Intern. Med.* 94:661, 1981.
16. Robbins, S.L., Cotran, R.S., and Kumar, V. *Pathologic Basis of Disease* (3rd ed.). Philadelphia: Saunders, 1984.
17. Salisbury, R.E., and Pruitt, B.A. *Burns of the Upper Extremity*. Philadelphia: Saunders, 1976.
18. Sauer, G.C. *Manual of Skin Diseases* (5th ed.). Philadelphia: Lippincott, 1985.
19. Shack, R.B., and Manson, P.N. Traumatic wounds. In F.J. Daghar (ed.), *Cutaneous Wounds*. Mt. Kisco, N.Y.: Futura, 1985.
20. Soter, N.A., and Baden, H.P. (eds.). *Pathophysiology of Dermatologic Diseases*. New York: McGraw-Hill, 1984.
21. Spittell, A.J. *Clinical Medicine*. Hagerstown, Md.: Harper & Row, 1982.
22. Steuber, K., and Spence, R.J. Pressure sores. In F.J. Daghar (ed.), *Cutaneous Wounds*. Mt. Kisco, N.Y.: Futura, 1985.

Unit Bibliography

Arndt, K. *Manual of Dermatologic Therapeutics* (3rd ed.). Boston: Little, Brown, 1983.

Balinsky, B.I. *An Introduction to Embryology* (5th ed.). Philadelphia: Saunders, 1981.

Baur, P.S., Parks, D.H., and Larson, D.L. The healing of burn wounds. *Clin. Plast. Surg.* 4:389, 1977.

Bickley, H. *Practical Concepts in Human Disease* (2nd ed.). Baltimore: Williams & Wilkins, 1980.

Binnick, S.A. *Skin Diseases: Diagnosis and Management in Clinical Practice*. Menlo Park, Calif.: Addison-Wesley, 1982.

Bryant, W. Wound healing. *Clin. Symp.* 29:1, 1977.

Carpenter, N.H., Gates, D.J., and Williams, H.T. Normal processes and restraints in wound healing. *Can. J. Surg.* 20:315, 1977.

Cohen, I.K., and Diegelmann, R.F. The biology of keloid and hypertrophic scars and influence of corticosteroids. *Clin. Plast. Surg.* 4:297, 1977.

Daghar, F.J. (ed.). *Cutaneous Wounds*. Mt. Kisco, N.Y.: Futura, 1985.

Dobson, R.L., and Abele, D.C. *The Practice of Dermatology*. Philadelphia: Harper & Row, 1985.

Domonkos, A.N., Arnold, H.L., and Odom, R.B. *Andrews' Diseases of the Skin*. Philadelphia: Saunders, 1982.

Epstein, E. *Controversies in Dermatology*. Philadelphia: Saunders, 1984.

Fry, L., Wojnaroska, F.T., and Shahrad, P. *Illustrated Encyclopedia of Dermatology*. Oradell, N.J.: Medical Economics, 1985.

Goldsmith, L.A. *Biochemistry and Physiology of the Skin*. New York: Oxford University Press, 1983.

Guyton, A.C. *Textbook of Medical Physiology*. (7th ed.). Philadelphia: Saunders, 1986.

Hayes, H., Jr. A review of modern concepts of healing of cutaneous wounds. *J. Dermatol. Surg. Oncol.* 3:188, 1977.

Kaplan, E.N. *Emergency Management of Skin and Soft Tissue Wounds*. Boston: Little, Brown, 1984.

Ketchum, L.D. Hypertrophic scars and keloids. *Clin. Plast. Surg.* 4:301, 1977.

Larson, C., and Gould, M. *Orthopedic Nursing* (9th ed.). St. Louis: Mosby, 1978.

Levene, G.M., and Calnan, D.C. *Color Atlas of Dermatology*. Chicago: Yearbook, 1974.

Levenson, S.M., and Seifter, E. Dysnutrition, wound healing, and resistance to infection. *Clin. Plast. Surg.* 4:375, 1977.

Lookingbill, D.P., and Marks, J.G. *Principles of Dermatology*. Philadelphia: Saunders, 1986.

Montandon, D., D'Andrian, G., and Gabbiani, G. The mechanism of wound contraction and epithelialization. *Clin. Plast. Surg.* 4:325, 1977.

Moschella, S., Pillsbury, D., and Hurley, H. *Dermatology* (2nd ed.). Philadelphia: Saunders, 1985.

Robbins, S.L., Cotran, R.S., and Kumar, V. *Pathologic Basis of Disease* (3rd ed.). Philadelphia: Saunders, 1984.

Rosen, K., Lanning, M., and Hill, M. *The Nurse's Atlas of Dermatology*. Boston: Little, Brown, 1983.

Salisbury, R., and Pruitt, B. *Burns of the Upper Extremity*. Philadelphia: Saunders, 1976.

Sana, J., and Judge, R. *Physical Assessment Skills for Nursing Practice*. Boston: Little, Brown, 1982.

Sauer, G.C. *Manual of Skin Diseases* (5th ed.). Philadelphia: Lippincott, 1985.

Solomons, B.E. *Lecture Notes on Dermatology* (5th ed.). Oxford: Blackwell, 1983.

Soter, N.A., and Baden, H.P. (eds.). *Pathophysiology of Dermatologic Diseases*. New York: McGraw-Hill, 1984.

Spittell, J.A. *Clinical Medicine*. Hagerstown, Md.: Harper & Row, 1982.

Wachtel, T.L., and Frank, D.H. *Burns of the Head and Neck*. Philadelphia: Saunders, 1984.

Williams, D.F., and Harrison, I.D. The variation of mechanical properties in different areas of a healing wound. *J. Biomech.* 10:633, 1977.

UNIT 15

Neural Control

Reet Henze / *Nervous System*

Cheryl Bean / *Pain*

The nervous system is incredibly complex and must be approached from an adequate basic knowledge of neural control. This approach considers the complicated system of connections and interconnections that allow for perception and movement. Through the advanced nervous system, individuals are capable of complicated thought and reasoning powers. This unit attempts to discuss neural pathology in sufficient depth for understanding without requiring a complete textbook on the topic.

Chapter 44 begins the discussion with the normal structure and function of the nervous system. Chapter 45 adds the normal and altered functions of the special senses. Chapter 46 details some alterations that affect higher cortical functions, especially cerebrovascular accident, aphasia, agnosia, and epilepsy. Chapter 47, which covers the physiologic phenomenon of pain, is adapted from material in *Trauma Nursing* by E. Howell, L. Widra, and G. Hill. Chapters 48, 49, and 50 detail traumatic alterations, tumors and infections, and degenerative alterations, respectively. Each chapter presents specific diagnostic tests that may be helpful in delineating these alterations.

The most useful approach to the nervous system is to show how alterations in specific areas can disrupt function. Frequently, the location of the alterations rather than their size finally determines the degree of functional difficulty. The reader is again encouraged to use the learning objectives to organize study and to acquire a firm grasp of the material in Chapter 44 before considering the pathophysiology of the nervous system. Study questions at the end of each chapter provide an opportunity to assess synthesis of chapter content. The unit bibliography provides further resources for learning.

CHAPTER 44

Normal Structure and Function of the Central and Peripheral Nervous Systems

CHAPTER OUTLINE

The Neuron

- Peripheral Axon Degeneration and Regeneration

Excitation and Conduction in Neurons

- Membrane Potential
- Resting Potential
- Action Potential
- Characteristics of the Action Potential
- Conduction Velocity in Nerve Fibers
- Factors Increasing Membrane Excitability
- Factors Decreasing Membrane Excitability

Receptors

- Characteristics of Receptors
- Receptor Potential

The Synapse

- Events at the Chemical Synapse
- Facilitation
- Presynaptic Inhibition
- Divergence and Convergence
- Neurochemical Transmitter Substances

The Central Nervous System

- Phylogenetic Development
- Protective Coverings of the Brain and Spinal Cord
- The Spinal Cord Processing System
  - *Reflex Arc*
- Low-Brain Processing System (Rhombencephalon)
  - *Medulla Oblongata*
  - *Pons*
  - *Cerebellar Processing*
- Midbrain Processing System (Mesencephalon)
- Diencephalon Processing System
  - *Thalamic Processing*
  - *Hypothalamic Processing*
  - *Basal Ganglia Processing*
- Forebrain (Prosencephalon)

The Peripheral Nervous System

- Afferent (Sensory) Division
- Efferent (Motor) Division
  - *Pyramidal and Extrapyramidal Systems*

The Autonomic Nervous System

- Sympathetic Division (Thoracolumbar)
- Parasympathetic Division (Craniosacral)
- Transmitter Substances of the Autonomic Nervous System
- Receptor Substances of the Effector Organs
- Stimulation and Inhibition of the Autonomic Nervous System
- Effects of Sympathetic and Parasympathetic Stimulation on Various Structures
  - *Lacrimal Glands*
  - *Eyes*
  - *Salivary Glands*
  - *Heart*
  - *Bronchi*
  - *Esophagus*
  - *Abdominal Viscera, Glands, and Vessels*
  - *Pelvic Viscera*
  - *Peripheral Vessels and Sweat Glands*
  - *Adrenal Medulla*
  - *Autonomic Reflexes*

The Ventricular and Cerebrospinal Fluid Systems

- Function of Cerebrospinal Fluid
- Formation and Absorption of Cerebrospinal Fluid
- Flow and Obstruction of Flow of Cerebrospinal Fluid
- Brain Barriers

Brain Blood Supply and Regulation

- Arterial and Venous Circulation
- Autoregulation and Vasomotor Control

LEARNING OBJECTIVES

1. Identify the components of the neuron.
2. Describe variations in neuron morphology.
3. Classify neurons according to function.
4. Explain the events occurring with axon injury and regeneration.
5. Define *membrane potential*.
6. Discuss the events of the action potential.
7. List the major types of nerve fibers and their characteristics.
8. Identify factors that influence conduction velocity in nerve fibers.
9. Identify factors that increase neuron membrane excitability.
10. Identify factors that decrease neuron membrane excitability.
11. Define *sensory receptors*.
12. Explain types of sensory receptors.
13. Discuss the phenomenon of receptor adaptation.
14. Contrast receptor potential and generator potential.
15. Define *synapse*.
16. Discuss the events occurring at the chemical synapse.
17. Discuss characteristics of neurotransmitters.
18. List the major structures of the central nervous system in hierarchic order from spinal cord to cerebral cortex.
19. Identify the major functions of the central nervous system structures.
20. Trace the major ascending and descending spinal tracts.
21. Identify the major information transmitted by the ascending and descending spinal tracts.
22. List the components of the peripheral nervous system.
23. Differentiate between structure and function of the somatic efferent and the visceral efferent fibers.
24. Contrast the functions of the sympathetic and parasympathetic divisions of the autonomic nervous system.
25. Differentiate between adrenergic and cholinergic effector organs.
26. Describe the function, formation, and flow of cerebrospinal fluid.
27. Discuss the function of the blood-brain barrier.
28. List the major arteries supplying blood to the brain.
29. Discuss the factors responsible for a constant cerebral blood supply in the healthy brain.

Humans interact with the environment through the nervous system, perceiving and responding to the stimuli that continually impinge on them. A complex system of connections and interconnections of nerve cells provides this perception, interim processing, and response. In addition, characteristics that endow humans with the ability to think, feel, reason, and remember evolve from these interacting neuronal networks of the brain.

The Neuron

The neuron is the structural and functional unit of nerve tissue, having the capability to generate and conduct electrochemical impulses (Fig. 44-1). Its cellular and cytoplasmic components and metabolic activities that maintain cell life are similar to those of other cells. The distinctive cellular shapes of neurons and their structural synapses

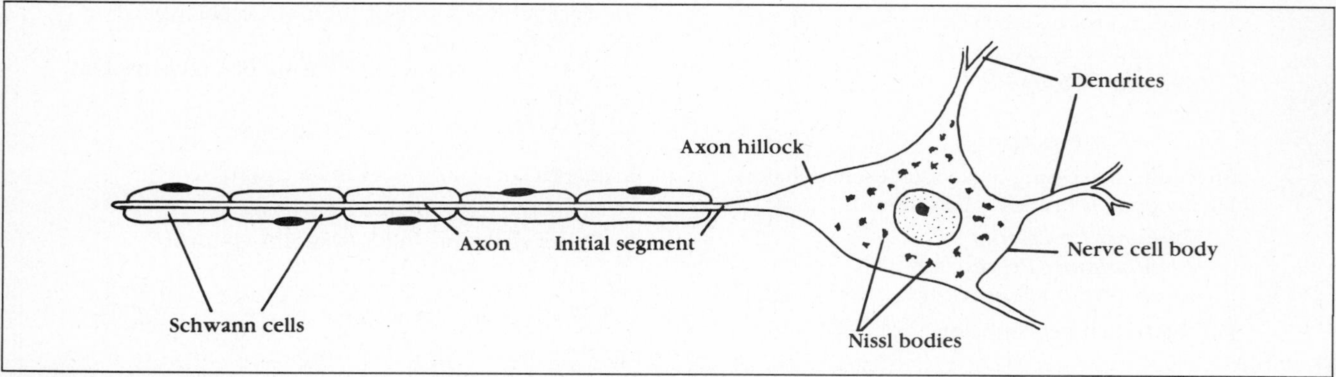

FIGURE 44-1 Neuron with myelinated axon. (From M. Borysenko et al., *Functional Histology* [2nd ed.]. Boston: Little, Brown, 1984.)

that allow transmission of impulses from one to another are unique to the nerve cells. Unlike other cells, mature neurons are unable to reproduce themselves. They lack centrosomes and therefore, are incapable of mitosis; if the cell body dies, the entire neuron dies. Under certain circumstances, however, *axons*, the processes of peripheral nerves, regenerate if the cell body is preserved.

Incoming signals to the neuron may be transmitted to dendrites directly by the cell body or to the axon by the axon of another neuron. The area of contact between neurons is known as the *synapse* (Fig. 44-2). Dendrites, together with the cell body, contain *Nissl bodies*, which synthesize cell protein and contain much of the ribonucleic acid (RNA) of the cytoplasm. Small vesicles and cisterns known as *Golgi apparatus* are present in the neuron and are thought to be involved in secreting neurotransmitters at the synapse [12].

A fibrous *axon*, or nerve fiber, originates from the *axon hillock* of the cell body (perikaryon) and transmits signals from the cell body to various parts of the nervous system. These long fibers differ from dendrites in their branching and in composition of their outer membrane. Some axons are myelinated while others have no myelin sheath. Myelin is a fatty layer that surrounds the nerve fiber and helps increase conduction of nerve impulses. The *myelin sheath* is interrupted by periodic gaps known as the *nodes of Ranvier*. Axon collaterals or fibers may emerge from these gaps. Exchange of metabolites takes place between the axon and the extracellular environment at the nodes. The nodes of Ranvier are present in both central and peripheral nervous system neurons; however, they are much easier to identify in the peripheral nervous system. *Schwann cells* are located along the peripheral axons and produce the myelin sheath of lipoprotein that encases the fiber. Some of these cells produce numerous concentric wrappings around the central core axon and give the axon its characteristic white color (Fig. 44-3). Unmyelinated fibers contain Schwann cells but lack the concentric wrappings. The outermost thin layer of myelin of the myelinated fibers is known as the *neurolemma* of the axon. This neurolemma is lacking in the myelinated fibers within the spinal cord and brain. Myelin provides protective, nutritive, and conductive functions for the axon.

In the central nervous system, *glial cells*, constituent cells to the neurons, protect, nourish, and support the neurons. Collectively, they are referred to as *neuroglia*. *Astrocytes*, *oligodendroglia*, *microglia*, and *ependymal*

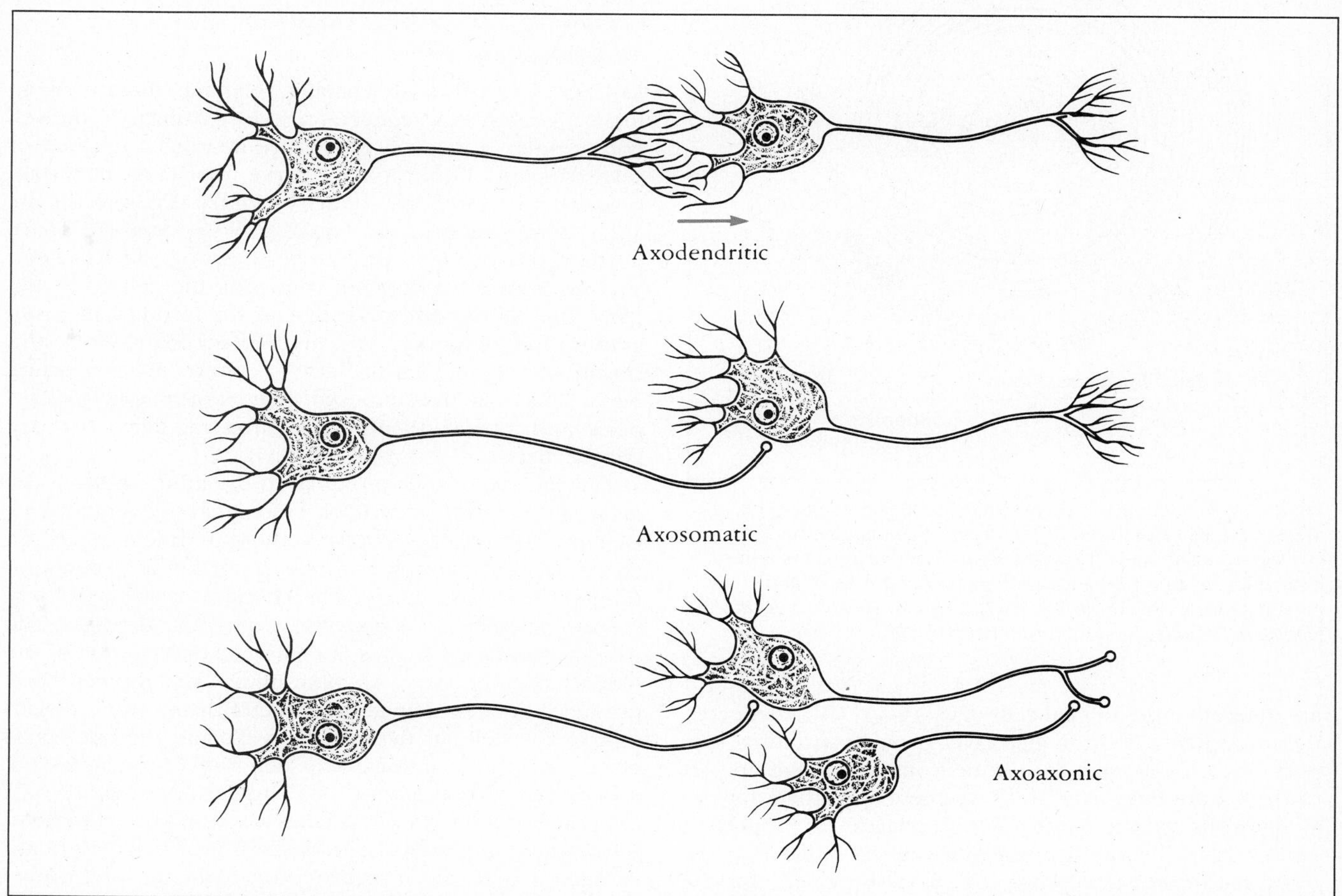

FIGURE 44-2 Examples of various types of synaptic connections. (From R.S. Snell, *Clinical Neuroanatomy for Medical Students*. Boston: Little, Brown, 1980.)

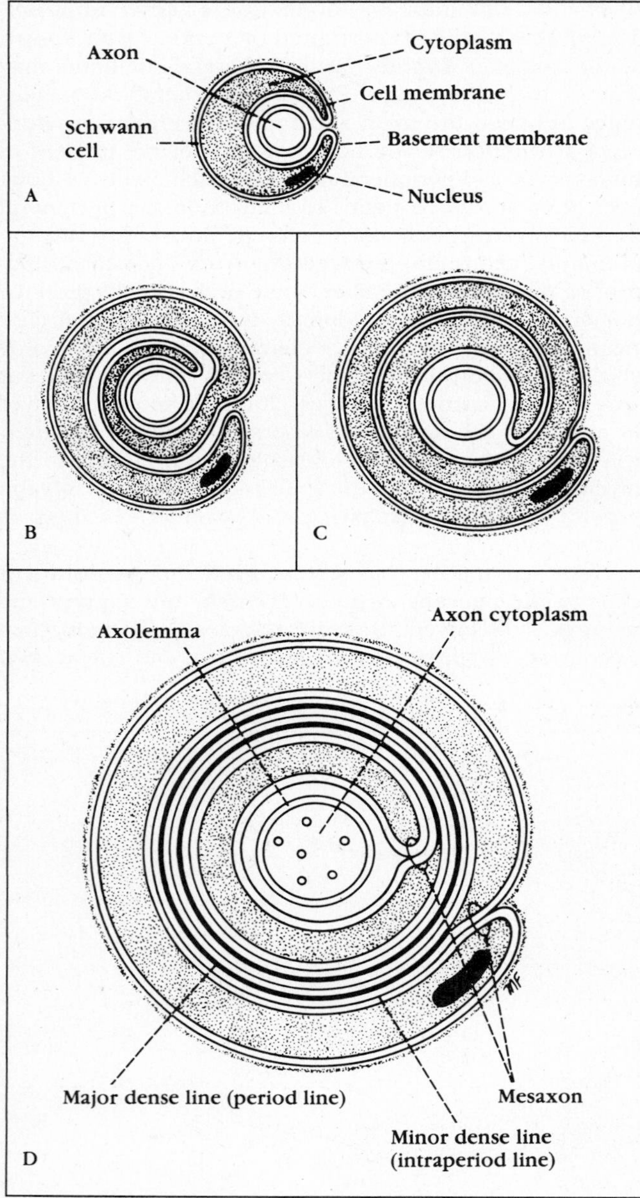

FIGURE 44-3 Schematic representation of evolution of the myelin sheath of an axon: (A) Schwann cell engulfs the axon, (B) surrounds it, and (C) wraps tight concentric layers around it (myelin sheath); (D) appearance of a mature axon and myelinated sheath. (From R.S. Snell, *Clinical Neuroanatomy for Medical Students*. Boston: Little, Brown, 1980.)

are different types of glial cells (Fig. 44-4) [10]. Astrocytes, the most plentiful of the glial cells, provide structural support, and nourishment for the neurons, and make up part of the blood-brain barrier. Oligodendroglia form myelin along axons and the microglia have phagocytic properties. Ependymal cells line the ventricles of the brain and central canal of the spinal cord, and in part, provide for the brain-cerebrospinal fluid barrier.

The billions of neurons in the nervous system may be identified according to their *morphology* and *function*. A variety of projections may arise from the body of the cell (Fig. 44-5).

Neurons can also be classified according to their general function. Sensory (*afferent*) neurons relay messages about internal and external body environmental changes to the central nervous system. Motor and secretory (*efferent*) neurons transmit messages from the central nervous system. Association (*internuncial* or *interneurons*) neurons relay messages from one neuron to another within the brain and spinal cord. The following diagram shows the relationship of the afferent, association, and efferent neurons and their fibers as sensations are perceived from the somatic and visceral tissue and transmitted to glands and muscles.

CNS

Somatic visceral tissue → Afferent fibers → [Interneurons] → Efferent fibers → Glands, muscles

Clusters of neurons within the central nervous system are called *nuclei*, or *gray matter*. Groups of neurons outside the central nervous system are known as *ganglia* (see page 736–737).

Peripheral Axon Degeneration and Regeneration

As long as its cell body remains relatively unharmed, an injured neuron may regenerate. Serious damage to the cell body results in death of the entire neuron. A crushed or severed axon of a peripheral nerve fiber triggers certain processes within a few hours of injury. Changes in the axon distal to the injury (*wallerian degeneration*) are particularly dramatic, because that portion has been severed from the metabolic control of the cell body. Initially, the distal portion swells and the terminal neurofilaments hypertrophy. The myelin sheath shrinks and retracts at the nodes of Ranvier where the remaining nerve fiber becomes exposed. The axon gradually disappears and myelin disintegrates into fragments that are phagocytized.

Changes also occur proximal to the injury, both in the axon and the cell body itself (retrograde degeneration). Degenerative changes similar to those in the distal portion of the axon occur at the proximal portion for a few millimeters from the injury. The changes in the cell body (chromatolysis) are in response to repair of damages. The extent of cellular changes is related to the location of the injury along the axon. An axon injury near the cell body produces greater changes in the cell than a more distant injury. The cellular cytoplasm swells and the nucleus is eccentrically placed toward the cell wall. Chromatolysis of basophilic substances (Nissl bodies), suggestive of increased protein synthesis, takes place and the number of mitochondria increases. Injured neurofibrils (delicate threads projecting into the axon from the cell body) attempt to grow back into their original placements and begin sprouting from the proximal portion of the injured axon within 7 to 14 days after injury. If the fibrils are suc-

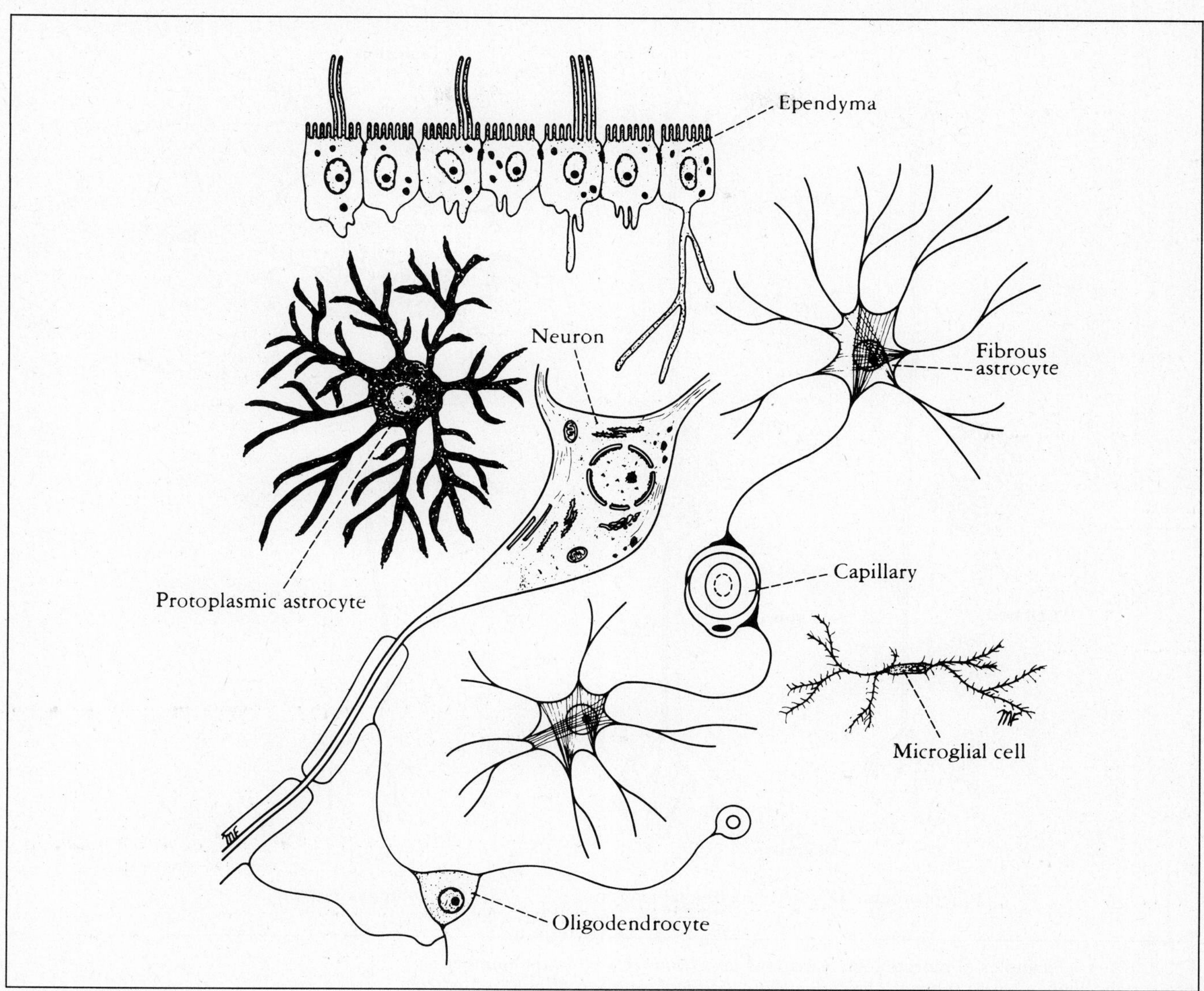

FIGURE 44-4 Different types of neuroglial cells. (From R.S. Snell, *Clinical Neuroanatomy for Medical Students*. Boston: Little, Brown, 1980.)

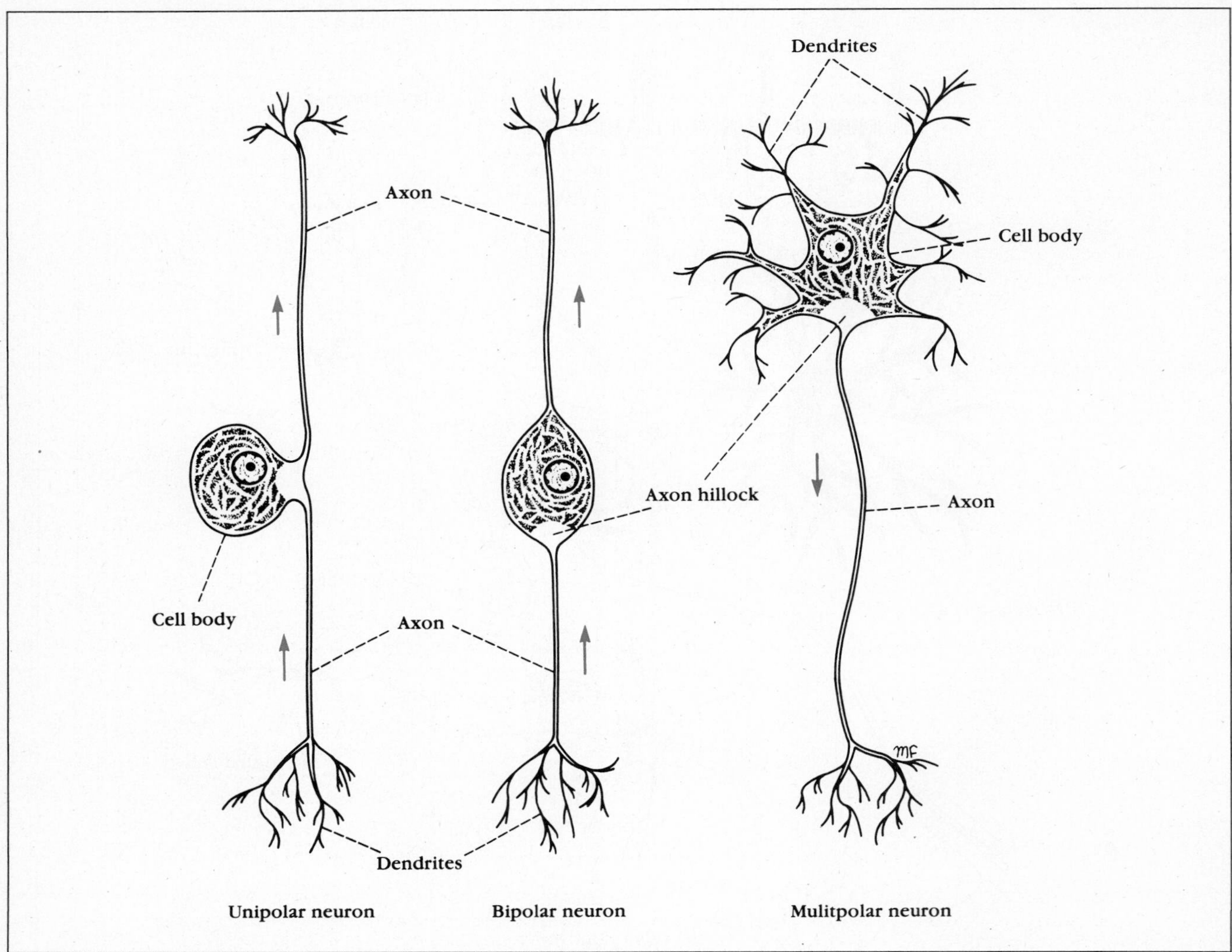

FIGURE 44-5 Examples of morphologic variations in neurons related to the number of projections evolving from the cell. (From R.S. Snell, *Clinical Neuroanatomy for Medical Students*. Boston: Little, Brown, 1980.)

cessful in finding their way into the neurolemma, they grow at a rate of 3 to 4 mm per day. The remaining Schwann cells form a sheet of myelin around the restored neurofibril, and the nodes of Ranvier are reformed as the nerve regenerates. Regeneration of injured nerves in the central nervous system is more difficult due to glial scarring, which frequently inhibits new fibrils from reaching their destinations.

Excitation and Conduction in Neurons

Membrane Potential

Membrane potentials are generated because of a disparity between cations and anions at the semipermeable cell membrane. Specific proteins at the cell membrane allow the movement of ions and facilitate the existence of the nerve cell potential and impulse propagation. These proteins include *cell membrane pumps* and *channels*. Pumps maintain appropriate ion concentrations in the cell side of the membrane by actively moving these ions against concentration gradients. Channel proteins provide selective paths for specific ions to diffuse across the cell membrane.

Resting Potential

During the resting potential the inner cell wall surface is negatively charged in relation to the positively charged outer surface (Fig. 44-6). The extracellular fluid has a higher sodium concentration than the intracellular fluid, whereas potassium concentration is higher within the cell. The inside of the cell also contains anions that are too large to pass across the cell membrane. These attract the positively charged sodium ions, some of which leak through the sodium channels. Should this movement continue unchecked, the influx of positively charged ions into

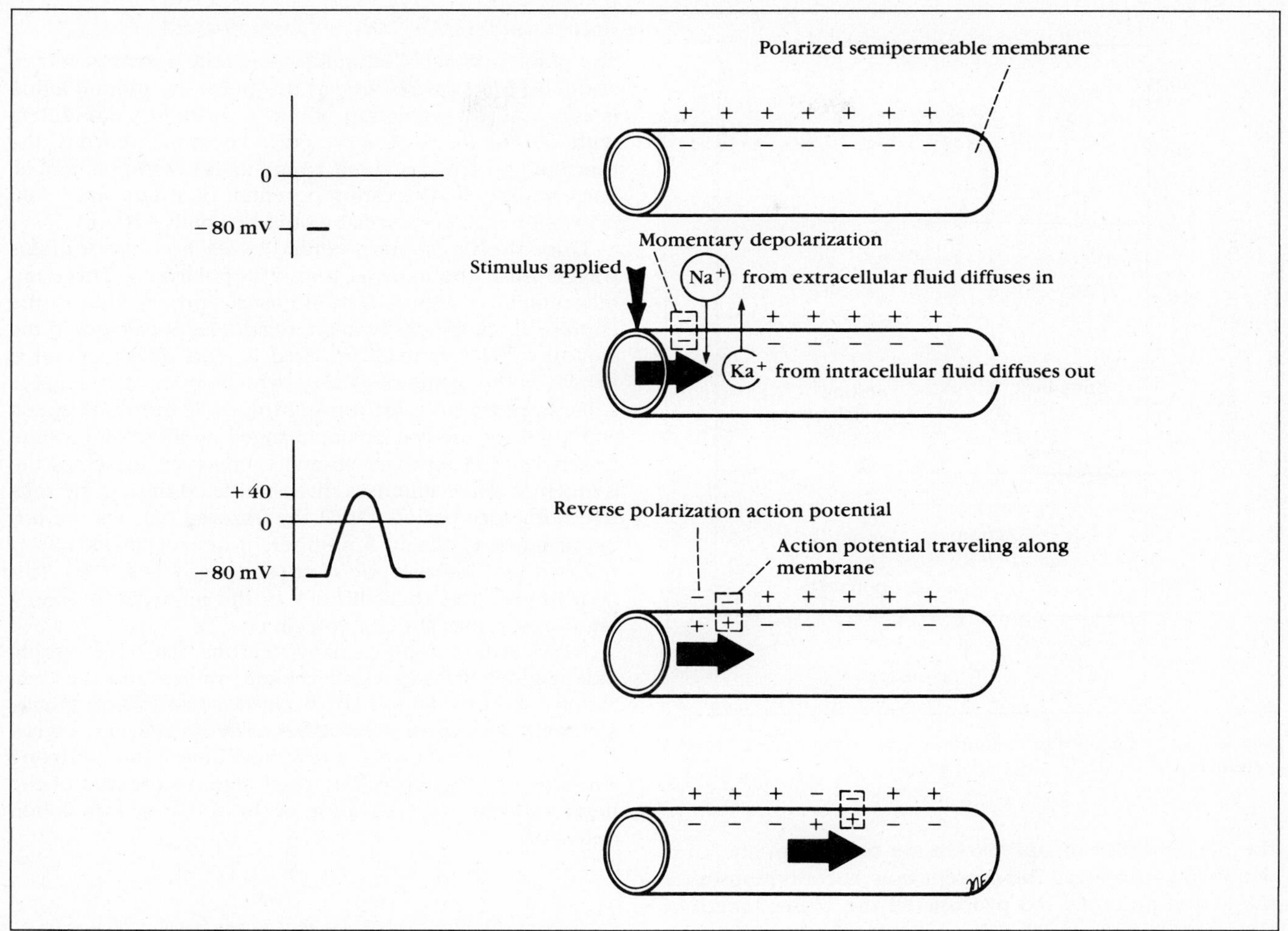

FIGURE 44-6 Summary of electrical changes occurring in the axon during an action potential. (From R.S. Snell, *Clinical Neuroanatomy for Medical Students*. Boston: Little, Brown, 1980.)

the cell would soon result in electroneutrality in the cell. To counterbalance this diffusion of ions, a strong active transport system (sodium pump) pumps out sodium that has leaked into the cell (see Chap. 1).

The resting membrane is more permeable to potassium ions, which results in a higher intracellular concentration of potassium ions. This higher concentration is maintained through passive movement of potassium and its attraction to the negative interior. A weaker potassium pump moves some potassium into the cell. Due to the higher intracellular concentration, some diffusion of potassium out of the cell occurs continuously. This movement of potassium from the cell leaves more negatively charged ions than positively charged ions in the cell [12]. Also contributing to the imbalance of charges at the cell membrane is a strong sodium pump that moves more sodium out of the cell than potassium is moved into the cell by the potassium pump. The inner surface remains electronegative and maintains a resting potential of approximately −70 to −90 mV. In this state the cell is said to be *polarized*. Lacking a stimulus, the resting potential can remain unchanged for a long period of time.

Action Potential

Unique to nerve, muscle, and gland cells is the change that can occur in a resting cell membrane potential when the cells are stimulated by electrical, chemical, or mechanical means. These stimuli can produce a sudden increase in cell membrane permeability to sodium, which results in a very brief, positive potential within the cell.

The sequence of physiochemical events that results in an alteration in the resting potential lasts a few millesec-onds (msec) and is called the action potential (see Fig. 44-6). In response to a stimulus, the cell membrane becomes much more permeable to sodium ions that rush into the cell through the opened sodium channels and cause the initial spike potential (Fig. 44-7). Due to the positive charges carried into the cell by sodium, a change in voltage occurs inside the cell from approximately −70 mV at resting potential to about +40 mV at the height of the spike. This phase of the action potential is identified as *depolarization*, is self-propagating, and travels in both directions along the entire fiber (Fig. 44-8). As the current flows along the adjoining resting membrane, it increases

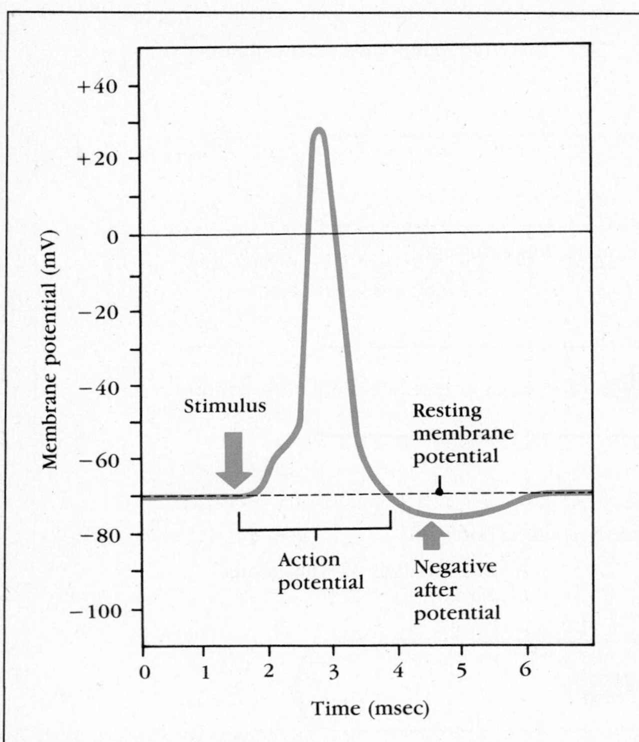

FIGURE 44-7 Changes in membrane potential during an action potential.

the permeability of the membrane to sodium and thus depolarizes this area. The current flow is continuous until the action potential has propagated the entire length of the axon, very much as a flame travels the fuse of a firecracker [11].

The influx of sodium is limited because permeability of the cell membrane to sodium is transient and the channels formerly open to it are closed. During a very brief time, called the *absolute refractory period*, the nerve cell responds to no further stimulus. After the absolute refractory period, the *relative refractory period* occurs during which time the cell gradually resumes its excitability and is able to respond to stronger than normal stimuli. As sodium permeability decreases, potassium permeability increases, and there is an efflux of potassium from the cell, resulting in a transient increase in extracellular potassium. This is reflected by the negative afterpotential (after-depolarization) shown in Figure 44-7. The efflux of potassium after the spike potential allows the inside of the cell to become more negative once again (after-hyperpolarization) [12]. The period of return to original potential is called the *repolarization phase*. The cell membrane becomes less permeable to potassium and the sodium pump transports sodium out of the cell. This pump is reflected by a positive afterpotential. Finally, potassium shifts into the cell through both membrane channels and pumps, returning the fiber to its resting potential [5].

Characteristics of the Action Potential

The point at which a stimulus can excite a fiber is known as the *threshold potential*. At this point the sodium influx is equal to the potassium efflux. Threshold value differs with various types of nerve cells. For most neurons, the threshold potential is about 15 mV above resting potential. For example, if the resting potential of a neuron is −80 mV, its threshold potential would be about −65 mV.

Once the threshold potential is reached, the stimulus travels until the axon is totally depolarized. The commencement of depolarization ensures propagation of the impulse along the entire axon, regardless of changes in the stimulus that originally initiated it. This phenomenon is known as the *all-or-none law*, which applies to excitable cells. Impulse propagation continues at the same speed and intensity and remains unchanged by increasing stimulus intensity. A stronger stimulus, however, increases the frequency of the impulses that is initiated during the relative refractory period. Once the impulse reaches the terminal bouton, one of a number of neurotransmitters is released into the synaptic cleft (see pages 715–718). This neurotransmitter then diffuses to the postsynaptic membrane and brings about a voltage change.

Nerve trunks contain many neurons that have varying independent threshold and velocity values, and the total action potential, known as the *compound action potential*, may depend on the number of neurons firing. A weak stimulus activates only a few neurons, while a strong stimulus excites more. The total action potential of the nerve trunk is the summation of the active neuron action potentials.

Conduction Velocity in Nerve Fibers

The velocity of nerve conduction is influenced by the myelinization and diameter of the axon. Myelin acts as an effective insulator and inhibits electrochemical conduction. Therefore, the current passes over the myelin and through the extracellular fluid, and enters the nodes of Ranvier at 1-mm to 2-mm intervals where the membrane is permeable to the ions. This type of current propagation is known as *saltatory conduction*, implying a leaping or hopping phenomenon (see Fig. 44-8A).

The myelin sheath enhances the velocity of current conduction as capacitance is reduced, which results in reduced numbers of charges propagating the length of the fiber. The heavily myelinated large motor fibers transmit impulses at approximately 100 m per second. In contrast, small unmyelinated fibers may conduct impulses as slow as 0.5 m per second.

The diameter of the fiber is an additional important factor contributing to nerve conduction velocity. Velocity is increased in large-diameter nerve fibers due to lower internal resistance and a quicker depolarization time. Table 44-1 presents the relationship of sheathing and diameter to conduction velocities in various types of nerve fibers.

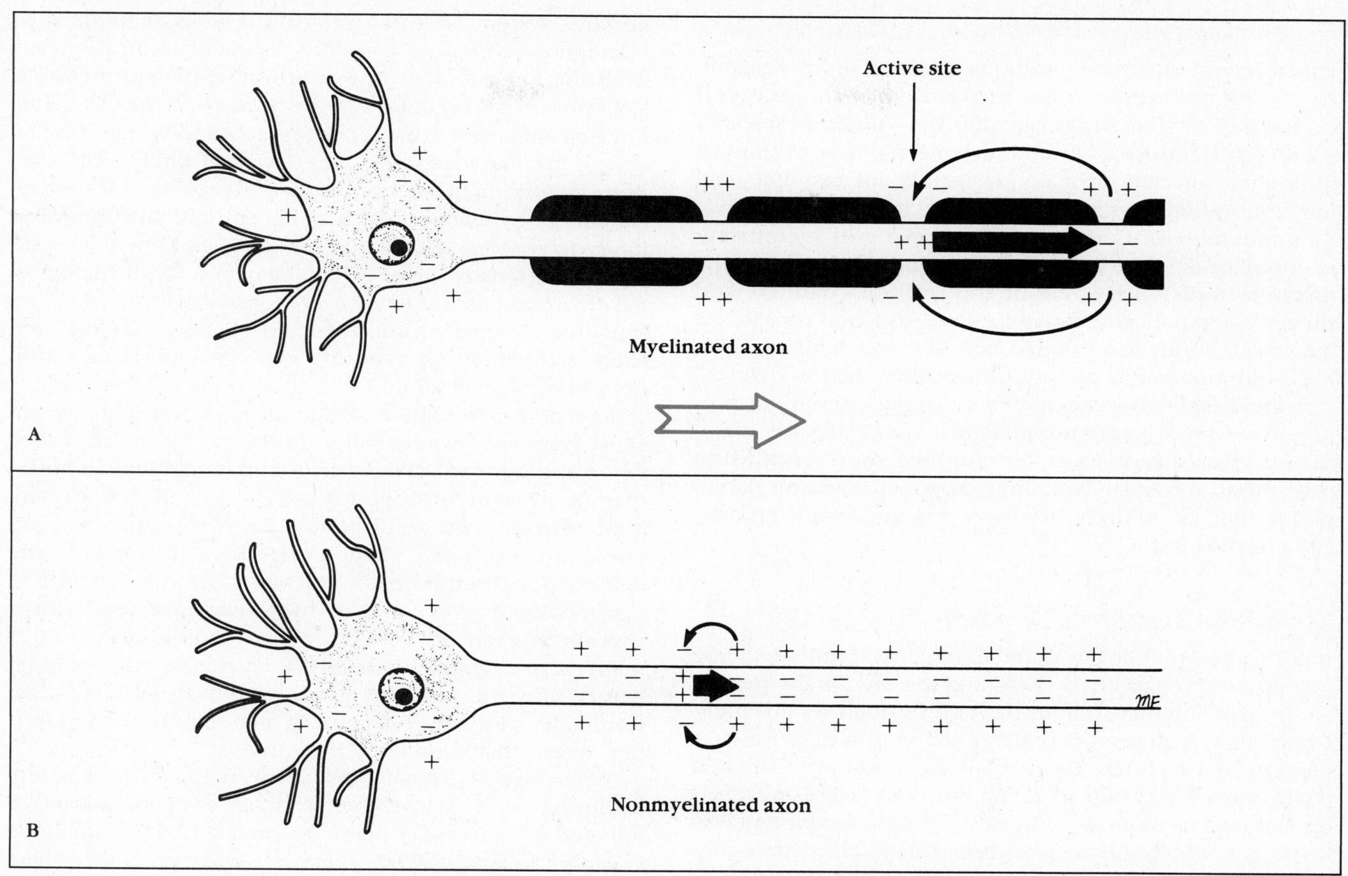

FIGURE 44-8 Propagation of the action potential along (A) myelinated and (B) unmyelinated axons. (From R.S. Snell, *Clinical Neuroanatomy for Medical Students*. Boston: Little, Brown, 1980.)

TABLE 44-1 Major Nerve Fiber Classification

Fiber type	Sheathing	Diameter (μm)	Conduction Speed (m/sec)	Function
A fibers				
Alpha α	Myelinated	10–18	60–120	Somatic motor, muscle proprioceptors
Beta β	Myelinated	5–10	38–70	Rapid sensory touch, pressure, kinesthesia
Gamma γ	Myelinated	1–5	15–45	Motor to muscle spindle, rapid sensory (touch, pressure)
Delta δ	Myelinated	2–5	5–30	Pain, temperature, pressure
B fibers	Thinly myelinated	3	3–15	Autonomic preganglionic transmission
C fibers	Unmyelinated	1–3	5–2	Autonomic postganglionic transmission

Factors Increasing Membrane Excitability

Extrinsic and intrinsic conditions affecting the permeability of the sodium ion can profoundly influence cell excitability. Certain drugs can alter the sodium permeability so that facilitory and inhibitory mechanisms of the cell no longer function normally. Diuretics, for example, can increase sodium loss and alter cell excitability.

A mechanism that increases nerve cell membrane excitability is low extracellular calcium level. Normally, calcium binds with some of the sodium channels and thereby reduces the movement of sodium across the membrane. With less calcium bound to the sodium channels, the movement of sodium becomes less restricted. The increased cell permeability to sodium results in progressively more excitable neuronal tissue. This is manifested clinically by a wide range of signs, including paresthesia, muscular twitching, carpopedal spasms, laryngeal stridor in children, bronchial spasms, tetanic spasms, and convulsions.

Factors Decreasing Membrane Excitability

Increased calcium levels in the extracellular fluid decrease membrane excitability by reducing the membrane permeability that inhibits sodium passage through its channels. Calcium has high protein-binding power as well as positive charges that facilitate its repulsion of sodium at the cell membrane. This results in an inhibitory or stabilizing effect on the cell membrane. Clinically, excess serum calcium levels are reflected by central nervous system depression.

Decreased levels of potassium in the extracellular fluids also decrease membrane excitability by increasing its resting potential. The resting potential is dependent on a constant concentration of potassium. A low extracellular potassium level is reflected clinically by depressed neuromuscular excitation, generalized weakness and fatigability of all muscles, diminished or absent reflexes, and paralytic ileus.

Local anesthetics such as lidocaine and tetracaine are other factors that can interfere with the initiation and transmission of the action potential. Depolarization is prevented by decreasing the membrane permeability to sodium, and the negative potential necessary for a propagated discharge does not develop or pass through the anesthetized area. The ease of achieving anesthesia is related to nerve fiber size. Small fibers associated with temperature and superficial pain sensations are most easily anesthetized. Large fibers that transmit sensation of deep pain, touch, and pressure are anesthetized with more difficulty.

Receptors

Characteristics of Receptors

Sensory receptors are specialized nerve cells that respond to specific information from the internal and external environments; the information is then transmitted by way of spinal or cranial nerves to specific areas of the central nervous system for interpretation. This is accomplished through conversion of various forms of natural energy from the environment into action potentials in neurons. Common to all receptors is this *transduction* of energy. Energy, converted by receptors, includes mechanical energy by *mechanoreceptors*, thermal energy by *thermoreceptors*, light energy by *photoreceptors*, and chemical energy by *chemoreceptors*. Receptors that respond to injury to physical and chemical tissues are known as *nociceptors*. *Exteroreceptors* give information about the external environment and *interoceptors* and *proprioceptors* are sensitive to internal impulses and changes. *Teleceptors*, such as those in the eyes and ears, provide information from more distant stimuli.

Receptor cells exhibit a wide range of morphologic and sensitivity differences (Fig. 44-9) [5]. Some have free nerve endings with coils, spirals, and branching networks; may be present throughout the body; and detect pain, cold, warmth, and crude touch. Some receptor cells are encased in variously shaped capsules and detect tissue deformation. Each receptor cell has adapted to respond to one specific type or modality of stimulus at a much lower threshold than do other receptors. This response is referred to as *adequate stimulus*. It remains the same no matter how the receptor is stimulated. Each nerve tract terminates at a specific point in the central nervous system where that stimulus is interpreted.

When a constant stimulus has been applied to a receptor for a period of time, the frequency of action potentials initiated in the sensory nerve decreases. This phenomenon is known as *adaptation*. There is a wide variation in sensory organ adaptation. The pressure applied to a pacinian corpuscle results in a receptor potential that adapts rapidly. The fast-adapting receptors are called *phasic* receptors. In contrast, the muscle spindles and receptors for pain adapt very slowly. These are known as *tonic* receptors.

Receptor Potential

The modalities of sensation are converted by specific receptors into electrical energy by action potentials through graded potential changes. The receptor responses are not an all-or-nothing event like the action potentials of neurons, but rather the magnitude is dependent on the intensity of the stimulus. As the magnitude of the stimulus is increased, the receptor potential increases. Receptor potentials are stationary, producing a local flow of current that spreads electrically to surrounding areas of the cell through a change of ionic conductance of the membrane of the nerve terminal. The ionic permeability change that initiates the receptor potential depends only on the stimulus, not on conductance changes through the function of the membrane potential as brought about in the action potentials. Because the receptor potential is not dependent on the membrane potential, it does not regenerate and remains stationary at the transducer area of the nerve terminal. If the receptor potential is great enough, the axon is depolarized and an action potential is triggered at the first node of Ranvier.

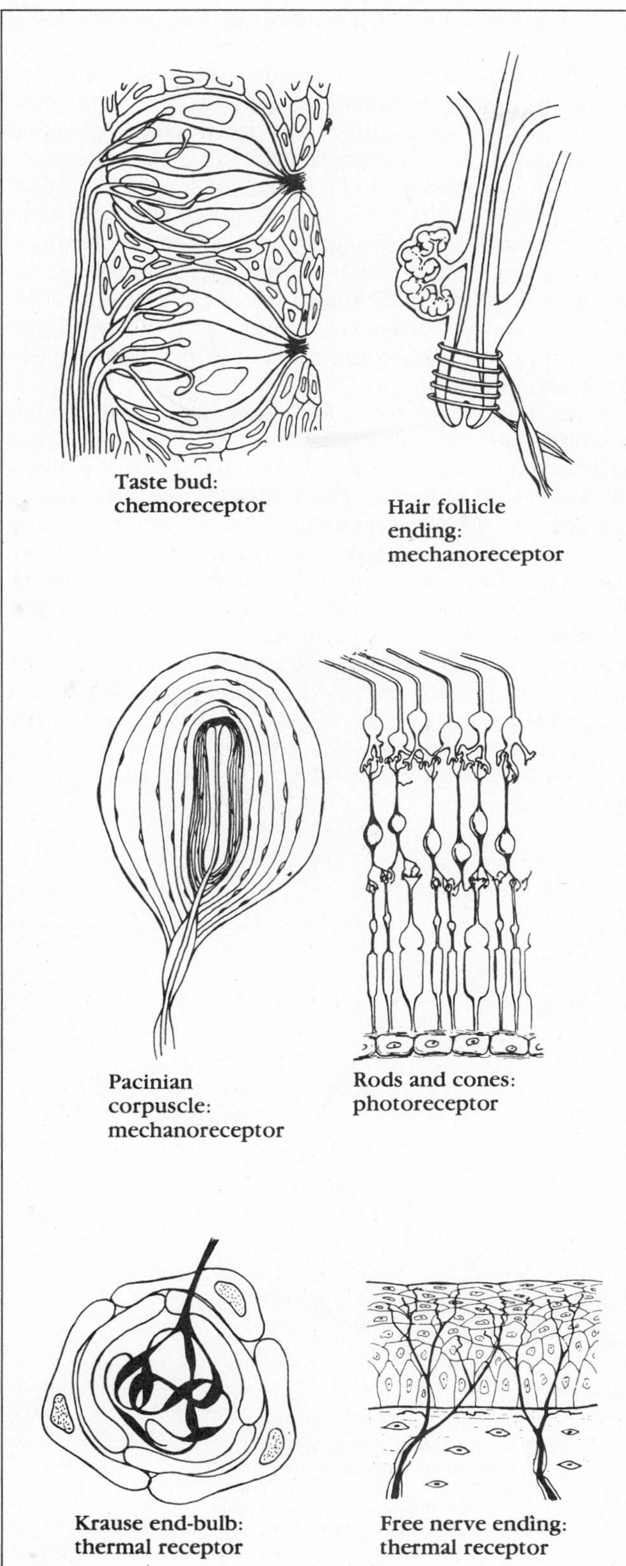

FIGURE 44-9 Examples of variation in morphologic composition of somatic sensory receptors. (From D.M. McKeough, *The Neuroscience Coloring Book*. Boston: Little, Brown, 1982.)

The mechanisms that generate receptor potentials vary with receptors [5]. For example, deformation generates receptor potential in the pacinian corpuscles, and chemicals initiate receptor potentials in the rods and cones of the eyes. Because most receptor terminals are minute in size and difficult to study, less information is available about their activity than about that of the action potentials.

The Synapse

Information concerning the environment is relayed through a succession of neurons in contact with each other. These areas of contact are known as *synapses*. The terminal portion of the presynaptic axon, the *bouton* or *knob*, may synapse with the cell body, dendrites, axons of other nerve cells, or effector cells of muscles or glands. Impulses at the synapse can be transmitted through chemical or electrical means. Chemical synapses, by far the most common, involve the release of a chemical substance (neurotransmitter) in response to a stimulus. This substance may have an excitatory or inhibitory effect on the postsynaptic cell membrane. The electrical synapses present in invertebrate and lower vertebrates are fused synapses to propagate uninterrupted impulses. The discussion here is limited to chemical synapses.

Electron microscopy has heightened our knowledge considerably of the synaptic characteristics and properties. The anatomic structure of synapses varies widely in different parts of the human nervous system. Similarly, numerous functional differences exist.

The presynaptic fiber terminates in an enlarged knob called the *synaptic bouton*, *knob*, *end-foot*, or *button*. This presynaptic bouton is divided from the postsynaptic membrane by a narrow cleft of about 200 to 300 angstoms (A) known as the *synaptic cleft*. The presynaptic bouton contains stored particles of a transmitter substance that is released at the synapse in response to a stimulus. Vesicles open and empty the transmitter substance that then excites or inhibits the postsynaptic neuron. Mitochondria in the presynaptic bouton provide adenosine triphosphate (ATP) for synthesizing the released substance that is continually regenerated. For example, the common transmitter substance acetylcholine is reduced to choline and acetic acid by the action of the enzyme cholinesterase. Choline and acetic acid are resorbed by the terminal bouton and, with the enzymatic assistance of choline acetylase, are resynthesized to acetylcholine, which is stored in the presynaptic vesicles until the next adequate stimulus.

Conduction of impulses through synapses is unidirectional. That is, impulses can be transmitted only through terminal boutons of presynaptic membranes to postsynaptic membranes.

Events at the Chemical Synapse

As previously noted, the presynaptic terminal bouton contains vesicles with packets of appropriate transmitter substances. A very low level of spontaneous release of this transmitter substance occurs in the resting synapse. This causes spontaneous mini-depolarizations at the synapse. When an action potential spreads to the presynaptic bouton, as shown in Figure 44-10, depolarization of the membrane triggers release of this transmitter substance. It is thought that the trigger release at the terminal bouton requires calcium ions. This theory is supported by observations that low extracellular calcium levels result in diminished amounts of transmitter substance being released. The neurotransmitter substance then attaches to the postsynaptic receptor sites and the postsynaptic membrane potential is modified. The neurotransmitter substance not taken up by the postsynaptic receptors may be taken up by the presynaptic bouton and stored or inactivated by monoamine oxidase (MAO). Some of the unattached neurotransmitter is inactivated at the synaptic cleft or at the postsynaptic membrane by enzymes. In addition, some of the free neurotransmitter is lost through extracellular diffusion.

The presynaptic release of an excitatory transmitter substance can initiate depolarizing response in the postsynaptic membrane that is referred to as the *excitatory postsynaptic potential* (EPSP) [4]. The EPSP is graded, nonpropagative, and the result of an increase in the permeability of the postsynaptic membrane to sodium, potassium, chloride, and calcium ions. Sodium ions flow in across the membrane and decrease the negativity of the postsynaptic cell. The threshold voltage change produced in a motoneuron during depolarization in an EPSP is approximately 13 mV, from a resting potential of −70 to −57 mV.

The activity of one terminal bouton is not significant enough to initiate an action potential in the postsynaptic cell. It requires many active terminals discharging spontaneously to elicit an action potential. This phenomenon is known as *summation* [11]. Thus, the amplitude of the EPSP depends on the number of activated synapses, and if sufficient numbers are firing, an action potential results.

It has been shown that threshold is lowest on the motoneuron at the axon hillock, and the thresholds of the cell body and dendrites are considerably higher. Therefore, action potentials initiated in most neurons originate in the axon hillock.

Some synapses release an inhibitory transmitter, thought to contain gamma-aminobutyric acid (GABA) at the postsynaptic membrane. This produces limited permeability to potassium and chloride. Potassium effluxes as chloride influxes, and no corresponding inflow of positive sodium ions occurs. This increases the negativity of the already negative postsynaptic cell, and a state of hyperpolarization results. This is called an *inhibitory postsynaptic potential (IPSP)* [4]. The permeability change is very brief as active transport of chloride out of the cell restores resting potential rapidly. Like the EPSP, the IPSP is graded and does not propagate. During the IPSP, the cell is less excitable as the membrane potential is more negative, and increased excitatory activity is needed to reach the threshold level.

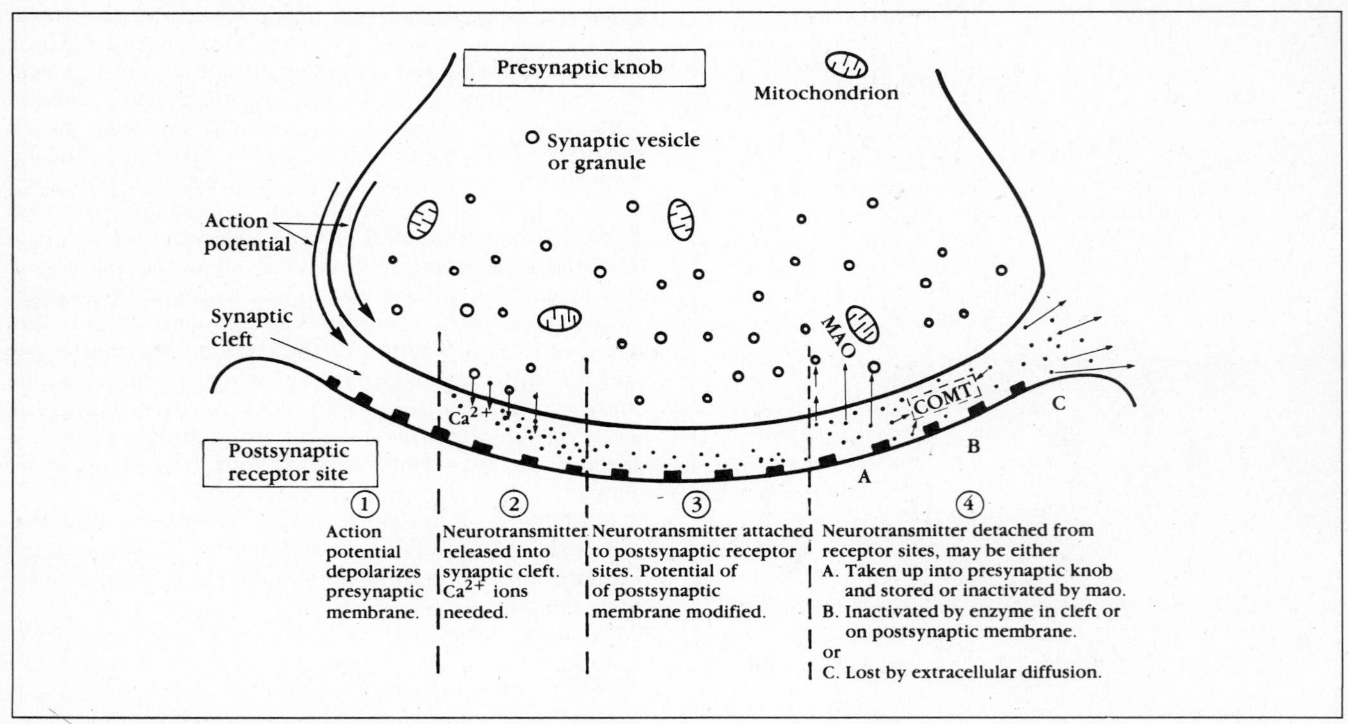

FIGURE 44-10 Events occurring at the chemical synapse. (From A. Lewis, *Mechanisms of Neurological Disease*. Boston: Little, Brown, 1976.)

Facilitation

Many presynaptic terminals converge on each postsynaptic neuron. A certain number of action potentials must be transmitted simultaneously for a sufficient amount of neurotransmitter to be released to produce an action potential in the postsynaptic membrane. If an insufficient amount of a neurotransmitter is released, the postsynaptic membrane is excitatory, although not to threshold level, and it is said to be facilitated. It is above resting potential but below threshold value, and thus very receptive to another stimulus that can activate it with ease.

Presynaptic Inhibition

In addition to the IPSP, another form of inhibition, called *presynaptic inhibition*, occurs throughout the nervous system. Although concentrated in the peripheral afferent fibers, this type of inhibition occurs at the presynaptic bouton and no change takes place in the postsynaptic membrane. An inhibitory terminal acts on the presynaptic bouton, which greatly reduces the voltage of the action potential, thus reducing the excitability in the membrane of the bouton by reducing the amount of transmitter substance released. It is thought that presynaptic inhibition provides for a control mechanism of sensory inflow, so that less important input is eliminated and the major signal is relayed more clearly to the central nervous system.

Divergence and Convergence

Extremely complex networks of neurons exist in the nervous system. Extensive interactions among neurons are mediated through highly organized circuit connections. As axons emerge from the cell body, they divide and subdivide into many collateral branches that synapse with various numbers of other neurons. This presynaptic division is known as divergence. For example, the fibers of afferent neurons entering the spinal cord generally divide and subdivide into collateral branches that supply terminal boutons to many other postsynaptic spinal neurons. As a result, no one fiber contributes to an action potential, but rather many fibers cooperatively produce the innervation. The repetitive subdivision strengthens the afferent information, which is made available to various parts of the central nervous system through the process of divergence.

Similarly, most postsynaptic neurons receive terminal boutons from presynaptic fibers. This postsynaptic anatomic phenomenon is known as convergence. Many axons may converge on a single neuron and the EPSP is dependent on sufficient amplitude of the active boutons converging upon it.

Neurochemical Transmitter Substances

Presynaptic bouton vesicles store specific chemical substances that, when released into the synaptic cleft, either excite or inhibit other cells. Some transmitter substances are present only in the specific parts of the nervous system, while others are widely dispersed. Table 44-2 lists a few neurochemical transmitters that have been identified with certainty, and it is thought that many more will be identified in the future. It has been very difficult to pinpoint these substances because of the complex structure of the nervous system fibers.

Table 44-2 Functions of Identified Neurotransmitters

Neurotransmitter	Function
Acetylcholine	Excitatory
Norepinephrine	Excitatory
5-Hydroxytryptamine (serotonin)	Excitatory
Gamma-aminobutyric acid (GABA)	Inhibitory
Glycine	Inhibitory
Glutamic acid	Excitatory
Dopamine	Excitatory

Substances are considered to be neurochemical transmitters if they have the following general characteristics [12].

1. Are released by the presynaptic bouton on stimulation
2. Contain an enzyme in the presynaptic bouton for transmitter synthesis
3. Produce excitation or inhibition in the postsynaptic cell
4. Have demonstrated a mechanism that diminishes the effects of the transmitter

Acetylcholine and norepinephrine are two well-established neurochemical transmitters [6]. This activity of acetylcholine at the neuromuscular junction is well understood. The terminal bouton of cholinergic nerve fibers contains vesicles, each of which contains about 10,000 molecules of acetylcholine. A vesicle fuses with the presynaptic membrane and results in the release of acetylcholine. This process is known as *exocytosis* (Fig. 44-11). It is thought that the fusion of the vesicle to the presynaptic membrane is brought about by a sudden, transient increase in the concentration of calcium ions in the terminal bouton. The nerve impulse at the terminal bouton opens calcium channels to allow their flow into the bouton to facilitate exocytosis. The exact mechanism of the calcium activity in exocytosis is unknown. When the fused vesicle has discharged its acetylcholine at the presynaptic membrane, it is reclaimed by the bouton and restored with acetylcholine for its future use. The synthesis of acetylcholine occurs in the bouton in the following manner [12]:

$$\text{Acetylcoenzyme A (acetate)} + \text{choline} \xrightarrow[\text{ATP}]{\text{choline acetyltransferase}} \text{acetylcholine}.$$

The acetylcholine that diffuses across the synaptic cleft binds with an acetylcholine receptor on the postsynaptic membrane. This receptor is a channel protein that, in the presence of acetylcholine, lowers its energy state to an open conformation, allowing passage of sodium and potassium ions. Thus, a postsynaptic potential or voltage change

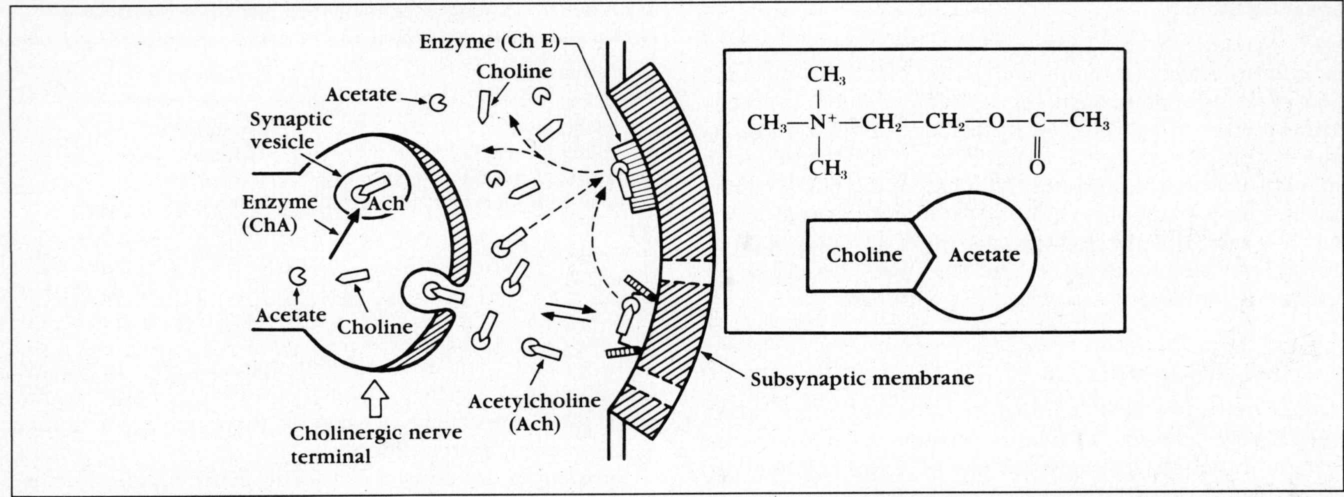

FIGURE 44-11 Acetylcholine (ACh) exocytosis. Acetylcholine is formed in presynaptic bouton through enzyme action of choline acetyltransferase on acetate and choline. It is removed from the cleft by action of enzyme cholinesterase (ChE), which is present in subsynaptic membrane. (From E. Selkurt, *Basic Physiology for the Health Sciences* [2nd ed.]. Boston: Little, Brown, 1982.)

is produced. The chemically gated postsynaptic potentials differ from action potentials of neurons in that their amplitude is smaller and their duration longer, and they are graded in accordance with the amount of transmitter released.

Within 2 or 3 msec of its release into the synaptic cleft, after it has depolarized the postsynaptic membrane, acetylcholine is hydrolyzed by the enzyme acetylcholinesterase:

$$\text{Acetylcholine} \xrightarrow[\text{water}]{\text{acetylcholinesterase}} \text{choline} + \text{acetate}.$$

Acetylcholinesterase is present abundantly in the membrane of the terminal bouton.

Insights into neurotransmitters and their inhibiting enzymes have been gained through the use of various pharmacologic agents that act on or compete with these substances. For example, the muscle relaxant curare competes with acetylcholine for receptor sites at the postsynaptic membrane. Thus, acetylcholine cannot bring about the membrane permeability for depolarization. Some drugs, such as nicotine, simulate acetylcholine action. Neostigmine and physostigmine inactivate the enzymatic action of acetylcholinesterase. Magnesium affects acetylcholine release. Elevated magnesium levels inhibit acetylcholine release by competing with the calcium ions that are necessary for the process.

Norepinephrine is the transmitter substance at all postganglionic sympathetic fibers except those innervating sweat glands and skeletal muscle vasculature. This substance is formed through a series of steps catalyzed by enzymes with the initial active transport of tyrosine from the circulation into the nerve terminals as follows [5].

$$\text{Tyrosine} \xrightarrow{\text{tyrosine hydroxylase}} \text{dopa} \xrightarrow{\text{dopa-decarboxylase}}$$

$$\text{dopamine} \xrightarrow{\text{dopamine beta-hydroxylase}} \text{norepinephrine}$$

$$\xrightarrow{\text{phenylethanolamine } N\text{-methyltransferase}} \text{epinephrine}.$$

A nerve impulse initiates the release of norepinephrine into the cleft. Norepinephrine activity at the receptor is terminated primarily through its uptake into the terminal bouton and transport back into the vesicles for reuse. In addition, a small amount of norepinephrine is inactivated by the activity of monoamine oxidase, and an additional small amount escapes the terminal bouton uptake and enters the systemic circulation, where it is primarily metabolized by the liver into vanillylmandelic acid (VMA) and excreted in the urine. Disease states exhibiting increased production of catecholamines characteristically show increased VMA urinary excretion. Minute amounts of released norepinephrine, which escape uptake and metabolic breakdown in the liver, appear unchanged in the urine.

The Central Nervous System

Phylogenetic Development

The human nervous system has a complex major processing system that lends control in a hierarchic manner. The highest level is the cerebral cortex, and the lowest, or most rudimentary, is the spinal reflex arc.

One can identify in the embryonic brain three distinct regions: the *rhombencephalon* or *hindbrain*, the *mesencephalon* or *midbrain*, and the *prosencephalon* or *forebrain* (Fig. 44-12). The most sophisticated activities and complex subdividing occur in the prosencephalon, which includes the cerebral hemispheres, basal ganglia, and olfactory tract. This portion of the brain is also called the *telencephalon* or *endbrain*. The "deep inside" component of the prosencephalon is the *diencephalon*. Optic tracts traverse the prosencephalon and terminate in the optic nerves of the retinae at the inferior surface of the forebrain. The diencephalon includes structures such as the thalamus, hypothalamus, subthalamus, and subthalamic nucleus. In addition, the pituitary complex evolves from the hypothalamus. The mesencephalon connects the forebrain with the hindbrain; anteriorly it comprises the cerebral peduncles and posteriorly the corpora quadrigemina (also known as superior and inferior colliculi).

Below the mesencephalon is the rhombencephalon, which surrounds the fourth ventricle and comprises the pons and medulla oblongata. Extending from the rhombencephalon posteriorly is the cerebellum; the spinal cord extends inferiorly.

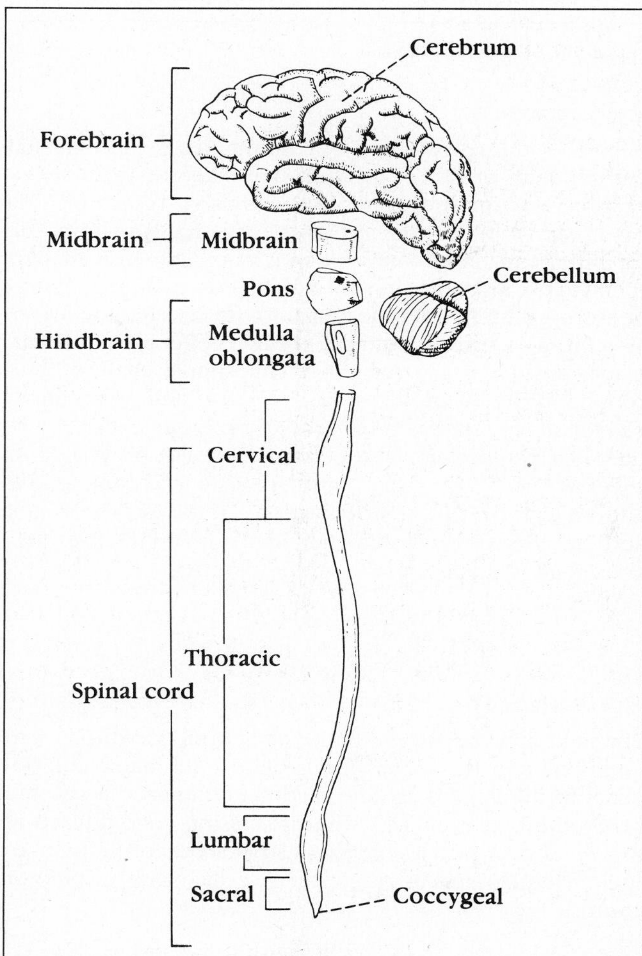

FIGURE 44-12 The brain develops from three regions: hindbrain, midbrain, and forebrain. (From R.S. Snell, *Clinical Neuroanatomy for Medical Students*. Boston: Little, Brown, 1980.)

Protective Coverings of the Brain and Spinal Cord

Protection is afforded the brain and spinal cord by bony coverings, the meninges, and cerebrospinal fluid. The brain is encased within the skull, which in the adult is a nonflexible structure composed of several fused bones. Three depressions in the base of the skull are known as the *anterior*, *middle*, and *posterior fossae*.

A major opening, the *foramen magnum*, is at the base of the skull and allows information to be processed between higher and lower centers (Fig. 44-13). At birth, openings within the skull known as the *fontanelles* can be noted. These generally close by 18 months of age.

The spinal cord is encased in the vertebral column that consists of 24 movable vertebrae: 7 cervical, 12 thoracic, and 5 lumbar, and fused 5 sacral and 4 coccygeal vertebrae (Fig. 44-14). Intravertebral disks separate each of the vertebrae. The central cartilaginous portion of the intervertebral disk is known as the *nucleus pulposus* and the outer fibrous capsule as the *anulus fibrosus*.

In addition, the brain and spinal cord are protected by three connective tissue membranes called the *meninges*: the *dura mater*, *arachnoid mater*, and *pia mater* (Fig. 44-15). The dura mater is a thick, tough, nonelastic, fibrous membrane that lies directly below the skull. Its extension between the cerebral hemispheres is known as the *falx cerebri*; and between the cerebrum and cerebellum it is known as the *tentorium cerebelli*. The dura mater together with the arachnoid and pia mater extends through the foramen magnum and lines the vertebral column. The *epidural space* is between the inner surface of the skull and the dura mater. The space between the dura and arachnoid is known as the *subdural space*. A network of small blood vessels traverses this space. The arachnoid, consisting of fibrous, weblike tissue, is the middle layer of the meninges wherein the cerebrospinal fluid circulates and is resorbed. The area below the arachnoid membrane containing the cerebrospinal fluid is known as the *subarachnoid* space. The innermost layer, the pia mater, is a delicate, vascular, lacelike membrane directly adherent to the brain and spinal cord. The arachnoid layer projects small extensions called *arachnoid villi* into the dura mater that resorb cerebrospinal fluid into the blood. Larger blood vessels lie in the subarachnoid space and branch into smaller vessels that pass through the pia mater as they enter the brain tissue.

The Spinal Cord Processing System

The spinal cord transmits more complex signals from higher centers and responds spontaneously to local sensory information with automatic motor responses called *reflexes*. It is approximately 42 to 45 cm long in the adult and is segmented into cervical, thoracic, lumbar, and sacral sections. Signals are received and transmitted

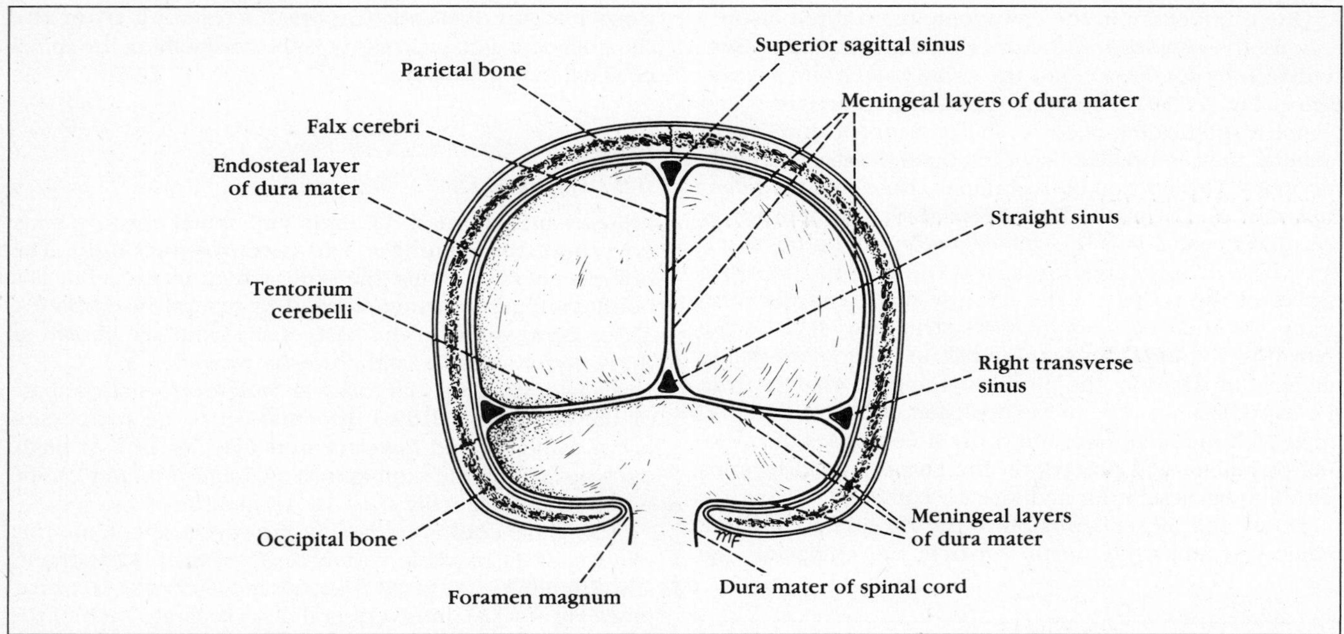

FIGURE 44-13 Relationship of intracranial contents with the foramen magnum. (From R.S. Snell, *Clinical Neuroanatomy for Medical Students*. Boston: Little, Brown, 1980.)

through 31 pairs of spinal nerves, which are named for their corresponding vertebral level. Segments of the spinal cord do not correspond with vertebral levels, however (see Fig. 44-14). The spinal cord is approximately 25 cm shorter than the vertebral canal and ends at the level of the first or second lumbar vertebra in the adult. It emerges from the base of the skull, the *foramen magnum*, and continues to the coccyx, where it ends in a tapered filament called the *filum terminale*. Together, the lumbosacral nerve roots are called the *cauda equina*.

The spinal cord enlarges at the lower cervical segments and again at the lower lumbar segments. These enlargements denote the origins of the *brachial* and *lumbar plexuses*, respectively. The brachial plexus innervates the upper extremities and the lumbar plexus innervates lower extremities. The cell bodies are located in the inner, butterfly-shaped, gray portion of the spinal cord, and the ascending and descending projection nerve fibers form the outer white area. Major ascending and descending tracts and their transmissions are presented in Table 44-3. A small opening in the middle of the spinal cord, the *central canal*, is lined by ependymal cells and contains cerebrospinal fluid. Spinal nerves enter the cord at the posterior horn (somatic sensory and visceral) and emerge at the anterior horn (motor and autonomic) (Fig. 44-16) [7]. The cell bodies of efferent motor fibers are located in the anterior horn and the cell bodies of the afferent sensory fibers are situated outside the spinal cord in the posterior root ganglion. Contact between the afferent and efferent fibers is made within the spinal cord through interneurons.

Reflex Arc. A fundamental component of the nervous system is the reflex, which, in its simplest form, occurs in the spinal cord. A stimulus from the external environment produces an immediate stereotypical reflex response from the central nervous system. For this response to occur, the following mechanisms must be functional: an afferent neuron with its receptor, an area for the synapse transmission to occur (one or more central neurons), and an efferent neuron with its effector organ. The impulse passes from receptor to effector and commands a quick organ response. This simple chain of neuronal activity is known as a reflex arc and, at its most elemental level, it is a monosynaptic process consisting of only one synapse and two neurons (see Fig. 44-16). Most reflexes result from many more synaptic interconnections and are referred to as *polysynaptic reflexes*. The reflex activity encountered at higher levels in the central nervous system is considerably more complex.

Low-Brain Processing System (Rhombencephalon)

The next level of processing in the central nervous system takes place in the rhombencephalon. The major components of this region are the medulla oblongata, pons, and cerebellum (Fig. 44-17). The processing encountered at this level occurs at the unconscious level and influences such vital activities as respiratory, cardiac, and vasomotor control.

Medulla Oblongata. The medulla extends directly from the cervical spinal cord at the level of the foramen magnum and lies below the pons and fourth ventricle (Fig. 44-18). The medulla is subdivided into three distinct sections, anterior, lateral, and posterior. Fissures and sulci

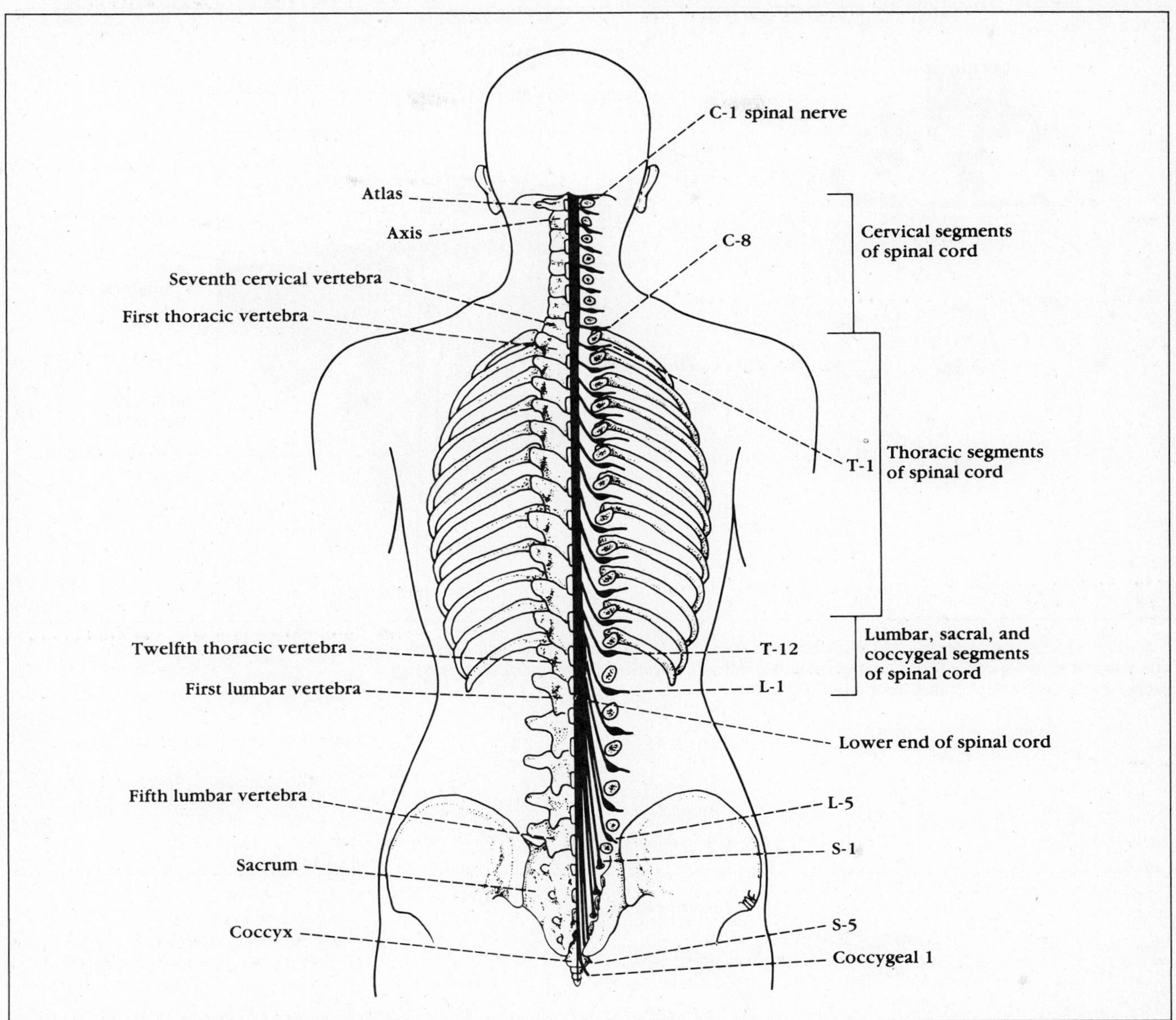

FIGURE 44-14 Relationship of vertebral segments of cord with actual vertebrae. (From R.S. Snell, *Clinical Neuroanatomy for Medical Students*. Boston: Little, Brown, 1980.)

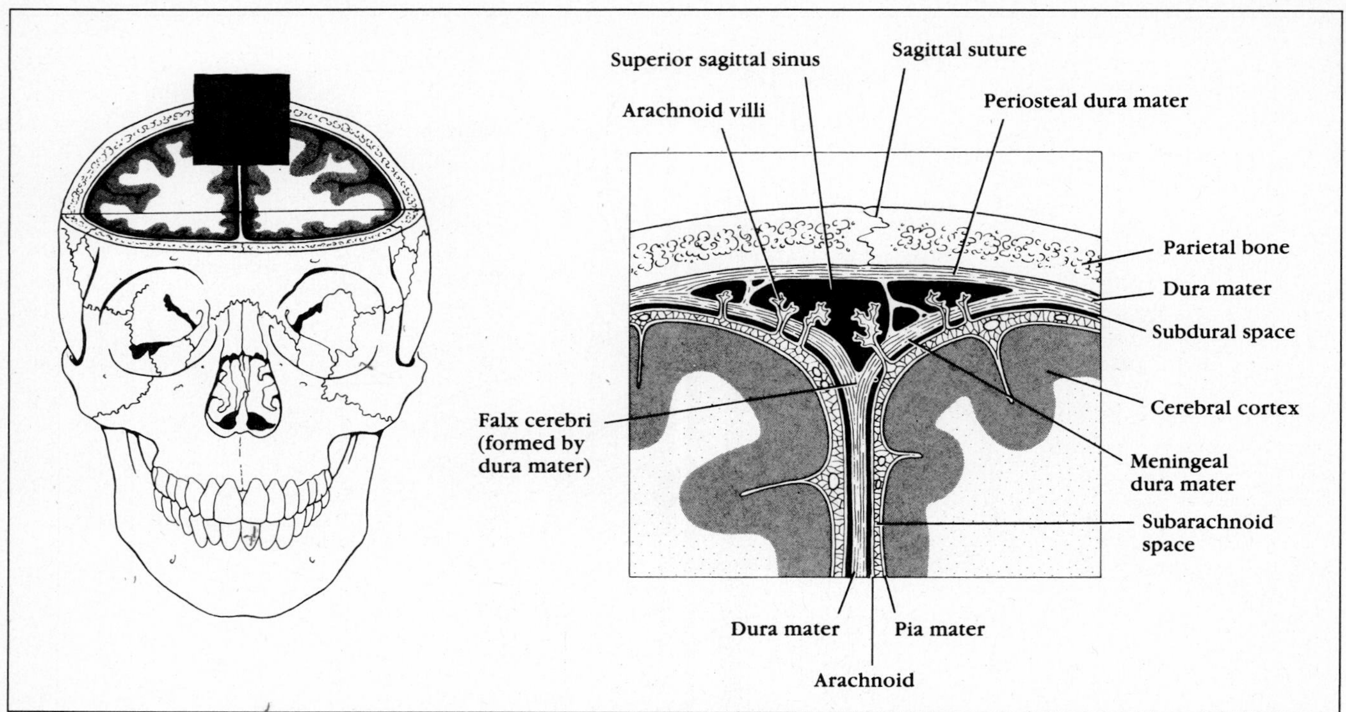

FIGURE 44-15 Frontal section showing the relationships of the dural venous sinuses, meninges, and subarachnoid space. (From A. Spence and E. Mason, *Human Anatomy and Physiology*. Menlo Park, Calif.: Benjamin/Cummings, 1979.)

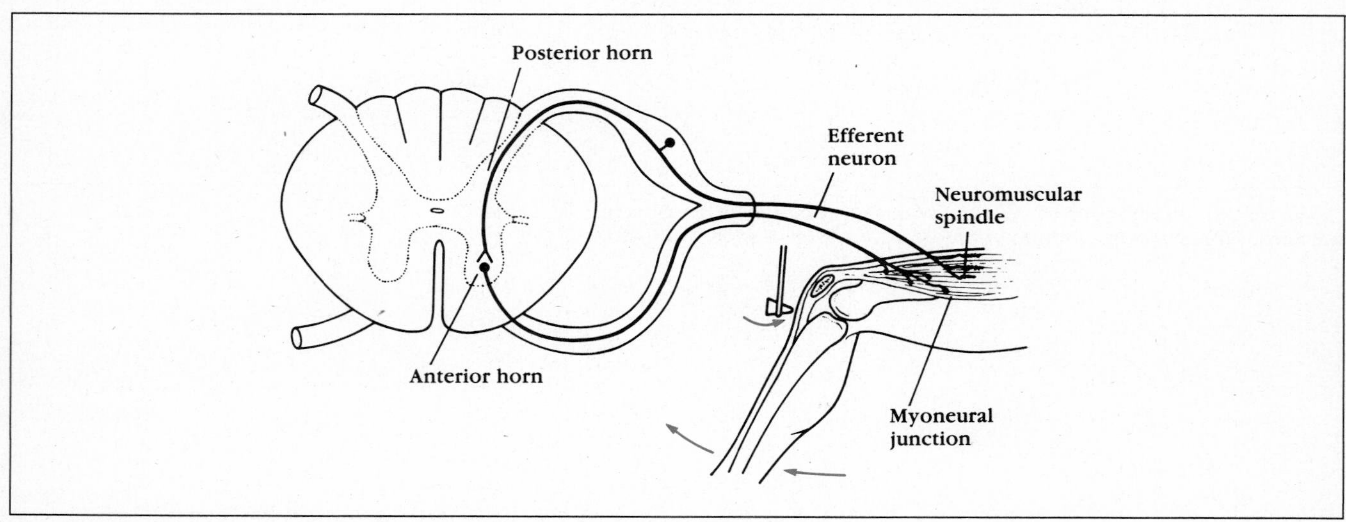

FIGURE 44-16 A monosynaptic reflex arc. (From R.S. Snell, *Clinical Neuroanatomy for Medical Students*. Boston: Little, Brown, 1980.)

TABLE 44-3 Major Ascending and Descending Spinal Tracts

Tracts	Major Transmission Information	Origin
Anterior white column		
Descending (motor)		
Ventral corticospinal	Voluntary movement	Pyramidal cells of motor cortex
Vestibulospinal	Posture and balance reflexes	Vestibular nuclei in medulla
Reticulospinal	Muscle tone controls activity of autonomic nervous system	Reticular of midbrain and medulla
Tectospinal	Audiovisual reflexes	Roof of the midbrain
Ascending (sensory)		
Ventral spinothalmic	Light touch and pressure	Opposite posterior column
Spinoolivary	Reflex proprioception	Anterior marginal zone of spinal column
Lateral white column		
Descending (motor)		
Lateral corticospinal	Voluntary movement	Contralateral pyramidal cells of motor cortex
Rubrospinal	Muscle tone, head and upper truck movement	Red nucleus of midbrain
Olivospinal	Facilitative and inhibitory reflexes	Inferior olivary nucleus
Ascending (sensory)		
Dorsal spinocerebellar	Reflex proprioception to cerebellum	Ipsilateral dorsal nucleus
Ventral spinocerebellar	Reflex proprioception to cerebellum	Posterior white column
Lateral spinothalamic	Pain temperature tactile sensations	Contralateral dorsal column
Posterior white column		
Descending (motor)		
Fasciculus interfascicularis	Integration and association	Intraspinal and dorsal root
Ascending (sensory)		
Fasciculus gracilis	Both transmit vibration, discriminative tactile senses, joint position, kinesthetic sensations	Posteromedian septum of low spinal cord
Fasciculus cuneatus		Posterior nerve roots of thoracocervical cord

Source: D. G. Chusid, *Correlative Neuroanatomy and Functional Neurology* (17th ed.). Copyright © 1979. Lange Medical Publishers. Reprinted by permission.

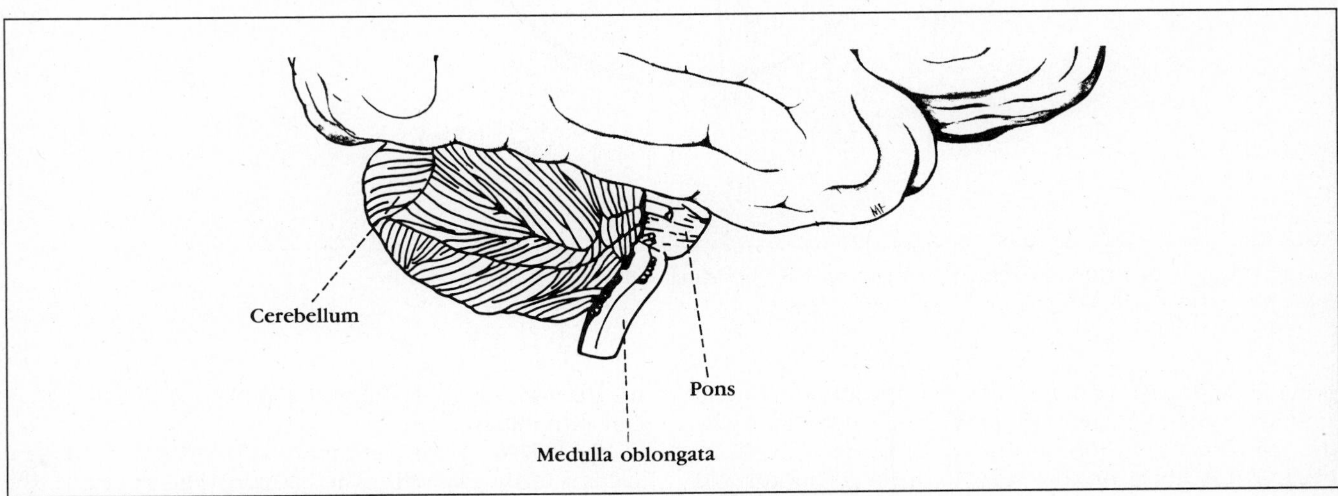

FIGURE 44-17 Low-brain processing system. (Adapted from R.S. Snell, *Clinical Neuroanatomy for Medical Students*. Boston: Little, Brown, 1980.)

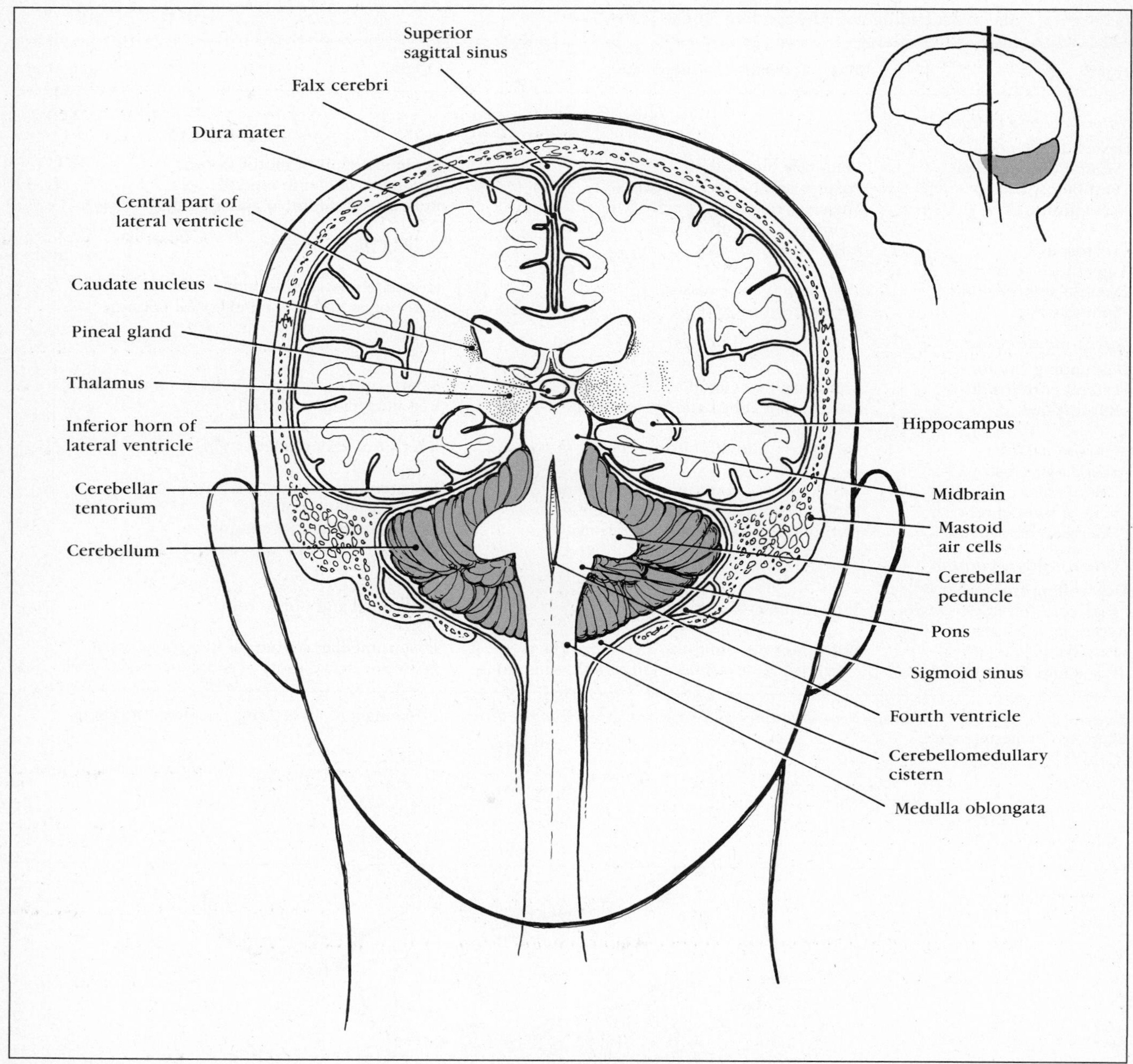

FIGURE 44-18 The structures of the rhombencephalon, consisting of the medulla oblongata, the pons, and the cerebellum.

provide landmarks that distinguish these divisions. The anterior portion contains two prominent ridges known as the *pyramids* that contain the *descending pyramidal tract*. These fibers project from the primary motor and somasthetic cortical areas and cross from one side to the other (pyramidal decussation) at the lower medulla before entering the spinal cord. By far the majority of these fibers decussate and descend as the *lateral corticospinal* tract. The fibers from the motor cortex that remain uncrossed descend into the spinal cord as the *anterior corticospinal* tract. Injury anywhere along the corticospinal tract above the decussation results in motor deficits of the contralateral extremities.

The *olive*, a prominent mass, is located in the lateral section of the medulla. This structure gives rise to the *inferior olivary nuclear complex*, which is important in controlling movement, postural change, locomotion, and equilibrium through an interconnecting network of fibers among the cerebral cortex, spinal cord, and cerebellum. This region contains nuclei for four cranial nerves: the twelfth (hypoglossal), eleventh (accessory), tenth (vagus), and ninth (glossopharyngeal). Cardiac and vasomotor control evolve from the reticular formation of this region. Respirations are controlled by the medullary center in coordination with the pneumotaxic center in the pons.

The posterior portion of the medulla forms a portion of the floor of the fourth ventricle. The ascending *medial lemniscus* tract arises here from the crossed-over fasciculi cuneatus and gracilis fibers (Fig. 44-19). The medial lemniscus is a major ascending brainstem tract that carries discriminative tactile information, proprioception, and vibration sensation to the sensory thalamic nucleus. Lesions in the medial lemniscus result in contralateral sensory deficits.

Pons. The pons is continuous with the medulla and midbrain, separated by the pontine sulcus from the medulla and the superior pontine sulcus from the midbrain. The pons lies ventral to the cerebellum and is divided into two parts: a *dorsal* portion, the pontine tegmentum, and a *ventral* portion, the pons proper [1]. The dorsal portion is continuous with the medullary reticular formation and, together with the medulla, forms the floor and lateral wall of the fourth ventricle. This portion also contains important ascending and descending tracts and cranial nerve nuclei for the fifth (trigeminal), sixth (abducens), seventh (facial), and eighth (acoustic) cranial nerves

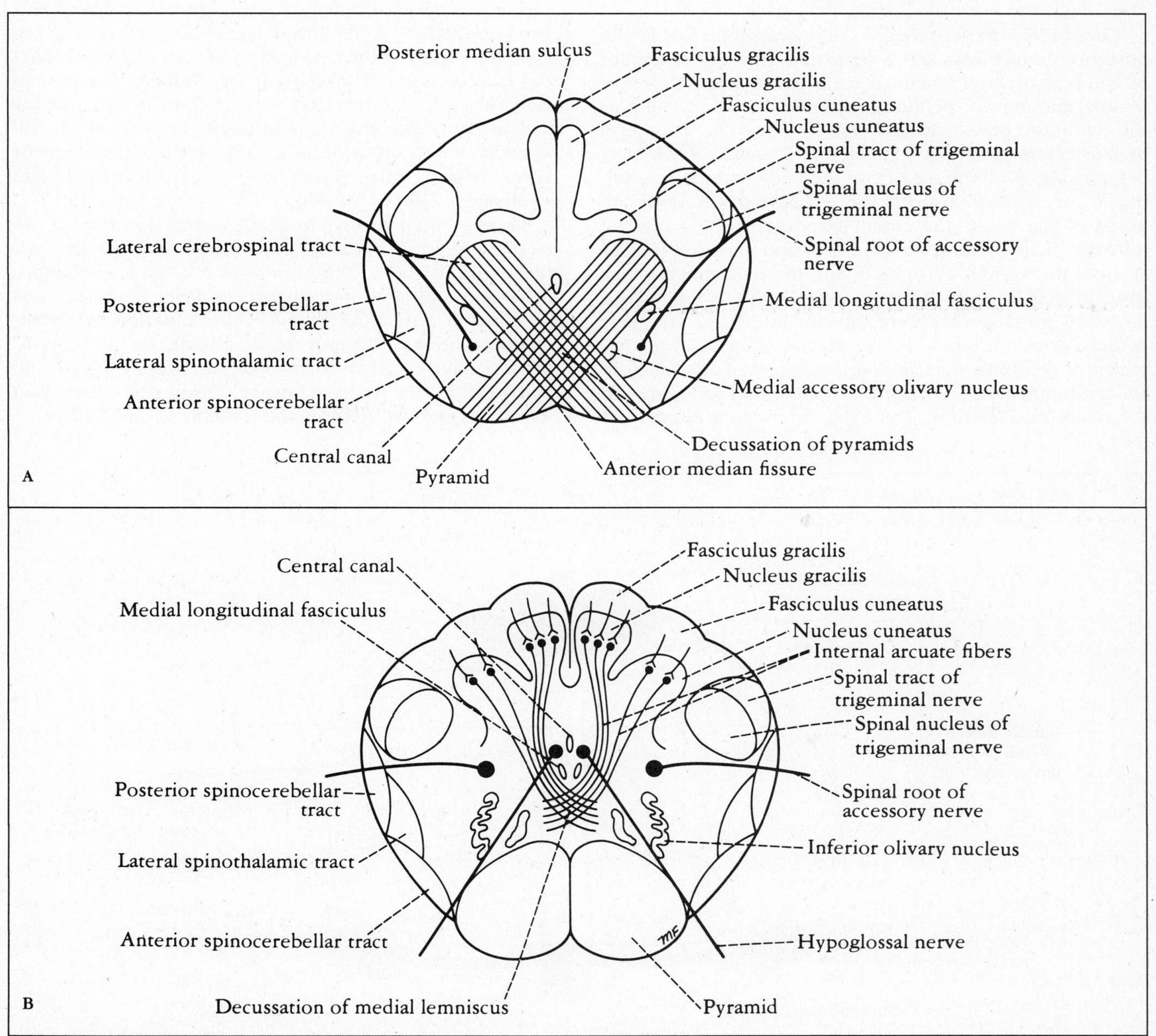

FIGURE 44-19 Transverse sections of the medulla oblongata. A. Level of decussation of the pyramids. B. Level of decussation of the medial lemnisci. (From R.S. Snell, *Clinical Neuroanatomy for Medical Students*. Boston: Little, Brown, 1980.)

(see Chap. 45). The pons regulates respiration through its pneumotaxic center.

The ventral portion of the pons consists of a large mass of orderly longitudinal and transverse fiber bundles that are interspersed with many pontine nuclei. The longitudinal fiber bundles traversing through this portion of the pons are the corticospinal, corticopontine, and corticobulbar. The ventral portion of the pons is an important relay center between the cerebral cortex and the opposite cerebellar hemisphere in providing smooth, coordinated movements. The transverse fibers arise from the pontine nuclei and cross to the opposite side to form the middle cerebellar peduncle.

Cerebellar Processing. The cerebellum lies in the posterior cranial fossa and is separated from the cerebrum by the tentorium cerebelli (see Fig. 44-18). The superior, middle, and inferior peduncles connect the cerebellum to the midbrain, pons, and medulla, respectively. The cerebellum exerts ipsilateral control: the right side of the cerebellum controls the right side of the body and the left side of the cerebellum controls the left side of the body. As noted in Fig. 44-20, the cerebellar structures are divided into two major lateral hemispheres and an intermediary section, the vermis. Fissures divide the hemispheres into three principal lobes: the *archicerebellum* (flocculonodular lobe), *paleocerebellum* (anterior lobe), and *neocerebellum* (posterior lobe). The archicerebellum is integrated with the vestibular system and is concerned with muscle tone, equilibrium, and position through its influence on the trunk musculature. The paleocerebellum consists of the cerebellum that lies anterior to the primary fissure, receiving most of the proprioceptive and interoceptive input from the head and body. It helps to maintain equilibrium and coordinate automatic movements, as well as to regulate muscle tone. The neocerebellum, phylogenetically the newest, consists of the cerebellum between the primary fissure and the posterior fissure. It coordinates voluntary movements and has extensive connections with the cerebral cortex.

The cerebellum processes and transmits information concerning current body movements, maintains posture, and regulates muscle tone. It does this through information it receives from the motor cortex of the cerebrum by way of the *corticocerebellar* pathway and from various sensory receptors by way of the *anterior* and *posterior spinocerebellar* tracts. Other significant tracts relaying this information to the cerebellum include the *spinoreticular* tract by way of the reticular area of the brainstem and the *spino-olivary* tract by way of the inferior olivary nucleus. Fiber-efferent tracts originate in various cerebellar nuclei and transmit information to the cerebral motor cortex, basal ganglia, red nucleus, reticular formation, and vestibular nuclei [5].

Because the pathways from the cerebral cortex to the cerebellum are not direct, descending motor tracts, disruption of cerebellar function does not hinder voluntary movement, although movement no longer is smooth and coordinated. Disruption of cerebellar function can result in ataxia, intention tremor, adiadochokinesia (inability to perform rapid alternating movements), dysmetria (inability to judge distances when reaching out toward an object), hypotonia, tremor, and asthenia.

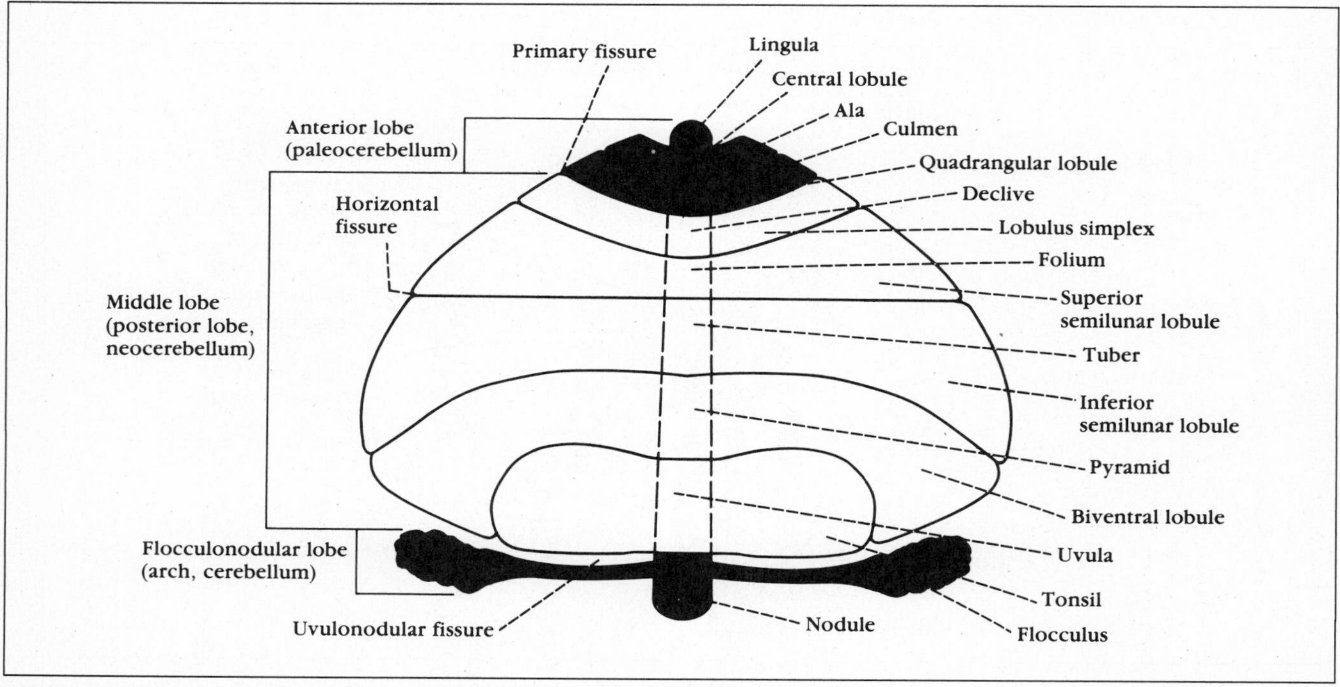

FIGURE 44-20 Main cerebellar lobes, lobules, and fissures. (From R.S. Snell, *Clinical Neuroanatomy for Medical Students*. Boston: Little, Brown, 1980.)

Midbrain Processing System (Mesencephalon)

The midbrain extends from the pons and projects briefly between the two cerebral hemispheres, connecting the lower centers with the diencephalon. It therefore is a major motor and sensory fiber pathway between the higher and lower centers. The nuclei for third and fourth cranial nerves originate in this region. The *cerebral aqueduct (aqueduct of Sylvius)*, a small channel between the third and fourth ventricles, lies in the midbrain. The midbrain *tegmentum* is located ventral to the cerebral aqueduct and is continuous with the pontine tegmentum. The reticular formation in this region contains the *substantia nigra* and the *red* nucleus.

The substantia nigra is a large pigmented mass containing neurotransmitters, particularly dopamine. It supports motor function through its connections with the thalamus, corpus striatum, and superior colliculus [1]. The red nucleus influences head and neck movement as well as motor control by the cerebellum. The *superior colliculus*, a relay center for the optic system, and the *inferior colliculus*, which relays information concerning auditory impulses, are also contained in this area. The superior and inferior colliculi (*corpora quadrigemina*) compose the tectum. The *crus cerebri* are masses on the ventral surface of the midbrain that comprise motor fibers originating in the cerebral cortex as well as corticobulbar fibers projecting to cranial nerve nuclei and reticular formation [1].

Diencephalon Processing System

The diencephalon arises from the midbrain and is considered to be a part of the forebrain. It lies between the cerebral hemispheres and encases the third ventricle. Included in this area are the epithalamus, thalamus, hypothalamus, and subthalamus.

Thalamic Processing. The thalamus, the largest portion of the diencephalon, is a major center for processing sensations and relaying these to higher stations of the brain. Input from all sensoria except that for olfaction is processed here. Numerous afferent nerve tracts from lower levels transmit information to the specific relay nuclei of the thalamus. The thalamus is divided into three sections, *lateral*, *medial*, and *anterior*, which are separated by the *internal medullary lamina*. Groups of nuclei within the internal medullary lamina are referred to as *intralaminar thalamic* nuclei. Sensory data are relayed through these nuclei.

The reticular activating system continues its upward projection to the thalamic nuclei. From the thalamic nuclei, fibers diffuse to all areas of the cerebral cortex. This system is known as the *diffuse thalamocortical system* (Fig. 44-21). This system, which is also referred to as the nonspecific thalamocortical system, activates the first two layers of neurons of the cortex by partially depolariz-

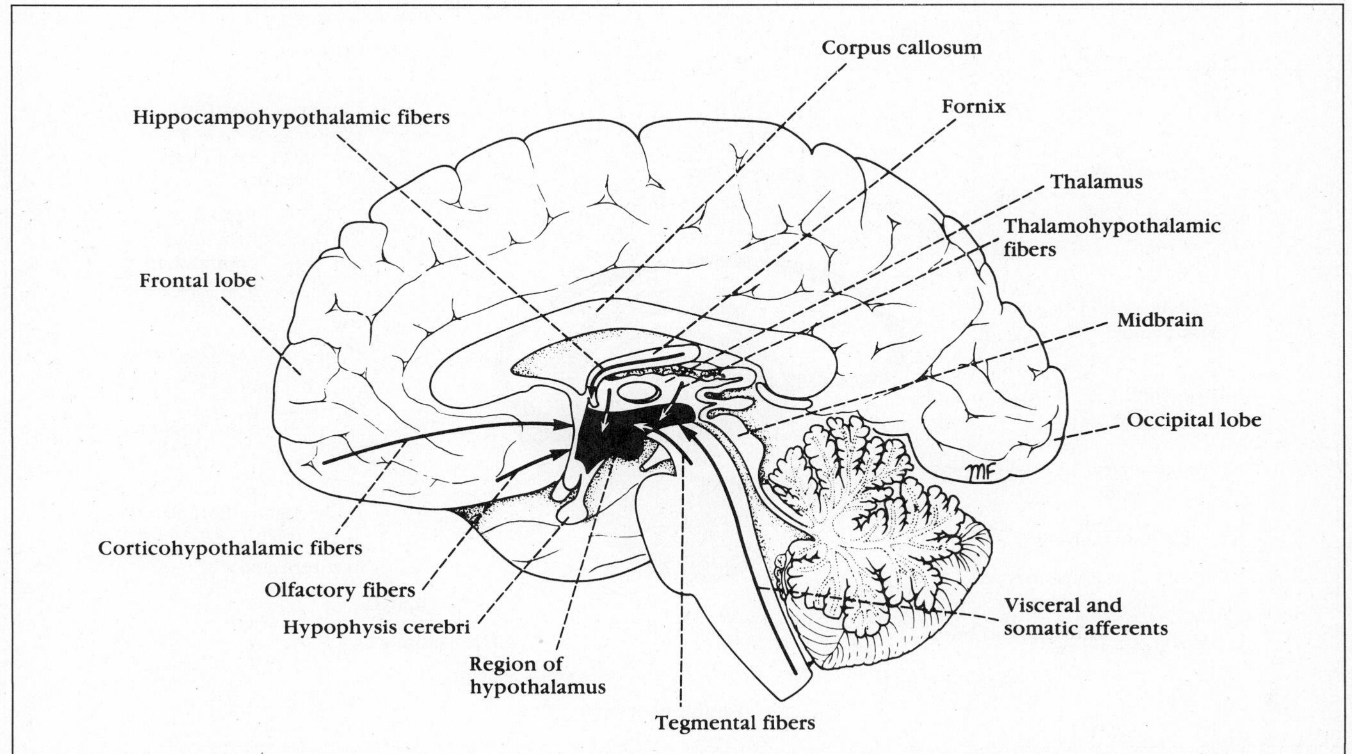

FIGURE 44-21 Sagittal section of brain showing main afferent pathways entering hypothalamus. (From R.S. Snell, *Clinical Neuroanatomy for Medical Students*. Boston: Little, Brown, 1980.)

ing superficial cortical dendrites, resulting in increased facilitation of the cortex [5]. The *paleospinothalamic pathway*, which transmits burning and aching sensations, terminates in the *diffuse thalamocortical system* (Fig. 44-22). Axons of the optic tract synapse in the lateral geniculate body, which projects from the thalamus. The fibers projecting from the lateral geniculate body pass posteriorly and terminate in the visual cortex.

Hypothalamic Processing. The hypothalamus lies below the thalamus and forms part of the walls and floor of the third ventricle. It consists of a group of nuclei with specific functions and is divided into the anterior and posterior portions. The pituitary stalk connects the hypothalamus to the pituitary gland, which provides the route for its neuroendocrine control.

Major processing of internal stimuli evoking the autonomic nervous system is concentrated in the hypothalamus. The functions that maintain the internal milieu processed by the hypothalamus include blood pressure, heart rate, respiratory rate, body temperature, water metabolism, and body fluid osmolality, feeding behavior, and neuroendocrine activity. The hypothalamus is a focal structure of the *limbic* system. Fig. 44-23 illustrates the structures of the limbic system, which, in concert with the hypothalamus, perform an important role in overall behavior and emotions. Because vital autonomic functions are

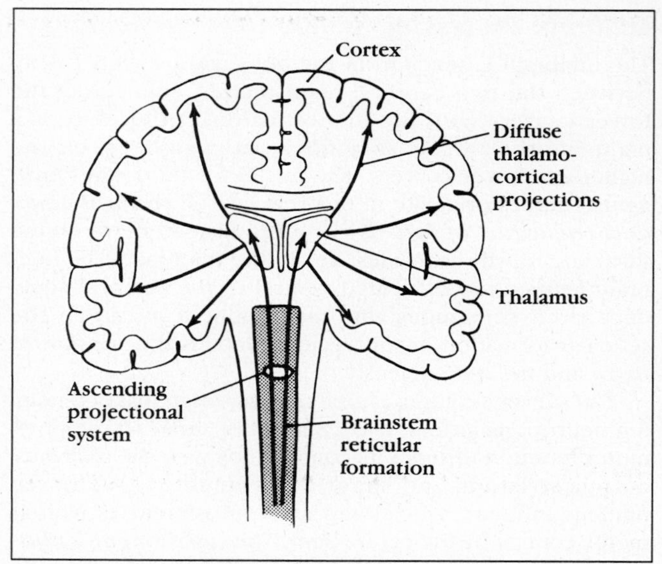

FIGURE 44-22 The diffuse thalamocortical system. (From J. Daube et al., *Medical Neurosciences: An Approach to Anatomy, Pathology, and Physiology by Systems and Level.* Boston: Little, Brown, 1978.)

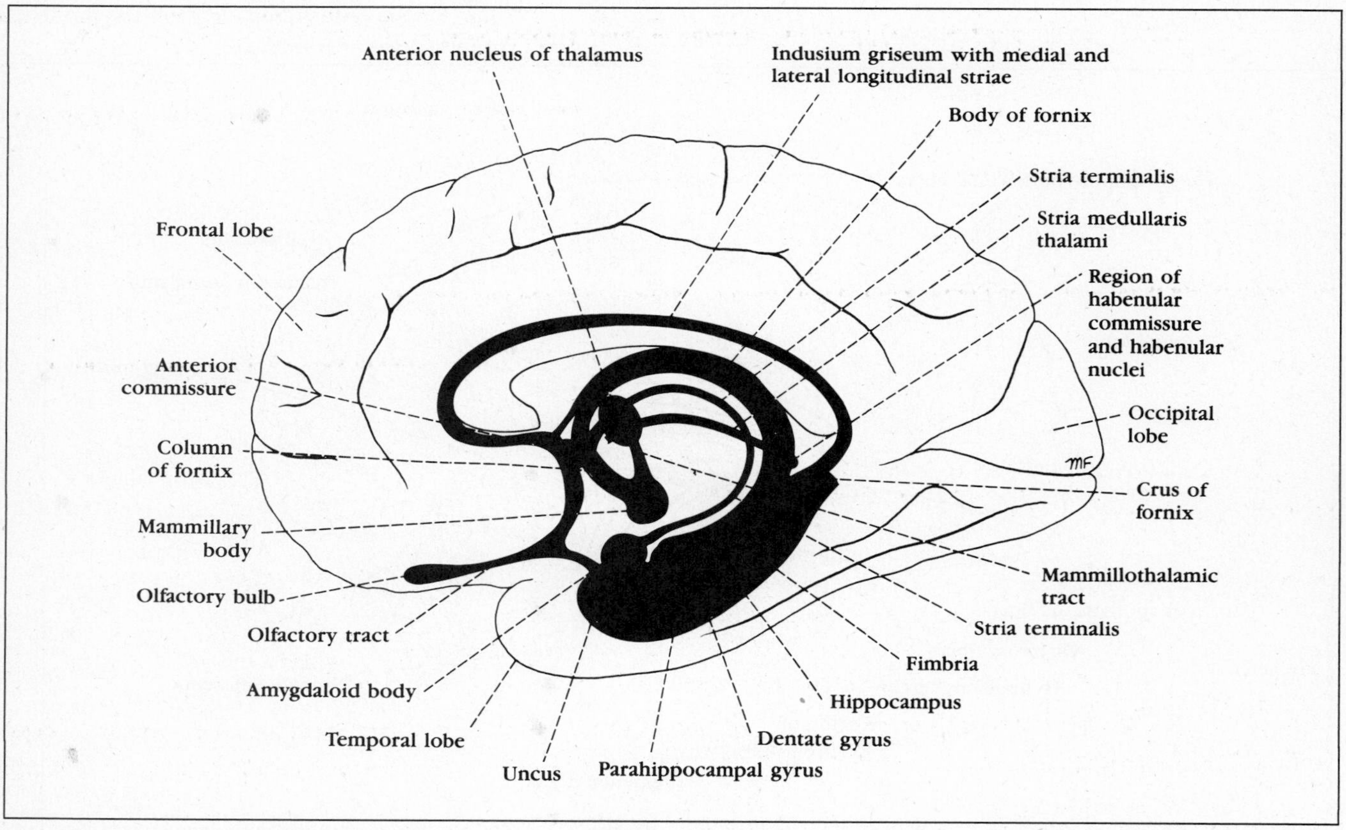

FIGURE 44-23 Key structures of the limbic system. (From R.S. Snell, *Clinical Neuroanatomy for Medical Students*. Boston: Little, Brown, 1980.)

processed here, destruction of the hypothalamus results in death. The majority of the hypothalamic activity occurs at an unconscious level, but excessive stimulation may evoke a conscious response. An example of this is a person who is chilled and consciously seeks warmth.

Responses to emotions of fear, anger, and excitement reflected by increased pulse rate, increased respiratory rate, increased gastric acidity, and sweating are communicated from the hypothalamus. Prolonged stimulation of the hypothalamus may result in hypertension or ulcers.

The *epithalamus* consists of the pineal body, habenular nuclei, stria medularis, and posterior commissure. It is located in the region above the thalamus and contains the roof of the third ventricle. Olfactory impulses are relayed through this region and visual reflexes are associated with certain fibers in the posterior commissure. The function of the pineal gland in the adult is uncertain. It becomes visible on skull films due to calcified material that accumulates with age, and it can provide useful information in the identification of space-occupying lesions.

Basal Ganglia Processing. The basal ganglia (Fig. 44-24), situated deep in the cerebral hemispheres, are responsible for motor control and information processing in the extrapyramidal system. The basal ganglia include the *caudate nucleus*, *putamen*, and *globus pallidus*. These nuclear masses have complex interconnections with the subthalamic nucleus, red nucleus, and substantia nigra. The claustrum and amygdaloid body, considered by some authors to be part of the basal ganglia, are not directly involved in motor control.

The basal ganglia are intimately related to the thalamus through circular neural pathways that control motor function. They inhibit muscle tone by transmitting inhibitory signals to the bulboreticular facilitory area and excitatory signals to the bulboreticular inhibitory area. Lesions in the basal ganglia result in an overactive facilitory area and underactive inhibitory area. Gross intentional movement that is performed without conscious thought is regulated by the caudate nucleus and putamen (collectively called the *striate body*).

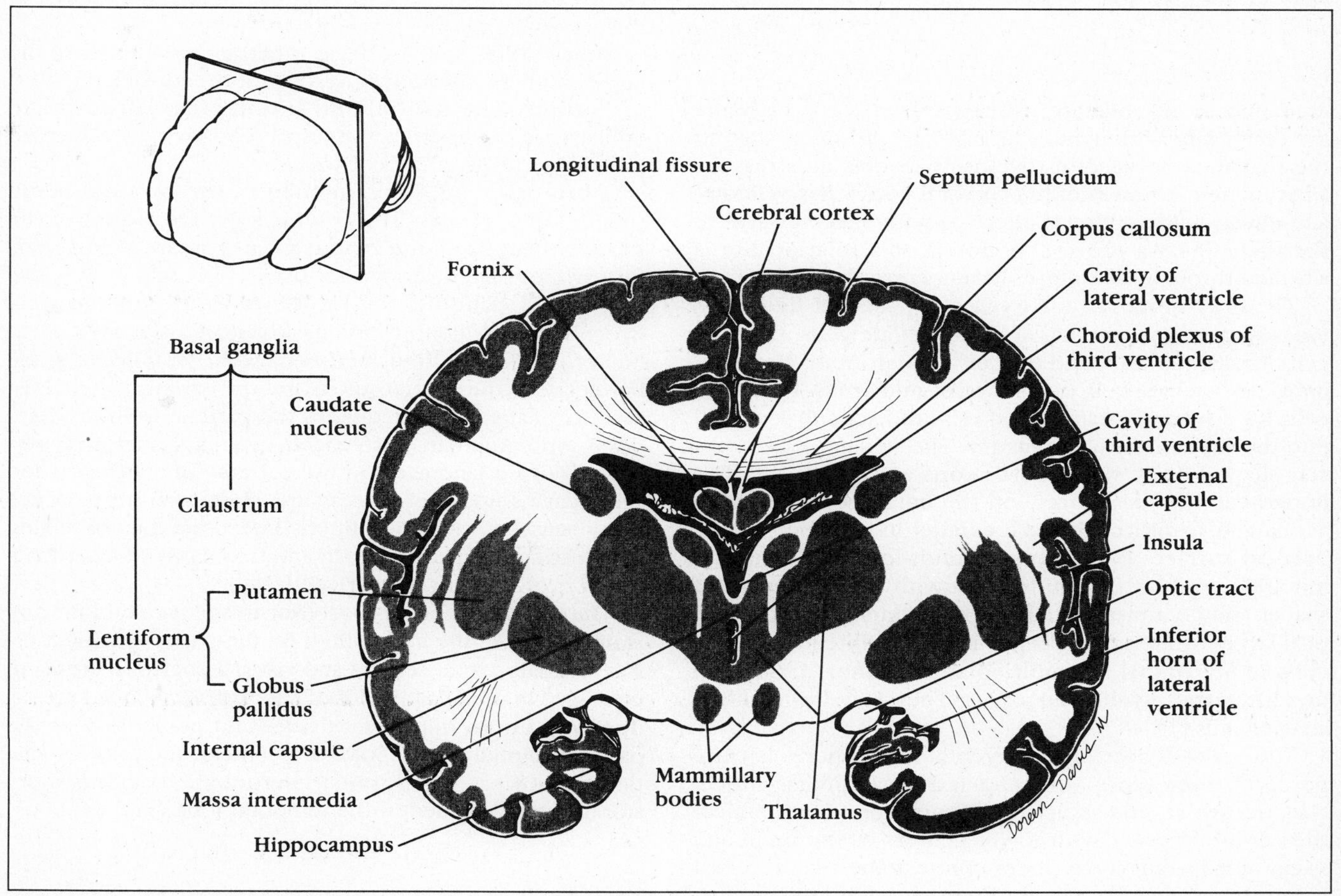

FIGURE 44-24 Frontal section of the cerebellum and diencephalon showing the cerebral cortex (gray matter) surrounding the white matter and the basal ganglia deep within the white matter. (From A. Spence and E. Mason, *Human Anatomy and Physiology*. Menlo Park, Calif.: Benjamin/Cummings, 1979.)

Striate body transmissions are sent to the globus pallidus and relayed on to the ventrolateral nucleus of the thalamus and then on to the cerebral cortex. From the cortex the information travels through the pyramidal and extrapyramidal tracts to the spinal cord. Other impulses travel to the globus pallidus and then on to the substantia nigra and on to the reticular formation, where the final route transmits down through the reticulospinal tract. The globus pallidus relays impulses through a similar feedback circuit to the ventrolateral nucleus of the thalamus and on to the cerebral cortex, and finally to the pyramidal and extrapyramidal tracts to the spinal cord. It also transmits by way of shorter circuits to the reticular formation and on to the reticulospinal tract of the spinal cord [5].

The subthalamus nucleus, red nucleus, and substantia nigra are closely related to the globus pallidus and striate body. Their interactions, which control and coordinate motor function, are extremely complex and extensive, and little is known of the exact interconnections.

The neurons transmitting to the globus pallidus and striate body from the substantia nigra are inhibitory through *dopamine* secretion [3].

Dysfunction or lesions in the region of the basal ganglia are manifested in involuntary tremor, athetosis, and torticollis (see Chap. 50).

Forebrain (Prosencephalon)

Anatomically, the highest and largest portion of the brain, the cerebrum, is thought to be phylogenetically related to the thalamus because of its closely associated structure and function. All areas of the cerebral cortex have afferent and efferent fibers interconnecting with specific areas of the thalamus. As previously noted, this relationship is affirmed through the diffuse thalamocortical system.

The gray cerebral cortex is composed of five basic types of neurons: pyramidal cells, stellate cells, fusiform cells, horizontal cells, and the cells of Martinotti. The pyramidal and stellate cells are the most numerous. Pyramidal cells have pyramid-shaped bodies with axons that extend into the subcortical white matter. The stellate cells have a star-shaped body with short axons and dendrites. The horizontal cells lie entirely on the horizontal plane with axons and dendrites that are parallel in direction to the cortical surface. Polymorph or multiform cells may be modified types of pyramidal cells with a wide variety of shapes and contours. Dendrites often extend into the cortical layers, while axons project into the white matter. The cells of Martinotti are multipolar with short branching dendrites and myelinated axons. They may be modified stellate cells [1].

The white matter of the cerebral hemispheres is composed of three types of myelinated nerve fibers: projection, transverse, and association. Projection fibers connect the cerebral cortex with lower centers of the brain and spinal cord, transverse fibers connect the two cerebral hemispheres, and association fibers provide interconnections within the same cerebral hemisphere.

The cerebrum appears as a series of convolutions (*gyri*) and grooves (*sulci*) that are instrumental in identifying the structural and functional geography of the cortex. The deeper grooves, called *fissures*, assist in establishing the major cerebral regional divisions; the *frontal*, *parietal*, *temporal*, and *occipital* lobes. Similarly, the two cerebral hemispheres are distinguished from each other by, the deep *longitudinal fissure* (Fig. 44-25). The cerebral hemispheres, which exhibit *contralateral* body control, are divided by continuation of the dura mater known as the *falx cerebri*, which projects into the longitudinal cerebral fissure. Directly inferior to the longitudinal cerebral fissure, the fibers of the corpus collosum join the hemispheres. In the great majority of the population the left hemisphere is dominant in the interpretive functions.

In addition to its anatomic superiority, the cerebral cortex maintains the highest level of information processing in the human. Some functional areas are localized; others are more general and widely dispersed. The significant localized functional areas include the primary motor projection and sensory projection areas. The motor projection area is located on the anterior wall of the central sulcus and adjacent to the precentral gyrus (Fig. 44-26). This area controls voluntary skeletal muscle movements of the contralateral body. The sensory projection area (somasthetic area) is located on the postcentral gyrus and receives input from the thalamus-projected sensations of the contralateral side of the body.

Other rather well-localized functions processed in the cortex include visual, hearing, olfaction, and somatic interpretations. The mental and intellectual activities in humans are processed and interpreted in widely dispersed association areas of the cortex.

A brief review of the function of the cerebral hemisphere lobes follows: The *frontal* lobe, the largest of the lobes, extends from the central sulcus (fissure of Rolando) forward and from the lateral fissure (fissure of Sylvius) upward. It contains the motor strip, premotor area, Broca's speech center, and association areas related to higher mental functions and behavior. The *parietal* lobe lies between the central sulcus and the parietooccipital fissure. The lateral fissure divides the parietal from the temporal lobe. Angular, postcentral, and supramarginal gyri are significant landmarks in the parietal lobe. Primary and secondary somasthetic areas are contained here, as are many sensory association fibers. Interpretations of feeling and hearing are made here. In addition, body image recognition evolves from the parietal lobe.

The *occipital* lobe lies posterior to the parietal lobe and is divided from the cerebellum by the parietooccipital fissure. Primary visual centers and visual association areas are contained in the occipital lobe. The *temporal lobe* extends downward from the lateral fissure and posteriorly to the parietooccipital fissure. Auditory centers, auditory association area (Wernicke's), smell interpretation, and memory storage are contained in the temporal lobe (Fig. 44-27).

The Peripheral Nervous System

The peripheral nervous system includes the nerve tissue outside the brain and spinal cord. It is composed of 31

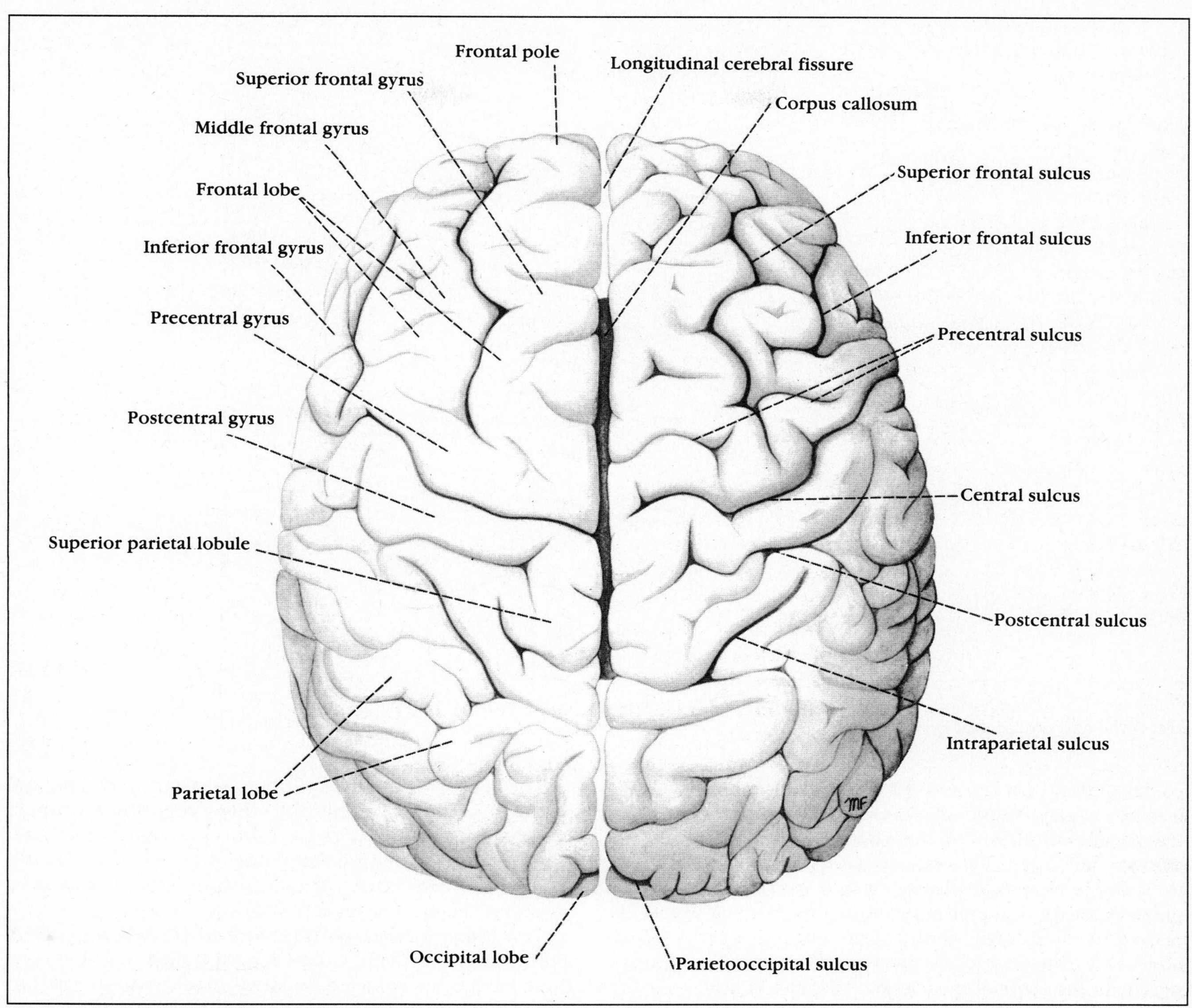

FIGURE 44-25 Superior view of cerebral hemispheres. (From R.S. Snell, *Clinical Neuroanatomy for Medical Students*. Boston: Little, Brown, 1980.)

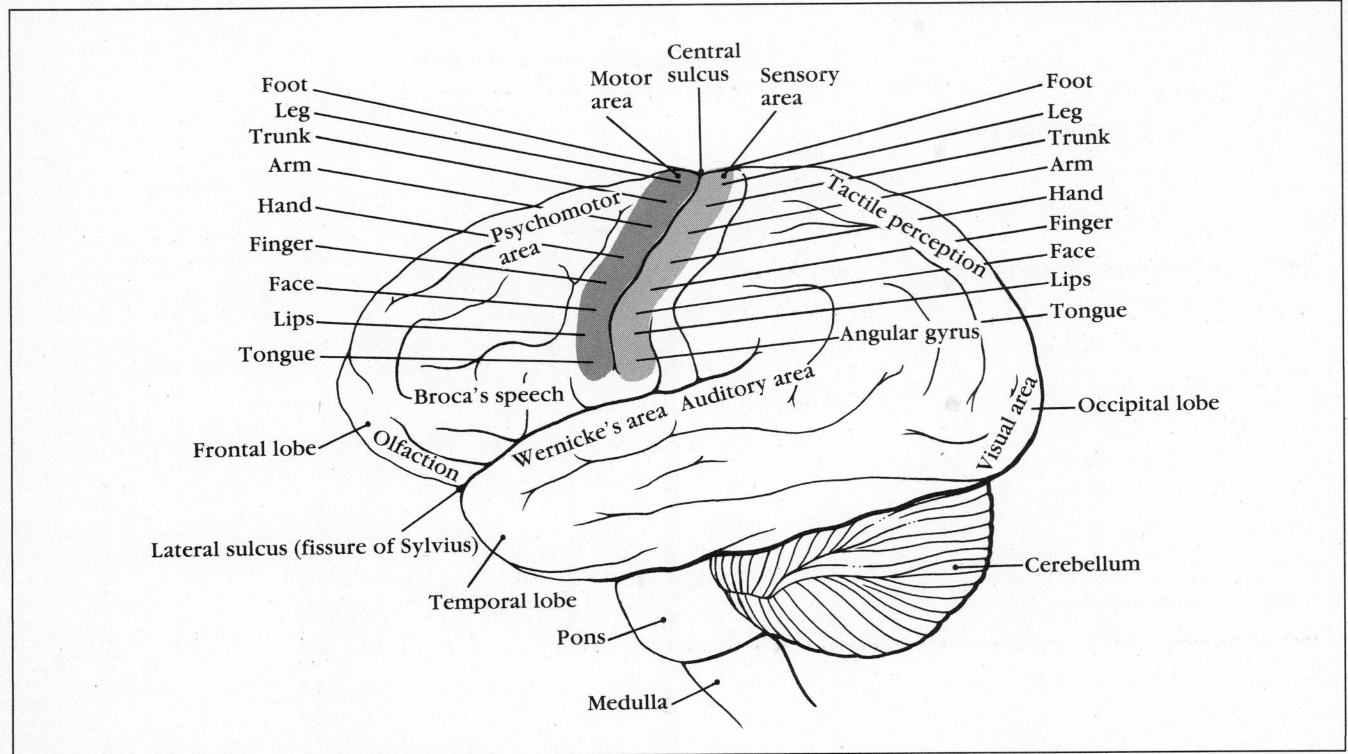

FIGURE 44-26 Topographic organization of functions of control and interpretation on the precentral and postcentral gyri.

paired spinal nerves and 12 cranial nerves, as well as numerous ganglia and plexuses. Every spinal nerve contains a dorsal (afferent) and ventral (efferent) root. The afferent nerve cells lie within the dorsal root ganglion and their fibers innervate through spinal nerves and through plexuses of the visceral nervous system. The efferent cell bodies lie within the ventral gray column of the spinal cord and innervate through ventral roots of all spinal nerves to the skeletal muscle and through ventral roots of spinal nerves of the thorax, upper lumbar, and middle sacral region to the viscera.

The cranial nerve nuclei are contained in the brainstem. The physiologic anatomy of the cranial nerves is not as clearly delineated as that of the spinal nerves. Some cranial nerves have only sensory components, some only motor components, and others contain both. Their names and general functions are presented in Table 44-4. Their functions and dysfunctions are further described in Chapter 48.

Afferent (Sensory) Division

The afferent, or sensory, division of the peripheral nervous system detects, transmits, and processes environmental information from internal and external sources through a variety of specific receptors. The *somatic afferent* fibers carry impulses from the skin, skeletal muscles, joints, and tendons to the central nervous system. The *visceral afferent* fibers carry impulses from the viscera to the central nervous system.

The receptors of afferent fibers transmit to the central nervous system by numerous converging fibers through peripheral nerves. As a result of this convergence of neurons, injury to a nerve fiber does not result in clearly defined sensory deficits. Rather, the area that responds in an altered manner is vaguely defined.

The areas in the skin innervated by specific spinal nerves are commonly called *dermatomes*. Traditionally, these have been arranged to correspond to the spinal cord segments. Thus, a rather loose topographic division of these segments includes the 8 cervical, 12 thoracic, 5 lumbar, and 5 sacral cord regions. Dermatomes are more specifically mapped according to the segmentation of individual dorsal roots (Fig. 44-28).

The afferent fibers carrying sensory data enter the spinal cord by way of the dorsal roots and become dispersed according to function. Fibers that transmit pain and temperature are anatomically related and ascend through the *lateral spinothalamic tract* to the posterior ventral nucleus of the thalamus. The *ventral spinothalamic tracts* contain fibers from receptors that are sensitive to touch and pressure (Fig. 44-29). From here they proceed to the somasthetic region of the cerebral postcentral gyrus. Impulses from muscles, tendons, ligaments, and joints (proprioceptive fibers) disperse in a variety of tracts. Some simply cross the cord to the anterior horn (stretch reflex). Others synapse with the posterior gray column and ascend the spinocerebellar tracts to the cerebellum, while yet others ascend by way of the posterior white

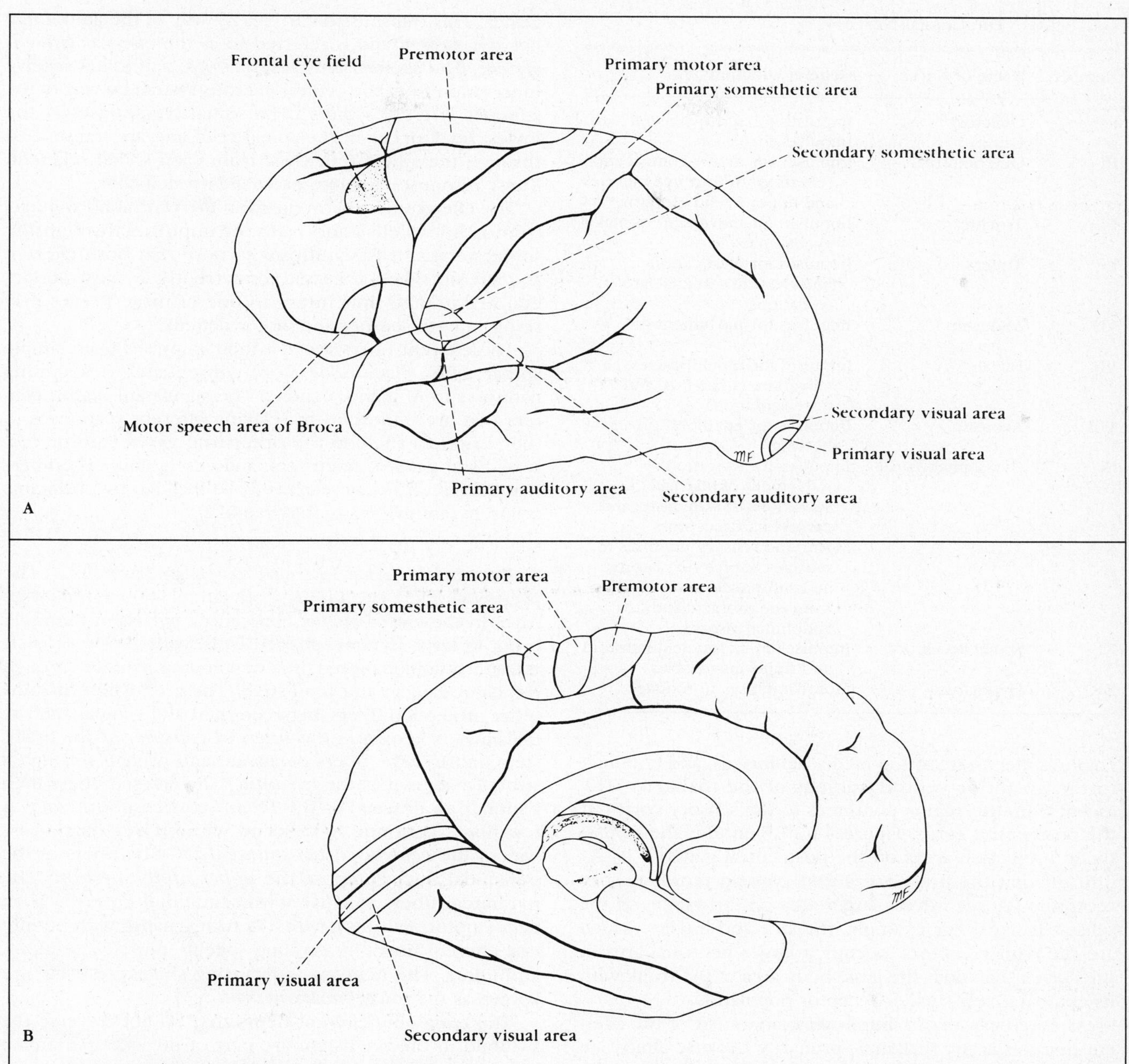

FIGURE 44-27 Functional localization of the cerebral cortex: (A) lateral view and (B) medial view of left cerebral hemisphere. (From R.S. Snell, *Clinical Neuroanatomy for Medical Students*. Boston: Little, Brown, 1980.)

TABLE 44-4 The Cranial Nerves

Number	Name of Nerve	General Function
I	Olfactory	Impulses for sense of smell
II	Optic	Impulses for vision
III	Oculomotor	Impulses for motor control and sensation for four eye muscles and upper eyelid elevator
IV	Trochlear	Impulses for movement of major eyeball muscle
V	Trigeminal	Impulses for mastication muscles and some facial sensations
VI	Abducens	Impulses for movement of eyeball
VII	Facial	Impulses for facial muscles, salivation, cutaneous, and taste sensations
VIII	Acoustic	Impulses for equilibration and hearing
IX	Glossopharyngeal	Impulses for salivation, movement of pharynx, sensations of skin, taste, and carotid baroreceptors
X	Vagus	Motor and sensory impulses to muscles of pharynx, larynx, and soft palate, and sensation from the thoracic and abdominal viscera.
XI	Spinal accessory	Impulses to sternocleidomastoid and trapezius muscles
XII	Hypoglossal	Motor impulses to tongue

columns, decussate at the medial lemniscus, and continue to the posterior ventral nucleus of the thalamus. The ascent from this region continues to the sensory cortex at the postcentral gyrus. Figure 44-27 identifies the somasthetic projection areas on the postcentral gyrus. It is significant that the body areas that contain more sensory receptors are accorded a larger area on the surface of the sensory cortex. For example, the face and fingers, which are rife with receptors, occupy a larger neuronal area in the cortex than does the large body area of the trunk with its comparatively smaller receptor population.

As noted earlier, an important component of the afferent division is the thalamus, primarily because almost all sensory systems convey impulses to its specific nuclei through either the dorsal column or anterolateral tract. Together with the thalamus, the cortex is concerned with conscious perception of sensory stimuli that occur distantly from it. The thalamus provides perception of touch and pressure, whereas more complex discrimination sensations such as texture, size, and weight of objects are interpreted by the cortex.

Efferent (Motor) Division

Voluntary and involuntary body activities initiated by the efferent division are transmitted as a response to the stimuli the central nervous system has received from the afferent division. These responses may be through the innervation of smooth muscles, cardiac muscle, and glands. This transmission arrives by way of the autonomic nervous system and is referred to as the *visceral efferent system*. The skeletal muscles, tendons, and joints receive innervation from the central nervous system by way of the *somatic efferent system*. The somatic responses at the lowest level occur in the spinal cord and are transmitted through the spinal reflex arc from each spinal segment. These responses are automatic and spontaneous.

The efferent fibers emerge from the ventral horn nuclei (motor horn cells) and transmit impulses through the spinal nerves. It is significant to note that both efferent and afferent fibers transmit concurrently in most peripheral nerves, and thus injury to one of these nerves may result in both sensory and motor deficits.

The efferent fibers receive their impulses from simple spinal reflex circuits or more complicated descending pathways from higher centers. The significant higher centers that are important in relaying efferent responses to the periphery include the precentral gyrus (motor cortex), basal ganglia, brainstem, and cerebellum. The fibers that transmit from these areas do so through two principal tracts, pyramidal and extrapyramidal.

Pyramidal and Extrapyramidal Systems. The pyramidal tract (Fig. 44-30), both lateral and ventral, originates in the motor cortex (precentral gyrus) of the cerebrum in large pyramid-shaped cells, called *Betz cells*. It transmits, uninterrupted, in a descending manner through the basal ganglia and brainstem. The area where it joins other projection fibers, between the basal ganglia and the thalamus, is known as the *internal capsule*. In the brainstem, most of the fibers decussate and project through a structure known as the *pyramid*. The crossed fibers then continue to descend as the *lateral corticospinal tract*. A few fibers continue to descend without decussation by way of the *ventral corticospinal tract*. The fibers of the pyramidal tract compose the *upper motor neuron*. The pyramidal fibers synapse with segmental anterior horn cells (motor neurons), which in turn synapse with peripheral efferent fibers innervating specific muscles, tendons, and joints. The neurons innervating skeletal muscle are known as the *lower motor neurons* [3].

The remaining efferent fibers that do not traverse the pyramid in the brainstem are part of the extrapyramidal systems. Unlike the pyramidal tract, the extrapyramidal tracts do not continue to the cord uninterrupted. The system is more complex and is considered by some authors to be a functional rather than an anatomic entity [1,2]. Many of the fibers descend from the cortex directly to specific areas in the basal ganglia and brainstem, while others make intermediate synapses. Several extrapyramidal tracts originate in the brainstem and are named for their site of origin. These include the *vestibulospinal tract* from the lateral vestibular nucleus in the medulla, the *rubrospinal tract* from the red nucleus in the midbrain, the *tectospinal tract* from the roof (superior colliculus) of the midbrain, and the *reticulospinal tract* from the reticular formation in the pons and medulla. The majority of extrapyramidal fibers decussate with the reticulospinal tract. In addition to the named tracts, important

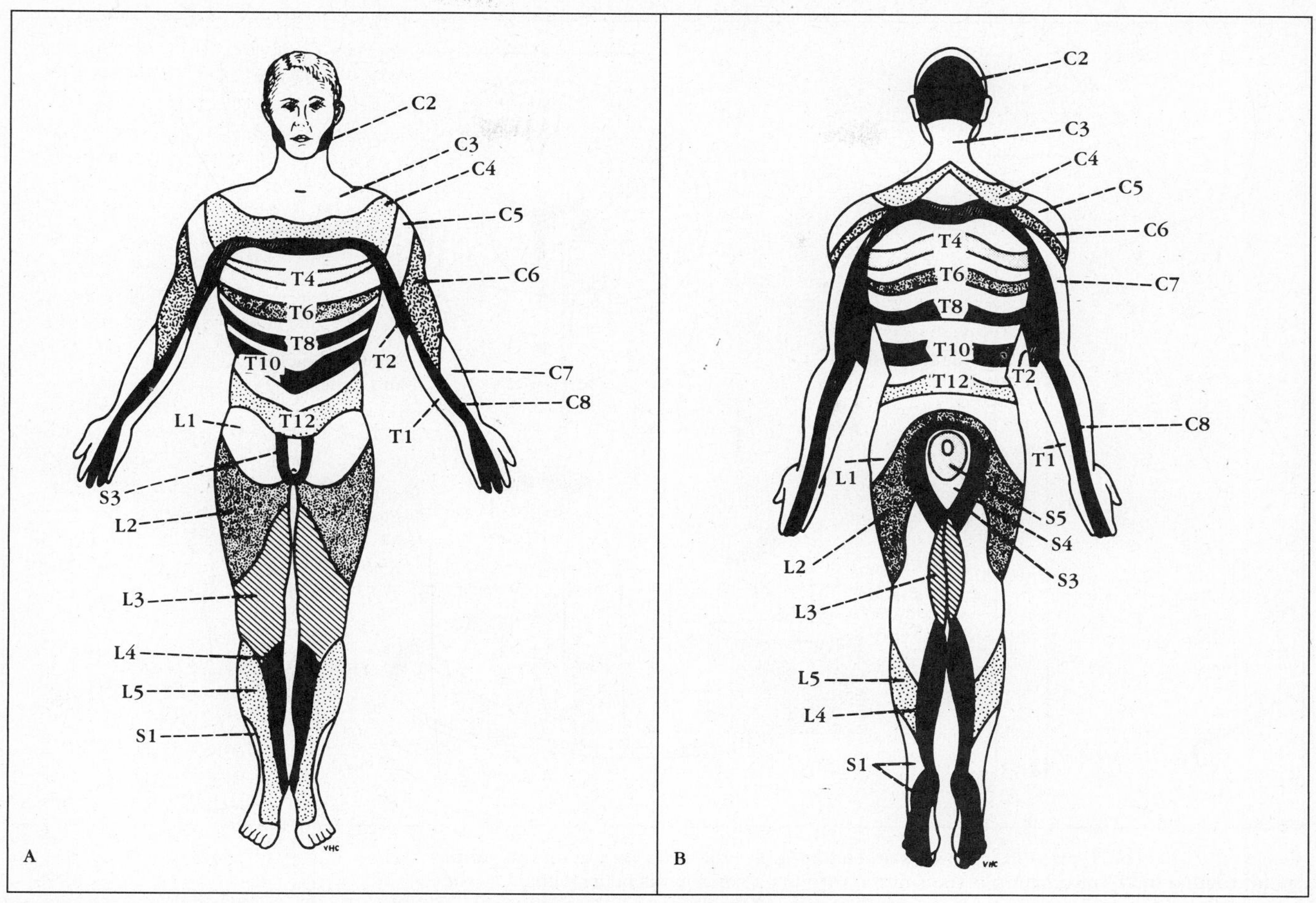

FIGURE 44-28 Dermatomes on (A) the anterior aspect and (B) the posterior aspect of the body. (From R.S. Snell, *Clinical Neuroanatomy for Medical Students*. Boston: Little, Brown, 1980.)

fibers of the extrapyramidal system originate in the cerebellum and the vestibular apparatus.

The pyramidal tract processes information regarding voluntary movement dealing with precise and specific activities of muscles, whereas the extrapyramidal tracts provide the "supporting" type of movement that accompanies the more precise movements afforded by the pyramidal tract. For example, the gross movements necessary to engage in the activity of writing are influenced by the extrapyramidal tracts. Included here are such movements as might be necessary for proper body positioning, particularly of the upper arm and shoulder. The more precise movement of holding the pencil effectively is controlled by the corticospinal tract.

The Autonomic Nervous System

Autonomic fibers project innervations from the central nervous system to smooth muscles, cardiac muscle, and glands in an involuntary manner to regulate activities related to respiration, cardiovascular function, digestion, excretion, body temperature, and sexual function. Centers in the hypothalamus, brainstem, and spinal cord transmit reflex responses to visceral organs to regulate the internal environment. Autonomic fibers differ from somatic efferent fibers in that they consist of a double neuron chain from the central nervous system to the visceral effectors, whereas the somatic efferents transmit through one neuron. Visceral efferent fibers transmit in spinal nerves and in several cranial nerves. Visceral efferent innervation frequently accompanies somatic efferent activity. For example, a jogger receives innervation from the somatic efferent fibers to provide the skeletal muscle responses required in the jogging activity, and simultaneously the somatic efferent system innervates the cardiac and smooth muscle. The somatic efferent responses can be observed readily, whereas the visceral efferent responses are less obvious.

In addition to the autonomic efferent fibers, certain afferent fibers are sometimes assigned to the autonomic nervous system. These are present in spinal nerves as well as in certain cranial nerves. They innervate receptors in the viscera, thorax, and walls of the blood vessels.

The autonomic nervous system consists of two functionally distinct divisions, *sympathetic* and *parasympa-*

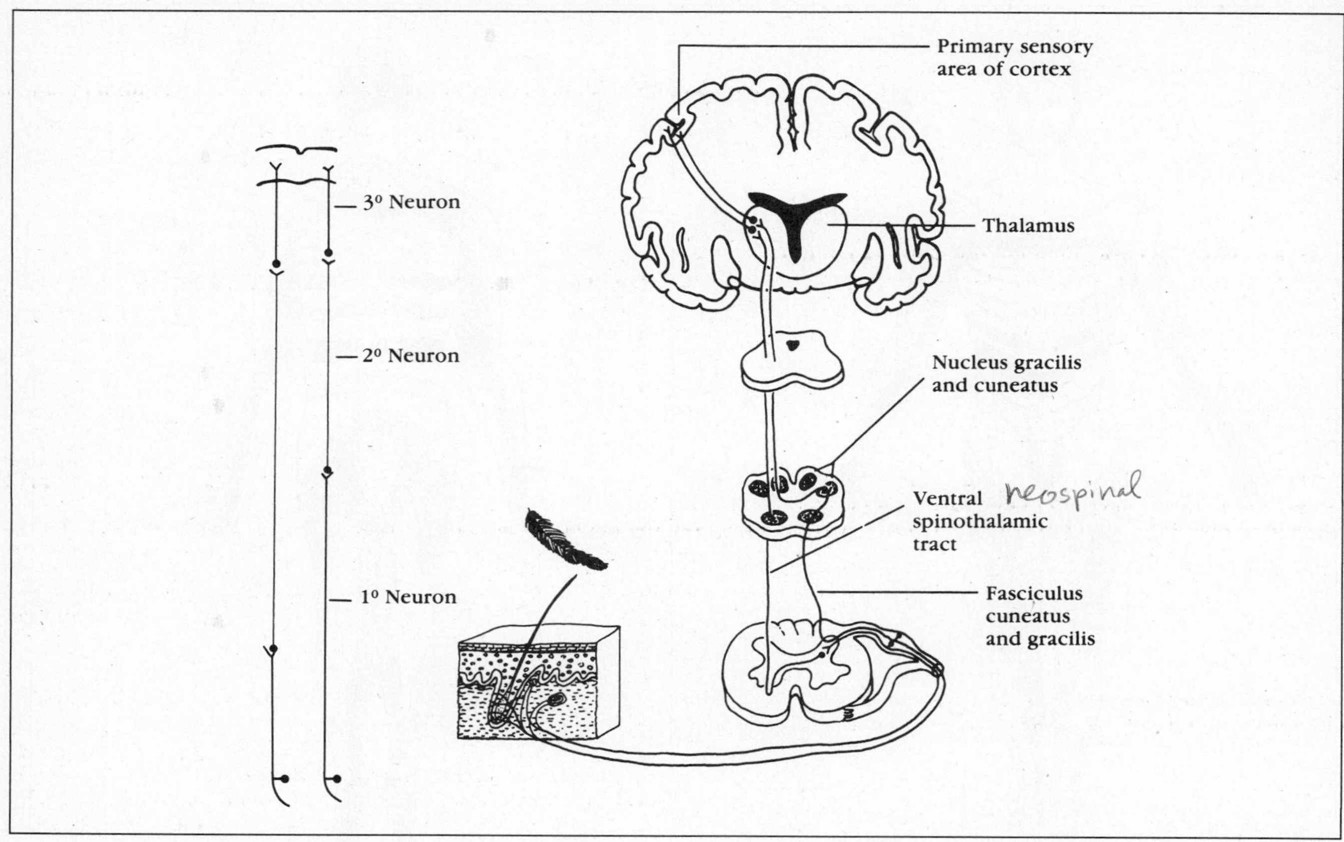

FIGURE 44-29 Touch-pressure pathways ascending to the thalamus by way of the ventral spinothalamic tract. Information is transmitted through a continuous neuron chain. (From L. Langley and F. Christensen, *Structure and Function of the Human Body*. Copyright © 1978. Burgess Publishing, an imprint of Burgess International Group, Inc., Edina, Minnesota. Reprinted by permission.)

thetic (Fig. 44-31). Many visceral effector organs have a dual nerve supply, one from each division. The sympathetic division assists the body into action during physiologic and psychologic stress by supportive activities such as increasing heart and respiratory rates and mobilizing glucose from glycogen stores to supply the skeletal muscles with additional energy. The parasympathetic division provides a counterbalance for the sympathetic division. Nerve cells of both divisions group outside the central nervous system in structures known as *autonomic ganglia*. Cell fibers that terminate with a synapse at these ganglia and retain the cell body within the central nervous system are the *preganglionic neurons*. Conversely, nerve cells having cell bodies in the ganglia and axons extending to the organs and glands are known as the *postganglionic neurons*.

The sympathetic system has a chain of paired ganglia on either side of the spinal cord (*paravertebral ganglia*), extending its full length. These ganglia are connected on each side by nerve trunks and together are referred to as the right and left *sympathetic chains*, or *sympathetic trunks*. In addition to these paired ganglia, single ganglia exist surrounding the abdominal aorta and its larger branches, where preganglionic neurons terminate without synapsing in the sympathetic chain. These are known as *collateral (prevertebral) ganglia* and include the celiac and superior and inferior mesenteric ganglia. The terminal ganglia are parasympathetic and are located in proximity to the effector organs.

Sympathetic Division (Thoracolumbar)

The cell bodies of the short preganglionic sympathetic neurons arise from the sympathetic motoneurons of the intermediolateral horns of the spinal cord between the first thoracic and second lumbar vertebrae (see Fig. 44-31). The fibers of these neurons pass through the intervertebral foramina in conjunction with respective spinal nerves. Shortly the sympathetic fibers (preganglionic) depart from the spinal nerve and enter a sympathetic chain through the white rami communicans (Fig. 44-32). They may synapse here immediately with a postganglion neuron or pass directly through the sympathetic chain to synapse with a single sympathetic ganglion, or pass up or down the sympathetic chain and synapse at a different level.

Some postganglionic sympathetic fibers, after having synapsed in the sympathetic chain, pass back into the

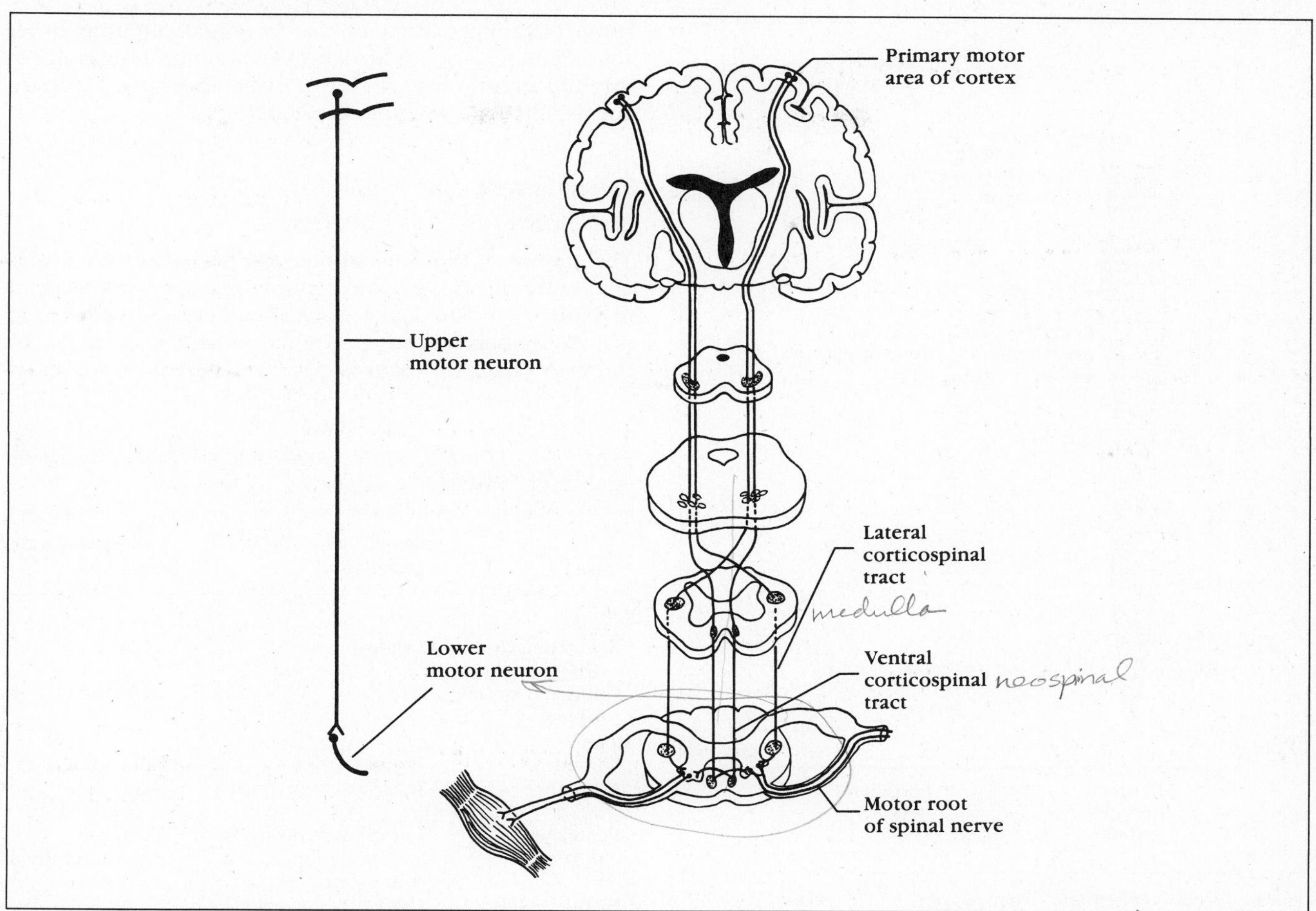

FIGURE 44-30 Pyramidal motor pathways originating at the primary motor area. The lateral corticospinal tract crosses at the level of the medulla and the ventral corticospinal tract descends uncrossed. The pyramidal tract is composed of the upper and lower motor neurons. (From L. Langley and F. Christensen, *Structure and Function of the Human Body*. Copyright © 1978. Burgess Publishing, an imprint of Burgess International Group, Inc., Edina, Minnesota. Reprinted by permission.)

spinal nerve through the gray rami communicans and accompany the spinal nerve to innervate blood vessels, sweat glands, and arrectores pilorum muscles in the skin.

Parasympathetic Division (Craniosacral)

The autonomic fibers that evolve from the cranial and sacral portions of the central nervous system compose the parasympathetic nervous system (see Fig. 44-31). Somatic efferent fibers in the cranial region arise in conjunction with the oculomotor (third), facial (seventh), glossopharyngeal (ninth), and vagus (tenth) nerves. The vagus transmits the majority of the parasympathetic impulses through its wide distribution in the thoracic and abdominal viscera. The remaining cranial nerves innervate organs of the head. The sacral fibers arise from the anterior roots of the second, third, and fourth sacral spinal nerves and innervate pelvic organs and the colon. Most of the preganglionic fibers transmit without interruption to the organs they innervate, where they synapse with the parasympathetic ganglia that are located in the area of the effector organ. In contrast to the sympathetic fibers, the parasympathetic preganglionic fibers are long and the postganglionic fibers short.

Transmitter Substances of the Autonomic Nervous System

Chemical mediation is necessary for neuronal transmission between neurons and between neurons and their effector organs. Excitation results from chemical release of transmitter substances between preganglionic and postganglionic neurons and their effectors in the autonomic nervous system. The transmitter substance in the autonomic nervous system from the preganglionic neurons to the postganglionic neurons in both the sympathetic and parasympathetic nervous systems is *acetylcholine (ACH)*. Acetylcholine continues to be the transmitter substance from the parasympathetic postganglionic neurons. Because of the secretion of ACh, these fibers are known as *cholinergic* and their receptors are *cholinoceptive*.

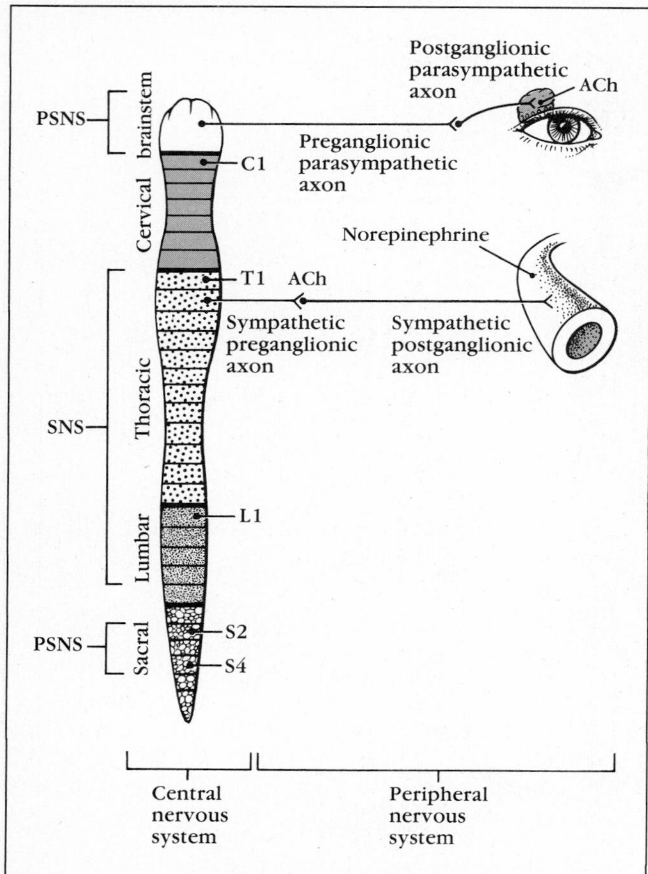

FIGURE 44-31 Schematic overview of the origins of sympathetic (SNS) and parasympathetic (PSNS) nervous systems with corresponding major transmitter substances at the synapses: acetylcholine (ACh) and norepinephrine (noradrenalin).

The primary transmitter substance secreted by the postganglionic fibers of the sympathetic nervous system to its effector organs is *norepinephrine (NE)*. The fibers are referred to as *adrenergic* and terminate on *adrenoceptive* receptors (alpha and beta). A few of the fibers of the postganglionic sympathetic nervous system secrete ACh at their terminal fibers, including fibers to sweat glands and postganglionic sympathetic vasodilator fibers to skeletal muscle vasculature [2]. A single postganglionic sympathetic nerve may innervate thousands of receptor sites. This is demonstrated by the diffuse response to the sympathetic nervous system excitation in contrast to the more localized responses characteristic of parasympathetic activity.

Receptor Substances of the Effector Organs

The effector organs secrete substances that react with terminal bouton secretions. The exact nature of these substances is uncertain. It has been theorized that the combination of the autonomic nervous system transmitter substance and receptor substances alters the permeability of the cell membrane to certain ions. This alteration may result in changes in membrane potential, eliciting either action potentials or tonic effects. In addition to changes in the cell membrane, receptor substances may initiate chemical reactions within the cell.

Stimulation and Inhibition of the Autonomic Nervous System

The actions of the sympathetic and parasympathetic nervous systems on various receptor organs are summarized in Table 44-5. The dual actions are a cooperative effort to maintain a constant internal environment in response to the ever changing external world. General responses of

TABLE 44-5 The Effects of Sympathetic and Parasympathetic Stimulation on Effector Organs

Organ	Sympathetic Stimulation	Parasympathetic Stimulation
Eye		
Radial muscle of iris	Dilates	
Sphincter muscle of iris		Constricts
Heart		
SA node	Increases rate	Decreases rate
Atria	Increases contractility	Decreases contractility
Ventricles	Increases contractility, conduction, automaticity	Decreases contractility
Blood vessels	Generally constricts, but may dilate coronary arteries	None
Lungs		
Bronchial muscle	Dilates (relaxes)	Constricts
Bronchial secretions	Decreases	Increases
Bronchial vessels	Constricts mildly	None
Skin		
Sweat glands	Copious generalized secretion	Slight localized secretion
Intestine		
Motility	Decreases	Increases
Sphincters	Contracts	Relaxes
Liver	Glycogenolysis	None
Gallbladder and ducts	Relaxes	Constricts
Pancreas		
Acini cells	None	Secrete
Islet cells	Inhibit alpha-receptors, stimulates beta-receptors to secrete	Secrete
Salivary glands	Thick secretions	Thin secretions
Fat cells	Lipolysis	None
Bladder		
Detrusor muscle	Relaxes	Contracts
Trigone	Contracts	Relaxes
Penis	Ejaculation	Erection
Basal metabolism	Increased	None
Adrenal medulla	Increased secretion	None
Mentation	Increased	None

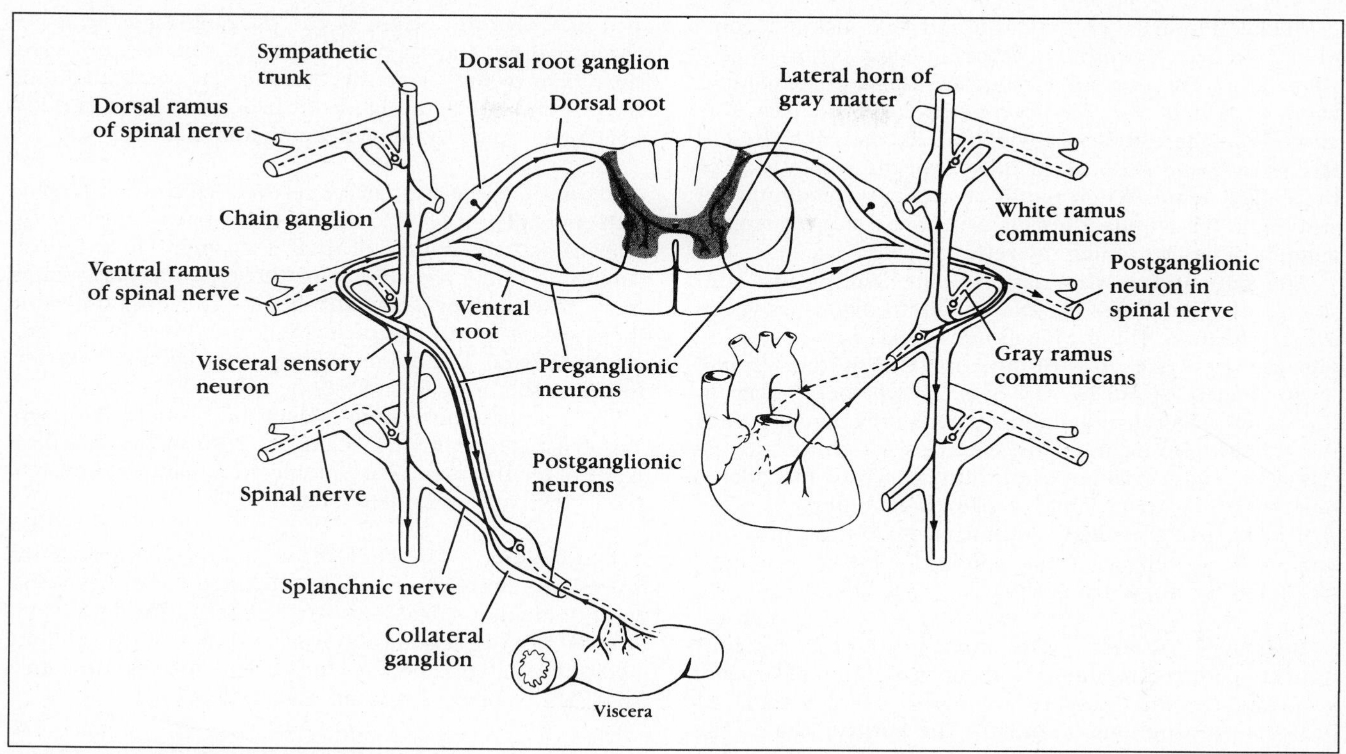

FIGURE 44-32 Sympathetic fibers emerge from the spinal cord in conjunction with respective spinal nerves and transmit to autonomic ganglia by way of white rami. (From A. Spence and E. Mason, *Human Anatomy and Physiology*. Menlo Park, Calif.: Benjamin/Cummings, 1979.)

the sympathetic nervous system are activated under emergency situations to make internal adjustments that facilitate an appropriate response by the body. For example, in response to stressful exercise, the cardiovascular system is stimulated by the sympathetic system to increase cardiac output by increasing heart rate and force, thus providing additional perfusion to skeletal muscle, brain, and liver, while simultaneously reducing the blood supply to the viscera. The parasympathetic system, in contrast, promotes activities that maintain body function from day to day, including digestion and elimination.

The visceral effectors that receive stimulation from both the sympathetic and parasympathetic systems generally receive antagonistic stimulation. An example of this includes the effect on bronchial secretions. Sympathetic stimulation decreases bronchial secretions and parasympathetic stimulation increases them. In another example, the sympathetic system dilates the pupils, while the parasympathetic system constricts them. The dual system does not function consistently in a cooperative balance, as some organs receive innervation primarily from only one system. Examples include the smooth muscles of the skin, hair, sweat glands, and cutaneous blood vessels, which are primarily innervated from the sympathetic system. The detrusor muscle of the bladder receives parasympathetic innervation only.

The inhibitory actions of the autonomic nervous system occur both directly and indirectly on the effector organs. For example, vagal stimulation (parasympathetic) slows the heart through a direct inhibitory action of the cholinergic postganglionic neurons on the sinoatrial node. On the other hand, vasodilation of the peripheral arterioles occurs indirectly through a decrease in impulse transmission in the sympathetic effector fibers.

While most organs and viscera receive innervation from both sympathetic and parasympathetic systems, one of these generally has an inhibitory effect and the other an excitatory effect. There is no consistent rule of thumb for guidance as to which system stimulates and which inhibits.

Effects of Sympathetic and Parasympathetic Stimulation on Various Structures

Lacrimal Glands. The parasympathetic system vasodilates and stimulates secretion of the lacrimal glands through the postganglionic axons from the sphenopalatine ganglion by way of the maxillary division of the fifth cranial nerve. The preganglionic axons originate in the superior salivatory nucleus and follow the route of the seventh cranial nerve. The sympathetic system has a vasoconstrictive effect on the lacrimal glands and transmits its impulses through preganglionic neurons, which originate from the intermediolateral cells in the thoracic spinal column, and through postganglionic neurons of the superior cervical ganglion; the impulses reach the glands by way of the maxillary division of the fifth cranial nerve [9].

Eyes. Pupillary constriction and near-vision accommodation are accomplished through parasympathetic stimulation. The oculomotor nucleus sends preganglionic axons by way of the oculomotor nerve to the ciliary ganglion. From here the postganglionic axons reach the ciliary muscle and constrictor muscle of the iris by way of the ciliary nerve. When pupils are reflexively stimulated with light, the pupillary openings decrease and reduce the amount of light reaching the retinae.

The sympathetic stimulation dilates the pupils, constricts vessels, elevates the eyelids, and provides far-vision accommodation. The preganglionic axons of fibers accomplishing these activities originate in the thoracic spinal segments and ascend by way of the sympathetic chain to the superior cervical ganglion where they synapse with the postganglionic neurons. The postganglionic axons travel through divisions of the fifth nerve to the dilator muscles of the irises (levator palpebrae superioris), and radial fibers of the ciliary muscles. Innervation of blood vessels of the retinae, orbits, and conjunctivae is accomplished in the same manner [8].

Salivary Glands. The superior salivary nucleus projects the preganglionic axons for the submaxillary and sublingual glands, and the inferior salivary nucleus projects preganglionic axons for the parotid gland. The axons from the superior salivary nucleus travel through a branch of the seventh cranial nerve to the submaxillary and sublingual ganglia, and those from the inferior salivary nucleus travel through a branch of the ninth cranial nerve to the otic ganglia. From the submaxillary and sublingual ganglia, axons project to their glands and from the otic ganglia to the parotid gland by way of the fifth cranial nerve. The parasympathetic system activates these glands to vasodilate and secrete.

The sympathetic system vasoconstricts and promotes secretion of salivary glands. Its preganglionic axons ascend from the upper thoracic spinal cord to the superior cervical ganglia to synapse with the postganglionic neurons. These axons reach the glands along the external carotid and external maxillary arteries [9].

Heart. The overall effects of the parasympathetic system on the heart are deceleration and coronary artery vasoconstriction. Its stimulation of the heart decreases its effectiveness; however, in the process it does slow the metabolism and oxygen requirements, and thus provides some rest for the cardiac muscle. The parasympathetic preganglionic fibers pass from the dorsal motor nucleus of the vagus and synapse with the postganglionic neurons through the vagal trunk at cardiac plexus ganglia in the atrial walls.

In contrast, the sympathetic system increases the overall activity of the heart, produces both positive chronotropic and inotropic effects, and dilates the coronary arteries. In essence, the sympathetic system makes the heart more effective, although it simultaneously increases workload and metabolic requirements. The upper thoracic spinal cord provides the origin of the preganglionic neurons, which project their axons from the ventral roots and white rami to the sympathetic chain. The postganglionic neurons emerge from higher thoracic and lower cervical ganglia and travel to the cardiac plexus [12].

Bronchi. The bronchi are constricted by the parasympathetic system. The origin of the parasympathetic neurons and the course of their preganglionic and postganglionic fibers are similar to those of the parasympathetic fibers innervating the heart. The preganglionic fibers synapse with the postganglionic fibers in the pulmonary plexus. The axons of the postganglionic cells terminate in the bronchi and blood vessels.

The sympathetic system dilates the bronchi. The neurons originate in thoracic segments 2 through 6 and their axons enter the pulmonary plexus in a manner similar to that of the parasympathetic system [5].

Esophagus. The parasympathetic system exerts the main autonomic influence over the function of the esophagus. Stimulation causes smooth muscle of the esophagus to constrict, increasing its overall activity in propelling ingested materials along its course. This stimulation comes from various branches of the vagus nerve [12].

Abdominal Viscera, Glands, and Vessels. Stimulation of the parasympathetic system promotes peristalsis and increases in secretion by the various gastrointestinal glands. The preganglionic fibers originate from the vagus and synapse with the postganglionic fibers of the various visceral organs in their intrinsic plexus.

In contrast, the sympathetic system inhibits peristalsis and enhances vasoconstriction. The lower thoracic and upper lumbar cord segments provide the origin of the preganglionic neurons. Their axons traverse the splanchnic nerves to synapse with the postganglionic neurons in the prevertebral ganglion plexus. Innervation is provided to the visceral smooth muscle and blood vessels [9].

Pelvic Viscera. Stimulation of the parasympathetic system assists in urination and defecation by contracting the bladder and lower colon. Penile erection is also facilitated by the parasympathetic system. The neurons that accomplish these functions originate in the sacral cord segments and their axons transmit to the various organs.

Stimulation of the sympathetic system promotes contraction of the vesicle sphincter, vasoconstriction, and ejaculation. The preganglionic neurons originate in the lower thoracic and upper lumbar segments and travel along the splanchnic nerves similarly to those of the abdominal viscera. The postganglionic fibers travel along the hypogastric nerves of the organs innervated [9].

Peripheral Vessels and Sweat Glands. The major effect of the autonomic nervous system on the peripheral and deep vessels is stimulation of the sympathetic system. This results in vasoconstriction of cutaneous vessels as well as deep visceral vessels. Sweat glands secrete in response to sympathetic stimulation. The postganglionic fibers to the sweat glands are cholinergic in contrast with other sympathetic fibers, which are adrenergic. For this reason, many sources classify sweat secretion as a sympathetic function [5].

Adrenal Medulla. In response to sympathetic stimulation, the adrenal medulla secretes epinephrine and norepinephrine into the circulating blood, which reaches all cells and produces an excitatory effect. This mechanism is part of the diffuse sympathoadrenal system, which is activated in response to stress. In addition to the stimulatory effect on the nervous system, epinephrine and norepinephrine affect metabolism through glycogenolysis in the liver and skeletal muscle and mobilization of fatty acids.

Distinct effects of circulating epinephrine and norepinephrine on heart function include increased force and rate of contraction, as well as increased excitability of the myocardium. Norepinephrine produces vasoconstriction in most organs, whereas epinephrine has a dilating effect on the vessels of the liver and skeletal muscle. Other effects observed in response to circulating epinephrine and norepinephrine include increased mental acuity, inhibition of the gastrointestinal tract, and pupillary dilation. Thus, the circulating catecholamines released by the adrenal medulla have functions similar to those of the adrenergic nerve discharges and, indeed, enhance their action. The effects of the circulating catecholamines linger, as their metabolism or removal from blood takes longer than it does in those released at the adrenergic nerve terminals [5].

Minimal secretion of epinephrine and norepinephrine occurs at basal conditions as in sleep; during increased activity and stress, or when adrenergic stimulation is increased in such conditions as pain, cold, hypoglycemia, and emotional excitement, secretion is considerably increased. This stimulation is transmitted to the adrenal medulla by way of the hypothalamic nervous centers as well as by direct sympathetic innervation of the medulla.

To distinguish the effects of epinephrine and norepinephrine on receptor cells, two receptor catecholamine substances have been identified. These are *alpha-adrenergic receptors*, which mediate vasoconstriction and are acted on by both norepinephrine and epinephrine, and *beta-adrenergic receptors*, which mediate vasodilation and actions to increase the rate and strength of the cardiac function. The latter are acted upon by epinephrine. Alpha-adrenergic receptors are dispersed widely in various organs but predominate in the precapillary sphincters of smooth muscles of blood vessels. Beta-adrenergic receptors predominate in the heart, coronary arteries, liver, and brain.

Autonomic Reflexes. In response to certain environmental conditions, autonomic reflexes maintain the internal environment appropriate to the demand, that of either action or repair. For the most part the actions occur at an unconscious level and involve functions such as control of pupillary size, cardiovascular status, and variations in respiratory, gastrointestinal, and genitourinary systems.

The Ventricular and Cerebrospinal Fluid Systems

Function of Cerebrospinal Fluid

The cerebrospinal fluid (CSF) that circulates in the subarachnoid space around the brain and spinal cord (Fig. 44-33) provides an important supportive and protective mechanism for the central nervous system. Together with support from blood vessels, nerve roots, and fine fibrous arachnoid trabeculae, the brain is directly encased within the subarachnoid cerebrospinal fluid and receives buoyancy from it that prevents the vessels and nerve roots from stretching in response to movements of the head. The average weight of the adult brain is approximately 1450 gm in the air, although in the buoyant CSF bath its weight is reduced to approximately 50 gm. This buoyancy allows for relatively effective suspension of the brain and assists in preventing lethal damage under everyday traumas.

Pneumoencephalography demonstrates the effects of CSF deficiency on the brain. This diagnostic procedure to visualize structural elements of the brain requires that CSF be removed and replaced by air. Thus, the weight of the brain rests on the vascular, nervous, and meningeal structures and results in a severe headache that is greatly intensified by the slightest jarring of the head.

In addition to its mechanical function, CSF provides a medium for passage of substances between blood and the extracellular fluid of the brain. It probably also nourishes brain tissues and removes the metabolites of nerve cell function.

Formation and Absorption of Cerebrospinal Fluid

The CSF is produced, circulated, and resorbed continuously. Its principal formation site is in the *choroid plexus* of the lateral ventricle, with most of the remainder being formed in the third and fourth ventricles (Fig. 44-34). The choroid plexus is a network of capillary tufts surrounded by cuboidal epithelium (Fig. 44-35). The fluid is produced through filtration, diffusion, and active transport from the blood. In the adult human, approximately 500 ml of fluid is produced per 24 hours and approximately 125 ml is circulating at any given time. Wide fluctuations may occur in the amount produced during any given 24-hour period (Table 44-6). Sodium ions are actively transported across the epithelial cells into CSF from blood. This results in a greater osmotic force in the CSF, so that to maintain osmotic equilibrium, water passively follows the ions. Thus, water is extracted from the capillaries and is responsible for the secretory function of the choroid plexus.

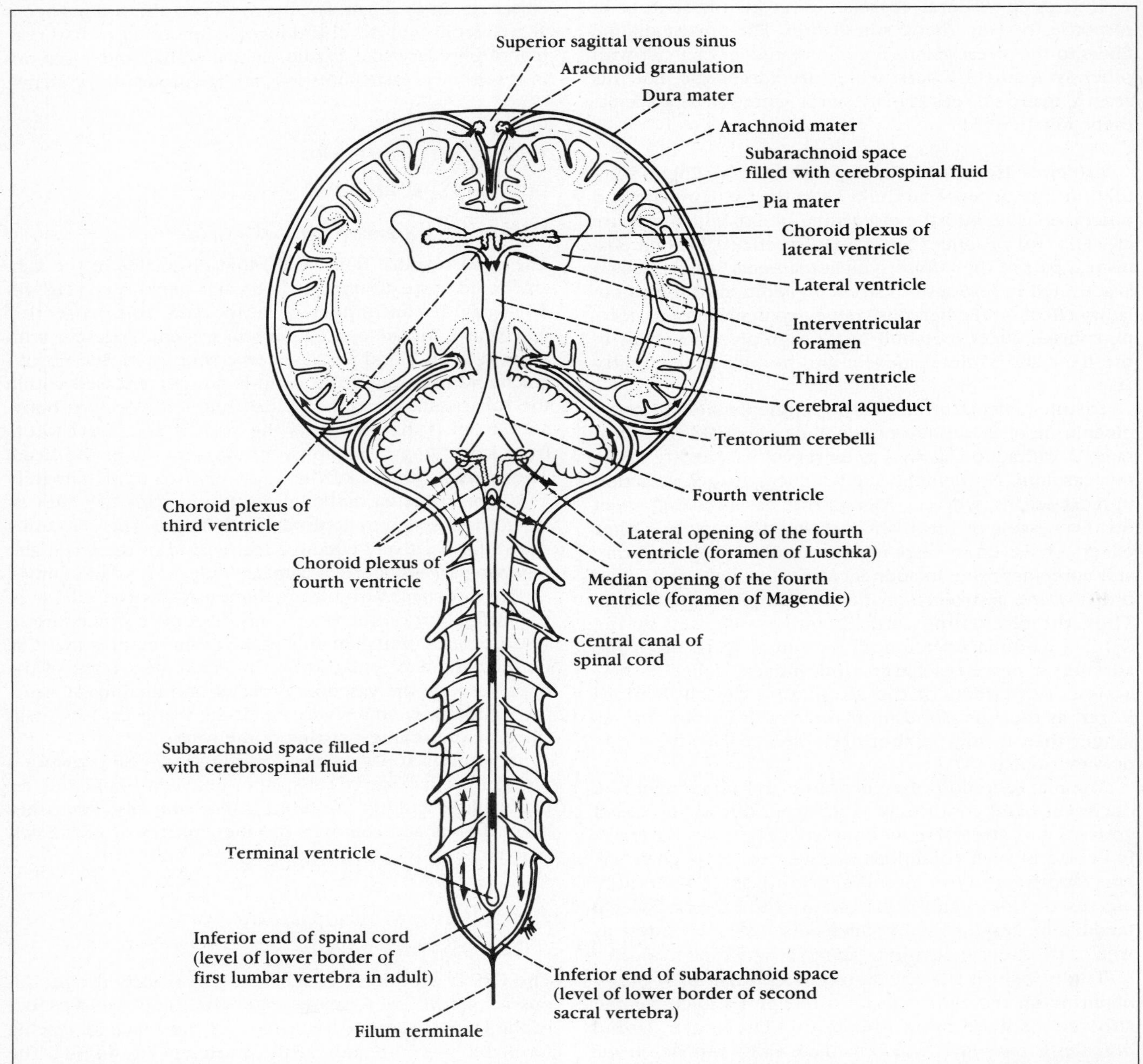

FIGURE 44-33 Formation and circulation of cerebrospinal fluid. (From R.S. Snell, *Clinical Neuroanatomy for Medical Students*. Boston: Little, Brown, 1980.)

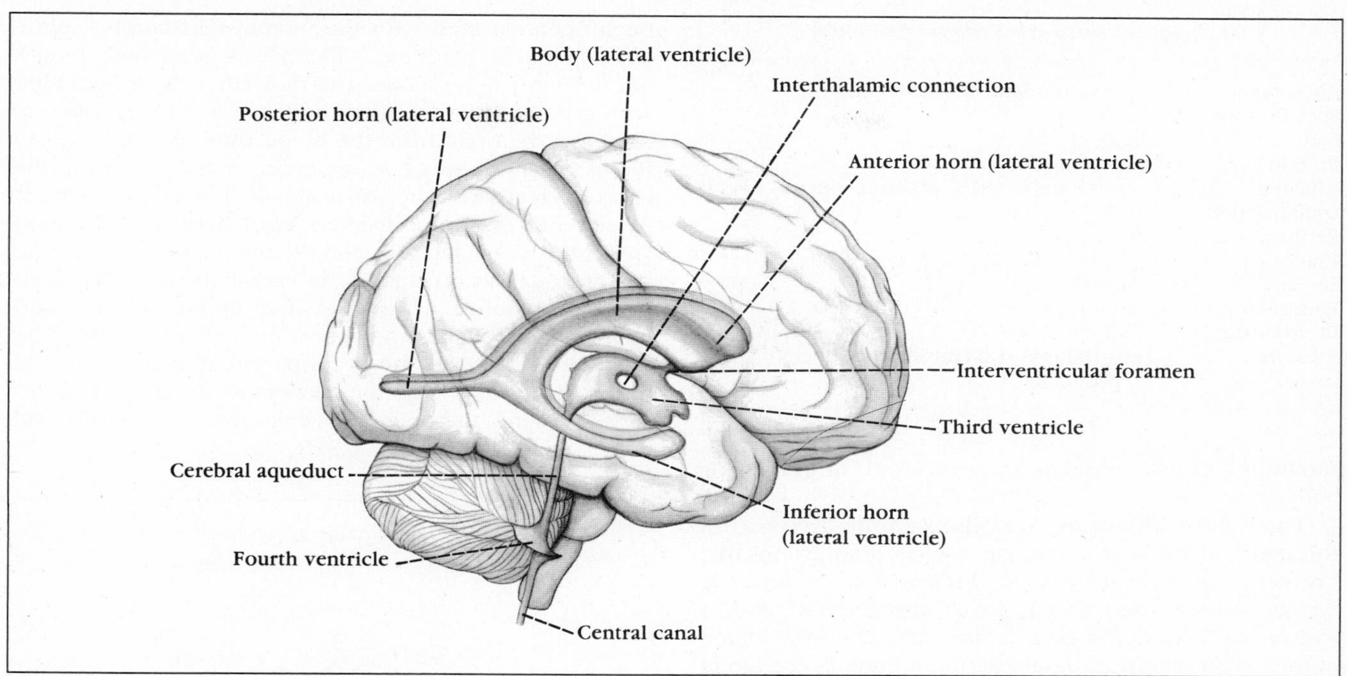

FIGURE 44-34 The lateral third and fourth ventricles. (From R.S. Snell, *Clinical Neuroanatomy for Medical Students*. Boston: Little, Brown, 1980.)

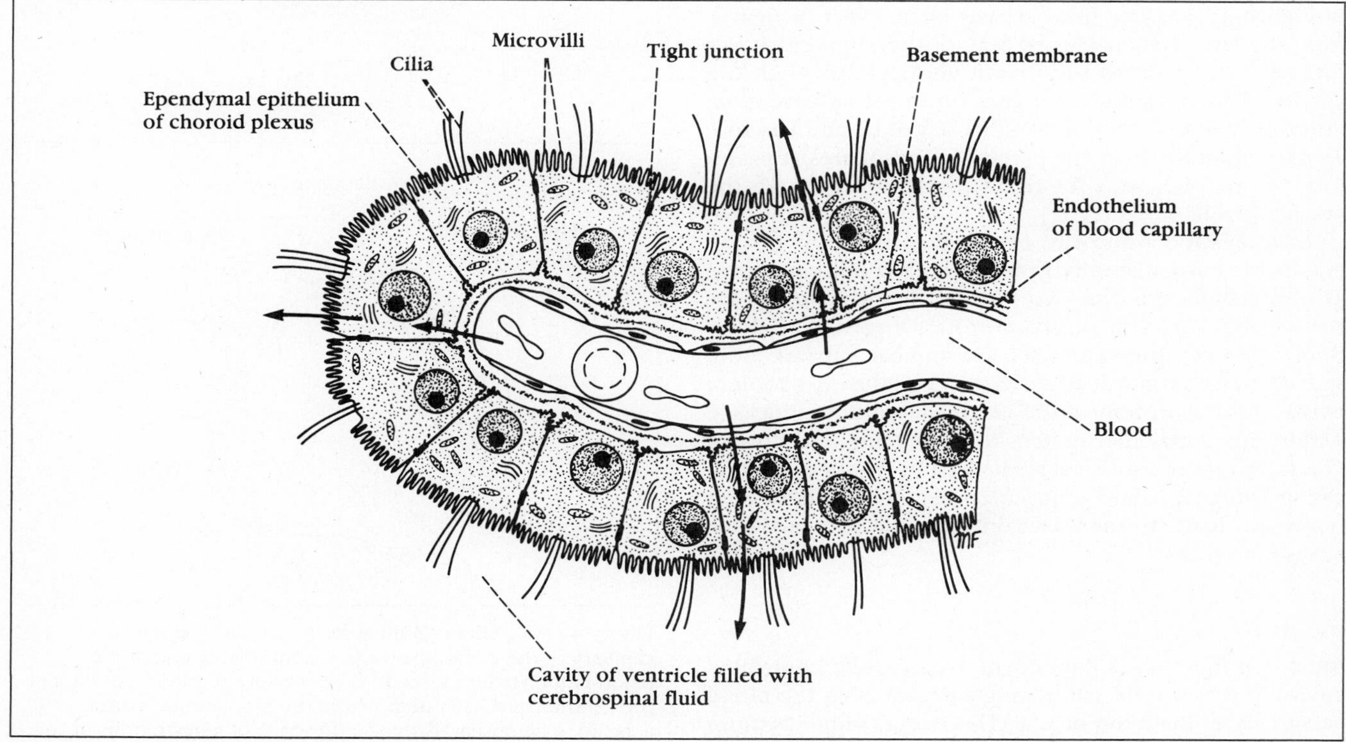

FIGURE 44-35 Microscopic structure of the choroid plexus. (From R.S. Snell, *Clinical Neuroanatomy for Medical Students*. Boston: Little, Brown, 1980.)

TABLE 44-6 Normal Values of Cerebrospinal Fluid

Appearance	Clear, colorless, odorless
Specific gravity	1.007
pH	7.35
Protein	14–45 mg/dl
Glucose	40–80 mg/dl (60% of serum glucose level)
Lymphocytes	0–5
Erythrocytes	0
Chlorides	120–130 mEq/L
Sodium	140 mEq/L
Potassium	3.0 mEq/L
Bicarbonate	23.6 mEq/L
Pressure	80–180 mm H_2O (in side recumbent position)

Facilitated diffusion allows transportation of glucose in both directions.

The CSF is absorbed into the venous circulation through *arachnoid villi* (see Fig. 44-15), granulations that project from the cerebral subarachnoid space into the venous sinuses. The CSF is passively absorbed because its hydrostatic pressure is greater than that of venous blood in the venous sinuses. Certain particles, such as red blood cells and creatinine, pass unimpeded through the arachnoid villi.

Flow and Obstruction of Flow of Cerebrospinal Fluid

The origin of CSF in the choroid plexus of the ventricles and its normal flow to the arachnoid villi are illustrated in Figure 44-33. The fluid arrives in the third ventricle from the lateral ventricles by way of the interventricular foramen, flows on to the fourth ventricle through the cerebral aqueduct, and then goes on to the subarachnoid cisterns by way of the foramina of Magendie and Luschka. As the fluid flows over the cerebral hemispheres, it passes into the sagittal sinus for rapid resorption through the arachnoid villi.

Interference along the pathway of the flow of CSF results in ventricular enlargement and a condition known as *hydrocephalus*. The two types of hydrocephalus are *communicating* and *noncommunicating*. If CSF flows freely between the ventricles and lumbar subarachnoid space, it is communicating hydrocephalus. A problem exists with resorption of CSF in this condition. Blockage within the ventricular system that prevents free flow of CSF from one or more ventricles results in noncommunicating hydrocephalus. Ventricular dilation results in both types and leads to increased intracranial pressure (see pages 820–822).

Brain Barriers

Brain cell function is dependent on a closely controlled environment. Not all circulating substances in the blood pass freely to the brain or CSF. This occurs either because their molecules are too large or the molecules they bind with are too large to cross the CNS membranes. This has been demonstrated with the injection of certain acidic dyes such as trypan blue, which stains other body tissues but not most brain tissue. The molecules these dyes bind with are too large to enter the brain or CSF. Substances pass into the brain from the blood through capillaries to the extracellular space of the brain, or by the way of the choroid plexus into the CSF from which small amounts are passed into the brain. Barriers exist between the blood and brain, blood and CSF, and the brain and CSF.

The materials separating the various cerebral compartments, in essence, are responsible for the entrance and exit of materials to and from the CSF and brain. The choroid plexus and the brain parenchyma (except the hypothalamus) provide the barriers to free movement of substances into the brain. Molecular size, charge, and lipid

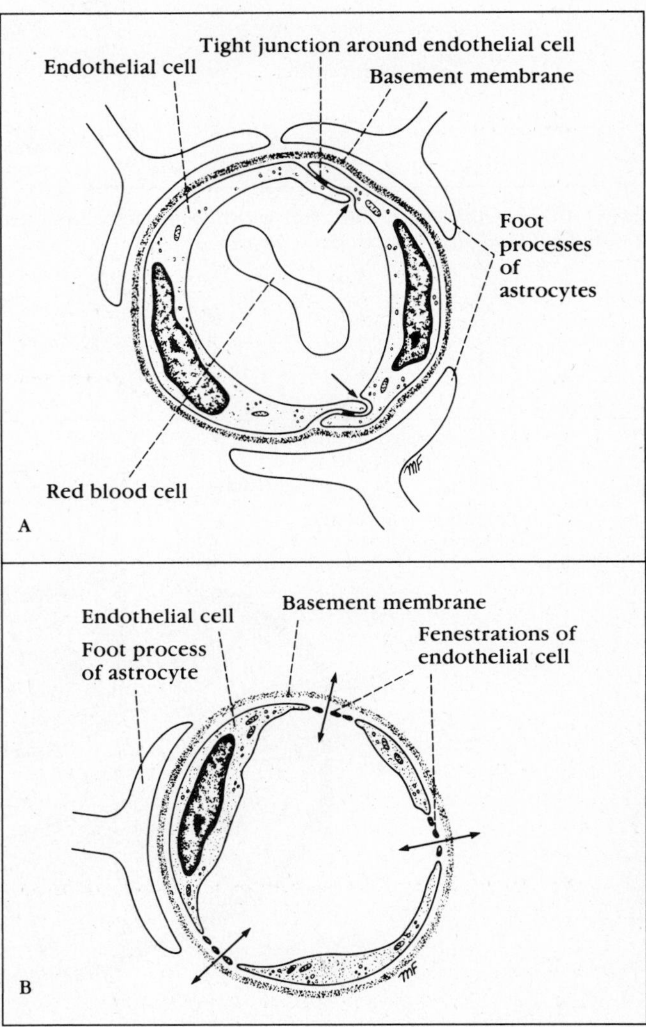

FIGURE 44-36 Blood-brain barrier. A. Cross section of blood capillary of the central nervous system in area where the blood-brain barrier exists. B. Cross section of blood capillary of the central nervous system where the blood-brain barrier appears to be absent. Note the presence of fenestrations in endothelial cells. (From R.S. Snell, *Clinical Neuroanatomy for Medical Students*. Boston: Little, Brown, 1980.)

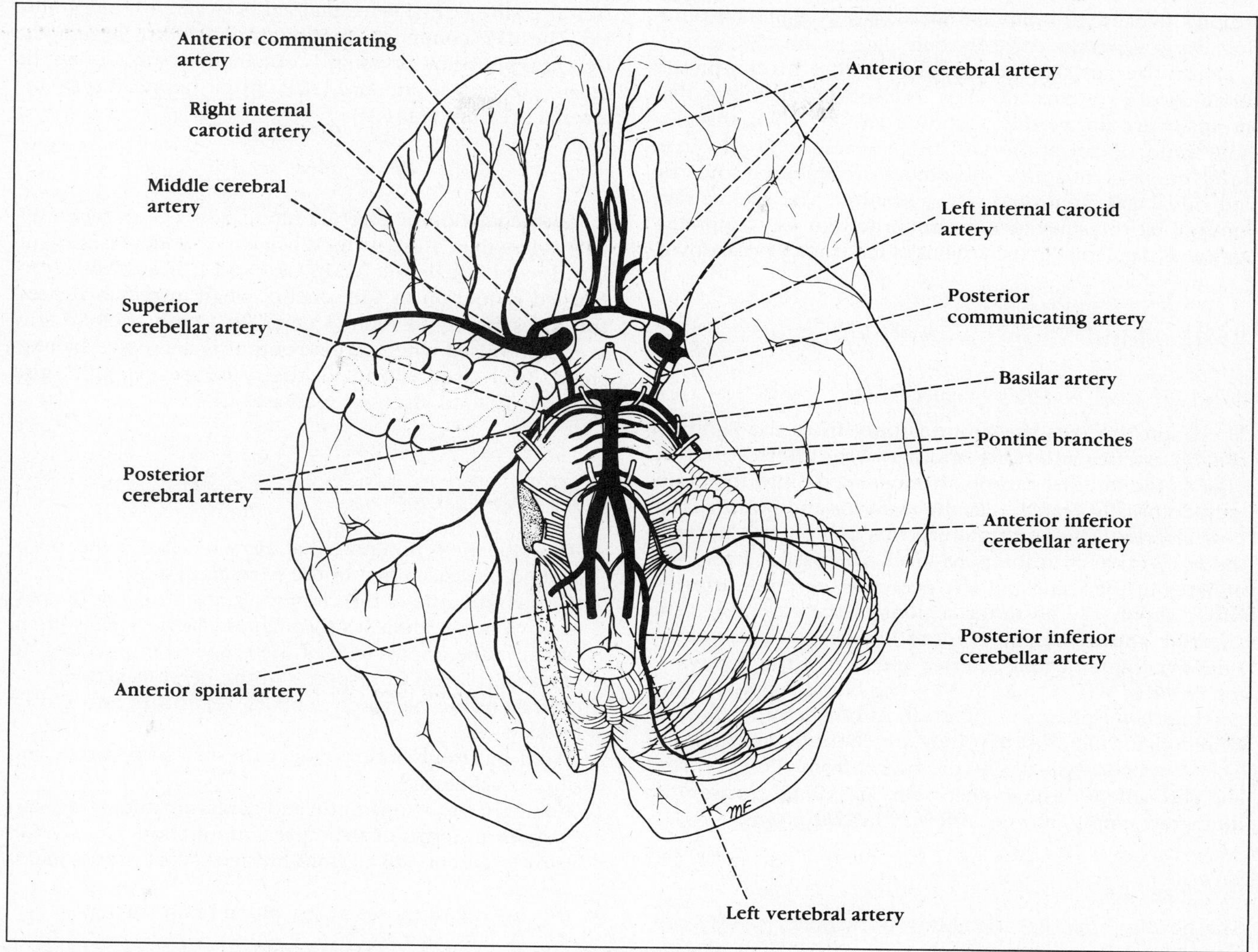

FIGURE 44-37 The arteries on the inferior surface of the brain. Note the formation of the circulus arteriosus (circle of Willis). (From R.S. Snell, *Clinical Neuroanatomy for Medical Students*. Boston: Little, Brown, 1980.)

solubility affect the rate of diffusion across the cerebral membranes and cells. Small molecules and lipid-soluble substances penetrate more rapidly than large molecules and water-soluble polar compounds. Plasma proteins are excluded from the central nervous system because of their large molecular size. Nonionized substances pass more readily into the brain and CSF than ionized substances. Substances that penetrate rapidly into the CSF and brain include water, carbon dioxide, and oxygen.

The endothelia of capillary cells of the brain overlap and are fused together by tight junctions, creating a common, thickened, basement membrane with adjacent glia and neurons. This dense basement membrane, in conjunction with an additional layer of neuroglial cells surrounding the capillaries, restricts diffusion of large-molecular substances between the blood and brain (Fig. 44-36). This capillary structure is equated with the blood-brain barrier. The blood-CSF barrier exists as a result of the secretory function of the choroid plexus. This is evidenced by different concentrations of certain substances in the CSF and in plasma indicating selective transport by the choroid plexus.

A weaker barrier is afforded by the brain-CSF barrier through the ependymal lining of the ventricular system and its adjacent glial cells. These structures provide some limitation in the transfer of fluids and chemical substances to the interstitial fluids from the CSF.

These barriers protect the brain by inhibiting potentially toxic substances from entering and facilitating entrance to those substances essential for its metabolism. Substances such as glucose and oxygen pass to the brain rapidly through the capillary system to maintain constant environment for the central nervous system neurons. Certain drugs penetrate the barrier with more ease than others. This is important in the treatment of central nervous system infections, as certain antibiotics, such as chlortetracyclines and penicillin, have very limited access to the brain; others, such as erythromycin and sulfadiazine, enter readily. Because proteins are not readily available for binding, drugs generally do not accumulate in the CSF.

Radiotherapy, infections, and tumors interrupt the brain barrier systems and allow transport of materials that normally are not readily accorded entrance. For this reason, tumor localization with brain scanning is effective. Intravenous radioactive substances are injected into the individual and monitored with a scanner. The gamma rays emitted by the substance are recorded on x-ray film and appear as dark areas in the regions of the barrier breakdown.

Brain Blood Supply and Regulation

Arterial and Venous Circulation

The brain receives the blood supply from the *internal carotid* arteries anteriorly and *vertebral* arteries posteriorly. As the internal carotid arteries ascend into the brain, they eventually branch into the *anterior* and *middle cerebral* arteries. The vertebral arteries ascend and become the *basilar* artery at the pons level. The basilar artery terminates in the right and left posterior cerebral arteries, which supply the posterior regions of the cerebrum. The anterior and posterior cerebral arteries are joined by smaller communicating arteries and form a ring known as the *circle of Willis* (Fig. 44-37). The blood supply to both cerebral hemispheres is identical. Although anomalies are common, for the most part they are clinically insignificant. The venous system drains the blood from the cerebrum and cerebellum through deep veins and *dural sinuses* that ultimately empty into the *internal jugular* veins.

Autoregulation and Vasomotor Control

The healthy brain has the ability to maintain a fairly constant blood flow (approximately 50 ml/100 gm/minute) even within widely fluctuating physiologic conditions. Significant factors influencing cerebral blood flow (CBF) constancy include chemical variations in carbon dioxide and oxygen levels and changes in systemic arterial blood pressure. Cerebral arteries dilate in response to increases in carbon dioxide tension and decreases in oxygen tension. This results in increased CBF. Vasodilation allows removal of excess carbon dioxide and may facilitate the restoration of oxygen levels toward normal. Hypercapnia and hypoxia have a significant effect on the vessel caliber and thus on the intrinsic control of cerebral blood flow.

Autoregulation of cerebral vessel size allows relatively constant blood flow in the presence of wide fluctuations in arterial blood pressure. Cerebral vessels constrict in response to increased systemic arterial pressure and dilate when the systemic pressure lowers. A mean systemic arterial blood pressure below 60 mm Hg results in decreased cerebral perfusion, whereas marked hypertension has essentially no effect on cerebral blood flow.

Other factors affecting cerebral blood flow include cerebral perfusion pressure, intracranial pressure, cardiac output, cerebral outflow, and blood viscosity. Normal cerebral blood flow is provided when the cerebral perfusion pressure (CPP) is maintained between 40 to 130 mm Hg. The CPP commonly ranges around 80 to 90 mm Hg. Cerebral perfusion pressure is obtained by subtracting the mean intracranial pressure (ICP) from the mean systemic arterial pressure (MAP):

$$\text{CPP} = \text{MAP} - \text{ICP}.$$

Autoregulation of cerebral blood flow ceases when the CPP is less than 40 mm Hg. When the ICP increases significantly and equals the MAP, CPP and CBF become zero. Marked reduction of CBF occurs when intracranial pressure rises rapidly to about 35 mm Hg. Cerebral blood flow is compromised when cardiac output is decreased by one-third. Increased blood viscosity decreases CBF, and decreased blood viscosity increases CBF.

Study Questions

1. Describe the action potential. How it is generated, propagated, and sustained in the nervous system?
2. Discuss the role of the chemical transmitters in the passage of nerve impulses throughout the nervous system.
3. What is the importance of the range from primitive to advanced levels of response in the nervous system?
4. Differentiate between sensory receptors and motor responses.
5. What pathways interconnect the cerebral cortex and the spinal cord?
6. Compare the sympathetic and parasympathetic nervous systems in terms of structure and function.
7. How is cerebrospinal fluid formed? What are its major functions?
8. Discuss the purposes of the blood-brain barrier.

References

1. Carpenter, M., and Sutin, J. *Human Neuroanatomy* (8th ed.). Baltimore: Williams & Wilkins, 1983.
2. Chusid, J. *Correlative Neuroanatomy and Functional Neurology* (19th ed.). Los Altos, Calif.: Lange, 1985.
3. Clark, R. *Essentials of Clinical Neuroanatomy and Neurophysiology* (5th ed.). Philadelphia: Davis, 1975.
4. Eccles, J. *The Understanding of the Brain*. New York: McGraw-Hill, 1973.
5. Guyton, A.C. *Textbook of Medical Physiology* (7th ed.). Philadelphia: Saunders, 1986.
6. Iverson, L. The chemistry of the brain. *Sci. Am.* 241:134, 1979.
7. Nauta, W., and Feirtag, M. The organization of the brain. *Sci. Am.* 241:88, 1979.
8. Peele, T. *The Neuroanatomic Basis for Clinical Neurology* (3rd ed.). New York: McGraw-Hill, 1977.
9. Ruch, T., and Patton, H. *Physiology and Biophysics* (19th ed.). Philadelphia: Saunders, 1965.
10. Snell, R.S. *Clinical Neuroanatomy for Medical Students*. Boston: Little, Brown, 1980.
11. Stevens, C. The neuron. *Sci. Am.* 241:54,
12. Willis, W., and Grossman, R. *Medical Neurobiology* (2nd ed.). St. Louis: Mosby, 1977.

CHAPTER 45

Adaptations and Alterations in the Special Senses

CHAPTER OUTLINE

Vision

- Structure and Function
- Visual Pathways
- Image Formation
- Accommodation
- Pupillary Aperture
- Physiology of Vision
- Color Vision
- Color Blindness
- Dark Adaptation
- Refraction Defects
- Measurement of Visual Acuity
- Other Disturbances of Vision
    - *Glaucoma*
    - *Cataracts*
    - *Retinal Detachment*
    - *Retinitis Pigmentosa*

Hearing

- Structure and Function
- Sound Conduction Through the Ear
- Hearing Pathways
- Hearing Loss
- The Vestibular System
    - *Vertigo*
    - *Meniere's Disease*
    - *Nystagmus*
    - *Labyrinthine Ataxia*
- Assessment of Hearing and Balance
- Sound Amplification

Taste

- Structure and Function
- Taste Pathways
- Taste Disturbances
- Taste Assessment

Smell

- Structure and Function
- Smell Disturbances
- Smell Assessment

LEARNING OBJECTIVES

1. Identify the structures of the eye.
2. State the normal intraocular pressure.
3. Trace the visual pathways from the optic disk to the occipital lobe.
4. Discuss the mechanism of image formation in the eye.
5. Define *refraction index*.
6. Explain the process of accommodation.
7. Discuss factors that influence the pupillary aperture.
8. Identify the functions of rods and cones.
9. Discuss the initiation of receptor potential of the retina.
10. Explain the trichromic theory of color vision.
11. Contrast myopia and hypermetropia.
12. Define *astigmatism*.
13. Discuss the pathologic basis of the hemianopsias.
14. Discuss the mechanisms maintaining normal intraocular pressure.
15. Identify conditions that lead to increased intraocular pressure.
16. Differentiate between chronic simple and acute glaucoma.
17. Identify the structures of the ear.
18. Trace sound conduction through the ear and the fiber pathways to the auditory cortex.
19. Differentiate between conduction deafness and sensorineural deafness.
20. Discuss the role of the vestibular system with respect to changes of position and movement.
21. Discuss common clinical findings associated with Meniere's disease.
22. Identify three tests that might be performed to detect hearing loss.
23. Locate the primary sensations of taste on the tongue.
24. Trace taste pathways from innervation of taste buds to cerebral cortex.
25. Discuss pathogenesis of taste disturbance.
26. Identify the receptor cell for the sense of smell.
27. Discuss adaptation of smell receptors.
28. Identify potential causes of anosmia.

The senses of vision, hearing, taste, and smell provide humans with the means to perceive the environment and respond in a way that supports adaptation and, at times, even survival. The receptors of the eyes, ears, tongue, and nose are stimulated and messages are transmitted to specific regions of the cerebral cortex for processing. Alterations in the function of these senses, particularly vision and hearing, can result in physiologic, psychologic, sociologic, and economic difficulties. Common alterations are described in this chapter, others can be found in specialized texts.

Vision

Structure and Function

The eye is a complex peripheral structure that transmits vision to the visual area of the occipital lobe of the cerebral cortex. It nestles in the orbit, a cone-shaped cavity with fragile walls composed of the frontal, maxillary, zygomatic, sphenoid, ethmoid, lacrimal, and palatine bones. The thinness of the orbital wall makes this area particularly susceptible to fractures. The eyeball occupies the anterior portion of the orbital cavity; its principal structures are identified in Figure 45-1. The area of the orbit not occupied by the eyeball is filled with fascia, fat, nerves, blood vessels, muscle, and the lacrimal gland. Six extrinsic muscles, most of which arise from the apex of the orbit and insert into the scleral lining, allow for the movement and rotation of the eyeball. These include the superior rectus, inferior rectus, medial rectus, lateral rectus, superior oblique, and inferior oblique muscles. Innervation for these muscles arrives from the third, fourth, and sixth cranial nerves.

The three layers of the eyeball are the *sclera*, *choroid*, and *retina*. The outermost supportive and protective layer, the sclera, is composed of dense fibrous tissue and forms a white, opaque membrane around the eyeball except at the cornea, where it becomes transparent. It is through this transparent area that light rays enter the eye to stimulate the rods and cones. The second, or middle, layer of the eyeball is the vascular choroid. Nutrients are exchanged in this heavily pigmented layer. The ciliary muscle, which is important in facilitating light and accommodation reflexes, lies between the sclera and choroid layers. The choroid also contains the *iris*, the center of which is the *pupil*. The sphincter and dilator muscles of the iris, together with the ciliary muscle, are known as the intrinsic muscles of the eye and control the amount of light admitted into the eye. Innervation to these muscles comes from the third cranial nerve and the superior cervical ganglion. The crystalline lens, which is suspended by the suspensory ligament from the inner surface of the ciliary body, bends the rays of light so that they are projected properly on the retina. The *anterior chamber* is a fluid-filled space anterior to the iris and lens. The *posterior chamber*, posterior to the iris and fluid-filled as well, together with the anterior chamber, assists in maintaining constant pressure in the eyeball. Normal intraocular pressure is between 10 and 22 mm Hg, with the most common pressures being 15 or 16 mm Hg. *Glaucoma* results if drainage of this aqueous humor through the canal of Schlemm is insufficient and intraocular pressure rises (Fig. 45-2). *Vitreous humor*, which is soft and gelatinous, fills the space behind the lens and helps maintain the shape of the eyeball.

The third layer of the eyeball, the retina, consists of two parts. The outer pigmented layer is attached to the choroid. The inner layer consists of a synaptic series of nervous tissue. The *macula lutea*, a yellowish spot near the center of the retina, encompasses a small depression in its center called the *fovea centralis*. This is an area consisting only of cones and projecting the most acute vision. Medial to the fovea centralis is the optic disk. It is at this whitish spot that the optic nerve exits from the eyeball. Because this area contains no sensory receptors, it is known as the *physiologic blind spot* of the retina. Increased intraocular pressure is reflected in the optic disk by its cupped shape, that is, the disk appears pushed backward. In contrast, increased intracranial pressure produces the opposite effect; that is, an optic disk that is pushed inward, called a choked disk, or *papilledema* (see Chap. 48).

The blood supply to the retina enters through the central artery, a branch of the ophthalmic artery, which enters the eyeball with the optic nerve and runs with it to the retina where it divides in the middle of the disk into superior and inferior branches. The veins in the eyeball are anatomically related to the arteries and empty into the ophthalmic veins.

Visual Pathways

The ganglionic cell axons of the retina emerge from the optic disk as the optic nerve. Axons from the nasal half of each eye cross in the optic chiasm and terminate in the opposite occipital lobe. Axons from the temporal half of each eye do not cross but terminate on their respective sides [3] (Fig. 45-3).

Image Formation

The refractive surfaces of the cornea and lens initiate the mechanism for image formation. These surfaces and the aqueous and vitreous humors provide varying densities for the light to pass through. This accounts for the refractive phenomenon. If a light ray passes into a denser medium, it is bent toward the perpendicular and the speed of transmission is slowed. A less dense medium bends the light ray away from the perpendicular and speeds its transmission. The degree of light impediment, or the power of a substance to bend light, is its *refractive index*. The refractive index of air is 1.0; of water, 1.33; of the cornea, 1.38; and of the crystalline lens, 1.40 [8].

Light strikes the cornea at different angles and is bent in different amounts, depending on the curvature and refractive indexes of the interposed structures. Refraction of light occurs at the corneal interface, aqueous humor, and crystalline lens, and is projected on the retina in an

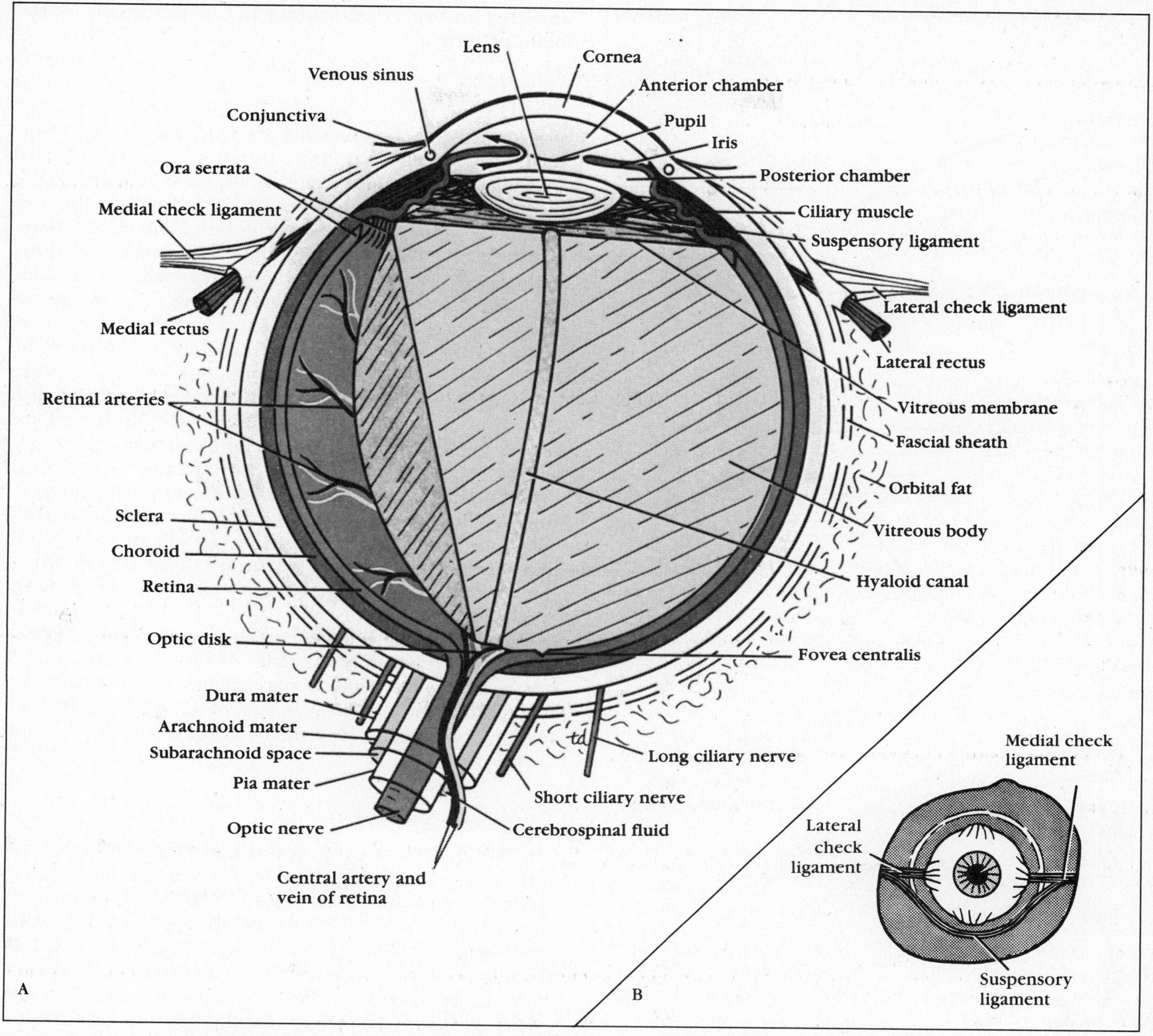

Figure 45-1 A. Horizontal section through eyeball and optic nerve. Note that central artery and vein of the retina cross the subarachnoid space to reach the optic nerve. B. The check ligaments and suspensory ligaments of the eyeball. (From R.S. Snell, *Clinical Anatomy for Medical Students* [2nd ed.]. Boston: Little, Brown, 1981.)

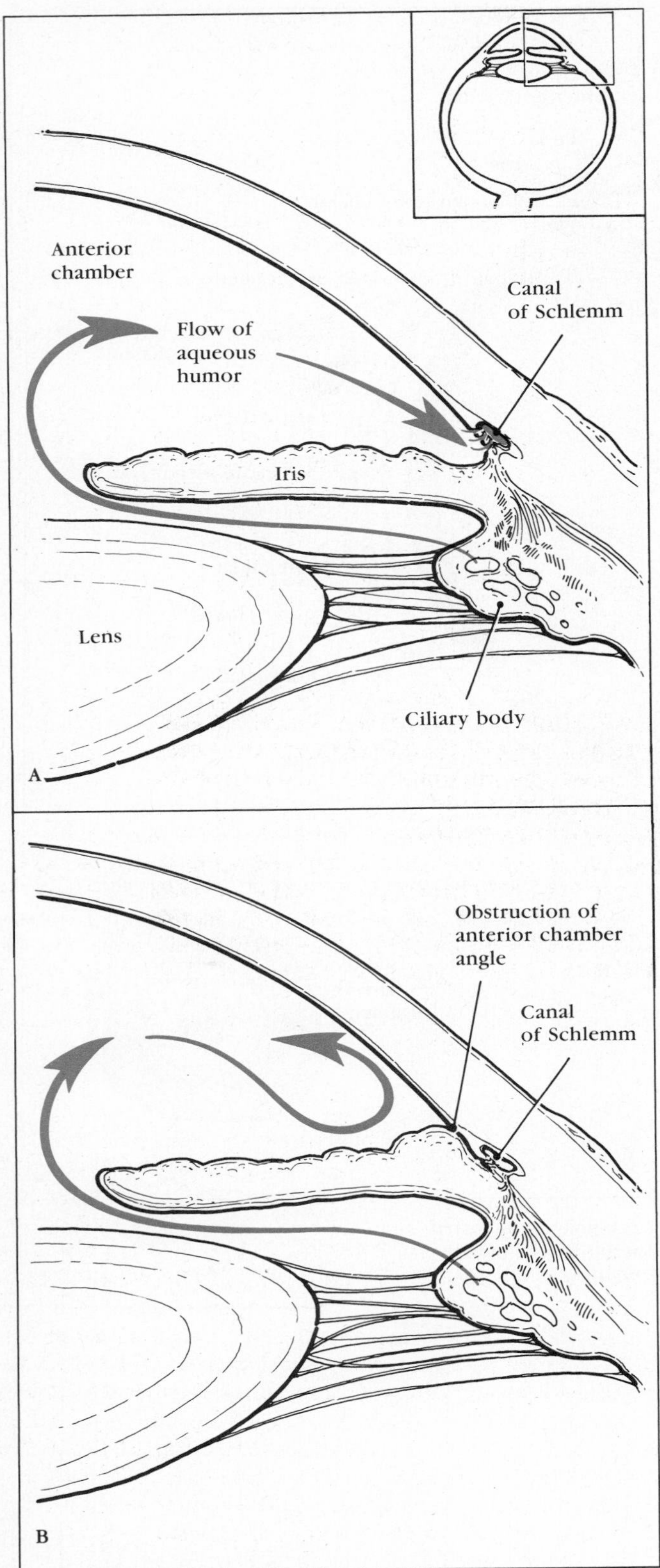

FIGURE 45-2 A. Normal flow of aqueous humor. B. Obstructed flow in acute (closed- or narrow-angle) glaucoma. (Adapted from M. Lechiger and F. Moya, *Introduction to the Practice of Anesthesia* [2nd ed.]. New York: Harper & Row, 1978.)

inverted and reverted manner that is perceived by the brain as upright.

Accommodation

Adjustments for distant vision are made by the lens. Normally, parallel light rays from distant objects are focused on the retina. The ciliary muscle contracts to increase the curvature of the lens to view objects closer to the eye. This is the process of *accommodation*. The closest point at which a person can clearly focus an object is called the *near point*. This point recedes with advancing age. For example, the near point for a normal eye of an 8-year-old is approximately 8.6 cm; for a 20-year-old it is 10.4 cm; and for a 60-year-old it is approximately 83 cm from the eye. Ocular convergence and pupillary constriction are associated with the accommodation reflex. The increased curvature of the lens increases its power, shortens focal length, and focuses near objects on the retina.

The accommodation reflex is mediated by the third cranial nerve through parasympathetic postganglionic fibers. The stimulus that triggers the accommodation response is perception of an image out of focus. The parasympathetic impulses on the ciliary muscle must therefore increase progressively to maintain the image in focus continually.

Progressive age reduces the efficiency of accommodation due to the loss of elasticity of the lens, and the eye may remain focused almost permanently on a constant distance. This deterioration is known as *presbyopia*. It is readily corrected with proper bifocal lenses for far and near vision.

Pupillary Aperture

The iris controls the amount of light that enters the eye through the action of its two sets of smooth muscles, the sphincter and dilator muscles. *Miosis* is accomplished through the contraction of the sphincter muscle, and *mydriasis* is facilitated through the contraction of the dilator muscle. Innervation for the sphincter muscles comes from the postganglionic parasympathetic neurons in the ciliary ganglion. The preganglionic neurons transmit to the ganglion by way of the third cranial nerve. Innervation for the dilator muscle arrives from the sympathetic postganglionic neurons of the superior cervical ganglion, and reaches the eye through a series of progressively smaller arteries.

The pupillary aperture in the human eye can vary from 1.5 to 8.0 mm in diameter. In normal eyes the aperture is a reflex response to change in light intensity. Pupils constrict in response to increased light intensities and dilate to decreased light intensities (pupillary light reflex). If illumination enters only one eye, both pupils constrict. This simultaneous constriction of the contralateral eye is referred to as the *consensual light reflex*. Photoreceptors of the retina, including rods and cones, are receptors for the light reflex.

Emotional states of alarm produce pupillary dilation. This reaction is initiated by stimulation of the sympathetic

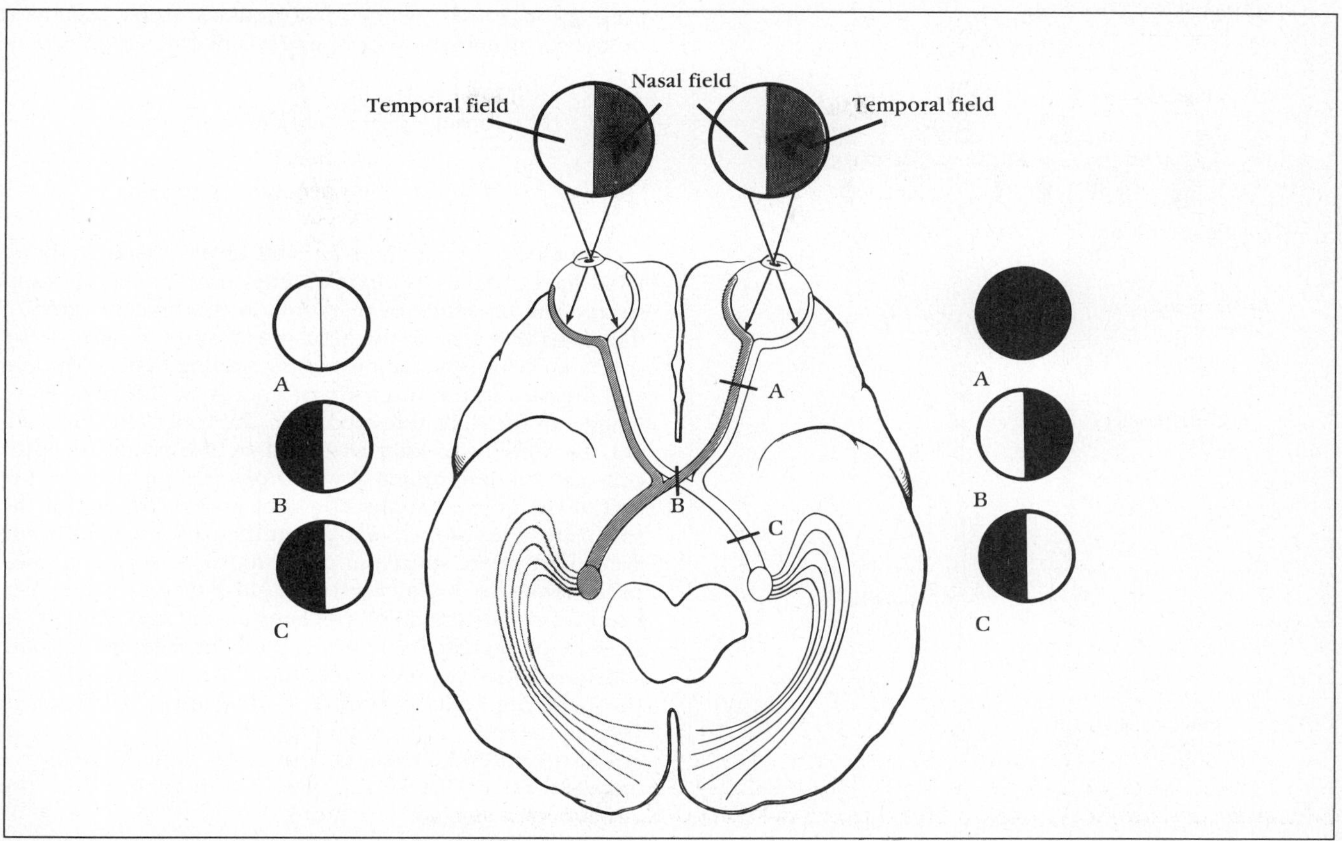

FIGURE 45-3 The visual pathway. On right and left are maps of visual fields with areas of blindness darkened to show the effects of lesions in each location. A. Lesion of optic nerve (loss of vision, right eye). B. Midline lesion of optic chiasm (bitemporal hemianopsia). C. Lesion of the right anterior optic tract; blindness for objects in left half of each field of vision (left homonymous hemianopsia). Lesions can occur at other locations along the visual pathway, causing a variety of patterns of visual field losses. (From J. Sana and R. Judge, *Physical Assessment Skills for Nursing Practice* [2nd ed.]. Boston: Little, Brown, 1982.)

fibers and inhibition of the parasympathetic fibers. Darkness inhibits the parasympathetic supply and results in pupil dilation.

Light reflex of the pupil and miosis of accommodation are not identical mechanisms and can occur independently of each other. An example of this occurs with the *Argyll Robertson* pupil, which may occur as a complication of syphilis. In this phenomenon the pupil remains constricted and unresponsive to light but does respond to the accommodation mechanism [2].

Physiology of Vision

Rods and *cones* are receptors of the retina and have distinctly different morphologic compositions and functions (Fig. 45-4). The cones mediate daylight vision, allowing perception of detail and color of objects. The rods mediate night vision, allowing visualization of outlines of objects without revealing color or detail. The rods, however, are very sensitive to movement of objects in the visual field.

The retina is formed by numerous layers of cells, fibers, and ganglia (Fig. 45-5). The nerve cells in the retina include bipolar cells, ganglion cells, horizontal cells, and amacrine cells. The rods and cones, which are adjacent to the pigment epithelium of the choroid, synapse with the bipolar cells, which in turn synapse with dendrites of the ganglion cells. Horizontal cells connect receptor cells (rods and cones), and amacrine cells connect ganglion cells to each other. The axons of the ganglion cells converge to form the fibers of the optic nerve, which is easily recognized on ophthalmoscopic examination of the optic disk. The fovea centralis is composed of tightly packed cones that connect individually to the optic nerve, whereas in other parts of the retina they share fibers with many other rods and cones. The pigmented layer of the retina is the outermost layer, which decreases light reflection. This pigment layer is directly adjacent to the choroid

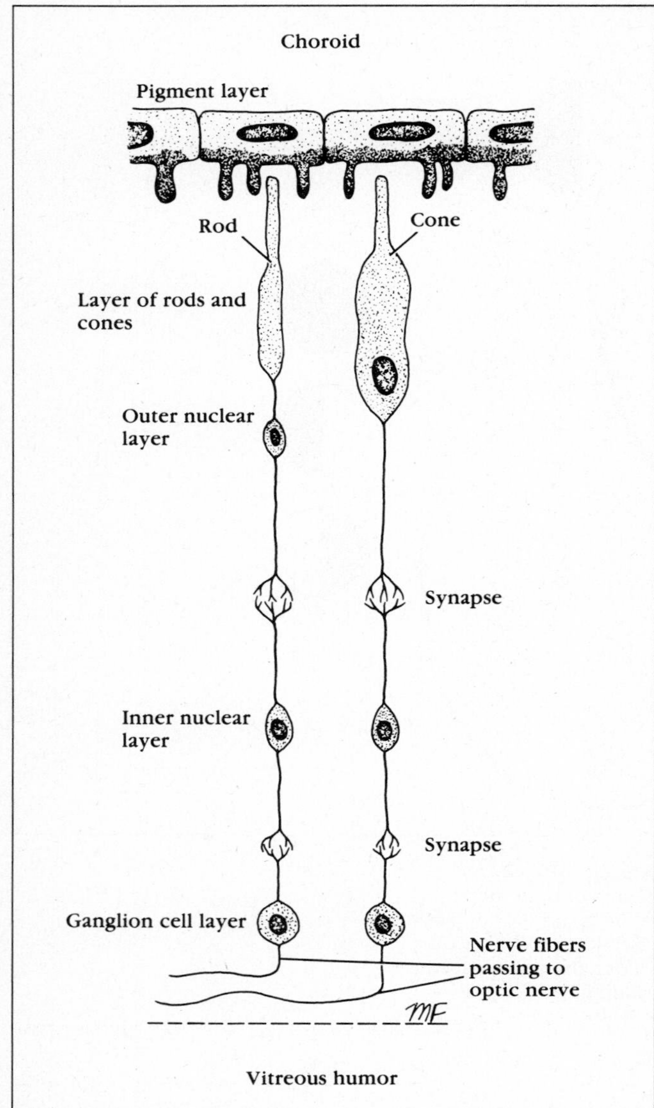

FIGURE 45-4 Rods and cones.

and receives much of its nutritive needs from the choroid vascular supply. Melanin is the black pigment that gives this layer its characteristic dark color.

As light passes through the layers of the retina to reach the light-sensitive portion of the rods and cones, light energy is absorbed by the pigment *rhodopsin*, or *visual purple*. Rhodopsin is a light-sensitive protein and aldehyde of vitamin A compound contained in rods that breaks down when light reaches it. This is the initial activity in producing the generator potential. The breakdown of rhodopsin can be visualized by the change in the dark-adapted retina from a dark purple to lack of color on exposure to light. The breakdown of rhodopsin results in the formation of a protein, *scotopsin*, and a carotene pigment, *retinene* [4]. In darkness, scotopsin and retinene recombine through a series of intermediary steps and form rhodopsin again, which once again is photoexcitable.

$$\text{Rhodopsin} \underset{\text{dark}}{\xrightarrow{\text{light}}} \text{retinene} + \text{scotopsin}$$

$$\longrightarrow \text{generator potential}$$

Knowledge about the pigments in the cones is somewhat speculative. Reflexion densitometry has demonstrated the presence of pigments in the foveal region of the retina that peak in the blue, green, and red parts of the spectrum. This is accomplished by shining light in the eye and measuring the intensity of energy at different wave lengths in the light reflected from the retina. In this manner the amount of light absorbed by the visual receptor cells can be determined. *Erythrolobe* is a pigment identified in the fovea that absorbs light in the red part of the spectrum; *chlorolobe* is a pigment that absorbs light in the green part of the spectrum in the fovea. A third cone pigment, *iodopsin*, a violet-sensitive substance, has been isolated from the retinae of chickens and is also thought to exist in the human eye cones. A pigment receptor for blue substances has also been identified. The composition of the cone pigments is similar to rhodopsin, although in varying degrees. Thus, cone pigments absorb a variety of colors to different extents, and color-dependent nerve impulses result. These impulses are interpreted by the visual cortex as color sensations.

The photochemical decomposition that occurs in response to light striking either the cones or rods produces a receptor potential that remains for the duration of the stimulus. The receptor potentials of the retina differ from other receptor potentials in that hyperpolarization is produced rather than depolarization. Each optic nerve fiber connects with many receptors by way of ganglionic cells. The number of receptor cells on the retina is much greater than the number in the optic nerve. This convergence on ganglionic cells allows summation to occur, so that light falling on different parts of the retina together may cause excitation. Thus, the more rods and cones that are excited, the more intense the signal. The ganglion cells receive the excitation impulses from the rods and cones through the bipolar cells.

The ganglionic cells produce synaptic depolarization and stimulate threshold spikes that are all or nothing and are propagated along their axons to the lateral geniculate body. Three types of responses are observed in ganglionic cells. One fires only in response to light stimulus on the retina and is known as the *on fiber*; another discharges only in response to light off and is known as the *off fiber*; the third, most numerous type, responds to both light on and off and is called the *on-off fiber*.

The horizontal cells transmit inhibitory impulses laterally from rods and cones to bipolar cells and become most important in detecting visual contrasts and color differentiations. Amacrine cells have a very transient inhibitory effect on the ganglionic cells in response to stimulation from bipolar cells and possibly rods and cones. Amacrine cells transmit, signaling a change in retinal illumination.

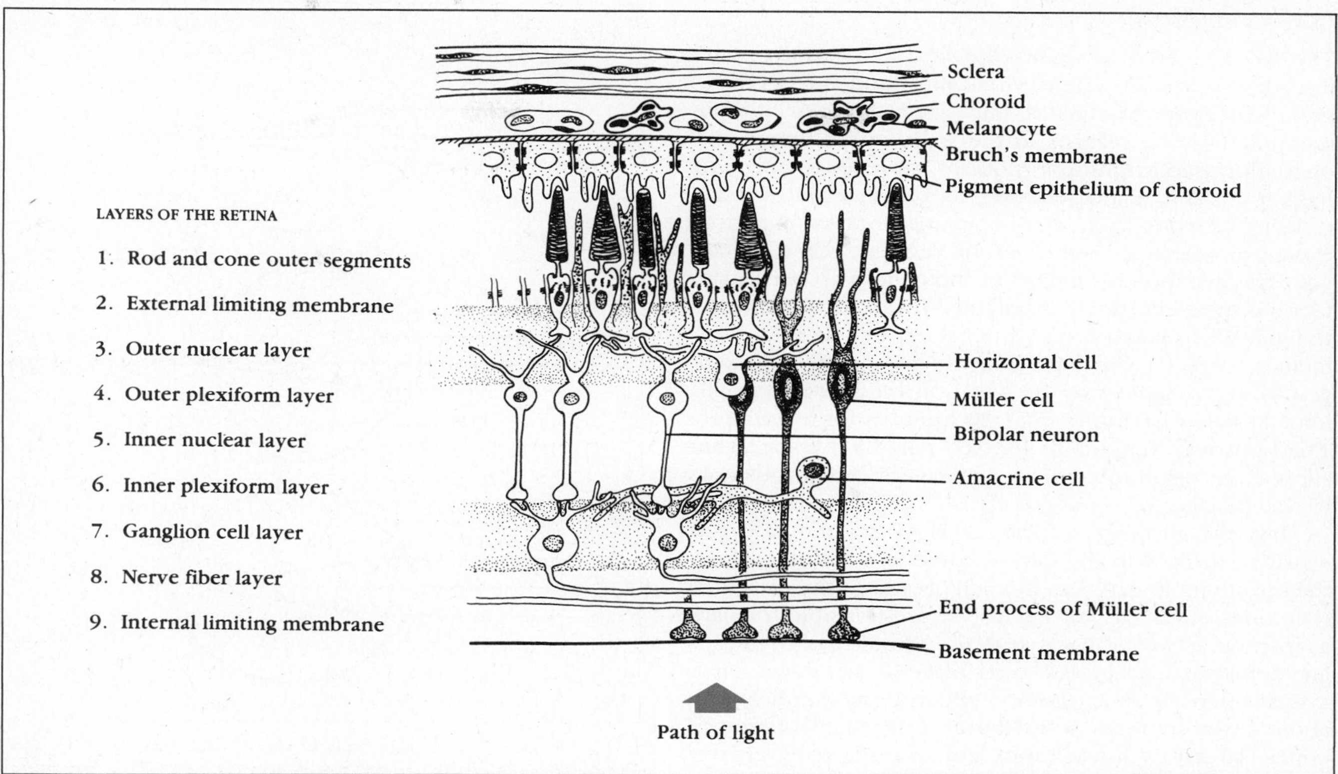

FIGURE 45-5 Highly schematic diagram showing the nine layers of the retina and their connections, using a few cells of each type as examples. Note that light must pass through the entire thickness of the retina before it finally triggers a photochemical reaction in the rod and cone outer segments. This "backward" retina is typical of all vertebrates. (From M. Borysenko et al., *Functional Histology* [2nd ed.]. Boston: Little, Brown, 1984.)

The neural pathways from the retina to the visual cortex are identified in Figure 45-3.

Color Vision

The differentiation of wave lengths of the visible spectrum allows the human eye to detect color in the environment. The precise mechanism that is responsible for color detection has been theorized by numerous researchers throughout the past century. Most of the investigation seems to be based on the *trichromatic theory*, which assumes that there are three variations in cones, each containing a different photochemical substance. One type of cone is responsible for red color, another for blue, and the third for green [4]. This theory, also known as the *Young-Helmholtz* theory, named after its originators over a century ago, is widely accepted today. Each of these cones gives rise to a distinct impulse that travels to the visual cortex of the occipital lobe. Red, blue, and green are colors that may produce any color in the spectrum by correct proportionate mixture. When all of the cones are stimulated equally, the sensation of white results. In contrast, when no stimulation of the three types of cones occurs, black is experienced. Other colors are perceived as a result of the combined stimulation of the three types of cones to varying degrees.

In summary, color vision evolves from the spectral sensitivity of cones and is most highly developed in the fovea where cones are concentrated. Each cone is maximally stimulated by a specific color. Color information is transmitted to the brain by common cone pathways of the optic fibers, and the transmission of specific colors is monitored by the stimulation of horizontal cells.

Color Blindness

Color blindness the inability to distinguish red from green. It may be hereditary or acquired. When a certain group of color receptors is not present in the retinae, all colors appear the same in the range of missing cones.

Individuals can be assessed for color blindness by numerous tests. Those most commonly used are the polychromatic charts and the yarn-matching tests. The former presents a chart, known as the *Ishihara* chart, with numerous look-alike, colored spots in a figuration that a person with normal vision can identify easily. The yarn-matching test involves asking the person to match a skein of yarn with strands from a pile of variously colored yarn.

Dark Adaptation

The eyes are said to be *dark adapted* after a period of time in darkness. This decline in visual threshold is at its maximum after approximately 20 minutes in the dark environment. When one returns to the light environment, the uncomfortable brightness requires the eyes to adapt to light again. This adaptation takes about five minutes and is called *light adaptation*. Dark adaptation occurs, in part, as rhodopsin stores are rebuilt in the rods and some similar, yet unknown, process occurs in the cones [4]. Dark adaptation is most effectively maintained by avoiding exposure to light. When visual acuity is necessary in a dark environment, such as for viewing a fluoroscopy screen and radiographs, red goggles may be worn on returning to bright light to avoid having to wait 20 minutes for adaptation. The light wavelengths in the red part of the spectrum allow cone vision to continue while stimulating rods only to a slight degree.

Only the periphery of the retina of the human eye is sensitive to light in the dark-adapted eye and, therefore, the sensitivity to darkness is much greater in the rods than the cones. Rods are not exclusively responsible for dark adaptation, however. Because of the presence of both rods and cones, dark adaptation takes place in two stages. First, a small increase in sensitivity, which is accomplished in about seven minutes, is attributed in dark adaptation of cones. After this, a less rapid, but quantitatively greater adaptation occurs in rods [5].

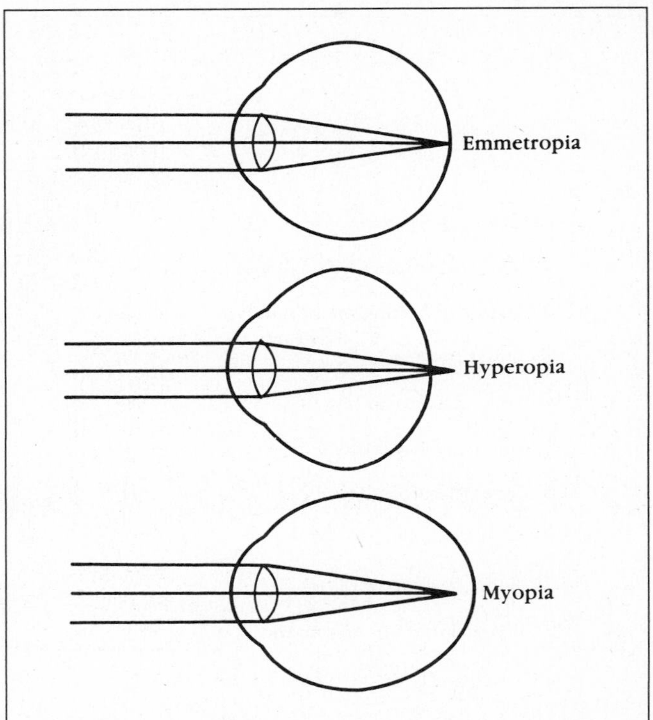

FIGURE 45-6 Common defects in the optical system of the eye. Emmetropia is normal refraction. A shortened eyeball gives rise to hyperopia (farsightedness). An abnormally long eyeball may characterize myopia (nearsightedness). Adjustments should be made in the lens selection on the ophthalmoscope for these anatomic differences. (From R. Judge, G. Zuidema, and F. Fitzgerald, *Clinical Diagnosis: A Physiologic Approach*. Boston: Little, Brown, 1982.)

Refraction Defects

Normal refraction (*emmetropia*) occurs when the relaxed eye is capable of clearly focusing distant parallel light rays on the retina (Fig. 45-6). Nearby vision requires contraction of the ciliary muscle to bring the object to focus. Defects of vision are present if the light rays converge either in front of or behind the retina, or if the eyeball is abnormally shaped [4].

Myopia (nearsightedness) is a result of an object focusing in front of the retina due to increased anteroposterior diameter (see Fig. 45-6). Myopic individuals cannot focus a distant object sharply, but as they move closer to the object, it becomes more focused and eventually falls on the retina. The excessive refraction of myopia is readily corrected by a *concave* diverging lens, which produces a longer than normal focal point.

Hyperopia (farsightedness) occurs with an abnormally short eyeball; the parallel light rays are focused beyond the retina in the relaxed eye (see Fig. 45-6). Through the mechanism of the accommodation, the hyperopic person can focus on distant objects. As objects move closer to the eye, images become blurred and accommodation can no longer compensate. The near point in this individual is abnormally distant. Hyperopia is corrected by using the refraction of light rays through a *convex* lens and shortening the normal focal point.

Astigmatism is a defect of the curvature of the cornea and lens that produces refractive errors where parallel light rays are imperfectly focused on the retina. Clear focusing requires a spheric cornea and lens on all meridians. In the presence of irregular curvature of these structures, light striking peripheral areas is bent at different angles and is not focused on a single point on the retina. Astigmatism can be corrected with lenses that are cut from a piece of cylindric instead of spheric glass. The axis of the cylinder is placed approximately in relation to the meridian of the eye lens.

Measurement of Visual Acuity

Individual visual acuity, the degrees to which a person can recognize contours and details of objects, can be readily measured by such instruments as the *Snellen letter chart*. The subject is asked to read the chart from the distance of 20 feet and identify the smallest line that can be seen. This is tested with each eye, one at a time. The results are recorded as a fraction, with 20 as its numerator for the distance from which the person views the chart. The denominator is the distance from which the smallest line is seen. Normal visual acuity is considered to be 20/20.

Visual acuity is dependent on a number of factors, including brightness of the stimulus, density of the receptor cells, state of the cones, contrasting illumination between background and the stimulus, and length of exposure to the stimulus.

Other Disturbances of Vision

Decreased visual acuity may be associated with various lesions, syndromes, drug therapies, and nutritional deficiencies. Specific types of impairments result from lesions in different locations along the visual pathways [3]. Some of these are identified in Figure 45-3.

Blindness in one-half of the visual field is known as *hemianopsia*. As there are many different types of hemianopsia, the term usually is localized, such as *bitemporal hemianopsia*, denoting blindness in the temporal visual fields of both eyes. *Unilateral hemianopsia* refers to blindness in one-half of the visual field in one eye; *homonymous hemianopsia* is loss of one-half of the visual field in both eyes, opposite the side of the visual pathway lesion in the brain.

Scotomas are abnormal blind spots in the visual field. These may exist with a person's knowledge (positive scotomas) or without his or her knowledge (negative scotomas). Scotomas may result from vascular disease, toxic effect of certain drugs, nutritional deficiencies, and glaucoma. Various visual field defects may result from *retrobulbar neuritis* involving the optic nerve. This defect is commonly associated with multiple sclerosis.

Papilledema (choked disk) is most common with increased intracranial pressure due to brain tumors, trauma, hemorrhage, infections, and other causes. Blindness can result very rapidly if the pressure is not relieved. *Diplopia*, double vision, results from an eye muscle imbalance between the eyes, resulting in image reception at different spots on each retina.

Optic atrophy results in decreased visual acuity. *Primary optic* atrophy such as that associated with multiple sclerosis or tabes dorsalis does not produce papilledema. *Secondary optic atrophy* resulting from neuritis, glaucoma, or increased intracranial pressure is associated with papilledema. *Degeneration of the retina* may result from drug therapy (particularly the phenothiazine group), from infections, and from various metabolic or endocrine disorders.

Cerebral tumors, aneurysms, vascular diseases, infections, and degenerative processes may lead to vision defects, producing a variety of symptoms associated with a specific region. Defects may result in ocular movement, visual acuity, or interpretation of what is seen.

Glaucoma. Increased intraocular pressure and loss in the visual field are hallmarks of glaucoma. Several underlying conditions can result in increased intraocular pressure. The most common of these is blockage or stenosis of aqueous outflow channels [7]. Normally the aqueous humor, which is produced by the ciliary epithelium, flows from the posterior chamber of the eye through the pupil into the anterior chamber. Aqueous humor then leaves the anterior chamber and returns to the venous system by passing through the trabecular mesh of the anterior chamber into Schlemm's canal. A balance between production and absorption of aqueous humor provides for normal intraocular pressure.

Other potential causes of increased intraocular pressure in glaucoma include increases in systemic vascular pressure, which is reflected in venous engorgement, and decreased drainage through aqueous drainage channels. Increased production of aqueous humor is thought to contribute to a small proportion of those suffering from glaucoma [7]. The increased intraocular pressure associated with glaucoma may result in atrophy and degeneration of the optic nerve.

Glaucoma is described as *chronic simple* (open-angle) or *acute* (closed-angle or narrow-angle). The angle refers to the area where the iris meets the cornea in the anterior chamber (see Fig. 45-2). Chronic simple glaucoma is thought to have a hereditary basis and is a common cause of blindness. It may be asymptomatic for years and finally reveal itself when the individual experiences peripheral vision loss, difficulty with dark adaptation, blurring of vision, seeing halos around lights, and difficulty focusing on near objects. Although the anterior chamber angle is open in chronic simple glaucoma, an obstruction exists for the flow of aqueous humor through the trabecular mesh. Once this type of glaucoma has been diagnosed, the existing visual defects cannot be corrected. Further deterioration can be controlled with miotic drugs.

Acute glaucoma is manifested when an obstruction, either complete or partial, in the flow of aqueous humor is produced by closure of the anterior chamber angle (see Fig. 45-2). This may result from an anteroposterior thickening of the lens or a forward movement of the lens that causes the iris to press against the lens capsule and prevent outflow of aqueous humor. Complete closure of the angle presents a dramatic clinical picture of severe eye pain, blurred or cloudy vision, halos around lights, a hard red eye with cloudy cornea, and nausea and vomiting. Intraocular pressure is elevated.

Glaucoma may be primary or secondary to eye conditions associated with infection, tumors, hemorrhage, and trauma. Diagnosis is based on clinical features and tonometry, tonography, and peripheral vision testing.

Cataracts. As noted earlier, the normal lens is clear and transparent, and acts as a major refractive structure. Certain conditions may cause clouding of the lens and result in loss of vision associated with cataracts. These may result from trauma to the eye, elevated glucose levels in the aqueous humor (diabetes mellitus), irradiation of the lens, viruses, chemicals, and amino acid or vitamin deficiencies. Occasionally, cataracts may be congenital, but more commonly they are associated with advancing age (*senile cataracts*). Also they have been associated with certain disease processes of the skin, skeleton, and nervous system, and chromosomal abnormalities.

Senile cataracts result from the aging process as the lens undergoes changes. New fibers develop continually in the lens and these slowly increase the lens size. Older lens fibers become dehydrated, compressed, and sclerosed, forming a yellowish brown pigment that becomes so dense as to result in nuclear sclerosis and decreased transparency. Cataracts may produce vision abnormalities as a result of decreased light transmission, abnormal morphology, or biochemistry and optical aberrations [7]. Diagnosis of cataracts is confirmed by the clinical features, usual eye tests, and ophthalmoscopic examination.

Retinal Detachment. The separation of the retina from the choroid is generally spontaneous, although it may occur secondary to trauma. Retinal detachment is common in older individuals, as aging may cause the vitreous body to shrink, resulting in retinal tearing. As the tear occurs in the retina, choroid vessels transudate and vitreous humor seeps under the retina, stripping it from the choroid.

The individual with a detached retina experiences "floaters" and lines in the visual field. In addition, flashes of light and blurred black spots appear suddenly in conjunction with defects in vision. If the macula is involved, severe vision loss results. The person often complains of a sensation of a curtain coming over the eye(s). Generally, there is no pain or redness of the eye.

Diagnosis of retinal detachment is made by clinical symptoms and ophthalmoscopy. A binocular indirect ophthalmoscope and scleral depressor are used to produce a three-dimensional view of the retina and its damage.

Retinitis Pigmentosa. Retinitis pigmentosa is a degenerative inherited disease of the eyes that manifests itself initially by night blindness. Persons may inherit the disease through an autosomal dominant, autosomal recessive, or X-linked gene [9]. Progression of symptoms may be so slow that it may be difficult to detail an accurate course of the disease. Visual field constriction, or tunnel vision, is commonly associated with the night blindness. Other symptoms include photophobia and disturbance in color vision. The disease may progress to total blindness, although some persons retain reading vision in a small central part of the visual field. Changes in the fundus may be identified early in the course of the disease by a disturbance in the pigment epithelium of the retina. Areas of hyperpigmentation and atrophy may be identified by angiography, although the hallmark of retinitis pigmentosa is degeneration of the rods and cones associated with loss of pigmentation [9]. The waxy-appearing optic disk, thinning of retinal arteries, and choriocapillary atrophy are other associated changes.

Diagnosis of retinitis pigmentosa is based on signs and symptoms of the disease, characteristic changes of the fundus, and a family history of the disease.

Hearing

Structure and Function

The ear is a mechanoreceptor; it is sensitive to rapid changes in pressure that are transmitted to its fluid medium. In essence, the ear is a mechanical transducer as sound at various frequencies is converted into nerve impulses that are transmitted into the central nervous system for interpretation. Sound is conducted through air, ossicles, and fluid, and is measured in number in vibrations per second, which are recorded as *cycles per second (cps)* or *Hertz (Hz)*. The human ear is able to perceive frequencies to 20,000 cps or Hz. Aging reduces the number of frequencies perceived. The greatest sensitivity of the human ear is in the range of 1000 to 4000 Hz.

In addition to the hearing function of the ears, their receptors mediate a sense of position and equilibrium.

Sound Conduction Through the Ear

The ear is anatomically segmented into the *outer*, *middle*, and *inner* areas (Fig. 45-7). The outer ear funnels sound waves to the *tympanic membrane* (eardrum). Its canal is an S-shaped, 3-cm tube that is supplied with ceruminous and sebaceous glands as well as hair follicles. The canal has resonance properties as sound waves are reflected from the tympanic membrane. It may enhance or dampen incoming waves. The external canal is lined with squamous epithelium, cartilage, and bone that provide support and maintain its patency.

At the terminal end of the external ear, the tympanic membrane separates it from the middle ear. This fibrous tissue vibrates freely with all audible sound frequencies and transmits these to the three auditory ossicles of the middle ear, the *malleus*, *incus*, and *stapes*. The middle ear with its three ossicles is situated in an air cavity of the temporal bone. It communicates with the nasopharynx by means of the auditory or eustachian tube; the mucous membrane that lines the middle ear continues to line the pharynx as well as the air cells of the mastoid. The auditory tube also equalizes pressure in the middle ear with that of atmospheric pressure. Swallowing and yawning open the tube; high atmospheric pressures tend to close the tube. Microorganisms from the oropharynx often travel through the auditory tube to the middle ear, causing infections in this area.

The manubrium of the malleus is attached to the tympanic membrane, and its short process articulates with the incus to produce vibratory movements in the stapes, which is attached to the walls of the oval window (Fig. 45-8). The *tensor tympani* and *stapedius muscles* of the middle ear prevent the bones from transmitting excessive vibrations by pulling on the bones to decrease contact with the tympanic membrane and oval window. The former is innervated by the fifth cranial nerve and the latter by the seventh.

The inner ear is encased in the petrous part of the temporal bone and mediates sound-induced nerve impulses, position orientation, and balance. It is composed of two labyrinths, one within the other. The outer labyrinth is bony and separated from the inner membranous one by perilymph fluid; it contains the cochlea, vestibule, and the three semicircular canals. The membranous labyrinth contains fluid called *endolymph*. The anterior portion of the membranous labyrinth contains the cochlea, which receives the sound waves from the oval window. The cochlea, a small, shell-shaped structure, is divided into three chambers by the *basilar* and *Reissner's membranes*.

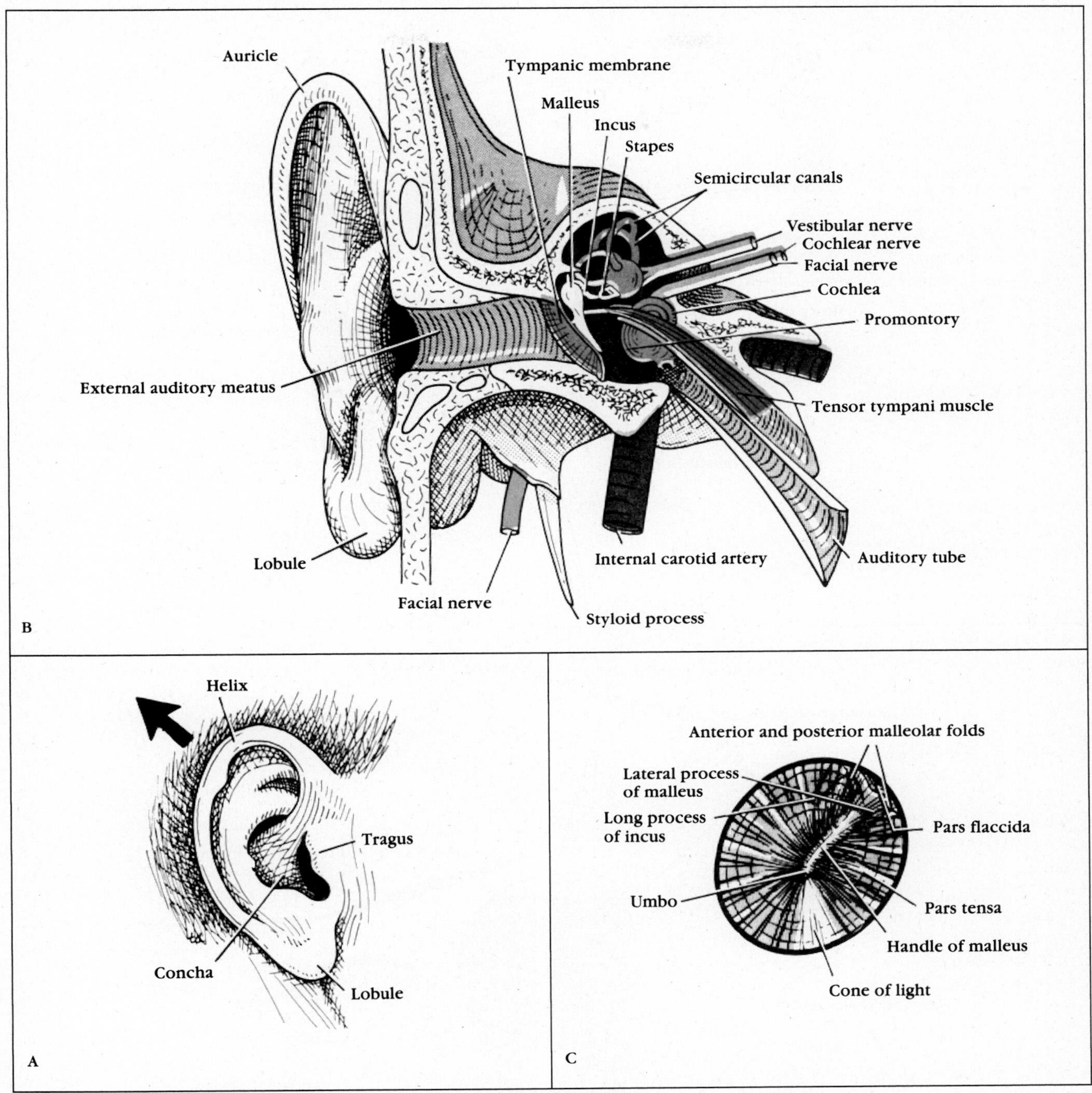

FIGURE 45-7 Parts of the ear. A. Outer or external ear. B. Middle ear components. C. Inner ear components. (From R.S. Snell, *Clinical Anatomy for Medical Students* [2nd ed.]. Boston: Little, Brown, 1981.)

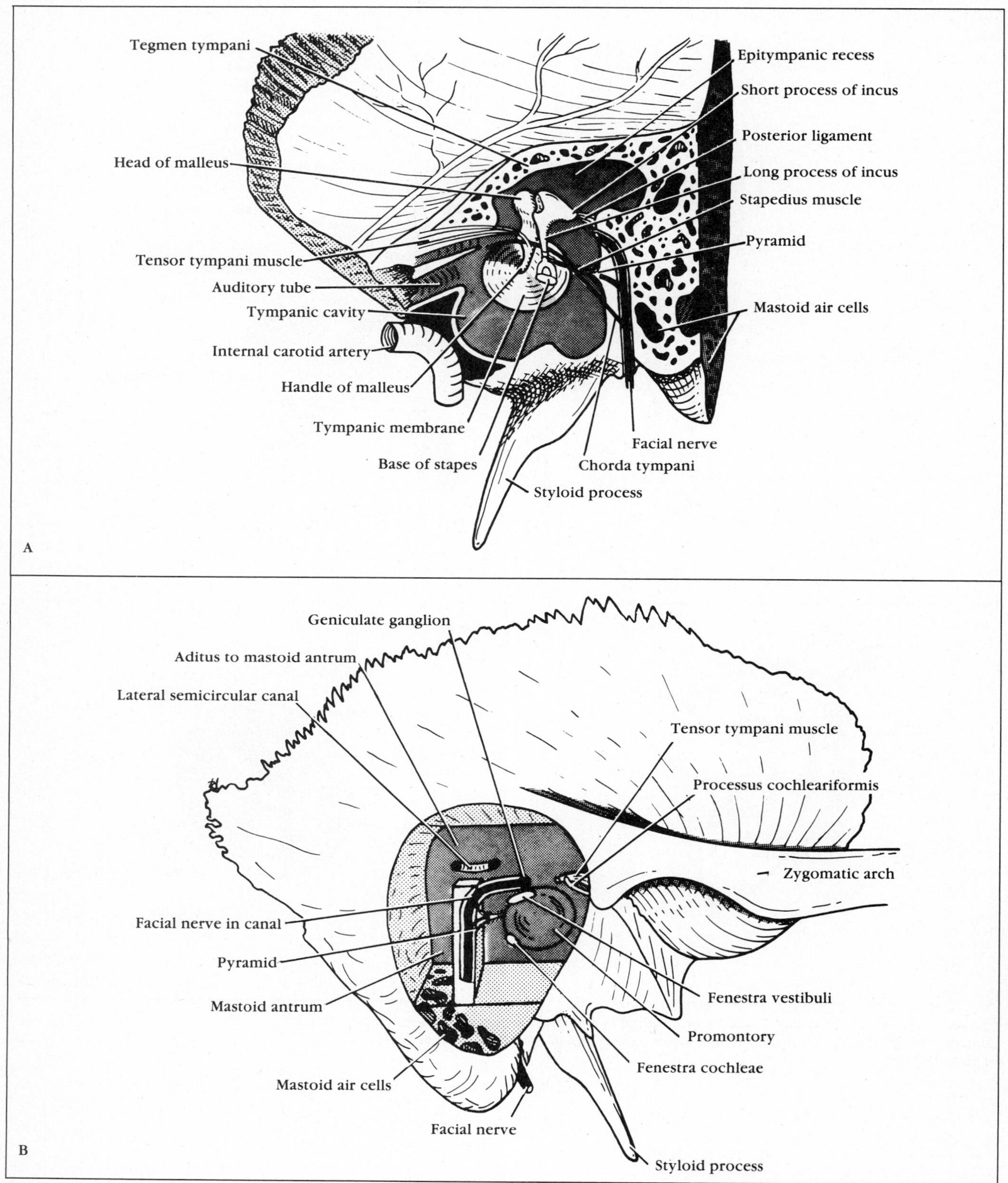

FIGURE 45-8 A. Lateral wall of right middle ear viewed from medial side. Note the position of ossicles and mastoid antrum. B. Medial wall of right middle ear viewed from lateral side. Note the position of the facial nerve in its bony canal. (From R.S. Snell, *Clinical Anatomy for Medical Students* [2nd ed.]. Boston: Little, Brown, 1981.)

These chambers are the *scala vestibuli*, *scala tympani*, and *cochlear duct*. Posteriorly, the cochlea opens into the osseous vestibule, which in turn extends to the three semicircular canals.

The *organ of Corti*, located on the basilar membrane, contains the receptor cells of audition. These are hair cells that generate nerve impulses in response to sound vibrations from the oscillations of the oval window. Impulses that arouse the dendrites of the cochlear division of the acoustic nerve are transmitted to the hearing center in the temporal lobe of the cortex. The various frequencies of sound generate different patterns of vibrations and allow sounds to be discriminated from each other. Subjective interpretation of the frequency of sound waves results in the recognition of *pitch*. The higher frequencies are identified as higher pitch. In addition to frequency, the location of the stimulation of cells on the basilar membrane affects pitch. Low-frequency sounds generate greater activity of the basilar membrane near the apex of the cochlea, and high-frequency sounds activate the basilar membrane near the base of the cochlea. Other frequencies fall between these extremes. This explanation of pitch discrimination is known as the *place theory*.

The amplitude of vibrations affects the perception of loudness at a constant frequency in that greater amplitude produces greater loudness. This does not hold true when two sounds of different frequency are contrasted simultaneously, however, as auditory sensitivity is a function of frequency. Thus, frequency and amplitude are both significant in determining the perception of loudness in two or more simultaneous sounds.

Hearing Pathways

The axons of bipolar neurons from the cochlea enter the pons and divide into the dorsal and ventral cochlear nuclei. Second-order neurons cross here and ascend by way of the lateral lemniscus to the inferior colliculus. From there they transmit to the medial geniculate body and on to the auditory cortex in the temporal lobe by way of the auditory radiations (Fig. 45-9).

The auditory cortex allows a person to recognize tone patterns, analyze characteristics of sound, and localize sound. Low-frequency tones are recognized anteriorly and high-frequency tones posteriorly in the auditory cortex. Neurons throughout the auditory cortex respond to onset, duration, and direction of stimulus.

The auditory association area lies inferior to the primary auditory center and is thought to associate auditory information with other sensations as well as different sound frequencies with each other. Lesions in this area prevent a person from comprehending the meaning of sounds heard; words can be heard but not understood. The origin (location) of a sound is determined by the sound's arrival to the two ears: one ear receives information before the other, and the ear that is closer to the sound source receives a louder sound.

Hearing Loss

Hearing loss can result from disorders of the central hearing mechanisms or the peripheral pathways. Peripheral hearing loss involves impairment of sound transmission in the external and middle ear and is referred to as *conduction deafness*. Lesions in the neural pathway produce *sensorineural deafness*.

Conduction deafness can result from obstruction of the external canal by cerumen or foreign objects, damage to the tympanic membrane, or immobility of the tympanic membrane or ossicles secondary to chronic otitis media. *Otosclerosis* results in conduction deafness by immobilizing of the stapes in the oval window.

Sensorineural deafness can be caused by long-term therapy with certain antibiotics in the mycin group, pathology of the hair cells of the cochlea, and disease processes in the auditory nerve pathway.

The Vestibular System

Disorders of coordination may result from the vestibular system through the labyrinthine and righting reflexes. Lesions may occur in the labyrinths, vestibular nerve, vestibular pathways within the brainstem, cerebrum, or cerebellum. Figure 45-10 shows the pathways of the vestibular nerve and its interconnections with the cerebellum, parts of the labyrinths, and the cerebrum. The vestibular system maintains equilibrium, preserves head position, and directs the gaze of the eyes.

The vestibular portion of the eighth nerve has its peripheral endings on the hair cells of the maculae of the *utricle* and *saccule* and on the cristae in the ampullae of the three *semicircular canals* (Fig. 45-11). The utricle and saccule record linear acceleration and static phenomena; and the semicircular canals record angular acceleration [6]. Recent evidence implies that the utricle may be more related to the semicircular canals' vestibular functions, while the saccule has a closer association with hearing.

The *utricle*, *saccule*, and *semicircular canals* function together to maintain equilibrium. These structures are housed in a bony labyrinth that contains a membranous labyrinth composed of the semicircular canals and the two chambers, the utricle and the saccule (Fig. 45-12). Within the utricle and saccule are maculae that provide sensory areas that detect the relationship of the head to gravitational pull and other forces. The maculae operate in conditions of acceleration and in static equilibrium. Internal and external hair cells synapse with a network of cochlear nerve endings, which terminate in the *cochlear nerve*. Within the semicircular canals endolymph flows and stimulates the sensory nerve fibers that join up with the vestibular nerve. Fluid flow in the opposite direction inhibits these sensory nerve fibers.

The ganglion cells of the vestibular division of the eighth nerve are in the internal auditory meatus, and the dendrites end in the specialized epithelium of the hair

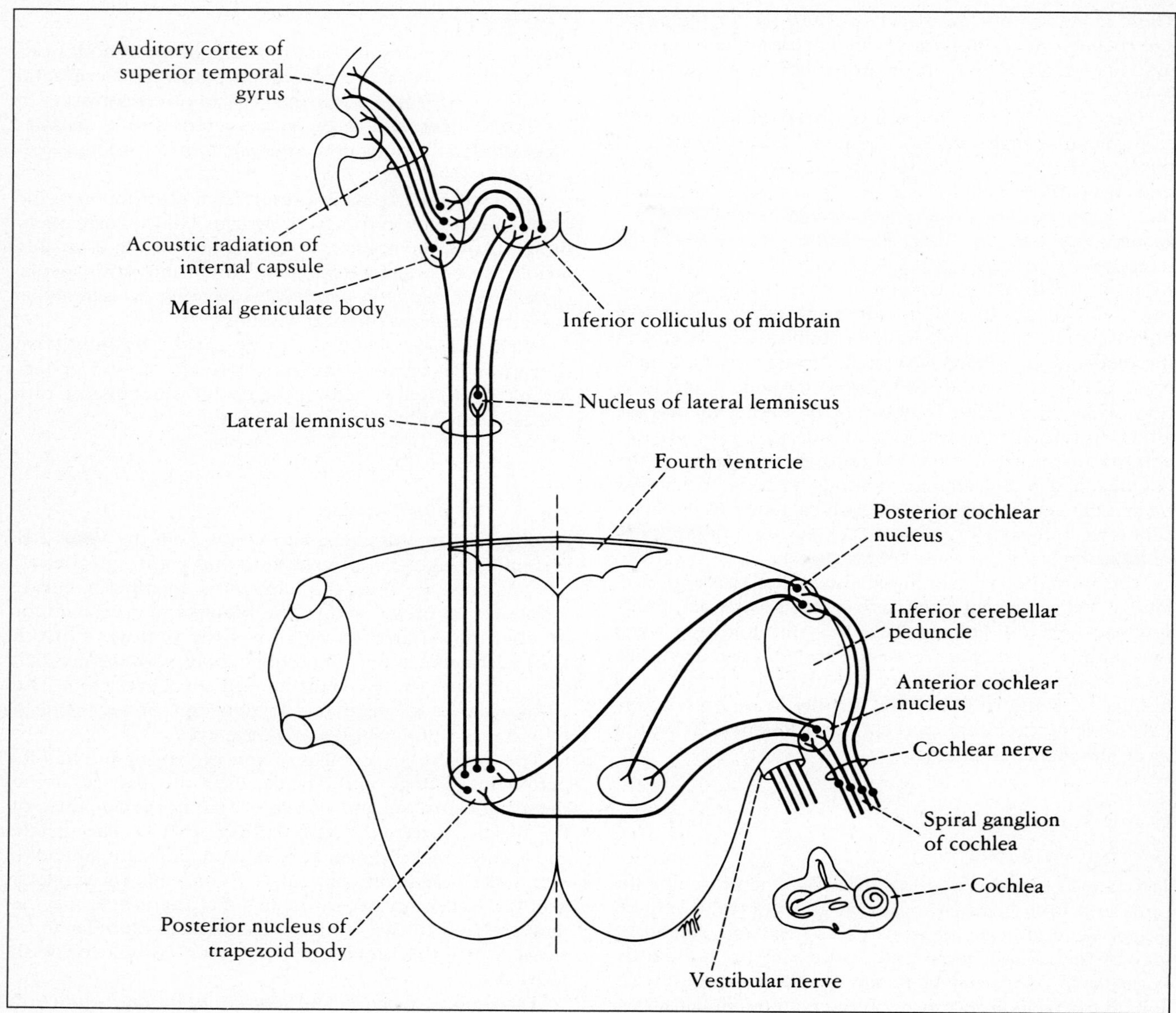

FIGURE 45-9 Cochlear nerve nuclei and their central connections. (From R.S. Snell, *Clinical Neuroanatomy for Medical Students*. Boston: Little, Brown, 1980.)

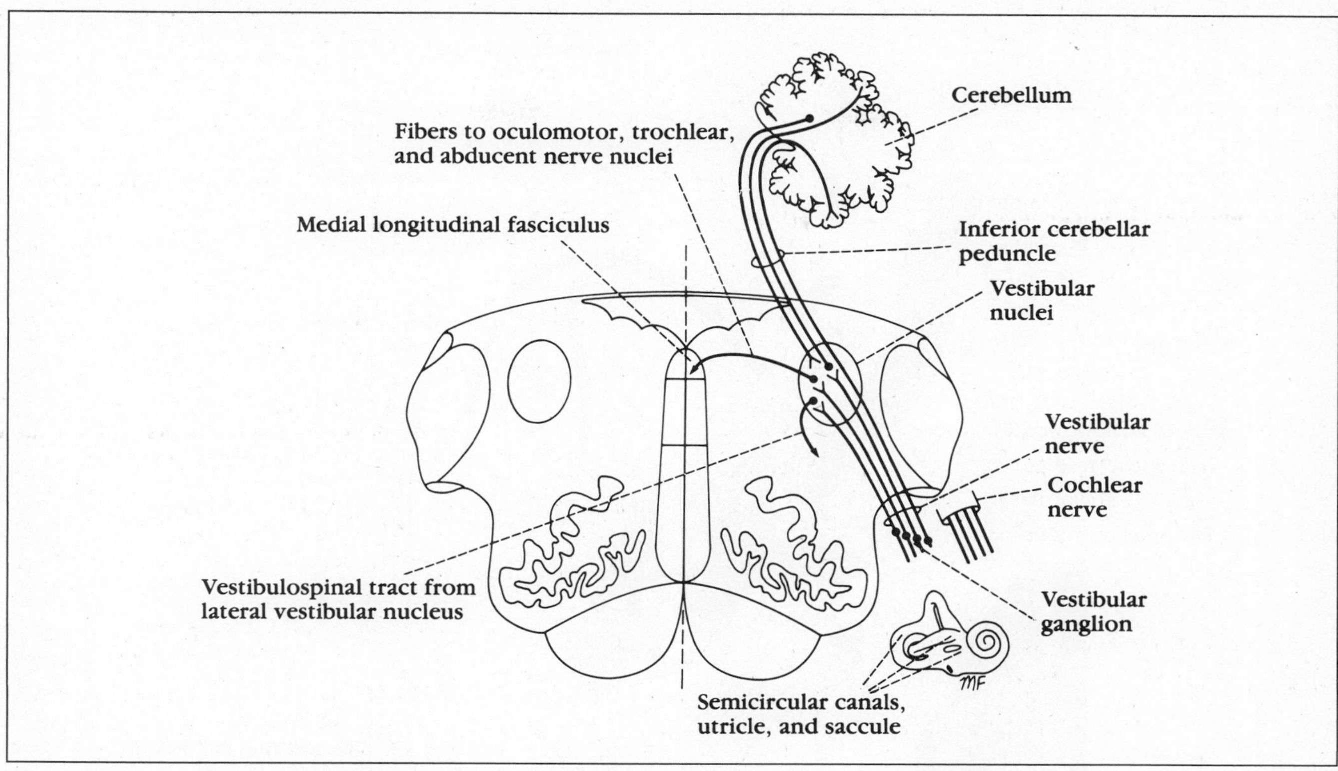

FIGURE 45-10 Vestibular nerve nuclei and their central connections. (From R.S. Snell, *Clinical Neuroanatomy for Medical Students*. Boston: Little, Brown, 1980.)

cells. The axons pass back to the upper medulla accompanied by the cochlear nerve. On entering the medulla, the fibers pass directly to the cerebellum and to four vestibular nuclei that communicate with the medial longitudinal fasciculus and communicate with the nuclei of the third, fourth, and sixth cranial nerves and the upper cervical and accessory nerves. This connection results in vestibular influence on movement of the neck, eyes, and head.

A close interrelationship exists between the vestibular nerves and the cerebellum. This relationship accounts for the equilibrium changes that occur with rapid changes in direction. The maculae of the utricle and saccule provide vestibular input to the cerebellum. The influence of the two-way input and output results in coordination of the muscles of the neck and in the coordination required for posture. Interconnection of vestibular nerves to the reticular system may account for the nausea, vomiting, and sweating that results when the vestibular system is stimulated.

Two vestibulospinal tracts arise from the vestibular nuclei. The lateral tract comes from the lateral vestibular nucleus and extends to the sacral level of the cord. The medial tract comes from the medial vestibular nucleus and extends through the cervical level. Impulses descending in these tracts assist in local myotactic (muscle stretching) reflexes and reinforce the tonus of the extensor muscles of the trunk and limbs, producing extra force to support the body against gravity and to maintain an upright posture.

Communication between the vestibular nuclei and the cerebral nuclei is not established but may exist, as vertigo and dizziness have resulted from cortical stimulation of posterior aspects of the temporal lobe. Disturbances of function of the vestibular system may result in vertigo, nystagmus, and ataxia.

Vertigo. Vertigo is a disturbance of equilibrium resulting in a sensation of whirling or rotation. Posture is maintained by the normal interaction of several structures—labyrinths, eyes, muscles, joints, and higher neural centers. Malfunction of the labyrinths results in vertigo. Causes of vertigo are multitudinous and include disorders of the labyrinth, vestibular nerve, vestibular nuclei, cerebellum, brainstem, eyes, and cerebral cortex.

There are several types of vertigo: acute paroxysmal, chronic, and benign positional. Acute paroxysmal vertigo is exemplified by sudden onset of acute movement, either rotatory and objective, or subjective. If rotatory and objective, external objects seem to be rotating while the person is stationary. If subjective, the person seems to be rotating in relation to the external environment. In addition to rotation, sensations of spinning, falling through space, or being pushed are experienced. Movement of objects or of oneself may appear in any plane—horizontal, oblique, or vertical.

Single attacks of vertigo may occur in acute labyrinthitis. Chronic vertigo is experienced as transient sensations

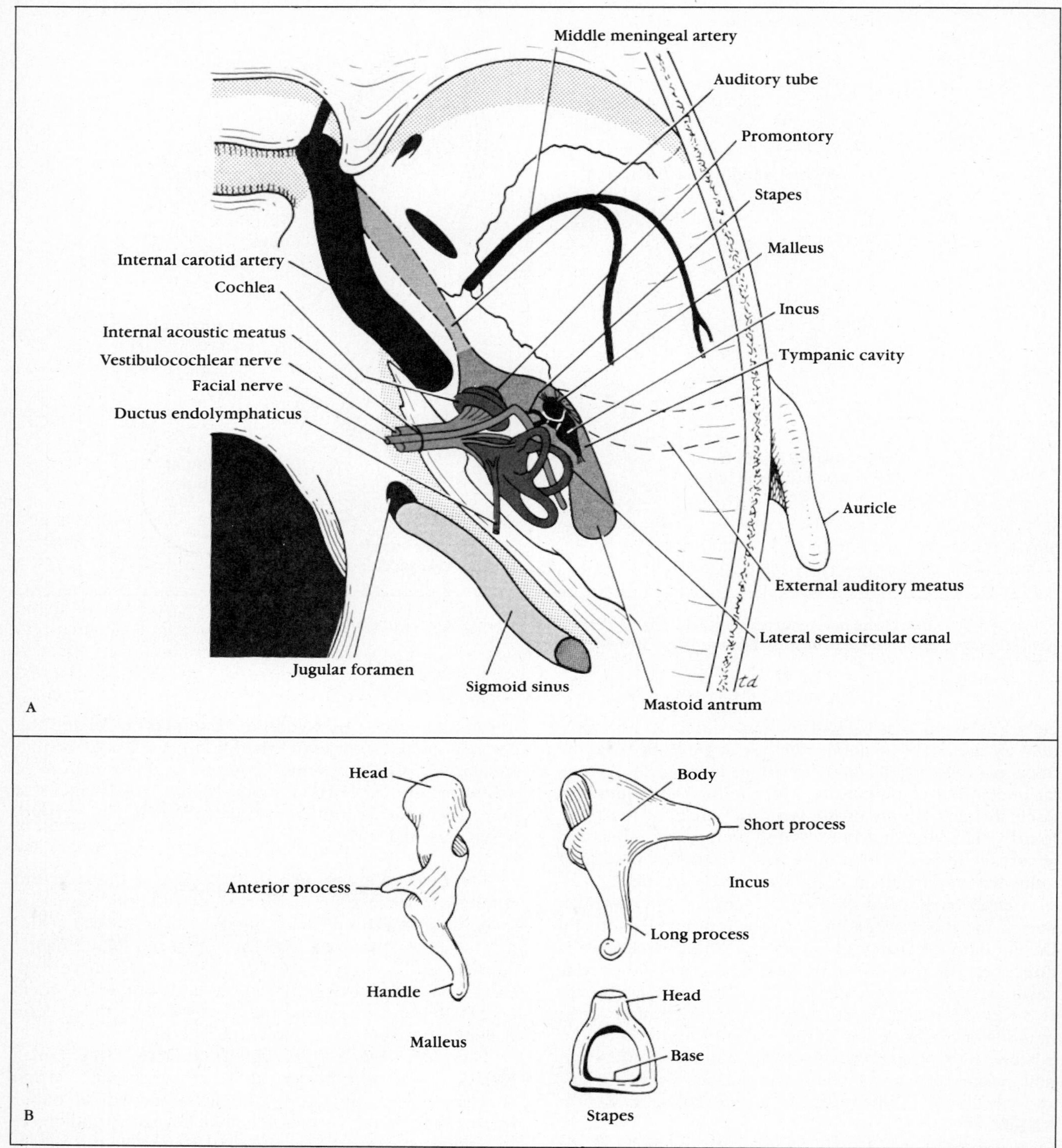

FIGURE 45-11 A. Parts of the right ear in relation to temporal bone as viewed from above. B. The auditory ossicles. (From R.S. Snell, *Clinical Anatomy for Medical Students* [2nd ed.]. Boston: Little, Brown, 1981.)

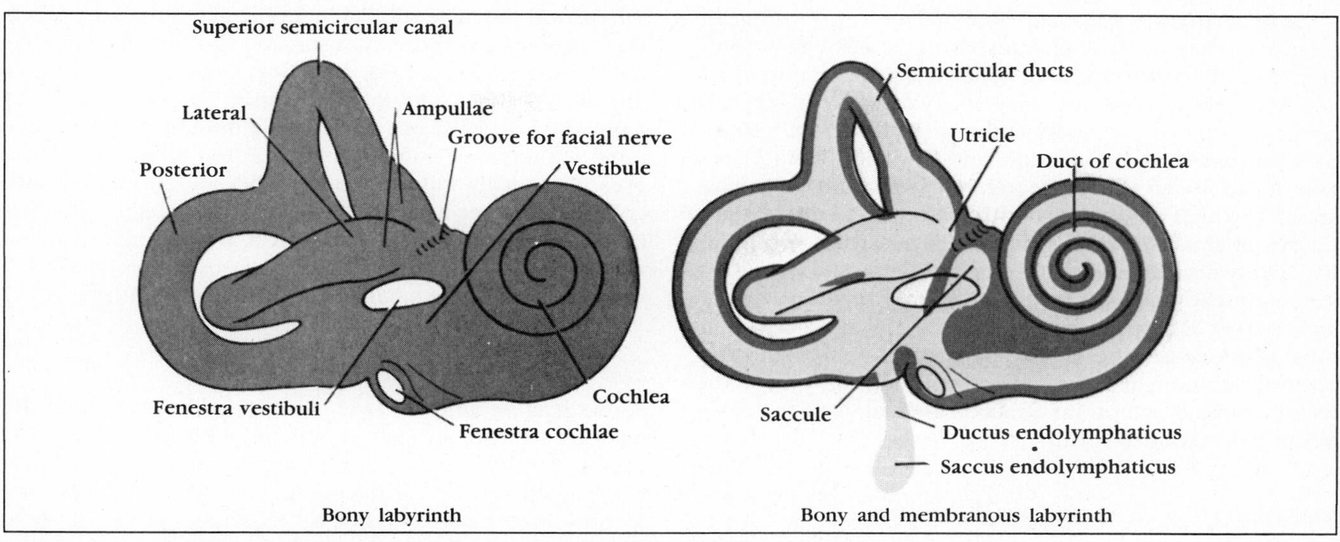

FIGURE 45-12 Bony and membranous labyrinths. (From R.S. Snell, *Clinical Anatomy for Medical Students* [2nd ed.]. Boston: Little, Brown, 1981.)

of rotation with sudden head turning. Another type of attack, which may persist for months, is a constant sense of imbalance. Benign positional vertigo occurs only when the head is in certain positions and ceases when the head is moved out of these positions. An attack may occur with the head in a forward or backward position, or turned to one side. Affected persons learn to avoid the particular posture that causes the attack.

Attacks of vertigo can be disabling, as the person may be thrown to the ground in reaction to false clues of movement. Nausea, vomiting, nystagmus, sweating, hypotension, and excessive salivation may accompany acute attacks of vertigo.

Rapid destruction of one labyrinth causes vertigo, nystagmus, and occasionally, temporary nausea and vomiting. The vestibular nuclei seem to work by comparing signals from both labyrinths. Whenever a labyrinth is destroyed, the other side overcompensates for the input. Bilateral destruction of the labyrinths does not cause nystagmus or vertigo, but the equilibrium may be disturbed for many months.

Meniere's Disease. Meniere's disease is a classic example of vertigo as a result of labyrinthine disease. It is characterized by recurrent attacks of vertigo associated with disordered autonomic activity and gradual loss of hearing. Vertigo appears abruptly and lasts from minutes to more than an hour. It is usually severe enough to cause the person to lie down. Nausea, vomiting, tinnitus, hypotension, sweating, and nystagmus may accompany the attacks. Considerable variation exists in the frequency and severity of the attacks. They may occur daily for a period and then go into remission for a considerable time.

The mechanism of vertigo is unknown at this time, although it is theorized that the autonomic nervous system control of the labyrinthine circulation is impaired. Caloric testing (irrigation of the ear canal) reveals dysfunction of thermally induced nystagmus on the involved side.

Nystagmus. Nystagmus is characterized by rhythmic oscillation of the eyes, and occurs both in physiologic and pathologic circumstances [1]. Nystagmus can be induced in healthy persons by irrigating the external auditory canal with hot or cold water or by rotation in a revolving chair. One form of physiologic nystagmus is ***opticokinetic nystagmus***, which is induced by having the person look at a repeating pattern passed in a horizontal or vertical direction in front of the eyes.

Pathologically, ***vestibular nystagmus*** occurs as a response to some disturbance of the synergistic action of the two vestibular organs or their central connection. The nystagmus is always phasic. There is a slow phase in one direction of the eyes and then an opposing quick phase. The direction of nystagmus is based on the direction of the fast component; if the slow phase is to the right and the quick one is to the left, the person is said to exhibit nystagmus to the left. The movement of the eye may be horizontal, vertical, or rotary. The rotary tendency is most prominent whenever a lesion involves the labyrinth.

Vestibular nystagmus is associated with vertigo and is increased on turning the head or eyes in the direction of the quick phase. This occurs in dysfunction of the semicircular canals or their peripheral neurons. It is limited in duration because central compensation occurs. If it should persist longer than a few weeks, it is usually because of change in the vestibular pathway [3]. Other causes of pathologic nystagmus are abnormal retinal and labyrinthine impulses, lesions of the cervical spinal cord, lesions involving the central paths concerned in ocular posture, weakness of the ocular muscles, and congenital abnormality of unknown etiology.

Labyrinthine Ataxia. Ataxia is often striking in vestibular disease. It is characterized by disturbances of equilibrium in standing and walking, and does not affect isolated limb movements. It has many features of cerebellar ataxia; such as the broad-based, staggering gait, leaning over backward or to one side, and deviation from direction of gait. It can usually be differentiated from cerebellar ataxia through association with nystagmus and vertigo. Causes of ataxias differ, some being caused by degenerative, demyelinating, or inflammatory lesions and others by lesions in the thalamus and subthalamic region near the main cerebellar and sensory pathways. The most common mixed ataxias are the cerebellar and vestibular, and the posterior column and cerebellar forms. In multiple sclerosis for example, symptoms of ataxia are mainly of the cerebellar and vestibular forms.

Assessment of Hearing and Balance

A single effective means of assessing hearing ability is to have the person cover one ear with the hand and whisper a few words softly near the opposite ear; this is repeated for the other ear. If the person is able to perceive these words, the hearing is probably normal. In addition, auditory loss can be determined through the use of equipment such as the tuning fork and audiometer. These tools can assist in distinguishing sensorineural hearing loss from conductive loss.

A simple test for conductive loss can be demonstrated through the use of a tuning fork. A vibrating tuning fork of 256 Hz is placed on the mastoid process until the individual no longer hears it and is then held in the air next to the external auditory meatus. This is known as the *Rinne test*; in persons with normal hearing, air conduction is acute and vibrations are heard after bone conduction has ceased. If vibrations are not heard in the air after bone conduction has ceased, the person has conductive deafness. If the vibrating tuning fork is heard at the ear canal after no longer being heard on the mastoid process, the conduction mechanisms through the middle ear are intact and the problem is in the inner ear or its transmissions; the person then has sensorineural loss.

Weber's test is also effective in identifying of hearing loss. A vibrating tuning fork is placed at the vertex of the head; normal perception of the sound is equal in both ears. If conductive loss is present, the sound is louder in the affected ear due to the masking effect of the environmental noise. In the presence of sensorineural damage, sound is heard better in the normal ear.

Audiometry tests the sensitivity of the ear to pure tones at different frequencies through earphones. The audiometer, which is an electronic oscillator, measures hearing objectively and plots it on a graph that represents the percentage of normal hearing based on the average threshold of normal hearing of a population. Conductive and sensorineural hearing impairments can be distinguished by this means.

The vestibular component of the eighth cranial nerve may be assessed if the person's history reveals vertigo with nausea and vomiting. Vestibular function is evaluated by the *caloric test*. The subject is supine at a 30-degree elevation; after ascertaining no observable defects of the external auditory canal, first cold and then warm water is introduced alternately into the canal. The ear is irrigated with water at 30°C and 44°C with a minimal pause of five minutes between irrigations [1]. Tonic deviation of the eyes is normally induced to the side being irrigated with cold water. After a short latent period, nystagmus occurs in the opposite side. Warm-water irrigation produces nystagmus in the irrigated side. An absent or decreased response indicates impairment of the vestibular system.

Sound Amplification

Sound may be amplified for some individuals through the use of a hearing aid. Some persons with hearing impairments may benefit more from a hearing aid than others. Those with middle ear disturbances generally receive the greatest improvement, while those with inner ear or nerve damage receive less. Hearing aids improve hearing through the mechanical amplification of sound. The person's ability to hear per se is not improved.

Taste

Structure and Function

The sense of taste is a specialized function that is concerned with identification of food. The four primary taste sensations are *sweet*, *sour*, *bitter*, and *salt*. The many others that humans perceive are combinations of the primary sensations together with the olfactory sensation. Specific areas of the tongue are more sensitive to particular sensations (Fig. 45-13).

Taste buds are the organs of taste (Fig. 45-14). These oval structures are located most numerously in the fungiform papillae of the tongue and are also present in the palate, pharynx, and epiglottis. Microvilli project from the buds to the surface and come into contact with the substances dissolved in the fluids of the mouth. This contact is thought to be the basis for the generator potentials. Innervation for the taste buds arrives from their base through small myelinated fibers. Each taste bud is innervated by several nerve fibers and each receives innervation from several taste buds. The life span of a taste bud is approximately five days. As buds degenerate, new ones are being formed and innervated.

In addition to taste buds, the sense of smell contributes significantly to taste perception. Odors of substances taken into the mouth pass to the nasopharynx and stimulate olfactory receptors. Consistency and temperature of ingested substances also contribute to overall taste perception.

Because taste affects what is consumed, it contributes significantly to the nutritional status and internal environment of the body. Nutritional needs are not solely dependent on taste, however. Researchers have shown that people tend to select foods and liquids containing substances in which they may be deficient. This is supported by studies on adrenalectomized animals, which tend to

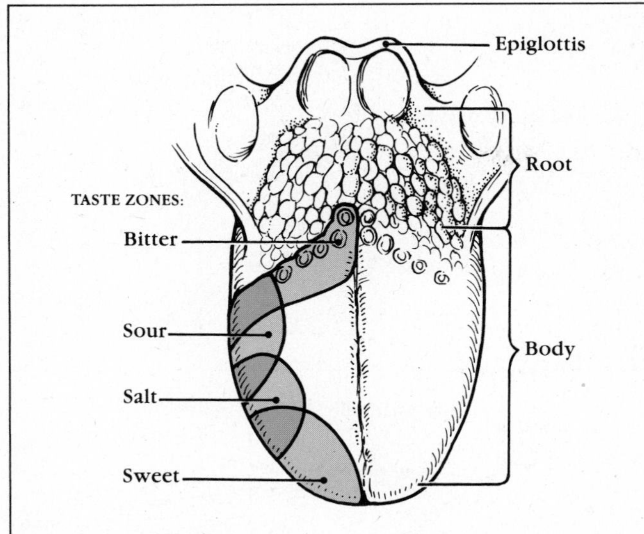

FIGURE 45-13 The dorsal surface of the tongue showing the areas for perception of sweet, sour, bitter, and salt tastes.

develop a preference for salty substances. Animals that have had the parathyroid gland removed usually show an increased appetite for calcium-containing substances [4].

Taste Pathways

Innervation from the taste buds to the central nervous system is through the seventh, ninth, and tenth cranial nerves. The taste buds of the anterior two-thirds of the tongue transmit by way of the chorda tympani branch of the seventh cranial nerve. The posterior one-third of the tongue transmits through the ninth cranial nerve, and the remainder of the areas are transmitted by the tenth cranial nerve. All three of these nerves terminate in the medulla oblongata and form the *tractus solitarius*. From this region, second-order neurons transmit to the thalamus and then on to the postcentral gyrus of the cerebral cortex, where taste sensation shares projection sites with other somatic sensations.

Taste Disturbances

The sense of taste may be diminished (hypogeusia) secondary to other underlying problems, such as dryness of the tongue, irradiation of the head, respiratory infections, and aging. It occurs with heavy smoking as well as unilaterally in accompaniment with Bell's palsy. Lesions of the thalamus and parietal lobe may result in impairment or loss of smell on the opposite side of the tongue, and parietal lobe seizures may be heralded by an aura of a specific taste. Certain medications may alter the interpretation of taste.

Idiopathic hypogeusia is a syndrome associated with hyposmia, dysomia, and dysgeusia in conjunction with diminished taste acuity. The smell and taste of food are most unpleasant for these people. They often experience

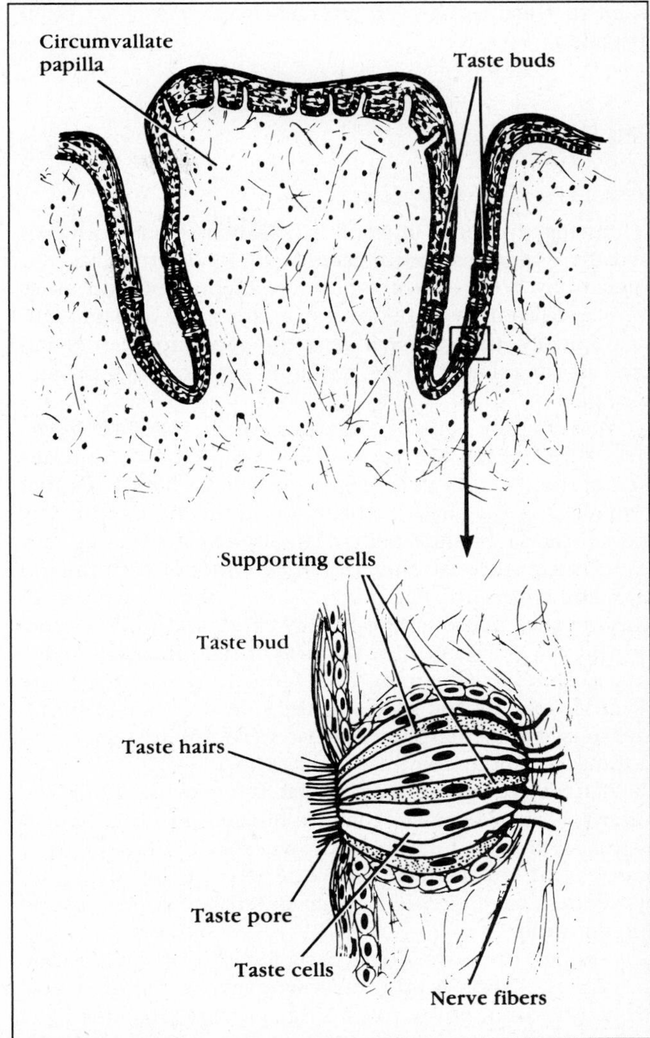

FIGURE 45-14 Microscopic appearance of a taste bud.

weight loss, depression, and anxiety. One identified cause is depression of zinc content in the parotid saliva [1].

Taste Assessment

To assess taste, one examines the function of the eighth, ninth, and tenth cranial nerves. The discrimination of taste in humans is relatively crude, and approximately a 30 percent concentration of a substance is necessary before discrimination is detected. Thresholds of response to substances vary and sensitivity to bitter tastes, in particular, is much higher than to other tastes. This protective mechanism is significant in that many poisonous alkaloids are characteristically bitter.

In assessing taste, substances that are sweet, sour, salty, and bitter are assembled. They are individually swabbed on the appropriate area of the tongue and the person is asked to identify the taste sensation. To prevent mixing of the substances applied to the tongue, the individual is asked to rinse the mouth after each sensation has been identified.

Smell

Structure and Function

In humans, the sense of smell is closely associated physiologically with the sense of taste. Many foods are perceived partially by both senses, which are chemoreceptors that are stimulated by substances in the nose and mouth. Anatomically, they differ in that the apparatus perceiving smell is not relayed to the thalamus or a cortical projection area.

The receptor cells of olfaction are the *bipolar olfactory cells*, which are located in the olfactory mucous membrane. Peripherally, these cells have dendrites that terminate on the surface of the mucus of the nasal cavity and project a group of cilia. The axons of the olfactory neurons pass through the *cribriform plate* of the ethmoid bone and enter the olfactory bulb. Here they synapse with second-order neurons, the *mitral cells*, and form a complex plexus of fibers called the *olfactory glomeruli*. Olfactory signals are transmitted from here through the olfactory tract of the axons of the mitral cells and terminate in two principal areas, the prepyriform area and parts of the amygdaloid complex (Fig. 45-15).

Olfactory receptors are stimulated by volatile lipid- and water-soluble substances that are inhaled into the mucosa of the nasal cavity. Little is known about the excitatory process of the individual receptor cells, although researchers have elicited several potentials in response to different odors.

Although the physiologic basis for odor discrimination and differentiation is still unknown, several theories have been proposed. Some physiologists have proposed the existence of primary odors that excite specific cells. An attempt to explain how this excitation takes place is proposed by the proponents of the *stereochemical* theory. They believe that the odor molecules fit into specifically shaped receptor sites on the surface of the olfactory microvilli membrane. Other theorists have attempted to explain odor discrimination by the physical properties of the stimulant such as its molecular vibrations. Electrophysiologic studies have ascertained that different odors stimulate different parts of the olfactory mucosa to varying degrees. On the basis of this, it would appear that olfactory receptors are not specific for a single odor, but rather for a variety of odors to a different degree.

Adaptation is quite rapid in the sense of smell, as receptors are readily fatigued by persistent odors. Newly appearing odors may be detected rapidly, however. It requires only a small amount of volatile substance to stimulate the olfactory receptors. Inhalation of irritating substances such as ammonium salts produces pain through stimulation of the trigeminal nerve. In addition, certain respiratory reflexes are initiated by its odors.

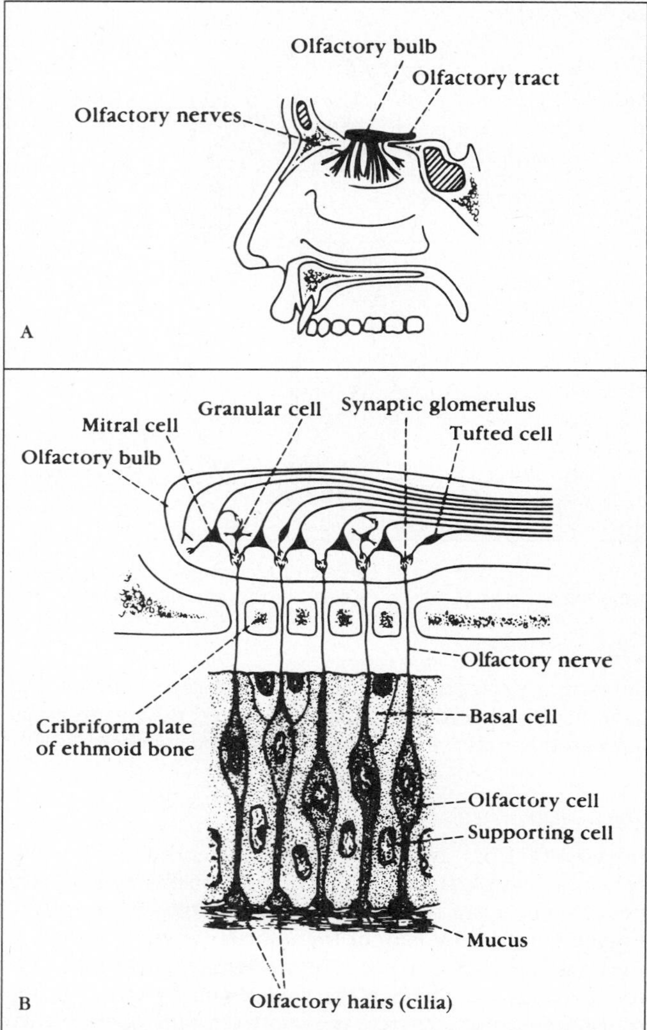

FIGURE 45-15 A. Distribution of olfactory nerves on lateral wall of the nose. B. Connections between olfactory cells and neurons of the olfactory bulb. (From R.S. Snell, *Clinical Neuroanatomy for Medical Students*. Boston: Little, Brown, 1980.)

Smell Disturbances

Anosmia, the loss of smell, may accompany such disorders as sinusitis, upper respiratory infections, and allergies. Facial injuries involving the cribriform plate and certain tumors involving the olfactory groove may result in the loss of smell. Hysteria may be accompanied by anosmia or *hyperosmia* (increased acuity of smell). Olfactory hallucinations may occur with certain mental illnesses. Specific smells may precede seizures arising from the uncal region.

Smell Assessment

The sense of smell can be assessed simply by requesting the individual to identify common aromatic substances such as coffee, vanilla, and cologne. When doing this, the person is asked to close his or her eyes and occlude the opposite nostril. Although the individual is requested to identify the odor if possible, this ability is less significant than the perception of the odor. Therefore, the individual is asked to identify when he or she initially perceives the odor. The procedure is then repeated for the other nostril and perception is compared.

Study Questions

1. Describe the sensory function of vision from the visual pathways to the interpretation of the object.
2. How does the eye adapt to light, distance, and color of viewed objects?
3. Discuss the basic eye dysfunctions of myopia, hypermetropia, and astigmatism.
4. How is normal intraocular pressure maintained?
5. Describe the sensory function of hearing from the eardrum to the auditory cortex.
6. How does the ear function in maintaining balance and position?
7. Describe the sensory functions of taste and smell. Define several causes of disorders of these functions.

References

1. Adams, R., and Mauria, V. *Principles of Neurology* (3rd ed.). New York: McGraw-Hill, 1985.
2. Carpenter, M., and Sutin, J. *Human Neuroanatomy* (8th ed.). Baltimore: Williams & Wilkins, 1983.
3. Clark, R.G. *Essentials of Clinical Neuroanatomy and Neurophysiology* (5th ed.). Philadelphia: Davis, 1975.
4. Guyton, A.C. *Textbook of Medical Physiology* (7th ed.). Philadelphia: Saunders, 1986.
5. Hubel, D.H., and Wiesel, T.N. Brain mechanisms of vision. *Sci. Am.* 241:150, 1979.
6. Hudspeth, A.J. The hair cells of the inner ear. *Sci. Am.* 248:59, 1983.
7. Moses, R. *Adler's Physiology of the Eye* (7th ed.). St. Louis: Mosby, 1981.
8. Nauta, W.J., and Feirtag, M. The organization of the brain. *Sci. Am.* 241:99, 1979.
9. Rose, F.C. *The Eye in General Practice*. Baltimore: University Park Press, 1983.

CHAPTER 46

Common Adaptations and Alterations in Higher Neurological Function

CHAPTER OUTLINE

Cerebrovascular Disease: Pathology and Related Clinical Signs
- Transient Ischemic Attacks
- Occlusive Cerebrovascular Disease
  - *Cerebral Thrombosis*
  - *Cerebral Embolism*
  - *Intracerebral Hemorrhage*
- Cerebral Aneurysms and Vascular Malformations
  - *Aneurysms*
  - *Arteriovenous Malformations (AVMs)*

Aphasia
- Wernicke's Aphasia
- Broca's Aphasia
- Global Aphasia
- Selective Disorders of Receptive or Expressive Activities of Spoken and Written Language

Apraxia

Agnosia
- Types of Agnosia
  - *Visual Agnosia*
  - *Tactile Agnosia*
  - *Auditory Agnosia*

Body Image
- Gerstmann's Syndrome

Epilepsy
- Electroencephalography in Epilepsy
- Classification of Seizures
- Generalized Seizures
  - *Absence Seizures (Petit Mal)*
  - *Tonic-Clonic Seizures (Grand Mal)*
  - *Myoclonic Seizures*
  - *Akinetic Seizures*
- Partial Seizures
  - *Focal Motor Seizures (Jacksonian Seizures)*
  - *Focal Sensory Seizures*
  - *Complex Partial Seizures (Psychomotor)*
- Secondary or Symptomatic Epilepsy

LEARNING OBJECTIVES

1. Discuss the two major classifications of cerebrovascular disease.
2. Describe the pathologic changes that occur with intracerebral hemorrhages, cerebral thrombosis, and embolism.
3. Locate and discuss cerebral aneurysms and arteriovenous malformations.
4. Relate the clinical manifestations of stroke to the underlying pathologic bases.
5. List clinical findings associated with occlusion of each of the major cerebral arteries.
6. Define *thrombotic stroke in evolution*.
7. List the etiologic factors of stroke.
8. Explain why bleeding is a common complication after initial rupture of an intracerebral aneurysm.
9. Describe the neurologic findings in each of the gradations of ruptured cerebral aneurysms.
10. Discuss the implications of vasospasm with ruptured cerebral aneurysms.
11. Draw or describe the appearance of arteriovenous malformation (AVMs).
12. Explain why AVMs rupture and the significance of the location of the bleeding.
13. Define *aphasia*.
14. Differentiate Wernicke's aphasia, Broca's aphasia, and global aphasia.
15. Define the disorders of speech: *anarthria*, *agraphia*, *alexia*, and *word-deafness*.
16. Define *apraxia*.
17. Define *agnosia*.
18. Discuss the various types of agnosia.
19. Define *Gerstmann's syndrome*.
20. Discuss the pathophysiology of epilepsy.
21. Differentiate between primary or idiopathic and secondary or symptomatic epilepsy.
22. Discuss partial versus generalized seizures.
23. List some precipitating factors that may initiate seizures.
24. Describe changes on the electroencephalogram that correlate with three different types of seizures.

Cerebrovascular disease leads to hospitalization for more persons than any other neurologic disorder. Cerebrovascular accidents are the third leading cause of death (after heart disease and cancer) in the United States. Major disabilities frequently remain in those who survive the initial assault. Paresis, aphasia, agnosia, and apraxia are among common associated impairments. Epilepsy is another major neurologic disorder. It ranks second only to cerebrovascular accidents in terms of numbers of persons with neurologic disease in the United States.

Cerebrovascular Disease: Pathology and Related Clinical Signs

As is the case with most neuropathology, the site of a lesion is more critical in the production of pathologic signs and symptoms than is its pathology. Most lesions that affect the motor cortex and its major pathways are vascular and result in either reversible or irreversible anoxic tissue damage. Cerebrovascular disease is commonly associated with hypertension and atherosclerotic disease. Both of these conditions are closely linked with other risk factors, including hypercholesterolemia, cigarette smoking, obesity, diabetes mellitus, physical inactivity, emotional stress, and family history of premature atherosclerosis. Intracerebral aneurysms are vascular malformations that, on enlargement or rupture, can cause the pathologic signs of stroke. Traumatic injuries, as detailed in Chapter 48, can cause significant alterations in consciousness and many signs equivalent to those of intrinsic cerebrovascular accidents.

Cerebrovascular disease may be classified according to two basic causes: hemorrhage and occlusion of cerebral arteries. Occlusive disease results from thrombosis and embolism. Hemorrhagic disease may result from intracerebral, subarachnoid, or arteriovenous malformation bleeding into the brain parenchyma or spaces. Whatever the cause, necrosis of the brain parenchyma may result.

The clinical features and course of the disease are variable. Neurologic impairments result from sudden disruption of blood supply to an area of the brain. This is referred to as a *cerebrovascular accident* (*CVA* or *stroke*). In addition to classifying strokes according to etiology (thrombosis, embolism, and hemorrhage), they are grouped according to onset and duration of symptoms: completed, progressing or evolving, and transient. A *completed stroke* is a major catastrophe when the blood supply has been suddenly cut off to a portion of the brain. Alterations in sensation, speech, vision, and muscle strength follow rapidly. *Progressing or evolving stroke* progresses over a period of hours and usually results from numerous embolizations to the same area of the brain. *Transient ischemic attacks* are strokes in which the neurologic defects last less than 24 hours.

Transient Ischemic Attacks

If tissue ischemia is reversible, the tissue changes are temporary, causing decreased blood supply to an area and focal ischemic clinical signs. These reversible signs are called transient ischemic attacks (TIAs). The result may be transient episodes of contralateral weakness (hemiparesis), sensory deficits (hemiparesthesias), or visual disturbances [5]. Involvement of the ophthalmic artery results in unilateral visual symptoms known as *amaurosis fugax*. The individual suddenly loses sight in one eye for two to three minutes as a result of transient ischemia of the retina.

Because intact circulation and a relatively constant flow of blood are required for continuous function of the cerebral cells, syncope (fainting) may result when the general circulation fails suddenly. Transient ischemic attacks are characterized by localized symptoms of cerebral dysfunction, often including syncope.

The symptoms of TIAs seem to result from a cerebral angiospasm or transient impairment of blood flow. The attacks usually last less than one hour and are followed by no neurologic impairment. Symptoms may include yawning, headache, vertigo, deafness, diplopia, ataxia, and motor or sensory deficits.

The TIAs also may be associated with collateral communications in the intracerebral arterial system that compensate in a short time for the deficits from occlusion of one arterial source. Many individuals who experience several TIAs have a completed stroke within five years.

Diagnosis of TIAs usually requires angiographic evaluation of the site, size, and pathologic processes in the cerebral arteries. Radiopaque substances are injected to outline the cerebral vasculature to locate areas of narrowing or disease.

Occlusive Cerebrovascular Disease

Occlusive cerebrovascular disease results from thrombosis and emboli formation in the cerebral vessels. The effects of occlusion vary with its extent, speed, and location (Table 46-1). In addition, the collateral vessels available to divert the remaining circulation affect the blood flow to a specific area of the brain. Obstruction of the flow to any region rapidly results in cell ischemia, and potentially irreversible necrosis and cerebral infarction.

Cerebral Thrombosis. Ischemic infarction in the brain is often due to cerebral thrombosis that occurs on an atherosclerotic plaque. Atherosclerotic thrombosis is the leading cause of the condition. The most common areas of thrombosis formation are those where atheromatous plaques have already resulted in narrowing of the vessels. The sites most frequently affected are the internal carotid artery in the region of the carotid sinus, the junction of the vertebral and basilar arteries, the bifurcation of the middle cerebral artery, the posterior cerebral artery in the area of the cerebral peduncle, and the anterior cerebral artery in the area of the corpus collosum [4].

Wide variations may be observed in clinical signs resulting from disruption of blood flow to specific regions of the brain. Occlusions of major arteries manifest the clinical findings given in Table 46-1. The resulting obstruction to blood flow causes infarction to the area

TABLE 46-1 Clinical Findings with Occlusion of Major Cerebral Arteries

Occluded Arteries	Associated Findings
Internal carotid system	Contralateral hemiplegia Aphasia with dominant side involvement Agnosia Hemianopia Cranial nerve deficits Contralateral anosognosia Bruit over occluded artery
Middle cerebral artery	Contralateral arm weakness or paralysis Contralateral leg weakness Homonymous hemianopia Eye deviation to opposite side Aphasia with dominant side involvement Left half anosognosia Contralateral sensory impairment Apraxia with nondominant side involvement
Anterior cerebral artery	Contralateral paralysis of leg and foot Contralateral arm paralysis (lesser degree) Bladder incontinence Sensory dificit in leg, foot, toes Akinetic mutism Gait impairment Mood disturbance, personality change
Vertebral-basilar system	Variations in level of consciousness Hemianopia Possible quadriplegia Eye muscle paralysis Headache Limb weakness Nystagmus Diplopia Mutism Ataxia Dysphagia Varying sensory deficits (numbness) Vertigo Varying cranial nerve deficits

supplied by the artery. This type of lesion is often called an *atherothrombotic brain infarction (ABI)*. The type of infarct produced depends upon the amount of hemorrhage that occurs into the area of ischemic necrosis.

Infarcts are often described as red (hemorrhagic) or white (anemic). In the first few days, the pale or white infarcts assume a muddy, mottled appearance that is associated with surrounding tissue edema. After about ten days, liquefaction of the area becomes evident from the release of neuronal lysosomes and other lytic substances into the brain parenchyma [5]. Scar tissue begins to form at the margins of the necrotic area. The necrotic tissue is removed and replaced by cystic scar tissue. Gliosis (proliferation of glial cells) around the area is characteristic and this is followed by polymorphonuclear leukocyte (PMN) exudation, leading to removal of the necrotic debris. Therefore, characteristic scar tissue is laid down after the acute inflammation subsides.

Red infarcts also cause tissue destruction. Red blood cells are broken down and removed. The necrotic parenchyma undergoes liquefaction, and characteristic scar tissue is formed at the margins of the affected area. Cerebral edema accompanies cerebral infarction and is maximal three to five days after an acute stroke [7]. It is a major cause of death after acute stroke.

The onset of cerebral thrombosis is usually gradual, with periods of progression and periods of improvement. This is apparently due to spread of the thrombus and is called a *thrombotic stroke in evolution*. This thrombosis causes the cerebral infarction, which may be associated with a hemorrhage into the brain parenchyma [2]. Symptoms often begin or are noted in the early morning. They may consist of headache, vertigo, mental confusion, aphasia, and focal neurologic signs, which may occur weeks to months before the actual evolved stroke. A full-blown stroke may cause a variety of clinical features (see Table 46-1).

Recovery is variable and depends on the location and the amount of intracerebral damage. Function in an affected leg usually is recovered prior to arm and hand function, which may not return at all.

Cerebral Embolism. Cerebral embolism is second only to thrombosis as a cause of stroke. The main source of an embolus is the heart. Heart conditions that predispose to cerebral embolization include atrial fibrillation, bacterial endocarditis, rheumatic endocarditis and the valvular diseases that may follow it, and congenital heart disease [4]. The embolus frequently lodges in the middle cerebral artery, which is a direct continuation of the carotid artery. Massive brain infarction occurs where a large embolus lodges in a major cerebral vessel. Frequently, however, large thrombi break into smaller clots that travel to occlude more distal branches.

The onset of embolic infarction is always very sudden and the effect is immediate. It usually has no warning signs. The clinical features depend on the artery affected and the amount and location of brain infarction.

Intracerebral Hemorrhage. Hypertension is the major cause of spontaneous bleeding into the brain parenchyma. The severity of the hemorrhage is related to the amount of blood extravasated and the region of the brain affected. Intracerebral bleeds generally tend to occur deep within the brain substance (Fig. 46-1A). The most common areas of bleed in the brain secondary to hypertension are the putamen and the adjacent internal capsule. These areas account for about 50 percent of cases [1]. Other potential areas include the central white matter of the temporal, parietal, and frontal lobes, the thalamus, cerebellum, and pons.

In large bleeds, such as in Figure 46-1, the extravasation of blood forms a circular type mass that disrupts and compresses surrounding brain tissue, resulting in infarc-

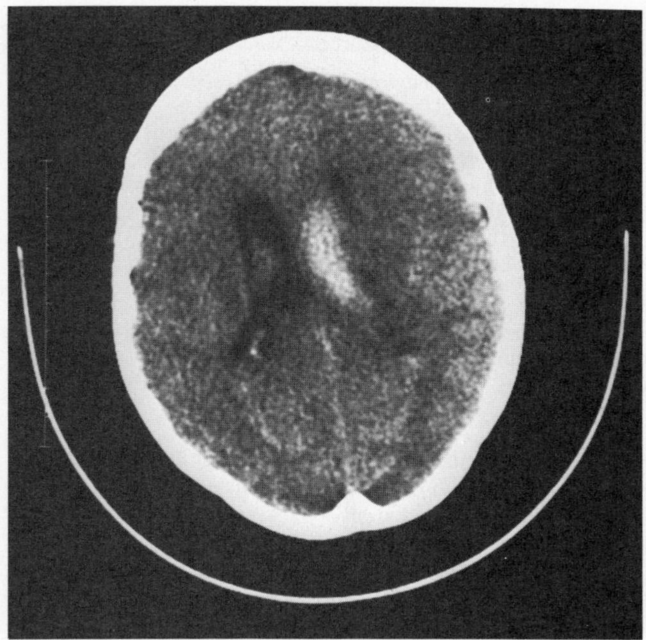

A

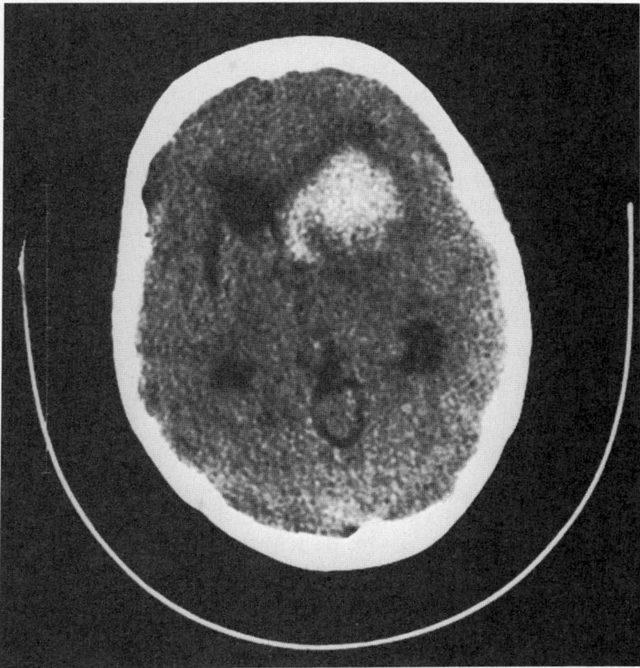

B

FIGURE 46-1 A. Large, right hemispheric, intracerebral bleed. B. Same bleed showing intraventricular involvement.

tion and tissue necrosis. These hemorrhages may displace midline structures that can compress vital centers, lead to coma, and eventually, death. Commonly, blood seeps into the ventricular system (Fig. 46-1B). Analysis of cerebrospinal fluid (CSF) reflects presence of blood in the great majority of those who have suffered large hemorrhages. Intracerebral hemorrhages may also be small, single bleeds or have several foci. Some may reflect no obvious neurologic deficits, whereas a large number of small hemorrhages in the parenchyma may result in severe neurologic impairment.

Intracerebral bleeds occur abruptly and the symptoms evolve rather rapidly. Prodromal symptoms are generally absent. Severe headache occurs fairly consistently. Other symptoms relate to the region of the brain involved.

Intracerebral hemorrhages commonly occur deep within the brain substance, in the region of the basal ganglia. The bleeding may be massive or have numerous foci. The blood in the parenchyma causes extensive neuronal destruction, and the central area of hemorrhage is often surrounded by small hemorrhages. The blood is treated like foreign material and eventually is broken down, phagocytized, and removed from the area. Many mechanisms appear to cause intracerebral hemorrhage, for example, a sudden elevation of blood pressure in the presence of diseased intracranial vessels that causes rupture of the vessels. The initial event may be ischemia produced from an arterial spasm, which may be followed by rupture of the diseased vessels. The most common cause of subarachnoid hemorrhage (bleeding into the ventricles and subarachnoid space) is rupture of an intracerebral aneurysm.

Cerebral Aneurysms and Vascular Malformations

Common sources of cerebral bleeding, which also contribute to the etiology of CVAs, are ruptured intracranial aneurysm and vascular malformation. Both frequently result in bleeding into the subarachnoid space and are clinically similar.

Aneurysms. The etiology of cerebral aneurysms is related to developmental defects and hypertensive atherosclerotic changes. Developmental defects involve a weakness in the middle coat (tunica media) of the vessel that results in a saccular out-pouching at the weakened area. These so-called *berry aneurysms* are by far the most common of these defects. Berry aneurysms can vary from one to several centimeters in size and generally have a well-defined neck that originates most often near bifurcations in the anterior vessels of the circle of Willis (Figs. 46-2 and 46-3) [6]. Berry aneurysms have the highest frequency of rupture in persons between 30 and 60 years of age, and both sexes are affected equally. Of individuals with developmental cerebral aneurysms, about one-fifth demonstrate numerous aneurysms.

Less common than developmental aneurysms are those associated with atherosclerotic degenerative changes of the cerebral vasculature. They are usually fusiform as a result of weakening of the tunica media from the degenerative atherosclerotic process. The arteries become thin and fibrous, often apparently as a result of long-term hypertension. Although fusiform aneurysms of cerebral

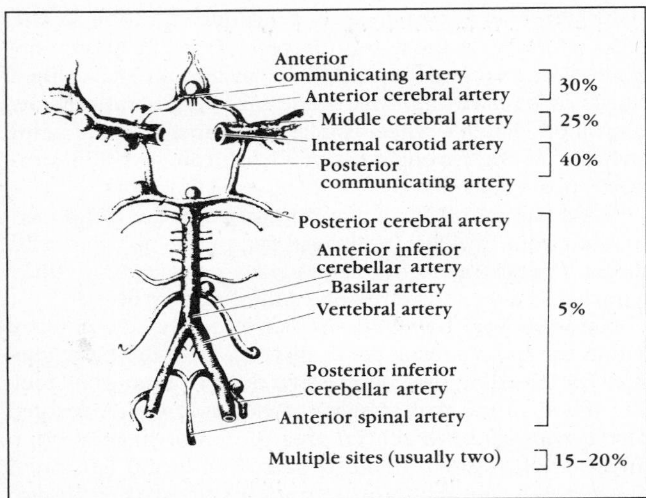

FIGURE 46-2 Common sites of aneurysms. (From J.H. Stein [ed.], *Internal Medicine*. Boston: Little, Brown, 1983.)

TABLE 46-2 Grades of Ruptured Cerebral Aneurysms

Grade	Neurologic Findings
I	Alert and oriented, mild headache, no neurologic deficits
II	Alert and oriented, moderate to severe headache, signs of meningeal irritation, minimal neurologic deficits
III	Drowsy and confused, pronounced focal neurologic deficits, signs of meningeal irritation
IV	Stuperous or unresponsive, major neurologic deficits may be present, mild decerebrate rigidity
V	Coma and decerebrate rigidity

arteries may occur in some younger individuals, they generally affect those over age 50 years.

Cerebral aneurysms can remain silent for many years, often going undetected throughout life and being discovered only on routine postmortem examination. They become evident during life when they rupture or compress adjacent nerve tissue, causing focal cerebral disturbances.

The signs and symptoms of subarachnoid bleeding from a ruptured aneurysm may be localized from the pressure exerted on surrounding tissue. Focal localizing signs are related to the region of the brain involved and may include visual defects, cranial nerve paralysis, hemiparesis, and focal seizures. Generalized signs of subarachnoid bleeding reflect meningeal irritation and include photophobia, fever, malaise, vomiting, abnormal mentation with disorientation, and nuchal rigidity. If conscious, the person complains of a severe headache of a different nature from any experienced previously. Transitory unconsciousness or extended coma may accompany bleeding from ruptured aneurysms. Initial and prolonged coma generally indicates an unfavorable outcome. It is common to assess ruptured cerebral aneurysms according to grade (Table 46-2).

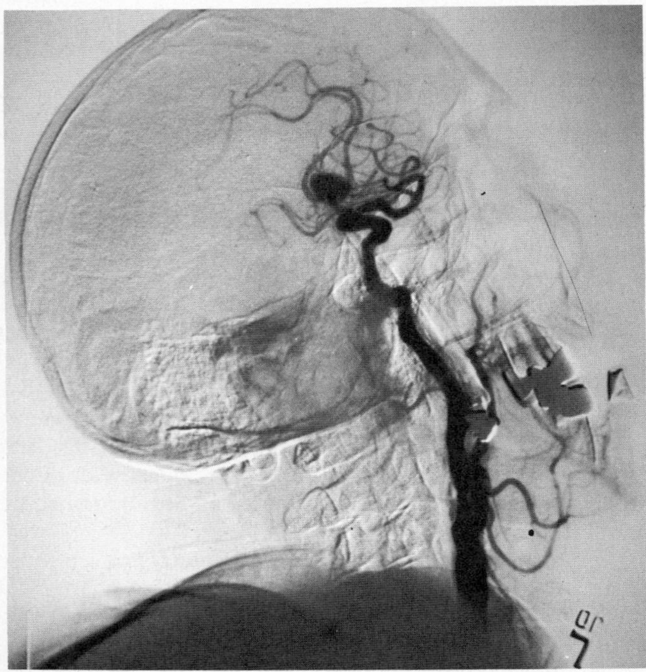

FIGURE 46-3 Arteriogram showing cerebral aneurysm involving the anterior communicating artery.

The aneurysm decreases in size after rupture and a fibrin clot forms over the site of the rupture. The individual is at risk of a recurrence of bleeding during the first few weeks after the initial bleed, during the period of clot lysis or breakdown. Recurrent bleeding in cerebral aneurysms considerably increases mortality risk.

Diagnosis of ruptured cerebral aneurysms is based on history, clinical examination, lumbar puncture, cerebral angiography, and computed axial tomographic (CAT) scans. Treatment is conservative initially in an effort to stabilize the pathologic processes. When stabilization has been accomplished, surgical intervention is generally necessary to resolve the aneurysm.

Vasospasm frequently accompanies ruptured cerebral aneurysms. It accounts for 50 percent of the morbidity and mortality of individuals who survive the initial bleed [3]. Because spasm develops within a week or two after the rupture, it results in narrowing of the vessel lumen. This may lead to cerebral ischemia and clinicially evident neurologic deficits. The precise cause of vasospasm is unknown but is thought to be related to certain intrinsic chemicals associated with lysis of the clot. These include substances such as serotonin, prostaglandins, catecholamines, histamine, angiotensin, and oxyhemoglobin [3]. In most cases, surgery is delayed until the spasm subsides.

Arteriovenous Malformations (AVMs). Vascular malformations that frequently cause a cerebral hemorrhage usually result from developmental defects of the cerebral veins, capillaries, or arteries in certain localized regions of the brain. These defects have very few distinguishing characteristics with respect to their location. The AVMs may also be secondary to trauma or injury.

The veins frequently appear to connect to the arteries without an intermediate capillary bed (Fig. 46-4). The vessel walls are very thin and lack the normal structure of arteries and veins. The malformations are referred to as arteriovenous malformations or, less appropriately, angiomas (Fig. 46-5). They are present most commonly on the surface of the cerebral hemispheres, although they may appear deeper within the cerebral lobes, brainstem, or spinal cord. Although AVMs are present from birth, they may not become evident until young adulthood or later. Their presence is manifested by symptoms of hemorrhage, seizures, headaches, or focal neurologic deficits. A bruit may be audible over the area of the malformation.

As the very thin walls of these vessels become engorged, the vessels are particularly vulnerable to rupture and bleeding. Bleeding most commonly occurs into the subarachnoid space and, therefore, the symptoms are similar to those observed with ruptured cerebral aneurysms. In addition, specific findings reflect the region of the brain that is involved.

Diagnosis of AVM is based on clinical findings and results of one or more of the following tests: cerebral angiography, lumbar puncture, CAT scan, electroencephalogram (EEG), and radioactive scan. Treatment is surgical ligation and excision of the feeder vessels into the area, whenever possible. If the location of the AVM does not permit surgical excision, embolization may be performed to occlude the feeder vessels in an attempt to reduce the blood flow to the AVM.

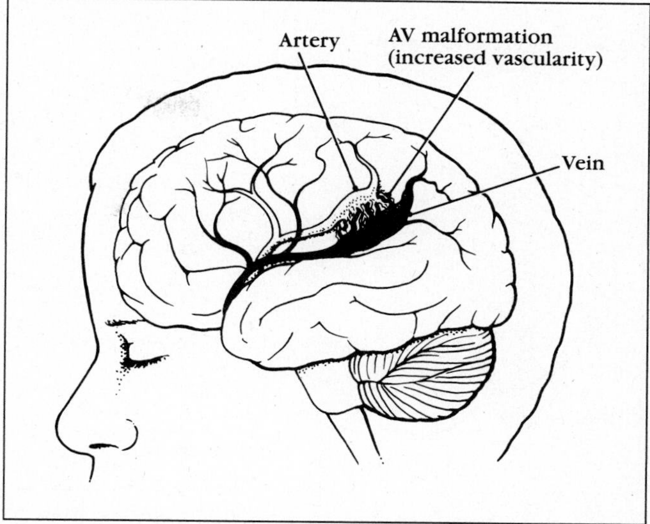

FIGURE 46-5 Appearance of superficial arteriovenous malformation. Vessels are dilated and tortuous.

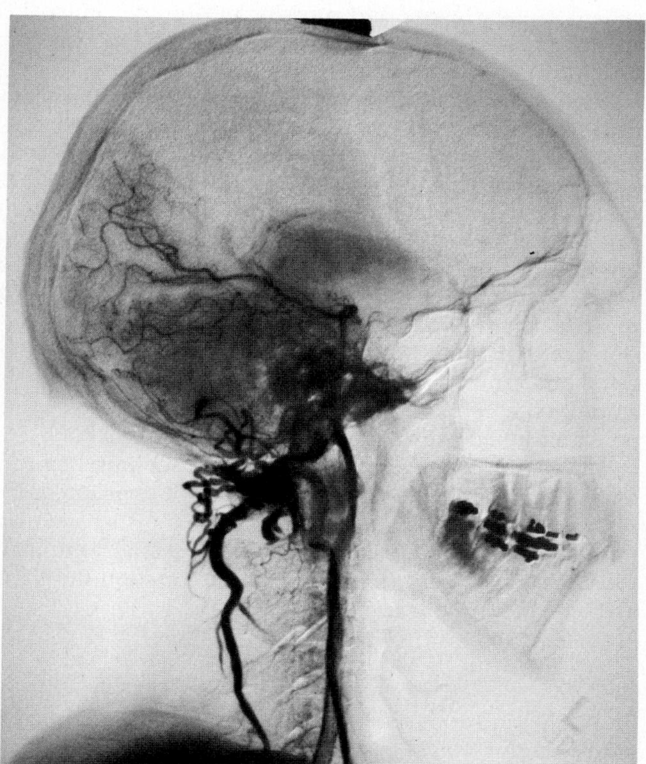

FIGURE 46-4 Arteriogram showing an arteriovenous malformation that is fed by the vertebral artery and drains into superficial veins and internal jugular vein.

Aphasia

Language is defined as audible, articulate human speech produced by the action of the tongue and adjacent vocal cords. *Speech* may be the act of speaking, the result of speaking, the utterance of vocal sounds that convey ideas, or the ability to express thoughts by words. Mechanisms of speech are accomplished through internal symbolization and thought. Language is dependent on retention, recall, visualization, and the integration of symbols. Speech depends on the interpretation of auditory and visual images, which reach the higher human processes during different states of consciousness and, to some degree, the lower states of consciousness.

Language is a function primarily of the left cerebral hemisphere. Figure 46-6 shows the approximate location of the speech centers in the brain. The ability to produce language is dependent on the normal function and integrity of the primary receptive areas in the temporal and occipital lobes and the expressive areas in the inferior part of the frontal lobe of the dominant hemisphere. To speak, one must initially formulate the thought to be expressed, choose appropriate words, and then control the motor activity of the muscles of phonation and articulation. Simultaneously, accurate recording of visual and auditory stimuli is necessary before the significance of the words used can be appreciated. Language and speech may become impaired in many ways. Regardless of the cause, the results are generally similar when the brain is damaged.

Aphasia is a neurologic defect in speech. The ability either to comprehend and integrate *receptive language* or

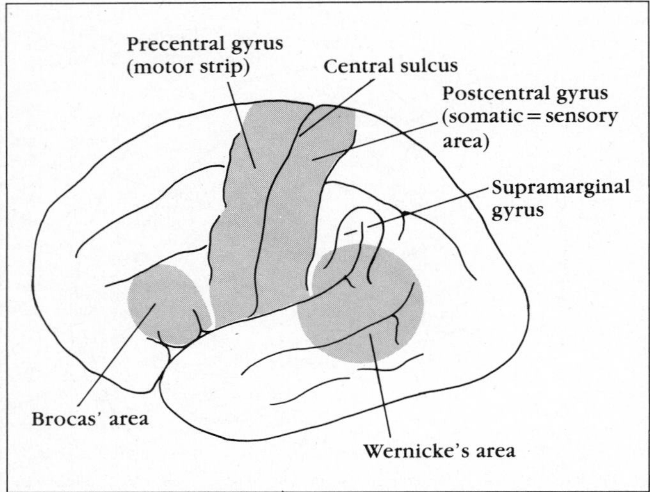

FIGURE 46-6 Speech involves many cortical activities. Two special areas have been identified: Wernicke's and Broca's. (From D. Dickson and W. Maue-Dickson, *Anatomical and Physiological Bases of Speech*. Boston: Little, Brown, 1982.)

to formulate and use *expressive language*, or both, is impaired. The receptive language modalities are *reading*, which requires visual integration and comprehension of the printed word, and *listening*, which necessitates auditory integration and comprehension of the verbal word. The expressive language modalities are *writing*, which requires visual-motor formulation and use of the printed word, and *speaking*, which requires oral-motor formulation and the use of verbal words. The aphasic individual usually has some impairment of all language modalities.

Aphasia is usually caused by organic disease of the brain that results from a lesion in the left cerebral hemisphere. This hemisphere is considered to be dominant in the reception and expression of language. Infrequently, aphasia has occurred in right-sided lesions associated with right-handed individuals; however, their right-handedness has sometimes been forced or induced. In left-handed persons, lesions of the left or of the right hemispheres may cause aphasia, most frequently the left.

When certain portions of the cortex and subcortical associated pathways of the dominant hemisphere are altered by lack of blood supply (loss of oxygen or hemorrhage to the brain tissue), speech patterns become altered, limited, or destroyed, depending on the magnitude of the pathology. Vascular disturbances are the most common cause of aphasia. Infarction, caused by thrombotic embolic occlusion of the middle cerebral artery or the left internal carotid artery, is the etiology in the majority of cases, and impairs both spoken and written language. Transitory ischemic attacks and migraine headache may trigger transitory speech disorders.

Space-occupying lesions, such as intracerebral hemorrhage, intracranial tumors, and infections, also may cause aphasia. Left hemisphere aphasia results from damage to a specific region of the brain, the first and second temporal gyri, the insula, and the posterior part of the third convolution. Visual and auditory impulses reach the cerebral cortex posteriorly by way of the occipital lobe and anteroinferiorly by way of the temporal lobe. There is extraction of the semantic value of the auditory and visual message and of the symbolic formation of the expressed message in the posterior portion of the temporal convolutions. The anterior part of the region is necessary for the motor realization of the expressed message. Many cortical areas and association pathways are concerned in the integration of the function of speech.

Many combinations of vascular, neoplastic, and traumatic causes and locations of lesions lead to different language patterns. Classifications have been developed to define prominent characteristics, to localize position and size of cerebral lesions, and to assess the language deficit pattern in each category of aphasia. The primary types of disorders are (1) Wernicke's aphasia, which causes disturbances of all language activities except articulation; (2) Broca's aphasia, involving disturbances in spoken and written language with dysarthria (disorder of articulation); and (3) selective disorders of receptive and expressive activities of spoken or written language.

Wernicke's Aphasia

The posterior one-third of the superior temporal convolution of the dominant hemisphere is called Wernicke's area (see Fig. 46-6). Wernicke's area influences the understanding and interpretation of word symbols. Lesions in other areas, particularly the posterior half of the dominant hemisphere, angular gyrus, and supramarginal gyrus, influence speech function through the involvement of association fibers.

Wernicke's aphasia is an impairment in comprehension of speech and includes central, receptive, cortical, sensory, auditory, semantic, and conduction aphasia. Affected persons have fluent, spontaneous speech with normal rhythm and articulation, but comprehension, repetition, and naming are impaired. Speech appears devoid of meaning despite the fluency and spontaneity. Expression is hindered by difficulty in the choice of words to speak and to write. Repetition, reading aloud, and writing from dictation are deranged. Understanding of spoken language is disturbed. The speech of others is heard, but the words are not comprehended. Speech lacks content and contains much meaningless expression.

Lesions in the Wernicke's area inhibit comprehension in spoken and written language because of their interconnections with the angular gyrus. Lesions of the angular gyrus and posteroinferior part of the parietal lobe may cause acalculia, autopanosia, and disorientation for right and left sides (Table 46-3).

Broca's Aphasia

The lesion in Broca's aphasia is located in the caudal part of the inferior frontal gyrus rostral to the motor area of the tongue, pharynx, or larynx, or involves the pathways carrying impulses from the temporal lobe to this area (see Fig. 46-6). Broca's aphasia includes disorders described as cortical motor, expressive, and verbal aphasias, and disor-

TABLE 46-3 Terms Used to Describe Some Disorders of Higher Cortical Function

Term	Definition
Acalculia	Inability to solve mathematical problems
Agnosia	Loss of comprehension of auditory, tactile, visual, or other sensations although the sensations and the sensory system are intact
Auditory agnosia	Inability to recognize auditory objects
Tactile agnosia	Inability to identify objects by touch
Visual agnosia	Inability to recognize objects seen
Verbal agnosia	Inability to recognize spoken language
Agrammatism	Inability to arrange words in grammatic sequence or to form a grammatic or intelligent sentence
Anosognosia	Lack of awareness of presence of disease, e.g., paralysis
Apraxia	Inability to carry out a voluntary movement, although the conductive systems are intact
Constructional apraxia	Inability to construct models with matchsticks, cubes, etc., to assemble puzzles, or to draw
Dressing apraxia	Inability to dress or undress
Autotopagnosia	Inability to orient various parts of the body correctly
Dysarthria	Disorder of articulation
Prosopagnosia	Inability to recognize faces and one's own face

ders in expression of spoken language. The person may not be able to utter a word or may have extremely limited speech. The speech is generally nonfluent, slow, and poorly articulated. Small words are frequently omitted from sentences. Simultaneously, the person fully comprehends the spoken word and obeys commands. Efforts to speak are frustrated by inability to find appropriate words. Agraphia, reduction of written language, coexists with aphasia and can be more severe in some individuals. Agrammatism, when present in spoken language, is present in written language (see Table 46-3). The individual is aware of the problem, and this frequently leads to feelings of frustration and depression.

Global Aphasia

Global aphasia is caused by large lesions involving both Broca's and Wernicke's areas of the dominant cerebral hemisphere. Commonly, the lesion is an occlusion of the left internal carotid artery or middle cerebral artery. Blood supply to the language areas of the brain is supplied almost exclusively through the middle cerebral artery.

As the term implies, global aphasia affects all aspects of speech. Individuals with global aphasia generally have hemiplegia and are unable to comprehend or speak. At best, they may be able to utter an occasional isolated word or well-known cliché. They are unable to repeat what is said to them and are unable to read and write.

Selective Disorders of Receptive or Expressive Activities of Spoken and Written Language

The pure disorders of receptive and expressive speech include anarthria, agraphia, alexia, and word-deafness.

In *anarthria*, reading aloud and voluntary speech repetition are disturbed, whereas understanding of spoken and written language and writing remain normal. It usually appears as a sequela of Broca's aphasia.

In *agraphia*, all forms of writing are defective. The lesion may be located in the posterior part of the second frontal gyrus.

Alexia severely impairs reading of words, and reading of letters is less obstructed. Language activities may be normal except for the recognition of written symbols. The lesion is located in the lingual and fusiform gyri.

Word-deafness is impairment in the understanding of spoken language, repetition, and writing from dictation, but all other speech activities are normal. The lesion is in the superior aspect of the temporal lobe.

Apraxia

Apraxia is the inability to carry out a voluntary movement, although the conductive systems are intact. The person is able to make the individual movements that comprise executing a certain act but cannot execute the total act. There is no paralysis, ataxia, abnormal movement, or sensory loss.

To execute a skilled movement, one must use a logical routine. First, the command is received at the primary auditory cortex and relayed to the auditory association areas for comprehension. The information is relayed by the association fiber systems to the motor association areas in the premotor cortex of the dominant hemisphere. From the dominant premotor cortex, information is conveyed to the premotor and motor cortexes of the nondominant hemisphere to enable the nondominant hand to perform the learned skilled movement.

Apraxia is caused by damage to the association areas or fibers concerned with voluntary motor activity. Lesions in these areas cause impairment in accordance with their locations. Those between the supramarginal gyrus and premotor regions of the dominant parietal lobe may produce bilateral apraxia (see Fig. 46-6). They usually also result in an aphasia. Lesions of the dominant premotor association areas may produce bilateral impairment in certain tongue and hand movements. Those of the anterior half of the corpus callosum result in an apraxia of the nondominant hand.

Apraxia of the lips and tongue is fairly common and may occur with lesions of the left supramarginal gyrus or the left motor association cortex, and frequently accompanies apraxia of the limbs. Apraxia of the limbs may be revealed as dressing apraxia (inability to dress or undress) and constructional apraxia (inability to construct models with matchsticks or cubes, assemble puzzles, or draw).

The location of lesions producing the various apraxias is somewhat controversial. All forms of apraxia frequently occur in cases of diffuse brain damage leading to dementia, which suggests that symptoms may be caused by the mass effect of a lesion rather than its location.

Agnosia

Perception occurs when sensory data originating at sensory receptors are forwarded by peripheral and spinal pathways to the primary sensory cortex for analysis and sorting. These data are dispatched to the association areas that contain the memory banks for higher-order interpretation, and there they are translated into codes and symbols of language. This process of recognizing the significance of sensory stimuli is known as *gnosia*. *Agnosia*, impairment of this faculty of recognition, is caused by lesions of the visual association areas of the cerebral cortex, although the primary sensory pathway is intact.

Types of Agnosia

Visual agnosia (inability to recognize objects seen), tactile agnosia (inability to identify objects by touch), and auditory agnosia (inability to recognize sounds although auditory sensation is intact) are the three types. A person with visual agnosia may not recognize a safety pin just by looking at it, but can name it instantaneously if it is placed in his hand. Conversely, one with tactile agnosia visually identifies the safety pin that she was unable to recognize when it was placed in her hand before she looked at it.

Visual Agnosia. Visual agnosia is caused by a lesion of the visual association areas. Lesions limited to these areas do not cause blindness. Objects are clearly seen but are not recognized or identified. Visual agnosia is characterized by inability to recognize any object or shape by sight, although it can be recognized through other senses, such as touch or smell. Categories include agnosia for (1) objects, (2) colors, and (3) physiognomies.

Persons suffering from the rare object agnosia are not able to recognize objects visually. Those with color agnosia are unable to recognize colors, a defect that may be confined to one-half of the visual fields (called *hemiagnosia* for colors). Agnosia for physiognomies, or prosopagnosia, renders the person unable to recognize faces, sometimes even his or her own face in the mirror. The individual is unable to recognize a familiar face but can identify the person once that person starts to speak.

Tactile Agnosia. Normal tactile recognition is the ability to identify an object by feeling without the help of other sensory information. Feeling movements provide impressions until the object is identified. Lesions of the parietal lobe posterior to the somesthetic area produce tactile agnosia, or the inability to identify objects by touch and feeling. It is often called *astereognosis*. Some previously acquired factual information is lost from the brain's memory stores. Therefore, one cannot compare present sensory phenomena with past experience.

Auditory Agnosia. Auditory agnosia is the inability to recognize sounds. The auditory sensation is intact, but the difficulty is in separating them from the sensory aphasias. The first temporal convolution and part of the second temporal convolution of the dominant hemisphere are considered important for auditory recognition.

From the descriptive point of view, auditory agnosia is the inability to recognize familiar concrete sounds, such as animal noises, a sounding bell, or the ticking of a clock (agnosia for nonlinguistic sounds). Other auditory perceptual disorders include verbal agnosia (the inability to recognize spoken language), sensory amusia (the inability to recognize music), and congenital auditory agnosia (primary retardation of speech development, usually associated with mental retardation).

Body Image

Humans build images of their bodies from sensory impulses from the special senses (skin, muscles, bones, and joints) that provide information of relationships with the body and the external environment. This concept of body image is stored in the association areas of the parietal lobes.

Lesions of the nondominant parietal lobe, particularly the inferior parietal lobe, may create abnormalities in concepts of body image. Lack of awareness of the left side of the body despite intact cortical and primary sensation is exhibited. Lack of awareness of hemiparesis may be noted. The person may perceive sensory stimuli applied independently to the two sides of the body, but if sensory stimuli are applied bilaterally simultaneously, one is generally ignored.

Gerstmann's Syndrome

Lesions of the left (dominant) parietal lobe, particularly the supramarginal and angular gyrus areas, may produce one or more of a complex of symptoms known as Gerstmann's syndrome (bilateral asomatognosia). It includes right-left disorientation, that is, inability to distinguish right from left. Finger agnosia is exhibited by failure to recognize one's fingers in the presence of intact sensation and is associated with constructional apraxia. Acalculia (inability to solve mathematical problems) and dyslexia (inability to read) are common when the lesion involves the angular gyrus.

Epilepsy

Epilepsy is a symptom, not a disease. An epileptic seizure is a sudden, disorderly, excessive discharge by neurons of electrical energy in the central nervous system within either a structurally normal or diseased cortex, cerebrum, brainstem, and spinal cord. The discharge may trigger a convulsive movement, interrupt sensation, alter consciousness, or lead to some combination of these disturbances. Seizures may originate from diverse factors that are metabolic, toxic, degenerative, genetic, infectious, neoplastic, traumatic, or unknown.

Epilepsy may be linked with increased local excitability, reduced inhibition, or a combination of both. Some neurons in focal lesions have been identified as hypersensitive and remain in a state of partial depolarization. Increased permeability of their cytoplasmic membranes makes these neurons susceptible to activation by hyperthermia, hypoglycemia, hyponatremia, hypoxia, repeated sensory stimulation, and even certain phases of sleep. Reduced inhibition may be caused by a lesion of the cortex.

Once the intensity of a seizure discharge has progressed sufficiently, it spreads to adjacent cortical, thalamic, and brainstem nuclei, and other brain areas. Excitement feeds back from the thalamus to the primary focus and to other parts of the brain. This process is evidenced by the high-frequency discharge shown on EEG. Within the process, a diencephalocortical inhibition intermittently interrupts the discharge and converts the tonic phase to the clonic phase (see p. 779). These discharges become less and less frequent until they cease.

Severe seizures may cause systemic hypoxia with accompanying acidosis from increased lactic acid, which may result from respiratory spasms, airway blockage, and excessive muscular activity that accompanies seizures. An extremely severe prolonged seizure can cause respiratory arrest or cardiac standstill. Metabolic needs increase markedly during a seizure, causing increased cerebral blood flow, glycolysis, and tissue respiration.

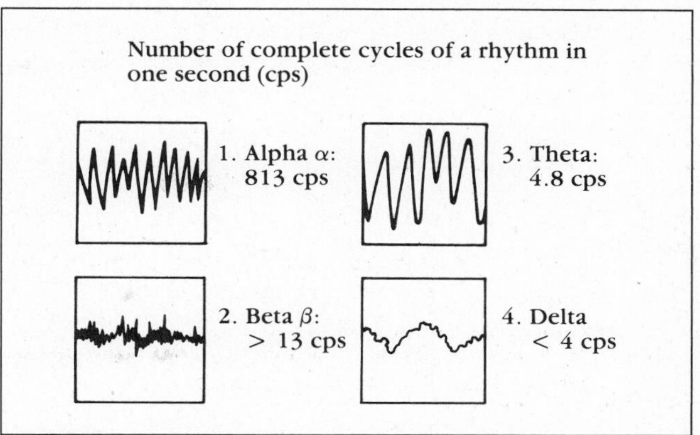

FIGURE 46-7 Frequency of brain waves.

Electroencephalography in Epilepsy

The EEG is the most sensitive tool for definitive diagnosis and clinical evaluation of epilepsy. The electrical discharges produced by the brain's electrical activity are called *brain waves* and are recorded by electrodes placed on the surface of the scalp. Because the EEG is a surface recording, it reflects the most superficial activity, especially that of the cerebral cortex. The waves are recorded while the person is awake and resting in a darkened room or with the eyes closed. Movements and external distractions should be minimized. During a recording of the brain's waves, the subject may be asked to hyperventilate. Provocative techniques, photic stimulation, and sleep deprivation may be useful in initiating abnormal electrical activity in some persons.

In the normal adult, dominant activity in the parietal occipital areas occurs at 8 to 13 cycles per second (cps), identified as alpha rhythm. In the frontal areas, the dominant activity is of lower amplitude and faster frequency, greater than 13 cps, and is known as beta rhythm. Slower frequencies than alpha rhythm are recognized as slow waves. Those 4 to 7 cps are theta rhythms, and 1 to 3 cps are delta rhythms (Fig. 46-7). Normal variations occur. Age differences are noted on the EEG (Figs. 46-8 and 46-9). An infant at 13 months has dominant awakened activity of 4 to 5 cps; at age 5 years, 6 to 7 cps; and at age 12 years, 8 to 9 cps (alpha rhythm) [2]. Two types of abnormalities are described.

Normally, amplitude and frequency should be relatively symmetric between the cerebral hemispheres. Type 1 abnormality is a difference between the hemispheres. There may be focal slow waves caused by focal cortical disorders such as an abscess, glioblastoma, meningioma, metastatic tumor, or infarction. Focal spikes indicating an irritable focus and having the quality of sudden excessive neuronal discharge correlate with partial, or symptomatic, seizures.

Type 2 abnormalities relate either to the frequency of the dominant awake activity or to the form of that activity. These abnormalities imply pathology of the cerebral cortex in a generalized or diffuse manner. A generalized slow wave may indicate a generalized cortical disorder or a metabolic, or toxic, state. Damage from encephalitis, hypoxia, or hepatic or renal failure may be deduced from generalized slow-wave activity. Electrical abnormalities are recorded as generalized bursts, 2.5 to 4.0 cps, which can be seen as spikes and slow-wave complexes. This type correlates with petit mal seizures.

Other generalized bursts consisting of polyspike slow-wave complexes correlate with myoclonic seizures. In infantile myoclonic spasms, the EEG demonstrates a continuous high amplitude generalized by often asynchronous spikes and slow waves. This pattern is called *hypsarrhythmia*. Repetitive fast spikes, 8 to 12 cps, correlate with generalized seizures, specifically grand mal seizures (Fig. 46-10).

Classification of Seizures

Seizures have been classified according to location of the focus, etiologic basis, and clinical features. The International Classification System has been adopted worldwide and is used in this chapter. It is based on clinical features and associated EEG findings in seizures that are generalized or partial. *Generalized seizures* have bilaterally symmetric epileptigenic foci originating within deep subcortical diencephalic structures, whereas partial seizures usually begin in a cortical focus, but may arise from subcortical structures. Seizures may be *primary* or *idiopathic* if their origin is unknown, or *secondary* or *symptomatic* if a definitive diagnosis is determined.

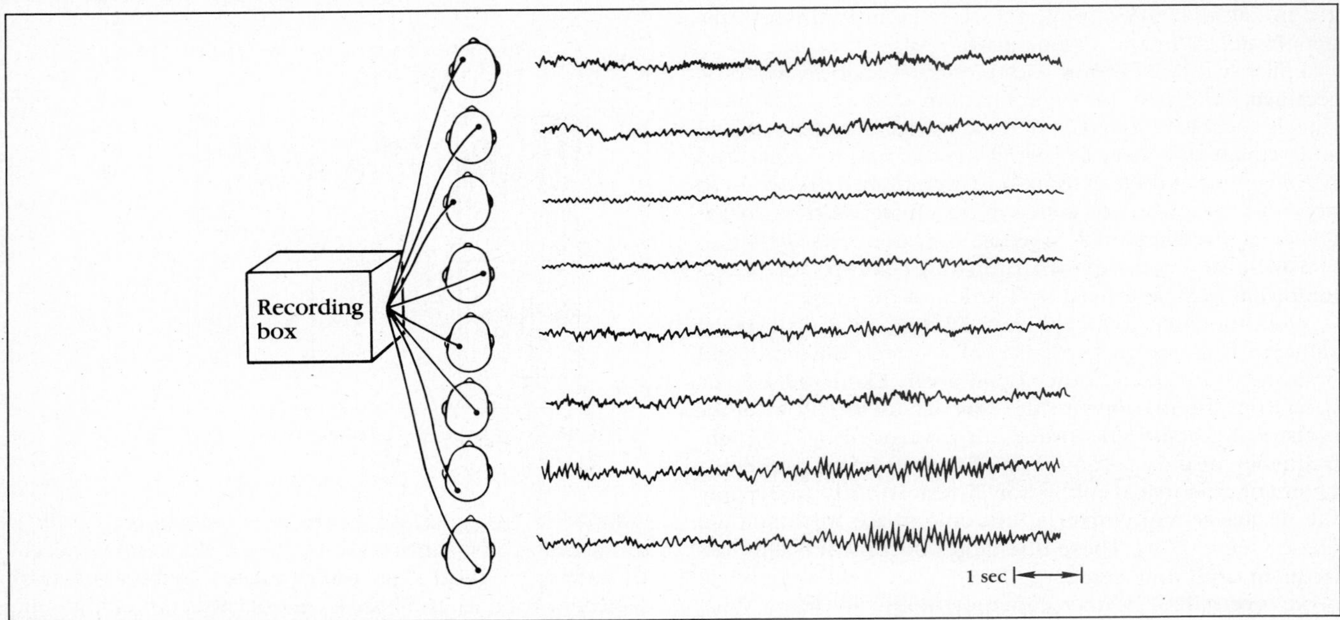

FIGURE 46-8 Normal electroencephalogram in an adult.

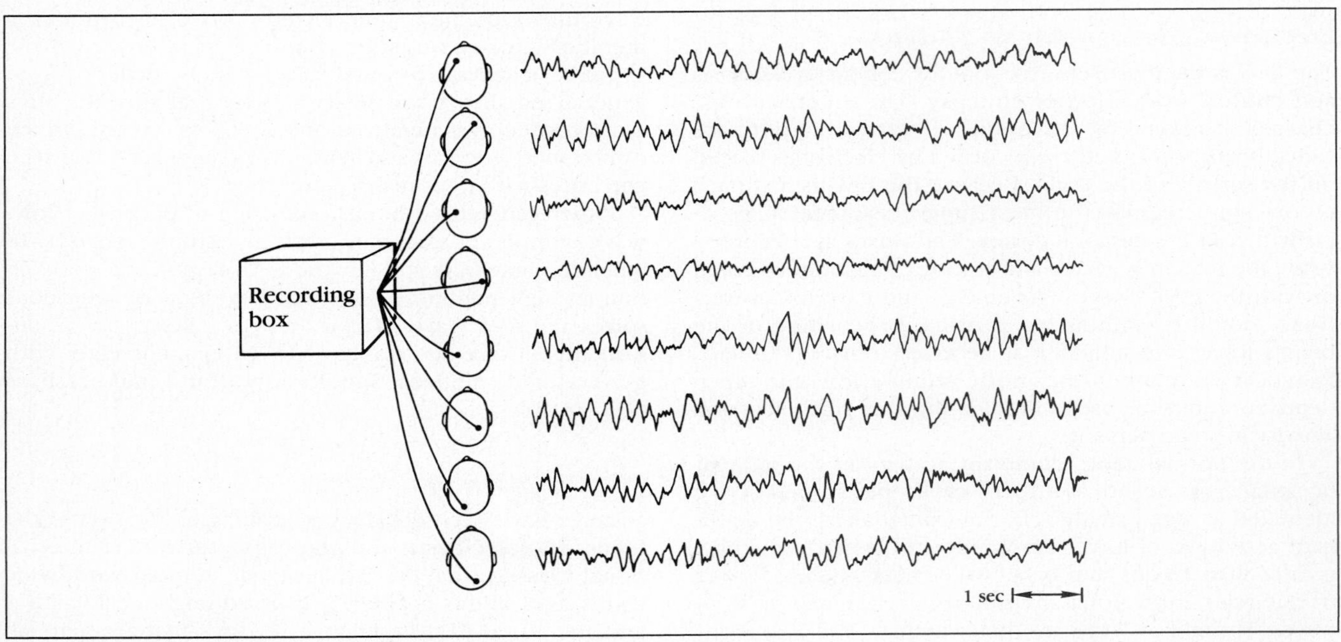

FIGURE 46-9 Normal electroencephalogram in a child.

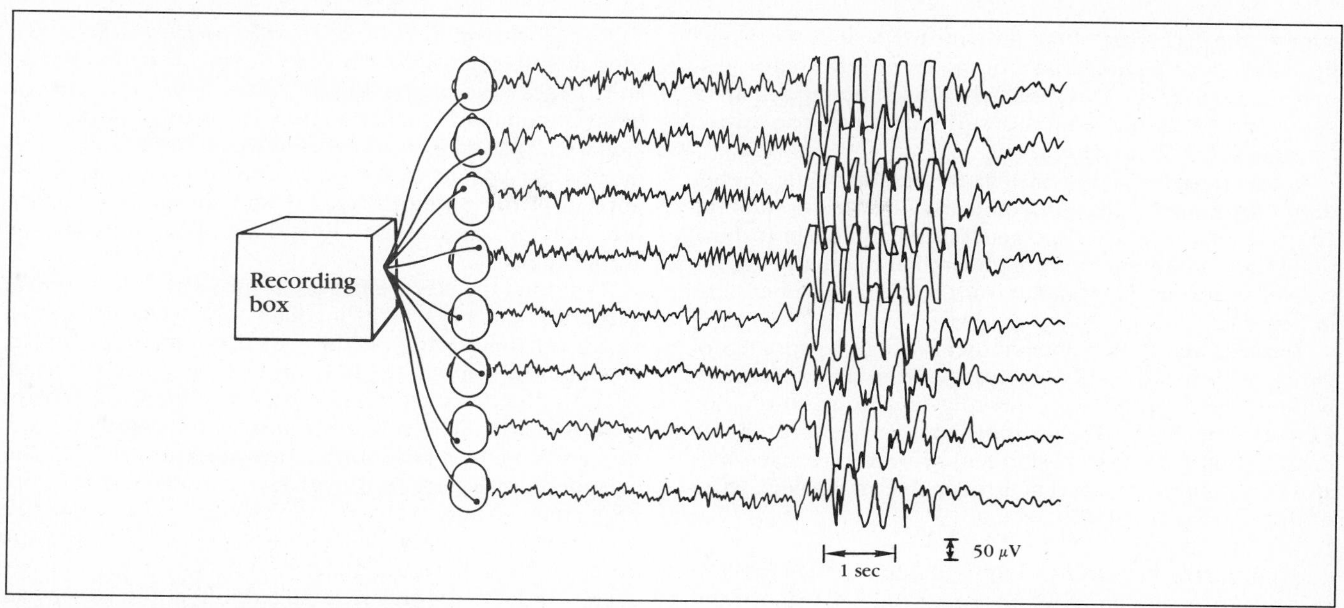

FIGURE 46-10 EEG appearance during a grand mal seizure.

Generalized Seizures

Generalized seizures involve both cerebral hemispheres and generally results in loss of consciousness, which may vary from a very brief episode to a more prolonged time. Anterograde and retrograde amnesia commonly accompany the loss of consciousness. The most common forms of generalized seizures are petit mal (absence) and grand mal (tonic-clonic). Generalized seizures also include myoclonic and akinetic types.

Absence Seizures (Petit Mal). These seizures exhibit a characteristic spike-and-wave pattern with 3 cps on the EEG. The term *absence seizure* is used because the person, although present physically, is absent with respect to higher cortical functions during the episode. The majority of such persons have normal intelligence and have no significant abnormal physical findings on neurologic examination. Onset is usually about age 5 years and attacks are most prevalent in childhood. Absence seizures are rare after puberty.

Petit mal seizures are characterized by a loss of awareness that may be accompanied by automatisms such as flicking of the eyelids, twitching of facial muscles, or staring into space while general postural tone is preserved. They may be precipitated by seeing bright or flashing lights or hearing loud noises, and may be preceded by hyperventilation. Attacks may recur numerous times during the day. They may last for 5 to 10 seconds, after which consciousness is abruptly restored and the interrupted activity is promptly resumed. Memory may be defective only through the seizure. As the person reaches adolescence, frequency decreases and the EEG may eventually show normal discharge. The individual may develop other types of seizures at any time.

Tonic-Clonic Seizures (Grand Mal). Electrical disruption with grand mal seizures originates anywhere in the forebrain and usually engulfs the whole forebrain. The epileptic discharge shows nonfocal changes of high amplitude and rapid synchronous bursts on the EEG (see Fig. 46-10). For several hours preceding the seizure, vague prodomal sensations such as epigastric distress or muscular twitching may occur. Commonly, a brief aura consisting of a specific movement or unnatural sensation usually is the last thing the individual remembers before the onset of the seizure.

After the aura, if present, the individual abruptly loses consciousness, falls to the ground, and suffers generalized tonic contractions followed by clonic contractions of all muscles. Muscle contraction in the tonic phase lasts for a few seconds. The entire body becomes rigid, with the arms and legs extended. The jaws become clenched, the head may be retracted, and the eyeballs are rolled backward. As air is forced through the closed vocal cords, a loud cry may emit. Breathing usually ceases during this time. Movements become jerky in the clonic phase as muscle groups contract and relax. The arms and legs contract and relax forcibly. Breathing becomes noisy and stertorous, and profuse perspiration is noted. Excessive salivation and loss of bladder or bowel sphincter control may also occur.

Contractions become slower, sometimes irregular, and then stop. The entire seizure may last up to 10 minutes. Spasms of the tongue and jaw may cause biting injuries to the tongue or cheeks. Unconsciousness for the entire seizure is characteristic and may continue up to one-half hour after the episode. As consciousness is regained, the individual is often briefly confused, fatigued, and drowsy, and complains of muscle soreness. The individual has no memory of the seizure attack, but usually remembers the aura. In the early part of the postseizure period, there may be reflex signs characteristic of upper motor neuron disorder (see p. 809). Paralysis may follow the attack for a short period of time and is described as postconvulsive (*postictal*) or *Todd's paralysis*.

Febrile grand mal convulsions frequently occur in children under age 5 years, predominantly between 6 months and 3 years of age. They are generalized and of short duration. These children have a high familial frequency of this type of seizure and may suffer from nonfebrile convulsions in later life.

Seizures that follow one another without restoration of consciousness are called *status epilepticus*, or seizures without interruption. This disorder is serious, producing exhaustion, hypoxia, acidosis, and other metabolic derangements. Hospitalization and prompt pharmacotherapy are required to prevent irreversible brain damage or death.

Myoclonic Seizures. Individuals with myoclonic seizures have sudden rapid flexion of the limbs and trunk singularly or repeatedly, with no loss of consciousness. Loud sounds or bright lights may precipitate the episodes. Intentional movement worsens them. These disorders occur with greatest frequency in childhood, but may continue after puberty. Bilateral, synchronous 3-cps discharges are noted on EEG during each episode.

Myoclonic spasms occurring in infancy are called massive spasms, are first noted at 6 to 9 months of age, and continue to age 2 or 3 years. There is usually associated retardation of psychomotor development, and the spasms may be related to other conditions such as phenylketonuria, perinatal brain damage, pyridoxine deficiency, and tuberous sclerosis. Myoclonic spasms may be generalized or multifocal and tend to disappear with growth, but other seizure patterns may emerge. In adults, myoclonic seizures may accompany dementia in conditions such as Creutzfeldt-Jacob disease and certain acute conditions such as acute viral encephalitis (see Chap. 49). A benign form of myoclonus has been described that is associated with sudden myoclonic jerks when falling asleep or awakening.

Akinetic Seizures. In these seizures, persons experience sudden loss of consciousness and fall to the ground without contraction or motion. Muscle tone is lost briefly, but stance is resumed almost immediately. A history of infantile spasms and mental retardation is often present.

Partial Seizures

Partial seizures arise from a focal area and progress in a manner consistent to the area of irritation. They are characterized by specific, repeated patterns of activity and are of two general types, *simple* or *elementary*, in which consciousness remains unimpaired, and *complex*, in which there is accompanying alteration in consciousness. Partial seizures may have a motor, sensory, or varied complex focus.

Focal Motor Seizures (Jacksonian Seizures). This disorder usually originates in the premotor cortex and causes involuntary movements of the contralateral limbs. A common manifestation is the turning of the individual's head and eyes away from the irritable focus. This may be the extent of the seizure, or it may start in one portion of the premotor cortex and spread gradually to the adjacent region; the clinical manifestations change accordingly.

Typically, the seizure begins in the distal portion of an extremity and progresses medially. For example, a focal motor seizure starting in the foot may move up the leg, down the arm, and to the face; or it may begin in the hand, spread to the face, and then to the leg. This is called *jacksonian march*. The seizure begins with a tonic contraction and rapidly progresses to a clonic movement. The episode may last 20 to 30 seconds without loss of consciousness. Conversely, it may spread to the opposite hemisphere attendant with loss of consciousness, thus becoming a generalized seizure. Despite the greater frequency of focal seizures in young children, the jacksonian march occurs most often in adults and adolescents; focal motor seizures may also occur in certain metabolic derangements.

Focal Sensory Seizures. A lesion in the postcentral or precentral convolution of the sensory cortex provokes focal sensory seizures. A simple, uniform, tactile, auditory, or visual experience with complaints of numbness, tingling, pins-and-needles sensation, coldness, or a sensation of water running over a portion of the body may be described. This type of seizure usually begins in the lips, fingers, and toes, and progresses to adjacent body parts. If the lesion is in the sensory association area, the experience is more complex and may be visual or auditory. If visual, sensations of light, darkness, or color may be experienced. If auditory, the person may complain of buzzing, roaring in the ears, or hearing voices or words. Consciousness and memory are preserved.

Complex Partial Seizures (Psychomotor). Temporal lobe structures, the medial surface of the hemispheres, and the limbic system are involved with this disorder; however, certain psychomotor seizures may arise from the frontal lobe. The person may exhibit bizarre behavior and exaggerated emotionality. These seizures may be characterized by slow, paroxysmal waves in either the anterior or posterior leads of the EEG. Episodic fluctuations in attitude, attention, behavior, or memory occur. Seizures may begin with an olfactory aura or an unpleasant smell or taste. On other occasions, the person may experience hallucinations or perceptual illusions; or perceive strange objects or people as familiar (*déjà vu*) and familiar objects and people as strange (*jamais vu*). The person appears to be in a dreamy state and may be unresponsive to vocal stimulation, but mechanically performs a task while the seizure is progressing. Abnormal movements and inappropriate speech may also be associated characteristics. Strong epigastric and abdominal sensations commonly occur.

Later, episodic recall is lost and the behavior is called automatic. Convulsive motor manifestations, when present, include chewing, smacking, licking of the lips, or clapping of the hands. Less frequently, the head and eyes may turn to one side, or tonic spasms of the limbs may occur. Some psychomotor seizures last about a minute, others may continue for hours, while still others may progress to tonic, tonic-clonic, or other forms of generalized seizures.

Secondary or Symptomatic Epilepsy

Secondary seizures are caused by some metabolic or structural underlying disorder. Metabolic disturbances can result from conditions such as renal failure, hypoglycemia, hypoxia, hyponatremia, hypernatremia, hypercalcemia, hepatic failure, or withdrawal of drugs.

Meningitis and encephalitis in children lead to strong convulsive tendencies. After recovery, there may be residual recurrent generalized, focal, or psychomotor seizures.

Many structural lesions are caused by disorders in cerebral blood supply, intracranial tumors, or scarring of the brain. These are described in other chapters in Unit 15.

Study Questions

1. Discuss the pathophysiology of cerebrovascular accidents. Relate the location of the causative lesion to the resulting clinical manifestations.
2. Describe the reaction of the brain to the rupture of an intracerebral aneurysm.
3. Locate and describe arteriovenous malformations.
4. Discriminate among the disorders of speech. Why are some of these truly considered to be aphasia while others are not?
5. Compare the different forms of seizures with regard to pathophysiologic mechanisms, symptoms, and EEG changes.

References

1. Adams, R., and Maurice, V. *Principles of Neurology* (3rd ed.). New York: McGraw-Hill, 1985.
2. Curtis, B. *An Introduction to the Neuro-Sciences*. Philadelphia: Saunders, 1972.
3. Jackson, L. Cerebral vasospasm after intracranial aneurysmal subarachnoid hemorrhage: A nursing perspective. *Heart Lung* 15:14, 1986.
4. Pallett, P., and O'Brien, M. *Textbook of Neurological Nursing*. Boston: Little, Brown, 1985.
5. Robbins, S.L., Cotran, R.S., and Kumar, V. *Pathologic Basis of Disease* (3rd ed.). Philadelphia: Saunders, 1984.
6. Stein, J.H. (ed.). *Internal Medicine*. Boston: Little, Brown, 1983.
7. Wall, M. Cerebral thrombosis: Assessment and nursing management of acute phase. *J. Neurosci. Nurs.* 18:36, 1986.

CHAPTER 47

Pain

CHAPTER OUTLINE

Definitions of Pain
Mechanisms of Pain

- Pain Receptors
- Transmission of Pain Signals
- Pain Without Nociception
- Pain Modulation
- Sources of Pain
  - *Cutaneous Pain*
  - *Deep Somatic Pain*
  - *Headache*
  - *Musculoskeletal Trauma*
  - *Visceral Pain*

Theories of Pain

- Affect Theory
- Specificity Theory
- Pattern Theory
- Gate-Control Theory
  - *Gate-Control System*
  - *Central Control System*
  - *Action System*
  - *Clinical Implications*
- Psychologic Theories

Acute Versus Chronic Pain
Variations in Pain Response and Reaction

LEARNING OBJECTIVES

1. Develop an encompassing definition of pain.
2. Describe the pain receptors through which pain perception is achieved.
3. Differentiate between fast or acute pain and slow or dull pain.
4. Define the purposes of the neospinothalamic and paleospinothalamic tracts.
5. Describe the spinoreticular system.
6. Describe the important chemical transmitters involved in pain modulation.
7. Discriminate between cutaneous pain and deep somatic pain.
8. Compare the affect, specificity, and pattern theories of pain.
9. Explain the gate-control theory.
10. List and describe at least three clinical implications for knowledge of the gate-control theory.
11. Discriminate between the causes of and reactions to acute as compared to chronic pain.
12. Using the understanding of factors affecting individual variations in pain response, describe the differences in at least four different populations of individuals

Pain is one of the most personal and private yet universal human experiences. It is a multidimensional and totally subjective perceptual phenomenon associated with actual or potential tissue damage, and influenced by emotional, cultural, environmental, and psychologic variables. Much has been learned about the neurophysiologic, biochemical, and psychologic substrates of pain since the 1960s; however, to date, many of the problems associated with pain remain unsolved.

Approximately 75 million Americans suffer from persistent or recurrent pain that requires medical therapy: 40 million with chronic recurrent headaches, about 15 million with low back pain, and almost 20 million with arthritis [45]. Moreover, one-third of persons with cancer undergoing active therapy and 60 to 90 percent of those with advanced disease experience moderate to severe pain [15].

Chronic pain is a malific force that imposes severe physical, emotional, social, and economic hardships on its victims, their families, and society. Its biopsychosocial effects are devastating. Moreover, it is remarkably resistant to conventional medical therapies and thus disables more people than any single disease entity [34]. Excluding the cost of human suffering and inflation, the annual cost of chronic pain—work days lost, health care expenses, compensation, and litigation—is conservatively estimated at between $80 and $90 billion [9].

Definitions of Pain

Pain is difficult to define because of its multidimensional and extremely complex nature. Despite extensive study and research, an accurate definition that can be applied by all the disciplines has eluded scientists and clinicians [29]. Consequently, pain must be defined and discussed in a variety of ways.

Pain is a common experience that is difficult to define in ordinary language [39]. It is not a single experience that can be specified in terms of defined stimulus conditions, but like vision and hearing, it is a complex perceptual experience [4].

Sensory psychologists and physiologists have primarily viewed pain as a separate sensation together with other cutaneous sensations. Pain stimuli are mechanical, electrical, thermal, and chemical, and responses measured are verbal, behavioral, and physiologic.

In light of the many and varied definitions, the International Association for the Study of Pain (IASP) compiled a taxonomy of terms and definitions and defined pain as "an unpleasant sensory and emotional experience associated with actual or potential tissue damage, or described in terms of such damage" [27, p. 250]. Recognizing the subjective nature of pain, the IASP incorporated pain's pathophysiologic and psychologic origins as well as sensory, affective, and motivational properties.

Mechanisms of Pain

The mechanisms of pain include (1) the peripheral receptors that monitor and mediate pain stimuli, (2) the pathways that transport impulses, (3) integration of the pain experience, and (4) highly personal and private reaction.

Pain Receptors

Pain is the result of the entire pattern of central input initiated at the dorsal horn level. Thus, because the quality of perceived pain depends on the class, size, depth, and arrangement of nerve fibers in a particular structure, it is necessary to view *pain receptor*, or *nociceptor*, more specifically. Figure 47-1 illustrates the factors involved in transmitting, modulating, and perceiving pain.

Pain receptors are free nerve endings of myelinated A-delta and unmyelinated C fibers that convert information about threatened tissue injury into a stimulus. When the proper threshold is reached, unspecialized free nerve endings (polymodal) as well as mechanoreceptors and thermoreceptors (unimodal) may contribute to pain perception [43].

For example, if heat greater than 45°C or cold lower than 10°C comes in contact with the skin, the thermoreceptor becomes a nociceptor. Strong mechanical pressure or deformation can also result in nociception [33]. The flexor withdrawal reflex occurs in response to nociception to protect the endangered tissue. Pain is experienced when nociceptive information is transmitted to the thalamus or forebrain by primary afferent fibers.

A-delta fibers are 2 to 5 μ in diameter and conduct rapidly at a rate of 12 to 30 meters per second. In contrast, C fibers are 0.4 to 1.2 μ in diameter and conduct at a rate of 0.5 to 2 meters per second [19].

Myelinated A-delta fibers are encased in a lipoprotein sheath produced by the Schwann cells. Intermittent gaps in the myelin sheath are known as the nodes of Ranvier. Some of the Schwann cells also wrap tight concentric layers of myelin sheath around the central core axons.

Myelin protects and nourishes nerve fibers. Because of low internal resistance in large-diameter nerve fibers, myelin also increases the velocity of nerve conduction. The increased velocity quickens depolarization time by decreasing the number of charges generated along the length of the nerve fiber.

Unmyelinated C fibers contain Schwann cells, but they lack the tight concentric wrappings around their central core axons. The absence of an insulating and protective coating makes the C fibers even more sensitive to mechanical, electrical, thermal, and biochemical stimulation [7,24].

Transmission of Pain Signals

Two types of pain comprise the initial and residual components of pain perception. *Fast* or *acute pain* is the first

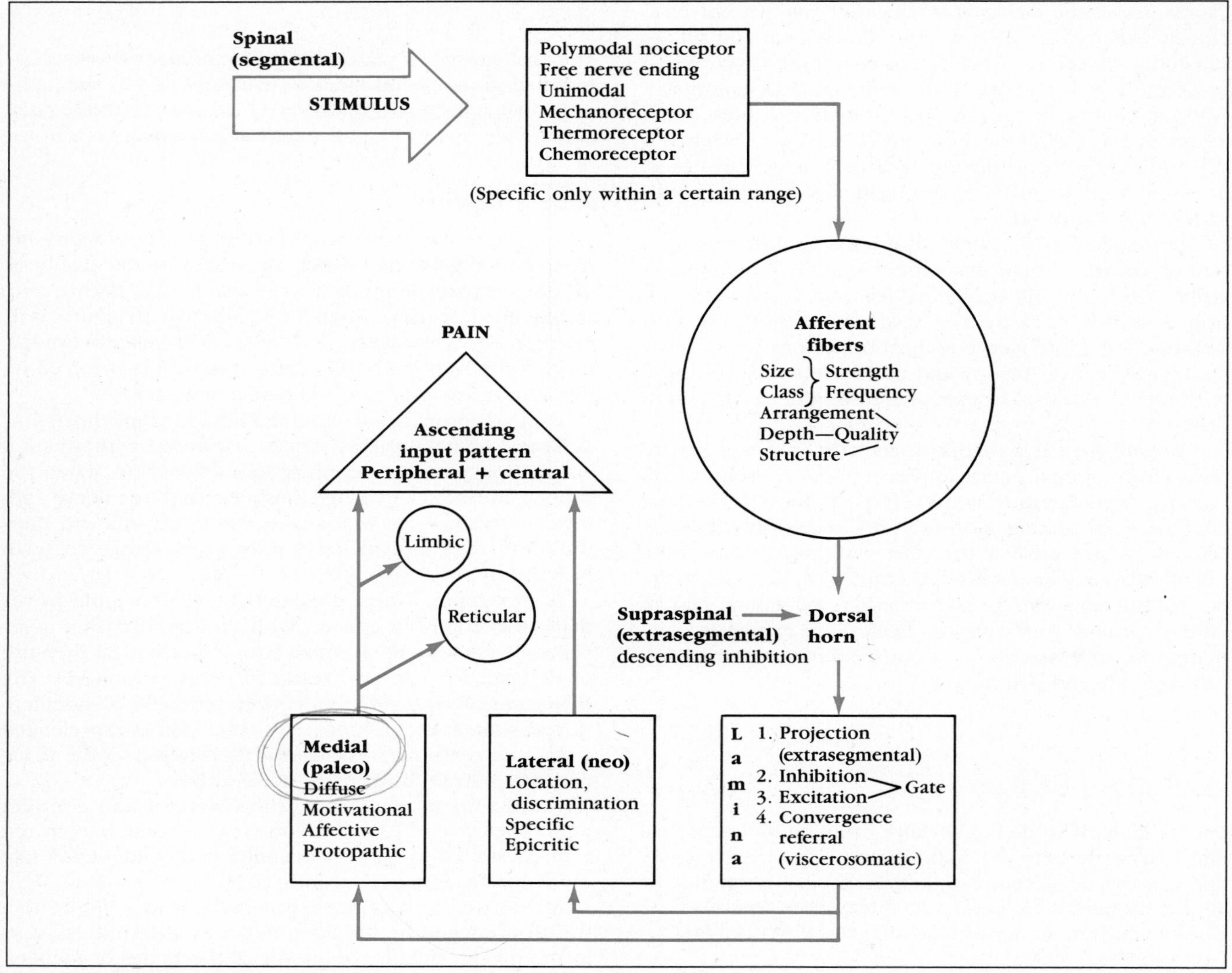

FIGURE 47-1 Factors involved in the transmission, modulation, and perception of pain. (From J. Mannheimer and B. Lampe, *Clinical Transcutaneous Electrical Nerve Stimulation*. Copyright © 1984. F.A. Davis. Reprinted by permission.)

component and is primarily carried by the A-delta fibers. Fast pain sensations are sharp, bright, and localized. They evoke the flexor withdrawal reflex.

Slow or *dull pain* follows, often beginning after the noxious stimulus has ceased, and is primarily carried by the C fibers. Dull pain sensations are burning, aching, diffuse, and unpleasant; moreover, they can continue for a long period of time and tend to become increasingly more painful over time [19]. Dull pain sensations have been implicated in the intolerable suffering associated with chronic pain [49].

Temporal separation of fast and slow pain sensations requires that the stimulus be distal to the brain. Thus, the most distal stimulus evokes the greatest temporal separation of fast and slow pain sensations.

Nociceptive information is transmitted by numerous classic systems. The main neural pathways of pain within the ascending spinothalamic tract are the neospinothalamic tract, paleospinothalamic tract, and spinoreticular system (Fig. 47-2) [9]. Information other than nociception is also transmitted along these pathways, however.

The *neospinothalamic tract* rapidly transmits the temporal, spatial, and intensity discrimination of pain from small, well-defined receptive fields. The tract gives rise to the perception of sharp, well-localized pain and a signal of possible progressive injury. Such information is termed phasic, or first pain sensation [7,9].

After synapsing at the segmental level, neurons project their axons into the spinothalamic tract of the opposite side of the spinal cord. The tract then travels to the lateral thalamus where the basic pain sensation occurs. The lateral thalamus and parietal lobe cortex interconnect and

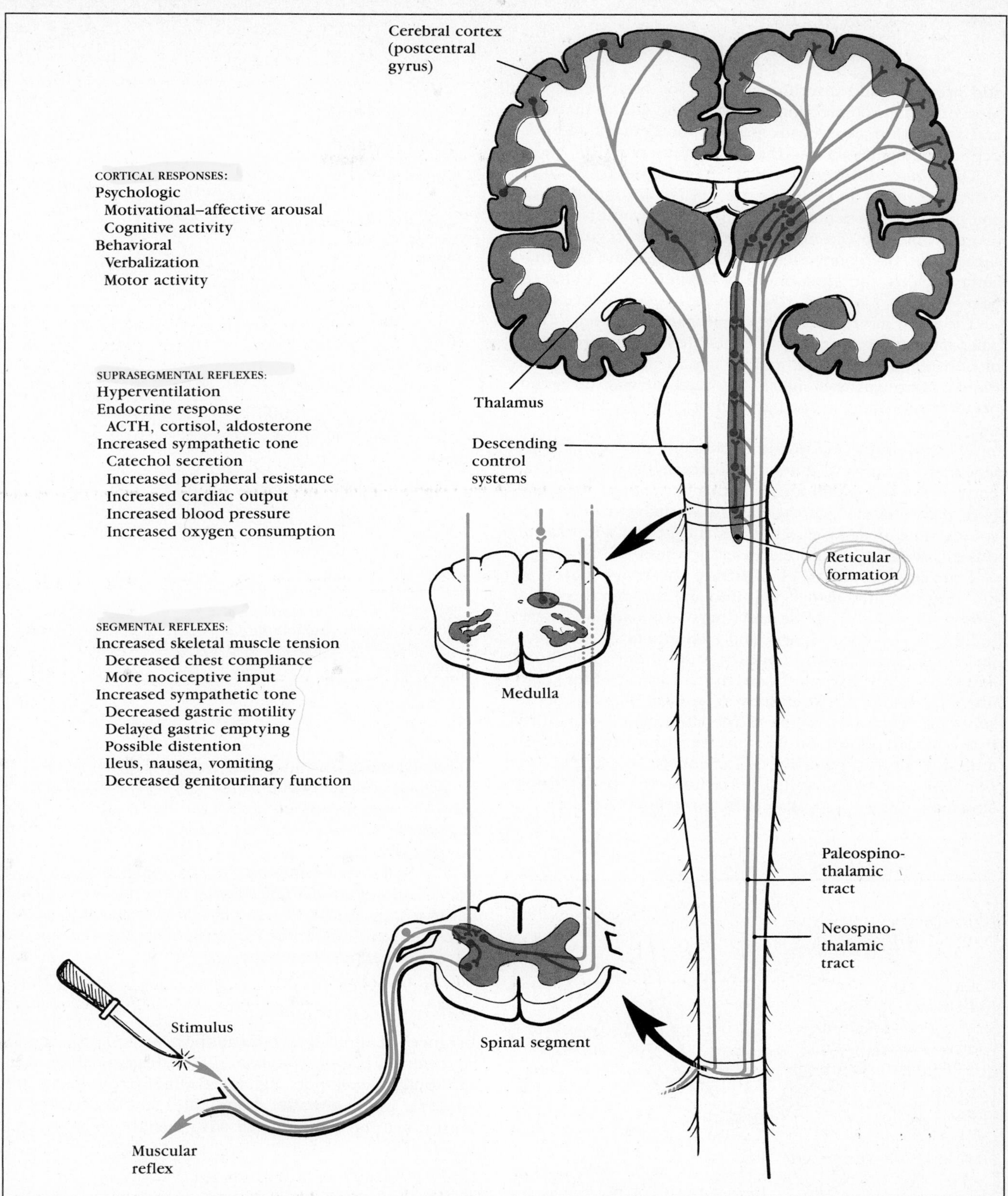

FIGURE 47-2 The CNS pathways. Sensory nerves transmit stimuli from pain receptors into the dorsal root ganglia. The impulses travel to the spinal cord, synapse, cross the cord, and ascend to either the neospinothalamic or paleospinothalamic branch of the spinothalamic tract. The tract rises to the medulla, where the paleospinothalamic projects a branch into the brainstem reticular formation. Branches also enter the pons and midbrain. The neospinothalamic branch proceeds directly into the cortex, synapsing in the midbrain and transmitting impulses into the postcentral gyrus, where pain is perceived. (Adapted from C. Chapman and J. Bonica, *Acute Pain*. Kalamazoo, Mich.: Scope, 1983.)

add precision and discrimination to the basic sensation. Moreover, interconnections between the lateral thalamus and association areas of the parietal lobe cortex add perception or significance to the pain experience [7].

The *paleospinothalamic tract* transmits from wide receptive fields and carries the diffuse autonomic and emotional components of pain. Because of multisynaptic projections into the midline-intrathalamic regions and subsequent interconnections with the limbic and hypothalamic regions, the component of hurtfulness is added to pain [7].

The tonic information, or second pain sensation, of the paleospinothalamic tract is responsible for the perception of burning, aching, dull, and poorly localized pain. The tonic component also signals the need for rest, care, and protection of the damaged area in order to facilitate healing [9].

The *spinoreticular system* is probably the most important tract in humans. It travels bilaterally from the spinal cord to the brainstem and reticular formation. Together with the collaterals of the paleospinothalamic tract, the spinoreticular system produces the flexor withdrawal reflexes at all levels and increases alertness.

Figures 47-3 and 47-4 illustrate the transmission of both fast and slow pain signals into and through the spinal cord to the brain. The fast pain fibers terminate in laminae I and V in the dorsal horns, and excite neurons that project immediately to the opposite side of the spinal cord and then upward to the brain. In contrast, the slow pain fibers terminate almost entirely in laminae II and III of the substantia gelatinosa. Most of the slow pain signals then pass through additional neurons, terminate in lamina V, and join the fast pain fibers. Instead of crossing to the opposite side of the spinal cord, however, some of the slow pain fibers pass ipsilaterally to the brain [19].

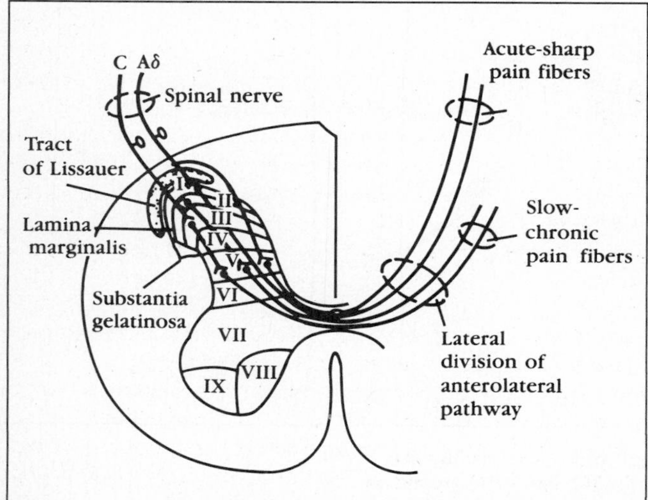

FIGURE 47-3 Transmission of acute and chronic pain signals through the spinal cord to the brainstem. (From A.C. Guyton, *Textbook of Medical Physiology* [7th ed.]. Philadelphia: W.B. Saunders Company, 1986. Reprinted by permission.)

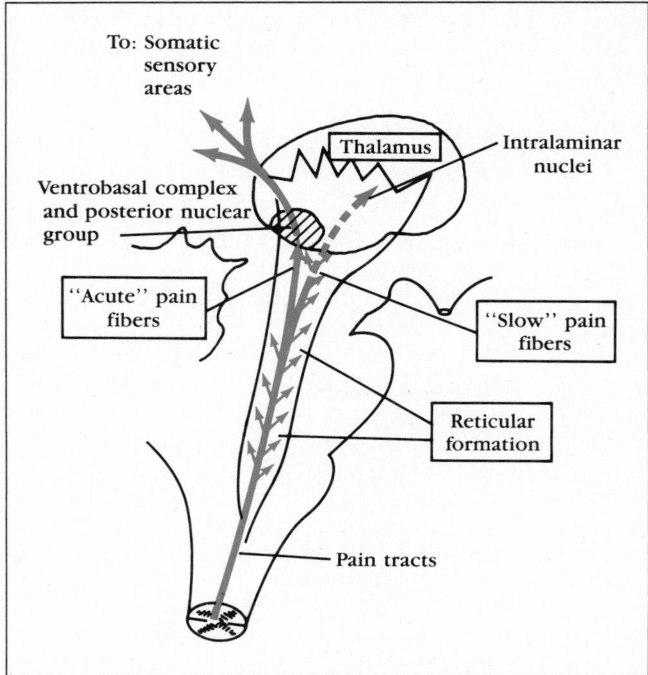

FIGURE 47-4 Transmission of acute and slow pain signals. (From A.C. Guyton, *Textbook of Medical Physiology* [7th ed.]. Philadelphia: W.B. Saunders Company, 1986. Reprinted by permission.)

Fast pain fibers terminate almost entirely in the reticular formation of the medulla, pons, and mesencephalon. In contrast, slow pain fibers terminate almost entirely in the brainstem reticular formation but relay signals upward to the thalamus [19].

The reticular activating system consists of both the brainstem reticular formation and the thalamus. Thus, because they excite the reticular activating system, slow pain fibers are essentially responsible for the activation of the entire central nervous system (CNS) [19].

Pain Without Nociception

Instances of clinically significant pain without nociception are referred to as *algodynia*. Classic trigeminal neuralgia and shingles exemplify algodynia. Other examples include phantom limb pain after amputation and deafferentation by trauma and hemialgesia with certain thalamic syndromes [9].

Pain Modulation

Afferent impulses initiated by nociceptive receptors are modulated by excitation or inhibition at all levels of the CNS before the signals reach higher brain centers. Psychologic factors further modify the complex perceptions from the incoming sensory information and continuous mental activity in the higher brain centers [9].

Mechanical, electrical, or thermal stimuli usually provoke nociceptive endings. Chemical or *algogenic* substances that occur naturally in the tissue environment of nociceptors also are known to alter microcirculation and generate or enhance nociception. Algogenic substances also induce as well as accompany inflammation. The chemical substances are amines, such as serotonin (5-HT) and histamine, and polypeptides such as bradykinin. The E group prostaglandins sensitize nociceptive endings [9].

Serotonin, histamine, and bradykinin are released during the early stage of inflammation. The inflammatory process then stimulates the formation of prostaglandins, which are thought to elicit or intensify inflammation. The prostaglandins, in turn, potentiate the effects of bradykinin on nociceptors. Algogenic potassium ions are also released from damaged cells. Thus, hyperalgesia, or excessive sensitivity to pain due to inflammation, is often attributed to the effects of chemical substances on free nerve endings [9].

Substance P, an 11-amino acid peptide present in synaptic vesicles of unmyelinated fibers, is a neurotransmitter that activates postsynaptic neuronal elements and subsequently, central nociceptive structures. The neuropeptide is released by electrical stimulation of peripheral unmyelinated fibers. For example, tooth pulp afferents contain substance P. Capsaicin, an algogenic substance, inactivates neurons containing substance P. Somatostatin, however, a peptide present in sensory fibers other than those containing substance P, is thought to inhibit nociceptive transmission. Somatostatin is released into cerebrospinal fluid after peripheral nerve stimulation [33].

Spinal reflexes may also affect the environment of nociceptive nerve endings and increase nociception. An injury may generate increased nociception by provoking efferent reflexes and subsequent muscle spasms in the injured area. Similarly, an injury may provoke sympathetic reflexes and increased nociception by decreasing microcirculation in the injured tissue and adjacent muscle with resultant ischemia. A sympathetic reflex may also produce vasospasms or other painful conditions unrelated to the injury by generating smooth muscle spasms [9].

A sympathetic reflex can alter the chemical environment of the free nerve endings at the injury site and intensify nociception as previously described. Hyperpathia, or painful overreaction and delayed aftersensation to a repetitive stimulus, occurs with reflex sympathetic dystrophies, probably as a result of the release of norepinephrine in the periphery [9,44].

The discovery of two independent peptidergic systems, the short-chain peptides called *enkephalins* and the long-chain peptides called *endorphins*, in the 1970s provided an entirely new dimension for pain research. Enkephalins are composed of a 5-amino acid chain and are located in the synapses between nerve fibers throughout the central and peripheral nervous systems. They serve as CNS neurotransmitters by binding to specific receptors and inhibiting the release of substance P with nociceptive stimulation. Enkephalins undergo rapid enzymatic degradation by aminopeptidase and carboxypeptidase, and thus have a short duration of action [9,33].

Methionine enkephalin and leucine enkephalin are derivatives of the morphinelike peptide. Both short-chain opioid peptides have half-lives of less than one minute. Methionine enkephalin is twice as strong as leucine enkephalin. Methionine enkephalin has opiate agonist properties [33].

Endorphins are abundant neuroactive peptides that are naturally secreted in the brain. While the action of enkephalins has been equated with that of neurotransmitters since they are weak and short-lasting in effect, the action of endorphins is so strong and widespread that they may be considered as hormones. Endorphins affect mood, endocrine function, respiration, and gastrointestinal motility in addition to pain. They are located in the cognitive areas of the brain as well as in the hypothalamus and amygdala, which regulate emotions; the periaqueductal gray and nucleus raphe magnus, which are thought to be the origin of descending control pathways that modify incoming sensory stimuli; and the substantia gelatinosa in the dorsal horns of the spinal cord. The plexuses of the gastrointestinal tract also contain endorphins [9,33].

The location of the opiate receptors in the brain areas associated with emotions supported the idea that rather than actually preventing pain, opiates relieve pain by altering pain perception. Endorphins are similar to brain receptors for the plant alkaloid morphine and other exogenous narcotic molecules, and are thought to combine with specific brain receptors to block the pain message and produce analgesia (Fig. 47-5) [3,58].

Beta-endorphin is a 31-amino acid chain peptide that is part of beta-lipotropin, a pituitary hormone. Beta-endorphin is more resistant to enzymatic degradation and thus has a half-life of at least two to three hours. Its action has been shown to be 48 times stronger than that of morphine.

Beta-endorphin is thought to initiate activity in the descending inhibitory system. High levels of endorphins are associated with elevated pain threshold and tolerance levels. Some chronic pain syndromes, such as trigeminal neuralgia, are associated with low levels of beta-endorphin in the cerebrospinal fluid (CSF), an indication that continuing pain may deplete beta-endorphin levels [54].

Other neuroactive peptides have also been isolated and may possess an even more powerful action than that of beta-endorphin. Neurotensin, bombesin, angiotensin, and dynorphin are examples [33]. Dynorphin, an extremely powerful opiate, is widely distributed in nervous tissue and interacts in vivo with its own opiate receptor. While it significantly inhibits beta-endorphin- or morphine-induced analgesia, dynorphin has no effect on enkephalin-induced analgesia. Thus, it may modulate analgesia [9].

Because endorphins, or "happiness peptides," sometimes produce euphoria and an overall sense of well-being, they probably affect the psychologic component of pain. Depression is also known to lower endorphin levels [58].

Stress and pain both stimulate the endorphin system. High endorphin levels may account for lower than expected levels of pain after injury during acute physical stress, such as under conditions of war and competitive sport [33,58]. Pregnancy is another stressful condition.

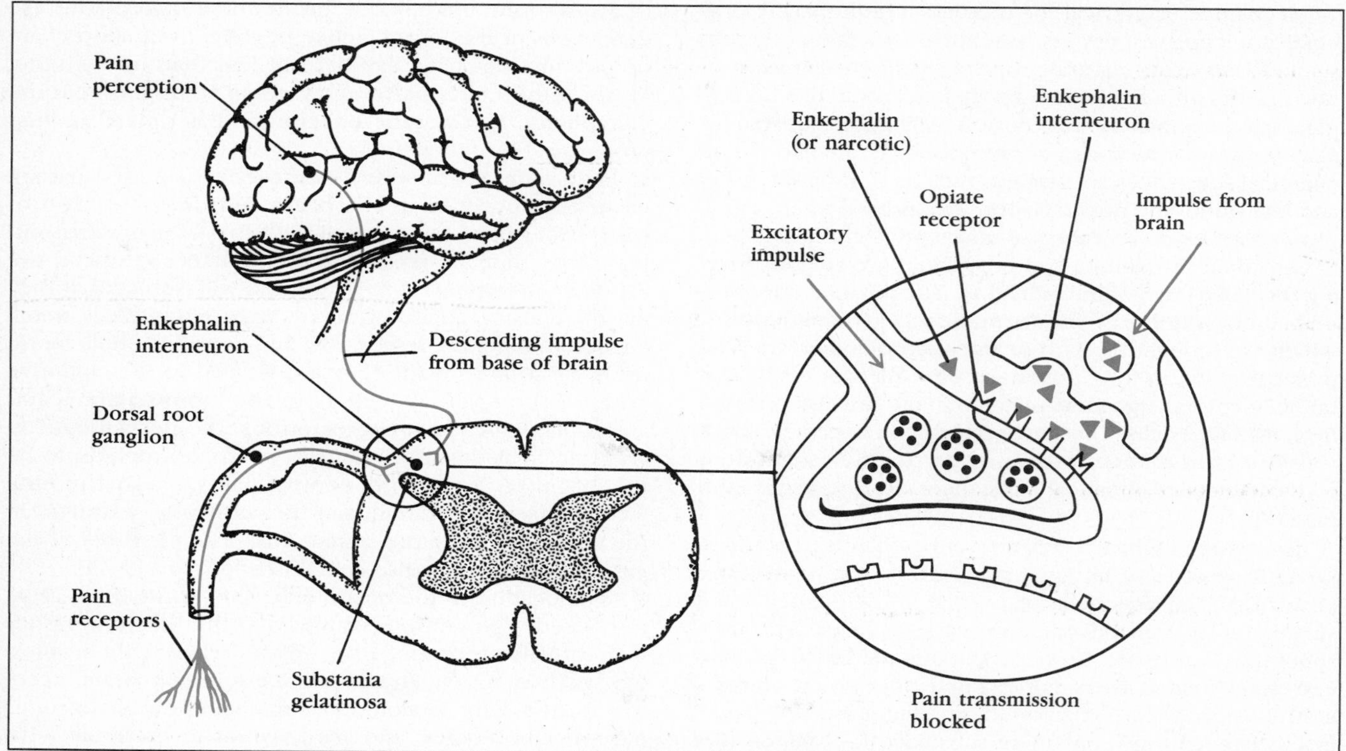

FIGURE 47-5 The biologic receptors of the endorphin system. (From K. Foley, *The Management of Cancer Pain: A Symposium*. New York: HP Publishing. Copyright © 1984. Reprinted by permission.)

Long labor may deplete endorphin levels and thus raise the pain sensitivity level.

Sources of Pain

Most pain is caused by injury or inflammation. Pain has its own sensory system, and its source determines its sensory characteristics. The three general sources are (1) *cutaneous system*, which consists of superficial somatic structures, such as skin and subcutaneous tissues; (2) *deep somatic system*, which includes periosteum, bone, nerve, muscle, tendons, joints, blood vessels, and their supporting tissues; and (3) *viscera*, which relate to body cavities and their respective organs [19,29]. Table 47-1 lists the characteristics of cutaneous, deep somatic, and visceral pain.

Because pain originates from deeper somatic structures, deep somatic and visceral pain are often collectively referred to as deep pain. Table 47-2 compares cutaneous, deep somatic, and visceral pain, while Table 47-3 lists their ascending transmission systems.

Cutaneous Pain. Skin has the greatest density of free nerve endings of any body tissue. A dense, subepithelial meshwork of thin unmyelinated nerve fibers innervates the skin and subcutaneous tissues, and smaller nerve endings pass upward and branch outward between the epithelial cells on the skin surface. The surfaces of the face, hands, and feet are the most highly sensitive areas [33].

Myelinated A-delta fibers throughout the rapidly conducting, lateral ascending system in the CNS primarily mediate cutaneous pain. Because of its rapid transmission, it is considered the first pain with nociceptive stimulation [33].

Cutaneous pain is often referred to as direct in that it can be directly perceived and precisely localized. Cutaneous pain is usually easy to diagnose since it originates in the area of the stimulus and increases with extent of the stimulus, such as with a large area of burn [9,29]. It can have an abrupt or slow onset and may be distributed along the dermatomes. *Dermatomes* are dermal segments, and each one is innervated by a specific spinal root (see page 732). Although the boundaries appear to be distinct, the nerve fiber distribution between the dermatomes actually overlaps. Thus, T-6 irritation results in pain being experienced in the T-5, T-6, and T-7 dermatomes [9]. Figure 47-6 illustrates the cutaneous distribution of dermatomes.

The three distinct skin layers produce different pain sensations. The epidermis produces itching and burning pain, and the dermis and the subcutaneous tissue produce superficial pain and aching pain, respectively [33].

Referred cutaneous pain does not occur with noxious stimulation but may occur with nonnoxious stimulation.

TABLE 47-1 Characteristics of Superficial, Deep Somatic, and Visceral Pain

Superficial (first, epicritic)	Deep Somatic (second, protopathic)	Visceral
Sharp Easily localized by patient Perceived at point of origin Easily palpated May result in loss of strength, reflexes, and sensory changes *Structures* Skin, superficial fascia, ligaments, tendon sheaths, periosteum	Dull ache Fairly well localized; tendency to be referred *Structures* Sensitivity — Threshold HIGH Periosteum LOW ↑ Ligaments ↑ Fibrous capsules of joints Tendons ↓ Fascia ↓ LOW Muscle HIGH Segmental reflexive changes can occur, indicative of ANS involvement such as cutaneous hyperalgesia	Dull ache Hard to localize by patient Perceived away from point of origin, referred to embryologically related dermatomes Difficult to palpate Rarely results in loss of strength, reflexes, sensation, but may cause segmental sudomotor, visceromotor, viscerocutaneous changes (rigidity, tenderness, hyperalgesia) *Structures* — Threshold Parietal serous membranes LOW Hollow visceral walls ↑↓ Parenchymatous organs HIGH

Source: From J. Mannheimer, and B. Lampe, *Clinical Transcutaneous Electrical Nerve Stimulation.* Copyright © 1984. F.A. Davis. Reprinted by permission.

TABLE 47-2 Characteristics of Pain as Commonly Related to Source of Pain

Source	Location	Intensity	Quality	Chronology
Cutaneous	Well localized	Correlates with intensity of stimulus.	Bimodal sensation may occur. Sharp, tingling, stinging. Abnormal surface sensations may occur.	Correlates with stimulus changes, tissue damage. May be steady or throbbing in inflamed tissues.
Deep somatic	Poorly localized. May localize with tendon, periosteum, ligament pain. May be referred to body surface.	Correlates with intensity of stimulus and with movement of involved area.	Vague, aching, boring, dull. Cutaneous tenderness may accompany.	May be steady or change in character with stimulus change or movement. Correlates with stimulus changes.
Visceral	Poorly localized. May localize as duration extends. May be referred to body surface.	May be severe with colic. May increase if not relieved. Correlates with intensity of stimulus.	Vague, dull, aching, burning. If continues may become sharper. If due to obstruction may be gripping, cramping, twisting.	Obstructive pain generally occurs in cycles. Untreated pain may mount. Correlates with stimulus changes.

Source: From A.K. Jacey, *Pain: A Source Book for Nurses and Other Health Professionals.* Boston: Little, Brown, 1977.

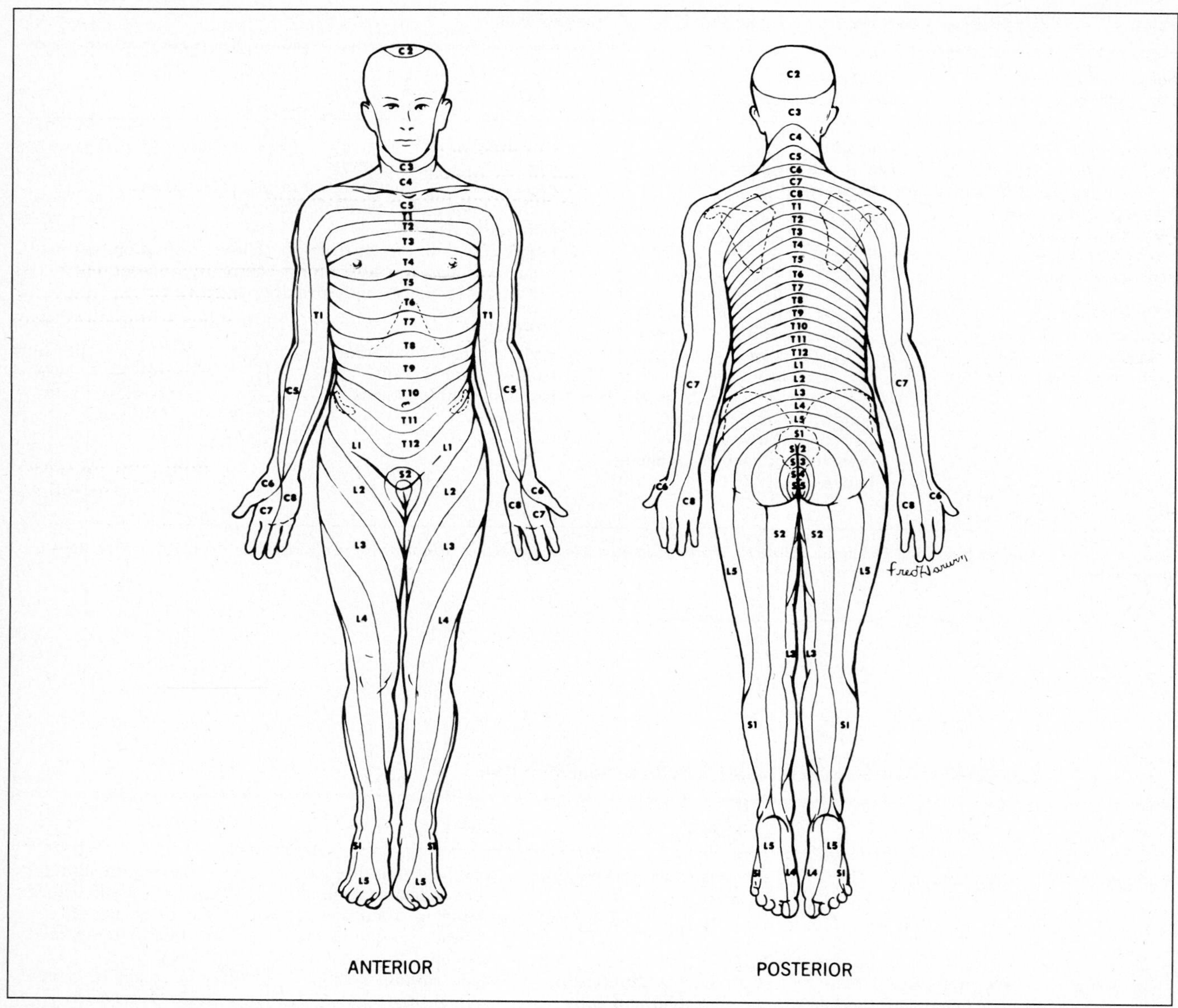

FIGURE 47-6 Anterior and posterior dermatomes. The cutaneous distribution of spinal segments (*right*) and peripheral nerves (*left*). (From J.F. Simpson and K.R. Magee, *Clinical Evaluation of the Nervous System.* Boston: Little, Brown, 1973.)

Referred cutaneous pain may result from a process of convergence in the spinal cord, CNS errors related to embryology, or some altered impulse pattern. Thus, referred cutaneous pain differs from that of visceral pain, which is referred to related dermatomes [33].

Deep Somatic Pain. Deep pain is synonymous with second pain in that it is transmitted primarily by unmyelinated C fibers through the slower-conducting medial ascending system in the CNS. In contrast to the dermatomes in cutaneous pain, deep somatic pain is poorly localized because the *myotomes* or *scleratomes* are less well-defined. Moreover, scleratomes do not have a corresponding skin segment [33]. Scleratomes are also the areas innervated by one posterior nerve root. Deep somatic pain frequently radiates from the primary nociceptive site along a nerve root, such as with lumbar disk pain traveling along the sciatic nerve [9].

Pain sensitivity varies by degrees in deep somatic structures. Tendons, deep fascia, ligaments, bone and joint periosteum, blood vessels, and nerves are extremely sensitive. The periosteum of bones and joints is the most sensitive. Tables 47-4 and 47-5 list musculoskeletal and nervous system structures that produce pain as a result of noxious stimulation. Cold, cutting, stretching, and handling induce pain in many blood vessels. Skeletal muscle

TABLE 47-3 Afferent Pain Transmission Systems

Superficial Pain	Deep Pain
Exteroreceptors	Interoreceptors
A-delta fibers (CNS)	B and C fibers (ANS and CNS)
Fast conduction by late-developing pathways (neospinothalamic)	Slow conduction by early pathways (paleospinothalamic)
Lateral ascending system	Medial ascending system
Postsynaptic dorsal column	Diffuse polysynaptic propriospinal system
Spinocervical tract	Spinoreticular system (diffuse limbic and reticular connections)
Few synapses (3)	Numerous synapses
Projects to lateral thalamic nuclei and localized by Somatosensory cortex	Projects to midline Intrathalamic regions
	Also conveys psychologic and motivational aspects of pain

Source: From J. Mannheimer and B. Lampe, *Clinical Transcutaneous Electrical Nerve Stimulation.* Copyright © 1984. F.A. Davis. Reprinted by permission.

sensitivity results from stretching, ischemia, or forceful or sustained contractile activity, and extreme pressures account for bone and cartilage pain.

Headache. A large proportion of headaches is caused by cranial nerves that are distorted by pulling, displacement, or distention. The most common form of headache results from muscle contraction about the head and neck, and includes the posttraumatic headache. The pain is dull, bandlike, and persistent [12]. Table 47-6 lists the characteristics of muscle contraction (tension) headaches.

Vascular headaches, most commonly of the migraine type, are thought to result from noxious stimulation, with a neurogenic vasomotor disorder involving the internal and external carotid arteries [1]. Constriction of the internal carotid artery produces local tissue acidosis, loss of vessel tone, and vasodilation of the external carotid artery. Subsequently, the periarterial inflammation and capillary permeability produce edema, stretching, and increased pulse amplitude that result in the pulsing, throbbing, migraine pain [12].

TABLE 47-4 Musculoskeletal Structures Producing Pain with Noxious Stimulation

Structure	Depth	Quality	Chronologic and Variant Factors	Localization	Referral Pattern
Skin	Epidermis ↓ Dermis	Itching, prickling Burning	Brief stimulus (noxious) Prolonged stimulus	Excellent	None
		Sharp	Nonnoxious stimulus	Good	Extrasegmental (dermatomal) Ipsilateral referral
Fascia Loose	Subcutaneous (adipose)	Sharp		Good	None
Compact	Intermuscular (deep) Septa + retinacula	Achy		Poor (diffuse)	Segmental (myotomal)
Tendon	Superficial	Sharp	Pain ↑ with movement and becomes diffuse with ↑ severity	Good	Segmental to distal extent of dermomyotome or tendon
Tendon Sheath		Burning, boring		Poor	
Muscle	Deep	Achy, dull Boring	Shape of muscle	Poor to fair (diffuse)	Segmental (myotomal)
	Superficial	Achy, dull Sharper	Permeated by superficial fascial planes	Fair to good	
Ligament	Superficial	Sharp	Pain ↑ with stretch	Fair	Segmental (sclerotomal)
	Deep	Achy, tender		Poor	
Bursae	Subcutaneous Subfascial Subtendinous Submuscular	Sharp ↓ Achy	Pain ↑ with movement (pinching) of communicating bursae (synovial membrane continuous with that of joint)	Fair	Segmental (sclerotomal)
Fibrous capsule	Deep	Ache	Bony attachment may be continuous with tendons & ligaments	Poor (diffuse)	Segmental (myotomal, sclerotomal)
Periosteum	Superficial	Sharp	Referral may be proximal or distal	Good	Sgmental (myotomal)
Bone joint	Deep	Dull		Poor (diffuse)	Segmental (sclerotomal)

Source: From J. Mannheimer and B. Lampe, *Clinical Transcutaneous Electrical Nerve Stimulation.* Copyright © 1984. F.A. Davis. Reprinted by permission.

TABLE 47-5 CNS Structures Producing Pain with Noxious Stimulation

Structure	Depth	Quality	Chronologic and Varient Factors	Localization	Referral Pattern
Dura mater	Deep	Dull, achy, boring, referred, paresthesia	Unilateral or bilateral	Poor to fair	Extrasegmental
Dural sleeve	Deep	Sharp, electric shock-like lancinating	Varies with foraminal encroachment	Fair	Segmental (dermatomal)
Nerve root	Deep	Irritation	Compression: no tenderness or pain, paralysis	Poor to fair	Segmental (myotomal)
Ventral		Tenderness, ache, cramp			
Dorsal	Superficial	Pins and needles, paresthesia	Compression: Numbness	Fair	Segmental (dermatomal)
Sympathetic component		↑ ANS signs	Compression: ↓ ANS signs	Poor	Sympathetic dermatome
Nerve trunk ↓ Peripheral nerve	Superficial ↓ Deep	Pins and needles Hyperesthesia Burning Background ache	Neurapraxia ↓ Axonotmesis Neurotmesis Numbness and paralysis	Fair to good	Course of nerve distally, sensory and/or motor loss
Spinal cord	Deep	Paresthesia, not pain	irritation or compression (Babinski, spasticity)	Poor	Bilateral extrasegmental

Source: From J. Mannheimer and B. Lampe, *Clinical Transcutaneous Electrical Nerve Stimulation.* Copyright © 1984. F.A. Davis. Reprinted by permission.

TABLE 47-6 Characteristics of Muscle Contraction Headaches

Characteristics	Description	Variables
Onset	Age — any Sex — females more than males Family history (−)	
Location	Bilateral occipital, frontal, temporal	Splenius capitis, SCM, upper trapezius, temporalis, masseter, scalenes, levator scapulae
Intensity	Not as severe as migrane or cluster	Psychogenic, mild to moderate
Quality	Nonthrobbing, dull, achy	Tight, pressure, heavy weight Delusion— crawling Depression — bandlike
Pattern	No prodromal symptoms, slow onset	Chronic — awaken with headache, ↑ + ↓ continuously throughout the day
Duration	Acute — 1–4 hours Chronic — with ongoing psychologic problems, months to years Anticipatory ↔ psychogenic	
Associated symptoms	Irritability	10% also have migraine, throbbing, nausea
Aggravating/easing factors	Relaxation ↓, alcohol ↓, anxiety ↑, poor posture ↑	
Precipitating/triggering factors	Posture, work, auto accident, tension, fatigue, eyestrain, emotional stress, bruxism, joint dysfunction (TM)	

Source: From J. Mannheimer and B. Lampe, *Clinical Transcutaneous Electrical Nerve Stimulation.* Copyright © 1984. F.A. Davis. Reprinted by permission.

Histamine, serotonin, (5HT), and bradykinin are involved in the mechanism of migraine. Intravenous histamine produces headaches in persons with migraine but not in healthy persons. The associated diarrhea or vomiting may be due to the release of 5-HT from normal blood platelets and the intestinal wall during the onset of migraine [1]. Administration of 1-tryptophan, a 5-HT precursor, decreases the frequency of migraine headaches. Bradykinin and 5-HT appear to potentiate each other and result in vasodilation [33]. Table 47-7 describes the characteristics of vascular or migraine headaches.

Musculoskeletal Trauma. Immediate, sharp, nociceptive pain after musculoskeletal trauma results from distortion of subcutaneous, perivascular, and periarticular nerve plexuses. A period of relative freedom from pain may follow certain severe injuries if there is marked associated mental stimulation or shock [63].

Deep, boring, persistent pain then begins and increases, often resulting from physical distention of the joint capsule or fascial compartments by blood or tissue fluid transudate. Pain occurs if pressure due to chronic ischemia and liberated neurotransmitters continues to increase within relatively rigid fascial compartments. Impairment of blood supply produces chronic ischemia, and liberated neurotransmitters activate the kinin and prostaglandin systems [63]. Subsequently, extravasated blood or necrotic tissue initiates phagocytosis and a sterile inflammatory response. A secondary release of neurotransmitters produces prolonged pain, as with, for example, sacral or tibial subperiosteal bruising. The persistence of pain at rest after resolution of the immediate effects of the injury may indicate a persistent inflammatory reaction.

Visceral Pain. Visceral, or splanchnic, pain originates in the viscera. In general, the viscera have only sensory receptors for pain [19]. Visceral pain also tends to be diffuse; however, if it persists, it may become localized. Because nerve fibers that follow the sympathetic or parasympathetic nerves into the spinal cord innervate body organs, autonomic responses often accompany visceral pain [29].

The parietal peritoneum and mesentary are sensitive to cutting, stretching, and handling. Most of the viscera are insensitive to these stimuli, but strong abnormal contractions, ischemia, and inflammation of the hollow viscera may induce severe pain [19].

Some typical causes of visceral pain include acute appendicitis, acute cholecystitis, biliary-pancreatic tract inflammation, gastroduodenal disease, cardiovascular disease, pleurisy, tubo-ovarian disorders such as acute salpingitis and ectopic pregnancy, and renal and ureteral colic [5].

Perforation of body organs and drainage of their contents into the peritoneal cavity may also induce abdominal pain. In descending order of irritation, the intraperitoneal fluids that may accumulate are (1) pancreatic enzyme fluid, (2) gastric or duodenal fluid, (3) fecal fluid, (4) bile, (5) urine, (6) blood, and (7) lymph.

General medical conditions that often cause acute abdominal pain include poorly controlled diabetes mellitus, sickle cell anemia, acute intermittent porphyria,

TABLE 47-7 Characteristics of Vascular or Migraine Headaches

Characteristics	Description
Onset	Childhood → puberty, plus family history
Location	70–80% temple or forehead Unilateral, spread to occiput, neck, shoulder Whole head; one side more painful
Intensity	Mild to severe
Quality	Throbbing, pulsing
Pattern	Stage I—Prodromal (aura) Stage II—Headache Scintillating scotoma Visual disturbances Paresthesia Dizziness Head noises
Duration	Stage I, 20–30 min; stage II, 12–24 hours
Frequency	Several times per day, week, or year
Associated symptoms	↑ urination, nervousness, colitis, abdominal pain, nasal symptoms, dyspepsia, diarrhea, constipation, sweating, exhaustion, pallor, fever, red, dull eyes, awaken 3–4 AM
Chronology	3–9% of population; onset as early as age 8 months; in children females and males are equal; 12% onset before age 40 years; more common in females
Aggravating/easing factors	Menstruation ↑, contraceptives ↑ Pregnancy ↓, tryptophan ↓
Precipitating factors	Food additives; MSG, caffeine, alcohol, tyranine, sodium nitrite, calcium propionate, histamine Glare, dust, odors, temperature changes, barometric pressure and humidity changes, stress—physical and psychologic, lack of oxygen, hunger, smoking, ↓ in blood serotonin

Source: From J. Mannheimer and B. Lampe, *Clinical Transcutaneous Electrical Nerve Stimulation.* Copyright © 1984. F.A. Davis. Reprinted by permission.

hyperlipemia, black widow spider and scorpion bites, opiate withdrawal, and lead poisoning. Intense physical exertion also can produce acute severe abdominal pain and vomiting, possibly as a result of splanchnic ischemia [5].

While both the parietal pleura and bronchi are very sensitive to pain because of innervation by the intercostal and phrenic nerves, the alveoli of the lungs and liver parenchyma are almost completely insensitive to any type of pain. The liver capsule is highly sensitive to both direct trauma and stretch. The bile ducts are also sensitive to pain. Localizing pain in the different viscera is difficult because sensations from the abdomen and thorax are projected to the CNS by either the true visceral pathway or the parietal pathway. True visceral pain is conducted primarily by C fibers of the autonomic system. The sensations are often referred in peculiar patterns to surface areas of the body [79].

The location of the referred pain on the body surface is in a dermatomal distribution embryologically related to the involved organ. For example, the pain in gallbladder disease may be experienced around and at the tip of the right shoulder. The pain of uterine contractions preceding childbirth is usually referred to lumbar areas of the back. Pain of esophageal or gastric origin is often confused with cardiac pain. Retroperitoneal structures, such as the kidneys, kidney pelvis, and ureters, receive most of their pain fibers directly from the skeletal nerves. Consequently, renal pain is better localized than the other visceral pains (Fig. 47-7 and Table 47-8) [19].

In contrast, sensations from the parietal peritoneum, pleura, and pericardium are carried directly into the local spinal nerves. Thus, parietal sensations are often localized directly over the irritated area. Because of the two pathways, pain from the viscera is frequently localized to two body surfaces. For example, pain impulses from an inflamed appendix project by way of the sympathetic chain into the spinal cord at T-10 or T-11 and are referred to the umbilical area. The pain is aching and cramping. Parietal pain impulses from an inflamed appendix pass through the spinal nerves into the spinal cord at L-1 or L-2. The pain is sharp and localized directly over the irritated peritoneum in the right lower abdominal quadrant (Fig. 47-8) [19].

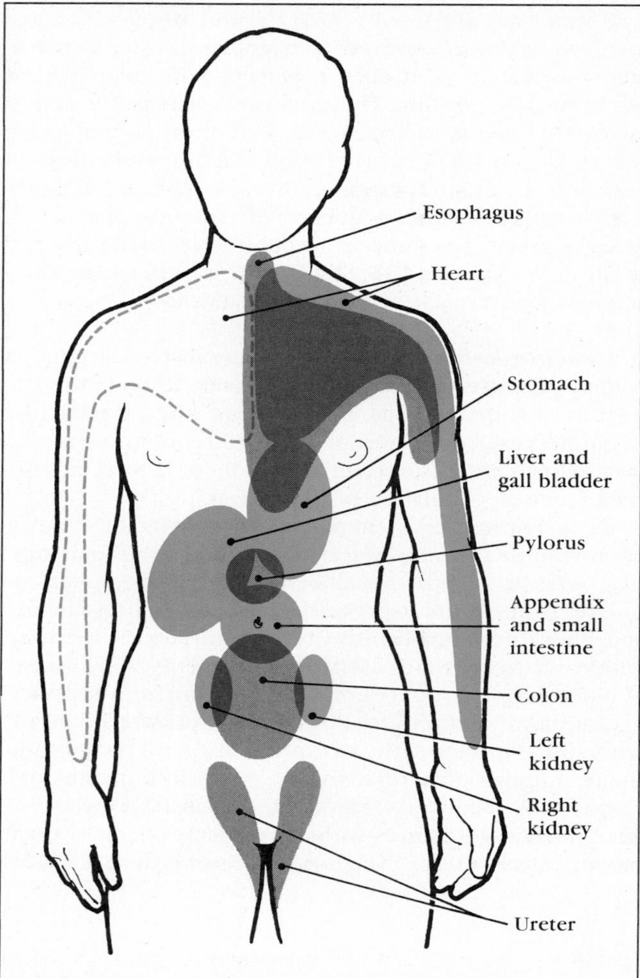

FIGURE 47-7 Surface areas of referred pain from visceral organs. (Adapted from A.C. Guyton, *Textbook of Medical Physiology* [7th ed.]. Philadelphia: W.B. Saunders Company, 1986. Reprinted by permission.)

TABLE 47-8 Localization of Referred Plan from Visceral Structure Damage

Visceral Structure Damage	Area of Skin Experiencing Pain
Diaphragm	Skin of ipsilateral shoulder and outer surface of upper arm
Heart	Dermatomes C-3–T-8, with resulting pain in left arm and hand, especially in distribution of ulnar nerve; shoulder, back, substernal region, neck, axilla, and jaw; occasionally stomach, with "indigestion" symptoms noted
Stomach	Dermatomes T-6–T-9; chest and substernal region
Ovaries	Dermatome T-10; periumbilical
Uterus	Dermatomes S-1–S-2, sometimes manifesting as pain in lower back
Prostate	Dermatomes T-10–T-12, manifesting as pain in periumbilical and inguinal areas, tip of penis, and occasionally scrotum
Kidneys	Dermatomes T-10–L-1; lower back and umbilical area
Rectum	Dermatomes S-2–S-4; low sacral back pain and sciatic pain in upper thigh or calf on dorsum of leg

Source: From N. Hendler, *Diagnosis and Nonsurgical Management of Chronic Pain.* Copyright © 1981, Raven Press, New York. Reprinted by permission of Raven Press.

Theories of Pain

The complexities of pain are reflected in the numerous theories that have evolved since the beginning of the cen-

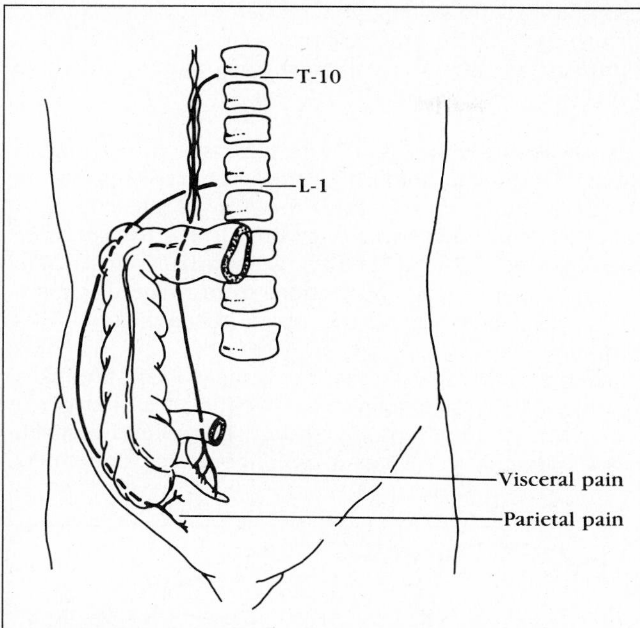

FIGURE 47-8 Visceral and parietal transmission of pain from the appendix. (From A.C. Guyton, *Textbook of Medical Physiology* [7th ed.]. Philadelphia: W.B. Saunders Company, 1986. Reprinted by permission.)

tury [50]. These theories are generally organized into five major perspectives: (1) *affect*, (2) *specificity*, (3) *pattern*, (4) *gate control*, and (5) *psychologic* [30].

Affect Theory

Dating back to Aristotle, who regarded pain as the antithesis of pleasure, the affect theory describes pain as an emotion rather than a sensation. The emotion of pain colors all sensations and motivates behavior to relieve it. The theory fails to describe pain systematically and explain why it is an emotion [30].

Specificity Theory

The specificity theory, first proposed by Max von Frey, gave rise to the expectation that a given form of therapy should be effective for all pains. Originating from Descartes's straight-through conception of pain in 1644, the specificity theory proposes that a mosaic of specific pain receptors in the skin projects impulses in a fixed, direct-line (stimulus-response) relationship to a pain center in the brain [40,41]. According to this theory, pain intensity is proportional to the severity of tissue damage. Thus, like hearing and smell, pain is a specific and immutable sensation with its own peripheral and central components [36].

Pain receptors are differentiated free nerve endings that generate pain impulses to a pain center in the thalamus. A-delta and C fibers in the peripheral nerves and the lateral spinothalamic tract in the spinal cord project the impulses [40].

The skin sensory system does contain highly specialized receptors and fibers that contribute to pain processes. There is no evidence, however, to substantiate the claim that special receptor-fiber units constitute an exclusive pain modality and a fixed, one-to-one relationship between stimulus and sensation. While sensations other than pain may also be produced, stimulation of pain-specific receptors and fibers with comparable stimuli does not always evoke pain or even the same intensity of pain within or among persons [40].

Pattern Theory

Several versions of pattern theory emphasize either stimulus intensity or central summation as the critical determinants of pain [40,41]. In contrast to specificity theory, the pattern theory proposes that there are no specific fibers or nerve endings for pain [39].

Intensive stimulation of nonspecific receptors produces temporal and spatial patterns of nerve impulses for pain. The patterns form codes that provide pain information. Pain results from the summation of the skin sensory input at the dorsal horn cells. The theory of nonspecific receptors ignores the physiologic evidence of highly specialized receptors and fibers in the skin sensory system [39–41].

Basically, pattern theory describes the existence of rapidly conducting, large cutaneous fibers that inhibit synaptic transmission in more slowly conducting, small cutaneous fibers that lead to pain awareness. Under pathologic conditions, the slow pain system dominates over the fast pain system, and the result is protopathic (undiscriminating) sensation, slow pain, diffuse burning pain, or hyperalgesia [40].

While the specificity and pattern theories appear to be mutually exclusive, they contain elements that supplement each other and contribute to an understanding of the pain phenomenon [41]. As with the specificity theory, the pattern theory fails to provide an adequate explanation for the psychologic processes of pain perception and response [30].

Gate-Control Theory

Melzack and Wall integrated the concept of physiologic specialization in the skin sensory system from the specificity theory and the concepts of central summation and patterning of input from the pattern theory in developing the gate-control theory [39]. In 1967 Melzack and Casey used the basic components of the theory to develop a new conceptual model of pain. According to the model, the pain experience consists of three interactive components [38].

The modulation of pain impulses in the neospinothalamic system serves as a neural basis for the *sensory-discriminative component* of pain. Subsequently, the brainstem reticular formation and limbic system become involved in the *motivational-affective component* of pain that influences aversive drive and affective reactions to pain [38]. Central control activities that are primarily cognitive functions selectively influence sensory processes or motivational mechanisms associated with *pain perception and response*. Present and past experiences are critical to the cognitive functions. Thus, pain perception and response are functions of the sensory, motivational, and cognitive processes [38].

The gate-control theory proposes that peripheral stimulation produces nerve impulses that are projected to three spinal cord systems: (1) the cells of the substantia gelatinosa (SG) in the dorsal horn, (2) the dorsal column fibers, and (3) the central transmission cells (T cells) in the dorsal horn (Fig. 47-9) [41]. The theory proposes that (1) the SG acts as a gate-control system to modulate the flow of nerve impulses from peripheral fibers to the central nervous system; (2) dorsal column fibers act as a central nervous system control trigger to stimulate selective brain processes (the central control system) that influence the gate-control system; and (3) T cells activate neural mechanisms (the action system) in the brain that are responsible for pain perception and response (Fig. 47-10). Pain phenomena result from the interactions among the three spinal cord systems [39,40].

Gate-Control System. The SG acts as a gating mechanism to modulate the flow of afferent nerve impulses. Its primary function is to inhibit the flow of afferent nerve impulses before they synapse to the T cells. Thus, it limits T cell activation by keeping the gate partially closed. The SG contains numerous projections from raphe magnus as well as substance P terminals, opiate receptors, and 5-HT terminals [9].

Afferent nerve fibers consist of three primary groups: A, B, and C. All class A fibers are myelinated and larger in diameter than the thinly myelinated class B and unmyelinated class C fibers. Class A fibers comprise alpha, beta,

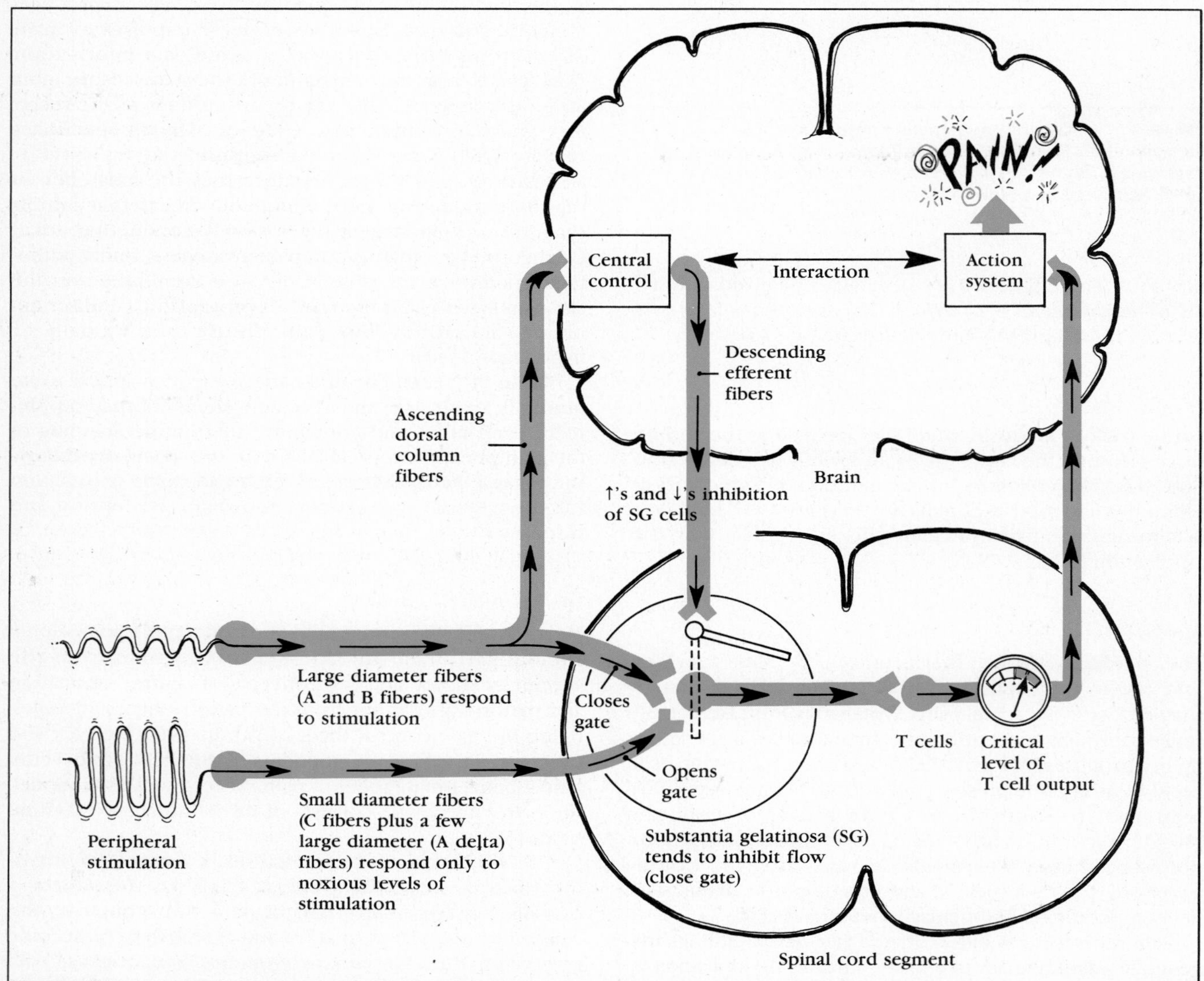

FIGURE 47-9 The gate-control theory of pain. (Adapted from J. Flynn and P. Heffron, *Nursing: From Concept to Practice*. Bowie, Md.: Brady, 1984.)

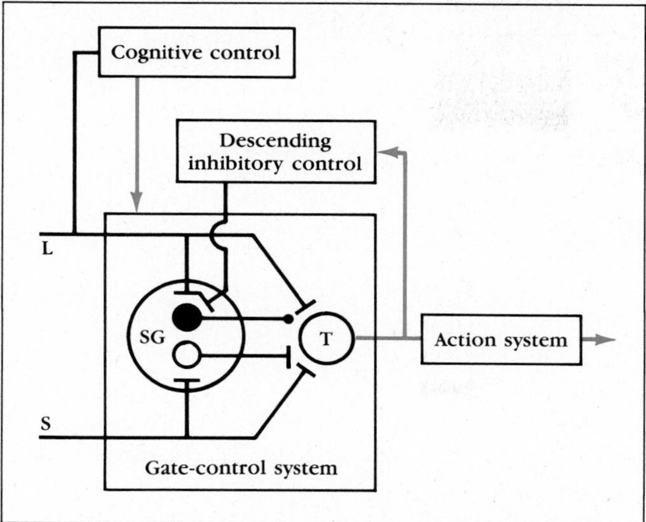

FIGURE 47-10 The gate-control theory. The SG contains both excitatory (*white circle*) and inhibitory (*black circle*) links. The action of the inhibitory link could be presynaptic, postsynaptic, or both (*round knob*). The brainstem inhibitory system is influenced by the sensory input after transmission through the gate and projects back to the dorsal horn. The system is a separate input to the gate. (From R. Melzack and P.D. Wall, *The Challenge of Pain*. Copyright © 1973 by Ronald Melzack. Copyright © 1982 by Ronald Melzack and Patrick D. Wall. Reprinted by permission of Basic Books, Inc., Publisher, and Penguin Books, Ltd., London.)

delta, and gamma subgroups. Except for the A-delta fibers, which carry noxious impulses created only by very strong stimuli, none of the other A fibers or the B fibers appear to transport nociceptive information. The function of C fibers is automatic postganglionic transmission. Thus, pain transmission is limited to subclasses of A-delta and C fibers [9].

Activation of the A-delta and C afferent nerve fibers decreases the inhibitory effect of the SG. While increased large fiber activity prevents pain awareness by partially closing the gate, increased small-fiber activity facilitates awareness by opening the gate wider and allowing more impulses to pass on to the T cells, aggregate, and mobilize the brain's action system [40,41].

Central Control System. The central control system consists of large-diameter, fast-conducting fibers that rapidly activate two cognitive subsystems in the brain. This activation selectively modulates or inhibits peripheral nerve impulses before they are projected to the brain. Specifically, the central control system activates the descending efferent fibers in the brainstem reticular formation and cortex [40].

While the reticular formation inhibits somatic, visual, and auditory input projected by the gate control system, the cortex, which subserves cognitive processes, affects the gate-control system. Specifically, the central control processes regulate activity in both the sensory-discriminative and motivational-affective systems [41]. Thus, central control activities, such as distraction, fear, and anxiety, may intervene between stimulus and response [35].

The central control processes occur before the synapse to the T cells and activation of the action system. The action system governs pain perception and response. Thus, a balance between the afferent nerve input and central control input to the gate-control system determines the presence or absence of pain.

Action System. The action system is often referred to as the pain reaction system. It is controlled by the central control system and is triggered only when the output of the T cells reaches or exceeds a critical level. The critical level consists of both temporal and spatial summation of the afferent impulses. The summation results in light pressure being distinguished from tissue damage and the identification of the body area being stimulated.

When activated, the T cells are projected to the brainstem reticular formation and cortex. Interaction between the action system and central control system influences pain perception and response. Thus, the interaction between the systems influences overt behaviors in response to noxious stimulation (Fig. 47-11).

In 1976 Wall made a general restatement of the gate-control theory. The concepts currently accepted include (1) peripheral nerves transmit information about an injury to the CNS; (2) A-delta and C fibers respond only to injury, while other fibers with lower thresholds increase their discharge frequency if the stimulus attains noxious levels; (3) other peripheral nerve fibers that transmit information about innocuous events also facilitate or inhibit cells that are excited by the injury signals; and (4) descending control systems originate in the brain and modulate the excitability of the cells.

Thus, peripheral stimulation and transmission as well as modulation occurring in the spinal cord and higher structures influence the perception of noxious stimuli and pain. Pain and pain control, therefore, must be viewed in terms of both afferent pain pathways and descending control systems that modify the sensory information [55].

Clinical Implications. The gate-control theory has numerous implications for clinical practice. McCaffery summarized its components (Table 47-9) [34]. The middle column of the table emphasizes three ways to close the gate partially or completely and hence to decrease the level of pain awareness. Accurate application of the gate-control theory to clinical practice requires that therapeutic modalities incorporate sensory, motivational, and cognitive interventions for pain relief.

The skin is richly endowed with large-diameter nerve fibers, activation of which may reduce or eliminate pain. Thus, while cutaneous stimulation by massage or vibration may partially or completely close the gate to pain, cutaneous stimulation through rhythmic rubbing of a painful body part can enhance distraction and relaxation strategies for pain relief [34]. Most distraction strategies, such as guided imagery, attempt to maximize sensory input to the reticular system in the brainstem so that the brainstem may project inhibitory impulses to close the gate to pain transmission. A decrease in anxiety, fear, or depression about pain and an increase in self-confidence and self-

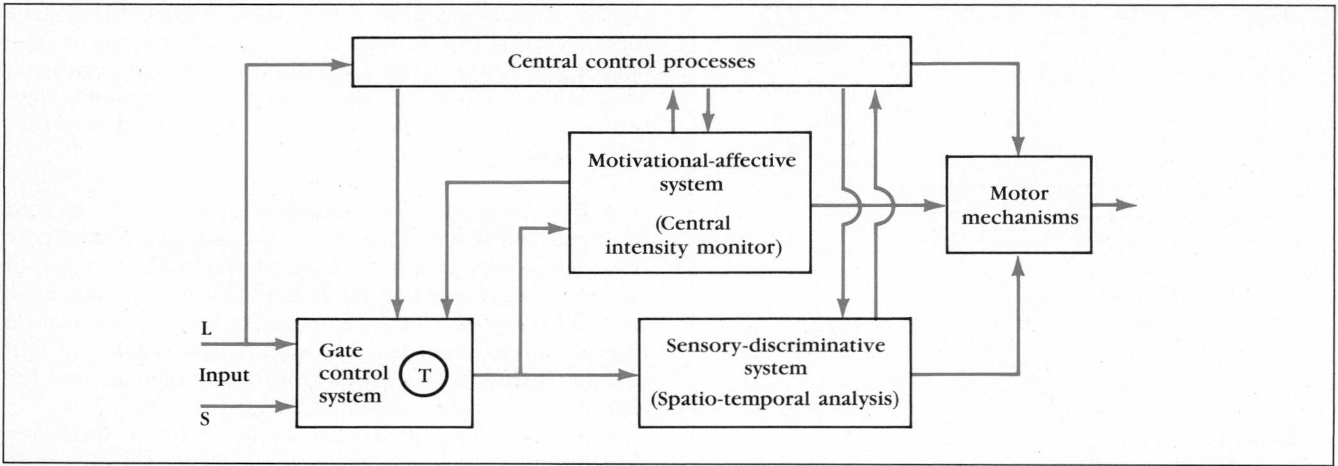

FIGURE 47-11 Conceptual model of the sensory, motivational, and central control determinants of pain. The sensory-discriminative system, motivational-affective system, and central control processes interact and project to the motor system. (From D. Kenshalo [ed.], *The Skin Senses,* 1978. Courtesy of Charles C. Thomas, Publisher, Springfield, Illinois.)

control also may relieve or alleviate pain by inhibiting signals from the cerebral cortex and thalamus [34].

Pain phenomena that are explained by applying concepts of the gate-control theory include (1) hyperalgesia with traumatic peripheral nerve lesions or postherpetic neuralgia; (2) congenital analgesia and referred pain; (3) spontaneous pain without stimulation, such as with peripheral nerve lesions; (4) pathologic pain syndromes where there are long delays between noxious stimulation and response; and (5) relief of phantom limb pain by gently tapping the stump with a rubber mallet. The gate-control theory also can be used to explain pain phenomena associated with, for example, alcoholic or diabetic neuropathy.

While the smaller peripheral nerve fibers in alcoholic or diabetic neuropathy are relatively intact, the large fibers are selectively destroyed. Normal presynaptic inhibition of stimuli by the gate-control system is absent. Intense pathologic pain results from an unchecked open gate. Also, long delays between stimulation and pain perception occur because of reduction in the total number of peripheral fibers projecting impulses to the T cells.

Psychologic Theories

While the physiologic theories describe and explain pain with bodily dysfunction, the psychologic theories account for pain when bodily dysfunction is minimal or absent

TABLE 47-9 Application of the Gate-Control Theory to Clinical Practice

Structures Involved	No Pain or Decreased Intensity of Pain	Pain
Spinal cord (?)	Results from closing the gate by	Results from opening the gate by
Nerve fibers	1. Activity in the large-diameter nerve fibers, e.g., caused by skin stimulation,	1. Activity in the small-diameter nerve fibers, e.g., caused by tissue damage,
Brainstem	2. Inhibitory impulses from the brainstem, e.g., caused by sufficient or maximum sensory input arriving through distraction or guided imagery, or	2. Facilitory impulses from the brainstem, e.g., caused by insufficient input from a monotonous environment, or
Cerebral cortex and thalamus	3. Inhibitory impulses from cerebral cortex and thalamus, e.g., caused by anxiety reduction based on learning when the pain will end and how to relieve it.	3. Facilitory impulses from the cerebral cortex and thalamus, e.g., caused by fear that the intensity of pain will escalate and will be associated with death.

Major contributions: (1) An integrated conceptual model for appreciating the many factors that contribute to individual differences in the experience of pain and (2) conceptualization of categories of activity that may form a theoretical base for developing various pain relief measures.
Nature of the gate: the transmission of potentially painful impulses to the level of conscious awareness may be affected by a gating mechanism, possibly located at the spinal cord level of the CNS.
Source: M. McCaffery, *Nursing Management of the Patient with Pain,* 2nd ed. Philadelphia: Lippincott/Harper & Row, 1979. Reprinted by permission.

[42]. The three primary psychologic theories are (1) pain as a consequence of hostility [13,57]; (2) the complaint of pain as a means of communicating and expressing emotion [13]; and (3) pain as a consequence of a threat to body integrity [52].

With regard to the last, the human body is an object of self-concern, and pain is considered psychogenic if the threat is not apparent to an external observer [52]. The three theories are not mutually exclusive as they attempt to deal with pain as a psychologic phenomenon in relation to the other psychologic phenomena that cause it.

Acute Versus Chronic Pain

Acute and chronic pain are quite distinct. They differ with regard to etiology, pathophysiology, symptomatology, diagnosis, and therapy and, thus, require individual consideration. Acute pain is a symptom of disease or injury; the pain itself in chronic pain is the disease [20]. Table 47-10 differentiates between acute and chronic pain.

Acute pain is usually a nociceptive event and, as such, is generally sharp, brief, and temporary; has a known physical cause; and subsides as healing takes place with or without treatment. A well-defined temporal pattern of onset is characteristic. It is a transitional period between coping with the cause of the tissue damage and preparing for recovery. The intensity of acute pain ranges from mild to severe [7,20,25].

As a protective or warning mechanism, acute pain signals the existence of actual or impending tissue damage or the need for convalescent rest. Although it is influenced by psychologic factors, it is rarely caused primarily by operant (environmental) factors or psychopathology [24,35].

Associated with acute pain are somatic, autonomic, psychologic, and behavioral responses. Changes in vital signs are common with autonomic responses; however, their magnitude and specificity are unpredictable. While sympathetic responses are common with pain of low to moderate intensity or superficial pain, parasympathetic or rebound responses often occur with intense or deep pain. Parasympathetic responses include pallor, decreased blood pressure and heart rate, nausea and vomiting, weakness and fainting, prostration, and possible loss of consciousness.

Anxiety often accompanies acute pain and occurs in a spectrum from specific to free floating (Fig. 47-12). Anxiety is normal when its intensity and character are appropriate in a given situation and when its effects are not disorganizing and maladaptive. The interaction of pain and anxiety is cyclic and results in more pain. Anxiety is associated with heightened arousal of attentional mechanisms and increases an individual's readiness for prompt and vigorous action. Anxiety usually subsides or disappears with pain relief [31,51].

Other possible emotional responses to acute pain include anger, fear, sadness, excitement, resentment, and denial. Anger, for example, may result from poor commu-

TABLE 47-10 Characteristics of Acute and Chronic Pain

Characteristic	Acute Pain	Chronic Pain
Onset	Recent	Continuous or intermittent
Duration	Short duration	6 months or more
Autonomic responses	Consistent with sympathetic fight-or-flight response[a] Increased heart rate Increased stroke volume Increased blood pressure Increased pupillary dilation Increased muscle tension Decreased gut motility Decreased salivary flow (dry mouth)	Habituation of autonomic responses
Psychologic component	Associated anxiety	Increased irritability Associated depression Somatic preoccupation Withdrawal from outside interests Decreased strength of relationships
Other types of responses		Decreased sleep Decreased libido Appetite changes

[a]Responses are approximately proportional to intensity of the stimulus.
Source: From C. Porth, *Pathophysiology: Concepts of Altered Health States*, 2nd ed., Philadelphia: Lippincott/Harper & Row, 1982. Reprinted by permission.

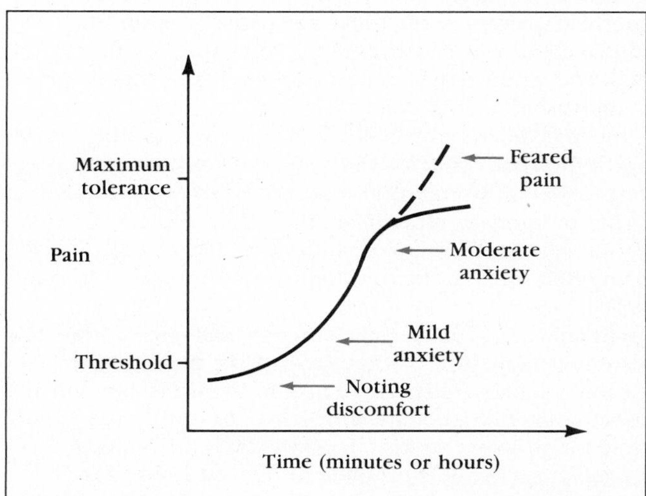

FIGURE 47-12 Sequence of reactions to acute pain. (From R. Sternbach, *Pain Patients: Traits and Treatment*. New York: Academic Press, 1974. Reprinted by permission.)

nication or unmet expectations [26]. Emotional responses have behavioral expressions that include withdrawal, irritability, restlessness, regression, inability to concentrate, difficulty in remembering, and egocentricity.

The physiologic and neuroendocrine responses and the typical psychologic reaction of anxiety associated with acute pain initially prepare individuals for an immediate response and assist them to cope with the disease or injury. Acute pain and the segmental, suprasegmental, and neuroendocrine reflex responses that develop after major surgery or major trauma, however, serve no useful biologic function, produce new nociceptive stimulation, and may cause death. If not promptly and adequately relieved, these responses produce progressively serious pathophysiologic reactions consistent with excessive adrenergic activity and hormonal changes indicative of stress. There is increased secretion of catabolic hormones with a subsequent decrease of anabolic hormones. The intense stress reaction is the primary source of subjective distress and colors the individual's description of the problem [20].

The pathophysiologic reactions, in turn, produce a marked increase in the cardiac workload, metabolism, and oxygen consumption. Gastrointestinal inhibition results in ileus, and genitourinary inhibition produces oliguria. The neuroendocrine stress response mobilizes substrate from storage to the central organs and traumatized tissue and ultimately produces a catabolic state with negative nitrogen balance. The combination of persistent skeletal muscle spasm, bronchial spasms due to cutaneovisceral and viscerovisceral reflexes, and the psychologic response of fear of aggravating the pain result in decreased chest wall compliance, vital capacity, and functional residual capacity. If unrelieved, these responses produce atelectasis, hypoxemia, and pneumonitis [20].

The pain and associated segmental and suprasegmental reflexes and cortical responses, especially excessive splanchnic vasoconstriction, in severe trauma are likely to initiate and sustain the vicious cycle of shock and may ultimately cause death [9]. Blocking nociceptive and sympathetic pathways with local anesthetics soon after the injury, however, can prevent or promptly eliminate the pain and its abnormal reflex responses and thus improve cardiovascular function [14].

Similar deleterious effects occur if there is not prompt and effective relief of the severe pain and associated responses of myocardial infarction, pancreatitis, renal colic, pulmonary embolism, and other acute pathologic processes. Furthermore, ineffective treatment of acute pain often leads to the development of chronic pain states [9].

In contrast to acute pain, chronic pain results from persistent dysfunction of the nociceptive pain system [20]. Chronic pain persists or recurs indefinitely beyond the usual course of an acute process or beyond a reasonable time for an injury to heal. It serves no clear biologic function and is a medical problem in its own right [25].

While the arbitrary figure of six months is often used to designate pain as chronic, the figure is, in fact, inappropriate since many acute processes heal in much less time. Thus, pain that is present three to four weeks after complete resolution of a disease process or injury must be considered chronic pain [20].

Chronic pain creates severe physiologic, psychologic, familial, and financial stresses. Psychologic and operant or environmental factors are often pivotal in chronic pain and the development of its associated behaviors [25]. Management therefore, must encompass treatment of both the cause if known and of the psychologic and social consequences.

The etiology of chronic pain may or may not be known, and its intensity can range from mild to severe. Somatic, autonomic, and affective behaviors commonly associated with acute pain are usually not manifested in chronic pain. These stress responses cannot continue for long periods of time or indefinitely without resulting physical harm to the body [24,25].

Habituation or tolerance to the sympathetic responses and the emergence of vegetative signs occur with chronic pain. Parasympathetic rebound or adaptation decreases the sympathetic responses and protects the body from physical harm [24]. Pain receptors evidence minimal, if any, adaptation. Chronic pain reactions tend to involve hormonal rather than neural processes [9].

Sleep disturbances and irritability are two of the most common complaints. Pain tolerance is lowered, and there is often a loss of appetite and weight loss. Frequently, motor activity decreases because of the fatigue and anergia of continued pain [49,50]. Sleep disturbances, lowered pain tolerance, and depression can result from depletion of central serotonin activity. Central serotonin activity is also part of the endogenous pain inhibitory processes. serotoninergic antidepressants, which are tertiary amine tricyclics may decrease or even reverse the vegetative signs [49].

While anxiety is a common response to acute pain, depression and despair often accompany chronic pain (Fig. 47-13). Depression may result from a sense of hope-

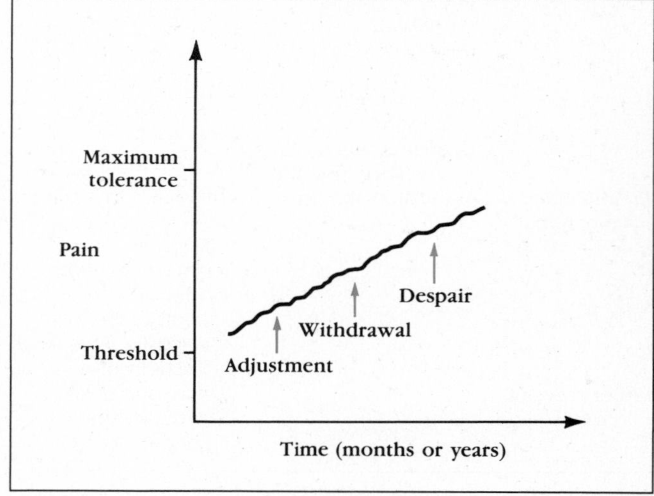

FIGURE 47-13 Sequence of reactions to chronic pain. (From R. Sternbach, *Pain Patients: Traits and Treatment*. New York: Academic Press, 1974. Reprinted by permission.)

lessness or helplessness, feelings of aloneness or isolation, loss of role in family, or loss of job, income, and self-respect. Compared to anxiety, depression is even more likely to exacerbate the pain response and reaction [26]. Pain and depression mutually accentuate each other and quickly establish a cycle of increasing distress. Depression is most prevalent in conditions that result in continuous sensations of pain.

Variations in Pain Response and Reaction

Figure 47-14 illustrates the numerous influences on the T cells in the CNS. It is evident that to change the pattern of output of the T cells, a multimodal approach that incorporates the simultaneous use of several pain relief strategies is necessary [41].

Despite the lack of research validation, the misconception of a uniform pain perception threshold persists [21,22]. *Pain perception threshold* (perception point) is the lowest or least intense stimulus value at which the sensation of pain is perceived [60]. It is an index of minimal pain. The theory of uniform pain perception threshold purports that the threshold is constant and that the duration and severity of pain are predictable. Thus, pain is the same for everyone.

While the theory describes pain as an indication of continuing tissue damage, some researchers have noted that pain may occur in the absence of tissue damage, such as with mechanical or thermal stimuli that do not damage tis-

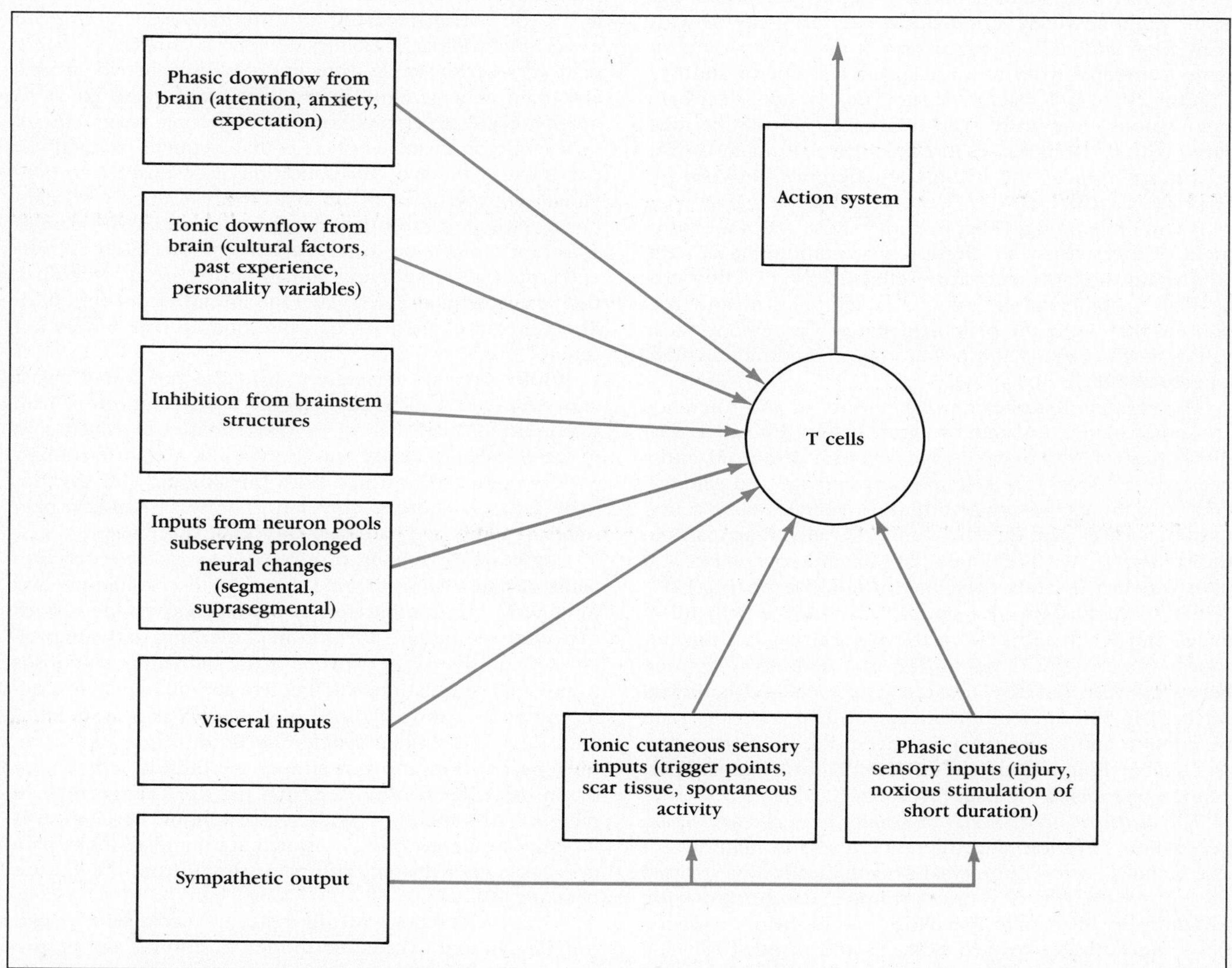

FIGURE 47-14 Diagram of the concept of many influences on the transmission (T) cells in the CNS. (From R. Melzack and P.D. Wall, *The Challenge of Pain*. Copyright © 1973 by Ronald Melzack. Copyright © 1982 by Ronald Melzack and Patrick D. Wall. Reprinted by permission of Basic Books, Inc., Publisher and Penguin Books, Ltd., London.)

sue. Accordingly, chronic pain would lack a physical explanation since it would have to correlate with massive tissue damage [11,17].

Constitutional variations in endorphins among individuals provide additional support for differences in pain perception. Thus, a high or low level of endorphins results in a high or low pain perception threshold, respectively [53,54].

Placebos also produce analgesia, in part by stimulating the release of endorphins [23,25,40]. Not only do they produce substantial relief in many individuals, they are a powerful adjunct to most forms of pain-relief therapy. Placebos enhance drug effects and may be critical in enhancing the effectiveness of other therapeutic interventions that, given alone, are relatively weak. Thus, they may be one of the most powerful available methods to combat pain [34].

Pain tolerance (end point) is an upper threshold; that is, the point at which an individual will terminate or withdraw from nociceptive stimulation. It may vary within the same individual from one nociceptive event to another. Pain tolerance and absence of suffering are not necessarily synonymous. Practically, pain tolerance can only be measured with serial increases in nociceptive stimulation. The *sensitivity range* is the arithmetic difference between the response variables [61].

It was once thought that pain threshold was a measurement of the sensory or physiologic components of pain, while pain tolerance primarily reflected the psychosocial, familial, cultural, and environmental factors. It is now recognized that while the proportions may vary among these values, both sensory and psychologic components affect all pain responses [61].

The results of studies on pain threshold and tolerance are somewhat inconsistent or inconclusive. A positive relationship was found between age and pain threshold, and a negative relationship was found between age and pain tolerance in the laboratory setting [62]. Females were found to have a lower pain threshold and tolerance than males in the laboratory, but the same relationship between sex and pain was not documented in the clinical setting [28]. White subjects showed a significantly higher pain tolerance than black subjects in the laboratory setting, but there was no significant difference in pain tolerance between white and black obstetric subjects in the clinical setting [56,59,62]. While anxiety and fear intensify pain perception and lower the pain threshold, the use of psychologic techniques, such as distraction, lowered pain perception and raised the pain threshold [2,6].

The *cultural belief system* strongly influences the pain perception threshold and tolerance levels in many latent and manifest ways. Zborowski systematically investigated the pain responses of ethnic groups and reported wide variations in overt pain behaviors due to ethnic expectations and attitudes toward sickness and health [64]. The variations also held constant through second and third generations. They were primarily with pain expression rather than pain sensation. Thus, a cultural group's response to pain may be similar irrespective of the underlying pathology.

One religion is dominant in most cultural groups, and individuals practicing within the religion selectively accept certain ethical principles and philosophical views. Religious attitudes influence the perception of the physical self and thus, may also color the pain reaction and response [37].

Individuals in pain display coping strategies and styles that reflect their self-images and perceptions of pain. *Victims* display coping inadequacy and see little need in trying to develop coping strategies. Their self-images are passive, and their locus of control is external. *Combatants* are fighters, and pain is an invading force. They expect others to help them to cope. Similarly, they also have minimal insight or experience with internal locus of control. *Responders* typically view pain as an encounter with impenetrable mystery and actively search for the meaning of the pain. They often continue to think about and analyze pain long after the experience. *Reactors* avoid pain and cope by anticipating and mentally rehearsing the experience before it occurs or recurs. *Interactors* view pain very seriously. As consumers with rights to acceptable pain management, interactors often go so far as to negotiate and develop contracts with people around them.

A common misconception is that frequent past experiences with pain favorably condition or desensitize an individual. On the contrary, increased experience with pain during childhood results in increased sensitivity to painful stimuli in adulthood. Adults are also more likely to perceive pain as threatening and to anticipate more pain if they experienced above average amounts during childhood. Anticipated pain can become an overwhelming threat [37,48].

While probably infrequent, it is also possible for past experiences as well as knowledge or observations of pain to condition the sensation. Psychic stimuli can trigger pain in the absence of peripheral stimulation. Memories of past experiences can produce both physiologic and psychologic arousal. There is correlation between chronic pain states in adults and painful childhood experiences [37].

Cognition or thought processes are important determinants of pain. These include memory, discrimination, and judgment; the comparison of present experiences with expectations; and the attribution of meaning to the experience. Cognitive style explains many individual responses to noxious stimulation. Nociceptive stimuli may evoke different perceptions if the thought processes associated with the experience are different. Because pain is a complex perception and not simply a stimulus sent to the brain, its experience depends on the integration of memory and cognition with sensory input. Perception is incomplete unless the emotional state and thought processes are coordinated with pain stimuli from the disease or injury [9].

While repressors typically react to threat with denial, repression, and avoidance modes of coping, sensitizers react with approaching, intellectualizing, and vigilant behaviors. Vigilance or selective attention allows efficient interaction with the environment through emotional arousal and stimulation of the autonomic nervous, central nervous, and endocrine systems [8,10]. Repressors also evidence a lower tolerance upon a second confrontation with pain than upon the first. The pain tolerance of sensitizers does not change from the first to second confrontation [46].

There is a basic human tendency for cognitive consistency between individuals and their environment. Cognitive dissonance results when two or more elements are psychologically inconsistent, and may produce a tension state that, in turn, motivates behavior [65]. Behavior that results in a reduction in dissonance is reinforced. The manipulation of cognitive processes with, for example, guided imagery or hypnosis, can reduce anxiety, restore a sense of control, and raise the pain threshold and tolerance levels.

Preexisting personality traits also influence the expression of, sensitivity to, and tolerance for pain. While certain features may change with advancing age, personality patterns probably continue throughout life. Pain as a pure conversion symptom is uncommon at any age [23].

Perceptual style explains why exposure to the same stimulus elicits varying estimations of its intensity. The three perceptual types are *reducers, augmenters*, and *moderates* [47]. Reducers tolerate pain well because they consistently underestimate its intensity; augmenters evidence a lower pain tolerance because they consistently overestimate the magnitude of the sensory data. Reducers are also intolerant of sensory isolation, which diminishes the sensory input even further, while augmenters tend to tolerate sensory isolation. Moderates neither increase nor decrease the magnitude of sensory input and are moderately tolerant of both pain and sensory isolation. Reducers, however, tend to tolerate pain for longer periods of time than do moderates [47].

Study Questions

1. How is pain perceived and why do responses to the same level of stimulus among individuals vary?
2. Specifically discuss the role of the endorphin system in pain modulation.
3. Explain the different forms of pain, including referred pain and deep somatic pain.
4. How do the various theories of pain causation and perception enhance understanding of pain?
5. Describe the clinical picture of acute and chronic pain reaction.
6. How do personality types and cultural, societal, and family reactions affect the individual's perception of pain?

References

1. Adams, R., and Martin, J.B. Headache. In E. Braunwald et al. (eds.), *Harrison's Principles of Internal Medicine* (11th ed.). New York: McGraw-Hill, 1987.
2. Barber, T. Toward a theory of pain: Relief of chronic pain by prefrontal leucotomy, opiates, placebos, and hypnosis. *Psychol. Bull.*, 56:430, 1959.
3. Barber, X., and Cooper, J. Effects on pain of experimentally induced and spontaneous distraction. *Psychol. Rep.*, 31:641, 1972.
4. Basbaum, A., and Fields, H. Endogenous pain control mechanisms: Review and hypotheses. *Ann. Neurol.*, 4:451, 1978.
5. Blendis, L. Abdominal pain. In P. Wall and R. Melzack (eds.), *Textbook of Pain*. Edinburgh: Churchill Livingstone, 1984.
6. Blitz, B., and Dinnerstein, A. Role of attentional focus in pain perception: Manipulation of response to noxious stimulation by instructions. *J. Abnorm. Psychol.*, 77:42, 1971.
7. Bonica, J. (ed.) *Considerations in Management of Acute Pain*. New York: HP, 1977.
8. Byrne, D. The repression-sensitization scale: Rationale, reliability, and validity. *J. Personality* 29:334, 1961.
9. Chapman, C., and Bonica, J. *Acute Pain*. Kalamazoo, Mich.: Scope, 1983.
10. Cohen, F., and Lazarus, R. Active coping processes, coping dispositions, and recovery from surgery. *Psychiatry in Medicine* 1:91, 1973.
11. Crue, B., Kenton, B., and Carregal, E. Neurophysiology of pain—Peripheral aspects. *Bull. Los Angeles Neurol. Soc.* 41:13, 1976.
12. Dalessio, D. Headache. In P. Wall and R. Melzack (eds.), *Textbook of Pain*. Edinburgh: Churchill Livingstone, 1984.
13. Engel, G. Primary atypical facial neuralgia: An hysterical conversion symptom. *Psychosom. Med.* 13:375, 1951.
14. Fine, J. Current status of the problem of traumatic shock. *Surg. Gynecol. Obstet.* 120:537, 1965.
15. Foley, K., and Sundaresan, N. The management of cancer pain. In V. DeVita, S. Hellman, and S. Rosenberg (eds.), *Cancer: Principles and Practice of Oncology*. Philadelphia: Lippincott, 1985.
16. Goodwin, J., Goodwin, J., and Vogel, A. Knowledge and use of placebos by house officers and nurses. *Ann. Intern. Med.*, 91:106, 1979.
17. Gorrell, R. The chronic pain patient: Victim or villain? *Ariz. Med.* 32:821, 1975.
18. Grevert, P., Albert L., and Goldstein, A. Partial antagonism of placebo analgesia by naloxone. *Pain* 16:129, 1983.
19. Guyton, A.C. Somatic sensations. II. Pain, visceral pain, headache, and thermal sensations. In A.C. Guyton, *Textbook of Medical Physiology* (7th ed.) Philadelphia: Saunders, 1986.
20. Halpern, L. Drugs in the management of pain: Pharmacology and appropriate strategies for clinical utilization. In C. Benedetti, C. Chapman, and G. Moricca (eds.), *Advances in Pain Research and Therapy* (Vol. 7). New York: Raven Press, 1984.
21. Hardy, J. The nature of pain. *J. Chron. Dis.* 4:22, 1956.
22. Hardy, J., Wolff, H., and Goodell, H. Studies on pain: A new method for measuring pain threshold: Observations on spatial summation of pain. *J. Clin. Invest.* 19:649, 1940.
23. Harkins, S., Kwentus, J., and Price, D. Pain and the elderly. In C. Benedetti, C. Chapman, and G. Moricca (eds.). *Advances in Pain Research and Therapy* (Vol. 7). New York: Raven Press, 1984.
24. Hendler, N. *Diagnosis and Nonsurgical Management of Chronic Pain*. New York: Raven Press, 1981.
25. Hendler, N., and Fenton, J. *Coping with Chronic Pain*. New York: Potter, 1979.
26. Holland, J. Psychological aspects of cancer. In J. Holland and E. Frei (eds.), *Cancer Medicine* (2nd ed.). Philadelphia: Lea and Febiger, 1982.
27. International Association for the Study of Pain Subcommittee on Taxonomy. Pain terms: A list with definitions and notes on usage. *Pain* 6:249, 1980.
28. Jacox, A., and Stewart, M. *Psychosocial Contingencies of the Pain Experience*. Iowa City: University of Iowa, 1973.
29. Johnson, M., and Eland, J. Pain. In J. Flynn and P. Heffron,

Nursing: From Concepts to Practice. Bowie, Md.: Brady, 1984.

30. Kim, S. Pain: Theory, research and nursing practice. *Adv. Nurs. Sci.* 2:43, 1980.
31. Lenehan, G. Psychiatric emergencies. In S. Sheehy and J. Barber, *Emergency Nursing: Principles and Practice* (2nd ed.). St. Louis: Mosby, 1985.
32. Levine, J., Gordon, N., and Fields, H. The mechanisms of placebo analgesia. *Lancet* 2:654, 1978.
33. Mannheimer, J., and Lampe, G. Differential evaluation for the determination of T.E.N.S. effectiveness in specific pain syndromes. In J. Mannheimer and G. Lampe, *Clinical Transcutaneous Electrical Nerve Stimulation*. Philadelphia: Davis, 1984.
34. McCaffery, M. Current misconceptions about the relief of acute pain. In B. Crue (ed.), *Chronic Pain.* Jamaica, N.Y.: Spectrum, 1979.
35. McCaffery, M. *Nursing Management of the Patient with Pain* (2nd ed.). Philadelphia: Lippincott, 1979.
36. McGuire, D. The perception and experience of pain. *Sem. Oncol. Nurs.* 1:83, 1985.
37. Meinhart, N., and McCaffery, M. *Pain: A Nursing Approach to Assessment and Analysis*. Norwalk, Conn.: Appleton-Century-Crofts, 1983.
38. Melzack, R., Casey, K. Sensory, motivational, and central control determinants of pain: A new conceptual approach. In D. Kenshalo (ed.), *The Skin Senses*. Springfield, Ill.: Thomas, 1968.
39. Melzack, R., and Wall, P. Pain mechanisms: A new theory. *Science* 150:971, 1965.
40. Melzack, R., and Wall, P. Psychophysiology of pain. In M. Weisenberg (ed.), *Pain: Clinical and Experimental Perspectives*. St. Louis: Mosby, 1975.
41. Melzack, R., and Wall, P. *The Challenge of Pain*. New York: Basic Books, 1982.
42. Merskey, H. Psychological aspects of pain. In M. Weisenberg (ed.), *Pain: Clinical and Experimental Perspectives*. St. Louis: Mosby, 1975.
43. Nathan, P. The gate control theory of pain: A critical review. *Brain* 99:123, 1976.
44. Nathan, P. Involvement of the sympathetic nervous system in pain. In H. Kosterlitz and L. Terenius (eds.), *Pain and Society*. Weinheim: Verlag-Chemie, 1980.
45. National Institutes of Health. *The Interagency Committee on New Therapies for Pain and Discomfort: Report to the White House*. Washington, D.C.: U.S. Government Printing Office, 1979.
46. Neufeld, R., and Davidson, P. The effects of vicarious and cognitive rehearsal on pain tolerance. *J. Psychosomat. Res.* 15:329, 1971.
47. Petrie, A., Collins, W., and Solomon, P. The tolerance for pain and sensory deprivation. *Am. J. Psychol.* 73:80, 1960.
48. Petrovich, D. The pain apperception test: Psychological correlates of pain perception. *J. Clin. Psychol.* 14:367, 1958.
49. Sternbach, R. Acute versus chronic pain. In P. Wall and R. Melzack (eds.), *Textbook of Pain*. Edinburgh: Churchill Livingstone, 1984.
50. Sternbach, R. Chronic pain as a disease entity. *Triangle* 20:27, 1981.
51. Sternbach, R. *Pain Patients: Traits and Treatment*. New York: Academic Press, 1974.
52. Szasz, T. *Pain and Pleasure: A Study of Bodily Feelings*. London: Tavistock, 1957.
53. Tamsen, A., et al. Postoperative demand for analgesics in relation to individual levels of endorphins and substance P in cerebrospinal fluid. *Pain* 13:171, 1982.
54. Terenius, L. Endorphins and pain. In L. Rees and T. Van Wimersma Greidanus (eds.), *Frontiers of Hormone Research* (Vol. 8). Basel: Karger, 1981.
55. Wall, P. Modulation of pain by nonspecific events. In J. Bonica and D. Albe-Fessard (eds.), *Advances in Pain Research and Therapy*. New York: Raven Press, 1976.
56. Weisenberg, M., et al. Anxiety and attitudes in black, white and Puerto Rican patients. *Psychosom. Med.*, 37:123, 1975.
57. Weiss, E. Psychogenic rheumatism. *Ann. Intern. Med.* 26:890, 1947.
58. West, B. Understanding endorphins: Our natural pain relief system. *Nurs. 81* 11:50, 1981.
59. Winsberg, B., and Greenlick, M. Pain response in Negro and white obstetrical patients. *J. Health Soc. Behav.* 8:222, 1967.
60. Wolff, B. Methods of testing pain mechanisms in normal man. In P. Wall and R. Melzack (eds.), *Textbook of Pain*. Edinburgh: Churchill Livingstone, 1984.
61. Wolff, B., and Langley, S. Cultural factors and the response to pain: A review. *Am. Anthropol.* 70:494, 1968.
62. Woodrow, K., et al. Pain tolerance and difference according to age, sex and race. *Psychosom. Med.* 34:548, 1972.
63. Yates, A., and Smith, M. Musculo-skeletal pain after trauma. In P. Wall and R. Melzack (eds.), *Textbook of Pain*. Edinburgh: Churchill Livingstone, 1984.
64. Zborowski, M. Cultural components in responses to pain. *J. Soc. Issues* 8:16, 1952.
65. Zimbardo, P., et al. Control of pain motivation by cognitive dissonance. *Science* 151:217, 1966.

CHAPTER 48

Traumatic Alterations in the Nervous System

CHAPTER OUTLINE

Consciousness

Alterations in Consciousness

- Coma
  - *Clinical Findings*
  - *Supratentorially Induced Coma*
  - *Infratentorially Induced Coma*
  - *Functional Disturbances Associated with Coma*
  - *Paralysis*
  - *Pupillary Responses in Altered States of Consciousness*
  - *Eye Movements in Altered States of Consciousness*
  - *Respiratory Patterns in Altered States of Consciousness*
  - *Recording Assessments*

Traumatic Head Injury

- Skull Fractures
- Concussions
- Contusions
- Vascular Injuries to the Brain
  - *Epidural Hematoma*
  - *Subdural Hematoma*
  - *Subdural Hygroma*
  - *Subarachnoid Hemorrhage*
  - *Intracerebral Hematoma*
- Cerebral Edema
- Initial Assessment and Management of Head Injuries

Assessment of Traumatic Disruption to Cranial Nerves

- Olfactory Nerve
- Optic Nerve
- Oculomotor, Trochlear, and Abducens Nerves
- Trigeminal Nerve
- Facial Nerve
- Vestibulocochlear Nerve
- Glossopharyngeal and Vagus Nerves
- Accessory Nerve
- Hypoglossal Nerve

Increased Intracranial Pressure

- Intracranial Shifts (Herniation Syndromes)

Spinal Cord Injury

- Morphologic Changes Associated with Irreversible Cord Damage
- Functional Alterations Related to Level of Injury
- Functional Alterations Related to Portion of Cord Injured
- Spinal Cord Transection
  - *Spinal Shock*
  - *Reflex Return in Cord Transection: Flexion-Extension Reflexes*
  - *Autonomic Reflexes*
- Intervertebral Disk Herniation
  - *Diagnosis and Management*

Diagnostic Studies of Nervous System Alterations

- Lateral and Posteroanterior Radiographs of Skull and Cervical Spine
- Cerebral Angiography
- Computerized Axial Tomography (CT)
- Magnetic Resonance Imaging
- Echoencephalography
- Brain Scan
- Pneumoencephalography
- Ventriculography
- Myelography
- Electroencephalography
  - *Types of Brain Waves*
  - *Evoked Potentials*

LEARNING OBJECTIVES

1. Explain the two aspects of consciousness.
2. Discuss the role of the reticular activating system in modulating consciousness.
3. Discuss alterations in the level of consciousness.
4. Explain the etiologic basis of coma.
5. Contrast coma of metabolic origin with coma of structural injury.
6. Discuss the bases of coma from supratentorial and infratentorial lesions.
7. Describe associated functional disturbances common in comatose persons, including altered motor and pupillary responses, respiratory patterns, and eye movements.
8. Differentiate between upper and lower motor neuron lesions.
9. Explain the various types of skull fractures.
10. Differentiate between cerebral concussion and contusion.
11. Discuss type of injury, early and progressive clinical signs and symptoms, and treatment of epidural hematomas, subdural hematomas, subdural hygromas, subarachnoid hemorrhage, and intracerebral hematoma.
12. Describe the effect produced by cerebral vasospasm associated with subarachnoid hemorrhage.
13. Differentiate between cytotoxic and vasogenic cerebral edema.
14. Discuss how traumatic injury may occur to each of the cranial nerves and the clinical findings associated with these injuries.
15. State the normal intracranial pressure.
16. Discuss the etiology of increased intracranial pressure.
17. Describe how intracranial pressure can be measured.
18. Discuss the major types of brain shifts that can occur with increased intracranial pressure.
19. Discuss the medical management of increased intracranial pressure.
20. Discuss the mechanisms of spinal cord injury.
21. Explain the morphologic changes associated with irreversible spinal cord damage.
22. Describe functional alterations in relation to the level of spinal cord injury.
23. Explain the basis for spinal shock and the associated clinical findings throughout its course.
24. Discuss the etiologic basis, physiologic changes, and immediate treatment of autonomic dysreflexia.
25. Describe injuries resulting in intravertebral disk herniation.
26. Identify regions of the vertebral column that are most commonly involved in disk herniation.
27. Discuss diagnosis and treatment of intravertebral herniated disk.
28. Describe the indications for and procedures performed in the following diagnostic studies in head and spine injuries: radiographs, angiography, computerized axial tomography (CT) scan, magnetic resonance imaging (MRI), echoencephalography, brain scan, pneumoencephalography, ventriculogram, myelography, and electroencephalography.

Trauma to the nervous system can result in major changes in physiologic and psychologic functioning. Damage secondary to a primary injury of the nervous system, such as cerebral edema and increased intracranial pressure, may be potentially more devastating than the original injury. Many structural and metabolic processes impinging on the brain lead to alterations in consciousness and varying degrees of brain dysfunction. This chapter begins with a focus on consciousness and its varying levels that is reflective of specific clinical findings.

Consciousness

The conscious state of human existence involves complex neural phenomena that provide for wakefulness and an awareness of self and environment. Two aspects of consciousness are *content of consciousness* and *arousal* [4]. The former relates to mental activities such as perception of self and memory, and the latter relates to wakefulness. The levels of function within the nervous system are related to varying levels of consciousness. In essence, when higher levels no longer function due to various disease or traumatic processes, the next lower level can be observed to function. Consciousness activities are carried out at the highest level, the cerebral cortex; the arousal phenomenon arises from a much lower level in the brainstem structures. The structures necessary for consciousness include the central structures of the diencephalon and projections from it, the thalamocortical system, and the reticular activating system of the brainstem. The cerebral cortex provides perception to the neural basis of consciousness that evolves from the lower levels of the brain.

The reticular activating system (RAS) is important in modulating wakefulness, arousal, and conscious perception of the environment. It evolves from the deep structures of the brain and brainstem to project onto the cortex. This portion of the RAS is known as the *ascending reticular activating* system. A portion of the reticular activating system bypasses the thalamus on its projectory route, whereas another part terminates in the specific nuclei of the thalamus and from these projects diffusely to the entire cortex. The former is referred to as the *non-*

specific or *diffuse thalamocortical system* and the latter as the *specific thalamocortical system* [2].

Peripheral stimulation is transmitted by the afferent pathways to projection areas on the cerebral cortex by way of the specific and nonspecific thalamic nuclei for the perception of consciousness. Chapter 44 details the important function of the thalamus in receiving sensory information from various parts of the body and then relaying it onto specific areas of the cortex. This relay involves a three-synapse transmission to its projection site on the cortex and is part of the specific thalamocortical system. Stimulation of the specific thalamic nuclei gives rise to localized primary responses that may not in themselves be sufficient to produce conscious perception.

The nonspecific thalamocortical system, on the other hand, does not project to specific nuclei of the thalamus, but rather bypasses the thalamus region in groups of nuclei, including the *midline nuclei*, *intralaminar nuclei*, and *reticular thalamic nucleus*. Nonspecific system conduction involves a multisynaptic path with indistinct boundaries and numerous interconnections with the specific thalamic nuclei, before finally projecting to widely distributed cortical receiving areas.

During sleep and anesthesia, transmission of the specific thalamic nuclei remains unchanged, whereas the nonspecific system becomes suppressed. In normal, wakeful brain functioning, a continuous activating flow from the nonspecific system controls the state of consciousness or wakefulness at any given time. This flow is known as the reticular activating system. As the activating afferent flow diminishes, sleep states ensue. Major damage to the reticular activating system anywhere rostral to the pons results in greatly diminished cortical activation, which affects the conscious state.

Investigators have applied electrical stimulation to different areas of the RAS in an attempt to understand its function better. Electrical stimulation of the upper brainstem portion of the RAS demonstrates immediate waking in the sleeping animal and general activation of the entire central nervous system. In contrast, electrical stimulation of the reticular activating system as it evolves from the thalamic nuclei results in more specific activation of the cortex, which allows for mental activities requiring a more direct focus. During sleep, the RAS may be activated by various external and internal stimuli. Some of these are more potent activators than others; pain is a strong activator.

In addition to stimulation of the reticular activating system from the afferent ascending system, stimulation may also descend from all areas of the cerebral cortex. Particularly strong stimulation arrives from the cortical motor projection areas. It is well known that activity such as walking wards off sleep, which might otherwise overtake the individual during sitting or reclining.

Alterations in Consciousness

The most effective indicator of brain function is level of consciousness. A wide range of consciousness, from alert to comatose, may be observed, and subtle changes that affect diagnosis and management can occur within short time spans.

A person with a normal level of consciousness is awake, aware, and interacting appropriately with the environment when not engaged in normal sleep. Therefore, alertness; orientation to time, place, and person; and general responses to the surroundings are evaluated frequently in individuals with cerebral neurologic disturbances. A person whose level of consciousness is deteriorating from normal interactions with the environment may lapse slowly or very rapidly to a totally unresponsive state, depending on the underlying neurologic pathology.

Slow deterioration of the level of consciousness reveals different levels of response that can be observed clinically. The *lethargic* person is somnolent and drowsy, and responds sluggishly to verbal and painful stimuli. Heightened stimuli may be necessary to evoke a response and the person may drift back into sleep soon after the stimulation. He or she may be oriented or exhibit occasional disorientation. As brain function deteriorates to lower levels, lethargy becomes *stupor*. Vigorous and persistent noxious stimuli are applied to evoke a response, as verbal stimuli generally produce little response. The attention span is very short and excessive motor responses may be exhibited.

Further deterioration of brain function is reflected in ensuing *coma*. The first sign is a *light coma* or *semicoma* in which no responses are made to ordinary verbal and tactile stimuli, but motor responses do occur in a reflexive manner to noxious stimuli. *Deepening coma* is observed when reflexive motor responses are no longer elicited in response to vigorous noxious stimulation, and flaccidity of the extremities predominates. Pupillary, pharyngeal, and corneal responses may be minimal or absent. Thermoregulatory mechanisms become erratic and respiratory patterns become irregular.

Coma

The importance of an intact and functioning ascending reticular activating system extending from the midbrain to the hypothalamus, thalamus, and finally to the cerebral cortex was discussed on p. 806. Disruption of the conscious state is commonly viewed from an etiologic basis of *structural* or *metabolic/toxic* origin. Uncommonly, coma has a psychogenic basis.

Persons who experience coma from structural processes have incurred physical damage to the brain, such as contusion, infection, intracerebral bleeding, tumor, edema, or infection. Coma results from structural causes when damage occurs to both cerebral cortices or the brainstem. Brain expansion such as that which occurs in the herniation syndromes may cause secondary damage to the structures necessary for consciousness and result in coma. The distinguishing characteristics of structurally induced coma are focal signs that reflect the area of the brain involved [7]. These focal signs are usually initially unilateral processes such as hemiparesis and unilateral pupillary dilation. Without intervention, the focal signs may become bilateral.

Toxic and metabolically induced coma results from ingestion of exogenous nervous system poisons (toxic) or from disease processes producing endogenous materials that interfere with normal brain metabolism [7].

In addition, coma may have psychogenic origins. These can be distinguished from organic basis by attempting to open an eyelid. Active resistance to eyelid opening occurs with psychogenic coma, whereas with true coma, the eyelid is readily opened, falls back into prior position slowly, and remains slightly open. The cold caloric test is another effective means to distinguish psychogenic from organic coma (see page 811). If nystagmus occurs during the test, the unresponsiveness is psychogenic [2]. The common causes of coma are summarized in Table 48-1.

Clinical Findings. Coma has been likened to sleep. Similarities do exist; for example, both lack conscious behavior, and electroencephalogram (EEG) recordings tend to show slow rhythms. Nevertheless, the differences are striking. Humans may be aroused from sleep, but those in profound coma cannot be. Eye movements are lacking in coma resulting from acute neurologic processes, and rapid eye movement (REM) sleep patterns are not present. As coma becomes chronic, some individuals display periods of restlessness that may be equated with sleep-wakefulness cycles.

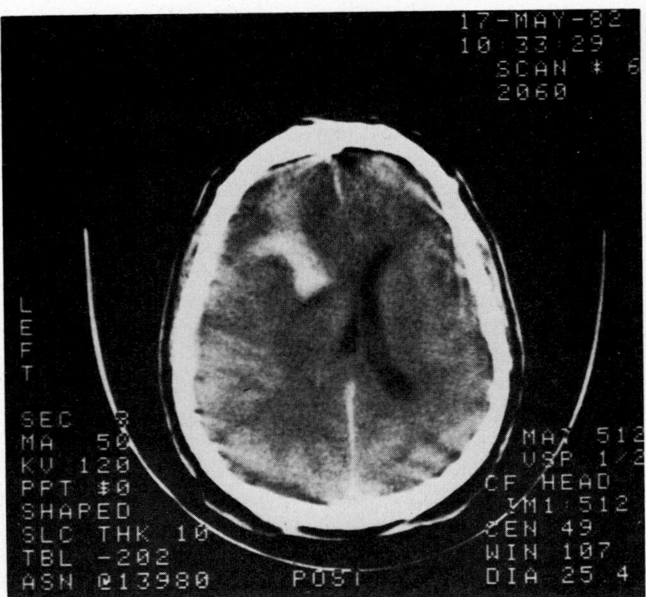

FIGURE 48-1 Intracerebral bleeding in left frontal lobe (*light area*) compression of left lateral ventricle with slight compression of midline structures.

Supratentorially Induced Coma. Isolated, small lesions of the cerebral hemispheres are not sufficient to cause coma as long as the ascending reticular activating system and its connections to the cortex are intact. With progressively larger hemispheric lesions in regions above the tentorium, behavior becomes dulled until maximum obliteration of the cortex occurs and no content of consciousness is preserved. Supratentorial hemispheric lesions produce coma by enlarging sufficiently to cross midline structures and compress the opposite hemisphere (Fig. 48-1) or by caudal compression of the diencephalon and midbrain. Dangerous manifestations of hemispheric compressions include herniations of the diencephalon or uncus through the tentorial notch, which results in aggravating vascular obstruction and accentuation of already present ischemia. Similarly, circulation of cerebrospinal fluid is blocked with transtentorial herniations, and the pressure in the cranium rises. Transtentorial herniation is also accompanied by brainstem hemorrhages and ischemia that is thought to be caused by the midbrain and pons stretching the medial branches of the basilar artery.

TABLE 48-1 Common Etiologic Bases for Coma

Structural processes	*Endogenous metabolic processes*
Supratentorial lesions	Renal failure (uremia)
Epidural hematomas	Diabetic ketoacidosis
Tumors	Electrolyte imbalances
Infections	Hyperosmolarity
Hemorrhage	*Acidosis*
Subdural hematomas	Hepatic encephalopathy
Contusions	Hypoxia
Edema	Hypercarbia
Infratentorial lesions	Hypoglycemia
Hemorrhage	*Exogenous toxic poisons*
Infarction	Sedative drugs
Aneurysms	Alcohol
Tumors	*Psychogenic disorders*
Contusions	Fainting
	Hysteria
	Catatonia

Infratentorially Induced Coma. Coma as a result of dysfunction or destruction of areas below the tentorium may evolve from within the brainstem structures and produce destructive effects on the paramedian midbrain-pontine reticular formation. Lesions external to the brainstem may result in compression of this reticular formation. Lesions of the brainstem may involve direct invasive destruction or compression of its blood supply, resulting in brainstem ischemia and eventual necrosis. The brainstem may be destroyed by cerebrovascular accident, neoplasm, nutritional deficiency, infectious processes, and head trauma.

Lesions external to the brainstem may produce compression by direct pressure on the tegmentum, which directly damages the neural tissue. This may compromise the vascular supply and result in ischemia. In addition, the mesencephalic tegmentum may be compressed through an upward herniation of the cerebellum and midbrain through the tentorial notch. This compression results in tissue distortion and vascular obstruction with eventual coma. Expanding lesions of the posterior fossa (cerebellum) are a common cause of upward herniation of structures through the tentorial notch. Downward compression of the brainstem may result from the herniation of the cerebellar tonsils through the foramen magnum. This results in compression and ischemia of the medulla with resultant circulatory and respiratory aberrations.

Functional Disturbances Associated with Coma. Certain clinical alterations in function often reflect the level and extent of underlying brain pathology. These include alterations in consciousness, motor responses, respiratory patterns, pupillary responses, and eye movements.

In evaluating level of consciousness, the individual's *motor responses* may be significant in relation to the extent of pathology and depth of coma. Limb movement also is a means of assessing asymmetry of function in the nervous system. A consistently justifiable correlation between the level of consciousness and motor responses should not be made, however, as each of these functions is controlled by separate pathways and stands apart. Nevertheless, lesions at certain levels within the central nervous system result in specific types of motor responses that are readily observable clinically and support the level of pathology.

If no response is elicited to verbal stimuli, other stimuli are used to arouse a response. The responses are significant in that they indicate the extent of damage by their appropriateness. Appropriate motor responses to noxious stimuli in the comatose person indicate that the sensory pathways and corticospinal pathways are functioning; an example is an attempt to push the noxious stimulus away. Inappropriate motor responses are stereotyped patterns that indicate the level of damage. *Decorticate* and *decerebrate* motor responses are examples of inappropriate involuntary responses (Fig. 48-2).

The decorticate response denotes supratentorial dysfunction commonly observed with the interruption of the corticospinal pathways by lesions of the internal capsule or cerebral hemisphere. It is clinically manifested by a flexion response of the upper extremities and an extension response of the lower extremities. The arms are adducted and in rigid flexion, with the hands rotated internally and fingers flexed. The decerebrate response is elicited in persons with extensive brainstem damage to the midpontine level as well as large cerebral lesions that compress the lower thalamus and midbrain. Severe metabolic disorders such as hypoglycemia, hepatic coma, and certain drug intoxications may diminish brainstem function and induce a decerebrate response. Characteristic musculoskeletal patterns include extension responses of both upper and lower extremities. Fully expressed, the decerebrate individual exhibits *opisthotonos* (head extended, body arched) posturing, with clenched teeth and arms rigidly extended, adducted, and hyperpronated. The legs are stiffly extended and feet plantar flexed. The extent of the decerebrate response correlates with severity of the pathology and is occasionally seen as wavering back and forth between decorticate and decerebrate, reflecting physiologic changes.

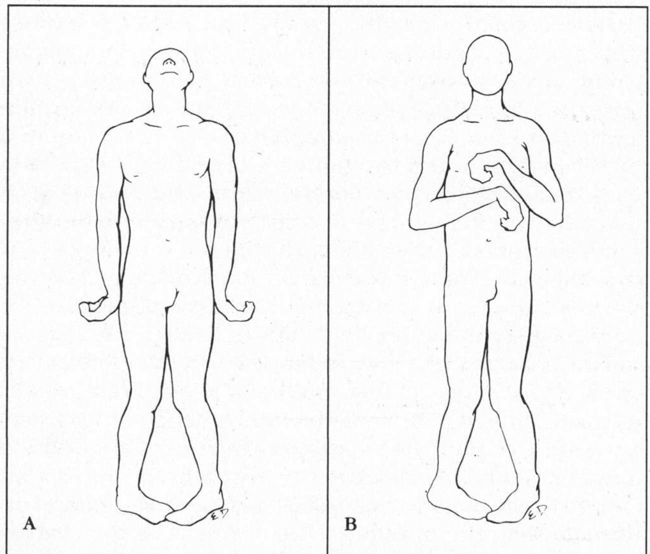

FIGURE 48-2 Abnormal posturing. A. Decerebrate position. B. Decorticate position. (From C.V. Kenner, C.E. Guzzetta, and B.M. Dossey, *Critical Care Nursing* [2nd ed.]. Boston: Little, Brown, 1981.)

Decerebrate responses of the upper extremities together with flaccidity of the lower extremities indicates more extensive brainstem damage extending even beyond the pons level. In certain persons, asymmetry of abnormal responses and normal responses may reflect underlying cerebral pathology. For example, a person may exhibit unilateral decorticate response, or decorticate response on one side and decerebrate on the other side.

Unilaterally absent motor responses to noxious stimuli indicates interruption in the corticospinal pathways, damage to the reticular activating system at the pontomedullary level, or psychogenic disruption. Hyperreflexia and the presence of Babinski's response support structural lesions of the central nervous system as the origin of the coma. Certain metabolic abnormalities, such as hypoglycemia and uremia, may exhibit the same signs but can be quickly confirmed by laboratory studies.

Paralysis. Paralysis, the loss of voluntary movement, is relatively common with trauma to the nervous system. Lesions involving the corticobulbar and corticospinal tracts are known as *upper motor neuron lesions* and result in *spastic paralysis* (Fig. 48-3). Lesions involving motor cranial nerves, whose cell bodies are in the brainstem nuclei, and spinal nerves, whose cell bodies are in the anterior horn of the spinal cord, are referred to as *lower motor neuron lesions* and result in *flaccid paralysis* (see Fig. 48-3). Motor and sensory losses may coexist, and indicate mixed motor and sensory nerve involvement or involvement of both the anterior and posterior roots.

The activity of the reflex arc provides the muscle with tone. Interruption of the arc associated with lower motor neuron lesions results in atony and soft, unresponsive muscle. Voluntary activity and reflex action cannot be elicited when the final common pathway of the lower motor neuron is severed. Deep tendon reflexes are absent also.

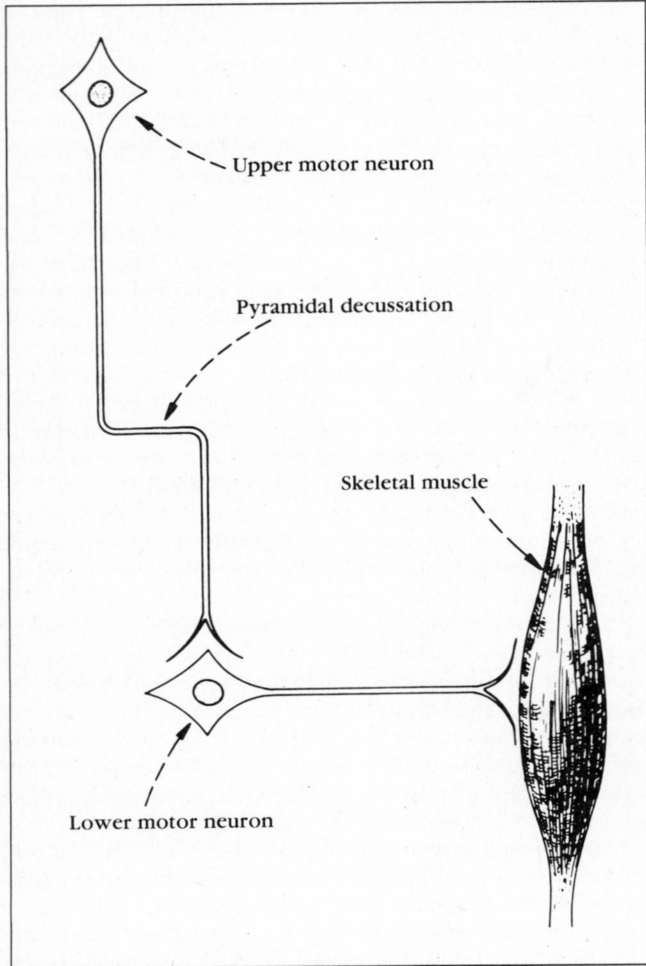

FIGURE 48-3 Traditional concept of motor control. Upper motor neuron lesions produce paralysis, hypertonia, and hyperreflexia. Lower motor neuron lesions produce paralysis, hypotonia, areflexia, and muscle wasting. (From M.A. Samuels, *Manual of Neurologic Therapeutics* [2nd ed.]. Boston: Little, Brown, 1982.)

In lesions of the upper motor neuron, the activity of the reflex arc remains intact, although voluntary control of movement is lost. The pyramidal tract and its collaterals, as well as other descending tracts that influence lower motor neurons, may be involved in the paralysis. The muscle feels hard, is very sensitive to stretch, and is said to be *hypertonic*. Deep tendon reflexes are increased after a period of areflexia immediately after this type of injury. The characteristics of upper and lower motor neuron lesions are summarized in Table 48-2.

TABLE 48-2 Characteristics of Upper Motor Neuron and Lower Motor Neuron Lesions

Upper Motor Neuron	Lower Motor Neuron
Spastic paralysis	Flaccid paralysis
Hyperreflexia (increased deep tendon reflexes)	Hyporeflexia (decreased deep tendon reflexes)
Unilaterally upgoing great toe (Babinski's sign)	Absent or normal plantar response
Minimal or no muscle atrophy	Significant muscle atrophy
Fasciculations absent	Fasciculations present

Pupillary Responses in Altered States of Consciousness. The close anatomic relationship of fibers that control pupillary reactions and consciousness provides a valuable guide to the location of the pathologic processes causing coma. Other origins of coma also may be assessed by the pupillary responses, as metabolic aberrations have little effect on the pupils whereas certain structural pathology produces distinct changes.

Pupillary responses are regulated by sympathetic and parasympathetic nervous systems. A balance is normally maintained by the two systems to produce a pupillary aperture appropriate to the prevailing environment. *Mydriasis* (dilation) is produced by the sympathetic nervous system and *miosis* (constriction) by the parasympathetic nervous system. The parasympathetic impulses arrive through the third nerve from the *Edinger-Westphal nuclei* in the midbrain; the sympathetic innervation arrives by way of a more complex route that originates in the hypothalamus, traverses the brainstem, and travels along with the internal carotid artery into the skull where it reaches the eye through the filaments of the ophthalmic artery and a division of the fifth nerve. Damage to specific areas of the brain produces characteristic pupillary responses that are valuable for diagnostic purposes.

Pupils' size, position, and response to bright light are observed in assessing the neurologic status of the comatose individual. Normal response to bright light in a partially darkened room is a brisk constriction. Other responses may indicate abnormal neurologic processes. In addition, simultaneous constriction occurs in the opposite pupil (*consensual reflex*). Pupils normally are at midposition and *conjugate* (equally coupled) at rest. Conjugated pupils can be noted by shining a bright light into both eyes simultaneously and observing the light reflection on the same area in each eye. In coma, eyes may exhibit slow, random, roving movements that may be conjugate or dysconjugate. These movements cannot be mimicked voluntarily, hence, are valuable in differential diagnosis.

Damage to the midbrain results in fixed pupils that are not reactive to light but do fluctuate in size. Pupils that react imply a functioning midbrain, as midbrain lesions generally impinge on both the sympathetic and parasympathetic eye pathways. Lesions affecting the midbrain most commonly result from transtentorial herniation. Other causes include neoplasms and vascular abnormalities affecting the midbrain. Involvement of the sympathetic fibers, either centrally between the hypothalamus and spinal cord or peripherally at the superior cervical ganglion, cervical sympathetic chain, or along the carotid artery, results in ipsilateral pupillary constriction, ptosis (drooping eyelids), and anhidrosis (absence of sweat) of the ipsilateral side of the face (*Horner's syndrome*). Pupillary light reflex remains intact with hypothalamic damage. The combinations of symptoms indicating Horner's syndrome with central involvement are significant in that they may lead to progressive neurologic deterioration resulting in transtentorial herniation (see page 821).

Pontine lesions interfere with descending sympathetic pathways and thus produce bilateral small pupils. Generally, pupils with pontine involvement react to light, but this may be difficult to discern without a magnifying glass.

Involvement of the third nerve may be observed in comatose persons when lesions compress the temporal uncus sufficiently to cause herniation and the resultant third nerve compression against the tentorium. Initially, a unilateral, dilated, nonreactive pupil is observed, which may progress to bilateral involvement with expanding cranial pathology.

In assessing pupillary size and reactivity to determine the origin of coma, awareness of certain pharmacologic effects may be useful. Heroin, morphine, and other opiates produce pupils characteristic of pontine lesions; that is, pinpoint and difficult to assess for light reactivity. Cocaine dilates pupils through interference with norepinephrine absorption by nerve endings. Ingestion of large amounts of atropine and scopolamine results in dilated, nonreactive pupils, which may give a false impression of a structural lesion. Glutethimide-produced (nonbarbiturate sedative, trade name Doriden) coma results in moderately dilated, nonreactive pupils.

Profound anoxia, usually secondary to severely diminished cardiac output, results in dilated, nonreactive pupils. Metabolically produced coma generally results in pupils that are reactive until the terminal stage and thus provide significant data in differential diagnosis of coma.

Eye Movements in Altered States of Consciousness. Vestibuloreflex pathways proximate areas controlling consciousness and therefore provide for a useful assessment guide. The *oculocephalic reflex (doll's head response)* is assessed by rotating the head from side to side with eyelids kept open. In the positive response, eyes deviate conjugatively opposite the head deviation. As the neck is extended, the eyes deviate to a downward gaze, and as it is flexed, the eyes deviate to an upward gaze. The precise physiologic mechanism responsible for this response remains obscure, although it is hypothesized that it involves either the vestibular system or the proprioceptive afferents from the neck, or both. The presence of the doll's head response indicates an intact brainstem and intact cranial nerves controlling eye movement. The oculocephalic reflex is tested in individuals whose voluntary eye responses cannot be tested due to coma. Absence of the doll's head response indicates severe brainstem dysfunction.

Oculovestibular reflex (cold caloric stimulation) is obtained by introducing cold water slowly into the intact, patent ear canal. Normal response implies that some intact brainstem function is present and is reflected by an intermittent tonic deviation of the eyes to the side of the irrigated ear.

Respiratory Patterns in Altered States of Consciousness. Because of the neurologic influences on respiration in various regions of the brain, respiratory patterns observed during coma are useful in diagnosis (Fig. 48-4). *Central neurogenic hyperventilation* is deep, rapid breathing that generally indicates dysfunction in the brainstem tegmentum between the midbrain and pons. Respiratory alkalosis is revealed by laboratory findings of low carbon dioxide tension and high pH. *Apneustic* breathing consists of a prolonged inspiratory phase followed by an expiratory pause. This pattern reflects pontine-level damage, most generally pontine infarctions secondary to basilar artery occlusions.

Ataxic breathing results from lesions in the reticular activating system of the dorsomedial portion of the medulla and is characteristically a very irregular breathing pattern with irregularly interspersed pauses. The respiratory center tends to be rather hyposensitive, and minimal depression, either with mild sedation or sleep, may lead to apnea. Generally, individuals with ataxic respirations who are apneic secondary to depressant drugs or sleep respond to verbal commands to resume breathing. In severe medullary compression or lesions, ataxic breathing is viewed as a preterminal event.

Cheyne-Stokes respiration consists of a regular crescendo-decrescendo pattern alternating with periods of apnea. It reflects bilateral hemispheric dysfunction with a brainstem that is essentially intact. The hemispheric disturbances resulting in Cheyne-Stokes respiration are generally deep within the brain, involving the basal ganglia and internal capsule. This respiratory pattern also accompanies disturbances of metabolic pathogenesis affecting similar

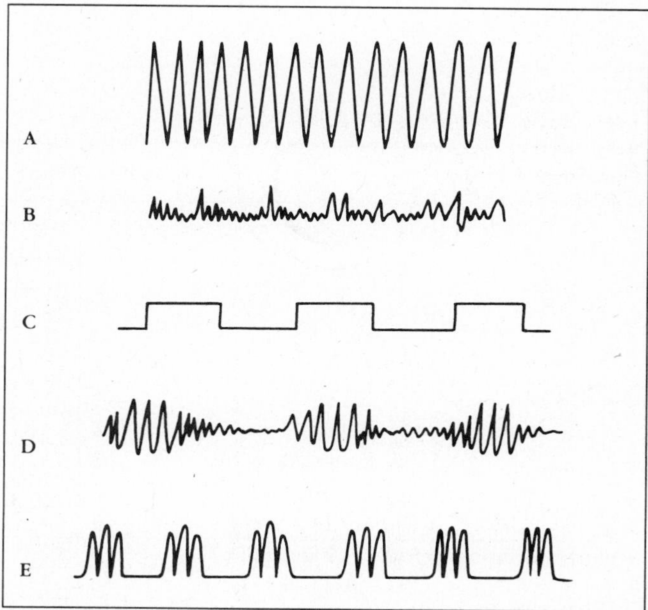

FIGURE 48-4 Respiratory patterns associated with cerebral dysfunction at various levels. A. Central neurogenic hyperventilation (diencephalon). B. Ataxic (medullary). C. Apneustic (pontine). D. Cheyne-Stokes (diencephalon). E. Cluster (high medulla, low pons).

cerebral regions, such as occurs with congestive heart failure. Cheyne-Stokes respiration results from an increased sensitivity to carbon dioxide levels, which leads to hyperpnea (increased respiratory rate). As a result, the blood carbon dioxide level falls to below the stimulatory level and results in a period of apnea. During the apneic period, the carbon dioxide again accumulates to the respiratory threshold level, and cyclic hyperpnea and apnea continue.

Cluster breathing, such as *Biot's* breathing, which is not associated with a regular pattern, may result from damage in the high medulla or low pons region. Lesions in the low brainstem also may lead to frequent yawning and hiccups. The underlying mechanism for this is not clearly understood.

Recording Assessments. Accurate neurologic assessment of the person in a coma is crucial to the correct treatment and best possible outcome. Initial assessment provides a comparative basis for subsequent observations. Changes in neurologic status are particularly important and may reveal serious pathologic processes within the nervous system.

The *Glasgow coma scale* is an assessment tool that has received wide acceptance in both the United States and Europe (Table 48-3). It provides an objective means for making and recording standardized observations with respect to eye opening, verbal responses, and motor responses. The best response in each of these categories is checked at regular time intervals and given a numeric value that, when totaled in all categories, can range from a low of 3 to 14 for healthy persons. It also provides a prognostic guide in that individuals with a Glasgow coma scale score of 7 or below generally have a guarded prognosis, and those having a score above 7 have a more favorable prognosis.

Traumatic Head Injury

Our highly mechanized society has created an appalling number of traumatic injuries, a great majority resulting from use of the automobile. Many of these injuries involve the head. The resulting mortality is associated with injury and compression of the brainstem, cerebral contusions and lacerations, large expanding hemispheric lesions, and cerebral edema.

The cranial vault affords protection to the brain with the hair, skin, bone, meninges, and cerebrospinal fluid. When force is applied, these protective encasements absorb energy that would normally be transmitted to the skull. When the force exceeds absorption capacity, it is transmitted to the cranial contents, and tissue damage results. The resultant injury frequently correlates with the amount of force applied to the cranial contents. The effect of head trauma may be a direct result of the injury or a secondary tissue response.

Head injuries with no obvious external damage but with an intact skull are referred to as *closed*. In contrast, *open head injuries* may reveal penetration of the scalp, skull, meninges, or brain tissue. Closed head injuries frequently result from sudden acceleration-deceleration accidents (Fig. 48-5). The cranial contents shift to the opposite side of the impact within the rigid skull. This is known as the *contrecoup* injury and may lead to contusions and lacerations as the semisolid brain moves over rough projections within the cranial cavity. In addition,

TABLE 48-3 Glascow Coma Scale

Coma Scale Criteria			Time (o'clock)																							
			7	8	9	10	11	N	1	2	3	4	5	6	7	8	9	10	11	M	1	2	3	4	5	6
Eyes open	Spontaneously	4																								
	To speech	3	×	×																						
	To pain	2			×																					
	None	1				×																				
Best verbal response	Oriented	5																								
	Confused	4	×	×																						
	Inappropriate words	3																								
	Incomprehensible sounds	2			×																					
	None	1				×																				
Best motor response	Obey commands	5	×	×																						
	Localize pain	4			×																					
	Flexion to pain	3																								
	Extension to pain	2				×																				
	None	1																								
Glascow coma score (Example findings)			12	12	8	4																				

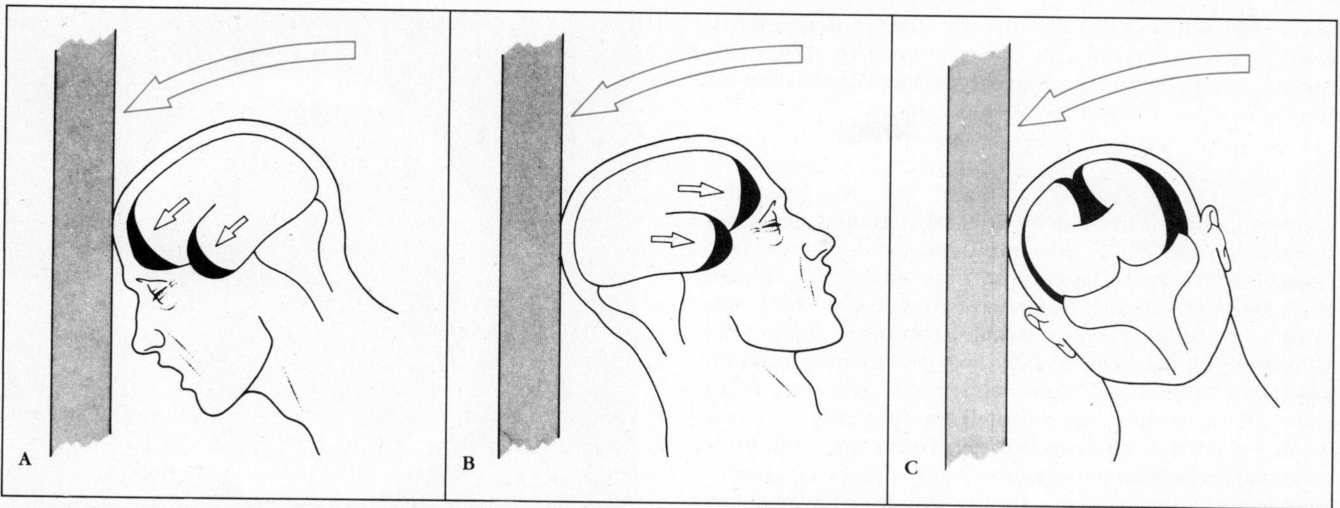

FIGURE 48-5 Cortical contusion with respect to direction of head movement. A. Head moving forward and striking stationary surface: major injury at tips of frontal and temporal poles. B. Head moving backward and striking stationary surface: major injury in frontal and temporal lobes (contrecoup). C. Head moving laterally and striking stationary surface: major injury on side opposite that which strikes surface (contrecoup). Medial surfaces of hemispheres are also injured by impingement on relatively rigid falx. (From S. Budassi and J. Barber, *Emergency Nursing Principles and Practice*. St. Louis: Mosby, 1981.)

the cerebrum may rotate with trauma, and result in damage to the upper midbrain as well as areas of the frontal, temporal, and occipital lobes.

Skull Fractures

A blow to the head may result in several types of skull fractures. Skull fractures may lack significance in themselves unless communication results, with the cranial contents or bone fragments driven into the neural tissue of the brain. These injuries show that a severe blow has occurred to the head and potentially severe injury has been incurred by the brain.

Skull fractures may be *linear*, *comminuted*, *compound*, and *depressed*. The most common linear fractures are simply line fractures without displacement or communication with cranial contents. Comminuted fractures are multiple linear fractures and have the same characteristics. Compound fractures provide communication of the cranial contents with the lacerated scalp and are more serious than linear and comminuted fractures. These require debridement and wound closure within 48 hours. Depressed skull fractures result in deformation of the cranial tissue by bone fragments. They decrease the volume of the cranial cavity and may produce uncal herniation. Venous return may be impeded, and secondary hemorrhages in the midbrain and pons may result. Cranial nerves may also be injured by skull fractures.

Basilar skull fractures involve the base of the skull at either the anterior, middle, or posterior fossa or combinations of the three regions. Although basilar skull fractures may be difficult to detect on radiographs, they do present some characteristic clinical signs. Fractures of the anterior and middle fossae in association with severe head trauma are more common than those of the posterior fossa. Persons with anterior fossa basilar skull fractures may exhibit periorbital ecchymosis, cranial nerve injury reflecting anosmia (first cranial nerve), and visual and pupil abnormalities (second and third cranial nerves). The presence of CSF rhinorrhea strongly suggests an anterior fossa basilar skull fracture. The signs of middle fossa basilar skull fractures include CSF otorrhea, hemotympanium, ecchymosis over the mastoid bone (Battle's sign), and facial paralysis (seventh cranial nerve injury). Involvement of the posterior fossa basilar skull may be indicated by signs of medullary failure.

Concussions

Concussions result in a transient and reversible injury to the brain caused by sudden movement of the brain. Damage may occur in many areas; however, involvement of the brainstem reticular activating system and certain subcortical areas may result in prolonged unconsciousness. This relatively minor injury in response to mild blows to the head leads to brief loss of consciousness due to the temporary physiologic disruption of the reticular activating system. The period of unconsciousness ranges from seconds to as long as a few hours or more. No anatomic injury is sustained, and the process is reversible when neuronal function returns.

Persons suffering concussions are amnesic to the accident and may appear confused for a short period after the accident. The length of amnesia is generally proportional to the severity of the concussion. The longer the period of amnesia the more severe the injury. Generally, neurologic signs return to normal rapidly and further deterioration does not result from the concussion after the initial impact. Invariably, headaches accompany concussions and may persist for a long time after the injury.

Contusions

Contusions result in brain tissue destruction at the area of the blow (*coup area*) or at the opposite side of the blow (*contrecoup area*). The cerebral hemispheres, particularly the basal portions, are frequently involved, as these areas slide over bony irregularities of the base of the skull. Blows to the back of the head may result in contrecoup injuries to frontal and temporal lobes. A variety of neurologic abnormalities may result from ***hemispheric contusions***, even though consciousness may be retained. In contrast, ***brainstem contusions*** result in loss of consciousness from tissue injury to the brainstem reticular activating system. The period of unconsciousness may range from hours to the individual's lifetime.

Visible bruising occurs with cerebral contusions due to the petechial hemorrhage that results from the blow to the head. The injured area swells and becomes visibly red and progressively purple due to venous obstruction and local edema. With large hemorrhages or clusters of small hemorrhages, intracranial pressure increases. The EEG recordings directly over an area of contusion reveal progressive abnormalities with the appearance of high-amplitude theta and delta waves. Regional hypoxia and acidosis may result in the contused area and produce hyperemia. Cerebral oxygen consumption is reduced by contusions, and cerebral lactate production is greatly increased, probably due to increased regional hypoxia and the resultant anaerobic metabolism.

Contusions may be partially reversible, depending on the severity of the blow and the amount of tissue injury. Lighter blows usually result in faster recovery.

Vascular Injuries to the Brain

Potentially catastrophic intracranial processes may result from hemorrhage into the cranial vault from epidural, subdural, subarachnoid, and intracerebral vascular sources. Individuals who are lucid for a period of time after trauma and then begin to deteriorate neurologically are in all probability suffering from cerebrovascular injury and bleeding into the cranial contents. Bleeding into the rigid cranium results in increased intracranial pressure, which is manifested by its localized or generalized effects on the brain (see pp. 821–822).

Epidural Hematoma. A serious sequela of head injuries is the epidural hematoma, venous or arterial bleeding into the extradural space resulting in compression of the brain toward the opposite side (Fig. 48-6). These bleeds can arise in various regions of the brain. Those occurring in the lateral brain tend to be most severe, running a course more rapid than other, more slowly developing epidural hematomas in the frontal and occipital areas. A common epidural bleed occurs as the

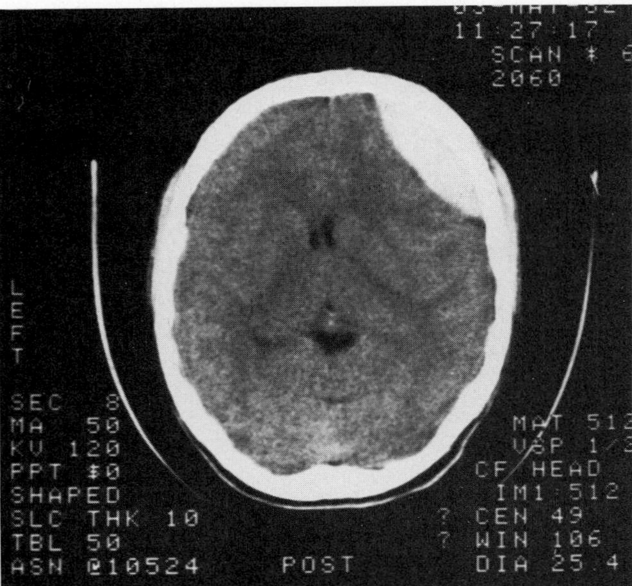

FIGURE 48-6 Epidural hematoma (*light area in well-contained round configuration*) in right frontal lobe.

result of middle meningeal artery injury in the parietotemporal area. This bleed is frequently accompanied by linear fractures of the skull at the temporal region over the groove of the middle meningeal artery. As the blood volume increases within the cranium, the brain is subjected to increasing pressure and distortion, which generally results in a fatal outcome within 24 hours without surgical intervention.

The individual with an epidural hematoma follows a rather predictable course. After the initial blow to the head, a lucid interval of varying length follows, although a brief period of unconsciousness frequently precedes the lucid interval, reflecting the concussive effects of head injury. The lucid interval may vary from 10 to 15 minutes to hours and rarely, days. During this period, a severe headache often occurs. Progressive loss of consciousness and deterioration in neurologic signs follow as a result of the expanding lesion and extrusion of the temporal lobe through the tentorial opening. ***Temporal lobe (uncal) herniation*** compresses the brainstem and presents a rather distinct clinical picture. Deterioration of the level of consciousness results from the compression of the brainstem RAS as the temporal lobe herniates on its upper portion. Contralateral motor deficiencies result due to compression of the corticospinal tracts that pass through the brainstem. Distinct ipsilateral pupillary changes can be observed as the nucleus of the third nerve originates in the brainstem and traverses upward through the tentorial opening. Without intervention, continual bleeding leads to progressive neurologic degeneration as evidenced by bilateral pupillary dilation, bilateral decerebrate response, and profound coma with irregular respiratory patterns.

Epidural hematomas are identified by the initial clinical picture, computed axial tomographic (CT) scan, roentgenograms, and EEG changes. The CT scans provide the most useful information. If a scanner is unavailable, carotid arteriography is used to outline the hematoma. Radiographs frequently reveal the linear fracture in the parietotemporal area and displacement of the pineal gland by the hematoma. The scan identifies any abnormal masses and structural shifts within the cranium. Electroencephalographic readings may reveal diffuse slowing in the waves over the hematoma, reflecting compression of the underlying structures.

Subdural Hematoma. Subdural hematomas are the most frequently encountered meningeal hemorrhages and occur in the *acute*, *subacute*, and *chronic* forms (Fig. 48-7). They may be unilateral or bilateral. Bleeding into the subdural space as a result of injury to vessels may result from either venous or arterial sources, although the venous source is more common.

Acute subdural hematomas result from severe head injuries and may accompany other manifestations of cerebral trauma such as contusions and lacerations; they may resemble epidural hematomas in their neurologic deficits, with rapid deterioration without prompt intervention. The person may be unconscious and rapidly deteriorate, or may be in a lucid state that deteriorates to drowsiness, agitation, stupor, and coma. Signs of brainstem compression may be evidenced by a unilaterally dilated pupil and contralateral hemiparesis. Acute subdural hematomas are identified in the same manner as epidural hematomas. Once diagnosed, they constitute a surgical emergency and must be treated promptly. The hematomas are generally evacuated through burr holes or by craniotomy. Unfortunately, acute hematomas carry a high mortality, even with surgical intervention.

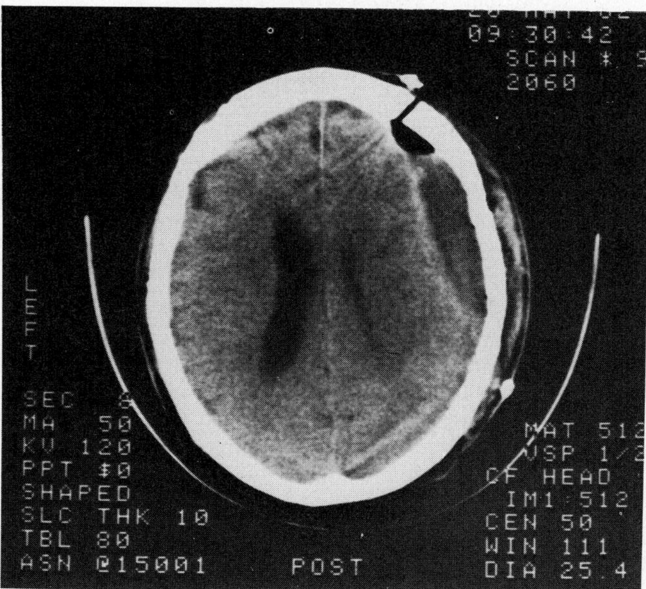

FIGURE 48-7 Subdural hematoma recurring after craniotomy (*darker area in right frontoparietal region*) showing compression of right ventricle.

Subacute subdural hematomas have an improved prognosis because the venous bleeding tends to be slower than in the acute form. The individual is usually lucid after the head injury; this state degenerates to drowsiness, stupor, and coma. The person may stabilize into a coma for a few days and not exhibit the steady deterioration that accompanies the epidural hematomas. The period of stability is followed by a period of fluctuating neurologic signs that progress to increasing intracranial pressure and eventual fatal outcome without surgical interventions. The presence of subacute subdural hematomas is established by the clinical signs and CT scans or roentgenograms.

Chronic subdural hematomas result from very slow bleeding with an insignificant injury. This type of injury is most common in infants, the elderly, and apparently demented or alcoholic individuals. Because the bleeding slowly accumulates as a clot within the subdural space, a period of hemolysis follows. Cerebrospinal fluid is attracted to the lysed blood through osmosis through the arachnoid membrane. The increasing size of the subdural hematoma impinges further on surrounding capillaries, tearing some of these and initiating more bleeding. This increases the osmotic force even further and contributes to the increase in the overall size of the hematoma. The hematoma may eventually form an encasing membrane around it that may calcify, or it may continue its slow bleed and, lacking proper intervention, result in transtentorial herniation and a fatal outcome.

An individual with chronic subdural hematoma may or may not recall injury to the head. A period of weeks may follow during which the person experiences headache, slowness of thinking, apathy, drowsiness, and confusion. He or she is usually conscious on admission to the hospital and may complain of a generalized dull headache. In the early stages, the individual may exhibit some hemiparesis on the contralateral side. With progressive changes, focal seizures, papilledema, homonymous hemianopsia, aphasia, and waxing and waning of the level of consciousness may develop.

Chronic subdural hematomas may be identified by the xanthochromic (yellow appearance) and relatively low protein content of the cerebrospinal fluid. The EEG may show increased slow activity in the theta and delta waves with diminished voltage in the region of the hematoma. Tomographic scans, radiographs, and arteriography may be helpful in confirming the presence of the hematoma. Chronic subdural hematomas are generally drained through burr holes, and this may be followed by turning a bone flap to remove any thickened membranes to diminish the possibility of recurrence. Small chronic subdural hematomas may be managed without surgery. The prognosis is considerably better when proper intervention has been instituted than for the more acute forms of this hematoma or the epidural hematoma.

Subdural Hygroma. Subdural hygroma is an excessive collection of fluid under the dura mater, which most commonly results from trauma. Subsequent tearing of the arachnoid allows cerebrospinal fluid to escape into the subdural space. Due to the vascularity of the arachnoid, some vessels are generally damaged, also allowing cerebrospinal fluid to mix with blood in the subdural space. This CSF-blood mix produces a highly osmotic fluid that continues to pull in fluid; it slowly expands in size.

The diagnosis is confirmed with certainty by burr hole skull opening, although these hygromas may be revealed by CT scan and other radiologic procedures. Developing signs and symptoms of subdural hygromas after trauma are very similar to those of the chronic subdural hematomas. Symptoms are relieved by draining the fluid if a large collection of fluid-produced neurologic deficits and other pathologic processes are not present.

Subarachnoid Hemorrhage. Subarachnoid hemorrhage refers to bleeding into the subarachnoid space (Fig. 48-8). It may occur spontaneously with a disruption in the vascular integrity, or most commonly, as a result of congenital malformations of cerebrovascular beds such as arteriovenous malformations or cerebral aneurysms. It may also result from trauma. Bleeding into the subarachnoid space originates from arterial sources and mixes freely with the circulating cerebrospinal fluid, irritating the contacting central nervous system structures.

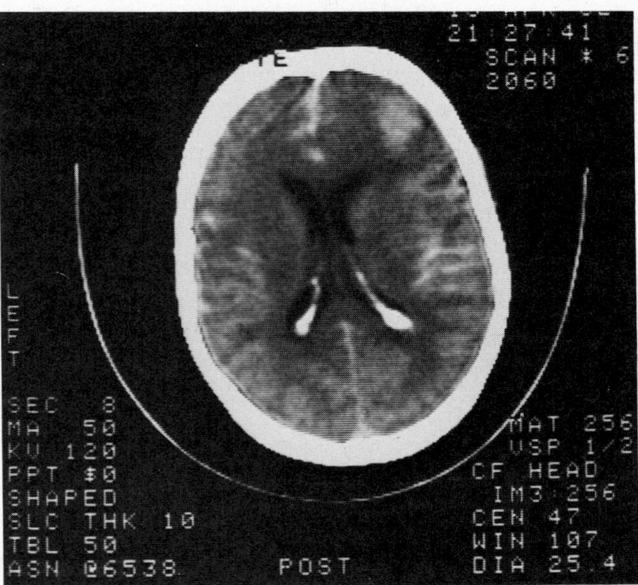

FIGURE 48-8 Subarachnoid bleeding (*light, diffuse areas throughout brain*).

The clinical signs in subarachnoid hemorrhage are generalized and do not focus in the area of involvement; therefore, they are not significant in localizing the site of hemorrhage. They include headache, which is frequently described as severe, violent, or excruciating. Some individuals retain consciousness initially, although about one-half experience a delayed-onset coma. Conscious individuals complain of visual disturbances such as photophobia or diplopia and deterioration of vision. Fever, malaise, vomiting, and nuchal rigidity may be additional clinical findings. Abnormal mentation with disorientation is not uncommon. The spinal fluid is grossly bloody and exhibits increased pressure. Xanthochromia is noted within a few hours of the bleed and persists for about 20 to 30 days. The spinal fluid also shows increased monocytes and protein. Other helpful diagnostic procedures are cerebral angiography and CT scan.

Cerebral vasospasm is a frequent and potentially serious complication associated with subarachnoid hemorrhage as a result of ruptured cerebral aneurysm. It may also accompany the hemorrhage from trauma, tumors, or arteriovenous malformations to a lesser degree. Cerebral vasospasm is the angiographically demonstrated narrowing of portions of the arteries comprising the circle of Willis and its major branches [4]. Symptomatic vasospasm becomes evident about 4 to 12 days after the hemorrhage and generally resolves within 3 weeks. The symptoms include worsening headache, low-grade fever, change in level of consciousness, aphasia, and hemiparesis. The focal deficits are related to the area involved. The exact cause of cerebral vasospasm remains unknown, but it is hypothesized that certain substances such as serotonin, prostaglandins, and catecholamines released from platelets and erythrocytes as well as histamine, oxyhemoglobin, and angiotensin have spasmogenic properties [4].

Subarachnoid hemorrhage may be treated surgically or conservatively, depending on the general overall condition of the individual. Those who are obtunded and experiencing significant vasospasm are generally not good surgical risks and are treated conservatively with strict bedrest until the condition improves or vasospasm decreases. Recurrence of bleeding is always a possibility, and much of the focus of care is directed at preventing this.

Intracerebral Hematoma. Traumatic disruption of cerebral vessels within the cerebral substance may result in neurologic deficits, depending on the location and amount of bleeding. The shearing forces resulting from brain movement within the skull frequently lead to laceration of the vessels and hemorrhage into the parenchyma. Common sites of intracerebral bleeding are the frontal and temporal lobes.

Individuals with intracerebral bleeding may be comatose or may have a lucid period before lapsing into a coma. Motor deficits may be present, and decorticate or decerebrate responses may occur. The bleeding site may be identified by CT scan, such as shown in Figure 48-1, or by cerebral arteriography. The cerebrospinal fluid pressure may be elevated and the fluid may appear bloody and xanthochromic.

Intracerebral hematomas may be treated by surgical decompression through burr holes or by removing a bone flap. Conservative treatment focuses on minimizing cerebral edema and increased intracranial pressure through medications, posture, and supportive therapy.

Cerebral Edema

A common and serious sequela of head injury is cerebral edema, wherein the water content in the brain parenchyma becomes excessive. In addition to head injury, cerebral edema may also occur with intracranial surgery, brain tumors, hypoxemia, infarctions, and infections. Two distinct types have been identified: *cytotoxic* and *vasogenic*. Cytotoxic cerebral edema reflects cellular dysfunction or injury and occurs secondary to conditions that produce cerebral hypoxia. The fluid collection is intracellular within most of the cell components of the brain. The sodium pump is not able to remove accumulating intracellular sodium due to adenosine triphosphate (ATP) deficiency that results from hypoxia. The accumulated intracellular sodium pulls water into the cell. Cytotoxic edema occurs with certain intoxications, hypoxia, some metabolic disorders, and water overload.

Vasogenic edema is a result of damage to or dysfunction in the cerebral blood vessels. The fluid forms intercellularly and its composition is very similar to plasma. This type of cerebral edema results from increased permeability of the capillary membranes and widening of the junctions between the cells. The widening of these normally tight junctions allows plasma proteins from the blood to pass into the extracellular spaces. Vasogenic edema occurs commonly with trauma, inflammatory processes, neoplasms, and vascular lesions.

It is thought that alteration in the blood-brain barrier occurs in both types of cerebral edema. The mechanism of the alteration is not known, but it has been proposed to be associated with loss of cerebral autoregulation. As a result of malfunction of the blood-brain barrier, the brain becomes more permeable to molecules that normally do not cross this barrier.

As cerebral edema increases within the nonflexible skull, clinical signs indicate increased intracranial pressure. If edema progresses, neurologic function continues to deteriorate due to intracranial shifts or herniations. The signs indicating increased intracranial pressure, brain shifts, and herniations are discussed on pages 820–822.

The morphologic changes in the edematous brain as seen at surgery or autopsy are characteristic and striking. The brain appears heavy and boggy. The gyri have lost their normal triangular appearance and the sulci have been obliterated. Brain sections reveal flattened ventricles and an indiscernible subarachnoid space [6].

Initial Assessment and Management of Head Injuries

After the initial ascertainment of an adequate airway, effective respiratory exchange, and absence of acute shock, a careful history is obtained. If possible, the nature of the accident is determined and the lapse of time since the accident is noted. This information may assist in localizing the site of injury and give some indication of its degree. Neurologic evaluation of the level of consciousness, pupillary responses, motor activity, respiratory patterns, and vital signs is obtained for a baseline assessment. In addition, the head is examined carefully to determine the presence of lacerations, foreign objects, or depressed skull fractures. The ear canals are evaluated for the presence of blood, and otoscopic examination of the tympanic membrane is carried out to assess for a bluish coloration indicating bleeding into the middle ear. The presence of ecchymosis over the mastoid area (*Battle's sign*) is evaluated and may indicate the possibility of a basilar skull fracture. Blood from the ear, if mixed with cerebrospinal fluid (*otorrhea*), will not clot and it leaves a halo effect at the periphery of the drainage on dressings or pillow. Drainage of mixed blood and cerebrospinal fluid from the nose (*rhinorrhea*) has characteristics similar to those of otorrhea.

Individuals with acute head injuries should be treated as if they also sustained a cervical spine injury until it is proved otherwise. Pain, if present, may be associated with the area of neck injury; however, this is not a totally reliable indicator of the presence of spinal cord injury, as pain may not be exhibited and cannot be verified in the unconscious person. Careful palpation of the neck and alignment of the spinous process at the midline of the posterior neck should be done to evaluate for possible cervical cord injury. The neck is immobilized with sandbags, cervical collars, or head straps until cervical radiographs indicate no abnormalities.

Vital signs reflect the status of the head-injured person and may support the late findings of increased intracranial pressure or the presence of shock. Elevated temperature may indicate small brainstem hemorrhages or trauma directly to the thermoregulatory mechanisms of the hypothalamus. Focal seizures may accompany acute head injuries and help to localize the site of the lesion. Observations of the nature and origin of the onset of the convulsions are invaluable to the overall assessment of the head-injured individual.

Assessment of Traumatic Disruption to Cranial Nerves

A person with a head injury may suffer partial or total loss of function of cranial nerves in the area of the lesion. If the individual is conscious, the function of each of the nerves can be assessed briefly. In addition, the integrity of several of the cranial nerves can be assessed grossly in the unconscious individual.

Olfactory Nerve

The first cranial nerve extends from the inferior surface of the frontal lobe and mediates the sense of smell. Disruption of the olfactory nerve may accompany acute head injury, particularly in the presence of basilar skull fractures involving the anterior fossa and fractures of the cribriform plate. Nerve filaments may be damaged in contrecoup injuries after trauma to the occipital or parietotemporal region. Other disorders responsible for disruption of the sense of smell (*anosmia*) include upper respiratory infections, rhinitis, tumors, meningitis, and subarachnoid hemorrhages.

The first cranial nerve can be assessed simply by requesting the individual to close his or her eyes and identify some common odors such as soap, coffee, and alcohol. Each nostril is tested individually and the person is asked to occlude one nostril while the other is being tested. First cranial nerve function cannot be evaluated in the unconscious individual.

Optic Nerve

The second cranial nerve is necessary for vision. Visual impulses originate in the photoreceptors of the retinas and are transmitted by way of the optic nerve to the optic chiasm and to the various parts of the occipital cortex for recognition and interpretation. Lesions from trauma or intrinsic origins anywhere along these pathways cause specific patterns of vision loss. Damage to the optic nerve generally results from force to the frontal area of the skull. Vision defects may also result from injury to the vessels supplying the optic nerve. Vision loss is maximal directly after injury. If vision is to be recovered, it may be anticipated within the first month after injury, as optic nerve atrophy begins within this time. Injury to the occipital lobe may also result in impaired vision; however, commonly pupillary light reflexes in this situation remain intact and prognosis generally is favorable.

Careful clinical evaluation of the visual fields can be very significant in determining the site of a lesion. The quadrants of each eye of the cooperative person can be examined individually by superimposing the examiner's eye directly in the visual field of the individual. The examiner closes the eye directly across from the individual's closed eye. The person is instructed to look directly into the examiner's eye and is asked to signal on first seeing the examiner's finger move into the visual field. This is repeated from each of the four quadrants—superior, inferior, temporal and nasal—of each eye. Assuming the examiner's vision to be normal, the injured person should see the finger at the same time the examiner does. A more rudimentary assessment is simply to ask the person to count the number of fingers the examiner is holding out. The unresponsive or uncooperative individual may respond with a blink to a threatened motion toward the head if visual fields are at least partially intact. An unconscious person's ability to perceive light can be assessed during examination of the direct light reflex, as the second cranial nerve forms the afferent nerve for this reflex arc.

A frequently encountered vision disturbance is *homonymous hemianopsia* in which corresponding halves of bilateral vision are lost. In addition to trauma, cerebral infarctions, tumors, and abscesses may cause homonymous hemianopsia. This defect can be recognized by having the individual count all 10 fingers held out by the examiner. Wide turning of the individual's head to visualize all fingers may indicate a homonymous hemianopsia.

Oculomotor, Trochlear, and Abducens Nerves

The third, fourth, and sixth nerves are generally examined together because of their cooperative function in controlling the movements of the eyes. In addition, the oculomotor nerve innervates the levator palpebrae superioris muscle, which mediates elevation of the eyelids, and the constrictor muscle of the iris, which alters pupillary aperture in accordance with the degree of illumination. Similarly, convergence and accommodation are mediated by the third nerve. Pupillary responses are more fully discussed on pages 810–811.

The nuclei of the oculomotor nerve are in the midbrain. The axons traverse ventrally to emerge from the midbrain at the level of the tentorial notch and pass through a portion of the cerebral peduncle. At this level, the nerve is particularly vulnerable to compression from other cerebral structures, and its encroachment is reflected by unilateral pupil change on the ipsilateral side. The third cranial nerve innervates the levator of the eyelid, superior and inferior recti, inferior oblique, and medial rectus. It moves the eyes up, down, obliquely, and medially. The nuclei of the trochlear nerve also are in the midbrain caudal to the oculomotor nucleus, and transmit impulses to the superior oblique muscle to move the eye down and out. The abducens nuclei are in the lower pons below the fourth ventricle floor and control lateral eye movements by innervating superior, inferior, and medial rectus muscles and the inferior oblique muscle.

Trauma of the frontal region of the skull may cause injury to the third, fourth, and sixth nerves. Brainstem trauma may result in difficulties with conjugate movement, and paralysis of individual nerves may ensue in some persons. Upward gaze and convergence and lateral eye movements may be interrupted with brainstem lesions. Numerous combinations of third, fourth, and sixth nerve palsies may accompany injuries to the nerves of the superior orbital fissure. Frequently these injuries are accompanied by diplopia.

In assessing extraocular eye movements, the eyes are observed for conjugate gaze. They are examined with respect to each other and should be aligned parallel in the visual axis when the individual is gazing straight ahead. Extraocular function is evaluated by asking the person to follow the examiner's finger in six cardinal positions. In the comatose individual spontaneous eye movement may be noted. Eye movement also may be noted by assessing the oculocephalic reflex (doll's head maneuver) (see page 811).

Trigeminal Nerve

The fifth cranial nerve is a mixed sensory motor nerve and mediates sensations from over the entire face and scalp to the vertex, the paranasal sinuses as well as the nasal and oral cavities, and the corneae. The motor component of the fifth nerve innervates the muscles of mastication. The sensory nuclei of the trigeminal nerve are in the gasserian ganglion anterior to the pons, and the motor nuclei arise in the midpons region.

The extracranial portions of the fifth nerve are most frequently involved in traumatic injuries. Scalp wounds or compression fractures of the supraorbital area may sever its supraorbital portion. This may be identified by the paresthesias, hyperesthesias, and neuralgic pain that lingers in the affected scalp and forehead. The infraorbital portion may also be severed and result in anesthesia of the affected cheek and upper lip.

Frequent causes of disruption of parts of the fifth nerve are tumors arising in the posterior fossa as well as generalized trauma to the cerebellopontile region or local trauma to the face. *Tic douloureux*, or *trigeminal neuralgia*, occurs primarily in women in their fifth and sixth decades and is manifested by excruciating, unpredictable, paroxysmal pain along part or all of the divisions of the fifth nerve. The cause of this condition remains obscure, but it has been known to be exacerbated by infections, emotional upset, facial movements, and drafts.

Three major divisions of the fifth nerve are the *ophthalmic*, *maxillary*, and *mandibular*. Each of these divisions is examined for touch perception and discrimination on both sides of the face. With the individual's eyes closed, the examiner tests areas with a wisp of cotton and a pin, asking the person to identify which area is touched. The afferent limb of the corneal reflex is mediated by the fifth cranial nerve. The *corneal reflex* is assessed by stroking the cornea with a wisp of cotton from the side while the person's eyes are turned to the opposite side to avoid an involuntary blink.

The motor component of the fifth nerve is examined by having the person clench the teeth and open the mouth while the examiner palpates the jaw. Deviation occurs to the affected side in presence of weakness.

Most of the assessment of the fifth cranial nerve requires cooperation by the person; however, a few aspects may be assessed in the comatose individual. The chin can be pushed down and resistance noted. The corneal reflex also can be assessed.

Facial Nerve

The seventh cranial nerve is a mixed motor and sensory nerve, although its primary innervation is motor control of the muscles of facial expression. Its sensory component mediates taste perception in the anterior two-thirds of the tongue and innervates the lacrimal and certain salivary glands. The nucleus for the seventh nerve is in the lower pons. Certain cortical innervation of the voluntary movement of the face is transmitted to portions of the seventh nerve nucleus by way of the corticobulbar tract. Some of these axons cross to the contralateral nuclei and others terminate in the ipsilateral nuclei. High face muscles are innervated by fibers from both contralateral and ipsilateral fibers, and the lower muscles are innervated by fibers from the contralateral cortex only. Weakness generated from the effects on the corticobulbar tract are of central origin (upper motor neuron) and cause only contralateral lower face weakness. Ipsilateral weakness of an entire side of the face is of peripheral origin (lower motor neuron) from a lesion at the nucleus or the peripheral axon of the seventh nerve.

Dysfunction of the seventh nerve may occur with basilar skull fractures, as its location traversing the temporal bone makes it particularly susceptible to injury. Fractures of the petrous portions of the temporal bone may result in injury to the seventh nerve and resultant facial paralysis. In such situations, the prognosis is generally favorable, and function returns with slow recovery that may last for months.

Proximity of the seventh nerve to the middle ear increases the injurious effects of middle ear infections and tumors of the region on the nerve. Central facial paralysis can result from infarctions, lesions, and abscesses of the contralateral cerebral cortex. *Bell's palsy* is an inflammatory response to infections and allergies affecting the seventh nerve within the temporal bone, which results in ipsilateral facial paralysis.

Assessment of the facial nerve includes examining facial tone and symmetry by requesting the person to wrinkle the forehead, smile, whistle, close the eyes, and show the teeth. The sensory component can be assessed by applying sweet, sour, salty, and bitter substances to the appropriate areas of the anterior tongue and having the person identify the tastes. The mouth is rinsed between applications of the substances.

In the comatose person the corneal reflex may be assessed as the efferent limb of the reflex is mediated by the facial nerve. In addition, facial grimacing can be noted in response to noxious stimulation.

Vestibulocochlear Nerve

The eighth cranial nerve is composed of the vestibular and cochlear divisions, the former mediating balance and equilibrium and the latter hearing. Nuclei of the acoustic nerve are in the lower pons (see Chap. 45).

Traumatic head injury may result in loss of hearing due to fractures extending through the middle ear. Severing of the nerve results in permanent deafness. Hemorrhage into the middle ear also compromises hearing; however, it does carry a prognosis of some recovery of hearing as the blood clot is absorbed. Edema and contusions of the eighth nerve result in hearing impairments that recover with the healing process. Vertigo results from edema or hemorrhage into the labyrinth, which is aggravated by head movement and associated with nausea and vomiting. Although vertigo may be resolved within two or three weeks, the person may continue to feel lightheaded and reveal signs of ataxia for months after the injury. True vertigo results from labyrinthine disease. The classic type is Meniere's disease (see page 763).

Hearing can be assessed simply by covering one of the person's ears and whispering softly near the other. This is repeated in the other ear. Ability to hear whispering is fairly indicative of normal hearing. Should whispering not be audible, further testing is indicated. The vestibular component is investigated primarily through a described history of vertigo, unsteadiness of gait, and nausea. Testing is undertaken on the basis of the presence of the above symptoms.

Hearing can be assessed grossly in the comatose individual by noting the response to noise or verbal stimuli. Lack of response may also indicate deep coma. The vestibular component may be assessed by the oculocephalic or oculovestibular reflexes.

Glossopharyngeal and Vagus Nerves

The ninth and tenth nerves are anatomically and structurally similar and therefore are examined together. The glossopharyngeal nerve innervates the muscles of the pharynx, posterior one-third of the taste sensation of the tongue, sensations of the tonsils, pharynx, and carotid sinuses, and carotid body. The vagus nerve has widespread innervation of the thoracic and abdominal visceral organs, as well as the larynx and pharynx. The nuclei of these nerves are in the medulla.

Traumatic injury to the lower brainstem, fractures of the posterior fossa, and vascular injuries at the base of the skull may injure the ninth and tenth nerves. This is reflected in dysphagia and a diminished or absent gag reflex.

Assessment of the ninth and tenth cranial nerves involves an initial inspection of the soft palate for symmetry. A gag reflex is elicited with a tongue blade in contact with the posterior oropharynx. Normally, the palate elevates and the pharyngeal muscles contract. The person is asked to swallow water, and the ability to do this without regurgitating is assessed. Speech is noted for signs of abnormal phonation and hoarseness. The gag and swallowing reflexes are routinely assessed in the comatose individual by noting the ability to handle secretions. This indicates gross function of the ninth and tenth cranial nerves.

Accessory Nerve

The eleventh cranial nerve nuclei are in the anterior gray column of the first few segments of the cervical spinal cord and transmit to innervate the sternocleidomastoid and trapezius muscles to allow lifting or shrugging of shoulders, head rotation, and neck extension. Low brainstem injuries and fractures of the posterior fossa and basilar skull may result in injury and paralysis of the eleventh nerve. In addition, trauma to the neck region may result in impairment of the spinal accessory nerve. Weakness on one side may be suggestive of a stroke, whereas bilateral weakness may support motor neuron diseases or neuromuscular problems.

The functioning of this motor nerve in innervating the sternocleidomastoid is evaluated by having the individual turn the head toward the shoulder while the examiner puts resistance on the movement and assesses the strength of the muscle. This test is repeated on the other side. The functioning of the trapezius is evaluated by having the person raise the shoulders against the resistance applied by the examiner. Assessment of this cranial nerve requires cooperation, and therefore its integrity cannot be determined in a comatose individual.

Hypoglossal Nerve

The twelfth cranial nerve is a motor nerve innervating the musculature of the tongue to allow normal articulation and food management in the mouth. Its nucleus is in the floor of the fourth ventricle. The function of the hypoglossal nerve may be jeopardized by trauma to the neck as well as to the regions described in the eleventh nerve injuries. Traumatic lesion here may result in unilateral tongue weakness, which is evidenced by deviation of the protruding tongue to the weak side. Bilateral tongue weakness is most commonly associated with disease processes such as amyotrophic lateral sclerosis and poliomyelitis.

The function of the hypoglossal nerve is evaluated by having the individual protrude the tongue and observing for any deviation. The strength of the muscles of the tongue is assessed by the examiner by pushing against the cheek that the person is pressing outward with the tongue. Notation is made of any difficulty with articulation during conversation. In the comatose individual one can note the position and movement of the tongue when the mouth is opened. The tongue normally lies in the midline and deviation to either side is abnormal.

Increased Intracranial Pressure

Head injuries frequently result in increased intracranial pressure due to expanding lesions and accumulation of edema. Without treatment, this may compromise neurologic function as well as life itself. Therefore, early diagnosis and treatment are essential.

In the adult, the cranial vault affords a nonflexible encasement around the brain tissue, extracellular fluid (primarily blood), and cerebrospinal fluid. Although total intracranial volume alters slightly, intracranial pressure remains relatively constant. Small increases in volume of one of the cranial components are compensated normally by a decrease in the volume of another (Monro-Kellie hypothesis). Intracranial cerebrospinal fluid may be shifted to the subarachnoid space of the spine, and the vascular bed of the brain may be reduced by shifting the blood to areas of less resistance. Intracranial compliance, the ability of the cranial contents to adapt to changes in volume, is determined by the volume and rate of displacement of intracranial tissue, blood, and CSF. During the period of compensation when the volume/pressure curves are increasing slowly, large intracranial volume increases can be tolerated without significant intracranial pressure changes. When the small margin of compensation within the cranium is exhausted, however, the intracranial pressure rises, and small increases in volume at this point result in large rises in intracranial pressure (Fig. 48-9). Without intervention, decompensation and death ensue.

Traditional clinical indicators of increased intracranial pressure include headache, recurrent vomiting, decreased level of consciousness, papilledema, pupillary dilation, peripheral motor changes, decreasing pulse, elevated systolic pressure, widening pulse pressure, and respiratory irregularities. The varying presence of these signs indicates the level of brain dysfunction that has occurred as a result of the pathologic process that led to the increased intracranial pressure. Generally, when the classic clinical indicators are present, the individual has reached a state of

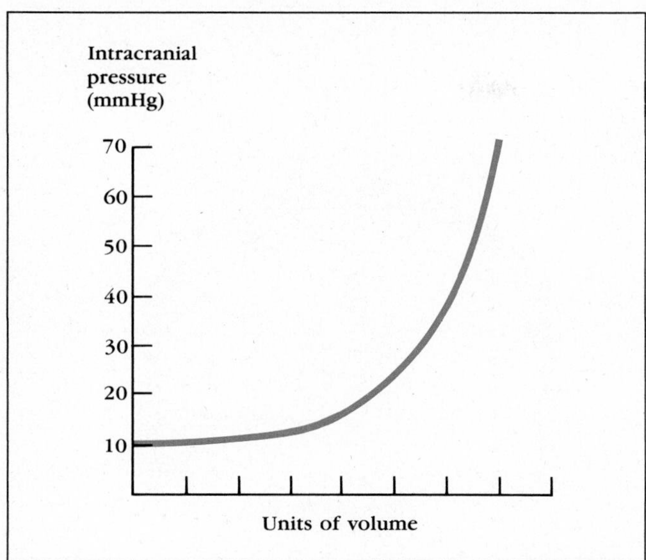

FIGURE 48-9 Compliance curve: intracranial volume/pressure relationship. Compensation rapidly falls as volume rises. (From B. Jennett, *An Introduction to Neurosurgery* [3rd ed.]. London: Heinemann, 1977.)

decompensation and has a poor prognosis for recovery. Treatment is most effective while the brain is in a compensatory state, because once compensatory mechanisms have been used up, the pressure within the cranium rises rapidly.

Intracranial monitoring provides a means to detect changes in pressure before clinical signs are evident. This is most conveniently done by measuring cerebrospinal fluid as pressure is equally transmitted in all directions in fluid. Changes in intracranial pressure (ICP) can be monitored by the use of a subdural screw, an epidural device, or through the lateral ventricles with an intraventricular cannula (Fig. 48-10). Normal intracranial pressures range from 0 to 13 mm Hg or 50 to 200 mm of water. Some fluctuations over the narrow normal range are common. The pressures measured by these methods are transmitted to a pressure transducer and recording instrument. The mechanical impulses transmitted to the transducer are converted into electrical impulses that appear on an oscilloscope as varying wave patterns (Fig. 48-11). The most significant of these are the plateau waves (A waves) that are recorded with advanced stages of increased intracranial pressure.

The pressure in the cranium may rise rather abruptly or insidiously. Severely head-injured individuals with rapidly increasing intracranial pressure and intracranial bleeding frequently have escape of blood into the cerebrospinal fluid, which results in an increased osmotic force, thus increasing cerebrospinal fluid volume. Increased intracranial pressure also occurs with infections, tumors, and hypercapnia. Tissue expands with inflammatory and neoplastic processes, and the cerebral vasculature increases in size in response to elevated carbon dioxide levels. Expansion of the volume of tissue and cerebrospinal fluid results in compression of cerebral vessels and, in turn, a reflexively higher arterial blood pressure, resulting in a lower pulse rate and shifting of cerebral structures. Supratentorial structural displacements result in characteristic clinical changes as previously uninvolved cerebral tissues are being encroached upon. With progressive expansion, the tissue eventually protrudes through the tentorial notch, which is the only opening available.

Intracranial Shifts (Herniation Syndromes)

Major brain shifts that can occur in response to expanding cerebral pathology are *cingulate herniation*, *transcalvarial herniation*, *central transtentorial herniation*, *uncal herniation*, and *cerebellar foramen magnum herniation* (Fig. 48-12). These develop as the cranial contents are subdivided by a rather rigid membrane, the dura. The falx cerebri divides the cerebral hemispheres, and the tentorium cerebelli divides the cerebrum from the cerebellum.

In cingulate herniation, lateral displacement of expanding cerebral lesions compresses the cingulate gyrus under the falx cerebri, which displaces the internal cerebral vein. This displacement results in the vessel compression and leads to ischemia, thus potentially further increasing the cerebral contents with the resultant edema. Transcalvarial herniation occurs with open head injuries where the brain tissue extrudes through an unstable fractured skull.

Central transtentorial herniation may result from supratentorial lesions; however, they are more commonly a result of diffuse increased intracranial pressure, such as in Reye's syndrome. Pressure is exerted centrally and downward displacement occurs, encroaching on the diencephalon and midbrain. Cingulate herniation may precede the central transtentorial herniation.

Clinical signs of central transtentorial herniation reflect increasing intracranial pressure and include changes in alertness and visual acuity. Papilledema results from optic nerve compression as interference occurs with venous return from the optic disk. As central expansion progresses caudally, brainstem compression is reflected clinically by a further deteriorating level of consciousness. With compression of the corticospinal tract, the Babinski's response is elicited and the extremities become rigid and deteriorate to a decorticate or a decerebrate response. Early central herniation exhibits pupillary constriction, which leads to moderate dilation without light reflex response as increasing pressure is exerted on the midbrain region. Wide, fixed dilation is a terminal sign. Respiratory patterns initially may be periodic with yawning and sighing interruptions. This changes to a persistent hyperventilation as central compression continues caudally and, in terminal stages, becomes an ataxic pattern prior to respiratory arrest.

Lesions in the lateral middle fossa or medial part of one temporal lobe result in *uncal herniation*. Crowding at the tentorial notch compresses the third nerve, which results in a unilaterally dilated pupil. This is the classic initial characteristic of uncal herniation. Neurologic deterioration may progress rapidly without successful intervention

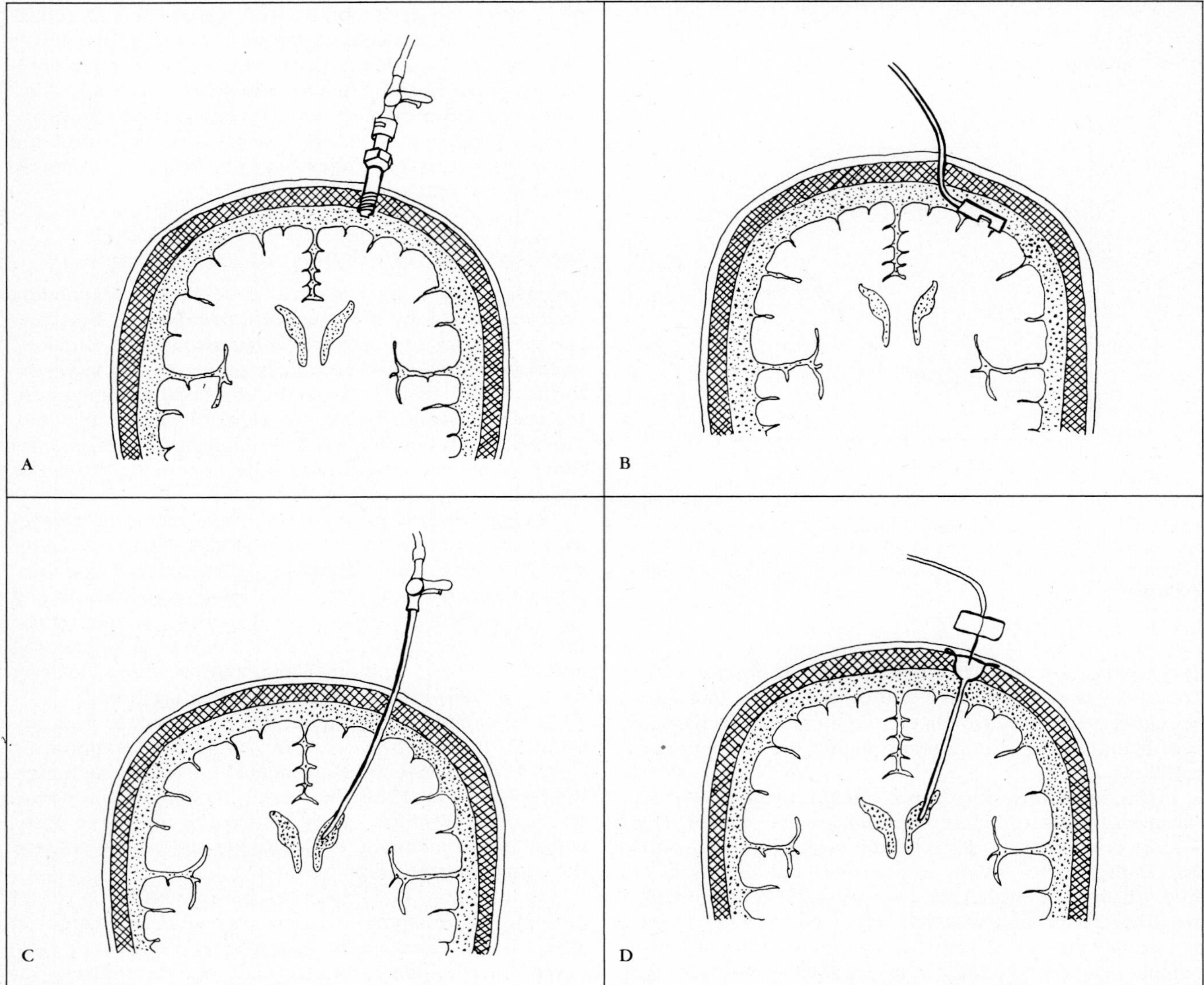

FIGURE 48-10 Devices used to measure intracranial pressure. A. Subdural screw. B. Epidural device. C. Intraventricular catheter. D. Intraventricular cannula. (From Massachusetts General Hospital Department of Nursing, *Manual of Nursing Procedures* [2nd ed.]. Boston: Little, Brown, 1980.)

after the initial pupillary dilation, to stupor, absence of extraocular movement (EOM), hemiplegia, and decerebrate posturing. Terminal stages of uncal herniation resemble central herniation.

Cerebellar foramen magnum herniation results from the expanding lesions of the cerebellum and may be unilateral or bilateral displacement. The expanding lesions may be caused by centrally placed frontal tumors or generalized brain swelling such as in Reye's syndrome, or arise in association with uncal herniation. The effects of cerebellar foramen magnum herniation and traumatic, rapidly expanding lesions below the tentorium result in rapid loss of consciousness and neurologic deficits indicating severe dysfunction. The dysfunction is caused by the direct effects on the vital centers in the brainstem and the inability of the subtentorial contents to compensate adequately. Motor responses vary from flaccidity to flexor to extension responses. Low brainstem breathing patterns such as apneustic and ataxic breathing predominate. Lesions of the medulla result in rapid neurologic deterioration, leading to death as centers controlling respiratory and vasomotor function become dysfunctional.

Spinal Cord Injury

Injuries of the spinal cord as a result of trauma are increasing every year due to the extensive use of the automobile and increased amount of time persons spend in recreation and sports activities. The extent and level of spinal cord

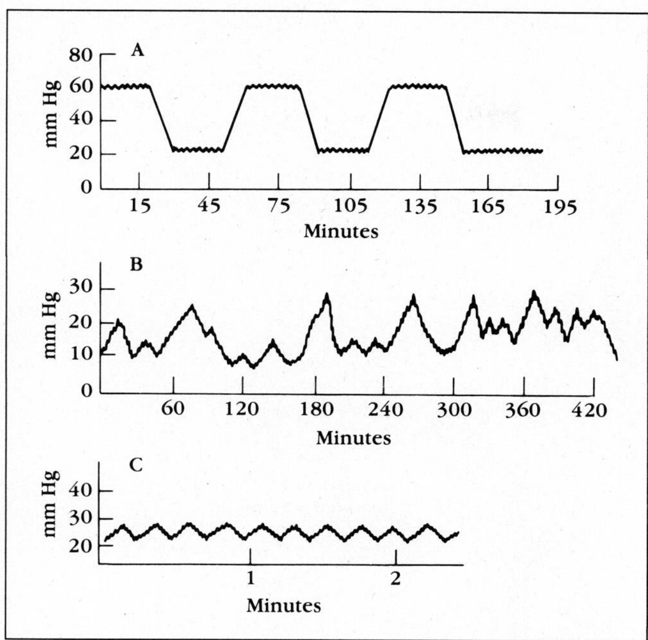

FIGURE 48-11 Generalized shapes of the three types of ICP waves: A, or plateau, waves (*top*), B waves (*middle*), and C waves (*bottom*). (From A. Hamilton, *Critical Care Nursing Skills.* New York: Appleton-Century-Crofts, 1981.)

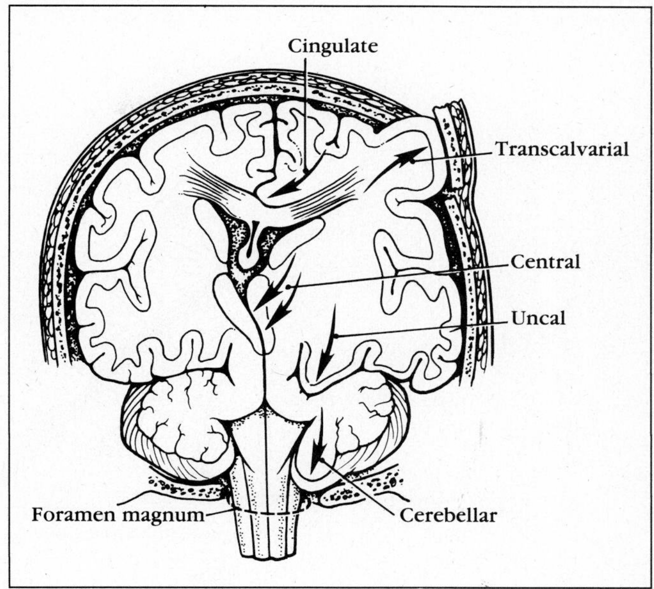

FIGURE 48-12 Major types of intracranial herniations.

injury vary widely. Whiplash may result in very minor discomfort from the mild flexion-extension type of cord injuries, whereas total quadriplegia may result from severe fracture dislocations of the cervical vertebral column and serious cord damage. Trauma to the spinal cord can occur at any level, although the areas most frequently damaged are the cervical spine and lower thoracic spine.

Common mechanisms of spinal cord injury from traumatic impact include the hyperextension or hyperflexion type of injury, frequently accompanied by rotational movement of the cord (Fig. 48-13). The resultant spinal cord damage may be transient or permanent depending on the extent of parenchymal damage. Injuries similar to those that occur to the brain can also occur to the spinal cord, including concussion, contusion, hemorrhage, lacerations, and compression. Associated vertebral injuries may lead to spinal cord damage in subluxation, compression fractures, and fracture dislocations as well as the other vertebral injuries noted in Figure 48-14. The extent of cord damage in vertebral injuries is related to the degree of bony encroachment or compression on the cord. Severe injuries result in partial or complete functional transection of the spinal cord.

Morphologic Changes Associated with Irreversible Cord Damage

Experimentally induced spinal cord injury in laboratory animals has provided insight into the structural changes occurring at varying times after injury. A force strong enough to result in irreversible total paraplegia causes severe edema and hemorrhage within a few hours, which then leads to massive necrosis and finally, parenchymal and vessel destruction.

Immediately after cord injury, focal hemorrhages begin in the gray matter and rapidly increase in size until the entire gray matter is hemorrhagic and necrotic. The hemorrhages in the white matter proximal to the gray matter do not coalesce but are associated with massive edema that envelops all of the white matter. It has been speculated that norepinephrine, which is released in large amounts by the traumatized cord, contributes to the hemorrhagic necrosis caused by direct physical damage [3]. The lesion is progressive for several hours. After the injury, the hemorrhage into the gray matter is present within 1 hour, fluid in between the axons is present in 15 minutes, and disintegration of the myelin sheath and axonal shrinkage occurs within 1 to 4 hours [6].

Functional Alterations Related to Level of Injury

Cervical spine injuries occurring above the fourth cervical segment (C-4) may be fatal, as innervation of the diaphragm and intercostal muscles may be obliterated by the injury and the individual dies from respiratory failure. With increasing sophistication of the public in knowledge and technique of cardiopulmonary resuscitation, increasing numbers of these victims arrive at emergency medical facilities. In addition, high cervical cord transection results in quadriplegia.

Persons with transection injuries below the fifth cervical segment (C-5) have full innervation of the sternocleidomastoid, trapezius, and other muscles, and therefore retain neck, shoulder, and scapula movement. Individuals with lesions at the sixth cervical segment (C-6) have the

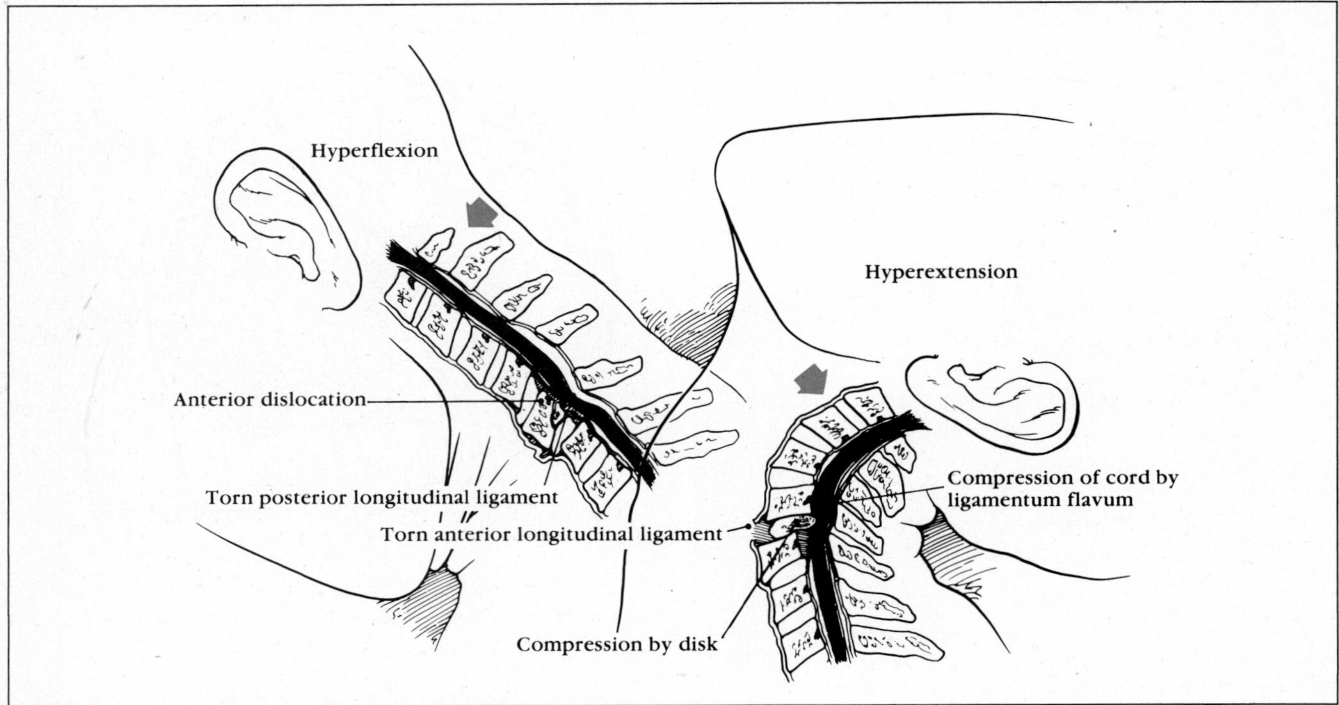

FIGURE 48-13 Mechanism of spinal injury. (From C.V. Kenner, C.E. Guzzetta, and B.M. Dossey, *Critical Care Nursing* (2nd ed.). Boston: Little, Brown, 1985.)

function of the shoulder and elbow, and partial function of the wrist. Complete innervation of the rotator muscles of the shoulder is retained and partial innervation is transmitted to the serratus, pectoralis major, and latissimus dorsi muscles. Wrist muscles and the biceps retain innervation allowing for elbow and wrist flexion.

Persons with these injuries at the seventh (C-7) and eighth (C-8) cord segments exhibit additional elbow, wrist, and hand function. Innervation is intact to the triceps and common and long finger extensors, enabling elbow extension and flexion, and functional, although weak, finger extension and flexion

Transection injuries to the region of the *thoracic* and *lumbar* cord render the victim paraplegic (Fig. 48-15). Those with high thoracic injury, of first thoracic segment (T-1), retain full innervation of upper extremity musculature. Injuries experienced at the sixth thoracic segment (T-6) allow the person to have an increased respiratory reserve as intercostal innervation is intact. Those experiencing twelfth thoracic segment (T-12) lesions have partial innervation to the lower extremities and may, in fact, regain ambulation when supported by long-leg braces and assisted by crutches.

Persons who sustain *low lumbar* and *sacral* cord lesions have full innervation to upper extremities and trunk, hip flexors and extensors, knee extensors, and ankle movement. Therefore, they are able to ambulate with minimal supportive devices.

Functional Alterations Related to Portion of Cord Injured

Central cord lesions (central cord syndrome) can occur at different levels of the spinal cord; symptoms vary with the extent of hemorrhage and edema as well as with the location. Motor weakness occurs with this syndrome in both upper and lower extremities, although it is greater in the upper extremities. Loss of pain and temperature sensations varies.

Brown-Séquard lesions (Brown-Séquard syndrome) are those that involve only one side of the cord (Fig. 48-16). The characteristic symptoms include paralysis and loss of position and vibratory sense ipsilaterally with contralateral pain and temperature perception loss. *Horner's syndrome* may accompany Brown-Séquard lesions at the cervical level ipsilaterally.

Anterior cord syndrome is reflected by loss of sensitivity to pain and of motor and temperature control below the level of the lesion. Touch, proprioception, and vibratory sense remain intact.

Spinal Cord Transection

Total spinal cord transection results in immediate loss of all voluntary movement from the segments below the transection. The skin and other tissues become permanently anesthetized. Initially, reflex activity is abolished;

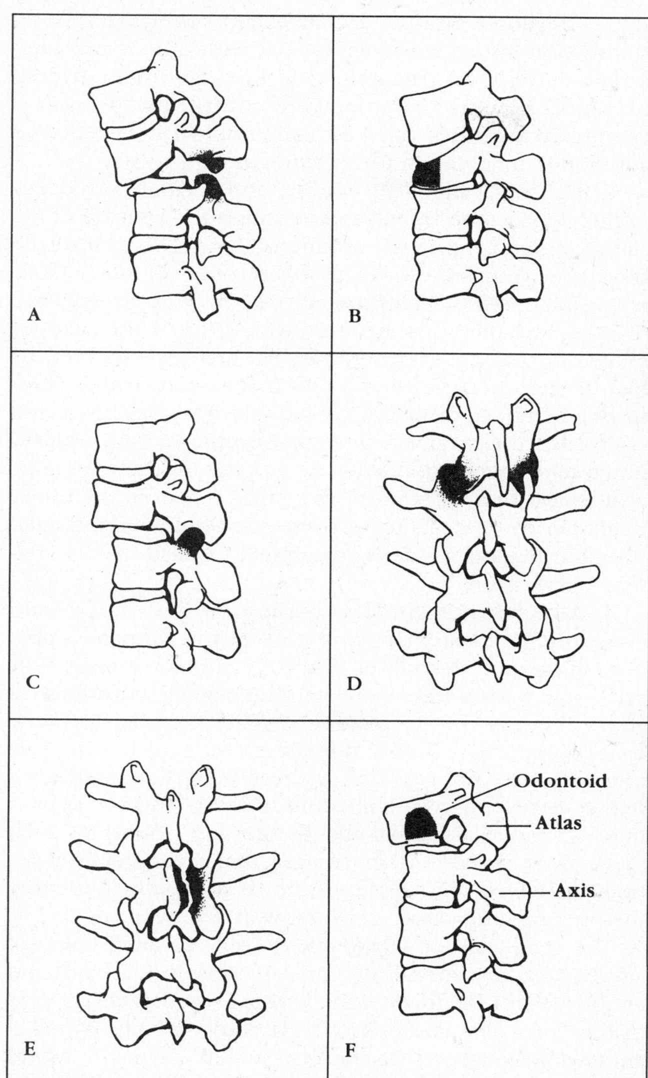

FIGURE 48-14 Common types of vertebral injury. A. Subluxation. B. Compression fracture. C. Bilateral fracture, joint dislocation. D. Unilateral facet joint dislocation. E. Posterior arch fracture. F. Odontoid fracture. (From R. Judge, G.E. Zuidema, and F. Fitzgerald, *Clinical Diagnosis: A Physiologic Approach*. Boston: Little, Brown, 1982.)

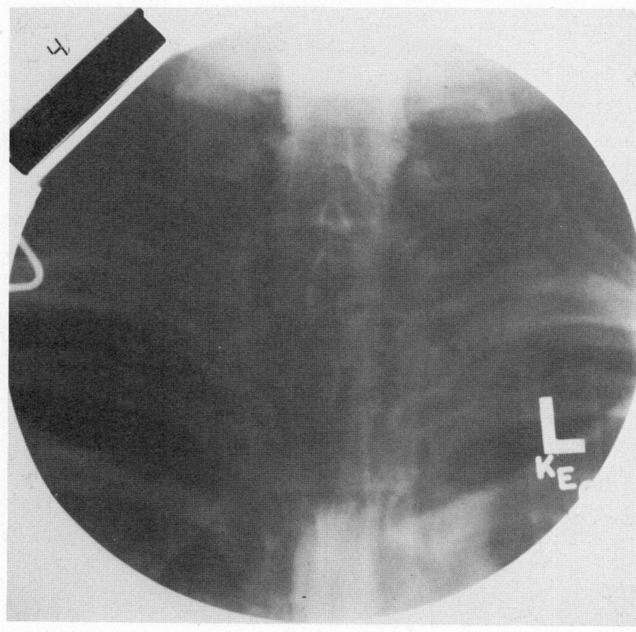

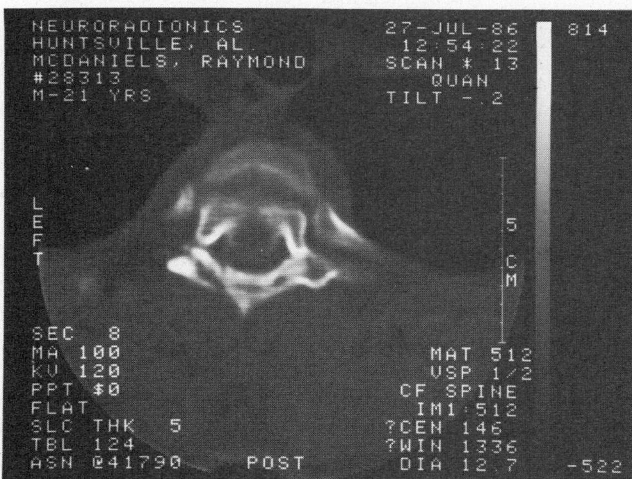

FIGURE 48-15 A. Myelogram showing cord injury at level T-2 and T-3. Area of decreased contrast shows cord contusion and edema. B. CT scan of same person showing numerous vertebral fractures and cord edema.

however, it does recover and eventually may become hyperactive.

Spinal Shock. The immediate depression of cord activity after transection is referred to as *spinal shock* or *posttransectional areflexia*. It results from the interruption of neural pathways with the remainder of the central nervous system. The exact mechanisms causing spinal shock and recovery of reflexes are still elusive. It has been speculated that the excitatory effects of alpha and gamma motoneurons on other spinal motoneurons have been lost due to transection of the descending pathways, and that inhibitory spinal internuncial neurons become disinhibited, thus resulting in diminished reflexes. Considerable variability of the duration of spinal shock exists in humans. Some reflexes may reappear as early as two or three days after transection whereas others may not return for six weeks. Spinal shock is more pronounced in the cord segments surrounding the lesion, and recovery of reflexes generally occurs last there.

In addition to areflexia in spinal shock, clinical signs include autonomic deficits, which are reflected in a lowered arterial blood pressure, bradycardia as well as loss of sweating, piloerection, and body temperature control

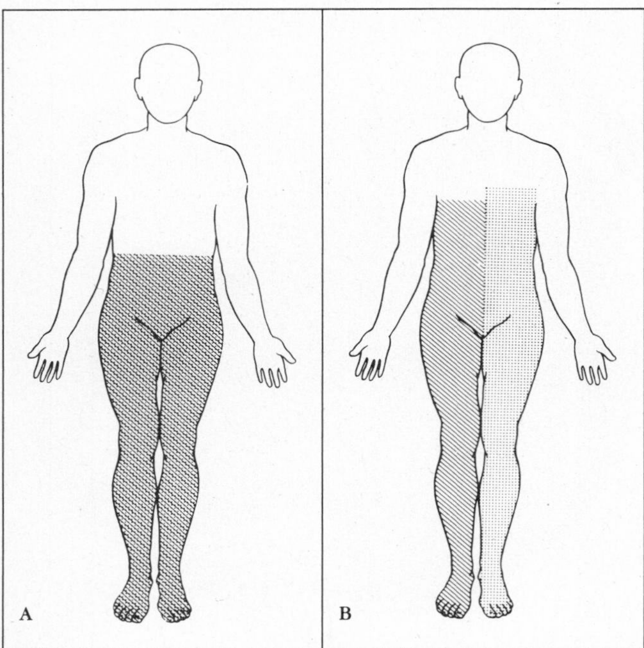

FIGURE 48-16 A. Complete transverse lesion of the spinal cord. B. Brown-Séquard syndrome: lesion of the left side of the spinal cord. (From J. Simpson and K. Magee, *Clinical Evaluation of the Nervous System*. Boston: Little, Brown, 1973.)

below the area of transection. The body tends to assume the temperature of the environment (poikilothermia). Because of depressed vasoconstrictive action below the level of the lesion by the sympathetic nervous system, individuals are susceptible to severe postural hypotension. Bowel and bladder reflexes from the sacrum are inhibited, and control over their functions is temporarily lost during spinal shock. Loss of sensation and flaccid paralysis occur below the transection site.

Reflex Return in Cord Transection: Flexion-Extension Reflexes. The first reflexes to recover from spinal shock, about two weeks after transection, are the stretch and flexion reflexes that are evoked by noxious cutaneous stimulation. An example of this withdrawal response is dorsiflexion of the great toe (Babinski's sign) in response to stimulation of the sole of the foot. Complications such as infection and malnutrition may delay the return of the flexor responses. As the flexor reflex recovers, it gradually becomes excited more readily from wider areas of the skin.

As recovery progresses after cord transection, flexor reflexes are interspersed with extensor spasms with ultimate progression to predominantly extensor activity. Individuals with partial cord transection generally exhibit strong extensor spasticity, whereas this seldom occurs with complete transection.

Autonomic Reflexes. The autonomic spinal reflexes include those that control reflexive action of vasomotor activity, diaphoresis, and emptying of the bladder and rectum. Vasomotor reflexes are abolished below the level of transection during spinal shock, but with time, tonic autonomic activity returns and wide fluctuations in arterial pressure diminish. Temperature control by the skin is essentially abolished for a time after spinal transection as autonomic innervation for sweating is suppressed.

Reflex emptying of the bladder and rectum does occur in individuals with spinal transections after a period of initial atony and increased sphincter tone. Dilation of the bladder with urine eventually overcomes sphincter resistance and overflow incontinence occurs. With progression of time, spontaneous, brief contractions of the bladder evolve into larger contractions that are accompanied by bladder sphincter opening and brief micturition. Thus, small amounts of urine are voided with varying amounts of residual urine retained. Sensory stimuli may be used to precipitate micturition, such as tapping on the abdomen, anal stimulation, or stroking the inner aspect of the upper thigh. Downward manual pressure on the lower abdomen over the bladder (Crede's maneuver) is also used to initiate micturition.

Autonomic dysreflexia or *autonomic hyperreflexia* constitutes a cluster of symptoms in which many spinal cord autonomic responses discharge simultaneously. This syndrome occurs in persons with high spinal cord injuries above the level of the sixth or seventh thoracic segment. Its occurrence is highly unpredictable and it can arise unexpectedly for years after the injury. The symptoms occur in response to a specific noxious stimuli, appear quickly, and may lead to life-threatening conditions such as seizures, cerebral hemorrhages, and myocardial infarction. Therefore, measures must be taken rapidly to identify the precipitating cause and remove it.

The symptoms of autonomic dysreflexia are a result of afferent sensory stimuli that travel to the spinal cord and are blocked at the level of the lesion as they travel upward in the cord. The resultant arterial spasm produces exaggerated sympathetic discharges, which cause the blood vessels of the skin and splanchnic bed below the level of the injury to vasoconstrict reflexively [5]. As a result, the individual may experience a pounding headache, blurred vision, and severe hypertension that may rise as high as 300 mm Hg systolic. The increased blood pressure distends the carotid sinus and aortic arch baroreceptors, which in turn, stimulate the vagus nerve to decrease the heart rate in an attempt to lower the blood pressure. Dilated vessels produce flushing and profuse diaphoresis above the level of the injury as a result of efferent impulses from the spinal cord sympathetic ganglia [5]. Because these impulses are blocked to the lower body, the vessels remain vasoconstricted and the individual exhibits *cutes anserina* (goose flesh) and pale skin below the lesion. Other symptoms include restlessness, nasal congestion, and nausea.

Precipitating factors leading to autonomic dysreflexia most commonly include bladder and bowel distention or manipulation. Other triggering stimuli may include decubitus ulcers, spasticity, stimulation of pain receptors, pressure on the penis, and strong uterine contractions.

When the symptoms occur, rapid intervention is necessary to lower the blood pressure. The head of the bed is elevated, as persons with high cord injuries usually have lower blood pressure in the sitting position. Next, the source of stimulation must be found and removed. If these measures are not successful in reducing hypertension, ganglionic-blocking agents or other antihypertensive drugs are given intravenously.

Intervertebral Disk Herniation

Herniation or rupture of the nucleus pulposus of the intervertebral disk is most commonly caused by minor or major trauma (Fig. 48-17). In many cases, however, onset is acute with no history of trauma. Sudden straining of the back in an unusual position and lifting while bending forward are frequently reported to be associated with disk herniation. Herniation of the nucleus pulposus produces pain, sensory loss, and paralysis by pressure on the spinal nerve roots or on the spinal cord. The most common injury is to the lumbosacral intervertebral disks, which reflects a clinical picture of sciatica. Herniations of the cervical disks occur occasionally, and those in the thoracic region are rare.

Clinical findings associated with ruptured or herniated disks are related to the size and location of the extruded material. Single nerve roots may be involved in small lesions; however, several roots may be compressed. The spinal cord may be compressed by large, centrally situated cervical disks, and symptoms are reflective of spinal cord tumors or degenerative diseases.

The vast majority of the *lumbosacral herniations* occur between the fourth or fifth lumbar and first sacral interspaces. Sciatic symptoms associated with lumbosacral herniation include pain in the lower back radiating down the posterior surface of one or both legs. In unilateral involvement, scoliosis occurs toward the opposite side of sciatic pain, and movement of the lumbar spine is limited. Paresthesias in the leg or foot are common. Tenderness is experienced on palpation along the course of the sciatic nerve. Motor weakness occurs in a small percentage of cases. Hypoesthesia to touch or pinprick is present in about one-half of cases. A decreased or absent ankle reflex is common with herniation of the lumbosacral disk. Coughing, sneezing, and straining may produce radiation of pain along the course of the sciatic nerve. Generally, symptoms are unilateral; however, with large central protrusions, they may be bilateral.

Herniation of the cervical disks occurs most commonly at the level of the fifth through seventh cervical roots. Displacement of the disk in this region causes stiffness of the neck and shoulder pain that radiates down the arm into the hand. Paresthesias may accompany the pain. Weakness and atrophy of the biceps and diminution of the biceps reflex may be present with sixth cervical root damage. Paresthesias and sensory loss in the index finger, weakness of the triceps muscle, and loss of triceps reflex are indicative of involvement of the seventh cervical root. Eighth cervical root compression reflects forearm pain along the medial side, as well as sensory loss along the medial cutaneous nerve of the forearm and ulnar nerve distribution in the hand.

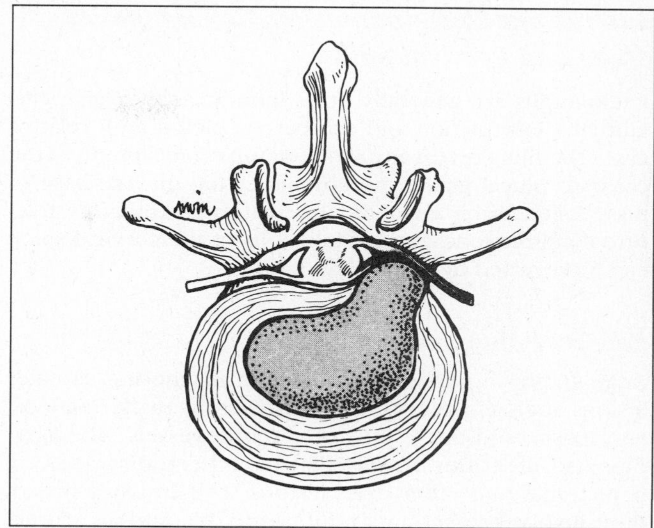

FIGURE 48-17 Herniated disk. (From R. Judge, G.E. Zuidema, and F. Fitzgerald, *Clinical Diagnosis: A Physiologic Approach*. Boston: Little, Brown, 1982.)

Diagnosis and Management. Radiologic findings supportive of a herniated disk show loss of normal curvature of the spine, scoliosis, and narrowing of intervertebral spaces. Diagnosis is most conclusively demonstrated by myelography, which reveals defects in outline of the subarachnoid space or interruption of the flow of the dye in the presence of herniated disks. In addition, CT scanning is effective in visualizing defective disks. Elevated protein content of cerebrospinal fluid is another supportive finding, and cerebrospinal fluid may be completely or partially blocked with extrusions in the thoracic or cervical regions.

Conservative treatment in the acute stage is focused on bedrest, local heat application, and analgesics. Traction to lower extremities may be applied initially with lumbosacral disk herniations. Cervical halter traction is indicated for cervical disk involvement. Surgical intervention is indicated if conservative modes of treatment fail and signs of cord compression develop. Simple removal of the disk is commonly performed to relieve the symptoms.

Diagnostic Studies of Nervous System Alterations

A variety of studies may be undertaken to support and expand the impression given by the clinical signs. The diagnostic studies commonly used are described in this section.

Lateral and Posteroanterior Radiographs of Skull and Cervical Spine

Radiographs are generally done initially as they give certain vital information and can be completed with relative ease. The films reveal any skull fractures and shifting of the calcified pineal gland, thereby indicating the presence of mass lesions such as subdural hematomas. Fractures, fracture compressions, and subluxations of the cervical spine can be revealed by plain films.

Cerebral Angiography

Angiography is particularly useful in diagnosing vascular lesions such as aneurysms, arteriovenous malformations, vasospasm, and occlusions of cerebral vessels. Angiography also identifies vessels that have been displaced by hematomas and other mass lesions. This invasive procedure involves injecting a radiopaque dye into an arterial blood vessel to allow visualization of the cerebral circulation. The material that passes through the intracranial and extracranial circulations outlines the arterial, capillary, and venous structures. Usual injection sites of the contrast media are the common carotid, femoral, and brachial arteries. The area of the suspected lesion largely influences the selection of the injection site.

Computerized Axial Tomography (CT)

Tomographic scanning is a very useful, effective, and rapid radiographic modality used for the diagnosis of nervous system lesions. The scans distinguish white matter from gray matter, identify the ventricles and sulci, and, with administration of intravenous contrast media, reveal major vessels of the brain. A narrow moving beam of x-ray is passed through successive layers of the head around a 360-degree axis. A small computer processes the accumulated data by calculating the differences in tissue density in contiguous tissue slices. Pathologic changes can be constructed from the density data in terms of shape, size, and position of structures of the brain. A wide variety of intracranial disorders may be demonstrated by the CT scan, including traumatic intracranial hematomas, neoplasms, cerebral infarctions, hydrocephalus, intracerebral hemorrhage, intracranial shifts, and brain abscesses. Certain spinal disorders, such as fractures, cord tumors, and disk abnormalities, can be effectively diagnosed by scanning.

As a neurodiagnostic tool, tomography has proved to be more efficient in many situations than conventional radiologic and air studies by virtue of its rapidity, noninvasiveness, and relative reliability in diagnosis.

Magnetic Resonance Imaging

Magnetic resonance imaging (MRI) is the most recently developed diagnostic tool. It provides views of the successive layers of the brain in any plane within a powerful magnetic field. Protons of brain tissue and CSF align themselves in the orientation of the magnetic field. A specific radio frequency is introduced into the field that causes protons to resonate and change their alignment. A computer analyzes the absorbed radio frequency energy and projects it as an image on a screen.

The MRI has some distinct advantages over the CT scan. It projects images more clearly in that the gray and white matter are more precisely distinguished, posterior fossa and brainstem tissues are viewed more accurately, and certain lesions involving white matter are more readily identified. Like the scan, MRI is noninvasive and poses no hazard to the individual. Due to its powerful magnetic field, however, the equipment requires special housing.

Echoencephalography

Echoencephalography is a safe, noninvasive neurologic diagnostic tool that involves the use of an ultrasound generator and receiver that display echo pulsations on an oscilloscope. Permanent recording is done through an attached camera. Echoes from deep within the skull visualize shifts in midline structures that may reflect intracranial trauma, cerebrovascular alterations, or space-occupying lesions. Lateral shifts of the pineal gland are also determined by echoencephalography as well as by plain radiographs. The echoencephalogram has been useful as an adjunct to more conventional and accurate neurodiagnostic studies such as the CT scan and angiography. The limitations in echoencephalography lie in the many chances for error in administering and interpreting the test.

Brain Scan

The brain scan is a safe neurodiagnostic technique used primarily to detect intracranial tumors, abscesses, and some subdural hematomas. A radioactive substance is injected intravenously and accumulates in abnormal areas of the brain as a result of breakdown of the blood-brain barrier. It is not particularly useful in diagnosis of acute head injury, as the radioactive substance must be injected one to two hours before scanning. This time span is excessive in persons who require rapid diagnosis and treatment. Positive brain scans result when scalp contusions are present. Because many acute head injuries are accompanied by scalp contusions, the scan findings may not present an accurate picture of the underlying brain pathology.

Pneumoencephalography

This procedure is used to diagnose space-occupying lesions and morphologic changes within the ventricular system. It is not feasible for diagnosis in acute head injuries because of its complex invasive nature. It is contraindicated in persons with papilledema and increased intracranial pressure.

This test involves replacing cerebrospinal fluid with air or oxygen by means of lumbar puncture or rarely, cisternal puncture. The air enters the ventricular system primarily through the foramen of Magendie, and serial films are taken to visualize the cerebral structures. This procedure is used infrequently, as it has been replaced by other diagnostic tests that are less invasive and allow adequate visualization of the cerebral structures.

Ventriculography

Ventriculography is a variation of the pneumoencephalogram in which CSF is replaced with air or oxygen directly in the lateral ventricles. This procedure is performed in the operating room through skull burr holes and under local anesthesia. The ventriculogram is done for the diagnosis of expanding intracranial lesions and cerebral anomalies, as it determines the patency of the ventricles.

Myelography

In myelography, radiopaque substance is introduced into the spinal subarachnoid space for the purpose of visualizing the vertebral canal. Prior to the injection of the contrast media, into the subarachnoid space through lumbar puncture, Queckenstedt's test may be done to determine patency of the spinal canal. This is performed by compressing the jugular veins when a lumbar puncture has been made. When the compression is maintained, the CSF pressure is elevated. Unilateral compression results in moderate elevation of CSF pressure, whereas bilateral compression shows an even higher rise. When the compression is terminated, the CSF pressure returns to normal. Failure of the pressure to rise and fall indicates some obstruction within the spinal canal above the lumbar puncture site.

Myelography is carried out in the radiology department on a tilt-table so that the person can be manipulated to allow the spinal canal to fill in several positions. With the person in position and lumbar puncture accomplished, approximately 10 ml of CSF is withdrawn and the radiopaque material is injected slowly. Serial films are then taken in various parts of the vertebral canal. On completion of the films, the contrast media is removed.

Myelography is most commonly used for the diagnosis of intravertebral disk protrusions of herniations. Abnormal results indicate incomplete canal filling with contrast media or total obstruction of its flow. In addition to disk abnormalities, tumors and adhesions encroaching on the spinal canal can be demonstrated.

Electroencephalography

The electroencephalogram (EEG) is recorded from the surface of the scalp and is a significant tool in assessing the continuing, spontaneous electrical activity of the cerebral cortex. Electrodes are placed on the skull and variations in potential are recorded between two cortical electrodes (bipolar record) or between a cortical electrode and an indifferent electrode usually placed on the ear (unipolar record). Simultaneous recordings from numerous portions of the cranium are accomplished by systematic electrode placement. The EEG activity reflects the graded potential changes in the cortical neurons. This cortical activity, in turn, is dependent on stimuli reaching it from deeper brain structures, as has been demonstrated by studies that indicate that the cerebral cortex separated from these structures lacks the normal EEG patterns. Additional support for deep structure effect on the EEG recording is the fact that both cerebral hemispheres generally demonstrate synchronous activity, suggesting a pacemaker mechanism in the deeper structures of the brain.

The changes observed in the EEG patterns in response to afferent stimulation are referred to as *desynchronization* of the EEG. This occurs whenever eyes are opened and alpha rhythm is replaced by a high-frequency, low-amplitude activity that exhibits no dominant pattern. Synchronized alpha activity indicates that many dendrite units are firing simultaneously, resulting in a rhythmic discharge. The frequency and amplitude of the EEG are affected by electrode placement, the activity or behavior and emotional status of the subject, and biochemical and structural status of the cortex. Oscillations vary from 1 to 50 Hz, and scalp voltage amplitude ranges widely according to internal and external environmental conditions.

Types of Brain Waves. The normal EEG depends on the integrity and normal functioning of the cerebral cortex as well as certain structures deep in the brain. Four principal wavebands are commonly recorded in the normal individual's brain function: alpha, beta, theta, and delta.

The *alpha waves* make up alpha rhythm, which ranges at frequencies of 8 to 13 per second but most commonly occurs at 9 to 10 per second (Fig. 48-18). Alpha waves are recorded symmetrically in most healthy adults from both the occipital and parietal regions. These are not fully developed until about age 13 years and may exhibit greater amplitude on the right side in younger individuals. Alpha waves are present only in the resting person whose eyes are closed. When eyes are open the alpha waves disappear and are replaced by an asynchronous rhythm of

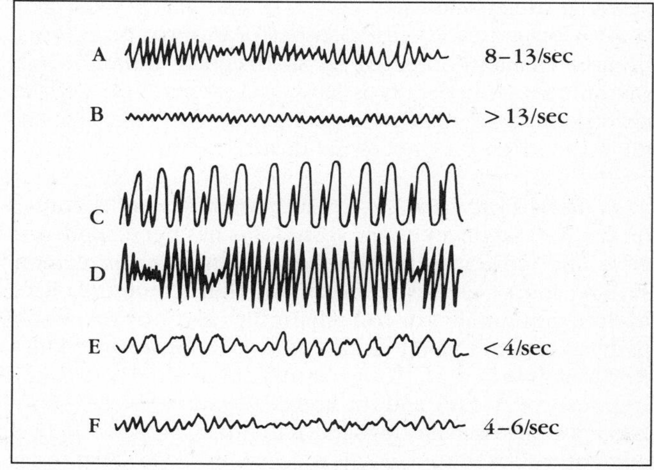

FIGURE 48-18 EEG waves. A. Alpha waves. B. Beta waves. C. Spike and dome waves during petit mal seizures. D. High-frequency spike waves during grand mal seizure. E. Delta waves. F. Theta waves.

low voltage. Metabolic aberrations such as anoxia and hypoglycemia slow alpha frequency.

Beta waves are recorded from the frontal lobe of the brain and represent activity of the motor cortex (see Fig. 48-18). Their frequency is above 13 cycles per second (cps) and the amplitude is generally low. Beta activity may predominate in some people and is seen to replace alpha waves in those who are tense and anxious. Voluntary movement can block beta wave activity. Closely related to beta waves and recorded from central regions of the brain are mu waves. These have a relatively high amplitude and a frequency of about one-half that of beta waves. Like beta waves, their activity is blocked by voluntary movement.

Theta waves project a frequency between 4 and 7 cps and an amplitude comparable to that of beta waves (see Fig. 48-18). These are recorded primarily in children and some adults in emotional distress from the parietal and frontotemporal regions of the brain. Visual attention may block theta wave activity.

Delta waves encompass all the electrical rhythms of less than 4 cps (see Fig. 48-18). This pattern is observed normally in individuals in deep stages of sleep and in young children, and is the dominant rhythm in infants. Presence of delta waves in the awake adult may signify organic brain pathology.

A significant correlation exists between an individual's level of arousal and the dominant frequency of the EEG. Waves appear at 3 or fewer per second in deep sleep states and, as sleep lightens, bursts of 10 to 12 waves per second begin to appear at shorter and shorter intervals until the waking state, when a continuous, more rapid frequency and lower-amplitude rhythm dominate. Thus, a direct correlation can be observed in the person's state of arousal and the cortical electrical activity recorded on the EEG.

The EEG evaluations are significant in contributing to the diagnostic process of persons with cranial neurologic conditions. Characteristic rhythms are observed with the various epileptic seizures as well as during the intervals between the attacks (see Fig. 48-18 and pages 776–781). Focal damage to the cortex, either of internal or external origin, is usually reflected by an irregular and abnormal rhythm, which generally is slow and asymmetric with its corresponding hemispheric position. The EEG is also useful in the diagnosis of cerebral death.

Evoked Potentials. Evoked potentials are recorded on the EEG when an external stimulus has been applied to a specific sense organ. These have been useful in demonstrating abnormal sensory organ function. Commonly used evoked potentials are to test the integrity of the visual pathways (pattern-shift visual evoked response, or PSVER), the brainstem (far field brainstem auditory evoked response, or BAER), and the somatosensory system (short-latency somatosensory evoked potentials, or SLSEP) [1]. A computer is used to average and maximize the responses.

The PSVER is particularly useful in diagnosing lesions of the optic nerve and its pathways. It is an effective test to detect optic neuritis, optic nerve compression, and demyelinization of the optic pathways such as is associated with multiple sclerosis. Each eye is tested separately as the individual views a pattern of light while recordings are made on the electroencephalograph.

The BAER tests auditory stimuli on the cerebral cortex and is useful for diagnosing peripheral hearing loss and lesions in the auditory tracts and brainstem. A series of clicks is administered to one ear through earphones while an electroencephalogram is recorded. This is repeated on the other ear. The ear that is not being tested at the time receives white noise.

The SLSEP diagnoses nerve conduction defects of the somatic sensory system. Peripheral nerves are stimulated by electrodes on overlying skin and EEG electrodes are placed peripherally and on the scalp. Common stimulation sites are the wrist and ankle. The SLSEP is most useful in diagnoses of lesions in spinal roots, posterior columns, and brainstem involvement such as may occur with Guillain-Barré syndrome and multiple sclerosis.

Study Questions

1. Explain the function of the reticular activating system.
2. Describe the etiology, pathophysiology, and clinical manifestations of coma.
3. Discriminate among epidural, subdural, subarachnoid, and intracerebral bleeding.
4. Why does cerebral edema occur when free blood escapes into brain tissue?
5. Why is increased intracranial pressure considered a life-threatening condition?
6. Discuss the etiology, pathophysiology, and clinical manifestations of the various levels of spinal cord injury.
7. Which diagnostic studies are best used with which injuries? Why?

References

1. Adams, R., and Victor, M. *Principles of Neurology* (3rd ed.). New York: McGraw-Hill, 1985.
2. Finkelstein, S., and Ropper, A. The diagnoses of coma: Its pitfalls and limitations. *Heart Lung* 8:1059, 1979.
3. Guyton, A.C. *Textbook of Medical Physiology* (7th ed.). Philadelphia: Saunders, 1986.
4. Jackson, L. Cerebral vasospasm after an intracranial aneurysmal subarachnoid hemorrhage: A nursing perspective. *Heart Lung* 1:14, 1986.
5. Lazure, L. Defusing the dangers of autonomic dysreflexia. *Nurs. 80* 8:52, 1980.
6. Lewis, A. *Mechanisms of Neurologic Disease*. Boston: Little, Brown, 1976.
7. Plum, F., and Posner, J. *The Diagnosis of Stupor and Coma* (3rd ed.). Philadelphia: Davis, 1980.

CHAPTER 49

Tumors and Infections of the Central Nervous System

CHAPTER OUTLINE

Tumors

- General Considerations
- Frequency
- Alterations in the Central Nervous System Due to Tumors
- Clinical Manifestations
- Diagnosis
- Tumors of the Neuroglial Cells (Gliomas)
  - *Astrocytomas*
  - *Glioblastoma Multiforme*
  - *Oligodendrogliomas*
  - *Ependymomas*
- Tumors of Neuronal Origin
- Tumors of Embryonic Origin
- Tumors of the Meninges
  - *Meningiomas*
  - *Meningeal Sarcomas*
- Tumors of the Pituitary Gland
- Tumors of the Cranial and Peripheral Nerves and Nerve Roots
- Tumors of the Blood Vessels
  - *Arteriovenous Malformations (AVMs)*
  - *Hemangioblastomas*
- Tumors of Developmental Defects
  - *Dermoids and Teratomas*
  - *Cholesteatomas*
  - *Chordomas*
  - *Craniopharyngiomas (Rathke's Pouch Tumors)*
- Tumors of Adenexal Structures
- Metastatic Tumors

Infections

- General Considerations
- Viral Infections
  - *Acute Encephalitis*
  - *Slow Virus Disease*
- Other CNS Viral Infections
  - *Aseptic Meningitis Complex (Benign Viral Meningitis)*
  - *Viruses Acquired Congenitally*
  - *Myelitis*
  - *Postinfectious/Postvaccinal Diseases*
- Bacterial Infections
  - *Pyogenic Infections*
  - *Tuberculous Infections*
  - *Neurosyphilis*
  - *Disorders Due to Bacterial Exotoxins*
- Fungal Infections
  - *Cryptococcus (Torulosis)*
  - *Coccidioidomycosis*
  - *Mucormycosis*
- Protozoal Infections
  - *Malaria*
  - *Toxoplasmosis*
  - *Amebiasis*
  - *Trypanosomiasis*
  - *Trichinosis*
- Metazoal Infections
  - *Cysticercosis*
  - *Echinoccosis (Hydatid Disease)*
- Rickettsial Infections

LEARNING OBJECTIVES

1. Identify the tissues from which central nervous system (CNS) tumors may originate.
2. Describe the classification systems for cranial and spinal tumors.
3. Compare the frequency and malignancy of brain and spinal tumors.
4. Describe CNS alterations that lead to focal disturbances and increased intracranial pressure.
5. State what is thought to be the basis for the localized cerebral edema that surrounds brain tumors.
6. Describe CNS alterations that lead to the development of papilledema.
7. State the body's compensatory mechanisms for dealing with increased intracranial pressure.
8. Describe the basis for the development of the classic triad of clinical manifestations associated with brain tumors.
9. Discuss the clinical manifestations associated with tumors of the frontal, temporal, parietal, and occipital lobes, cerebellum, and brainstem.
10. Discuss clinical manifestations associated with the various types of spinal tumors, as well as with different levels of compression by spinal tumors.
11. Describe techniques used to diagnose brain and spinal tumors.
12. Compare and contrast characteristics of the CNS tumors: tissue type, appearance, rate of growth, invasive qualities, CNS alterations, and pertinent clinical manifestations.
13. State the two most common primary sites from which metastasis occurs to the brain.
14. State the various routes by which microorganisms reach the CNS.
15. List the ways in which viruses gain access to the body.
16. State the ways in which viruses invade the CNS.
17. Compare and contrast characteristics of the CNS infections: routes of infection, CNS alterations, pertinent clinical manifestations, and prognosis.

Tumors of the central nervous system and the invasion of this system by infectious organisms are discussed in this chapter. Frequency, alterations within the central nervous system, resultant clinical manifestations, and relevant diagnostic studies are reviewed. The topic is vast, and the reader is referred to special texts for additional information and study of the subject.

Tumors

General Considerations

Tumors of the central nervous system (CNS) include both benign and malignant neoplasms within the brain as well as the spinal cord. The location, size, invasiveness, and rate of growth of these tumors are frequently more crucial to the ultimate course of the disease than the degree of malignancy. Virtually all brain tumors are potentially life threatening. They can arise from the glial cells, blood vessels and connective tissue, meninges, pituitary gland, and pineal gland (Fig. 49-1). Metastatic tumors from primary sites throughout the body are also encountered within the CNS.

With their variety and complexity, classification of intracranial tumors becomes a problem. An adaptation of the Kernahan and Sayre classification is found in Table 49-1. It is based on naming the tumor with respect to cells present in the adult nervous system, vascular tissue, and developmental defects. A single tumor may contain more than one cell type. A malignancy grading of I to IV is also included, with I being the least malignant.

Intraspinal tumors are classified in accordance with their location in relation to the dura and spinal cord as well as histologic type. Thus, two groups are generally considered: *extradural*, those arising from the extradural space or vertebral bodies, and *intradural*, those arising from the blood vessels, meninges, or nerve roots (extramedullary), and those arising from within the substance of the spinal cord itself (intramedullary). Intramedullary tumors are intradural, while extramedullary tumors can be either extradural or intradural.

Generally speaking, the location, size, and invasive quality of intracranial and intraspinal neoplasms are responsible for certain neurologic symptoms. The destruction and displacement of tissue, in addition to increased intracranial pressure, cause specific symptoms (Fig. 49-2). Morbidity and mortality associated with intracranial tumors are high, but advancements in diagnostic techniques, medical therapeutics, and neurosurgical techniques have improved the prognosis. Spinal cord tumors are more easily removed surgically than brain tumors. Thus, if recognized early and removed, prognosis for persons with intraspinal tumors is quite favorable.

Frequency

Primary CNS tumors are not rare. As an intracranial disease, they are second in frequency only to stroke. They occur in all age groups and in both sexes.

Although it is difficult to establish accurate incidence of primary tumors in the general population, Table 49-1 presents widely accepted percentages of occurrence for the various types of intracranial neoplasms. The brain and its coverings are also involved by neoplasm in 20 percent of all persons who have cancer [1]. Furthermore, 1.2 percent of all autopsies indicate the presence of tumors of the CNS, dura, or meninges [6].

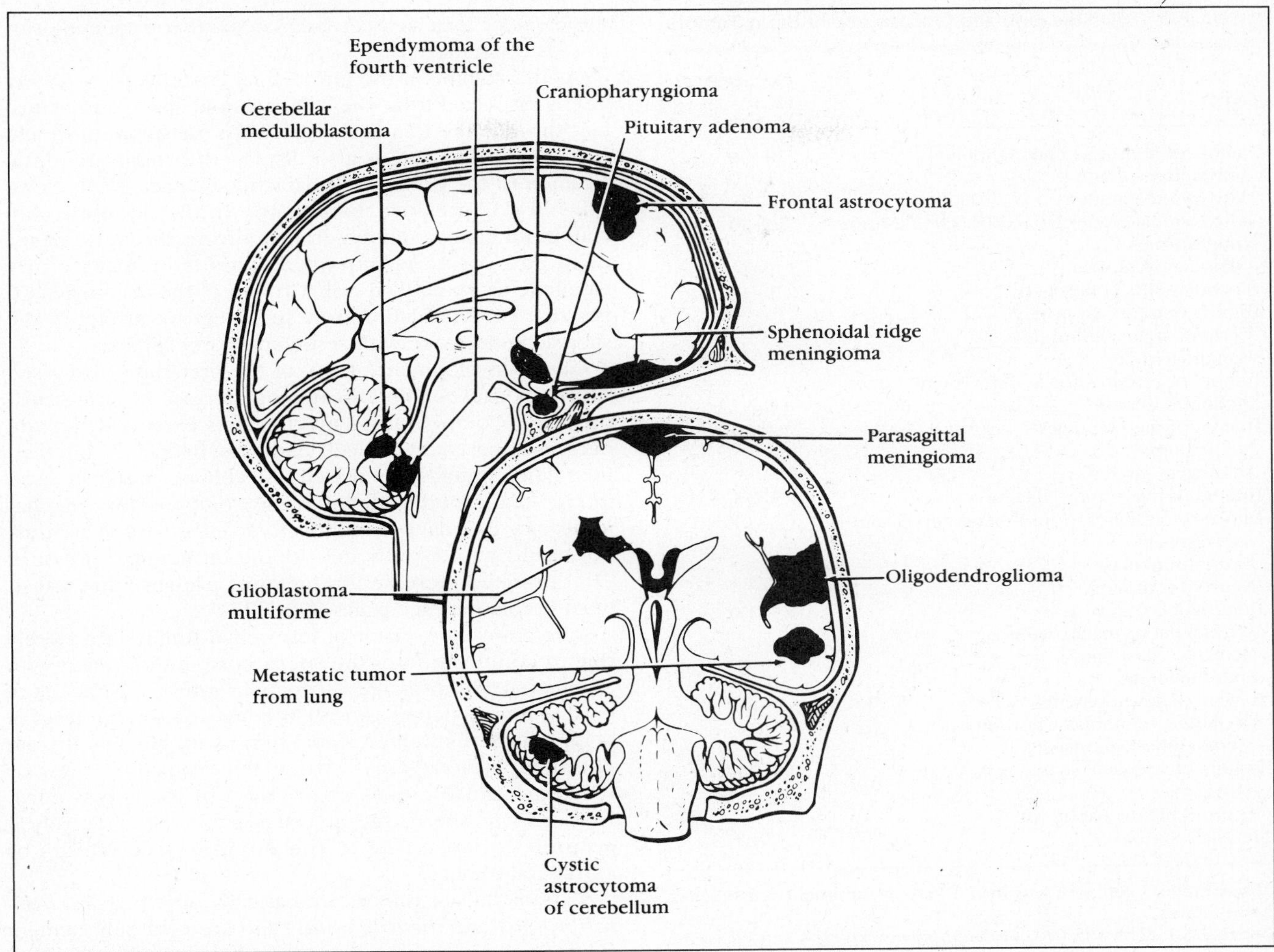

FIGURE 49-1 Common intracranial tumors and the positions in which they frequently occur. Metastatic tumors may localize anywhere. (From M. Snyder and M. Jackle, *Neurologic Nursing: A Critical Care Nursing Focus*. Bowie, Md.: Brady, 1981.)

Although intracranial tumors can occur at any age, their frequency seems to be increased in young children and again in the fifth and sixth decades of life. Between ages 6 and 15 years, brain tumors are the second most common malignancy and from birth to 5 years the third most common [2]. The most common brain tumors of childhood include craniopharyngiomas, ependymomas, medulloblastomas, cerebellar and cerebral astrocytomas, brainstem gliomas, optic path gliomas, and pinealomas. In adults, gliomas account for 45 percent of all tumors [4]. Pituitary adenomas, acoustic neuromas, and meningiomas are prevalent during adulthood and almost completely absent during childhood.

Intraspinal tumors occur less frequently than those that involve the brain and are rare in children. Of 8784 primary CNS tumors in a Mayo Clinic series, only 15 percent were within the spine [8]. Twenty-five percent of intraspinal tumors are extradural and are generally metastatic. Seventy-five percent are intradural. Of these, extramedullary lesions are more frequent than intramedullary lesions. Extramedullary tumors are usually meningiomas or neurofibromas and are easily removed surgically. Intramedullary tumors have the same cellular origins as intracranial tumors and generally infiltrate surrounding tissue. These intramedullary tumors are frequently gliomas (particularly ependymomas), which commonly arise from the cauda equina and lumbar areas. Astrocytomas, oligodendrogliomas, glioblastomas, hemangioblastomas, and medulloblastomas occur less frequently and can arise in any of the spinal segments.

Alterations in the Central Nervous System Due to Tumors

Brain tumors may be benign or malignant with regard to histology and morphology of their cellular components. It must be remembered, however, that all tumors of the brain are potentially harmful due to their relationship to vital structures. Thus, malignant or harmful effects may be produced by histologically benign lesions.

TABLE 49-1 Classification and Occurrence of Brain Tumors

Tumor	Occurrence (%)
Tumors of neuroglia cells (gliomas)	40–50
Astrocytoma grade I	5–10
Astrocytoma grade II	2–5
Astrocytoma grades III and IV (glioblastoma multiforme)	20–30
Oligodendroglioma	1–4
Ependymoma grades I–IV	1–3
Tumors of neuronal origin[a]	
Cerebral neuroblastomas	
Gangliogliomas	
Tumors of primitive or undifferentiated cells	
Medulloblastoma	3–5
Tumors of the meninges	12–20
Meningioma	
Meningeal sarcomas	
Tumors of the pituitary gland	5–15
Tumors of cranial and peripheral nerves and nerve roots	3–10
Neurilemmomas	
Neurofibromas	
Tumors of blood vessels	0.5–1.0
Arteriovenous malformations	
Hemangioblastomas	
Endotheliomas	
Tumors of developmental defects	3–8
Dermoids, teratomas, chordomas, craniopharyngiomas	
Tumors of adenexal structures	0.5–0.8
Pinealomas	
Choroid plexus papillomas	
Metastatic tumors	5–10

[a]These tumors compose less than 1–3% of the total occurrence of brain tumors.
Source: S. I. Schwartz (ed.), *Principles of Surgery* (2nd ed.). New York: McGraw-Hill, 1974.

Brain tumors rarely metastasize to extraneural tissue; however, they infiltrate into surrounding nervous tissue, into the meninges, or through the ependymal layer into the ventricles. Once the tumor gains access to the subarachnoid space or ventricular system, and thus the cerebrospinal fluid (CSF) pathways, it may spread throughout the entire CNS. This may include the spinal cord and peripheral nerve roots [5].

Within the confined space of the skull, a growing tumor alters the normally stable volume of the brain, blood, and CSF. Thus, as the mass grows, compression of brain tissue as well as alterations in blood and CSF circulation lead to focal disturbances and increased intracranial pressure. More specifically, tumor growth can produce any of several alterations. Compression of brain tissue and invasion of brain parenchyma cause destruction of neural tissue. Blood circulation may be decreased to such an extent that necrosis of brain tissue occurs. Compression, infiltration of neural tissue, and decreased blood supply may also lead to altered neural excitability with resultant seizure activity. Elevation of capillary pressure, due to compression of venules in the area adjacent to the tumor, is thought to be the basis for localized cerebral edema that frequently surrounds the tumor.

As the volume of the intracranial contents is increased, CSF is displaced from the subarachnoid space and ventricles through the foramen magnum to the spinal subarachnoid space. The CSF is also displaced through the optic foramen to the perioptic subarachnoid space. With elevations in CSF pressure, particularly in the perioptic subarachnoid space, venous drainage from the optic nerve head and retina is impaired. This is manifested by papilledema, or choked disk. Growth of the mass may also obstruct CSF circulation from the lateral ventricles to the subarachnoid space with resultant hydrocephalus.

Rapid development of any of the previously discussed situations causes a life-threatening increase in intracranial pressure. Compensatory mechanisms exist and include decreased parenchymal cell numbers, decreased intracellular fluid contents, decreased CSF volume, and decreased intracranial blood volume. These compensatory mechanisms may take days or months to be effective and are thus not useful with rapidly developing intracranial pressure [7]. Untreated increased intracranial pressure may cause brain herniation (see pages 820–822).

Alterations as a result of intraspinal tumors are largely due to compression of the spinal cord, interference with circulation, and pressure on veins or arteries. Ischemia of cord segments occurs as well as edema below the level of compression. Extradural spinal tumors usually result from extraneural metastases, particularly from the breast or lung, and cause rapid compression of the spinal cord. Hemorrhage due to the metastases as well as vertebral column collapse add to the compressive effects of extradural tumors.

Extramedullary tumors are basically of two types, *neurofibromas* and *meningiomas*, and are generally benign. Neurofibromas grow in the nerve root and often form an hourglasslike expansion that extends into the extradural space. Meningiomas grow from the arachnoid membrane. These tumors are commonly present in the posterolateral aspect of the cord. They often result in the Brown-Séquard syndrome, due to the compressive damage to one-half of the spinal cord (see Chap. 48).

As mentioned previously, intramedullary tumors are histologicallly the same as intracranial tumors. These lesions damage sensory fibers that cross each other in the center of the cord. They also destroy neurons. There is a frequent association between intramedullary tumors and syringomyelia [1].

Clinical Manifestations

The symptoms produced by intracranial tumors are extremely variable and depend on characteristics of the neoplasm, invasive qualities, location, and rate of growth. Because these tumors eventually give rise to an increase in intracranial pressure, a classic triad of symptoms usually occurs: headache, vomiting, and papilledema.

Headache is a common symptom of intracranial tumors. Early in the course of tumor growth, headache is thought to result from local displacement and traction of pain-

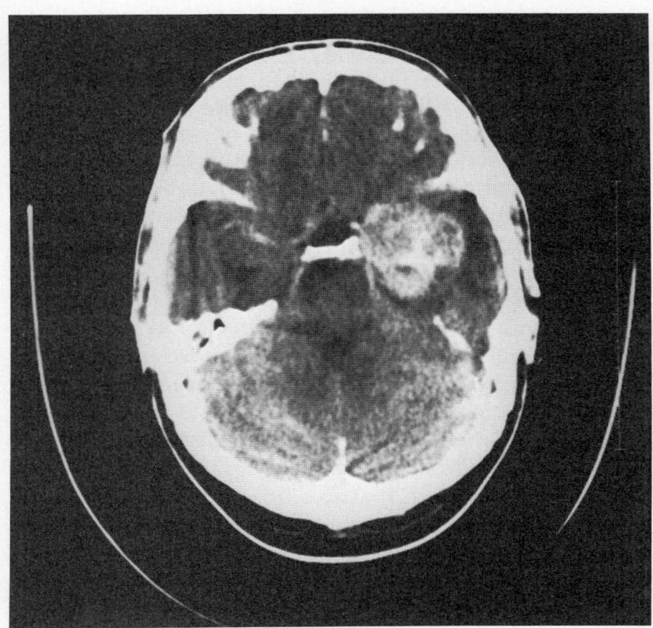

A

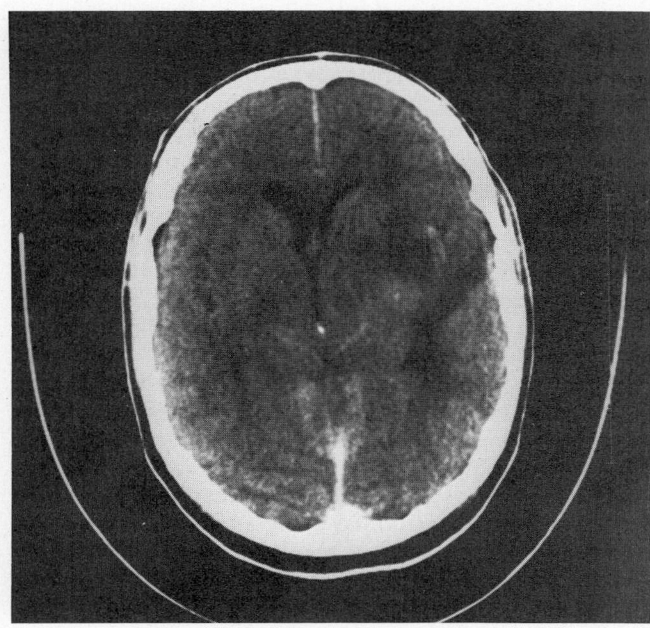

B

Figure 49-2 A. Contrast-enhanced CT scan showing right cerebral metastatic tumor. B. View of compression and shift of midline structures by same tumor.

sensitive structures within the skull—cranial nerves, arteries, veins, and venous sinuses. As the tumor grows, the pain is reflective of generalized increased intracranial pressure. The headache may be dull and is usually temporary, although it may be severe, dull or sharp, and intermittent. It is generally most severe on awakening and tends to improve through the day. Typically, it is aggravated by stooping, coughing, or straining to have a bowel movement. In general, the headache has little localizing value with regard to tumor site.

Vomiting is also experienced by many persons with intracranial tumors, particularly those who suffer from tumors of the posterior fossa. It is a result of stimulation of the emetic center in the medulla. Vomiting associated with tumors is not necessarily preceded by nausea and is not related to ingestion of food. It often occurs before breakfast and is frequently projectile.

Papilledema may not be present in the early stages of tumor growth but occurs as intracranial pressure increases. In some persons papilledema does not develop even when the intracranial pressure becomes greatly elevated. Hemorrhages may be noted around the optic disk in association with papilledema. Complaints of blurred vision and halos around lights with enlargement of a blind spot and fleeting moments of dimmed vision (amaurosis fugax) may be elicited.

Other than the classic triad of symptoms, local effects of intracranial tumors occur due to irritation, destruction, or compression of neural tissue in the location of the tumor. Generally speaking, supratentorial lesions give rise to paralysis, seizures, memory loss, visual field defects, and impairment in consciousness; infratentorial lesions give rise to cranial nerve dysfunction and ataxia.

Frontal lobe tumors cause disturbed mental status, speech disturbances, generalized or focal seizures, hemiparesis, and ataxia. Mental symptoms are manifested by progressive apathy, mild dementia with impairment of memory and intellect, decreased judgment, altered social adaptation, labile emotions, and depression. Aphasia or apraxia may occur when the left or dominant frontal lobe is affected. Pressure on motor areas produces hemiparesis and may result in jacksonian seizures, which may progress to generalized seizures. The unsteady gait associated with frontal lobe tumors may resemble cerebellar ataxia.

Involvement of the dominant temporal lobe may cause sensory aphasia, which begins with difficulty in naming objects. The individual has difficulty comprehending the spoken word and speaks in jargon. Tinnitus occurs as a result of irritation to the adjacent cortex or temporal auditory receptor. Anterior temporal lobe tumors cause visual field changes that may progress to complete hemianopsia. Psychomotor seizures may occur.

Parietal lobe involvement may include motor-sensory focal seizures, agnosia, hypoesthesia (decreased sensibility to touch), paresthesia, and dyslexia. Visual defects may also occur. Tumors of the parietal lobe in the dominant hemisphere may result in difficulty comprehending language. Those in the nondominant hemisphere parietal lobe may interfere with awareness of contralateral body parts.

Involvement of the occipital lobe may produce visual field disturbances in the form of homonymous hemianopsia and quadratic defects. This may be associated with visual agnosia (loss of comprehension of visual sensation) on the dominant side, hallucinations, and convulsive seizures that are preceded by an aura.

Cerebellar tumors produce disturbances in equilibrium and coordination. The specific disorder depends on the location and size of the tumor. Disorders of movement may include nystagmus, adiadochokinesis (inability to make rapid alternative movements); asynergia (incoordination of muscle groups), dysmetria (abnormal force of muscular movements), intention tremor, and deviation from a line of movement [3]. Hypotonia may be present. Speech disturbances may be noted, with tendency toward staccato or scanning speech. Papilledema often occurs with a cerebellar tumor. Cerebellar tumors may exert pressure on the brainstem and result in cranial nerve deficits.

Brainstem involvement produces varied effects. There is increasing paralysis of the cranial nerves with paralysis of eye movements, loss of facial sensation, and difficulty swallowing. Motor deficits reflect involvement of the descending and ascending motor tracts. Lesions of the hypothalamus may produce diabetes insipidus, obesity, disturbances of temperature regulation, and somnolence.

Clinical manifestations associated with spinal cord tumors depend on the type of lesion and the level at which the lesion occurs (Table 49-2). Generally speaking, a soft, slow-growing mass causes gradual compression of the spinal cord with gradually increasing neurologic signs. Malignant and metastatic tumors cause rapid compression of the spinal cord and destruction of the neural tissue.

Extradural tumors usually result from metastasis from primary tumor sites. Local, dull pain is often the first symptom; it is intensified with movements of the spine. Later, due to rapid growth, the spinal cord becomes compressed and severe pain occurs. Early signs of cord compression include loss of joint position sense, loss of vibration, and spastic weakness below the level at which the lesion occurs. Without surgical removal of the tumor, irreversible damage that may include irreversible paraplegia occurs.

Extramedullary lesions, primarily neurofibromas and meningiomas, are usually benign and early in their growth involve the periphery of the cord. There is pain in the back and along the spinal roots. The pain is worse at night and is aggravated by movement or straining. Posteriorly situated tumors produce sensory losses including paresthesia and loss of proprioceptive sense. Sensory loss first occurs below the level of the lesion. Anterior compression of the cord causes severe motor dysfunctions. Lateral cord compression may produce the Brown-Séquard syndrome, in which there is ipsilateral motor weakness and deep sensory loss, as well as contralateral loss of pain and temperature perception below the level of the lesion. Early diagnosis and surgical removal produce good prognoses.

Intramedullary tumors tend to be more histologically benign, are slow growing, and have a more benign course than similar intracranial tumors. There is usually a dull, aching pain in the area of the lesion. A dissociated sensory loss occurs in which there is a bilateral sensory loss of pain and temperature that extends through all involved segments; however, the senses of touch, motion, position, and vibration are usually preserved. Intramedullary tumors may extend through several spinal cord segments, making surgical removal difficult.

The various levels of compression by spinal cord tumors are as follows: foramen magnum, cervical region, thoracic region, lumbar-sacral region, and cauda equina. A summary of signs and symptoms of common root lesions appears in Table 49-3.

A tumor in the area of the foramen magnum compresses intracranial contents, nerve roots, and the spinal cord. This causes suboccipital pain. Dermatomes C-2 and C-3 are compressed, which produces weakness of the head and neck. As the tumor extends into the intracranial cavity, increased pressure is produced as well as pressure on the cerebellum and cranial nerve nuclei.

Tumors in the cervical region produce motor and sensory losses in the shoulders, arms, and hands. Bicep, tricep, and brachioradial tendon reflexes may be lost, and varying motor and sensory deficits of the upper extremities arise if the lesion occurs in the lower cervical region.

TABLE 49-2 Common Symptoms of Spinal Cord Tumors

Symptom	Description
Pain in spine, neck, back	Usually gradual onset; may occur suddenly with sudden movement or injury; aggravated by Valsalva maneuver; nocturnal pain predominates due to recumbency (patient may prefer to sleep upright).
Radicular pain	Occurs in the distribution of segmental innervation; aggravated by movement that alters anatomic relationships; causes diagnostic confusion (T-8 root involvement may be misinterpreted as ulcer disease).
Medullary referred pain	Shooting or burning over peripheral areas; often bilateral; not influenced by Valsalva maneuver; appears at different sites.
Motor disturbances	Motor deficits are caused by lesions of the pyramidal or corticospinal tracts, causing spasticity and increased reflexes and spastic gait; weakness may present as a limp in the guise of muscle stiffness or rigidity.
Nonspecific sensory disturbances	Numbness; tingling; coldness.

Source: From F. McQuat, The insidious spinal cord tumor. Reprinted with permission from *Journal of Neurosurgical Nursing* 13:18, 1981. By permission of the American Association of Neuroscience Nurses.

TABLE 49-3 Symptoms and Signs of Common Root Lesions

Root	Location of Pain	Sensory Loss	Reflex Loss	Weakness and Atrophy
C-5	Lower neck, tip of shoulder, arm	Deltoid area (inconsistent)	Biceps	Shoulder abductors, biceps
C-6	Lower neck, medial scapula, arm, radial side of forearm	Radial side of hand, thumb, index finger	Biceps	Biceps
C-7	Lower neck, medial scapula, precordium, arm, forearm	Index finger, middle finger	Triceps	Triceps
C-8	Lower neck, medial arm and forearm, ulnar side of hand, fourth and fifth fingers	Ulnar side of hand, fourth and fifth fingers		Intrinsic hand muscles
L-4	Low back, anterior and medial thigh	Anterior thigh	Quadriceps	Quadriceps
L-5	Low back, lateral thigh, lateral leg, dorsum of foot, great toe	Great toe, medial side of dorsum of foot, lateral leg, and thigh		Toe extensors, ankle dorsiflexors, and evertors
S-1	Low back, posterior thigh, posterior leg, lateral side of foot, heel	Lateral foot, heel, posterior leg	Achilles	Ankle dorsiflexion and plantar flexion

Source: J. Simpson and K. Magee, *Clinical Evaluation of the Nervous System.* Boston: Little, Brown, 1970.

High cervical tumors compress the diaphragmatic nerves and result in paralysis of the diaphragm.

Thoracic lesions may produce pain and tightness across the chest and abdomen. Lower-extremity paresthesia may develop with the loss of abdominal reflexes when the lesion is in the lower thoracic area. Paralysis of the intercostal muscles results at the involved region.

Upper lumbar lesions cause hip flexion weakness, lower leg spasticity, loss of knee jerk reflexes, brisk ankle reflexes, and bilateral Babinski's signs. With extensive involvement of the high lumbar cord, movement and sensation are lost in the lower limbs. Sensory deficits result in the area of the perineum.

Lower lumbar and upper sacral lesions cause weakness of perineal, calf, and foot muscles. There is often loss of the Achilles reflex. Lower sacral lesions cause sensation losses in the buttocks and perianal area. Bladder and bowel control may be impaired. Lesions in the cauda equina region cause impotence and loss of sphincter control; pain in the sacral and perineal areas often radiates to the legs.

Diagnosis

Two basic steps are used to in diagnose CNS tumors. First, a detailed history is elicited and careful neurologic examination is performed. Second, radiologic investigations are performed depending on the findings of the neurologic examination. Films of the skull do not visualize the brain itself but reflect changes caused by chronically increased intracranial pressure. These changes include erosion of the sella turcica, calcification of the pineal body or of a lesion, increased density of surrounding bone, and destruction of vertebrae associated with spinal tumors.

Air encephalography (AEG) performed through a lumbar puncture is useful in outlining tumors that impinge on CSF pathways or displace and distort the ventricles. *Ventriculography* is used to outline the ventricular system through the use of contrast material or air introduced directly into the lateral ventricle. This procedure is useful especially for persons with increased intracranial pressure in whom a lumbar puncture for the AEG could cause a cerebellar foramen magnum herniation. *Angiography* detects displacement of vessels from their normal position due to tumor growth. It also provides information concerning the intrinsic vasculature of the tumor.

Isotopes injected intravenously break down the blood-brain barrier, which allows an abnormal amount of radioactive material to accumulate in the area of the tumor. With isotope scanning, blood supply to the tumor is important and avascular or small tumors may not be detected. The *computerized axial tomography* (CT) scan is the screening procedure of choice because it is noninvasive and nonpainful. It involves the use of a computer, which because of various absorptive characteristics of brain tissue, blood, CSF, cyst fluid, and tumors, can process numerous high-speed films to produce a pictorial print of transverse sections of the body.

The newest diagnostic tool used to identify central nervous system abnormalities is *magnetic resonance imaging* (MRI). It views the brain in successive layers within a powerful magnetic field. Images are clear and more precisely identified than with CT scanning (see Chap. 48). An *electroencephalogram (EEG)* gives valuable information concerning altered neuron excitability in the region of the tumor and shows abnormalities in 75 percent of tumors [3]. An *echoencephalogram* shows shifts in intracranial contents. A *myelogram* is useful in localizing tumors of the spinal cord.

Lumbar puncture may be performed to examine the CSF. In the presence of tumors, this test usually reveals a normal CSF glucose, an elevated protein level, and sometimes tumor cells. During lumbar puncture *Queckenstedt's jugular compression test* can demonstrate a spinal subarachnoid block (see p. 829). Due to the danger of brain herniation, lumbar puncture is not performed when there is obvious evidence of increased intracranial pressure.

Finally, to make a diagnosis, tumor histology must be determined. This usually requires surgery and tumor tissue examination.

Tumors of the Neuroglial Cells (Gliomas)

The glial cells provide support and protection for nerve cells and include astrocytes, oligodendroglia, and ependymal cells. The tumors are named and classified according to cell type: astrocytomas, oligodendrogliomas, and ependymomas. Gliomas may invade any area of the central nervous system and are infiltrating by nature. They may also spread from one area of the brain or spinal cord to another.

Astrocytomas. Astrocytomas develop from astrocytes. These spider- or star-shaped cells infiltrate brain tissue and are frequently associated with cysts of various sizes. Their invasive nature usually makes surgical removal difficult. An exception is the pilocytic astrocytoma that grows in the cerebellum and optic nerve and has a good prognosis after removal [5].

Astrocytomas have varying degrees of malignancy. Most are well-differentiated and grow slowly for many years. Some are susceptible to change over time and become mixed astrocytomas and glioblastomas. Gross inspection usually reveals poorly defined, gray-white, infiltrative masses that enlarge and distort underlying CNS tissue. The initial symptom frequently is seizures. Headaches, mental disturbances, and signs of increased intracranial pressure may develop several years later.

Other astrocytomas are very poorly differentiated, anaplastic tumors that have a rapid rate of growth. On gross inspection, they are large, infiltrative lesions. Their prognosis is dismal, with death occurring within months to a few years after diagnosis.

Due to variations in anaplasia, a malignancy grading system of I to IV is used. Differentiated astrocytomas are referred to as grade I or II, anaplastic astrocytomas as grade III, and glioblastoma multiforme as grade IV. Rating systems are highly subjective and their clinical usefulness is limited.

Glioblastoma Multiforme. Glioblastoma multiforme is an extremely malignant, highly vascular glioma that frequently arises from undifferentiated astrocytomas. The appearance on gross inspection varies according to the region of the brain in which it arises. Some appear white and firm while others appear yellow and soft [5]. Glioblastomas grow very rapidly, are invasive, and are resistant to various combinations of surgery, radiotherapy, and chemotherapy. Tissue necrosis and brain edema are characteristic, thus prognosis is poor. Ninety percent of these patients die within two years after diagnosis [5].

Oligodendrogliomas. Oligodendrogliomas arise from oligodendroglia, a neuroglia with vinelike processes present sporadically throughout the CNS. Gross examination usually reveals well-defined, gray, globular masses. These may contain cystic foci, calcifications, and hemorrhagic areas [6]. These tumors are similar in behavior to astrocytomas in that they generally grow slowly. On occasion, however, rapid growth occurs and these tumors may imitate the glioblastomas. Distinction may be made only on histologic examination. Oligodendrogliomas also have a tendency to form focal calcification.

Ependymomas. Ependymal cells line the ventricular walls and form the central canal in the spinal cord. Generally, cranial ependymomas appear as fairly well-defined masses that grow by expansion [5]. Ependymomas tend to form small canals (rosettes) within the tumor. The tumor cells also align themselves around blood vessels (pseudorosettes). Those that arise from ependymal cells lining the walls of the ventricular system fill and obstruct the ventricles and invade adjacent tissue. This can obstruct CSF passage and lead to the development of hydrocephalus. The most common site of ependymomas is the fourth ventricle.

Ependymomas that arise within the spinal cord represent a large percentage of intraspinal gliomas. Symptoms are related to the spinal level at which they occur. The location of these tumors often makes them inaccessible to removal by surgery. Thus, even though they grow slowly, the prognosis is poor and death occurs in a few years.

Variants of ependymomas include subependymomas and myxopapillary ependymomas. Subependymomas arise from neuroglial tissue beneath the ependymal lining and are composed of astrocytic and ependymal elements. These small, hard, lobular tumors rarely grow large enough to cause symptoms. Myxopapillary ependymomas are composed mostly of ependymal cells arising almost exclusively in the filum terminale.

Tumors of Neuronal Origin

Cerebral neuroblastomas arise in precursor cells of neurons. Gross examination reveals well-defined, gray, granular masses that may contain areas of necrosis, hemorrhage, and cysts [5]. Neuroblastomas are rare and usually occur during the first decade of life. Their rate of growth is rapid and they commonly recur after surgery.

Gangliogliomas are very rare tumors composed of neuroglial tissue. Gross inspection reveals well-defined masses with granular surfaces. Calcifications and small cysts may be present within the mass. These tumors are most common in children and young adults. If the location permits surgical excision, the prognosis is good.

Tumors of Embryonic Origin

Medulloblastomas arise predominantly from primitive cells in the cerebellum. Thus, they have the potential to develop along neuronal or neuroglial lines. Gross inspection generally reveals fairly well-demarcated, gray-white masses with indistinct edges [5]. Medulloblastomas occur almost exclusively in children but have been found in adults in rare situations up to the sixth decade of life. They most frequently affect males. They are highly malignant, grow rapidly, and infiltrate throughout the subarachnoid space with resultant widespread meningeal foci. The CSF pathways become blocked and signs of increased intracranial pressure develop. These tumors are associated with increasing ataxia, headaches, and forceful vomiting. The prognosis is dismal, but combinations of surgery, radiotherapy, and chemotherapy can prolong survival.

Tumors of the Meninges

Meningiomas. Meningiomas are primary tumors arising from the meninges. They are most common in females and occur generally in the seventh decade of life [6]. Meningeal constituents that may be involved include arachnoid cells, fibroblasts, and blood vessels. Gross inspection tends to reveal tough, gray-white, irregular to round, lobular masses [5]. Meningiomas are quite vascular and are seen readily on radioisotope scans. They are usually well circumscribed, encapsulated, and press into surrounding tissue. The tumors may penetrate adjacent bone, but widespread infiltration of surrounding nervous tissue is not common. Most of these tumors are benign and grow slowly so that initial symptoms may be overlooked. As they continue to grow, symptoms include seizures, headache, visual impairment, hemiparesis, and aphasia. If they are diagnosed early and are in an area accessible to surgery, complete excision is possible and a good prognosis results. If these tumors are not completely resected, they may recur.

Meningeal Sarcomas. Spindle-cell sarcomas may arise in the meninges. These malignant lesions are very anaplastic and may metastasize to sites outside the nervous system, particularly to the lungs and lymph nodes [5].

Tumors of the Pituitary Gland

Pituitary adenomas are a special group of nervous system tumors that produce neurologic signs and symptoms when they put pressure on the hypothalamus, optic chiasm, third ventricle, and medial temporal lobe. The initial symptoms are hormonal disturbances or visual field defects. These tumors arise from the three cell types in the anterior pituitary: basophil cells, which stain blue; eosinophil cells, which stain red; and chromophobe cells, which do not stain. Although pituitary tumors have usually been classified according to cell type, it is more accurate to identify them as functioning (secreting a hormone) or nonfunctioning (nonsecreting). They usually contain a predominant cell type, however, and the chromophobe cells give rise to these tumors most frequently (see Chap. 32). Prognosis depends on the success of treatment, which may include irradiation, hypophysectomy, and/or hormone replacement. Treatment is considerably more successful when the tumor is still confined to the sella.

Adrenocorticotropic hormone (ACTH)-producing pituitary adenomas are primarily composed of basophil cells and are usually so small that adjacent tissue is not compressed. They have powerful effects, however, due to hypersecretion of ACTH, which is one of several mechanisms that produce Cushing's syndrome. Symptoms of Cushing's syndrome include weakness, emotional lability, moon face, obesity of the torso, hypertension, salt and water retention, diabetes mellitus, glycosuria, osteoporosis, skin striae over the abdomen, hirsutism, and amenorrhea (see Chap. 33).

Pituitary adenomas inducing gigantism and acromegaly are primarily composed of acidophilic cells, and are small and rather slow-growing. They cause an increase in the output of growth hormone. If they develop before bone growth is complete, gigantism results. Tumor development after bone growth has stopped produces the clinical picture called *acromegaly*. These adenomas may grow to such size that they press on the optic chiasm, causing bitemporal hemianopsia or other visual disturbances.

Nonsecreting pituitary adenomas are the most common pituitary tumors and are composed primarily of chromophobe cells. Although these cells have no known special function, tumors arising from them are rather large and produce symptoms by compressing the pituitary gland, optic chiasm, hypothalamus, and adjacent brain tissue. These tumors usually produce hypopituitarism. Signs and symptoms include a sallow appearance, loss of body hair, weakness, amenorrhea, loss of sexual desire, low basal metabolism, hypoglycemia, hypotension, and electrolyte disturbances. As the tumor presses on the optic chiasm, bitemporal hemianopsia is produced and blindness may result (see Chap. 32).

Tumors of the Cranial and Peripheral Nerves and Nerve Roots

Neurilemmomas (schwannomas) and neurofibromas arise from cells that ensheath cranial nerves, peripheral nerves, cauda equina, and nerve roots. The three types of cells within the nerve sheaths include Schwann cells, perineural cells, and fibroblasts in the epineurium and endoneurium. Although the three cells are similar morphologically, Schwann cells are generally the primary source of tumors.

Neurilemmomas (schwannomas) are tumors that arise from the Schwann cells and occur on any of the nerves or nerve roots. The tumors are firm, circumscribed, well-encapsulated, and white to gray [5]. Many lesions may be present on the same nerve or throughout the body. They often involve the vestibulocochlear division of the acoustic (eighth) nerve (acoustic neuroma), most frequently at the cerebellopontile angle, or where the acoustic nerve enters the internal auditory meatus. Bilateral involvement of the acoustic nerve occurs in *von Recklinghausen's neurofibromatosis*.

Acoustic neuromas produce the following symptoms due to position and/or disruption in function: impaired hearing; tinnitus; vertigo; balance and coordination difficulties; ataxia; loss of caloric vestibular reactivity with horizontal nystagmus; palsies of the third, fifth, and seventh cranial nerves; and signs of increased intracranial pressure as the normal flow of CSF is obstructed. Complete surgical removal is usually attempted to prevent recurrence of the tumor, but this often produces cranial nerve dysfunctions such as deafness or facial paralysis.

Neurofibromas arise primarily from Schwann cells and fibroblasts and generally tend to be multiple and encapsulated. Gross examination reveals enlargement of the affected nerve or nerve root. Numerous tumors are often present, especially when associated with the hereditary disease, von Recklinghausen's neurofibromatosis.

Tumors of the Blood Vessels

Blood vessel tumors include arteriovenous malformations, hemangioblastomas, and endotheliomas. They account for only a very small percentage of brain tumors.

Arteriovenous Malformations (AVMs). These malformations consist of an abnormal collection of blood vessels in which arteries join veins directly rather than through capillaries. The majority of angiomas are in the posterior half of the cerebral hemispheres. The abnormal vessels are present at birth and enlarge with the passage of time. Thus, symptoms may not occur for years although manifestations are often noted between ages 10 and 30 years. As the vessels grow, they may compress the normal brain, and weak walls may bleed into the cerebral or subarachnoid spaces. Hemorrhage may be fatal, but in 90 percent of cases bleeding stops and the person survives [1]. Recurrence of hemorrhage is a constant danger and various modes of treatment have been used. Symptoms vary according to the region of involvement and size of the AVM. In some cases there are no clinical symptoms and the AVM is found only on autopsy.

Hemangioblastomas. Hemangioblastomas are neoplasms made up of an aggregation of blood vessels that may also be cystic. These arise most commonly in the cerebellum, but may occur in the cerebrum. Symptoms include ataxia, dizziness, and signs of increased intracranial pressure. Because erythropoietin is often secreted from these tumors, polycythemia may be exhibited. If the cerebellar cyst can be opened and the hemangioblastomatous nodule excised, the prognosis is good. A combination of cerebellar hemangioblastoma in association with cysts of the kidneys and pancreas, together with angiomatosis of the retinas, is known as *von Hippel-Lindau syndrome*.

Tumors of Developmental Defects

Developmental tumors arise from cells that have developed abnormally and persist throughout prenatal growth. They include dermoids, teratomas, cholesteatomas, chordomas, and craniopharyngiomas.

Dermoids and Teratomas. Dermoids and teratomas may occur anywhere in the CNS but frequently arise in the ventricular system. They may obstruct the third ventricle, the aqueduct of Sylvius, or the fourth ventricle. As a result of embryonic displacement of tissue, these tumors may contain bits of hair, primitive teeth, or other material.

Cholesteatomas. These relatively rare growths are also known as epidermoid tumors or cysts and occur most commonly in the young adult. They consist of encapsulated epithelial debris and are most frequently located in the cerebellopontile angle. They simulate acoustic neuromas when located there. Other areas that may give rise to cholesteatomas include the fourth ventricle, supraseller region, and the pineal recession. Although they are benign tumors, they may enlarge and cause erosion of adjacent bones.

Chordomas. These are rare, congenital, malignant tumors that are derived from remnants of the primitive notochord. They are jellylike, gray-pink growths and grow near the sella turcica, at the base of the brain, at the cervical or the sacrococcygeal areas. These tumors erode the bone and invade the dura. Total surgical removal is impossible due to their highly invasive nature. Symptoms of congenital tumors usually develop within the first 10 years of life and depend on the size and location of the lesion.

Craniopharyngiomas (Rathke's Pouch Tumors). These are tumors derived from Rathke's pouch, a pouch in the embryonic membrane that develops into the anterior lobe of the pituitary. They are most often located above the sella turcica. This tumor is encapsulated and grows as a solid mass or more frequently as a cyst. The cyst often contains thick, brown, oily fluid and often has some degree of calcification. Rupture of the cystic fluid into the subarachnoid space may cause recurrent bouts of "sterile" meningitis or, in some cases, bacterial meningitis. As the craniopharyngioma grows, pressure is applied to the pituitary gland, the optic chiasm, and sometimes the base of the brain. Erosion of the sella wall may occur. Symptoms most commonly occur in children and young adults, and reflect signs and symptoms of pituitary hypofunction, hydrocephalus, visual disturbances, and diabetes insipidus. Surgical removal is possible if the site is accessible.

Tumors of Adenexal Structures

Pinealomas are rare tumors composed of large epithelial cells present in the adult pineal gland. Cell differentiation divides pinealomas into pinecytomas and pineablastomas. Pinealomas cause symptoms by compressing the aqueduct of Sylvius, causing hydrocephalus and increased intracranial pressure. Treatment may include a combination of surgery, atrioventricular shunt, and radiotherapy.

Choroid plexus papillomas are rare tumors that occur primarily in children. Gross inspection reveals well-defined, cauliflowerlike, papillary masses that often protrude into the fourth ventricle [6]. Although histologically benign, they may cause intraventricular bleeding, papilledema, hydrocephalus, and increased intracranial pressure. Treatment includes surgery followed by radiotherapy.

Metastatic Tumors

Metastases most commonly occur from primary sites in the breasts and lungs, but neoplasms of the gastrointestinal tract, genitourinary tract, bone, thyroid gland, and nasal sinuses can also metastasize to the brain and spinal cord. Metastatic tumors are generally solid, circumscribed masses that are surrounded by vasogenic edema. They may be solitary tumors or multiple small masses scattered throughout the central nervous system. Signs and symptoms vary with the location, size, and number of lesions. Intracranial metastases most often appear in individuals who already have symptoms of far-advanced cancers, but occasionally produce the initial symptoms. Even with combinations of surgery, radiotherapy, and chemotherapy, prognosis is poor.

Infections

General Considerations

Central nervous system tissue is not immune to viral, bacterial, or other infections. The infections usually arise initially in another region of the body. Organisms can gain access to the CNS in several ways: (1) by spread from adjacent structures—nasal sinuses, skull, middle ear; (2) by entrance through penetrating wounds; and (3) through the bloodstream. Once infectious organisms enter the CNS, they can spread rapidly by way of the CSF, leading to widespread, devastating results.

Diagnosis of any CNS infections depends on evidence of the infective organism together with changes in pressure, glucose, and protein levels of the CSF. The CNS alterations and clinical manifestations vary according to the type of infection.

Viral Infections

Viruses may gain access to the body orally, through the respiratory system, by animal or mosquito bites, or across the placenta to the fetus. Once inside the body, they make their way to the CNS through the hematogenous route by way of the cerebral capillaries and the choroid plexus. Other entry routes include the peripheral nerves and possibly, penetration of the olfactory mucosa [1].

Within the CNS, viruses apparently affect specific, susceptible cells; thus the pathologic effects are considerably different. Damage to the CNS may be due to direct viral invasion of cells with subsequent lysis (acute encephalitis), due to selective lysis with resulting demyelination (progressive multifocal leukoencephalopathy), due to immune responses to viral antigens (acute disseminated encephalomyelitis), and in some cases, due to cellular destruction without apparent inflammatory or immune response. Viruses may also remain latent in cells for months or years until circumstances trigger acute infections (see Chap. 8).

Innumerable viruses are known to invade the nervous system, and only a representative sample of the most frequently encountered viruses is presented in the following section.

Acute Encephalitis. Encephalitis is a general term that encompasses infections of the brain parenchyma in which a wide range of symptoms is manifested. Although encephalitis may be caused by bacteria, rickettsia, parasites, and fungi, viral infections are most common. Symptoms include headache, high fever, confusion, convulsions, and restlessness that progresses to stupor and coma. There may also be focal CNS impairment such as hemiparesis, asymmetry of tendon reflexes, Babinski's sign, involuntary movements, ataxia, and difficulty in speaking or understanding. Brainstem involvement may be manifested by facial weakness or ocular palsies. Analysis of CSF usually reveals increased numbers of lymphocytes, normal to slightly increased pressure, slightly increased protein, normal glucose, and normal chloride levels. A comatose state may persist for days, weeks, or months after the acute infection. Residual effects may include behavior and personality changes, mental deterioration, parkinsonism, paralysis, and persistant seizures. The specific signs and symptoms that predominate depend on the causative organism. A wide variety of viruses causes encephalitis and a discussion of the more common ones follows.

Arthropod-Borne (ARBO) Virus Encephalitis. This large group of viruses commonly causes encephalitis. The organisms seem to occur in certain geographic locations and during certain seasons. Except for tick-borne arboviruses, all of these viruses have vertebrate hosts with mosquito vectors. The principal site of infection is the brain. Clinical manifestations among the different arboviruses are similar; however, they may vary with the age of the afflicted individual. For example, onset of fever and convulsions is most abrupt in children.

Eastern equine encephalitis, occurring primarily in the eastern states, is an infrequent cause of encephalitis. It is the most serious of the arboviruses because it causes extensive destruction of the cerebral cortex and white matter. When there is clinical evidence (1 in 19 cases) of encephalitis due to this virus, mortality is close to 80 percent [5]. Those who survive often have residual effects that include blindness, deafness, mental retardation, emotional disorders, and hemiplegia. The greatest change in CSF is large numbers of polymorphonuclear leukocytes.

Western equine encephalitis may involve the upper spinal cord as well as large portions of the brain. It is most common in the western region of the country. Fever, stupor, dizziness, confusion, and headache are common factors. Mortality is lower than with eastern equine encephalitis. Postencephalitic parkinsonism is a frequent sequela of this type of ençephalitis.

St. Louis encephalitis is a milder form of the disease and may involve both the brain and spinal cord. It occurs primarily in the central and western states. Prominent meningeal involvement accompanies St. Louis encephalitis. Other findings include fever, athetosis, drowsiness or stupor, tremors, and, more commonly, seizures. Any age group may develop this infection and recovery is generally good.

California encephalitis affects children more frequently than adults. Its onset is insidious and its signs include headache, fever, vomiting, mental confusion, seizures, and stupor that may deteriorate to coma.

Although recovery from the acute episode is common, residual learning difficulties, emotional lability, and seizures may remain as long-term problems.

Herpes Simplex. Herpes simplex is a very serious and common form of encephalitis that may produce illness in any age group. This type of encephalitis has been reported in all parts of the world. Most frequently the disease is associated with type I herpes simplex virus, which is also the common cause of oral mucosal lesions. The virus may be introduced from a primary lip infection to the brainstem by the trigeminal nerve. Type II herpes simplex virus causes genital infection and, when present in the mother, produces acute encephalitis in the neonate; acquired during passage through an infected birth canal [1].

Alterations in the CNS are more common in the medial and inferior portions of the temporal lobes and orbital gyri of the frontal lobes. The lesions include hemorrhagic necrosis, inflammation, and perivascular infiltrates. The CSF reveals an increased pressure, increased protein level, increased number of lymphocytes, and the presence of red cells due to the hemorrhagic nature of the lesions. Serologic tests and brain biopsy confirm a diagnosis of herpes simplex encephalitis. Clinical manifestations include acute onset with headache, fever, convulsions, confusion, stupor, and coma, in addition to focal disturbances related to lesions in specific portions of the temporal and frontal lobes. Mortality is estimated to be almost 70 percent, but early treatment with the antimetabolite adenine arabinoside A (Ara-A) has reduced mortality to about 28 percent [9].

Rabies. Clinical cases of rabies in humans are rare, but once the disease is established, it is almost always fatal. This dreaded viral disease can affect anyone who has sustained a bite through the skin by a rabid animal (usually dogs, cats, bats, foxes, raccoons, or skunks). Its incubation period varies from 14 days to 3 months. Survival of inoculated victims depends on specific postexposure prophylaxis.

The virus makes its way from the wound to the CNS through the peripheral nerves, producing degenerative changes in these neurons. Alterations in the CNS include brain edema, neuron degeneration, and vascular congestion. Inflammatory reactions seem to be greatest in the basal nuclei, midbrain, and medulla. The spinal cord, sympathetic ganglia, the dorsal root ganglia may also be involved. Negri bodies, which are oval-shaped, eosinophilic, cytoplasmic inclusions, are a characteristic histologic feature of rabies.

Clinical manifestations occur in stages, beginning with generalized malaise, apathy, fever, and headache. These general symptoms, together with pain and numbness in the area of the wound, are diagnostic of the illness in its early stage. Within 24 to 72 hours after the general symptoms, there is an excitement phase marked by extreme fear, violent spasms of the larynx when swallowing that lead to hydrophobia, and dysphagia that leads to salivating with frothing from the mouth. Heightened sensitivity to external stimuli can produce localized twitching and generalized seizures. Facial numbness, dysarthria, hallucinations, and a confusional psychosis accompany this phase. Finally, there are alternating periods of stupor and mania, high fever, flaccid paralysis, coma, and respiratory failure. Death usually occurs from respiratory center failure within two to seven days after the onset of neurologic symptoms.

Slow Virus Disease. Unlike the acute encephalitides, the slow virus diseases go through a long latent period lasting from months to years before they manifest symptoms. Once symptoms have appeared, these diseases tend to progress at a slower pace. Two general types of slow infections are (1) true slow virus infections, which include subacute sclerosing panencephalitis (SSPE), progressive multifocal leukoencephalopathy (PML), and progressive rubella panencephalitis; and (2) unconventional agent infections (spongiform), which include Jacob-Creutzfeldt disease and kuru [1]. The former are caused by known, conventional viruses; and the latter by yet unidentified agents that have some resemblance to viruses but do not produce an immune reaction in the host.

Subacute Sclerosing Panencephalitis (SSPE). This illness usually occurs in children and is related to a prior infection by the measles virus. Granular regions, areas of focal destruction, and proliferation of neuroglial cells are present in the CNS. The CSF reveals increased protein, increased gamma globulin fraction, and high levels of measles antibody. There is also evidence of measles antigen in neurons and glial cells. Bursts of high-voltage and sharp waves are noted on EEG examination. The illness occurs in stages over several years: (1) initially, personality changes occur; (2) intellectual deterioration, seizures, and visual disturbances follow; and (3) rigidity, progressive unresponsiveness, and signs of autonomic dysfunction cause death within a few months or years.

Progressive Multifocal Leukoencephalopathy (PML). This condition most often occurs in middle-aged persons who have a chronic debilitating disease such as rheumatoid arthritis, acquired immunodeficiency syndrome (AIDS), or neoplastic disease, or in those who are receiving immunosuppressive therapy. Opportunistic viruses cause CNS alterations, including widespread demyelinization of white matter, particularly of the cerebral hemispheres, brainstem, cerebellum, and rarely, the spinal cord. The CSF usually remains normal. Diagnosis of lesions may be facilitated by computerized axial tomography [1]. Symptoms of PML include hemiparesis, visual field defects, aphasia, ataxia, dysarthria, confusion, and eventually coma. Death occurs within three to six months after onset of symptoms.

Progressive Rubella Panencephalitis. This type of encephalitis, associated with rubella either of congenital or childhood origin, appears after a long latent period and continues on a progressive course. Initial symptoms are subtle changes in behavior and intellectual performance. Seizures arise in association with progressive mental deterioration, motor incoordination and spasticity; mutism, quadriplegia, and ophthalmoplegia mark the terminal stages of the disease. Progressive rubella panencephalitis seems to affect the white matter primarily, destroying nerve cells and attracting lymphocytes and mononuclear cells.

Subacute Spongiform Encephalopathy (Jacob-Creutzfeldt Disease, Transmissible Viral Dementia). This rare, rapidly progressive disease, which usually occurs in late middle age, produces CNS alterations mainly in the cerebral and cerebellar cortices and occasionally the basal ganglia. Alterations include neural degeneration, gliosis, and a spongelike condition in affected areas. Although serologic studies and CSF are normal, there is usually an associated, distinctive EEG pattern of diffuse nonspecific slowing, which changes to sharp waves or spikes on an increasingly flat background [1].

The early clinical manifestations include personality changes, memory loss, visual abnormalities (distortions of shape, decreased visual acuity), and delirium. These symptoms are followed rapidly by dementia, myoclonic contractions, dysarthria, and ataxia, which eventually give way to stupor and coma, although myoclonic contractions continue. To date there is no effective treatment. Death usually occurs within one to two years after onset of symptoms.

Kuru. Kuru, the first slow viral infection documented in humans, occurs in the Fore natives of Papua-New Guinea. The disease is associated with cannibalism in this tribe. Although the CNS alterations are similar to those associated with subacute spongiform encephalopathy, in kuru the spongelike conditions are more prominent in the corpus striatum and cerebellum [6]. Clinical manifestations include progressive cerebellar ataxia, shivering tremors, abnormal extraocular movement, incontinence, progression to complete immobility, and dementia in the terminal stage. After the onset of symptoms, death usually occurs within three to six months.

Other CNS Viral Infections

Aseptic Meningitis Complex (Benign Viral Meningitis). These are general names for disorders in which there is evidence of meningeal irritation, although pyogenic organisms, parasites, or fungi are not present in CSF. Lymphocytes are commonly present in the CSF in individuals with aseptic meningitis. A virus is expected to be the causative agent, and the following viruses have been found in over one-third of the individuals with aseptic meningitis complex: mumps, herpes simplex, Coxsackievirus, lymphocytic choriomeningitis virus, and ECHO virus. The symptoms are mild, and most individuals recover from these illnesses without significant residual effects.

Viruses Acquired Congenitally. Viruses are capable of crossing the placenta to reach the fetus, especially during the first trimester of pregnancy. They often produce devastating effects on the fetus. Although it is possible for many types of viruses to infect the fetus, the most common ones are *rubella* and *cytomegaloviruses (CVM)*.

Congenital rubella often occurs during the first 10 weeks of gestation. The virus invades the fetus's brain and contributes to the establishment of severe mental retardation, seizures, and motor defects. Other manifestations may include low birth weight, abnormally small eyeballs, pigmentary retinal degeneration, glaucoma, cloudy cornea, cataracts, neurocochlear deafness, enlarged liver and spleen, jaundice, and patent ductus arteriosus or intraventricular septal defects [1]. These severe effects are preventable by ensuring that women receive the rubella vaccine prior to becoming pregnant.

Cytomegaloviruses usually infect the fetus early during the first trimester of pregnancy and may produce cerebral malformation. Later, although the brain is normally formed, CMV may produce inflammatory necrosis in various parts of the brain. Nervous system effects of this infection may include mental defects, convulsions, microcephaly, and often hydrocephalus. Other manifestations include enlarged liver and spleen, jaundice, melena, hematemesis, and petechiae [1]. Whether a fetus has been infected by CMV cannot be determiined until birth (and in some cases, several years after birth) because the infection is not apparent in pregnant women.

Myelitis. Poliomyelitis and herpes zoster are the two principal types of myelitis (inflammation of the spinal cord).

Poliomyelitis. Since the advent of the Salk vaccine in 1955 and the oral Sabin vaccine in 1958, cases of paralytic poliomyelitis are uncommon. The synonym for poliomyelitis is "infantile paralysis"; however, the disease occurs in all age groups. The disease is known to occur throughout the world and peak frequency is during the summer months.

The human intestinal tract is the main viral reservoir for the ribonucleic acid (RNA) virus, which infects through the fecal-oral route. Incubation lasts from one to three weeks. The virus then penetrates intestinal walls, invades the bloodstream, and is carried throughout the body.

Alterations in the CNS include destruction of nerve cells, as well as cellular infiltration, edema, and severe inflammatory processes that produce tissue necrosis and hemorrhages. Experimental inoculation of the nerve cell with the poliomyelitis virus has produced cytoplasmic swelling, chromatolysis, and nuclear displacement [5]. Although the entirie CNS may be involved, the predominant site of alterations is the anterior horn of the spinal cord. Examination of CSF usually shows no evidence of the virus during the clinical disease; but protein levels are elevated, glucose level is normal, and the numbers of lymphocytes is increased.

The majority of persons infected with the virus experience no symptoms, or only a vague illness because of the failure of the virus to invade the CNS. Even after CNS invasion, however, clinical effects range from a mild, nonparalytic form of the disease to a severe, paralytic form. This variation in symptoms is related to the severity of the inflammatory response and to the degree to which nerve cells are injured.

Nonparalytic poliomyelitis produces general symptoms of fever, headache, listlessness, anorexia, nausea, vomiting, sore throat, and aching muscles. At this point, the disease may be resolved. With increasing irritability, restlessness, muscle tenderness and spasms, neck and back pain, and neck stiffness, in addition to Kernig's and Brudzinski's signs, the paralytic form of the disease is often imminent.

Paralytic poliomyelitis is often divided into three types: *spinal*, *bulbar*, and *encephalitic*. This division is primarily useful as a descriptive mechanism, since these types are often combined during the course of the disease. Spinal involvement may include muscle weakness with fasciculations, diminished reflexes in association with progressive abdominal and limb muscle weakness, eventual paralysis (the level varying among different age groups), and muscle atrophy. Bulbar involvement impairs the ability to swallow, disturbs respiration and vasomotor control, and progressively slows respirations. Cyanosis and hypertension may occur, followed by hypotension and circulatory collapse. Mortality is as high as 75 percent when there is accompanying paralysis of phrenic and intercostal muscles [1]. Involvement of the high brainstem and hypothalamus produces encephalitic symptoms that include restlessness, confusion, and anxiety initially, progressing to stupor and coma [1].

Herpes Zoster (Shingles). Herpes zoster infection, caused by the varicella zoster virus, occurs most commonly in adulthood, particularly with advancing age, and in persons with underlying systemic diseases such as the leukemias or lymphomas. The development of this illness is not completely understood. It is thought that herpes zoster infection represents a reactivation of varicella virus infection that persists in the nerve ganglia after a primary infection with chickenpox. Individuals who have herpes zoster infection usually have a past history of chickenpox. Nervous system alterations include congested, edematous, and hemorrhagic dorsal root ganglion. There is also disintegration of ganglion cells. Painful, vesicular skin eruptions, which harbor varicella zoster virus, are associated with involvement of the corresponding dorsal root ganglion or *gasserian* ganglion. The most frequently involved dermatomes are T-5 to T-10; however, any dermatome may be involved. In some cases accompanying sensory loss and motor palsies occur. Although most individuals recover, the process is often slow and painful. The pain may persist for months or even years, causing much despair for the person.

Postinfectious/Postvaccinal Diseases. Acute disseminated (postinfectious) encephalomyelitis, acute inflammatory polyradiculoneuropathy (Guillain-Barré syndrome), and Reye's syndrome often occur during or shortly after viral infection, or rarely after vaccinations for smallpox, rabies, or typhoid. These conditions often require individual susceptibility to the virus or viral effects.

Acute Disseminated (Postinfectious) Encephalomyelitis. Postinfectious encephalomyelitis develops two to four days after a rash and is thought to be an autoimmune response to myelin, which is triggered by a virus [5]. Demyelination occurs in the region of the brainstem and spinal cord. In addition, the meninges are infiltrated by inflammatory cells. Clinical manifestations include headaches, stiffness of the neck, lethargy, and eventually coma. One-third to one-half of affected persons die in the acute phase of the illness. Neurologic residual effects are severe in those who survive.

Guillain-Barré Syndrome (Acute Idiopathic Neuropathy). This syndrome is thought to be the result of an autoimmune reaction triggered by a virus in the peripheral nerves. Nervous system alterations include inflammatory infiltrate around vessels throughout the cranial and spinal nerves, demyelination, and axon destruction. The CSF reveals an elevated protein level and pleocytosis. Clinical manifestations include proximal and distal weakness or paralysis of extremities, hypotonia, areflexia, pain, and paresthesias. Weakness that progresses to total motor paralysis of respiratory muscles can result in death. Autonomic dysfunction may occur with resultant sudden fluctuations in blood pressure and heart rate, orthostatic hypotension, and cessation of sweating. Individuals who survive the acute phase of the disease usually recover completely; however, some have residual motor or reflex deficits (see pp. 857–858).

Reye's Syndrome. Reye's syndrome seems to occur after viral infections such as chickenpox or a respiratory virus, although the relationship between the virus and pathologic changes is not understood. Whether the condition results from the viral infection or from treatment with *aspirin* is under investigation. The probability is high that the syndrome is produced in concert with aspirin ingestion [6]. Many factors, including genetic and environmental, apparently function together in the production of this catastrophic disorder. It occurs predominantly in children between ages 6 months and 15 years [5]. It is characterized by the onset of acute encephalopathy 10 days to 2 weeks after a viral infection. Cerebral edema is produced, as well as fatty changes in the liver and renal tubules. The disease is also characterized by hypoglycemia and increased serum ammonia levels. Clinical manifestations include persistent vomiting, delirium, seizures, stupor, and eventual coma. Full-blown disease with encephalopathy and liver involvement carries 40 to 60 percent mortality, but this appears to be improving due to earlier diagnosis and supportive treatment.

Bacterial Infections

Pyogenic Infections. The brain or its coverings can be infected by pyogenic (pus-forming) microorganisms.

The most common organisms that are responsible for bacterial infections are normally harbored in the nasopharynx in the general population. Bacteria enter the CNS by spread from adjacent cranial structures, through the bloodstream; in a few unfortunate cases the infection is iatrogenic, for example, from a lumbar puncture or contaminated scapel. It is frequently difficult to determine the exact entry route of the organism. Once within the CNS, the effects of pyogenic microorganisms may be disastrous.

Bacterial Meningitis (Leptomeningitis). The leptomeninges and subarachnoid space are primary targets for invasion by pyogenic microorganisms. Once an infection enters any part of the subarachnoid space, it spreads quickly throughout CSF pathways in the brain and spinal cord. Thus, an inflammatory reaction is set up in the pia and arachnoid, and in the ventricles. Any microorganisms entering the body may cause meningitis, however, some bacteria are more prominent and seem to be more prevalent in certain age groups. *Pneumococcus* organisms are commonly cultured in very young patients and adults over 40 years of age, *Escherichia coli* in the neonatal period, *Hemophilus influenzae* in infants and young children, and *Neisseria meningitidis* in adolescents and young adults [5]. Spinal fluid cultures usually reveal the causative agent.

Meningococcal infections develop more rapidly and distinctly than other forms of meningitis. They may occur singularly or in epidemics where overcrowding exists. The organism is spread by droplet infection from those who harbor the meningococcus in their nasal passages. Disease onset is heralded by a distinctive petechial or purpuric rash. A particularly disastrous event (Waterhouse-Friderichsen syndrome) may occur after any bacterial meningitis, although it is most commonly associated with fulminant meningococcemia. This condition is manifested by overwhelming bacteremia, adrenocortical necrosis, and vasomotor collapse. *Hemophilus influenzae* meningitis commonly follows ear and upper respiratory infections in the young. Pneumococcal meningitis can be related to prior infections in the lungs, nasal sinuses, and heart valves.

Alterations occurring with the various bacterial infections include swelling and congestion of the brain and spinal cord, as well as exudate within the subarachnoid space. In severe cases, inflammatory cells can occlude vessels that penetrate the brain, resulting in areas of necrosis. The CSF reveals elevated protein, decreased glucose, and decreased chloride levels, elevated pressure (above 180 mm of water), and the presence of large numbers of leukocytes.

Clinical manifestations of acute pyogenic meningitis are fever, headache, pain with eye movement, photophobia, neck and back stiffness, positive Kernig's and Brudzinski's signs, generalized convulsions, drowsiness, and confusion. Focal signs may be observed with some bacterial infections as a result of occlusion of vessels and regional brain necrosis. Stupor, followed by coma and death may occur without prompt and adequate treatment.

Residual effects are also a danger due to destruction or fibrotic thickening of the meningeal framework. Potential residual effects include optic arachnoiditis, meningomyelitis, and chronic meningoencephalitis with hydrocephalus. Again, with prompt diagnosis and antibiotic therapy, these residual effects are less common than they once were.

Brain Abscess. Approximately one-half of all brain abscesses are secondary to infection in the nasal cavity, middle ear, and mastoid cells. The remaining cases are due to primary focus of infection elsewhere in the body, particularly the lungs or pleura, heart, and distal bones (Fig. 49-3). Streptococci, staphylococci, and pneumococci are often the causative organisms.

An abscess is formed when an inflammation, caused by an invading organism, liquifies and begins to accumulate white blood cells. A fibrous capsule is formed in an effort to contain the pus. As the abscess expands, nerve tissue is compressed and destroyed. Chronic inflammation and pronounced edema surround the abscess. The CSF reveals a normal glucose level, increased protein level, and increased white cell count. The CSF pressure is often moderately elevated early in the abscess formation and markedly elevated in the later stages. If the abscess ruptures into the subarachnoid space or ventricles, organisms can be cultured from CSF. Other diagnostic techniques that may be used are skull films, CT scans, EEG, and ventriculography.

The most frequent initial clinical manifestation is headache, with other symptoms being similar to those produced by growing masses within the brain. Notably, the increased intracranial pressure and focal complaints related to the location of the abscess are important. In addition, a brain abscess can rupture and lead to other complications such as sinus thrombosis, ventriculitis, or meningitis. Mortality from brain abscesses has been greatly reduced due to successful combinations of antibiotic therapy and surgery.

Subdural Empyema. Empyema refers to pus in a body cavity; thus, subdural empyema is a suppurative process in the subdural space. It usually occurs between the dura's inner surface and the outer surface of the arachnoid. The most common causative organisms are *Staphylococcus aureus* and streptococci. Infective organisms usually travel to the subdural space by spread from thrombophlebitis or by erosion through bone or dura from the frontal sinuses, ethmoid sinuses, middle ear, or mastoid cells. Exudate is present on the undersurface of the dura. As the empyema grows, pressure is applied to the underlying cerebral hemisphere. Thrombophlebitis of cerebral veins that are near the subdural empyema can contribute to ischemic necrosis of the cortex. The CSF reveals elevated pressure, increased protein and normal glucose levels, and an increased number of lymphocytes.

Many affected persons have a history of chronic mastoiditis or sinusitis. Clinical manifestations indicating that the infection has spread to the subdural space include fever, general malaise, a localized headache that becomes

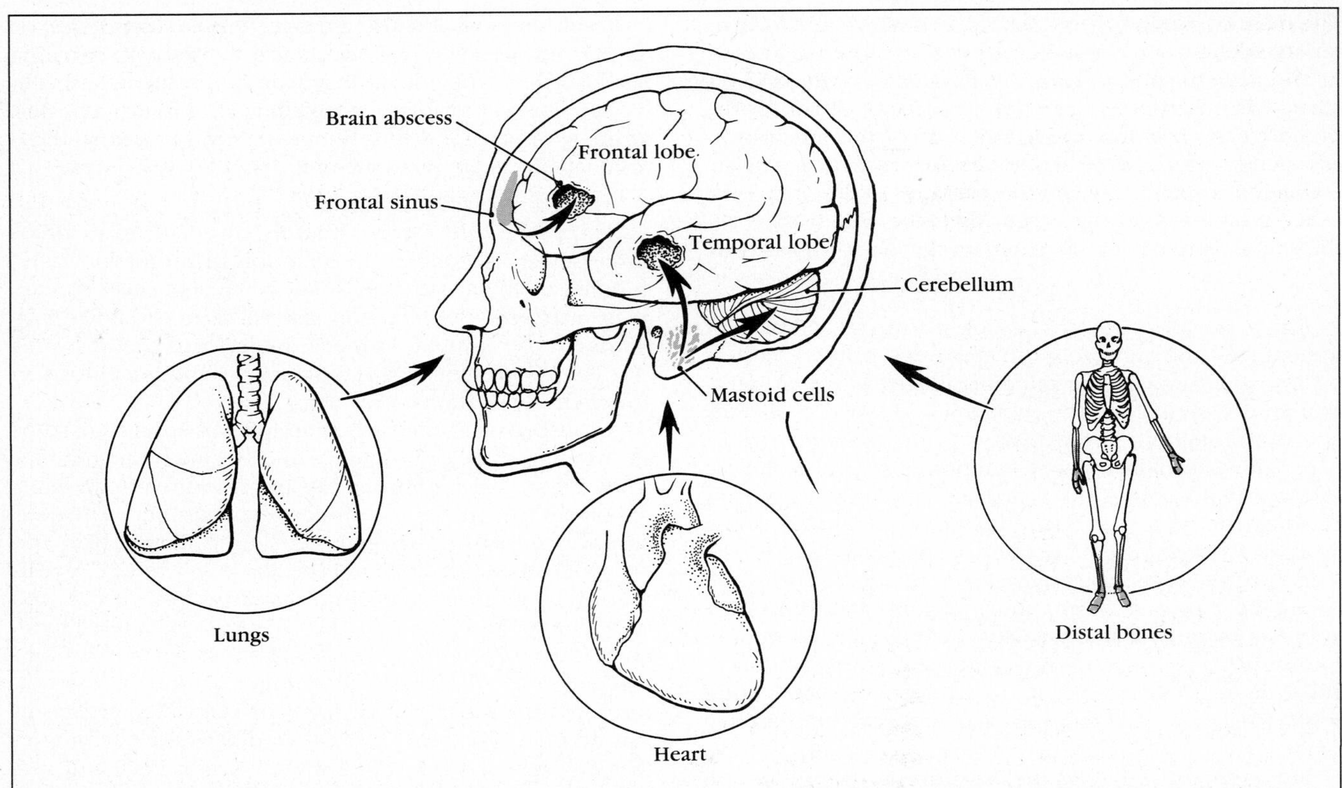

FIGURE 49-3 Origins and locations of cerebral abscesses.

generalized, associated vomiting, and neck stiffness. As the empyema enlarges, focal neurologic signs, lethargy, and coma develop. Prognosis depends on the success of surgery and antibiotic therapy, as well as the extent to which neurologic deficits have occurred.

Tuberculous Infections. Tuberculous meningitis and tuberculomas of the brain and spinal cord are usually secondary to a tuberculous focus in another part of the body. Thus, as better public health measures and modern therapy help control the frequency of tuberculosis, the frequency of tuberculous meningitis and tuberculomas of the brain and cord are decreased.

Tuberculous Meningitis. Tuberculous meningitis occurs in areas of high tuberculosis prevalence, primarily in young children. In low-frequency areas it occurs mostly in the elderly population as a result of reactivation of dormant organisms. Tuberculous meningitis is caused by *Mycobacterium tuberculosis*. This condition has a slower onset and more chronic course than pyogenic meningitis.

The base of the brain and the spinal cord become compressed by shaggy, necrotic, fibrinous, yellow exudate. There may also be large areas of caseation and tiny tubercles around the blood vessels [5]. The CSF reveals increased pressure, elevated protein and decreased glucose levels (but not as low as values observed in pyogenic meningitis), and the presence of polymorphonuclear leukocytes and lymphocytes. With careful technique in obtaining a specimen, tubercle bacilli may be recovered from CSF.

Clinical manifestations depend on the chronicity of the disease and the extent of pathologic processes. In general, adults have headache, fever, lethargy, confusion, neck stiffness, positive Kernig's and Brudzinski's signs, weight loss, and night sweats. Young children frequently experience vomiting, irritability, and seizures.

Due to the slow onset of this illness, neurologic damage may be present before treatment is sought. Then, even though the person survives, there may be lasting effects, such as recurrent seizures, retarded intellectual development, mental disturbances, visual disturbances, deafness, and hemiparesis.

Tuberculomas of Brain and Spinal Cord. Tuberculomas (tuberculous granulation masses), although rare in the United States, constitute from 5 to 30 percent of all intracranial space-occupying lesions in underdeveloped countries [1]. Tuberculomas may be single or multiple and contain a core of caseation necrosis surrounded by a fibrous capsule. Within the brain and spinal cord they produce neurologic effects similar to those of other expanding intracranial and intraspinal lesions. The CSF reveals increased protein levels and a small number of lymphocytes. Tuberculomas of the brain and spinal cord have been known to calcify while still small before any neurologic changes have occurred. These are often found at autopsy.

Neurosyphilis. The frequency of neurosyphilis (tertiary stage of syphilis) has decreased in the last several decades due to prompt diagnosis and treatment of early syphilis. The overall frequency of syphilis is increasing, however, particularly in young persons and homosexuals.

Treponema pallidum is a spiral, motile organism that causes syphilis. Once this organism is introduced into the body, it usually invades the CNS within 3 to 18 months. Neurosyphilis is progressive in the large majority of individuals and includes several forms: asymptomatic neurosyphilis, meningovascular syphilis, general paresis, and tabes dorsalis (see Chap. 55).

Meningitis is the initial event in all forms of neurosyphilis, but the severity of symptoms varies among the different forms and it may remain asymptomatic for several years. The CSF is the most accurate, sensitive indicator that an active neurosyphilitic infection is present. Changes in CSF include positive serologic tests—the Venereal Disease Research Laboratory (VDRL) slide test, Kolmer test, fluorescent treponemal antibody absorption (FTA/ABS) test, and treponema immobilization (TPI) test; increased protein level; presence of increased lymphocytes, plasma cells, and mononuclear cells; and an abnormal colloidal gold curve.

Asymptomatic Neurosyphilis. As the name *asymptomatic neurosyphilis* implies, there are usually no physical signs or symptoms of the meningitis. This form of the disease is recognized by the changes in CSF listed above. Treatment prevents further development of the disease.

Meningovascular Syphilis. This form of neurosyphilis commonly develops six to seven years after the original infection. The CNS alterations include infiltration of meninges and blood vessels with plasma cells and lymphocytes, inflammation of arteries, and fibrosis that leads to occlusion of vessels. The vascular lesions are referred to as Heubner's arteritis. Miliary gummas may also be seen in the meninges.

Clinical manifestations are similar to those of low-grade meningitis as well as cerebrovascular accident and mental derangement. Unless treated, neurologic deficits continue to progress.

General Paresis. This form of neurosyphilis usually develops 15 to 20 years after the original infection. Early treatment of syphilis has decreased the frequency of general paresis. In this form of neurosyphilis, the parenchyma of the brain is involved due to the presence of spirochetes. There is a diffuse destruction of cortical neurons and proliferation of astrocytes. Plasma cells and lymphocytes accumulate around blood vessels.

Clinical manifestations are those of progressive mental and physical deterioration. Initially, slight memory loss, changes in behavior, and decreased ability to reason occur. Later, the individual develops a severe dementia with elaborate delusional systems and disregard for moral and social standards. Physically, the individual experiences dysarthria, tremor of the tongue and hands, myoclonic jerks, muscular hypotonia, hyperactive tendon reflexes, Babinski's signs, seizures, and Argyll Robertson pupils. Without treatment, the prognosis is poor and death occurs in a few years.

Tabes Dorsalis. Tabes dorsalis, like general paresis, occurs many years after the onset of infection. This form of neurosyphilis is also uncommon now due to improved, early treatment with penicillin.

The CNS alterations include degeneration of the posterior columns, fibrosis around the posterior roots, and destruction of proprioceptive fibers in the radicular nerves. These changes produce various symptoms, the most common being ataxia. Other features of this type of neurosyphilis are lightening pains (sudden sharp pains lasting only a portion of a second), ataxia due to sensory defects, and urinary incontinence. Visceral symptoms include vomiting and bouts of sharp epigastric pain that extends around the body. Other clinical manifestations may include Argyll Robertson pupils, Charcot's joints due to repeated injury to insensitive joints, absence of a vibration sense, and deep tendon reflexes, as well as Romberg's sign. Romberg's sign is the inability to maintain balance with the eyes closed and the feet together. Although treatment with penicillin can arrest the disease process, residual effects such as urinary incontinence, lightening pains, visceral crises, and Charcot's joints may persist indefinitely.

Disorders Due to Bacterial Exotoxins. Bacterial exotoxins can have powerful effects on the CNS and can result in life-threatening motor problems. The major diseases produced by these toxins are tetanus, diphtheria, and botulism.

Tetanus. Clostridium tetani produces tetanus after contaminating penetrating wounds or the umbilical cord of the newborn with spores. These anaerobic, spore-forming bacilli produce two exotoxins: a tetanolysin and a tetanospasmin. Neurotoxic effects are produced by tetanospasmin. Most of the toxin enters the peripheral endings of motor neurons from the bloodstream, travels up the fibers to the spinal cord and brainstem, and crosses the synaptic cleft to the inhibitory neurons, where it prevents the release of glycine. Glycine is a neuromuscular transmitter secreted mainly in the synapses of the spinal cord, and it acts as an inhibitor. The action of tetanospasmin is through an affinity for the sympathetic nervous system, the medullary centers, the anterior horn cells of the spinal cord, and the motor end plates in skeletal muscle. It produces uninhibited motor responses that lead to the typical muscle spasm.

The incubation period varies from several days to several months. Usually, symptoms occur within two weeks after wound contamination. The initial manifestation is usually difficulty opening the jaw (trismus); thus, the synonym "lockjaw." There is generalized muscle stiffness with eventual muscle spasms (tetanic seizures or convulsions). These convulsions are very painful and can occur spontaneously or in response to the slightest stimuli. Facial spasms produce a characteristic sardonic smile (risus sardonicus). Contractions of back muscles produce a forward arching of the back (opisthotonos). Spasms of glottal, laryngeal, and respiratory muscles cause difficulty in breathing and frequently lead to death due to asphyxia. In established clinical cases of tetanus, overall mortality is 50 percent [1]. The toxin is not able to cross the blood-brain barrier, which accounts for the normal mentation in these individuals [5]. The disease is prevented with active immunization with tetanus toxoid. Also, prompt administration of antitoxin may prevent progression of symptoms.

Diphtheria. Corynebacterium diphtheriae produces an acute infection, diphtheria. Although open wounds in any part of the body can provide entry for this organism, the usual portal of entry is the oral cavity. The incubation period is one to seven days. During this time the organism becomes established and proliferates at the site of implantation, usually the throat and trachea. The bacteria produce exotoxin that is absorbed by the blood and carried to the CNS and heart. Early general manifestations of the disease are fever, sore throat, chills, and malaise. Local neurologic manifestations occur within 5 to 12 days and include vomiting, dysphagia, possible cranial nerve involvement, and nasal voice due to palatal paralysis. Blurred vision and loss of accommodation occur in the second or third week due to ciliary paralysis. Between the fifth and sixth weeks, weakness and paralysis of the extremities may occur. Most neurologic disturbances disappear slowly, and individuals usually improve completely if respiratory obstruction or cardiac failure does not supervene. The disease is prevented by immunization; prompt administration of antitoxin may prevent clinical manifestations.

Botulism. Clostridium botulinum can contaminate and produce exotoxins in food such as fruits, vegetables, and meats that are kept for long periods of time without refrigeration. When ingested, the toxin resists gastric digestion, is absorbed by the blood, and then travels to the nervous system. The botulinus toxin acts only on the presynaptic endings of neuromuscular junctions and autonomic ganglia. It prevents the release of acetylcholine and therefore causes symptoms resembling those of myasthenia gravis. The result is a descending form of paralysis from the cranial nerves downward [5]. Symptoms occur within 2 to 36 hours after ingestion of the contaminated food. Neural symptoms may or may not be preceded by nausea and vomiting. The individual may develop cranial nerve palsies, blurred vision, diplopia, ptosis, strabismus, hoarseness, dysarthria, dysphagia, vertigo, deafness, constipation, and progressive muscle weakness. Tendon reflexes may be absent. Sensation remains intact and the person is conscious throughout the illness. Even with prompt administration of antitoxin, death occurs in more than 20 percent of cases due to paralysis of respiratory muscles and respiratory infections. Those who survive generally recover completely with effective supportive care over a long, slow course.

Fungal Infections

Fungi infect the CNS less commonly than bacteria and viruses. Their effects can be similar to bacterial infection, but more difficult to treat. Fungal infections may produce brain abscesses, meningitis, meningoencephalitis, and thrombophlebitis of vessels within the CNS. As with other infections, fungal infections of the CNS are usually secondary to a primary source of infection elsewhere in the body. In addition, they may be a complication of another disease process, such as cancer, or related to immunosuppressant drugs.

Fungi usually spread to the CNS by way of the bloodstream. Once within the CNS, they cause an inflammatory reaction, and a purulent exudate involves the meninges. In some cases, invasion of vessel walls results in vasculitis and thrombosis with subsequent nervous tissue infarction. The process develops slowly over a period of days or weeks. Clinical manifestations are similar to those of tuberculous meningitis. In addition, hydrocephalus is a frequent related complication. The CSF reveals elevated pressure, increased protein and decreased glucose levels, moderate pleocytosis (increased number of lymphocytes), and often the isolation of the infective organism.

Many types of fungi may invade the CNS; the most common infections are candidiasis, cryptococcosis, coccidioidomycosis, and mucormycosis.

Cryptococcosis (Torulosis). Common in soil and bird droppings, cryptococci are the most frequent cause of fungal infection of the CNS. The fungus is transmitted to humans through the respiratory tract. Cryptococcosis, which usually arises secondary to a pulmonary infection, produces cysts and granulomas in the cortex and occasionally in the deep white matter and basal ganglia. These cysts contain large numbers of organisms. *Cryptococcus neoformans* is recovered from spinal fluid. Mortality, even in the absence of preexisting diseases (lymphomas and Hodgkin's disease), is nearly 40 percent [1]. Clinical features are similar to those of subacute meningitis or encephalitis.

Coccidioidomycosis. *Coccidioides immitis* produces a relatively mild, flulike illness involving the respiratory organs. Common in the southwestern United States, coccidioidomycosis may become a chronic, diffuse, granulomatous disease that spreads throughout the body. The meninges and CSF become involved with resultant pathologic and clinical manifestations similar to those of tuberculous meningitis. When the meninges become involved, treatment is difficult. Amphotericin B is the only effective drug, and even with this treatment, the disease is often fatal.

Mucormycosis. Mucormycosis, caused by one of the mucorales, is a rare opportunistic infection occurring in very debilitated persons. One of the primary sites of invasion is the nasal sinuses. From the nasal sinuses the organism may spread along invaded vessels to periorbital tissue and the cranial vault. Nervous tissue infarctions occur as a result of vascular occlusion. Once the mucorales organism has invaded the brain, prognosis is very poor.

Protozoal Infections

Malaria. *Plasmodium vivax* produces the most common form of malaria. This organism does not actually invade brain tissue, but the parasitized red blood cells block microcirculation, thus leading to tissue hypoxia and ischemic necrosis. The vessel blockage within the brain leads to glial necrosis, which causes drowsiness, confusion, and seizures. Quinine is used for treatment and is helpful unless the cerebral symptoms are far advanced.

Plasmodium falciparum produces a form of malaria that has more severe symptoms. The parasite fills capillaries, and Dürck's nodes (small foci of necrosis surrounded by glia) are present in brain tissue. The CSF reveals elevated pressure and contains white blood cells. Clinical manifestations include focal neurologic signs, headache, seizures, aphasia, cerebellar ataxia, hemiplegia, hemianopsia and, eventually, coma. Cerebral malaria due to *P. falciparum* is usually rapidly fatal.

Toxoplasmosis. *Toxoplasma gondii* produces an infection that is either acquired or congenital. The organism is transmitted by eating raw beef or by contact with cat feces.

Acquired toxoplasmosis that produces clinical effects is rare. In clinical cases the white and gray matter contain necrotic lesions that harbor *T. gondii*. Symptoms are similar to meningoencephalitis. Acquired toxoplasmosis is observed rather frequently in persons with acquired immune deficiency syndrome (AIDS).

Congenital toxoplasmosis causes much destruction of the neonatal brain. Signs of infection are fever, rash, seizures, and enlarged liver and spleen that may be present at birth. Slow psychomotor development becomes evident early in life. In some cases, clinical manifestations of the illness are not present for days, weeks, or months. These clinical effects include hydrocephalus, retardation, cerebral calcification, and chorioretinitis.

Amebiasis. Infection with amebae may occur after swimming in lakes or ponds. The causative organisms are usually of the *Naegleria* genus, and there is a prevalence of cases in the southeastern United States.

The CNS alterations include abscesses in the cortex and purulent exudate involving the meninges. The CSF findings are similar to those of bacterial meningitis. The disease is rapidly progressive with the symptoms of nausea, vomiting, fever, neck stiffness, focal neurologic signs, seizures, and eventually coma. This illness is usually fatal within a week of onset due to the resistance of *Naegleria* to treatment.

Trypanosomiasis. Several strains of *Trypanosoma brucei* produce African sleeping sickness, which is transmitted by the tsetse fly. Two epidemiologic patterns are described: Gambian (Middle and West African) and Rhodesian (East African). The Rhodesian type is more severe, with intercurrent infections and myocarditis dominating the clinical picture. Within two years after infection with the Gambian form, trypanosomes produce meningoencephalitis, with thickening of the meninges and cerebral edema. Symptoms range from somnolence to convulsions and coma. Mortality depends on the effectiveness of treatment and the degree of CNS involvement.

Trypanosoma cruzi produces Chagas' disease in Central and South America, rarely in North America. The organism is transmitted by biting bugs commonly called assassin bugs. Chagas' disease is either acute or chronic. The acute form is prevalent in children and produces fever, enlarged liver and spleen, myocardial involvement with congestive failure, and eventually involvement of the lungs, meninges, and brain. Months or years after an acute attack, the chronic form may develop with subsequent meningoencephalitis. Pentavalent arsenicals have shown some success in the treatment of both types of trypanosomiasis.

Trichinosis. *Trichinella spiralis* enters the body when raw or insufficiently cooked pork is eaten. Within two to three days, early symptoms of the disease are apparent and are mainly due to the invasion of muscle by larvae, producing mild gastroenteritis, muscle weakness, and tenderness. Three to six weeks after ingestion, larvae invade the nervous system. Lymphocytic and mononuclear infiltration of the meninges, as well as focal gliosis, occurs. Symptoms of CNS involvement include headache, confusion, neck stiffness, seizures, and occasionally coma. Although trichinosis is usually not fatal, seizures and neurologic deficits may continue indefinitely.

Metazoal Infections

Cysticercosis. Ingestion of encysted eggs of pork tapeworm, *Taenia solium*, produce cysticercosis. This disease is most common in South American countries. The larvae spread throughout the body and develop cysts in any body tissue. Cystic nodules within the brain produce symptoms similar to those of brain tumors. Jacksonian seizures are common manifestations. Prognosis depends on the extent of neurologic damage and effective therapy with praziquantel, an antihelminthic agent.

Echinococcosis (Hydatid Disease). This disease is caused by the ingestion of larvae of the canine tapeworm, *Echinococcus granulosus*. The larvae invade the liver, lungs, bones, and less frequently, the brain. The larvae become encysted and are at first microscopic. Within five or more years the cysts may grow to massive sizes of

10 cm or more [5]. Thus, within the brain, symptoms are similar to those associated with brain tumors. The amount of local destruction throughout the body determines the prognosis.

Rickettsial Infections

Rickettsial infections are relatively rare in the United States. They are caused by microorganisms that are obligate intracellular parasites with multiplication occurring only within living cells of susceptible hosts. Their cycle involves an animal reservoir and an insect vector (ticks, fleas, lice, mites, and humans). Epidemic typhus involves only a cycle with lice and humans.

Major rickettsial diseases include epidemic (primary) typhus, louse-borne; murine (endemic) typhus, flea-borne; scrub typhus or tsutsugamushi fever, mite-borne; Rocky Mountain spotted fever, tick-borne; and Q fever, tick- and airborne. Within the CNS, rickettsial diseases can produce lesions in the gray and white matter. Focal gliosis together with mononuclear leukocytes produce characteristic typhus nodules.

All the rickettsial diseases except Q fever have similar pathologic and clinical effects. A 3- to 15-day incubation period is followed by the abrupt onset of high fever, chills, headache, and weakness followed by a generalized macular rash. During the second week after the onset of fever, the CNS becomes involved, producing apathy, dullness, intermittent episodes of delirium, and eventually stupor and coma. Occasionally, in untreated cases there are focal neurologic manifestations and optic neuritis. The CSF may be completely normal. Q fever is not accompanied by a rash and produces symptoms similar to those of low-grade meningitis.

Mortality due to typhus is greatest during epidemics. Early antibiotic therapy has reduced fatality rates to less than 10 percent for typhus and 3 to 10 percent for Rocky Mountain spotted fever. Fatalities are rarely associated with scrub typhus and Q fever [5].

Study Questions

1. Describe the etiology, pathophysiology, and clinical manifestations of the various types of brain tumors.
2. How does location affect the prognosis and morbidity for different tumors?
3. Discuss the source of brain metastasis and the resulting clinical manifestations.
4. Compare the clinical course of viral, bacterial, fungal, and protozoal infections that affect the CNS.
5. Select one common infection and map its course from onset to disease production and resolution.

References

1. Adams, R., and Victor, M. *Principles of Neurology* (3rd ed.). New York: McGraw-Hill, 1985.
2. Hausman, K. Brain tumors in children. *J. Neurosurg. Nurs.* 10:8, 1978.
3. McDonald J., et al. *Central Nervous System Tumors in Clinical Oncology for Medical Students and Physicians: A Multidisciplinary Approach* (5th ed.). New York: American Cancer Society, 1978.
4. Nelson, G. Current approaches in the treatment of malignant gliomas of the brain. *J. Neurosurg. Nurs.* 6:109, 1974.
5. Robbins, S.L., Cotran, R.S., and Kumar, V. *Pathologic Basis of Disease* (3rd ed.). Philadelphia: Saunders, 1984.
6. Russell, D., and Rubinstein, L. *Pathology of Tumors of the Nervous System* (4th ed.). Baltimore: Williams & Wilkins, 1977.
7. Schwartz, S.I. (ed.). *Principles of Surgery* (3rd ed.). New York: McGraw-Hill, 1979.
8. Sloof, J., Kernohan, J., and Mallarty, C. *Primary Intramedullary Tumors of the Spinal Cord and Fillum Terminale*. Philadelphia: Saunders, 1964.
9. Whitley, R., et al. Adenine arabinoside therapy of biopsy-proved herpes-simplex encephalitis: National Institute of Allergy and Infectious Diseases collaborative antiviral study. *N. Engl. J. Med.* 297:289, 1977.

CHAPTER 50

Degenerative and Chronic Alterations in the Nervous System

CHAPTER OUTLINE

Progressive Neurologic Disabilities
- Primary Disabilities
- Secondary Disabilities
- Disability Versus Handicap

Paralyzing Developmental or Congenital Disorders
- Spina Bifida
- Syringomyelia
- Hydrocephalus
  - *Pseudotumor Cerebri*
- Cranial Malformations
- Cerebral Palsy

Disorders Characterized by Progressive Weakness or Paralysis
- Myasthenia Gravis
- Subacute Combined Degeneration of the Cord
- Guillain-Barré Syndrome (Acute Idiopathic Polyneuritis)
- Multiple Sclerosis
- Amyotrophic Lateral Sclerosis

Disorders Characterized by Abnormal Movements
- Parkinson's Disease (Paralysis Agitans)
- Drug-Induced Dyskinesias and Dystonias
- Torticollis
- Huntington's Chorea

Disorders Characterized by Memory and Judgment Deficits
- Atherosclerotic Dementia
- Alzheimer's Disease
- Pick's Disease
- Neurosyphilis

LEARNING OBJECTIVES

1. Contrast the terms *disability* and *handicap*.
2. Differentiate between primary and secondary disabilities.
3. Identify examples of developmental, congenital, and degenerative alterations in the nervous system.
4. Explain why the site of a neurologic alteration has a greater impact on the production of clinical signs than does the nature of the lesion.
5. Identify examples of congenital and developmental alterations in the motor areas of the brain and cord.
6. Identify examples of developmental and degenerative alterations in the upper voluntary motor areas of the nervous system leading to progressive weakness, tremor, and/or spastic paralysis.
7. Contrast upper and lower motor neuron paralysis.
8. Describe alterations in the lower voluntary motor areas of the nervous system leading to transient or permanent sensory or motor changes, and/or flaccid paralysis.
9. Describe the structural basis for signs and symptoms of bulbar palsy.
10. Explain the physiologic basis for medical treatment of muscle weakness and fatigue related to inadequate transmission of impulses across the myoneural junction.
11. Describe pathologic changes in the extrapyramidal motor system resulting in the loss of normal automatic or spontaneous body movements.
12. Describe pathologic changes in the extrapyramidal system resulting in the generation or facilitation of abnormal movements.
13. Identify examples of structural alterations affecting higher cerebral functions such as memory and judgment.
14. Define prognostic terms such as *recovery*, *stabilization*, *progression*, *recurrence*, *remission*, and *exacerbation*.

Progressive Neurologic Disabilities

Primary Disabilities

A primary disability is a structural and functional alteration that results directly from a pathologic process. Primary disabilities may be due to congenital disorders, genetic disorders, injuries, or disease, and, unlike cardiovascular or skeletal disorders, are usually referred to in terms of the functional, rather than structural, alteration. For example, terms such as *spastic quadriplegia* or *right homonymous hemianopsia* are more frequently used than such phrases as *demyelination of the... tracts* or *anoxia of the... branch of the... nerve*.

A reason for referring to primary neurologic alterations in functional terms is that often the nature of the lesion is very hard to identify early in the course of the disease. Also, the description of the dysfunction helps to pinpoint the site of the lesion, even if it does not give much evidence as to its nature. The location of changes in the nervous system dictate the expression of signs and symptoms no matter whether the lesion that interrupts the generation of transmission of nerve impulses is developmental, infectious, degenerative, vascular, neoplastic, or traumatic. Therefore, a lesion that interrupts the pyramidal tracts in the brain or cord tends to produce spastic paralysis whether it is due to neuronal anoxia or to an inborn metabolic defect in the nerve cells. Similarly, an imbalance between the neurotransmitters in the basal ganglia results in abnormalities of movement whether it is due to degeneration of dopamine-projecting neurons after carbon monoxide poisoning, or to the dopamine-blocking or binding effects of phenothiazine drugs.

The degenerative and other neurologic disorders selected as examples in this chapter share common signs and symptoms because they cause structural or chemical alterations in common locations in the brain. Because their etiologies vary greatly, their treatment and prognosis are quite different, even when initial symptoms seem identical.

Secondary Disabilities

Secondary disabilities are caused by restrictions or conditions imposed due to presence or treatment of a primary neurologic disability. These secondary conditions may arise from forced inactivity, such as a muscle contracture that occurs in a paralyzed limb. They also may arise from injury; for example, when a paralyzed extremity is not supported properly, its weight may cause subluxation of the associated joint. Most of the secondary disabilities associated with primary neurologic disease are progressive and may be threatening to function and indeed, to life, even if the primary disorder is resolved. Secondary disabilities often are as preventable as they are crippling.

Organic disease of the nervous system tends to be long-term and does not always end with recovery. If a person does recover from a neurologic disease, such as neurosyphilis, full function may not be regained, even though the causative agent has been eliminated. Residual primary damage or secondary disabilities may linger or become permanent. Even if recovery is possible or when a disorder such as Guillain-Barré syndrome is self-limiting, it usually takes considerable time for full function to return.

Disability Versus Handicap

Because the word *disability* simply means deficit or impairment, health care providers usually prefer it over the older term, *handicap*, which carries the connotation of disadvantage. Whether the alteration is as common as senile atherosclerotic dementia or as rare as amyotrophic lateral sclerosis, individuals, families, and health care providers all find it difficult to sustain motivation and to marshal resources when the prognosis for function and for life itself is poor.

Paralyzing Developmental or Congenital Disorders

Developmental disorders occur when neurologic structures fail to develop to full size or mature function, or when they develop abnormally. Usually their causes are not known. Congenital diseases are those present at birth; the classification includes clinically apparent genetic disease and that which occurs during fetal life as a result of infection, anoxia, malnutrition, or some other traumatic or toxic factor.

Spina Bifida

Spina bifida is a developmental disorder of the vertebral arches. During embryogenesis, the bony arch of the canal fails to close completely. If this is the only defect, it is called *spina bifida occulta* because there are no signs of neurologic deficit to advertise its presence. The bony defect is only identifiable by radiographs or palpation. Occasionally, the site of the lesion may be marked by dimpling and wisps of hair on the skin surface. The cause of this defect is unknown, although various theories link it with prenatal infection, prenatal drug usage, or heredity [13].

Unfortunately, spina bifida is often associated with a defect in the closure of the neural tube (Fig. 50-1). This can range from a closed but dilated central cord canal (*syringomyelocele*) to a sac protruding through the bony defect containing meninges (*meningocele*) and/or, more commonly, elements of the spinal cord (*meningomyelocele*). These sacs may leak cerebrospinal fluid (CSF) if the skin covering is incomplete. Other defects such as abnormal neural tissue or a fistula also may be associated with this type of spina bifida. Occasionally, in the occipital area, brain elements may protrude through a defect in the skull; this impairment is referred to as an *encephalocele*.

Spina bifida occulta may occur with no clinical signs or symptoms. It is possible, however, for late signs such as persistent or intermittent eneuresis (the most common

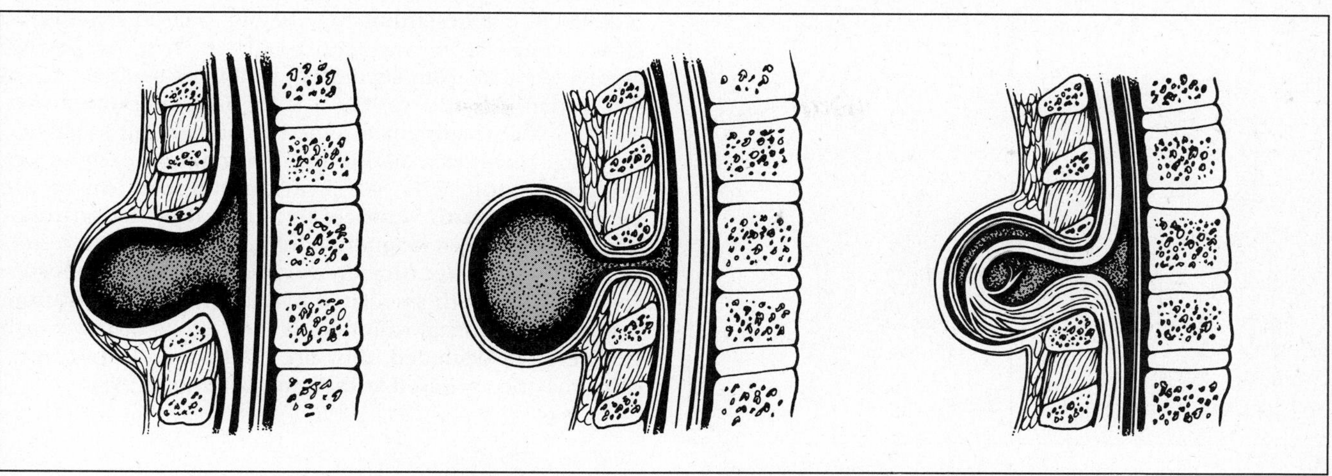

FIGURE 50-1 Types of spina bifida: syringomyelocele, meningocele, and meningomyelocele.

symptom), late walking, or even chronic cold feet to be traced to a previously undetected lesion.

Several forms of spina bifida can be diagnosed in utero by amniocentesis and ultrasound, or at birth by the presence of the sac protruding through the defect in the vertebral arch. If the sac is a meningocele, it is possible for the infant to show no signs of neurologic deficit, although hydrocephalus may occur after surgical repair. The meningomyelocele is accompanied by signs of neurologic damage, the extent of which is dependent on the size and level of the lesion and the presence of dysplastic neural tissue. If the defect occurs in the lumbosacral area, flaccid paralysis of the lower limbs and absence of sensation below the level of the lesion are usual. Sphincter control is also affected in both bowel and bladder. These neurologic deficits occur because the defect and abnormal tissue often involve all or most of the lumbosacral spinal cord together with the nerve roots entering and exiting in the lumbosacral area. Alteration in blood supply due to pressure, trauma, or infection may also contribute to the interruption of the reflex arcs in the area. If the tip end of the conus terminalis is intact, some external bowel sphincter control may be present due to an intact reflex arc [13]. The frequency of accompanying mental retardation with severe developmental spinal defects is high.

Prognosis for life and function are excellent with spina bifida occulta and after surgical repair of a meningocele, especially in the absence of hydrocephalus. Surgical repair is commonly undertaken with serious developmental spinal defects in order to avoid the dangerous complication of ascending meningitis. Approximately 50 percent of children who survive surgical treatment for meningomyelocele reach adulthood, and some may learn to walk with braces and crutches. The primary disabilities of meningomyelocele may be resolved, but complications result from secondary disabilities, especially from immobility.

Syringomyelia

The cause of primary syringomyelia remains unknown, although considerable attention has been given to its origin as a congenital neural tube defect. Unlike spina bifida, syringomyelia is characterized by the onset of progressive motor symptoms in the adult. Weakness and spastic paralysis as well as alterations in sensory function all may progress steadily or intermittently throughout the remainder of life.

Syringomyelia is considered to be a developmental disorder involving enlargement of affected segments of the spinal cord and development of tubular fluid cavities. It may be a developmental defect involving disruption of CSF flow through the outlets of the fourth ventricle. It is present throughout embryogenesis but does not become symptomatic until the normally microscopic central canal of the spinal cord balloons and forms fluid-filled cavities in the nervous tissue of the cord itself (Fig. 50-2). A pathologic cavity caused by retained cerebrospinal fluid, called a *syrinx*, results, thus the name syringomyelia.

Syringomyelia may occur in association with other developmental defects such as spina bifida, Chiari malformation, or hydrocephalus. Secondary syringomyelia may accompany tumors, infections, trauma, bleeding, and infarction in the central nervous system. Usually, signs and symptoms of syrinx formation occur sometime after age 30 years, although they may begin at any age. The nature of the clinical signs depends on the level and size of the cavities, and which structures are affected. Typically, the syrinx develops from the center of the cord outward in the direction of the dorsal gray horns (Fig. 50-3). Because pain and temperature fibers cross immediately in the cord and are relayed by the cells in the dorsal gray horns of the cord, the loss of these sensations with analgesia, thermoanesthesia, and preservation of the touch sensation are early signs of the onset of syringomyelia. Accompanying

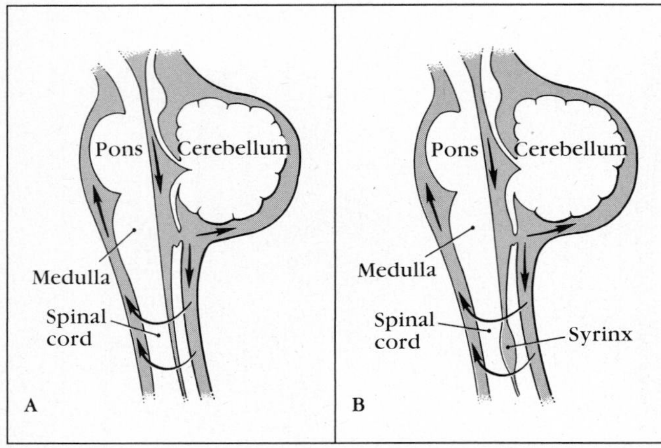

FIGURE 50-2 Syringomyelia. A. Normal circulation. B. Presence of syrinx in the spinal column.

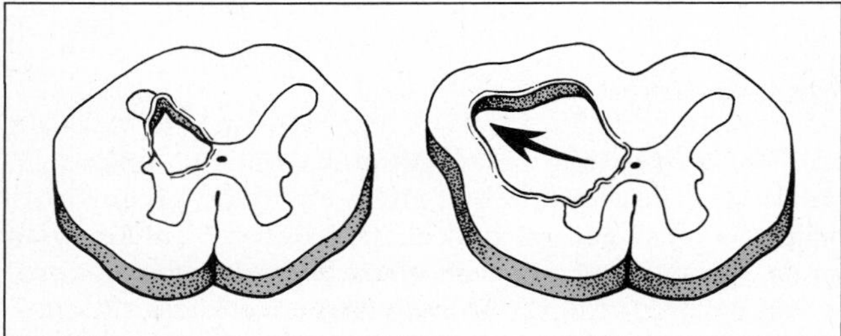

FIGURE 50-3 Development of a syrinx from the center outward into the dorsal gray horns.

these early signs are weakness and wasting of hands and arms. If the syrinx spreads anteriorly toward the anterior horn cells, signs of lower motor neuron damage with small-muscle atrophy occur. Signs and symptoms develop asymmetrically at first, but cord compression may become so severe that complete paraplegia results.

The lower cervical and upper thoracic areas of the cord most frequently develop syrinx-related alterations. If the brainstem is affected initially or by extension, it is termed *syringobulbia*. Characteristic symptoms of medullary involvement result from cranial nerve damage and include weakness of facial and palatal muscles, laryngeal palsy, wasting and weakness of the tongue, loss of pain and temperature sensation, and onset of trigeminal pain. Occasionally dizziness may occur. Severe medullary involvement may be lethal.

In primary syringomyelia, the cerebrospinal fluid remains normal unless its circulation becomes obstructed. The protein content is high in CSF of syringomyelia associated with tumor growth. The cord enlarges in the areas of syrinx formation, and signs and symptoms may be suggestive of spinal cord tumor, multiple sclerosis, or amyotrophic lateral sclerosis. Later, manifestations of poorly healed, painless injuries with trophic skin lesions confirm the diagnosis of syringomyelia.

Clinical manifestations may be stationary for years, or slow progression may lead to death from brainstem involvement or from secondary problems such as extensive decubitus ulcers, renal infection, or pneumonia. Symptomatic treatment is aimed at preventing lethal and crippling secondary disabilities. If attempted early in primary syringomyelia, surgical decompression of the medulla and fourth ventricle by removal of the posterior rim of the foramen magnum has yielded promising results in arresting and occasionally reversing the sensory losses. Some persons with associated hydrocephalus benefit from ventriculoperitoneal shunting. If the outlets in the fourth ventricle are occluded, they are opened; and the central canal may be aspirated at the time of surgery [3].

Hydrocephalus

The word *hydrocephalus* refers to an increased quantity of CSF within the ventricles of the cerebrum. If CSF pressure is normal or only sporadically increased with gradual cortical atrophy, the symptoms tend to begin slowly and relate to memory and judgment deficits, speech disorders, alterations in gait, some spasticity, incontinence, and the signs of progressive dementia. If the pressure is elevated due to excess formation, faulty circulation, or inadequate resorption of CSF, the symptoms tend to be more abrupt in onset and more severe.

The most common cause of hydrocephalus is obstruction to the flow of CSF (Fig. 50-4). In the fetus or neonate, the obstruction may result from cerebellar dysplasia, tumor, subarachnoid hemorrhage, and infectious or developmental abnormalities of the cerebellar tonsils, medulla, cerebral aqueduct, or fourth ventricle. In the older person, obstruction may be due to trauma, infection, or tumor. If the obstruction is within the CSF pathways, the disorder is classified as *noncommunicating*, or *obstructive*, *hydrocephalus*. If CSF can gain access to the subarachnoid space and is then not absorbed by the arachnoid villi, it is classified as a *communicating hydrocephalus*. This type of hydrocephalus may be associated with postmeningitic or posthemorrhagic states. Excess formation of cerebrospinal fluid is rare and may be caused by choroid plexus tumors. Noncommunicating hydrocephalus due to faulty circulation or obstruction results in enlargement of the ventricular system. This eventually leads to signs of increased intracranial pressure in adults and to bulging fontanelles and an enlarged head in infants. The treatment of choice is removal of the obstruction. Prognosis depends on the cause and the severity of the obstruction and on the timing and effectiveness of treatment.

Clinical manifestations of hydrocephalus depend on the age and rapidity of onset, as well as on the nature and success of the treatment. A newborn infant who exhibits a grossly enlarged head, widely separated cranial sutures, and protruding eyes usually has irreversible signs of prolonged pressure, such as blindness from optic atrophy, paralysis, and mental retardation. In other infants, rapidly increasing head circumference, feeding problems, irritability, delayed motor skills, high-pitched cry, or turned down (setting sun) eyes are signs of progressive hydrocephalus

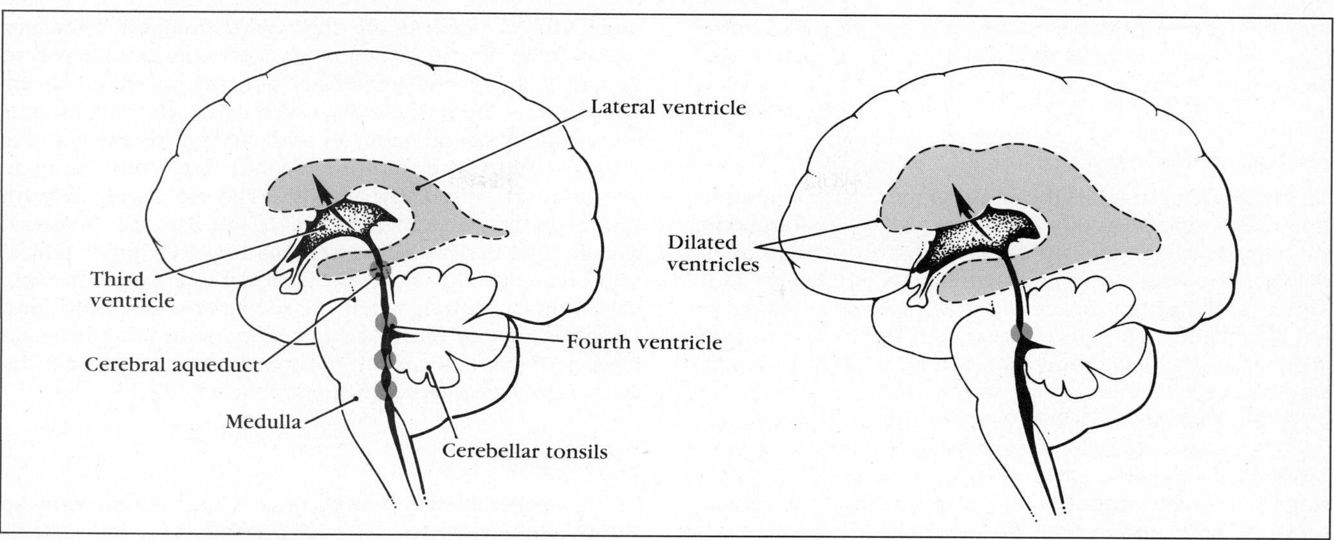

FIGURE 50-4 Schematic representation of areas of possible obstruction to spinal fluid and resulting ventricular enlargement.

(Fig. 50-5). Because cerebral expansion is permitted by the open sutures and fontanelles in infancy, classic signs of increasing intracranial pressure such as headache, vomiting, and altered vital signs are usually minimal or absent. In older children or adults whose cranial sutures have closed, headache and vomiting are often early signs and develop with much less trapping of CSF and greater increases in CSF pressure.

Diagnosis is based on clinical observation of head circumference increase in infants and by demonstration of dilated ventricles. Computerized axial tomography (CT) scan often demonstrates the ventricular dilatation and the cause. In the absence of available CT scanning, a combination of skull films, angiography, and/or air studies can identify hydrocephalus.

Pseudotumor Cerebri. This condition, which occurs most frequently in young, obese women, is related to hydrocephalus in that the volume of CSF increases. Intracranial pressure is greatly elevated, usually to 250 to 400 mm of water, and may be as high as 600 mm of water. Persons with this benign intracranial hypertension have headache and papilledema. Focal signs and other neurologic deficits generally are absent. Treatment focuses on serial lumbar punctures to drain cerebrospinal fluid to maintain intracranial pressure near normal. In many

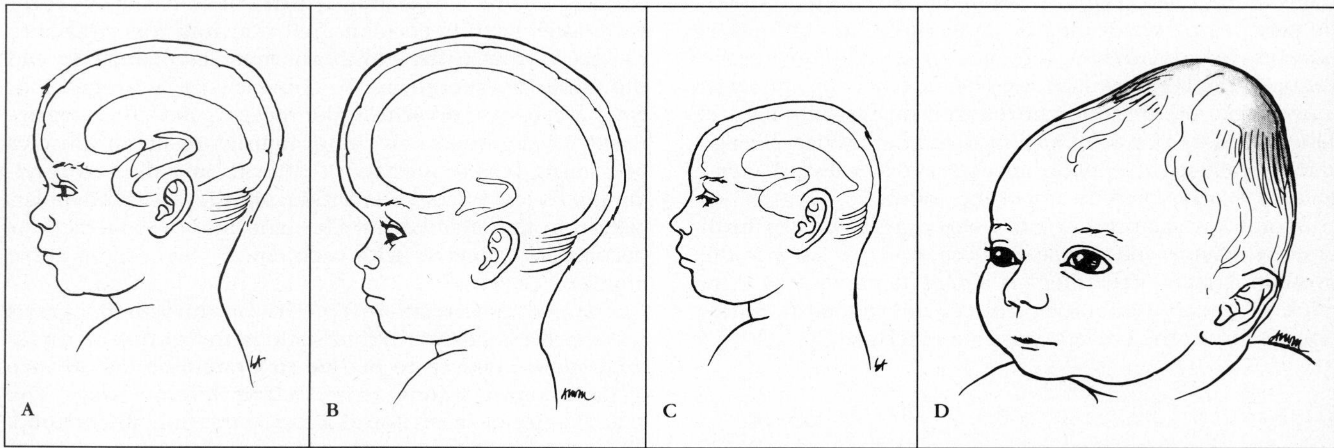

FIGURE 50-5 Some cephalic shapes. A. Normal. B. Hydrocephalus. C. Microcephalus. D. Molding. (From R. Judge, G. Zuidema, and F. Fitzgerald, *Clinical Diagnosis: A Physiologic Approach*. Boston: Little, Brown, 1982.)

instances these persons recover after repeated lumbar punctures have restored the balance of CSF formation and absorption.

Cranial Malformations

Arrested brain growth is the cause of the cranial malformation called *microcephaly vera*, or small head. Premature suture closure frequently associated with microcephaly results from arrested brain growth and is not a cause of it. This is an inherited defect of the autosomal recessive or sex-linked gene. There is no treatment for the severe mental retardation of microcephaly, which is often accompanied by cerebral palsy and/or seizure activity.

Craniostenosis is early closure and ossification of one or more of the sutures in the skull that occurs before brain growth is arrested. Early recognition and immediate surgery to create artificial sutures are necessary to decompress the brain and to limit the extent of neurologic damage caused by increasing intracranial pressure. If treatment is absent or delayed, this pressure can cause exophthalmos, optic atrophy, seizures, and mental retardation.

Cerebral Palsy

The term *cerebral palsy* is used to include a wide variety of nonprogressive brain disorders that occur during intrauterine life, during delivery, or during early infancy. Cerebral palsy, by definition, is a syndrome of motor disabilities, although it may be accompanied by mental retardation and/or seizure disorders. Causes are many and include cerebral developmental disorders such as microcephaly, intracranial hemorrhage, and cerebral anoxia, and poisoning by toxins such as excessive bilirubin in the blood (kernicterus).

Clinical manifestations of cerebral palsy (CP) depend on the areas of the brain that sustain damage. Three main groups of CP have been described according to the dominant signs. The *paralytic cerebral palsies* are the result of damage to the cortical motor cells and the pyramidal tracts in the brain. Typically, these are manifested as spastic paraplegias, quadriplegias, or hemiplegias. The *dyskinetic cerebral palsies* are caused by damage to the extrapyramidal system and are characterized by abnormal movements of athetoid, choreiform, or dystonic nature. The *ataxic cerebral palsies* indicate cerebellar damage and typically involve incoordination and gait disturbances. Mixed CP may combine any of the above.

Symptoms are present and nonprogressive from birth or early infancy, and diagnosis is usually made early in the preschool years. Treatment is aimed at preventing crippling secondary disabilities and providing special education to ensure the greatest possible function.

Disorders Characterized by Progressive Weakness or Paralysis

Progressively paralyzing neurologic disorders affect the pyramidal system of the brain or cord, or the final common pathway between the cord and the muscle. They may result from dietary deficiencies, autoimmune disorders, genetic defects, and infectious diseases, or they may be idiopathic. If the reflex arc remains intact, the usual sign is a spastic paresis or paralysis with normal or hyperactive reflexes. If the lower motor neuron or final common pathway is interrupted, the result is flaccid paralysis with diminished or absent reflexes. If the damage is spread throughout the motor system, as in amytrophic lateral sclerosis, spasticity is present until the final common pathway is interrupted, when characteristic flaccidity and atrophic wasting of muscles predominate. Prognosis and treatment depend on the nature of the disease and the availability and use of treatment.

Myasthenia Gravis

This chronic disease, which occurs most commonly in young adults and progresses with remissions and exacerbations, is characterized by activity induced abnormal muscle fatigability. The fatigue results in typical drooping of eyelids (ptosis) and jaw, nasal voice, slurred speech, and weakness of the proximal extremities; all symptoms worsen during the day, but improve with rest or with the use of anticholinesterase drugs such as neostigmine. Eventually, muscle fibers may degenerate, and weakness, especially of the muscles of the head, neck, trunk, and limbs, may become irreversible. Hyperplasia of the thymus is frequently associated, and approximately 12 percent of persons with myasthenia gravis have a thymoma. Reflexes may remain normal or reflect fatigue, decreasing with each repeated test. There appears to be no sensory alteration.

Several primary muscle disorders cause clinically similar fatigue in the muscles, but myasthenia gravis is the only one that responds to anticholinesterase drugs. Myasthenia gravis involves progressive failure of impulse conduction at the neuromuscular junction. It is an autoimmune disease with cellular and humoral factors playing a part. The triggering mechanism for the autoimmune response remains elusive. Circulating acetylcholine (ACh) receptor antibodies have been identified that link themselves to receptor sites in the voluntary muscles, damaging and blocking the receptors. In some cases, aggregates of lymphocytes are present in the muscles and other organs. Postsynaptic membrane abnormalities result in muscles becoming less responsive to nerve impulses. Acetylcholine is less effective in producing the desired depolarization in the affected muscles, and muscle contractions become less effective with each rapidly succeeding nerve impulse.

The observed relationship between myasthenia gravis and disorders of the thyroid such as thyroiditis or thyrotoxicosis is believed to be due to a common disturbance of the immune system, expressed in different ways. The exact nature of these disturbances is not fully understood, nor is their relationship clear. Many experts postulate that genetic characteristics may constitute risk factors for autoimmune disorders such as myasthenia gravis, thyroiditis, and even diabetes mellitus [2].

During the early active stage of myasthenia gravis, while the characteristic remissions and exacerbations are occurring and before muscle atrophy sets in, some individuals may respond well to surgical removal of the thymus. It is believed by many that early thymectomy may decrease the level of autoimmune activity before much permanent damage is sustained by the acetylcholine receptor sites in the voluntary muscles. Plasmapheresis is another method of treatment aimed at removing anti-acetylcholine receptor antibodies from the blood to decrease the autoimmune activity [2]. Steroids are usually given to suppress the production of antibodies. Other immune-suppressive drugs such as azathioprine have been beneficial in some cases. Anticholinesterase drugs are administered to prevent the breakdown of the acetylcholine at the myoneural junction. Too much anticholinesterase drug activity may produce skeletal muscle weakness that resembles the myasthenic defect. This phenomenon is called *cholinergic crisis* or *depolarization block* [1]. It is hard to differentiate clinically between a cholinergic crisis and a myasthenic crisis, or disease exacerbation. Most individuals in a crisis state are treated for cholinergic crisis, withdrawn from the anticholinesterase drugs, and maintained on assisted respiration until the type of crisis can be identified.

The course of myasthenia gravis is variable. Some persons do not develop other symptoms than the initial ocular muscle fatigue and weakness. Others, who exhibit more generalized symptoms, respond well to standard treatment for years. A small percentage suffer the acute, fulminating disease accompanied by muscle atrophy and have poor response to all treatment. Death from myasthenia gravis usually occurs within the first 5 to 10 years of onset, when the disease is most acute. Lethal crises do not usually occur late in the disease, and the damage sustained tends to remain constant or to be compensated for by other muscles. Death occurring after many years is usually due to the secondary problem of immobility, resulting in pneumonia.

Myasthenic mothers who pass the antibodies to their infants experience spontaneous recovery of the myasthenia symptoms, whereas others persist with the disease for their lifetime.

Subacute Combined Degeneration of the Cord

Vitamin B_{12} deficiency, usually occurring as a part of pernicious anemia (see Chap. 15), can lead to degeneration of the white matter in the lateral and posterior spinal cord, as well as peripheral polyneuropathy and slight cerebral atrophy. Neurologic manifestations begin gradually and usually are accompanied by the classic megaloblastic anemia. Unusual sensations such as tingling, numbness, and pain are often the first symptoms of neurologic degeneration. These paresthesias are followed by motor signs of weakness and incoordination. The paresthesias and motor signs both tend to begin in the lower limbs and move to the upper limbs and trunk as the disease spreads up the posterior and lateral cord. With progressive and untreated degeneration of the cord, sensory ataxia and either spastic paralysis with hyperactive reflexes or flaccid paralysis with absent reflexes may occur in all four limbs, being the most severe in the lower limbs. If degeneration is confined to the posterior columns, incoordination is predominant. If it is more lateral, weakness and paralysis are most characteristic. The nature of the paralysis is influenced by the presence or absence of peripheral neuropathy and the status of the reflex arc. In addition to these motor signs, individuals may suffer optic atrophy and/or nystagmus if the second or third cranial nerve is affected. The other cranial nerves are rarely affected. Cerebral atrophy may result in impaired memory, confusion, paranoid behavior, irritability, or depression.

Eventually, the damaged peripheral nerves can regenerate, with improvement in sensory symptoms, coordination, and reflexes, but spasticity and signs of cerebral atrophy are likely to disappear, since central nervous system damage is not reversible. Early diagnosis is important, as the condition is treatable and reversible if symptoms have been present for only a short duration.

Clinically similar disorders such as neurosyphilis and multiple sclerosis must be ruled out by gastric acid evaluation, blood tests for megaloblastic anemia, and bone marrow evaluation for abnormalities of red cells. Serum B_{12} may be evaluated or tests may be made of vitamin B_{12} absorption using radioactive vitamin B_{12}.

Guillain-Barré Syndrome (Acute Idiopathic Polyneuritis)

This acute, frequently postinfectious polyneuritis may be due to an allergic response or some type of hypersensitivity reaction. The specific triggering mechanism for this disturbance in the immune response remains unknown. The onset usually occurs a few days or weeks after a febrile illness, vaccination, injury, or surgery. Guillain-Barré syndrome has no predilection for any age group, sex, or race, and when an infectious etiology, generally respiratory or gastrointestinal, can be demonstrated, it is usually viral. It has also occurred after immunizations.

Demyelination and degeneration of the myelin sheath and axon occur in the segmental peripheral nerves and the anterior and posterior spinal nerve roots. Cranial nerve involvement is often observed. Lymphocytes and macrophages infiltrate the myelin sheath initially, and later, if disease progression continues, the axon is involved. Inflammation, edema, and damaged nerves result in both sensory and motor dysfunction.

Initial clinical symptoms are general bilateral weakness, first manifested by difficulty in walking. These symptoms become progressive and accompanied by parethesias and possibly pain in the back. The symptoms progress in an ascending fashion to involve the muscles of the trunk, upper extremities, and cranial nerves. Complete flaccid paralysis may or may not occur. Maximum manifestations of the disease occur in about three weeks, though the rate of spread varies. In severe cases, total paralysis develops rapidly, and serious respiratory involvement requires artificial ventilation. Generally the sensory involvement is less profound than the motor involvement. Proprioception and vibratory sense are the most commonly observed sensory deficits, but deficits in light touch, pinprick, muscle sensitivity, and temperature sensations may occur.

Variant autonomic dysfunction may occur and may include postural hypotension, tachycardia, diaphoresis, and other manifestations. Reflexes are usually diminished or lost, but occasionally remain normal even with severe muscular weakness. When the onset of flaccid paralysis is sudden and symmetric, and when it is accompanied by sensory changes, diagnosis of Guillain-Barré syndrome can be made by clinical observation and history alone. Muscular atrophy is not common but may result when axon loss is severe. Electrodiagnostic studies show slowing of nerve conduction in most affected individuals. Cerebrospinal fluid protein level becomes markedly elevated after the first few days of illness, while the cell count remains negative (albuminocytologic dissociation).

When death occurs, it is usually due to respiratory arrest or pneumonia. For survivors of respiratory problems, the prognosis for life and for eventual recovery of function is good. Eighty-five percent make a complete recovery in four to six months, but others may have severe residual disabilities. Treatment with steroids, adrenocorticotropic hormone (ACTH), or other immunosuppressant drugs may or may not be beneficial in altering the course of the disease.

Multiple Sclerosis

Multiple sclerosis (MS) is a relatively common chronic and progressive inflammatory, demyelinating disease of the central nervous system that results in diverse manifestations of neurologic alteration. Its basic cause or causes are unknown, but it probably is an autoimmune disorder influenced by a genetic susceptibility. While no single virus has been incriminated in its causation, MS has been associated with HLA (human leukocyte) antigens, particularly HLA-B7 and HLA D2/DR2 [9]. This suggests the possibility that a latent viral infection precipitates the disease. Dietary deficiencies and acute viral infections have also been studied as etiologic agents. Stress and trauma seem to play a role in precipitating the onset of MS or in exacerbating the symptoms. Multiple sclerosis is most common in colder climates and its onset generally is between ages 20 and 40 years. Females have a higher incidence than males [10].

The disease usually begins rather suddenly with the occurrence of a set of focal symptoms of visual disturbance or of motor dysfunction in one or two limbs. The causative lesion or plaque is present predominantly in the white matter of the central nervous system, and the myelin sheaths that normally act as insulation around nerve fibers are lost. Loss of myelin slows, blocks, or distorts transmission of nerve impulses. During the course of the disease, some of the myelinated fibers may regenerate and associated symptoms disappear. Eventually, gliosis occurs in the lesions and scar tissue replaces myelin and may replace the axis cylinders themselves. From this gliosis comes the term *sclerosis*, meaning induration or scarring. Oligodendrocytes disappear and astrocytes proliferate.

Initial symptoms may be transient and are frequently followed by complete, or nearly complete, recovery as the myelin is replaced. Periods of remission are common. Later alterations become permanent, with remissions and exacerbations limited to new symptoms superimposed on a baseline of disability. This permanence in symptoms is due to eventual disruption and destruction of the nerve cells themselves, even though this is initially a disease of the myelin sheath rather than of the cells.

If the lesions are predominantly in the pyramidal tracts of the cerebrum and/or spinal cord, the symptoms are motor. If they affect the lateral spinothalamic or posterior tracts of the cord, sensory changes are noted. Weakness or spastic paralysis of the limbs and sphincters with hyperactive reflexes is common. Sexual dysfunction, with impotence in males and alteration in vaginal sensations in females, is a common and disturbing aspect of sensorimotor changes. Paresthesias such as pain, numbness, or tingling may be noted in the limbs and/or the face. Emotional changes may range from lability to sustained euphoria or severe depression.

Brainstem lesions often contribute to emotional lability and also produce symptoms of cranial nerve injury. The optic, oculomotor, trochlear, and abducens nerves and the vestibular branch of the auditory nerve are especially common sites of damage. Visual signs and symptoms range from nystagmus to diplopia to visual dimness to patchy or complete blindness. Occasionally, pupillary abnormalities may be noted. Dizziness may be mild, or it may be severe and associated with nausea and vomiting. Speech may be difficult due to spastic weakness of facial and speech muscles. Dysphagia makes eating difficult, with increased danger of aspiration. Cerebellar lesions also affect speech, producing slurred, uncoordinated articulation. Other signs such as intention tremor of the hands, head tremor, and/or staggering gait are indicative of cerebellar lesions.

Although early clinical manifestations may be limited to effects of alteration in the cerebellar area, the brainstem, or the cerebrum, late multiple sclerosis usually affects all parts of the central nervous system. The classic triad of Charcot described in 1868, which occurs late in the disease, includes nystagmus, intention tremor, and speech disorders [10]. Spastic paraplegia, incontinence, and extreme emotional lability are also typical of the late stages of MS.

The diagnosis is based on clinical features, observing the pattern of remission and exacerbation of symptoms, and ruling out other diseases such as subacute combined degeneration of the cord. Studies of antibodies in the blood or cerebrospinal fluid often show gammaglobulin abnormalities in those with established MS. The most consistent CSF finding is the presence of oligoclonal bands of IgG [9]. These bands are immunoglobulins directed against the various antigens of the measles virus, but no specific antigen has been isolated in MS [10]. Other changes in the CSF are inconsistent and nonspecific.

The prognosis varies from progression to death in less than 6 months or a benign course for over 20 years without shortening or altering productive life. Even when the person survives to old age, however, the last years are often spent as a spastic paraplegic, with visual disorders, incontinence, dysarthria, and lack of emotional control. Death is often due to secondary disorders such as pneumonia or septic decubitus ulcers.

Treatment for MS is generally symptomatic and focused on preventing complications. Special high-vitamin, low-fat diets, steroids, and core-cooling of the body have failed to influence the course of the disease consistently. Immunosuppression using plasma exchange, steroids, azathioprine, and cyclophosphamide have provided encouraging results [6].

Amyotrophic Lateral Sclerosis

Amyotrophic lateral sclerosis (ALS, or progressive muscle atrophy) is another primary neurologic disease that affects motor function and results in alterations of gait and paralysis. It is a noninflammatory disease of the upper and lower motor neurons, with demyelination secondary to axon degeneration. Unlike MS, which classically is characterized by remissions and exacerbations, ALS usually steadily progresses to death within two to six years of diagnosis [10]. Premature aging of nerve cells due to some environmental or genetic factor, nutritional deficiencies, heavy metal poisoning, an automimmune response, metabolic defects, and even a dormant virus have all been identified as possible causes or contributors to ALS.

Loss of the motor cells in the cerebral cortex can result in signs of upper motor neuron damage, with weakness or spastic paralysis and hyperactive reflexes. This is especially likely to occur in the lower limbs. Damage to cranial nerves in the medulla produces signs of ***bulbar palsy***, either of the spastic or flaccid type. Bulbar palsy refers to weakness or paralysis of the muscles supplied by the motor cranial nerves. Commonly, upper and lower motor neuron damage are mixed in ALS. Lower motor signs predominate in the upper extremities and upper motor signs predominate in the lower limbs. When reflexes are interrupted, muscles atrophy secondary to denervation and loss of muscle tone. In these areas, diminished reflexes or flaccid paralysis occurs. Muscle atrophy is often present in the upper limbs and tongue.

Degeneration may occur anywhere within the pyramidal system, the anterior motor cells of the spinal cord, and/or the ventral nerve roots. It does not characteristically affect peripheral nerves. The muscle fasciculations or twitching frequently seen in the upper limbs and/or tongue are believed to be due to accumulating excessive neurotransmitter at the myoneural junction, rather than being caused by abnormal spontaneous discharges of degenerating nerve cells [5].

The onset of ALS usually occurs after age 50 years, with 2:1 occurrence in men over women. One common early sign may be muscle fasciculations of the tongue when the brainstem is involved. Fasciculations may also be seen in the hands or upper limbs, and are small local muscle contractions that occur when a muscle is tapped or moved passively [5]. Whenever the brainstem is affected, slurred speech and weakness of the palate and facial muscles may occur. Reflexes may be normal, hyperactive, or diminished, depending on whether there is lower motor neuron damage. If lower motor neuron damage is present, muscle wasting occurs in the tongue or other muscles. Eventually, swallowing is affected and speech may become unintelligible.

Weakness and clumsiness are first noted in the distal portions of the upper limbs, and wasting of the muscles of the hand is characteristic. Sexual dysfunction, such as impotence, is an early sign; bowel and bladder sphincters are not usually affected until late in the disease. Lower extremity function is retained longer than upper extremity function, but as the disease progresses, the latter also is lost. Characteristically, there is no sensory alteration in ALS. Paralysis of the trunk and respiratory muscles occurs late in the course of the disease if bulbar palsy does not cause death first. Death is often due to pneumonia or respiratory failure.

Diagnosis is based on characteristic clinical signs such as upper limb weakness, wasting of hand muscles, and muscle fasciculations. Disorders such as syringomyelia, cord tumors, and neurosyphilis may cause similar clinical signs, but usually have pain and sensory changes associated with them. The absence of muscle atrophy and lack of muscular response to edrophonium hydrochloride rules out a diagnosis of myasthenia gravis. Biopsy of muscle and electromyograms show denervation atrophy in ALS.

Prognosis is worst when the brainstem is affected first. Life expectancy is best when the degeneration remains confined to the lower motor neurons of the middle and lower spinal cord. It is rare for individuals to survive longer than 10 years after onset, however, and death can occur within a year. Treatment is symptomatic, with no beneficial effects from antiinflammatory and immunosuppressive drugs.

Disorders Characterized by Abnormal Movements

Abnormal movements often indicate alterations in the extrapyramidal motor system. This system is not clearly understood, so that the relationship of the pathology and structural alterations with the clinical manifestations is not clear. Abnormal movements often result from alterations and reflect a disturbance in the balance between the excitatory and inhibitory neurotransmitters in the basal ganglia. The neurotransmitters involved apparently are dopamine, acetylcholine, and gamma-aminobutyric acid (GABA). The basal ganglia most often affected are the four that make up the corpus striatum: caudate, putamen, globus pallidus, and claustrum. In some disorders, such as early parkinsonism, conscious effort can suppress these movements temporarily, but typically they return when the person relaxes or is distracted.

The abnormal movements that result are of different types but may be painful or incapacitating. Abnormal movements range from the fine, rhythmic quivering of tremor to the violent, irregular jerking or twisting movements of ***ballismus***. ***Dyskinesias***, or alterations in voluntary muscle movement, and *dystonias*, or alterations in muscle tone (such as rigidity), are both classified as abnormalities of movement. *Fixed* or *intermittent muscle spasms*, such as are characteristic of torticollis, may be included unless they are due to muscle rather than nerve damage. *Choreas* are irregular muscle twitchings that may become so severe that they contribute to death from exhaustion. *Athetosis*, or athetoid movements, are slow, repeated, purposeless muscle movements that may affect only the digits or the entire body.

There are many causes of extrapyramidal dysfunction. Cerebral anoxia and/or trauma in utero or during delivery may produce an athetoid cerebral palsy, spastic cerebral palsy, or both. The characteristic tremors of parkinsonism may be produced by therapy with the major tranquilizers of the phenothiazine family or by carbon monoxide poisoning. The exhausting muscle twitchings of chorea may be due to a genetic defect or to an infectious disease. As with all neurologic disorders, abnormal movements give more clues about which structures are damaged than about what has damaged them. Therefore, a very complete physical examination and a thorough family history may be more important than laboratory test results in identifying the source of the problem.

Parkinson's Disease (Paralysis Agitans)

When the levels of dopamine in the corpus striatum are decreased, a primary neurologic disorder called parkinsonism or a parkinsonian syndrome may result. Parkinson's disease refers to parkinsonism of unknown etiology that occurs between ages 50 and 80 years.

Dopamine is one of the chemical transmitters in the brain. This monoamine transmitter appears to be concentrated in areas such as the substantia nigra, where dopamine-containing neurons project to the corpus striatum through fibers called the nigrostriatal pathway. In the corpus striatum, dopamine, together with acetylcholine, is important in controlling complex movements. Dopamine acts as an inhibitory transmitter while acetylcholine acts as an excitatory transmitter.

The clinical signs of Parkinson's disease apparently arise from progressive degeneration of the pigmented cells of the substantia nigra (Fig. 50-6) [10]. The underlying cause of this cellular destruction is unknown. The dopaminergic cells synthesize and secrete the neurotransmitter dopamine, and their degeneration results in a subsequent decrease of dopamine transmitted to the corpus striatum. As a result, the striatal cells, under the predominance of acetylcholine, initiate action potentials more rapidly as the counterbalance of dopamine is decreased or absent. If the dopamine fibers projecting to the corpus striatum degenerate, permanent or progressive muscle rigidity and/or the tremors of parkinsonism result. If the dopamine in the corpus striatum is blocked or bound temporarily by a drug such as chlorpromazine, the typically reversible rigidity and/or tremors of the parkinsonian syndrome occur.

Parkinson's disease is characterized by tremor, rigidity, and akinesia. Other signs and symptoms include a masklike facial expression and infrequent blinking due to diminished automatic movements. Speech is quiet and monotonous. Cognitive and perceptual abilities reflect deterioration in memory and problem solving in many individuals. Spontaneous, automatic movements, such as swinging the arms when walking, also diminish and cease. The body posture becomes stooped, with apparent flexion of the limbs. The characteristic gait progresses with small, shuffling steps that pick up speed as the person travels. The individual suffers increasing muscle rigidity in both extensor and flexor muscles that may cause jerky or spastic movements. Rather than losing voluntary function, the person finds it increasingly difficult to initiate voluntary acts (akinesia) and the actions tend to be slow and clumsy.

The tremor of parkinsonism commonly occurs in the hands initially, and then progresses to involve the ankles, head, and/or mouth. The tremor is most prominent during periods of rest. It can be suppressed with conscious effort for brief periods and usually disappears with sleep. If the index finger and thumb are both involved, the tremor may be described as "pill-rolling." Intention tremor, which refers to a tremor occurring during the performance of a precise movement, can also occur. Both resting and intention tremors become worse under emotional stress, although extreme provocation may result in the quick, efficient performance of complex motor functions. Other symptoms such as heat intolerance and excessive salivation are due to autonomic system dysfunction.

If the symptoms of parkinsonism are due to dopamine binding or blocking by drugs such as chlorpromazine, they usually disappear when the drug is withdrawn or decreased. If the symptoms are due to a discrete episode of cerebral anoxia or trauma, such as carbon monoxide poisoning or head injury, they may stabilize. Most cases, however, are characterized by progressive disability until death occurs from secondary problems such as pneumonia in 10 or more years after onset of the disease. Diagnosis is based on the signs and symptoms and by ruling out other diseases with muscle rigidity or tremor, such as multiple sclerosis and neurosyphilis.

Drug-Induced Dyskinesias and Dystonias

The major tranquilizers have many effects on the extrapyramidal nervous system. Besides the drug-induced parkinsonian syndrome, which usually occurs early in therapy, there may be a number of other effects, some of which are reversible and some permanent. Dyskinesias are embarrassing, rhythmic, involuntary movements such as chewing or smacking. Dystonias are spasms that jerk the face, head, or limbs in a painful and/or frightening way. Both can occur alone or in association with more typically parkinsonian symptoms soon after major tranquilizer therapy is begun. Usually they respond well to anticholinergic therapy and are probably caused by a relative increase in cholinergic activity in the presence of a sudden reduction in the level of dopamine in the basal ganglia. The anticholinergic therapy seems temporarily to restore the balance [11]. *Akathisia*, or a feeling of restlessness in the muscles, is more difficult to treat and may require dosage reduction or a change in drugs [4].

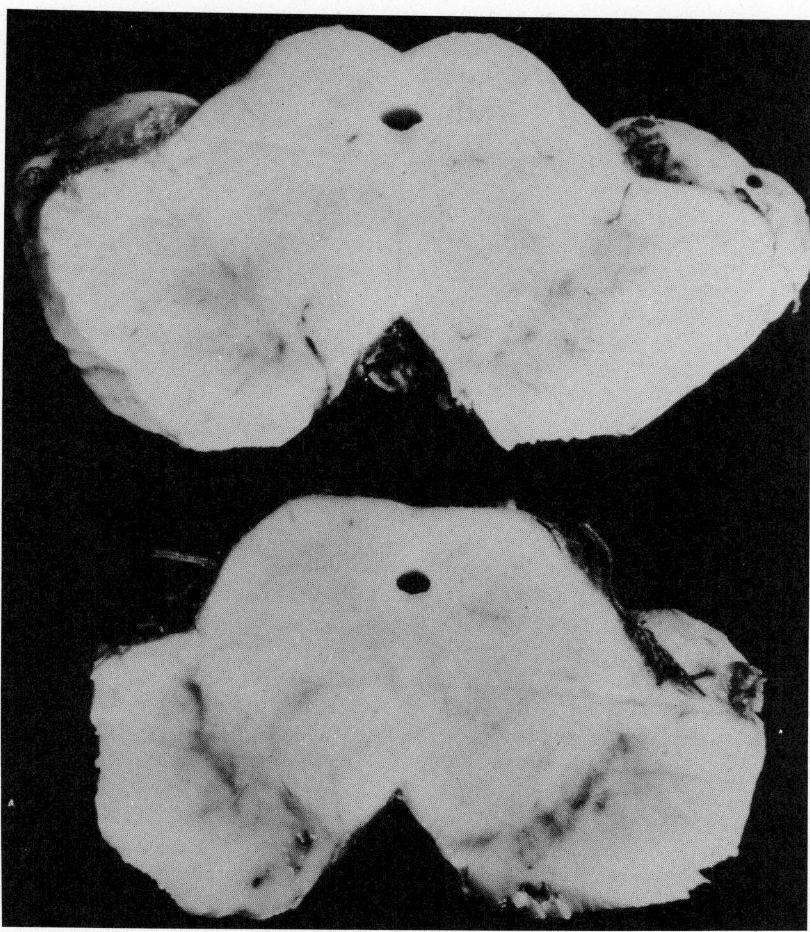

FIGURE 50-6 Brainstem in parkinsonism. Pigmentation is decreased in the substantia nigra as compared to normal (below). (From F. Miller, *Peery and Miller's Pathology* [3rd ed.]. Boston: Little, Brown, 1978.)

Dyskinesias and dystonias also may occur during levodopa therapy. They usually disappear as the drug is decreased. Unfortunately, these symptoms may appear before the tremor of parkinsonism is under control, which means that if the dosage of levodopa is increased enough to control the tremor, the dyskinesias or dystonias may become intolerable. If the dosage is decreased to eliminate the dystonias, the tremor may become much worse.

When dyskinesias occur late in tranquilizer therapy or appear after the drug has been discontinued (tardive dyskinesias), they may be evidence of permanent, irreversible change in the extrapyramidal nervous system. This change may be in the dopamine receptors themselves. Tardive dyskinesias do not respond well to anticholinergic therapy, as do early dyskinesias, although they also seem to be due to a disturbed balance in the brain between acetylcholine and dopamine [11].

Torticollis

Torticollis, or wry neck, is an intermittent or sustained dystonic contraction of the cervical muscles on one side of the neck due to hysteria, drug therapy, or organic neurologic disease. It may occur as one of the painful dystonias in early phenothiazine therapy or, rarely, it may accompany primary parkinsonism. When it occurs in association with primary or secondary parkinsonism, it may be due to a relative increase in cholinergic activity in the brain associated with a striatal dopamine deficiency [11].

The angle of head rotation depends on which muscles are affected; the affected muscles often hypertrophy in response to the constant or frequent powerful muscle contractions. The muscles most commonly involved are the scalene, sternocleidomastoid, and trapezius. The spasm may occur suddenly and painfully, which is characteristic of the drug-induced dystonias and hysteria. The contraction also can occur very slowly. Primary muscle fibrosis after trauma and abnormalities of the cervical spine must be ruled out as the cause of this disorder. If major tranquilizers are being used, reduction in dose and/or anticholinergic therapy may prove useful. Psychotherapy and/or relaxation therapy may be helpful for hysterical torticollis. Unfortunately, if the cause is a lesion in the corpus striatum, the prognosis for cure is poor [14]. In severe cases the only successful treatment is to section the upper anterior cervical roots and spinal accessory nerves.

Huntington's Chorea

Huntington's chorea is an inherited autosomal dominant disorder that is characterized by a progressive degeneration of the cerebral cortex as well as of the basal ganglia, particularly the caudate nucleus and putamen. In addition to the dramatic choreiform movements for which it is named, there is progressive deterioration of higher intellectual functions such as memory and judgment, to the point of severe dementia and death.

In Huntington's chorea the neurotransmitter GABA is markedly reduced in the degenerating areas of the brain. Acetylcholine also seems to be reduced, resulting in an imbalance among the three transmitters, GABA, acetylcholine, and dopamine. When dopamine predominates, chorea results, indicating heightened dopamine sensitivity of the striated receptors [12]. When chorea is the major motor symptom, degenerative lesions are especially common in the caudate. In those occasional persons in whom rigidity and tremor predominate, lesions seem to be more likely in the putamen. In many cases of Huntington's chorea, however, lesions are common throughout the corpus striatum and in the thalamus as well [14]. As is usual with extrapyramidal disorders, the full significance of these lesions is not fully understood.

It is believed that GABA is an inhibitory transmitter and the neurons that degenerate in the corpus striatum are inhibitory neurons [7]. As a result, increasingly violent choreiform movements begin to occur in the face, neck, and arms during middle age, and may be the first signs of neurologic disease. In addition to the chorea or less commonly, widespread muscle rigidity and tremors, dementia develops that is characterized by impulsiveness, paranoia, neurosis, emotional outbursts, loss of judgment and memory, irritability or apathy, delusions or hallucinations, and suicidal tendencies. The dementia seems to result from atrophy of the cerebral cortex, especially over the frontal and parietal lobes [14].

When a family history of Huntington's chorea exists, diagnosis is made by this history and confirming physical examination. With a negative family history, diseases such as neurosyphilis must be ruled out. Usually, Huntington's chorea progresses to death from pneumonia or heart failure in 10 to 20 years. No treatment is known to have any effect on the progression of the disease. Drugs that stimulate GABA and acetylcholine synthesis have proved ineffective in treatment of this disease.

Disorders Characterized by Memory and Judgment Deficits

Dementia refers to an organically caused syndrome of impaired intellectual functions. There is widespread deterioration in the cerebral cortex, especially in the frontal lobes. Characteristically, decreasing quality of judgment, loss of abstract thinking and reasoning, and diminished memory are accompanied by emotional changes ranging from apathy to lability, decreasing personal cleanliness, increasing impulsiveness, and confusion and disorientation.

There are many causes of dementia, but there is no theory for the etiology or pathophysiology for most of these diseases [10]. The examples presented here have been selected because dementia is the prime symptom and demonstrates similarity among vascular, infectious, and other types of lesions. No cure exists, but the pathologic process may be arrested with subsequent therapy for residual symptoms.

Atherosclerotic Dementia

Cerebral atherosclerosis may contribute to the development of transient ischemic attacks or cerebrovascular accidents of a focal nature (see pages 769–771). Cerebral atherosclerosis can also produce the symptoms of dementia secondary to diffuse, small, cerebral infarctions and widespread cerebral anoxia. About 15–20 percent of dementias are attributed to cerebral atherosclerosis [15]. The term *senile dementia* may be used for the results of diffuse cerebral atherosclerosis; generally it refers to a condition of decreasing intellectual capability with increasing disorientation and emotional lability beginning in the aged individual. Most frequently, the disorder seems to be due to a decreasing blood supply and cerebral anoxia resulting in cortical degeneration. Sensory deprivation and overmedication in the institutionalized elderly may also be contributing factors to the progression of senile dementia.

Alzheimer's Disease

This common, progressive, cerebral degeneration begins to be symptomatic during middle age, usually after age 40 years, being most common between 50 and 65 years of age [10]. The etiologic basis for Alzheimer's disease remains unknown. Much research has been conducted in an attempt to understand this devastating disease better. Several models have been proposed as basis for the disease, including decreased acetylcholine, genetics, abnormal protein, infectious agents, toxins, and inadequate blood flow [15]. Future research may elucidate a cause of and appropriate therapy for this condition.

Pathologic changes include cortical degeneration that is most marked in frontal, temporal, and parietal lobes. Characteristic degeneration includes a decrease in neurons most pronounced in regions of the brain that are responsible for cognition, memory, and other thought processes. Neurons accumulate characteristic fiberlike strands, and the blood vessels contain and are surrounded by amorphous aggregates of protein. In addition, deposits of cellular debris and amyloid (neuritic plaques) are present throughout the brain. Finally, there is marked reduction in the production of neurotransmitters, particularly acetylcholine [15].

Early symptoms include loss of memory, carelessness about personal appearance, speech disturbances that progress to complete disorientation, severe deterioration in speech, incontinence, and stereotyped, repetitive movements. Depression is common as the individual recognizes the cognitive decline that is occurring. Progression to severe dementia is relentless and occurs over a period of 5 to 10 years, although the rate of progression varies. Death may result from secondary causes such as septic decubitus ulcers, dehydration, and pneumonia. Diagnosis of Alzheimer's disease is usually made after other conditions that can cause dementia have been ruled out. No treatment seems to have a significant effect on the course of the disease.

Pick's Disease

This degenerative neurologic disease of the fourth and fifth decades is thought to be passed on by an autosomal dominant gene. It affects women more than men and may occur in families [10]. The clinical picture is similar to that of Alzheimer's disease. Degeneration occurs, with atrophy of the frontal and temporal lobes. The first three cortical layers are most severely involved, and the gyri are dramatically atrophied so as to give this area of the brain the appearance of a dried walnut [7]. The unaffected cells frequently swell and contain cytoplasmic filamentous inclusions known as *Pick bodies* [10].

The initial signs and symptoms reflect personality changes that, unlike Alzheimer's disease and Huntington's chorea, elude the person's awareness. The behavioral deterioration is evidenced by disinterest in surroundings, forgetfulness, confusion, cognitive sluggishness, and apathy and dementia. As the disease progresses, language deteriorates to echolalia (parrotlike repetition of words) and stereotyped words and phrases to incomprehensible jargon and finally, to mutism. Motor deterioration begins with gait disturbances, weakness, and rigidity, and progresses to flexion contractions and paraplegia.

There is no known effective treatment of Pick's disease. Supportive and symptomatic treatment is the mainstay of care at present. Death occurs after a 2- to 10-year course with the disease [10].

Neurosyphilis

Neurosyphilis is very rarely seen, except in primitive cultures [10]. It is believed that the causative spirochete, *Treponema pallidum*, reaches the nervous system during the second stage of a syphilitic infection, although neurologic symptoms may not occur for months or years. If neurologic symptoms appear within a few years of the initial infection, they tend to be focal and respond well to antibiotic therapy. When the onset of neurologic symptoms is delayed for a longer period of years, the earliest signs reveal widespread pathology and do not respond as well to therapy.

In the second stage of syphilis, the symptoms of neurosyphilis are transient and vague, including headache and intermittent pains in the trunk and limbs. Rarely, acute meningitis or encephalitis occurs and may result in seizures and/or coma [14]. A few years after this early stage, inflammation of arterial walls and meningitis often occur, occasionally manifesting a communicating hydrocephalus. Symptoms of the vascular pathology and meningitis include seizures, headache, anxiety, and signs of cranial nerve damage such as palsies, neuralgia, dizziness, and deafness [14].

Blood tests for syphilis are usually positive in secondary and early tertiary neurosyphilis. The CSF is positive for *T. pallidum*, and generally the serum protein level and mononuclear cell count are elevated. These tests, used to confirm the diagnosis of neurosyphilis and to monitor the response to antibiotic therapy, indicate success when cell count falls, the protein content decreases, and changes eventually occur in the VDRL test.

General paresis develops approximately 20 years after the initial infection, and the spirochetes seem to invade the brain parenchyma and cord tissue rather than staying in the meninges and blood vessels. As a result, lesions are spread diffusely over the cerebral cortex, basal ganglia, and sometimes the cerebellar cortex. Early symptoms include impaired memory and concentration. Later, characteristic personal carelessness, impulsiveness, incontinence, and signs of both receptive and expressive aphasia develop. Seizures are common, as are irregular and miotic pupils. Pupils' reaction to light is diminished or absent even though they may accommodate to distance changes; this condition is called *Argyll Robertson pupils*, which signifies midbrain damage. It is especially suggestive of neurosyphilis, although similar pupil changes may be seen in other disorders, such as alcoholic polyneuropathy. Because of damage to the cortical motor cells and pyramidal tracts, voluntary motor function decreases, and reflexes become hyperactive unless the cord is invaded, in which case reflexes may diminish or disappear. The untreated end result of general paresis is usually a bedridden, incontinent, confused, hallucinating person who is susceptible to all the secondary problems of immobility. Penicillin and erythromycin are curative for syphilis, and no tolerance to the drugs appears to be developed by the organism.

Study Questions

1. Describe the following common congenital or development disorders: spina bifida, syringomyelia, hydrocephalus, and cerebral palsy.
2. Discuss the defect that causes myasthenia gravis and explain why it is believed to be an autoimmune disorder.
3. Relate the clinical course of multiple sclerosis to its pathologic processes.
4. Describe the etiology, pathophysiology, and clinical manifestations of Parkinson's disease.
5. Using Alzheimer's disease as a model, describe the clinical picture of dementia.

References

1. Albanese, J.A. *Nurses' Drug Reference*. New York: McGraw-Hill, 1982.
2. Anchi, T. Plasmapheresis as a treatment of myasthenia gravis. *J. Neurosurg. Nurs.* 13:23, 1981.
3. Haerer, A., and Currier, R.D. *Neurology Notes* (5th ed.). Jackson, Miss.: University of Mississippi Medical School, 1974.
4. Harris, E. Extrapyramidal side effects of antipsychotic medication. *Am. J. Nurs.* 81:1324, 1981.
5. Hartley, F.D. A nurse's view: Amyotrophic lateral sclerosis. *J. Neurosurg. Nurs.* 13:89, 1981.
6. Hartshorn, I. Immunosuppresive treatment of multiple sclerosis. *J. Neurosurg. Nurs.* 16:275, 1984.
7. Iverson, L. The chemistry of the brain. *Sci. Am.* 9:141, 1979.
8. Lannon, M., et al. Comprehensive care of the patient with Parkinson's disease. *J. Neurosurg. Nurs.* 18:121, 1986.
9. Lewis, S. Viral and immunopathology in multiple sclerosis. *J. Neurosurg. Nurs.* 15:346, 1983.
10. Robbins, S.L., Cotran, R.S., and Kumar, V. *Pathologic Basis of Disease* (3rd ed.). Philadelphia: Saunders, 1984.
11. Rosal-Greif, V. Drug-induced dyskinesias. *Am. J. Nurs.* 82:66, 1982.
12. Stripe, J., et al. Huntington's disease. *Am. J. Nurs.* 79:1428, 1979.
13. Vigliarolo, D. Managing bowel incontinence in children with meningomyelocele. *Am. J. Nurs.* 80:105, 1980.
14. Walton, J.N. *Brain's Diseases of the Nervous System* (8th ed.). New York: Oxford University Press, 1977.
15. Wurtman, R. Alzheimer's disease. *Sci. Am.* 252:62, 1985.

Unit Bibliography

Adams, R., and Maurice, V. *Principles of Neurology* (3rd ed.). New York: McGraw-Hill, 1985.

Appel, S.H., et al. Amytrophic lateral sclerosis. *Arch. Neurol.* 3:234, 1986.

Bartol, G.J. Psychological needs of spinal cord-injured person. *J. Neurosurg. Nurs.* 10:171, 1981.

Blanco, K. The aphasic patient. *J. Neurosurg. Nurs.* 14:28, 1982.

Boltshauser, E., et al. Permanent flaccid paraplegia in children with thoracic spinal cord injury. *Paraplegia* 19:227, 1981.

Bracken, M.B., et al. Psychological response to acute spinal cord injury: An epidemiological study. *Paraplegia* 19:271, 1981.

Butterworth, J.F., et al. Flaccidity after head injury: Diagnosis, management and outcome. *Neurosurgery* 9:242, 1981.

Byers, V., and Guthrie, M. The limbic system and behavior. *J. Neurosurg. Nurs.* 16:80, 1984.

Carpenter, M., and Sutin, J. *Human Neuroanatomy* (8th ed.). Baltimore: Williams & Wilkins, 1983.

Conway, B. *Pediatric Neurologic Nursing*. St. Louis: Mosby, 1977.

Davis, J., and Mason, C. *Neurological Critical Care.* New York: Van Nostrand Reinhold, 1979

de la Torre, J.C. Spinal cord injury: Review of basic and applied research. *Spine* 6:315, 1981.

Dodson, J. The slow death: Alzheimer's disease. *J. Neurosurg. Nurs.* 16:270, 1984.

Dudas, S., and Stevens, K. Central cord injury: Implications for nursing. *J. Neurosurg. Nurs.* 16:84, 1984.

Dunant, Y., and Maurice, I. The release of acetylcholine. *Sci. Am.* 252:58, 1985.

Dye, O.A., et al. Long-term neuropsychological deficits after traumatic head injury with comatosis. *J. Clin. Psychol.* 37:472, 1981.

Easton, K.C. Emergencies in the home: Head, neck and back injuries. *Br. Med. J.* 282:2099, 1981.

Feiring, E. (ed.). *Brock's Injuries of the Brain and Spinal Cord and Their Coverings* (5th ed.). New York: Springer, 1974.

Findelstein, S., and Ropper, A. The diagnoses of coma: Its pitfalls and limitations. *Heart Lung* 8:1063, 1979.

Fischer, R.P., et al. Postconcussive hospital observation of alert patients in primary trauma center. *J. Trauma* 21:920, 1981.

Foo, D., et al. Post traumatic acute anterior spinal cord syndrome. *Paraplegia* 19:201, 1981.

Ganong, W.F. *Review of Medical Physiology* (12th ed.). Los Altos, Calif.: Lange, 1985.

Ginnity, S.W. Assessment of cervical cord trauma by the nurse practitioner. *J. Neurosurg. Nurs.* 10:193, 1981.

Gudeman, S.K., et al. Computed tomography in the evaluation of incidence and significance of post traumatic hydrocephalus. *Radiology* 141:397, 1981.

Guttmann, L. *Spinal Cord Injuries: Comprehensive Management and Research* (2nd ed.). Oxford: Blackwell, 1976.

Guyton, A.C. *Textbook of Medical Physiology* (7th ed.). Philadelphia: Saunders, 1986.

Hachinski, V., and Norris, J. *The Acute Stroke*. Philadelphia: Davis, 1985.

Hanneman, E. Brain resuscitation. *Heart Lung* 15:3, 1986.

Harthorn, J. Immunosuppressive treatment of multiple sclerosis. *J. Neurosurg. Nurs.* 16:275, 1984.

Hudspeth, A. The hair cells of the inner ear. *Sci. Am.* 284:54, 1983.

Jackson, L. Cerebral vasospasm after intracranial aneurysmal subarachnoid hemorrhage: A nursing perspective. *Heart Lung* 15:14, 1986.

King, L.R., et al. Pituitary hormone response to head injury. *Neurosurgery* 9:229, 1981.

Kunkel, J., and Wiley, J. Acute head injury: What to do when . . . and why. *Nurs. 79* 9:22, 1979.

Lannon, M., et al. Comprehensive care of the patient with Parkinson's disease. *J. Neurosci. Nurs.* 18:121, 1986.

Leina's, R. Calcium in synaptic transmission. *Sci. Am.* 247:56, 1983.

Leverenz, J., and Sumi, S. Parkinson's disease in patients with Alzheimer's. *Arch. Neurol.* 7:662, 1986.

Levin, H.S., et al. Ventricular enlargement after closed head injury. *Arch. Neurol.* 38:623, 1981.

Lewis, S. Viral and immunopathology in multiple sclerosis. *J. Neurosurg. Nurs.* 15:346, 1983.

Lindgren, S., et al. Acute head injuries: Cooperative efforts in clinical assessment. *J. Neurosurg.* 25:32, 1981.

Mitchell, S., and Yates, R. Extracranial-intracranial bypass surgery. *J. Neurosurg. Nurs.* 17:288, 1985.

Moses, R. (ed.). *Adler's Physiology of the Eye* (7th ed.). St. Louis: Mosby, 1981.

Peele, T. *The Neuroanatomic Basis for Clinical Neurology* (3rd ed.). New York: McGraw-Hill, 1977.

Pierce, D., and Nickel, V. (eds.). *The Total Care of Spinal Cord Injuries*. Boston: Little, Brown, 1977.

Plum, F., and Posner, J. *The Diagnosis of Stupor and Coma* (3rd ed.). Philadelphia: Davis, 1980.

Polhpek, M. Stroke: An update on vascular disease. *J. Neurosurg. Nurs.* 12:81, 1980.

Powner, D. (ed.). Coma: Cessation of therapy and decision making process. The University of Pittsburgh School of Medicine symposium. *Heart Lung* 8:1057, 1979.

Richmond, T. A critical care challenge: The patient with a cervical spinal cord injury. *Focus* 12:23, 1985.

Rimel, R.W. A prospective study of patients with central nervous system trauma. *J. Neurosurg. Nurs.* 13:132, 1981.

Rimel, R.W., et al. Disability caused by minor head injury. *Neurosurgery* 9:221, 1981.

Robbins, S.L., Cotran, R.S., and Kumar, V. *Pathologic Basis of Disease* (3rd ed.). Philadelphia: Saunders, 1984.

Rockswold, G.L. Evaluation and resuscitation in head trauma. *Minn. Med.* 64:81, 1981.

Sipkins, J.H., et al. Severe head trauma and acute renal failure. *Nephron* 28:36041, 1981.

Spencer, P.S., and Schaumberg, H.H. *Experimental and Clinical Neurotoxicology*. Baltimore: Williams & Wilkins, 1980.

Stone, J.L., et al. Traumatic subdural hygroma. *Neurosurgery* 8:542, 1981.

Swann, I.J., et al. Head injuries at an inner-city accident and emergency department. *Injury* 12:274, 1981.

Taylor, J. Increased intracranial pressure. *Nurs. 83* 13:44, 1983.

Taylor, J., and Ballenger, S. *Neurological Dysfunction and Nursing Interventions*. New York: McGraw-Hill, 1980.

Wald, M. Cerebral thrombosis: Assessment and nursing management of the acute phase. *J. Neurosci. Nurs.* 18:36, 1986.

Wang, C., et al. Brain injury due to head trauma. *Arch. Neurol.* 6:570, 1986.

Weisberg, L. Subdural empyema. *Arch. Neurol.* 5:49, 1986.

Wurtman, R. Alzheimer's disease. *Sci. Am.* 252:62, 1985.

Wurtz, R., Goldberg, M., and Robinson, D. Brain mechanisms in visual attention. *Sci. Am.* 246:124, 1982.

Yanoff, M., and Fine, B. *Ocular Pathology* (2nd ed.). Philadelphia: Harper & Row, 1982.

Yashon, D. *Spinal Injury*. New York: Appleton-Century-Crofts, 1978.

Young, M.S. A bedside guide to understanding the signs of intracranial pressure. *Nurs. 81* 11:59, 1981.

Zuidema, G., Rutherford, R., and Ballenger, W. *The Management of Trauma* (4th ed.). Philadelphia: Saunders, 1985.

UNIT 16

Reproduction

Sharron P. Schlosser

Unit 16 discusses male and female reproductive physiology and the common pathologic problems associated with them. Chapter 51 provides an overview of the anatomy and physiology of the male reproductive system. Chapter 52 presents common alterations in male function, including the prostate, penis, scrotum, testes, and epididymis. Chapter 53 discusses normal female anatomy and physiology together with laboratory and diagnostic aids in the examination of the female system. Chapter 54 details some of the common alterations in female function, including menstrual problems, infections, and benign and malignant conditions. Chapter 55 discusses sexually transmitted diseases, including gonorrhea and syphilis as well as herpes and AIDS.

The reader is encouraged to use the learning objectives as a study guide outline and the study questions as a review. The unit bibliography gives direction for further research.

CHAPTER 51

Normal Male Function

CHAPTER OUTLINE

Anatomy
- Testes
- Epididymis
- Vas Deferens
- Seminal Vesicles
- Ejaculatory Ducts
- Prostate Gland
- Urethra
- Bulbourethral Glands
- Penis

Male Reproductive Functions
- Spermatogenesis
- Fertility
- Male Function in the Sex Act
- Hormonal Regulation of Male Sexual Function
- Gonadotropic Hormonal Control of Male Sexual Function

Physical, Laboratory, and Diagnostic Tests
- Physical Examination
- Testosterone Measurement
- Semen Examination
- Testicular Biopsy

LEARNING OBJECTIVES

1. Describe the development and function of the male sex organs.
2. List three functions of the male reproductive system.
3. Discuss the process of spermatogenesis.
4. List and discuss the factors involved in determining male fertility.
5. List and discuss the stages of male response in the sex act.
6. Identify the functions of testosterone.
7. Describe the production and degradation of testosterone.
8. Discuss the influence of the hypothalamus and anterior pituitary on the production of testosterone and spermatogenesis.
9. Describe briefly three diagnostic tests used to determine alterations in male reproductive function.

Reproductive function is an integral facet of the human being. Survival of the species is dependent on proper functioning of the reproductive system. This chapter provides an overview of normal male reproductive physiology and function.

Anatomy

The male reproductive system includes both essential and accessory organs (Fig. 51-1). The essential organs are the testes, which produce sperm; accessory organs include the epididymis, vas deferens, seminal vesicles, ejaculatory ducts, prostate gland, and urethra. The supporting structures of the scrotum, penis, and spermatic cords are also considered to be accessory organs.

Testes

The testes are two ovoid glands suspended in the scrotum by attachment to both scrotal tissue and spermatic cords. The testes consist of many lobules, each of which contains the *seminiferous tubules* and *interstitial cells of Leydig*. Spermatogenesis occurs in the seminiferous tubules, and the interstitial cells secrete testosterone, the male hormone (see p. 875).

Epididymis

The epididymis is a tortuous genital duct that serves as a passageway for spermatozoa. It is located on top of the testes and is divided into three parts: (1) head, which is connected to the testes; (2) body, and (3) tail, which is

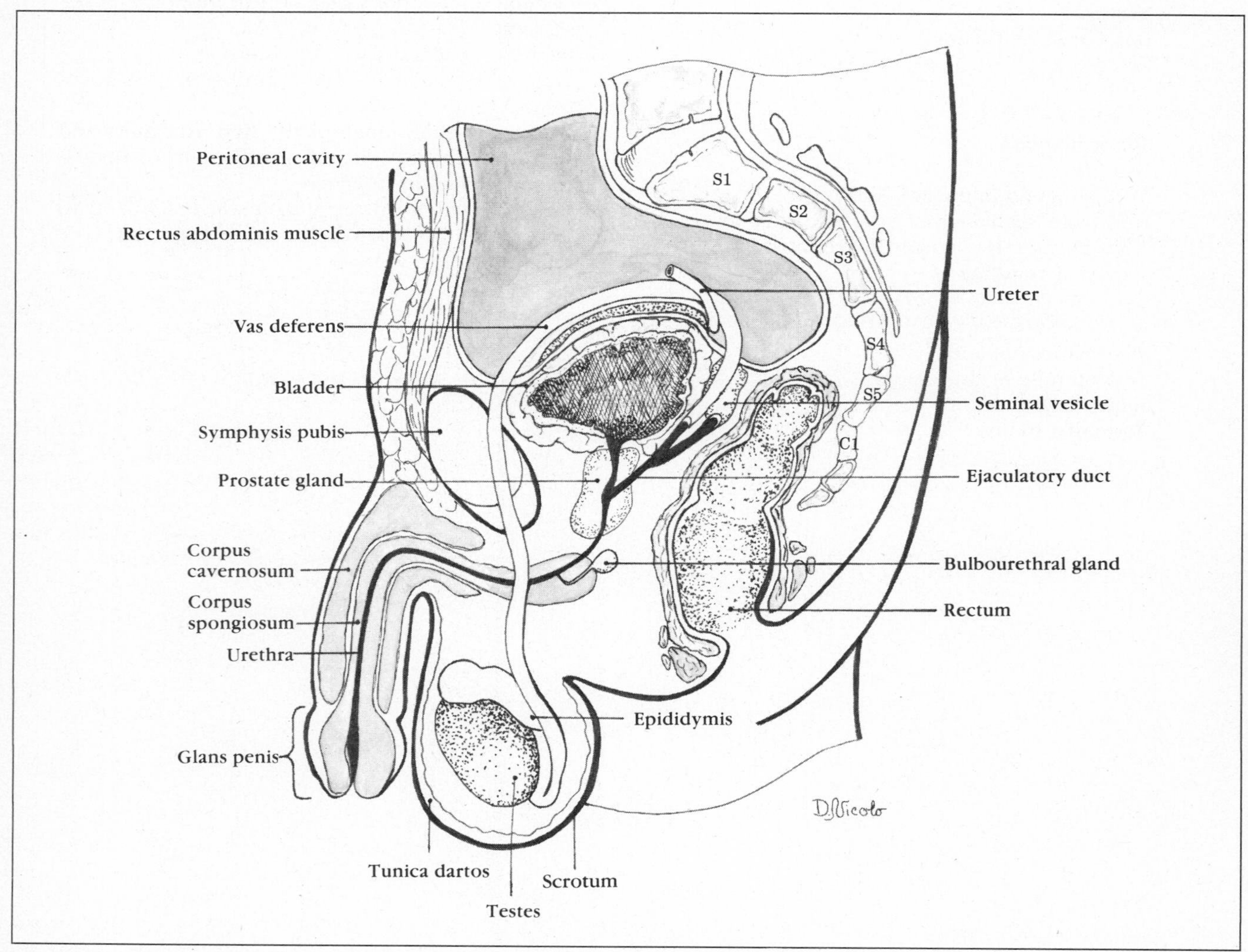

FIGURE 51-1 Side view of male genitourinary anatomy. (From M.A. Miller and D.A. Brooten, *The Childbearing Family: A Nursing Perspective* [2nd ed.]. Boston: Little, Brown, 1983.)

continuous with the vas deferens (Fig. 51-2). Sperm are stored in the epididymis from 18 hours up to 10 days. During this time they mature, develop the power of motility, and become capable of fertilizing an ovum.

Vas Deferens

The vas deferens is an uncoiled tube or duct that is an extension of the tail of the epididymis. This duct ascends from the scrotum into the abdomen where it passes over the bladder. On the posterior of the bladder the duct enlarges into the ampulla of the vas deferens and joins with the duct from the seminal vesicle to form the ejaculatory duct (Fig. 51-3).

The vas deferens stores the majority of the sperm. During the storage period, sperm metabolism continues, and large amounts of carbon dioxide are formed and secreted into the surrounding fluid. The resulting acidic pH inhibits activity of the sperm during storage. On release to the exterior, the sperm again exhibit the power of motility [1].

Seminal Vesicles

The seminal vesicles are two pouches that are lined with secretory epithelium and are located directly behind the urinary bladder (see Fig. 51-3). They produce a viscous, alkaline fluid that makes up about 30 percent of the seminal fluid volume. This fluid is rich in fructose, an energy source for sperm metabolism. Fluid from the seminal vesicles also contains citric acid, five amino acids, and prostaglandins.

Ejaculatory Ducts

The ejaculatory ducts are two short tubes that descend through the prostate gland and terminate in the urethra. As previously mentioned, they are formed by union of the vas deferens and seminal vesicle ducts.

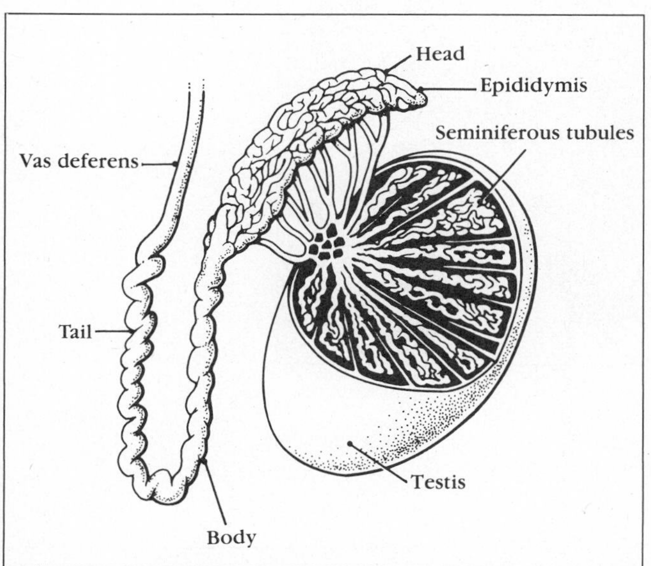

FIGURE 51-2 The vas deferens in relationship to the tubules of the testis and epididymis.

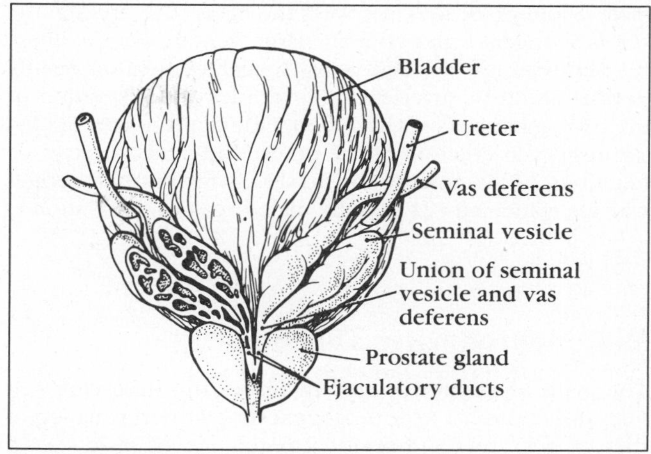

FIGURE 51-3 The seminal vesicles, union with the vas deferens, and entrance into the prostate gland.

Prostate Gland

The prostate is a walnut-sized gland located just below the bladder. It surrounds the ejaculatory duct and about an inch of the urethra. Its primary function is to secrete a thin, milky, alkaline fluid that comprises about 60 percent of seminal fluid volume. This fluid is discharged into the urethra during emission and helps to neutralize the acidic fluid of the male urethra and female vagina.

Urethra

The urethra is the terminal portion of the seminal fluid passageway. It is about 18 to 20 cm long and passes through the prostate gland and the penis, terminating at the external urethral orifice. Located along the urethra are the glands of Littre, which supply mucus. The urethra also receives alkaline fluid from the bulbourethral glands.

Bulbourethral Glands

The bulbourethral glands are two pea-sized glands located just below the prostate. The alkaline secretions from these glands constitute less than 5 percent of seminal fluid volume.

Penis

The penis is covered by a loose layer of skin and contains three compartments of erectile tissue: two corpora cavernosa and the corpus spongiosum (see Fig. 51-1). Corpora cavernosa are large and parallel to each other. The corpus spongiosum is smaller, lower than the corpora cavernosa, and contains the urethra. Distally, the corpus spongiosum expands to form the glans penis. In the uncircumcised male, a fold of loose skin covers the glans. The erectile tissue is spongelike and contains large venous sinuses interspersed with arteries and veins. Sexual stimulation results in dilation of the arteries and arterioles and distention of the cavernous spaces with blood. Filling of the erectile tissue results in erection of the penis. The penis serves two functions: (1) it contains the urethra, which is the passageway for urine and (2) it is the male organ of copulation.

Male Reproductive Functions

The male reproductive system serves the following primary functions: (1) spermatogenesis, (2) performance of the sex act, and (3) hormonal regulation of male sexual function.

Spermatogenesis

The seminiferous tubules of the newborn male's testes contain primitive sex cells called *spermatogonia*. They are located in two to three layers in the outer border of the tubular epithelium (Fig. 51-4). At approximately age 13 years, spermatogenesis begins in all the seminiferous tubules. This develops as a result of stimulation by the adenohypophyseal (anterior pituitary) gonadotropic hormones (see pages 490–491).

During spermatogenesis, a series of meiotic divisions occurs. The primary spermatocyte divides into two secondary spermatocytes, which subsequently divide and produce four spermatids (Fig. 51-5). During this process each cell retains one of each pair of 23 chromosomes. Of the 23 chromosomes, 1 is the sex chromosome.

In the process of spermatid production, each cell loses most of its cytoplasm and elongates into a sperm, which

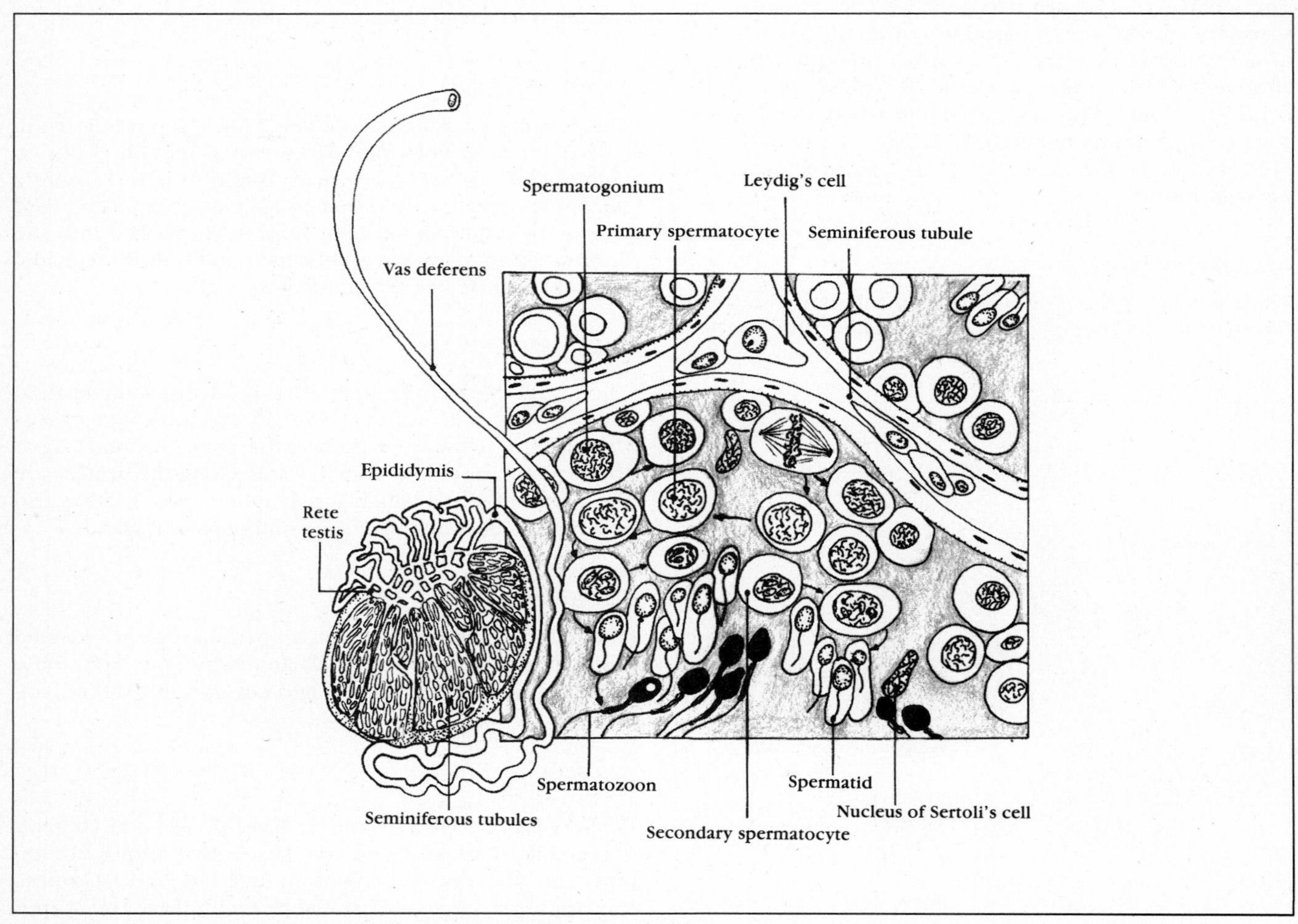

FIGURE 51-4 Male ductal system and developing reproductive cells. The detail on the right shows spermatogenesis and the seminiferous tubule. (From M.A. Miller and D.A. Brooten, *The Childbearing Family: A Nursing Perspective* [2nd ed.]. Boston: Little, Brown, 1983.)

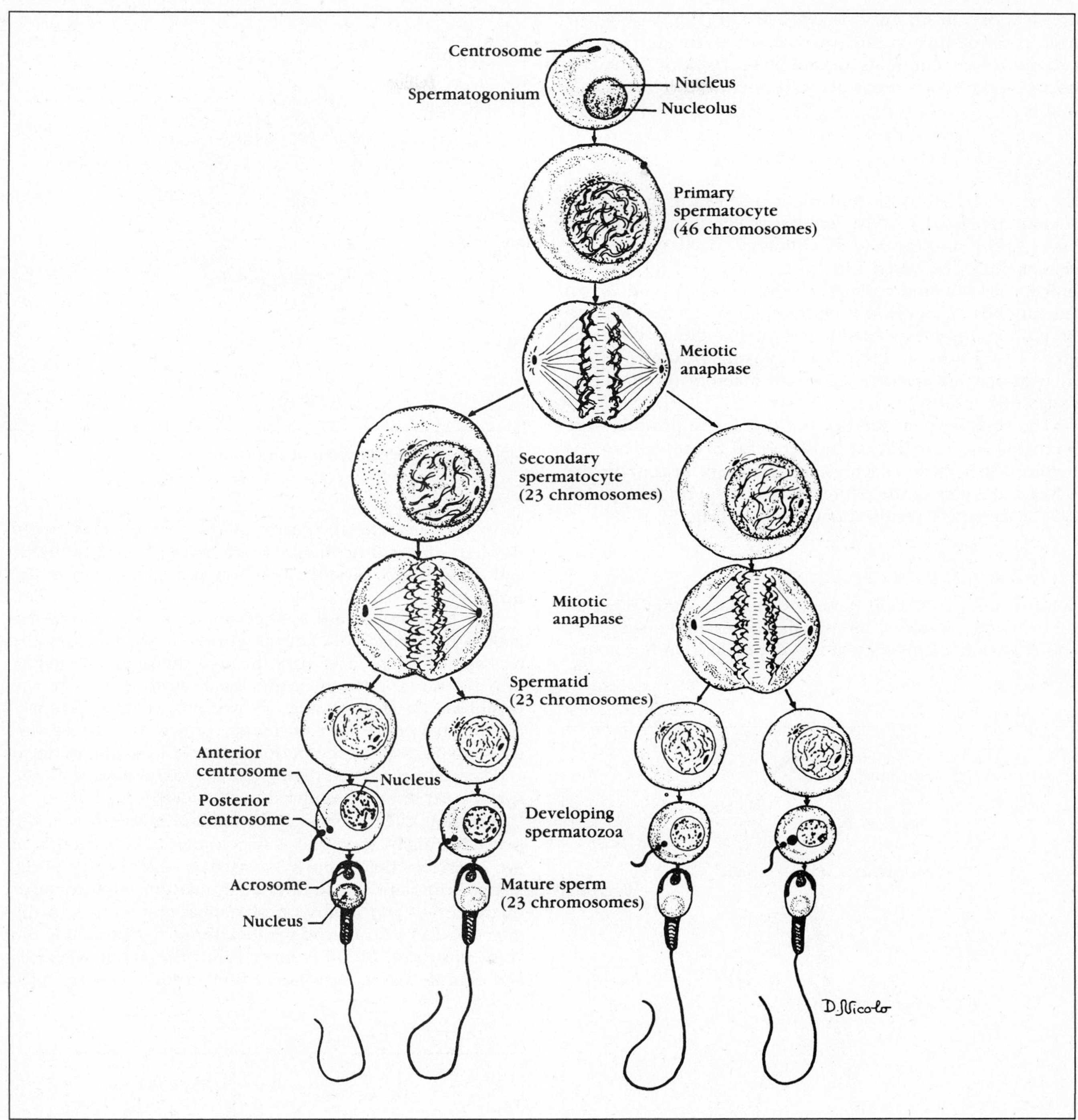

FIGURE 51-5 Maturation of male reproductive cells. (From M.A. Miller and D.A. Brooten, *The Childbearing Family: A Nursing Perspective* [2nd ed.]. Boston: Little, Brown, 1983.)

consists of a head, neck, body, and tail (Fig. 51-6). The head is formed when nuclear material rearranges and the cell membrane contracts around it. This part of the sperm fertilizes the ovum while the tail portion provides rapid motility.

Fertility

Actual male fertility is dependent on (1) the quantity of semen ejaculated, (2) the number of sperm per milliliter, and (3) the motility and morphology of the sperm. The seminal fluid ejaculated with each coitus averages 400 million sperm in a fluid volume of approximately 3 ml. When the number of sperm in each milliliter drops below 20 to 50 million, *infertility* (defined as the inability to conceive after 12 months of adequate exposure in unprotected intercourse) or *sterility* (absolute inability to conceive) frequently results.

The acrosome on the head of the sperm produces the enzymes *hyaluronidase* and several proteinases. It is believed that these enzymes are necessary to remove the outer cell layers of the ovum. Only one sperm is responsible for the actual fertilization, however (Fig. 51-7).

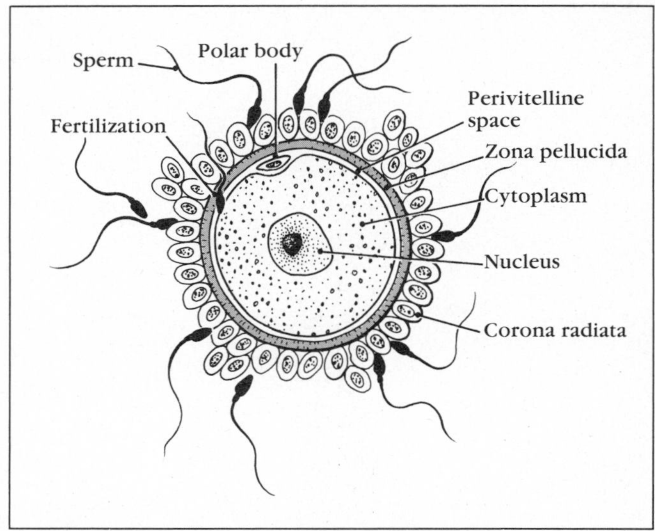

FIGURE 51-7 Fertilization of an ovum.

Male Function in the Sex Act

With respect to sexual behavior, humans differ from all other living creatures. In animals, for example, sex drive and behavior are instinctual and dependent on hormones. With humans, the initiation of the sex act may begin through physical or mental stimulation. Erotic thoughts and dreams may produce erection and ejaculation in the male.

The most important area of sexual stimulation in the male is the glans penis. Sexual sensations produced by the massage of intercourse pass through the pudendal nerve, into the sacral portion of the spinal cord, and on to the cerebrum. Physical stimulation may also occur with touching the anal epithelium, perineum, or scrotum. These sexual sensations enter the pudendal nerve from the perineal and scrotal nerves and then enter the sacral portion of the spinal cord to be transmitted to the cerebrum.

The first effect of sexual stimulation is *erection* of the penis. Normally, the penis is flaccid due to constriction of the arterioles that supply its vascular spaces (Fig. 51-8). Sexual stimulation results in a stimulation of parasympathetic nerves and inhibition of sympathetic nerves to the arterioles. As a result, the penile arterioles dilate while the veins constrict. Blood is forced into the vascular spaces and erectile tissue. The blood flow, under pressure, pro-

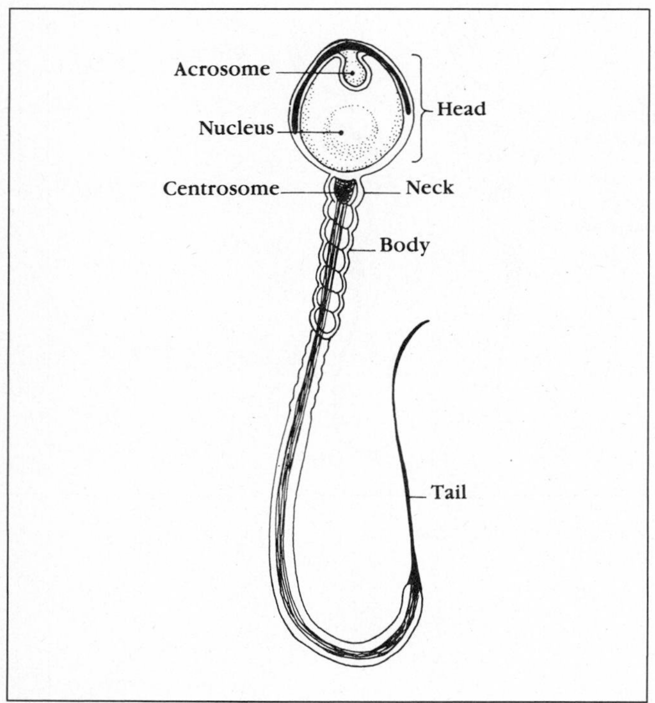

FIGURE 51-6 The mature sperm, consisting of a head, neck, body, and tail. (From M.A. Miller and D.A. Brooten, *The Childbearing Family: A Nursing Perspective* [2nd ed.]. Boston: Little, Brown, 1983.)

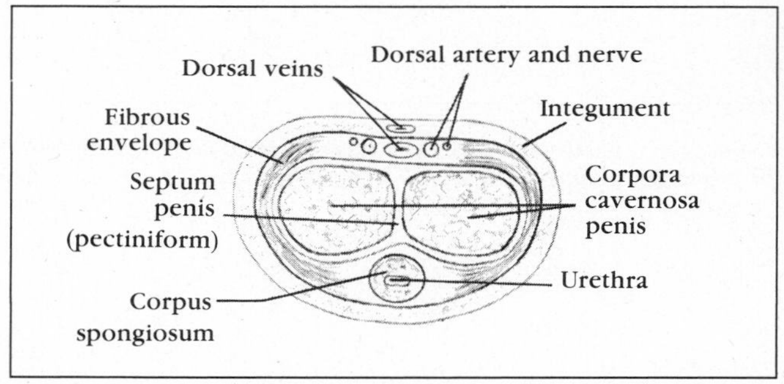

FIGURE 51-8 Vascular supply to penis. (From W.H. Masters and V.E. Johnson, *Human Sexual Response*. Boston: Little, Brown, 1966.)

duces a ballooning effect of the erectile tissue and results in a hard, elongated penis.

During this first stage of the male sexual response, lubricating fluid is discharged from the bulbourethral glands and the glands of Littre, a result of parasympathetic stimulation.

The second stage involves two processes: *emission* and *ejaculation*. Emission is initiated when sympathetic impulses are emitted by reflex centers in the spinal cord, which pass to the smooth muscle of the genital ducts, producing contractions and forcing the sperm and seminal fluid into the internal urethra. Filling of the internal urethra then initiates impulses that result in contractions of the skeletal muscle at the base of the penis. During these contractions, the sphincter at the base of the bladder constricts, preventing the expulsion of urine, as seminal fluid and sperm are expelled through the external urethral orifice. This ejaculation represents a parasympathetic response and culminates the sex act for the male.

Hormonal Regulation of Male Sexual Function

Testosterone is the active male hormone secreted by the testes. It is produced by the *interstitial cells of Leydig*, which are located between the seminiferous tubules. The testosterone released by these cells circulates in the bloodstream only 15 to 30 minutes before it is fixed in tissues to perform intracellular functions or is degraded by the liver. Once testosterone enters the cells it is converted to *dihydrotestosterone*. Dihydrotestosterone combines with nuclear protein, promotes messenger ribonucleic acid (RNA) synthesis, which then enhances cellular protein production. Testosterone not fixed in tissues is converted in the liver into androsterone and dehydroepiandrosterone. These forms are conjugated into glucuronides or sulfates and are excreted in bile or urine as 17-ketosteroids (Fig. 51-9). The inactivation process for testosterone accounts for the ineffectiveness of oral administration of this hormone. Testosterone has the following functions: (1) it controls development of male secondary sex characteristics, (2) it regulates metabolism, (3) it affects fluid and electrolyte balance, and (4) it inhibits anterior pituitary secretion of gonadotropins.

Testosterone primarily accounts for the distinguishing male characteristics. As early as the second month of embryonic life, chorionic gonadotropin from the placenta stimulates production of small amounts of testosterone, which is believed to effect the development of the penis, scrotum, prostate gland, seminal vesicles, and genital ducts in the fetus. During childhood, virtually no testosterone is produced until puberty, at which time secretion increases rapidly. After puberty and continuing until maturity at approximately age 20 years, testosterone stimulates enlargement of the penis, scrotum, and testes.

Testosterone also stimulates protein anabolism, which is directly responsible for virilization of the male. The sec-

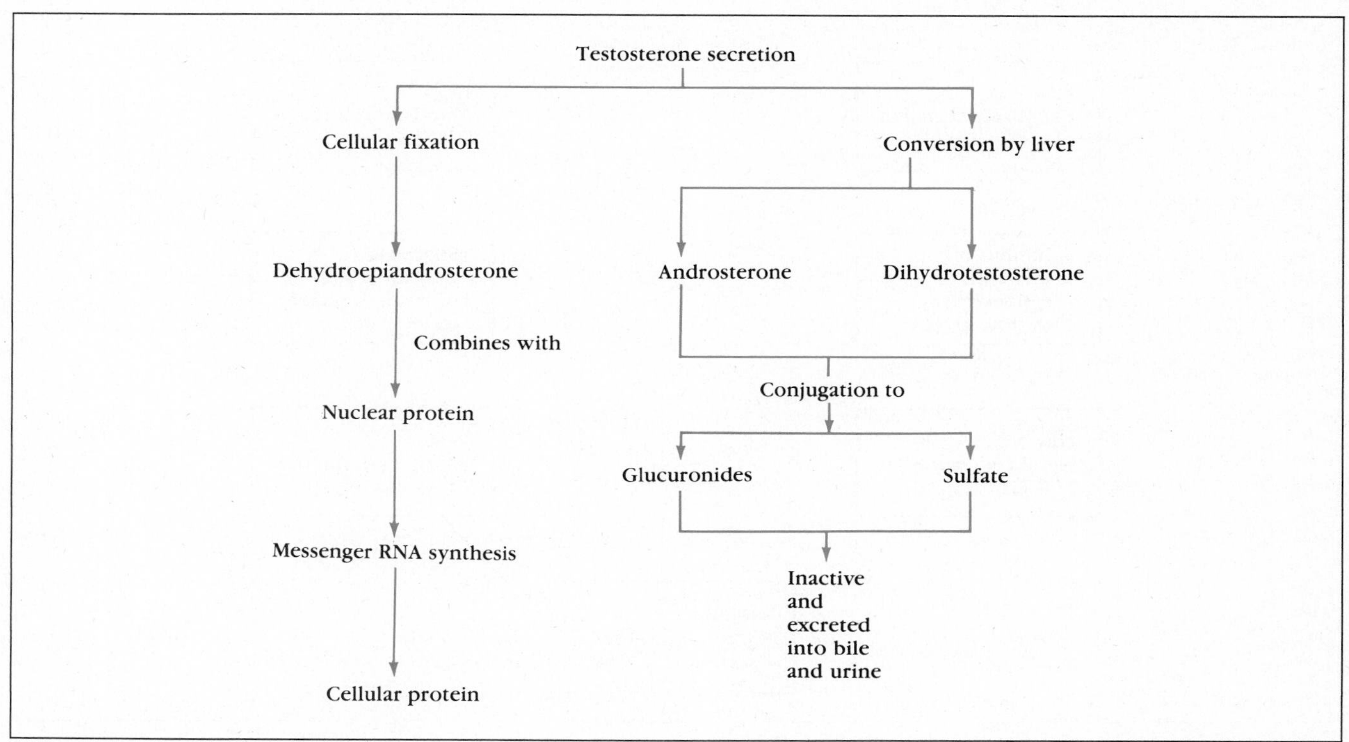

FIGURE 51-9 Paths of testosterone after secretion by testes. Part of the hormone becomes fixed in tissues to perform intracellular functions and part is degraded by the liver.

ondary sex characteristics—muscular development and strength; hair growth on the face, axillae, and chest; bone growth; and deepening of the voice—are manifestations of this process. In affecting bone growth, testosterone also functions in early uniting the epiphyses and shafts of long bones, which stops the growth process. The basal metabolic rate (BMR) increases under the influence of this hormone.

Testosterone secondarily increases retention of sodium, potassium, calcium, and water. The hormone levels can affect the fluid balance through influencing iron retention by the kidneys. It is a method to retain substances necessary to effect the anabolic process. High levels of testosterone inhibit secretion of gonadotropins by the anterior pituitary.

Gonadotropic Hormonal Control of Male Sexual Function

In the male, the anterior pituitary secretes two sex hormones: follicle-stimulating hormone (FSH) and interstitial cell-stimulating hormone (ICSH); also referred to as the luteinizing hormone (LH).

The latter stimulates Leydig cells to produce testosterone. A rise in the blood level of testosterone provides negative feedback to the anterior pituitary, thus reducing the levels of FSH and ICSH. A drop in ICSH level inhibits secretion of testosterone. As testosterone levels drop, the anterior pituitary is again triggered to secrete ICSH (Fig. 51-10). In the fetus, chorionic gonadotropin has properties like those of ICSH. Thus, it stimulates the interstitial cells in the testes, the production of testosterone, and the development of the penis, scrotum, prostate gland, seminal vesicles, and genital ducts.

Follicle-stimulating hormone converts spermatogonia into sperm. Without FSH, spermatogenesis does not occur, and without testosterone the sperm do not mature. The secretion of FSH and ICSH is controlled not only by testosterone but by follicle-stimulating hormone-releasing factor (FSHRF) and luteinizing hormone-releasing factor (LHRF). These releasing factors are secreted by the hypothalamus and conducted through the blood flow channels, called the hypothalamicohypophyseal portal system, between the hypothalamus and the pituitary. Stress and emotions affect secretions by the hypothalamus and usually decrease secretion of the releasing factor.

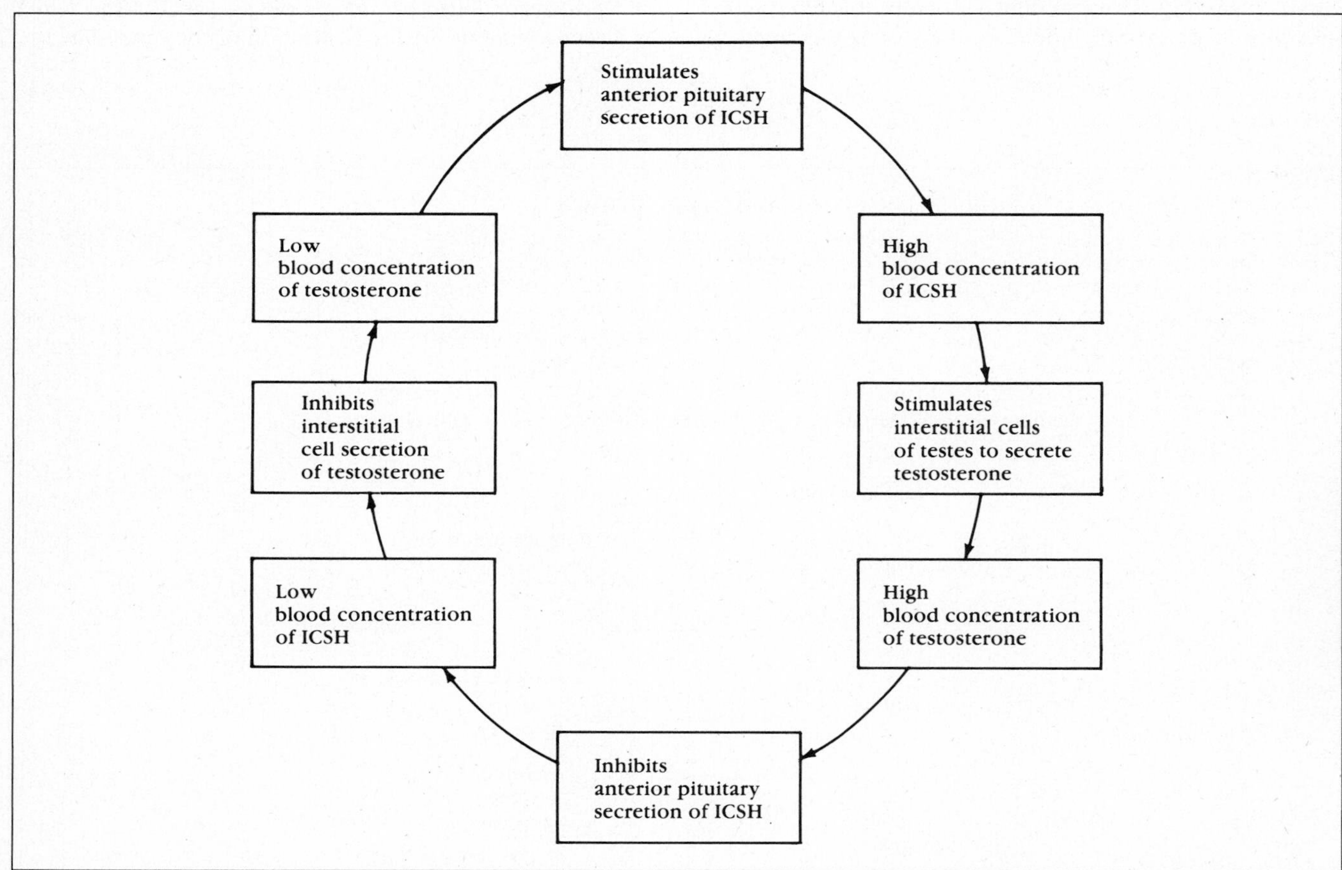

FIGURE 51-10 Illustration of negative feedback mechanism for the secretion of ICSH and interstitial cell secretion of testosterone. (From C. Anthony, *Textbook of Anatomy and Physiology*. St. Louis: Mosby, 1979.)

Physical, Laboratory, and Diagnostic Tests

In study of the male reproductive system, both physical examination and laboratory evaluation are important. The former detects redness, swelling, discharge, or abnormal masses, while the latter centers on testicular function. Primary laboratory studies include measurement of testosterone secretion and examination of seminal fluid.

Physical Examination

The physical examination includes inspection and palpation of the external genitalia and a rectal examination. After visual examination of the external genitalia, the examiner palpates the scrotal contents for abnormal masses. A rectal examination is performed to detect the size and texture of the prostate or the presence and location of masses. Prostatic massage may also be performed to obtain a sample of prostatic secretions.

Testosterone Measurement

Testosterone, a 19-carbon hormone that affects the development of male sex characteristics, degrades into androsterone and dehydroepiandrosterone, which can be measured as ***17-ketosteroids***. Approximately one-third of 17-ketosteroid excretion in the male can be attributed to testosterone and its products.

Testosterone levels, measured directly, are particularly helpful in assessment of hypogonadism, impotence, cryptorchidism, and pituitary gonadotropin functions in the male. Male hypogonadism and Kleinfelter's syndrome can be associated with a decreased testosterone level.

In women, testosterone measurement may assist in the diagnosis of ovarian and adrenal tumors. Adrenal neoplasms, benign and malignant ovarian tumors, adrenogenital syndrome, and Stein-Leventhal syndrome with virilization are frequently associated with an increased testosterone level. Table 51-1 depicts normal laboratory values for testosterone production; these values may vary slightly.

Levels of 17-ketosteroids may be high in testicular tumors or adrenal cortical hyperplasia. Prior to puberty, spermatogenesis rarely occurs as a result of testosterone production.

Semen Examination

Semen evaluation is of particular importance in evaluating infertility. Seminal fluid for examination is best collected through masturbation, which provides a complete specimen of ejaculate. This method also protects sperm morphology and motility, which may be affected by rubber condoms.

Both the sperm and the quantity of fluid are examined. Semen viscosity and morphology and motility of the sperm are assessed. The normal sperm count varies widely. Most authorities consider greater than 50 to 60 million sperm per ml to be normal; however, pregnancies have been documented with lower levels. The normal volume of ejaculate is 3 to 5 ml. Infertility has been associated with both lower and higher volumes.

The morphology and motility of sperm may be factors in infertility even when the count is normal. High percentages of inactive or abnormally formed sperm are associated with infertility [2]. Viscosity of seminal fluid may vary. Initially thick, the fluid must liquify to allow normal motility of the sperm. This liquefaction is usually complete in 15 to 20 minutes. Normal semen test results are summarized in Table 51-2.

Testicular Biopsy

Testicular biopsy may be indicated if the semen examination reveals no sperm or if a tumor is suspected. Biopsy may disclose abnormalities of the epididymis or vas deferens that block the emission of normal sperm. It also aids in the diagnosis of testicular atrophy.

TABLE 51-1 Normal Hormone Levels

Hormone	Age	Blood	Urine
Testosterone			
Male	Adult	0.3–1.0 gm/dl (average = 0.7)	47–156 gm/24 hours (average = 70)
	Adolescent	0.10 gm/dl	
Female	All ages	0–0.1 gm/dl (average = 0.04)	0–15 gm/24 hours (average = 6)
17-Ketosteroids			
Male and female	All ages	25–125 gm/dl	
Male	10 years		1–4 mg/24 hours
	20–30 years		6–26 mg/24 hours
	50 years		5–18 mg/24 hours
	70 years		2–10 mg/24 hours
Female	10 years		1–4 mg/24 hours
	20–30 years		4–14 mg/24 hours
	50 years		3–9 mg/24 hours
	70 years		1–7 mg/24 hours
Chorionic gonadotropin			
Male			0

TABLE 51-2 Semen Examination

Test	Normal Results
Sperm count	50–60 million/ml
Volume	3–6 ml
Morphology	60% of sperm motile; 50% of normal morphology
Liquefaction	Complete in 15–20 minutes

Study Questions

1. Explain all the factors necessary for the male reproductive function to occur.
2. How is testosterone formed? What controlling influences are necessary for its regulation?
3. Discuss the influence of testosterone on various bodily activities.
4. What features are necessary in sperm for fertilization to occur?
5. Briefly describe the significance of the 17-ketosteroid level.

References

1. Guyton, A.C. *Textbook of Medical Physiology* (7th ed.). Philadelphia: Saunders, 1986.
2. Yen, S.S.C., and Jaffe, R.B. *Reproductive Endocrinology; Physiology, Pathophysiology and Clinical Management* (2nd ed.). Philadelphia: Saunders, 1986.

CHAPTER 52

Alterations in Male Function

CHAPTER OUTLINE

Prostate

- Degeneration
- Prostatitis
- Benign Prostatic Hyperplasia
- Cancer

Penis

- Phimosis
- Hypospadias
- Epispadias
- Balanitis
- Carcinoma

Scrotum, Testes, and Epididymis

- Hydrocele
- Varicocele
- Torsion of the Testis
- Cryptorchidism
- Testicular Tumors
- Orchitis
- Epididymitis
- DES Exposure

LEARNING OBJECTIVES

1. Differentiate prostatitis, benign prostatic hyperplasia, and carcinoma of the prostate.
2. Discuss the staging of prostatic carcinoma.
3. Define *phimosis*, *hypospadias*, *epispadias*, *balanitis*, *hydrocele*, *varicocele*, *torsion of testis*, and *cryptorchidism*.
4. Describe the four types of testicular germ-cell tumors.
5. List and describe the three major stages of testicular tumors.
6. Discuss the possible influence on male offspring of in utero exposure to DES.

Alterations in male function may be very disturbing as they often represent a threat to how a man feels about himself and his ability to reproduce. Alterations can occur in any reproductive organ at virtually any age. Some of the congenital anomalies, infections, and malignancies are discussed in relation to the various reproductive organs affected.

Prostate

Alterations in prostate function generally occur in adult life and include (1) degeneration, (2) prostatitis, (3) benign prostatic hyperplasia, and (4) carcinoma.

Degeneration

The prostate gland maintains its normal adult size until approximately age 40 to 50 years. At this point, in some men it begins to decrease in size. This atrophy is associated with a decrease in testosterone level and usually produces no symptoms.

Prostatitis

Prostatitis is inflammation of the prostate gland that may result from (1) ascending infection of the urethra; (2) descending infection from the bladder or kidneys; (3) hematogenous spread from teeth, skin, gastrointestinal, or respiratory systems; or (4) lymphogenous spread from rectal bacteria. This condition also occurs in three different forms: (1) acute bacterial, (2) chronic bacterial, and (3) chronic abacterial (also called prostatosis).

Manifestations of acute bacterial prostatitis include chills and fever, dysuria, urinary frequency and urgency, and hematuria. It may also be associated with suprapubic, perineal, or scrotal pain and purulent urethral discharge. On rectal examination the prostate is enlarged and tender. The seminal vesicles may also be palpated, as infection of these organs frequently accompanies prostatitis. Pus cells and bacteria are present in the urine, with specific organisms such as gonococci and staphylococci being identified. Appropriate antibiotics, analgesics, and sitz baths, if instituted early, usually resolve the condition. The infection may become chronic if it is not treated adequately.

Chronic bacterial prostatitis may represent a continuation of acute prostatitis that did not completely respond to antibiotics. Clinical manifestations may include low-grade fever, dull perineal pain, nocturia, and dysuria. The condition may also be asymptomatic. The infection is resistant to antibiotic therapy and prostate massage may be implemented to help drain the bacteria.

Abacterial chronic prostatitis is the most common form of prostatitis [5]. Symptoms are usually mild and include low back pain, and urinary frequency and urgency with rectal, urethral, or perineal discomfort. Physical examination reveals a nontender prostate with normal urine and prostate fluid. Abacterial chronic prostatitis may be related to excessive alcohol or caffeine intake.

Benign Prostatic Hyperplasia

Benign prostatic hyperplasia (BPH) is a common condition. Its incidence gradually increases in men over 50 years of age and occurs in about 95 percent of men over the age of 70 years [5]. Hyperplasia occurs in the periurethral glands, producing adenomas that appear as large, fairly discrete nodules, located in the median and lateral lobes.

Enlarging nodules compress the prostatic portion of the urethra producing symptoms of urinary obstruction. The man may experience difficulty in starting the urinary stream, which is then smaller and less forceful than normal. He may also experience frequency and nocturia. In addition, the median lobe enlarges and pushes upward on the bladder. Bladder muscle thickening and diverticula may develop, which results in incomplete emptying of the bladder and urinary stasis. Compression of the urethrovesical junction leads to reflux. Hydroureter and/or hydronephrosis also may occur and eventually may cause renal insufficiency.

The cause of BPH is unknown, but it is not always progressive. It may be associated with an increase in estrogen from the adrenal gland as the testosterone levels decline with age.

Diagnosis is based on history, physical exam, x-ray examinations, laboratory studies, and instrumentation examination. Prior to any diagnostic studies or examinations, a complete history of any specific signs or symptoms is obtained. A rectal exam is especially useful in determining the size and condition of the gland. Both an intravenous pyelogram (IVP) and voiding cystourethrogram help to determine the condition of the kidneys and degree of bladder emptying. Specific laboratory studies include routine urinalysis, culture and sensitivity, and renal function studies [i.e., blood urea nitrogen (BUN) and creatinine]. Instrumentation studies include catheterization for residual urine and cystoscopy, which allows the examiner to visualize the urethra and bladder. Bladder tone and diverticula may be noted and the size of the prostate estimated. The usual treatment is surgical removal of enlarged tissues. More conservative treatment may include prostatic massage, hot sitz baths, chemotherapy, catheterization, and urethral dilation.

Cancer

Cancer of the prostate is among the leading cancers in men. It ranks third in cause of death from cancer in all men, with only lung and colorectal cancers having higher frequency [1]. In men over age 75 years, it is the leading cause of death. It occurs primarily after age 50 years, but when it arises in younger men, it usually is an aggressive tumor.

Adenocarcinoma is the usual form of prostate cancer. It occurs most frequently in the posterior lobe; hard fixed nodules can be palpated on rectal examination. In the early stages, it produces no symptoms. For this reason, metastasis is common, with the most frequent sites being bones, lungs, lymph nodes, and liver. Early symptoms are those of urethral obstruction, and at this time it is usually associated with metastasis.

The most accepted classification of prostatic adenocarcinoma divides the disease into four stages [2]. Stage A represents a small localized lesion. It is clinically unsuspected and not detectable on rectal examination. This stage is most frequently found at autopsy or during surgery for benign prostatic hyperplasia. Stage B represents a localized lesion palpable rectally. In both stages, the acid phosphatase levels are usually normal, but they may be somewhat elevated in stage B. Stage C indicates extracapsular extension of the lesion. It is palpable on rectal examination and may involve the seminal vesicles. The acid phosphatase level may be elevated. In stage D, metastases to various organs, pelvic nodes, and distant lymph nodes have occurred. Bone metastasis results in elevation of alkaline phosphatase levels.

Probably the most beneficial of all diagnostic tools is the rectal examination. It should be performed in annual examination of all men over age 40 years. Because most tumors arise in the posterior lobe, palpation is usually easy. Additional diagnostic studies include measuring levels of acid phosphatase and alkaline phosphatase, biopsy of detectable lesions of the posterior lobe, and bone scans or radiographs of the spine and pelvis if scans are unavailable. Cystoscopy and lymphangiography also aid in diagnosing the extent of the disease.

Treatment depends on the stage of the disease, the person's age, and symptoms. It generally consists of (1) radiation therapy; (2) radical prostatectomy, transurethral resection, or orchiectomy; (3) chemotherapy; or (4) hormone therapy. The five-year survival in prostatic cancer has improved from 50 to 63 percent [1].

Penis

Phimosis

Phimosis is a condition in which the prepuce is too small to retract over the glans penis. Frequently it is congenital, but it may occur after infection or injury. It predisposes the man to secondary infection and scarring, as secretions and smegma accumulate under the prepuce and cannot be cleaned away. Forcible retraction of the foreskin may lead to constriction, swelling, and pain of the glans penis. Circumcision is the treatment of choice.

Hypospadias

At about 7 to 8 weeks' gestation, the embryo develops a genital tubercle and two genital swellings. In the male fetus the genital tubercle develops into the penis. The two swellings develop into two folds (urethral and scrotal), which descend and fuse. This fusion closes the urethra in the penis and forms the scrotum. Failure of these folds to fuse on the ventral side results in the congenital anomaly of hypospadias. The urethral orifice is located on the underneath side of the penis. The condition is also associated with undescended testicles and chordee, or curvature of penis. If the anomaly is so severe that the infant's sex is questionable, chromosomal studies are initiated. Surgical repair is aimed at straightening the penis and forming a urethra that terminates as centrally as possible.

Epispadias

Epispadias results from failure of the dorsal side of the penis to fuse. The urethral opening is located on this surface rather than in the center. Epispadias occurs less frequently than hypospadias and is often associated with exstrophy of the bladder. Surgical repair is aimed at establishing a normally functioning urethra and penis.

Balanitis

Balanitis is an inflammation of the glans penis. It occurs most frequently in uncircumcised males who exercise poor hygiene. It also may result from venereal disease. Clinical manifestations include redness, swelling, pain, and purulent drainage. Infection may cause adhesions and scarring. Cultures and sensitivity are performed to diagnose the organism so as to initiate antibiotic therapy. Circumcision may be indicated in uncircumcised males.

Carcinoma

Carcinoma of the penis is an extremely rare condition that progresses slowly. The prepuce and glans are primarily affected and onset is often associated with chronic infection. Early circumcision seems to prevent development of the squamous cell carcinoma, which first appears as a gray, crusted papule. The papule gradually enlarges and produces necrotic ulceration in the center. Early diagnosis may result in a cure by local excision and circumcision, if necessary. Larger lesions involving the shaft of the penis and/or the inguinal nodes may require penile resection or amputation. Radiation therapy and chemotherapy are used increasingly as palliative and curative treatments.

Scrotum, Testes, and Epididymis

Hydrocele

A hydrocele is an accumulation of clear or straw-colored fluid within the tunica vaginalis sac that encloses the testicle. It is the most common cause of scrotal enlargement [5]. Frequently it develops without a known cause, but may occur after epididymitis, orchitis, injury, or neoplasm. In the newborn, it results from late closure of the tunica vaginalis. The condition may be asymptomatic or cause pain or tension in the scrotal sac. Treatment may include aspiration or incision if the hydrocele is large or uncomfortable or if the testis cannot be palpated. The condition must be differentiated from a testicular mass, which is usually demonstrated by a translucent rather than an opaque mass on transillumination.

Varicocele

Varicocele refers to the abnormal dilation of the venous plexus of the testis. Onset is usually between 15 and 25 years of age and usually affects the left side. Occurrence on the right side is strongly suggestive of a tumor obstructing a vein above the scrotum. Palpation reveals dilated and tortuous veins often described as "a bag of worms." Clinically, the primary concern relates to possible subfertility. Both motility and numbers of sperm are decreased because of the increased warmth created by vascular engorgement. The condition is usually asymptomatic, but the person may complain of a dragging sensation or a dull pain in the scrotum. Surgical ligation of the internal spermatic vein is reserved for severe conditions or to increase sperm count.

Torsion of the Testis

Torsion of the testis is an infrequent cause of testicular enlargement. It results from rotation of the testis within the tunica vaginalis, which cuts off the blood supply to the testis. It occurs primarily during adolescence and usually occurs after physical exercise. With twisting of the spermatic cord and testis, venous obstruction results in vascular engorgement and sometimes extravasation of blood into the scrotal sac.

The first symptom is usually sudden onset of severe pain in the testicular area. It is unrelieved by rest or support and may radiate into the groin. Other manifestations include scrotal edema, testicular tenderness, and perhaps nausea and vomiting. If the torsion cannot be reduced, surgery must be performed immediately to preserve fertility.

Cryptorchidism

Cryptorchidism is the term given to incomplete or maldescent of the testis. The testis may remain in the abdomen or may be arrested in the inguinal canal or at the puboscrotal junction. It may be unilateral or bilateral, and when unilateral, is somewhat more common on the right [5].

The cause of cryptorchidism is unknown; however, it has been associated with a shortened spermatic cord, testosterone deficiencies, narrowed inguinal canal, and adhesions of the pathway. It is necessary to correct the condition if sterility is to be avoided, because after puberty, the testes atrophy progressively. Spermatogenesis decreases and the cells may be replaced by collagenous fibrous tissue. Because there is a direct relationship between cryptorchidism and testicular cancer, surgical placement in the scrotum is recommended.

Testicular Tumors

Tumors are the most common cause of testicular enlargement. They occur primarily between ages 15 and 30 years, are predominantly malignant, often metastasize before diagnosis, and arise from germ cells in 95 percent of cases [5]. The benign tumors usually arise from the interstitial cells of Leydig or Sertoli.

Four types of testicular germ-cell tumors have been identified: (1) seminoma, (2) embryonal carcinoma, (3) teratoma and teratocarcinoma, and (4) choriocarcinoma [3]. Seminomas are the most common and appear as gray-white, fleshy masses. Most seminomas remain localized until late in the course of the disease, when metastases occur to regional and aortic lymph nodes. Because of their sensitivity to irradiation, seminomas are best treated with this modality.

Embryonal carcinomas are highly malignant tumors that exhibit a wide variety of cell types. They may occur in both adults and children. Small, gray-white nodules are formed, which do not usually invade the entire testis. Metastasis to the lymph nodes, liver, lungs, and bones is frequent. Elevated serum levels of alpha-fetoprotein (AFP) and/or chorionic gonadotropin help to differentiate these from other testicular tumors [5].

Teratoma and teratocarcinoma are tumors with various cellular types. Testicular enlargement and invasiveness are less frequent than with seminomas, but more frequent than with embryonal carcinomas. Metastases generally follow the lymphatic system but may involve many other structures.

Choriocarcinomas are small, gray tumors that may not be palpable. Characteristically, they produce both cytotrophoblastic and syncytiotrophoblastic cells identical to those formed in the placenta. These cells secrete chorionic gonadotropins, which, when found, aid in the diagnosis of choriocarcinoma. Early, distant metastasis usually causes death within a year of diagnosis.

Four stages of testicular progression have also been identified. Stage 1 is subdivided into stage 1A, which includes tumors confined to one testis without evidence of metastasis, and stage 1B, in which the iliac or paraaortic nodes are involved. Stage 2 requires clinical or radiographic evidence of metastasis to lymph nodes below the diaphragm. Stage 3 includes lymph nodes above the diaphragm or metastasis to other body organs such as lungs and liver [4].

Palpation provides the most important diagnostic aid, and most testicular tumors can be identified relatively early in the course of the disease. Once a mass has been identified, a biopsy is necessary to determine if it is malignant. In addition to chemotherapy and radiation therapy, orchiectomy may be performed.

Orchitis

Orchitis is an inflammation of the testes. It most commonly occurs as a complication of mumps, as the mumps virus is excreted through the urine. Orchitis may also be acquired as an ascending infection of the genital tract. Treatment includes bedrest, scrotal support, warm compresses, and antibiotics, if indicated. Clinical manifestations include pain, swelling, chills, and fever. It may be bilateral or unilateral and may result in sterility or impotence.

Epididymitis

Epididymitis occurs when disease-producing organisms in the urine, urethra, prostate, or seminal vesicles spread to the epididymis. Acute epididymitis may result from a sexually transmitted organism, such as *Neisseria gonorrhoeae*. It also occurs as a complication of prostatectomy. Symptoms include pain, chills, fever, and malaise, with scrotal swelling so great that it interferes with ambulation and produces congestion of the testes. Necrosis and fibrosis may occlude the genital ducts and result in sterility. Treatment includes bedrest, scrotal elevation, sitz baths, hot or cold applications, and antibiotics appropriate for the organism.

DES Exposure

The use of diethylstilbesterol (DES) in the treatment of threatened spontaneous abortion increased rapidly from the late 1940s through the 1960s. The effects of in utero exposure of the female fetus to this drug has been known and publicized for years. However it was not until the late 1970s that evidence associating in utero exposure of the male fetus to DES with certain reproductive anomalies began to emerge.

Reported anomalies include abnormalities of the urethra, epididymis, testes and semen. Urethral anomalies include meatal stenosis and hypospadius. There has also been increased incidence of epididymal cysts, varicoceles, and decreased fertility. Cryptorchidism has also been associated with DES exposure. The possible link between DES exposure in males and reproductive cancer is still under study.

Study Questions

1. What conditions can cause acute and chronic prostatitis?
2. Discuss the significance of benign prostatic hyperplasia and how it can be differentiated from prostatic carcinoma.
3. Relate the diagnostic tests for prostatic carcinoma to the condition's prognosis.
4. Why is repair of cryptorchidism considered essential?
5. Identify the stages of testicular carcinoma and relate them to the different forms of these diseases.

References

1. American Cancer Society. *Cancer Facts and Figures*. New York: American Cancer Society, 1986.
2. American Joint Committee in Cancer Staging and End Result Reporting. *Manual for Staging of Cancer, 1983*. Philadelphia: Lippincott, 1983.
3. Dixon, F.J., and Moore, R.A. Testicular tumors: Clinicopathological study. *Cancer* 6:427, 1953.
4. Maier, J.G., et al. An evaluation of lymphadenectomy in the treatment of malignant testicular germ cell neoplasms. *J. Urol.* 101:356, 1969.
5. Robbins, S.L., Cotran, R.S., and Kumar, V. *Pathologic Basis of Disease* (3rd ed.). Philadelphia: Saunders, 1984.

CHAPTER 53

Normal Female Function

CHAPTER OUTLINE

Anatomy
- Ovaries
- Uterus
- Fallopian Tubes
- Vagina
- Bartholin's Glands
- Skene's Glands
- Mammary Glands
- External Genitalia

Female Reproductive Functions
- Hypothalamic Influence
- Pituitary Influence
- The Menstrual Cycle
  - *The Menstrual Phase*
  - *The Proliferative Phase*
  - *Ovulation*
  - *Oogenesis*
  - *Secretory Phase*
- Production of Female Hormones
  - *Estrogen*
  - *Progesterone*
  - *Androgens*
  - *Prolactin*
  - *Prostaglandins*
- Female Response in the Sex Act
- Gestation
- Menopause

Laboratory and Diagnostic Aids
- Gynecologic Examination
- Hormone Levels
  - *Progesterone*
  - *Estrogen*
- Smears
  - *Papanicolaou Smear*
  - *Wet Smear*
- Biopsy
  - *Endometrial Biopsy*
  - *Cervical Biopsy*
  - *Cone Biopsy*
  - *Open Breast Biopsy*
  - *Needle Biopsy*
  - *Vulvar Biopsy*
- Radiography
  - *Hysterosalpingogram*
  - *Mammography*
- Other Procedures
  - *Culposcopy*
  - *Laparoscopy and Culdoscopy*
  - *Ultrasound*
  - *Schiller's Test*
  - *Cultures*
  - *Thermography*
  - *Rubin's Test*
  - *Huhner Test*

LEARNING OBJECTIVES

1. Describe the development and function of the female sex organs.
2. List the functions of estrogen, progesterone, prolactin, and prostaglandins.
3. Describe hypothalamic and pituitary influence on the menstrual cycle.
4. List and discuss the three phases of the menstrual cycle.
5. Describe the phases involved in the female response in the sex act.
6. Discuss the process of oogenesis.
7. Describe the processes of fertilization and implantation.
8. Define *menopause* and discuss the physiologic basis for the associated symptoms.
9. Define the various diagnostic tests used in diagnosis of female reproductive alterations.
10. Give the normal values for laboratory tests used in the diagnosis of alterations in female reproduction.

This chapter provides an overview of the anatomy and physiology fundamental to understanding alterations in female reproductive function.

Anatomy

The female reproductive organs include both essential and accessory organs. The essential organs are the ovaries, which produce ova. The accessory organs include the fallopian tubes, uterus, and vagina, which serve as ducts (Fig. 53-1); Bartholin's, Skene's, and mammary glands; and external genitalia (Fig. 53-2).

Ovaries

These essential reproductive organs of the female are two nodular glands located on either side of the uterus. Each ovary is attached by three ligaments: mesovarium, ovarian, and suspensory (Fig. 53-3). The mesovarium ligament attaches the ovary to the back of the broad ligament, while the ovarian ligament attaches the ovary to the uterus. The suspensory ligament is an extension of the broad ligament beyond the fallopian tubes. The ovaries perform the vital functions of ovulation and hormone secretion, functions discussed in more depth later in this chapter.

The ovary is covered with germinal epithelium and consists of three portions: cortex, medulla, and hilum (Fig. 53-4). The outer portion is the cortex, which is composed of fine areolar stroma, blood vessels, and follicles containing ova at various stages of development. The medulla is the central portion and is composed of stroma or connective tissue, smooth muscle, blood and lymph vessels, and nerves. The innermost portion is the hilum, which is composed of nerves, blood vessels, connective tissue, and the hilar cells, which secrete steroid hormones.

Uterus

The uterus is a pear-shaped organ consisting of three parts: (1) the fundus, located above the entrance of the tubes; (2) the corpus, or body, located below the entrance of the tubes; and (3) the cervix, which is the lowest and narrowest portion (Fig. 53-5). It is important in the processes of menstruation, pregnancy, and labor.

The uterine walls are composed of three layers: endometrium, myometrium, and peritoneum, also known as the perimetrium. The endometrium is the mucous membrane lining of the body of the uterus. It consists of three layers of tissue: stratum compactum, stratum spongiosum, and stratum basale. The *stratum compactum* is the surface layer and consists of partially ciliated simple columnar epithelium. The *stratum spongiosum* is the spongy middle layer of loose connective tissue. Both the stratum compactum and stratum spongiosum slough during menstruation and after delivery. The *stratum basale* is the dense inner layer that attaches to the myometrium.

The myometrium is the thick middle layer consisting of three layers of smooth muscle fibers supported by connective tissue. This layer blends into the endometrium and provides great strength for the uterus. The myometrial layer is thickest in the fundus, which allows for more force during the contractions of labor, aiding in delivery.

The third layer of the uterine wall, the peritoneum, consists of a serous membrane covering almost all of the uterus. On the anterior surface, the peritoneum is reflected onto the bladder below the internal os of the cervix.

The uterus is supported mainly by the levator ani muscles and eight ligaments, which include two broad ligaments, two uterosacral ligaments, a posterior, an anterior, and two round ligaments. The round ligaments are fibromuscular cords that extend from the upper outer portion of the uterus through the inguinal canals and terminate in the labia majora. The outer ligaments are extensions of the peritoneum (Fig. 53-6).

Two of these ligaments are of particular importance because of the pouches they form. The posterior ligament forms the rectouterine pouch (or cul-de-sac of Douglas) as it extends from the posterior surface of the uterus to the rectum (see Fig. 53-1). This is the lowest point of the pelvic cavity.

The anterior ligament forms the uterovesical pouch as it extends from the anterior uterus to the posterior bladder. This pouch is not as deep as the rectouterine pouch.

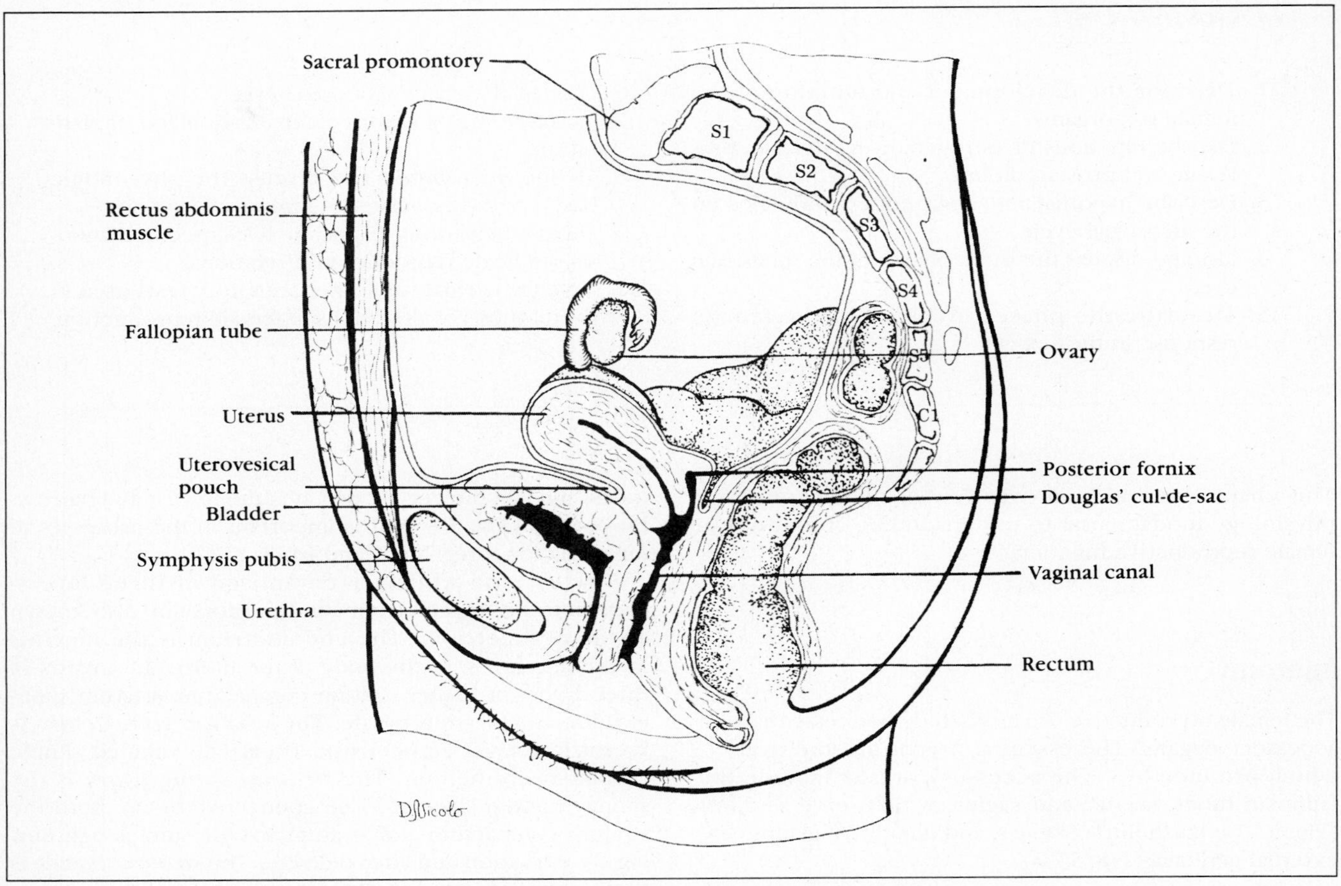

FIGURE 53-1 Side view of female genitourinary anatomy. (From M.A. Miller and D.A. Brooten, *The Childbearing Family: A Nursing Perspective* [2nd ed.]. Boston: Little, Brown, 1983.)

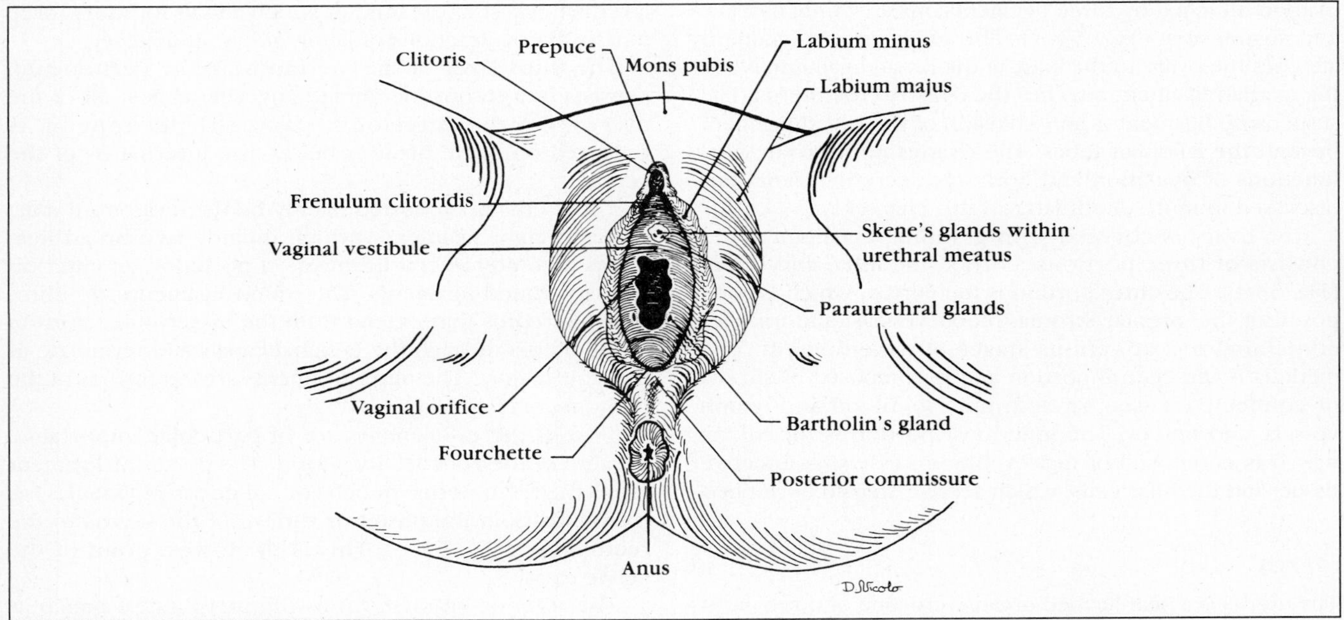

FIGURE 53-2 External female genitalia. (From M.A. Miller and D.A. Brooten, *The Childbearing Family: A Nursing Perspective* [2nd ed.]. Boston: Little, Brown, 1983.)

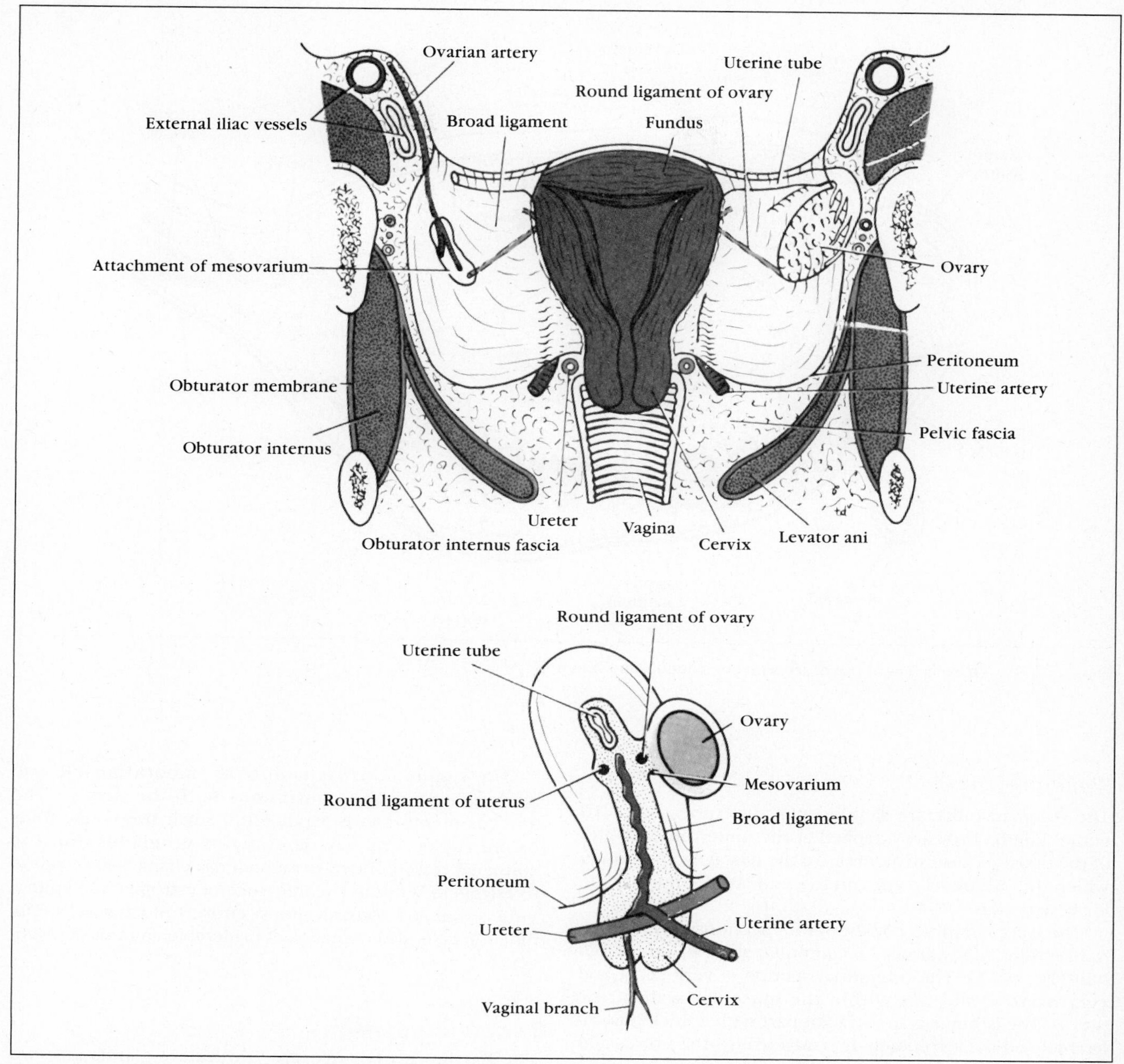

FIGURE 53-3 Coronal section of pelvis, showing uterus, broad ligaments, and right ovary on posterior view. The left ovary and part of the left uterine tube have been removed. Below, uterus on lateral view. Note structures that lie within broad ligament. (From R.S. Snell, *Clinical Anatomy for Medical Students* [2nd ed.]. Boston: Little, Brown, 1981.)

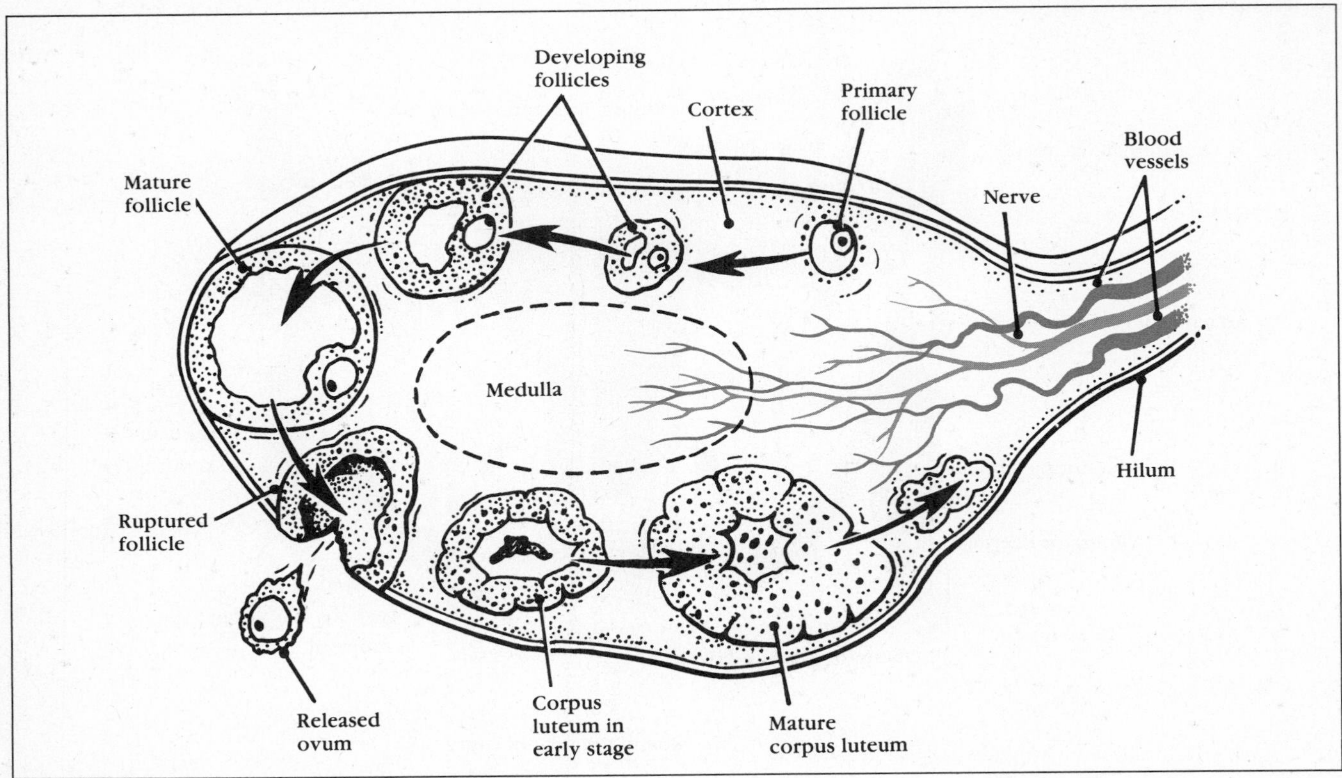

FIGURE 53-4 Three layers of the ovary: cortex, medulla, and hilum.

Fallopian Tubes

The fallopian tubes are slender muscular tubes about 10 cm in length. They are attached at the upper outer angles of the uterus. These structures are the passageway through which the ova travel to the uterus, and are the normal site for conception.

The fallopian tubes consist of four sections: (1) interstitial section, (2) isthmus, (3) ampulla, and (4) infundibulum (Fig. 53-7). The interstitial section is very short and very narrow, and lies within the muscular wall of the uterus. The isthmus is the straight part with a thick muscular wall and narrow lumen. It is adjacent to the uterus and is the usual site for tubal ligation. The ampulla is the dilated lateral section, which is thin-walled with a highly folded lining. The wide distal opening near the ovary is the infundibulum, or fimbriated end. Through muscular action, the fimbriae wave back and forth to create a current that moves ova toward the infundibulum.

Vagina

The vagina is a musculomembranous canal located between the rectum and urethra. It extends upward from the vulva to the midpoint of the cervix. It is the passageway both for menstrual flow and the fetus during delivery and is the recipient for the penis during sexual intercourse.

The vagina consists mainly of smooth muscle and mucous membrane continuous with the uterus. The mucous membrane is arranged in small transverse folds called rugae. The vagina contains no glands, but the epithelial cells of the mucosa undergo changes in response to estrogen. Without the influence of estrogen, the epithelium is thin and consists almost entirely of basal cells. The mucosal cells also contain a considerable amount of glycogen.

Bartholin's Glands

The Bartholin's (or greater vestibular) glands are two bean-shaped mucus-secreting glands located on each side of the vaginal orifice (see Fig. 53-2). Secretion is increased during sexual excitement and moistens the inner surfaces of the labia in preparation for intercourse. The duct may become obstructed or infected, particularly by gonococci, and Bartholin's cyst or abscess may be formed.

Skene's Glands

Skene's glands are tiny mucus-secreting glands located just posterior to the external urethral meatus (see Fig. 53-2). The mucus from the Skene's glands, together with mucus from glands in the urethra, keeps the urethral opening moist and lubricated. The Skene's glands are also suscepti-

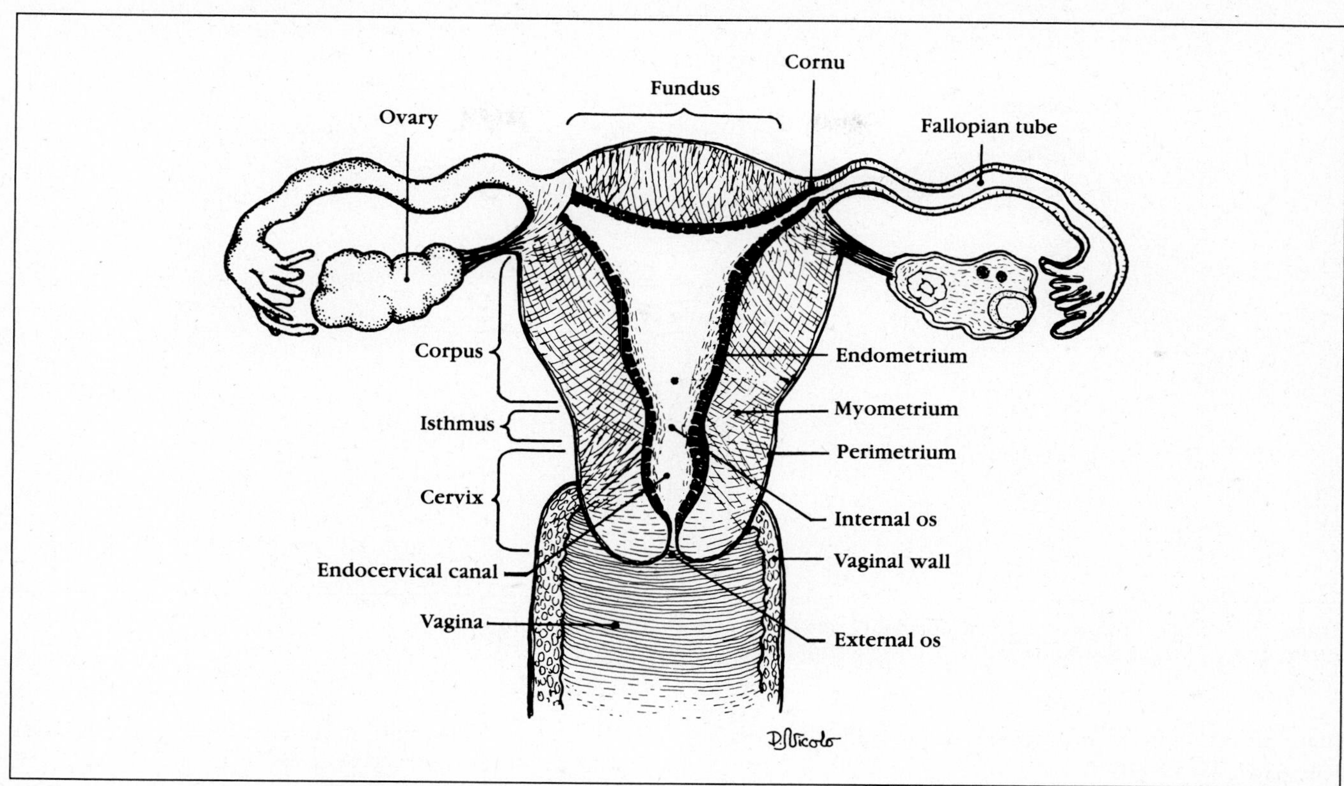

FIGURE 53-5 Internal female reproductive organs. (From M.A. Miller and D.A. Brooten, *The Childbearing Family: A Nursing Perspective* [2nd ed.]. Boston: Little, Brown, 1983.)

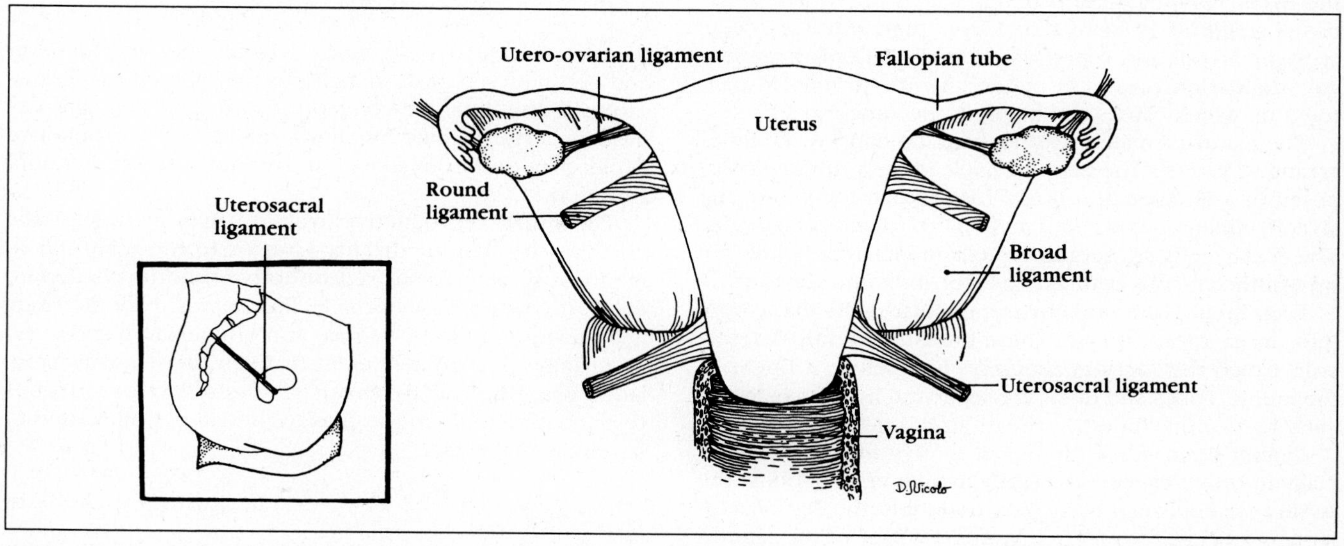

FIGURE 53-6 Ligaments supporting the uterus in the pelvic cavity. (From M.A. Miller and D.A. Brooten, *The Childbearing Family: A Nursing Perspective* [2nd ed.]. Boston: Little, Brown, 1983.)

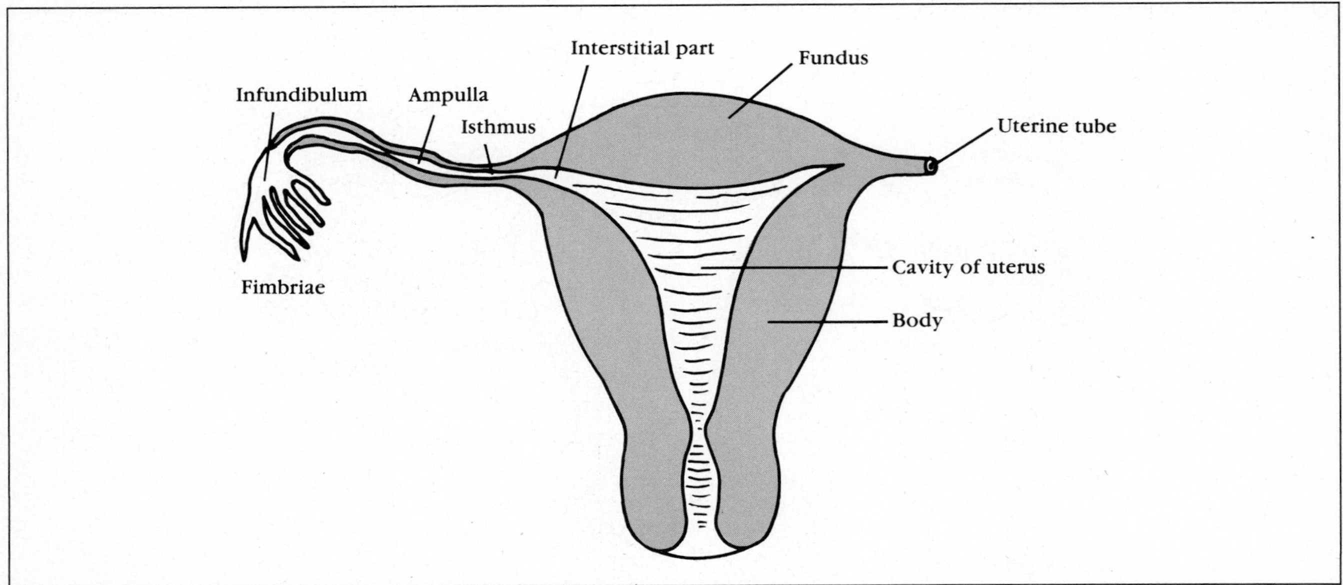

FIGURE 53-7 Different parts of the fallopian tube and uterus. (From R.S. Snell, *Clinical Anatomy for Medical Students* [2nd ed.]. Boston: Little, Brown, 1981.)

ble to infection by gonococci, which are difficult to eradicate from this location.

Mammary Glands

The mammary glands, or breasts, are two skin glands located over the pectoral muscles and attached by a layer of connective tissue. Each consists of a nipple and surrounding areola, lobes, ducts, and fibrous and fatty tissue (Fig. 53-8). The function of the breast is to secrete milk to nourish the newborn infant.

The nipple, a cylindric projection near the center of the breast, is located approximately in the fourth intercostal space. It is surrounded by a pigmented, circular area, the areola, and is perforated by ductal openings. Sexual stimulation results in engorgement and muscle contraction, which causes the nipple to become erect.

The mature female breast is made up of 15 to 20 lobes arranged around the nipple. Each lobe is further composed of a number of lobules. Inside each lobule are the alveoli, which contain both myoepithelial and acinar cells. The acinar cells are secretory cells in lactation, while the myoepithelial cells contract to force milk into the ducts.

Each lobule is drained by intralobular ducts that empty into the lactiferous duct. These ducts dilate into a reservoir, called the *lactiferous sinus*, just before it opens in the nipple. Lobes and ducts are separated by fibrous tissue. Fatty tissue contributes to breast size.

Lymph drainage of the breast is very important, especially in breast cancer. Generally, lymph vessels follow the lactiferous ducts and eventually drain into the central axillary nodes (Fig. 53-9). This creates drainage of the superficial and areolar as well as glandular parts of the breast.

During puberty, breast development is controlled by estrogen and progesterone production. Estrogen causes the gland and ducts to grow while progesterone stimulates development of the secreting cells.

External Genitalia

The external genitalia, commonly called the vulva, consists of the mons pubis, labia majora, labia minora, clitoris, urinary meatus, vaginal orifice, and vestibule (see Fig. 53-2). Bartholin's glands are sometimes considered part of the vulva.

Female Reproductive Functions

Female reproductive functions, which begin with puberty and end with menopause, fall into two phases: (1) preparation of the body for conception and gestation, and (2) gestation. The specific functions include the reproductive cycle, production of female hormones, the sex act, and gestation.

The female reproductive cycle involves many periodic changes throughout the life span or from menarche to menopause. Successful reproductive function is dependent on changes that occur in the ovaries, endometrium, myometrium, breasts, vagina, and endocrine glands, and on changes in body temperature. Even the woman's emotions are affected by these changes. Various organs respond differently to the changes but all can be related to the menstrual cycle.

Hypothalamic Influence

Cyclic changes in the reproductive cycle begin with hormonal changes initiated by the hypothalamus, which is considered to be a part of both the nervous and endocrine

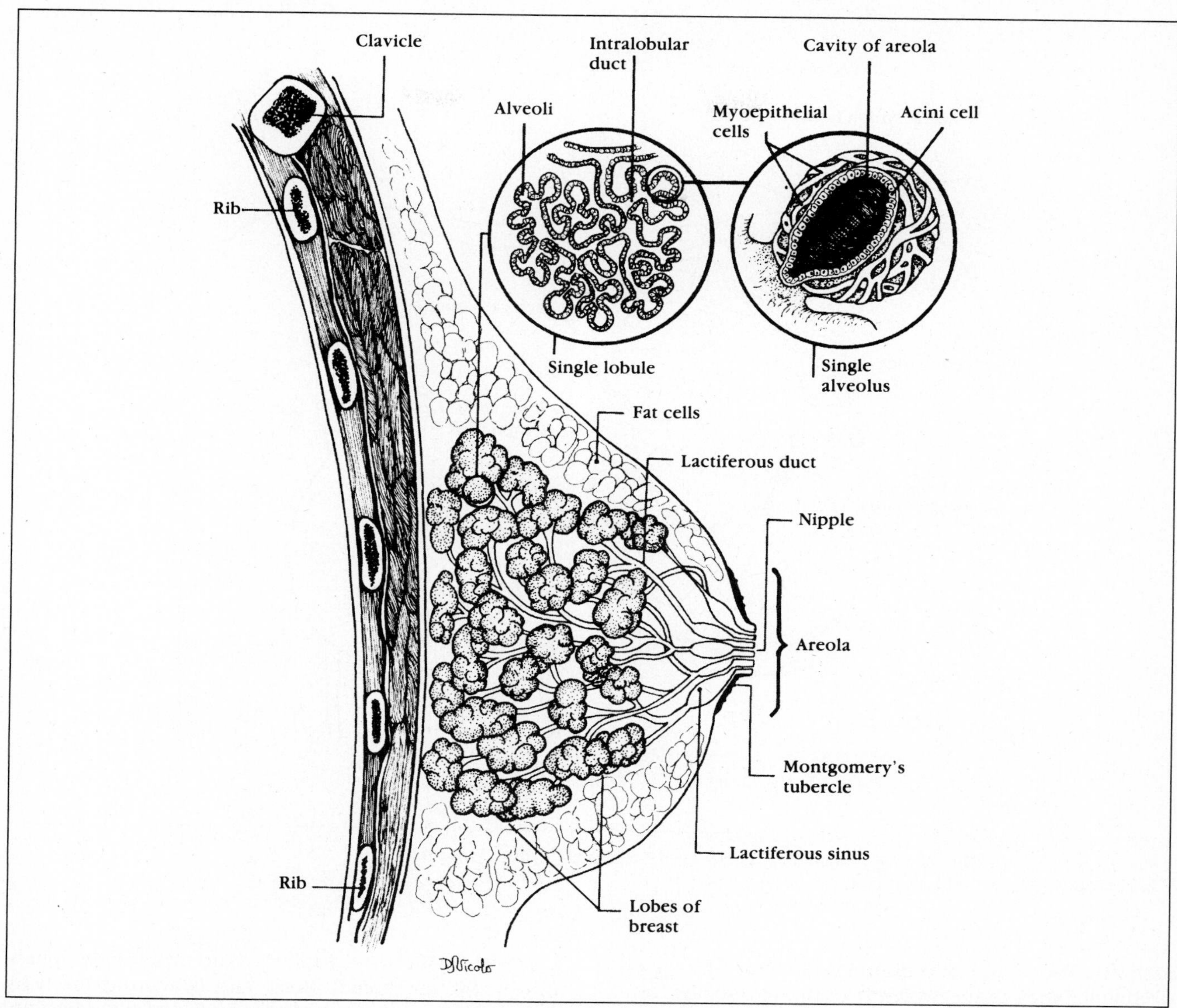

FIGURE 53-8 Breast and ductal system. (From M.A. Miller and D.A. Brooten, *The Childbearing Family: A Nursing Perspective* [2nd ed.]. Boston: Little, Brown, 1983.)

systems. Both physical and emotional stressors can affect menstrual regularity through the nervous control of the hypothalamus. Depending on the messages it receives, the hypothalamus then secretes hormones called *releasing* or *inhibiting factors*, which act directly on the pituitary gland. Neurosecretory substances that are secreted by the hypothalamus and transported through the hypothalamicohypophyseal portal system to the anterior pituitary include (1) follicle-stimulating hormone-releasing factor, (2) luteinizing hormone-releasing factor, and (3) luteotropic hormone-inhibiting factor. These factors act on the anterior pituitary to control the gland's secretion. *Oxytocin*, secreted by the posterior pituitary but formed in the hypothalamus, increases uterine contractions during labor and moves milk from breast glands to nipples during suckling.

Pituitary Influence

The anterior pituitary secretes two hormones that directly influence reproductive function: follicle-stimulating hormone (FSH) and luteinizing hormone (LH). Together with estrogen and progesterone, FSH and LH act directly on the ovaries to control ovulation. The release of FSH and LH is regulated by feedback effects of estrogen and progesterone on the hypothalamus. The anterior pituitary also secretes *prolactin*, also called luteotropic hormone, or LTH. Prolactin acts on the breasts to control lactation after

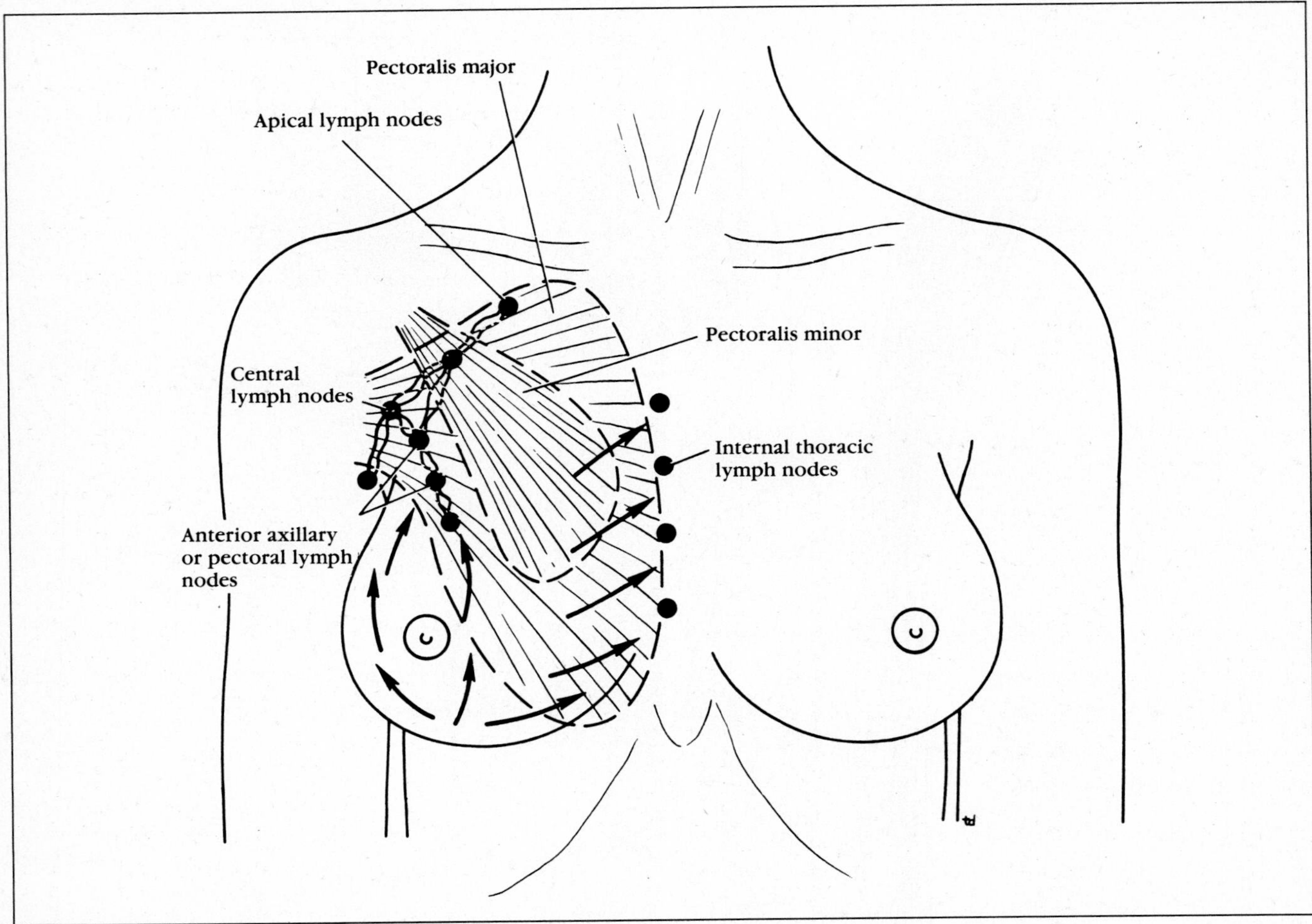

FIGURE 53-9 Lymphatic drainage of mammary gland. (From R.S. Snell, *Clinical Anatomy for Medical Students* [2nd ed.]. Boston: Little, Brown, 1981.)

delivery. The release of prolactin is prevented by the prolactin-inhibiting factor, which is controlled by high levels of estrogen and/or progesterone. Suckling and low estrogen levels stimulate prolactin production.

The Menstrual Cycle

The menstrual cycle involves regular changes that are repeated approximately every 28 days. This process may vary some in individual women but has three phases: menstrual, proliferative, and secretory. The proliferative and secretory phases are separated by ovulation.

The Menstrual Phase. The menstrual phase begins with the onset of the menses and lasts approximately five days. Average blood loss is 30 to 150 ml, the amount varying widely among individuals. During the menstrual phase the blood levels of both estrogen and progesterone are low. This phase also involves degeneration and sloughing of the stratum compactum and most of the stratum spongiosum.

The Proliferative Phase. The proliferative phase follows the menstrual phase and is accompanied by changes in the ovaries, endometrium, and myometrium. The cyclic changes result from changes in gonadotropin and estrogen levels.

Low levels of estrogen in the menstrual phase signal the production of FSH by the anterior pituitary. In the ovaries, FSH production then stimulates the primary follicles. At this time a number of follicles begin to mature. Soon only one, the *graafian follicle*, begins to dominate while the others recede. This follicle gradually moves to the surface of the ovary (Fig. 53-10). The follicle contains the ovum and is surrounded by a layer of granulosa cells, which are further surrounded by specialized cells called the *theca interna* and *theca externa*. Estrogen is secreted by the theca interna, and the granulosa cells supply nutrition for the ova.

As the follicle enlarges, fluid begins to collect inside, pushing the ovum to one side. It is surrounded on the outside by granulosa cells called the cumulus oophorus. A clear membrane also develops and surrounds the ovum.

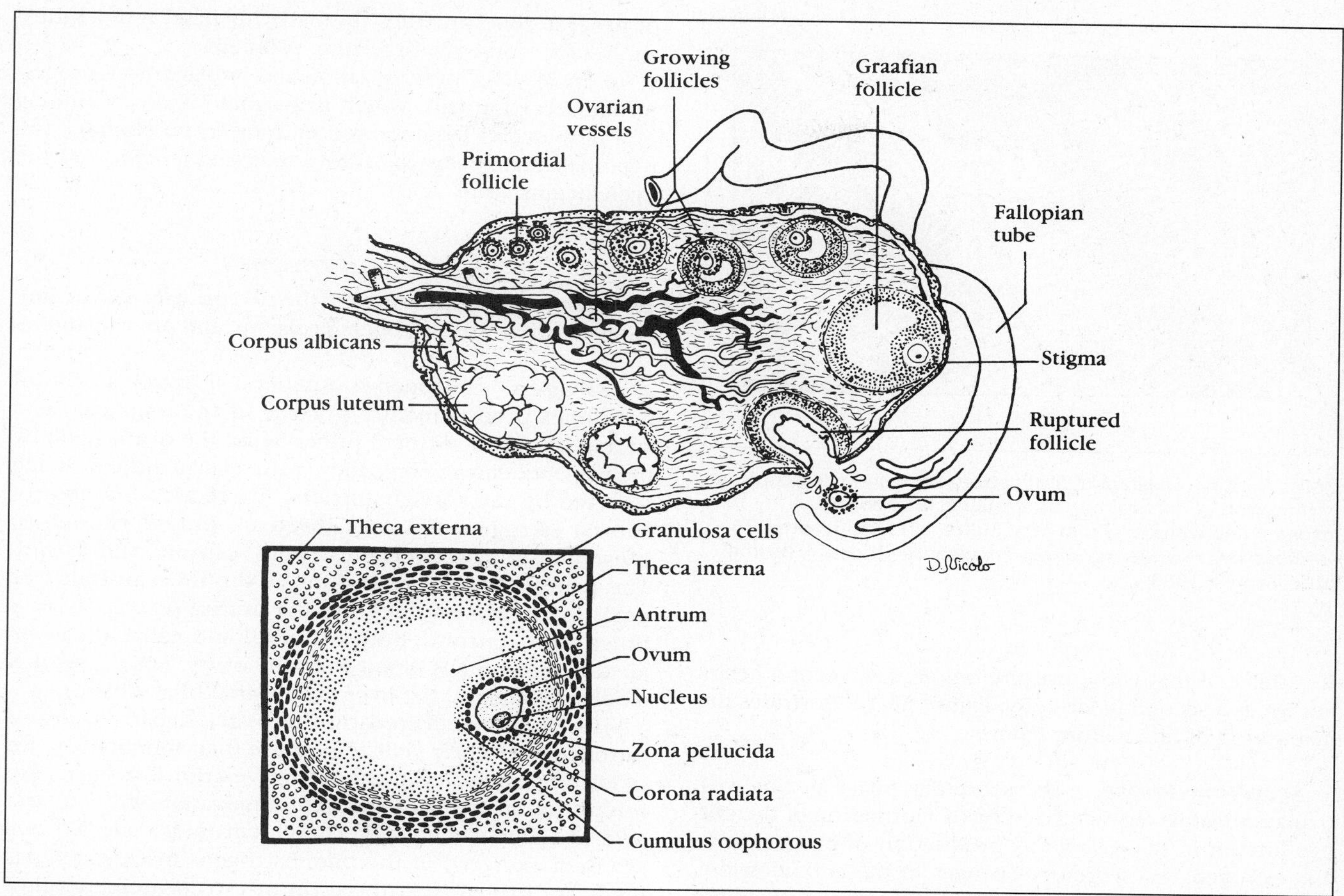

FIGURE 53-10 The ovary, showing maturation and release of ovum. Inset shows a developing graafian follicle. (From M.A. Miller and D.A. Brooten, *The Childbearing Family: A Nursing Perspective* [2nd ed.]. Boston: Little, Brown, 1983.)

This inner surrounding is termed the zona pellucida. Outside the zona pellucida and inside the cumulus oophorus is a single layer of cells called the zona radiata. While these changes are occurring within the follicle, the anterior pituitary also begins gradual secretion of LH, which stimulates the follicles to increase estrogen production. High levels of estrogen then signal the hypothalamus to stop producing FSH-releasing factor. Production of LH continues, resulting in a surge of LH about 12 hours prior to ovulation. This increase triggers ovulation within 1 to 24 hours. The mature ovum is then extruded from the ovary with both the zona pellucida and corona radiata surrounding it.

During this same period, changes also occur in the endometrium and myometrium. These changes are controlled primarily by blood levels of estrogen. The endometrium thickens as the endometrial cells and arterioles grow longer and more coiled. The water content of the endometrium and contractions of the myometrium also increase.

Ovulation. Ovulation divides the proliferative and secretory phases of the menstrual cycle and usually occurs 14 days before the onset of the next menstrual cycle. In a number of women it is accompanied by low abdominal pain, termed *mittelschmerz*. The escape of fluid or blood from the follicle is believed to produce peritoneal irritation that causes the pain.

Ovulation is also accompanied by changes in cervical mucus. Cervical mucus increases in amount as it becomes clear and thin. Under the influence of high estrogen levels, it forms a ferning pattern when allowed to dry on a slide (Fig. 53-11).

Oogenesis. Unlike spermatogenesis, which continuously produces many sperm, oogenesis is the cyclic production of a single ovum. Immediately prior to ovulation the primary oocyte undergoes its first meiotic division, resulting in a secondary oocyte containing 23 chromosomes and most of the cytoplasm. A second body is formed and is referred to as a first polar body. This first polar body receives 23 chromosomes but little cytoplasm. In the event of fertilization, the secondary oocyte undergoes a mitotic division. Both cells again contain 23 chromosomes but only one receives the majority of cytoplasm.

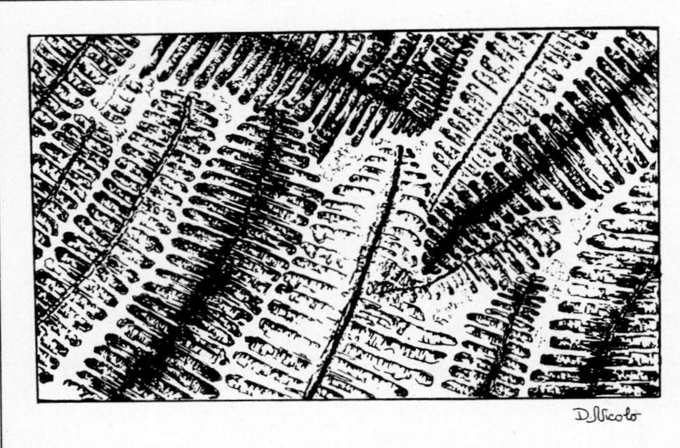

FIGURE 53-11 Diagram of fern pattern seen on microscopic examination of cervical mucus at midcycle in normal menstruating women. (From M.A. Miller and D.A. Brooten, *The Childbearing Family: A Nursing Perspective* [2nd ed.]. Boston: Little, Brown, 1983.)

It is this cell that is the *mature ovum*. The second cell is known as a second polar body. Figure 53-12 illustrates the maturation of one mature ovum.

Secretory Phase. The secretory phase begins with ovulation and is characterized by (1) formation of the corpus luteum in the ovary, (2) production of progesterone and estrogen, (3) secretory changes in the endometrium, and (4) decreased contractions in the myometrium. In the ovary, follicle walls now collapse with some hemorrhage into the cavity, forming a corpus hemorrhagia. Under the influence of LH, the granulosa cells hypertrophy, take on a yellow color, and become known as luteal cells. This golden body, the corpus luteum, continues to function for about seven to eight days. Its primary function is to secrete progesterone and some estrogen. In the absence of fertilization, luteal cells begin to degenerate, causing a decrease in estrogen and progesterone levels. Eventually the corpus luteum is converted into the corpus albicans, which moves to the center of the ovary and finally disappears.

The production of progesterone by the corpus luteum leads to secretory changes in the endometrium that create a favorable environment for pregnancy. Increase in the endometrium at this time is believed to be due to swelling from increased water content rather than cellular proliferation. The endometrium becomes more vascular, with coiled spiral arteries located close to the surface. The changes produce a thick, succulent environment, rich in glycogen and ideal for implantation of the fertilized ovum.

Progesterone is also associated with a decrease in myometrial contractions. In addition, women may notice fluid retention, breast tenderness and fullness, as well as moodiness and premenstrual tension from the high levels of progesterone. Increased levels of progesterone also create the increase in basal body temperature during the secretory phase of the menstrual cycle. This characteristic of progesterone provides the basis for basal temperature studies for women with fertility problems.

In the absence of fertilization and implantation, progesterone secretion falls, which is a signal for the beginning of a new cycle. Degenerated endometrium sloughs, the hypothalamus begins to secrete releasing factors, and the cycle begins again.

Production of Female Hormones

Estrogen and progesterone are the two primary female hormones. Others are androgen, prolactin, and prostaglandins.

Estrogen. Estrogen is a general term for a class of hormones predominantly present in the female. It is a steroid hormone secreted primarily by the ovaries and by the placenta during pregnancy, with a small amount being secreted by the adrenal cortices. There are a number of natural estrogens but only three are potent enough to cause physiologic effects: estradiol, estrone, and estriol. The major estrogen, estradiol, is the most potent (12 times more than estrone), but the ovaries secrete about 4 times more estrone. Both estradiol and estrone can be identified in venous blood from the ovary, while estriol is oxidized mainly in the liver from estradiol and estrone.

After being secreted by the ovaries, estradiol and estrone either enter cells to perform their functions or are oxidized principally in the liver to estriol. Estrogens are inactivated in the liver through conjugation with sulfuric acid and glueuronic acid. The glucuronides and sulfates are then excreted in the bile. Estrogens in extracellular fluids are primarily in the form of estroprotein, another process accomplished in the liver. This inactivation process accounts for the ineffectiveness of the natural estrogens when administered orally. Conditions that depress liver function may also be associated with increased estrogen levels because of the absence of the inactivation process.

In the clinical setting two other forms of estrogen may be used: synthetic and conjugated. The synthetic estrogens are of particular importance because of their potency when administered orally. Estrogen affects cell proliferation and development of the female secondary sex characteristics as well as the previously described effect on the menstrual cycle.

Throughout childhood very small quantities of estrogen are produced, but at puberty the levels increase greatly. As a result of estrogen influence, the sex organs, including external genitalia, breasts, ovaries, fallopian tubes, uterus, and vagina, increase in size [5]. Vaginal epithelium thickens and differentiates into layers that increase the resistance of the vagina to injury and infection. The epithelium also increases its glycogen levels, which are acted on by Döderlein's bacilli to create an acidic pH. Estrogens also affect the fat deposits in the vulva and mons pubis, growth of the pelvis, and distribution of axillary and pubic hair.

The onset of puberty is associated with a very rapid growth rate in the female. Estrogens cause early uniting of the epiphyses and shafts of the long bones, causing female growth to cease earlier than male growth. They also affect

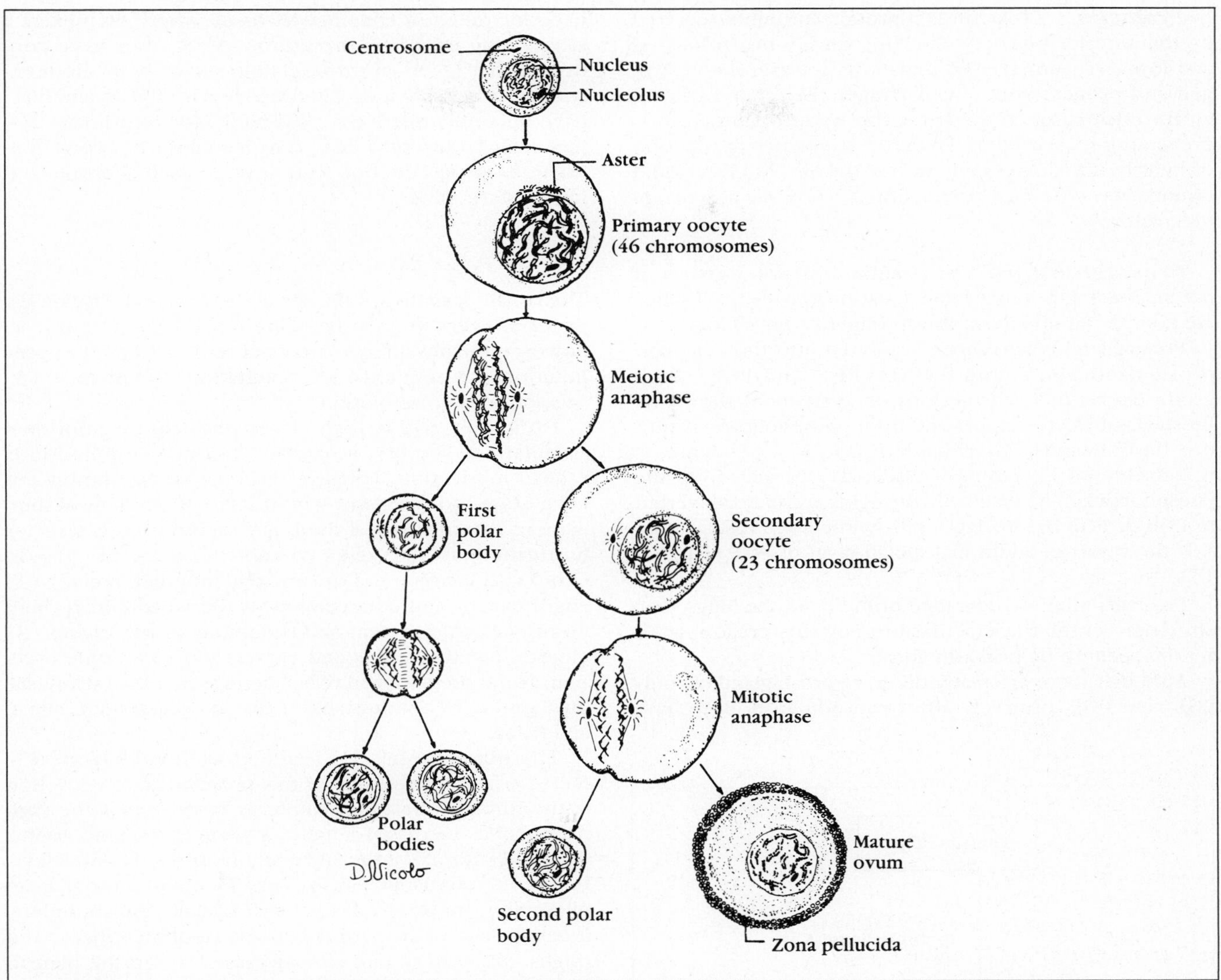

FIGURE 53-12 Maturation of female reproductive cells resulting in formation of one mature ovum. (From M.A. Miller and D.A. Brooten, *The Childbearing Family: A Nursing Perspective* [2nd ed.]. Boston: Little, Brown, 1983.)

calcium and phosphate retention, which is important in menopause when estrogen levels are greatly reduced.

Estrogens influence the skin and capillary walls. With increased levels of estrogen, the skin becomes soft, smooth, and thicker than that of a child. It is also more vascular. For this reason women may bleed more when cut or note increased skin warmth. In addition, the capillary walls become stronger. When estrogen levels are low there is a greater tendency toward bruising.

Progesterone. Progesterone is often considered the hormone of pregnancy because of its effect on the endometrium and myometrium (see page 894). It is produced almost exclusively by the corpus luteum in the nonpregnant female and by the placenta during pregnancy. Chemically, natural progesterone is very similar to estrogen. It is less potent than estrogen and it is secreted in larger amounts. Shortly after secretion it is degraded to pregnanediol and is excreted in this form in the urine.

In addition to its uterine effects, progesterone affects the breasts. While estrogen is responsible for breast growth, progesterone is responsible for maturation of lobules and alveoli so that they may become secretory when stimulated by prolactin.

Androgens. Female androgens are secreted in very small amounts by the adrenal glands and ovaries [5]. In disruptions of female function, the amount of secretions can become significant and result in masculine hair distribution, acne, and deepening of the voice.

Prolactin. Prolactin is a protein hormone secreted by the anterior pituitary. Suckling during breast-feeding and low estrogen levels stimulate its release. High estrogen and progesterone levels trigger the release of prolactin inhibiting factor from the hypothalamus, thus preventing its secretion. Prolactin stimulates production of milk by the acinar cells in the alveoli. Pituitary gland tumors can cause milk production, even in the absence of pregnancy.

Prostaglandins. Prostaglandins are a group of potent lipids that function as local hormones [2,7]. They are considered important in reproductive physiology.

Prostaglandins have been separated into three groups: prostaglandin A, E, and F (PGA, PGE, and PGF). Each group exerts different actions on systems of the body. Prostaglandins are synthesized from phospholipids in various body tissues [3]. Phospholipase A, an enzyme, is responsible for liberation of essential fatty acids from the phospholipids. The essential fatty acids are then converted to PGE or PGF by prostaglandin synthetase. Prostaglandin A is the result of additional metabolism of PGE (Fig. 53-13).

Prostaglandins are degraded primarily in the lungs soon after they enter the circulation. For this reason, their actions seem to be primarily local.

Although there are many different prostaglandins, only PGE_2 and PGF_2 primarily affect reproduction. Both have been identified in endometrial tissue where they exert a stimulating effect on the uterus [4]. Studies have confirmed that levels of prostaglandins vary with the menstrual cycle (Table 53-1). Elevated levels of PGE_2 and PGF_2 have been identified as a possible factor in primary dysmenorrhea. Currently, PGE_2 is used to induce uterine contractions for intrauterine fetal death, missed abortion, and hydatidiform mole.

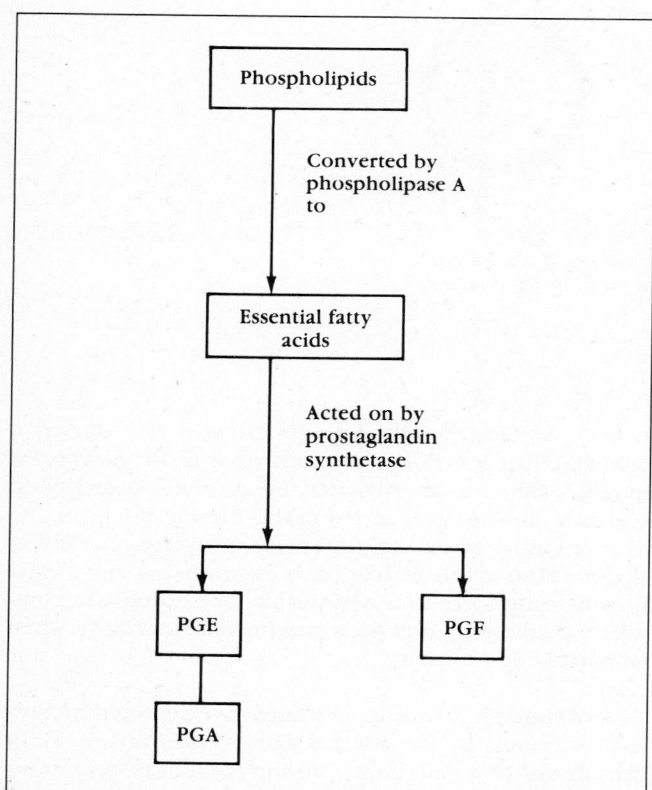

FIGURE 53-13 Synthesis of prostaglandins.

Female Response in the Sex Act

The female response in the sex act is a normal physiologic process. Every woman has different levels of response; however, the physiologic events of response tend to occur in an orderly sequence: (1) excitation, (2) plateau, (3) orgasm, and (4) resolution.

Excitation begins with either physical or emotional stimulation. The first response to sexual stimulation is vaginal lubrication. This is a result of vasodilatation and congestion and can occur within 10 to 30 seconds of stimulation. Transudation of fluid, not secretion, accounts for lubrication, as the vagina contains no secretory glands. Other characteristics of the excitement phase include (1) engorgement and enlargement of the labia, clitoris, and uterus, (2) enlargement and ballooning of the vagina, (3) elevation of the uterus and cervix, and (4) nipple erection. Blood pressure and pulse increase and the "sex flush" may appear as a measleslike rash on epigastrium, chest, and throat.

The plateau phase is reached as sexual arousal is increased. Characteristics of this phase include retraction of the clitoris against the symphysis, narrowing of the vaginal opening, increased length and diameter of the vagina, deep red coloring of the labia minora, and complete elevation of the uterus. Breast size may increase in the plateau phase and the sex flush may spread over the shoulders, inner surface of arms, and perhaps, abdomen, back, and thighs. Respiratory rate also increases late in the plateau phase.

During orgasm, vasocongestion reaches its maximum and stimulates the reflex stretch mechanism. As a result, rhythmic contractions occur in the clitoris, uterus, outer one-third of the vagina, and perhaps the rectal sphincter. Rhythmic contractions may also be noted in the arms, legs, abdomen, and buttocks.

TABLE 53-1 Levels of Prostaglandins in Different Phases of the Menstrual Cycle (ng/100 ng tissue)

Prostaglandin	Proliferative Phase	Midluteal Phase	Menses
PGE_2	13–26	13–26	52
$PGF_{2\alpha}$	10–25	67	67, maintained

Sources: H. J. Clithroe and V. R. Pickles, The separation of the smooth muscle stimulants in menstrual fluid. *J. Physiol.* (Lond.) 156:225, 1961; and J. Downie, N. L. Poyser, and M. Wunderlick, Levels of prostaglandins in the human endometrium during the normal menstrual cycle. *J. Physiol.* (Lond.) 236:456, 1974.

During resolution, the final phase of sexual response, the body returns to its preexcitement phase. Within 10 to 15 seconds the clitoris returns to normal and normal color returns to the labia minora. Ten to 15 minutes are required for the vagina to return to normal, and the cervical os remains open for about 30 minutes. Unlike the male, who experiences a refractory period during resolution when he is incapable of sexual stimulation, some women are capable of several orgasms without dropping below the plateau phase. Resolution then follows the last orgasm.

Gestation

Gestation begins with fertilization of the ovum and continues throughout the development of the fetus. This normal process is the basis of many complete and comprehensive texts. Therefore, this discussion is limited to gestation from conception through placental formation to provide the basis for a discussion of the alterations in normal pregnancy, some of which are discussed in Chapter 54.

Conception generally occurs in the outer one-third of the fallopian tube and mitotic divisions begin immediately. Cellular division continues and after approximately three to four days the cell mass is referred to as a *morula*. At this point it enters the uterus where it remains free but moves toward the site of implantation. The morula consists of both an inner and an outer cell mass. The inner cell mass develops into the embryoblast and finally the embryo, while the outer cell mass forms the trophoblast and finally the placenta. As cellular division continues, the embryoblast becomes located at one pole while the trophoblast forms the outer wall (Fig. 53-14). The zygote is now referred to as a blastocyst.

After about seven days the trophoblasts are in direct contact with the endometrium and the process of implantation begins. The trophoblast consists of two layers: cytotrophoblast, or inner layer, and syncytiotrophoblast, or outer layer. This outer layer of syncytial cells has the ability to erode the endometrial tissue (now referred to as decidua) producing enlarged areas which become filled with blood. The stromal cells also become enlarged and contain increased cytoplasmic amounts of lipids and glycogen [1]. Cytotrophoblastic cells begin to send out fingerlike projections producing chorionic villi. Fetal capillaries also form in the chorionic villi so that maternal-fetal exchange can occur. As pregnancy continues, villi beneath the embryo continue to grow while those on the other side degenerate and form the chorion. This process continues until implantation and placental formation are complete.

Menopause

Menopause, the cessation of menstruation, marks the final phase of female reproductive function. The transition or gradual change in ovarian function is termed *climacteric*. The average age of menopause for women in the United States is 50 years, but it may occur before the age of 45 or after 50. Menopause is complete when the woman has experienced no menstrual periods for one year.

In some women, menopause occurs abruptly with complete cessation of menstruation after normal periods. In others, gradual cessation is characterized by decreased amounts of bleeding with monthly cycles, periods of amenorrhea, and finally complete cessation of normal periods. Menopause is accompanied by decreased estrogen levels and reversal in estrogen forms. The production of all estrogens by the ovaries decreases. The primary estrogen in menopause is estrone, which is derived from androstenedione and fat conversion.

Menopause is frequently associated with other physiologic changes and symptoms. These include hot flashes, changes in reproductive organs, cardiovascular disease, osteoporosis, and nervousness and psychologic problems [3]. The most common symptom is hot flashes. It begins as a feeling of warmth in the chest and progresses upward over the neck and face. It may be accompanied by flushing of the skin in these areas and profuse diaphoresis. The exact cause has not been determined, but it appears related to estrogen withdrawal.

Changes in reproductive organs include atrophy of the labia; dryness and thinning of vaginal walls; decreased support of bladder, rectum, and uterus; and decreased size of the uterus and cervix. The changes are all associated with lower estrogen levels and account for such complaints as dyspareunia, stress incontinence, and vaginal itching and burning.

Evidence supports increased frequency of hypertension, stroke, and heart disease after menopause [6]. Decreased estrogen levels are also linked to osteoporosis and increased bone fragility. Estrogen administration has been shown to halt the process in young women who undergo surgical removal of the ovaries.

Psychologic symptoms associated with menopause include nervousness, depression, headache, insomnia, decreased sex drive, memory loss, vertigo, and a feeling of worthlessness and hopelessness [8]. No connection has been identified between these symptoms and estrogen levels. Therefore, basic personality and cultural influences are of more importance in determining treatment.

Laboratory and Diagnostic Aids

Gynecologic Examination

The most important of all diagnostic tools available is the physical examination. Gynecologic examination of the female reproductive system involves three steps: (1) external examination, (2) speculum examination, and (3) bimanual examination. External examination includes inspection and palpation of the breasts, palpation of the abdomen, and inspection of the external genitalia. With these procedures, one can detect masses, redness, and swelling or lesions of the breasts and external genitalia.

The speculum examination allows for visualization of the cervix and vaginal wall and detection of redness, lesions, swelling, or unusual discharge. Specimens for laboratory tests, including Pap smear, wet smear, gonorrhea cultures, and biopsies, may also be collected at this time.

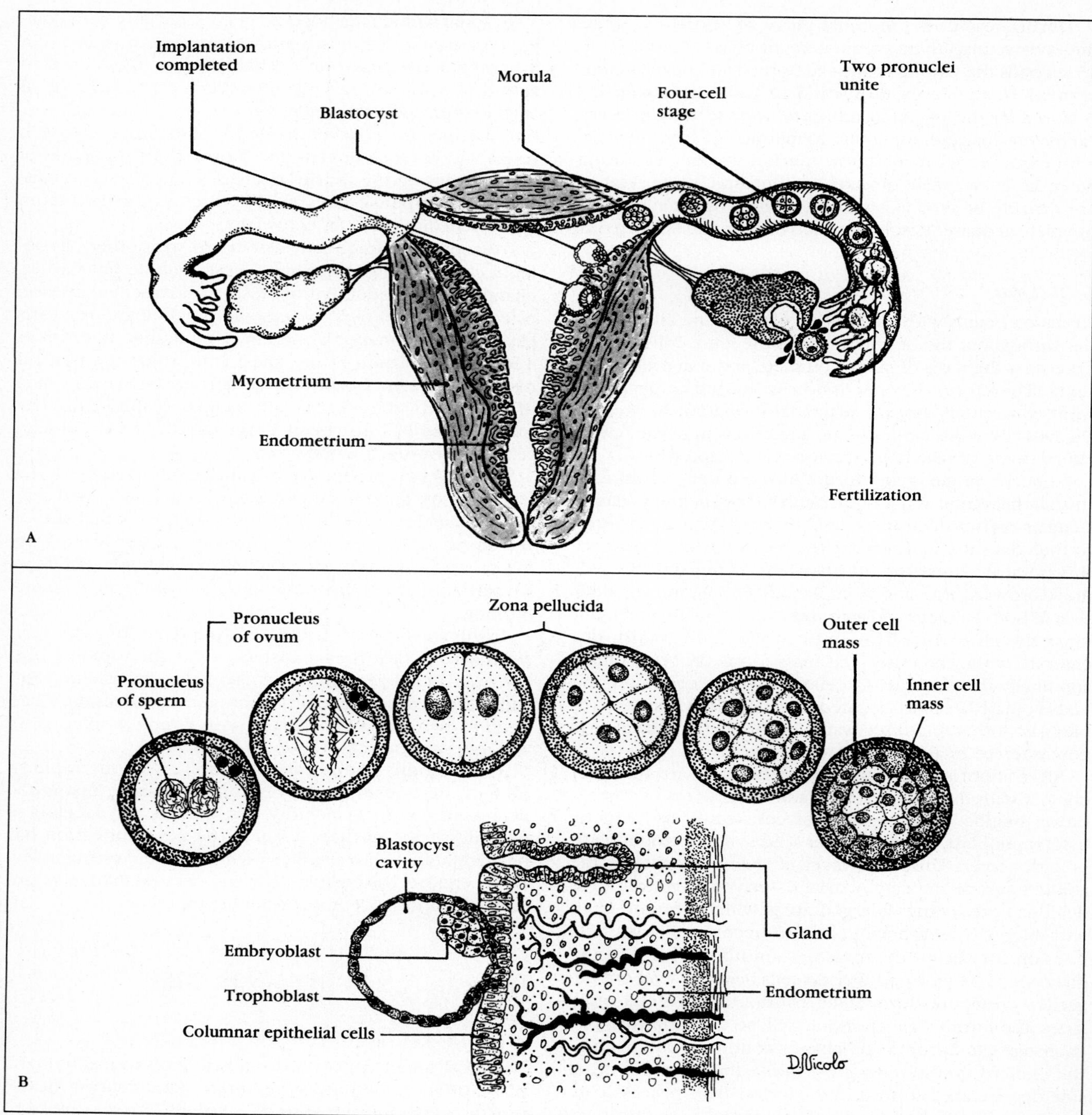

FIGURE 53-14 Implantation of the blastocyst. A. Serial representation of ovum from ovulation to implantation. B. Blastocyst beginning implantation (zona pellucida has been lost). (From M.A. Miller and D.A. Brooten, *The Childbearing Family: A Nursing Perspective* [2nd ed.]. Boston: Little, Brown, 1983.)

The final step is the bimanual examination, in which the uterus, ovaries, and fallopian tubes are palpated. It also generally involves either a rectal or rectovaginal examination, by which the examiner is able to palpate such pelvic structures as the posterior surface of the uterus, the uterosacral ligaments, and the cul-de-sac of Douglas.

Hormone Levels

Both bioassay and chemical methods are available for determining ovarian hormone levels. These are time consuming, difficult to perform or to standardize, and expensive. Therefore, most of the studies to detect hormone levels are indirect.

Progesterone. Progesterone is a steroid that is degraded shortly after secretion. Most of this degradation occurs in the liver, with the major end product being pregnanediol. Because pregnanediol is excreted in the urine, its rate of excretion can be used to estimate progesterone formation. This estimation must be done by chemical means, as pregnanediol exerts no progesteronic effects. Results are difficult to standardize, but the generally accepted normal values are summarized in Table 53-2.

Increased levels of progesterone may be associated with luteal cysts of the ovary, arrhenoblastoma of the ovary, and hyperadrenocorticism. Decreased levels may occur in amenorrhea, threatened abortion, fetal death, and toxemia of pregnancy.

Indirect methods of determining progesterone levels include endometrial biopsy and basal body temperature. An endometrial biopsy is useful in determining the stage of the menstrual cycle and therefore infers the level of hormone production. In studying basal body temperature charts, a sustained rise of 1°F implies that ovulation has taken place and that progesterone secretion is adequate.

TABLE 53-2 Normal Hormone Levels

Hormone	Blood	Urine
Pregnanediol		
Male		<1.5 mg/24 hours
Female		
Proliferative phase		0.5–1.5 mg/24 hours
Luteal phase		2–7 mg/24 hours
Postmenopausal		0.2–1.0 mg/24 hours
Estrogens (total)		
Male		4–25 μg/24 hours
Female		4–60 μg/24 hours with increase in pregnancy
Prolactin	<20 ng/ml	
Progesterone		
Proliferative phase	<1.0 ng/ml	
Luteal phase	<2.0 ng/ml	
FSH		6–50 mouse uterine units/24 hours
Luteinizing hormone		
Proliferative phase	<70 mIU/ml	
Luteal phase	>70 mIU/ml	
Estriol		10–20 mg/24 hours

Estrogen. One very useful laboratory test in the study of estrogen levels is measurement of 24-hour urinary estriol excretion. Because estriol is produced by the placenta, it represents both fetal and placental activity. A significant drop (40% less than the mean of three previous values) may indicate that the fetus is in jeopardy, as urinary estriol excretion increases as pregnancy progresses. Incomplete 24-hour urine specimens as well as pyelonephritis have been known to affect the results. Normal findings are 10 to 20 mg per 24 hours.

Changes in cervical mucus and epithelial cells of the vagina are good indicators of estrogen production. Cervical mucus undergoes very definite changes in response to estrogen and progesterone production. Spinnbarkeit and ferning are two characteristics of cervical mucus that can easily be studied. Spinnbarkeit refers to the elasticity of cervical mucus at the time of ovulation that allows the examiner to draw it out into a long thin thread of 15 to 20 cm. During minimal estrogen production, threads only reach 1 to 2 cm.

Ferning refers to the pattern created when cervical mucus, under the influence of estrogen, dries (see Fig. 53-11). Ferning results when sodium chloride in the mucus crystallizes. Estrogen secretion increases the sodium chloride content of cervical mucus while progesterone decreases it. Therefore, the level of estrogen without progesterone determines the presence of a ferning pattern. This pattern is fullest and most complete at the time of ovulation.

Vaginal smears are also useful in determining estrogen levels because the vaginal cells also undergo cyclic changes. Estrogen thickens the vaginal epithelium. Glucose excretion also corresponds to estrogen secretion. Both are highest at the time of ovulation.

Smears

Papanicolaou Smear. A specimen for Papanicolaou (Pap) smear is best collected from the cervical canal and the squamocolumnar junction near the external os during the speculum examination. Dry cotton swabs are used to collect cervical canal secretions while a small wooden spatula is used for the squamocolumnar specimen. The specimen is then transferred to a glass slide where it is fixed for staining and microscopic examination. The primary purpose of a Pap smear is to screen for abnormal cervical cells and indicate the need for more extensive testing. It may also help detect cancer of the endometrium and vagina.

Classification of Pap smear results varies widely from institution to institution. The original system identified five classes of smears ranging from I, which was normal, to V, definitely malignant. A more recent method uses three major classifications: (1) benign, (2) precancerous, and (3) malignant. The precancerous classification includes the cervical intraepithelial neoplasia (CIN), also referred to as dysplasia. Other clinicians use a verbal description to indicate their findings. A summary of the various classifications is shown in Table 53-3.

Wet Smear. Wet smears are especially beneficial in diagnosing the cause of vaginitis. In this procedure a specimen of vaginal discharge is placed on a slide, mixed with a drop of saline solution or potassium hydroxide, and examined under the microscope for *Candida*, *Trichomonas*, or other organisms. It is not conclusive for gonorrhea.

Biopsy

Endometrial Biopsy. To take an endometrial biopsy, a curet is inserted through the cervix, placed against the uterine wall, and slowly withdrawn. It is best to repeat the procedure on different walls of the uterus in order to obtain enough tissue to represent a major portion of the uterus.

Endometrial biopsy is especially useful in evaluating dysfunctional bleeding. It may be helpful in diagnosis of endometrial cancer; however, there is a chance that scattered growths may be missed. Another use for endometrial biopsy is in infertility studies. It is best performed just prior to onset of menses or day 22 of the menstrual cycle. It can interfere with pregnancy if conception has occurred.

Cervical Biopsy. A punch biopsy instrument is used in the physician's office to obtain samples of cervical tissue. This can aid in more precise diagnosis of questionable lesions. It is also helpful in removing small polyps.

Cone Biopsy. Cone biopsy, also referred to as conization, is a hospital procedure. It involves removing a cone-shaped specimen of cervical tissue, any visible lesions, and tissue specimens of the squamocolumnar junction and cervical canal. It may be used as follow-up to Pap smear or punch biopsy.

Open Breast Biopsy. Breast biopsy is surgical intervention to remove a lump. A frozen section can be examined for immediate classification, while more extensive pathologic studies require more time.

Needle Biopsy. The physician inserts a needle into a breast lesion and aspirates its contents. This procedure may be performed in the office and is followed up as necessary.

Vulvar Biopsy. Punch biopsy forceps can be used to obtain vulvar tissue. Frequently, the gross appearance is normal, and staining procedures must be used to identify pathology.

Radiography

Hysterosalpingogram. Hysterosalpingogram is a radiographic examination of the uterus and fallopian tubes. A small cannula is inserted through the cervix and radiopaque dye is injected into the uterus and fallopian tubes. Filling of the uterus and tubes can be observed on the fluoroscopy screen. Spot films may also be made. Hysterosalpingogram is especially useful in noting the size and shape of the uterus and tubes as well as tubal obstruction.

Mammography. Mammography is a radiologic examination of the breasts. It is useful to detect early lesions that cannot be palpated and the exact location of deep tumors. It may be useful in predicting malignancy. Radiation exposure occurs and the procedure is not recommended for routine screening except in women over age 35 years, when the risk of developing a malignancy increases.

Other Procedures

Colposcopy. The colposcope is a binocular diagnostic instrument that provides a magnified (10–20 X) view of the cervix and vaginal walls. It is mounted on a tripod and maintains no contact with the person. Colposcopy is useful in follow-up of abnormal results of Pap smears, to identify abnormal areas for biopsy, and to examine lesions on the vulva. Colposcopy is also recommended in follow-up of women whose mothers took DES (diethylstilbestrol) during pregnancy; it may also be employed for women with dyspareunia and bleeding with intercourse. Each procedure involves the following five observations: (1) vascular pattern, (2) color tone, (3) intercapillary distance, (4) borderline versus normal tissue, and (5) surface pattern [4].

Laparoscopy and Culdoscopy. Both laparoscopy and culdoscopy are surgical procedures that allow the physician to visualize the pelvic area through a lighted tube. The procedures are performed to note the condition and position of the various organs, as well as scarring,

TABLE 53-3 Classifications of Pap Smear Findings

Class	Original	CIN System	Category	Other Descriptive Terms
I	Absence of atypical or abnormal cells	Normal	Benign	Negative
II	Atypical cytologic picture, but no evidence of malignancy	Inflammatory	Benign	Atypical
III	Cytologic picture suggestive of, but not conclusive for, malignancy	Mild CIN	Mild CIN	Mild dysplasia
IV	Cytologic picture strongly suggestive for malignancy	Severe CIN	Severe CIN	Carcinoma in situ
V	Cytologic picture conclusive for malignancy	Cancer	Malignant	Invasive cancer

presence of endometrial tissue, and infection. A tubal ligation may also be performed through the laparoscope.

Ultrasound. Ultrasound, also referred to as sonography, is a noninvasive technique particularly useful in providing pictures of soft tissues of the body. Little preparation is necessary for pelvic ultrasound except that the individual must have a full bladder. The bladder distended with 200 to 400 ml of urine is used as a reference point and to displace the pelvic organs for better visualization. Overdistention can distort the findings.

An ultrasound transducer serves both as a transmitter and receiver. It converts an electrical signal into ultrasound energy, which is transmitted into the body and then reflected from tissues of different densities. These reflections of ultrasound energy are then received by the transducer and converted again to electrical energy for recording. The procedure is completely painless and requires from 5 minutes to 30 minutes or more for completion.

Ultrasound has become a valuable diagnostic tool in both obstetrics and gynecology. In obstetrics, it is especially useful to confirm pregnancy, to establish or confirm dates or placental location, to rule out large or small size for gestational age, to determine fetal position, and to detect hydrops. Gynecologists use ultrasound to assist in the diagnosis of uterine malformations, hydatidiform mole, malignancies, ovarian masses, pelvic inflammatory disease, tubal malformations, and pelvic abscess or hematoma.

Schiller's Test. The Schiller's test is a very simple procedure that involves painting the cervix with Schiller's solution or similar iodine solution. A normal cervix, which contains glycogen, appears mahogany brown from absorption of the iodine. Abnormal areas that contain no glycogen remain a light brown. The primary usefulness of the test is to locate exact areas for biopsy (Fig. 53-15).

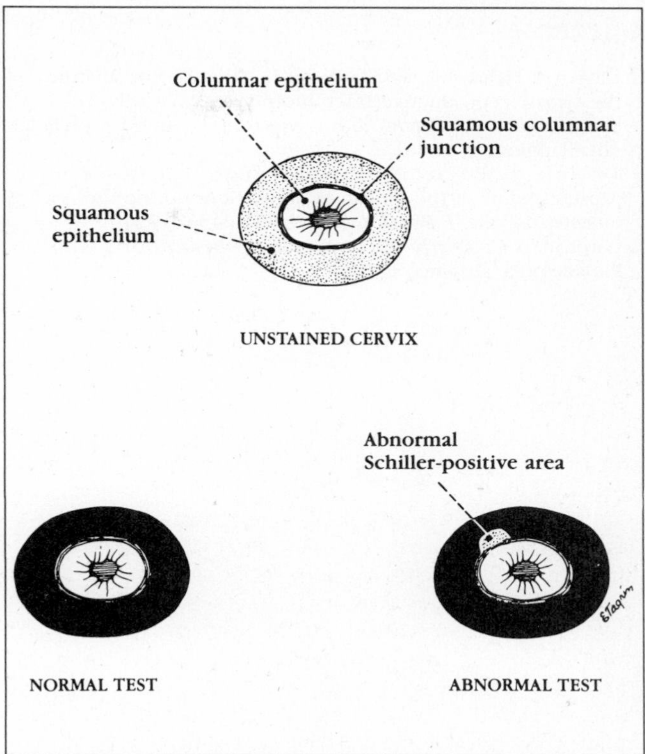

FIGURE 53-15 Schiller's test. (From T.H. Green, Jr. and R.C. Knapp, Gynecology. In G.L. Nardi and G.D. Zuidema [eds.], *Surgery: A Concise Guide to Clinical Practice* [4th ed.]. Boston: Little, Brown, 1982.)

Cultures. Cultures are most helpful in the diagnosis of the specific organism responsible for an infection. A specimen is collected from the infection site with a sterile cotton swab and placed immediately in an appropriate medium. The specimen is then incubated and checked for growth and sensitivity. If gonorrhea is suspected, special precautions should be undertaken to ensure an anaerobic environment. Special media may also be used to reduce growth of other bacteria.

Thermography. Thermography is the photographic display of infrared rays from skin temperature over the breast. Skin temperature is elevated in breast cancer because of increased blood flow in the tumor area. This procedure does not always detect early cancers and false positive results are quite common.

Rubin's Test. In the Rubin's test, carbon dioxide is injected through a cannula into the uterus. If one or both fallopian tubes are open, the woman feels referred shoulder pain. The value of this test is to determine the patency of at least one tube.

Huhner Test. Huhner test, also frequently called postcoital test, is an examination of cervical mucus. Ideally it is performed during ovulation and within several hours of intercourse. Cervical mucus is collected with an eyedropper or cotton swab and examined under a microscope. It is a simple procedure used in screening for infertility, as the examiner can note the characteristics of the cervical mucus as well as the numbers and activity of sperm present.

Study Questions

1. Discuss the functions of the female hormones in regulating the normal monthly cycle.
2. How do the hypothalamus and pituitary glands influence female characteristics and menstrual cycles?
3. Describe the process of conception.
4. What are the inherent problems that result from menopause?
5. Describe briefly the different types of biopsies done to diagnose alterations in the female reproductive system.

References

1. Davies, J. Hafez, J.S., and Ludwig, H. Microscopic anatomy of the female reproductive tract and pituitary. In D.N. Danforth and J.R. Scott, *Obstetrics and Gynecology* (5th ed.). Philadelphia: Lippincott, 1986.
2. Downie, J., Poyser, N.L., and Wunderlick, M. Levels of prostaglandins in the human endometrium during the normal menstrual cycle. *J. Physiol.* (Lond.) 236:456, 1974.
3. Guyton, A.C. *Textbook of Medical Physiology* (7th ed.). Philadelphia: Lippincott, 1986.
4. Kistner, R.W. *Gynecology: Principles and Practice* (4th ed.). Chicago: Yearbook, 1986.
5. Kolodny, R.C., et al. *Textbook of Human Sexuality for Nurses*. Boston: Little, Brown, 1979.
6. London, S.N., and Hammond, C.B. The climacteric. In D.N. Danforth and J.R. Scott, *Obstetrics and Gynecology* (5th ed.). Philadelphia: Lippincott, 1986.
7. Selkurt, E.E. (ed.). *Basic Physiology for the Health Sciences* (2nd ed.). Boston: Little, Brown, 1982.
8. Stewart, F.H., et al. *My Body, My Health: The Concerned Woman's Guide to Gynecology*. New York: Wiley, 1979.

CHAPTER 54

Alterations in Female Function

CHAPTER OUTLINE

Menstrual Problems

Endometriosis
Premenstrual Syndrome
Dysmenorrhea
Abnormal Uterine Bleeding
Dysfunctional Uterine Bleeding
Amenorrhea

Reproductive Tract Infections

Atrophic Vaginitis
Cervicitis
Toxic Shock Syndrome
Pelvic Inflammatory Disease

Benign Conditions of the Female Reproductive Tract

Uterine Fibroids
Functional Ovarian Cysts
Benign Neoplastic Tumors of the Ovaries
Benign Breast Alterations

Premalignant and Malignant Conditions

Trophoblastic Disease
Hydatidiform Mole
Chorioadenoma Destruens
Choriocarcinoma
Endometrial Carcinoma
Cervical Cancer
DES Exposure
Ovarian Cancer
Breast Cancer

LEARNING OBJECTIVES

1. Define *endometriosis*.
2. List the clinical manifestations of endometriosis and its pathologic basis.
3. Distinguish between primary and secondary dysmenorrhea.
4. Discuss the role of prostaglandins in dysmenorrhea.
5. Define *dysfunctional uterine bleeding*.
6. Distinguish between primary and secondary amenorrhea.
7. Compare and contrast the forms of vaginitis with respect to causative organisms, clinical manifestations, and diagnostic studies.
8. Distinguish between cervical erosion and eversion.
9. Define *toxic shock syndrome* and give its clinical manifestations.
10. Compare and contrast uterine fibroids and cancer.
11. Distinguish functional ovarian cysts, benign neoplastic tumors of the ovary, and ovarian cancer.
12. Compare and contrast the three types of trophoblastic disease.
13. Discuss the sequential process of cellular proliferation of cervical cancer.
14. Describe the effects of diethylstilbestrol administration on mothers and offspring.
15. Describe the staging systems of cancer of the ovary, breast, cervix, and endometrium.
16. List the three influences on breast cancer currently under study.

For many women, alterations in female function represent a threat to body image and self-concept. Alterations may occur in all reproductive organs and with no consideration of age.

Menstrual Problems

Endometriosis

Endometriosis refers to the abnormal location of endometrial tissue. Two types of endometriosis, internal and external, are described. *Internal endometriosis*, or adenomyosis, refers to the location of aberrant endometrial tissue within the myometrium. *External endometriosis* refers to the location of endometrial tissue outside the uterus. Sites for external endometriosis include the outer surface or perimetrium of the uterus, fallopian tubes, ovaries (most common site), bladder and rectal surfaces, uterine ligaments, cul-de-sac, rectovaginal septum, appendix, and bowel. On occasion, aberrant tissue may also be found in laparotomy scars, vulva, vagina, and umbilicus (Fig. 54-1). In this chapter the term *adenomyosis* is used to refer to the internal and *endometriosis* to the external conditions.

Endometriosis is characterized by functional aberrant endometrium that responds to hormonal stimulation as normal uterine endometrium does. This tissue grows and thickens under cyclic hormonal influence; as estrogen and progesterone are withdrawn, it reacts with bleeding. Early lesions appear as tiny red-blue spots surrounded by puckered scar tissue. Larger masses may form when the smaller lesions coalesce. These are usually located on the serosal layer of the involved organs. In the ovaries, lesions may take the form of *endometriomas*, cystic lesions lined with functioning endometrium. Bleeding within the cysts results in thick, chocolate-colored fluid, thus the term *chocolate cysts* (Fig. 54-2). Adhesions result when bleeding occurs into the peritoneal cavity and lead to fixation of involved pelvic structures. Infertility has been reported in 40 percent of women diagnosed with endometriosis [10].

The exact cause of endometriosis is unknown, but two primary theories are accepted: retrograde menstruation and metaplasia. The *retrograde menstruation* theory, known as Samson's theory, states that during menstruation, endometrial tissue is regurgitated through the fallopian tubes into the pelvic cavity where it implants. The *metaplasia theory* suggests that the undifferentiated coelomic epithelia of the embryo remain dormant until menarche. This tissue then begins to respond to estrogen and progesterone in a similar way as other endometrial tissue.

Clinical manifestations are dependent on the locations of lesions. The most common symptom is low abdominal

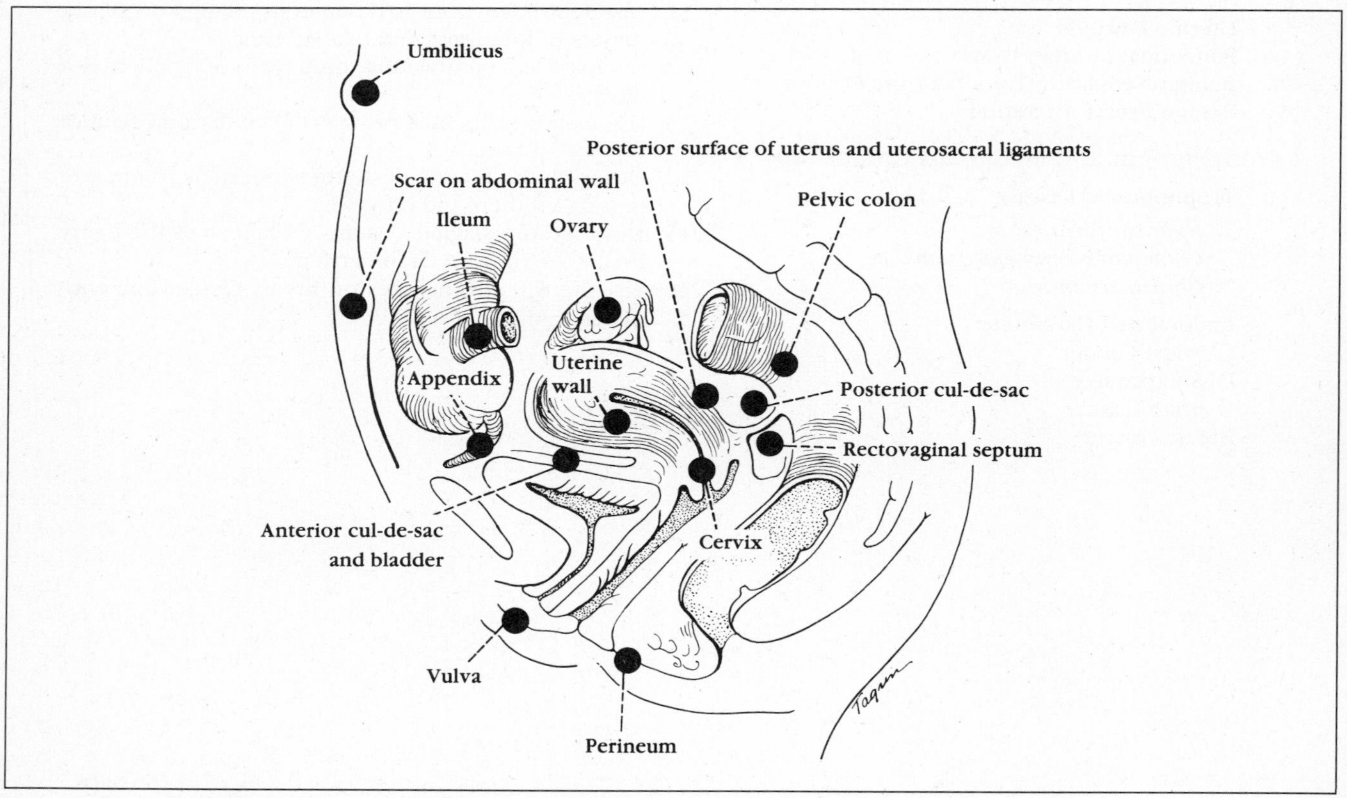

FIGURE 54-1 Sites of occurrence of endometriosis. (From T.H. Green, Jr., *Gynecology: Essentials of Clinical Practice* [3rd ed.]. Boston: Little, Brown, 1977.)

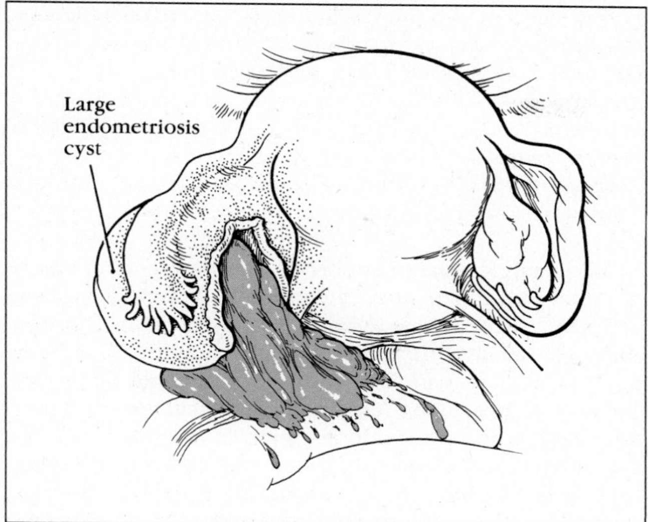

FIGURE 54-2 Endometriomas with cyst formation.

and/or pelvic pain associated with the menstrual period, such as backache and cramps beginning just prior to or with the onset of menses. The pain increases throughout menstruation and subsides afterward. It is commonly described as a dull, bearing-down type of pain. Its cause is irritation from hemorrhage of the aberrant tissue or distention. Occasionally, a chocolate cyst may rupture with signs of acute abdomen. Sterility and/or infertility may result from extensive scarring of the ovaries and tubes. Dyspareunia reflects uterine involvement, dysuria reflects bladder involvement, and pain on defecation occurs with rectal involvement.

No specific laboratory test is available for diagnosis of endometriosis. Physical examination may reveal small nodular masses on pelvic organs that enlarge during menstruation and are rarely movable (Fig. 54-3). Laparoscopy and exploratory surgery are the most beneficial as they allow direct visualization of the lesion.

Treatment depends on the woman's symptoms, age, and childbearing desires. In early endometriosis, treatment consists of analgesia and regular follow-up care. With severe symptoms, surgery is indicated. Surgery in women desiring children is usually aimed at removing as much endometrial tissue as possible while preserving the uterus and ovaries. Hormone therapy that prevents ovulation or produces pseudopregnancy may also help in the younger woman.

In adenomyosis, endometrial tissue has invaded the myometrium. The invasion may be diffuse or localized and results in enlarged uterus (Fig. 54-4). This buried endometrium is usually nonfunctional. Symptoms include menorrhagia, dyspareunia, dysmenorrhea, and generalized pelvic discomfort. The usual treatment is hysterectomy, which is indicated by symptoms.

Premenstrual Syndrome

Premenstrual syndrome is a term used to cover collectively the discomforts noted prior to the onset of menses.

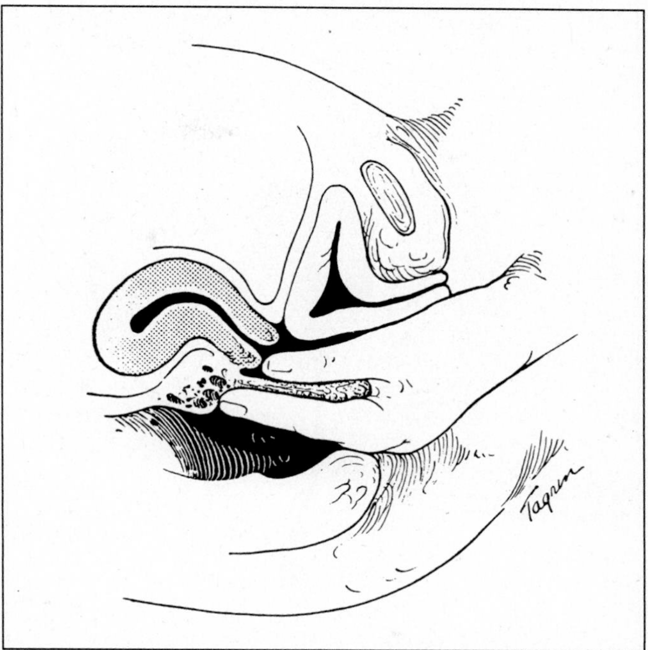

FIGURE 54-3 Rectal examination in the patient with typical pelvic endometriosis. The tender nodularity of the uterosacral ligaments and cul-de-sac and the fixed retroversion of the uterus are almost diagnostic of the disease. (From T.H. Green, Jr., *Gynecology: Essentials of Clinical Practice* [3rd ed.]. Boston: Little, Brown, 1977.)

The symptoms vary with individuals but most frequently include headache, breast tenderness, abdominal heaviness and bloating, edema, weight gain, backache, nervous irritability, mood changes, crying spells, depression, insomnia, and anxiety. These symptoms become worse 7 to 10 days prior to menses and subside when the menstrual flow is well established. The exact cause of premenstrual discomfort is unknown; however, it is believed to be associated with estrogen and progesterone levels.

Treatment is symptomatic and varies with individuals. The most frequently employed treatments include diuretics, dietary restriction of sodium, tranquilizers, and sedatives.

Dysmenorrhea

Dysmenorrhea may occur as a single entity or as part of the premenstrual syndrome. Dysmenorrhea means painful menstruation and is commonly referred to as cramps. There are two types of dysmenorrhea: primary and secondary. *Secondary dysmenorrhea* is caused by organic pelvic disease such as cancer of the uterus, bladder, or intestinal tract. Primary dysmenorrhea refers to painful menses unrelated to an obvious physical cause. It usually begins with the establishment of the ovulatory cycle. Spasmodic primary dysmenorrhea is usually characterized by sharp cramping sensations the first day or two of menses. It may improve as cycles are reestablished after pregnancy. Congestive primary dysmenorrhea frequently occurs in association with premenstrual syndrome. It is

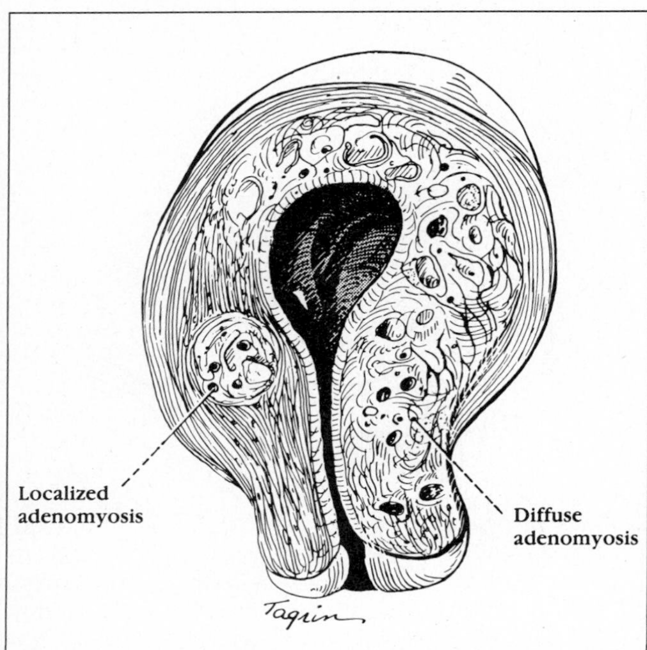

FIGURE 54-4 Adenomyosis of the uterus. Diffuse involvement of the uterine wall (*right*) and the localized form, the so-called adenomyoma (*left*). (From T.H. Green, Jr., *Gynecology: Essentials of Clinical Practice* [3rd ed.]. Boston: Little, Brown, 1977.)

characterized by a dull, aching pain prior to onset of menses.

The cause of primary dysmenorrhea remains unknown. One theory attributes it to the secretion of prostaglandins, especially PGE_2, which have a stimulating effect on uterine muscle. Nausea, vomiting, and diarrhea associated with dysmenorrhea have also been attributed to prostaglandins [6]. Other possible factors include acute anteflexion of the uterus, estrogen-progesterone imbalance, and hypersensitivity of the individual to pain.

The most common treatments include hormones, analgesics, prostaglandin synthetase, optimum health maintenance, and psychotherapy. Hormone therapy is aimed at preventing ovulation, as anovulatory cycles are rarely painful. Antiprostaglandins, such as aspirin, indomethacin, naproxen, and ibuprofen, may be administered prior to the onset of menses to inhibit prostaglandin synthesis. The drugs may not only inhibit prostaglandin synthesis, but block its action. Mild analgesics may also be administered.

Abnormal Uterine Bleeding

Abnormal uterine bleeding is usually a symptom of some underlying disease process rather than a disease entity itself. Several descriptive terms are used to describe abnormal uterine bleeding:

Metrorrhagia or intermenstrual bleeding—bleeding between periods
Menorrhagia or hypermenorrhea—excessive menstrual flow
Polymenorrhea—abnormally frequent menstrual bleeding
Oligomenorrhea—abnormally infrequent menses
Hypomenorrhea—deficient menstrual flow
Amenorrhea—absence of menstrual flow
Perimenopausal bleeding—irregular bleeding prior to menopause
Postmenopausal bleeding—bleeding occurring one year or more after menopause

The many causes of abnormal uterine bleeding can be grouped into four major categories: (1) complications of pregnancy, (2) organic lesions, (3) constitutional diseases, and (4) true dysfunctional uterine bleeding. Complications of pregnancy include abortion, trophoblastic disease, and ectopic pregnancy. Organic lesions include conditions associated with pelvic diseases such as infections, tumors, and polyps. Constitutional diseases are conditions such as hypertension, blood dyscrasias, and hormonal dysfunction. No pelvic disease is present, but symptoms are reflected through abnormal uterine bleeding. The last category represents abnormal bleeding associated with endocrine dysfunction.

Dysfunctional Uterine Bleeding. The term *dysfunctional uterine bleeding* is frequently used interchangeably with anovulatory bleeding. It refers to abnormal bleeding that is the result of endocrine dysfunction. It is associated with absence of ovulation. Therefore, no corpus luteum is formed, no progesterone produced, and no secretory changes occur in the endometrium. The endometrium becomes hyperplastic. As estrogen levels decrease from degenerating follicles, withdrawal bleeding occurs. Occasionally, dysfunctional uterine bleeding results from inadequate production of progesterone after ovulation.

Psychogenic uterine bleeding may be included in dysfunctional uterine bleeding when both organic and constitutional causes have been ruled out. The influence of emotional stimulation on the hypothalamus and the resultant influence on the gonadotropic hormones are discussed in Chapter 53. Emotions may also directly affect the uterine blood vessels and produce bleeding.

Diagnosis is made after a complete and thorough menstrual history. Physical examination reveals pelvic lesions and aids in the diagnosis of constitutional diseases. Laboratory studies include thyroid function, complete blood count (CBC), and platelet count to rule out blood dyscrasias. Studies to determine the presence of ovulation include measurements of estrogen and progesterone levels, endometrial biopsy, and spinnbarkeit and ferning studies of cervical mucus. During the climacteric, both cytologic studies and biopsy are important to rule out cancer.

Amenorrhea. Amenorrhea is not a disease entity. It may indicate a very serious condition or be completely normal, as in pregnancy. It may be either primary or secondary. *Primary amenorrhea* refers to a failure to begin menstrual cycles. *Secondary amenorrhea* occurs after a variable period of normal function. Causes of amenorrhea may be physiologic, anatomic, genetic, endocrinologic, constitutional, or psychogenic. Physiologic causes include pregnancy, lactation, menopause, and adolescence. Anatomic factors include congenital anomalies, hysterectomy, and endometrial destruction. Genetic factors include Turner's syndrome and hermaphroditism. Dysfunction of the hypothalamus, pituitary, ovary, thyroid, or adrenal glands may also produce amenorrhea. Malnutrition, obesity, drug addiction, diabetes, and anemia are all constitutional problems that can prevent menstrual periods. Psychogenic factors include psychosis and anorexia nervosa.

Specific diagnostic tools, in addition to history and physical examination, include thyroid function studies, serum prolactin level, buccal smear, skull radiographs, progesterone challenge test, and hormone values.

Reproductive Tract Infections

Atrophic Vaginitis

Atrophic vaginitis refers to inflammation of the atrophied epithelium in postmenopausal women. It produces an irritating vaginal discharge, with pruritus and swelling, and secondary dyspareunia and dysuria. Red strawberry spots may be noted on the vaginal wall. Bleeding may occur from trauma to the thin epithelium, but malignancy must be ruled out as its cause. Estrogen therapy is used to convert the epithelium to the more normal thick, stratified squamous layer.

Cervicitis

Cervicitis refers to inflammation of the cervix, which may be acute or chronic. Acute cervicitis usually occurs with other acute reproductive tract infections. Causative organisms include *Gonococcus*, *Staphylococcus*, and *Streptococcus*, species and *Escherichia coli*. Speculum examination reveals an edematous, congested cervix with purulent discharge. Symptoms may include dyspareunia, backache, dull pain in lower abdomen, and urinary frequency and urgency. Pain may be noted on palpation. Cultures and smears identify the causative organism, and appropriate antibiotic therapy is then instituted.

Many women exhibit some form of chronic cervicitis. It may occur after acute infections, childbirth trauma, or abortion. The cervical canal is primarily affected, but there are no characteristic findings of the cervix. The only symptom may be a mucopurulent vaginal discharge or occasionally, paracervical or low back pain. Abnormal bleeding is rare and often indicates cervical cancer. Physical examination may reveal cervical erosions, cervical eversions, or nabothian cysts.

Cervical erosion refers to an area of the surface of the cervix in which the surface epithelia are partially or totally absent. It appears red and raw. Columnar cells are more likely to exhibit this characteristic than squamous cells, and they are not as curable. *Cervical eversion* refers to a portion of the cervix in which columnar epithelium of the cervical canal extends outward (Fig. 54-5). The characteristic squamocolumnar junction is then located along the outer edge of the lesion. Eversion occurs most frequently in women taking oral contraceptives, young women who have never been pregnant, and the daughters of women who took diethylstilbestrol during pregnancy. There is an increase in mucoid secretions. In an attempt to repair the eversion, the squamous cells begin to grow inward. As this invasion progresses, the mucus-secreting glands are obliterated. Their secretions are then trapped beneath the epithelium, producing *nabothian cysts*. These cysts are filled with normal mucus, are not infected, and produce no symptoms.

The primary concern in diagnosing cervicitis is screening for cervical cancer because the lesions are not easily differentiated by the naked eye. In addition to cultures, Pap smear, colposcopy, and biopsy are the most important screening aids.

Silver nitrate, douches, and antibiotics are relatively ineffective methods of treatment because of the depth of the lesions. Small areas may be treated with thermal cautery or cryosurgery. Entire areas are treated in depth; healing and reepithelialization then take place. The sloughing cervical tissue produces an annoying discharge that may be treated with antibiotic creams for 7 to 10 days. Complete healing may take six to eight weeks.

Toxic Shock Syndrome

Toxic shock syndrome (TSS) is a relatively new entity first recognized and reported in 1978 [9]. At that time it was thought to be related to *Staphylococcus aureus*. Since then it has gained notoriety as a condition occurring most often in menstruating women who use tampons. Nonmenstrual TSS has been associated with vaginal and cesarean delivery, therapeutic abortion, and infected wounds and

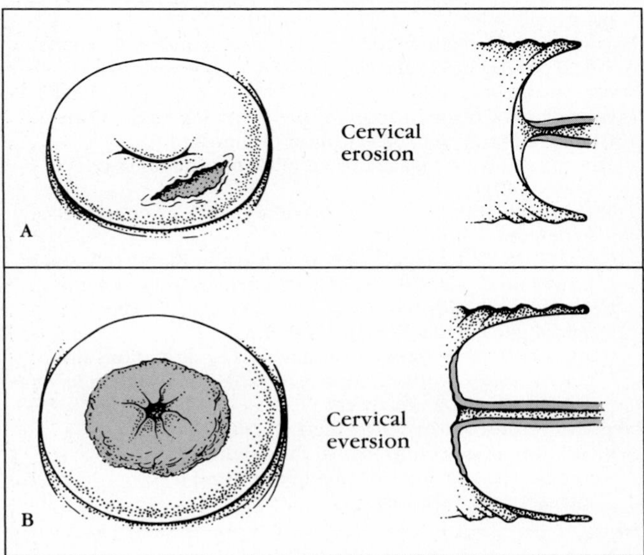

FIGURE 54-5 A. Cervical erosion. B. Cervical eversion.

skin lesions. The causative agent is believed to be a toxin produced by *S. aureus*.

The link with tampons is most interesting, as the unused tampons of women developing TSS contained no *S. aureus* [2]. Two theories support the tampon link. One states that bacteria are nourished by carboxymethyl cellulose, which is present in many tampons [2]. The other indicates that conditions for bacterial growth are improved through use of superabsorbent tampons [5].

Clinical manifestations of TSS include (1) elevated temperature, sudden in onset, (2) vomiting and diarrhea, and (3) an erythematous macular rash, which is present especially on palms of hands and soles of feet. The sunburnlike rash progresses to peeling of palms and soles about 10 days later. Renal dysfunction may develop, with decreased urinary output. Hypotension and shock may develop. Laboratory studies usually reveal elevated blood urea nitrogen (BUN), serum creatinine, bilirubin, and creatine phosphokinase levels. Additional complications associated with TSS include disseminated intravascular coagulation, shock lung, and acidosis. Table 54-1 summarizes criteria for diagnosis.

Treatment varies depending on extent of symptoms. It may include antibiotics (penicillinase-resistant penicillin) or cephalosporins, intravenous colloid to prevent fluid loss from blood vessels, ventilation therapy, heparin, blood transfusion, and correction of acid-base imbalance.

Pelvic Inflammatory Disease

Pelvic inflammatory disease (PID) is a general term used to refer to any infection of the upper reproductive tract (above the cervix). More precise terms such as endometritis, endoparametritis, salpingitis, oophoritis, and pelvic peritonitis indicate specific areas of involvement. Common causes of PID include *Gonococcus*, *Staphylococcus*, and *Streptococcus* species, and *Chlamydia trachomatis* (see Chap. 55). It often occurs after delivery or abortion, or in women using intrauterine devices (IUD) as a means of contraception.

Symptoms include the sudden onset of severe pelvic pain, chills and fever, nausea, vomiting, and a heavy, purulent vaginal discharge with foul odor. Vaginal bleeding may also be present.

One of the most important diagnostic tools in PID is a complete and thorough history. Specific information of most importance relates to previous reproductive tract infection, delivery, abortion, pelvic surgery, onset of pain, date of last menses, sexual history, and type of contraceptive used. Specific diagnostic tests include cultures of any discharge, CBC, and possibly ultrasound studies if pelvic abscess is suspected.

Medical regimen depends on the cause, acuteness, and extent of the infection. Hospitalization with bedrest and appropriate intravenous antibiotics may be indicated. Analgesics may be ordered for pain. Removal of an IUD is indicated when one is present. Surgical drainage is usually recommended for an abscess. The importance of follow-up care cannot be overemphasized. Untreated or inadequately treated PID may result in infertility and/or sterility.

TABLE 54-1 Toxic Shock Syndrome Case Definition

Fever (temperature ≥38.9°C [102°F]
Rash (diffuse macular erythroderma)
Desquamation, 1–2 weeks after onset of illness, particularly of palms and soles
Hypotension (systolic blood pressure ≤90 mm Hg for adults or <fifth percentile by age for children <16 years old, or orthostatic syncope)
Involvement of three or more of the following organ systems:
- GI (vomiting or diarrhea at onset of illness)
- Muscular (severe myalgia or creatine phosphokinase level ≥2 × ULN)
- Mucous membrane (vaginal, oropharyngeal, or conjunctival) hyperemia
- Renal (BUN or Cr ≥2 × ULN or ≥5 white blood cells/high-power field—in the absence of a urinary tract infection)
- Hepatic (total bilirubin, SGOT, or SGPT ≥2 × ULN)
- Hematologic (platelets ≤100,000/μl)
- Central nervous system (disorientation or alterations in consciousness without focal neurologic signs when fever and hypotension are absent)

Negative results on the following tests, if obtained:
- Blood, throat, or cerebrospinal fluid cultures
- Serologic tests for Rocky Mountain spotted fever, leptospirosis, or measles

ULN = upper limits of normal.
Source: Centers for Disease Control, *Morbidity and Mortality Weekly Report* 29:442, 1980.

Benign Conditions of the Female Reproductive Tract

Uterine Fibroids

Uterine fibroids, also referred to as *leiomyomas*, *myomas*, or *fibromyomas*, are second only to pregnancy as the most common cause of uterine enlargement. Twenty to fifty percent of women between ages 30 and 50 years have some evidence of these growths. They are very common in black women [8]. Actually, fibroids are masses of muscle and connective tissue that are stimulated by estrogen. Diagnosis is most often made on the basis of physical examination. Ultrasound, radiographs, and dilatation and curettage may aid in the diagnosis.

The tumors occur singly or in groups. Size varies from the size of peas to that of an apple or cantaloupe. They are firm, smooth, and spheric. Sectioning of a fibroid tumor reveals a pinkish white, whorled, and lined muscle bundle.

Position in the uterine wall determines the type or classification of fibroids (Fig. 54-6). Intramural or interstitial tumors are present in central portions of the uterine wall; these are the most common. Submucosal tumors are located between the endometrium and uterine lining. Projection into the uterine cavity with subsequent distortion and enlargement of the endometrium may cause excessive menstrual bleeding and habitual abortion. Subserous fibroids lie beneath the serous lining of the uterus and project outward into the abdominal cavity. If a subserous tumor extends outward on a stalk, it is called *pedunculated*.

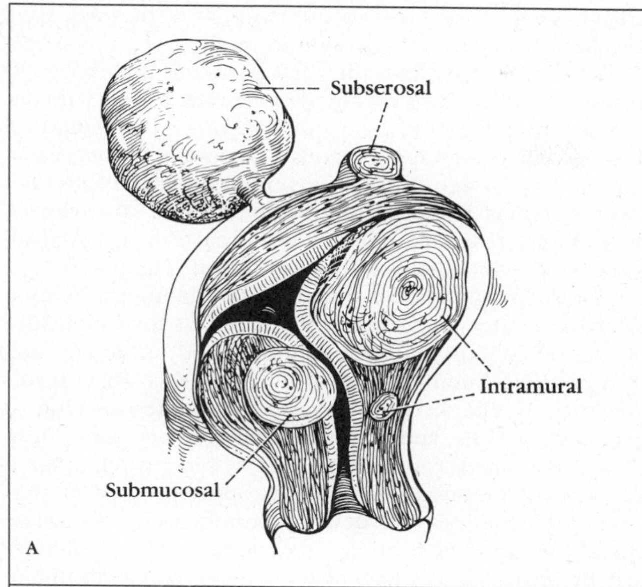

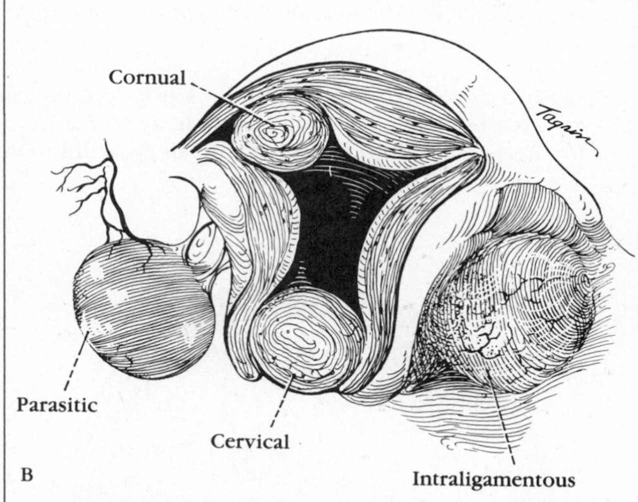

FIGURE 54-6 Uterine fibroids. A. Types. B. Various locations. (From T.H. Green, Jr., *Gynecology: Essentials of Clinical Practice* [3rd ed.]. Boston: Little, Brown, 1977.)

Many fibroids are asymptomatic. As they enlarge, the woman may experience excessive or prolonged bleeding during regular monthly cycles, urinary frequency, constipation, abdominal fullness, low abdominal pain, dysmenorrhea, and infertility. Abnormal bleeding usually occurs with submucous tumors because of the increased amount of endometrium to build and slough. Enlargement of fibroids can produce pressure on the bladder, urethra, rectum, or nerves. Infertility and habitual abortion occur most frequently with submucous tumors because of distortion of the endometrium and uterine cavity. Enlarging fibroids have also been known to interfere with delivery of a full-term baby.

The course of treatment is determined by age, parity, symptoms, and condition of the individual. No treatment at all is needed for asymptomatic persons. Women approaching menopause are usually observed at regular intervals, as withdrawal of estrogen results in a stationary or decreasing size of the fibroids. Hysterectomy may be indicated for the woman desiring no additional children or with bleeding problems.

Functional Ovarian Cysts

Functional ovarian cysts are the result of normal ovarian function and account for more than 50 percent of ovarian enlargements. A functional follicular cyst results when a maturing follicle fails to rupture an ovum. Instead it continues to enlarge and produce estrogen. A corpus luteum cyst occurs when the corpus luteum fails to degenerate normally. It continues to grow and produce progesterone.

Ordinarily, functional ovarian cysts produce no symptoms. They may be noted on periodic examination and usually disappear after the next menstrual cycle. Occasionally, when a functional cyst ruptures it tears an ovarian vessel. Intraperitoneal bleeding occurs, and the extent of symptoms is related to the amount of hemorrhage. With excessive bleeding, abdominal pain may be severe in onset, requiring hospitalization and surgery.

Benign Neoplastic Tumors of the Ovaries

Benign neoplasms are more important than functional cysts, although they occur less frequently. They may grow to be quite large and secrete hormones. Classification is by cellular origin: (1) germ cell, (2) germinal epithelium, (3) gonadal stroma, and (4) nonspecialized stroma. Three of the most common benign neoplasms are cystic teratomas or dermoid cysts, serous cystadenomas, and mucinous cystadenomas.

Dermoid cysts represent about 15 to 20 percent of all ovarian neoplasms and arise from germ cells. They are most frequent in women 18 to 35 years of age. The tumor is gray, smooth, and contains tissue from all three germ layers, commonly skin, hair, and sebaceous glands.

Benign serous cystadenomas arise from germinal epithelium and, with mucinous cystadenomas, account for about 50 percent of benign ovarian neoplasms. They most frequently affect women between 40 and 50 years of age. The tumors may be unilateral or bilateral. Tumors are pearly gray, lobulated, and filled with a clear, yellow fluid that becomes brown if there is bleeding in the cyst. *Psammoma bodies*, which are small, calcified granules, may be present in the cell wall. Papillary serous cystadenomas may develop into malignancies.

Mucinous cystadenomas also arise from germinal epithelium and are usually unilateral. They are usually larger than serous cystadenomas, contain no psamma bodies, and contain thick, straw-colored fluid.

Most ovarian tumors are asymptomatic and are noted on routine pelvic examination. Once they are enlarged enough to produce pressure, the woman may complain of pain on defecation, dyspareunia, heaviness, and sterility. Increased enlargement may result in abdominal distention, dyspnea, and anorexia. Menstrual irregularities, masculinization, and feminization may occur if hormones are produced. Complications include rupture, hemorrhage, possible infection, and torsion of pedicle cyst. The treatment of choice is surgical removal, as the tumors increase in size and may undergo malignant changes.

Benign Breast Alterations

The two most common benign breast alterations are fibrocystic disease and fibroadenoma. Fibrocystic disease is the most common of all female breast lesions, affecting approximately 1 in 20 women. Characteristically, the lesion becomes nodular from fibrous thickening. It may be tender, especially prior to menstruation, and exhibit cystic formation. Complaints of dull, heavy pain and a sense of fullness that increase prior to menstruation are characteristic. Aspiration may be used to aid in diagnosis. The exact cause is unknown, but it is thought to result from abnormal or exaggerated response of breast tissue to cyclic hormonal stimulation. It is a benign neoplasm consisting of proliferative ductal epithelium and fibrous stroma.

The second most common benign breast tumor is fibroadenoma. Physical examination reveals a well-outlined, solid, firm lump that moves freely. It occurs most often in women 15 to 40 years of age, being the most common breast lesion in the adolescent female. The cause of this condition is unknown, but estrogen stimulation is suspected as it occurs primarily in younger women and rarely after menopause. Treatment is surgical removal of the lump. Recurrence is common.

Premalignant and Malignant Conditions

Trophoblastic Disease

The term *trophoblastic disease* refers to three complications of uterine pregnancy: hydatidiform mole, chorioadenoma destruens, and choriocarcinoma. Hydatidiform mole is usually benign with malignant potential, while choriocarcinoma is a highly aggressive malignancy.

Hydatidiform Mole. Hydatidiform mole represents a malformation of the placenta. It is characterized by absence of embryo development, conversion of the chorionic villi into marked vesicles with clear, thick, sticky fluid, and production of human chorionic gonadotropin (HCG).

Clinical manifestations include intermittent bleeding, excessive increase in uterine size, no evidence of fetal development, markedly elevated HCG levels, and spontaneous abortion. The woman may experience intermittent bleeding after amenorrhea. A dark brown vaginal discharge may be accompanied by passage of watery fluid containing the characteristic vesicles. Even by the sixteenth to twentieth week, no fetal heart tones are noted and no fetal movement is felt; ultrasound reveals no fetal skeleton. Levels of HCG levels may be as much as 10 times higher than those associated with normal pregnancy [6]. Hyperemesis gravidarum, bilateral ovarian cysts, and toxemia of pregnancy prior to the twenty-fourth week have also been noted with hydatidiform mole.

Diagnostic tools include dilatation and curettage (D and C), histologic studies, measurement of HCG levels, and sonography. Histologic studies can be performed on tissue that is passed spontaneously or obtained from dilatation and curettage. Curettage scrapings usually include both superficial and deep tissue to determine invasiveness. Sonography reveals a characteristic pattern of hydatidiform mole, which helps in differentiation (Fig. 54-7).

Treatment of choice is evacuation of the uterus as soon as possible after diagnosis. Possible means for evacuation of uterine contents include dilatation and curettage, suction curettage, and hysterectomy. After this, HCG levels are initially checked every week, gradually moving to every other week, and finally monthly for one year. Ordinarily, HCG levels return to normal within a week or so. If they are still elevated at four weeks, approximately 50 percent of affected persons develop choriocarcinoma unless chemotherapy is instituted. Occasionally, chemotherapy may be instituted as a prophylactic measure. Chemotherapeutic agents include the folic acid antagonists methotrexate and actinomycin D.

Chorioadenoma Destruens. Chorioadenoma destruens is an invasive hydatidiform mole. It is characterized by the presence of chorionic villi deep within the

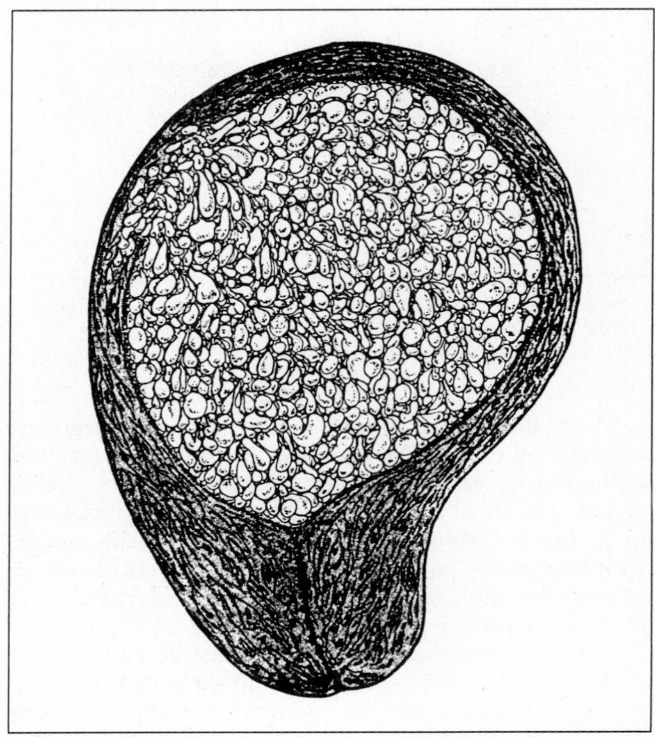

FIGURE 54-7 Hydatidiform mole. (From M.A. Miller and D.A. Brooten, *The Childbearing Family: A Nursing Perspective* [2nd ed.]. Boston: Little, Brown, 1983.)

myometrium. Penetration of the uterine wall with rupture and hemorrhage is possible.

Curettage may not be successful in removing the lesion because of the depth of invasion. Chemotherapy with methotrexate or actinomycin D is usually initiated. Levels of HCG levels are measured regularly until they return to normal. Thereafter, they are measured at monthly intervals for one year.

Choriocarcinoma. Choriocarcinoma is a malignant tumor of the trophoblast occurring most frequently in the uterus. It is characterized by sheets of immature cells (cytotrophoblasts and syncytiotrophoblasts) that invade the uterine wall and produce necrosis and hemorrhage. Chorionic villi are not present. Occasionally, choriocarcinoma may occur in the ovaries.

The only symptom noticed may be irregular bleeding or continual bleeding after a delivery or abortion. Frequently, the first symptoms are related to metastasis. Because the most common site of metastasis is the lung, hemoptysis may be the first complaint. Other metastatic sites include the vagina, brain, liver, and kidneys. Levels of HCG remain markedly elevated.

Prior to the use of chemotherapeutic agents, the prognosis for a woman with choriocarcinoma was extremely grim, with death within one to two years. The 1986 Cancer Facts and Figures lists choriocarcinoma among 14 cancers that are being cured primarily because of chemotherapy [1]. Among the agents used are methotrexate, actinomycin D, chlorambucil, and vincristine. The response of lung metastasis is also very good, but lesions in the brain and liver respond poorly. Prognosis continues to be directly related to degree of metastasis, duration of disease, and HCG titer.

Endometrial Carcinoma

During the last 40 years, uterine cancer, including endometrial and cervical, has decreased over 70 percent. Its frequency is surpassed by cancer of breast, colon, and rectum, and tied with lung cancer in women [1]. It affects primarily postmenopausal women, with peak occurrence around 55 years of age.

Experimental evidence has linked endometrial cancer with ingestion of exogenous estrogens. Endogenous estrogen production unbalanced by progesterone may contribute to its frequency in early menopause. Additional factors that seem to increase the risk of endometrial cancer include history of infertility, obesity, diabetes, hypertension, and family history of uterine cancer [3]. It is also prevalent among white women in high socioeconomic levels [8].

In many cases, malignant changes are preceded by abnormal cell maturation. Adenomatous hyperplasia has been known to occur both spontaneously and as a result of estrogen drugs. If untreated, the process progresses to an in situ lesion in which the cells are larger and more disoriented. Nuclei may be present in different locations with varying size and staining characteristics. About 85 percent of endometrial malignancy is adenocarcinoma. Cells may be well-differentiated as in in situ lesions or so undifferentiated that no glandular pattern is evident. The lesion represents a slow-growing tumor with late metastasis. Metastasis occurs first to the cervix and myometrium, and later involves the vagina, pelvis, and lungs.

Staging or extension of lesion from the site of origin and grading of cellular differentiation of endometrial cancer are possible only after removal of the uterus and subsequent pathologic studies. Therefore, grading is of little value in determining initial therapy. The grades of endometrial cancer are I through III, with grade I representing well-differentiated cells and grade III undifferentiated. The Federation Internationale de Gynecologie et Obstetrique (FIGO) has adopted a system of five major stages (Table 54-2).

The first sign of endometrial cancer is abnormal uterine bleeding. It may range from light irregular bleeding with intermenstrual spotting to heavy prolonged periods when it occurs prior to menopause. After menopause any bleeding should be suspicious. Another early sign may be marked leukorrhea. Both reflect erosion and ulceration of the endometrium. Later signs include cramping, pelvic discomfort, lower abdominal or bladder pressure, bleeding after intercourse, and swollen lymph nodes.

The most important diagnostic tool is probably dilatation and curettage, as it allows the most comprehensive study. Routine Pap smears have limited usefulness unless metastasis has occurred. Both endometrial biopsy and washing may reveal abnormal endometrial tissue.

Stage 0 endometrial cancer is considered curable with hysterectomy. Stage I and II disease is treated with radiation and surgery. Chemotherapy is quite ineffective. Progesterone therapy may be used, especially in recurrent disease.

Cervical Cancer

The frequency of cancer in the cervix continues to decline. No longer is it the second most prevalent female cancer. It occurs generally between ages 30 and 50 years, in women (1) who began intercourse prior to age 20 years, (2) of low socioeconomic status, (3) who are black, (4) who received DES during pregnancy, (5) who have

Table 54-2 Stages of Endometrial Carcinoma as Devised by the Federation Internationale de Gynecologie et Obstetrique (FIGO)

Stage	Description
0	carcinoma in situ
I	tumor confined to the corpus uteri
II	tumor involves both the corpus and cervix
III	tumor extends outside the uterus, but not outside the true pelvis
IV	tumor involves bladder and/or rectum, or extends outside the true pelvis

had many sexual partners, or (6) who are multiparous. There also seems to be an emerging link with the sexually transmitted diseases, especially genital herpes infection. Chronic cervicitis and unrepaired cervical lacerations seem to predispose to malignancy [7].

Cancer of the cervix is most frequently of the squamous cell type and represents a sequential process of cellular proliferation. It usually begins in the transformation zone of the squamocolumnar junction as a basal cell hyperplasia. As the hyperplasia extends toward the surface, it becomes known as dysplasia, which refers to the disorderly cellular arrangement in the upper layers of the epithelium. The nuclei of the these cells are enlarged and stain darkly. Some cells may be multinucleated. The number of atypical cells determines the classification: (1) mild, (2) moderate, or (3) severe.

The next stage in the sequential process is carcinoma in situ. This stage represents an involvement of the entire epithelial cell layer and is referred to as intraepithelial neoplasm. The term *cervical intraepithelial neoplasia* (*CIN*) is currently used to refer to all dysplasia and carcinoma in situ, as the potential for progression and metastasis exists.

There are three forms of invasive cervical cancer: fungating, ulcerative, and infiltrative. The fungating tumor is a nodular thickening of the epithelium that may project above the mucosa. The ulcerative lesion represents a sloughing necrosis of the central portion of the tumor. Infiltrative invasion represents downward growth into the stroma. As metastasis continues, there is spread to the bladder, rectum, and lymph nodes; eventually the lungs, bones, and liver may be involved. The slow process of metastasis is believed to take as long as 10 years after the diagnosis of carcinoma in situ. In more rapidly growing lesions, invasion can occur in three to four years.

Because early cervical cancer is asymptomatic, early diagnosis and staging of the lesion are essential (Table 54-3). Routine Pap smears have probably done more than any other diagnostic tool to detect early cervical cancer. Early CIN can also be detected by Pap smears. Colposcopy, cervical biopsy, and conization can confirm the diagnosis.

Laser surgery, electrocautery, and cryosurgery are procedures aimed at removing the lesion in early stage cancer. Total hysterectomy, radical hysterectomy, radiation therapy, or pelvic exenteration may be indicated as the extent of malignancy increases.

TABLE 54-3 FIGO Recommendations for Staging Cervical Cancer

Stage	Description
0	carcinoma in situ
I	carcinoma limited to the cervix
II	carcinoma extends beyond the cervix and involves the upper two-thirds of the vagina
III	carcinoma involves the lower one-third of the vagina and has become fixed to the pelvic wall
IV	carcinoma involves the rectum and/or bladder, or extends beyond the true pelvis

DES Exposure

The first synthetic estrogen was released in the 1940s. It was used to prevent miscarriage and lactation after delivery, and as hormone therapy for dysfunctional uterine bleeding after menopause. In the late 1960s it became linked with adenocarcinoma of the vagina, vaginal adenosis, squamous cell carcinoma of the cervix and vagina, and cervical dysplasia, as well as congenital abnormalities of both male and female offspring and impaired sperm production.

Cancer of the vagina is a very rare condition, most frequently occurring in women over age 50 years. It usually is the squamous cell type, but adenocarcinoma has been identified in a number of adolescent girls whose mothers received DES during pregnancy.

Vaginal adenosis is a benign condition in which the transformation zone of the squamocolumnar junction extends over the vaginal portion of the cervix and may involve the vaginal walls. This condition is extremely common in daughters of mothers who took DES and may predispose them to adenocarcinoma. A question also arises as to whether adenosis may progress to squamous cell cancer of the cervix and/or vagina [3].

Lowered fertility rates have been identified in both male and female offspring of mothers who took DES. Irregular or infrequent menstrual periods occur in females. Low sperm counts, abnormally shaped sperm, and decreased ejaculate volume have been noted in males. Congenital anomalies in males include undescended as well as underdeveloped testicles, testicular cysts, and abnormal meatal openings.

The most important factor in treatment of DES problems is identification of those exposed and follow-up care every 6 to 12 months. Children of women known or suspected of DES exposure should have regular examinations beginning at puberty. Routine procedures should include Pap smears and colposcopy. Precancerous cell changes can be found early and appropriate therapy initiated.

Ovarian Cancer

Ovarian cancer is the most lethal of all pelvic cancer in women; however, it accounts for only 5 percent of cancer deaths in women [1]. The reason for its lethality is the advanced stage when diagnosis is made. It occurs most frequently in women around 50 years of age.

There is no diagnostic tool for early detection of ovarian cancer. If detected early it is by chance and on routine periodic examinations. Any ovarian enlargement in the postmenopausal woman and any ovary larger than 5 cm in diameter regardless of age should be suspected.

Ovarian cancer is difficult to diagnose from gross inspection until it invades the ovarian wall or seeds tumor cells in the peritoneal cavity. The epithelial form is usually cystic, while the appearance is a solid form when it involves the stroma and connective tissue [11].

Initial treatment in any woman with ovarian cancer is surgical. Total hysterectomy with bilateral salpingo-oophorectomy and omentectomy is recommended. Supplementary therapy when indicated includes irradiation and chemotherapy. Chemotherapeutic agents include aklylating drugs such as busulfan, chlorambucil, cyclophosphanide, and melphalan.

Grading and staging systems are also used in ovarian cancer. The tumors are graded I through IV from well-differentiated to undifferentiated (Table 54-4).

Breast Cancer

The most frequent site of cancer in the woman is in the breast. This disease is now second only to lung cancer as a cause of death from cancer in women. The cause is not known, but three theories have been put forth: (1) viral influence, (2) hormonal influence, and (3) genetic influence.

It has been discovered that mouse mammary tumor virus (MMTV) can be transmitted through mother's milk and produce cancer in suckling mice. The enzyme reverse transcriptase, present in oncogenic virus particles, has also been identified in human milk samples with viruslike particles. The hormonal influence receives some support from the risk factors associated with breast cancer: (1) early menarche and/or late menopause, (2) no children or children born after age 30 years, and (3) history of fibrocystic disease. All of these women are exposed to long periods of ovarian function with high estrogen levels. Having a history of breast cancer increases one's risk factor and also supports the theory of genetic influence [4].

Breast cancer is usually discovered by the woman. She notes a single lump that is painless, nontender, and movable. It most frequently is found in the upper outer quadrant. The tumor may arise in either the ducts or lobules and may be either infiltrating or noninfiltrating. As the condition progresses the tumor becomes adherent to the pectoral muscles and fixed. Dimpling and retraction of the skin may develop. *Peau d'orange* skin may be noted, with dimpling that resembles the skin of an orange in the area of tumor involvement. Metastatic sites include lymph nodes, lungs, bones, adrenals, brain, ovaries, and liver.

Breast self-examination is widely taught to detect lumps in the breast. Mammography, thermography, and ultrasound may be used for diagnosis. Mammography is a major diagnostic tool, as it detects breast masses before they are palpable. Biopsy confirms the diagnosis.

The treatment for breast cancer is highly individualized. Surgical procedures ranging from lump removal to radical mastectomy are employed depending on the individual situation. Supplementary therapy includes radiation, endocrine therapy, and chemotherapy. A grading system for breast cancer is important in comparing the effectiveness of various treatments. Table 54-5 provides a summary of the widespread grading system.

TABLE 54-4 An Accepted Staging Classification for Ovarian Carcinoma

Stage	Description
I	tumor limited to one or both ovaries
II	tumor involves one or both ovaries with pelvic extension
III	tumor growth with widespread intraperitoneal metastasis
IV	tumor growth involves metastasis outside the peritoneal cavity

TABLE 54-5 Staging and TNM Classification for Breast Malignancy

Stage	Class	Description
1	T_1	Tumor 2 cm or less
	N_0	No palpable axillary nodes
	M_0	No evident metastasis
2	T_0	No palpable tumor
	T_1	Tumor 2 cm or less
	T_2	Tumor less than 5 cm
	N_1	Palpable axillary nodes with histologic evidence of breast malignancy
	M_0	No evidence of metastasis
3	T_3	Tumor more than 5 cm; may be fixed to muscle or fascia
	N_1 or N_2	Fixed nodes
	M_0	No evidence of metastasis
4	T_4	Tumor any size with fixation to chest wall or skin; presence of edema, including peau d'orange; ulceration; skin nodules; inflammatory carcinoma
	N_3	Supraclavicular or intraclavicular nodes or arm edema
	M_1	Distant metastasis present or suspected

Source: W. J. Phipps, B. C. Long and N. F. Woods, *Medical-Surgical Nursing* (2nd ed.). St. Louis: Mosby, 1983.

Study Questions

1. Differentiate between premenstrual syndrome and dysmenorrhea.
2. Compare the different types of malignancies of the female reproductive system in reference to etiology, pathology, clinical manifestations, and prognosis.
3. Discuss the staging systems of the types of malignancies.
4. How does toxic shock syndrome develop?
5. Compare the results of DES administration on male and female offspring.

References

1. American Cancer Society. *Cancer Facts and Figures*. New York: American Cancer Society, 1986.
2. Centers for Disease Control. Follow-up on toxic-shock syndrome. *Morbidity and Mortality Weekly Report* 29:441, 1980.

3. Creasman, W.T. Malignant lesions of the corpus uteri. In D.N. Danforth and J.R. Scott, *Obstetrics and Gynecology* (5th ed.). Philadelphia: Lippincott, 1986.
4. Donegan, W.L. Diseases of the breast. In D.N. Danforth and J.R. Scott, *Obstetrics and Gynecology* (5th ed.). Philadelphia: Lippincott, 1986.
5. Gold, M. Toxic shock. *Science* 80:8, 1980.
6. Robbins, S.L., Cotran, R.S., and Kumar, V. *Pathologic Basis of Disease* (3rd ed.). Philadelphia: Saunders, 1984.
7. Rutledge, F.N. Gynecologic malignancy: General considerations. In D.N. Danforth and J.R. Scott, *Obstetrics and Gynecology* (5th ed.). Philadelphia: Lippincott, 1986.
8. Stewart, F.N., et al. *My Body, My Health: The Concerned Woman's Guide to Gynecology*. New York: Wiley, 1979. P. 356.
9. Todd, J. Toxic-shock syndrome associated with phage-group I staphylococci. *Lancet* 2:1116, 1978.
10. Wedell, M.A., Billings, P., and Fayez, J.A. Endometriosis and the infertile patient. *J. Obstet. Gynecol. Neonat. Nurs.* 14:280, 1985.
11. Zaloudek, C., Tavassoli, F.A., and Kurman, R.J. Malignant lesions of the ovary. In D.N. Danforth and J.R. Scott, *Obstetrics and Gynecology* (5th ed.). Philadelphia: Lippincott, 1986.

CHAPTER 55

Sexually Transmitted Diseases

CHAPTER OUTLINE

Primary Sexually Transmitted Diseases

- Gonorrhea
- Syphilis
- Genital Herpes
- Chancroid
- Granuloma Inguinale
- Lymphogranuloma Venereum

Sexually Transmitted Infections

- Trichomonal Vaginitis
- Candidiasis
- *Hemophilus vaginalis* Vaginitis
- *Chlamydia trachomatis*
- Condylomata Accuminata

Acquired Immune Deficiency Syndrome

LEARNING OBJECTIVES

1. Identify the causative organism for each of the sexually transmitted diseases (STDs).
2. Discuss the clinical manifestations of each STD.
3. Identify the three most prevalent STDs.
4. Discuss the impact of each STD on the fetus and/or neonate.
5. Discuss the appropriate treatment for each STD.

Sexually transmitted disease (STD) is a relatively new term used to refer to those conditions that can be transmitted through sexual intercourse or intimate contact. For many years these conditions were referred to as venereal disease and included primarily gonorrhea and syphilis. The term STD, however, is more inclusive and refers to as many as 14 conditions so classified by the Centers for Disease Control (CDC).

In addition to gonorrhea and syphilis, primary STDs include genital herpes, chancroid, granuloma inguinale, and lymphogranuloma venereum. The term *STD* has also been used to refer to several infections involving the reproductive organs. Among these are trichomonal and candidal infections, those caused by *Hemophilus vaginalis* and *Chlamydia trachomatis*, and condylomata accuminata. The most recent alteration in male and female reproductive function to be classified as STD is acquired immune deficiency syndrome (AIDS).

Conditions recognized by the CDC as STDs and not discussed in this chapter include scabies, pediculosis pubis, and hepatitis B; and the enteric infections amebiasis and giardiasis, and those caused by *Campylobacter jejuni*, and *Shigella* species [2].

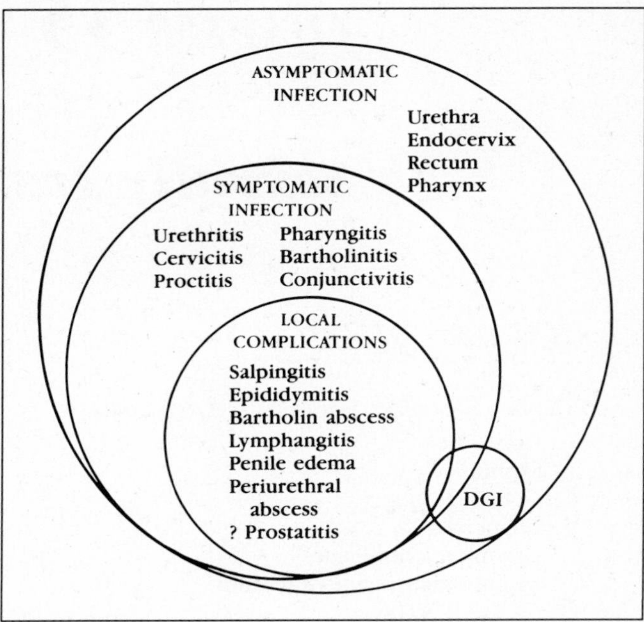

FIGURE 55-1 Spectrum of gonococcal manifestations. (DGI = disseminated gonococcal infection.) (From K.K. Holmes et al., *Sexually Transmitted Diseases*, NY: McGraw-Hill, 1984, p. 207.)

Primary Sexually Transmitted Diseases

Gonorrhea

Gonorrhea is the most common of all the primary sexually transmitted diseases. It is occurring in epidemic proportions in the United States, affecting 2 million citizens in 1984 [4]. The clinical spectrum of gonococcal infection is illustrated in Figure 55-1.

The causative organism in gonorrhea is *Neisseria gonorrhoeae*, which is a gram-negative diplococcus. This organism thrives in the warm, moist environment of mucous membranes. It may spread rapidly during menstruation because of the favorable environment produced by the blood. It does not survive well outside the body and exhibits increasing resistance to penicillin. It is almost exclusively a sexually transmitted disease, but it can be contracted by an infant during delivery or by persons who have skin breaks that come in contact with contaminated discharge. Occasionally, it may occur in the throat, eyes, or rectum.

Women who contract gonorrhea are frequently asymptomatic. When symptoms are present, they may include green or yellow vaginal discharge, dysuria, urinary frequency, pruritus, and red swollen vulva. Rectal discharge may be noted with rectal infection. Both Skene's glands and Bartholin's glands may be involved.

Within 2 to 10 days of exposure, urethritis occurs, with the male noting a purulent discharge from the urethral meatus. The discharge is clear at first but soon becomes white or even green. It may be accompanied by itching, burning, and pain of the meatus, especially during voiding. Ten to 20 percent of males with gonorrhea may have no symptoms. In the absence of prompt treatment, infection is likely to spread to involve the prostate, seminal vesicles, and epididymis. With chronic or prolonged infection, abscesses, tissue destruction, and scarring may result. Urethral strictures may lead to hydronephrosis, while epididymitis may cause sterility. Other complications that may occur from gonococcal bacteremia include suppurative arthritis, acute bacterial endocarditis, and suppurative meningitis.

Conclusive diagnosis must be made on the basis of cultures because there are no serology tests for diagnosis. Culture media usually contain antibiotics to inhibit other bacterial growth and should be placed in an atmosphere of increased carbon dioxide. Bacterial growth should be apparent within 24 to 48 hours if gonorrheal organisms are present.

Treatment with penicillin is instituted immediately and is usually curative. In persons sensitive to penicillin or with gonococcal strains resistant to penicillin, other antibiotics such as tetracycline may be used. Cultures should be repeated after treatment to ensure the eradication of the gonococcus organism. Sexual partners should be treated concurrently and intercourse should be avoided until repeat cultures indicate a cure. Single infection with the gonococcus organism does not confer immunity.

Syphilis

Syphilis is less common than gonorrhea but more serious. Serologic screening has been successful in detecting syphilis, resulting in a dramatic decline of the disease in the 1950s. It is estimated that 70 percent of the cases remain unreported. In 1984, 90,000 cases were reported [4].

The causative organism in syphilis is the spirochete *Treponema pallidum*. Due to its size, the spirochete is visible only with darkfield microscopy. It is sensitive to both drying and temperature and normally enters the skin through moist mucous membranes. It has also been known to enter through breaks in the skin. Transmission may be through sexual contact, by personal contact, or by an infected mother to her unborn fetus.

The course of untreated syphilis progresses in three stages: primary, secondary, and tertiary. Within 24 hours after the spirochete has entered the body, it spreads throughout. Primary syphilis develops after an incubation period of 10 days to 3 months. The first symptom, a chancre, appears at the site of entry. The chancre is usually a painless, hardened lesion that may resemble a pimple (Fig. 55-2). It may go undetected at this stage, and results of serology tests are normal. Infection is highly contagious at this time and the chancre usually disappears within two to six weeks with or without treatment. At this point blood remains contagious. Diagnosis is based on identification of the spirochete from the ulceration.

The second stage appears at variable times up to six months later. It begins with the development of a generalized, usually maculopapular rash, especially on the palms of the hands and soles of the feet. Other lesions may be follicular, pustular, or scaling. Large elevated plaques, termed *condylomata lata* (wartlike, flattened areas), develop on the genitalia. Secondary syphilis may also be characterized by fever, headaches, loss of appetite, sore mouth, and loss of hair. Generalized lymphadenopathy also occurs. Spirochetes are present in all lesions, especially condylomata lata. Syphilis in this stage remains highly contagious and spirochetes may even cross the placenta to an unborn baby. Approximately 4 to 12 weeks after the beginning of the second stage, all symptoms disappear and the disease enters a latent period. Results of serology tests at this time are usually positive. After the latent period, syphilis may be cured spontaneously, remain latent permanently, or enter the third stage.

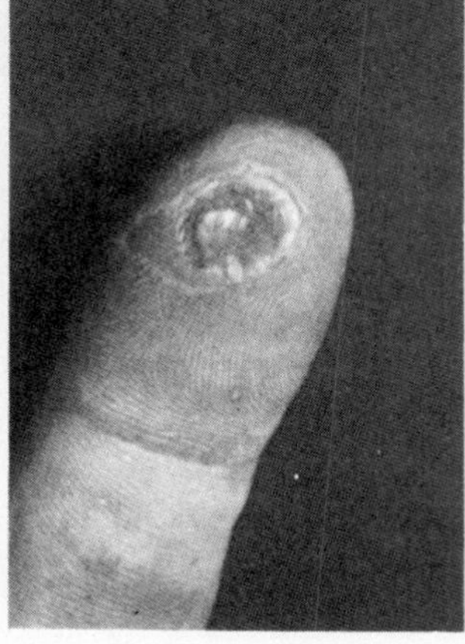

A B

FIGURE 55-2 A. Primary stage syphilis chancre on the penis. B. Primary chancre on a finger. (From *Sexually Transmitted Diseases* by D. Barlow, photographed by Tom Treasure. Published by Oxford University Press. © 1979 by David Barlow. Printed with permission of Oxford University Press.)

After a period of several years the condition progresses to tertiary syphilis and eventually is no longer contagious. About two-thirds of infected persons remain symptom-free; however, results of serology tests may remain positive and the spirochetes can affect an unborn fetus if an infected woman becomes pregnant. For the other one-third, the disease progresses and develops into late clinical syphilis. It can affect any body part, especially the heart and central nervous system. Chronic inflammation of bones and joints may also occur. Gummas, large necrotic areas, may develop in the liver, bones, and testes. Gummatous lesions in the central nervous system are rare, but meningovascular syphilis commonly causes infiltration of the meninges and blood vessels by lymphocytes and plasma cells [5]. Neurosyphilis involves the loss of cortical neurons due to large numbers of spirochetes throughout the brain parenchyma. The effect of neurosyphilis is dementia and behavioral changes that progress to psychotic behavior and ataxic paresthesias. Finally, loss of position, deep pain, and temperature sensation occur. The average interval from infection to symptomatic neurosyphilis is 20 to 30 years.

Infection with *T. pallidum* confers immunity on the infected person. Both syphilitic reagin and treponemal immobilizing serum antibodies are produced after one to four months. Treponemal immobilizing antibodies are specific and probably account for the active immunity. Syphilitic reagin is the basis for both the complement fixation and flocculation diagnostic tests.

In the early stages diagnosis is made only by darkfield microscopy. After the antigen-antibody reaction has occurred, serology tests such as the VDRL, FTA-ABS (fluorescent treponemal antibody-absorption), TPI (*Treponema pallidum* immobilization), TPHA (*Treponema pallidum* hemoagglutinin assay), and RPR (rapid plasma reagin) can be used. The VDRL is the most widely used because of cost and simplicity; however, both false positive and false negative results are likely to occur with this test. The next most favorable is the PTA-ABS. The TPHA and RPR are used for screening large populations.

The treatment of choice for syphilis is penicillin. It must be given in doses appropriate to the stage of disease. In persons with known sensitivity to penicillin, the choice is tetracycline. Because of its teratogenic effect, tetracycline should not be administered to pregnant women. In these cases, the treatment of choice becomes erythromycin. Treatment should be initiated at any point of diagnosis during pregnancy to prevent additional damage to the fetus.

Genital Herpes

Genital herpes, the second most common of the primary sexually transmitted diseases, is a highly contagious condition caused by the herpesvirus hominis (HVH) type 2, one of the herpes simplex viruses. Type 1 refers to the common cold sore or fever blister that occurs primarily above the waist. After incubation of 3 to 7 days, HVH type 2 produces single or multiple vesicles that rupture spontaneously after 24 to 72 hours. Painful, reddened ulcers develop that eventually scab, heal, and disappear (Fig. 55-3). The virus then remains dormant in the nerve cells, and sores appear whenever it is triggered to multiply. Factors known to trigger outbreak of symptoms include colds, fever, severe sunburn, menstruation, gastrointestinal upset, and stress.

The first attack of genital herpes is usually the worst and is characterized by small, extremely painful blisters. Prior to the appearance of blisters, the individual may notice a tingling or burning sensation possibly followed by intense itching. In the male, lesions of 0.5 to 1.5 cm are present on the glans penis, prepuce, buttocks, and inner thighs. Secondary infection may occur when the blisters rupture. In both sexes the initial infection may be accompanied by fever, swelling, enlarged painful lymph nodes, and in the male, dysuria. Fever and enlarged lymph nodes are less likely to occur with subsequent attacks.

There is no known cure for herpes. Several agents have been used with varying success. These include iodine solutions, chloroform, immunotherapy, bacillus Calmette-Guerin vaccine, nitrous oxide, ether, and photoinactivation with a light-sensitive dye and fluorescent light. The most frequently used drug at the present time is acyclovir (Zovirax). Alone it is inactive. When in contact with the virus it is converted to an active form by an enzyme, thymidine kinase, produced by the virus. It hastens healing and decreases transmissibility, but has no effect on recurrence.

Herpes infection can be painful and annoying to the man or woman; however, it can represent a life-threatening situation to an unborn fetus. This disease can produce abortion or premature delivery. Genital herpes is highly contagious when the vesicles rupture, and delivery through an infected vagina increases the chance that the infection will be passed to the infant. Herpes infection in a newborn can produce brain damage or death. Therefore, a cesarean birth is advisable in any woman with active genital herpes. Another primary concern for women with herpesvirus is the increased risk of cervical cancer. It is now suspected that herpes may be a factor in the development of cervical cancer [6].

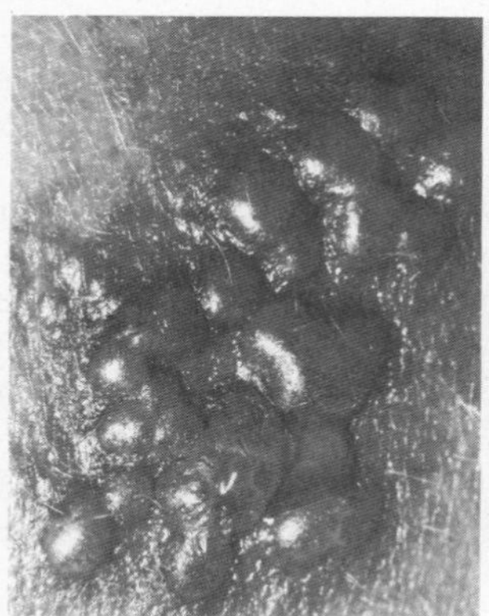

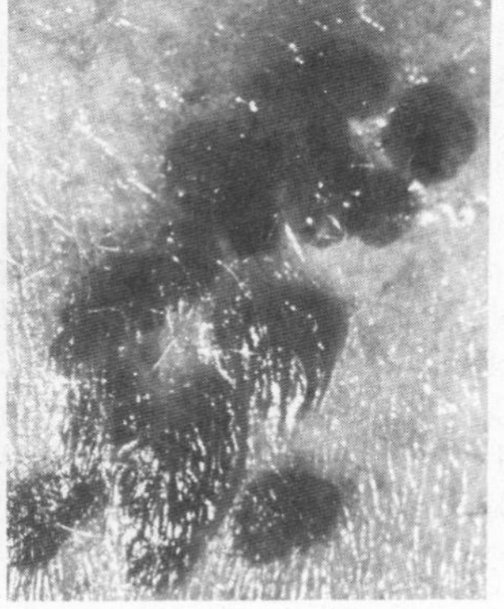

A B

Figure 55-3 A. Genital herpes blisters before treatment. B. Blisters after four days of treatment with intravaginal and topical 2-deoxy-D-glucose. (From H. Blough and R. Giuntoli, "Successful Treatment of Human Genital Herpes with 2-deoxy-D-Glucose," *Journal of the American Medical Association* 241:2798–2801, 1979, p. 2799, figure 2. Copyright 1979, American Medical Association.)

Chancroid

Chancroid is an acute disease process that produces a soft chancre, or shallow, ragged ulcer, after an incubation period of up to 10 days. This condition is prevalent worldwide, especially in Southeast Asia, Africa, and South America. It is caused by the gram-negative bacillus, *Hemophilus ducreyi*. Regional lymph nodes may become swollen and tender. Suppuration from lymph nodes and the necrotic chancre occur. Gram's stain of exudate, culture, and biopsy aid in diagnosis. Erythromycin or sulfisoxazole (Gantrisin) and good hygiene allow healing in two to four weeks.

Granuloma Inguinale

Granuloma inguinale is a chronic disease process caused by the gram-negative bacillus *Donovania granulomatis*. It begins as a papule and progresses to a spreading necrotic ulcer with extensive scarring. It has a low degree of infectivity and progressively involves the skin and lymphatics of the groin and inguinal areas. Smears and biopsy aid in differentiation from other STDs. Antibiotic treatment with tetracycline usually results in complete healing. Gentamycin and chloramphenicol have also been used in treatment of granuloma inguinale.

Lymphogranuloma Venereum

This condition is caused by a strain of *Chlamydia* organisms. It is characterized by a small, painless papule or vesicle that appears after an incubation of less than three weeks. Spontaneous healing usually occurs after several days. Within two to eight weeks painful lymphatic involvement occurs with possible obstruction. Malaise, fever, and headache may also be noted. In addition to history and physical examination, aspiration of lymph for complement fixation and skin test with Frei antigen may be performed to confirm the diagnosis. Treatment of lymphogranuloma venereum includes erythromycin and tetracycline.

Sexually Transmitted Infections

Trichomonal Vaginitis

Trichomoniasis is a vaginal infection caused by the single-celled protozoan *Trichomonas vaginalis* (Fig. 55-4A). The organism may remain dormant for extended periods of time and prefers a basic vaginal pH. It has been identified in the male urethra and prostate, so sexual contact serves as a frequent source of reinfection for the female.

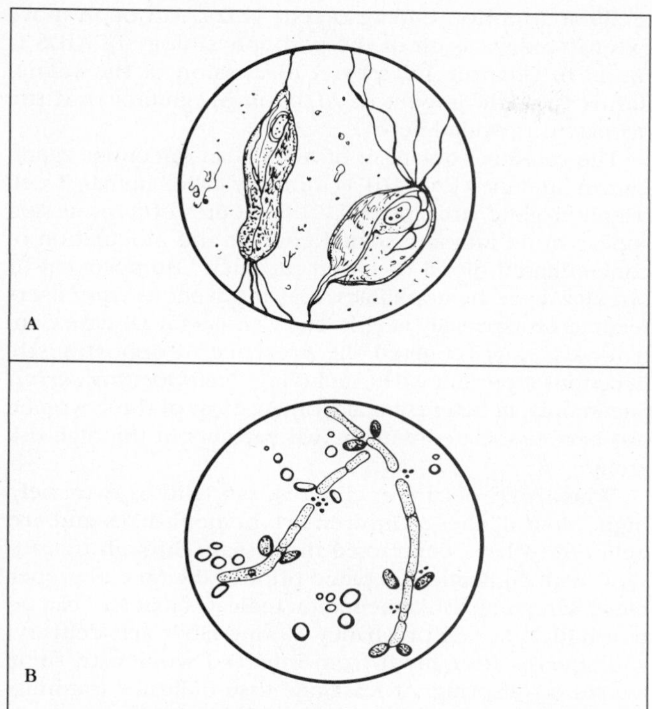

FIGURE 55-4 Fresh vaginal smear preparations. A. Microscopic appearance of *Trichomonas vaginalis* organisms. B. Microscopic picture in candidal vaginitis. (From T.H. Green, Jr., *Gynecology: Essentials of Clinical Practice* [3rd ed.]. Boston: Little, Brown, 1977.)

The frequency of *Trichomonas* infection is highest in women with many sexual partners.

The organism produces an intense itching and burning of the vulva and vagina. It is accompanied by a moderate to profuse discharge that is thin, frothy, greenish yellow to greenish white with a foul odor. Examination of the cervix may reveal small, deep, red spots referred to as strawberry spots. Microscopic examination of a wet smear reveals the one-cell protozoan with four flagellae. Cultures are rarely done to confirm the diagnosis.

The treatment of choice is a trichomonacidal drug, metronidazole. It is effective in eradicating the organism in 90 percent of cases. It may be accompanied by severe side effects and should be used only after confirmed diagnosis of *Trichomonas*. Side effects of the drug include leukopenia, nausea, diarrhea, headache, and alcohol intolerance. The drug has been found to produce cancer in mice and birth defects in guinea pigs and mice. Therefore, its use is avoided in pregnant women or those suspected of being pregnant. Alternative treatment includes AVC cream or suppositories, Aci-Jel, and iodoquinol.

Candidiasis

Candidiasis is a vaginal infection produced by the fungus *Candida albicans* (Fig. 55-4B). It is also referred to as moniliasis, thrush, and yeast infection. The organism normally is present on the skin and in the digestive tract and may colonize the vagina of some asymptomatic women. Symptoms arise when there is an overgrowth of the organism, which occurs most frequently during pregnancy, after antibiotic therapy, in diabetics, and in women taking oral contraceptives. Infants may become infected at delivery and develop thrush. In pregnant women and those taking oral contraceptives, estrogen levels are high, resulting in high glycogen levels that produce a favorable environment for fungal growth. It is believed that systemic antibiotics also suppress the normal bacterial flora in the vagina, and in diabetics the vaginal environment is "sweeter," both of which encourage fungal growth. The yeast infection produces a heavy, white, cottage cheeselike discharge that is odorless. Complaints of severe itching, dysuria, dyspareunia, and perineal burning are common. The vulva appears erythematous and inflamed. Speculum examination may reveal white plaques on the vaginal wall. Diagnosis is confirmed by wet smear examination with potassium hydroxide.

Antifungal preparations such as nystatin, miconazole, and clotrimazole are the treatments of choice. These medications are used as topical drugs and inserted into the vagina where they exert a local action on the organism. Absorption is poor from the skin and mucous membrane in the vagina. Gentian violet swabs and suppositories may also be used, but they produce staining and sometimes allergic reactions. Taking lactobacillus tablets and eating yogurt may be helpful in restoring the normal bacterial flora after antibiotic therapy.

Hemophilus vaginalis *Vaginitis*

Hemophilus vaginalis, formerly referred to as *Gardnerella*, has now been identified as one causative organism in vaginitis previously referred to as nonspecific vaginitis. It is a gram-negative bacillus similar to *Corynebacterium vaginalis*. It is spread through sexual contact and elimination of the infection requires treatment of both sexual partners.

The most outstanding symptom is a thin, heavy, gray discharge with the presence of only mild irritation. Diagnosis is made by identifying cells dotted with small, short bacilli. Cultures may be done for additional confirmation. Ampicillin or tetracycline may be administered orally for systemic effect. Milder cases may be treated with sulfonamide creams or suppositories such as sulfathiazole, sulfisoxazole or nitrofurazone. Metronidazole may also be used.

Chlamydia trachomatis

Chlamydia are the most common sexually transmitted organisms in the United States today, having surpassed even gonorrhea. It has been estimated that as many as 3 to 4 million persons suffer from chlamydial infections [1]. It has been noted most often in the younger population, especially in sexually active adolescents.

The causative organism in chlamydial infections is *Chlamydia trachomatis*, an intracellular bacterial parasite. Definitive diagnosis is based on cultures, which are time consuming and expensive to perform. Clinical diagnosis is more often based on documentation of urethritis with discharge or symptoms of cervicitis when gonorrhea has been ruled out. Gram's stains may indicate the presence of polymorphonuclear leukocytes.

The most outstanding symptoms involve the genitourinary system. Males are most likely to have urinary symptoms. Symptoms in the female include lower abdominal pain, vaginal discharge, dysuria, and vaginal bleeding. Some females may be asymptomatic. Discharge, when present, may be very heavy, with a fishy odor. The discharge is gray-white and creamy, and is usually not accompanied by itching or irritation. Examination of the cervix may reveal congestion, mucopurulent discharge, or ectopy. Acute salpingitis, conjunctivitis, and repeated sore throats may be noted in females.

Chlamydial infections are usually controlled with antibiotics, including erythromycin and tetracycline, but not penicillin. If left untreated, they can result in pelvic inflammatory disease with salpingitis. The newborn may acquire the disease through contact with an infected birth canal. The disease in the newborn may result in conjunctivitis or pneumonia. Treatment for chlamydial infection also requires treatment of the sexual partner. Lack of treatment in the partner may result in reinfection of the woman.

Condylomata Accuminata

Condylomata accuminata is also referred to as venereal warts. The causative organism is *human papillomavirus*. Symptoms include cauliflowerlike lesions on the introitus, vulva, or rectum. Anyone with external growths should be examined for lesions within the vagina, cervix, or rectum.

Diagnosis is based upon clinical appearance and/or history of sexual contact with an infected individual. Biopsy may be performed to rule out vulvar tumors and a VDRL test may be performed to rule out the condylomata lata found in secondary syphilis.

Condylomata accuminata lesions are treated with podophyllin (20–25%) in tincture of benzoin. This solution should be applied to all lesions at weekly intervals until the lesions are resolved. Podophyllin is a corrosive solution and should be washed off within two to four hours of the initial application. Length of application may be increased with subsequent treatments provided there is no adverse effect. Vaseline may be used to protect the surrounding normal tissue. Cautery or surgical excision may be performed depending on size of the lesions. Concurrent treatment of sexual partners may help prevent recurrence.

Acquired Immune Deficiency Syndrome

The multiplicity of transmission routes has contributed to the controversy over the status of acquired immune deficiency syndrome (AIDS) as a sexually transmitted disease. This syndrome, first identified in 1979, has received much medical attention during recent years. Although more extensive discussion of the pathophysiology of AIDS is found in Chapter 11, a brief discussion of the sexual nature and the impact of AIDS on pregnancy and the neonate is provided here.

The causative organism of AIDS is an infectious agent, human immune virus (HIV) (formerly called human T cell lymphotrophic virus, or HTLV III). Routes of transmission appear to be intimate sexual contact and inoculation of contaminated blood or blood products. Homosexual or bisexual men, hemophiliacs, and intravenous drug users seem to be especially at risk. The Centers for Disease Control have now reported the presence of opportunistic infections typical of AIDS, including *Pneumocystis carinii* pneumonia, in heterosexual women. Most of these women had been associated with sexual partners in the high-risk group.

When AIDS occurs in children, mortality is extremely high. Most of these children are hemophiliacs and are believed to have contracted the disease through transfusions with contaminated blood prior to the time of proper blood screening. Documentation indicates that HIV can be transmitted during pregnancy, during labor and delivery, and shortly after birth from infected women to their fetuses or offspring. At least one case indicates transmission of the virus through breast milk [3]. Additional studies are needed to identify the true rate and route of perinatal transmission.

Study Questions

1. Compare the causative agents, clinical manifestations, and courses of gonorrhea and syphilis.
2. Describe the appearance of genital herpes and explain how recurrences can be triggered. What is the effect of this condition on the unborn fetus?
3. How do infections caused by fungi and protozoa differ in general from those caused by bacteria?
4. List some precipitating causes of chronic vaginal infection.
5. Discuss the causative agent and transmission of AIDS.

References

1. Centers for Disease Control. *Chlamydia trachomatis* infections: Policy guidelines for prevention and control. *Morbidity and Mortality Weekly Report Supplement* 34(3S):4, 1985.
2. Centers for Disease Control. 1985 STD treatment guidelines. *Morbidity and Mortality Weekly Report Supplement* 34(4S):10, 1985.
3. Centers for Disease Control. Recommendations of human T-ymphotropic virus type III/lymphadenopathy associated virus and acquired immunodeficiency syndrome. *Morbidity and Mortality Weekly Report* 34:721, 1985.
4. An epidemic of sex diseases. *Newsweek on Health* 4:16, 1985.
5. Robbins, S.L., Cotran, R.S., and Kumar, V. *Pathologic Basis of Disease* (3rd ed.). Philadelphia: Saunders, 1984.
6. Tyler, S.L., and Woodall, G.M. *Female Health and Gynecology: Across the Lifespan*. Bowie, Md.: Brady, 1982.

Unit Bibliography

American Cancer Society. *Cancer Facts and Figures*. New York: American Cancer Society, 1986.

Athey, P.A., and Hadlock, E.P. *Ultrasound in Obstetrics and Gynecology*. St. Louis: Mosby, 1981.

Beacham, D.W. and Beacham, W.D. *Synopsis of Gynecology* (10th ed.). St. Louis: Mosby, 1982.

Benson, R.C. *Current Obstetric and Gynecologic Diagnosis and Treatment* (5th ed.). Los Altos, Ca.: Lange Medical Publications, 1984.

Bettoli, E.J. Herpes: Facts and fallacies. *Am. J. Nurs.* 82:924, 1982.

Brown, R.B. *Clinical Urology Illustrated*. New York: ADIS Press, 1982.

Campbell, C.E., and Herten, R.J. VD to STD: Redefining venereal disease. *Am. J. Nurs.* 81:1629, 1981.

Clark, A.L., Affonso, D.D., and Harris, T.R. *Childbearing: A Nursing Perspective* (2nd ed.). Philadelphia: Davis, 1979.

Conklin, M., et al. Should health teaching include self-examination of the testes? *Am. J. Nurs.* 78:2073, 1978.

Danforth, D.N. and Scott, J.R. *Obstetrics and Gynecology* (5th ed.). Philadelphia: Lippincott, 1986.

DiSala, P.J. and Creasman, W.T. *Clinical Gynecologic Oncology* (2nd ed.). St. Louis: Mosby, 1984.

Downie, J., Poyser, N.L., and Wunderlich, M. Levels of prostaglandins in the human endometrium during the normal menstrual cycle. *J. Physiol.* 236:465, 1974.

Dwyer, J.M. *Human Reproduction: The Female System and the Neonate.* Philadelphia: Davis, 1976.

Edwards, M.S. Venereal herpes: A nursing overview. *J. Obstet. Gynecol. Neonat. Nurs.* 7:7, 1978.

Green, T.H., Jr., *Gynecology: Essentials of Clinical Practice* (3rd ed.). Boston: Little, Brown, 1977.

Guyton, A.C. *Textbook of Medical Physiology* (7th ed.). Philadelphia: Saunders, 1986.

Himmell, K. Genital herpes: The need for counseling. *J. Obstet. Gynecol. Neonat. Nurs.* 10:446, 1981.

Jones, A.G., and Hoeft, R.T. Cancer of the prostate. *Am. J. Nurs.* 82:826, 1982.

Kistner, R.W. *Gynecology: Principles and Practice* (4th ed.). Chicago: Yearbook, 1986.

Kolodny, R.C., et al. *Textbook of Human Sexuality for Nurses*. Boston: Little, Brown, 1979.

Lipshultz, L.I., and Howards, S.S. *Infertility in the Male*. Edinburgh: Churchill Livingstone, 1983.

Martin, L.L. *Health Care of Women*. Philadelphia: Lippincott, 1978.

Masters, W.H., and Johnson, V.E. *Human Sexual Response*. Boston: Little, Brown, 1966.

Miller, M.A., and Brooten, D.A. *The Childbearing Family: A Nursing Perspective* (2nd ed.). Boston: Little, Brown, 1983.

Pardue, S.F. Hydatidiform mole: A pathological pregnancy. *Am. J. Nurs.* 77:836, 1977.

Parsons, L., and Sommers, S.C. *Gynecology* (2nd ed.). Philadelphia: Saunders, 1978.

Pritchard, J.A., MacDonald, P.C., and Gant, N.F. *William's Obstetrics* (7th ed.). Norwalk, Conn.: Appleton-Century-Crofts, 1985.

Robbins, S.L., Cotran, R.V., and Kumar, V. *Pathologic Basis of Disease* (3rd ed.). Philadelphia: Saunders, 1984.

Romney, S.L., et al. *Gynecology and Obstetrics: The Health Care of Women*. New York: McGraw-Hill, 1975.

Schuster, C.S., and Ashburn, S.S. *The Process of Human Development: A Holistic Approach* (2nd ed.). Boston: Little, Brown, 1986.

Selkurt, E.E. (ed.). *Basic Physiology for the Health Sciences* (2nd ed.). Boston: Little, Brown, 1982.

Simpson, J.L. *Disorders of Sexual Differentiation: Etiology and Clinical Delineation*. New York: Academic, 1977.

Sloane, E. *Biology of Women*. New York: Wiley, 1980.

Smith, D.R. *General Urology* (11th ed.). Los Altos, Ca.: Lange Medical Publishers, 1984.

Stewart, F.H., et al. *My Body, My Health: The Concerned Woman's Guide to Gynecology*. New York: Wiley, 1979.

Sutton, H.E. *An Introduction to Human Genetics* (2nd ed.). New York: Holt, Rinehart & Winston, 1975.

Thompson, H.E., and Bernstine, R.L. *Diagnostic Ultrasound in Clinical Obstetrics and Gynecology*. New York: Wiley, 1978.

Tobiason, S.J. Benign prostatic hypertrophy. *Am. J. Nurs*. 79:286, 1979.

Walsh, P.C., et al. *Campbell's Urology* (5th ed.). Philadelphia: Saunders, 1986.

Whaley, L.F., and Wong, D.L. *Nursing Care of Infants and Children*. St. Louis: Mosby, 1979.

Widmann, F.K. *Clinical Interpretation of Laboratory Tests* (8th ed.). Philadelphia: Davis, 1979.

Willson, J.R., and Carrington, E.R. *Obstetrics and Gynecology* (6th ed.). St. Louis: Mosby, 1979.

Wroblewski, S.S. Toxic shock syndrome. *Am. J. Nurs.* 81:82, 1981.

Yen, S.S.C., and Jaffe, R.B. *Reproductive Endocrinology: Physiology, Pathophysiology and Clinical Management*. Philadelphia: Saunders, 1978.

Ziegel, E.E., and Cranley, M.S. *Obstetric Nursing* (7th ed.). New York: Macmillan, 1978.

UNIT 17

Aging

Gretchen S. McDaniel

Aging is not a disease process but is the result of yearly wear and tear on the systems of the body. It is associated, perhaps inevitably, with an increase in disease. The development of disease in the aged is highly individualized and related to predisposing factors such as heredity, culture, race, and nutritional status. Chapter 56 presents some of the theories of aging and a summary of biologic effects of aging on the body systems. The timetable of changes varies with individuals, but as age progresses, certain general alterations occur almost universally.

This disucssion of aging organizes pathologic processes that occur in the aged person. Each of these changes is discussed in greater depth in other units in the text. Readers are encouraged in their study of the learning objectives to refer to other chapters in the book that discuss each pathologic process. Study questions at the end of the chapter allow for synthesis of learning concepts.

CHAPTER 56

Aging

CHAPTER OUTLINE

Biologic Theories of Aging

- Free Radical Theory
- Waste Product Theory
- Immunologic Theory
- Cross-Link Theory
- Genetic Aging Theory

Biologic Effects of Aging on Body Systems

- General Effects
- Nervous System
- Cardiovascular System
    - *Anatomic Changes*
    - *Physiologic Changes*
    - *Conduction System Changes*
    - *Arterial Changes*
    - *Venular Changes*
    - *Hypertension*
- Respiratory System
    - *Anatomic Changes*
    - *Functional Changes*
- Genitourinary System
    - *Anatomic Changes in the Kidneys*
    - *Physiologic Changes in the Kidneys*
    - *Diseases and Problems with Aging Kidneys*
    - *Bladder Changes*
    - *Gynecologic Changes in the Elderly Woman*
    - *Sexual Changes in the Elderly Man*
- Gastrointestinal System
    - *Normal Anatomic Changes*
    - *Esophageal Changes*
    - *Stomach Changes*
    - *Colon Changes*
- Musculoskeletal System
    - *Characteristic Changes in Anatomic Structure and Function*
    - *Joint Changes*
    - *Osteoporosis*
    - *Fractures and Risk of Falling*
- Skin and Dermal Appendages
    - *Changes in the Skin, Nails, and Hair*
- Sensory System
    - *Vision Changes*
    - *Hearing Changes*
    - *Other Sensory Changes*

Drugs and the Elderly

Aging and Cancer

LEARNING OBJECTIVES

1. Discuss important research on the aging process.
2. Describe the biologic cellular theories: free radical, waste product, cross-link, immunologic, and genetic aging theories.
3. List the general effects of aging.
4. Describe the causes and effects of nervous system alterations.
5. Relate anatomic alterations in the cardiovascular system to the resultant physiologic changes.
6. Describe how the arterial changes in the elderly alter blood flow and pressure.
7. Discuss causes and effects of hypertension in the elderly.
8. Describe the physiologic result of respiratory changes due to aging.
9. Explain why elderly persons are at risk for the development of respiratory failure after stressful situations.
10. Compare renal function of the young adult with that of the elderly.
11. List common organisms that can cause bladder infection in the elderly.
12. Describe the effects of lack of estrogen in postmenopausal women.
13. Describe the effects of hormone changes in elderly men.
14. Discuss briefly the many factors that cause digestive disturbances in the elderly.
15. Characterize the alterations in body movement that occur as a consequence of aging.
16. Explain the factors that lead to increased risk of bone fractures in the elderly.
17. List the joint changes that are common in the elderly, at what age they begin, and when they become symptomatic.
18. Describe the characteristic changes in skin, nails, and hair associated with aging.
19. Explain how sensory alterations affect adjustment in the aging process.
20. Discuss the factors associated with aging that cause alterations in drug metabolism.
21. List at least two cancers that are more common in the elderly than in the younger population.

The causes of aging have been investigated for centuries, yet no researcher has been able specifically to identify any single causative factor. More questions are being asked and research has intensified as people live to an older age. It is very difficult to define what aging is or to establish the facts about the process. Much of the confusion arises from the difficulty of distinguishing between normal aging and changes secondary to disease. Health and longevity are affected by a number of factors, such as heredity, culture, race, and nutrition.

Science and medicine have concentrated on preventing and curing illness in the earlier stages of life, which has resulted in an increased life expectancy in the United States. Worldwide, however, the lifespan of human beings has not increased. The variability of life span seems to be a function of genetic and environmental factors. Total life span seems to be limited to 90 to 105 years, however, regardless of mitigating circumstances. This limitation supports the belief that aging is an innate process.

In the elderly, more often than not, several problems are present simultaneously. Degenerative changes and certain diseases worsen with age and can be superimposed one on the other. Two of these age-related changes are altered temperature response and pain perception. In the older person, elevation in temperature may not occur or may occur late in the presence of an acute infection. Pain, may be looked on as a burden of old age and not as an important indicator of disease.

Elderly persons are more prone to infections than are younger persons because of alterations in the circulatory system and insufficiencies in immune factors. The production of antibodies that fight disease is depressed partially because their production is somewhat dependent on nutritional supply. Many elderly persons do not have a nutritious diet and therefore do not have optimal nutritional reserves for antibody production. Also important in lowered resistance to infection are the degenerative changes that occur in the immune system with advancing years [25]. The elderly are susceptible to an increased frequency of various infectious diseases and have a higher mortality as a result.

Biologic Theories of Aging

Until the nineteenth century, most of the interest in the aging process was concerned with ways to prevent it. The ancient Egyptians tried to find the fountain of youth. Hippocrates (c. 460–377 B.C.) perceived aging as stemming from a decrease in body heat, a natural, irreversible, and unavoidable phenomenon. Galen (c. 130-201 A.D.) had a similar theory postulating that the increased coldness and dryness of aging resulted from changes in body humor. Leonardo da Vinci stimulated later development of theories of biologic aging through his descriptions and drawings [10].

One of the main problems encountered in researching theories is the fact that so many of them were developed with the biases of several disciplines, rather than with an objective, interdisciplinary approach. Biology, sociology, and psychology all arrived at different explanations for the changes that occur with the aging process. Some theories have been thoroughly researched and verified, whereas others do not enjoy the support of clinical testing or the acceptance of the medical community.

Humans age biologically, psychologically, and sociologically [3]. To understand differences among theories of aging it is necessary to examine these processes that take place within the aging organism. Of importance to research is the number of times cells replicate themselves [24]. Findings that have since been confirmed have shown that the number of times normal diploid human fibroblasts can replicate themselves in vitro is limited. Hayflick reported, "The sum of population doublings undergone by normal fetal human fibroblasts both before and after preservation is always equal to 50 ± 10" [24]. Cells isolated from older persons show progressively fewer doublings before finally stopping.

Other researchers noted that the homeostatic mechanisms that govern immunity and cell replication decrease as a person grows older. Both cell division and ribonucleic acid (RNA) synthesis of protein slow down. There is also increasing heterogenicity of cells in terms of size, shape, and mitotic capabilities.

Common in metabolism of the older person is increased collagen cross-linking. Cross-linkages are stable molecules that prevent deoxyribonucleic acid (DNA) strands from dividing in the normal cell reproductive cycle. Cross-linkage molecules accumulate and affect proteins in elastin and collagen, resulting in cell death. The cell death results in decreased elasticity of blood vessels and skin [17].

This section describes three biologic cellular theories. No one theory answers all the questions, but each provides a clue to the aging process and certain interrelationships that do appear to exist.

Free Radical Theory

The free radical theory has been described as a unitary approach to the study of the phenomena of aging. It proposes that free radicals serve as central agents in the changes observed with aging at the tissue, cellular, and subcellular levels [25]. Free radicals are parts of molecules that have broken off or molecules that have had an electron stripped from their structure. Free radicals are a normal part of metabolic reactions that form part of a structural system and are not free to diffuse within the cells. Diffusible free radicals damage or alter the original structure or function of other molecules by attaching themselves to them [25]. The free radical theory has been linked to the idea of oxygen toxicity. Oxidation of protein, fat, carbohydrate, and other elements in the body results in the formation of these free radicals [11]. Diffusible free radical end products and compounds can cause cellular disruption. In the aging process, the number of free radical compounds appears to increase faster than body cells can repair the damage. Some scientists consider the cell membrane as the key to survival and believe that the greatest damage could be perpetrated by free radicals at this level [14].

When DNA is irradiated, for example, it responds with free radical formation and establishes aberrant cellular development. Vitamin E and coenzyme Q are thought to protect the mitochondria from the hazards of the free radical activity. Vitamin E may function as an antioxidant and binding agent in the antioxidation process, which supports the use of antioxidants such as vitamin E in an attempt to delay cellular aging [32].

Free radical activity is also fostered in the body by such environmental factors as smog, by-products of the plastics industry, gasoline, and atmospheric ozone. The human body appears to be bombarded from both external and internal sources of free radicals. If this theory is as fundamental to aging as proponents believe, careful monitoring of the environment and proper food selection should lead to better health in old age.

Waste Product Theory

The waste product theory is derived as a result of observing increased pigment in aging cells. The pigment, called *lipofuscin*, is a dark, irregular, granular inclusion within cells [11]. There is some evidence that lipofuscin occurs in cells as a result of a variety of processes such as autophagocytosis, oxidation of lipids, and copolymerization of organic molecules [36]. It has been suggested that lipofuscin forms as an end product of free radical-induced lipid peroxidation. This suggestion provides a connection between oxygen consumption, free radicals, lipofuscin, and aging [37]. The actual effect of lipofuscin on cell function is not known.

Immunologic Theory

The immunologic theory asserts that aging is an autoimmune process. The body's immune system fails to recognize its own cells as the cells change with age. Autoimmune responses damage or destroy cells, leading to cell death [17]. Tissue damage and increased susceptibility to infection may be caused by the presence of autoantibodies and decreased numbers of immunocompetent cells (see Unit 5). Whether or not the diminished capacity for immune responses is a cause of aging is not known, but it certainly is the source of many of the disease problems of the aged, such as increased frequency of autoimmune disease, cancer, and infections of all types.

Aging affects all parts of the immune system, but especially the T cells. A decline in T cell-dependent immune function begins at sexual maturity with the onset of involution of the thymus gland. This factor is associated with increased frequency of diseases such as cancer and autoimmune diseases. Macrophages that play a major role in protecting the body against infection do not seem to diminish in number as the body ages. The B cell number remain elevated, but responsiveness to stimulation by antigens decreases markedly, probably because of dependence on T cell stimulation.

The involution of the thymus gland appears to be the key to the aging of the immune system. Whether it is caused by the changing hypothalmic regulation or factors intrinsic to the cells of the gland itself remains unknown.

Cross-Link Theory

"The cross-link theory, sometimes called the collagen theory, suggests that strong chemical reactions create strong bonds between molecular structures that are normally separate. Cross-link agents are so numerous and varied in the diet and in the environment that they are impossible to avoid" [14]. Connective tissue changes are an indicator that cross-linkage has occurred. Collagen, which makes up a large part of the proteins of the body, is the substance that maintains strength, support, and structural form. As a result of the chemical action of cross-linkage, aging collagens become more insoluble and rigid, resulting in inhibition of cell permeability. Passage of nutrients, metabolites, antibodies, and gases through the blood vessel walls is inhibited. The linings of the lungs and gastrointestinal tract are also affected.

Elastin, another of the fibrillar proteins present in connective tissue, is very prone to cross-linkage. It differs from collagen on the basis of its chemical composition and physical properties. Both elastin and collagen respond to cross-linkage in the same manner. Aging elastin becomes frayed, fragmented, and brittle, leading to many changes in connective tissue throughout the body. A good example of this is skin changes, such as loss of turgor, elasticity, and tone, and dryness. Cross-linkage also affects cell division because its molecules prevents division of the strands of the DNA. If only one strand is affected, no damage results. If the cross-link molecule attaches itself to both sides of the DNA, the cell dies because division is prevented. Such cell death has a profound effect on the elasticity of blood vessels and skin. As a result of the changes in collagen and elastin, cross-linkage is thought to be a primary cause of aging.

Genetic Aging Theory

The genetic aging theory is based on the belief that the life span is programmed before birth into the genes in the DNA molecule. This means that a person fortunate enough to have long-lived parents or grandparents has a life expectancy longer than it would have been with short-lived parents. Gender also makes a difference in predicting longevity, as built-in genetic material seems to favor the female. In all countries of the world women live longer than men by approximately six years. Race is also a factor in predicting longevity. Whites of both sexes have a longer life expectancy than blacks [19].

Biologic Effects of Aging on Body Systems

Many physical and chemical changes that occur as a person ages have been identified through research, even though the exact causes of aging cannot be isolated. Some of the changes are harmful in that they interfere with the healthy function of cells and tissues. Others have not been found to be harmful.

Aging leads to a gradual diminution in the functional capacity of the organ systems. It must be realized, however, that the process is extremely variable among different individuals. Chronologic age, therefore, is a poor index of physiologic age or of performance, and advancing years are not necessarily equated with illness. If one problem is identified, however, others must be looked for because several diseases are characteristic of the elderly [29].

General Effects

The appearance of the aging person characteristically is altered. Stature is lost, body proportions are changed, skin is dry and wrinkled, hair is thinning and gray, and there are changes in body movement characterized by slowness, stiffness, and diminished coordination and balance. The intervertebral disks become thin, as do the vertebrae themselves, leading to reduction in height. The thoracic curve of the vertebral column increases, resulting in a kyphosis. This plus changes in lung elasticity result in increased anterioposterior diameter of the chest. The cervical curve increases to compensate for the thoracic curve, causing a tilting of the head. Height loss, therefore, is in the trunk. The length of the long bones is unchanged. Thus the effect is a short trunk and long limbs, which is just the opposite of that of the child (Fig. 56-1).

The total body composition is altered. Lean body mass is reduced, which includes fat-free body tissues such as nerves, organ parenchyma, and skeletal muscle. Increased amounts of fat are laid down in mesenteric or perinephritic areas rather than in subcutaneous fat. Decreased subcutaneous fat leads to increased skin folding. Amounts of total body potassium, water, and intracellular fluid decrease; however, there is no change in the amount of

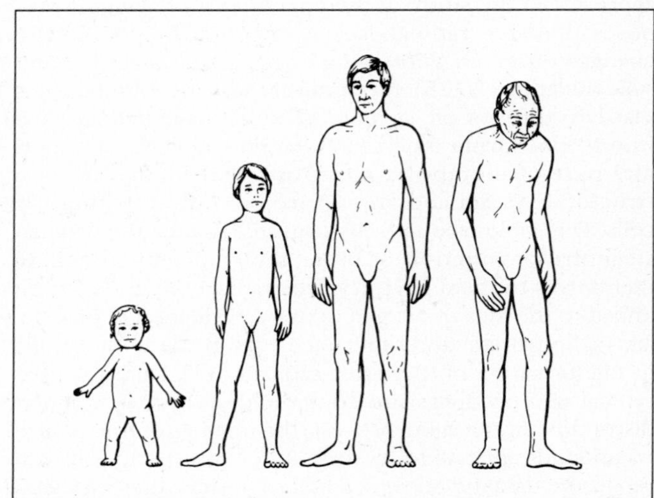

FIGURE 56-1 Changes in body proportions throughout the life span.

extracellular fluid. The bone mineral mass is reduced, with increased bone porosity (Fig. 56-2). The total effect of these losses is reduced total body density.

Weight changes are characteristic. In men, the average maximum weight is 172 pounds at ages 35 to 54 years. This falls to 166 pounds at ages 55 to 64. In women, the average maximum weight is 152 pounds at 55 to 64 years, 146 pounds at ages 65 to 74, and 138 pounds at ages 75 to 89 (Table 56-1). Women's weight declines less proportionately than men's [31].

Visible changes in movement are primarily due to alterations in the nervous system, with diminished muscle strength and joint mobility contributing only minimally. Movement is an extremely complex activity requiring integration of many portions of the nervous system. Intact sensory information going to the brain must be coupled with integration of cortical, basal ganglionic, and cerebellar function. The extrapyramidal system is subject to early changes in function due to diminished presence of neurotransmitters. Vascular supply to all portions of the brain is critical to coordinated function for movement. Locomotion becomes increasingly precarious with aging.

Fasting blood sugar, blood volume, serum pH, red blood cell count, and osmotic pressure are unchanged with aging in the absence of disease. The ability to respond to severe stresses is altered, however. For example, normal pH may be well maintained under normal circumstances, but should ventilatory failure or metabolic acidosis occur, the elderly person takes much longer to restore normal pH. Responses to events such as infection may be diminished or slowed. An elderly person may have an infectious illness with subnormal or normal temperature and a normal heart rate.

Table 56-1 Average Heights and Weights by Age and Sex: U.S. Health Examination Study 1960–62

	Males		Females	
Age (yrs)	Height (in.)	Weight (lbs.)	Height (in.)	Weight (lbs.)
18–24	68.7	160	63.8	129
25–34	69.1	171	63.7	136
35–44	68.5	172	63.5	144
45–54	68.2	172	62.9	147
55–64	67.4	166	62.4	152
65–74	66.9	160	61.5	146
75–79	65.9	150	61.1	138

Based on a nationwide probability sample of 7,710 persons. Averages and fiftieth percentiles were quite equal. Both secular trends and aging changes are mirrored by such measures as the three-inch difference in height of younger and older males.

Source: Public Health Service Publication 1000, Series 11, No. 8. Washington, D.C.: Government Printing Office, 1965.

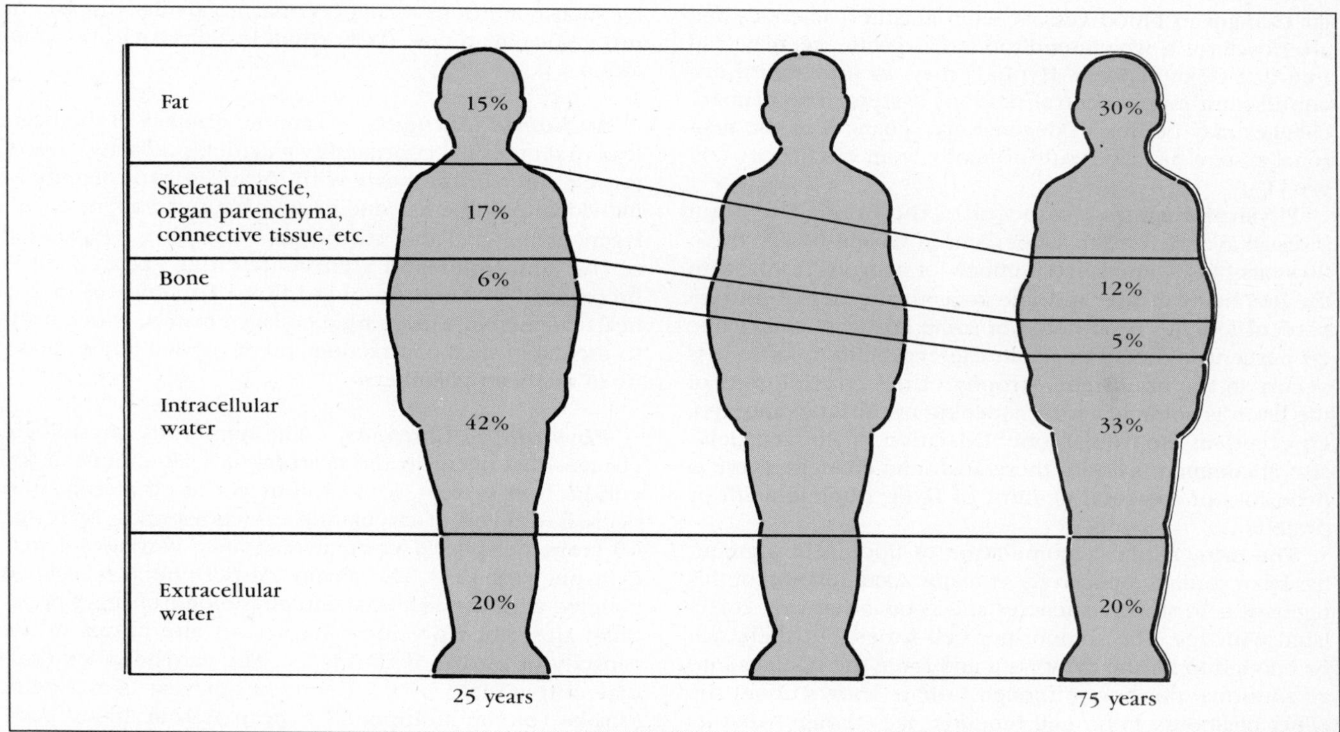

Figure 56-2 Changes in major body components with the aging process.

Nervous System

The general integrative effects of aging are strongly affected by alteration in the central nervous system. Because of its dependency on oxygen, the central nervous system responds to change in the circulatory system, such as arteriosclerosis, which can lead to decreased oxygen supply. A decreased oxygen supply to the brain leads to changes in mental acuity, sensory interpretation, and movement, and a generally reduced capacity to cope with numerous environmental events. The onset of such changes is extremely variable from one individual to another.

The transmission strength of signals from the brain to the body parts decreases as a result of the dwindling number of neurons and the degenerating myelin sheath with age. The signals become slightly blurred and the threshold for arousal of an organ system may be altered. Adaptation to physiologic stressors does not occur as rapidly in the elderly as in younger persons. The increased recovery time within the autonomic system causes an organ to take longer to return to base level activity after stressful situations.

The muscular weakness frequently seen in the aged is due mostly to disuse atrophy or may be due to pharmacologic side effects and decreased hormone secretion. Nerve impulses decrease their rate of conduction by about 10 percent, which may lead to ischemia, generally lower basal metabolism, and temperature changes in nerve fibers [7].

The reasons for change in function of the central nervous system are not specifically known. The cardiovascular changes in blood vessels, such as atherosclerosis and arteriosclerosis, which tend to increase with age, may lead to a degree of hypoxia. Hypoxia may, in turn, cause disequilibrium in the central nervous system. The primary changes may be due to degenerative changes in the neuronal system or may result primarily from circulatory failure [17].

Physical changes also occur in the brain. The brain loses an average of 5 to 10 percent in weight by age 80 to 90 years [34]. Diminished numbers of neurons result, with the loss being greater in some areas than others. Up to 45 percent loss has been noted in some cortical areas, while 25 percent loss may occur in the cerebellum. Little loss occurs in the brainstem. Atrophy of the convolutions of the brain is common, with widening of the sulci and gyri, especially in the frontal lobe. Dilatation of the ventricles also is common. Despite these anatomic changes, there is little loss of the total amount of DNA, nucleic acid, or protein.

The intracellular accumulation of lipofuscin pigment has been studied extensively. A major accumulation of this pigment is in storage vacuoles and is quantitatively correlated with age. The amount per cell varies, but there can be enough to fill the cytoplasm and force the nucleus into an abnormal position. Although little is known about the effect of lipofuscin on cell function, it is thought that its accumulation can hamper oxygen use [5].

Because of physiologic and metabolic changes in the brain and the reduced oxygen consumption, less intracellular energy is produced; glucose use is diminished and cerebral blood flow is reduced. The electroencephalogram (EEG) of the older adult remains within the normal limits of other age groups except that it is about one cycle slower.

Substantial metabolic changes within the synaptic complexes are related to neurotransmitter production. Changes in neurotransmitter effects are known to be related to many brain functions related to neuroendocrine events such as sleep, temperature control, and especially mood. Depression is associated with reduced levels of norepinephrine in the brain, a common occurrence in elderly persons. Despite these changes, intellectual function in the older adult seems to be sustained.

The effects of general changes in the brain are associated with the common characteristics of aging. These include decreasing motor strength; lack of dexterity and agility; difficulties in association, retrieval, and recall; diminished memory and cognitive ability and change in affect; and often depression. The behavior resulting from these changes causes concern to the person and family.

Cardiovascular System

Under normal circumstances, the aging heart adapts and allows the person to maintain an average level of activity. Anatomic and physiologic changes cause reduced stroke volume and cardiac output. The heart begins to have difficulty adapting to the workload, especially when unusual demands are made on it. Also, if the workload is increased by such conditions as hypertension, valvular disease, or myocardial infarction, it can result in altered cardiac adaptation.

Anatomic Changes. Anatomic changes in the heart lead to diminished contractility and filling capacity. Loss of muscle fiber in the heart with localized hypertrophy of individualized fibers is due to an increased amount of collagenous material that surrounds every fiber. Thickening of the semilunar and atrioventricular valves causes increased resistance to blood flow. The end result is a heart encased in a more rigid collagen matrix, which leads to the diminished contraction and decreased filling capacity of the heart chambers.

Physiologic Changes. The numerous physiologic changes that occur in the heart include alterations in the conduction system, loss of contractile efficiency, and decreased levels of circulating catecholamines. After age 60 years, peripheral vascular resistance increases 1 percent per year [23]. The change in peripheral resistance coupled with the anatomic and physiologic changes previously described produces numerous alterations in the capacity of cardiac performance. The cardiac index (cardiac output) falls by 0.79 percent per year. Heart work (stroke volume multiplied by mean systolic blood pressure) decreases at the rate of 0.5 percent per year [26]. The heart rate increase that occurs in response to stress is less effective, and the range of optimal heart rate narrows.

Mild tachycardia or bradycardia may lead to a significant deficit in blood flow in vital organs.

All these factors combined result in a heart that no longer has the capacity to meet all the demands that it met in earlier years. Excessive fluid load, excessive workload (as in shock or hemorrhage), and insult to the heart muscle, such as ischemia or infarction, are met by a heart muscle less able to compensate. Output may be inadequate relative to demands, which leads to many circulatory problems, such as cardiogenic shock and congestive heart failure. Even in situations of mild stress, all organs are less well perfused and therefore function inadequately.

Conduction System Changes. The changes in the conduction system of the heart of the elderly are due to alterations in the conduction system per se and to ischemia due to interrupted blood supply through the coronary arteries. Disturbances of the autonomic nervous system and the local chemical (ionic) environment of the pacemaker cells may initiate dysrhythmias. The conduction impulses may be blocked as a result of increased fibrous tissue and fat in the myocardium, as well as loss of fibers in the bifurcating main bundle of His and the junction of the main bundle and its left fascicles [6]. Parts of the system may become irritable and susceptible to irregular discharge. Digitalis administration is a common cause of dysrhythmias in the elderly that can be potentiated by low serum potassium levels. A real danger exists when potassium-depleting diuretics are used in association with digitalis. Cardiac dysrhythmias contribute to poor cardiac output and may result in cardiac arrest.

Arterial Changes. Blood vessels are markedly affected by degenerative changes in aging, particularly the arteries. Basic to the problems of all arteries is the progressive stiffness due to the cross-linkage effect on elastin and smooth muscle with an increase in the amount of collagen present. This generalized problem in the arteries leads to increased peripheral resistance. The major arteries demonstrate these changes as follows [26]:

1. The tunica intima becomes thickened and less smooth as arteriosclerotic streaks are accumulated.
2. In the tunica media, muscle fibers are replaced with collagen or connective tissue and calcium material.
3. The ability to expand or stretch decreases due to the changes of the intimal layers.
4. Higher blood pressures become common in the older adult, resulting from the decreased interior diameter of the arteries and diminished stretchability.
5. The aorta and its branches tend to dilate and become tortuous.

In addition, *atherosclerosis* develops. Fatty streaks in the intima have been found to be present in the first year of life. These may or may not be related to the subsequent development of atherosclerotic changes. As a person ages, the number of atheromatous plaques increases, resulting in raised areas with a central core of degenerative lipid on the tunica intima. These plaques are most numerous in the major arteries, particularly the aorta and iliac, coronary, and carotid arteries. They also occur frequently in the renal and femoral arteries. Pathologically they cause two problems: (1) thrombosis and occlusion in the lumen of the artery and (2) destruction of the tunica media leading to aneurysm. Aneurysms occur most typically in the abdominal or thoracic aorta.

Arterial changes are widespread and result in diminished circulation to all organs and tissues. Of particular consequence is reduced circulation to the brain and to the kidneys. Renal plasma flow is reduced approximately 10 percent for each decade of life, from 600 ml per minute per kidney in early adulthood to 300 ml per minute per kidney by age 80 years [25].

Venular Changes. The thin-walled veins have valves formed from the internal layer that assist the blood to flow toward the heart, but prevent a reversal of the flow. Veins constrict and enlarge, store large quantities of blood and make it available when it is required by the circulation, and can actually propel blood forward [22].

Because muscle contractions in the legs provide the upward propelling force for venous return, every time the legs are moved or the muscles are tensed a certain amount of blood is propelled toward the heart. Varicose veins occur when the valves of the venous system are destroyed. They are quite common in older persons, and are usually caused by inactivity, constricting clothing, and crossing legs at the knees. The venous stasis that occurs with varicose veins further complicates the circulatory problems.

A major vascular problem of aging is that of venous thrombosis and pulmonary emboli. One study speculates that 10 to 25 percent of all persons reaching age 65 years will have had venous thrombosis of some type [40]. Immobilization from increased time spent sitting and in bed enhances the risk of thrombosis.

Hypertension. Hypertension substantially increases in frequency with age, even though it is not an essential aspect of aging. The systolic pressure gradually increases with age due to decreased aortic elasticity. The increase in diastolic pressure is less marked and results from increased resistance in the peripheral blood vessels. The diastolic pressure tends to level off in later life. Cardiac output and blood volume are also factors in the regulation of blood pressure. Blood pressure is elevated through increased resistance to blood flow due to arteriolar constriction. Blood pressure lowers when arteriolar relaxation reduces resistance to blood flow.

Benign essential hypertension is the most common type in persons over 70 years, with more than 90 percent of all cases being in this category [38]. Elevated pressure usually develops slowly with little untoward effect in benign essential hypertension. Malignant hypertension occurs in individuals who exhibit an accelerated course and a diastolic pressure of 110 mg Hg and a systolic pressure of 200 mm Hg [18]. This type of hypertension is rare in persons over 70 years of age. Those with either type of elevated pressure may develop cardiovascular, renal, or cerebral problems due to secondary organ damage. Complications due to hypertension account for a significant number of the deaths in the United States.

Hypertension contributes considerably to diseases of the cardiovascular system. It is associated with increased frequency of coronary artery disease and myocardial infarction, and with hemorrhagic problems and infarcts in the brain. It is also associated with major hemorrhage from cerebral arteries and resultant strokes.

The frequency of cerebrovascular disease increases with age. There are two major sources of serious damage to the brain through the vascular system. One is infarction of areas of the brain due to occlusion of cerebral arterial vessels. The other is hemorrhage. Infarction is by far the more common, but hemorrhage has a more grave prognosis. Events that may precipitate a cerebrovascular accident are (1) marked or sudden reduction in blood pressure, (2) decreased cardiac output, (3) diminished circulating blood volume, (4) anemia, and (5) increased blood viscosity [28].

Transient cerebral ischemic attacks may occur prior to major strokes. These attacks are due to arterial occlusion or hypotension. The occlusive phenomena occur most frequently in the carotid artery. The signs are hemiparesis, hemianopsia, aphasia, and loss of vision in one eye. The vertebral artery is more often involved with hypotensive states, causing the person to fall forward on the knees without loss of consciousness, vertigo, vomiting, dysarthria, visual blurring, or diplopia [9].

The baroreceptors in the aorta and carotid arteries become less sensitive to pressure changes, and sudden changes in position may cause dizziness or syncope. Pressure on the carotid sinus may cause serious slowing of the heart rate and may be elicited by twisting and turning of the head.

Respiratory System

Alterations in the respiratory system in the aged impose many limitations that are not always obvious when the person is at rest but appear with exertion or stress. Under usual circumstances, older persons are capable of maintaining usual daily activities, but various changes make them more susceptible to pulmonary infections. Among aged individuals, influenza and pneumonia are the fourth leading causes of death, with bronchitis, emphysema, and asthma ranking eighth [15].

Anatomic Changes. Loss of elasticity affects the older person's pulmonary compliance and results from increased cross-linkage in collagen and elastin fibers around the alveolar sacs. Pressure builds up within the alveolar sacs during inspiration, some of which tends to be retained during expiration, and finally results in an increased residual air volume. In addition, there is a decrease in the quantity of air that can be taken in during normal breathing. This is also affected by the older person's tendency to take shallower and more frequent breaths than a younger persons [34].

Changes in the costal cartilage result in a diminution of chest wall compliance, which is further complicated by skeletal deformities of the thorax and postural changes such as stooped shoulders. In the older adult the changes in the muscular system lead to a decline in the strength of muscles that assist respiration. Degeneration of the intervertebral disks of the thoracic spine results in increased anterioposterior diameter of the chest and a chest wall that is less compliant during respiration.

The end result of the loss of elasticity, the muscle weakness, and changes in the structure of the chest is difficulty in expiration of air. Results of pulmonary function studies are altered as a result of this reduced capacity to empty the lungs. Total lung capacity is changed little, but vital capacity is gradually and progressively reduced. The forced expiratory volume and maximum breathing capacity are both reduced, while the residual volume and functional residual capacity of the lungs are increased. The residual volume increases 50 percent between ages 30 and 90 years. The maximum breathing capacity is diminished by 60 percent between ages 20 and 80 years [19]. Actual air flow is reduced 20 to 50 percent throughout the adult years.

Functional Changes. The partial pressure of arterial oxygen gradually falls with aging. With the structural and mechanical changes described above, the bases of the lungs are ventilated less and less. The part of the lungs that is well perfused is the part of the lungs not being ventilated. Blood must be shunted to the ventilated upper portions of the lungs. The redistribution of blood is usually insufficient to compensate, and the arterial partial pressure of oxygen falls. The condition becomes worse when the elderly person lies down, and nocturnal hypoxemia may be a major cause of confusion. The partial pressure of arterial oxygen (PaO_2) declines with age, averaging 77 mm Hg in the seventh decade [12]. The partial pressure of carbon dioxide (PCO_2), however, remains the same unless disease is superimposed on the diminished ventilation; this is probably due to the higher rate of diffusion of carbon dioxide.

The main functional respiratory problems in the elderly person without pulmonary disease are reduced ventilation of all alveoli, especially at the bases of the lungs, and reduced oxygen partial pressure in the arterial blood. This deficit may not impair function under baseline conditions with minimal physical exertion. Changes in the capacity to increase the work of breathing due to structural changes in the chest wall, and the structural changes that reduce the maximum breathing capacity, however, put the elderly person at risk. The need to increase oxygen intake rapidly or to blow off carbon dioxide rapidly due to acidemia may cause decompensation and rapid respiratory failure in an elderly person with no respiratory disease per se. Sudden increases in physical activity or sudden psychologic stress may overwhelm a respiratory system that handles moderate stress well.

In addition to these changes, which are normal alterations with aging, most persons in modern Western society have lung changes due to chronic environmental pollution. Inhalants such as smoke, various industrial end products, and the end products of combustion of petrochemicals have a profound effect on respiratory function. They cause decreased ciliary action, increased mucus production, and deposition of foreign materials in the functional alveoli and in intercellular spaces. These pollutants have two main effects: (1) they increase the obstructive component in lung function and (2) they decrease the compliance of the lung tissue through deposits of foreign material increasing its stiffness. The latter is common among miners and industrial workers who constantly inhale coal dust, asbestos, and the like.

The predominant clinical problem is the presence of an increased obstructive component. Smoking, being around smokers, bronchial constriction due to exposure to a wide variety of irritants, and chronic bronchitis with large increases in mucus production all cause increased obstruction in the airways, contributing to trapping of air in the alveoli, structural changes (emphysema), and markedly diminished ventilation. In addition, the unevenness of the changes results in perfusion difficulties in that some pulmonary arterial blood receives oxygen and some does not.

The aging effects and environmental effects on lung function interact and cannot be separated. Aging is continuous, and environmental effects on the lungs are long-term and continuous. One has to assume that all elderly persons have some degree of diminished ventilation together with alterations in ventilation and perfusion.

An elderly person with little previous difficulty may develop respiratory failure rather rapidly after stress such as surgery, excessive exercise, a sudden rise in environmental pollution (as in smog crises), or infection such as pneumonia. The assumption must be made that all elderly individuals are at risk for respiratory failure. Respiratory failure is evidenced by a diminishing PaO_2 and a rising $PaCO_2$ associated with a drop in arterial pH.

Potential causes of respiratory failure are surgery, the use of depressant drugs, lung infections, bedrest, pulmonary edema due to circulatory problems, and pulmonary embolism. Pulmonary embolism occurs frequently in elderly patients who are immobilized due to bone fractures or other conditions requiring bedrest. Any acute condition such as trauma, burns, or myocardial infarction in the elderly may be complicated by respiratory failure. The potential of unrecognized pulmonary changes, particularly those due to environmental effects, is present in all persons over age 40 years. Pulmonary function tests on middle-aged or elderly persons facing elective surgery are necessary to be prepared to prevent respiratory failure during the postoperative period (see also Chap. 27).

Genitourinary System

Genitourinary conditions in older adults are common problems that many of these individuals are reluctant to discuss. In addition to causing embarrassment, they are bothersome and frequently thought of as another sign of growing old. Renal dysfunctions are potentially life-threatening and become more so because of delay in detection and treatment.

Anatomic Changes in the Kidneys. The urinary tract undergoes many changes with age. The kidneys are affected by involutional processes and normal age-related changes occur in renal vascular anatomy and function independent of disease. The nephrons begin to degenerate and disappear by the seventh month in utero. The normal young adult has approximately 800,000 to 1 million nephrons in each kidney [22]. These gradually degenerate and their number is reduced by one-third to one-half by the seventh decade [19]. Changes in kidney size, volume, and filtering surface over the life span are shown in Table 56-2 [21].

In addition to the loss of nephrons, there is some degeneration of the remaining nephrons. The degeneration starts as a sclerosis or scarring of the glomeruli, followed by atrophy of the afferent arterioles. The glomeruli, deep in the cortex of the kidney, retain one capillary that enlarges and acts as a shunt between the afferent and efferent arterioles. The compensation that does occur results from enlargement of the remaining nephrons. Despite enlargement of the nephrons, the net weight of each kidney decreases by about 30 percent [25].

Physiologic Changes in the Kidneys. Due to the loss of nephrons or functional units of the kidneys, a decline in function is to be expected with age. The kidneys do not concentrate urine as well because of the loss of nephrons. Under normal circumstances, however, the kidneys are capable of maintaining acid-base balance.

The renal filtration rate decreases about 6 percent per decade as the general circulation decreases. As general arteriosclerosis occurs throughout the body, the arterioles in the kidneys are also affected. The result is that some of the blood is diverted to other parts of the body and does not pass through the glomerular filtration system [17].

These physiologic alterations result in slower renal adaptation to sodium restriction and excess acid or alkaline loads in the elderly [2]. Even minor stress can cause disruption in kidney function, and aged kidneys have difficulty in restabilizing.

TABLE 56-2 Change in Kidney Size, Volume, and Filtering Surface Across the Life Span.

	At birth	Young adult	Over 65 years	Percentage loss
Kidney mass (gm)	50	270	185	31
Kidney volume (ml)	20	250	200	20
Filtering surface area (sq m)	0.02	1.6	0.9	43

Diseases and Problems with Aging Kidneys. Renal function in the elderly may be compromised by one or more of the following: (1) inadequate fluid intake, (2) fluid loss due to vomiting or diarrhea, (3) shock due to hemorrhage, (4) acute or chronic cardiac failure, (5) septicemia due to gram-negative bacteria, and (6) injudicious use of diuretics [36]. Any one of these may result in renal ischemia and acute renal shutdown if not promptly corrected.

The minimum urinary output should be 400 ml daily. Output of 20 ml per hour or less may herald acute renal failure. Acute renal failure (ARF) frequently arises in the elderly and carries a mortality in persons 70 years and over of 80 percent. The dangers of ARF include (1) fluid overloading, leading to congestive heart failure and pulmonary edema, and (2) rising serum potassium level, which may cause cardiac arrest.

Diseases of the kidneys, regardless of the cause, create long-term problems. In addition to the various pathologic events associated with such diseases, the elderly also must adapt to the normal changes of aging. The most frequent chronic kidney disease in the elderly is pyelonephritis. Associated physiologic conditions are hypertension, sodium and water retention, marked sodium or water loss, retention of potassium, and loss of serum protein. The greatest concern is inability of the kidneys to handle changing concentrations of hydrogen ion. The responses to increased hydrogen ion concentration are slowed and diminished, leading to metabolic acidosis.

Several antibiotics often used in infections of the elderly are nephrotoxic, including tetracycline, cephaloridine, and gentamycin. Occasionally, penicillin also has this effect. It is not uncommon for an elderly person who develops an infection and is treated by one of these antibiotics to have septic shock and renal shutdown. It is difficult to ascertain under such circumstances whether renal failure is caused by the antibiotic or by the shock associated with the infection. Indiscriminate use of antibiotics may produce more renal failure than the sepsis for which the agents are prescribed [30].

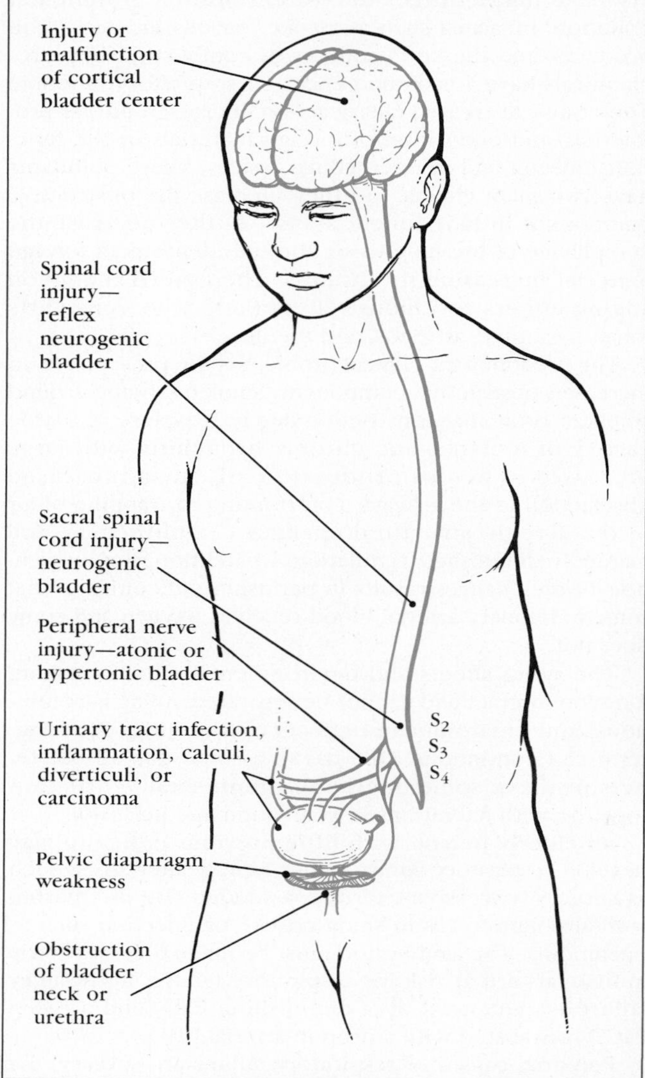

FIGURE 56-3 Stresses that contribute to urinary incontinence.

Bladder Changes. Two of the most common and bothersome problems the elderly encounter are nocturnal frequency of micturition and urinary incontinence. Among changes that contribute to these problems are loss of muscle tone that results in relaxation of the perineal muscles in the female, prostatic hypertrophy in the male, bladder diverticuli, sphincter relaxation, and altered bladder reflexes (Fig. 56-3). Frequently bladder capacity is reduced. Incomplete emptying of the bladder predisposes the elderly person to residual urine and infection.

Escherichia coli is the most frequent cause of bladder infection in women, while *Proteus* species are the most common in men [11]. Bladder infections can result from poor hygienic practices or from anything that impedes urinary flow, such as neoplasms, strictures, or a clogged indwelling catheter. Urine may become alkaline in the presence of an infection, leading to the formation of small inorganic salt calculi. Hematuria, gross and/or microscopic, may occur with urinary tract infections (see Chap. 29).

Gynecologic Changes in the Elderly Woman. In the elderly woman, objective gynecologic findings are directly related to the effects of estrogen deprivation. General atrophy occurs in the reproductive system, causing a reduction in the size of the uterus and cervix; thinning of the vaginal walls; changes in mucous secretions; and greater friability and susceptibility of vaginal tissue to irritation and infection. Due to diminished secretions, the vagina loses normal flora that create its protective acid environment. Atrophic changes result in a vulva that is pallid and has a loss of subcutaneous fat accompanied by a flattening and folding of the labia. Breast tissue thins and sags as a result of replacement of atrophying glandular tissue with fat.

Sexual Changes in the Elderly Man. Physiologic changes in the elderly man are also due to lowered hormone production and occur much more gradually than in the female. The testes undergo cellular change with no significant change in size. Fat content increases in testicular cells, accompanied by a decrease in the number of cells. The number of sperm ejaculated decreases by up to 50 percent by age 90 years. Sperm change in size and shape and lose their fertilization ability [3]. Androgen production begins to decline at age 30 and continues to decline until age 90 years [17].

Most elderly men have some benign prostatic hyperplasia, which is considered to be a normal aging change. The changes result in a prostate that is more fibrous and has irregular thickening. The frequency of prostatic cancer also increases with age (see Chaps. 30 and 52).

Gastrointestinal System

Normal Anatomic Changes. The gastrointestinal system is the source of many diseases in the elderly that range from simple dyspepsia to carcinomas. Contributing to the prevalence of these conditions are many normal features of aging (Table 56-3). The grinding surfaces of the molars have worn down, and many elderly persons have lost most or all of their teeth. With the loss of chewing ability, they may eat soft food, thereby developing gum and digestive problems. Altered taste sensation due to a decline in numbers of taste buds fosters a poor appetite, and this can result in malnutrition.

TABLE 56-3 Gastrointestinal Changes of Aging

Change	Complication or Association
Loss of teeth	Poor intake, large bolus
Loss of tongue papilla, taste, and smell	Poor appetite, weight loss
Reduced salivary ptyalin	Slightly reduced carbohydrate digestion
Reduced esophageal peristalis; Irregular nonperistalitic esophageal waves; Poor relaxation of esophageal sphincter	Delayed emptying, presbyesophagus
Hiatal hernia	Esophagitis, bleeding
Thinned gastric mucosa and muscularis; Decreased gastrin, gastric acid, pepsin, intrinsic factor	Atrophic gastritis, iron deficiency anemia, pernicious anemia, ulcer, carcinoma
Decreased colonic muscle tone; Decreased colonic motor function	Constipation
Diverticulosis	Diverticulitis
Reduced liver weight and blood flow	None
Decreased liver inducible enzymes	Altered drug metabolism
Reduced serum albumin	Weakness, weight loss
Increased globulin	None
Cholelithiasis	Cholecystitis

Source: Morgan, Thomas, and Schuster, Gastrointestinal System. In M. O'Hara-Devereaux, L.H. Andous, and C.D. Scott (eds.), *Eldercare: A Practical Guide to Clinical Geriatrics.* New York: Grune & Stratton, 1981. P. 100.

Esophageal Changes. Changes in esophageal motility begin to occur with aging. Degenerative changes in smooth muscle that lines the lower two-thirds of the esophagus result in a delay in esophageal emptying, dilatation of the esophagus, and an increase in nonpropulsive contractions [7]. Obstructive phenomena can occur as a result of tumors, rings, or strictures.

The risk of hiatal hernia in persons over 50 years of age may be as high as 40 to 60 percent. Small hiatal hernias are so common that they are frequently considered a normal finding or radiographs [39]. Difficulty in swallowing is one of the primary symptoms. Hiatal hernias can mimic pulmonary distress and angina; therefore, radiographs should be performed to verify the diagnosis.

Stomach Changes. The stomach mucosa becomes thinner, and less hydrochloric acid and enzymes are produced. Pernicious anemia is common in the elderly because vitamin B_{12} is dependent on the gastric intrinsic factor for its absorption (see Chap. 36). Cell changes in the stomach lining result in atrophic gastritis in 50 percent of individuals by age 70 years [17]. The prevalence of peptic ulcers increases over age 60 years, but associated epigastric pain is not as acute in older persons as it is in younger persons.

Colon Changes. The elderly person is particularly at risk for constipation because of decreases in physical exercise, food and water intake, and low-residue diets.

Diverticulosis is considered a disease of aging. The majority of diverticuli occur in the sigmoid colon and are asymptomatic. A high percentage of cancer in aged persons occurs in the colon.

Constipation is one of the most frequent complaints of the elderly. In a large percentage, constipation is due to cultural eating patterns, decreased exercise, decreased gastric mobility due to vascular changes, low fluid intake, and the ingestion of drugs such as antihypertensives and sedatives. Constipation in the elderly is compounded by the abuse of purgatives, laxatives, and enemas, which are employed to resolve constipation—a vicious cycle is created.

Musculoskeletal System

One of the most visible characteristics of aging is the change in patterns of movement. Successful portrayal of an old person by an actor nearly always includes certain features of body movement, such as stooped posture, muscular rigidity, slow movement, and lack of coordination and stability. Alterations in neuromuscular function result from the combined effect of changes in the muscles, the peripheral motor neurons, the myoneural synapses, and the central nervous system. Diet, heredity, and hormonal balances also are influences.

Characteristic Changes in Anatomic Structure and Function. General wasting of skeletal muscles occurs due to loss of muscle fibers. Muscle strength, endurance, and agility are affected by the decrease in muscle mass. All muscle activity in the elderly is affected by the degree of oxygen supply and its alterations, which are due to reduced circulatory and respiratory function. The peripheral motor neurons also have some decrease in protein synthesis, with thickening at the myoneural junction and decrease in acetylcholine levels.

The general decrease in movement, coupled with muscle stiffness and slowness particularly in initiating movement, is attributable primarily to changes in the extrapyramidal system. A resting tremor may also be present. These changes are considered normal. If the extrapyramidal function becomes severely impaired, Parkinson's syndrome, chorea, or dystonia of various types may appear.

In addition to the wasting of skeletal muscles, loss of minerals causes the bones to become more brittle. Some joints stiffen and lose motion, while others become more mobile because of stretching of the ligaments. Reduction in height results from hip and knee flexion, kyphosis of the dorsal spine, and shortening of the vertebral column.

Joint Changes. Joint changes in the elderly include (1) erosion of the cartilaginous surface of the joints, (2) degenerative changes of the soft tissue in the joints, and (3) calcification and ossification of the ligaments, especially those around the vertebrae. The name given to the degenerative processes of the joints is *osteoarthritis*. Once again, it is difficult to determine how much of this process is normal aging because it is present in all persons to some degree. It may begin at age 20 years, and by age 50 years radiologic changes may be present [19].

The cartilage of the joints loses elasticity, becomes dull and opaque, and then softens and frays, denuding the underlying bone. The underlying bone develops a proliferation of fibroblasts, and new bone is formed. At the joint margins, extensive proliferation produces bony outgrowths, or spurs. When spurs project into the joint, they can cause considerable pain and limitation of motion. Pieces of cartilage and bone may break off to form loose bodies in the joint that require surgical removal.

Changes in joints are probably the result of long-term trauma. Alterations resulting from osteoarthritis are easily seen in the fingers with the development of Heberden's and Bouchard's nodes (Fig. 56-4). When overgrowth of the bone margins occurs on the fingers, most often in women, it may be unsightly but is generally not painful. When bone overgrowth occurs about the hip, the femoral head may become trapped, painful and immobile. Hip replacement surgery may be required [17]. The cartilaginous disks that exist between the vertebrae undergo the same pathologic changes that take place in the other joints. The degenerative changes are contributed to by the predisposing factors of aging, extensive involvement in physical activities leading to injury, excessive use of the joint, and obesity. These pathologic changes are accompanied by pain and limitation of motion.

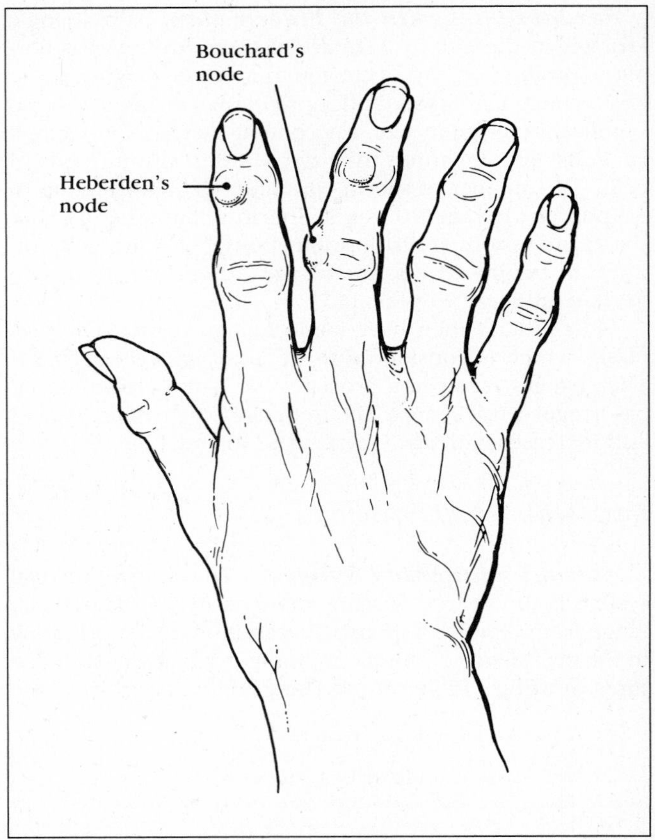

FIGURE 56-4 Heberden's and Bouchard's nodes in elderly individual. Note the lateral deviation of the third and ring fingers.

Osteoporosis. Osteoporosis is basically caused by an increase of bone absorption over bone formation. This primarily affects trabecular bone and also the cortices of long bones. The outer surfaces of long bones continue to grow slowly throughout life, but with osteoporosis, the inner surfaces are resorbed at a slightly faster rate. The end result is a long bone that is slightly longer in external diameter but with thinner walls and with markedly diminished trabecular bone in its ends. Vertebral bodies, which have a larger percentage of trabecular bone, are severely affected by this process [1].

In osteoporosis, there is evidence of decreased calcium absorption from the gastrointestinal tract. Also, the disease has some relationship with gonad deficiency, as its frequency is greatly increased in postmenopausal women. Immobilization and lack of weight bearing on the skeletal system causes osteoporosis at any age. Also elevated levels of cortisone, either exogenous or endogenous, cause the condition. Regardless of the underlying pathologic process, osteoporosis occurs to a degree in all elderly persons, but is much more marked in women.

Of primary concern in osteoporosis is the tendency for bone fracture, most frequently of the vertebrae and the femurs. Studies in the elderly show that 34 percent of fractures of the femur are due to accidents [3]. Twenty-five percent are due to a "drop attack," which is a sudden fall due to postural instability that results from changes in the hindbrain and cerebellum. The person suddenly falls to the ground without warning or with momentary vertigo. In examining all the causes of falls for 384 persons evaluated in one study, the most frequent cause was tripping, the second most frequent was loss of balance, and the third most frequent was drop attack [3]. Forty-three percent of the total sample had neurologic disease.

Kyphosis, or curvature of the spine, in older persons frequently occurs as a result of osteoporosis of the vertebrae. Vertebral atrophy also occurs. Due to the progressive degeneration, the number of cells diminishes, the water content decreases, and the tissues lose turgor and become friable. The combined changes in the vertebrae and disks result in curvature of the spine. Kyphosis causes decreased respiratory capacity of the chest wall and conditions due to impingement on various spinal nerves from the narrowed disks and vertebral changes. These problems are most often related to the lumbar and cervical spine. Compression fractures of the spine are also common.

Fractures and Risk of Falling. Cerebrol vascular disease is a major cause of disability and difficulty in locomotion of the elderly. Arteriosclerosis of the carotid and vertebral arteries resulting in ischemia may cause transient paralysis or lightheadedness, poor balance, and falling episodes. When such events occur, the person becomes anxious and tense about moving, and coordination is reduced even further. Older persons who fear falling tend to take fewer and fewer risks; the result is increased immobility. Individuals who have had cerebrovascular accidents tend to have hemiparesis or hemiplegia. Those who recover from such episodes tend to have some motor disability that creates difficulty in walking, postural changes both in sitting and standing, residual spasticity, and footdrop. These factors put the person at risk for falling.

Injury from falling is a very real problem for the elderly. Fractures of the hip and wrist are frequent, as is head injury. The subsequent hospitalization and surgery also carry high risk [4].

The bone becomes increasingly vulnerable to injury through mechanical stress. Osteoporosis and osteoarthritis occur as a natural course of events in aging. As in all the other systems, it is difficult to know where natural aging ends and disease begins. The nature of the changes and the fact that they occur in most all persons who live long enough lend credence to the belief that they are inevitable with aging.

Skin and Dermal Appendages

Changes in the Skin, Nails, and Hair. Next to alterations in the musculoskeletal system, changes in the integument are the most obvious with aging. With loss of elasticity, wrinkles, lines, and drooping eyelids occur. Exposed areas such as the hands develop age spots, or excessive skin pigmentation. The skin becomes dry, thin, fragile, and prone to injury. Nails become dry and brittle. Toenails become susceptible to fungal infection and appear thickened; there is a lifting of the nail plates. The rate of change is very individual and is dependent on such factors as nutrition, genetics, emotions, and environment. Changes that occur in the various layers of the skin are depicted in Figure 56-5.

Numerous problems occur due to the changes in the skin. The loss of water, which is the basis for many problems in the elderly, results from atrophy of all skin layers, with diminished vascularity and decreased elasticity. Lack of water leads to pruritus and decubitus ulcers. Lesions such as tumors, warts, and keratoses may arise with no pain; however, lesions such as herpes zoster may be very painful.

Sebaceous and sweat glands become less active and contribute to the dry skin. The older person frequently has overgrowths of epidermal tissue, which cause cosmetic problems but rarely require surgical excision. *Senile telangiectasias*, small scarlet growths scattered over the skin, increase in number after middle age. *Hyperkeratotic warts*, raised brown or black epidermal overgrowths, also develop in increased numbers with age. These two types of lesions, together with others that occur less frequently, have no clinical significance and do not require removal unless irritated by clothing or jewelry [25].

Another inevitable change is the loss of hair pigment, or graying; its onset and degree vary greatly. There is also generalized thinning of the hair, contributed to by a decrease in the density of hair follicles. In older females, the hair appears finer and more sparse; some axillary and pubic hair is lost. Often an increase in facial hair is noted due to decreased estrogen production after menopause. Older males frequently have hair growth in ears and nares, and the eyebrows grow more bushy. Men are more susceptible to alopecia than women, with genetics playing a part in the degree and rapidity of balding.

Sensory System

Few persons escape sensory deficits as they age. They become more vulnerable to injury, more isolated from society, and less able to care for their personal needs as these deficits occur. Deficits are greatest in sight, hearing, taste, smell, and touch, and interfere with the ability to communicate.

Vision Changes. With age, changes take place in both the structural and functional aspects of the eyes. Eyelids become thinner and wrinkled, and skin folds result from loss of orbital fat, leading to proptosis. Inversion or eversion of the lids is common, and the conjunctivae are thinner and more fragile.

Arcus senilis, a bluish gray ring, may surround the corneal limbus and be visible against the darker pigments of the eyes. Arcus senilis is a harmless change and does not affect visual acuity. Light brown patches may occur in the

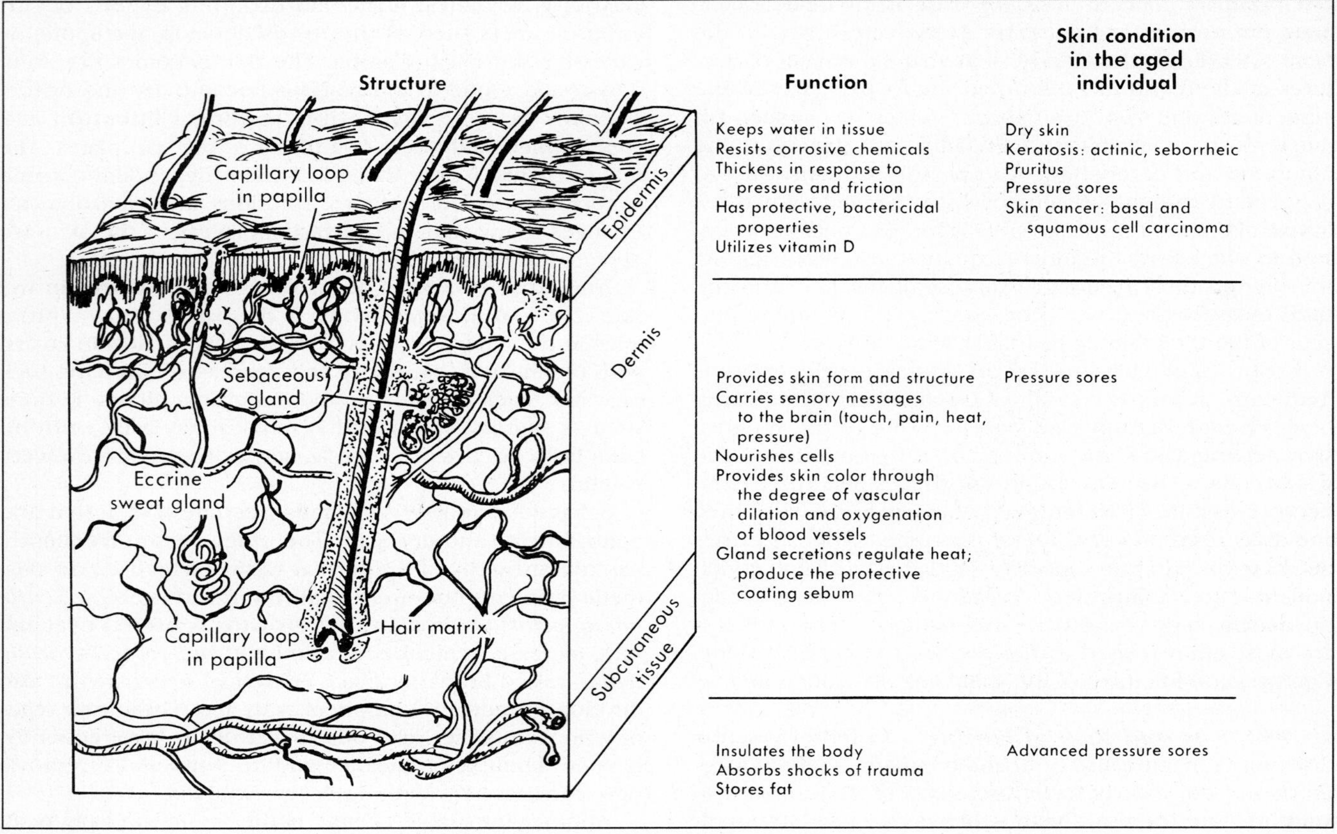

FIGURE 56-5 How structure and function of the skin change with age. (Reproduced by permission from P. Ebersole and P. Hess, *Toward Healthy Aging* (2nd ed.). St. Louis: The C.V. Mosby Co., 1985.)

irides, changing their appearance but not their ability to regulate pupil size. The lenses may develop changes that cause vision problems such as loss of elasticity, or presbyopia (see Chap. 45).

Cataracts may develop as a result of loss of soluble proteins, with loss of lens transparency. The cloudy, hazy lens results in visual loss. Reduced transmission of light causes distant objects to become hazy. Surgical excision may become necessary if the cataracts become too dense.

Glaucoma is another major eye problem that affects the aged. Glaucoma accounts for about 10 percent of all blindness in the United States [15]. Intraocular pressure rises rapidly in acute glaucoma and slowly in chronic glaucoma. Peripheral vision and night vision are both affected. The decline in peripheral vision may occur slowly, and interferes with driving ability. Medications and surgery are now available to treat glaucoma. Early treatment is essential because the blindness that results is irreversible.

Hearing Changes. With aging, changes may develop in the functional ability of the ears as well as their external appearance. Population studies indicate that beginning in the third decade of life, hearing gradually deteriorates [16].

The external ears undergo very little change other than some slight elongation of the lobes. Cerumen decreases in amount but contains a greater amount of keratin, which easily becomes impacted and difficult to remove. Impacted cerumen can block sound waves and cause temporary hearing loss until it is removed.

Sclerosis or atrophy of the tympanic membrane affects the middle ear usually by reducing the number of high frequency sound waves reaching the inner ear. Loss of cells at the base of the cochlea leads to retrocochlear loss of efficiency. The ability to hear high-frequency sounds is reduced first, and is followed by loss of ability to hear lower frequencies. The term used to describe progressive hearing loss in the aging is *presbycusis*. This bilaterally symmetric perceptive hearing loss starts at about the fourth decade, but the effects are usually not noticeable at their outset.

Exposure to excessive noise, recurrent otitis media in younger years, trauma to the ears, and certain drugs contribute to hearing loss. Persons living or working in highly industrialized areas experience more hearing loss than those in nonindustrial areas.

Other Sensory Changes. The aging process does not have as dramatic an effect on taste, smell, and touch as it does on vision and hearing, but these senses are also reduced. There is an obvious decrease in ability to taste sweet and salty flavors due to a decrease in the number of taste buds. Diet becomes an important factor because the aging person tends to eat more sweets and to salt food more heavily. The sweets lead to obesity and increased dental problems, and the salt may aggravate hypertension when it exists. Olfactory function may diminish, resulting in inability to smell, which also interferes with appetite. It also can present a hazard in the case of fire or smoke.

A decrease in tactile sensation may be noted by difficulty discriminating temperature changes. Older persons tend to burn themselves because of this change. Minor injuries occur as a result of occasional unawareness of pain or pressure.

Drugs and the Elderly

Aged persons use one-third of all prescribed drugs in this country. Most take several drugs and also use over-the-counter agents frequently [3,20]. All drugs can pose risks to elderly persons and can decrease the mental, physical, and functional status [27]. Nutritional status may be impaired by long-term use of certain drugs.

The elderly are the least able to tolerate injudicious use of drugs because many physiologic changes make them respond to medication in more variable ways than young adults. These physiologic changes result in a system that is less able to distribute, metabolize, and excrete drugs. The liver, kidneys, and heart are most involved with drug excretion and metabolism. Because they may have lost some of their efficiency, compounds may accumulate and cause toxicity. The cumulative effects of trauma, prior illnesses, accidents, and disabilities further reduce the aging person's ability to handle drugs.

Pharmacokinetic (drug disposition in the body) factors have been studied in relationship to absorption in the gastrointestinal tract, which would theoretically be reduced in the elderly as a result of changes in intestinal mucosa, blood flow, and motility. At present, however, there is no convincing evidence that alterations in absorption actually occur [8]. With age, the total body composition changes, with a higher percentage of fat tissue and less lean tissue and water. The disposition of drugs that are selectively used in different tissues is affected. Also, body size decreases, and thus the concentration of the drug in the body is higher for standard dosages. Plasma binding by albumin in the elderly decreases 20 percent. Drugs that are normally plasma focused are therefore increased in concentration in the tissues.

Metabolism of drugs by the liver is diminished in the elderly by poor circulation to the liver, by a reduction in the hepatic mass, and by the possible decrease in hepatic enzymes. Any disease of the liver will aggravate this considerably. Some of the most common drugs metabolized by the liver that have increased half-life in the elderly are the antidepressants diazepam (Valium) and chlordiazepoxide (Librium).

Another problem is reduced excretion due to diminished renal function. Renal reserve is markedly reduced as people age, and the ability to excrete drugs is also markedly reduced. Drug action in the elderly is also altered by changes in tissue responses. There may be an increased threshold to the drug's actions. Also, there may be a decrease in the number of receptive sites for the drug, coupled with a decrease in the necessary enzymes. A summary of alterations in the pharmacokinetic variables in the elderly is presented in Table 56-4.

Listed high among drugs that can be dangerous to the elderly are antibiotics such as tetracyclines and gentamycin. Antibiotics are excreted by the kidneys, and reduced kidney function can lead to toxic accumulation of the agents. Mental disturbances, gastrointestinal side effects, and rashes are some toxic effects [8]. When diuretics, which cause potassium loss, are given in combination with digoxin, the danger of dysrhythmias is greatly increased. The effect of digitalis on the conduction system is enhanced by low serum potassium levels. Many of the antihypertensive agents have diverse side effects, but they all possess the ability to cause hypotension. Orthostatic hypotension can lead to falls and fractures. Elderly persons should be warned of this possibility, and when taking antihypertensives they should be cautioned not to rise too rapidly from a supine or sitting position.

The elderly person does not display the toxic effects of digoxin, such as gastrointestinal and ocular symptoms, that usually arise in younger adults. This makes digoxin one of the drugs that places the older individual at grave risk. Digoxin blood levels are not always a good guide to toxicity because the elderly person reacts in a different fashion. Electrocardiogram changes and confusion appear more readily in the elderly and should be anticipated with digoxin.

TABLE 56-4 Alteration of Pharmacokinetic Values in the Elderly, Including Clinical Importance

Factor	Altered Physiology	Clinical Importance
Absorption	Elevated gastric pH Reduced GI blood flow ? Number of absorbing cells ? GI motility	Studies have not supported any loss absorptive ability.
Distribution	↓ Total body water ↓ Lean body tissue mass/kg body weight Increased body fat	Higher concentration of drugs distributed in body fluids ? Longer duration of action of fat-soluble drugs
Protein binding	↓ Serum albumin concentrations	↑ Unbound plasma concentrations of highly protein-bound drugs
Metabolism	↓ Hepatic blood flow; ↓ hepatic mass; ? ↓ enzyme activity	↓ Hepatic clearance Drugs will have ↓ clearance.
Elimination	↓ GFR ↓ Renal plasma flow Altered tubular function	↓ Renal clearance of drugs and metabolites

Many elderly persons develop nutritional problems from long-term use of medications such as laxatives. Mineral oil can interfere with absorption of nutrients and vitamins in the intestinal tract, and its use should be discouraged.

Aging and Cancer

Cancer is a serious problem, regardless of age. The prevalence of cancer and aging advance together until age 80 years [17]. Even though the prevalence of cancer is higher in older persons, certain types are diagnosed less frequently, including cervical cancer and sarcoma. Several factors are associated with cancer, although the exact etiology is unknown. Constant irritation from smoking a pipe can cause oral cancers, chewing tobacco can result in cancer of the mouth, and smoking cigarettes can lead to carcinoma of the lung. The percentage of lung cancer was once highest in men, but the disease is increasing in women due to the increase in number of women who smoke.

Environmental factors such as air pollution, food additives, asbestos, and certain chemicals are carcinogenic. According to the National Research Council, evidence indicates that most common cancers are influenced by diet, although there are no precise estimations of the impact of foods on cancer. Support exists for a viral cause of certain malignancies (see Chap. 14).

Chemical carcinogens produce different effects at different periods of life. Chemical carcinogenesis occurs most readily in the aged. The assumption is that there is either an accumulated effect on the DNA of the cell or an accumulated risk for a cell to become malignant.

The majority of persons with carcinoma of the colon are in the older age group. This cancer is usually very slow-growing and remains localized for a long period of time [13]. Early surgical removal is beneficial.

Cancer of the prostate is the most common tumor of men over age 85 years [19]. The disease is known to metastasize to the pelvis, vertebrae, and other bony sites, as well as to the brain. Breast cancer is a serious problem in elderly women and is often discovered during examination for other conditions.

Chronic lymphocytic leukemia, lymphosarcoma, and myeloma are malignancies with a high frequency in the elderly population. Hodgkin's disease tends to run a rapid course in the aged, while malignancies of the lung, oral cavity, larynx, and gastrointestinal tract seem to have a similar prognosis in young and old [35].

Study Questions

1. Compare the different biologic cellular theories of aging.
2. Describe the usual changes in each of the organ systems of the body, caused by aging in the absence of disease.
3. Why do elderly individuals have a higher frequency of infection than younger individuals?
4. What physiologic alterations of aging cause greater tendencies toward such conditions as renal, respiratory, and cardiac failure?
5. Discuss the development and consequences of osteoporosis in the elderly individual.
6. Why do elderly individuals develop cancers more readily than their younger counterparts?
7. Discuss the general alterations in drug metabolism in the elderly. How can these changes affect an individual who is poorly nourished and protein-depleted?

References

1. Barzel, U. Common metabolic disorders of the skeleton in aging. In W. Reichel (ed.), *Clinical Aspects of Aging* (2nd ed.). Baltimore: Williams & Wilkins, 1983.
2. Bichet, D., and Schrier, R. Renal function and disease in the aged. In R. Schrier (ed.), *Clinical Internal Medicine in the Aged*. Philadelphia: Saunders, 1982.
3. Birren, J.E., and Schaie, K.W. (eds.). *Handbook of the Psychology of Aging*. New York: Van Nostrand Reinhold, 1977.
4. Brockehurst, J.C., et al. Fracture of the femur in old age: A two-centre study of associated clinical factors and the cause of the fall. *Age Ageing* 7:7, 1978.
5. Burggraf, V., and Donlon, B. Assessing the elderly. *Am. J. Nurs.* 85:976, 1985.
6. Caird, F., Dall, J., and Williams, B. The cardiovascular system. In J.C. Brockehurst (ed.), *Textbook of Geriatric Medicine and Gerontology* (3rd ed.). New York: Churchill Livingstone, 1985.
7. Carnevali, D.L., and Patrick, M. *Nursing Management for the Elderly*. Philadelphia: Lippincott, 1979.
8. Carruthers, S. Pharmacokinetics. In I. Rossman (ed.), *Clinical Geriatrics* (3rd ed.). Philadelphia: Lippincott, 1986.
9. Carter, A. The neurologic aspects of aging. In I. Rossman (ed.), *Clinical Geriatrics* (3rd ed.). Philadelphia: Lippincott, 1986.
10. Clark, K. *Leonardi da Vinci*. London: Cambridge University Press, 1939.
11. Davies, I. Biology of aging—Theories of aging. In J.C. Brockehurst (ed.), *Textbook of Geriatric Medicine and Gerontology* (3rd ed.). New York: Churchill Livingstone, 1985.
12. Dhar, S., Shastri, S., and Robalgi, L. Aging·and the respiratory system. *Med. Clin. North Am.* 60:1121, 1976.
13. Donovan, M.I., and Pierce, S.G. *Cancer Care Nursing* (2nd ed.). New York: Appleton-Century-Crofts, 1984.
14. Ebersole, P., and Hess, P. *Toward Healthy Aging* (2nd ed.). New York: Van Nostrand Reinhold, 1985.
15. Eliopoulos, C. *Gerontological Nursing*. Hagerstown, Md.: Harper & Row, 1979.
16. Fisch, L. Special senses—The aging auditory system. In J.C. Brockehurst (ed.), *Textbook of Geriatric Medicine and Gerontology* (3rd ed.). New York: Churchill Livingstone, 1985.
17. Forbes, E.J., and Fitzsimons, V.M. *The Older Adult: A Process for Wellness*. St. Louis: Mosby, 1981.
18. Futrell, M., et al. *Primary Health Care of the Older Adult*. Duxbury, Mass.: Duxbury Press, 1980. Pp. 301–305.
19. Gioiella, E., and Bevil, C. *Nursing Care of the Aging Client: Promoting Healthy Adaptation*. Norwalk, Conn.: Appleton-Century-Crofts, 1985.
20. Goldberg, P.B. How risky is self-care with OTC medicines? *Geriatr. Nurs.* 1:279, 1980.
21. Goldman, R. Aging of the excretory system. In C. Finch and E. Schneider (eds.), *Handbook of the Biology of Aging* (2nd ed.). New York: Van Nostrand Reinhold, 1985.

22. Guyton, A.C. *Textbook of Medical Physiology* (7th ed.). Philadelphia: Saunders, 1986.
23. Harris, R. Cardiac problems: Treating the geriatric patient. In E.W. Busse (ed.), *Theory and Therapeutics of Aging*. New York: Medcom, 1973.
24. Hayflick, L. Current theories of biological aging. *Fed. Proc.* 34:9, 1975.
25. Kenney, R. *Physiology of Aging: A Synopsis*. Chicago: Yearbook, 1982.
26. Kohn, R. Heart and cardiovascular system. In C. Finch and E. Schneider (eds.), *Handbook of the Biology of Aging* (2nd ed.). New York: Van Nostrand Reinhold, 1985.
27. Lamy, P.P. Drugs and the elderly: A new look. *Fam. Comm. Health* 5:34, 1982.
28. Locke, S., and Galaburda, A. Cerebrovascular disorders in later life. In W. Reichel (ed.), *Clinical Aspects of Aging* (2nd ed.). Baltimore: Williams & Wilkins, 1983.
29. Malasanos, L., et al. *Health Assessment* (3rd ed.). St. Louis: Mosby, 1982.
30. Parsons, V. What decreasing renal function means to aging patients. *Geriatrics* 32:93, 1977.
31. Rossman, I. Anatomic and body composition changes with aging. In C. Finch and E. Schneider (eds.), *Handbook of the Biology of Aging* (2nd ed.). New York: Van Nostrand Reinhold, 1985.
32. Sacher, G.A. Life table modification and life prolongation. In C. Finch and E. Schneider (eds.), *Handbook of the Biology of Aging* (2nd ed.). New York: Van Nostrand Reinhold, 1985.
33. Schneck, S.A. Aging of the nervous system and dementia. In R.W. Schrier, *Clinical Internal Medicine in the Aged*. Philadelphia: Saunders, 1982.
34. Schrock, M.M. *Holistic Assessment of the Healthy Aged*. New York: Wiley, 1980.
35. Serpick, A.A. Cancer in the elderly. *Hosp. Pract.* 13:101, 1978.
36. Shapiro, W., Parish, J., and Kohn, A. Medical renal diseases in the aged. In W. Reichel (ed.), *Clinical Aspects of Aging* (2nd ed.). Baltimore: Williams & Wilkins, 1983.
37. Sohal, R., and Allen, R. Relationship between metabolic rate, free radicals, differentiation and aging: A unified theory. In A. Woodhead, A. Blachett, and A. Hollaender (eds.), *Molecular Biology of Aging*. New York: Plenum Press, 1985.
38. Williams, G.H. and Braunwald, E. Hypertensive vascular disease. In E. Braunwald et al., *Harrison's Principles of Internal Medicine* (11th ed.). New York: McGraw-Hill, 1987.
39. Winsberg, F. Roentgenographic aspects of aging. In I. Rossman (ed.), *Clinical Geriatrics* (3rd ed.). Philadelphia: Lippincott, 1986.
40. Wright, I. Venous thrombosis and pulmonary embolism. In W. Reichel (ed.), *Clinical Aspects of Aging* (2nd ed.). Baltimore: Williams & Wilkins, 1983.

Index

Abdominal wall, 375
Abducens nerve, 734, 818
Abetalipoproteinemia, 49
ABO blood groups, 170, 220
Abrasions, 136
Abscess, 141
  of brain, 845
  of pancreas, 554
Absorption, 568, 573–576
  disorders of, 585–587
Acalculia, 774, 775
Acanthosis nigrans, 176
Accessory nerve, 734, 820
Accommodation reflex, 750
Acetylcholine, 23, 624, 717
Acetyl coenzyme A, 10, 717
Achalasia, 578
Achlorhydria, 581
Acids
  burns from, 697–698
  stomach. *See* Gastric secretions
  titratable, 93
  volatility of, 89
Acid-base balance, 88–97
  acidosis. *See* Acidosis
  alkalosis. *See* Alkalosis
  buffer system regulation of, 89–91
  normal, 88–94
  in renal failure, 471
  renal regulation of, 89, 92–93, 96, 442
  respiratory regulation of, 91–92, 96, 391–392
Acidemia, 95
Acidosis, 94–96
  anion gap in, 96–97
  compensation for, 96
  diabetic ketoacidosis, 546, 549
  differential diagnosis of, 97
  lactic acid
    in diabetes, 548, 549
    in pancreatitis, 553
    in shock, 111
  metabolic, 94–95
    in renal failure, 471
  renal tubular, 452
  respiratory, 94, 386, 390–391, 418–419
Acini
  of lungs, 416
  of pancreas, 531, 552, 602
Acne, 685
Acoustic nerve, tumors of, 839
Acquired Immune Deficiency Syndrome (AIDS), 125, 164–166, 920
Acromegaly, 498, 500, 839
ACTH secretion, 490
  circadian rhythms and, 67, 492, 504
  and cortisol secretion, 504
  deficient, 496
  excessive, 498
  in pituitary adenoma, 839
  in stress, 67, 104, 504
Actin, 23, 25, 622, 624, 625
Action potentials, 26, 711–712
  of cardiac muscle, 267, 283
  refractory periods of, 28, 712
  of smooth muscle, 628
  of striated muscle, 624
Active transport, 21–22
Adaptation, 65
Adaptation—*Continued*
  cellular, 52
  of eyes to light and dark, 750, 754
  general adaptation syndrome, 64–65
  local adaptation syndrome, 65
  of sensory receptors, 714
Addison's disease, 176, 511
Adenocarcinoma, 192. *See also* Carcinoma
Adenohypophysis. *See* Pituitary gland, anterior
Adenoids, 383
Adenomas, 192
  parathyroid, 528
  pituitary, 498, 500–501, 839
  of renal cortex, 459
  thyroid, 521
Adenomatous polyps, intestinal, 521
Adenomyosis, 904, 905, 906
Adenosine diphosphate (ADP), 10
Adenosine triphosphate (ATP), 8, 10, 627
Adrenal gland, 503–513
  anatomy of, 503–504
  cortex of, 504–510
    in androgenital syndromes, 510
    in aldosteronism, 509–510
    hyperplasia of, 510
    hormones secreted by, 504, 506–507
    hyperfunction of, 507–510
    hypofunction of, 510–511
  medulla of, 511–513
    autonomic regulation of, 741
    hormones of, 511
    tumors of, 513
  in stress response, 65, 66
  tumors of, 512–513
Adrenalin. *See* Epinephrine
Adrenergic (adrenoceptive) receptors, 738, 741
Adrenocorticotrophic hormone. *See* ACTH secretion
Adult respiratory distress syndrome (ARDS), 111, 112, 381, 401, 409–410
Aflatoxins, 195
Afterload, 272
Agammaglobulinemia, 44, 162
Agglutination, 220
Aging, 926–940
  Alzheimer's disease in, 862–863
  blood volume in, 213
  cancer in, 940
  cardiovascular system, 930–932
  cell replication in, 927
  collagen cross-linking in, 927, 928
  diabetes in, 540
  drug-induced disorders of, 939–940
  free radical activity as cause of, 927
  gastrointestinal system, 935
  general effects of, 928–929
  genetic factors affecting, 928
  hearing changes in, 938
  immune system in, 927–928
  musculoskeletal system, 928–929, 935–936
Aging—*Continued*
  nervous system, 930, 935–936
  reproductive system, 932–933
  respiratory system, 932–933
  sensory system, 937–939
  skin, nails, hair in, 937
  theories of, 926–928
  urinary system, 933–934
  vision in, 750, 755, 937–938
Agnosia, 775, 776
Agranulocytes, 229
Agrammatism, 775
Agraphia, 775
AIDS, 125, 164–166, 920
AIDS-related complex, 125, 165
Air encephalography, 837
Airways. *See also* Respiratory tract
  anatomy of, 372–373
  defenses of, 381–384
  deposition of particulates in, 383
  laminar and turbulent flow in, 379
  obstructive diseases of, 412–414
  reflexes of, 383–384
  resistance to air flow in, 380
  size changes during ventilation, 379–380
Akathisia, 860
Akinesia, 860
Alarm stage in stress response, 65
Albers-Schönberg's disease, 651
Albinism, 42
Albright's osteodystrophy, 527–528
Albright's syndrome, 652
Albumin, 75, 83, 596, 607
  hypoalbuminemia, 599, 600
  synthesis of, 596
Alcohol abuse
  birth defects and, 48
  carcinogenesis in, 195, 197
  cirrhosis in, 612–613
  liver and, 597, 608
  hepatitis and, 612
  pancreatitis in, 551, 552
Aldosterone
  aldosteronism, 351, 509–510
  in blood pressure regulation, 101
  and fluid and electrolyte balance, 74–75, 507
  in heart failure, 305, 306
  renal tubules and, 439, 440
  in stress response, 65, 68
Alexia, 775
Algodynia, 786
Algor mortis, 59
Alkalemia, 95
Alkali burns, 697–698
Alkaline phosphatase, 599, 600
Alkalosis, 94, 95–96
  compensation for, 96
  metabolic, 95
  respiratory, 94, 386, 390–391
Alkaptonuria, 42
Alkylating agents as carcinogens, 195
Alleles, 35, 39
Allergens, 174
  dermatitis and, 173, 686
Allergic reactions. *See* Hypersensitivity and allergic reactions
Alpha cells, pancreatic, 532
Alpha rhythm, 777, 829
Aluminum intoxication, 474
Alveoli
  age changes in, 932
  anatomy of, 373, 374
  in emphysema, 416, 417
  macrophage activity in, 382–383, 384
  pulmonary edema and, 403
  surfactant in, 380–381, 408, 409
Alzheimer's disease, 862–863
Amaurosis fugax, 769
Amebiasis, 132
  nervous system disorders in, 849
Amenorrhea, 906–907
Amines as carcinogens, 195
Amino acids, 594, 596
  deamination of, 596, 597
  metabolism of, 426, 596
  synthesis of, 594, 596
  transamination of, 597
  transport of, 575
γ-Aminobutyric acid, 717
  in Huntington's chorea, 862
Ammonia, 93, 596
Amnesia, 779, 813
Amoebae, 130
Amoeboid locomotion, 23, 233
Amphiarthroses, 641
Amylase
  gastric, 572
  pancreatic, 604
  salivary, 564, 570
Analbuminemia, 44
Anal canal and rectum, 576
  carcinoma of, 591–592
  hemorrhoids of, 590
Anaphase, 17
Anaphylaxis, 110–111, 168–169
Anaplasia, 188–189
Anarthria, 775
Anasarca, 607
Androgen. *See also* Testosterone
  adrenal secretion of, 504, 507
    in androgenital syndromes, 510
    in Cushing's syndrome, 509
  in females, 895
  formation of, 154
  functions of, 507
Anemia, 221–226
  acquired immune hemolytic, 223
  aplastic, 222–223
  in blood loss, 225–226
  classification of, 222
  dilutional, 225
  folic acid, 225
  hemolytic, 170, 223–224
    autoimmune, 170, 176, 223
  iron-deficiency, 225
  in malaria, 132
  pernicious, 176, 225, 227
  in renal failure, 472, 475
  sickle cell, 44, 224, 606
  thalassemias, 224–225
Aneurysms
  aortic, 359–361
  cerebral, 361, 771–772
  ventricular, 327
Angina pectoris, 321–322
Angioedema, 683
Angiogenesis, 143

Angiography, 367
aortic, 367
cardiac, 329
cerebral, 828, 837
lymphangiography, 366
of peripheral arteries, 367
Angiotensin, 787
in blood pressure regulation, 101
in heart failure, 305, 306
in shock, 103
and renal tubule resorption, 439
Anion gap, 96–97
Anisocytosis, 222
Ankylosing spondylitis, 657–658
Anorexia-cachexia syndrome, 202–203
Anosmia, 766
Anosognosia, 775
Anovulatory bleeding, 906
Antibodies, 150, 154. *See also* Immunoglobulins
coagulation factors and, 251
cold antibody disease, 171, 223
deficiency of, 162–164
warm antibody disease, 171, 223
Anticoagulation factors, 248
Antidiuretic hormone (ADH)
in ascites, 687
blood pressure regulation and, 101
deficiency of, 499
effects of, 492–493
and fluid and electrolyte balance, 74
hypersecretion of, 500
regulation of, 493–494
shock and, 103
in stress response, 67–68
and water resorption, 440
Antigenic determinants, 150
Antigens, 150, 152, 157
histocompatibility, 155
on red cell membrane, 219–220
thymus-independent, 157
tumor-specific, 200–201
Antithrombin III, 248
Antitoxins, 848
α_1-Antitrypsin, 381, 416
Aorta, 278
aneurysms of, 359–361
coarctation of, 345, 352
blood volume in, 280
Aortic valve, 262
blood flow impedance at, 280
pressure gradient at, 334
regurgitation of, 335–336
stenosis of, 334–336
Aphasia, 773–775
Aplastic anemia, 222–223
Apneustic breathing, 811
Apneustic center, 376
Apoferritin, 218
Aponeuroses, 31
Appendix, 570
Appetite, 564, 616, 617
in diabetes, 546
Apraxia, 775–776
Arachidonic acid metabolites, 139–140
Arachnoid mater, 719
Arbovirus, 125
ARC, 125, 165
Arcuate blood vessels, 434
Arcus senilis, 937–938
ARDS, 111, 112, 381, 401, 409–410
Areflexia, 825
Arenavirus, 125
Areolar tissue, 31
Argyll Robertson pupil, 751, 863
Arrhythmias. *See* Dysrhythmias
Arteries. *See also* Blood vessels
anatomy of, 262, 264, 277, 278
disorders of, 346–363
Arteriography. *See* Angiography
Arterioles, 277, 278
Arteriolosclerosis, 361
Arteriosclerosis obliterans, 358–359, 840, 937
Arteriovenous malformations, cerebral, 772–773, 840
Arteritis, 356
Arthritis, 656–658
osteoarthritis, 658, 936
rheumatoid. *See* Rheumatoid arthritis
Arthropod-borne encephalitis, 841
Arthus reaction, 172
Articulations. *See* Joints
Asbestos
carcinogenesis by, 195, 196
lung damage from, 407
Aschoff body, 329
Ascites, 607
Ascorbic acid. *See* Vitamin C
Aspiration pneumonia, 401
Asterixis, 610
Asthma, 169, 176, 412–414
Astigmatism, 754
Astrocytes, 707, 838
Astrocytoma, 838
Ataxia, 764, 819
Ataxic breathing, 811
Atelectasis, 396
Atheroma, 357, 541
Atherosclerosis, 356–358
in aging, 862, 931
aneurysms in, 359
dementia in, 862
in diabetes, 541
hypertension and, 353
pathogenesis of, 320–321, 356–357
pathology of, 357, 358
plaque formation in, 356–357
risk factors for, 319–320, 357
Athetosis, 860
Athlete's foot, 131, 545, 688
Atopic dermatitis, 686
Atopy, 168–169
ATP
aerobic and anaerobic synthesis of, 8, 10
in muscle contraction, 627
Atrioventricular (AV) block, 299–300
Atrioventricular dissociation, 302
Atrioventricular node, 264, 266
Atrioventricular valves, 260, 262
Atrium, 258, 273
ectopic beats from, 293–295
septal defects of, 342, 343
Atrophy, 630–631
disuse, 55, 631
optic, 755
physiologic, 55
Attitudes, and stress-induced disease, 69
Audiometry, 764
Auditory cortex, 759
Aura, epileptic, 779
Autocoids, 139
Autoimmune disorder(s), 150, 174–178
Addison's disease, 176
aging as, 927–928
allergic rhinitis, 176
asthma, 169, 176, 412–414
bullous pemphigoid, 176
cirrhosis, 176, 556, 611–613
diabetes mellitus, 176, 537–550
Goodpasture's disease, 171, 176, 447
Autoimmune disorder(s)—*Continued*
Graves' disease, 176, 177, 520–521
Hashimoto's disease, 176, 523–524
hemolytic anemia, 170, 176, 223
hepatitis, 176
hypoparathyroidism, 176, 526–527
lupus erythematosus, 175, 176, 177
Meniere's disease, 176, 763
myasthenia gravis, 176, 856–857
neutropenia, 142, 176, 235
osteosclerosis, 176, 475
pemphigus, 176
penicious anemia, 176, 225, 227
premature ovarian failure, 176
rheumatoid arthritis, 175, 176, 177–178
Sjögren's syndrome, 176
spontaneous infertility, 176
thrombocytopenic purpura, 176, 223
ulcerative colitis, 591
vitiligo, 176
Autolysis, 12, 59
Automaticity, cardiac, 267–268, 287, 288
after myocardial infarction, 326
Autonomic nervous system, 735–741. *See also* Parasympathetic nervous system; Sympathetic nervous system
cardiac activity and, 99–100, 274, 276
functions of, 738–741
and insulin secretion, 533
receptor substances in, 738
in spinal cord injury, 826
transmitter substances in, 734
Autoregulation of fluid volume, 100, 280
Autosomal inheritance, 38–41
dominant, 39–40
recessive, 40–41
Autotopagnosia, 775
Avulsion, 136
Axonemes, 13
Axons, 707
degeneration and regeneration of, 708–709
Azotorrhea, 554

Babinski sign, 826
Bacteremia, 128
Bacterial cultures, 901
Bacterial infections, 126–130. *See also* names of specific strains
of bone, 128, 654–655
of central nervous system, 844–848
of genitourinary tract, 446–449
of heart, 336–338
pathogenesis of, 126, 130
of prostate, 880
of respiratory tract, 397–400, 423
of skin, 688
toxins produced in, 109–110, 847–848
Bacteriophages, 122
Baker's cyst, 659
Balance. *See* Vestibular system
Balanitis, 881
Balantidium coli, 130
Ballismus, 859
Baroreceptors, 100, 102, 276
Bartholin's glands, 888
Basal cell carcinoma, 690
Basal ganglia, 729–730
Basilar artery, 746
Basilar membrane, 756
Basophils, 229, 230, 231
functions of, 233
quantitative alterations of, 235
Battle's sign, 817
Bell's palsy, 819
Bence Jones proteinuria, 664
Beta cells, pancreatic, 532
Beta rhythm, 777, 829, 830
Bicarbonate ion
in CO_2 transport, 387
in gastric secretions, 576
ratio to carbonic acid, 90
renal resorption of, 92
Bile
composition of, 598–599
in gallbladder, 601
synthesis in liver, 598–599
Bile salts, 598–599
Biliary tract, 601
in cirrhosis, 611–612
Bilirubin, 598
conjugation of, 598
hyperbilirubinemia, 170
jaundice and, 606
measurement of, 599, 600
unconjugated, 598
Biorhythms. *See* Circadian rhythms
Biot's breathing, 812
Black lung disease, 407
Bladder, 442
age-related changes in, 934
infections of, 446–447
micturition reflex in, 442
Blastomas, 193
Bleeding. *See* Hemorrhage
Bleeding time, 248, 249
Blindness
color, 752
in diabetes, 543
partial, 755
from pituitary tumors, 839
Blood, 212–227
coagulation of. *See* Coagulation
composition of, 213
erythrocytes in. *See* Erythrocytes
hematologic values, 226
hematopoiesis, 214–215, 217
laboratory tests of, 226–227, 548–549
leukocytes in. *See* Leukocytes
and metastasis, 199–200
oxygenation of, 213–214
paraneoplastic alterations of, 202
physical characteristics of, 214
types of, 170, 220
and erythroblastosis fetalis, 220
and transfusion reactions, 170
in uremic syndrome, 475
volume of, 212–213
Blood-brain barrier, 744–745
Blood gas values, 94, 96
in heart failure, 315
Blood pressure
age-related changes in, 931
diastolic, 277
elevated. *See* Hypertension
factors affecting, 279–280, 348–350
pulse, 277, 278–279
regulation of, 99–101
systolic, 277
Blood vessels
age-related changes in, 862, 931
anatomy of, 277, 278
arterial disorders, 356–363

Blood vessels—*Continued*
of bones, 637
cerebral, 746
in diabetes, 541
diagnostic tests of, 366–367
of heart, 262–264
of kidney, 434
of liver, 594
peripheral. *See* Peripheral blood vessels
resistance in, 280
of respiratory tract, 375
of skin, 679
of stomach, 567
spasms. *See* Vasospasms
venous disorders, 363–365
Bloom's syndrome, 237
Body image, disorders of, 776
Boils, 688
Bombesin, 787
Bone(s), 32
age-related changes in, 936–937
avascular necrosis of, 654
blood supply to, 637
cancellous (spongy), 32, 33, 637–638
compact, 32, 33, 637
of ear, 756
fibrous dysplasia of, 651
flat, 638
formation of, 634–635
growth of, 491–492, 638–640
infections of, 654–655
irregular, 638
long, 637–638
marble, 651
marrow of, 214, 222–223, 227, 661–662
medullary, 637
nerves in, 637
osteogenesis imperfecta of, 650
osteomalacia of, 653–654
osteomyelitis of, 654–655
osteopetrosis of, 651
osteoporosis of, 653
Paget's disease of, 652
parathyroid hormone and, 525
physical stress on, 640
rickets of, 653–654
in scoliosis, 655
in scurvy, 654
short, 638
strength of, 634
structure of, 33, 635–637
in syphilis, 655
tuberculosis of, 655
tumors of, 659–664
von Recklinghausen's disease of, 652–653
woven, 635
Bone marrow, 214
in aplastic anemia, 222–223
laboratory studies of, 227
red and yellow, 214
tumors of, 661–662
Botulism, 848
Bouton, synaptic, 715
Bowman's capsule, 432
Bradycardia, 290, 292
Bradykinin, 111, 139
Brain. *See also* Cerebellum; Cerebrovascular disorders; Cerebrum; Medulla
abscess of, 848
age-related changes in, 930
blood supply to, 746
barriers in, 744–746
diencephalon, 719, 727–730
embryonic development of, 719
forebrain, 719, 730
herniations of, 814, 821–822, 823
Brain—*Continued*
hindbrain, 719, 720, 723, 724–726
in hypertension, 353
infections of, 841–848
isotope scans of, 828
kernicterus of, 170, 606
lobes of, 730, 814
midbrain, 719, 727
protective barriers of, 719
tuberculomas of, 846
tumors of, 834–837
clinical manifestations of, 834–836
diagnosis of, 837–838
increased intracranial pressure in, 834
metastatic, 840–841
waves, 777, 829–830
Breast(s), 890, 934
biopsy of, 900
cancer of, 913
fibroadenoma and fibrocystic disease of, 910
radiography of, 900
self-examination of, 913
Breathing. *See* Ventilation
Broca's aphasia, 774–775
Bromosulphalein test, 600
Bronchi, 372–373
autonomic regulation of, 740
Bronchial circulation, 375
Bronchiectasis, 414
Bronchitis, 412, 415
Bronchoconstriction reflex, 384
Brown lung disease, 407
Brown-Séquard lesions, 824, 826
Bruises, 54
Bruton-type agammaglobulinemia, 162
Buerger's disease, 362–363
Buffer systems, 89–91
Bulbar palsy, 859
Bulbourethral glands, 871
Bullous pemphigoid, 176
Bundle branches, 264
block of, 300–301
Bundles of His, 266
Burns, 691–698
chemical, 697–698
degrees of, 692
electrical, 696–697
full-thickness, 693
partial-thickness, 691, 693
shock caused by, 106
skin changes from, 692, 693–694
systemic changes from, 694–696
Bursae, 642, 658
Bursitis, 658–659
Byssinosis, 407

Cachexia, 202–203
Calcification, 54
arterial, 361
of cardiac valves, 330, 334
in uremic syndrome, 474
Calcitonin, 81, 517–518, 525, 526, 640
Calcium
abnormal deposits of, 54, 330, 334, 361, 474
absorption of, 576
in bone, 634, 637
and calcitonin secretion, 81, 517–518, 525, 526
in calculi, 458
and cardiac contraction, 264
functions of, 80–81
hypercalcemia, 79, 81–82, 452
hypocalcemia, 79, 81
in multiple myeloma, 240
Calcium—*Continued*
in muscle contraction, 625
and pancreatitis, 552, 553
and parathyroid secretion, 81, 525
renal resorption of, 472
serum levels of, 78–79
and phosphate levels, 81
and serum pH, 81, 96
Calculi
cholelithiasis, 615–616
renal, 456–459
composition of, 458–459
staghorn, 456, 457, 458
Caloric test, 764
Canaliculi, 594, 636
Cancer. *See also* Carcinogenesis; Carcinoma; Sarcoma; Tumors
aging and, 940
epidemiology of, 191
immunosuppressive therapy for, 164
stress and, 940
Candida albicans infections, 131, 688, 919
Capillaries
anatomy of, 277, 278
in burns, 694
colloid osmotic pressure of, 596
hydrostatic pressure of, 75
in edema, 83
permeability of, 83
Carbaminohemoglobin, 387–388
Carbohydrates
absorption of, 575
digestion of, 604
intolerance to, 473
metabolism of
insulin and, 535
by liver, 597
thyroid hormones and, 518
Carbon dioxide
alveolar, 387–388
blood levels of, 387–388, 390
and acid-base balance, 89–91
hypercapnia, 418, 427, 746
narcosis, 427
transport of, 219, 387–388
Carbonic anhydrase, 92, 572
Carbuncles, 141, 688
Carcinogenesis, 194–196
chemical agents of, 195
life-style factors in, 197
physical agents in, 195–196
theories of, 194
viruses and, 196
Carcinoma, 192
basal cell, 690
cervical, 911–912
colon, 591–592
embryonal, 882
esophageal, 580
gastric, 584–585
hepatic, 613–614
laryngeal, 423
pancreatic, 554–555
parathyroid, 528
penile, 881
prostatic, 880
renal, 690
of skin, 690
squamous cell, 425, 580, 690, 912
testicular, 882
thyroid, 524
uterine, 910–912
Cardiac catheterization, 106–107, 329
in aortic regurgitation, 336
in aortic stenosis, 335
in heart failure, 311, 315
Cardiac catheterization—*Continued*
in mitral regurgitation, 333
in myocardial infarction, 325
Cardiac cycle
electrical events in, 268, 270–271
mechanical events in, 272
phases of, 272–274
Cardiac index, 107
Cardiac muscle, 629–630
Cardiac output, 99, 279–280, 931
Cardiac tamponade, 338, 339
Cardiogenic shock, 106–108, 315, 326
Cardiomyopathies, 315–317
Cardiovascular system. *See* Blood vessels; Heart; Myocardium
Carotid arteries, 746
Cartilage, 31, 32
Cataracts, 755
in diabetes, 543
of elderly, 938
Catecholamines
in blood pressure regulation, 101
production and secretion of, 511
Catheterization, cardiac, 106–107, 311, 315, 325, 329, 333, 335, 336
CAT scan. *See* Computerized axial tomography
Cauda equina, 720, 837
Caveolae, 623, 627
CCK. *See* Cholecystokinin
Cecum, 570
Celiac enteropathy (sprue), 585–586
Cell(s), 6–32. *See also* specific cell types
adaptive or lethal changes of, 52–59
adhesion of, 185–186
anaplastic, 188–189
atrophy of, 55
of bone, 635
calcification in, 54
communication among, 186–187
differentiation of, 188
dysplasia of, 55–56
epithelial, 28, 29, 381
glycogen in, 54
hyaline infiltration of, 54–55
hyperplasia of, 56
hypertrophy of, 56
labile, 17, 142
life cycle of, 17–18, 184
lipids in, 53–54
locomotion of, 23–26
membrane of, 7–8
defects of, 44–45
electrical properties of, 26–28
in neoplasia, 185–187
transport across, 21–22
metaplasia of, 56–57
muscle, 622–624
organization of, 28–33
organelles of, 6–16
permanent, 17, 142
pigmentation of, 54
recognition mechanism of, 137, 185, 233
regeneration of, 17
reproduction of, 16–17, 927
stable, 17, 142
swelling of, 53
Cell-mediated immunity, 158–159, 163, 172–173
Cellular exchange, 18, 20–23
Cellulitis, 141
Central nervous system (CNS), 718–730. *See also* Brain; Spinal cord

Central nervous system (CNS)—*Continued*
age-related changes in, 930
bacterial endotoxins affecting, 847–848
depression of, 405
infections of, 841–850
pain generation in, 792
pathways of, 785
phylogenetic development of, 718–719
renal failure affecting, 474
tumors of, 832–841
Centrioles, 13–14
Centromere, 18
Cerebral arteries, 746
Cerebral palsy, 856
Cerebrospinal fluid, 719, 741–746
endorphins in, 787
flow of, 742, 744
formation of, 741
function of, 741
in hydrocephalus, 854
lumbar puncture for, 837
in pseudotumor cerebri, 855–856
Cerebrovascular disorders, 769–775
in aging, 931–932
aneurysms, 361, 771–772
aphasia in, 773–775
arteriovenous malformations, 774
cerebral edema in, 816–817
embolism, 770
hemangioblastomas, 840
hematomas and hygromas, 814–816
hemorrhage, 770–771, 816
in hypertension, 353
risk factors for, 769
thrombosis and ischemic infarction, 769
transient ischemia, 769, 932
traumatic, 822–827
vasospasms, 772
Cerebrum, 730
cortex of, 733
consciousness and, 806
disorders of
agnosia, 776
aphasia, 773–775
apraxia, 775–776
body image in, 776
edema, 816–817
Gerstmann's syndrome, 776
seizures in, 776–781
traumatic, 812–817
hemispheres of, 731
lobes of, 730
Cervicitis, 907
Cervix (cervix uteri), 885
biopsy of, 900
cancer of, 911–912
erosions of, 907
eversion of, 907
inflammation of, 907
mucus of, 893, 899, 901
Cestodes, 132, 133
Chagas' disease, 849
Chalones, 187
Chancre, 917
Chancroid, 918
Charcot's joints, 544
Chemical burns, 697–698
Chemoreceptors, 714
and cardiac activity, 276
respiratory, 376–377
Chemotaxis, 137, 156, 232
Chest
deformities of, 409
trauma to, 403–404

Chest—*Continued*
Cheyne-Stokes respiration, 811
Chicken pox, 124, 686
Chief cells, 566
Chlamydia, 918, 919–920
Chloride ion
functions, 82
hypochloremia, 79, 82
intestinal absorption of, 576
serum levels of, 79, 82
Chloride shift, 219, 387
Choked disc, 748, 755, 835
Cholecystitis, 615–616
Cholecystokinin (CCK), 570, 573
gallbladder response to, 601
pancreatic response to, 603
Cholelithiasis, 615–616
Cholesteatomas, 840
Cholesterol. *See also* Lipoprotein
in adrenocortical hormone synthesis, 506
and atherosclerosis, 319, 357
in gallstones, 615
Cholinesterase, 624
Chondroblastoma, 660
Chondrocytes, 31
Chondrosarcomas, 661
Chordae tendineae, 840
Chordomas, 840
Chorea, 860
Huntington's, 862
Chorioadenoma destruens, 910–911
Choriocarcinoma
testicular, 882
uterine, 911
Choroid of eye, 748
Choroid plexus
cerebrospinal fluid formation in, 741, 743
papilloma of, 840
Christmas disease, 249
Chromaffin cells, 351
Chromatids, 17
Chromatin, 14
Chromosomes, 14, 15, 37
numeric aberrations of, 45–46
sex, 36, 47
structural aberrations of, 46–47
Chronic obstructive pulmonary disease (COPD), 414–416
Chvostek's sign, 81, 527
Chylomicrons, 575
Chyme, 567, 570, 572
Cicatrization, 143
Cigarettes. *See* Smoking
Cilia, 13, 132
Circadian rhythms, 67, 492, 504
Circle of Willis, 360, 746
Circulation, 258–280
arterial, 277, 279
disorders of, 356–363
failure of, 305
overloaded. *See* Congestive heart failure
pulmonary. *See* Pulmonary circulation
venous, 262
disorders of, 363–365
Circus movement, 287
Cirrhosis, 176, 556, 611–613
and cystic fibrosis, 556
Cisternae, 11
Citric acid cycle, 8
Claudication, intermittent, 358
Cleft, synaptic, 715
Clitoris, 890, 896
Clostridium botulinum, 848
Clostridium tetani, 129, 847
Clots. *See also* Coagulation; Embolism
composition of, 247

Clots—*Continued*
formation of, 247, 248
intravascular, 59
lysis of, 247–248
retraction of, 247, 249
Clotting factors, 244–246, 553, 608
Clubbing, in emphysema, 418
Clubfoot, 655
Cluster breathing, 811
CNS. *See* Central nervous system
Coagulase, 126
Coagulation
anticoagulation factors, 248, 251
clot formation, 247, 248
clotting factors, 244–246, 553, 608
disorders of
disseminated intravascular clotting, 111–112, 250–251, 599
fibrinolysis, 251
hemophilia, 249–250
hypercoagulation, 252
in liver disease, 608
in pancreatitis, 553
platelet disorders, 251–252
in uremia, 475
vitamin K deficiency, 250
enzymatic complexes involved in, 245–246
laboratory tests of, 248–249
pathways of, 244
platelets and, 242–243
Coal worker's pneumoconiosis, 407
Coarctation of aorta, 345, 352
Coccidioidomycosis, 131
of central nervous system, 848
Cochlea, 759
Coenzyme Q, 920
Cold, common, 423
Cold sores, 124, 686
Colic, biliary, 616
Colitis, ulcerative, 591
Collagen, 31, 142, 674
cross-linking in aging, 927, 928
Collagenase, 198
Colloid osmotic pressure, 75, 83, 596, 607
Colon. *See* Large intestine
Color vision and blindness, 752–753
Colposcopy, 900
Coma, 807–812
clinical findings in, 808
diabetic, 546–548
etiology of, 808
eye movements in, 811
focal signs of, 807
Glascow measurement of, 812
infratentorial lesions and, 808–809
metabolic or toxic origin of, 808
motor responses in, 809
myxedema, 522–523
psychogenic, 807, 808
pupillary response in, 810–811
respiration patterns in, 811–812
structural origin of, 807
supratentorial lesions and, 808
Comedones, 685
Compartmental syndromes, 650
Compensation, 65
Complement system, 138, 150
deficiency of factors in, 163–164
Compliance
of lung and chest wall, 377–378
myocardial, 272
Computerized axial tomography (CAT or CT scan), 601, 828, 837

Concussion, 815–816
Conduction
impulse. *See* Impulse conduction
of sound, 756, 759
Condyloma acuminatum, 687, 920
Condyloma lata, 917
Cones of retina, 751–752
Congenital disorders
adrenal hyperplasia, 510
AIDS, 920
aortic aneurysm, 359
cerebral palsy, 856
cranial malformations, 856
cytomegalovirus infections, 843
heart disease. *See* Congenital heart disease
herpes simplex, 918
hydrocephalus, 854
immune disorders, 161–164
mitral valve prolapse, 332–333
of penis, 881
of renal tubules, 452
rubella, 843
spina bifida, 852–853
syphilis, 917
syringomyelia, 853–854
Congenital heart disease, 340–346
atrial septal defects, 342, 343
consequences of, 342
embryology of, 340
patent ductus arteriosus, 342
tetralogy of Fallot, 344–345
transposition of vessels, 345
ventricular septal defects, 342, 344
Connective tissue, 31–33
Conn's syndrome, 509
Consciousness, 806–807
alterations in, 807–812
Contact dermatitis, 685–686
Contraction, muscular, 23–26, 624–627
action potentials in, 624, 628
of cardiac muscle, 25, 268–274
energy requirements of, 627
isometric and isotonic, 627
and oxygen debt, 627
sliding filament theory of, 624–625
of smooth muscles, 25–26, 628–629
of striated muscles, 23, 25, 624–626
"walk-along" mechanism of, 625
Contracture, 144
Contrecoup head injury, 812–813
Contusion, 136
cerebral, 814
Conus artery, 262
Convulsions. *See* Seizures
Coomb's test, 223–224
Coordination. *See* Vestibular system
Corium, 673
Cornea, 748
reflex testing of, 819
Coronary arteries, 262–264
arteriography of, 322
Coronary veins, 264
Cor pulmonale, 423
Corpus luteum, 894
Corticospinal tracts, 734
Corticosteroids. *See* Steroids
Corticotropin. *See* ACTH secretion
Cortisol, 506–507
Corynebacterium diphtheriae, 129, 848
Cough reflex, 383
Countercurrent mechanism, 138–139
Coxsackieviruses, 125
Cramps

Cramps—*Continued*
menstrual, 905–906
muscular, 630
Cranial nerves, 734
assessment of, 817–821
tumors of, 838
Craniopharyngioma, 501, 840
Craniostenosis, 856
Creatine phosphate, 627
Creatine phosphokinase, 631
Creatinine, 473
Crede's maneuver, 826
Cretinism, 522
Crigler-Najjar syndrome, 606
Crohn's disease, 586–587
Cryptococcosis, 848
Crypts of Lieberkühn, 568
Cryptorchidism, 882
CT scan. *See* Computerized axial tomography
Cushing's disease, 351, 498, 508, 509
Cushing's syndrome, 507–509
Cushing's ulcers, 70
Cyanocabalamin. *See* Vitamin B_{12}
Cyanosis. *See also* Hypoxia
in bronchitis, 415
in emphysema, 418
in Raynaud's disease, 362, 363
Cysts
Baker's, 659
ovarian, 904, 909
Cystadenocarcinoma, 555
Cystadenoma of ovary, 909
Cysticerocosis, 849
Cystic fibrosis, 45, 414–415, 555–558
clinical manifestations of, 558
diagnosis of, 415, 558
frequency of, 555–556
pathogenesis of, 556–558
Cystine stones, 458–459
Cystinuria, 45, 458
Cystitis, 446
Cytokinesis, 18
Cytomegalovirus infections, 124, 843
Cytoplasm, 6
of neoplastic cells, 187–188
Cytotoxic hypersensitivity, 170–171

Dandruff, 686
Dane particle, 614
Deafness, 759
platelet disorders and, 253
Death
cellular changes in, 59
rigor mortis, 59
Decerebrate response in coma, 808
Decorticate response in coma, 808
Decreased venous return, 106–108
Decubitis ulcers, 698–700
Defecation, 570, 576
Defenses. *See* Immune response; Immunity
Degenerative conditions
of joints, 656–658
of prostate, 380
of retina, 755
of spinal cord, 857
Deglutition. *See* Swallowing
Dehiscence of wounds, 144
Dehydration, 74, 105–106
Delta cells, pancreatic, 532
Delta rhythm, 777, 829, 830
Dementia, 862–863
from dialysis, 474
viral, 843
Dendrites, 707
Depolarization of cells, 26–27, 711

Dermatitis
atopic, 169, 686
contact, 173, 685–686
seborrheic, 686
Dermatomes, 732, 735, 788, 790
Dermis, 673–674
Dermoid tumors, 840, 909
DES exposure, 883, 912
Diabetes insipidus, 499
Diabetes mellitus, 537–550
adult-onset, 540–541
autoimmune mechanisms in, 539–540
classification of, 538
clinical course of, 548
complications of, 546–548
coma in, 546–548, 549
factors affecting, 540–541
hypertension in, 349–350
incidence and etiology of, 539
infections and, 539–540, 545
insulin-dependent, 539–540
insulin-resistant, 176, 540
insulin secretion in, 538–539
insulin therapy in, 540, 548
juvenile-onset, 176, 539–540
ketoacidosis in, 546, 549
kidney involvement in, 541, 543
laboratory findings in, 548–550
lactic acidosis in, 548, 549
liver changes in, 545
muscle changes in, 545
noninsulin-dependent, 540–541
nervous system pathology in, 543–544
in obesity, 540
pancreas involvement in, 541
pathophysiology of, 545–546
skin changes in, 544–545
stages of, 538–539
vascular disorders in, 541, 542
Dialysis dementia, 474
Diapedesis, 232
Diaphragm, 375, 579
Diaphysis of bone, 637
Diarthroses, 641, 659
Diastole, 272, 277
DIC (Disseminated intravascular coagulation), 111–112
Diencephalon, 719, 727–730
Diet
age-related changes in, 935
amino acids essential in, 594
and atherosclerosis, 319
and breast cancer, 197
causing cellular injury, 52
celiac disease, 585–586
and colon cancer, 197, 592
in diabetes, 540
and fatty liver, 607
and goiter, 522
and liver cancer, 613
and obesity, 616
and stomach cancer, 584
Diethylstilbesterol (DES) exposure, 883, 912
Differentiation, cellular, 188
Diffusion, 18, 20
facilitated, 21, 22, 535
DiGeorge syndrome, 163
Di Guglielmo's disease, 238
Digestion. *See* Gastrointestinal system
2,3-Diphosphoglycerate, 104–105
Diphtheria, 129, 848
Diplopia, 755
Disability assessment, 852
Disk, choked optic, 748, 755, 835
Disk, herniated intervertebral, 827
Disseminated intravascular coagulation, 111–112, 250–251, 599

Diverticula, 589–590
Diverticulitis, 590
Diverticulosis, 590, 635
DNA, 8, 16
Doll's head reflex, 811
Dominant gene, 39
Donor-recipient tissue matching, 174
Dopamine, 717, 730, 860
Doppler ultrasound, 366
Down syndrome, 45, 46, 237
Dressler's syndrome, 327
Drop attacks, 937
Drowning and near-drowning, 401
Drug-induced conditions
cancer, 195
cardiac dysrhythmias, 291
dyskinesias and dystonias, 860–862
in elderly, 939–940
gout, 658
hemolysis, 606
hypersensitivity reactions, 44, 171
leukopenia, 235
liver injury, 611
osteoporosis, 653
Parkinsonism, 860–861
renal diseases, 451
serum sickness, 121–122
thrombocytopenia, 252
thrombophlebitis, 364
Duchenne's muscular dystrophy, 631
Ducts of Santorini and Wirsung, 531
Duodenum, 567
absorption in, 575
reflux in, 552
ulcers of, 583–584
Dura mater, 719
Dürck's nodes, 849
Dust exposure, 406–407
Dwarfism, 496
Dynorphin, 787
Dysarthria, 775
Dysentery, 587
Dyskinesias, 859–861
drug-induced, 860–861
Dysmenorrhea, 905–906
Dysphagia, 578, 579, 580
Dysplasia, 55–56
fibrous, of bone, 651
Dyspnea
in emphysema, 416
in mitral valve disorders, 331
paroxysmal nocturnal, 331
Dysreflexia, 826
Dysrhythmias, cardiac, 287–302
abnormal automaticity, 287, 288
atrial fibrillation, 294–295
atrial flutter, 294, 295
atrial tachycardia, 294
atrioventricular block, 299–300
bifascicular block, 301
bundle branch block, 300–301
classification of, 290–302
conduction disturbances, 298–302
dissociation, 301
ectopic, 293–298
etiology of, 288
hemodynamic effects of, 290
intraventricular blocks, 300–301
junctional rhythms, 295–296
after myocardial infarction, 327
preexcitation, 302
premature contractions, 293
premature ventricular contraction, 296
sick sinus syndrome, 290
sinoatrial block, 298
sinus arrest, 293

Dysrhythmias, cardiac—*Continued*
sinus bradycardia, 290, 292
sinus dysrhythmias, 290, 292
sinus tachycardia, 290, 292
tachydysrhythmias, 287
trifascicular block, 301
ventricular fibrillation, 298, 326
ventricular standstill, 302
ventricular tachycardia, 302
Dystonias, 860–861
Dystrophy, muscular, 406, 631

Ears, 756–764
age-related changes in, 938
anatomy of, 756–759, 762
assessment of, 764
bleeding from, 817
hearing function, 756, 759
aids for, 764
disturbances of, 759
sound conduction in, 756, 759
vestibular function of, 759–763
Echinococcosis, 849–850
Echocardiography, 328–329, 335, 340
Echoencephalography, 828, 837
Ectoproteins, 7
Eczema. *See* Dermatitis
Edema, 82–84
angioedema, 683
in arteriosclerosis, 358
in ascites, 607
brawny, 365
in bronchitis, 415
in burns, 694
capillary hydrostatic pressure in, 83
capillary permeability in, 83
cerebral, 816–817
colloid osmotic pressure in, 83
distribution of, 84
in hypothyroidism, 522–523
laryngeal, 423
in lymphatic obstruction, 83–84
myxedema, 522–523
in nephrosis, 450
papilledema, 748, 755, 835
pitting and nonpitting, 84
pulmonary, 311, 401–403
sodium and water retention in, 84
Edinger-Westphal nuclei, 870
Ejaculation, 875
Ejaculatory ducts, 871
Elastance, 377–378
Elastic connective tissue, 31
Elastin, 674
age-related changes in, 674, 928
Electrical burns, 696–697
Electrical properties of cells, 26–28
action potentials of. *See* Action potential
refractory period of, 28
resting potentials of, 26, 710–711
Electrocardiography, 270–272, 275, 282–303
in angina pectoris, 321–322
exercise, 321–322
lead position in, 282–284
in myocardial infarction, 284, 325
normal, 285–289
in pericarditis, 338
R wave progression, 282
in valvular heart disease, 328, 331, 333, 334
Electroencephalography, 777, 778, 829–830, 837
evoked potentials in, 830
in seizures, 777, 779, 780

Electrolytes, 88
balance of. *See* Fluids, electrolyte balance
gastrointestinal absorption of, 575–577
growth hormone affecting, 492
Electromyography, 631
Embden-Meyerhof pathway, 10
Embolism, 58
in atherosclerosis, 357
in myocardial infarction, 326–327
pulmonary, 421–423
saddle, 357
Embryology. *See* Fetus
Emission, penile, 875
Emotions, 729
and asthma, 413
and coma, 807, 808
and gastric secretions, 573
and megacolon, 589
in menopause, 897
in multiple sclerosis, 859
and pain, 798–799
and peptic ulcer, 583
and sweat production, 676
and tortocollis, 861
and uterine bleeding, 906
Emphysema, 415–418
Empyema, 404
subdural, 845–846
Encephalitis, 841–842
Encephalocele, 852
Encephalography, air, 837
Encephalomyelitis, 844
Encephalopathy
hepatic, 609–611
uremic, 474
viral spongiform, 843
Endbrain, 719, 730
Endocarditis, 336–338
Endocardium, 258
Endochondroma, 661
Endocrine glands, 482–558
adrenal, 501–513
carcinogenic effects of disorders of, 197
circadian patterns affecting, 492
location of, 483
neoplasia of, 550–551
pancreas, 531–558
paraneoplastic syndromes of, 202
parathyroid, 515, 525–528
pituitary, 482–501
thyroid, 515–524
Endocytosis, 23
Endolimax, 130
Endolymph, 756
Endometriomas, 904, 905
Endometriosis, 904–905
Endometrium, 885, 904–905
biopsy of, 900
carcinoma of, 910–912
changes of, in menstrual cycle, 893–894
Endomysium, 622
Endoplasmic reticulum, 10–11
Endoproteins, 7
Endorphins, 787–788, 802
Endosteum, 638
Endotoxins, 109, 126
Enkephalins, 787
Entamoeba, 130, 132
Enteritis, 586–587
Enterobacter-Klebsiella, 127
Enteromonas, 130
Enterobiasis, 133
Enterogastric reflex, 573
Enterokinase, 603
Environment
allergens in, 173, 174, 686
interaction with genetic factors,
Environment—*Continued*
47–49
and lung disease, 383
Enzymes, 8, 10. *See also* names of specific enzymes
cardiac, 324–325
in coagulation, 245, 247
epidermal, 673
gastric, 572
intestinal, 574
in liver, 599
pancreatic, 531–537, 602–604
restriction, 45
salivary, 564, 570
Eosinophils, 229, 230, 231
functions of, 234
quantitative alterations of, 142, 235
Eosinophilia, 142, 235
Ependymal cells, 707–708
Ependymomas, 838
Epicardium, 258
Epidermis, 670–673
Epididymis, 870–871
Epididymitis, 883
Epidural hematoma, 814–815
Epilepsy. *See* Seizures
Epimysium, 622
Epinephrine, 511–512, 741
in stress response, 65, 66
Epiphysis of bone, 637
Epispadias, 881
Epithalamus, 729
Epithelial cells, 28, 29
ciliated, 381
Epithelialization, 142
Epithelioid cells, 401
Epstein-Barr virus, 124, 236
Equilibrium maintenance. *See* Vestibular system
Erb's sign, 527
Erection, penile, 874
Erosion, cervical, 907
Erysipelas, 128
Erythroblasts, 217
Erythroblastosis fetalis, 170
Erythrocytes, 217–227
in anemia, 221–226
antigenic properties of, 219–220
aplasia of, 223
development of, 217–218
energy production in, 219
hematocrit measurement of, 226
hemoglobin concentration in, 226
hemolytic reactions, 170, 606
jaundice and, 606
laboratory studies of, 226–227
life span of, 220
mean corpuscular volume of, 226
in oxygen and CO_2 transport, 219, 388
oxygen extraction from, in heart failure, 306
production of, 217–221
defective, 606
factors influencing, 219
increased, 221
substances needed for, 218–219
sedimentation rate of, 226
in inflammatory response, 142
structure of, 217
Erythrocytosis, 221
Erythropoiesis, 217–221, 606
Erythropoietin, 219, 221, 475
Escape rhythms, 295–296
Eschar, 693
Escherichia coli infections, 127, 586
in genitourinary tract, 446
Esophagitis, 579
Esophagus, 564, 566
achalasia of, 578
age-related changes in, 935
autonomic regulation of, 740
carcinoma of, 580–581
in gastroesophageal reflux, 579
in hiatal hernia, 579
sphincter of, 564, 566
swallowing by, 571
varices of, 608
Estrogens (Estradiol, Estriol, Estrone), 891, 894–895
plasma levels of
age-related changes in, 455, 894
and bone formation, 639
and fern pattern of cervical mucus, 899
measurements of, 899
in menopause, 897
in menstrual cycle, 892–894
Eversion, cervical, 907
Evisceration, 144
Evoked potentials in EEG, 830
Ewing's sarcoma, 661–662
Excitability
cardiac muscle, 268
membrane, 714
Exercise
anformation, 640
electrocardiography in, 321–322
oxygen debt from, 627
Exfoliation, 672
Exhaustion, in stress response, 65
Exocytosis, 23, 717
Exophthalmos, 519, 521
Exotoxins, 126, 847–848
shock from, 109
Extracellular fluids
cellular exchange and, 18, 20
composition of, 6
imbalances in, 77–79
Extrapyramidal system, 734–735, 936
Exudates, 140, 141
Eyes, 748–756
accommodation of, 750
adaptation to light and dark, 750, 754
in coma, 810–811
anatomy of, 748, 749
age-related changes in, 750, 937–938
assessment of, 818, 830
autonomic regulation of
color vision by, 752–753
in diabetes, 543, 544
diseases of, 748, 755–756
hypertension and, 353
hyperthyroidism and, 519, 521
image formation mechanism in, 748, 750
intraocular pressure in, 748
movements of
in altered states of consciousness, 811
nystagmus, 763
nervous system of, 748, 749
physiology of, 751–753
pigments of, 751–752
pupillary aperture of, 750–751, 810–811
refraction defects of, 754
rheumatoid arthritis and, 657
stroke affecting, 769
Facial nerve, 734, 819
Factors, blood, 244–246, 553. *See also* Fibrinogen; Hageman factor; Prothrombin
Fallopian tubes, 888
Fallot, tetralogy of, 344–345
Falx cerebri, 719, 730
Farsightedness, 754
Fascia, renal, 432
Fascicles, 264, 622
Fasciculations, 630
Fasting, 6
blood sugar levels, 548–549
Fat. *See also* Obesity
absorption of, 575
digestion of, 603–604
metabolism of, 492, 555, 597
Fatty streak, 357
Fecaliths, 590
Feces, 570, 576
Female reproductive system, 885–913
Ferning, 893, 899
Ferritin, 218
Fertility
male, 874
of offspring of DES mothers, 883, 912
Fertilization, 897
oxytocin affecting, 494
Fetal alcohol syndrome, 48
Fetus
bone formation in, 635
central nervous system in, 719
circulation of, 341
development of, 897
and congenital heart disease, 340, 342
environmental alterations in, 47–49
spina bifida in, 852
syringomyelia in, 853
tumors in, 840
viral infections in, 843
Fever, 141–142
Fibrillation, 630
atrial, 294–295
ventricular, 298, 326
Fibrin, 242, 247
Fibrinogen
in coagulation, 244, 245
deficiency of, 599, 600
degradation products of, 247
synthesis in liver, 596
Fibrinolysis, 247, 251
Fibrinous exudate, 141
Fibrin threads, 248
Fibroadenoma of breast, 910
Fibroblasts, 674
Fibrocystic disease
of breast, 910
of pancreas. *See* Cystic fibrosis
Fibrocytes, 31
Fibroids, uterine, 908–909
Fibromatosis, 659
neurofibromatosis, 839
Fibromyomas, 908
Fibrosis
of pancreas, 541. *See also* Cystic fibrosis
pulmonary, 407
Fibrothorax, 404
Fibrous dysplasia of bone, 651–652
Fight or flight response, 65–66
Filiariasis, 83
Fissures, cerebral, 730
Flagella, 13, 131
Flagellates, 130
Flail chest abnormality, 404
Fluid mosaic membrane, 8
Fluids. *See also* Acid-base balance; Edema
absorption of, 575–576
depletion of, 74
electrolyte balance
and active transport, 21–22
in burns, 694–695
and cellular exchange, 18, 20–23

Fluids, electrolyte balance—*Continued*
    regulation of, 74–82, 440
    in renal failure, 471–472
  extracellular, 6, 18, 75
  hypertonic and hypotonic, 21
  interstitial, 75
  intestines and, 575
  intracellular, 6, 75
  isotonic, 21
  renal tubular resorption of, 92, 437
  sweating and, 675–676
  volume, intravascular, 100–101
Flukes, 132, 133
Flutter, atrial, 294, 295
Folic acid, 219
Follicles
  graafian, 892
  hair, 676–678
Follicle-stimulating hormone (FSH), 490
  in females, 891–893
  in males, 876
Folliculitis, 688
Fontanelles, 641, 719
Food. *See* Diet; Gastrointestinal system
Foot
  club, 655
  fibromatosis of, 659
  tinea infection of, 131, 545, 688
  warts on, 687
Foramen magnum, 687
  tumors of, 719, 720
Forebrain, 719, 730
Fossae, 719
Fovea centralis, 748, 751
Fractures, 644–650
  avulsion, 644
  classification of, 644
  comminuted, 644
  and compartmental syndromes, 650
  compression, 644
  compound and simple, 644
  delayed union of, 648
  depressed, 644
  in elderly, 937
  fat embolization from, 423, 648
  healing of, 645, 647–649
  impacted, 644
  infections in, 648
  malunion of, 648
  nerve trauma in, 648, 649–650
  nonunion of, 648
  pathologic, 644
  of ribs, 403–404
  of skull, 813
  soft tissue interposition in, 648
  symptoms of, 644
  vertebral, 823
  visceral damage in, 650
Frank-Starling law, 272, 273, 306
Fröhlich's syndrome, 496
Frontal lobe, 730
Fungal infections, 130, 131. *See also* names of specific strains
  of central nervous system, 848–849
  of skin, 131, 688
Funnel chest, 407
Furuncles, 141, 688

Gag reflex, 820
Galactosemia, 43
Gallbladder, 601–602
  disorders of, 615–616
Gallstones, 615–616
  and pancreatitis, 551
Gamma globulin deficiencies, 44, 162
Ganglia
  autonomic, 736
  basal, 729–730
  collateral (paravertebral), 736
Gangliogliomas, 838
Gangrene, 58, 59
  in arteriosclerosis, 358
Gastric secretions, 536, 571–573
  achlorhydria, 581
  bicarbonate ion in, 576
  enzymes in, 572
  in gastritis, 581
  and peptic ulcer, 581, 583
  pH of, 572
  reflux of, 579
  and stress ulcers, 581
  in Zollinger-Ellison syndrome, 550, 584
Gastrin, 572–573
Gastrinoma, 550
Gastritis, 581
Gastroesophageal reflux, 579
Gastroesophageal sphincter, 564, 566
Gastrointestinal system, 564–576. *See also* Esophagus; Hemorrhage, gastrointestinal; Large intestine; Oral cavity; Small intestine; Stomach; Ulcer(s)
  age-related changes in, 935
  anatomy of, 564–570
  in cystic fibrosis, 556
  in pancreatitis, 553
  paraneoplastic syndromes of, 202
  parathyroid hormone affecting, 525–526
  peristalsis, 564, 570, 576, 628, 740
  pharynx in, 564
  physiology of, 570–576
  stress-induced conditions of, 581
  in uremic syndrome, 474
Gaucher disease, 44
General adaptation syndrome, 64–65
Genes, 14, 16, 35
Genetic disorder(s)
  albinism, 42
  alkaptonuria, 42
  atherosclerosis as, 319
  autosomal, 38
  Bloom's syndrome, 237
  cell membrane defect, 44–45
  chromosomal, 36, 45–47
  classification of, 36
  of collagen, 45
  cystic fibrosis, 45, 556
  cystinuria, 44
  diabetes, 540
  Down syndrome, 45, 46, 237
  drug sensitivities, 44
  galactosemia, 43
  Gaucher disease, 44
  glucose-6-phosphate dehydrogenase deficiency, 43, 224
  glycogen storage diseases, 43
  Graves' disease, 177, 521
  hemophilia, 44, 249–250
  Huntington disease, 45, 862
  immunodeficiency disorders, 162–163
  Klinefelter syndrome, 47
  leukemia as, 237
  lipid storage disease, 44
  lysosomal storage disease, 43
  Marfan syndrome, 45, 359
  multifactorial, 36, 47
Genetic disorder—*Continued*
  osteodystrophy, Albright's, 527–528
  osteogenesis imperfecta, 45, 650
  osteopetrosis, 651
  peptic ulcer as, 583
  phenylketonuria, 42–43
  Pick's disease, 863
  porphyrias, 44
  protein deficiencies, 44
  retinitis pigmentosa, 756
  sex chromosome aberrations, 47
  sickle cell anemia, 44, 224, 606
  single-gene, 36–45
  stress-induced diseases as, 69
  Tay-Sachs disease, 44
  thalassemia, 44, 224–225
  Turner syndrome, 47
  vitamin D-resistant riekets, 45
  von Gierke disease, 43
  von Willebrand disease, 44, 249, 252
  Werner's syndrome, 550
  X-linked, 38
Genetics
  and carcinogenesis, 194, 584
  interaction with environmental factors, 47–49
  and life span, 928
  and predisposition to disease, 69
  and skin pigmentation, 673
Genitalia. *See* Reproductive system
Genotype, 39
German measles, 688
Gerstmann's syndrome, 776
Gestation, 897
Ghon complex, 401
Giant cells, 233–234
Giant cell tumors
  of bone, 662
  of lungs, 425
Giardia, 130
Gigantism, 498, 500
  pituitary tumor and, 839
Gilbert's syndrome, 606
Gingiva
  inflammation of, 578, 686
  overgrowth of, 578
Gingivitis, 578
Gingivostomatitis, herpetic, 686
Glascow coma scale, 812
Glaucoma, 748, 755, 938
Glial cells, 707, 838
Glioblastoma multiforme, 838
Gliomas, 838
Globin, 218, 598
Globulins, 44, 162, 599, 600
Globus pallidus, 729, 730
Glomerular basement membrane, 432
  antibodies to, 447–448
Glomerular diseases, 447–452
  glomerulonephritis, 128, 351, 447–450
  glomerulosclerosis, 450, 546
  immune disorders, 447–448
  membranous nephropathy, 450
  minimal change (lipoid nephrosis), 450
Glomerular filtration, 465–466
Glomerulonephritis, 128, 351, 447–450
Glomerulosclerosis
  in diabetes, 543
  focal, 450
Glossopharyngeal nerve, 734, 820
Glucagon, 532, 537, 597
Glucocorticoids, 75, 504, 506, 507, 640
Gluconeogenesis, 597
Glucose
  blood levels of, 537
Glucose—*Continued*
    in diabetes, 545–546
    fasting, 548–549
    and glucagon secretion, 537, 597
    and glucocorticoid activity, 507
    and insulin secretion, 532, 534
    regulation of, 537
    two-hour postprandial, 549
  in cerebrospinal fluid, 744
  hyperglycemia, 546
  hypoglycemia, 548
    rebound, in insulin therapy, 548
  insulin response to, 535–536
  metabolism of, 536, 597
    growth hormone affecting, 492
  in muscle cells, 536
  tolerance test, 49
  in urine, 549
Glucose-6-phosphate dehydrogenase deficiency, 43, 224
Glutamic acid, 717
Glutamic pyruvic transaminase test (SGPT), 599, 600
Gluten intolerance. *See* Sprue
Glycine, 717
Glycogen storage disorders, 43, 54
Glycolipids, 7
Glycolysis, 10
Glycoproteins, 7
Goiter, 519
  endemic, 522, 523
  nontoxic, 524
  toxic, 176, 521
Golgi complex, 11, 707
Gomphosis, 641
Gonadotropins, 496. *See also* Follicle-stimulating hormone; Luteinizing hormone
Gonorrhea, 129, 916
Goodpasture's disease, 171, 176, 447
Gout, 658
Graafian follicle, 892
Graft rejection, 174
Graft-versus-host disease, 161, 162
Gram-negative bacteria, 109, 126
Gram-positive bacteria, 122, 126
Granulation tissue, 142–143
  exuberant, 144
Granulocytes, 229
  formation of, 230–231
  functions of, 233–234
  life span of, 231
  phagocytosis by, 232, 233–234
  qualitative alterations of, 235
  quantitative alterations of, 229
Granuloma
  inguinale, 918
  in tuberculosis, 141, 401
Granulomatous disease, 234
Granulomatous inflammation, 141
Graves' disease, 177, 520–521
Growth hormone, 490
  deficiency of, 496
  excessive, 498, 500
  functions of, 490–492
Guillain-Barré syndrome, 406, 844, 857
Gums, 578
Guthrie bacterial-inhibition assay, 42–43
Gynecologic examination, 897, 899
Gyri, cerebral, 730, 732

Hageman factor, 139, 245

Hair, 676–678
  age-related changes in, 937
Hamartoma of lung, 426
Hamman-Rich syndrome, 407
Hand, fibromatosis of, 659
Haptens, 157
Haptoglobin, 220
Hashimoto's disease, 176, 523–524
Haversian system, 636
Headache, 791–793
  in brain abscess, 845
  in brain tumors, 834–835
  migraine, 791, 793
Head injuries, 812–822
  closed and open, 812
  concussions and contusions, 813–814
  contrecoup, 812–813
  cranial nerve assessment in, 817–820
  intracranial pressure in, 820–822
  management of, 817
  spinal cord injury caused by, 822–827
  vascular injury caused by, 814–817
Healing, 142–145
  aberrant, 144–145
Hearing. *See* Ears
Heart. *See also* Electrocardiogram
  action potentials in, 267, 283
  age-related changes in, 930–931
  automaticity of, 267–268
  autonomic regulation of, 100, 305, 740
  blood supply to, 262–264
  cardiogenic shock and, 315
  catheterization of. *See* Catheterization, cardiac
  conduction system of, 264, 265
  contractility of, 266–267, 273–274
  cor pulmonale, 423
  cycle, 268–274
  endocarditis, 336–338
  failure. *See* Heart failure, congestive
  Frank-Starling law, 272, 273
  in hypertension, 353
  hypertrophy of, 306–307, 630
  inotropic state of, 272
  ischemic disease of, 286, 321
  muscles of, 629–630
  myocardium. *See* Myocardium
  myxedema, 521–523
  pericarditis, 327, 338–339
  physiology of, 266–276
  rate, 272
  reserve, 307
  sounds. *See* Heart sounds
  tamponade, 338–339
  thrombosis in, 57–58
  in uremic syndrome, 474
  valvular disease of, 327–336
  ventricles. *See* Ventricles
Heart failure, congestive, 305–315
  anaerobic metabolism in, 306
  and cardiogenic shock, 315
  causes of, 305
  compensatory mechanisms in, 305–307
  diagnosis of, 311, 314, 315
  dilatation of heart in, 307
  edema in, 84
  Frank-Starling effect, 306
  left-sided, 307–311
    causes of, 307, 309
    effects of, 308
    pathophysiology of, 307–308, 310
    signs and symptoms of, 308, 311
Heart failure, congestive—*Continued*
  myocardial hypertrophy in, 306–307
  in myocardial infarction, 307, 326, 327
  oxygen extraction from erythrocytes in, 306
  pathophysiology of, 305–307
  pulmonary edema in, 311, 402–403
  radiologic evidence of, 311, 314
  renin-angiotensin-aldosterone system in, 305, 306
  right-sided, 311–313, 314
  sympathetic response to, 305
  in uremic syndrome, 474
Heart sounds, 274
  in aortic valve disorders, 336
  Austin Flint murmur, 336
  in endocarditis, 336
  in mitral valve disorders, 331, 333
  in pulmonary edema, 413
Heights, table of, 929
Helminths, 132–133
Hemangioblastomas, 840
Hemangioma, 460, 690
Hematocrit, 226
Hematologic values, 226
Hematology. *See* Blood; specific types of blood cells
Hematoma
  dissecting, 359
  epidural, 814–815
  fracture, 645
  intracerebral, 816
  subdural, 815
Hematopoiesis, 214–217
  bone marrow in, 214
  spleen in, 215–217
  stem cell theory of, 214
Heme, 218, 598
Hemianopsia, 755
Hemoconcentration, 221
Hemodynamic homeostasis. *See* Blood pressure
Hemoglobin, 218, 385
  as blood buffer, 90
  concentration of, 226
  glycosylated, 549
  in iron deficiency anemia, 225
  laboratory studies of, 226
  recycling by macrophages, 234
  reduced, 385
  in sickle cell anemia, 44, 224
  synthesis of, 218–219
  in thalassemias, 44, 224
Hemolysis, 170, 225
  and anemia, 170, 176
  in cold antibody disease, 171, 223
  drug-induced, 171, 606
  in erythroblastosis fetalis, 170
  jaundice from, 606
  in transfusion reactions, 170, 606
  in uremic syndrome, 475
  in warm antibody disease, 171, 223
Hemophilia, 44, 245
Hemophilus ducreyi, 918
Hemophilus influenzae, 127
Hemophilus pertussis, 127
Hemophilus vaginalis, 919
Hemorrhage
  anemia caused by, 225–226
  in cystitis, 446
  exudate in, 141
  gastrointestinal
    esophageal varices and, 580, 608
    hemorrhoids, 590
Hemorrhage, gastrointestinal—*Continued*
    in portal hypertension, 608
    in ulcers, 581, 583
    in uremic syndrome, 474
  in head trauma, 814–816
    from ear and nose, 817
  intracerebral, 770–771
    in aneurysm rupture, 772
    in arteriovenous malformations, 773
    subarachnoid, 770–771, 816
  in pancreatitis, 551, 553
  retinal, in diabetes, 543
  shock after, 104–105
  in spinal cord injuries, 823
  uterine, 906
Hemorrhoids, 590
Hemosiderosis, 54
Hemostasis, 242–244
  platelet function in, 243–244
  vasoconstriction in, 242
Hemothorax, 404
Henderson-Hasselbalch equation, 91
Hepatitis
  alcoholic, 612
  chronic active, 176
  viral, 614–615
    delta, 615
    non-A, non-B, 125, 615
    type A, 125, 614
    type B, 125, 614–615
Hepatobiliary system, 594–617. *See also* Biliary tract; Liver
Hepatorenal syndrome, 608
Hepatotoxins, 597–598, 611
Hering-Breuer reflex, 376
Hernias, 589
  hiatal, 579–580, 935
  incarcerated, 589
  reducible, 589
  strangulated, 589
Herniations
  cerebral, 821–822, 823
    temporal lobe, 814
  intervertebral disk, 827
Herpes simplex, 686
  genital, 124, 918
  gingivostomatitis from, 686
  and neonatal encephalitis, 842
  type 1, 124
  type 2, 124, 918
    cervical cancer associated with, 686
Herpes zoster, 124, 687, 844
Heterozygote, 39
Hidradenitis suppurativa, 685
High-density lipoproteins, 70, 319
Hindbrain, 719, 720, 723, 724–726
Hip, congenital dislocation of, 656
Hirschsprung's disease, 589
Histamine
  in anaphylaxis, 111
  in inflammatory response, 140
  and gastric secretions, 573
Histiocytes, 156
Histocompatability antigens, 155
Histoplasmosis, 131
Hives, 682–683
Hodgkin's disease, 238–239
Homozygote, 39
Hookworm, 133
Hormones, 482–483. *See also* Endocrine glands; names of specific hormones
Horner's syndrome, 811, 824
Host-parasite relationships, 120
Huhner test, 901
Human immunodeficiency virus, 125
Humoral immunity, 157–158
Hunger, 564–565
Huntington's disease, 45, 862
Hyaline infiltration, 54–55
    of pancreas, 541
Hyaline membrane disease, 409
Hyaluronidase, 874
Hydatid disease, 849–850
Hydatidiform mole, 910–911
Hydrocarbons, carcinogenic effects of, 195
Hydrocele, 881
Hydrocephalus, 854
Hydrochloric acid. *See* Gastric secretions
Hydrogen ion concentration, 88–89, 440. *See also* pH
Hydrostatic pressure, 75
Hydrothorax, 404
Hygroma, subdural, 815–816
Hyperbilirubinemia, 170
Hypercalcemia, 79, 81–82, 452
Hypercapnia, 418, 427, 764
Hypercholesterolemia, 44
Hyperemia, 280
Hyperglycemia, 546, 549
Hyperinsulinism, 550
Hyperkalemia, 78, 80, 469
Hyperlipidemia, 44, 552, 553
Hypermagnesemia, 82
Hypermetropia, 754
Hypernatremia, 77, 78
Hyperosmia, 766
Hyperparathyroidism, 528
Hyperphenylalaninemia, 42–43
Hyperphosphatemia, 82
Hyperpituitarism, 497–499
Hyperplasia, 56
Hyperplastic polyps, 591
Hyperpolarization, 27
Hyperprolactinemia, 498
Hyperreflexia, 826
Hypersensitivity and allergic reactions
  Arthus reaction, 172
  asthma, 169, 176, 412–414
  basophils in, 234
  celiac sprue, 585–586
  delayed, 172–173
  dermatitis in, 173, 686
  drug-induced, 171
  eosinophils in, 234
  Goodpasture's disease, 171
  graft rejection, 174
  Guillain-Barré syndrome, 857
  hemolytic, 170–171
  serum sickness, 171–172
  in transfusions, 170
  types of, 168–173
Hypertension, 348–357
  in aging, 348, 931–932
  in aldosteronism, 351
  atherosclerosis and, 319, 351
  benign, 348
  borderline, 348
  and cerebrovascular disorders, 353
  clinical manifestations of, 352–353
  in coarctation of aorta, 352
  Cushing's disease and, 351
  in diabetes, 349–350
  diagnosis of, 353–354
  etiology of, 348–349, 350
  and kidney, 350, 351, 353
  labile, 348
  malignant, 348, 353
  pathophysiology of, 350–353
  in pheochromocytoma, 351
  portal, 607–608
  pulmonary, 423
  renin-angiotensin-aldosterone system in, 350–351, 474
  secondary, 348, 350

Hypertension—*Continued*
sustained, 348
Hyperthyroidism, 519–521
Hypertonic fluids, 21
Hypertrophy, 56, 630
cardiac, 306–307, 630
Hyperuricemia, 452
Hyperventilation, 94, 811
Hypervolemia, 77, 78
Hypocalcemia, 79, 81
Hypochloremia, 79, 82
Hypogeusia, 765
Hypoglossal nerve, 734, 820
Hypoglycemia, 548, 549, 550
Hypogonadism, 496
Hypokalemia, 78, 80, 95–96, 452
Hypomagnesemia, 79, 82
Hypomenorrhea, 906
Hyponatremia, 77, 78
Hypoparathyroidism, 176, 526–527
Hypophosphatemia, 79, 82
Hypophysis. *See* Pituitary gland
Hypopituitarism, 496–497, 839
Hypospadias, 881
Hypothalamic-hypophyseal-portal system, 485, 486, 489
Hypothalamus, 719, 728–729
and female reproductive system, 890–891
hunger center in, 564
and male reproductive system, 876
pituitary and, 488–489, 493
Hypothyroidism, 521–524
Hypotonic fluids, 21
Hypoventilation, 391
Hypovolemia, 77, 78
shock and, 104–106
Hypoxemia, 385
in aging, 932
in emphysema, 418
erythrocytosis in, 221
in heart failure, 315
in pulmonary edema, 403
in respiratory failure, 427
Hypoxia, 385, 418
of brain, 418
cellular injury in, 52, 53, 57–59
in emphysema, 418
Hypsarrythmria, 777
Hysterosalpingography, 900

Icterus, 606
gravis, 170
Ileum, 567
absorption in, 576
Crohn's disease of, 586–587
Ileus, 588
Immune disorders, 161–166. *See also* Autoimmune disorders
AIDS, 164–166
complement disorders, 163–164
Di George's syndrome, 163
hypogammaglobulinemia, 44, 162
IgA deficiency, 162–163
opportunistic infections in, 165
primary, 161–164
secondary, 164–166
severe combined, 44, 161
Immune response, 150–159
in neoplasms, 200–201
to respiratory infections, 384–385
specificity of, 154
in stress, 65, 68, 70
Immunity, 149–166. *See also* Hypersensitivity and allergic reactions; Immune response
cell-mediated, 158–159
humoral, 157–158

Immunity, humoral—*Continued*
complement activation in, 158
disorders of, 163
primary response in, 158
secondary response in, 158
organs of, 150–151
Immunocompetent cells, 150
Immunogens, 157
Immunoglobulins
deficiency of, 162–163
Fab and Fc portions of, 153
IgA, 153–154
deficiency of, 162–163
in respiratory defense mechanisms, 384
IgD, 153, 154, 384
IgE, 153, 154, 384
in allergic response, 110, 234
in asthma, 412
IgG, 153, 384
IgM, 153, 384
heavy chain of, 153
light chain of, 153
regions of, 154
specificity of, 153
Immunosuppressive therapy, 164
Immunosurveillance, 159
Impetigo, 688
Impulse conduction, 710–714
action potentials. *See* Action potential
age-related changes in, 931
in autonomic nervous system, 737–738
facilitation of, 717
in heart, 264, 265, 268, 270–271
after myocardial infarction, 326
disturbances of, 298–302
and membrane excitability, 714
neurotransmitters in, 717–718, 737–738
presynaptic inhibition of, 717
in reflex arc, 720
resting potential in, 26, 710–711
saltatory, 712
at synapses, 715–716
velocity of, 712
Incisions, 136
Incisurae, 274
Incus, 756
Infant respiratory distress syndrome, 381, 408–409
Infarction, 57, 58
cerebral, 769–770
pulmonary, 421
myocardial. *See* Myocardial infarction
Infectious diseases
bacterial. *See* Bacterial infections
of bones, 654–655
of central nervous system, 841–850
defenses against. *See* Immune response
fungal. *See* Fungal infections
helminthic, 132–133
metazoal, 849–850
opportunistic, 165
protozoal, 130, 132, 849
of reproductive tract, 916–920
of respiratory tract, 397–401
rickettsial, 122, 126, 850
of skin, 131, 688
urinary tract, 127, 128, 131, 446–447, 934
viral. *See* Virus infections
Infertility, male, 176, 874
Inflammation
acute, 136–141
cellular phase of, 136–137

Inflammation—*Continued*
chronic, 141
effects of, 141–142
exudates in, 140–141
mediators of, 140
resolution of, 142–145
vascular phase of, 136, 137
Influenza, 125
Infratentorial lesions, 808–809
Inheritance, 35. *See also* Genetics
Inotropic state, 272
Insufficiency, valvular, 364, 366
Insulin, 532
hypersecretion of, 550, 616
metabolic effects of, 535–537
secretion of, 532–534
therapy, 538–539
reactions to, 548
resistance to, 540
Insulinomas, 550
Intercostal muscles, 375
Interferon, 122, 155, 385
Interphase, 17
Interstitial cells of Leydig, 870, 875
Interstitial cell stimulating hormone. *See* Luteinizing hormone
Interstitial fluids, 75
Intestines. *See* Gastrointestinal system; Large intestine; Small intestine
Intracellular fluids
and cellular exchange, 18, 20
composition of, 6
imbalances in, 77, 78, 79
Intracranial pressure increase, 820–822
in brain tumors, 834
in hydrocephalus, 854
Intraocular pressure, 748
Intraventricular shock, 300–301
Iodamoeba, 130
Iodine
and goiter, 522–523
thyroid and, 516
IRDS, 381, 408–409
Iris, 748
Iron
absorption of, 576
deficiency of, 225
in hemoglobin synthesis, 219
Ischemia, 57, 112
cardiac, 286, 321
cerebral, 769
infarction from, 57
of lower extremities, 541
renal, 466–467
Volkmann's, 650
Ishihara chart, 753
Islets of Langerhans, 531–533
and diabetes, 541
diseases of, 550–551
Isocitrate dehydrogenase (ICD) test, 599, 600
Isometric and isotonic muscular contractions, 627
Isotonic fluids, 21
Isotope scans. *See* Radioisotope scans
Isovolumic contraction and relaxation of heart, 273, 274

Jacob-Creutzfeld disease, 843
Jacksonian seizures, 780
Janeway lesions, 338
Jaundice, 606–607
Jejunum, 567
absorption in, 575
Jock itch, 688
Joints, 640–643

Joints—*Continued*
age-related changes in, 936
degeneration of, 658. *See also* Arthritis
gout and, 658
movements of, 643
synovial, 641–642
tumors of, 659
types of, 640–643
Jugular vein, 746
pressure, 314
Junctional rhythms, 295–296
Juxtaglomerular apparatus, 439
tumors of, 460

Kaposi's sarcoma, 197
Kallikrein, 140
Karyotype, 35
Keloid scars, 144
Keratoacanthoma, 690
Keratosis, 689–690
Kernicterus, 170, 606
Ketoacidosis, 546, 549
Kidneys
and acid-base balance, 89, 92–93, 96
acute failure of, 351, 353, 465–470
in aging, 934
causes of, 465–466
prognosis of, 470
stages of, 469–470
tubular factors in, 466–468
age-related changes in, 933–934
anatomy of, 432–435
blood supply to, 434
calculi in, 456–459
chronic failure of, 470–473
causes of, 449, 451, 470
complications of, 471–473
stages of, 470
uremic syndrome in, 473–475
congenital disorders of, 452–453
in diabetes, 541, 543
filtration by, 435–437
and fluid and electrolyte balance, 74
glomerular diseases, 447–452, 541, 543
in heart failure, 305
in hepatorenal syndrome, 608
in hypertension, 350, 351, 353
nephrons of, 432–434, 436, 933
nerves of, 435
in osteodystrophy, 473, 528
paraneoplastic syndromes of, 202
parathyroid hormone affecting, 525, 528
physiology of, 435–442
pyelonephritis, 447, 451
in response to shock, 104
tubules of, 443–442
disorders of, 451–452
distal convoluted, 434, 439–440
necrosis of, 466–469
proximal convoluted, 433, 437–439
resorption in, 437, 439–440
tumors of
benign, 459–460
classification of, 460
malignant, 460–462
Kimmelstiel-Wilson lesions, 543
Kinins, 139
Klinefelter syndrome, 47
Korotkoff sounds, 277, 279
Krebs cycle, 8
Kupffer cells, 156, 234, 594
functions of, 597

Kuru, 843
Kyphoscoliosis, 407
Kyphosis in aging, 937

Labia, 890, 934
Labyrinth of ear, 756, 763
destruction of, 764, 819
Lacerations, 136
Lacrimal glands, autonomic regulation of, 739
Lactation, 890, 892
oxytocin secretion and, 494
Lactic acidosis
in diabetes, 548, 549
in pancreatitis, 553
in shock, 111
Lactic dehydrogenase (LDH) test, 599, 600, 631
Laennec's cirrhosis, 612–613
Lamellae, 636
Langerhans cells, 672
Language and speech disorders, 773–775
Lanugo, 676
Laparoscopy, 900–901
Large-cell carcinoma, 425
Large intestine
absorption in, 575–576
age-related changes in, 935
anatomy of, 570
carcinoma of, 591–592
diseases of, 588–592
diverticula of, 589–590
ileus of, 588
obstructions of, 588
Laryngitis, 423
Larynx
carcinoma of, 424
edema of, 423
Lectin, 186
Legg-Calvé-Perthes disease, 654
Leiomyomas, 193
uterine, 908
Leishmania, 130
Leptomeningitis, 845
Lethargy, 807
Leukemia, 195, 236–238
acute, 237
chronic, 237
clinical manifestations of, 237–238
genetic factors in, 237
environmental factors in, 237
prognosis, 238
types of, 237–238
viruses associated with, 237
Leukocytes, 220–240. *See also* specific types of white cells
classification of, 232
count in peripheral blood, 229–230
life span of, 231–232
malignancies of, 236–240
nonmalignant disorders of, 234–236
phagocytosis by, 232–234
polymorphonuclear, 152
types of, 229, 230
Leukocytosis, 142
basophilic, 235
eosinophilic, 142, 235
neutrophilic, 234
Leukoencephalopathy, multifocal, 842
Leukopenia, 235
Leukoplakia, 690
Leukotrienes, 111, 139
Leydig cells, 870, 875
Ligaments, 31, 643
ovarian, 885
uterine, 885, 889
Limbic system, 728
Lipase
gastric, 572
pancreatic, 603–604
Lipids. *See also* Lipoproteins
hyperlipidemia, 44, 552, 553
intracellular accumulation of, 53–54
metabolism of
by liver, 597
in obesity, 616–617
thyroid hormones and, 518–519
Lipid storage disease, 44
Lipochrome, 54
Lipodystrophy, 545
Lipofuscin, 54, 927, 930
Lipoid nephrosis, 450
Lipomas, 460
Lipoproteins, 597, 616–617
high-density, 70, 349
serum levels in atherosclerosis, 357
serum levels in hypertension, 349
types of, 349
Lithiasis. *See* Calculi
Liver, 594–601
anatomy of, 594, 595
bile synthesis in, 598–599
biopsy of, 600–601
biotransformation in, 597
blood supply to, 594
carbohydrate metabolism in, 597
carcinoma of, 613–614
cirrhosis of, 556, 611–613
coagulation diseases and, 608
coagulation factors synthesized in, 245, 596
drug metabolism in, 597
encephalopathy from diseases of, 609–611
failure, 608–609, 610
fat metabolism in, 597
fatty changes of, 607–608
in diabetes, 545
function tests of, 599–601
hepatitis, 614–615
in hepatorenal syndrome, 608
insulin effect on, 535–536
jaundice, 606
lobules of, 596
phagocytosis in, 597
physiology of, 594, 596–599
protein synthesis and metabolism in, 594, 596–597
scanning of, 600
sinusoids of, 594, 597
toxins and, 597–598, 611
Livor mortis, 59
Local adaptation syndrome, 65
Lockjaw, 129, 847–848
Loop of Henle, 433, 438–439
Low-brain processing, 719, 720, 723, 724–726
Lown-Ganong-Levine syndrome, 302
Lumbar puncture, 837
Lungs. *See also* Airways; Ventilation
air-related changes in, 932–933
anatomy of, 373–374
blood supply to, 373, 375
capacity measurements of, 392–393
compliance and elastance of, 377–378
defenses of, 381–385
embolism in, 421–423
fibrosis of, 407
function testing of, 391–393
gas exchange in, 373, 385–390
Lungs—*Continued*
obstructive diseases of, 414–418
particulates deposited in, 383
restrictive diseases of, 396–410
shock and, 104
tumors of, 424–426
uremic, 474
volume of, 380
work done by, 380
Lupus erythematosus, 175, 176, 177
Luteinizing hormone (LH), 490
in females, 891, 893
in males, 870
Luteotrophic hormone. *See* Prolactin
Lymphadentitis, 141, 365
Lymphadenopathy, 141, 236
Lymphangiography, 366
Lymphangitis, 141, 365, 366
Lymphatic system, 150–151, 277
diseases of, 365–366
in dissemination of neoplasms, 198–199
in fluid volume regulation, 76–77
functions of, 365
obstruction of, 83–84
of stomach, 568
Lymphedema, 365–366
Lymph nodes, 150–151
Lymphocytes, 229–231
B cells, 152–154, 232, 236
in aging, 927
as memory or plasma cell, 154
in respiratory defense mechanisms, 384
response to neoplasms, 201
deficiency of, 236
disorders of, 235–238
functions of, 234
life span of, 232
T cells, 154–156, 232
age-related changes in, 927
in cell-mediated immunity, 158–159
in diabetes, 539
helper, 155
in hypersensitivity reactions, 172–173
killer, 155
in respiratory defense mechanisms, 384
response to neoplasms, 201
in skin, 672–673
suppressor, 155–156
Lymphocytolysis, cell-mediated, 159
Lymphocytosis, 235–236
Lymphogranuloma, 918
Lymphokines, 155, 156, 158, 172
in inflammatory response, 140
Lymphoma
classification of, 238–239
Hodgkin's, 238–239
origins of, 239
Lymphopenia, 236
Lymphoreticular organs, 238
Lysosomes, 11–12, 58
Lysosomal storage disease, 43
Lysozyme, in gastric secretions, 572

Macrophages
alveolar, 156, 382–383, 384
in dermis, 674
heme oxidase activity of, 234
in immune response, 121, 156
in mononuclear phagocytosis system, 233–234
peritoneal, 156
in shock response, 109
Macula lutea, 748
Magnesium
functions of, 82
hypermagnesemia, 82
hypomagnesemia, 79, 82
pH changes in serum and, 96
serum levels of, 79, 471–472
Magnetic resonance imaging, 828, 837
Major histocompatability complex, 155
Malabsorption diseases, 585–586
Maladaptation, 65
and disease development, 68
Malaria, 130, 132, 849
Male reproductive system, 870–873
Malleus, 756
Mallory's bodies, 612
Mammary glands. *See* Breast(s)
Mammography, 900
Marble bones, 651
Marfan syndrome, 45, 359
Margination, in inflammatory response, 136
Marie-Strümpell disease, 657–658
Mast cells, 674
Measles, 687–688
German, 688
and panencephalitis, 842
Meckel's diverticulum, 590
Medulla oblongata, 720, 724, 725
Medulloblastomas, 838–839
Megacolon, 589
Meiosis, 35, 36
Melanin, 54, 673
Melanocytes, 673
Melanoma, 690–691
Membrane potential, 26–28, 710
Memory disorders, 862–863
Memory, immune, 150
Meniere's disease, 176, 763
Meninges, 719
Meningiomas, 834, 839
Meningitis, 129
bacterial, 845
tuberculous, 846
viral, 843
Meningocele, 852, 853
Meningococcemia, 129
Meningomyelocele, 853, 856
Menopause, 897
perimenopausal and postmenopausal bleeding, 906
Menorrhagia, 906
Menstrual cycle, 892–894
disorders of, 904–907
menstrual phase of. *See* Menstruation
premenstrual syndrome, 905
proliferative phase of, 892–894
secretory phase of, 894
Menstruation, 892
abnormal, 906
cessation of, 897
dysmenorrhea, 905–906
retrograde, and endometriosis, 904
Merkel cells, 672
Mesencephalon, 719, 727
Metabolism
anaerobic, 306, 315, 627
carbohydrate, 518, 535, 597
drug, 597
fat, 492, 555, 597
glucose, 492, 536, 597
by liver, 535–536, 594, 596–597
in obesity, 616–617
protein, 492, 507, 518, 535, 594, 596–587
Metals, carcinogenesis by, 195
Metaphase, 17

Metaphysis, 638
Metaplasia, 56–57
Metastasis, 192, 198–200
  to brain, 840–841
  to liver, 814
  to spinal cord, 840–841
Metazoal infections of central nervous system, 849–850
Metrorrhagia, 906
Micelles, 575
Microcephaly, 855, 856
Microglia, 156, 707
Microtubules, 12–13
Micturition, 442, 826
Midbrain, 719, 727
Migraine, 791, 793
Mineralocorticoids, 504, 505, 507
Minimal change disease, renal, 450
Miosis, pupillary, 750, 810
Mitochondria, 8
  ATP formation in, 8–10
Mitosis, 17–18, 19, 36, 671
Mitral valve, 260
  prolapse of, 333–334
  regurgitation by, 332–333
    and stenosis of, 333
  stenosis of, 330–332
Mittelschmerz, 893
Mobitz AV block, 299–300
Mole, hydatidiform, 910–911
Mönckeberg's sclerosis, 361
Monilia. See Candida albicans infections
Monocytes, 156, 229, 230, 231
  abnormalities of, 235
  functions of, 233–234
Mononeuropathy, 543
Mononucleosis, 236
Morula, 897
Mosaics, chromosome, 47
Motor system
  disorders of, 630. *See also* Movement disorders
  efferent nerves in, 734–735
  neurons of, 734
    lesions of, 809
Mouth. *See* Oral cavity
Movement disorders, 859–862
Mucociliary transport, 381–382
Mucopolysaccarides, 43
Mucormycosis, 848–849
Mucosal neuroma syndrome, 551
Mucoviscidosis. *See* Cystic fibrosis
Mucus, 382
  cervical
    ferning pattern of, 893, 899
    Huhner test of, 901
  gastric secretion of, 570, 572
Multiunit smooth muscle, 628
Mumps, 125
  and orchitis, 882
Murmurs. *See* Heart sounds
Muscles, 28, 30–31
  action potentials in, 624, 628
  age-related changes in, 935–936
  atrophy of, 630–631
  cardiac, 629–630
    cellular structure of, 30
    contraction of, 23–26, 266–267
    metabolism in, 267
  contraction. *See* Contraction, muscular
  cramps, 630
  in diabetes, 545
  disorders of, 630
  dystrophies of, 406, 631
  eye, 750
  fasciculations of, 630
  fibrillation of, 630
  hypertrophy of, 630
  insulin effects on, 536–537
  in myasthenia gravis, 631
  myoclonus of, 630
Muscles—*Continued*
  oral, 564
  respiratory, 375
  smooth, 25–26, 30, 627–629
  spasms of. *See* Spasms, muscular
  strains of, 630
  stress and, 71
  striated, 13, 25, 30, 624–627
  tetany of, 630
  tics of, 630
  tone, 627, 810
  tumors of, 631
  twitches of, 630
Muscular contractions, 23–26, 624–627
Muscular dystrophy, 406, 631
Myasthenia gravis, 177, 631, 856–857
Mycobacterium leprae, 129
Mycobaterium tuberculosis, 129, 401
Mycoplasma, 400
Mycoses, 130, 131
Mydriasis, 750, 810
Myelin, 707, 783
Myelitis, 843–844
Myelography, 829, 837
Myeloma, multiple, 239–240, 663–664
Myocardial infarction
  and cardiogenic shock, 106
  complications of, 326–327
  diagnosis of, 283, 287, 324–326
  heart failure in, 307
  in hypertension, 353
  locations of, 300, 323
  pathophysiology of, 322–324
Myocarditis, 317
Myocardium, 258
  action potentials in, 267
  anatomy of, 629–630
  cellular structure of, 264, 266
  circus movement in, 287
  contraction of, 266–267
  disorders of,
    cardiomyopathy, 315–317
    hypertrophy, 306–307
    infarction. *See* Myocardial infarction
    ischemia, 321
    rupture of, 327
  metabolism in, 267
  in shock, 103
Myoclonus, 630, 780
Myofibrils, 622
Myoglobin, 622
Myokymia, 630
Myomas, uterine, 908
Myometrium, 885
Myoneural junction, 624, 629
Myopia, 754
Myosin, 23, 25, 622, 624, 625
Myotomes, 790
Myxedema, 521–523
Myxovirus, 125. *See also* Rubella; Rubeola

Naegleria, 849
Nails, 678–679
  age-related changes in, 937
Narcosis, in respiratory failure, 427
Nasopharyngitis, 397
Nearsightedness, 754
Necrobiosis lipoidica epidermis, 544
Necrosis, 59, 112
  of bone, 654
  of kidney, 466–469, 543
Neisseria infections, 129
  gonorrhoeae, 129, 883, 916
Nematodes, 132, 133
Neoplasia. *See* Tumors
Neospinothalamic tract, 784
Neovascularization, 143
Nephritic glomerular disease, 447–449
Nephritis, analgesia, 451
Nephrolithiasis, 456
Nephrons, 432–434, 436
  age-related changes in, 933
Nephrosis, 450
Nephrotic glomerular disease, 449–451
Nephrotoxins, 451–452, 466, 934
Nervous system, 705–863
  age-related changes in, 930, 935–936
  autonomic. *See* Autonomic nervous system
  of bone, 637, 649–650
  central. *See* Central nervous system
  cerebral disorders of, 817–821
  in cerebral palsy, 856
  and cerebrospinal fluid system, 741–746
  cranial malformations and, 734, 817–821
  in dementia, 862–830
  in diabetes, 543–544
  diagnostic tests for, 828–830
  disabilities caused by, 852
  drug-induced disorders of, 860–862
  fibers of, 713
  in Guillain-Barré syndrome, 406, 844, 857
  hepatic encephalopathy and, 609–611
  Huntington's disease and, 45, 862
  in hydrocephalus, 854
  in hypocalcemia, 79, 81
  hypothalamic-pituitary, 488–489
  impulse conduction in. *See* Impulse conduction
  infections of, 841–850
  of kidney, 435
  in myasthenia gravis, 856–857
  neurons of. *See* Neurons
  pain and, 783–786
  paraneoplastic syndromes of, 202
  parasympathetic. *See* Parasympathetic nervous system
  in Parkinsonism, 860
  peripheral. *See* Peripheral nervous system
  receptors of. *See* Sensory receptors
  of respiratory tract, 375–376, 406
  sclerosis of, 755, 858–859
  of skin, 679
  of stomach, 567
  of special senses
    hearing, 759, 760, 819–820
    smell, 766, 819
    taste, 765, 819, 820
    vision, 748, 749, 818
  in spina bifida, 852–853
  in spinal cord. *See* Spinal cord
  in stress response, 65–66
  sympathetic. *See* Sympathetic nervous system
  synapses of, 707, 714–718
  tissue of, 31
  trauma to, 822–827
  tumors of, 832–841
  vestibular, 761
Neuralgia, trigeminal, 819
Neurilemmomas, 839
Neuroblastomas, cerebral, 838
Neurofibromas, 834, 840
Neurofibromatosis, von Recklinghausen's, 839
Neurogenic shock, 108
Neuroglial cells, 707
Neurohypophysis. *See* Pituitary gland, posterior
Neurolemma, 707
Neuromas, acoustic, 839–840
Neuromuscular junction
  in smooth muscle, 629
  in striated muscle, 624
Neurons, 31, 706–714
  components of, 700–701
  in diabetes, 543
  excitation and conduction in, 710–714
  motor, 734
    lesions of, 809
  postganglionic, 736
  preganglionic, 736
  types of, 708
Neurophysin, 489
Neurosyphilis, 847, 863
Neurotensin, 787
Neurotransmitters, 717–718
  of autonomic nervous system, 737–738
Neutropenia, 142, 176, 235
Neutrophils, 229
  in inflammatory response, 140
  life span of, 231
  quantitative alterations of, 234–235
Nevi, pigmented, 691
Nissl bodies, 707
Nitrosamines, as carcinogens, 195
Nociceptors, 783
Nodes of Ranvier, 707
Norepinephrine (noradrenalin), 717–718
  secretion of, 511–512
    in stress response, 65, 66
    and vasoconstriction, 741
Normoblasts, 218
Nose
  deposition of particulates in, 383
  drainage of blood and CSF from, 817
  and smell sensation, 766–767
Nuclear imaging. *See* Radioisotope scans
Nucleolus, 14
Nucleoplasm, 6, 188
Nuclei, 14, 16–17
Null cells, 156–157
Nutrition. *See* Diet
Nystagmus, 763

Oat-cell carcinoma, 425
Obesity, 616–617
  and atherosclerosis, 319
  in Cushing's syndrome, 509
  and diabetes, 540
  interstitial fatty infiltration in, 53–54
  lipid metabolism in, 616–617
  respiratory disorders from, 408
Occipital lobe, 730
Oculocephalic reflex, 811, 818
Oculomotor nerve, 734, 818
Oculovestibular reflex, 817
Olfactory nerve, 734, 766, 817
Oligodendroglia, 707, 838
Oligodendrogliomas, 838
Oligomenorrhea, 906
Oliguria, 467–468, 469
Oncotic pressure. *See* Colloid osmotic pressure
Oogenesis, 893–894
Opisthonotonos, in coma, 808
Opportunistic infections, 120, 165

Opsonin, 137
Opsonization, 233
Optic nerve, 748, 749, 818
Oral cavity, 564
herpes infection of, 124
inflammations of, 578
mucosal changes in, 578
secretions of, 570–571
Orchitis, 882
Organelles, 6–16, 623
Organ of Corti, 756
Organotropism, 120
Orgasm, 875, 896
Orthopnea, 308
Ortolani's click, 656
Osgood-Schlatter disease, 654
Osler's nodes, 336, 338
Osmoreceptors, 493
Osmosis, 20
Osmotic pressure, 21, 75. *See also* Colloid osmotic pressure
Ossicles, 756
Ossification, 635
Osteitis fibrosa,
cystica, 652–653
in uremic syndrome, 474
Osteoarthritis, 658, 936
Osteoblasts, 635
Osteoblastoma, 659–660
Osteochondroma, 660
Osteochondrosis, 654
Osteoclasts, 635
Osteocytes, 635
Osteodystrophy
Albright's hereditary, 527–528
renal, 473, 528
Osteogenesis imperfecta, 45, 650
Osteomas, 659–660
Osteomalacia, 653–654
in uremic syndrome, 474
Osteomyelitis, 654–655
staphylococcal, 128
Osteons, 636
Osteopetrosis, 651
Osteophytes, 658
Osteoporosis, 653
in aging, 936–937
Osteosarcoma, 660
Osteosclerosis, 176, 475
Otorrhea, 817
Otosclerosis, 759
Ovary
anatomy of, 885, 893
benign tumors of, 909
cancer of, 912–913
cysts of, 904, 909
in menstrual cycle, 892–894
Ovulation, 893
premature failure of, 176
Ovum
fertilization of, 897
production of, 891, 895
Oxalate stones, 458
Oxidative phosphorylation, 8
Oxygen
and aging, 927
in arterial blood, 213, 385
consumption by heart, 267
consumption by lungs, 380
debt, 10, 627
deficiency of. *See* Hypoxemia; Hypoxia
and muscular contraction, 627
tissue levels, 385, 387
transport, 219, 385
Oxyhemoglobin, 219, 385
dissociation curve, 385–386
Oxytocin, 494, 891

Paget's disease, 652
Pain, 783–803
acute vs. chronic, 783, 799–801
Pain—*Continued*
angina pectoris, 321
cutaneous, 788–790
deep somatic, 789–791
defined, 783
endorphins and, 787–788, 802
fast, 783
headache, 791–793, 834–835, 845
mechanism of, 783–794
modulation of, 786–787
perceptual style and, 803
receptors, 783
response to, 801–803
slow, 784
sources of, 788–794
theories of, 794–799
threshold of, 801
tolerance to, 802
transmission of, 783–786, 790
in trauma, 793
visceral, 793–794
Paleospinothalamic tract, 785
Palsy
Bell's, 819
bulbar, 859
cerebral, 856
Pancreas, 531–558
abscesses of, 554
anatomy and physiology of, 531–537
carcinoma of, 554–555
in cystic fibrosis, 45, 414–415, 555–558
in diabetes, 537–550
endocrine functions of, 531–550
enzymes of, 531–537, 602–604
exocrine functions of, 602–604
insulinomas of, 550
insulin secretion. *See* Insulin
islet cells of, 531–533
diseases of, 550
pancreatitis, 554
regulation of, 603
in Zollinger-Ellison syndrome, 550, 584
Pancreatitis, 551–554
acute, 551–553
chronic, 554
diagnosis of, 554
Panencephalitis
rubella and, 842–843
sclerosing, 842
Panhypopituitarism, 496
Pannus formation, 657
Papanicolaou smear, 899
Papilledema, 748, 755, 835
Papillomas, 192
choroid plexus, 840
Papovirus, 124
Paraaminohippurate, 440
Parafollicular cells, 516
Paralysis, 809–810
agitans, 860
in amyotrophic lateral sclerosis, 859
in cerebral palsy, 856
facial, 819
flaccid, 809
in Guillain-Barré syndrome, 844
in multiple sclerosis, 858
in poliomyelitis, 843–844
spastic, 809
in spina bifida, 853
in spinal cord degeneration, 857
in syringomyelia, 854
Todd's, 780
Paraneoplastic syndromes, 202
Parasitic infections, 132–133
Parasympathetic nervous system, 274, 276, 737
actions of, 738–741, 875
influence on cardiac activity,
Parasympathetic nervous system—*Continued*
100, 740
of respiratory tract, 375
Parathyroid gland, 515
anatomy of, 525
functions of, 525–526
hyperparathyroidism, 527
hypoparathyroidism, 526–528
pseudohypoparathyroidism, 527–528
pseudopseudohypoparathyroidism, 528
secretion of hormone, 81, 525
Parenchyma, 373
Parenchymal cells, 6
Paresis, general, 847, 863
Parietal cells, 566
Parietal lobe, 730
Parkinsonism, 860
Partial thromboplastin time, 248
Passive transport, 18, 20–21
Pavementing of leukocytes, 137
Pectus carinatum, 407, 654
Pectus excavatum, 407
Pelvic inflammatory disease (PID), 908
Pemphigus, 176
Penis, 871–872
disorders of, 881
in sex act, 874–875
Pepsin, 572
Pepsinogen, 566
Peptic ulcers, 550, 581–584
Perfusion, 385, 388–390, 403
Pericarditis, 327, 338–339
Pericardium, 338
Peridontitis, 578
Perimysium, 622
Periosteum, 638
Peripheral blood vessels
arterial disorders, 356–363
autonomic regulation of, 740–741
diagnostic studies of, 366–367
resistance of, 99, 280
venous disorders, 363–365
Peripheral nervous system, 730, 732, 734
afferent (sensory) division of, 732, 734
efferent (motor) division, 734–735
pyramidal and extrapyramidal tracts in, 734–735
Peristalsis, 564, 570, 576, 628, 740
Peritoneum of uterus, 885
Peritonitis, 589, 590
Pernicious anemia, 176, 225
Personality
and atherosclerosis, 319, 357
changes in, in hepatic encephalopathy, 610
and stress-induced diseases, 69
type A, 69
Peyer's patches, 151
pH, 81, 88
Phagocytes, 232. *See also* Macrophages; Neutrophils
functions of, 233–234
Phagocytosis, 23, 137–138, 232
disorders of, 235
in liver, 597
Phagosome, 232
Pharyngitis, 423
streptococcal, 128
Pharynx, 564
Phenotype, 39
Phenylketonuria, 421
Pheochromocytoma, 351, 512–513
Phimosis, 881
Phlebitis, 359, 363, 364
Phlebothrombosis, 364
Phosphate ion
in bone, 639
function of, 82
hyperphosphatemia, 82
hypophosphatemia, 79, 82
serum levels of, 79
and calcium serum levels, 81
in renal failure, 472, 474
Phosphocreatine, 627
Phospholipids, 7
Pia mater, 719
Pick's disease, 863
Pickwickian syndrome, 408
Picornavirus, 125
Pigeon breast, 407, 654
Pigmentation
eye, 751–752
intracellular accumulation of, 54
skin, 673
Pineal gland, 729
Pinealomas, 840
Pinocytosis, 23, 233
Pinworm, 133
Pitch discrimination, 756
Pituitary gland, 482–501
anatomy of, 483, 485, 486
anterior
and female reproductive function, 891–892
functions of, 490–492
and male reproductive function, 876
histology of, 485–488
hormones of, 485, 487, 490, 492–494
hyperpituitarism, 497–499
hypopituitarism, 496–497, 839
hypothalamus and, 488–489
pars intermedia of, 488
pathology of, 494–501
posterior, 492–494
tumors of, 498, 500–501, 839
Pityriasis rosea, 689
Placenta, 897
structure of, 340
Plantar warts, 687
Plaque, atherosclerotic, 356–357, 541
Plasma, 212–213. *See also* Colloid osmotic pressure; Proteins, plasma
Plasma cell myeloma, 239–240
Plasmin, 247
Plasmodium, 130, 132, 849
Platelets
count of, 248, 249
hyperfunction of, 252–253
plug formation by, 242–243
structure of, 243
thrombocytopenia, 251
thrombocytosis, 251
Pleura, 373, 374
effusions of, 404–405
in pancreatitis, 553
Plummer's disease, 521
Pneumococcal pneumonia, 398
Pneumoconioses, 406–407
Pneumoencephalography, 741, 828–829
Pneumomediastinum, 416
Pneumonia
aspiration, 401
bacterial, 128, 398–400
mycoplasmal, 400
viral, 400
Pneumotaxic center, 376
Pneumothorax, 404–405, 416
Poikilocytosis, 222
Polarization and depolarization of cells, 26–27
Poliomyelitis, 843–844
Poliovirus, 125
Pollutants, inhalation of, 424

Polyarteritis nodosa, 356
Polycythemia, 221, 222
  in emphysema, 418
  vera, 221
Polydipsia, 543
Polymenorrhea, 906
Polymorphonuclear leukocytes, 152
Polyneuropathy, 543
Polyps, 192
  of large intestine, 591
Polyphagia, 546
Polyribosomes, 11
Polyuria,
  in renal failure, 470, 471
  in diabetes, 546
Pons, 725
Pores of Kohn, 373, 397
Porphyria, 44
Portal vein, 607, 608. *See also* Hypertension, portal
Port-wine stain, 690
Potassium
  absorption of, 576
  excretion of, 442
  functions of, 79, 712, 714
  hyperkalemia, 78, 80
  hypokalemia, 78, 80, 452
  renal resorption of, 439–440
  serum levels of, 78
    and aldosterone secretion, 504, 506, 509
    in heart failure, 315
    pH changes and, 95
    in renal failure, 471
Potentials
  membrane, 26–28, 710
    action, 26, 267, 283, 624, 628, 711–712
    resting, 710–711
  postsynaptic, 716
  of sensory receptors, 714
Pott's disease, 655
Pox viruses, 124
Preexcitation, 302
Pregnancy, 897
  AIDS and, 920
  chlamydia infections and, 920
  chorioadenoma destruens in, 910–911
  choriocarcinoma in, 911
  complications of, 906
  cytomegalovirus infections in, 843
  DES use during, 883, 912
  diabetes caused by, 541
  herpes infections and, 918
  hydatidiform mole in, 910
  oxytocin secretion in, 494, 891
  pituitary complications of, 495, 496, 497
  progesterone secretion during, 895
  rubella and, 688
  syphilis and, 917
  trophoblastic disease in, 910–911
  ultrasonography of, 901
  uterine bleeding in, 906
Preload, 272
Premenstrual syndrome, 905
Prenatal period. *See* Fetus
Presbycusis, 938
Presbyopia, 750
Pressure sores, 698–700
Proerythroblast, 217
Progesterone, 891, 892, 895
  measurement of, 899
  in menstrual cycle, 894
  in pregnancy, 895
Projectile wounds, 136
Prolactin, 490, 891–892, 895
  deficiency of, 496
Prolactin—*Continued*
  hypersecretion of, 498
Prolapse of mitral valve, 333–334
Prophase, 17
Prosencephalon, 719, 730
Prosopagnosia, 775
Prostaglandins
  and female reproductive system, 896
  and fluid and electrolyte balance, 75
  in inflammatory response, 139
  in renal failure, 469
  in shock, 105, 111
Prostate, 871, 880–881
  age-related changes in, 935
  benign hyperplasia of, 455–456, 880
  carcinoma of, 880–881
  degeneration of, 880
  infection of, 880
Protein-calorie malnutrition (PCM), 54
Proteins
  absorption of, 575
  Bence Jones, 664
  deficiencies of, 44
  digestion of, 603
  metabolism of
    cortisol affecting, 507
    growth hormone affecting, 492
    insulin affecting, 535
    by liver, 594, 596–597
    pancreas and, 603
    thyroid hormones affecting, 518
  plasma, 75, 83, 596, 607
    in burns, 694
    concentration of, 75
    in liver disease, 599, 600
    synthesis by liver, 596–597
  in protoplasm, 7
  synthesis of, 16–17
Proteus infections, 127, 459
Prothrombin, 244–247, 596, 599
Prothrombin time, 248, 599
Protoplasm, 6
Protozoal infections, 130, 132
Psammoma bodies, 909
Pseudocysts, pancreatic, 553–554
Pseudohypoparathyroidism, 527–528
Pseudomonas aeruginosa, 127
Pseudopodium, 23
Pseudopod movement, 130, 132
Pseudopseudohypoparathyroidism, 528
Pseudotumor cerebri, 856
Psoriasis, 689
Psychogenic conditions. *See also* Emotions
  coma, 807, 808
  uterine bleeding, 906
Ptyalin, 564, 570
Puberty, 894
Pulmonary circulation, 375, 388–390
Pulmonary edema. 311, 401–403
Pulmonary embolism, 421–423
Pulmonary hypertension, 423
Pulmonary system. *See* Lungs
Pulmonary valves, 262
Pulse, 277, 278–279
  arterial, in arteriosclerosis, 358
  deficit in, 295
  water-hammer (Corrigan's), 336
Pulsus alternans, 308
Pulsus paradoxus
  in asthma, 413
  in pericarditis, 338
Puncture wounds, 136
Pupil, 748, 810–811
Pupil—*Continued*
  reflexes of, 750–751, 810–811
Purkinje network, 264
Purpura
  idiopathic thrombocytopenic, 176
  in renal failure, 472
  thrombotic thrombocytopenic, 253
Purulent exudate, 141
Putamen, 729
Putrefaction, 59
Pyelonephritis, 447, 451
Pyramids, renal, 432
Pyramidal system, 734–735
Pyrogens, 141
Pyruvic acid, 10

Q fever, 126, 850
QRS waves, 270
Queckenstedt's test, 837

Rabies, 125, 842
Radiation exposure
  and birth defects, 48
  carcinogenic effects of, 195–196, 524, 690
  and immunodeficiency disorders, 164
  and osteoporosis, 653
  wounds from, 136
Radioisotope scans
  of brain, 828, 837
  of heart, 322, 326, 339
  of liver, 600
Radiology
  of brain, 837
  of breast, 900
  of cervical spine, 829
  of heart, 311, 314, 328, 331
  of skull, 828
  of uterus and fallopian tubes, 900
Rathke's pouch tumor, 501, 840
Raynaud's disease and phenomenon, 71, 362, 363
Receptors, sensory, 714–715
  baroreceptors, 100, 102, 276
  chemoreceptors, 276, 376–377, 714, 715
  exteroreceptors, 714
  interoreceptors, 714
  mechanoreceptors, 714, 715
  nociceptors, 783
  olfactory receptors, 493
  osmoreceptors, 493
  photoreceptors, 714, 715
  potential of, 714
  proprioceptors, 714
  in retina, 751
  teleceptors, 714
  thermoreceptors, 714, 715
Recessive genes, 39
Recognition mechanism, 137, 233
Rectum, 576. *See also* Anal canal and rectum
Red cells. *See* Erythrocytes
Reflex arc, 720
Reflexes, 719
  autonomic, 741, 826
  bronchoconstriction, 384
  corneal, 819
  cough, 383
  enterogastric, 573
  flexion-extension, 826
  gag, 820
  Hering-Breuer, 376
  micturition, 442, 826
  in motor neuron lesions, 809
  oculocephalic, 811, 818
  oculovestibular, 811
Reflexes—*Continued*
  pupillary, 750–751, 810–811
  respiratory, 383–384
  sneeze, 383
  in spinal cord injuries, 826–827
  swallowing, 820
Reflux
  bile, 552
  of duodenal secretions, 552
  gastroesophageal, 579
  vesicoureteral, 446
Refractive index, 748
Refractory periods, 28
Regeneration of cells, 142
Regurgitation, 327
  aortic, 335–336
    with stenosis, 336
  mitral, 332–333
    with stenosis, 333
  venous, 364, 366
Reissner's membrane, 756
Rejection, tissue, 124
Renal system. *See* Kidneys
Renin
  and aldosteronism, 510
  in blood pressure regulation, 101, 350–351
  in heart failure, 305, 306
  in hypertension, 350, 351, 474
  and oliguria, 469
  and renal tubules, 439
  in shock response, 103
Rephosphorylation, 10
Replication, 17
Repolarization of cells, 27
Reproductive system
  in cystic fibrosis, 558
  female, 885–913
    age-related changes in, 934
    anatomy of, 443, 885–890
    disorders of, 904–913
    hormonal regulation of, 894–896
    laboratory studies of, 897, 899–901
    menstrual cycle, 892–894
    normal function of, 890–897
  male, 870–883
    age-related changes in, 935
    anatomy of, 444, 870–872
    disorders of, 880–883
    hormonal regulation of, 875–876
    laboratory studies of, 877–878
    normal function of, 872–876
  sexually transmitted diseases of, 916–920
Resistance stage, in stress response, 65
Resorption, 92, 437, 439–440
Respiratory centers, 376
Respiratory distress syndromes
  adult, 111, 112, 381, 401, 409–410
  infant, 381, 408–409
Respiratory failure, 426–427
Respiratory insufficiency, 426
Respiratory tract, 372–393. *See also* Alveoli, Lungs
  acid-base regulation by, 91–92, 96, 390–391, 418–419
  age-related changes in, 932–933
  airway resistance in, 379–380
  anatomy of, 372–376
  blood supply of, 373, 375
  breathing mechanism in, 378–380
  central nervous system depression and, 405
  coma and, 811–812
  cystic fibrosis and, 556, 558

Respiratory tract—*Continued*
defense mechanisms of, 381–384
edema in, 311, 401–403
failure of, 426–427
function testing of, 391–393
Guillain-Barré syndrome and, 406
hypertension and, 423
infectious diseases of, 397–401, 423
insufficiency of, 426
muscles of, 375, 379
muscular dystrophy and, 406
nervous control of, 375–377
obesity and, 408
obstructive diseases of, 412–418
particulates deposited in, 383
reflexes of, 383–384
restrictive diseases of, 396–410
stress and, 71
thoracic deformities and, 407–408
tissue resistance in, 380
trauma of, 403–404
tuberculosis and, 400–401
ventilation-perfusion relationships in, 388–390, 403
Resting potentials, 26, 710–711
Restriction enzymes, 45
Restrictive pulmonary diseases, 395–410
Reticular activating system, 806–807
Reticulocytes, 218, 226, 227
Reticulospinal tract, 734
Reticulum
endoplasmic, 10–11
sarcoplasmic, 623
Retina, 748, 751–752
blind spot of, 748
degeneration of, 755
detachment of, 756
in diabetes, 543, 544
Retinitis pigmentosa, 756
Reye's syndrome, 844
Rhabdomyosarcoma, 631
Rhabdovirus, 125
Rheumatic fever, 128, 329
Rheumatoid arthritis, 656–657
autoimmune reactions in, 175–178, 658
juvenile, 657
Rheumatoid factor, 175
Rhinitis, 423
allergic, 176
Rhinorrhea, 817
Rhinovirus, 125
Rhodopsin, 752
Rhombencephalon, 719, 720, 723, 724–726
Rh system of blood typing, 220
Rhythmicity, cardiac, 268
Ribs, fractures of, 403–404
Ribosomes, 11, 16
Rickets, 653–654
vitamin D-resistant, 45
Rickettsial diseases, 122, 126
in central nervous system, 850
Rigor mortis, 59, 631
Ringworm, 131, 688
Rinne test, 764
RNA, 14, 16, 492
Rocky mountain spotted fever, 122, 126, 850
Rods and cones, 751
Rosenthal's disease, 250
Roth's spots, 338
Rubella, 125, 688
panencephalitis from, 842–843
in pregnancy, 688, 843
Rubeola, 687–688
Rubin's test, 901
Rubor, 358, 362, 363
Rubrospinal tract, 734
Rugae
gastric, 566
vaginal, 888

Saccules, 759
Saliva, 564, 570, 765
Salivary glands, 564, 566
autonomic regulation of, 740
in cystic fibrosis, 556
Salmonella, 127
Sarcoidosis, 407
Sarcolemma, 622
Sarcomas, 192, 193
of bone, 660, 661
meningeal, 839
synovial, 659
Sarcomeres, 622, 623
Sarcoplasm, 623
Satiety, 564
Scalae of ear, 759
Scalene muscle, 375
Scar formation, 142–144
after myocardial infarction, 324
keloid, 144
Scarlet fever, 128
Schiller's test, 901
Schilling test, 227
Schistosomiasis, 133
and bladder cancer, 196
Schmidt's syndrome, 511
Schwann cells, 707
Schwannomas, 839
Scintiscans. *See* Radioisotope scans
Sclera of eye, 748
Scleratomes, 790
Sclerosis
amyotrophic lateral, 859
arteriolosclerosis, 361
arteriosclerosis, 358–359, 840, 937
atherosclerosis. *See* Atherosclerosis
of bone, 474, 659, 759, 764
Mönckeberg's, 361
multiple, 755, 858–859
Scoliosis, 655
Scotomas, 755
Scrotum, 881
Scurvy, 654
Sebaceous glands, 676, 685
Seborrheic dermatitis, 686
Seborrheic keratosis, 689
Sebum, 676
Secretagogues, 573
Secretin, 573, 603
Seizures, 776–781
absence attacks in, 779
akinetic, 780
aura in, 779
classification of, 777
déjà vu and jamais vu in, 780
electroencephalography of, 777, 779, 780, 829, 830
focal motor (Jacksonian), 780
focal sensory, 780
generalized, 777, 779
grand mal, 779–780
myoclonic, 630, 780
partial, 780
petit mal, 779
primary (idiopathic), 777
secondary (symptomatic), 777, 781
temporal lobe psychomotor (complex partial), 780
tonic-clonic, 779–780
Sella turcica, 483, 495
Semicircular canals, 759
Semilunar valves, 262
Seminal fluid, 875, 877–878
Seminal vesicles, 871
Seminiferous tubules, 870
Seminomas, 882
Sensory system
afferent peripheral nerves in, 732, 734
age-related changes in, 937–939
hearing, 759, 760, 819–820
smell, 766, 817
taste, 765, 819, 820
touch, 679–680
vision, 748, 749, 818
Septic shock, 109
Serotonin, 140, 717
Serous exudate, 141
Serum sickness, 121–122
Sex chromosomes, 36, 47
Sexuality and carcinogenesis, 197
Sexually transmitted diseases, 916–920
Sexual response
female, 896
male, 875
Sheehan's syndrome, 496, 497
Shigella, 127
Shingles. *See* Herpes zoster
Shock
anaphylactic (allergic), 110–111, 168–169
causes of, 104–111
cardiogenic, 106–108, 315, 326
complications of, 111–112
hemorrhagic, 104–105
hyperdynamic, 109
hypodynamic, 110
hypovolemic, 104–106
irreversible, 103, 104
neurogenic, 108
nonprogressive, 102–103
normodynamic, 109–110
progressive, 103–104
septic (toxic), 109–110
spinal, 825–826
stages of, 104, 315
vasogenic, 108–111
Sickle cell anemia, 44, 224, 606
Sickle cell trait, 44, 224
Sick euthyroid syndrome, 522
Sick sinus syndrome, 290
Silicosis, 406
Sinoatrial block, 298
Sinus arrest, 293
Sinusitis, 423
Sinus (SA) node, 264
dysrhythmias of, 290, 292, 293–298
Sinusoids, of liver, 594, 597
Sjögren's syndrome, 176
Skeletal muscle. *See* Striated muscle
Skeletal system. *See* Bones; Bursae; Joints; Ligaments; Tendons
Skene's glands, 888
Skin, 670–700
acne and, 685
age-related changes in, 937
in angioedema, 683
bacterial infections of, 688
blood supply to, 679
burns of, 691–698
chemical properties of, 673
and cutaneous pain, 788–790
dermatitis of, 685–686
dermis, 673–674
eczema of, 685
epidermal appendages, 675–679
functions of, 671, 674, 675
fungal diseases of, 131, 688
hidradenitis suppurativa of, 685
hypersensitivity and allergic reactions and, 169, 686
inflammation of, 682–683, 684–685
Skin—*Continued*
lesions of, 683, 684
nerve supply to, 679
pigmentation of, 673
scaling disorders of, 689
stress and, 71
subcutaneous layer of, 674–675
trauma of, 691–700
tumors of, 688–691
ulcerations of, 358, 698–700
in uremic syndrome, 475
urticaria of, 682–683
viral infections of, 686–688
vitamin D synthesis in, 680
Skull fractures, 813
Sleeping sickness, 849
Slow virus disease, 842–843
Small-cell carcinoma, 425
Small intestine
absorption in, 568, 573, 575
anatomy of, 567–570
in Crohn's disease, 586–587
cystic fibrosis and, 556
disorders of, 585–586
secretions of, 573, 574
Smell, 766–767
age-related changes in, 939
assessment of, 766–767, 817
disturbances of, 766
Smoking
and atherosclerosis, 319, 357
and birth defects, 48
and cancer, 195, 197
and hypertension, 349
and laryngeal disorders, 423, 424
and lung disorders, 424, 933
Smooth muscles, 30, 627–629
contraction of, 25–26, 628
Sneeze reflex, 383
Snellen chart, 754
Sodium ion, 77–79
absorption of, 576
daily intake of, 77
extracellular, 77, 79, 712
functions of, 77
hypernatremia, 77, 78, 79
hyponatremia, 77, 78
membrane permeability and, 712
renal resorption of, 439
serum levels of, 78
and aldosterone secretion, 504, 506, 507
in heart failure, 315
in renal failure, 471
Sodium-potassium pump, 21–22
Somatostatin, 532, 537
Somatotropin. *See* Growth hormone
Sonography. *See* Ultrasonography
Sound conduction in ear, 756, 759
Spasms
bronchial, 412, 413
muscular, 630, 860
in tetanus, 847–848
in tetany, 630
vascular. *See* Vasospasms
Specificity of immune response, 150
Speech disorders, 773–775
Spermatogenesis, 872–874
Spermatogonia, 872
Spherocytosis, hereditary, 223
Sphincter
anal, 570
gastroesophageal, 564, 566
of Oddi, 531
Spina bifida, 852–853
Spinal cord, 719–721
ascending and descending tracts of, 723

Spinal cord—*Continued*
degeneration of, 857
infections of, 841–850
protective coverings of, 719
tracts to brain, 726, 785–786
trauma of, 822–827
anterior and central cord syndromes in, 824
functional alterations due to, 823–824
morphologic changes in, 823
reflex return after, 826–827
shock in, 825–826
transection, 824–825
tuberculoma of, 846
tumors of, 832–839
clinical manifestations of, 836–837
diagnosis of, 837–838
metastatic, 840–841
neurologic alterations in, 833–834
Spinal nerves, 720, 721
Spinal shock. *See* Neurogenic shock
Spine. *See* Vertebral column
Spinnbarkeit, 899
Spinoreticular system, 786
Spleen, 151
and hematopoiesis, 215–217
marginal zone of, 215
red and white pulp of, 151, 215
Spondylitis, ankylosing, 657–658
Spotted fever, 126
Sprue, 585–586
Squamous cell carcinoma
of cervix, 912
of esophagus, 580
of lungs, 425
of skin, 690
Staghorn calculi, 456, 457, 458
Staging, of neoplasms, 198–199
Stapes, 756
Staphylococcal infections, 127, 336
of bone, 654
Starling's equation, 401–402
Steatorrhea, 550, 554
Stem cells, 230, 231
deficiency of, 161
Stenosis, 144
aortic, 334–335
with regurgitation, 336
mitral, 330–332
with regurgitation, 333
Sterility, 874
Sternberg-Reed cells, 238
Sternomastoid muscle, 375
Steroids, 482
hypersecretion of, 507–510
hyposecretion of, 510–511
physiologic activity of, 507
synthesis of, 506
transport of, 506
Stomach
age-related changes in, 935
anatomy of, 566–567
carcinoma of, 584–585
digestion in, 572–573
in hiatal hernia, 519–520
inflammation of, 581
motility of, 572
movement of food to, 571
nerve supply to, 567
secretions of. *See* Gastric secretions
ulcers of, 581–583
Stones. *See* Calculi
Stools, 570, 576
Strains, muscular, 630
Streptococcal infections, 128–129
endocarditis, 336
glomerulonephritis, 448
lymphangitis, 366

Streptococcal infections—*Continued*
lymphedema and, 366
of respiratory tract, 397, 398
and valvular heart disease, 329
Streptokinase, 247
Stress, 63–71
ACTH secretion in, 67
aldosterone levels in, 68
antidiuretic hormone secretion in, 67–68
cardiovascular response to, 65, 66, 69–70
cancer and, 71
defined, 64
and disease development, 68–71, 319
epinephrine secretion in, 65, 66
and general adaptation syndrome, 65
and Graves' disease, 521
immune response in, 65, 68, 70
and local adaptation syndrome, 65
musculoskeletal changes in, 71
physiologic effects of, 65, 71
respiratory effects of, 71
skin changes during, 71
thyroid-stimulating hormone secretion in, 67
ulcers from, 70–71, 581
Stressors, 64
Striated muscles, 30
anatomy of, 622–624
contraction of, 23, 25, 624–627
physiology of, 624–627
sarcoma of, 631
Stroke, 769. *See also* Cerebrovascular disorders
Struvite stones, 459
Stupor, 807
Subarachnoid hemorrhage, 770–771, 816
Subcutaneous tissues, 674–675
Subdural hematomas and hygromas, 815–816
Substance P, 787
Substantia nigra, 727
Sulci, cerebral, 730
Sun exposure
and skin pigmentation, 673
and skin tumors, 196, 691
Suppurative exudate, 141
Supratentorial lesions, 808
Surfactant, alveolar, 380–381
deficiency of, 408, 409
Swallowing, 571
reflex, 820
Swan-Ganz catheterization. *See* Cardiac catheterization
Sweat, 558, 675–676
Sweat glands
apocrine, 676
autonomic regulation of, 740–741
eccrine, 675
Sympathetic nervous system, 274, 736–737
actions of, 738–741
in blood pressure regulation, 350, 351
in heart failure, 305
in heart regulation, 100, 740
of respiratory tract, 375
in shock response, 102
in stress response, 66, 67–68
Symphysis, 555
Synapses, 707, 714–718
facilitation of impulse transmission at, 717
neurotransmitters in, 717–718
and presynaptic inhibition of impulses, 717

Synarthroses, 641
Synchondrosis, 641
Syncope, in aortic stenosis, 334
Syndesmosis, 641
Synovial joints, 641
sarcoma of, 659
Syphilis, 129
Argyll Robertson pupil in, 751, 863
and aortic aneurysms, 360–361
of bone, 655
diagnostic tests for, 917
meningovascular, 847
neurologic symptoms of, 847, 863
primary, 917
secondary, 863, 917
tertiary, 847, 863, 917
ulcers in, 917
Syringobulbia, 854
Syringomyelia, 853–854
Syringomyelocele, 853
Systems theory, 64
Systole, 272, 277

Tabes dorsalis, 847
Tachycardia
atrial, 294
sinus, 290, 292
ventricular, 297
Tachydysrhythmias, 287
Taenia, 133, 849
Takayasu's disease, 356
Talipes, 655
Tamponade, cardiac, 338, 339
Tapeworms, 132, 133, 849
Taste, 570, 571, 764–766
age-related changes in, 935, 938–939
assessment of, 765–766, 819
disturbances of, 765
pathways of, 765
Taste buds, 564, 764
Tay-Sachs disease, 44
Tectospinal tract, 734
Teeth, 564, 935
Telangiectasias, 937
Telencephalon, 719, 730
Telophase, 17
Temporal lobe, 730
herniation of, 814
Tendinitis, 630
Tendons, 31, 643, 659
Tenosynovitis, 659
Teratocarcinoma, 882
Teratogens, 48
Teratomas, 193, 840, 882
Testes, 870, 935
biopsy of, 877
diseases of, 882
torsion of, 882
tumors of, 882
Testosterone, 510, 875–876
and bone formation, 639
plasma levels of
male, 877
in prostatic hyperplasia, 455
Tetanus, 129, 847–848
Tetany, 630
Thalamocortical system, 727–728, 806–807
Thalamus, 719, 727–728
consciousness and, 806–807
pain sensation and, 784
Thalassemias, 44, 224–225
Thermography, 901
Theta rhythm, 777, 829, 830
Thirst, 74
Thorax. *See* Lungs; Ribs
Threadworm, 133
Thrombin, 242
Thromboangiitis obliterans,

Thromboangiitis obliterans—*Continued*
362–363
Thrombocytopenia, 257–258
Thrombocytopenic purpura, 176, 253
Thrombocytosis, 252
Thromboembolism. *See* Embolism
Thrombophlebitis, 359, 363, 364
Thromboplastin time, partial, 248
Thrombosis, 57–58
in atherosclerosis, 357
cerebral, 769–770
venous, 363–364
Thrush, 131, 688, 919
Thymic hormones, 151
Thymomas, 856
Thymopoietin, 151
Thymus, 151, 154
age-related changes in, 927–928
in stress response, 65
Thymus-independent antigens, 157
Thyrocalcitonin. *See* Calcitonin
Thyroglobulin, 516
Thyroglossal duct, 516
Thyroid gland, 515–524
anatomy of, 515
carcinoma of, 524
enlargement of. *See* Goiter
Hashimoto's disease, 176, 523–524
hormones secreted by, 516–519, 640
hyperthyroidism, 519–521
hypothyroidism, 521–524
iodide uptake by, 516
physiology of, 516–517
Thyroiditis, autoimmune, 523–524
Thyroid-stimulating hormone, 490
deficiency of, 496
and stress response, 67
Thyroid storm, 520
Thyrotoxicosis. *See* Hyperthyroidism
Thyrotropin. *See* Thyroid-stimulating hormone
Thyroxine (T4), 68, 516, 519
Tic douloureux, 819
Tics, 630
Tinea infections, 131, 688
Titratable acids, 93
Tissues, types of, 28–33
Todd's paralysis, 780
Tolerance to antigens, 150
Tongue, 564. *See also* Taste
Tonsils, 151, 383
Tophi, in gout, 650
Torsion of testes, 882
Torticollis, 861–862
Torulosis, 848
Touch, 679–680
age-related changes in, 939
Toxic shock, 907–908
Toxins, bacterial, 109
central nervous system disorders from, 847–848
Toxoplasmosis, 132, 849
Trabeculae, 636
Transcription of RNA, 16
Transferrin, 218
Transfusions, hemolytic reactions to, 170
Translation, 16
Transplantation, rejection of, 174
Transport
active, 21–22
passive, 18, 20–21
Transudates, 403
Trauma
to chest wall, 403–404
fractures in. *See* Fractures
to head, 812–822

Trauma—*Continued*
pain caused by, 793
shock caused by, 106
to skin, 691–700
to spinal cord, 822–827
types of wounds in, 136
Trematodes, 132, 133
Treponema pallidum, 129, 847, 863, 917
Trichinosis, 133
central nervous system disorders from, 849
Trichomonas infections, 130
vaginitis from, 918–919
Tricuspid valve, 260
Trigeminal nerve, 734, 818–819
Triiodothyronine (T3), 516
Trisomy 21, 45, 46
Trochlear nerve, 734, 818
Trophoblast, 897
Trophoblastic disease, 910–911
Tropomyosin, 25, 264, 622, 624, 625
Troponin, 25, 264, 622, 624, 625
Trousseau's sign, 81, 527
Trypanosoma infections, 130, 849
Trypsin, 603
Trypsin inhibitor, 603
Trypsinogen, 603
Tsutsugamushi fever, 850
Tuberculomas, 846
Tuberculosis, 59, 129, 400–401
granuloma formation in, 141, 401
meningeal, 846
skeletal, 655
Tubules
renal. *See* Kidneys, tubules of
seminiferous, 870
Tubulin, 12
Tumor angiogenesis factor, 197
Tumors, 192–203. *See also* specific anatomic sites and tumor types
adrenal, 512–513
benign, 184, 192, 193
blood vessel, 840
bone, 659–664
brain, 832–839
breast, 910, 913
and carcinogens, 194–196
causes of, 194–196
cellular alterations in, 193–194, 196
cervical, 911–912
classification of, 193
clinical manifestations of, 201–203
developmental, 840
esophageal, 580–581
establishment and proliferation of, 200
growth of, 197
immune response to, 200–201
of joints, 659
kidney, 459–462
of large intestine, 591–592
laryngeal, 424
liver, 613–614
lung, 424–426
malignant, 184, 192, 193–194
of meninges, 839
metastasis of. *See* Metastasis
multiple endocrine, 513
muscle, 631
nerve, 839
in obesity, 617
ovarian, 909–910, 912–913
pancreatic, 550–551, 554–555
parathyroid, 528
of penis, 881
pineal, 840
pituitary, 500–501, 839

Tumors—*Continued*
of placenta, 910–911
precancerous, 197
prostate, 880–881
skin, 689–691
of spinal cord, 832–839
staging of, 197–198
stomach, 584–585
testicular, 882
thyroid, 524
uterine, 908–909, 911
of vagina, 912
viruses associated with, 196, 237, 686
Turner syndrome, 47
Twitches, 630
Tympanic membrane, 756
Typhoid fever, 127
Typhus, 126, 850

Ulcers
burn-induced, 696
cutaneous
in arteriosclerosis, 358
decubitus, 698–700
duodenal, 71, 583–584
peptic, 550, 581–584
stomach, 71, 581–584
stress-induced, 70–71, 581
Ulcerative colitis, 591
stress and, 71
Ultrasonography
in obstetrics and gynecology, 901
of vascular system, 367
Ultraviolet exposure. *See* Sun exposure
Urea, 473
Urease, gastric, 572
Uremic syndrome, 473–475
Ureters, 441, 442
Urethra, 442, 444, 871
Uric acid
hyperuricemia, 452
gout and, 658
stones, 458
Urinary tract. *See also* Bladder; Kidneys
age-related changes in, 933
anatomy of, 443, 444
calculi in, 456–459
infections in, 446–447
bacterial, 127, 128
fungal, 131
obstruction of, 455–462
tumors of, 459–462
ureters, 441, 442
urethra, 442, 444, 871
Urination
age-related changes in, 933
micturition reflex, 442, 826
Urine
bilirubin in, 599
formation of, 435–442
glucose in, 549
oliguria, 467–468, 469
physical characteristics of, 440
polyuria, 470, 471, 506
supersaturation of, and stone formation, 457
volume of, 435
Urobilinogen, 599–600
Urolithiasis, 456
Urticaria, 682–683
Uterus, 885, 887, 889. *See also* Cervix uteri; Endometrium
abnormal bleeding from, 906
carcinoma of, 911–912
fibroids of, 908–909
oxytocin and, 494
in pregnancy, 897, 898
Utricles, 759

Vaccinia virus, 124
Vagina, 888, 934
adenosis of, 912
cancer of, 912
infections of, 918–920
wet smears of, 899, 900, 919
Vaginitis, 907
Vagus nerve, 376, 734, 820. *See also* Parasympathetic nervous system
Valvular heart disease, 327–336. *See also* specific valves
diagnosis of, 328–329
rheumatic fever and, 329
Varicella virus, 124, 686
Varices, esophageal, 580, 608
Varicocele, 882
Varicose veins, 364–365
Variola virus, 124
Vas deferens, 871
Vascular system. *See* Blood vessels
Vasoconstriction, 242
Vasogenic shock, 108–111
Vasopressin. *See* Antidiuretic hormone
Vasospasms
of cerebral artery, after rupture of aneurysm, 772
of coronary artery, 70
in Raynaud's disease, 362
in thromboangiitis obliterans, 362
Veins, 262. *See also* Blood vessels
anatomy of, 277
circulation of, 280
coronary, 264
diseases of, 363–364, 366
insufficiency of, 364, 366
varicose, 364–365
Vellus hairs, 676
Vena cava, 262
Venereal disease, 916–920
Ventilation
at apex and base of lung, 389, 390
collateral, 373
dead space in, 390
hyperventilation, 94, 811
hypoventilation, 391
measurements of, 400–401
muscles of, 375
phases of, 378–379
and perfusion, 388–390, 403
shunting in, 390
splinting effect in, 375
Ventricles, cardiac
anatomy of, 258, 260
aneurysms of, 327
diseases of, 305–317
filling and contraction of, 273–274
hypertrophy of, 306–307
rhythms of, 296–298
rupture of, 327
septum of, 260
defects of, 342, 344
Ventricles, cerebral
cerebrospinal fluid in, 741, 744
in hydrocephalus, 854
Ventriculography, 829, 837
Verrucae, 329, 687
Vertebral column, 719, 721
age-related changes in, 937
ankylosing spondylitis of, 657–658
fractures of, 823
herniation of disks of, 827
kyphosis of, 407, 937
Pott's disease of, 655
scoliosis of, 655
Vertebral vein plexus, 199
Vertigo, 761, 763, 819
Vesicoureteral reflux, 446

Vestibular system, 759–763
assessment of, 764
ataxia in, 764
nystagmus in, 763
vertigo in, 761, 763
Vestibulocochlear nerve, 734, 819–820
Vestibulospinal tract, 734
Villi
arachnoid, 719, 744
intestinal, 568, 569
Virions, 121
Virulence, 120
Virus infections, 120–122, 124–125
of central nervous system, 841–844
hepatitis, 125, 614–615
neoplasms associated with, 196, 237, 686
Paget's disease and, 652
pathogenesis of, 121–122
of respiratory tract, 397, 400, 423
of skin, 686–688
Visceral pain, 793–794
Visceral smooth muscle, 628
Viscous metamorphosis, 242
Vision. *See* Eyes
Vitamin A, and bone formation, 640
Vitamin B_6, and amino acid transport, 575
Vitamin B_{12}
absorption of, 576
deficiency of, 176, 225, 227, 857
in erythropoiesis, 219
Vitamin C
and bone formation, 640
deficiency of, 654
and iron absorption, 576
Vitamin D
and bone formation, 640
and calcium absorption, 81, 639
deficiency of, 45, 654
dietary sources of, 525
metabolism in renal failure, 472, 474
synthesis in skin, 680
Vitamin E, as antioxidant, 927
Vitamin K
in blood clotting, 250, 608
synthesis of, 576
Vitamins
absorption of, 576
metabolism of, 519
Vitiligo, 176
Vocal cords, 423
Volkmann's canal, 636
Volkmann's ischemia, 650
Von Gierke disease, 43
Von Hippel-Lindau syndrome, 840
Von Recklinghausen's disease, 652–653
Von Recklinghausen's neurofibromatosis, 839
Von Willebrand disease, 44, 249, 252
Vulva, 890, 934
biopsy of, 900

Wallerian degeneration, 708
Warts, 329, 687
hyperkeratotic, 937
on valve leaflets, in rheumatic fever, 329
venereal, 920
Water. *See* Fluids
Waterhouse-Friderichsen syndrome, 845
Weak-organ theory, 69

Weber's test, 764
Weight(s)
  age-related changes in, 928–929
  diabetes and, 540
  table of, 929
Wenckebach AV block, 299
Werner's syndrome, 550–551
Wernicke's aphasia, 774
Wheezing, 412, 413
Whiplash injury, 823
Whipple's syndrome, 551
White cells. *See* Leukocytes
Whooping cough, 127
Wilms' tumor, 461–462
Wolff-Parkinson-White syndrome, 342
Wolff's law, 647
Word deafness, 775
Worm infestations, 132–133
Wounds, 136
  healing of, 142–145
    aberrant, 144–145
Wounds—*Continued*
  types of, 136
Wright's stain, 229
Wry neck, 861–862

Xanthomas, 545, 612
X-linked inheritance, 38
  and agammaglobulinemia, 162
  dominant, 41
  recessive, 41–42
X rays. *See* Radiology

Yeast infection. *See Candida albicans*

Zinc, affecting taste sensation, 765
Zollinger-Ellison syndrome, 550, 584
Zymogen, 245